PERSPECTIVES ON *Pathophysiology*

PERSPECTIVES ON
Pathophysiology

Lee-Ellen C. Copstead, *PhD, ARNP, NCC*

Associate Professor
Intercollegiate Center for Nursing Education
Spokane, Washington

W.B. Saunders Company
A Division of Harcourt Brace & Company

Philadelphia / London / Toronto / Montreal / Sydney / Tokyo

W.B. SAUNDERS COMPANY
A Division of Harcourt, Brace & Company

The Curtis Center
Independence Square West
Philadelphia, PA 19106

Library of Congress Cataloging-in-Publication Data

Perspectives on pathophysiology / [edited by] Lee-Ellen C.
Copstead.
    p.   cm.
    ISBN 0–7216–3846–5
    1. Physiology, Pathological.   I. Copstead, Lee-Ellen C.
    [DNLM: 1. Pathology.   2. Disease.   QZ 4 P467 1995]
    RB113.P45   1994
    616.07—dc20
    DNLM/DLC   94–21277

PERSPECTIVES ON PATHOPHYSIOLOGY   ISBN 0–7216–3846–5

Printed in the United States of America

Last digit is the print number: 9 8 7 6 5 4 3 2

Dedicated to

MY MOTHER,
Ellen Lillian Mathilda Landstrom Copstead,
for her sensitivity and grace;

and to

MY FATHER,
Ernest Arnold Copstead,
for his guiding wisdom and common sense.

Preface

*T*he title, **Perspectives on Pathophysiology,** represents the varied and unique perspectives of the many contributors who agreed that the goal was worthwhile and put their expertise into writing the text.

Perspectives on Pathophysiology is a comprehensive text and reference presented in a clear, well-organized, concise manner. The information integrates content, emphasizing **concepts** rather than descriptions. Within every chapter **key concepts** are identified every few pages and shown in short bulleted lists that help readers check their understanding frequently and make the best use of study time. To help students master the new vocabulary of pathophysiology, **key terms** are defined at the beginning of each chapter and appear in boldface within the chapter. Chapter opening outlines also serve as a study aid for students.

Perspectives on Pathophysiology incorporates current research developments and delineates areas where future research is needed. Bibliographies are comprehensive and include references from classic and current literature.

The scientific basis of pathophysiology is rapidly expanding. Accelerated progress in human genetics and the use of electron microscopy have dramatically altered perceptions of disease. As genetic research and research into immunologic mechanisms advance, new theories are generated almost daily. Research papers and reviews are being published in many specialty journals, monographs, and symposia proceedings. To educate and excite the reader about some of these advances, units in this text open with a futuristic perspective. **Frontiers of Research**—short essays that highlight examples of this cutting edge technology—give a foretaste of some of the state-of-the-art findings germane to each unit and, where possible, speculate about future research trends.

Broadly speaking, the sixteen units of this book may be conceptually organized into four parts that build upon one another:

Part I—Introduction

Part II—Cells and Tissues

Part III—Organs and Systems

Part IV—Multisystems

An understanding of normal structure and function of the body is necessary for any detailed understanding of its abnormalities and pathophysiology. The first chapter or section of each unit includes a discussion of normal physiology.

Changes in structure and function as a result of normal development and aging are addressed where appropriate. **Changes due to the aging process** are highlighted for the student.

Part I—Introduction

Chapter 1 (Unit I) sets the stage for understanding major elements of the pathophysiological processes in individuals and population groups. The purpose of this chapter is to **give students an appreciation for the complex nature of disease and illness, including sociocultural influences.** Students are given a basis for understanding that the disease process represents a disruption in homeostasis and a breakdown of normal integration of form and function. The unifying concepts of pathophysiological processes—etiology, pathogenesis, clinical manifestations, and implications for treatment of disease—are carefully explained. Common terminology that helps students understand pathogenic mechanisms are defined and used in an appropriate context. Discussion of epidemiology provides a basic understanding of how the patterns of disease development affect population groups.

Part II—Cells and Tissues

Chapters 2 through 6 (Unit II) address **cellular mechanisms.** Chapter 2 describes normal cells to give students an insight into how normal cells look and behave. Discussion of cell transport mechanisms, membrane potentials, and gated channels is carefully explained. Chapter 3 discusses **cellular pathology,** or the basic pathologic processes of cellular injury, aging, and death. Many diseases occur from birth, and thus Chapters 4 and 5 describe **genetic development** and how birth defects ensue from faulty development. Current information about DNA replication and protein synthesis is explained using clear, unintimidating language. Chapter 6 describes the **cellular pathology of neoplasia.** Such basic cellular processes underlie diseases that occur in various organ systems. These chapters, and subsequent ones, also describe what attempts can be made to interrupt the natural course of disease.

Chapters 7 through 11 (Unit III) address **tissue pathology,** including the basic processes of *stress and adaptation, infectious disease, inflammation, immunity,* and *lymphoproliferative disorders.* Because of new research, the entire area of immunology is experiencing explosive change. Great care was taken in the development of Chapters 7 through 11 to build step by step for readers an explanation of these related processes. A detailed and current explanation of nonspecific versus specific immunity is provided in Chapter 9, and comprehensive discussion of HIV is presented in Chapter 10.

Chapters 12 through 15 (Unit IV) cover **alterations in tissue oxygenation.** Red blood cell alterations and alterations in oxygen transport, hemostasis and blood coagulation, alterations in blood flow and blood pressure are all included.

Part III—Organs and Systems

The largest part of this text, Chapters 16 through 53 (Units V through XV) survey body **systems** and the pathology that commonly occurs in patients who must be hospitalized. Occasionally, unusual disorders are discussed to illustrate fundamental mechanisms.

The biophysical properties of the various organs of the human body, complex and heterogeneous as they are, appear to be more than a simple sum of the properties of individual molecules. The **bio-psychosocial interactions of the human body** are reviewed throughout the text and emphasized in chapters where such content seems especially relevant. This approach gives students studying one aspect of pathophysiology a view of the human body in toto.

Part IV—Multisystems

Chapters 54 through 56 (Unit XVI) reinforce concepts presented previously in the text and specifically cover **multisystem organ involvement,** such as that encountered in *shock, burn,* and *malnutrition.* Although most diseases affect multiple organ systems, the conditions of shock, burn, and malnutrition can cause multisystem organ failure (MSOF). Some of the most complex patients encountered in the health care delivery system are those experiencing failure of more than one organ.

Nutritional alterations in critical illness are emphasized in this unit, but nutritional concerns, where relevant, are also integrated into individual chapters throughout the entire text.

The final chapter of the text provides a bridge between disease and its treatment, emphasizing human considerations especially relevant in critical care or emergent care units. This chapter takes the student into the urgent atmosphere of critical care units, emphasizing the multiple stresses that are encountered in these environments and their effects upon the body and upon family and other social systems.

Instructor's Manual

Students of pathophysiology are expected to comprehend a multitude of individual structures, functions, and dysfunctions. The text focuses on major degenerative, neoplastic, metabolic, immunologic, and infectious diseases. Discussions of advanced biochemistry and basic sciences have been simplified. To be clinically relevant and useful to health care professionals and educators, a text must be able to "pull together" this information.

The companion **Instructor's Manual** has been written to help unify information. A **lecture guide,** which can also serve as a **notetaking guide for students,** facilitates organization of content. Chapter **key questions** that correspond to the text key concepts stimulate critical thinking. **Case scenarios** provide fruitful material for discussion and motivate students to master not only a new vocabulary, but also a new conceptual understanding of the dynamics of disease. A **test bank** of relevant questions, a **comprehensive final examination,** a **sample syllabus,** and **transparency masters** that amplify key points are also included with the Instructor's Manual.

Acknowledgments

Many individuals deserve acknowledgment. Without the support of Dr. Jacquelyn L. Banasik, this book would never have happened. Dr. Banasik—chapter author par excellence, creator of key concepts used throughout the text, and author of the Instructor's Manual—has my heartfelt thanks. Her decade of experience as a teacher of pathophysiology and her willingness to share this expertise helped ensure that all chapters were well organized, internally consistent, and accurate.

I would also like to respectfully acknowledge the significant efforts of expert nurse educator and clinical specialist Dr. Lorna Schumann, whose chapters regarding normal and abnormal respiratory function helped provide the initial impetus for this project. As a professional colleague, I am personally grateful for her consistent support and interest from the beginning of the endeavor and throughout the book's progress.

Certainly grateful appreciation is extended to *all* of the contributing authors—recognized experts in clinical practice—who gave exhaustively of their time to write chapters and create illustrations. In particular, I would like to recognize three individuals who not only wrote chapters but also contributed additional content. Sincere thanks to clinical specialist Faith Peterson, who created the aging process boxes in an effort to help students understand critical differences between normal aging and pathophysiological processes; to clinical specialist Cleo Richard for her excellent contributions regarding urinary tract pain in Chapter 27 and diuretic medication in Chapter 28; and to clinical specialist Mary Sanguinetti-Baird for her carefully written content regarding epilepsy in Chapter 44.

Editing this book has been an interactive process; most chapters have been helpfully commented on, added to, and criticized by a variety of colleagues and external reviewers. I am indebted to the many thoughtful clinical specialists who gave of their time to read and critique manuscripts and help ensure excellence in chapter content throughout the text. Special thanks to nursing consultant Donna Ignatavicius for her formative critique and advice in the initial stages of the work.

Thanks also to pharmacist Terri Levien of the Washington State University Drug Information Center for her critical reading of the pharmacology content in Chapters 52 and 53; and to physician William Dittman of Sacred Heart Medical Center, Hematology Department, Spokane, for his helpful review of blood films in Chapter 11.

No project of this magnitude could ever be accomplished without wonderfully supportive colleagues and students who provided a source of continual motivation and encouragement. I am most keenly aware of the inspiration provided by the Intercollegiate Center for Nursing Education in Spokane. Many sincere thanks to Dean Thelma L. Cleveland, members of the administrative team, faculty, staff, and nursing students, for the energy, enthusiasm, patience, and care extended throughout this endeavor. Special thanks also to librarians Mary Wood and Robert Pringle of the Betty M. Anderson Library, whose many talents proved to be an invaluable resource. To Linda Jones, Kathy Thistle, Marguerite Clinton, and Beverly Mahrt, special acknowledgment for excellent secretarial services.

Grateful recognition is extended to photographers Kathleen Kelly, Rachael DeHaan, and Elizabeth Green, whose captivating pictures added clarity and interest. Thanks also to all the Inland Northwest health care agencies who allowed access to their sites.

To Dr. Michael J. Kirkhorn, acknowledgment and thanks for the provocative and thoughtfully crafted essays that begin each unit.

Many creative and unique efforts grace the pages of this work. Truly, it is exceedingly difficult to know how best to recognize everyone. Writing a text such as this has only been possible because of a tremendous volume of data, comments, and criticism provided by a great number of committed individuals. Thanks to all who helped.

Grateful recognition to the staff and associates of the W. B. Saunders Company, to editorial assistant Marie Thomas, to JAK Graphics for their excellence in computer-generated art, and to Joan Sinclair and Peggy Gordon for editorial and production excellence.

Special thanks to Michael Brown, who began the project with me and who supported my efforts in the initial and formative stages of the book's development. Finally, thanks to Senior Nursing Editor Ilze Rader for seeing the project through to its completion—for believing in the integrity of the work and for helping to give the book shape, direction, and guidance.

Developmental editors Martha Tanner and Sue Bredensteiner deserve special recognition for their superb efforts, for their exquisitely sensitive care about detail in the illustrations and tabular presentations, and for their meticulous concern for accuracy in references and bibliographic citations.

LEC

Contributors

Jacquelyn L. Banasik, PhD, RN
Associate Professor
Intercollegiate Center for Nursing Education
Spokane, Washington
Chapter 2, Cell Structure and Function
Chapter 3, Cell Injury, Aging, and Death
Chapter 4, Genetic Control—Inheritance
Chapter 5, Genetic and Developmental Disorders
Chapter 6, Neoplasia
Chapter 16, Cardiac Function
Chapter 17, Alterations in Cardiac Function
*Chapter 18, Heart Failure and Dysrhythmias: Common
    Sequelae of Cardiac Diseases*

Barbara Bartz, MN, CCRN, RN
Nursing Instructor
Yakima Valley Community College;
Staff Nurse
Saint Elizabeth Medical Center
Yakima, Washington
*Chapter 39, Mechanisms of Endocrine Control and Metab-
    olism*
Chapter 57, Human System Response to Special Care Units

Linda Belsky-Lohr, MSN, ARNP, FNP, OCN
Private Practice
Internal Medicine Associates
Yakima, Washington
Chapter 11, Lymphoproliferative Disorders

Tim Brown, MD
Yakima Valley Memorial Hospital
Saint Elizabeth Medical Center
Yakima, Washington
*Chapter 37, Alterations in Function of the Gallbladder and
    Exocrine Pancreas*

Karen Carlson, MN, CCRN, RN
Clinical Instructor
Department of Physiological Nursing
University of Washington;
Critical Care Clinical Nurse Specialist
Group Health Cooperative of Puget Sound
Seattle, Washington
Chapter 28, Renal Failure

Arnold Cohen, MD, FACP, FACG
Assistant Clinical Professor of Medicine
University of Washington Medical School;
Staff (Attending) Physician
Deaconess Medical Center
Sacred Heart Medical Center;
Consulting Physician
Valley Hospital and Medical Center
Holy Family Hospital
Spokane, Washington
Chapter 38, Liver Disease

Lee-Ellen C. Copstead, PhD, ARNP, NCC
Intercollegiate Center for Nursing Education
Spokane, Washington
Chapter 1, Complex Nature of Disease
Chapter 11, Lymphoproliferative Disorders
*Chapter 40, Alterations in Endocrine Control of Growth
    and Metabolism*
Chapter 44, Chronic Disorders of Neurologic Function
Chapter 45, Alterations in Special Sensory Function
*Chapter 52, Structure and Function of the Integumentary
    System*
Chapter 53, Alterations in the Integument

Roberta Emerson, PhD, CCRN, RN
Assistant Professor
Intercollegiate Center for Nursing Education
Spokane, Washington
Chapter 14, Alterations in Blood Flow

Leslie A. Clark Evans, MSN, RN
Clinical Nurse Specialist/Pain Consultant
University of California–San Diego Medical Center
San Diego, California
Chapter 46, Pain

Linda Felver, PhD, RN
Associate Professor
School of Nursing
Oregon Health Sciences University
Portland, Oregon
*Chapter 24, Fluid and Electrolyte Homeostasis and Imbal-
    ances*
Chapter 25, Acid-Base Homeostasis and Imbalances

Jane M. Georges, PhD, RN
Assistant Professor
College of Nursing
Ohio State University
Columbus, Ohio
Chapter 32, Structure and Function of the Female Reproductive System
Chapter 33, Alterations in Structure and Function of the Female Reproductive System
Chapter 34, Sexually Transmitted Diseases
Chapter 35, Gastrointestinal Function
Chapter 36, Gastrointestinal Disorders

Karen Groth, CSMN, RN
PhD Candidate
Washington State University
Pullman, Washington;
Instructor
Intercollegiate Center for Nursing Education
Spokane, Washington
Chapter 56, Nutritional Alterations in Critical Illness

Christine Henshaw, MN, RN
Nursing Program Coordinator
Highline Community College
Des Moines, Washington;
Staff Nurse
Highline Community Hospital
Burien, Washington
Chapter 15, Alterations in Blood Pressure

Jo Annalee Irving, MS, ARNP, CS
Assistant Professor
University of Florida
College of Nursing
Gainesville, Florida
Chapter 47, Neurobiology of Psychotic Illness
Chapter 48, Neurobiology of Nonpsychotic Illness

Debby Kaaland, MN, RN
Education Director
Providence Medical Center
Yakima, Washington
Chapter 39, Mechanisms of Endocrine Control and Metabolism

Michael J. Kirkhorn, PhD
Associate Professor and Director
Journalism Program
Gonzaga University
Spokane, Washington;
Adjunct Professor
Union Institute
Cincinnati, Ohio
Frontiers of Research Essays

Marie Kotter, PhD, MS, CLS, BS
Professor of Clinical Laboratory Science
Weber State University
Ogden, Utah
Chapter 12, Alterations in Oxygen Transport

Melva Kravitz, PhD, CCRN, RN
Director of Nursing Research
Yale–New Haven Hospital
New Haven, Connecticut
Chapter 55, Burn Injuries

LCDR Rick Madison, MN, RD
Nurse Corps, U.S. Navy
Division Officer
Medical/Surgical/Pediatric Unit
Naval Hospital
Great Lakes, Illinois;
Chairman, Nursing Management Council;
Relief, Department Head In-Patient Nursing
Chapter 23, Other Respiratory Disorders

Anne Roe Mealey, PhD, RN
Professor of Nursing
Intercollegiate Center for Nursing Education
Spokane, Washington
Chapter 47, Neurobiology of Psychotic Illness
Chapter 48, Neurobiology of Nonpsychotic Illness

David Mikkelsen, MD
Clinical Practice
Deaconness Medical Center
Sacred Heart Medical Center
Spokane, Washington
Chapter 30, Structure and Function of the Male Genitourinary System
Chapter 31, Alterations in Structure and Function of the Male Genitourinary System

Susan Osguthorpe, MS, CNA, RN
Clinical Associate Professor
University of Utah;
Acting Chief of Nursing Service
V.A. Medical Center
Salt Lake City, Utah
Chapter 12, Alterations in Oxygen Transport

Faith Young Peterson, MPA, MSN, CS, RN
Medical–Surgical Clinical Nurse Specialist
Saint Luke's Regional Medical Center
Boise, Idaho
Chapter 8, Infectious Processes
Chapter 9, Inflammation and Immunity
Chapter 10, Alterations in Immune Function
Aging Process Boxes

Maryann F. Pranulis, DNSc, RN
Director of Nursing Research and Education
University of California–San Diego Medical Center
San Diego, California
Chapter 7, Stress, Adaptation, and Coping

Mark Puhlman, MSN, ARNP, CCRN
Clinical Research Coordinator
Heart Institute
Spokane, Washington
Chapter 8, Infectious Processes

Edith Randall, MS, CCRN, RN
Clinical Nurse Specialist
Saint Luke's Medical Center
Phoenix, Arizona
Chapter 13, Alterations in Hemostasis and Blood Coagulation

Bridget Recker, EdM, RN
Clinical Coordinator
Department of Pediatrics
Maimonides Medical Center
Brooklyn, New York
Chapter 40, Alterations in Endocrine Control of Growth and Metabolism

Cleo Richard, MSN, RN
Clinical Consultant
Missoula, Montana
Chapter 26, Renal Function

Mary Sanguinetti-Baird, MN, ARNP, CNRN
Adjunct Faculty
Saint Martin's College;
Nurse Practitioner
Northwest Neuromuscular Associates
Olympia, Washington
Chapter 42, Neural Development and Cortical Function
Chapter 43, Acute Disorders of Brain Function

Lorna Schumann, PhD, ARNP, CCRN, RNCS
Associate Professor in Nursing
Intercollegiate Center for Nursing Education;
Critical Care Staff Nurse
Valley Hospital and Medical Center
Spokane, Washington
Chapter 19, Respiratory Function
Chapter 20, Obstructive Pulmonary Disorders
Chapter 21, Restrictive Pulmonary Disorders
Chapter 22, Ventilation and Respiratory Failure
Chapter 23, Other Respiratory Disorders

Billie Severtsen, PhD, RN
Associate Professor
Intercollegiate Center for Nursing Education
Spokane, Washington
Chapter 7, Stress, Adaptation, and Coping

Jacqueline Siegel, MN, ARNP, CDE
Diabetes Nurse Educator
Saint Joseph Hospital and Health Care Center
Tacoma, Washington
Chapter 41, Diabetes Mellitus

Gary Smith, PhD, OCS, PT
Chair and Assistant Professor
Department of Physical Therapy
Eastern Washington University
Cheney, Washington;
Vice President
Eagle Rehabilitation
Spokane, Washington
Chapter 49, Structure and Function of the Musculoskeletal System
Chapter 50, Alterations in Musculoskeletal Function: Trauma, Infection, and Disease
Chapter 51, Alterations in Musculoskeletal Function: Rheumatic Disorders

Martha J. Snider, EdB, RN
Associate Professor
University of Florida
College of Nursing
Gainesville, Florida
Chapter 47, Neurobiology of Psychotic Illness
Chapter 48, Neurobiology of Nonpsychotic Illness

Pam Springer, MS, RN
Director, Associate of Science Program
Department of Nursing
Boise State University
Boise, Idaho
Chapter 9, Inflammation and Immunity

Patti Stec, MSN, MN, RN
Clinical Instructor
Intercollegiate Center for Nursing Education;
Trauma Coordinator
Holy Family Hospital
Spokane, Washington
Chapter 27, Intrarenal Disorders
Chapter 29, Disorders of the Bladder

Gail Summers, RN
BFcN Candidate
York University
Toronto, Canada;
Manager, Nursing Services, CCU, ICU, MSS

Centenary Health Centre
Scarborough, Ontario, Canada
Chapter 54, Cardiogenic, Hypovolemic, Septic, Anaphylactic, and Neurogenic Shock

Julie Symes, MN, RN
Huron, South Dakota
Chapter 9, Inflammation and Immunity

Lorie Rietman Wild, MN, RN
Clinical Nurse Specialist, Acute Pain Management
University of Washington Medical Center
Seattle, Washington
Chapter 46, Pain

Debra Winston-Heath, MN, CCM, CNRN, RN
Auxiliary Faculty
University of Washington
School of Nursing
Seattle, Washington;
Staff Nurse
Department of Veterans Affairs
Medical Center
American Lake
Tacoma, Washington;
Neuroscience Clinical Specialist
Overlake Hospital Medical Center
Bellevue, Washington
Chapter 44, Chronic Disorders of Neurologic Function
Chapter 45, Alterations in Special Sensory Function

Reviewers

Catherine F. Bennett, MS, MSN, BSN, RNC
School of Nursing
Lansing Community College
Lansing, Michigan

Edward Butler, MD
Chief of Staff
Lawrence Memorial Hospital
Medford, Massachusetts

Evelyn Chatmon, CHN, RN
St. Jude Medical Center
Tulsa, Oklahoma

Sara E. Connor, EdD, MSN, RNCS
School of Nursing
Armstrong State College
Savannah, Georgia

Lawrence E. Cornett, PhD, BS
College of Medicine
University of Arkansas for Medical Sciences
Little Rock, Arkansas

Jean J. Cuppett, MSN, RN
School of Nursing
Saint Francis College
Loretto, Pennsylvania

Marilyn B. Damato, CNRN, MS, RN
St. Joseph's Hospital and Medical Center
Paterson, New Jersey

Julia K. Dattolo, MN, CCRN, RN
University of California
San Diego Medical Center
San Diego, California

Judy E. Davidson, MS, CNE, CCRN, RN
University of California Medical Center
San Diego, California

E. Dean, PhD, PT
School of Rehabilitation Medicine
University of British Columbia
Vancouver, British Columbia

Angela Demman-Treinen, MN, OCN, RN
Kenneth Norris Comprehensive Cancer Center
Los Angeles, California

Mary Edwards, PhD, RNC
School of Nursing
University of Texas Medical Branch
Galveston, Texas

Mary Beth Egloff, CCRN, MSN, RN
Sharp Memorial Hospital
San Diego, California

Katherine Elliott, MA, BS, RN
Coosa Valley Medical Center
Sylacauga, Alabama

Lou Ann T. Emerson, DNS, RN
School of Nursing
University of Cincinnati
Cincinnati, Ohio

Margaret M. Farrell, BA, RN
Frederick Memorial Hospital
Frederick Cancer Research Development Center
National Cancer Institute
Frederick, Maryland

Vickie K. Fieler, MS, RN
University of Rochester Cancer Center
Rochester, New York

Geraldine G. Flaherty, MSN, RN
School of Nursing
Wayne State University
Detroit, Michigan

Carol Fountain, MS, ONC, RN
School of Nursing
Boise State University
Boise, Idaho

Susan L. Gatto, MSN, RNP
School of Nursing
University of Central Arkansas
Conway, Arkansas

Martha J. Morrow, MSN, RN
School of Nursing
Shenandoah University
Winchester, Virginia

Elizabeth Olson, EdD, CRRN, RN
School of Nursing
Western Connecticut State University
Danbury, Connecticut

Jan Ellin Olson-Zeringue, MSN, FNP, RNC
School of Nursing
University of Alabama
Huntsville, Alabama

Anna Omery, DNSc, RN
School of Nursing
University of the City of Los Angeles
Los Angeles, California

Marilyn N. Pase, MSN, RN
School of Nursing
New Mexico State University
Las Cruces, New Mexico

Marie Rafalowski, MSN, CCRN, RN
School of Nursing
Georgia State University
Atlanta, Georgia

Edwina Gaylene Reichlin, MS, BS, RN
School of Nursing
Mesa State College
Grand Junction, Colorado

Patricia Sagan, MSN, RN
School of Nursing
University of Southern Mississippi
Long Beach, Mississippi

Olive A. Santavenere, PhD, MS, RN
School of Nursing
Southern Connecticut State University
New Haven, Connecticut

Richard R. Schmidt, PhD
Department of Anatomy
Thomas Jefferson Medical College
Philadelphia, Pennsylvania

Beverly J. Sedlacek, MSN, RN
School of Nursing
Kent State University
Ashtabula, Ohio

William A. Sodeman, Jr., MD
Medical College of Ohio
Toledo, Ohio

Teresa J. Stallcop, MSN, CCRN, RN
Saint Francis Hospital
Tulsa, Oklahoma

Christopher P. Steidle, MD
Northeast Indiana Urology, P.C.
Fort Wayne, Indiana

Jean Stewart, MSN, CEN, CNRN, RN
University of California Medical Center
San Diego, California

Nancy A. Stotts, EdD, RN
School of Nursing
University of California
San Francisco, California

Janice M. Sylakowski, MS, RN
School of Nursing
University of Buffalo
Buffalo, New York

Karen L. Then, BN, RN
School of Nursing
University of Calgary
Calgary, Alberta, Canada

Bette Doolan Titus, MSN, RN
School of Nursing
Armstrong State College
Savannah, Georgia

Agnes Urbas-Llewellyn, MS, CETN, RN
Virginia Medical Center
Martinsburg, West Virginia

Connie B. Varn, MN, RN
School of Nursing
Orangeburg-Calhoun Technical College
Orangeburg, South Carolina

Jennifer Vonnahme, MA, OCN,
Home Intensive Care, Inc.
Cincinnati, Ohio

Marge Whitman, BS, ONS, RN
Ellis Fischel Cancer Center
Columbus, Missouri

Brief Contents

Detailed Contents

Special Features

PERSPECTIVES ON *Pathophysiology*

U N I T   I
Central Concepts of Pathophysiology

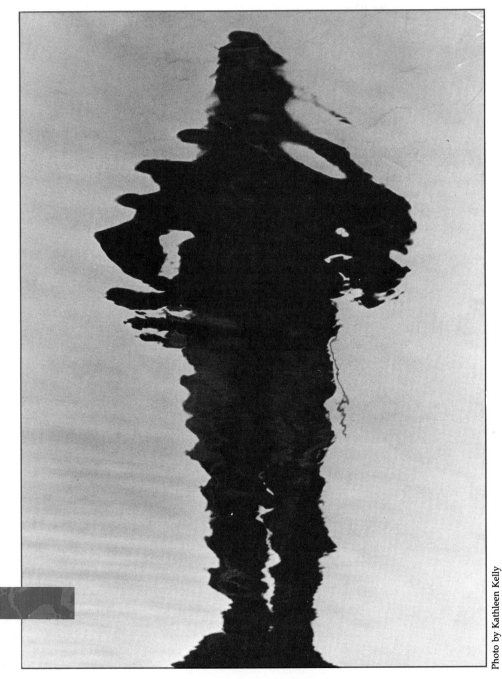

Reflected image of a person symbolizes distortions of the disease process. Just as water creates ripples, disease affects cells, tissues, organs, systems, and multiple systems simultaneously.

Photo by Kathleen Kelly

At one time people could afford to hold fairly simple beliefs about disease. Good health was a blessing, disease a curse. Disease was seen, quite sensibly, as an unwanted deviation from good health. Health was a state of wellness, fitness, movement, energy and an absence of bothersome or disabling symptoms. Disease was the underminer.

Deep inside, many people still believe these simple precepts. They feel lucky when they are healthy and unlucky when they are not, as though health were a natural state of goodness and disease an unexpected evil.

The truth is different. Or maybe we should say our current approximation of the truth differs from the folklore of disease and health, for all we ever know is what we know at the time. When we have available even an approximate truth about conditions as complicated and deeply intertwined as those of disease and health, we will have as much certainty as humans ever enjoy. Nature is never simple, and while we may like to think that disease is very nearly a deliberate violation of nature's preferences, the concept of disease is a much more challenging proposition to a student of disease and health. As Lewis Thomas has said, disease "usually results from inconclusive negotiations for symbiosis, an overstepping of the line by one side or the other, a biological misinterpretation of borders." It's a matter of delicate balance, timing, close calls.

We make progress. We now know—and our understanding increases steadily—more about the processes of disease than we have ever known before. The revelations produced by the broad advances in genetic research signal the most dramatic of the directions in which research is carrying us. We also steadily acquire information about cultural, age, and sex differences and other factors that allow us to see disease not as an evil visitor but an inherent factor in the spectrum of possibilities presented to each human being at birth. We also know more and more about the effects of outside factors such as environmental pollution and tobacco smoking, which may turn a likelihood—a susceptibility or inherited weakness—into actual illness.

We search outside the single diseased body for patterns of disease in human communities. Epidemiologists, who study those patterns, continue to teach us more about the occurrence of disease. This science is important in determining the causes of disease when environmental agents are suspected—contaminants with which the miners of radioactive materials have been brought into contact, for example, or lung disorders in places with heavy air pollution. Epidemiologists also remind us to keep a clear sense of balance when we think about disease. Some diseases are highly publicized, often for good reason and with beneficial effects, but a good local epidemiologist will notice that a community may suffer as much or more when its older citizens encounter an epidemic of a mundane illness such as flu.

We remain troubled by common terms such as "normal" or "abnormal." Perhaps we should allow ourselves to be troubled because the determining of norms in health and disease often involves the assessment of individuals who vary greatly in their susceptibilities and in their ability to withstand, cope, and even thrive while they are in what is considered a diseased state.

The balance that we find in those enjoying good health, or in people with disease who have settled at plateaus of stability, however impaired, is called homeostasis. That balance is as precious in those suffering from disease as it is for those who have no affliction. But the natural human optimism that glories in good health and detests disease conveys an inadequate sense of the actual symbiosis, in which the agents of disease and health struggle or commingle or quietly ignore each other in the body.

FRONTIERS OF RESEARCH
Ecology of Human Disease
Michael J. Kirkhorn

Those interested in disease will find guidance in history. Medical historian Logan Clendening found the first written descriptions of disease in Egyptian papyri almost 3,000 years old. Some of the ancient remedies, diagnoses, and treatments from early Egyptian, Greek, and Arabic medicine sound plausible today. So do some of the aphorisms of Hippocrates, if only because his observations invoke that valuable commodity, common sense: "When sleep puts an end to delirium, it is a good symptom," Hippocrates said, and, "In every movement of the body, whenever one begins to endure pain, it will be relieved by rest."

Our time is one in which the understanding of the nature of disease, and therefore of health, seems to be proceeding with unusual speed and confidence. Researchers expect that in the near future genetic research could produce a number of astonishing cures as well as new kinds of diagnosis, immunization, prevention, anticipation of disease, and preemptive therapy.

The genetic research into the nature of disease, in which so much hope is being placed, promises exactitude. It promises to locate precisely the origin of many diseases, allowing us either to prevent or to correct them with therapies unavailable to past generations. It promises to decode our physical nature and reveal the qualities that we associate with defects of the body, mind, or spirit. So disease is tracked to its most secret refuge, where it is naturally present in the body. The findings of genetic research are most rewarding when they relieve people of the diseases that trouble us most—severe acute or chronic diseases—but they promise a range of responses to lesser ailments.

The current research also promises reliable prevention of the particularly tragic diseases that cause agony because they kill prematurely, such as breast cancer. Some current research indicates that through T-cell vaccines and T-cell therapy the cancer patient's own immune system can be strengthened in ways that fight cancer and offer possible lifelong protection against relapse.

Hippocrates would have been impressed.

CHAPTER 1
Complex Nature of Disease

LEE-ELLEN COPSTEAD

KEY TERMS

acute: A condition with relatively severe manifestations but running a short course.

chronic: A condition that lasts for a long period of time.

complication: A new or separate process that may arise secondarily because of some change produced by the original entity. For example, bacterial pneumonia may be a complication of viral infection of the respiratory tract.

convalescence: The stage of recovery after a disease, injury, or surgical operation.

disease: Sum of the deviations from normal structure or function of any part, organ, or system (or combination thereof) of the body manifested by a characteristic set of symptoms and/or signs and whose etiology, pathogenesis, and prognosis may be known or unknown.

epidemic: Disease occurring suddenly and affecting numbers of people clearly in excess of normal expectancy.

etiology: The assignment of causes or reasons for phenomena.

exacerbation: A relatively sudden increase in the severity of a disease or any of its signs and symptoms.

intercurrent: Occurs during the course of an already existing disease.

morphologic changes: The structural and associated functional alterations in cells or tissues that are either characteristic of the disease or diagnostic of the etiologic process.

pandemic: Epidemics that affect large geographic regions, perhaps spreading worldwide.

pathogen: An agent that causes disease.

pathogenesis: The development or evolution of the disease. A description of the pathogenesis includes everything that happens in the body from the initial stimulus to the ultimate expression of manifestations of the disease.

pathophysiology: The science of disordered function.

prognosis: A forecast about the probable outcome of a disease; the prospect of recovery from a disease indicated by the nature, signs, and/or symptoms of the case.

remission: An abatement or decline in severity of the signs and symptoms of a disease. If a remission is permanent, we say that the person is "cured."

sequela: A condition caused by and following a disease (plural, sequelae).

sign: Objectively identifiable aberration of the disease. Fever, reddening of the skin, and a palpable mass are *signs* of disease.

symptom: Subjective feeling of discomfort that can be reported by the affected individual to an observer. Nausea, malaise, and pain are *symptoms* of disease.

syndrome: A collection of different signs and symptoms that occur together.

---

*T*he foundation for understanding the concepts of disease and illness begins here. A discussion of the complex nature of disease—what constitutes disease, and how disease and illness are manifested—is especially relevant to a pathophysiology text. Sociocultural influences that affect our perceptions concerning disease and illness, key elements of pathophysiologic processes, and an agreed common terminology are important to the discussion.

Physiology is the study of the specific characteristics and functions of a living organism and its parts; *patho-* comes from the Greek *pathos,* which means suffering or disease. Together, as **pathophysiology,** these terms refer to the disorder or breakdown of the human body's function. Most people recognize what it is to be "healthy," and would define disease or illness as a change from or absence of that state. But under closer scrutiny, the concept of health is difficult to describe in simple, succinct terms; correspondingly, the concepts of disease and illness are also complex.

Concepts of Disease and Illness

The negative dimension of health can be described as ill health. However, a straightforward determination of how ill health is experienced by an individual often is not possible. The **physical, mental,** and **social** facets are inextricably intertwined[1]: serious or troublesome physical illness, for example, may lead to mental ill health (a state of depression or anxiety) or social impairment; likewise, mental illness may result in physical ill health (an injury arising from failed suicide) or social handicap. Indeed, these facets may damage other aspects of health: for instance, low socioeconomic status is associated with a wide range of physical and mental health problems.[2] Thus, ill health can refer to disease, injury, illness, disability, or handicap, occurring singly or in various combinations and experienced over long or short periods of time.

Although disease and illness are often used synonymously, they are not the same. Disease is a technical term that represents a medically defined condition that is identifiable as similar to that suffered by others. Someone may feel ill for a variety of reasons: illness as a result of a diagnosed disease, from situational depression, or simply from an adverse drug reaction. On the other hand, disease may be present without any manifestation of illness. This situation may arise with some skin conditions that first appear as rashes, or even with a presymptomatic cancer. Nevertheless, within the context of physical, mental, and social facets of ill health, disease and illness distort normal life processes.

Disease and Illness as Abnormal States

One common notion is that disease and illness represent abnormal states, or at least an extension or distortion of the normal life processes going on in the individual. According to *Dorland's Illustrated Medical Dictionary*, 27th edition, disease is[3]

> . . . *any deviation from or interruption of the normal* structure or function of any part, organ, or system (or combination thereof) of the body that is manifested by a characteristic set of symptoms and signs and whose etiology, pathogenesis, and prognosis may be known or unknown [italics added].

Disease is actually the *sum* of the deviations from normal. Even in the case of an obviously infectious disease, where the body is literally invaded, the infectious agent does not constitute the disease but only evokes the changes in the subject that ultimately manifest as disease. One way of looking at disease is to see it as an external entity with its own life cycle, course, manifestations, and cure. However, in the example of the invasive infectious agent, attempted treatment with antibiotics alone may not be a sufficient cure if proper attention is not directed toward the intrinsic bodily processes and the external environment of the affected individual.

In order to understand and adequately treat disease, one must take into account the normal processes that have been altered, the nature of the disturbances, and the effects that such disturbances have on other vital processes.

By means of a variety of clinical and laboratory tests it is possible to measure characteristics of normalcy as well as deviations from it. In the healthy state, a certain value is consistently obtained for a particular factor, within specific laboratory definitions. This range of values or indices is considered to be **within normal limits,** given the constraints of laboratory variables. Deviations from this range are usually considered abnormal.

Factors Affecting Determination of Normality

Genetic Variations

There is no absolute normal for any biologic parameter. What is usual for one person may be different for another because of genetic variations. For example, a blood pressure of 120/80 mm Hg is a common value. Other people consistently have a blood pressure of 90/70 mm Hg, yet are in good health. This value represents their normal blood pressure. By sampling a large number of people, an "average normal" and a range of normal can be determined.

An occasional person may consistently show a value outside the usual range for the factor and yet be functioning well. Although the person may be abnormal for that characteristic in terms of the population as a whole, the unusual value may be normal for that individual.

Cultural Considerations

To place the above considerations in perspective, it should be noted that the notion of what constitutes

normalcy and even *illness* is, to a certain extent, arbitrary and influenced by culture as well as genetics. Each culture defines health and illness in a manner that reflects its previous experience.[4] Cultural factors determine which signs, symptoms, or behaviors are perceived as abnormal.[5] A person from a literate culture, for example, with a significant reading disability would be labeled as having an *abnormality*, whereas the same defect would not be identified in a nonliterate culture. Further, a trait such as very short stature is average and thus *normal* in a population of Japanese elders, yet it would be considered distinctly *abnormal* in a population of United States National Basketball Association players. An infant from an impoverished culture with "normal" chronic diarrhea and poor weight gain would be viewed as abnormal in a progressive culture such as a well baby clinic in Sweden. Given cultural variations that affect definitions of normal and abnormal, the resulting pattern of behaviors or clinical manifestations is what the culture labels as illness.[6]

Age Differences

Many biologic factors vary with age, and the normal value for a person at one age may be abnormal at another. A number of physiologic changes, such as hair color, skin turgor (tension), and organ size, vary with age. In general, most organs shrink—exceptions are the male prostate and the heart, which enlarge with age. Gray hair, wrinkled skin, and receding gums, normal in an elderly person, are abnormal in a child. Special sensory changes, such as diminished near sight, high-tone hearing loss, and loss of taste discriminations for sweet and salty, are normal in an elderly adult and abnormal in a middle-aged adult or child. There are fewer sweat glands and less thirst perception in an elderly person than in a young adult or child. Elderly persons have diminished temperature sensations and can, therefore, sustain burn injuries—from a heating pad or bathwater—because they do not perceive heat with the same intensity as a middle-aged adult. A resting heart rate of 120 beats per minute is normal for an infant, but not for an adult.

Gender Differences

Some laboratory values, such as levels of sex hormones and growth hormones, show gender differences. The complete blood cell count shows differences by gender in hematocrit, hemoglobin, and red blood cell (RBC) count.[7] For example, the normal range of hemoglobin concentration for adult women is lower than that for adult men. For adult women the normal range is 12–15 g/100 mL of blood; for adult men the normal range is 14–17 g/100 mL of blood.[8] Blood calcium ranges are slightly higher in adult women than in adult men.[9] There are also gender differences in large granular lymphocytes[10] and in the erythrocyte sedimentation rate (ESR). The ESR is a nonspecific laboratory test of the speed at which erythrocytes settle. In this test, blood to which an anticoagulant has been added is placed in a long, narrow tube, and the distance the RBCs fall in 1 hour is the rate, or ESR. Normally, in males, it is less than 10 mm/hr[8]; it is slightly higher in females. There are also differences by gender in creatinine values. For females, the normal serum creatinine is 0.4–1.3 mg/dL, for males, the normal range is 0.6–1.5 mg/dL.[8] Research into gender differences also suggests that, on average, males snore more than females,[11–13] have longer vocal cords, have better daylight vision, have higher metabolic rates, and are more likely to be left-handed. Research also suggests that females and males have different communication styles and respond differently to similar conditions.[14]

Situational Differences

In some cases, a deviation from the usual value may occur as an adaptive mechanism, and whether the deviation is considered abnormal or not depends on the situation. For example, the RBC count increases when a person moves to a high altitude.[15] This increase is a normal adaptive response to the decreased availability of oxygen at a high altitude and is termed **acclimatization.** A similar increase in the RBC count at sea level would be abnormal.

Time Variations

Some factors vary according to the time of day; i.e., they exhibit a **circadian rhythm** or **diurnal variation.** In interpreting the result of a particular test, it may be necessary to know the time at which the value was determined. For example, body temperature and plasma concentrations of certain hormones (such as growth hormone and cortisol) exhibit diurnal variation. Reflecting fluctuation in plasma levels, the peak rate in urinary excretion for a particular steroid (17-ketosteroid) occurs between 8 A.M. and 10 A.M. and is about two to three times greater than the lowest rate, which occurs between midnight and 2 A.M.[8] The urinary excretion of ions (such as potassium) also exhibits diurnal variation. Figure 1–1 illustrates circadian rhythms of several physiologic variables.

Laboratory Conditions

Some clinical and laboratory measurements vary according to methods used. For example, the prothrombin time is sensitive to the *reagent* used in the procedure. In order to determine a prothrombin time, the **reagent**—a substance composed of thromboplastin and calcium—is added to decalcified plasma to create a reaction—in this case, clot formation. The prothrombin time is determined by measuring the length of time it takes for clotting to occur after this reagent is added.

In the United States alone, there are several different reagent companies and a variety of lot numbers representing each reagent. Although a given laboratory may keep the same lot number for up to a year,

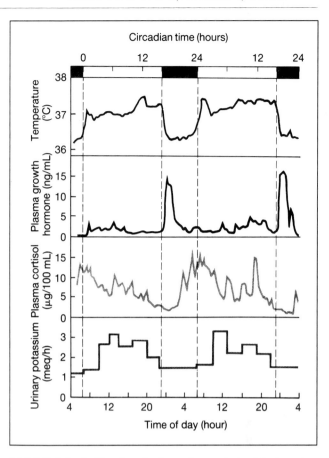

FIGURE 1–1. Circadian rhythms of several physiologic variables in a human subject depict the effect of light and dark. In an experiment with lights on (open bars at top) for 16 hours and off (black bars at top) for 8 hours, temperature, plasma growth hormone, plasma cortisol, and urinary potassium levels exhibit diurnal variation. (From Vander et al: *Human Physiology,* 5th ed. New York, McGraw-Hill, 1990; as adapted from Moore-Ede MC, Sulzman FM, Fuller CA: *The Clocks That Time Us: Physiology of the Circadian Timing System.* Cambridge, Harvard University Press, 1982. Reproduced by permission of McGraw-Hill.)

the reagent that is used in specific testing situations likely varies between laboratories.

Whenever a new reagent is obtained, a corresponding range of normal values must be calculated. For example, in order to determine the range of normal for a particular reagent, a **normal study** using a minimum of 30 specimens—carefully controlled for age and sex and excluding all drugs, including nicotine—is conducted. The values obtained from this study determine what are called the **population mean** and the **reference range.** Figure 1–2 illustrates hypothetical examples of different reagent sensitivities in determining the prothrombin time.

Disturbances of the internal environment occur in disease, altering a variety of measurable factors. Prolongation of the clotting time, for example, could be related to a wide variety of clinical variables, including liver disease, vitamin K deficiency, or anticoagulant therapy. Values obtained in laboratory tests are useful in assessing a person's state of health or disease.

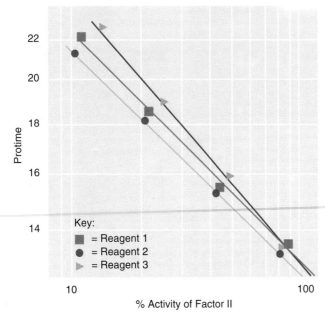
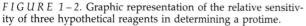

F I G U R E 1 – 2. Graphic representation of the relative sensitivity of three hypothetical reagents in determining a protime.

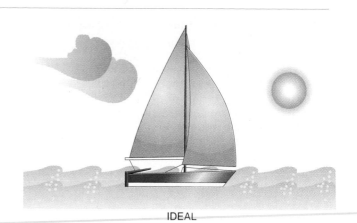

IDEAL

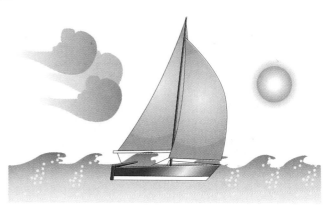

NORMAL

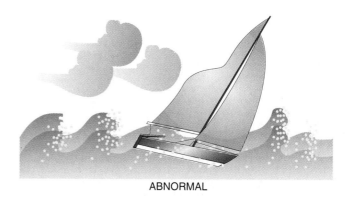

ABNORMAL

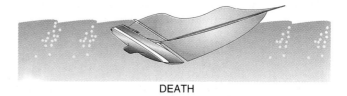

DEATH

F I G U R E 1 – 3. Example of physiologic oscillation. The movement of a sailboat at sea represents the fluctuation of a physiologic variable around ideal conditions. A disturbance in either direction could move the sailboat into danger—for our purposes, the disease state. If the disturbance is so extreme that the boat sinks, death results.

Baseline Evaluations

Often, when assessing a person's health status, a *change* in some value or factor is more significant than the actual value of the particular factor. A blood pressure of 90/70 mm Hg may not be significant if that is the usual value for a particular person. If a person usually has a blood pressure of 120/80 mm Hg, however, a reading of 90/70 mm Hg would be very significant. Deviation from the usual value can be indicative of disease, especially if it is accompanied by other signs and symptoms.

Because of these considerations, determining a normal range of variation from an average value is a complex matter. This complexity includes knowing the degree of physiologic oscillation of a particular measurement, accounting for the degree of variation among normal individuals under **baseline** conditions, and figuring the precision of the measurement method. Finally, the biologic significance of the measurement must be estimated. Single measurements, observations, or laboratory results that seem to indicate abnormality must always be judged in the context of the entire health picture of the individual. One slightly elevated blood glucose level does not mean clinical diabetes, a single high blood pressure reading does not denote hypertension, a temporary feeling of hopelessness does not indicate clinical depression, and a single hemoglobin value lower than the average does not define anemia. The concept of physiologic oscillation may be depicted schematically as a sailboat moving at sea, fluctuating around "ideal" conditions (Fig. 1–3).

Disease and Illness as Disordered or Disrupted States

A crucial notion in both illness and disease is that of upset or disorder. We can partly understand this if we think of the human body as a machine, in which various processes (such as digestion and excretion, maintenance of a certain temperature, inhaling of oxygen) necessary to its maintenance and smooth working are carried out, and through which the person whose body it is carries out his or her actions. In this model, an upset or disorder represents a failure in the system that prevents the machine from working properly. What is "wrong" or "bad" is precisely this interference with the machine's normal working.

Disease and Illness as Incapacitating States

Discomfort

The above mechanistic model of ill health is only partly satisfactory. For one thing, it does not accommodate *pain* and other subjective symptoms, such as nausea, feeling faint, and so on. These subjective symptoms are essentially inward feelings and non-mechanistic in that they do not interfere with the actual working of the bodily mechanism.[16] This is not to say, though, that the subjective symptom may not constitute a disorder. *Pain*, for example, may constitute a disorder that must be addressed. If severe, it will psychologically interfere with the sufferer's activities. Even when it does not, pain is still a matter for medical attention.[17] Thus a person in pain, from apparent cause or not, is regarded, in American culture, as ill or not well.

So far, then, we have two kinds of abnormal phenomena that constitute ill health: what may be termed mechanical failure, and discomfort. One possible connection between these two phenomena is that both pain and malfunction are unpleasant things for those who have them. This assertion would, of course, need a little qualification. Some pain, in some circumstances, can be pleasant, as any athlete knows, and illness can be positively welcome—if, for example, it allows the youngster to skip school, missing a day of grueling tests. But, in general terms, pain is unpleasant, and in general, being incapacitated prevents people from doing whatever they want to do—at least with normal plans and projects. Thus, the disorder that characterizes illness and disease, and that takes the form both of discomfort and of mechanical failure, is to be described as a (physical) condition that is in general unpleasant or prevents people from doing what they want.

Disability and Deformity

Deformity is analogous to illness because it represents a disorder that health professionals treat—or, better, try to prevent. It should be noted that deformity, un-like some illness and disease, is not incompatible with good health.[18] Of course, there are some deformities, such as congenital heart anomalies, that produce mechanical failures, and a sufferer from these is said to be in poor health. But a child who is born deaf is not therefore unhealthy. This is difficult to understand if ill health is depicted solely as uncomfortable or frustrating abnormalities of a system. However, if ill health is viewed within the context of culture and self, it is somewhat more comprehensible. It is true that a person who is severely handicapped by deafness might hesitate before stating on a form that he or she is in perfect health, but, broadly speaking, such a handicap is not thought of as impairing health.

An alternative view, not unknown in history, holds that disease is actually a new form of life, a sort of possession of the body by an outside invader. From this notion, it would follow that surgery or medicine—warfare directed at eradicating the invader—are proper therapies for disease. In such cases one can always sensibly ask whether the sufferer is getting better or worse. Being ill is essentially an unstable situation. The deaf child, by contrast, is fixed in disability, and so is not regarded as unhealthy because there is nothing untoward going on in him or her. But the fact that the deaf child is not unhealthy does not mean that health professionals remain unconcerned with trying to prevent cases of childhood deafness or to alleviate disability.

Injury

Some of the points that apply to deformity also apply to injury.[19] Sometimes people who have been badly injured are described as ill, and when this is so they are suffering from the same kinds of incapacity that attend other illness—weakness, faintness, unconsciousness, and so forth. But if the lack of capacity is simply the essential result of the injury, then the sufferer might in one sense be in good health. A skier who has broken a leg cannot walk, but may be in glowing health. The doctor's task here may be described as the restoration not of health but of wholeness. But injury is in one respect more like illness than deformity: it can progress in that it can heal.

This account of physical ill health may be summarized by saying that ill health can occur in episodes or over long periods, that it can manifest in illness or disease, and that these overlapping concepts can be linked if they are seen on the model of abnormal, disordered or disrupted, or incapacitating states of a biologic system (Fig. 1–4).

Health and Disease

Prevention of ill health is too narrow to be the goal of health care. Needed instead is some notion of positive health or physical "wholeness" that includes not only what is implied by the absence of ill health but additional elements. The World Health Organization (WHO) defines health as complete physical, mental,

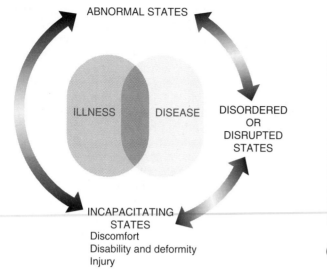

FIGURE 1–4. Illness and disease are overlapping concepts linked on the model of abnormal, disordered or disrupted, or incapacitating states of a biologic system.

and social well-being, and not merely the absence of disease or infirmity.[20] For some, health implies the ability to do what they regard as worthwhile and conduct their lives as they want. Figure 1–5 depicts examples of healthy aging.

KEY CONCEPTS

- Pathophysiology is the study of abnormalities or alterations in body function. Disordered function is often, but not always, due to an identifiable disease process. Disease and illness may be manifested by perceptions of discomfort or by deformity, disability, or injury.

- Disease and illness are complex phenomena. Environment, genetic constitution, socioeconomic status, life-style, and previous physical health all affect the timing and ultimate expression of disease in a particular individual.

- Variations in physiologic processes may be a result of factors other than disease or illness. Age, sex, genetic and ethnic background, geographic area, and time of day may influence various physiologic parameters. Care must be taken to interpret "abnormal" findings in light of these possible confounding factors. In addition, the potential for spurious findings always exists. Thus, trends and changes in a particular individual are more reliable than single observations.

Concepts of Homeostasis

Physiologically, all cells in the body need a balance of oxygen and nutrients for their continuing survival and also require an environment which affords such things as narrow ranges of temperature, water content, acidity, and salt concentration. Walter Cannon defined this balance as **homeostasis**—the sum of the processes by which the body maintains itself at a relatively constant composition.[21] Yet even Cannon's definition is oversimplified. Research with a variety of radioisotopes has since demonstrated that homeostasis does not mean "constant composition." The concept of homeostasis as a *dynamic steady state* is much more accurate. The fat or protein content of the body, for example, may not vary much from day to day, but the substances that make up the fat and protein—fatty acids and amino acids—can vary widely.[22] The enzymes in a healthy person are constantly synthesizing and breaking them down. The

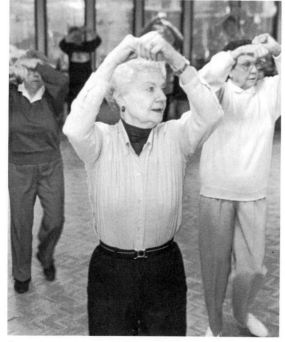

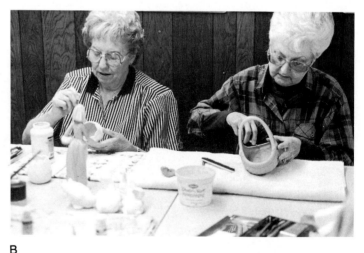

FIGURE 1–5. Healthy aging. Healthy elders exercising in an aerobics class (**A**) and working with ceramics (**B**) illustrate the concept that aging and disease are not synonymous. (Photographer: Kathleen Kelly, Spokane, WA.)

process of synthesis and breakdown of all bodily substances is known as **turnover.** Hence, homeostasis is more accurately defined as a *dynamic steady state, representing the net effect of all the turnover reactions.* Maintenance of internal homeostasis is an essential feature of the normal body.

Disruption of Homeostasis

One of the most revealing and readily measurable concepts of disease and illness (mental, physical, and social) is that of *imbalance.* Family, other caregivers, friends, or spiritual counselors affect the balance between requirements of daily living and the resources necessary to meet them (Fig. 1–6).[23] Financial stress, impaired ability to perform activities of daily living, or family or caregiver conflicts may disrupt the balance.

Under conditions of health, we are in balance with the antagonistic forces of our environment. Since neither we nor our environment are static, this is a constantly shifting balance—a state of dynamic equilibrium. Sometimes these balancing forces are equal and cancel each other through direct reaction, one against the other. At other times, the balance of opposing forces is like that which exists between the mainspring and the hairspring of a watch: the second is necessary to control the first. In disease, offsetting controls fail and imbalances prevail, and cells, tissues, organs, and systems are altered because of it (Fig. 1–7).

When some of the structures and functions of the body deviate from the norm to the point that homeostasis is destroyed or threatened or the individual can no longer meet the environmental challenges, **disease** is said to exist. The upper and lower limits of homeostasis are illustrated in Figure 1–8. Here, the safe range, or the range over which homeostasis is maintained, is bounded at the lower limits by the minimal physiologic requirement and at the upper limits by the maximal physiologic tolerance. These limits become progressively narrowed in disease.[24] As the degree of functional impairment progresses, minimal requirements tend to increase while maximal tolerances tend to decrease (Fig. 1–8). It follows that if homeostasis is disrupted, cells, tissues, organs, systems, or an affected individual cannot function optimally.

The origin of disease actually lies within the adaptive machinery of the body itself. The very same machinery that renders the body immune to infection also evokes reactions such as hay fever and asthma in the presence of certain environmental agents. Similarly, the machinery of cellular renewal that repairs wounds and constantly replenishes cell populations in tissue may morbidly proliferate, giving rise to cancer. If the demands made on the body are too great, the homeostatic mechanisms may be inadequate to compensate.

The body's vital equilibrium is maintained by a mechanism of **self-regulation,** so broad in its scope as to include most of the complex, sensitive functions that characterize life. The ability of the body to "self-regulate" or "return to normal" to maintain homeostasis is a critically important concept in modern physiology and also serves as a basis for understanding mechanisms of disease.

Homeostatic Control Mechanisms

Each cell of the body, each tissue, each organ, and each system plays an important role in homeostasis. These diverse regulatory systems employ feedback and feedforward mechanisms that far surpass our most brilliant electronic achievements. If circumstances occur that require changes or more intense regulation in the internal environment, the body must have appropriate control mechanisms available to respond to the change and must also be able to restore and maintain normalcy. Regardless of the body func-

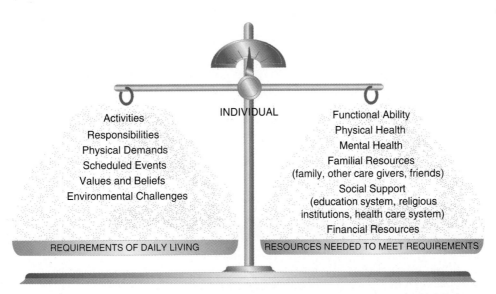

FIGURE 1–6. A scale symbolizes the concept of *balance* between the requirements of daily living and the resources necessary to meet those requirements.

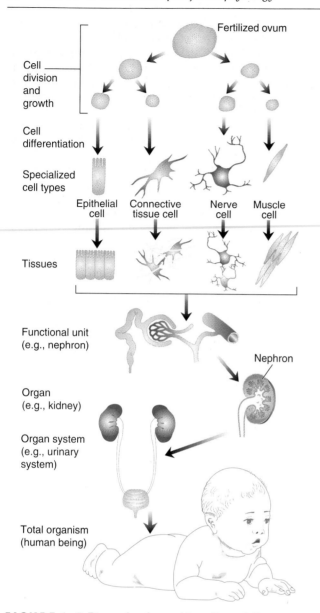

F I G U R E 1 – 7. Disease has far-reaching effects. Cell, tissue, and organ system involvement are illustrated as structural levels of organization.

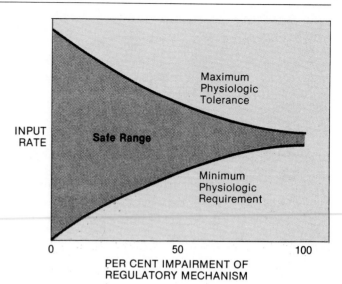

F I G U R E 1 – 8. Upper and lower limits of homeostasis. The safe range, or the range over which homeostasis is maintained, is bounded at the upper limits by the maximum physiologic tolerance and at the lower limits by the minimum physiologic requirements. Impairment of the regulating mechanism by disease narrows the safe range. (From Wyngaarden JB, Smith LH Jr (eds): *Cecil Textbook of Medicine*, 18th ed. Philadelphia, WB Saunders, 1988. Used with permission.)

be able to identify the outlier and to respond to it. A variable is considered to be an outlier if it deviates from the normal set point or set point range. The level or magnitude of the variable's deviation is calculated by comparing the outlier to the normal "set point" level that must be maintained for homeostasis. If a deviation occurs, the sensor generates a response such as a neural or hormonal signal to the integration or control center, which notifies the center that homeostasis is being threatened.

When the control center (often a discrete area of the brain) receives this message, it analyzes the input and integrates it with input from other sensors in order to decide upon a specific action. If significant deviation exists, the integration/control center will send its own specialized signal to the third component of the control loop—the effector mechanism.

Effectors are the targets that directly influence control of physiologic variables. For example, it is effector action that ultimately increases or decreases variables such as body temperature, heart rate, blood pressure, or blood sugar concentration to keep them within their normal range. The activity of effectors is regulated by feedback of information to sensors, which in turn evaluate the effects on variable control.

Negative Feedback Systems

Homeostatic systems tend to be **negative feedback systems** and regulate deviations from normal by *negating* any attempts toward radical excess or deficiency (Fig. 1–9).

To comprehend how a system of negative feedback operates within the body, a mechanical model

tion being regulated or the mechanism of information transfer (nerve impulse or hormone secretion), communication is managed through the same feedback loop, which includes three basic components: (1) a sensor mechanism, (2) an integrating or control center, and (3) an effector mechanism. Feedforward regulation *anticipates* changes in a regulated variable (internal body temperature, for example) and improves the speed of the body's homeostatic responses, minimizing fluctuations in the level of the variable being regulated.

The process of regulation and the concept of "return to normal" first require that the body be able to "sense" or identify the outlying variable. Specialized nerve cells or hormone-producing (endocrine) glands frequently act as homeostatic sensors. A sensor must

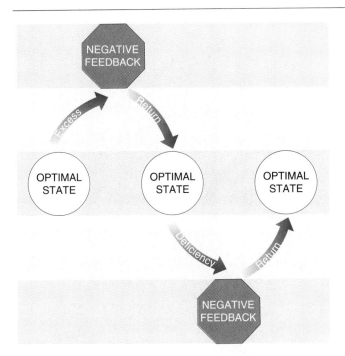

FIGURE 1-9. Homeostatic systems tend to be *negative feed-back* systems and regulate deviations from normal, leading the organism back to an optimal state and thereby negating any attempts toward radical excess or deficiency.

will be used for purposes of explanation. Although mechanical models are helpful for understanding how the system of negative feedback operates within the body, they can also be misleading because they tend to greatly oversimplify the biologic activities and processes that they represent. The ideas expressed by feedback mechanisms provide a way of thinking about the control of physiologic mechanisms, but they do not actually represent distinct physiologic processes.

One major type of negative feedback mechanism is a thermostat-like regulator. Thermostat-like regulators are distinguished by two features. First, these mechanisms operate by correcting deviations from a definite predetermined goal or "setting." Second, thermostat-like regulators operate intermittently rather than continuously, turning off and on as needed to correct errors. The system is triggered whenever an error is signaled, toward that activity which will return it to the range of function normal for it. Figure 1–10 illustrates the concept of heat regulation by comparing the thermostat-like mechanism in the home with that of the human body.

In disease, the set point or reference level may be altered, just as a thermostat may be set too high or too low. Consequently, negative feedback regulates temperature at abnormal levels. The set point is altered, for example, in fever. Here, the internal "thermostat" is set too high and there is a corresponding elevation in temperature.

In the example of temperature regulation, homeostatic regulation for a particular variable is controlled by one negative feedback system. Some variables, for example blood pressure, may be under the control of several different feedback systems, which must all function so they complement each other.

A second major type of negative feedback is the continually fluctuating mechanism. With the continually fluctuating mechanism, the reference point is continually fluctuating and the system is in continuous motion rather than shutting off and on. Control of blood glucose levels within the body is an example of a continually fluctuating mechanism. Other examples of continually fluctuating mechanisms are the controls that involve endocrine balance and hormonal regulation. (See also Chapter 39, Mechanisms of Endocrine Control and Metabolism.)

Sometimes outside intervention is required to maintain homeostasis. For example, control mechanisms may fail. An example is when the pancreas fails to secrete insulin, a necessary hormone, necessitating injection of insulin.

Positive Feedback Systems

Although negative feedback systems are by far the most common homeostatic systems in the body, there is another type of feedback, known as **positive feedback.** With positive feedback, an initial disturbance in a system sets off a chain of events that increases the disturbance even further. Positive feedback does not favor stability and often abruptly displaces a system away from its steady-state operating point. Only a few positive feedback examples operate in the body under normal conditions. However, events that lead to a simple "sneeze," the birth of a baby, and formation of a blood clot involve several important positive feedback relationships. (See Chapter 13, Alterations in Hemostasis and Blood Coagulation, for a further discussion of the physiology of blood clotting.)

Homeostasis as a Unifying Concept

The concept of homeostatic balance represents an ideal. Actually, in every self-regulating system there is always some degree of deviation from what is optimum or normal for that system. Overmire writes, "Homeostatic regulators can never be expected to function perfectly, since control is achieved only through adjustment of error."[25]

Knowledge of homeostatic mechanisms has nevertheless contributed greatly to the study of physiology and pathophysiology, and to the general dynamics of living. The field of physiology has benefited from the concept of homeostasis in several ways. Homeostasis has engendered a sense of order and unity to the study of biologic processes. Bodily changes and adjustments that formerly seemed to conflict can now be better understood as adaptive or compensatory manifestations of homeostasis and as functions related to the total needs of the individual. The concept of homeostasis has elucidated the interdependence of the body's systems. For example, the circulatory, endocrine, and nervous systems are no longer regarded as isolated units, operating independently of

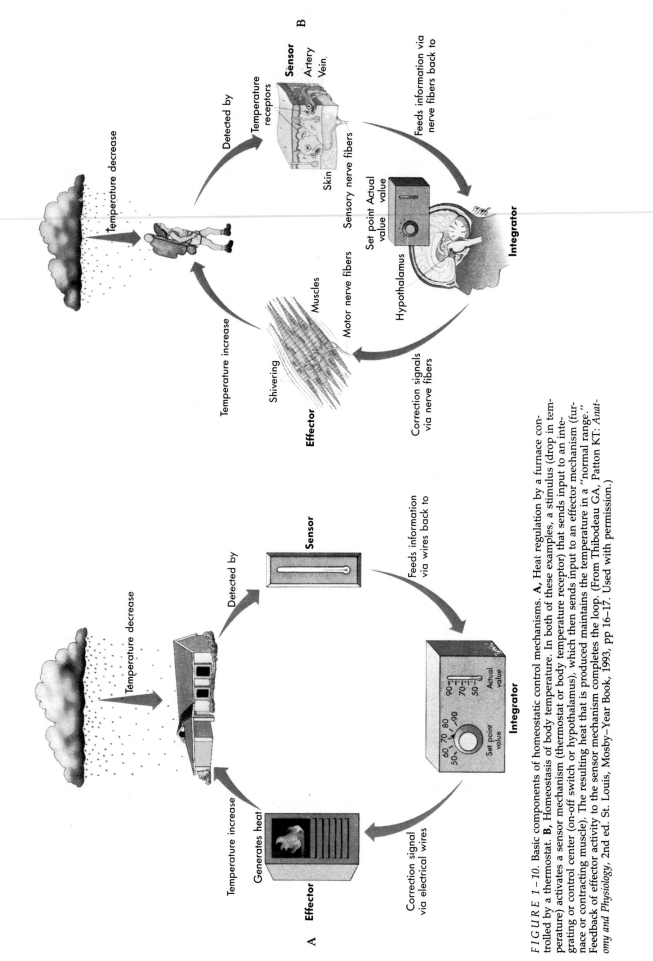

FIGURE 1–10. Basic components of homeostatic control mechanisms. **A,** Heat regulation by a furnace controlled by a thermostat. **B,** Homeostasis of body temperature. In both of these examples, a stimulus (drop in temperature) activates a sensor mechanism (thermostat or body temperature receptor) that sends input to an integrating or control center (on-off switch or hypothalamus), which then sends input to an effector mechanism (furnace or contracting muscle). The resulting heat that is produced maintains the temperature in a "normal range." Feedback of effector activity to the sensor mechanism completes the loop. (From Thibodeau GA, Patton KT: *Anatomy and Physiology,* 2nd ed. St. Louis, Mosby–Year Book, 1993, pp 16–17. Used with permission.)

each other. Rather, they are part of a functioning whole, working together to enable the individual to survive emergencies and everyday stresses. Homeostasis has enabled us to see physiology as a dynamic process of continuous self-regulation and self-adjustment. Consequently we can better understand the many fluctuations and oscillations that occur constantly within the body. In light of these factors, it is not surprising that many scientists believe homeostasis is the single most important concept in human physiology.

KEY CONCEPTS

- Homeostasis refers to the body's tendency to maintain a steady state in the face of continual environmental variation. Parameters such as temperature, cardiac output, blood pressure, oxygen and carbon dioxide levels, acid-base balance, fluid volume, and electrolyte composition are closely regulated to maintain homeostasis.

- Most homeostatic control mechanisms in the body function on the principle of negative feedback. The variable to be controlled must be "sensed" in order to be regulated. Sensory neurons and endocrine glands are primary homeostatic sensors. Sensors then feed back to a regulatory center (usually the brain), which integrates all relevant input and initiates a response. The response is carried out by effectors (muscles and glands).

- Disease can be viewed as a disturbance of homeostasis. Homeostasis can be disrupted by processes that interfere with the function of homeostatic sensors, regulatory centers, or effectors.

Concepts of Epidemiology

Differences among *individuals* are, of course, very important in determining the diseases to which they are susceptible and their reactions to the diseases once they contract them. But the study of *patterns of disease*, involving large groups of people, provides yet another important dimension (Fig. 1–11).

Epidemiology is the study of the occurrence, distribution, and transmission of diseases in human *populations*. A disease that is native to a local region is called an **endemic disease.** If the disease spreads to many individuals at the same time, the situation is called an **epidemic. Pandemics** are epidemics that affect large geographic regions, perhaps spreading worldwide. Because of the speed and availability of human travel around the world, pandemics are more common than they once were. Almost every flu season, a new strain of influenza virus quickly spreads from one continent to another.

Factors Affecting Patterns of Disease

Principal factors affecting human populations include the following: (1) age (i.e., time in the life cycle), (2) ethnic group, (3) gender, (4) socioeconomic factors and life-style considerations, and (5) geographic location.

Age

In one sense, there is an entirely different life during the first 9 months of existence. The structures and functions of tissues are different; they are primarily dedicated to differentiation, development, and growth. Certainly the environment is different; the individual is protected from the light of day, provided with predigested food—even preoxygenated blood, suspended in a fluid buffer, and maintained at incubator temperature. This is fortunate, for the developing embryo and fetus has relatively few homeostatic mechanisms to protect it from environmental change. The factors that produce disease **in utero** are discussed in Unit II. Diseases that arise during the **postuterine** period of life and affect the **neonate** include immaturity, respiratory failure, birth injuries, congenital malformations, nutritional problems, metabolic errors, and infections. These conditions are discussed in separate chapters.

Accidents, including poisoning, take their toll in **childhood.** Infections of children reflect their increased susceptibility to agents of disease. Consideration of other childhood diseases is addressed in each chapter as appropriate. The study of childhood processes and changes that occur in this period of life is the domain of *pediatrics.*

Specific diseases that occur during **maturity** (ages 15–60) are the primary emphasis of this text.

The term *atrophy* is used to describe the wasting effects of age. In addition to structural atrophy, the functioning of many physiologic control mechanisms also decreases and becomes less precise as age advances. The changes in function that occur during the early years of life are termed **developmental processes.** Those that occur during **maturity and postmaturity** (age 60 and beyond) are called **aging processes.** The study of aging processes and other changes that occur during this period of life is called *gerontology.* The effects of aging on selected body systems are so important physiologically that they receive separate consideration throughout the text. The immune system, cardiac, respiratory, musculoskeletal, neurologic, special sensory, endocrine, gastrointestinal, and integumentary systems are all affected by the process of aging.

Ethnic Group

It is difficult to differentiate sharply between the effects of ethnic group on patterns of disease and those

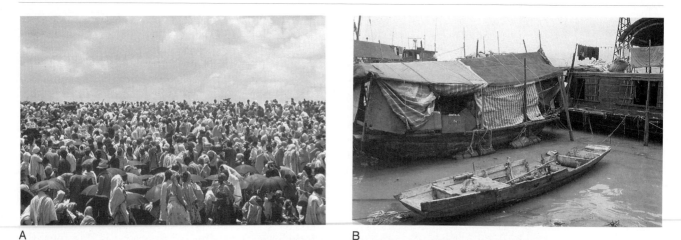

A   B

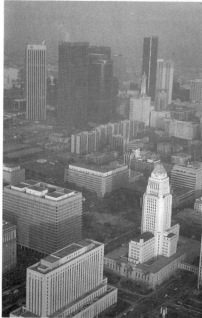

C

FIGURE 1–11. The aggregate focus in disease. **A,** Overcrowding. **B,** Contaminated water. **C,** Air pollution. **D,** Global environmental dangers (Antarctic ozone hole). (Phototake, New York.)

socioeconomic factors, customs, and geographic considerations that are inseparably bound to them. For example, carcinoma of the penis is virtually unknown among Jews and Moslems who practice circumcision at an early age (avoiding the carcinogenic stimulus that comes from accumulation of smegma about the glans penis).

However, ethnic group comparisons reveal significant differences between groups in certain disease states that seem to be more closely related to genetic predisposition than to environmental factors. For example, sickle cell anemia is almost exclusively limited to blacks, whereas pernicious anemia occurs more frequently among Scandinavians and is rare among blacks.

The study of racial and ethnic group variation in disease states is the domain of *medical anthropology*. Volumes have been written about disease-specific differences that relate to racial or ethnic group differences. In clinical practice, recognition of diversity in

disease risk by racial or ethnic group is useful in disease diagnosis, prevention, and treatment. Ethnic group–specific differences, where important, are presented in individual chapters.

Gender

Particular diseases of the genital system obviously show important differences between the sexes; men do not have endometriosis, nor do women have hyperplasia of the prostate, and carcinoma of the breast is more common in women than in men. Pyelonephritis is commoner in younger women than in men of comparable age (before they develop prostatic hyperplasia) because the external urethral orifice of women is more readily contaminated, and bacteria can more easily travel up a short urethra than up a long one. Less obviously related to the reproductive system, the onset of severe atherosclerosis in women is delayed some 20 years or so over that in men, presumably because of the protective action of estrogenic hormone. Current research into cardiovascular disease (described in Chaps. 17 and 18) points up the importance of sex as a physiologic variable. It should be noted that females were excluded from some earlier studies of cardiac pathophysiology[26]—a major investigative oversight.

There are also sex-specific factors that defy explanation. For example, systemic lupus erythematosus is much more common in women.[27] Both toxic goiter and hypothyroidism are also commoner in women.[28] Rheumatoid arthritis is more common in women, but osteoarthritis affects men and women with equal frequency.[29] Thromboangiitis obliterans (a chronic, recurring, inflammatory peripheral vascular disease) occurs more commonly in men.[3] Sex differences in predisposition to cancer and other diseases are presented throughout the text.

Socioeconomic Factors and Life-Style Considerations

The environment and the political climate of countries determine how people live and the health problems that are likely to ensue. The importance of poverty, malnutrition, overcrowding, and exposure to adverse environmental conditions such as extremes of temperature is obvious. Again, volumes have been written about the effects of socioeconomic status on disease. *Sociologists* study the influence of these factors. Social class influences education, and also the type of occupation one is likely to have.

Occupational exposure to such agents as coal dust, noise, or extreme stress affects the type of disease one is likely to contract.[30] The quantity and quality of medical care are also influenced by socioeconomic factors.

Closely related to socioeconomic factors are *life-style considerations*. People living in the United States, for example, consume too much food, alcohol, and tobacco and do not exercise enough. Arteriosclerosis, cancer, diseases of the kidney, liver, and lungs, and accidents cause most deaths in the United States. By contrast, people living in developing nations suffer and frequently die from undernutrition and infectious diseases.

Infectious disease is not limited to developing countries. After decades of decline, the incidence of tuberculosis in the United States has increased annually since 1985. In 1990, more than 25,000 cases were reported, a 9.4% increase over the previous year's total. The AIDS epidemic, inner city homelessness, poverty, and the influx of immigrants from endemic areas explain much of the increase.[31]

The incidence of many parasitic diseases is closely tied to socioeconomic factors and life-style considerations. Worm infections, for example, are related to the use of human feces as fertilizer. In some areas, for example Africa and tropical America, the frequency of schistosomiasis (a parasitic infestation with blood flukes) is tied directly to the widespread use of irriga-tion ditches that harbor the intermediate snail host.[32] The fact that children play in the ditches, or that clothes are washed there, gives adequate opportunity for human infection (Fig. 1–12).

Trichinosis (a disease caused by the ingestion of *Trichinella spiralis*) comes almost entirely from eating inadequately cooked infected pork. People who are fond of raw meat and inadequately cooked sausage are at highest risk.

Sometimes education is effective in changing life-style patterns that contribute to disease. In Tokyo, Japan, for example, mass public education about minimizing the use of sodium—a common ingredient in most traditional Japanese cooking—has been effective in changing current dietary practices and thus affecting the control of hypertension.

Examples of educational efforts directed toward life-style modification in the United States are numerous.[33,34] Antidrug, antismoking, and pro-fitness messages fill the media. Choosing healthy alternatives to unhealthy ones is made easier through positive peer pressure and support groups.

Geographic Location

Patterns of disease vary greatly by geographic location. Certainly there is considerable overlap with ethnicity, socioeconomic factors, and life-style choices, but physical environment is also an important aspect. Obviously, frostbite in Antarctica and dehydration in the Sahara Desert are examples of disorders that are more prevalent *between* geographic settings. But there are also important patterns of disease *within* individual countries. For example, the incidence and kind of

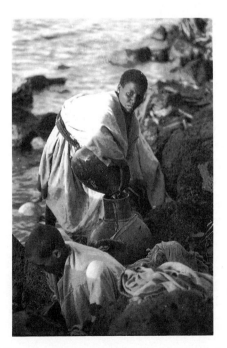

FIGURE 1–12. High-risk factors in the development of schistosomiasis. (Phototake, New York.)

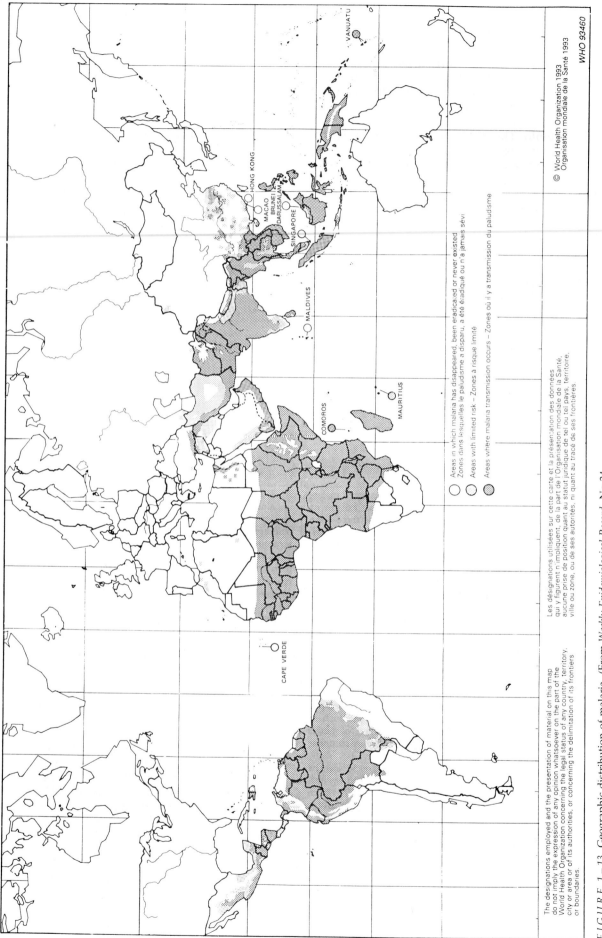

FIGURE 1–13. Geographic distribution of malaria. (From *Weekly Epidemiological Record*, No 34, August 20, 1993. © 1993, World Health Organization. Used by permission.)

malnutrition vary tremendously by geographic region.

Many diseases have a geographic pattern for reasons that are clear. Malaria, for example, an acute and sometimes chronic infectious disease due to the presence of protozoan parasites within RBCs, is transmitted to humans by the bite of an infected female *Anopheles* mosquito. The *Anopheles* mosquito can live only in certain regions of the world (Fig. 1–13).[35]

Fungal diseases are more frequent and more serious in hot, humid regions. But some infectious diseases are highly limited geographically for reasons that are not well understood. Bartonellosis, for example, also called Carrion's disease, is found only in Peru, Ecuador, Chile, and Colombia.[3] This disease resembles malaria superficially in that the minute rickettsia-like organisms invade erythrocytes and destroy them. Humans are infected by the bite of the sandfly. Although conditions in other parts of the world should be favorable for this disease, it remains limited geographically.

Taking a world view, there is widespread recognition of the importance of geographic factors in influencing human disease.[36] The World Health Organization and the National Institutes of Health have been deeply concerned with geographic problems in disease.

KEY CONCEPTS

- Although some aspects of disease causation may be studied in individual persons, additional information is gained by examining the occurrence, transmission, and distribution of diseases in large groups of people or populations.
- Epidemiology is the study of patterns of disease in human populations. Age, ethnicity, sex, life-style, socioeconomic status, and geographic location are epidemiologic variables that influence the occurrence and transmission of disease. Understanding the epidemiology of a disease is essential for effective prevention.

Pathophysiologic Processes

Four aspects of a disease process that form the core of pathophysiology are its cause (**etiology**), the mechanisms of its development (**pathogenesis**), including the structural alterations induced in the cells and organs of the body (**morphologic changes**), the functional consequences of the morphologic changes (**clinical manifestations**), and **implications for treatment** (Fig. 1–14). Structure is an expression of altered chemistry, and dysfunction is an inevitable consequence. Structure, composition, and function are inseparably related.

Etiology

Etiology, in its most general definition, is the assignment of causes or reasons for phenomena.[37] *Staphylo-*

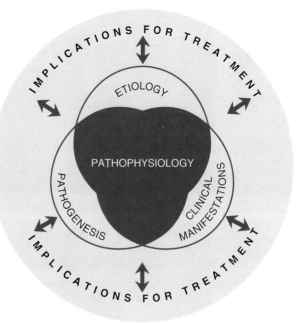

FIGURE 1–14. Four interrelated aspects of a disease process form the core of pathophysiology: (1) its cause (etiology), (2) the mechanisms of its development (pathogenesis), including the structural alterations induced in the cells and organs of the body (morphologic changes), (3) the functional consequences of the morphologic changes (clinical manifestations), and (4) implications for treatment.

coccus aureus, a pathogen, is designated as the etiologic agent of an infection. Other etiologic factors in the development of the disease that influence the course of the infection include the age, health, and general nutritional status of the person. It is important to repeat that even in the case of an infectious disease such as a staphylococcal infection, the agent itself does not constitute the disease. Rather, the *result of all of the responses to that agent,* all of the abnormalities of biologic processes, constitutes the disease.

A description of etiology includes the identification of those causal factors that, acting in concert, provoke the particular disease or cause traumatic injury. When the cause is unknown, a condition is said to be **idiopathic.**

Inheritance and Environment

In the etiology of a particular disease, physical, chemical, infectious, or nutritional factors in the environment as well as a variety of intrinsic characteristics of the person are important considerations. The influence of environmental factors in producing the barrel-shaped chests of natives of the Andes Mountains, for example, is extremely significant. Here, the altered chest shape represents not a genetic difference between them and their lowland compatriots, but rather an irreversible acclimatization induced during the first few years of their lives by exposure to the low oxygen environment of high altitude. The altered chest size—an adaptive response to the environment—re-

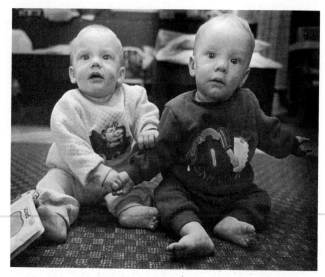

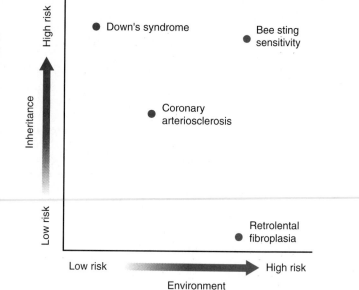

F I G U R E 1 – 15. Identical twins, produced by division of one fertilized egg, have virtually identical genetic endowments and similar appearance. Even as infants, however, characteristics visibly distinguish them. Yet their *invisible* traits, including IQ, temperament, and tendency to develop behavioral disorders, are either predetermined by genetics or subject to environmental modification. (Photographer: Kathleen Kelly, Spokane, WA.)

F I G U R E 1 – 16. Relative contributions of inheritance and environmental factors to the development of four disorders. Retrolental fibroplasia requires the unusual environment of premature birth and high oxygen concentration; this combination causes damage to the retina, resulting in blindness. In contrast, Down's syndrome, an inherited condition, is expressed in all environments. Bee sting sensitivity requires a high-risk genotype as well as exposure to a high risk environmental factor. Coronary arteriosclerosis is a common disease involving many genotypes and a variety of environmental agents. (From Martin G, Hoehn H: *Human Pathology.* Philadelphia, WB Saunders, 1974. Redrawn and used with permission.)

mains even though the individual moves to the lowlands later in life and stays there. Lowland persons who have suffered oxygen deprivation from heart or lung disease during their early years show precisely the same chest shape, further demonstrating the importance of environmental factors.

The relative impact of genes and environment varies with each disease (Fig. 1–15). Some diseases, for example Down's syndrome, an entirely genetic disorder resulting from an extra chromosome, occur in all environments. New research into the etiology of certain diseases, for example schizophrenia, reveals a greater relative impact of genetic control than previously understood. By comparison, retrolental fibroplasia (vasoconstriction of the immature retinal vessels resulting from exposure of a premature newborn to a high oxygen concentration) has an entirely environmental basis. Further, a hypersensitivity disease can result when a bee sting occurs; both genetic predisposition and exposure to venom are required for the disease. Finally, coronary arteriosclerosis results from many predisposing genetic and environmental factors. This widely occurring disease has multiple causes. Figure 1–16 depicts one way of describing the relative contribution of inheritance (genotypes) and environmental factors in determining four disorders.

Note that agents present in one environment may be hurtful to some but not all people. Unfortunate combinations and instances of hereditary factors may combine with environmental factors. For example, the abnormal hemoglobin of sickle cell anemia—an inherited condition that causes red cells to form sickle shapes when the oxygen concentration is low—leads to headaches, dizziness, and pain in the abdomen

when the sickled erythrocytes plug small blood vessels in the brain and liver.[38] With exposure to low oxygen concentrations, unconsciousness may be induced in affected persons, yet no harm results to the unaffected (Fig. 1–17).

In short, the cause of human disease is intimately linked with two factors: genetic makeup and environmental interaction. Some regard disease as a means by which nature judges the desirability of an individual's genetic makeup in a given environment. "Survival of the fittest," the theme of Darwinian evolution, or the struggle between nature (genetic makeup or inheritance) and nurture (environment), is ongoing.[39] This struggle is encompassed by the term **ecogenetics.**

Classification of Disease

Myriad etiologic agents can initiate disease. Figure 1–18 depicts one way of representing these agents in broad, general terms.

No single etiologic classification is truly comprehensive. Some diseases fall into multiple categories, and many diseases have unknown etiologies. Some diseases may actually receive different designations in the future, as further research reveals new data. Table 1–1 summarizes the etiologic classification of diseases.

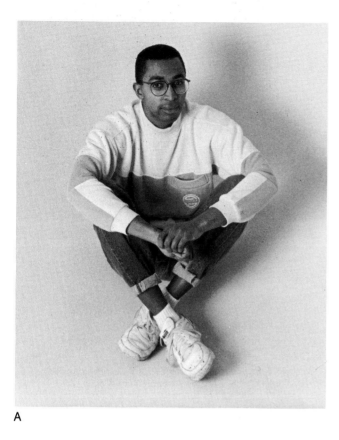

A

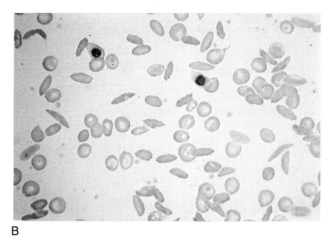

B

FIGURE 1–17. Sickle cell disease. Many African-Americans carry the same genetic protection against malaria that baffled early European Caucasian explorers in West Africa, nearly all of whom died from "the fever." However, the gene responsible for this protection can be deadly: a double dose of it produces a variant blood protein known as hemoglobin-S, which induces sickle cell anemia. The abnormal hemoglobin causes red blood cells to form sickle shapes when the oxygen concentration is low. When the sickled erythrocytes plug small blood vessels in the brain and liver, serious headache, dizziness, and abdominal pain result. (Photographer: Kathleen Kelly, Spokane, WA. Blood film courtesy of Pamela G. Kidd, M.D., Department of Laboratory Medicine, University of Washington, Seattle, WA.)

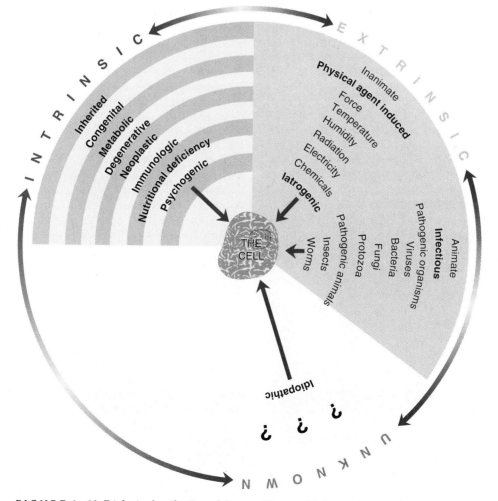

FIGURE 1–18. Etiologic classification of disease. Illustrated here are the contributions of intrinsic, extrinsic, and unknown factors to disease causation.

21

TABLE 1–1. Etiologic Classification of Diseases

Inherited diseases	Infectious diseases
Congenital (inborn) diseases or birth defects	Physical agent–induced diseases
Metabolic diseases	Nutritional deficiency diseases
Degenerative diseases	Iatrogenic diseases
Neoplastic diseases	Psychogenic diseases
Immunologic diseases	Idiopathic diseases

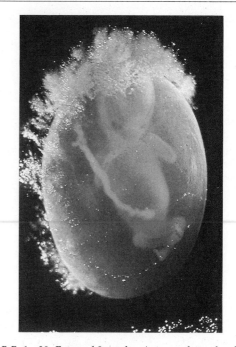

FIGURE 1–20. Fetus of 9 weeks. As an embryo develops into a fetus, genetic controls orchestrate the workings of countless genes such as those determining sex and influencing physiologic features. Some genes operating during fetal development remain active into adult life. Others operate only during the period of intrauterine development and are normally silent thereafter. (Phototake, New York.)

The reader will find more detailed information on each of these categories in the subsequent chapters of this book; cross-references to those chapters or units are provided here for the reader's convenience. A brief explanation of the etiologic categories presented in Table 1–1 follows.

Inherited Diseases. Altered or *mutated* genes can cause abnormal proteins to be made. These abnormal proteins often do not perform their intended function, resulting in the absence of an essential function. In other cases such proteins may actually perform an abnormal, disruptive function. Either case poses a potential threat to the body's internal homeostasis.[40]

Previously, emphasis has been placed on the fact that inheritance provides certain conditions for diseases that are induced by environmental agents (Fig. 1–19). Many abortions are caused by mutations induced by chemicals or radiation. Most mutations are lethal, but other mutations cause problems only when the person is exposed to certain environmental agents. Other mutations cause problems without any environmental contribution. Chapter 4 discusses genetic control and inheritance.

Congenital Diseases. Prenatal influences are responsible for most neonatal deaths. **Prenatal** denotes the period of in utero life, whereas **neonatal** denotes the first 2 months of life (Fig. 1–20). During infancy, the first 2 years of life, birth defects arising from the pregnant mother having taken drugs, such as thalido-

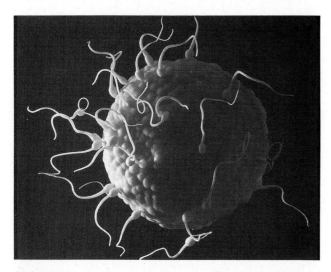

FIGURE 1–19. Sperms covering egg. One sperm will eventually penetrate the egg. The sperm and egg each carry a random selection of parental genes, and their fusion determines genetic endowment. (Phototake, New York.)

mide, or viral infection are major causes of death. These agents can deform the brain or other organs. (See Chapter 5, Genetic and Developmental Disorders.)

Metabolic Diseases. Metabolic diseases arise from abnormalities in the chemistry of the body. Over 100 deficiencies of vital enzymes have genetic bases.[41] Screening for metabolic disorders, such as phenylketonuria (PKU), is an important aspect of preventive medicine for childhood. Children having the enzyme deficiency of PKU suffer brain damage when toxic chemicals accumulate in the brain. Phenylketonuria must be diagnosed and the infant placed on a special diet before reaching the age of 1 year.[42] Abnormalities in the genes that affect metabolism are further discussed in Chapter 5.

Degenerative Diseases. By means of many still unknown processes, tissues sometimes break apart, or *degenerate*. Although a normal consequence of aging, degeneration of one or more tissues as a result of disease can occur at any time. The degeneration of tissues associated with aging is discussed in nearly every chapter of this book. Degenerative diseases associated with the aging process are increasing in frequency as persons are living beyond the fifth decade. Heart attacks and strokes combined account for over one-half of all deaths in the United States.[43] Other degenerative diseases, including cirrhosis of the liver and emphysema of the lungs, cause chronic illness and numerous deaths. These diseases are discussed in further detail in Chapter 38, Liver Disease, and Chapter 20, Obstructive Pulmonary Disorders.

Aging and degeneration have been linked to excessive caloric intake, radiation, the winding down of biologic clocks, errors in gene function, and a loss of immunologic vigor. Most medicine practiced in the United States is conducted in hospitals and clinics that diagnose and treat individuals with degenerative diseases. The average life span in the United States of 75.4 years[43] is not likely to be extended much because degenerative and neoplastic diseases are difficult to prevent and cure.

Neoplastic Diseases. Neoplastic diseases (tumors), especially the malignant variety (see Chap. 6), are a menace: one in five persons dies of cancer. Cancers cause death when they spread from their site of origin. Generally, cancers are signaled by a lump, an increase in the size of an ulcer, loss of weight, anemia, or pain.

Of the deaths attributable to the hundred different types of cancer, more than 60 percent are caused by a few common types involving the breast, lung, colon, stomach, and uterus.[44]

Cancer probably arises from mutagenic agents such as chemicals, viruses, sunlight, irradiation, and chronic irritation. The clustering of cancer in selective geographic areas also implicates environmental factors as possible etiologic agents. For example, Burkitt's malignant lymphoma, a rare cancer, is confined almost exclusively to tropical Africa, where specific humidity, temperature, and altitude may provide an optimal environment. Burkitt's lymphoma is also associated with the presence of Epstein-Barr virus, a lymphotropic herpesvirus. The precise role of this virus in the development of Burkitt's lymphoma remains unclear.[45]

Immunologic Diseases. The immune system provides protection against inflammation, infection, and cancer. In some instances, the immune system may attack one's own body (*autoimmune response*) or overreact (*hypersensitivity reaction*) or underreact (*AIDS*). (See Unit III, Alterations in Defense.) Anaphylactic immunologic reactions to allergens such as bee venom could be lethal in hypersensitive persons. Immunologic reactions are responsible for allergies, AIDS, asthma, rheumatic heart disease, and many kidney, skin, and endocrine diseases.

Infectious Diseases. Many important diseases are caused by **pathogens,** or disease-causing organisms, that damage the body in some way. Any organism that lives in or on another organism to obtain its nutrients is called a **parasite.** The presence of microscopic or larger parasites may interfere with normal body functions of the **host,** causing disease. Besides parasites, there are organisms that poison or otherwise damage the human body to cause disease. An in-depth discussion of infectious disease caused by pathogenic organisms is provided in Chapter 8, Infectious Processes. Some of the major pathogenic organisms are briefly described in Table 1–2. Figure 1–21 illustrates these pathogens.

Diseases Induced by Physical Agents. Agents such as toxic or destructive chemicals, extreme heat or cold, mechanical injury, and radiation can affect the body.[46] Examples of tissues damaged by burn injury is discussed in Chapter 55. Violent injury (trauma) or death from mechanical, chemical, or physical agents are common among young people. Traffic accidents, homicide, suicide, and trauma from accidents at home, work, and war are examples. In addition, some genetically predisposed persons react adversely to certain drugs or chemicals.[47] Such persons may injure their skin, lungs, intestinal tract, liver, and kidneys from adverse drug reaction. The liver and kidneys are often damaged because these organs concentrate and excrete toxic drugs and chemicals. (See also Chapters 27 and 38.)

Within the body, mechanical failures can occur. An intestinal loop can slip through a defect in the abdominal wall and become trapped. This is called a *hernia.* The intestine can also become twisted or telescoped within itself. Pain in the abdomen and urinary tract infection occur when a blood vessel or stricture blocks the flow of urine. Similarly, gallstones commonly form in the gallbladder; they can pass into the bile ducts and mechanically obstruct them, caus-

TABLE 1–2. Major Pathogenic Organisms

Organism	Description
Viruses	Intracellular parasites that consist of a DNA or RNA core surrounded by a protein coat and, sometimes, a lipoprotein envelope. They invade human cells and cause them to produce viral components.
Bacteria	Tiny, primitive cells that lack nuclei. They cause infection by parasitizing tissues or otherwise disrupting normal function.
Fungi	Simple organisms similar to plants but lacking the chlorophyll pigments that allow plants to make their own food. Since they cannot make their own food, fungi must parasitize other tissues, including those of the human body.
Protozoa	*Protists,* or one-celled organisms larger than bacteria and whose DNA is organized into a nucleus. Many types of protozoa parasitize human tissues.
Pathogenic animals	Large multicellular organisms, such as insects and worms. Such animals can parasitize human tissues, bite or sting, or otherwise disrupt normal body function.

Data from Thibodeau GA, Patton KT: *Anatomy and Physiology,* 2nd ed. St. Louis, Mosby–Year Book, 1993, pp 28–29.

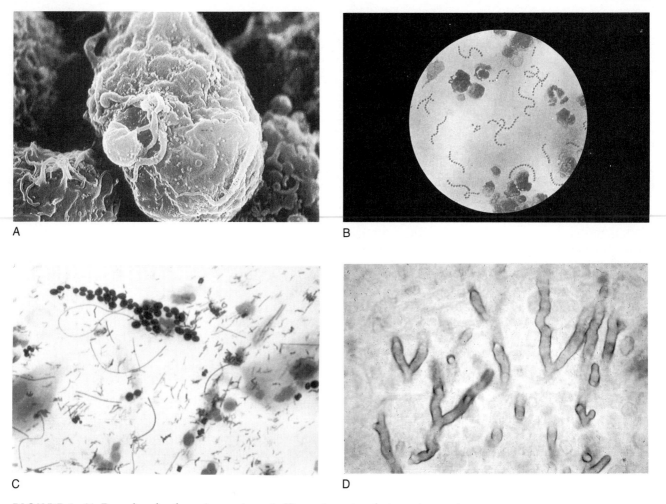

F I G U R E 1 – 21. Examples of pathogenic organisms. **A,** Viruses (scanning electron micrograph of HIV-I–infected T4 lymphocytes showing virus budding from the plasma membrane of the lymphocytes). **B,** Bacteria (group A β-hemolytic *Streptococcus pyogenes* in short chains from pus; Pappenheim's stain, ×900). **C,** Fungi—yeast cells (candidiasis, vaginal discharge; Gram stain). **D,** Fungi—mold (aspergillosis, lung tissue; hematoxylin-eosin).

ing abdominal pain, nausea, and vomiting. (See also Unit X, Alterations in Gastrointestinal Function.)

Nutritional Deficiency Diseases. Deficiencies in nutrients are responsible for many diseases. On a worldwide basis, deficiencies of proteins, calories, and vitamins are rampant; over 300 million preschool-aged children are malnourished and vulnerable to infectious diseases.[44] In developing countries, tuberculosis and malnutrition are the most common causes of death. Also, deficiencies in vitamins or iodine may induce nutritional deficiency diseases.[44] Chapter 56 focuses on nutritional alterations in critical illness.

Iatrogenic Diseases. Many diseases are caused by a physician or health professional; such diseases are **iatrogenic** in origin. The first dictum of health care is to do no harm; violation of this dictum results in iatrogenic disease. Five percent of patients entering a hospital, for instance, become infected from a procedure performed on them.[44] The slip of a surgeon's knife or an incorrect diagnosis can cause disease.

Moreover, numerous drugs cause disease. For example, pregnant women threatened with spontane-

ous abortions were once given the drug diethylstilbestrol. Approximately 20–25 years later, many young women born of these pregnancies developed vaginal cancer.

A subcategory of drug-induced iatrogenic disease is growing in importance. Approximately 2 percent–5 percent of hospitalized patients are ill because of a drug-induced disease.[44] In addition, preliminary data from a 1993 study[48] show that 15 percent of elderly patients experience adverse reactions to drugs while being treated in the hospital. Allergy to penicillin resulting in a rash is a common example.

The misuse of radiation by those not realizing its potential danger has resulted in the development of cancers of the liver, skin, thyroid gland, and blood.

Psychogenic Diseases. Psychogenic or emotional factors contribute to many diseases. Moreover, psychogenic factors are extremely important in determining the course of the disease. Many diseases are encompassed by psychosomatic medicine, the discipline involving the physiologic impact of psychic stress on the emergence of disease. Chapter 7 addresses stress

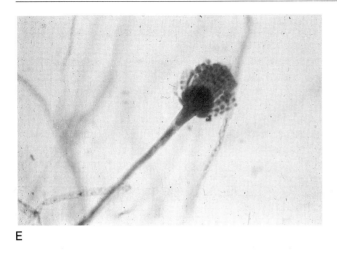

E

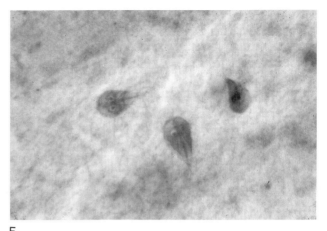

F

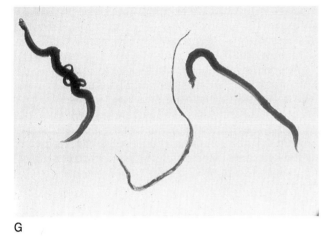

G

FIGURE 1-21 Continued. **E,** Fungi—mold (*Aspergillus fumigatus* conidiophore; ×750). **F,** Protozoans (*Giardia lamblia,* trophozoite; chlorozol black E stain, ×1150). **G,** Pathogenic animals—schistosome (male and female). (Centers for Disease Control, Atlanta, GA.)

and adaptation. A variety of gastrointestinal disorders, such as peptic ulcer, ulcerative colitis, and spastic colon may be aggravated by psychic stress. (See Unit X, Alterations in Gastrointestinal Function.) In addition, asthma and dermatitis have important psychological components, which are explained in subsequent chapters.

Idiopathic Diseases. The term **idiopathic** means undetermined cause. Although it is tempting to suggest that much is known about the etiology of disease, most diseases are idiopathic!

Examples of diseases with unknown causes abound. One example is hypertension. Persistent elevation of blood pressure to above 140/90 mm Hg is a sign of underlying disease. Only 10 percent of people with hypertension have an identifiable cause; approximately 90 percent have no discernible cause for hypertension.[49] They have *idiopathic hypertension* (see Chap. 15).

Pathogenesis

Pathogenesis refers to the development or evolution of a disease.[50] A description of the pathogenesis of a staphylococcal infection, for example, would include the *mechanisms* whereby invasion of the body by the pathogen ultimately led to the observed abnormalities. The study of pathogenesis—from the initial stimulus to the ultimate expression of the manifestations of the disease—remains one of the main domains of pathophysiology and is addressed for each disorder in subsequent chapters throughout the text.

It is difficult to characterize the mechanism of disease development in general terms because pathogenesis varies with the causative agent and with the type of cell, tissue, and organ affected. Nevertheless, some common manifestations of the immediate response to injury include depression and/or stimulation of cells. Stimulation of cells is expressed as increased metabolism and, frequently, an increase in the size or number of cells. Stimulation, also expressed as hyperfunction, may be shown by increased secretion (e.g., excessive mucous production) or by an increase in some mechanical function (e.g., muscle spasm). Depression, by comparison, is expressed as decreased metabolism, hypofunction, or a reduction in the size or number of cells. The type and degree of response are determined by the specific causative agent, its virulence, the quality, quantity, and duration of exposure, and the unique characteristics of the affected cells, tissues, and organs. Following the immediate action, the counteraction is almost always complex and indirect.

It is the result of many combined factors acting over a period of time.

Consider, for example, a severe bacterial infection causing an abscessed tooth. First, there is local invasion of cells by the bacteria and their products, and an immediate direct action expressed as cellular degeneration. Then changes occur in circulation and in vascular permeability, which are important in development of the inflammatory process. Connective tissue also plays a role. After this, mixed responses develop—depression and stimulation of cells, with repercussions that go far beyond the local area of infection and inflammation. These reactions include fever, an increased white blood cell count, an accelerated heart rate, accelerated respiratory rate, and altered blood chemical constituents. There are widespread morphologic effects as well: hyperplasia of the spleen, lymph nodes, and bone marrow, and cellular changes in the liver, kidneys, and heart. Refer to Unit III for an in-depth look at the processes of infection, inflammation, and immunity.

To take another example, consider hypertension. As a result of a causative agent, mechanisms are set into operation that produce spasm of arterioles throughout the body. This results in increased resistance to arterial blood flow. The left ventricle of the heart responds to the stress of an increased work load, first by slight dilation, then by increased forcefulness of the heartbeat. This counteracts the increased peripheral resistance and restores circulation to normal—a homeostatic mechanism. If the stress increases, the complex pattern of counteraction will develop further, and it is likely that a failure of adaptation will occur—a gross break in the constantly shifting balance to maintain stability—and heart failure may result. This brings a variety of manifestations such as epigastric tenderness and abdominal discomfort (from congestion of the liver, spleen, and intestines), dyspnea (i.e., difficult, labored breathing, from pulmonary venous congestion), edematous swelling of the feet and ankles (from increased capillary filtration pressure and sodium retention), and a host of other functional, chemical, and structural changes. Units IV and V provide the background for understanding the complexities of altered cardiac function. All of this action and counteraction, a dynamic, ever-changing process, describe **pathogenesis** of disease.

Factors Affecting Pathogenesis

Some of the factors that influence pathogenesis include time, quantity, location, and morphologic changes.

Time. In the case of an infectious disease, the *time* the body is invaded by a pathogen and the amount of its exposure have an important effect on the reaction, qualitatively as well as quantitatively. The time at which a diseased patient is examined influences what one sees to such an extent that different stages of a disease often appear quite unrelated unless the succession of events that led from one stage to the next

in time is appreciated. One must always ask the questions: Is the disease in its early or late stages? Is the process acute or chronic?

Quantity. *Quantity* is often as important in invasion, action, and counteraction as quality. "How much?" may be the crucial question, even more important than "What?" Although it is often difficult to measure precisely bodily reactions or tissue lesions, in the case of tissue trauma, one can give at least a semiquantitative indication by using such terms as slight, moderate, or marked. Further, the **virulence** or strength of the pathogen—as in the case of infectious disease—may be measured by its ability to induce serious disease.[3]

Location. The *location* of invasion and reaction is also of great importance. An invasion, such as a tumor, that is trivial if received in one part of the body (a benign skin tag) may be lethal if received in another (an inoperable brain tumor). Furthermore, different cells have their own peculiar patterns of reaction. (See Chapter 6, Neoplasia.)

Morphologic Changes. **Morphologic changes** refer to the structural and associated functional alterations in cells or tissues that are either characteristic of the disease or diagnostic of the etiologic process.[51] The cell is the structural unit of the body, and the significance of cellular abnormality in disease can hardly be overemphasized. Morphologic changes are described in detail in Chapters 3–6.

Clinical Manifestations

Signs and Symptoms

As certain biologic processes are encroached upon, the person begins to feel subjectively that something is wrong. These subjective feelings are termed **symptoms** of disease. By definition, symptoms are subjective and can only be reported by the affected individual to an observer. When, however, the manifestations of the disease involve objectively identifiable aberrations, these are termed **signs** of the disease. Nausea, malaise, and pain are symptoms, while fever, reddening of the skin, and a palpable mass are signs of disease. Although *sign* and *symptom* are distinct terms, they are often used interchangeably.

A **syndrome** is a collection of different signs and symptoms that occur together.

A demonstrable structural change produced in the course of a disease is referred to as a **lesion.** Lesions may be evident at a gross or a microscopic level.

Stages

Early in the development of a disease, the etiologic agent or agents may provoke a number of changes in biologic processes that can be detected by laboratory analysis even though there is no recognition by the patient that these changes have occurred. Thus, many diseases progress through several stages. The interval between exposure of a tissue to an injurious agent and the first appearance of signs and symptoms may be called a **latent period,** or, in the case of infectious diseases, an **incubation period.** The **prodromal period,** or **prodrome,** refers to the appearance of the first signs and symptoms indicating the onset of a disease. Prodromal symptoms often are nonspecific, such as headache, malaise, anorexia, and nausea. During the **stage of manifest illness,** or the **acute phase,** the disease reaches its full intensity, and signs and symptoms attain their greatest severity. Sometimes during the course of a disease, the signs and symptoms may become mild or even disappear for a time. This interval may be called a **silent period** or **latent period.** For example, in the total body radiation syndrome, a latent period may occur between the prodrome and the stage of manifest illness. Another example is syphilis, which may have two latent periods: one occurring between the primary and secondary stages, and another occurring between the secondary and tertiary stages.

A number of diseases have a **subclinical** stage during which the patient functions normally even though the disease processes are well established. It is important to understand that the structure and function of many organs provide a large reserve or safety margin, so that functional impairment may become evident only when disease has become quite advanced anatomically. For example, chronic renal disease could completely destroy one kidney and partly destroy the other before any symptoms related to decreased renal function would be perceived. Health care professionals, therefore, need to be especially sensitive to the fact that many of their patients will not exhibit any indication of illness, even though they may be quite diseased.

Some diseases (e.g., some types of leukemia) follow a course of alternating **exacerbations** and **remissions.** An **exacerbation** is a relatively sudden increase in the severity of a disease or any of its signs and symptoms. A **remission** is an abatement or decline in severity of the signs and symptoms of a disease. If a remission is permanent, we say that the person is "cured."

Convalescence is the stage of recovery after a disease, injury, or surgical operation. Occasionally a disease produces after-effects. A condition caused by and following a disease is called a **sequela** (plural, **sequelae**). For example, the sequela of an inflammatory process in a given tissue might be a scar in that tissue. The sequela of acute rheumatic inflammation of the heart might be scarred, deformed cardiac valves. A **complication** of disease is a new or separate process that may arise secondarily because of some change produced by the original entity. For example, bacterial pneumonia may be a complication of viral infection of the respiratory tract.

Acute or Chronic Disease

Disease processes are often classified as **acute** or **chronic.** An **acute** condition has relatively severe man-ifestations but runs a short course. A **chronic** condition lasts for a long period of time. Sometimes chronic disease processes begin with an acute phase and become prolonged when the body's defenses are unable to overcome the causative agent or stressor. In other cases, chronic conditions develop insidiously and never have an acute phase. An **intercurrent** condition is one that occurs during the course of an already existing disease.

Implications for Treatment

Environmental and cultural influences that are brought to bear upon people will also affect the disease. The availability of warm housing, clean drinking water, and nutritious food determines recovery from certain diseases. Cultural influences affect not only the disease, but also the methods the individual uses to seek treatment.[52] In some Native American cultures in the United States, for example, tribal elders are cared for within the context of a closely knit extended family using alternative healing practices. In other cultures within the United States, hospitals and nursing homes are surrogates for the extended family, and healing is practiced exclusively within the context of traditional Western medicine.

Levels of Prevention

Epidemiologists suggest that treatment implications fall into categories called **levels of prevention.** There are three levels of prevention: primary, secondary, and tertiary. **Primary prevention** is prevention of disease by altering susceptibility or reducing exposure for susceptible individuals. **Secondary prevention** (applicable in early disease, i.e., preclinical and clinical stages) is the early detection, screening, and treatment of the disease. **Tertiary prevention** (appropriate in the stage of advanced disease or disability) includes rehabilitative and supportive care and attempts to alleviate disability and restore effective functioning.[53]

Primary Prevention. Prolongation of life has resulted largely from decreased mortality from infectious disease. Primary prevention in terms of improved nutrition, economy, housing, and sanitation of persons living in developed countries is also responsible for increased longevity. Certain childhood diseases—measles, poliomyelitis, pertussis (whooping cough), and neonatal tetanus—are decreasing, owing to a rapid increase in coverage by immunization programs. Cardiovascular diseases in developed countries (except those in Eastern Europe) are on the wane, thanks to the spread of health education and promotion. Infant and child mortality rates and the overall death rate are continuing to decrease globally.

Education about safe sex and ways to say no to drugs and alcohol are other examples of primary prevention making a difference in the lives of people. Primary prevention also includes adherence to safety precautions such as wearing seat belts, observing the posted speed limit on highways, and taking precautions in the use of chemicals and machinery. Violent crimes involving dangerous weapons must be stopped in order to prevent traumatic or fatal injuries caused by them.

Environmental pollutants poison the organs. Some experts fear an epidemic of cancer due to carcinogenic chemicals blighting the environment.[54] Public health measures to ensure clean food, air, and water prevent many diseases, including cancer. As air, water, and soil quality is improved, the risk of exposure to harmful carcinogens is minimized.

Secondary Prevention. Yearly physical examinations can lead to the early diagnosis of disease and, in some cases, cures. The routine use of Papanicolaou (Pap) smears has led to a decline in the incidence of invasive cancer of the uterine cervix.[55] Also, more women are examining their own breasts monthly for cancer; thus earlier diagnoses are achieved.

Prenatal diagnosis of certain genetic diseases is possible (see Chap. 4). New diagnostic laboratory techniques provide definitive information for the genetic counseling of parents. This information can aid in predicting chances of involvement or noninvolvement of offspring for a given genetic disorder, for example, mongolism. One technique, *amniocentesis,* consists of removing a small amount of fluid from the amniotic sac that surrounds the fetus and analyzing the cells and chemicals in the fluid. Blood samples can also be obtained from the fetus by amniocentesis; the amniotic fluid and fetal blood are then studied for defects in enzymes, to determine sex, and to measure substances associated with defects in the spinal cord and brain.

Tertiary Prevention. Once a disease becomes established, treatment—at least within the context of traditional Western medicine—generally falls into one of the following two major categories: **medical treatment** (including such measures as physical therapy, pharmacotherapy, psychotherapy, radiation therapy, chemotherapy, immunotherapy, and experimental gene therapy) or **surgery.** Numerous other subspecialties of medicine and surgery have also evolved to focus on a given organ or technique. In a clinical setting,

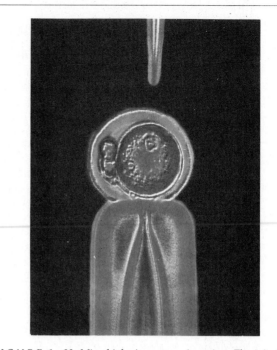

FIGURE 1–23. Microbiologic systems in action. The injection of foreign DNA into a mammalian egg engineers genetic changes faster than natural selection, surmounting natural barriers that normally prevent genetic exchange between species. In this image, from the cutting edge of genetic engineering, a mouse egg is held by suction against a micropipette. An even smaller pipette approaches, laden with artificially assembled DNA that carries a selected foreign gene. (Phototake, New York.)

there is a large array of professional caregivers who will be providing rehabilitative and supportive services to the diseased individual. Every professional brings the perspective of his or her discipline to the caregiving situation. Each will make clinical judgments about the needs, problems, goals, and intervention strategies that should be employed to be most helpful.

Nursing integrates the perspectives of other disciplines, as well as the perspective of the patient, in a holistic approach that is clinically sound and grounded in an understanding of biology, psychology, sociology, spirituality, cultural diversity, and cultural uniqueness. The influence of integrated interpretation is evident in the development of nursing knowledge, and this influence is expressed in the caregiving situation.

Future Possibilities

An explosion in knowledge of DNA, especially in the last three decades, has virtually transformed definitions of the living world and has permeated every branch of biologic science (Figs. 1–22 and 1–23).[56] The benefits of this new biology have been awesome—a deeper understanding of evolution, greater insights into the immune mechanisms, and nearly every advance against cancer and against AIDS (Fig. 1–24). But genetic manipulation also raises sensitive and complex ethical and moral questions that didn't even

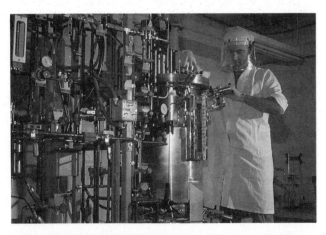

FIGURE 1–22. Macrobiologic systems in action. A biologic fermentation tank, part of a bioreactor complex, coddles genetically engineered bacteria and harvests their products for biologic and pharmaceutical research. (Phototake, New York.)

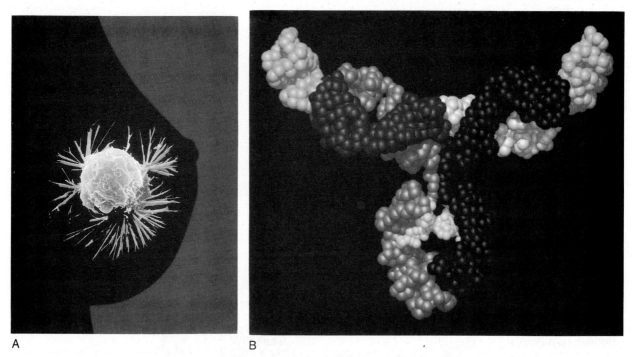

A   B

FIGURE 1–24. **A,** Mammogram showing a breast tumor, a potentially deadly collection of cancerous cells. By acquiring mutations in vital control genes, this tumor evades normal constraints and thus threatens the life of the host. One new molecular weapon in the war against breast cancer is the IgG antibody, which can be tailored by genetic engineering to recognize and attack a particular protein—the product of the Her-2/neu gene—whose unusual abundance in certain cancer cells sets them apart from normal body cells. **B,** Model of such an antibody. (**A,** Phototake, New York. **B,** courtesy of Drs. Len Presta and Mark Sliwkowski, Genentech, Inc.)

exist half a century ago. Scientists are now able to crack and manipulate the genetic code. They can experiment with what genes do and how they do it. This will dramatically alter medical practice, especially the treatment of inherited diseases.

This new ability has led to experimental treatments such as gene therapy—molecular surgery powerful enough to cure and alter the next generation. When gene therapy is perfected as a biomedical technique, and when its attendant ethical and moral dilemmas have been resolved, the routine diagnosis and treatment of genetic defects will be commonplace.

KEY CONCEPTS

- Pathophysiologic processes are generally studied by examining etiology, pathogenesis, clinical manifestations, and implications for treatment.
- Etiology refers to the proposed cause or causes of a particular physiopathology. Etiology is a complex notion because most diseases are multifactorial, resulting from an interplay between genetic constitution and environmental influences.
- Pathogenesis refers to the proposed mechanisms whereby a disease or disorder leads to typically observed clinical manifestations. Pathogenesis describes the direct effects of a particular disorder as well as the usual physiologic responses and compensatory mechanisms.

- Clinical manifestations describe the signs and symptoms that typically accompany a particular pathophysiologic process. Manifestations may vary depending on the stage of the disorder, individual variation, and acuity or chronicity.
- Treatment for pathophysiologic disorders is "implied" by the etiology, pathogenesis, and clinical manifestations. Prevention is more desirable than treatment. Education, regular examinations, and life-style management are important factors for all levels of prevention.

Summary

Given the complexity of disease and illness, determining a person's level of ill health is not the straightforward activity implied by the day-to-day work of the health care professional. Within the context of physical, mental, and social facets of ill health, there are two major concepts that govern our understanding of disease and illness: (1) disease and illness distort normal life processes, and (2) disease and illness disrupt homeostasis. In the future it is likely that more energy will be directed toward the homeostatic aspects of an individual's health with the goal of recognizing disease and controlling its incipient forms before the body's autoregulative mechanisms are stretched to the breaking point. Until then, there is still much to learn about manifest disease, which all too often runs a fatal course because it is not fully understood.

Major elements of pathophysiology—etiology, pathogenesis, clinical manifestations, and implications for treatment—have been presented. When we consider the totality of human disease, the sheer numbers of etiologic factors and separately named diseases seem endless. Fortunately, the numbers don't tell the whole story. The response mechanisms of the body are finite. Disease A differs from disease B because of variations in pathologic action. Thus, the understanding of a controlled number of responses permits understanding of many seemingly different diseases. Given etiologic classification of diseases applicable to each organ or system, the best model seeks to cope with disease by identifying causal factors, pathogenic mechanisms, clinical manifestations that include structural and molecular abnormalities, and treatment implications.

Disease is *dynamic* rather than static. The nature of the disease process includes the interplay between injury and reaction to injury, a kaleidoscopic series of actions and counteractions. The signs and symptoms of disease in a given person may change daily as biologic equilibriums shift and compensatory mechanisms are brought into play. Every disease has a *range* of manifestations and a *natural history* that varies from individual to individual.

Sheldon points out that disease "is the pattern of response of a living organism to some form of injury."[44] But to the affected individual, disease means discomfort, or exactly what the word says, *dis-ease*. Throughout this text, a recurrent theme is that disease is not a monstrous entity from without, but rather the inevitable expression of conflict between unique individuality and adverse environmental force.

REFERENCES

1. Moore LG, et al: *The Biocultural Basis of Health: Expanding Views of Medical Anthropology.* Prospect Heights, IL, Waveland Press, 1980.
2. Wilson WJ: *The Truly Disadvantaged: The Inner City, the Underclass, and Public Policy.* Chicago, University of Chicago Press, 1987.
3. *Dorland's Illustrated Medical Dictionary,* 27th ed. Philadelphia, WB Saunders, 1988, p 481.
4. Zatzick DF, Dimsdale JE: Cultural variations in response to painful stimuli. *Psychosom Med* 1990;52:544–557.
5. Trueba HT: Notes on Cultural Acquisition and Transmission, in Trueba HT (ed): *Anthropol Educ Q* 1990;22(3):279–280.
6. Bennett MJ: Towards ethnorelativism: A developmental model of intercultural sensitivity, in Paige RM (ed): *Cross-Cultural Orientation: New Conceptualizations and Applications.* Lanham, MD, University Press of America, 1986, pp 27–69.
7. Harper P, Wadstrom C, Cederblad G: Carnitine measurements in liver, muscle tissue, and blood in normal subjects. *Clin Chem* 1993;39(4):592–599.
8. Normal reference values. *N Engl J Med* 1992;327:718–724.
9. Gafter U, Malachi T, Barak H, Levi J: Red blood cell calcium level is elevated in women: Enhanced calcium influx by estrogens. *J Lab Clin Med* 1993;121(3):486–492.
10. Iwantani Y, Amino N, Kabutomori O, Tamaki H, Aozasa M, Motoi S, Miyai K: Effects of different sample preparations of enumeration of large granular lymphocytes (LGLs) and demonstration of a sex difference of LGLs. *Am J Clin Pathol* 1988;90(6):674–678.
11. Weissbluth M, Davis AT, Poncher J: Night waking in 4- to 8-month old infants. *J Pediatr* 1984;104(3):477–480.
12. Partinen M, Telakivi T: Epidemiology of obstructive sleep apnea syndrome. *Sleep* 1992;15(suppl 6):S1–S4.
13. Ancoli IS, Kripke DF, Klauber MR, Mason WJ, Fell R, Kaplan O: Sleep-disordered breathing in community dwelling elderly. *Sleep* 1991;14(6):486–495.
14. Davis DL, Low SM: *Gender, Health, and Illness: The Case of Nerves.* New York, Hemisphere Publishing, 1989.
15. Grover RF, Weil JV, Reeves JT: Cardiovascular adaptation to exercise at high altitude. *Exerc Sport Sci Rev* 1986;14:269–302.
16. Good BJ, Good MD: The meaning of symptoms: A cultural hermeneutic model for clinical practice, in Eisenberg L, Kleinman A (eds): *The Relevance of Social Science for Medicine.* Dordrecht, Holland, Reidel Publishing, 1981, pp 165–196.
17. Wall PD, Melzack RE: *Textbook of Pain.* Edinburgh, Churchill Livingstone, 1984.
18. Feinstein AR, et al: Scientific and clinical problems in indexes of functional disability. *Ann Intern Med* 1986;105:413–420.
19. World Health Organization: *International Classification of Impairments, Disabilities, and Handicaps.* Geneva, World Health Organization, 1980.
20. World Health Organization: *Proceedings of an International Conference on Primary Care (Declaration of Alma-Ata).* Geneva, World Health Organization, 1978.
21. Cannon WB: Stresses and strains of homeostasis. *Am J Med Sci* 1935;189:1–14.
22. Dickman SR: *Pathways to Wellness.* Champagne, IL, Life Enhancement Publishers, 1988.
23. Carnevali D, Reiner A: *The Cancer Experience: Nursing Diagnosis and Management.* Philadelphia, JB Lippincott, 1990.
24. Andreoli TE: Disorders of fluid volume, electrolyte, and acid-base balance, in Wyngaarden JB, Smith LH Jr (eds): *Cecil Textbook of Medicine,* 18th ed. Philadelphia, WB Saunders, 1988, p 528.
25. Overmire TG: Homeostatic regulation. Pamphlet 9, American Institute of Biological Sciences Curriculum Study, September 1963.
26. Young RF, Kahena E: Gender, recovery from late life heart attack, and medical care. *Women Health* 1993;20(1):11–31.
27. Robinson DR: Systemic lupus erythematosus, in Rubenstein E, Federman DD (eds): *Scientific American Medicine.* New York, Scientific American, 1993, chapt. 15, sect. IV, pp 1–17.
28. Federman DD: Thyroid, in Rubenstein E, Federman DD (eds): *Scientific American Medicine.* New York, Scientific American, 1991, chapt. 3, sect. I, pp 9–15.
29. Rodman GP, Schumacher HR, Zvaifler NJ: *Primer on the Rheumatic Diseases,* 8th ed. Atlanta, Arthritis Foundation, 1983.
30. An evaluation of chemicals and industrial processes associated with cancer in humans based on human and animal data: IARC monographs, vols 1–20. *Cancer Res* 1980;40:1–12.
31. Simon HB: Infections due to Mycobacteria, in Rubenstein E, Federman DD (eds): *Scientific American Medicine.* New York, Scientific American, 1993, chapt. 7, sect. VIII, pp 1–3.
32. Tropical diseases research. *World Health,* June–July–August 1990, pp 1–31.
33. Davis RM: Current trends in cigarette advertising and marketing. *N Engl J Med* 1987;316:725–732.
34. MacMahon B, Copley G, Fraumeni JF Jr, et al: Populations at low risk of cancer: A workshop held in Snowbird, Utah, August 23–25, 1978. *JNCI* 1980;65:1049.
35. Liisberg E: World malaria situation (editorial). *World Health,* September–October 1991, p 6.
36. Smith MN, Whitney GM: Caring for the environment: The ecology of health, in Chinn P (ed): *Anthology on Caring.* New York, National League for Nursing Press, 1991, pp 59–69.
37. Burkitt DP: Relationship as a clue to causation. *Lancet* 1970;2:1237–1240.
38. Dean J, Schechter AN: Sickle cell anemia: Molecular and cellular bases of therapeutic approaches. First of 3 parts. *N Engl J Med* 1978;299:752–763.
39. Copeland DD: Concepts of disease and diagnosis. *Perspect Biol Med* 1977;20:528.
40. Dick HM: HLA and disease. *Br Med Bull* 1978;34:271.
41. Cahill GF: Genetics and inborn errors of metabolism, in Rubenstein E, Federman DD (eds): *Scientific American Medicine.* New York, Scientific American, 1987, vol 2, pp 1–17.

42. Scriver CR: Treatment in inborn errors of metabolism: The nature-nurture argument specified, in Crawford MDA, Gibbs DA, Watts RWE (eds): *Advances in the Treatment of Inborn Errors of Metabolism.* New York, John Wiley & Sons, 1982, pp 289–303.

43. National Center for Health Statistics: Health United States, 1992. Hyattsville, MD, US Public Health Service, 1993.

44. Sheldon H (ed): *Boyd's Introduction to the Study of Disease,* 10th ed. Philadelphia, Lea & Febiger, 1988, pp 79–86.

45. Baird SB, McCorkle R, Grant M: *Cancer Nursing: A Comprehensive Textbook.* Philadelphia, WB Saunders, 1991, p 555.

46. Kilbourne EM, Choi K, Jones TS, Thacker SB: Risk factors for heatstroke. *JAMA* 1982;247:3332–3336.

47. Lasagna L: The diseases drugs cause. *Perspect Biol Med* 1964;7:457–470.

48. Baker D, et al: Washington State University study of iatrogenic drug interactions among elderly: Preliminary data. Seattle, Washington State University, 1993.

49. Perry HM Jr, Miller JP: Difficulties in diagnosing hypertension: Implications and alternatives. *J Hypertens* 1992;10:88–97.

50. Scriver CR: Window panes of eternity: Health, disease, and inherited risk. *Yale J Biol Med* 1982;55:487–513.

51. O'Toole M (ed): *Miller-Keane Encyclopedia & Dictionary of Medicine, Nursing, & Allied Health,* 5th ed. Philadelphia, WB Saunders, 1992.

52. Borkan JM, Neher JO: A developmental model of ethnosensitivity in family practice training. *Fam Med* 1991;23:212–217.

53. Mausner JS: *Epidemiology: An Introductory Text,* 2nd ed. Philadelphia, WB Saunders, 1985.

54. Dockery DW, et al: An association between air pollution and mortality in six U.S. cities. *N Engl J Med* 1993;329:1752–1759.

55. Fink DJ: Change in American Cancer Society checkup guidelines for detection of cervical cancer. *CA* 1988;38:127–128.

56. Levine J, Suzuki D: "The Secret of Life." Boston, WGBH Educational Foundation, 1993.

BIBLIOGRAPHY

American Cancer Society: American Cancer Society report on the cancer-related health check-up. *CA* 1980;30:194.

Barsley AJ: The paradox of health. *N Engl J Med* 1988;318:414.

Boring CC, Squires TS, Tong T: Cancer statistics, 1992. *CA* 1992;42:19.

Cannon WB: Stresses and strains of homeostasis. *Am J Med Sci* 1935;189:1–14.

Castiglioni A: *A History of Medicine.* New York, Knopf, 1947.

Craighead JE, Mossman BT: The pathogenesis of asbestos-associated disease. *N Engl J Med* 1982;306:1446.

Dubos RJ: Infection into disease. *Perspect Biol Med* 1957;1:425.

Eibl-Eibesfeldt I: *Human Ethology.* New York, Aldine de Gruyter, 1989.

Eisenberg L: Disease and illness: Distinctions between professional and popular ideas of sickness. *Culture Med Psychiatry* 1977;1:9–23.

Engel GL: The need for a new medical model: A challenge for biomedicine. *Science* 1977;196:129.

Fabrega H Jr: Concepts of disease: Logical features and social implications. *Perspect Biol Med* 1972;15:583.

Fabrega H Jr: The need for an ethnomedical science. *Science* 1975;189:969–975.

Feinstein AR, et al: Scientific and clinical problems in indexes of functional disability. *Ann Intern Med* 1986;105:413–420.

Gardner ID: The effect of aging on susceptibility to infection. *Rev Infect Dis* 1980;2:801.

Gould GM: A system of personal biologic examinations: The condition of adequate medical and scientific conduct of life. *JAMA* 1900;35:134.

Hearing problems of elderly people (editorial). *Br Med J* 1989;299:1415.

Hoar SK, Blair A, Holmes FF, et al: Agricultural herbicide use and risk of lymphoma and soft-tissue sarcoma. *JAMA* 1986;256:1141.

Kleinman A: The cultural meanings and social uses of illness: A role for medical anthropology and clinically oriented social science in the development of primary care theory and research. *J Fam Pract* 1983;16:539–545.

Kohn RR: Cause of death in very old people. *JAMA* 1982;247:2793.

Levine J, Suzuki D: "The Secret of Life." Boston, WGBH Educational Foundation, 1993.

Long CA, Holden R, Mulkerrin E, et al: Opportunistic screening of visual acuity of elderly patients attending outpatient clinics. *Age Ageing* 1991;20:392.

Major RH: *Classic Descriptions of Disease,* 3rd ed. Springfield, IL, Charles C Thomas, 1948.

Mann GV: The influence of obesity on health. *N Engl J Med* 1974;291:178.

Moss NH, Mayer J: Food and nutrition in health and disease. *Ann NY Acad Sci* 1977;300.

National Center for Health Statistics: *Health, United States, 1992.* Hyattsville, MD, US Public Health Service, 1993.

Osborn JE: The AIDS epidemic: Multidisciplinary trouble. *N Engl J Med* 1986;314:779.

Osler Sir W: *The Evolution of Modern Medicine.* New Haven, Yale University Press, 1921.

Paffenbarger RS, et al: Physical activity, all cause mortality, and longevity of college alumni. *N Engl J Med* 1986;314:605.

Pariza MW: A perspective on diet, nutrition, and cancer. *JAMA* 1984;251:455.

Patrick DL, Erickson P: What constitutes quality of life: Concepts and dimensions. *Clin Nutr* 1988;7:53–63.

Petersen P: A perspective of infection and infectious disease. *Perspect Biol Med* 1980;23:255.

Polednak AP: *Racial and Ethnic Differences in Disease.* New York, Oxford University Press, 1989, pp 288–293.

Rosenberg CE: The therapeutic revolution: Medicine, meaning and social change in 19th century America. *Perspect Biol Med,* May 26, 1978.

Roueché B: *Eleven Blue Men and Other Tales of Medical Detection.* Boston, Little, Brown & Co, 1954.

Schatzkin A, Jones DY, Hoover RN, et al: Alcohol consumption and breast cancer in the Epidemiologic Follow-up Study of the First National Health and Nutrition Examination Survey. *N Engl J Med* 1987;326:1169.

Schistosomiasis from tropical diseases research. *World Health,* June–July–August 1990.

Scrimshaw NS, Behar M: Malnutrition in underdeveloped countries. *N Engl J Med* 1965;272:137.

Smith CE: The Broad Street pump revisited. *Int J Epidemiol* 1982;11:99.

Smoking and Health: A Report of the Surgeon General. US Department of Health, Education, and Welfare, DHEW Publication No (PHS) 79-50066. Washington, DC, US Government Printing Office, 1979.

Sontag S: *Illness as Metaphor.* New York, Farrar, Straus & Giroux, 1978.

Stults BM: Preventive health care for the elderly. *West J Med* 1984;141:832.

Thibodeau GA, Patton KT: Mechanisms of disease, in *Anatomy and Physiology,* 2nd ed. St. Louis, Mosby–Year Book, 1993, pp 28–34.

Twaddle AC: Sickness and the sickness career: Some implications, in Eisenberg L, Kleinman A (eds): *The Relevance of Social Science for Medicine.* Dordrecht, Holland, Reidel Publishing, 1981.

Vander AJ, Sherman JH, Luciano DS: *Human Physiology: The Mechanisms of Body Function,* 5th ed. New York, McGraw-Hill, 1990.

Vetter NJ, et al: The relationship between symptoms of chronic disease and dependence. *Int Disabil Stud* 1990;12:22–27.

Willett WC, MacMahon B: Diet and cancer—an overview (pt 1). *N Engl J Med* 1984;310:633.

Willett WC, Stampfer MJ, Colditz GA, et al: Dietary fat and the risk of breast cancer. *N Engl J Med* 1987;316:22.

Wood PHN: Measuring the consequences of illness. *World Health Stat Q* 1989;42:115–121.

World Health Organization: *International Classification of Impairments, Disabilities, and Handicaps.* Geneva, World Health Organization, 1980.

World malaria situation. *World Health,* September–October 1991.

Wyngaarden JB, Smith LH Jr (eds): *Cecil Textbook of Medicine,* 18th ed. Philadelphia, WB Saunders, 1988.

UNIT II
Alterations in Cellular Function

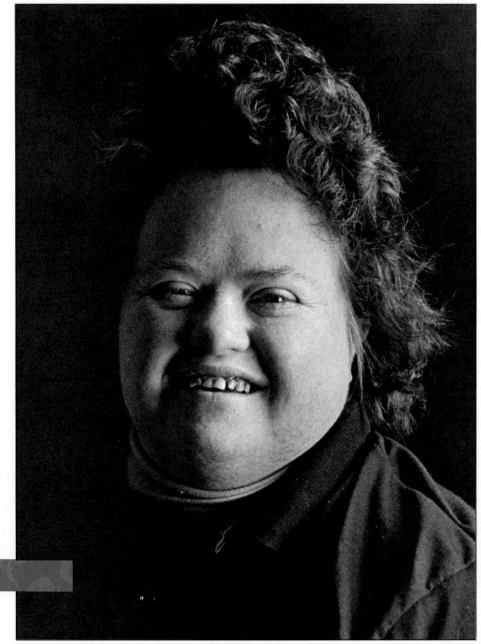

Down's syndrome, a chromosomal abnormality in which there is a triplet of chromosomes 21 rather than the usual pair, produces distinctive anatomical features in affected individuals. Notice characteristic features of folds around the eyes, flattened nose, and round face.

Photo by Kathleen Kelly

More than we might ordinarily suppose, insights we take for granted depend on our ability to decipher inherited mysteries. Most of this work falls to specialists, trained decipherers who use their skill, judgment, and intuition to find keys to lost or undiscovered languages. So the decoded Rosetta Stone revealed the language of ancient Egypt and the Dead Sea Scrolls yielded their secrets to scriptural scholars. In national emergencies cryptographers decode enemy messages. Decoding protects us, illuminates lost ages, and unriddles mysteries that defied other generations.

Today researchers are decoding the secret language of the human body to diagnose and perhaps prevent and cure diseases by discovering exactly what their causes are and how the body responds to the threat of disease. For medical decipherers decoding takes on a meaning beyond the languages with which humans communicate thoughts, desires, and purposes. The vocabulary and syntax of medical research are the ever more closely observed processes of the human body.

The human body is an ancient cryptogram. For countless millennia its codes have been concealed in the genetic makeup of the body's molecules. Thousands of generations have lived and died according to unvarying processes hidden in the body's molecules without having any way of understanding or explaining them except to invoke the "mystery of life." Now, as the mysteries are disclosed, life is less mystifying though no less wondrous.

In the past half-century researchers have ventured closer and closer to an understanding of the molecular language. Drawing on increasingly exact genetic research and employing new methods of observation, such as imaging, they have grasped elements of the vocabulary and used their discoveries to begin deciphering diseases formerly beyond comprehension.

So far they have lacked the cipher book that decoders use to understand encrypted messages—the source of keys to the language. Now cellular research promises to provide the code book that will lead to the prevention and cure of many diseases.

Cellular research pervades medical research. It lends plausibility to the popular view of medical research as a detective story, highlighted with dramatic "breakthroughs" when the culprit is found. Research has its dramatic moments, but it often takes much longer to find the exact cause of a disease than it does to track down a gang of bank robbers or arsonists. And although research has its superstars—Jonas Salk comes to mind—instead of one private eye walking warily along the mean streets of a threatening city, a number of researchers are always at work in different settings on the same fundamental problems.

When they manage to triumph over a disease, or a combination of diseases, deciphering often is the key. The cipher then can be shared, converted to techniques of immunization or therapy that can save humans from death and misery.

The work is exacting in ways unprecedented in medical research. One of two 1993 Nobel prizes in chemistry was awarded to Kary B. Mullis for research in genetics that in its minute understanding of the processes of life—and therefore the processes of disease—required an understanding of, as the *New York Times* said, "vanishingly small" units of matter.

Scientists' ability to work efficiently with vanishingly small particles depends today in part on Mullis's discovery of the polymerase chain reaction (PCR), which accelerated scientists' ability to swiftly copy many gene fragments, thus

FRONTIERS OF RESEARCH
Genes and Genetic Diseases
Michael J. Kirkhorn

profoundly accelerating the rate of cellular research. Like many discoveries, Mullis's came as a revelation following a long period of strenuous investigation. In 1983, when he was employed by the Cetus Corporation, he came up with the idea for PCR while driving one night from the San Francisco Bay area to his cabin in Medocino. His idea made it possible to quickly and efficiently carry on DNA replication in volumes never before achieved.

The perfection of amplification techniques allowed PCR to be applied to genetic diseases. Cystic fibrosis, a recessive genetic disease, was the first newly discovered defective gene whose mutation was confirmed by PCR. Without PCR the cloning and sequencing necessary to identify the defective gene might have taken years, even decades. With PCR, in a few days the researchers found that two copies of the gene deletion they suspected of causing the disease were present in about 70 percent of the patients they tested who had cystic fibrosis, a defect involving the exocrine glands, especially those secreting mucus, and resulting in pancreatic insufficiency, chronic pulmonary disease, abnormally high sweat electrolyte levels, and, in some cases, cirrhosis of the liver. Incomplete forms led to variations in the clinical manifestations. Having identified defective genes, medical scientists can hope to replace them.

PCR is only one of the technological developments that is contributing to the development of the human genome project, which intends to reveal a wealth of new biological information by producing genetic maps of the human body and by determining the DNA sequence of the human genome and of several model organisms. The genome project already has led to the isolation of genes associated with diseases such as Huntington's disease, amyotrophic lateral sclerosis, neurofibromatosis types 1 and 2, myotonic dystrophy, and fragile X syndrome. Other research has sharpened medical understanding of the predisposition to breast cancer, colon cancer, hypertension, diabetes and Alzheimer's disease. And this is only the beginning.

CHAPTER 2
Cell Structure and Function

JACQUELYN L. BANASIK

KEY TERMS

amphipathic: A molecule with portions having different characteristics. For example, membrane lipids are partly hydrophobic and partly hydrophilic, and hence are amphipathic.

eucaryotic: Cells that have a true nucleus bounded by a nuclear membrane.

glycolysis: The anaerobic process of breaking down sugars into simpler molecules, with the net production of two ATP molecules per glucose molecule.

procaryotic: Cells that do not have a membrane-bound nucleus or other membrane-bound organelles.

second messenger: An intracellular signal that is produced in response to an extracellular signal.

A basic principle of biology states that the cell is the fundamental unit of life. As more diseases are understood on the cellular and molecular level, it appears that the cell is also the fundamental unit of disease. Currently, a knowledge explosion is occurring in the fields of cell and molecular biology, leading to a better understanding of human physiology and the cellular aspects of disease. Detailed knowledge of cellular dysfunction has led to the development of more specific and appropriate prevention and treatment modalities for many disease processes. An understanding of cellular mechanisms is essential for health care providers and fundamental to the discussions of pathophysiology presented throughout the remainder of this text.

Cells are complex, membrane-bound units packed with a multitude of chemicals and macromolecules. They are able to replicate and thus form new cells and organisms. The very first cell on earth probably arose from the spontaneous association of organic (carbon-containing) and inorganic molecules about 3.5 billion years ago.[1-3] Over billions of years, the self-replicating molecules now known as DNA and RNA are believed to have evolved by chance association and natural selection. Evolution of the cell membrane created a closed compartment that provided a selective advantage for the cell and accomplished the first separation of life (inside) from nonlife (outside). In this protected environment, the cell continued to evolve and develop. Today, a number of different cell types exist, but many of the basic biochemical mechanisms of these cell types are remarkably similar. Scientists believe that all modern cells, from bacteria to human neurons, evolved from a single primordial cell.[4] It is therefore possible to unlock many of the secrets of human cellular physiology by studying easily grown and rapidly proliferating cells such as yeasts and bacteria.

Much of our knowledge of cell physiology has derived from study of the class of cells known as **procaryotic,** which includes bacteria. Procaryotic cells were the first to evolve and are simpler than eucaryotic cells, having no defined nucleus or cytoplasmic organelles. Fungi, plants, and animals belong to the **eucaryotic** class of cells, which possess a membrane-bound nucleus and a host of cytoplasmic organelles (Fig. 2–1). In this chapter, the essentials of eucaryotic cell structure, physiology, and metabolism are reviewed.

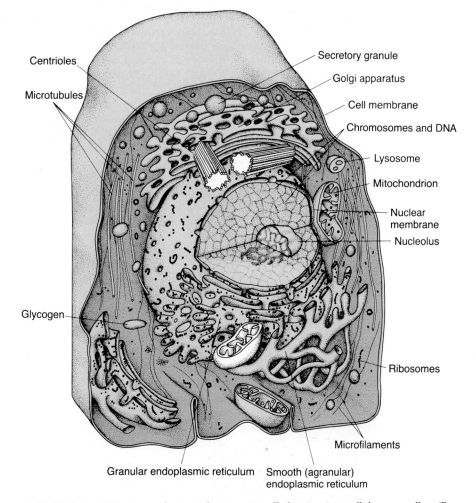

Centrioles

Microtubules

Glycogen

Secretory granule

Golgi apparatus

Cell membrane

Chromosomes and DNA

Lysosome

Mitochondrion

Nuclear membrane

Nucleolus

Ribosomes

Microfilaments

Granular endoplasmic reticulum   Smooth (agranular) endoplasmic reticulum

FIGURE 2–1. Structure of a typical eucaryotic cell showing intracellular organelles. (From Guyton AC: *Textbook of Medical Physiology,* 8th ed. Philadelphia, WB Saunders, p. 10. Reproduced with permission.)

Plasma Membrane

Membrane Structure

All cells are enclosed by a barrier composed primarily of lipid and protein and called the **plasma membrane** (plasmalemma). This cell membrane is a highly selective filter that shields internal cell contents from the external environment. The plasma membrane is an important structure that performs a variety of functions, including transport of nutrients and waste products, the generation of membrane potentials, and cell recognition, communication, and growth regulation. The cell membrane is a sensor of signals that enables the cell to respond and adapt to changes in its environment.

According to the **fluid mosaic model,** described in the 1960s by Singer and Nicolson,[5] the plasma membrane is a dynamic assembly of lipid and protein molecules. Most of the lipids and proteins are able to move about in the fluid structure of the membrane. As shown in Figure 2–2, the lipid molecules are arranged in a double layer, or **lipid bilayer,** which is highly impermeable to most water-soluble molecules. A variety of proteins embedded or "dissolved" in the lipid bilayer serve a number of cell functions. Some **membrane proteins** are involved in the transport of specific molecules into and out of the cell; others function as enzymes or respond to external signals; and some serve as structural links that connect the plasma membrane to adjacent cells. The specific structures and functions of the cell membrane and its constituents are described in the following sections.

Lipid Bilayer

The bilayer structure of all biological membranes is related to the special properties of lipid molecules which cause them to spontaneously assemble into bilayers.[6] The three major types of membrane lipids are cholesterol, phospholipids, and glycolipids. All three have a molecular structure that is **amphipathic;** that is, they have a hydrophilic (water-loving) polar end and a hydrophobic (water-hating) nonpolar end.

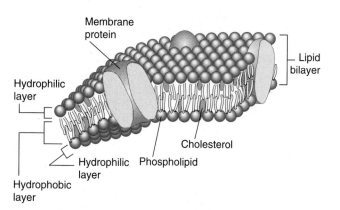

FIGURE 2–2. Section of the cell membrane showing the lipid bilayer structure and integral membrane proteins.

This amphipathic nature causes the lipids to form bilayers in aqueous solution. A typical phospholipid molecule is shown in Figure 2–3. The hydrophobic nonpolar tails will tend to associate with other hydrophobic nonpolar-tail groups in order to avoid association with water molecules. The hydrophilic polar-head groups preferentially interact with the surrounding aqueous environment. A bilayer, with tails sandwiched in the middle, allows both portions of the lipid molecules to be chemically "satisfied." Additionally, the lipid bilayers tend to close on themselves, forming sealed, spherical compartments (Fig. 2–4). If the membrane is punctured or torn it will spontaneously reseal itself to eliminate contact of the hydrophobic tails with water.

Until the late 1960s, the cell membrane was viewed as a rather rigid structure. It is now recognized to behave in a fluid-like manner, with individual lipid and protein molecules able to diffuse freely and rapidly within the bilayer.[7] The degree of membrane fluidity depends on the lipid composition.[8–10] Saturated lipids tend to stiffen the membrane, whereas lipids with unsaturated hydrocarbon tails tend to increase fluidity. Cholesterol is another important determinant of membrane fluidity. Eucaryotic cells contain large amounts of cholesterol, which serves to decrease membrane permeability and fluidity. The importance of cholesterol in maintaining mechanical stability and flexibility is suggested by mutant animal cell lines that are unable to synthesize cholesterol. These cells rapidly break open (lyse) unless cholesterol is added to the culture medium in which they are growing. This suggests that abnormalities in membrane cholesterol content could result in more fragile, less resilient cells.

The lipid composition of the cell membrane is important to the function of membrane proteins as well.[11,12] In addition to cholesterol and glycolipids, human cell membranes contain a variety of phospholipids that differ in the size, shape, and charge of the polar-head groups. Figure 2–5 shows the structures of the four most prevalent membrane phospholipids: phosphatidylethanolamine, phosphatidylserine, phosphatidylcholine, and sphingomyelin. It is likely that some membrane proteins must have specific phospholipid head groups present in order to function.[11]

Glycolipids contain one or more sugar molecules at the polar head region. Interestingly, glycolipids are found only in the outer half of the lipid bilayer, with the sugar groups exposed at the cell surface (Fig. 2–6). The functional significance of membrane glycolipids remains largely a mystery. They are thought to be involved in cell recognition and cell-to-cell interactions.[13]

Membrane Proteins

Approximately 50 percent of the mass of a typical cell membrane is composed of protein. These membrane proteins carry out most of the functions of the membrane. The specific types of membrane proteins will

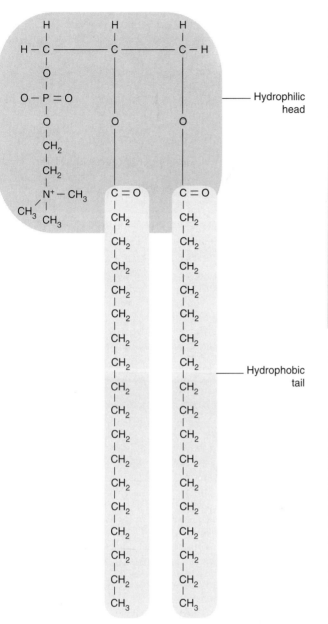

FIGURE 2–3. Schematic drawing of a typical membrane phospholipid molecule showing the amphipathic nature of the structure.

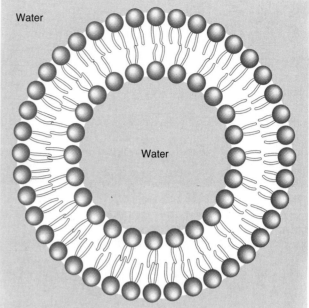

FIGURE 2–4. The amphipathic nature of membrane lipids results in bilayer structures that tend to form spheres.

For example, a kidney tubule cell has a large proportion of transmembrane proteins, which are necessary to perform the kidney's function of electrolyte and nutrient reabsorption. In contrast, the human red blood cell contains mainly peripheral proteins attached to the inner surface of the membrane.[15] One of these proteins, spectrin, has a long, thin, flexible rodlike shape that forms a supportive meshwork or **cytoskeleton** for the cell. It is this cytoskeleton that enables the red cell to withstand the membrane stress of being forced through small capillaries.

Although proteins and lipids are generally free to move within the plane of the cell membrane, many cells are able to confine certain proteins to specific areas. Using the example of the kidney tubule cell again, it is important for the cell to keep transport proteins on its luminal side in order to reabsorb filtered molecules (Fig. 2–8). This segregation of particular proteins is thought to be accomplished by intercellular connections called **tight junctions,** which restrict protein movement.[16] Some of the other types of membrane proteins will be described later in this chapter.

KEY CONCEPTS

- The plasma membrane is composed of a lipid bilayer that is impermeable to most water-soluble molecules but permeable to lipid-soluble substances.
- Proteins embedded in the lipid bilayer carry out most of the membrane's functions, including transport and signal transduction.

vary according to cell type and environmental conditions. Some membrane proteins, called **transmembrane proteins,** are known to extend across the membrane bilayer.[14] Transmembrane proteins serve a variety of functions, including transport of charged and polar molecules into and out of cells and transduction of extracellular signals into intracellular messages. Other **peripheral** membrane proteins are less tightly anchored to the membrane. The common structural orientations of membrane proteins are shown in Figure 2–7.

The type of principal membrane proteins of a particular cell depends on the cell's primary functions.

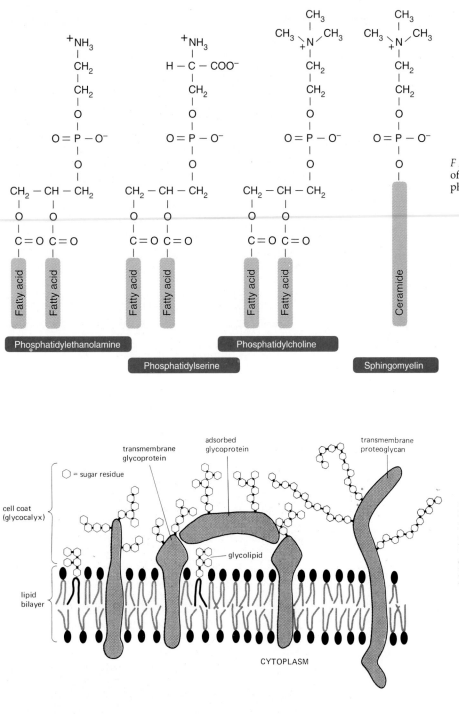

FIGURE 2-5. Chemical structures of the four most common membrane phospholipids.

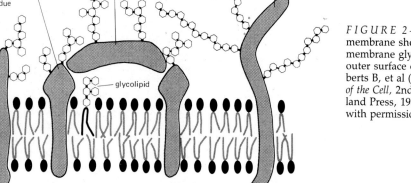

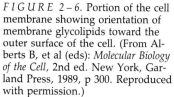

FIGURE 2-6. Portion of the cell membrane showing orientation of membrane glycolipids toward the outer surface of the cell. (From Alberts B, et al (eds): *Molecular Biology of the Cell,* 2nd ed. New York, Garland Press, 1989, p 300. Reproduced with permission.)

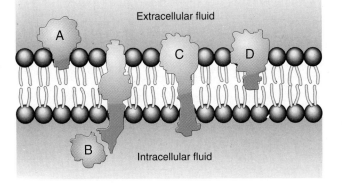

FIGURE 2-7. Structural orientation of some proteins in the cell membrane. *A,* membrane protein with noncovalent attachment to plasma lipids; *B,* membrane protein with noncovalent attachment to another membrane protein; *C,* transmembrane protein extending through the lipid bilayer; *D,* covalently attached peripheral membrane protein.

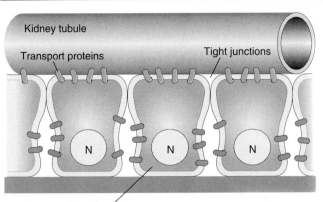

FIGURE 2–8. Transport proteins may be confined to a particular portion of the cell membrane by tight junctions. Segregation of transport proteins is important for the absorptive functions of the kidney epithelial cells. *N*, nucleus.

Organization of Cellular Compartments

Cytoskeleton

Eucaryotic cells have a variety of internal compartments, or **organelles,** which are membrane bound and carry out distinct cellular functions. The cell's organelles are not free to float around haphazardly in the cytoplasmic soup; rather, they are elaborately organized by a protein network called the **cytoskeleton** (Fig. 2–9).[17] The cytoskeleton maintains the cell's shape, allows cell movement, and directs the trafficking of substances within the cell. Three principal types of protein filaments make up the cytoskeleton: actin filaments, microtubules, and intermediate filaments. **Actin filaments** play a pivotal role in cell movement. As one might expect, muscle cells are packed with actin filaments, which allows the cell to perform its primary function of contraction. However, nonmuscle cells also possess actin filaments that are important for complex movements of the cell membrane, such as cell crawling and phagocytosis. Such movements of the cell membrane are mediated by dense networks of actin filaments that cluster just beneath the plasma

FIGURE 2–9. Schematic of the cytoskeleton showing two of the major protein structures, actin and intermediate filaments. (From Hirokawa N, Heuser JE: *J Cell Biol* 1981;91:399–409. Reproduced by copyright permission of the Rockefeller University Press. Micrograph produced by Dr. John Heuser, Washington University, St. Louis.)

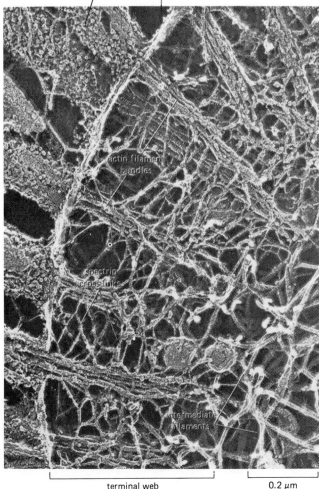

membrane and interact with specific proteins embedded in it.

Organization of the cytoplasm and its organelles is achieved primarily by **microtubules.** In animal cells, microtubules originate at the cell center, or **centrosome,** near the nucleus and radiate out toward the cell perimeter in fine lacelike threads. Microtubules guide the orderly transport of organelles in the cytoplasm as well as the equal distribution of chromosomes during cell division (see Chap. 4). **Intermediate filaments,** so named because their size is between that of microtubules and actin filaments, are the least well characterized. Their primary function seems to be mechanical support of the cell.[17] A variety of intermediate filaments have been identified that differ from tissue to tissue. Continued research will no doubt reveal important specific functions for this class of cytoskeletal proteins.

Nucleus

The largest cytoplasmic organelle is the **nucleus,** which contains the genetic information for the cell in the form of **deoxyribonucleic acid (DNA).**[18] The nuclear contents are enclosed and protected by the **nuclear envelope,** which consists of two concentric membranes. The inner membrane forms an unbroken sphere around the DNA and contains protein-binding sites that help to organize the chromosomes inside. The outer nuclear membrane is continuous with the endoplasmic reticulum (ER) (see below) and closely resembles it in structure and function (Fig. 2–10). The nucleus contains many proteins that help mediate its functions of genetic control and inheritance. These proteins, including histones, polymerases, and regu-

latory proteins, are manufactured in the cytosol and transported to the nucleus through holes in the membrane called **nuclear pores.** The nuclear pores are very selective as to which molecules are allowed access to the nuclear compartment and in this way protect the genetic material from enzymes and other molecules in the cytoplasm. The nuclear pores also mediate the export of products such as RNA and ribosomes that are synthesized in the nucleus but function in the cytosol. A major function of the nucleus is to protect and preserve genetic information so that it can be replicated exactly and passed on during cell division. However, the nucleus is continuously functioning even when the cell is not actively dividing. The nuclear DNA controls the production of cellular enzymes, membrane receptors, structural proteins, and other proteins that define the cell's type and behavior. (The structure and function of DNA are discussed in Chapter 4.)

Endoplasmic Reticulum

The ER is a membrane network that extends throughout the cytoplasm and is present in all eucaryotic cells (see Fig. 2–9).[19] The ER is thought to have a single continuous membrane that separates the lumen of the ER from the cytosol—it could be likened to the "GI tract" of the cell. The ER plays a central role in the synthesis of membrane components, including proteins and lipids, for the plasma membrane and cellular organelles, as well as in the synthesis of products to be secreted from the cell. The ER is divided into rough and smooth types based on its appearance under the electron microscope. The **rough ER** is coated with ribosomes along its outer surface. **Ribosomes** are complexes of protein and RNA; they are formed in the nucleus and transported to the cytoplasm. Their primary function is the synthesis of proteins (see Chap. 4). Depending on the destination of the protein to be created, ribosomes may float free in the cytosol or may bind to the ER membrane. Proteins synthesized by free-floating ribosomes stay within the cytosol of the cell. When a protein is to be transported into the ER, the ribosome responsible for its synthesis will bind to the ER membrane. The protein is then translocated through the ER membrane and eventually transported to the appropriate organelle or secreted at the cell surface.

Regions of ER that lack ribosomes are called **smooth ER.** The smooth ER is involved in lipid metabolism. Most cells have very little smooth ER, but cells specializing in the production of steroid hormones or lipoproteins may have significant amounts of smooth ER. For example, the hepatocyte (liver cell) has abundant smooth ER containing enzymes responsible for the manufacture of lipoproteins as well as the detoxification of harmful lipid-soluble compounds such as alcohol. The cellular smooth ER can double in surface area within a few days if large quantities of drugs or toxins enter the circulation.

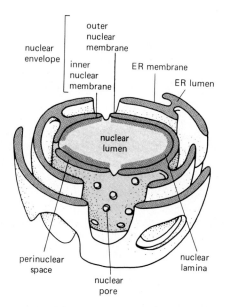

FIGURE 2–10. Structure of the double membrane envelope that surrounds the cell nucleus. (From Alberts B, et al (eds): *Molecular Biology of the Cell,* 2nd ed. New York, Garland Press, 1989, p 422. Reproduced with permission.)

Golgi Apparatus

The **Golgi apparatus** or Golgi complex is composed of a stack of smooth membrane–bound compartments resembling a stack of hollow plates (Fig. 2–11). These compartments or *cisternae* are organized in a series of at least three processing compartments. The first compartment (*cis* face) lies next to the ER and receives newly synthesized proteins and lipids by way of ER transport vesicles. The proteins and lipids then move through the middle compartment (medial) to the final compartment (*trans* face), where they depart for their final destination. As the lipid and protein molecules pass through the sequence of Golgi compartments, they are modified by enzymes that attach sugar molecules to them. After specific rearrangement of these sugars has occurred, the lipids and proteins are packaged into Golgi transport vesicles. The particular configuration of sugar molecules on the lipid or protein is thought to serve as an "address label," directing them to the correct destination within the cell. Golgi vesicles transport their contents primarily to the plasma membrane and to lysosomes.

Lysosomes and Peroxisomes

Transport of Golgi vesicles to the membrane-bound bags of digestive enzymes known as **lysosomes** has been well described and provides a model for Golgi sorting and transport to other destinations. Lysosomes are filled with over 40 different acid hydrolases, which are capable of digesting organic molecules, including proteins, nucleotides, fats, and sugars.[19] Lysosomes obtain the materials they digest from three main pathways.[20,21] The first is the pathway used to digest products taken up by endocytosis. In this pathway, endocytotic vesicles bud off from the plasma

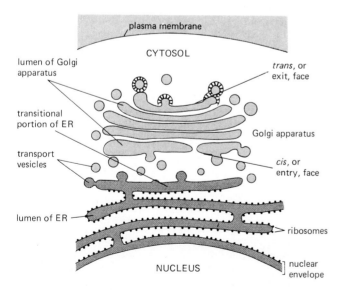

FIGURE 2–11. Schematic of the endoplasmic reticulum (ER) and its relationship to the Golgi apparatus. (From Alberts B, et al (eds): *Molecular Biology of the Cell,* 2nd ed. New York, Garland Press, 1989, p 434. Reproduced with permission.)

membrane to form endosomes, which then fuse with a **primary** (inactive) lysosome. This fused endolysosome converts to a **mature** lysosome by an unknown mechanism, the pH inside the lysosome acidifies, and active digestion occurs. The second pathway is **autophagy,** whereby damaged and obsolete parts of the cell itself are destroyed. Unwanted cellular structures are enclosed by membrane from the ER, which then fuses with the lysosome, leading to autodigestion of the cellular components. Autophagy may also occur during cell starvation or disuse, leading to a process called **atrophy,** in which the cell becomes smaller and more energy efficient. The third pathway providing materials to the lysosomes is present only in specialized phagocytic cells. White blood cells, for example, are capable of ingesting large particles, which then form a **phagosome** capable of fusing with a lysosome. The final products of lysosomal digestion are simple molecules such as amino acids, fatty acids, and sugars, which can be utilized by the cell or secreted as cellular waste at the cell surface.

Discovery of the mechanism for sorting and transport of lysosomal enzymes was aided by studying patients suffering from the **lysosomal storage diseases.**[22] Patients with **I-cell disease,** for example, accumulate large amounts of debris in lysosomes, which appear as spots or "inclusions" in the cells. These lysosomes lack nearly all of the hydrolases normally present and thus are unable to perform lysosomal digestion. However, all the hydrolases missing from the lysosomes can be found in the patient's bloodstream. The abnormality results from "missorting" by the Golgi apparatus, which erroneously packages the enzymes for extracellular secretion rather than sending them to the lysosomes. Studies of this rare genetic disease resulted in the discovery that all lysosomal enzymes have a common marker, mannose-6-phosphate, which normally targets the enzymes to the lysosomes. Persons with I-cell disease lack the enzyme responsible for attaching this marker.

Peroxisomes (**microbodies**), like lysosomes, are membrane-bound bags of enzymes that perform degradative functions. They are particularly important in liver and kidney cells, where they detoxify various substances such as alcohol. In contrast to lysosomes, which contain hydrolase enzymes, peroxisomes contain **oxidative enzymes.** These enzymes use molecular oxygen to break down organic substances by an oxidative reaction that produces hydrogen peroxide. The hydrogen peroxide is then used by another enzyme (catalase) to break down other organic molecules, including formaldehyde and alcohol. Catalase also prevents accumulation of excess hydrogen peroxide in the cell by converting it to water and oxygen.

Mitochondria

The **mitochondria** have been aptly called the "powerhouses of the cell" because they convert energy to forms that can be used to drive cellular reactions. A distinct feature of mitochondria is the large amount of membrane they contain. Each mitochondrion is bounded by two specialized membranes. The **inner membrane** forms an enclosed space, called the **matrix,** which contains a concentrated mix of mitochondrial enzymes. The highly convoluted structure of the inner membrane (Fig. 2–12) provides a large surface area for the important membrane-bound enzymes of the **respiratory chain.** These enzymes are essential to the process of oxidative phosphorylation, which generates most of the cell's **adenosine triphosphate (ATP).** The **outer membrane** is very porous, having large aqueous channels much like a sieve. Large molecules, including protein, can pass freely through the outer membrane, such that the space between the outer and inner membranes is chemically similar to the cytosol. The inner membrane, however, is quite impermeable even to small molecules and ions. Specific protein transporters are required to shuttle the necessary molecules across the inner mitochondrial membrane.

The number and location of mitochondria differ according to cell type and function. Cells with high energy needs, such as cardiac or skeletal muscle, have many mitochondria. These mitochondria may pack between adjacent muscle fibrils such that ATP is delivered directly to the areas of unusually high energy consumption. The details of mitochondrial energy conversion are discussed in the next section.

KEY CONCEPTS

- The cytoskeleton is made up of actin, microtubules, and intermediate filaments. These proteins regulate cell shape, movement, and the trafficking of intracellular molecules.
- The nucleus contains the genomic DNA. These nuclear genes code for the synthesis of proteins.
- The endoplasmic reticulum and the Golgi apparatus function together to synthesize proteins and lipids for transport to organelles or to the plasma membrane.
- Lysosomes and peroxisomes are membrane-bound bags of digestive enzymes that degrade intracellular debris.
- Mitochondria contain tricarboxylic acid and respiratory chain enzymes necessary for oxidative phosphorylation to produce adenosine triphosphate.

Cellular Metabolism

All living cells must continually perform essential cellular functions such as movement, ion pumping, and synthesis of macromolecules. Many of these cellular activities are energetically unfavorable—i.e., they are unlikely to occur spontaneously. Unfavorable reac-

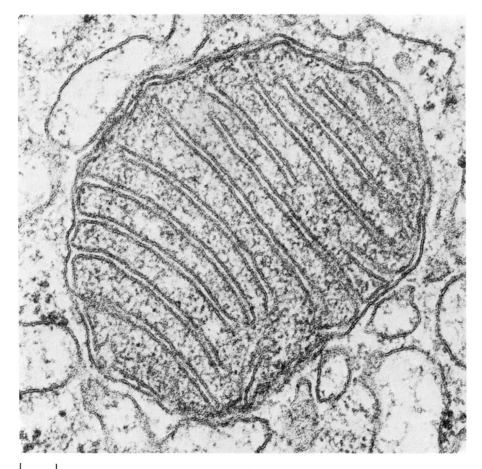

FIGURE 2–12. Electron micrograph of the mitochondrial structure. The highly convoluted inner membrane provides a large surface area for membrane-bound metabolic enzymes. (From Alberts B, et al (eds): *Molecular Biology of the Cell,* 2nd ed. New York, Garland Press, 1989, p 344. Micrograph courtesy of Daniel S. Friend.)

100 nm

tions can be driven by linking them to an energy source such as ATP. ATP is a molecule that contains high-energy phosphate bonds. Approximately 7 kilocalories of energy per mole of ATP is liberated when one of the phosphate bonds is hydrolyzed (broken with the aid of water) in a chemical reaction. Enzymes throughout the cell are able to capture the energy released from ATP hydrolysis and use it to break or make other chemical bonds. In this way, ATP serves as the "energy currency" of the cell. A specific amount of ATP is "spent" to "buy" a specific amount of chemical work. Most cells contain only a small amount of ATP, sufficient to maintain cellular activities for just a few minutes. Because ATP cannot cross the plasma membrane, each cell must continuously synthesize its own ATP to meet its energy needs. ATP is synthesized from the breakdown of glycogen and fat. An average adult has enough glycogen stores (primarily in liver and muscle) to supply about 1 day's needs, but enough fat to last for a month or more. After a meal, the excess glucose entering the cells is used to replenish glycogen stores or to synthesize fats for later use. Fat is stored primarily in adipose tissue and is released into the bloodstream for other cells to use when needed. When cellular glucose levels fall, glycogen and fats are broken down to provide glucose and fatty acyl molecules, which are ultimately metabolized to provide ATP. During starvation, body proteins can also be used for energy production by a process called gluconeogenesis.

Cellular **metabolism** is the biochemical process whereby foodstuffs are utilized to provide cellular energy and biomolecules. Cellular metabolism includes two separate and opposite phases: anabolism and catabolism. **Anabolism** refers to *energy-using* metabolic processes or pathways that result in the synthesis of complex molecules such as fats. **Catabolism** refers to the *energy-releasing* breakdown of nutrient sources such as glucose to provide ATP to the cell. Both of these processes require a long, complex series of enzymatic steps. The catabolic processes of cellular energy production are briefly discussed below. (See Chapter 39 for a detailed discussion of metabolism.)

Glycolysis

The catabolic process of energy production begins with the intestinal digestion of foodstuffs into small molecules: proteins into amino acids, polysaccharides into sugars, and fats into fatty acids and glycerol. The second stage of catabolism occurs in the cytosol of the cell, where sugar molecules are further degraded by **glycolysis** into pyruvate (3-carbon atoms).[23] Glycolysis involves nine enzymatic steps to break the 6-carbon glucose molecule into two 3-carbon pyruvate molecules (Fig. 2–13). Glycolysis requires the use of two ATP molecules in the early stages but produces four ATP molecules in the later steps, for a net gain of two ATP per glucose molecule. The production of

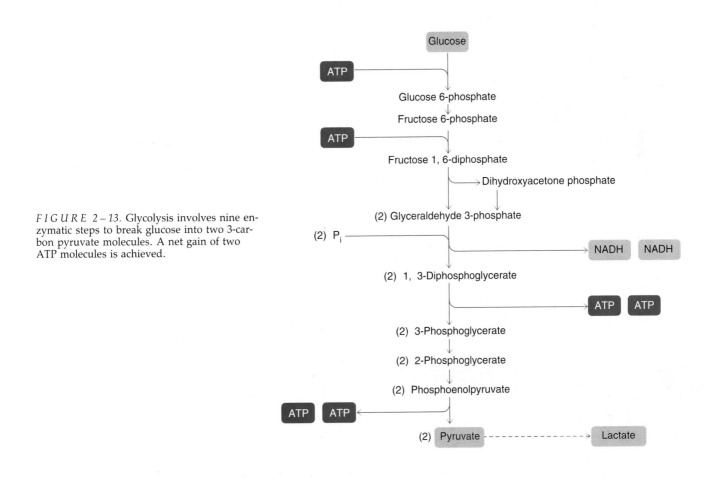

FIGURE 2–13. Glycolysis involves nine enzymatic steps to break glucose into two 3-carbon pyruvate molecules. A net gain of two ATP molecules is achieved.

ATP through glycolysis is relatively inefficient, and the pyruvate end-products still contain substantial chemical energy that can be released by further catabolism in stage three. However, glycolysis may be an important provider of ATP under **anaerobic** conditions because oxygen is not required. Cells, such as red blood cells, that do not contain mitochondria must rely totally on glycolysis for cellular ATP production. ATP production by glycolysis also becomes important during conditions of reduced cellular oxygenation, which may accompany respiratory and cardiovascular disorders. The pyruvate that accumulates during prolonged anaerobic conditions is converted to lactate and excreted from the cell into the bloodstream. **Lactic acidosis** is a dangerous condition that may result from excessive lactate production due to severe or prolonged lack of oxygen (see Chap. 12).

Citric Acid Cycle

For most cells, glycolysis is only a prelude to the third stage of catabolism, which takes place in the mitochondria and results in the complete oxidation of glucose to its final end products, CO_2 and H_2O. The third stage begins with the **citric acid cycle** (also called the **Krebs cycle** or the **tricarboxylic acid cycle**) and ends with the production of ATP by oxidative phosphorylation.[24] The purpose of the citric acid cycle is to break, by oxidation, the C—C and C—H bonds of the compounds produced in the second stage of catabolism. These compounds (pyruvate and fatty acyl groups) enter the citric acid cycle in the form of acetyl coenzyme A (Fig. 2–14). In the first reaction of the cycle,

the 2-carbon acetyl group is transferred from coenzyme A to a 4-carbon oxaloacetate molecule. This results in the formation of the 6-carbon molecule, citrate, for which the cycle is named. In a series of enzymatic oxidations, carbon atoms are cleaved off in the form of CO_2 (Fig. 2–15); this CO_2 is free to diffuse from the cell and be excreted by the lungs as a waste product. Two carbon atoms are removed to form two CO_2 molecules for each complete turn of the cycle. Molecular oxygen is not required for the citric acid cycle to function because the extra oxygen molecules needed to create CO_2 are provided by the surrounding H_2O.

Although the citric acid cycle directly produces only one ATP molecule (in the form of guanosine triphosphate) per cycle, it captures a great deal of energy in the form of **activated hydride ions** (H^-). These high-energy ions combine with larger carrier molecules, which transport them to the electron transport chain in the mitochondrial membrane. Two important carrier molecules are **NAD⁺** (nicotinamide adenine dinucleotide), which becomes NADH when reduced by H^-, and **FAD** (flavin adenine nucleotide), which becomes $FADH_2$ when reduced by H^-. The energy carried by these molecules will ultimately be used to produce ATP through a process called oxidative phosphorylation.

Oxidative Phosphorylation

Oxidative phosphorylation follows the processes of glycolysis and the citric acid cycle and results in the formation of ATP by the reaction ADP + Pi → ATP.[25] The energy to drive this unfavorable reaction is provided by the high-energy hydride ions (H^-) derived from the citric acid cycle. This energy is not used to form ATP directly; a series of energy transfers is required. In eucaryotic cells, this series of energy transfers occurs along the **electron transport chain** on the inner mitochondrial membrane. The transport chain consists of three major enzyme complexes and two mobile electron carriers that shuttle electrons between the protein complexes (Fig. 2–16). The hydrogen molecules and their associated electrons are transported to the electron transport chain by the carrier molecule NADH. The path of electron flow is NADH → NADH dehydrogenase complex → ubiquinone → b–c_1 complex → cytochrome c → cytochrome oxidase complex. As the electrons pass from one complex to the next they transfer energy, which is used to pump hydrogen ions (H^+) out of the mitochondrial matrix. At the very end of the transport chain, low-energy electrons are finally transferred to O_2 to form H_2O. Oxidative phosphorylation is called **aerobic** because of this oxygen-requiring step.

Thus far, no ATP synthesis has been accomplished. However, the enzymes of the transport chain have harnessed energy from the transported electrons in the form of a proton (H^+) gradient. Finally, the proton gradient is used to power the synthesis of ATP. Special enzymes in the inner mitochondrial membrane (ATP synthetase) allow protons to flow back

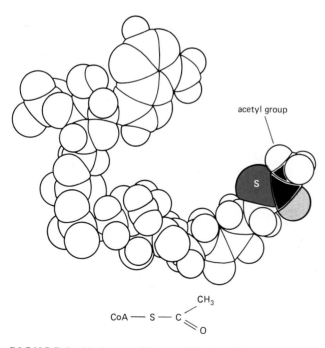

CoA — S — C ⟨ CH₃ / O

F I G U R E 2 – 14. A space-filling model of acetyl coenzyme A. (From Alberts B, et al (eds): *Molecular Biology of the Cell,* 2nd ed. New York, Garland Press, 1989, p. 345. Reproduced with permission.)

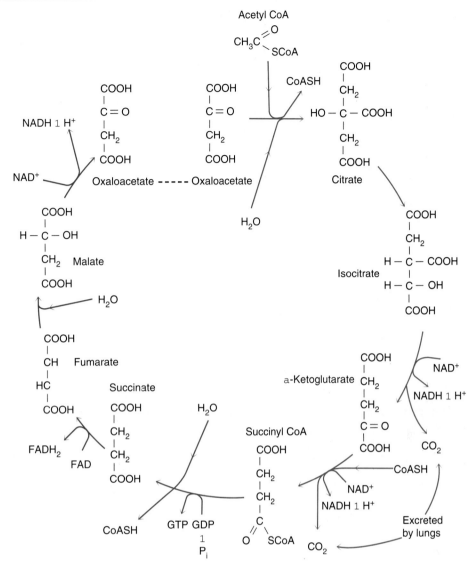

FIGURE 2-15. Chemical structures of the compounds of the citric acid cycle (Krebs cycle). In a series of enzymatic reactions, carbon atoms are cleaved to form CO_2 and high-energy hydride ions which are carried by FAD and NAD.
(Adapted with permission from Alberts B, et al (eds): *Molecular Biology of the Cell,* 2nd ed. New York, Garland Press, 1989, p 348.)

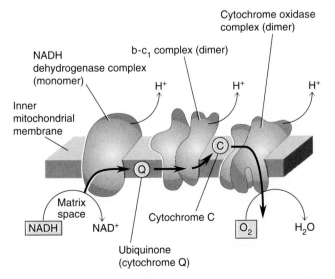

FIGURE 2-16. A representation of the electron transport chain located in the inner mitochondrial membrane. High-energy electrons are passed along the chain until they combine with oxygen to form water.

into the mitochondria down their concentration gradient. The energy of the proton flow is used to drive ATP synthesis (Fig. 2–17).[26] A total of 36 to 38 ATP molecules are formed from the complete oxidation of glucose into CO_2 and H_2O. Two of these are from glycolysis, two from the citric acid cycle (in the form of guanosine triphosphate), and 32 to 34 more are from oxidative phosphorylation. The ATP formed within the mitochondria is transported to the cytosol by protein transporters in the mitochondrial membrane. The ATP is then available to drive a variety of energy-requiring reactions within the cell.

KEY CONCEPTS

- Energy-requiring reactions within cells are driven by coupling to ATP hydrolysis.
- ATP is not stored and must be continuously synthesized by each cell to meet the cell's energy needs.
- Glycolysis is an anaerobic process that produces two ATP molecules and two pyruvate molecules per glucose molecule.

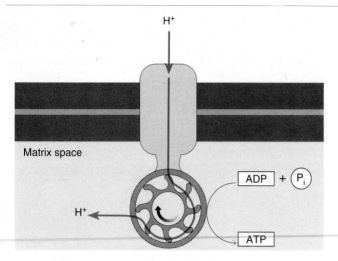

FIGURE 2–17. The inner mitochondrial ATP-synthetase captures the potential energy of the H^+ gradient in a manner similar to a turbine. The proton gradient drives the synthesis of ATP from adenosine diphosphate (*ADP*) and phosphate (*P_i*). (Adapted with permission from Alberts B, et al (eds): *Molecular Biology of the Cell*, 2nd ed. New York, Garland Press, 1989, p 357.)

• The function of the tricarboxylic acid cycle and the respiratory chain enzymes is dependent on the availability of molecular oxygen (O_2) and produces 34 to 36 ATP molecules per glucose molecule.

Functions of the Plasma Membrane

Membrane Transport of Macromolecules: Endocytosis and Exocytosis

The transport of large molecules such as proteins and polysaccharides across the plasma membrane cannot be accomplished by the membrane transport proteins discussed above. Rather, macromolecules are ingested and secreted by the sequential formation and fusion of membrane-bound vesicles. **Endocytosis** refers to cellular ingestion of extracellular molecules.[27] The process of cellular secretion is called **exocytosis.** There are two types of endocytosis, which are differentiated by the size of the particles ingested. **Pinocytosis,** or "cellular drinking," is the method of ingesting fluids and small particles and is common to most cell types. **Phagocytosis,** or "cellular eating," involves the ingestion of large particles such as microorganisms and is practiced mainly by specialized phagocytic white blood cells. Endocytosis begins at the cell surface by the formation of an indentation or "pit" in the plasma membrane, which is coated with special proteins, including clathrin (*coated pit*). The indentation invaginates and then pinches off a portion of the membrane to become a **vesicle** (Fig. 2–18). Each vesicle thus formed is internalized, sheds its coat, and fuses with an **endosome.** The contents of these

endocytic vesicles generally end up in **lysosomes,** where they are degraded.

Endocytosis of certain macromolecules is regulated by specific receptors on the cell surface.[28] These receptors bind the molecules (ligands) to be ingested and then cluster together in coated pits. The receptor-ligand complexes are internalized by the invagination process described above. The vesicles generally fuse with lysosomes, where the ligand is removed from the receptor for processing by the cell. The receptor may be degraded in the lysosome or may be recycled to the cell surface to be used again. **Receptor-mediated endocytosis** allows the cell to be selective about the molecules ingested and to regulate the amount taken into the cell. The cell can produce greater numbers of cell surface receptors in order to ingest more ligand.

An example of receptor-mediated endocytosis is cellular uptake of cholesterol.[29] The process of cholesterol uptake by cells is shown in Figure 2–19. Most cholesterol in the blood is transported by protein carriers called **low-density lipoproteins (LDLs).** The cell can regulate the number of LDL receptors on its cell surface in order to increase or decrease the uptake of cholesterol. Once the LDL binds to its receptor, this complex is rapidly internalized in a coated pit. The coated vesicle thus formed sheds its coat and fuses with an endosome. In the endosome, the LDL receptor is retrieved and recycled to the cell surface to be used again. The LDL is transported to lysosomes and degraded to release free cholesterol, which the cell uses for synthesis of biomolecules such as steroid hormones.

Dangerously high blood cholesterol levels occur in some individuals who lack functional LDL receptors. These individuals inherit defective genes for making LDL receptor proteins and are incapable of taking up adequate amounts of LDL. Accumulation of LDL in the blood predisposes these individuals to development of **atherosclerosis** (hardened arteries) and heart disease (see Chap. 17).[30]

Exocytosis is essentially the reverse of endocytosis. Substances to be secreted from the cell are packaged in membrane-bound vesicles and travel to the inner surface of the plasma membrane. There the vesicle membrane fuses with the plasma membrane and the contents of the vesicle arrive at the cell surface. Some secreted molecules may remain embedded in the cell membrane, others may be incorporated into the extracellular matrix, and still others may enter the extracellular fluids and travel to distant sites. Many substances synthesized by the cell, including new membrane components, are continuously packaged and secreted.[31] This continuously operative and unregulated pathway is termed **constitutive.** In some specialized cells, selected proteins or small molecules are packaged in **secretory vesicles,** which remain in the cell until the cell is triggered to release them. These special secretory vesicles are typically regulated by stimulation of cell surface receptors. For example, the **mast cell,** a special type of white blood cell, releases large amounts of histamine when its cell surface receptors are activated.

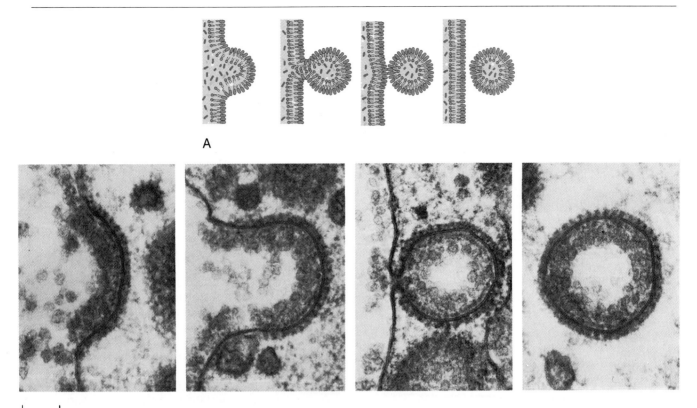

A

B

FIGURE 2-18. **A**, A representation of the steps of endocytosis. An invagination of the membrane occurs and pinches off to form a vesicle. Exocytosis progresses in essentially the reverse. **B**, Electron micrograph showing the steps of endocytosis. (**B** from Perry M, Gilbert A: Yolk transport in the ovarian follicle of the hen (*Gallus domesticus*): Lipoprotein-like particles at the periphery of the oocyte in the rapid growth phase. *J Cell Sci* 1979;39:257–272. Reproduced by permission of the Company of Biologists, Ltd.)

FIGURE 2-19. Steps in the process of receptor-mediated endocytosis of cholesterol. Cholesterol is carried in the blood by low-density lipoproteins (LDLs). The uptake of LDL with its associated cholesterol is mediated by a specific LDL receptor protein on the cell surface. Once internalized, the cholesterol is removed from the LDL-receptor complex and used by the cell. (Adapted with permission from Alberts B, et al (eds): *Molecular Biology of the Cell*, 2nd ed. New York, Garland Press, 1989, p 329.)

Membrane Transport of Small Molecules

All cells must internalize essential nutrients, excrete wastes, and regulate intracellular ion concentrations. However, the lipid bilayer is extremely impermeable to most polar and charged molecules. Transport of small water-soluble molecules is achieved by specialized transmembrane proteins called **transporter proteins**.[32] Most membrane transporters are highly specific—a different transporter protein is required for each type of molecule to be transported. Only water and nonpolar molecules can permeate the lipid bilayer directly by simple diffusion.

There are two major kinds of membrane transport proteins, **channel proteins** and **carrier proteins.** Channel proteins form a water-filled pore through the lipid bilayer. These pores are able to open and close to allow molecules (usually ions) to pass through the membrane. The particular structure of the protein channel ensures that only ions of a certain size and charge can move through. Carrier proteins, on the other hand, bind to the solute to be transported and move it through the membrane by undergoing a structural, or **conformational,** change. Carriers, which transport ions as well as nonelectrolyte molecules

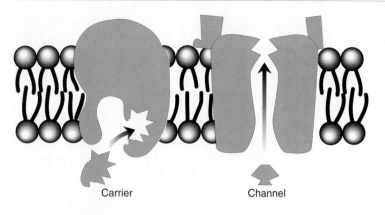

F I G U R E 2 – 20. Carrier and channel proteins in the plasma membrane are highly selective about the type of molecule allowed to pass through.

such as glucose and amino acids, are also specific (Fig. 2–20).

Figure 2–21 describes the mechanisms of solute and water movement across biological membranes. Water and lipid-soluble particles can cross the lipid bilayer directly by **osmosis** (water) or **simple diffusion.** Diffusion occurs passively due to an **electrochemical gradient.** The electrochemical gradient exists because of differences in intracellular and extracellular charge and/or concentration of chemicals. **Passive transport** does not require life and is governed by laws of physics. (See Chapter 24 for a discussion of electrolyte chemistry.) Polar or charged molecules must cross the membrane via protein channels or carriers. Transport through membrane proteins may be a passive or an active process. Passive transport through membrane proteins is called **facilitated diffusion.** All channel proteins and some carrier proteins allow particles to move down their electrochemical gradient passively by facilitated diffusion.

Active transport is the process whereby carrier proteins move or "pump" solutes across the membrane against an electrochemical gradient. Active transport requires metabolic energy, which may be supplied by ATP hydrolysis or by an ion gradient. The molecular details of carrier transport mechanisms are unknown, but carrier proteins are thought to undergo reversible conformational (shape) changes that alternately expose the solute-binding site on one side and then on the other side of the membrane (Fig. 2–22).[33]

There are a large number of membrane transporter proteins which continually function to maintain the ionic and nutrient balance within the cell. Some of the more common transporters are discussed below.

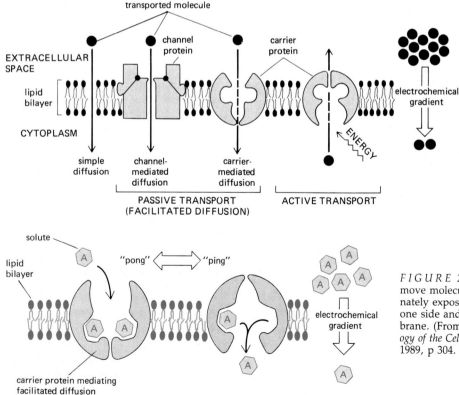

F I G U R E 2 – 21. Schematic diagram of the modes of passive and active transport across biological membranes. Passive transport occurs when molecules are allowed to move down an electrochemical gradient, whereas active transport is required to move molecules against a gradient. (From Alberts B, et al (eds): *Molecular Biology of the Cell,* 2nd ed. New York, Garland Press, 1989, p 303. Reproduced with permission.)

F I G U R E 2 – 22. Carrier proteins are thought to move molecules across the membrane by alternately exposing the solute-binding site first on one side and then on the other side of the membrane. (From Alberts B, et al (eds): *Molecular Biology of the Cell,* 2nd ed. New York, Garland Press, 1989, p 304. Reproduced with permission.)

Sodium Ion/Potassium Ion Pump

The Na$^+$/K$^+$ pump is present in the plasma membranes of virtually all animal cells. It serves to maintain low Na$^+$ and high K$^+$ concentrations within the cell.[33-35] The Na$^+$/K$^+$ transporter must pump ions against a steep electrochemical gradient. Almost one third of the energy use of a typical cell is consumed by the Na$^+$/K$^+$ pump. ATP hydrolysis provides the energy to drive the Na$^+$/K$^+$ transporter. The Na$^+$/K$^+$ pump actually behaves as an enzyme in its ability to split ATP to form adenoside diphosphate (ADP) and phosphate (P), leading to the protein being termed Na$^+$/K$^+$-ATPase.

Transport of sodium and potassium ions through the Na$^+$/K$^+$ carrier protein is **coupled:** the transfer of one ion must be accompanied by the simultaneous transport of the other ion. Actually, the transporter moves three sodium ions *out* of the cell for every two potassium ions moved *into* the cell (Fig. 2–23). The Na$^+$/K$^+$ pump is important in maintaining cell volume. It controls the solute concentration inside the cell, which in turn affects the osmotic forces across the membrane. If Na$^+$ is allowed to accumulate within the cell, the cell will swell and may burst. The role of the Na$^+$/K$^+$ pump can be demonstrated by treating cells with ouabain, a drug that inhibits Na$^+$/K$^+$-ATPase. Cells thus treated will indeed swell and often burst.

Membrane Calcium Transporters

Numerous important cellular processes such as cell contraction and growth initiation are dependent on the intracellular calcium concentration. Intracellular calcium concentration is normally very low and tightly

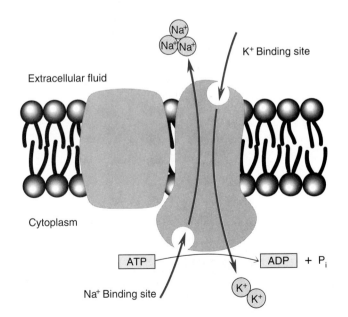

FIGURE 2–23. Schematic drawing of the sodium-potassium transport protein, which uses ATP to pump Na$^+$ out of the cell and K$^+$ into the cell against steep electrochemical gradients.

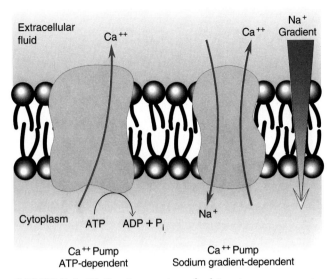

FIGURE 2–24. Two transporters of calcium ions are present in some cell membranes. One uses ATP as the energy source to pump calcium against a gradient. The other captures the potential energy of the sodium gradient to pump calcium out of the cell.

regulated. Two types of calcium pumps present in the plasma membrane function to extrude excess calcium from the cell.[36,37] Both calcium transporters are energy-requiring carrier proteins, but each utilizes a different energy source.

One of these transporters utilizes ATP as its energy source, much as the Na$^+$/K$^+$ transporter does (Fig. 2–24). The other Ca^{++} transporter utilizes an electrochemical gradient to power the transport of Ca^{++} out of the cell. In animal cells, a very steep Na$^+$ gradient exists across the cell membrane. The potential energy of this Na$^+$ gradient is used to "power" the pumping of calcium ions (Fig. 2–24). The dependence of this calcium transporter on the sodium gradient helps explain the cardiotonic effects of a commonly prescribed drug, **digitalis.** Digitalis is a cardiac glycoside that inhibits the Na$^+$/K$^+$ pump and allows the accumulation of intracellular Na$^+$. The Na$^+$ gradient across the membrane is thus decreased, leading to less efficient calcium removal by the Na$^+$-dependent Ca^{++} pump. A more forceful cardiac muscle contraction results from the increased intracellular Ca^{++}.

Other Carrier Proteins

In animal cells, the Na$^+$ gradient created by the Na$^+$/K$^+$ pump is used to power a variety of transporters in addition to the calcium pump described above (Fig. 2–25).[38-40] The **Na$^+$/H$^+$ exchange carrier** uses the Na$^+$ gradient to pump out excess hydrogen ions to help maintain intracellular pH balance. The Na$^+$ gradient also can be used to bring substances into the cell. For example, **glucose** and **amino acid** transport into epithelial cells is coupled to Na$^+$ entry. As Na$^+$ moves through the transporter, down its electrochemical gradient, the sugar or amino acid is "dragged" along.

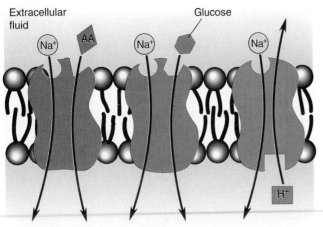

Extracellular fluid

Glucose

Na$^+$

AA

Na$^+$

Na$^+$

H$^+$

Cytoplasm

FIGURE 2-25. The sodium gradient is used by some cell types to provide the energy to transport amino acids (*AA*) and glucose and to exchange sodium ions for hydrogen ions.

Entry of the nutrient will not occur unless Na$^+$ also enters the cell. The epithelial cells that line the gut and kidney tubules have large numbers of these nutrient transporters present in the luminal (apical) surfaces of their cell membranes. In this way, large amounts of glucose and amino acids can be effectively absorbed.

Membrane Channel Proteins

In contrast to carrier proteins, which bind molecules and move them across the membrane by a conformational transformation, channel proteins form water-filled pores in the membrane. Nearly all of the channel proteins are involved in transport of ions and may be referred to as **ion channels.** Ions can flow through the appropriate channel at very high rates (10^6 ions per second); this is much faster than carrier-mediated transport.[41] However, channels are not linked to an energy source, so ions must flow passively down an electrochemical gradient. The channel proteins in the plasma membranes of animal cells are highly selective, permitting only a particular ion or class of ions to pass. Over 50 different types of ion channels have been described thus far. Ion channels are particularly important in allowing the cell to respond rapidly to a variety of external stimuli. Most channels are not continuously open, but they open and close according to membrane signals. Ion channels may be stimulated to open or close in three principal ways. **Voltage-gated** channels respond to a change in membrane potential; **mechanically gated** channels respond to mechanical deformation; and **ligand-gated** channels respond to the binding of a signaling molecule (a hormone or neurotransmitter) to a receptor on the cell surface. In addition, some channels open without apparent stimulation and are referred to as **leak channels.** Specific examples of ion channels are discussed in the next section.

Cellular Membrane Potentials

Animal cells typically have a difference in the electrical charge across their plasma membranes. There is a slight excess of negative ions along the inner aspect of the membrane and extra positive ions along the outer membrane. This separation of charges creates a **membrane potential** that can be measured as a voltage. Positive and negative ions separated by the plasma membrane have a strong attraction to each other that can be utilized by the cell to perform work, such as the transmission of nerve impulses. A relatively large membrane potential is created by the separation of a very small number of ions along the membrane (Fig. 2–26).

Resting Membrane Potential

The major determinant of the membrane potential is the potassium concentration gradient across the mem-

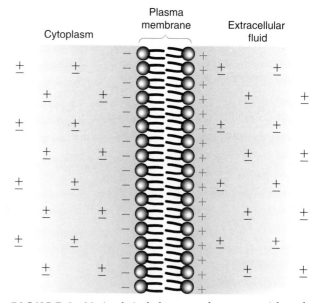

Cytoplasm

Plasma membrane

Extracellular fluid

FIGURE 2-26. A relatively large membrane potential results from the separation of a very small number of ions across the plasma membrane.

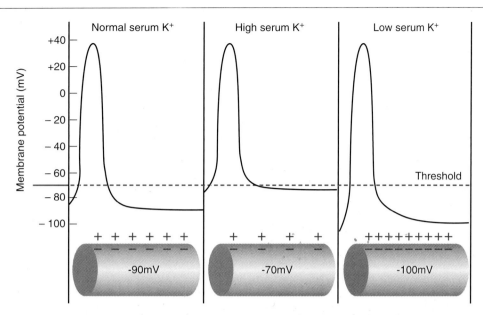

FIGURE 2–27. The effects of changes in extracellular K$^+$ on the resting membrane potential. High serum K$^+$ results in a depolarization of the membrane. Low serum K$^+$ results in membrane hyperpolarization. With high serum K$^+$, the resting membrane potential is closer to threshold, making it easier to achieve an action potential. Low serum K$^+$ moves the resting membrane potential away from threshold, making it more difficult to achieve an action potential.

brane.[42] As mentioned earlier, the concentration of potassium inside the cell is much greater (about 30 times greater) than the extracellular potassium concentration. This huge difference exists even though the cell membrane is highly permeable to potassium ions via potassium leak channels. Potassium ions remain inside the cell because of the attraction of fixed intracellular anions—negatively charged organic molecules such as proteins that cannot diffuse out of the cell. Because the cell membrane is impermeable to Na$^+$ and Ca^{++}, only K$^+$ is available to balance these negative intracellular ions. Thus, two opposing forces are acting on the potassium ion. The negative cell interior attracts K$^+$ into the cell, whereas the huge K$^+$ concentration gradient favors movement of K$^+$ out of the cell. When the cell is at rest and not transmitting impulses, these forces are balanced, and there is no net movement of potassium. The equilibrium condition is termed the **resting potential.***

Changes in extracellular K$^+$ concentration can have profound effects on the resting membrane potential. For example, a typical nerve cell has a normal resting potential of about −85 millivolts (mV). If the extracellular K$^+$ level is increased, fewer K$^+$ ions will leave the cell, owing to the reduced concentration gradient. These extra positive intracellular ions will

neutralize more of the negative cellular anions, and the cell will **depolarize,** or become less negative. Conversely, if extracellular K$^+$ levels fall, more K$^+$ will exit the cell, owing to a greater concentration gradient. Fewer intracellular anions will be neutralized, and the cell interior will become more negative, or **hyperpolarized** (Fig. 2–27).

The membrane potential is described by the potassium equilibrium potential because the cell is relatively impermeable to other ions. Under certain conditions, the membrane may become highly permeable to an ion other than potassium. The membrane potential will reflect the equilibrium potential of the most permeant ion.

Long-term maintenance of the potassium concentration gradient across the cell membrane is accomplished primarily by the Na$^+$/K$^+$ pump. The Na$^+$/K$^+$ pump also contributes to the negative resting membrane potential in that it extrudes *three* Na$^+$ for every *two* K$^+$ brought into the cell. However, this pump can be inhibited for minutes to hours in some tissues with little effect on the resting membrane potential.

Action Potential

Nearly all animal cells have negative resting membrane potentials, which may vary from −20 to −200 mV, depending on the cell type and organism. The cell membranes of some specialized cell types, mainly nerve and muscle, are capable of rapid changes in their membrane potentials. These cells are electrically "excitable" and can generate and propagate **action potentials.** Action potentials are rapid, self-propagating electrical excitations of the membrane that are me-

---

* The numerical value of the resting potential can be calculated from the ratio of K$^+$ outside the cell to K$^+$ inside the cell using the **Nernst equation:**

$$M \text{ (millivolts)} = -61 \log \frac{[\text{K}^+ \text{ outside}]}{[\text{K}^+ \text{ inside}]},$$

where M is the membrane potential and −61 is a constant derived from the gas constant, absolute temperature, Faraday's constant, ion valence, and a logarithm conversion factor.

diated by ion channels that open and close in response to changes in voltage across the membrane (**voltage-gated ion channels**).[41,43–47] An action potential is triggered by membrane depolarization.

In nerve and muscle cells, the usual trigger for depolarization is binding of a neurotransmitter to cell surface receptors. Transmitter binding causes channels or pores in the membrane to open, allowing ions (primarily Na^+) to enter the cell. This influx of positive ions results in a shift in the membrane potential to a less negative value, resulting in depolarization. **Threshold** is reached when the membrane becomes sufficiently depolarized (approximately −65 mV in animal neurons) to activate voltage-gated sodium channels in the membrane. At threshold, these channels open rapidly and transiently to allow the influx of Na^+ ions. A self-propagating process therefore occurs, whereby Na^+ influx causes membrane depolarization, which activates Na^+ channels, allowing more Na^+ to enter the cell.[48] This process repeats over and over again as the action potential proceeds along the length of the cell (Fig. 2–28). In this way, action potentials can transmit information rapidly over relatively long distances.

A typical neuronal action potential is shown in Figure 2–29. The various changes in membrane potential during the time course of the action potential are attributable to the flow of ions through membrane ion channels. The steep upstroke of the action potential corresponds to Na^+ influx through "fast" sodium channels as described above. Fast channels are so termed because they open and close rapidly—the entire process lasting less than a millisecond. This phase of rapid depolarization is terminated when the fast Na^+ channels close and the **repolarization** phase begins. Fast Na^+ channels are interesting in that they can assume at least three conformations (forms).[49] In addition to the open and closed conformations, the fast Na^+ channel has a **refractory** form during which the channel will not open again in response to another depolarizing stimulus (Fig. 2–30).

Two major factors contribute to cellular repolarization: sodium conductance (inflow) is stopped by closing Na^+ channels, as described above, and K^+ conductance (outflow) through voltage-gated K^+ channels increases. These K^+ channels respond to depolarization of the membrane in the same manner as fast Na^+ channels, but they take much longer to open and close. When K^+ channels open, K^+ will flow out of the cell, owing to the concentration gradient and the loss of intracellular negativity that accompanies Na^+ influx. The loss of positive intracellular potassium ions returns the membrane potential to a negative value.

Action potentials in muscle cells are more complex than the neuronal ones just described. Recall that muscle contraction depends on the presence of intracellular calcium ions. Since Ca^{++} carries a charge, its entry into the cell will be reflected in the membrane potential. In skeletal muscle, most of the free cytosolic calcium comes from intracellular stores (sarcoplasmic reticulum) that are released when the cell is depolarized. In cardiac muscle cells, Ca^{++} entry through voltage-gated channels in the plasma membrane is also important. Calcium conductance into the cell tends to prolong the action potential, resulting in a **plateau phase** (Fig. 2–31).[50] This is of functional importance in cardiac tissue, as it allows time for muscular contraction before another impulse is conducted and prevents the potentially disastrous condition of cardiac muscle tetany. (For a thorough discussion of cardiac electrophysiology, see Chapter 16.)

Intercellular Communication and Growth

Cell Signaling Strategies

Cells in multicellular organisms need to communicate with one another and respond to changes in the cellular environment. Coordination of growth, cell division, and the functions of various tissues and organ systems is accomplished by three principal means: (1) through gap junctions that directly connect the cytoplasm of adjoining cells, (2) by direct cell-to-cell contact of plasma membranes or the extracellular molecules associated with the cell (extracellular matrix), and (3) by secretion of chemical mediators that influence cells some distance away (Fig. 2–32).[51]

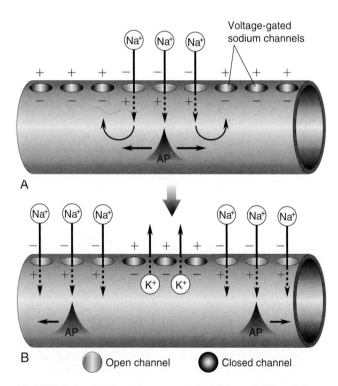

FIGURE 2–28. The action potential (*AP*) in excitable cells is propagated along the membrane by the sequential opening of voltage-gated sodium channels in adjacent sections of membrane. **A,** An action potential is initiated by the opening of sodium channels in a section of membrane. **B,** The action potential is regenerated in adjacent sections of membrane as more sodium channels open. The initial segment repolarizes as sodium channels close and potassium ions move out of the cell.

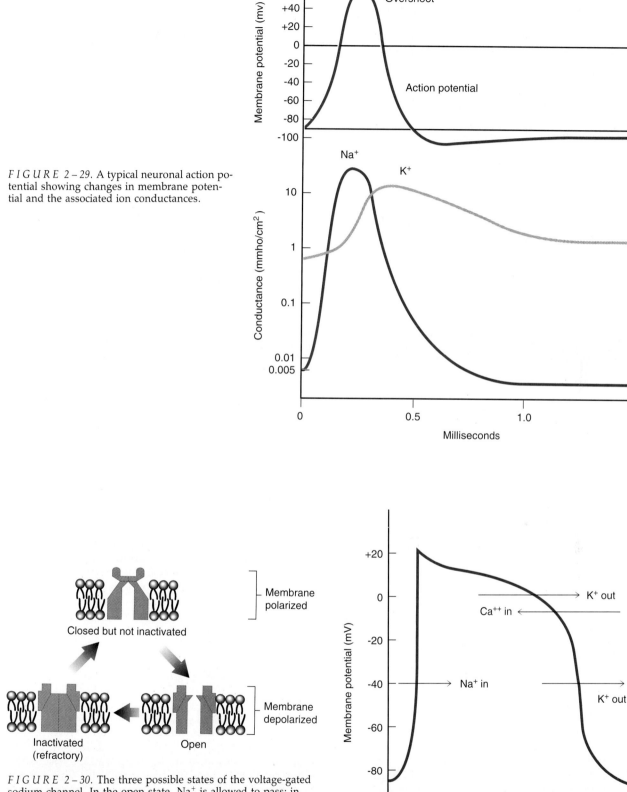

FIGURE 2–29. A typical neuronal action potential showing changes in membrane potential and the associated ion conductances.

FIGURE 2–30. The three possible states of the voltage-gated sodium channel. In the open state, Na$^+$ is allowed to pass; in the inactivated state the channel is closed and refractory and will not open in response to a depolarizing stimulus. In the closed state the channel will open in response to a membrane depolarization. (Adapted with permission from Alberts B, et al (eds): *Molecular Biology of the Cell*, 2nd ed. New York, Garland Press, 1989, p 317.)

FIGURE 2–31. A typical cardiac muscle cell action potential showing the ion fluxes associated with each phase.

REMOTE SIGNALING BY SECRETED MOLECULES

CONTACT SIGNALING BY PLASMA-MEMBRANE-BOUND MOLECULES

CONTACT SIGNALING VIA GAP JUNCTIONS

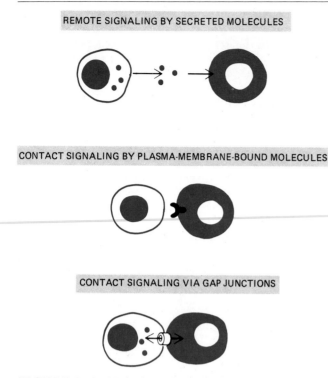

F I G U R E   2 – 3 2. Methods used for intercellular communication. (From Alberts B, et al (eds): *Molecular Biology of the Cell*, 2nd ed. New York, Garland Press, 1989, p 681. Reproduced with permission.)

Gap junctions are found in large numbers in most tissues. They are connecting channels between adjacent cells that allow the passage of small molecules from one cell to the next. These junctions are formed by special transmembrane proteins that associate to form pores of about 1.5 nanometers (nm) width. Small molecules such as inorganic ions, sugars, amino acids, nucleotides, and vitamins may pass through the pores, whereas macromolecules (proteins, polysaccharides, and nucleic acids) are too large to pass through. Gap junctions are particularly important in tissues where synchronized functions are required, such as cardiac muscle contraction and intestinal peristaltic movements. Gap junctions appear to be important in embryogenesis as well. Cellular differentiation may be mediated in part through chemical signaling through gap junctions. (See Chapter 4 for a discussion of the development and differentiation of tissue types.)

Signaling by **direct contact of cell membranes** is poorly understood at present. Signaling molecules present on the cell surface are thought to influence other cells that come into contact with them. Glycolipids and glycoproteins may be such signaling molecules. Contact-dependent signaling appears to be important for the development of the immune response. Such cell-to-cell contact during fetal development is thought to allow the cells of the immune system to discriminate between foreign and self tissues and develop self-tolerance.[52] If cell-to-cell contact does not occur during fetal life, the immune cells may later attack the body's own cells, leading to the develop-

ment of autoimmune diseases. (See Chapter 10 for a discussion of autoimmunity.)

The best understood form of cell communication is signaling through **secreted molecules or ligands.** Three strategies of chemical signaling have been described, relating to the distances over which they operate. **Synaptic signaling** is confined to the cells of the nervous system and occurs at specialized junctions between the nerve cell and its target cell. The neuron secretes a chemical neurotransmitter into the space between the nerve and target cell; the neurotransmitter then diffuses across and binds receptors on the postsynaptic cell. Synaptic signaling occurs over very small distances (50 nm) and involves only one or a few postsynaptic target cells. In **paracrine signaling,** chemicals are secreted into a localized area and are rapidly destroyed, so that only cells in the immediate area are affected. Growth factors, for example, act locally to promote wound healing without affecting the growth of the entire organism. **Endocrine signaling** is accomplished by specialized endocrine cells that secrete **hormones** that travel via the bloodstream to target cells widely distributed throughout the body. Endocrine signaling is slow in comparison to nervous signaling because it relies on diffusion and blood flow to target tissues. **Autocrine signaling** occurs when cells are able to respond to signaling molecules that they secrete. Autocrine stimulation is thought to be a mechanism in some forms of cancer (see Chap. 6).

Target cells respond to all three methods of ligand signaling through specific protein **receptors** (see further discussion below). Cells can respond to a particular ligand only if they possess the appropriate receptor. For example, all cells of the body are exposed to thyroid-stimulating hormone (TSH) as it circulates in the blood, but only thyroid cells will respond because they alone possess TSH receptors. On the other hand, cells that possess the same receptor may respond very differently to a particular ligand. Binding of acetylcholine to its receptor on a glandular cell, for example, may induce secretion, while binding to the same receptor on a cardiac muscle cell will decrease contractile force. The cellular response to signaling molecules is regulated not only by the array of receptors the cell carries, but also by the internal machinery to which the receptors are linked.

Cell Surface Receptor–Mediated Responses

Most hormones, local chemical mediators, and neurotransmitters are water-soluble molecules and are unable to pass through the lipid bilayer of the cell. These ligands exert their effects through binding with a receptor on the surface of the target cell, which then changes or transduces the external signal into an intracellular message. There are at least three classes of cell surface receptor proteins: channel linked, catalytic, and G-protein linked.[53–55]

Channel-linked receptors bind neurotransmitters, causing specific ion channels in the membrane to open or close. This type of signaling is prevalent in the nervous system, where rapid synaptic signaling between neurons is required. **Catalytic receptors** behave as enzymes when they are activated by appropriate ligands. Nearly all catalytic receptors function as **protein kinases;** that is, they mediate the transfer of phosphate groups from ATP (or GTP) to proteins and thus affect the activity of those proteins. The insulin receptor is an example of a catalytic protein kinase receptor; it transfers phosphate groups from ATP to particular intracellular proteins. Many receptors are **G-protein linked.** G-protein-linked receptors act indirectly through a membrane protein "middleman" that binds and hydrolyzes GTP. The activated G-protein then activates other enzymes or ion channels within the membrane (Fig. 2–33). The end result of most ligand-receptor interactions is the generation of one or more intracellular mediators, or **second messengers.**

Two common second messengers are **cyclic AMP (cAMP)** and **Ca^{++}**.[56–60] Cyclic AMP is formed from ATP when the enzyme **adenylate cyclase,** located in the plasma membrane, is activated. Similarly, Ca^{++} is a universal intracellular signal. Ca^{++} enters the intracellular solution or cytosol in two principal ways: (1) by influx through open membrane channels and (2) by release from intracellular compartments. Both cAMP and Ca^{++} lead to changes in cellular behavior. For example, cAMP causes glycogen breakdown in liver cells, increases contractile force in heart muscle, and stimulates secretion in glands. Calcium regulates muscle contraction, cell growth, and exocytosis of vesicles. Cells respond differently to the same second messengers because of differences in the particular set of enzymes and molecules present within the cell.

Intracellular Receptor–Mediated Responses

A small number of hormones are lipid soluble and can pass directly through the cell membrane to inter-act with receptors *inside* the cell.[61] These receptors are usually located in the cell cytosol or may be associated with the cell nucleus. Intracellular receptors are specific for a particular ligand, just as surface receptors are. Binding of the ligand causes the receptor to become activated. The activated receptor then travels to the nucleus, where it binds with specific genes and regulates their activity. Since lipid-soluble ligands enter the cell directly, no second messengers are needed. **Steroid** and **thyroid** hormones are members of this class of signaling molecules. **Aldosterone** is an example of a steroid hormone that binds intracellular receptors and affects kidney tubule cells by increasing their production of Na$^+$/K$^+$ transporter proteins.

Regulation of Cellular Growth by Extracellular Ligands

In multicellular organisms such as humans, the growth of cells and tissues must be strictly controlled to maintain a balance between cell birth rate and cell death rate. The system must be able to rapidly increase growth of a particular tissue to replace cells lost to injury and normal wear and tear while simultaneously inhibiting unwanted growth of other cells. Special intracellular communication systems function to regulate the replication of individual cells in the body. The details of these mechanisms remain sketchy at present, but two important strategies of growth control have been described. First, a variety of **protein growth factors** are required in specific combinations for growth of particular cell types.[62] Second, cells respond to **spatial signals** that indicate how much room is available for growth.[63]

In order to respond to a particular growth factor, a cell must have the corresponding growth factor receptor on its cell surface. Many cells in the body synthesize and secrete growth factors, which then influence the growth of other cell types in a paracrine or endocrine fashion. **Platelet-derived growth factor (PDGF)** was one of the first growth factors to be discovered. It is secreted by platelets when they form blood clots in response to an injury.[64] PDGF stimulates fibroblasts and smooth muscle cells in the damaged area to divide and replace cells lost to the injury. Currently, about 30 different protein growth factors have been identified. A general rule of growth factor regulation is that a particular cell type does not secrete growth factors for which it has complementary receptors. This would allow the cell to stimulate its own growth and release it from the control systems of the rest of the body. Some types of cancer cells may operate in this way (see Chap. 6).

The shape of a cell as it spreads over its immediate space also appears to be important in the control of cell division. Surrounding cells and the extracellular scaffold or **matrix** provide the cell with information about the need for more cells. The more spread out the cell becomes, the more likely it is to grow and divide.

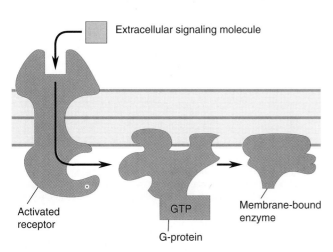

Extracellular signaling molecule

Activated receptor

GTP

G-protein

Membrane-bound enzyme

F I G U R E 2 – 33. Schematic of the proposed role of guanosine triphosphate *(GTP)*-binding proteins in the transduction of extracellular signaling messages.

KEY CONCEPTS

- The resting membrane potential (RMP) is negative in all cells. The ratio of intracellular to extracellular K^+ determines how negative the RMP is. Changes in serum K^+ can have profound effects on the RMP.
- Cells with voltage-gated ion channels are excitable and can produce and conduct action potentials. An action potential results from the opening of "fast" Na^+ channels, which allows Na^+ to rush into the cell.
- Repolarization is due to closure of Na^+ channels and efflux of K^+ from the cell. In cardiac muscle, repolarization is prolonged, owing to Ca^{++} influx through "slow" Ca^{++} channels.
- Intercellular communication is accomplished by three principal means: (1) gap junctions, which directly connect the cytoplasm of adjoining cells; (2) direct cell-to-cell surface contact; and (3) secretion of chemical mediators (ligands).
- Binding of a ligand to a cell surface receptor usually results in the production of second messengers (Ca^{++}, cAMP) within the target cell.

Summary

Detailed knowledge of cell physiology is essential to understanding disease processes. Cells are complex, membrane-bound units that perform a variety of functions necessary to the maintenance of life. The major cell components and their functions are summarized in Table 2–1. The cell membrane is an important cellular structure that protects the cell interior and mediates information transfer to and from the extracellular environment. Proteins embedded in the membrane lipid bilayer perform most of the membrane functions, including transduction of extracellular messages, membrane transport, electrical excitation, and cell-to-cell communication. Human and animal cells also have several important intracellular organelles. These include the cytoskeleton, which organizes the intracellular compartment; the nucleus, which holds the cell's genetic material and directs the day-to-day activities of the cell; the endoplasmic reticulum and the Golgi apparatus, which produce, package, and transport proteins and lipids to the plasma membrane and lysosomes; the lysosomes and peroxisomes, which perform the task of intracellular digestion of organic waste; and the mitochondria, which produce cellular energy in the form of ATP. The energy released by ATP hydrolysis is used by the cell to drive the many energetically unfavorable reactions necessary to maintain cellular functions.

TABLE 2–1. Structure and Function of Major Cellular Components

Cellular Structure	Functions
Plasma membrane	Protective barrier, separates life from nonlife
	Extracellular message transduction
	Transport of materials into and out of the cell
	Maintenance and transmission of membrane potentials
	Cell-to-cell recognition, interaction
Cytoskeleton	Maintenance of cell shape
	Cell movement
	Trafficking within the cell
Nucleus	Protection of genetic material
	Regulation of cell type and function through control of protein synthesis
Endoplasmic reticulum	Protein and lipid synthesis
	Lipid metabolism and detoxification
Golgi apparatus	Protein and lipid modification and sorting
	Transport of proteins and lipids to appropriate destinations
Lysosomes	Hydrolytic breakdown of organic waste
Peroxisomes	Oxidative breakdown of organic waste
Mitochondria	Cellular energy production (ATP)

REFERENCES

1. Ferris JP, Usher DA: Origins of life, in Zubay G (ed): *Biochemistry*, 3rd ed. Dubuque, IA, William C Brown Communications, 1993, pp 1120–1151.
2. Miller SM, Orgel LE: *The Origins of Life on the Earth.* Englewood Cliffs, NJ, Prentice Hall, 1974, pp 219–223.
3. Schopf JW, Hayes JM, Walter MR: Evolution of earth's earliest ecosystems: Recent progress and unsolved problems, in Schopf JW (ed): *Earth's Earliest Biosphere: Its Origin and Evolution.* Princeton, Princeton University Press, 1983, pp 361–384.
4. Vidal G: The oldest eukaryotic cells. *Sci Am* 1984;250(2):48–57.
5. Singer SJ, Nicolson GL: The fluid mosaic model of the structure of cell membranes. *Science* 1972;175:720–731.
6. Storch J, Kleinfeld AM: The lipid structure of biological membranes. *Trends Biochem Sci* 1982;10:418–421.
7. Edidin M: Rotational and lateral diffusion of membrane proteins and lipids: Phenomena and functions. *Curr Top Membr Transport* 1987;29:91–127.
8. Chapman D: Lipid dynamics in cell membranes, in Weissmann G, Claiborne R (eds): *Cell Membranes: Biochemistry, Cell Biology and Pathology.* New York, HP Publishing Co, 1975, pp 18–22.
9. Chapman D, Benga G: Biomembrane fluidity—studies of model and natural membranes, in Chapman D (ed): *Biological Membrane Series.* London, Academic Press, vol 5, 1985, pp 1–56.
10. McElhaney RN: The concept of fluidity in lipid bilayers, in Kates M, Manson LA (eds): *Biomembranes.* New York, Plenum Press, 1984, vol 12, p 250.
11. Carruthers A, Melchoir DL: How bilayer lipids affect membrane protein activity. *Trends Biochem Sci* 1986;11:331–335.
12. deKruif B, et al: Lipid polymorphism and membrane function, in Martonosi AN (ed): *The Enzymes of Biological Membranes*, 2nd ed. New York, Plenum Press, 1985, vol 1: *Membrane Structure and Dynamics*, pp 131–204.
13. Hakomori S: Glycosphingolipids. *Sci Am* 1986;254(5):44–53.
14. Unwin N, Henderson R: The structure of proteins in biological membranes. *Sci Am* 1984;250(2):78–94.
15. Shen BW, Josephs R, Steck TL: Ultrastructure of the intact skeleton of the human erythrocyte membrane. *J Cell Biol* 1986;102:997–1006.
16. Simons K, Fuller SD: Cell surface polarity in epithelia. *Annu Rev Cell Biol* 1985;1:243–288.
17. Alberts B, Bray D, Lewis J, Raff M, Roberts K, Watson J: The cytoskeleton, in Alberts B, Bray D, Lewis J, Raff M, Roberts K, Watson J (eds): *Molecular Biology of the Cell*, 2nd ed. New York, Garland Press, 1989, pp 613–676.
18. Alberts B, Bray D, Lewis J, Raff M, Roberts K, Watson J: The cell nucleus, in Alberts B, Bray D, Lewis J, Raff M, Roberts K,

Watson J (eds): *Molecular Biology of the Cell,* 2nd ed. New York, Garland Press, 1989, pp 481–546.
19. Alberts B, Bray D, Lewis J, Raff M, Roberts K, Watson J: Intracellular sorting and the maintenance of cellular compartments, in Alberts B, Bray D, Lewis J, Raff M, Roberts K, Waton J (eds): *Molecular Biology of the Cell,* 2nd ed. New York, Garland Press, 1989, pp. 405–479.
20. Mayer RJ, Doherty F: Intracellular protein catabolism: State of the art. *FEBS Lett* 1986;198:181–193.
21. Helenius A, Mellman I, Wall D, Hubbard A: Endosomes. *Trends Biochem Sci* 1983;8:245–250.
22. Kornfeld S: Trafficking of lysosomal enzymes in normal and disease states. *J Clin Invest* 1986;77:1–6.
23. Alberts B, Bray D, Lewis J, Raff M, Roberts K, Watson J: Small molecules, energy and biosynthesis, in Alberts B, Bray D, Lewis J, Raff M, Roberts K, Watson J (eds): *Molecular Biology of the Cell,* 2nd ed. New York, Garland Press, 1989, pp 41–58.
24. Krebs HA: The history of the tricarboxylic acid cycle. *Perspect Biol Med* 1970;14:154–170.
25. Hatefi Y: The mitochondrial electron transport and oxidative phosphorylation system. *Annu Rev Biochem* 1985;54:1015–1070.
26. Mitchell P: Coupling of phosphorylation to electron and hydrogen transfer by a chemi-osmotic type of mechanism. *Nature* 1961;191:144–148.
27. Steinman RM, Mellman IF, Muller WA, Cohn ZA: Endocytosis and recycling of plasma membrane. *J Cell Biol* 1983;96:1–27.
28. Goldstein JL, Anderson RGW, Brown MS: Coated pits, coated vesicles and receptor-mediated endocytosis. *Nature* 1979;279:679–685.
29. Brown MS, Goldstein JL: A receptor-mediated pathway for cholesterol homeostasis. *Science* 1986;232:34–48.
30. Brown MS, Goldstein JL: How LDL receptors influence cholesterol and atherosclerosis. *Sci Am* 1984;251(5):58–66.
31. Burgess TL, Kelly RB: Constitutive and regulated secretion of proteins. *Annu Rev Cell Biol* 1987;3:243–294.
32. Stein WD: *Transport and Diffusion Across Cell Membranes.* Orlando, Academic Press, 1986, p 35.
33. Stein WD: *Channels, Carriers and Pumps: An Introduction to Membrane Transport.* New York, Harcourt Brace Jovanovich, 1990, p 263.
34. Cantley LC: Structure and mechanisms of the (Na, K) ATPase. *Curr Top Bioenerg* 1981;11:201–237.
35. Sweadner KJ, Goldin SM: Active transport of sodium and potassium ions: Mechanism, function and regulation. *N Engl J Med* 1980;302:777–783.
36. Hasselbach W, Oetliker H: Energetics and electrogenicity of the sarcoplasmic reticulum calcium pump. *Annu Rev Physiol* 1983;45:325–339.
37. Schatzman HJ: The red cell calcium pump. *Annu Rev Physiol* 1983;45:303–312.
38. Scott DM: Sodium cotransport systems: Cellular, molecular and regulatory aspects. *Bioessays* 1987;7:71–78.
39. Wright JK, Seckler R, Overath P: Molecular aspects of sugar: Ion transport. *Annu Rev Biochem* 1986;55:225–248.
40. Grinstein S, Rothstein A: Mechanisms of regulation of the Na$^+$/H$^+$ exchanger. *J Membr Biol* 1986;90:1–12.
41. Hille B: *Ionic Channels of Excitable Membranes,* 2nd ed. Sunderland, MA, Sinauer Associates, 1992, pp 329–351.
42. Kutchai HC: Ionic equilibria and resting membrane potentials, in Berne RM, Levy MN (eds): *Principles of Physiology.* St. Louis, CV Mosby, 1990, p 23.
43. Hodgkin AL: *The Conduction of the Nervous Impulse.* Liverpool, England, Liverpool University Press, 1971.
44. Baker PF, Hodgkin AL, Shaw T: The effects of changes in internal ionic concentrations of the electrical properties of perfused giant axons. *J Physiol* 1962;164:355–374.
45. Hodgkin AL, Huxley AF: Currents carried by sodium and potassium ions through the membrane of the giant axon of Loligo. *J Physiol* 1952;116:449–472.
46. Hodgkin AL, Huxley AF, Katz B: Measurement of current-voltage relations in the membrane of the giant axon of Loligo. *J Physiol* 1952;116:424–448.
47. Hodgkin AL, Katz B: The effect of sodium ions on the electrical activity of the giant axon of the squid. *J Physiol* 1949;108:37–77.
48. Hodgkin AL, Huxley AF: A quantitative description of membrane current and its application to conduction and excitation in nerve. *J Physiol* 1952;117:500–544.
49. Catterall WA: Molecular properties of voltage-sensitive sodium channels. *Annu Rev Biochem* 1986;55:953–985.
50. Kutchai HC: Generation and conduction of action potentials, in Berne RM, Levy MN (eds): *Principles of Physiology.* St. Louis, CV Mosby, 1990, p 34.
51. Alberts B, Bray D, Lewis J, Raff M, Roberts K, Watson J: Cell signaling, in Alberts B, Bray D, Lewis J, Raff M, Roberts K, Watson J (eds): *Molecular Biology of the Cell,* 2nd ed. New York, Garland Press, 1989, p 681.
52. Nossal GJV: Cellular mechanisms of immunologic tolerance. *Annu Rev Immunol* 1983;1:33–62.
53. Kahn CR: Membrane receptors for hormones and neurotransmitters. *J Cell Biol* 1976;70:261–286.
54. Snyder SH: The molecular basis of communication between cells. *Sci Am* 1985;253(4):132–140.
55. Gilman AG: G proteins: Transducers of receptor-generated signals. *Annu Rev Biochem* 1987;56:615–649.
56. Schramm M, Selinger Z: Message transmission: Receptor controlled adenylate cyclase system. *Science* 1984;225:1350–1356.
57. Casperson GF, Bourne HR: Biochemical and molecular genetic analysis of hormone-sensitive adenylate cyclase. *Annu Rev Pharmacol Toxicol* 1987;27:371–384.
58. Rodbell M: The role of hormone receptors and GTP-regulatory proteins in membrane transduction. *Nature* 1980;284:17–22.
59. Levitzki A: From epinephrine to cyclic AMP. *Science* 1988;241:800–806.
60. Carafoli E: Intracellular calcium homeostasis. *Annu Rev Biochem* 1987;56:395–433.
61. Alberts B, Bray D, Lewis J, Raff M, Roberts K, Watson J: Cell signaling, in Alberts B, Bray D, Lewis J, Raff M, Roberts K, Watson J (eds): *Molecular Biology of the Cell,* 2nd ed. New York, Garland Press, 1989, p 690.
62. Deuel TF: Polypeptide growth factors: Roles in normal and abnormal growth. *Annu Rev Cell Biol* 1987;3:443–492.
63. Folkman J, Moscona A: Role of cell shape in growth control. *Nature* 1978;273:345–349.
64. Ross R, Raines EW, Bowen-Pope DF: The biology of platelet-derived growth factor. *Cell* 1986;46:155–169.

BIBLIOGRAPHY

Aidley DJ: *The Physiology of Excitable Cells,* 3rd ed. Cambridge, Cambridge University Press, 1989.
Alberts B, Bray D, Lewis J, Raff M, Roberts K, Watson J: *Molecular Biology of the Cell,* 2nd ed. New York, Garland Press, 1989.
Badwey JA: Transmembrane signaling, then and now: The decade of the eighties. *J Bioenerg Biomembr* 1991;23(1):1–5.
Berne RM, Levy MN: *Principles of Physiology.* St. Louis, CV Mosby, 1990.
Bergethon PR, Simons ER: *Biophysical Chemistry: Molecules to Membranes.* New York, Springer-Verlag, 1990.
Beyenbach KW: *Cell Volume Regulation.* New York, S Karger, 1990.
Ciba Foundation: *Interactions Among Cell Signaling Systems.* New York, John Wiley & Sons, 1992.
Fiskum G: *Cell Calcium Metabolism: Physiology, Biochemistry, Pharmacology, and Clinical Implications.* New York, Plenum Press, 1989.
Freier S: *The Neuroendocrine-immune Network.* Boca Raton, CRC Press, 1990.
Gayford C: *Energy and Cells.* Hampshire, England, Macmillan, 1986.
Gordon JL: *Vascular Endothelium: Interactions With Circulating Cells.* Amsterdam, Elsevier, 1991.
Hardie DG: *Biochemical Messengers: Hormones, Neurotransmitters, and Growth Factors.* London, Chapman & Hall, 1991.
Hille B: *Ionic Channels of Excitable Membranes,* 2nd ed. Sunderland, MA, Sinauer Associates, 1992.
Jou D, Llebot JE: *Introduction to the Thermodynamics of Biological Processes.* Englewood Cliffs, NJ, Prentice Hall, 1990.
Kemp BE: *Peptides and Protein Phosphorylation.* Boca Raton, CRC Press, 1990.
Koretsky AP: Investigation of cell physiology in the animal using transgenic technology. *Am J Physiol* 1992;262(2 pt 1):C261–C275.

Latorre R, Bacigalupo J, Delgado R, Labarca P: Four cases of direct ion channel gating by cyclic nucleotides. *J Bioenerg Biomembr* 1991;23(4):577–597.

Montgomery R, Conway TW, Spector AA: *Biochemistry: A Case-Oriented Approach*, 5th ed. St. Louis, CV Mosby, 1990.

Nahorski SR: *Transmembrane Signaling, Intracellular Messengers, and Implications for Drug Development*. New York, John Wiley & Sons, 1990.

Stein WD: *Channels, Carriers and Pumps: An Introduction to Membrane Transport*. New York, Harcourt Brace Jovanovich, 1990.

Tsien RY: Intracellular signal transduction in four dimensions: From molecular design to physiology. *Am J Physiol* 1992;263(4 pt 1):C723–C728.

Wong PY-K, Serhan CN: *Cell-Cell Interactions in the Release of Inflammatory Mediators: Eicosanoids, Cytokines, and Adhesion*. New York, Plenum Press, 1991.

Zubay G: *Biochemistry*, 3rd ed. Dubuque, IA, William C Brown Communications, 1993.

CHAPTER 3
Cell Injury, Aging, and Death

JACQUELYN L. BANASIK

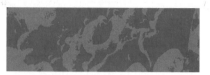

KEY TERMS

atrophy: Cellular shrinkage and reduction of function.

endotoxin: Toxin contained in the cell walls of some bacteria that is released with bacterial cell lysis.

exotoxin: Toxin secreted by bacterial cells.

free radical: An excessively reactive compound that avidly makes molecular bonds with other compounds.

gangrene: Cellular death involving a large area of tissue; may be characterized as wet, dry, or gas gangrene.

hypertrophy: Increased cell mass accompanied by augmented functional capacity.

ischemia: Insufficient blood flow to tissues, resulting in inadequate delivery of oxygen.

mutation: A permanent change in genetic material that may be transmitted to daughter cells during cell division.

necrosis: Death and degradation of body cells or tissues.

rigor mortis: Stiffened muscles throughout the body after death due to formation of permanent actin-myosin crossbridges.

D isease and injury are cellular phenomena. While pathophysiology is often presented in terms of systemic effects and manifestations, ultimately it is the *cells* that make up these systems that are affected. Even complex multisystem disorders such as cancer are due to alterations in cell function. Increasingly, the mysterious mechanisms of diseases are being understood on the cellular and molecular level, allowing better methods of treatment and prevention. This chapter presents the general characteristics of cellular injury, adaptation, aging, and death that underlie the discussions of system pathophysiology in later chapters of this text.

Cells are confronted by many challenges to their integrity and survival and have efficient mechanisms for coping with an altered cellular environment. Cells respond to environmental changes or injury in three general ways: (1) If the change is mild or short-lived, the cell may withstand the assault and completely return to normal. This is called a **reversible cell injury.** (2) The cell may adapt to a persistent but sublethal injury by changing its structure or function. Generally, **adaptation** also is reversible. (3) **Cell death** may occur if the injury is too severe or prolonged. Cell death is irreversible. At present it is not possible to determine the exact point at which a reversible injury becomes irreversible.

Reversible Cell Injury

Regardless of the cause, reversible injuries and the early stages of irreversible injuries often result in cellular swelling and the accumulation of excess substances within the cell. These changes reflect the cell's inability to perform normal metabolic functions, owing to insufficient cellular energy in the form of adenosine triphosphate (ATP) or dysfunction of associated metabolic enzymes. Once the acute stress or injury has been removed, by definition of a reversible injury, the cell returns to its preinjury state.

Hydropic Swelling

Cellular swelling due to accumulation of water, or **hydropic swelling,** is the most common manifestation of reversible cell injury.[1] Hydropic swelling results from malfunction of the sodium/potassium (Na^+/K^+) pumps that normally maintain ionic equilibrium of the cell. Failure of the Na^+/K^+ pump results in accumulation of sodium ions within the cell, creating an osmotic gradient for water entry. Since Na^+/K^+ pump function is dependent on cellular ATP, any injury that results in insufficient energy production will result in hydropic swelling (Fig. 3–1).[2] Hydropic swelling is characterized by a large, pale cytoplasm, dilated endoplasmic reticulum, and swollen mitochondria. With severe hydropic swelling, the endoplasmic reticulum may rupture and form large water-filled vacuoles. Generalized swelling in the cells of a particular organ will cause the organ to increase in size and weight.

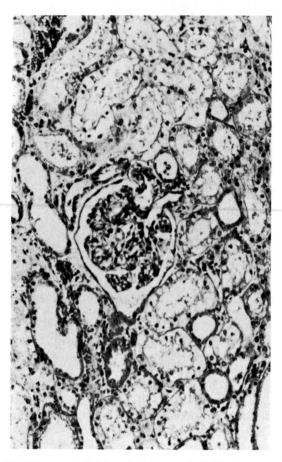

FIGURE 3–1. Cellular morphology typical of hydropic swelling. (From Cotran RS, Kumar V, Robbins SL (eds): *Robbins Pathologic Basis of Disease,* 4th ed. Philadelphia, WB Saunders, 1989, p 16. Reproduced with permission.)

Organ enlargement is indicated by the suffix *-megaly.* An enlarged spleen is splenomegaly, an enlarged liver is hepatomegaly, and so on.

Cellular Accumulations

Excess accumulations of substances within cells may result in cellular injury because the substances are toxic or provoke an immune response, or merely because they occupy space necessary for cellular functions. In some cases, accumulations do not in themselves appear to be injurious, but rather are indicators of cell injury. Intracellular accumulations may be categorized as (1) excessive amounts of normal intracellular substances such as fat, (2) accumulation of abnormal substances produced by the cell because of faulty metabolism, and (3) accumulation of pigments and particles that the cell is unable to degrade.

Normal intracellular substances that tend to accumulate in injured cells include lipids, carbohydrates, glycogen, and proteins. Faulty metabolism of these substances within the cell results in excessive intracellular storage. In some cases, the enzymes necessary for breaking down a particular substance are absent or abnormal as a result of a genetic defect. In other cases, altered metabolism may be due to excessive intake, toxins, or other disease processes.

A common site of intracellular lipid accumulation is the liver, where many fats are normally stored, metabolized, and synthesized. **Fatty liver** is often associated with excessive intake of alcohol.[3] The mechanism whereby alcohol causes fatty liver remains unclear, but it is thought to result from direct toxic effects as well as the preferential metabolism of alcohol instead of lipid. Lipids may also accumulate in blood vessels, kidney, heart, and other organs. Fat-filled cells tend to compress cellular components to one side and cause the tissue to appear yellowish and greasy (Fig. 3–2). There are several genetic disorders in which the enzymes necessary to metabolize lipids are impaired. These include Tay-Sachs disease and Gaucher's disease, in which lipids accumulate in neurologic tissue.

Glycosaminoglycans (mucopolysaccharides) are large carbohydrate complexes that normally make up the extracellular matrix of connective tissues. Connective tissue cells secrete most of the glycosaminoglycans into the extracellular space, but a small portion remains inside the cell and is degraded by lysosomal enzymes. The **mucopolysaccharidoses** are a group of genetic diseases in which the enzymatic degradation of these molecules is impaired and they collect within the cell. Mental retardation and connective tissue disorders are common.

Like other disorders of accumulation, excessive **glycogen storage** can be due to inborn errors of metabolism, but the most common cause is diabetes mellitus.[2,4] Diabetes mellitus is associated with impaired cellular uptake of glucose, which results in high serum and urine glucose levels. Cells of the renal tubules reabsorb the excess filtered glucose and store it intracellularly as glycogen. The renal tubule cells are also a common site for abnormal accumulations of **proteins.**

Normally, very little protein escapes the bloodstream into the urine. However, with certain disorders, renal capillaries become leaky and allow proteins to filter through. Renal tubule cells recapture the escaped proteins through the process of endocytosis.

In some cases, the accumulated substances cannot be metabolized by normal intracellular enzymes. In diabetes, for instance, high serum glucose levels result in excessive glucose uptake by neuronal cells. Neurons possess an enzyme that converts the glucose to sorbitol.[5] The sorbitol cannot be metabolized by normal glycolytic enzymes and thus accumulates in the cell. Excessive neuronal sorbitol is believed to interfere with nerve impulse conduction and contribute to altered sensation in the person with diabetes.

Finally, a variety of **pigments** and **inorganic particles** may be present in cells. Some pigment accumulations are normal, such as the accumulation of **melanin** in tanned skin, while others signify pathophysiologic processes. Pigments may be produced by the body (endogenous) or may be introduced from outside sources (exogenous). In addition to melanin, the iron-containing substances hemosiderin and bilirubin are endogenous pigments that indicate disease processes when present in excessive amounts. **Hemosiderin** and **bilirubin** are pigments derived from hemoglobin. Excessive amounts may indicate abnormal breakdown of hemoglobin-containing red blood cells (RBCs), prolonged iron administration, and hepatobiliary disorders. Inorganic particles that may accumulate include calcium, tar, and mineral dusts such as coal, silica, iron, lead, and silver. Mineral dusts are generally inhaled and accumulate in lung tissue (Fig. 3–3). Inhaled dusts cause chronic inflammatory reactions in the lung, which generally result in destruction of pulmonary alveoli and capillaries and the formation of scar tissue. Over many years the lung may become stiff and difficult to expand because of extensive scarring.

Deposits of calcium salts occur in conditions of altered calcium intake, excretion, and metabolism. Impaired renal excretion of phosphate may result in the formation of calcium-phosphate salts that are deposited in the tissues of the eye, heart, and blood vessels. Calcification of the heart valves may cause obstruction to blood flow through the heart or interfere with valve closing. Calcification of blood vessels may result in narrowing of vessels and insufficient blood flow to distal tissues. Dead and dying tissues often become calcified (filled with calcium salts) and appear as dense areas on x-ray films. For example, lung damage due to tuberculosis is often apparent as calcified areas called tubercles.

With the exception of inorganic particles, the intracellular accumulations are generally reversible if the causative factors are removed.

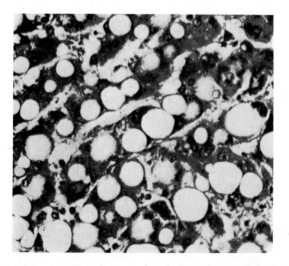

FIGURE 3–2. Fatty liver. Accumulations of intracellular lipids result in a yellowish, greasy appearance. (From Cotran RS, Kumar V, Robbins SL (eds): *Robbins Pathologic Basis of Disease,* 5th ed. Philadelphia, WB Saunders, 1994. Reproduced with permission.)

KEY CONCEPTS

- **Hydropic swelling is an early indicator of cell injury. It results from Na⁺/K⁺ pump dysfunction at the cell membrane.**

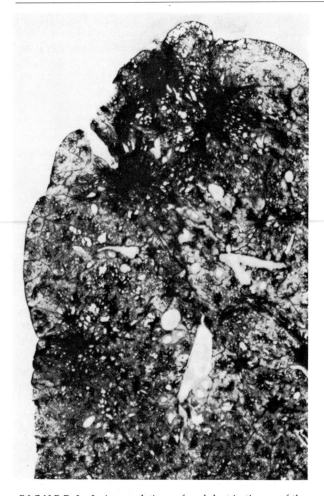

F I G U R E 3 – 3. Accumulations of coal dust in tissues of the lung. (From Cotran RS, Kumar V, Robbins SL (eds): *Robbins Pathologic Basis of Disease*, 4th ed. Philadelphia, WB Saunders, 1989, p 475. Reproduced with permission. Photograph courtesy of Dr. Werner Laquer, Dr. Jerome Kleinerman, and the National Institute of Occupational Safety and Health.)

Atrophy

Atrophy occurs when cells shrink and reduce their differentiated functions in response to a variety of normal and injurious factors. The general causes of atrophy may be summarized as (1) disuse, (2) denervation, (3) ischemia, (4) nutrient starvation, (5) interruption of endocrine signals, (6) persistent cell injury, and (7) aging. Apparently, atrophy represents an effort by the cell to minimize its energy and nutrient consumption by decreasing intracellular organelles and other structures.

A common form of atrophy is due to a reduction in functional demand, sometimes called **disuse atrophy.** For example, immobilization, by bed rest or casting of an extremity, results in shrinkage of skeletal muscle cells. On resumption of activity, the tissue resumes its normal size. Denervation of skeletal muscle results in a similar decrease in muscle size due to loss of nervous stimulation. Inadequate blood supply to a tissue is known as **ischemia.** If the blood supply is totally interrupted, the cells will die, but chronic sublethal ischemia usually results in cell atrophy. The heart, brain, kidneys, and lower leg are common sites of ischemia. Atrophic changes in the lower leg due to ischemia include thin skin, muscle wasting, and loss of hair. Atrophy also is a consequence of chronic nutrient starvation, whether due to poor intake, absorption, or distribution to the tissues. Many glandular tissues throughout the body depend on growth-stimulating (trophic) signals to maintain size and function. The adrenal cortex, thyroid, and gonads, for example, are maintained by trophic hormones from the pituitary gland and will atrophy in their absence. Atrophy due to persistent cell injury is most commonly related to chronic inflammation and infection.

The biochemical pathways that result in cellular atrophy are imperfectly known; however, lysosomal activity increases as intracellular structures are digested.[2] Certain substances are apparently resistant

---

• **Intracellular accumulations of abnormal endogenous or exogenous particles indicate a disorder of cellular metabolism.**

Cellular Adaptation

The cellular response to persistent, sublethal stress reflects the cell's efforts to adapt. Cellular stress may be due to an increased functional demand or a reversible cellular injury. Although the term *adaptation* implies a change for the better, in some instances an adaptive change may not be beneficial. The common adaptive responses are atrophy (decreased cell size), hypertrophy (increased cell size), hyperplasia (increased cell number), metaplasia (conversion of one cell type to another), and dysplasia (disorderly growth) (Fig. 3–4). Each of these changes is potentially reversible when the cellular stress is relieved.

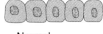
Normal

Atrophy
(decreased cell size)

Hypertrophy
(increased cell size)

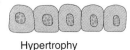
Hyperplasia
(increased cell number)

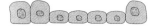
Metaplasia
(conversion of one cell
type to another)

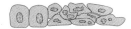
Dysplasia
(disorderly growth)

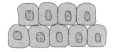

F I G U R E 3 – 4. The adaptive cellular responses of atrophy, hypertrophy, hyperplasia, metaplasia, and dysplasia.

to degradation and remain in the lysosomal vesicles of atrophied cells. For example, lipofuscin is an age-related pigment that accumulates in residual vesicles in atrophied cells, giving them a yellow-brown appearance.

Hypertrophy

Hypertrophy is an increase in cell mass accompanied by an augmented functional capacity. Cells hypertrophy in response to increased physiologic or pathophysiologic demands. Cellular enlargement results primarily from a net increase in cellular protein content.[6] Like the other adaptive responses, hypertrophy subsides when the increased demand is removed; however, the cell may not entirely return to normal because of persistent changes in connective tissue structures. For example, an increase in skeletal muscle mass and strength in response to repeated exercise is due to hypertrophy of individual muscle cells. Physiologic hypertrophy occurs in response to a variety of trophic hormones in sex organs—the breast and uterus, for example. Certain pathophysiologic conditions may place undue stress on some tissues, causing them to hypertrophy. Liver enlargement in response to bodily toxins and cardiac muscle enlargement in response to high blood pressure (Fig. 3–5) represent hypertrophic adaptations to pathologic conditions. Hypertrophic adaptation is particularly important for cells such as muscle cells that are unable to undergo mitotic division.

Hyperplasia

Cells that are capable of mitotic division will generally increase their functional capacity by increasing the number of cells (**hyperplasia**) as well as by hypertrophy. Hyperplasia generally results from increased physiologic demands or hormonal stimulation. Persistent cell injury also may lead to hyperplasia. Examples of demand-induced hyperplasia include an increase in RBC number in response to high altitude, and liver enlargement in response to drug detoxification. Trophic hormones induce hyperplasia in their target tissues. Estrogen, for example, leads to an increase in endometrial and uterine stromal cells.

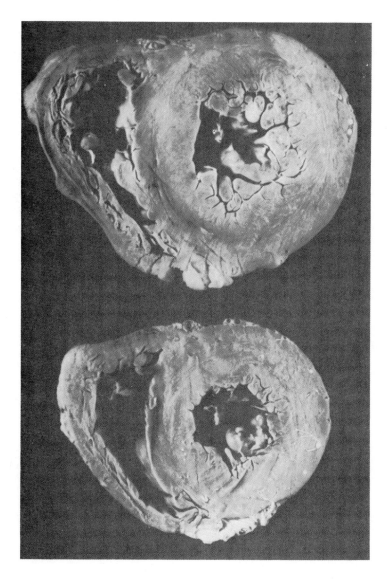

FIGURE 3–5. Hypertrophy of cardiac muscle in response to chronic high blood pressure (*top*) is compared to a normal heart (*bottom*). (From Rubin E, Farber J: *Essential Pathology*. Philadelphia, JB Lippincott, 1990, p 7. Reproduced with permission.)

Chronic irritation of epithelial cells often results in hyperplasia. Calluses and corns, for example, result from chronic frictional injury to the skin. The epithelium of the bladder commonly becomes hyperplastic in response to the chronic inflammation of cystitis.

Metaplasia

Metaplasia is the replacement of one differentiated cell type with another. This almost always occurs as an adaptation to persistent injury, with the replacement cell type better able to tolerate the injurious stimulation.[2] Metaplasia is fully reversible when the injurious stimulus is removed.[1] Metaplasia often involves the replacement of glandular epithelium with squamous epithelium. Chronic irritation of the bronchial mucosa by cigarette smoke, for example, leads to the conversion of ciliated columnar epithelium to stratified squamous epithelium. Metaplastic cells generally remain well differentiated and of the same tissue type, although cancerous transformations can occur. Some cancers of the lung, cervix, stomach, and bladder appear to result from areas of metaplastic epithelium.

Dysplasia

Dysplasia refers to the disorganized appearance of cells because of abnormal variations in size, shape, and arrangement. Dysplasia occurs most frequently in hyperplastic squamous epithelium, but it may also be seen in the mucosa of the intestine. Dysplasia probably represents an adaptive effort gone astray. Dysplastic cells have significant potential to transform into cancerous cells and are usually regarded as preneoplastic lesions.[1] (See Chapter 6 for a discussion of cancer.)

KEY CONCEPTS

- Adaptive cellular responses indicate cellular stress due to altered functional demand or chronic sublethal injury.
- Hypertrophy and hyperplasia generally result from increased functional demand. Atrophy results from decreased functional demand or chronic ischemia. Metaplasia and dysplasia result from persistent injury.

Irreversible Cell Injury

Cellular death occurs when an injury is too severe or prolonged to allow cellular adaptation or repair. Death and degradation of body cells or tissues is called **necrosis.** Necrotic cells demonstrate typical morphologic changes, including a shrunken (pyknotic) nucleus that is subsequently degraded (karyolysis), a swollen cell volume, dispersed ribosomes, and disrupted plasma and organelle membranes (Fig. 3–6). The disruption of the permeability barrier of the plasma membrane appears to be a critical event in the death of the cell.[7] Cell death is not reversible.

Localized injury or death of tissue is generally reflected in the entire system as the body attempts to clear away dead cells and works to compensate for loss of tissue function. There are several manifestations indicating that the system is responding to cellular injury and death. A general inflammatory response

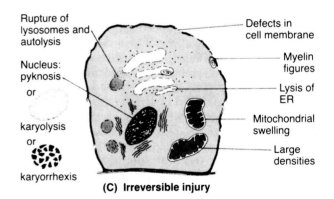

FIGURE 3–6. Cellular features of cell necrosis (**C**) compared with a normal cell (**A**) and a reversibly injured cell (**B**). (From Cotran RS, Kumar V, Robbins SL (eds): *Robbins Pathologic Basis of Disease,* 5th ed. Philadelphia, WB Saunders, 1994. Reproduced with permission.)

is often present, with general malaise, fever, increased heart rate, increased white blood cell (WBC) count, and loss of appetite. With the dissolution of necrotic cells, intracellular contents are released and often find their way into the bloodstream. The presence of specific cellular enzymes in the blood is used as an indicator of the location and extent of cellular death. For example, an elevated serum α-amylase level would indicate pancreatic damage, and an elevated creatine kinase (MB isoenzyme) level would indicate myocardial damage. The location of pain due to tissue destruction may also aid in the diagnosis of cellular death.

Four different types of tissue necrosis have been described: coagulative, liquefactive, fat, and caseous (Fig. 3–7). They differ primarily in the type of tissue affected. **Coagulative necrosis** is the most common. Manifestations of coagulative necrosis are the same, regardless of the etiology of cell death. In general, the steps leading to coagulative necrosis may be summarized as follows: (1) irreversible cellular injury, leading to (2) loss of the plasma membrane's ability to maintain electrochemical gradients, which results in (3) influx of calcium ions, and (4) the appearance of coagulative necrosis. The common morphologic changes that accompany cell death can be attributed to the accumulation of calcium within the dead cells. The area of coagulative necrosis is composed of denatured proteins and is relatively solid. The coagulated area is then dissolved by proteolytic enzymes and often replaced with scar tissue.

When the dissolution of dead cells occurs very quickly, a liquefied area of lysosomal enzymes and dissolved tissue may result and form an abscess or cyst. This type of necrosis, called **liquefactive necrosis,** may be seen in the brain, which is rich in degradative enzymes and contains little supportive connective tissue. Liquefaction may also result from a bacterial infection that triggers a localized collection of WBCs. The phagocytic WBCs contain potent degradative enzymes that may completely digest dead cells, resulting in liquid debris.

Fat necrosis refers to death of adipose tissue and usually results from trauma or pancreatitis. The process begins with the release of activated digestive enzymes from the pancreas or injured tissue. The enzymes attack the cell membranes of fat cells, which releases their stores of triglycerides. Pancreatic lipase can then hydrolyze the triglycerides to free fatty acids, which precipitate as calcium soaps. Fat necrosis appears as a chalky white area of tissue.

Caseous necrosis is characteristic of lung tissue damaged by tuberculosis. The areas of dead lung tissue are white, soft, and fragile, resembling clumpy cheese. Dead cells are walled off from the rest of the lung tissue by inflammatory WBCs. In the center, the dead cells lose their cellular structure, but are not totally degraded. Necrotic debris may persist indefinitely.

Gangrene is a term used to describe cellular death involving a large area of tissue. Gangrene usually results from interruption of the major blood supply to a particular body part, such as the toes, leg, or bowel. Depending on the appearance and subsequent infection of the necrotic tissue, it is described as dry gangrene, wet gangrene, or gas gangrene. **Dry gangrene** is a form of coagulative necrosis characterized by blackened, dry, wrinkled tissue that is separated from adjacent healthy tissue by an obvious line of demarcation (Fig. 3–8). It generally occurs only on the extremities. Liquefactive necrosis may result in **wet gangrene,** which is typically found in internal organs, appears cold and black, and may be foul-smelling, due to the invasion of bacteria. Rapid spread of tissue damage and the release of toxins into the bloodstream make wet gangrene a life-threatening problem. **Gas gangrene** is characterized by the formation of bubbles of gas in damaged muscle tissue. Gas gangrene is due to the infection of necrotic tissue by anaerobic bacteria of the *Clostridium* family. These bacteria produce toxins and degradative enzymes that allow the infection to spread rapidly through the necrotic tissue. Gas gangrene may be fatal if not treated rapidly and aggressively.

The cell death and tissue necrosis described in this section are examples of pathophysiologic processes. However, in some cases cell death may be a normal physiologic response. The selective destruction of cells during embryonic development and the involution of glands in the absence of trophic signals are examples of physiologic processes that result in cellular death.[8]

KEY CONCEPTS

- Cell death or necrosis occurs when the injury is too severe or prolonged to allow adaptation.
- Local and systemic indicators of cell death include pain, elevated serum enzyme levels, inflammation (fever, elevated WBC count, malaise), and loss of function.
- Different tissue types exhibit necrosis of different types: heart (coagulative), brain (liquefactive), lung (caseous), and pancreas (fat).
- Gangrene refers to a large area of necrosis which may be described as dry, wet, or gas gangrene. Gas gangrene and wet gangrene may be rapidly fatal.

Etiology of Cellular Injury

Cellular injury and death result from a variety of cellular assaults, including lack of oxygen and nutrients, infection and immune responses, chemicals, and physical and mechanical factors. The extent of cell injury and death depends in part on the duration and severity of the assault and in part on the prior condition of the cells. Well-nourished and somewhat adapted cells may withstand the injury better than cells that are not. Common causes of cellular injury include hypoxic injury, nutritional injury, infectious and immunologic injury, chemical injury, and physical and mechanical injury.

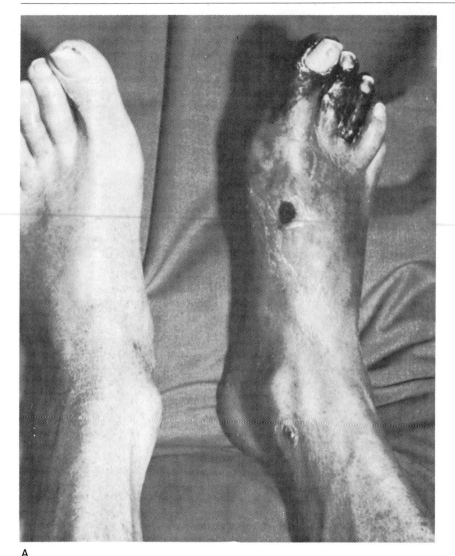

A

FIGURE 3–7. The four primary types of tissue necrosis. **A,** Coagulative.

Hypoxic Injury

Living cells must receive a continuous supply of oxygen to produce ATP to power energy-requiring functions. Lack of oxygen, or **hypoxia,** results in power failure within the cell. Tissue hypoxia is most often due to **ischemia,** or the interruption of blood flow to an area, but it may also result from heart disease, lung disease, and RBC disorders. The cellular events that follow oxygen deprivation are shown in Figure 3–9. Decreased oxygen delivery to the mitochondria causes ATP production in the cell to stall and ATP-dependent pumps, including the Na^+/K^+ and Ca^{++} pumps, to fail.[9] Sodium accumulation within the cell creates an osmotic gradient favoring water entry, resulting in hydropic swelling. Excess intracellular calcium collects in the mitochondria, further interfering with mitochondrial function. A small amount of ATP is produced by anaerobic glycolytic pathways, which break down cellular stores of glycogen. The pyruvate end products of glycolysis accumulate and are converted to lactate, causing cellular acidification. Cellular proteins and enzymes become progressively more dysfunctional as the pH falls. Up to a point, ischemic injury is reversible, but when the plasma and mitochondrial membranes are critically damaged, cell death ensues. A number of mechanisms have been postulated to cause irreversible membrane damage; however, none has been proved. One theory suggests that cellular hypoxia leads to the release of mitochondrial calcium into the cytoplasm, activating membrane phospholipases and causing membrane lipids to be digested.[10]

Three potentially harmful molecules—superoxide (O_2^-), peroxide (H_2O_2), and hydroxyl radicals $(OH\cdot)$—have been implicated in ischemic membrane injury.[11] All three are forms of **partially reduced oxygen,** which are highly reactive with other molecules. Cellular injury due to activated oxygen may actually occur after the blood supply to the area has been restored—a so-called reperfusion injury.[12,13] The buildup of adenosine diphosphate (ADP) and pyru-

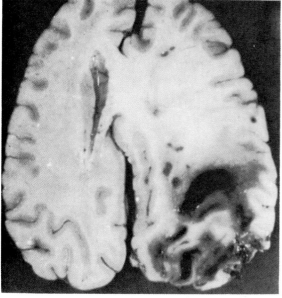

B

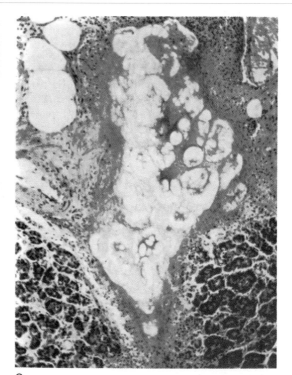

C

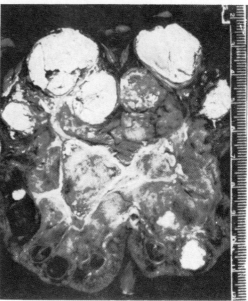

D

F I G U R E 3 – 7 Continued **B,** Liquefactive. **C,** Fat. **D,** Caseous. (**A** from Crowley L: *Introduction to Human Disease,* 3rd ed. © 1992. Boston: Jones & Bartlett Publishers, p 270. Reprinted by permission. **B** from Rubin E, Farber J: *Essential Pathology.* Philadelphia, JB Lippincott, 1990, p 185. **C** from Cotran RS, Kumar V, Robbins SL (eds): *Robbins Pathologic Basis of Disease,* 5th ed. Philadelphia, WB Saunders, 1994. **D** from Cotran RS, Kumar V, Robbins SL (eds): *Robbins Pathologic Basis of Disease,* 4th ed. Philadelphia, WB Saunders, 1989, p 19. Reproduced with permission.)

vate during ischemia apparently results in rapid production of electrons when the oxygen supply is reestablished. Partially reduced oxygen molecules are formed when the electrons are transferred to oxygen. The activated oxygen molecules may injure cell membranes by stealing hydrogen molecules and by forming abnormal molecular bonds. Partially reduced oxygen molecules are also produced by phagocytic WBCs in the inflammatory reactions that follow cell death (Fig. 3–10).

Nutritional Injury

Adequate amounts of fats, carbohydrates, proteins, vitamins, and minerals are essential for normal cellular function. Most of these essential nutrients must be obtained from external sources because the cell is unable to manufacture them. The cell is unable to synthesize many of the 20 amino acids necessary to form the proteins of the body. Likewise, most vitamins and minerals must be obtained from exogenous

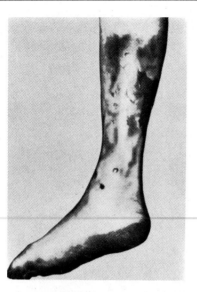

F I G U R E 3 – 8. Dry gangrene. (From Robbins SL, Cotran RS, Kumar V (eds): *Pathologic Basis of Disease,* 3rd ed. Philadelphia, WB Saunders, 1984, p 17. Reproduced with permission.)

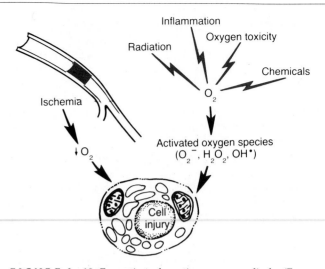

F I G U R E 3 – 10. Formation of reactive oxygen radicals. (From Cotran RS, Kumar V, Robbins SL (eds): *Robbins Pathologic Basis of Disease,* 5th ed. Philadelphia, WB Saunders, 1994. Reproduced with permission.)

sources. Cell injury results from deficiencies as well as excesses of essential nutrients.[14]

Certain cell types are more susceptible to injury from particular nutritional imbalances. Iron deficiency, for example, will primarily affect RBCs, whereas vitamin D deficiency affects bones. All cell types must receive glucose for energy, and fatty acid and amino acid building blocks to synthesize and repair cellular components. Nutritional deficiencies result from poor intake, altered absorption, impaired distribution by the circulatory system, or inefficient cellular uptake. Nutritional excesses primarily result from excessive intake, although deficient cellular uptake by one cell type may contribute to excess nutrient delivery to other cell types. For example, in the condition of diabetes mellitus, some cell types have deficient receptors for insulin-dependent glucose uptake, which causes excessive amounts of glucose to remain in the bloodstream. As a result, cells that do not require insulin to take in glucose, such as neurons, may reach abnormally high intracellular glucose levels.

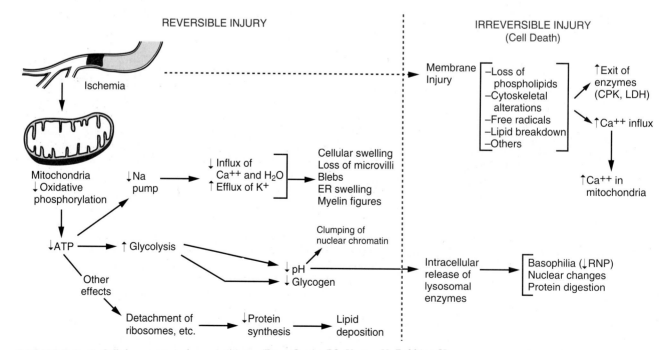

F I G U R E 3 – 9. Cellular events in hypoxic injury. (From Cotran RS, Kumar V, Robbins SL (eds): *Robbins Pathologic Basis of Disease,* 5th ed. Philadelphia, WB Saunders, 1994. Reproduced with permission.)

Infectious and Immunologic Injury

Bacteria and viruses are common infectious agents that may injure cells in a variety of ways.[15] The virulence of a particular biological agent depends on its ability to gain access to the cell and on its success in altering cellular functions. (See Chapter 8 for a detailed discussion of infectious processes.) Some of the injurious effects are directly due to the biological agent, but added injury may be done indirectly by triggering the body's immune response.

Bacteria are too large to gain entry into the cell and so accomplish their injurious effects from the outside. Some bacteria produce and secrete powerful destructive enzymes that digest cellular membranes and connective tissues. Collagenases and lecithinases, for example, are produced by the bacterium *Clostridium perfringens*. Other bacteria produce **exotoxins,** which interfere with specific cellular functions when released from the bacterium. *Claustridium botulinum* and *Claustridium tetani,* for example, produce life-threatening toxins that disrupt normal neuromuscular transmission. Cholera and diphtheria are well-known examples of exotoxin-related diseases. Exotoxins are primarily proteins and are generally susceptible to destruction by extremes of heat. Certain gram-negative bacteria contain another type of toxin, *endotoxin,* in their cell wall. On lysis of the bacteria, the endotoxin is released, causing fever, malaise, and even circulatory shock.

The indirect cellular injury due to the bacteria-evoked immune response may be more damaging than the direct effects of the infectious agent. White blood cells secrete many enzymes and chemicals meant to destroy the invading organism, including histamines, kinins, complement, proteases, lymphokines, and prostaglandins. Normal body cells may be exposed to these injurious chemicals because they are too close to the site of immunologic battle.

Viruses are small bits of genetic material that are able to gain entry into the cell. They may be thought of as intracellular parasites that use the host cell's metabolic and synthetic machinery to survive and replicate. Viral infections tend to follow two distinct pathways. In some cases the virus remains within the cell for a considerable time without inflicting lethal injury. In other cases the virus causes rapid lysis and destruction of the host cell. The mechanisms that determine which course the virus will take are poorly understood.

The polio virus is an example of a virus that is **directly cytopathic:** it kills the host cell directly without immune system participation. The polio virus is made up of RNA, which the cell recognizes as any other messenger RNA molecule and translates into viral proteins. Some of the virally coded proteins insert into the plasma membrane of the cell, forming pores or channels that allow ions to diffuse across. The cell dies as the vital ion gradients are dissipated.

Other viruses remain within the cell for long periods of time, unobtrusively making and releasing viral copies of themselves without causing lethal cell injury. The virally infected cells may not escape death, however, because they express cell surface proteins that are foreign to the host's immune system. The hepatitis B virus is an example of such an **indirectly cytopathic** virus that causes immune-mediated cell death. The hepatitis B virus consists of double-stranded DNA that gets incorporated into the host cell's nucleus, where it can be transcribed by the normal DNA polymerases. The mRNA transcripts of the viral genes are transported to the cytoplasm and translated into structural proteins and enzymes, which are used to make more copies of the virus. Such virally infected cells may remain functional virus factories until they are destroyed by the host's immune system.

Chemical Injury

Toxic chemicals or poisons are plentiful in the environment. Some toxic chemicals cause cellular injury directly, while others become injurious only when they are metabolized into reactive chemicals by the body. Carbon tetrachloride (CCl_4) is an example of the latter.[16] **Carbon tetrachloride,** a formerly used dry-cleaning agent, is converted to a highly toxic **free radical,** CCl_3^-, by liver cells. The free radical is very reactive, forming abnormal chemical bonds within the cell and ultimately destroying the cellular membranes of liver cells, causing liver failure. In high doses, **acetaminophen,** a commonly used analgesic, may have similar toxic effects on the liver.

Many toxins are inherently reactive and do not require metabolic activation to exert their effects. Common examples are **heavy metals** such as lead and mercury, **toxic gases, corrosives,** and **antimetabolites.** Some toxins have an affinity for a particular cell type or tissue, while others exert widespread systemic effects. Carbon monoxide, for example, binds tightly and selectively to hemoglobin, preventing the red cell from carrying sufficient oxygen. Lead poisoning, on the other hand, has widespread effects, including effects on nervous tissue, blood cells, and the kidney. Extremely acidic or basic chemicals are directly corrosive to cellular structures. Certain chemicals interfere with normal metabolic processes of the cell. Some of these antimetabolites have been put to use in the form of cytotoxic agents for the treatment of cancer (see Chap. 11).

Physical and Mechanical Injury

Injurious physical and mechanical factors include extremes of temperature, pressure, and mechanical deformation, electricity, and electromagnetic radiation.[17]

Extremes of cold result in the **hypothermic injury** known as frostbite. Prior to actual cellular freezing, severe vasoconstriction and increased blood viscosity may result in ischemic injury. With continued exposure to cold, a vasodilatory response may occur, leading to intense swelling and peripheral nerve damage. The cytoplasmic solution may actually freeze, resulting in the formation of intracellular ice crystals and rupture of cellular components. Frostbite generally affects the extremities, ears, and nose and is often complicated by gangrenous necrosis.

Extremes of heat result in **hyperthermic injury** or burns. High temperatures cause microvascular coagulation and may speed up metabolic processes within the cell. Burns result from direct tissue destruction by high temperatures and are classified according to the degree of tissue destruction. Burns are discussed in Chapter 55.

Abrupt changes in **atmospheric pressure** may result from high altitude flying, deep sea diving, and explosions. Pressure changes may interfere with gas exchange in the lungs, cause the formation of gas emboli within the bloodstream, collapse the thorax, and rupture internal organs. A well-known example of pressure injury is the condition of "the bends," which afflicts deep sea divers who surface too quickly. The rapid decrease in water pressure results in the formation of bubbles of nitrogen gas in the blood, which may block the circulation, causing ischemic injury.

Destruction of cells and tissues due to **mechanical deformation** ranges from mild abrasion to severe lacerating trauma. Cell death may result from direct trauma to cell membranes, resulting blood loss, or obstruction of blood flow and hypoxia. Nonpenetrating trauma generally results from physical impact with a blunt object such as a fist, car steering wheel, or the pavement. Common causes of penetrating trauma are knives and guns. Trauma-induced inflammatory swelling may further compromise injured tissues.

Electrical injury may occur when the cells of the body act as conductors of electricity. The electrical current damages tissues in two ways: by disrupting neural and cardiac impulses, and by hyperthermic destruction of tissues. Resistance to the flow of electrons results in heat production, which damages the tissues. The current tends to follow the path of least resistance—through neurons and body fluids—causing violent muscle contractions and thermal injury and coagulation in blood vessels. In general, greater electrical injury is suffered with high-voltage alternating current applied to a low-resistance area (wet skin).

There are many forms of **electromagnetic radiation,** ranging from low-energy radiowaves to high-

energy gamma rays or photons (Fig. 3–11). Radiation is capable of injuring cells by three general mechanisms: direct breakage of chemical bonds, ionization, and heat production.[18] Cellular DNA is particularly susceptible to damage from radiation exposure.[19-21] A **direct hit** of the radiant energy on the DNA molecule may result in breakage of the chemical bonds holding the linear DNA together. This type of direct bond breakage generally results from the high-energy forms of radiation like x-rays and gamma rays. The molecular bonds of DNA may also be indirectly disrupted by **ionizing radiation.** Ionization refers to the ability of the radiant energy to split water molecules by knocking off orbital electrons (**radiolysis**). Radiolysis creates activated oxygen molecules that behave as free radicals, stealing electrons from other molecules and disrupting chemical bonds. Many forms of radiation are capable of ionization, but the medium-energy alpha and beta particles that result from decay of atomic nuclei are especially destructive. Low-energy electromagnetic radiation such as that from microwaves, ultrasound, computers, and infrared light is unable to break chemical bonds but causes rotation and vibration of atoms and molecules.[22] The rotational and vibrational energy is then converted into heat. It is probable that the resulting **localized hyperthermia** may result in cellular injury. Unfortunately, definitive research on the effects of low-energy radiation is lacking.

At the cellular level, radiation has two primary effects: genetic damage and acute cell destruction (Fig. 3–12). The vulnerability of a tissue to **radiation-induced genetic damage** depends on its rate of proliferation. Genetic damage to the DNA of a long-lived, nonproliferating cell may be of little consequence, whereas tissues with rapid cellular division have less opportunity to repair damaged DNA before passing it on to the next generation of cells.[23] (Genetic mutation is discussed in Chapter 5.) Hematopoietic, mucosal, gonadal, and fetal cells are particularly susceptible to genetic radiation damage.

Radiation-induced cell death is attributed primarily to the radiolysis of water, with resulting free radical damage to the plasma membrane. Whole-body exposure to sufficiently high levels of radiation (>300 rad) results in acute radiation sickness with hematopoietic

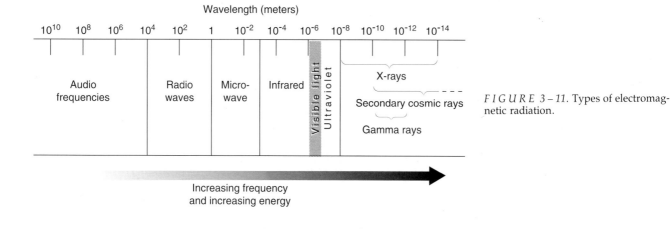

F I G U R E 3 – 11. Types of electromagnetic radiation.

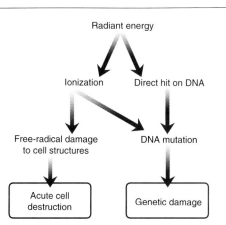

F I G U R E 3 – 12. The mechanism of radiation-induced genetic and cell injury.

failure, destruction of the epithelial layer of the gastrointestinal tract, and neurologic dysfunction. The high levels of irradiation that cause acute radiation sickness are associated with events such as nuclear accidents and bombings. Radiation exposure from diagnostic x-rays, cosmic rays, and natural radiant chemicals in the earth are far below the level that would result in acute radiation sickness. The signs and symptoms of acute radiation sickness are shown in Figure 3–13. The ability of radiation to kill proliferating cells is used to advantage in the treatment of some forms of cancer. **Radiation therapy** may be used when a cancerous growth is confined to a particular area. Injury associated with radiation therapy is generally localized to the irradiated area. Small arteries and arterioles in the area may be damaged, leading to blood clotting and fibrous deposits that compromise tissue perfusion.

KEY CONCEPTS

- Hypoxia is an important cause of cell injury that usually results from poor oxygenation of the blood (hypoxemia) or inadequate delivery of blood to the cells (ischemia).
- Reperfusion injury to cells may occur when circulation is restored, owing to the production of partially reduced oxygen molecules that damage cell membranes.
- Cellular damage due to infection and immunologic responses is common. Some bacteria and viruses damage cells directly, others stimulate the host's immune system to destroy the host's cells.
- Chemical, physical, and mechanical factors injure cells in various ways. Chemicals may interfere with normal metabolic processes in the cell. Injury due to physical factors, such as burns and frostbite, causes direct destruction of tissues. Radiation-induced cell death is primarily a result of radiolysis of water, with resulting free radical damage to the cell membrane.

Cellular Aging

The inevitable process of aging and death has been the subject of interest and investigation for centuries. Despite scientific study and the search for the fountain of youth, neither the mechanisms that result in cellular aging nor methods for halting the aging process have been revealed. The maximum human life span has remained constant at about 110 years, despite significant progress in the treatment of diseases.[24] It seems apparent that aging is entirely distinct from

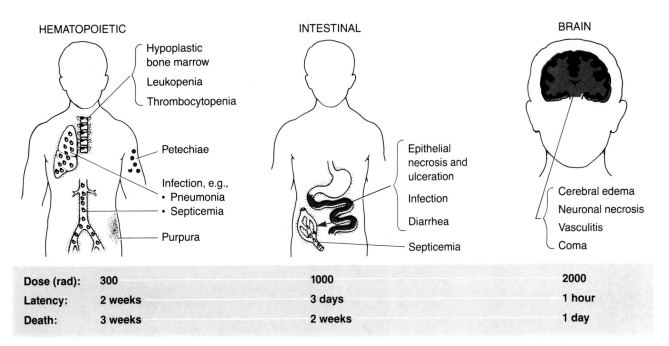

Dose (rad):	300	1000	2000
Latency:	2 weeks	3 days	1 hour
Death:	3 weeks	2 weeks	1 day

F I G U R E 3 – 13. Signs and symptoms of acute radiation sickness. (From Rubin E, Farber J: *Essential Pathology.* Philadelphia, JB Lippincott, 1990, p 188. Reproduced with permission. Artist: Dimitri Karetnikov.)

disease, and that the life span is limited by the aging process itself rather than by the ravages of disease. Although the elderly are certainly more vulnerable to diseases, the aging process and disease processes are generally viewed as entirely different phenomena. In practice, the distinction between aging and disease may be difficult to make. For example, the aging skeleton normally loses some bone mass, but too much bone loss results in osteoporosis—a disease process. Likewise, a loss of blood vessel elasticity is generally viewed as a normal aging change, but at what point does too much "hardening of the arteries" become abnormal? This confusion results from the continued inability to identify the irreversible and universal processes of cellular aging as separate from the potentially reversible effects of disease.

Cellular Basis of Aging

The two major schools of thought regarding aging hold that it is caused either by **extrinsic** events that progressively damage cells or by **intrinsic** genetic programs of the cells themselves.[24] Evidence supporting each of the theories of aging is scant and mostly circumstantial, and no theory has gained general acceptance. Each of the following theories of aging has been proposed to explain certain manifestations of the aging process: the somatic mutation theory, the free radical theory, the immunologic theory, the error theory, the neuroendocrine theory, and the programmed senescence theory.

The **somatic mutation theory** is based on the idea that chronic exposure to normal background environmental radiation results in random genetic damage in cells. The cell dies when genetic damage becomes extensive enough to impair critical functions. This theory was proposed to explain the observation that chronic irradiation shortens the life span of experimental animals. This theory suggests that people living in places with increased levels of background radiation, such as at high altitude, would age more quickly. No such difference has yet been reported.

The **free radical theory** was prompted in part by the observation that larger animals, which have slower metabolic rates, generally have longer life spans.[25,26] Metabolic rate, in turn, determines the production of activated oxygen free radicals. Aging is thought to result from the cumulative and progressive damage to cell structures, particularly the cell membrane by these oxygen radicals. The accumulation of lipofuscin pigment, the brown aging pigment, in older cells is taken as evidence of the progressive destruction of membrane lipids by the free radicals. However, no evidence of increased free radical production with aging has been found.

The functional capacity of the immune system declines with age, and the ability to distinguish between self tissue and foreign tissue appears to become impaired. Autoimmune disorders, in which the immune system attacks the body's own cells, are more prevalent in the elderly. The **immunologic theory of aging** maintains that aging is due to failure of the immune system, resulting in the progressive destruction of body cells. The immune theory does not explain the process of aging in simple animals that do not have a well-developed immune system.

The **error theory** of aging is based on the idea that random errors in the translation of key cellular proteins will eventually lead to cell death.[27,28] This theory holds that if errors occur in transcriptional and translational enzymes, which control their own synthesis, the errors will be multiplied with time until an "error catastrophe" results in cell death. Although this theory has drawn much interest, it has accumulated little supportive evidence.

The invariable sequence of cell death in certain tissues and organs during embryogenesis has suggested to some researchers that aging is controlled by some intrinsic genetic program. The **neuroendocrine theories** suggest that the hypothalamic-pituitary system, as the master timekeeper of the body, controls the aging process.[29] Age-related changes in the structure and function of certain hormones have been reported.

The **programmed senescence theory** also holds that aging is the result of an intrinsic genetic program.[30] Support for the theory of a genetically programmed life span comes primarily from studies of cells in culture. In classic experiments by Hayflick, fibroblastic cells in culture were shown to undergo a finite number of cell divisions. Fibroblasts taken from older individuals underwent fewer cell divisions than those from younger individuals. Given an adequate environment, the information encoded in the cellular genome is thought to dictate the number of possible cell replications, after which damaged or lost cells are no longer replaced.

Physiologic Changes of Aging

All of the body systems show age-related changes, which can be generally described as a decrease in functional reserve or inability to adapt to environmental demands.[31] An overview of the tissue and systemic changes of aging is presented in Table 3–1. The details of age-related changes in the various body systems are described in later chapters of this book.

KEY CONCEPTS

- Aging is distinct from disease. The life span is limited by the aging process itself, rather than by the ravages of disease.
- Aging theories are of two general schools. According to the first school, aging is caused by extrinsic events that progressively damage cells. Aligned with this school are the somatic mutation theory, the free radical theory, and the immunologic theory of aging. According to the second school, aging is caused by intrinsic genetic programs. Representa-

TABLE 3-1. Overview of the Physiologic Changes of Aging

System	Physiologic Changes
Cardiovascular	↓ Vessel elasticity due to calcification and connective tissue (↑ pulmonary vascular resistance) ↓ No. of heart muscle fibers with ↑ size of individual fibers (hypertrophy) ↓ Filling capacity ↓ Stroke volume ↓ Sensitivity of baroreceptors Degeneration of vein valves
Respiratory	↓ Chest wall compliance due to calcification of costal cartilage ↓ Alveolar ventilation ↓ Respiratory muscle strength Air trapping and ↓ ventilation due to degeneration of lung tissue (↓ elasticity)
Renal/urinary	↓ Glomerular filtration rate due to nephron degeneration (↓ 1/3 to 1/2 by age 70) ↓ Ability to concentrate urine ↓ Ability to regulate H^+
Gastrointestinal	Muscular contraction ↓ Esophageal emptying ↓ Bowel motility ↓ Production of HCl, enzymes, and intrinsic factor ↓ Hepatic enzyme production and metabolic capacity Thinning of stomach mucosa
Neurologic/sensory	Nerve cells degenerate and atrophy ↓ of 25%–45% of neurons ↓ Neurotransmitters ↓ Rate of conduction of nerve impulses Loss of taste buds Loss of auditory hair cells and sclerosis of eardrum
Musculoskeletal	↓ Muscle mass Bone demineralization Joint degeneration, erosion, and calcification
Immune	↓ Inflammatory response ↓ In T cell function due to involution of thymus gland
Integumentary	↓ Subcutaneous fat ↓ Elastin Atrophy of sweat glands Atrophy of epidermal arterioles causing altered temperature regulation

tives of this school are the neuroendocrine theories and the programmed senescence theory.
- Age-related changes in body systems can generally be described as a decrease in functional reserve and a reduced ability to adapt to environmental demands.

Somatic Death

Death of the entire organism is called **somatic death.** In contrast to localized cell death, there is no immunologic or inflammatory response in somatic death. The general features of somatic death include the absence of respiration and heartbeat. This definition of death is insufficient, however, because in some cases breathing and cardiac activity may be restored by resuscitative efforts. Within several minutes of cardiopulmonary arrest, the characteristics of irreversible somatic death become apparent. Body temperature falls, the skin becomes pale, and blood and body fluids collect in dependent areas. Within 6 hours, the accumulation of calcium and the depletion of ATP result in perpetual actin-myosin crossbridge formation in muscle cells. The presence of stiffened muscles throughout the body after death is called **rigor mortis.** Rigor mortis gives way to limpness or flaccidity as the tissues of the body begin to deteriorate. Tissue deterioration or putrefaction becomes apparent 24 to 48 hours after death.[32] Putrefaction is associated with the widespread release of lytic enzymes in tissues throughout the body, a process called postmortem autolysis.

The determination of "brain death" has become necessary because of technological ability to keep the heart and lungs working through artificial means even though the brain is no longer functional. Criteria for determining brain death as proof of somatic death may vary by geographic area but generally include unresponsiveness, flaccidity, absence of brain stem reflexes (swallowing, gagging, pupil and eye movements), absence of respiratory effort when the subject is removed from the mechanical ventilator, absence of electrical brain waves, and lack of cerebral blood flow.

KEY CONCEPTS

- Somatic death is characterized by the absence of respirations and heartbeat. Definitions of brain death have been established to describe death in instances when heartbeat and respiration are maintained mechanically.
- After death, body temperature falls, blood and body fluids collect in dependent areas, and rigor mortis ensues. Within 24 to 48 hours the tissues begin to deteriorate and rigor mortis gives way to flaccidity.

Summary

Cells and tissues face many challenges to survival, including injury from lack of oxygen and nutrients, infection and immune responses, chemicals, and physical and mechanical factors. Cells respond to environmental changes or injury in three general ways: (1) If the change is mild or short-lived, the cell may withstand the assault and return to its preinjury status. (2) The cell may adapt to a persistent but sublethal injury by changing its structure or function. (3) Cell death or necrosis may occur if the injury is too severe or prolonged. Characteristics of reversible cell injury include hydropic swelling and the accumulation of abnormal substances. Cell necrosis is characterized by irreversible loss of function, release of cellular enzymes into the bloodstream, and an inflammatory response. The disruption of the permeability barrier of the plasma membrane appears to be a critical event in cellular death.

Aging is a normal physiologic process characterized by a progressive decline in functional capacity and adaptive ability. The biological basis of aging remains largely a mystery, but several theories have been proposed to explain certain aspects of the process. At present, most sources differentiate between the biological alterations of aging and the alterations consequent on disease processes. In practice, however, the distinction may be difficult to make.

REFERENCES

1. Rubin E, Farber J: Cell injury, in Rubin E, Farber J (eds): *Essential Pathology*. Philadelphia, JB Lippincott, 1990.
2. Cotran RS, Kumar V, Robbins SL: Cellular injury and adaptation, in Cotran RS, Kumar V, Robbins SL (eds): *Robbins Pathologic Basis of Disease*, 4th ed. Philadelphia, WB Saunders, 1989.
3. Geokas MC, Lieber CS, French S, Halsted CH: Ethanol, the liver and the gastrointestinal tract. *Ann Intern Med* 1981;95(2):198–211.
4. Stanbury J: *The Metabolic Basis of Inherited Disease*, 5th ed. New York, McGraw-Hill, 1983.
5. Craighead J: Diabetes, in Rubin E, Farber J (eds): *Essential Pathology*. Philadelphia, JB Lippincott, 1990.
6. Zak R: Cardiac hypertrophy: Biochemical and cellular relationships. *Hosp Pract* 1983;18(3):85–97.
7. Farber JL, Chien KR, Mittnacht S Jr: Myocardial ischemia: The pathogenesis of irreversible cell injury in ischemia. *Am J Pathol* 1981;102(2):271–281.
8. Searle J, Kerr JF, Bishop CJ: Necrosis and apoptosis: Distinct modes of cell death with fundamentally different significance. *Pathol Annu* 1982;17(2):229–259.
9. Cowley R, Trump B: *Pathophysiology of Shock, Anoxia, and Ischemia*. Baltimore, Williams & Wilkins, 1981.
10. Farber JL: Biology of disease: Membrane injury and calcium homeostasis in the pathogenesis of coagulative necrosis. *Lab Invest* 1982;47(2):114–123.
11. Freeman BA, Crapo JD: Biology of disease: Free radicals and tissue injury. *Lab Invest* 1982;47(5):412–426.
12. Bolli R, Patel BS, Jeroudi MO, Lai EK, McCay PB: Demonstration of free radical generation in (stunned) myocardium of intact dogs. *J Clin Invest* 1988;82(2):476–485.
13. Burton KP, Massey KD: Alterations in membrane phospholipids, mechanisms of free radical damage and antioxidant protection during myocardial ischemia and reperfusion, in Singal PK (ed): *Free Radicals in the Pathophysiology of Heart Disease*. Boston, Martinus Nijhoff, 1987.
14. Cotran RS, Kumar V, Robbins SL: Nutrition disease, in Cotran RS, Kumar V, Robbins SL (eds): *Robbins Pathologic Basis of Disease*, 4th ed. Philadelphia, WB Saunders, 1989.
15. Hewlett EL: Toxins and other virulence factors, in Mandell GL, Douglas RG Jr, Bennett JE (eds): *Principles and Practice of Infectious Disease*, 3rd ed. New York, Churchill Livingstone, 1990.
16. Farber J: Xenobiotics, drug metabolism and liver injury, in Farber E, Phillips MJ, Kaufman N (eds): *Pathogenesis of Liver Disease*. Baltimore, Williams & Wilkins, 1987.
17. Cotran RS, Kumar V, Robbins SL: Environmental pathology, in Cotran RS, Kumar V, Robbins SL (eds): *Robbins Pathologic Basis of Disease*, 4th ed. Philadelphia, WB Saunders, 1989.
18. Pizzarello D, Witcofski R: *Basic Radiation Biology*, 2nd ed. Philadelphia, Lea & Febiger, 1975.
19. Dalrymple G: *Medical Radiation Biology*. Philadelphia, WB Saunders, 1973.
20. Hutchinson F: The molecular basis for radiation effects on cells. *Cancer Res* 1966;26:2045–2052.
21. Mettler FA Jr, Moseley RD Jr: *Medical Effects of Ionizing Radiation*. Orlando, Grune & Stratton, 1985.
22. Wrenn F, Mays C: Characteristics of ionizing radiation, in Rom W (ed): *Environmental and Occupational Medicine*. Boston, Little, Brown & Co, 1983.
23. M.D. Anderson Hospital and Tumor Institute: *Cellular Radiation Biology*. Eighteenth Symposium on Fundamental Cancer Research (Houston, 1964). Baltimore, Williams & Wilkins, 1965.
24. Warner H, Butler R, Sprott R, Schneider E: *Modern Biological Theories of Aging*. New York, Raven Press, 1987.
25. Pryor W: The free-radical theory of aging revisited: A critique and a suggested disease-specific theory, in Warner HR, Butler R, Sprott R, Schneider E (eds): *Modern Biological Theories of Aging*. New York, Raven Press, 1987.
26. Harman D: Aging: Role of free radicals in aging and disease, in Johnson H (ed): *Aging: Relations Between Normal Aging and Disease*. New York, Raven Press, vol 28, 1985.
27. Orgel L: The maintenance of the accuracy of protein synthesis and its relevance to aging. *Proc Natl Acad Sci USA* 1963;49:517–521.
28. Orgel L: The maintenance of the accuracy of protein synthesis and its relevance to aging: A correction. *Proc Natl Acad Sci USA* 1970;67:1476.
29. Everitt A, Burgess J: *Hypothalamus, Pituitary and Aging*. Springfield, Charles C Thomas, 1976.
30. Hayflick L: The biology of human aging. *Adv Pathobiol* 1980;7(2):80–99.
31. Cotran RS, Kumar V, Robbins SL: Diseases of aging, in Cotran RS, Kumar V, Robbins SL (eds): *Robbins Pathologic Basis of Disease*, 4th ed. Philadelphia, WB Saunders, 1989.
32. Shennan T: *Postmortems and Morbid Anatomy*, 3rd ed. Baltimore, William Wood, 1935.

BIBLIOGRAPHY

Beyreuther K, Schettler G: *Molecular Mechanisms of Aging*. Berlin, Springer-Verlag, 1990.
Cotran RS, Kumar V, Robbins SL (eds): *Robbins Pathologic Basis of Disease*, 4th ed. Philadelphia, WB Saunders, 1989.
Dillman VM: *The Neuroendocrine Theory of Aging and Degenerative Disease*. Pensacola, FL, Center for Bio-Gerontology, 1992.
Emerit I, Chance B: *Free Radicals and Aging*. Boston, Birkhauser Verlag, 1992.
Fabris N, Harman D, Knook DL, Steinhagen-Thiessen E, Zs-Nagy I: *Physiopathological Processes of Aging: Towards a Multicausal Interpretation*. New York, New York Academy of Sciences, 1992.
Mandell EL, Douglas RG Jr, Bennett JE: *Principles and Practice of Infectious Disease*, 3rd ed. New York, Churchill Livingstone, 1990.
Mettler FA Jr, Moseley RD Jr: *Medical Effects of Ionizing Radiation*. Orlando, Grune & Stratton, 1985.
National Institute of Aging/National Institute of Health: Bethesda, MD, National Institutes of Health, 1992.
Reichardt JK: Genetic basis of galactosemia. *Hum Mutat* 1992; 1(3):190–196.
Rubin E, Farber J: *Essential Pathology*. Philadelphia, JB Lippincott, 1990.
Singal PK: Oxygen-radicals in the pathophysiology of heart disease, in *Symposia on Oxygen-radicals in Heart Pathophysiology*, Winnepeg, Manitoba—1987. Boston, Kluwer Academic, 1988.
Warner H, Butler R, Sprott R, Schneider E: *Modern Biological Theories of Aging*. New York, Raven Press, 1987.
Welch WJ: Mammalian stress response: Cell physiology, structure/function of stress proteins, and implications for medicine and disease. *Physiol Rev* 1992;72(4):1063–1081.
Welch WJ, Kang HS, Beckmann RP, Mizzen LA: Response of mammalian cells to metabolic stress: Changes in cell physiology and structure/function of stress proteins. *Curr Top Microbiol Immunol* 1991;167:31–55.
Yang SS, Warner HR: *The Underlying Molecular, Cellular, and Immunological Factors in Cancer and Aging*. New York, Plenum Press, 1993.

CHAPTER 4
Genetic Control—Inheritance

JACQUELYN L. BANASIK

KEY TERMS

allele: One of two or more alternative forms of a gene located at the same site on homologous chromosomes.

autosome: Any ordinary paired chromosome, as distinguished from a sex chromosome.

chromosome: A linear thread of nuclear DNA that becomes visible under the microscope during cell mitosis.

exon: The portion of an RNA message that remains after unwanted sections have been removed from the primary transcript.

gene: A linear section of DNA that serves as a template for synthesis of a particular RNA sequence.

genotype: The genetic constitution of an individual, often described by listing the allele types at a certain gene locus.

heterochromatin: A type of chromatin (DNA) that is tightly compacted and genetically inactive.

intron: The portion of a primary RNA transcript that is removed prior to translation of the RNA message.

meiosis: A method of cell division which results in daughter cells with one half the normal number of chromosomes. Meiosis occurs in gonadal germ cells.

mitosis: A method of cell division which results in daughter cells with chromosomes which are identical to the parent cell. Mitosis occurs in somatic cells.

phenotype: The physical, biochemical, and biological makeup of an individual, expressed as recognizable traits.

transcription: The process by which a segment of DNA is used as a template to produce a complementary sequence of mRNA.

translation: The formation of a polypeptide chain in a sequence dictated by mRNA.

The science of genetics developed from the premise that invisible, information-containing elements, called **genes,** exist in cells and are passed on to daughter cells when a cell divides. The nature of these elements was at first difficult to imagine: what kind of molecule could direct the day-to-day activities of the organism and also be capable of nearly limitless replication? The answer to this question was discovered in the late 1940s and was almost unbelievable in its simplicity. It is now common knowledge that genetic information is stored in long chains of stable molecules called **deoxyribonucleic acid** (**DNA**). The information necessary to produce over 50,000 different proteins is encoded by only four different molecules. These are the deoxyribonucleotides containing the bases **adenine** (**A**), **cytosine** (**C**), **guanine** (**G**), and **thymine** (**T**). Genes are composed of varying sequences of these four **bases,** which are linked together by sugar-phosphate bonds. By serving as the templates for the production of body proteins, genes ultimately affect all aspects of an organism's structure and function. Some knowledge of the basic principles of genetics and inheritance is therefore prerequisite to understanding a variety of disease processes. This chapter examines the biochemistry of genetics (molecular genetics), concepts of regulation of gene expression, the processes of tissue differentiation, and the basic principles of inheritance.

Molecular Genetics

Structure of DNA

DNA carries genetic information in long unbranched polymers (chains) of nucleotides.[1] A nucleotide consists of a 5-carbon sugar (deoxyribose), a phosphate group, and one of the four nucleotide bases (Fig. 4–1). The nucleotide bases are divided into two types based on their chemical structure. The **pyrimidines,** cytosine and thymine, have single-ring structures. The **purines,** guanine and adenine, have double-ring structures (Fig. 4–2). DNA polymers are formed by the chemical linkage of these nucleotides. The linkages, called **phosphodiester bonds,** join the phosphate group on one sugar (attached to the 5' carbon) to the 3' carbon of the next sugar (see Fig. 4–1). The four kinds of bases (A C G T) are attached to the repeating sugar-phosphate chain as if they were four kinds of beads strung on a necklace. The bases of one strand of DNA form weak bonds with the bases of another strand of DNA. These noncovalent **hydrogen bonds** are specific and complementary (Fig. 4–3). The bases G and C bond together and the bases A and T bond together. Nucleotides that are able to bond together are called **base pairs.**

In the early 1950s, Watson and Crick proposed that the structure of DNA was a **double helix.**[2] In this model, DNA can be envisioned as a twisted ladder, with the sugar-phosphate bonds as the sides of the ladder and the bases forming the rungs (see Fig. 4–3).

SUGAR-PHOSPHATE BACKBONE OF DNA

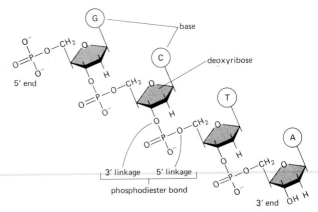

FIGURE 4–1. A nucleotide consists of a sugar (deoxyribose), a phosphate group, and one of the four nucleotide bases. Nucleotides are joined by repeating sugar-phosphate bonds to form long chains called polymers. (From Alberts B, et al (eds): *Molecular Biology of the Cell,* 2nd ed. New York, Garland Press, 1989, p 99. Reproduced with permission.)

The two strands of DNA must be complementary in order to form the double helix—that is, the bases of one strand must pair exactly with their complementary bases on the other strand. The discovery of the double helix model was profound, as it immediately suggested how information transfer could be accomplished by such simple molecules. Because each DNA strand carries a nucleotide sequence that is exactly complementary to the sequence of its partner, both strands can be used as **templates** to create an exact

FOUR BASES AS BASE PAIRS OF DNA

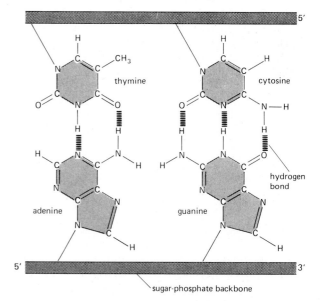

FIGURE 4–2. The two types of DNA bases are the single-ring pyrimidines and the double-ring purines. Thymine and cytosine are pyrimidines and adenine and guanine are purines. (From Alberts B, et al (eds): *Molecular Biology of the Cell,* 2nd ed. New York, Garland Press, 1989, p 99. Reproduced with permission.)

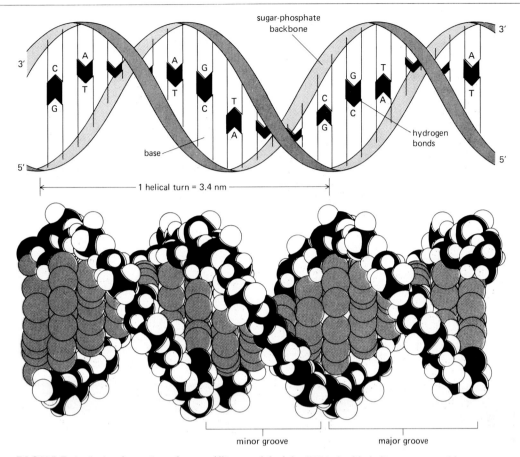

FIGURE 4–3. A schematic and space-filling model of the DNA double helix as proposed by Watson and Crick. The pairing of bases is specific and complementary: C always pairs with G, and A always pairs with T. (From Alberts B, et al (eds): *Molecular Biology of the Cell*, 2nd ed. New York, Garland Press, 1989, p 99. Reproduced with permission.)

copy of the original DNA double helix. When a cell divides to form two daughter cells, each daughter cell must receive a complete copy of all the parent cell's DNA. The process of DNA **replication** begins with separation of the DNA double helix by breaking the hydrogen bonds between the base pairs. Specific replication enzymes then direct the attachment of the correct (complementary) nucleotides to each of the single-stranded DNA templates. In this way two identical copies of the original DNA double helix are formed and passed on to the two daughter cells during cell division.

DNA Replication

Although the underlying principle of gene replication is simple, the cellular machinery required to carry out the replication process is complex, involving a host of enzymes and proteins.[3] This enzyme structure is often referred to as a "replication machine." The DNA double helix must first separate so that new nucleotides can be paired with the old DNA template strands. The DNA double helix is normally very stable: the base pairs are locked in place so tightly that they can withstand temperatures approaching the boiling point. Special enzymes called **DNA helicases**

are needed to rapidly unwind and separate the DNA strands, while **helix-destabilizing proteins** (also called single-strand DNA-binding proteins) bind to the exposed DNA strands to keep them apart until replication can be accomplished (Fig. 4–4).

Once a portion of the DNA double helix has been separated, special enzymes called **DNA polymerases** bind the single strands of DNA and begin the process of forming a new complementary strand of DNA. The polymerases match the appropriate base to the template base and catalyze the formation of the sugar-phosphate bonds that form the backbone of the DNA strand. Replication proceeds along the DNA strand in one direction only: from the 3' end toward the 5' end. The ends of the DNA strands are labeled 3' and 5' according to the exposed carbon atom at that end. DNA bases located in the 5' direction are "downstream"; those toward the 3' end are "upstream." Replication is semiconservative, as each of the two resulting DNA double helices contains one newly synthesized strand and one original (conserved) strand (Fig. 4–5). The polymerase also has an ability to proofread the new strand for errors in base pairing. If an error is detected, the enzyme will back up and remove the incorrect nucleotide and replace it with the correct one. The fidelity of copying during DNA replication

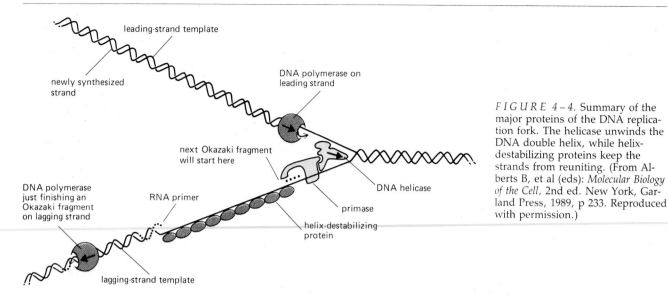

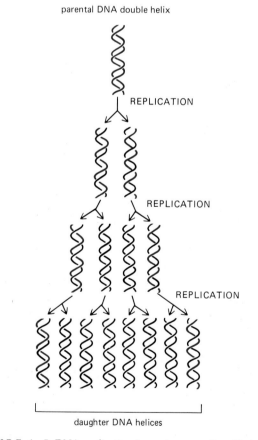

FIGURE 4–4. Summary of the major proteins of the DNA replication fork. The helicase unwinds the DNA double helix, while helix-destabilizing proteins keep the strands from reuniting. (From Alberts B, et al (eds): *Molecular Biology of the Cell,* 2nd ed. New York, Garland Press, 1989, p 233. Reproduced with permission.)

is such that only about one error is made for every 10^9 base pair replications.[4] The self-correcting function of the DNA polymerases is extremely important because errors in replication will be passed on to the next generation of cells.

Genetic Code

How do an organism's "genes" influence its structural and functional characteristics? The prevailing theory in biology holds that genes direct the synthesis of proteins and enzymes in cells. It is the presence (or absence) and relative activity of various structural proteins and enzymes that produce the characteristics of the cell. Proteins are composed of one or more chains of **amino acids** (polypeptides) that fold into complex three-dimensional structures. The body contains 20 different types of amino acids that join together in a particular sequence to form a particular protein (Table 4–1). Each type of protein has a unique sequence of amino acids that dictates its structure and activity.

If genes are to direct the synthesis of proteins, the information contained in just four kinds of DNA nucleotide bases must, in some way, code for 20 different amino acids.[5] This so-called **genetic code** was deciphered in the early 1960s.[6] It was determined that a series of three nucleotides (triplet) was needed to code for each of the 20 amino acids. Because there are four different bases, there are 4^3 or 64 different possible triplet combinations. This is far more than needed to code for the 20 known amino acids. Three of the nucleotide triplets or **codons** do not code for amino acids at all, and are called non-sense or **stop codons** because they signal the end of a protein code. The remaining 61 codons all code for one of the 20 amino acids (see Table 4–1). Obviously, some of the amino acids are specified by more than one codon. For example, the amino acid arginine is determined by six different codons. The code has been highly conserved during evolution and is essentially the same in organisms as diverse as humans and bacteria.

Several intermediate molecules are involved in the process of DNA-directed protein synthesis, including the complex protein-synthesizing machinery of the ribosomes and **ribonucleic acid (RNA)**. With few exceptions, the flow of information transfer is from DNA to RNA to protein. RNA is structurally similar to DNA

FIGURE 4–5. DNA replication is semiconservative. Each of the new DNA double helices contains one newly synthesized strand and one original strand. (From Alberts B, et al (eds): *Molecular Biology of the Cell,* 2nd ed. New York, Garland Press, 1989, p 100. Reproduced with permission.)

TABLE 4-1. RNA Codons for the Different Amino Acids and for Start and Stop

Amino Acid	RNA	Codons				
Alanine	GCU	GCC	GCA	GCG		
Arginine	CGU	CGC	CGA	CGG	AGA	AGG
Asparagine	AAU	AAC				
Aspartic acid	GAU	GAC				
Cysteine	UGU	UGC				
Glutamic acid	GAA	GAG				
Glutamine	CAA	CAG				
Glycine	GGU	GGC	GGA	GGG		
Histidine	CAU	CAC				
Isoleucine	AUU	AUC	AUA			
Leucine	CUU	CUC	CUA	CUG	UUA	UUG
Lysine	AAA	AAG				
Methionine	AUG					
Phenylalanine	UUU	UUC				
Proline	CCU	CCC	CCA	CCG		
Serine	UCU	UCC	UCA	UCG	AGC	AGU
Threonine	ACU	ACC	ACA	ACG		
Tryptophan	UGG					
Tyrosine	UAU	UAC				
Valine	GUU	GUC	GUA	GUG		
Start (CI)	AUG					
Stop (CT)	UAA	UAG	UGA			

From Guyton AC: *Textbook of Medical Physiology*, 8th ed. Philadelphia, WB Saunders, 1991, p 27. Reproduced with permission.

except that the sugar molecule is ribose rather than deoxyribose, and one of the four bases is different: **uracil** replaces thymine. Because of the biochemical similarity of uracil and thymine, both are able to form base pairs with adenine.

Several functionally different types of RNA are involved in protein synthesis. **Ribosomal RNA (rRNA)** is found associated with the ribosome (see Chap. 2) in the cell cytoplasm. **Messenger RNA (mRNA)** is synthesized from the DNA template in a process termed **transcription** and carries the protein code to the cytoplasm where the proteins are manufactured. The amino acids that will be joined together to form proteins are carried in the cytoplasm by the third type of RNA, **transfer RNA (tRNA)**, which interacts with mRNA and the ribosome in a process termed **translation.** In addition to the usual four RNA bases, tRNA also contains over 30 different modified bases such as inosine and ribothymidine. The function of these unusual bases is not presently understood.

Transcription

Transcription is the process whereby mRNA is synthesized from a single-stranded DNA template.[7] The process is similar to DNA replication. Double-stranded DNA must be separated in the region of the gene to be copied, and specific enzyme complexes (**RNA polymerases**) orchestrate the production of the mRNA polymer. Only one of the DNA strands contains the desired gene sequence and serves as the template for the synthesis of mRNA. This strand is called the *sense strand.* The other strand is termed the

non-sense or *anti-sense strand* and is not transcribed into an RNA message.

Some genes are continuously active in certain cells, while others are carefully regulated in response to cellular needs and environmental signals. Special sequences of DNA near a desired gene may enhance or inhibit its rate of transcription. In general, a gene is transcribed when the RNA polymerase-enzyme complex binds to a **promoter** region near the start of the gene. The RNA polymerase directs the separation of the DNA double helix and catalyzes the synthesis of the RNA message by matching the appropriate RNA bases to the DNA template (Fig. 4–6). The RNA message is directly complementary to the DNA sequence except that uracil replaces thymine.

In higher organisms, the DNA template for a particular protein is littered with stretches of bases that must be removed from the RNA message before it can be translated into a protein. These unwanted areas, called **introns,** are removed in the nucleus by a complex splicing process, resulting in an RNA message that contains only the wanted segments, called **exons.** Introns range from 65 to 100,000 nucleotides in length. A single gene may contain as many as 50 of them.[8] The function of introns remains largely a mystery, although they are believed to be important in the evolution of new genetic information and in the regulation of gene activity during embryonic development. The removal and splicing of the RNA message is mediated by a group of small RNA-protein complexes located in the nucleus. These so-called **snurps,** or **small nuclear ribonucleoproteins,** attach to the native mRNA, making it too large to escape the nuclear envelope until all of the necessary splicing has been accomplished.[8]

The processed mRNA is finally transported to the cell cytoplasm, where it directs the synthesis of a protein in cooperation with tRNA and the ribosomes. Each mRNA may serve as a template for thousands of copies of protein before it is degraded.

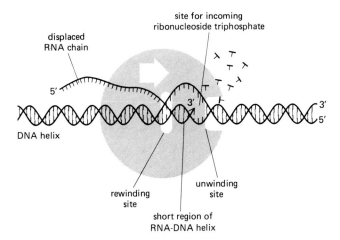

FIGURE 4–6. A moving RNA polymerase complex unwinds the DNA helix ahead of it while rewinding the DNA behind. One strand of the DNA serves as the template for the formation of mRNA. (From Alberts B, et al (eds): *Molecular Biology of the Cell,* 2nd ed. New York, Garland Press, 1989, p 204. Reproduced with permission.)

Translation

Translation is the process whereby the RNA message is used to direct the synthesis of a protein. The mRNA is read in linear fashion from one end to the other, with each set of three nucleotides serving as a codon for a particular amino acid. The codons in the mRNA do not directly recognize the amino acids. Intermediary molecules or "translators" are required. These intermediaries are the transfer RNA molecules. A tRNA molecule resembles the letter L, with a codon reading area at one end (the **anticodon**) and an amino acid attachment at the other (Fig. 4–7). Recognition of the codon is accomplished by the same complementary base pairing as was described for DNA. The complex machinery of the ribosome is needed to line up the tRNA on the mRNA and to catalyze the peptide bonds that hold the amino acids together. **Ribosomes** are large complexes of protein and RNA. Each ribosome is composed of two subunits. The smaller subunit binds the mRNA and the tRNA, while the larger subunit catalyzes the formation of peptide bonds between the incoming amino acids.[9] The ribosome must first find the appropriate starting place on the mRNA to set the correct reading frame for the codon triplets. Then the ribosome moves along the mRNA, translating the nucleotide sequence into an amino acid sequence, one codon at a time (Fig. 4–8). The newly synthesized protein chain is released from the ribosome when a "stop codon" signaling the end of the message is reached.

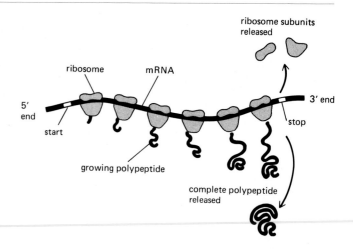

FIGURE 4–8. Synthesis of a protein by the ribosomes attached to an mRNA molecule. Ribosomes attach near the start and catalyze the formation of the peptide chain. (From Alberts B, et al (eds): *Molecular Biology of the Cell*, 2nd ed. New York, Garland Press, 1989, p 104. Reproduced with permission.)

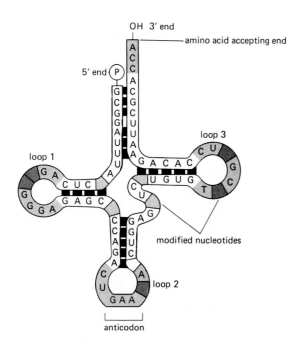

FIGURE 4–7. A schematic drawing of a transfer RNA. Each transfer RNA binds a specific amino acid which corresponds with the three-base sequence at the anticodon end. (From Alberts B, et al (eds): *Molecular Biology of the Cell*, 2nd ed. New York, Garland Press, 1989, p 206. Reproduced with permission.)

KEY CONCEPTS

- The structure of DNA can be envisioned as a twisted ladder, with the sugar-phosphate bonds as the sides of the ladder and the four nucleotide bases (adenosine, cytosine, guanine, and thymine) forming the rungs. The nucleotides form complementary base pairs, C with G and A with T.

- The DNA double helix must separate into single strands to provide a template for synthesizing new, identical DNA strands that can be passed on to daughter cells during cell division. DNA replication is accomplished by the enzyme complex, DNA polymerase.

- A linear sequence of DNA that codes for a particular protein is called a gene. During transcription, genes provide a template for the synthesis of mRNA by the enzyme complex, RNA polymerase.

- After appropriate cutting and splicing of the RNA transcript, the mRNA is translated into a protein. Each nucleotide triplet (codon) in the mRNA codes for a particular amino acid. Protein synthesis is accomplished by ribosomes, which match the mRNA codon with the correct tRNA and then catalyze the peptide bond to link amino acids together into a linear protein.

Regulation of Gene Expression

The **genome** contains all the genetic information of the cell and ultimately determines its form and function. Because all the cells of a particular cell type in a multicellular organism contain the same DNA, some of the cellular DNA must be actively transcribed while other genes remain quiescent. In addition, the cell must be able to change the expression of certain genes in order to respond and adapt to changes in the cellular environment. Some basic principles about the mechanisms that control gene expression are beginning to emerge, but much remains to be determined. There is evidence that gene expression can be regulated at each of the steps in the pathway from DNA to RNA to protein synthesis.[10] The proteins made by a cell can be controlled in the following ways: (1) regulating the rate and timing of gene transcription; (2) controlling how the mRNA is spliced; (3) selecting which mRNAs are transported to the cytoplasm; (4) selecting which mRNAs are translated by ribosomes; (5) selectively destroying certain mRNAs in the cytoplasm; or (6) selectively controlling the activity of the proteins after they have been produced.[10]

For most genes, the most important regulators of gene expression are the transcriptional controls. Animal cells contain DNA-binding proteins that are able to enhance or inhibit gene expression. These **gene regulatory proteins** recognize and bind only particular DNA sequences and thus are specific to the genes they regulate.[11] A cell contains many gene regulatory proteins, each of which works in combination with others to control numerous other genes. Additionally, there appear to be master gene regulatory proteins that have decisive control over the cell's structure and function. Disruption of a master regulatory protein may result in dramatic alterations in cellular development. For example, the absence of a single master regulatory protein in humans (the testosterone receptor) causes a male genotype (XY) to develop as an almost perfect female.

Transcriptional Controls

The gene regulatory proteins described in the preceding paragraphs are thought to control gene transcription by binding near the promoter sequence of DNA, where the RNA polymerase must attach to initiate transcription of the gene.[12] Binding of the regulatory protein may either enhance or inhibit RNA polymerase binding and subsequent transcription of the gene. This is sometimes referred to as "turning on" or "turning off" a gene. Gene regulatory mechanisms are best characterized in bacteria, particularly *E. coli*. Similar regulatory strategies have been demonstrated in eucaryotic cells as well. One of the first regulatory systems to be elucidated explained the ability of *E. coli* to alter its metabolic enzymes in response to a change in its nutrient supply. This example of gene regulation will be briefly described as a general model for transcriptional regulation.

E. coli growing in a mixture of glucose and lactose preferentially uses up all of the glucose before beginning to metabolize the lactose. The switch to lactose utilization is accompanied by the appearance of an enzyme that breaks down lactose (β-galactosidase). The appearance of this enzyme indicates that the gene coding for the enzyme has been activated, or "turned on." But how does the genome "know" that the glucose has been depleted and that it now needs to me-

tabolize lactose? In 1959, it was determined that the gene for the lactose-metabolizing enzyme is usually repressed or turned off in *E. coli*, and soon after that, the **lactose repressor protein** was identified.[13] The lactose repressor protein binds near the promoter region for the lactose enzyme and prevents the RNA polymerase from beginning transcription. However, when lactose (allolactose) is present in the cell, it binds the repressor protein, changing its shape and causing it to lose its grip on the DNA promoter area. In this way, lactose removes the inhibitor protein and allows the lactose-metabolizing enzyme to be transcribed only when lactose is present.

This is a form of **negative regulation,** in which the gene regulatory protein inhibits transcription. There are also examples of **positive regulation** by **gene activator proteins.** Even when the DNA promoter regions are not being actively inhibited by repressor proteins, they may be too weak to initiate transcription. In this case, a gene activator protein may be used to enhance the rate of transcription. This is true for the lactose-metabolizing gene just described, which needs an activator protein called **CAP (catabolite activator protein)** in order to be turned on. The activity of CAP in the cell is regulated by glucose. When glucose levels are high, CAP is unable to bind the lactose enzyme gene. As glucose levels fall, CAP is available to bind the promoter, and the lactose-metabolizing enzyme is transcribed. In this way the bacteria are able to respond to changes in the environment by altering gene transcription.

This example is a simple model of the ways in which gene regulatory proteins are thought to function. In higher organisms, the strategies for gene regulation are more complex. Gene regulatory proteins often bind DNA segments far from the gene being regulated. A variety of controls may be used to regulate the activity of gene regulatory proteins. Most higher eucaryotic genes appear to be regulated by nearby promoters *and* distant enhancers: the binding of several gene regulatory proteins in combination is often necessary.

KEY CONCEPTS

- All the cells in an individual have essentially the same DNA; however, cells differ greatly in structure and function. This occurs because genes are selectively expressed in particular cells.

- Gene expression can be regulated at any step in the pathway from DNA to RNA to protein synthesis. The most important regulators are transcriptional controls.

- Transcription is controlled by a large number of proteins that specifically bind to DNA. The presence of certain DNA-binding proteins at specific sites can enhance or inhibit the transcription of a particular gene.

Differentiation of Tissues

Cell Diversification and Cell Memory

The cells of a multicellular organism tend to specialize to perform particular functions in coordination with other cells and tissues of the body. Cells must not only become different during development, they must also remain different in the adult, after the original cues for cell diversification have disappeared. The differences among cell types are ultimately due to the differentiating influences experienced in the embryo. Differences are maintained because the cells somehow remember the effects of those past influences and pass the memory on to their descendants. When a skin cell divides to replace lost skin cells, the daughter cells are also skin cells; when a liver cell divides, its daughter cells are liver cells, and so on. The behavior of cells of higher organisms is governed not only by their genome and their present environment, but also by their developmental history.

There is substantial evidence that the differences in tissue structure and function in a particular organism are not due to deletions or additions to the genome.[14] All the cells of an organism contain the same genes. There appear to be about 30,000 genes that are expressed in nearly all cell types, the so-called **housekeeping genes** that code for proteins essential for cell viability. It is the expression of a relatively few number of **tissue-specific genes** that results in differences among cell types.[12] The exact mechanisms leading to the stable expression of tissue-specific genes in particular cells are unknown; however, differences in DNA packaging may be involved. It is apparent that in order for a gene to be expressed, it must be accessible to the transcriptional machinery of the nucleus. The DNA in human cells is extensively packaged, so that 40 inches of linear DNA can be compacted to fit into the cell nucleus. The DNA double helix is first wound around special protein complexes called **histones** and then further twisted into coils and supercoils (Fig. 4–9).

Some regions of DNA, called **heterochromatin,** are so condensed that they are never open to transcription. These regions of heterochromatin are common among all the organism's cell types. Other areas of DNA that are condensed in a manner similar to heterochromatin have been noted to differ in various cell types. Embryonic cells have very little of this condensed DNA, called **facultative heterochromatin,** whereas highly specialized cells have a great deal. This suggests that as a cell develops into a highly differentiated form, more and more of its cellular genes are inactivated because they are packaged in a condensed form that is resistant to transcription. This condensed packaging is apparently passed on to the progeny cells, thus creating a sort of cell memory.

An example of this mechanism is the inactivation of one of the X chromosomes in females.[15] In mammals, all female cells contain two X chromosomes (XX), whereas male cells contain an X chromosome and a Y chromosome (XY). One of the X chromosomes

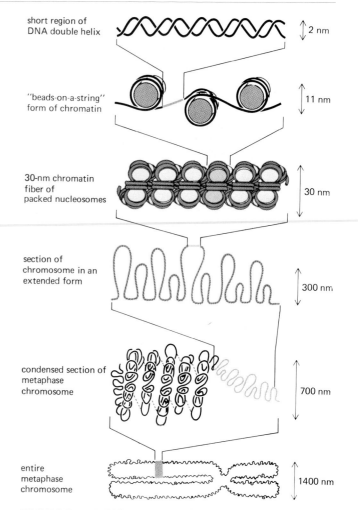

short region of DNA double helix — 2 nm

"beads-on-a-string" form of chromatin — 11 nm

30-nm chromatin fiber of packed nucleosomes — 30 nm

section of chromosome in an extended form — 300 nm

condensed section of metaphase chromosome — 700 nm

entire metaphase chromosome — 1400 nm

F I G U R E   4 – 9. DNA is extensively packaged by wrapping around protein complexes called histones and then coiled extensively to form a condensed package. (From Alberts B, et al (eds): *Molecular Biology of the Cell,* 2nd ed. New York, Garland Press, 1989, p 504. Reproduced with permission.)

in females is permanently inactivated early in development by packaging as facultative heterochromatin. This apparently occurs to prevent a double dose of the X gene products. Which of the two X chromosomes is inactivated in a particular cell is a random event. However, the same X chromosome will be inactive in all of the cell's progeny. The pattern of inactivated genes in a particular cell type is "remembered" in subsequent generations of cells and may explain how differentiated tissues remain differentiated in the adult.

Mechanisms of Development

Despite recent advances in developmental biology, many details of human development and tissue differentiation remain a mystery. Several strategies have been proposed to explain the process of cell diversification during embryonic development, but no comprehensive theory has yet emerged. Three of these strategies—cell-to-cell interactions, chemical gradients, and the extracellular matrix—are described below.

After fertilization, the mammalian egg begins a series of divisions to become a cluster of cells. Until the eight-cell stage, these cells are identical and may be rearranged or even separated (as in the case of identical twins) without interfering with the development of the individual. Soon after, however, the cells begin to show differences. These early differences are a result of the **cell-to-cell contacts** in the cell cluster. The region of the cell surface that is in contact with other cells remains smooth, whereas free cell membrane develops projections called microvilli. The cell also rearranges its internal components in an asymmetric way, such that the next cell division results in two daughter cells that are no longer identical (Fig. 4–10). Experiments have shown that it is the cell-to-cell contacts that govern the asymmetric distribution of cells.[16] The fate of each cell continues to be governed by interactions with neighboring cells throughout the early stages of development. This strategy is highly regulative, since there is continuous communication back and forth between groups of cells. The nature of these cell-to-cell communication signals is largely unknown.

Cells in the developing embryo must have information about their location with regard to other cells in order to behave appropriately. The future head must be distinguished from the tail, the front from the back, and so forth. One mechanism for transmitting this information is the creation of **chemical gradients.**[17] A particular area is specialized to be the source of the chemical—for example, the head region. The chemical will be progressively degraded as it diffuses through the neighboring tissue, such that the chemical will have a higher concentration close to the source. Because the concentration of the chemical progressively decreases with increasing distance from the source, a particular cell will have information regarding its proximity to the head region based on the surrounding concentration of the chemical. Chemicals that control the patterning of fields of nearby tissue in this way are termed **morphogens.** Morphogens are thought to be effective only over small distances. Thus the gross distinctions—between head and tail, for example—must be made very early in the embryo, and therefore morphogens can provide only a general pattern for future development. Successive levels of detail can be filled in later by other positional signals. This strategy requires that cells "remember" earlier signals even after they are no longer exposed to the original morphogens.

The organization of molecules surrounding the cell surface also provides positional information. The **extracellular matrix** is composed of a large meshwork of molecules that is produced locally by cells in the area. Some common components include the proteins collagen and elastin, long polysaccharide chains called glycosaminoglycans, and a variety of peptides, growth factors, and hormones. The extracellular matrix is highly organized, with components binding to each other and to the cell membrane in specific ways. The extracellular matrix is thought to be important in cell development through its ability to screen or modulate the transport of molecules such as growth factors to the cell membrane, and through direct contacts with the cell membrane that bring about changes in cell structure and function.[18] The term *dynamic reciprocity* has been used to describe the continuous interaction between the cell and its extracellular matrix. The cell produces, structures, and restructures the extracellular matrix, which in turn influences the cell's structure, biochemistry, and gene expression. There appears to be continuous crosstalk between the cell and its extracellular matrix that is important for appropriate cellular growth and differentiation.

The extracellular matrix surrounding the cells in different locations may provide positional information to other cells that must migrate to their final destination.[18] In vertebrates, connective tissue cells appear to provide most of this positional information. As the migratory cell travels through the connective tissue, it may continually "test" the surroundings, searching for cues to guide it. Migratory cells with specific cell surface receptors may interact differentially with the extracellular matrix in different areas. In this way the migratory cell can be guided along particular paths and induced to settle in particular areas. Once the migratory cell has settled, local extracellular matrix molecules may further affect the cell's growth rate, differentiation, and likelihood of survival. The molecular details of these mechanisms are not known.

The steps leading to the development of differentiated tissues in a multicellular organism are such that once differentiated, a cell type generally cannot revert back to earlier forms. Some tissues are said to be **terminally differentiated** and have no capacity to change form. Other tissues maintain less differentiated **stem cells** that are able to develop into a variety of cell types, depending on environmental cues. Highly differentiated cells usually lose the capacity to divide

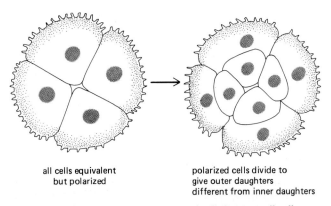

all cells equivalent
but polarized

polarized cells divide to
give outer daughters
different from inner daughters

FIGURE 4–10. In the early stages of cell division, all cells are equivalent. Surface contact with other cells in the group results in asymmetric distribution of cell contents. The next cell division results in daughter cells that are no longer identical. (From Alberts B, et al (eds): *Molecular Biology of the Cell,* 2nd ed. New York, Garland Press, 1989, p 897. Reproduced with permission.)

and thus cannot be replaced when they are lost to disease or injury.

Differentiated Tissues

The over 200 different cell types in the adult human are generally classified into four major categories: epithelium, connective tissue, muscle, and nerve. These tissue types with some of their subtypes are summarized in Table 4–2. Most of the organ systems of the body are combinations of these four tissue types mixed together in a highly organized and cooperative manner.

Epithelial Tissue

Epithelial cells cover the majority of the external surfaces of the body and line the glands, blood vessels, and internal surfaces.[19] Epithelial cells adopt a variety of shapes and functions, depending on their locations. The **stratified epithelium** that makes up the epidermis of the skin, for example, is several layers thick and is primarily protective in function. New epithelial skin cells are formed in the deepest part of the epidermis, where it contacts the basal lamina. As cells mature, they move outward toward the surface until they be-

come keratinized and finally flake away (Fig. 4–11). Keratin is a tough protective protein present in large quantities in the outer skin layers of flattened, dead epithelial cells.

In addition to stratified epithelium, the epithelium may be characterized as simple or pseudostratified, according to the number and arrangement of cell layers (Fig. 4–12). **Simple epithelium** consists of a single layer of cells, all of which contact the basement membrane. Simple epithelium is found in the lining of blood vessels and body cavities, in many glands, and in the alveoli of the lungs. The simple epithelium that lines the blood vessels is called **endothelium.** Simple epithelium also forms the kidney tubules and lines the intestine, where absorption is its primary function. **Stratified epithelium** consists of two or more layers of epithelial cells and is found in mucous membranes, such as the mouth, and in the skin, as mentioned above. Epithelium that appears to be more than one layer thick because of a mixture of cell shapes, but is actually a single layer, is called **pseudostratified epithelium.** The linings of the respiratory tract and some glands contain pseudostratified epithelium.

Epithelial cells may also be classified according to cell shape. The three basic cell shapes are squamous, cuboidal, and columnar. **Squamous** cells are thin in comparison to their surface area and have a flattened appearance. **Cuboidal** cells are approximately equal in width and height, similar to a cube. **Columnar** cells are a bit taller than they are wide, resembling a rectangular column. Several classifications of epithelial tissue are given in Table 4–2 using both shape and layering as criteria.

Connective Tissue

Connective tissue is the most abundant and diverse tissue in the body, including cell types as different as bone, fat cells, and blood cells.[20] Connective tissue commonly functions as a scaffold on which other cells cluster to form organs, but it does much more than hold tissues together. Connective tissue cells often form an elaborate extracellular matrix which is thought to be important in the maintenance of cell differentiation (Fig. 4–13). Connective tissue cells play an important part in the support and repair of nearly every tissue and organ in the body. Three major classifications of connective tissue are commonly identified: loose connective tissue, dense or supportive tissue, and hematopoietic tissue.

Loose connective tissue appears unstructured, with a fair amount of space between fibers of the extracellular matrix. The matrix contains a number of cell types and an elaborate meshwork of protein and other molecules (Fig. 4–14). The primary protein constituents are collagen, elastin, and reticular fibers. Collagen is composed of tough, nonelastic bundles of protein fibers that are secreted by fibroblasts. It gives structural strength to skin, tendons, ligaments, and other tissues. The ability of a structure to withstand deforming and stretching forces is due, in large part,

T A B L E 4–2. Major Categories and Locations of Body Tissues

Tissue Type	Locations
Epithelium	
Simple squamous	Lining of blood vessels, pulmonary alveoli, Bowman's capsule
Simple cuboidal	Thyroid, sweat, and salivary glands; kidney tubules
Simple columnar	Lining of intestine, glandular ducts
Pseudostratified (mixed cell shapes)	Male urethra, respiratory passages
Stratified squamous	Skin, mucous membranes
Stratified columnar	Epiglottis, anus, parts of pharynx
Stratified transitional (layers of different cell shapes)	Bladder
Connective Tissue	
Loose	Widespread locations, dermis of skin, adipose tissue, organs
Dense/supportive	Cartilage, bone, tendons, joints, fascia surrounding muscles
Hematopoietic	Bone marrow, lymph tissue, plasma
Muscle	
Skeletal	Voluntary muscles of the body
Cardiac	Heart (myocardium)
Smooth	Intestine, blood vessels, bladder, uterus, airways
Myoepithelial	Mammary, sweat, and salivary glands
Nervous	
Neurons	Central and peripheral nerves
Neuroglia	Primarily central nervous system

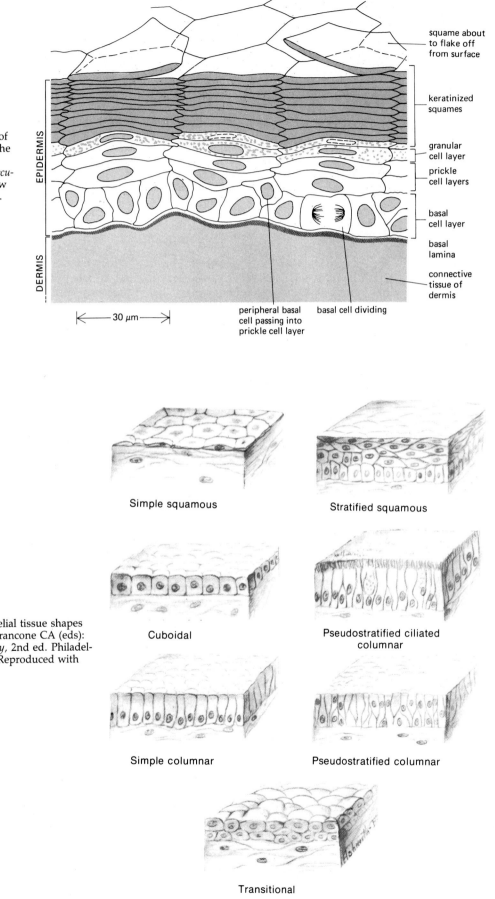

squame about to flake off from surface

keratinized squames

granular cell layer

prickle cell layers

basal cell layer

basal lamina

connective tissue of dermis

EPIDERMIS

DERMIS

|← 30 μm →|

peripheral basal cell passing into prickle cell layer

basal cell dividing

FIGURE 4–11. Organization of epidermal skin layers, showing the flattened keratinized outer layer. (From Alberts B, et al (eds): *Molecular Biology of the Cell*, 2nd ed. New York, Garland Press, 1989, p 970. Reproduced with permission.)

Simple squamous

Stratified squamous

Cuboidal

Pseudostratified ciliated columnar

Simple columnar

Pseudostratified columnar

Transitional

FIGURE 4–12. Various epithelial tissue shapes and layering. (From Jacob SW, Francone CA (eds): *Elements of Anatomy and Physiology*, 2nd ed. Philadelphia, WB Saunders, 1989, p 34. Reproduced with permission.)

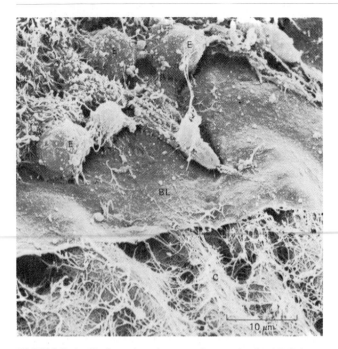

F I G U R E 4 – 13. Scanning electron micrograph of epithelial cells (*E*) attached to the basal lamina (*BL*) in the cornea of a chick embryo. Note the underlying network of loose connective tissue (*C*). (From Alberts B, et al (eds): *Molecular Biology of the Cell,* 2nd ed. New York, Garland Press, 1989, p 819. Micrograph courtesy of Robert Trelstad. Reproduced with permission.)

to elastin, which is able to return to its original length after being pulled, in the manner of a rubber band. Elastin is important to the function of structures such as the aorta, which must expand to accept the blood ejected from the heart during systole and bounce back to its original shape during diastole. Reticular fibers are short branching fibers that provide networks for

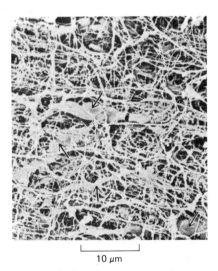

F I G U R E 4 – 14. Scanning electron micrograph of fibroblasts (*arrows*) in the connective tissue of a chick embryo cornea. The matrix is composed primarily of collagen fibers. (From Alberts B, et al (eds): *Molecular Biology of the Cell,* 2nd ed. New York, Garland Press, 1989, p 803. Micrograph courtesy of Robert Trelstad. Reproduced with permission.)

the attachment of connective tissue to other cell types, such as epithelial cell attachments in glands, hematopoietic cells in bone marrow, and the parenchymal cells (functional cells) in organs. Cell types associated with loose connective tissue include the fibroblasts, mast cells, and adipocytes (fat cells).

Dense or supportive connective tissue is rich in collagen, which gives strength to structures such as cartilage, tendon, bone, and ligaments. The collagen fibers are more organized and densely packed than in loose connective tissue. Cartilage cells or chondrocytes may be found in the trachea, joints, nose, ears, vertebral disks, organs, and the young skeleton. Once formed, the collagenous extracellular matrix structures need little maintenance and do not receive a blood supply. Bone is a very dense form of connective tissue composed of a mixture of tough collagen fibers and solid calcium phosphate crystals in approximately equal proportions. Throughout the bone's hard extracellular matrix are channels and cavities occupied by living cells (osteocytes) (Fig. 4–15). These cells incessantly model and remodel their bony environment, responding to unknown signals. These osteocytes are of two kinds: the cells that erode old bone are called **osteoclasts,** while the cells that form new bone are called **osteoblasts.** Osteoblasts somehow "know" when a bone is subjected to a greater load stress and will adapt by strengthening the bone mass. Conversely, when the load is removed, as during bed rest, the osteoclasts busily digest the bone away, often resulting in some of the common complications of immobility. Osteocyte activity is essential, however, for bone growth and the repair of bone injuries. (See Chapter 49 for a detailed description of the musculoskeletal system.)

The blood-forming organs of the body are formed by a specialized type of connective tissue called **hematopoietic tissue.** The blood cells include the red cell, or **erythrocyte,** which is specialized for the transport of oxygen; the platelet, or **thrombocyte,** which is important in blood coagulation; and a host of white cells, or **leukocytes,** which mediate immune function. Blood-forming tissue is located in the bone marrow, spleen, and lymphatic tissue. Hematopoietic cells are necessarily nomadic, traveling to distant areas of the body, sometimes settling in a particular organ, sometimes continuously moving (Fig. 4–16). Blood cells have a short life span in comparison to other cells and must continually be replenished. This is accomplished by the hematopoietic stem cells. Stem cells reside primarily in the bone marrow and are pluripotent; they may differentiate into any of the blood cell types. This results in a system that is able to respond quickly to the changing needs of the body.

Muscle Tissue

The term *muscle* refers to tissues that are specialized for contraction. Muscle cells, or **myocytes,** are usually long and thin and packed with the proteins **actin** and **myosin,** which make up the contractile apparatus.[21]

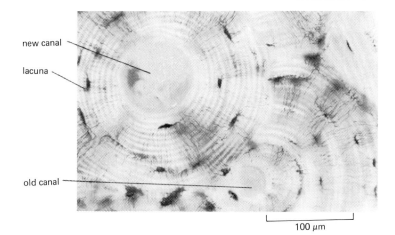

F I G U R E 4 – 15. Photomicrograph of a section of compact bone showing circular networks formed by the action of osteoclasts and osteoblasts as they remodel the bone. The osteocytes occupy the lacunae and canals. (From Alberts B, et al (eds): *Molecular Biology of the Cell,* 2nd ed. New York, Garland Press, 1989, p 993. Reproduced with permission.)

In mammals, there are four main categories of muscle cells: skeletal, cardiac, smooth, and myoepithelial (Fig. 4–17).[22] Contraction in all four types depends on intracellular calcium and occurs because of interactions between actin and myosin filaments. Actin and myosin filaments differ among cell types with regard to amino acid sequence, arrangement within the cell, and the mechanisms that control contraction. The mechanism of muscle contraction has been called the **sliding filament hypothesis** or **crossbridge theory.** These terms describe the interactions of the actin and myosin filaments as they form bonds and pull past each other, causing the muscle cell to shorten. Contraction is initiated by an increase in intracellular free calcium and requires energy in the form of ATP.

Skeletal muscle is responsible for nearly all voluntary movements. Skeletal muscle cells can be huge, up to a half meter in length, and are often referred to as muscle fibers because of their long, thin shape. The actin and myosin proteins in skeletal muscle are aligned in orderly arrays, giving the tissue a striped appearance under the microscope, which in turn has

led to the term, **striated muscle.** Skeletal muscle contracts in response to stimulation from the motor neurons of the nervous system. As in other types of muscle, stimulation results in an increase in free calcium within the cell. In skeletal muscle, the calcium comes from internal storage sites in the sarcoplasmic reticulum. Contraction is initiated when the calcium binds **troponin,** a regulatory protein attached to the actin filament. Because of the high energy requirements of contracting skeletal muscle, the cells are packed with energy-producing mitochondria.

Like skeletal muscle, **cardiac muscle** also has a striated appearance due to the systematic organization of its actin and myosin filaments. Cardiac muscle cells are linked by special structures called *intercalated disks* that cause the tissue to behave as a **syncytium:** all the cells contract synchronously. Cardiac muscle contracts in response to autonomic innervation and blood-borne chemicals, but it also has the special property of automaticity. **Automaticity** refers to the inherent ability of the cell to initiate a contraction without outside stimulation. The contractile mechanisms of cardiac muscle are similar to those of skeletal muscle, requiring free calcium to interact with troponin, resulting in the formation of actin-myosin crossbridges. In cardiac muscle, some of the free calcium comes from the sarcoplasmic reticulum, but diffusion into the cell through channels in the cell membrane is also necessary. These membrane calcium channels represent an important difference from skeletal muscle, as they can be manipulated by drugs (calcium channel blockers) without disrupting skeletal muscle control. Unfortunately, cardiac muscle cells are unable to replicate, so any damage results in permanent loss of tissue. (Cardiac muscle is discussed in Chapter 16.)

Smooth muscle comprises a diverse group of tissues located in organs throughout the body. Smooth muscle generally is not under voluntary control and therefore is called *involuntary muscle.* Some types of smooth muscle are able to contract intrinsically, and most are influenced by the autonomic nervous system. Smooth muscle is found in blood vessels and in the walls of hollow organs such as the gastrointestinal tract, uterus, and large airways.

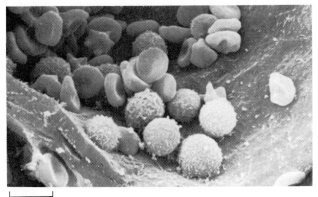

F I G U R E 4 – 16. Scanning electron micrograph of red and white blood cells in the lumen of a blood vessel. Red cells are smooth and concave, while white cells are rough and rounded. (From Kessel RG, Kardon RH: *Tissues and Organs: A Text-Atlas of Scanning Electron Microscopy.* San Francisco, WH Freeman and Co, 1979, p 37. Copyright © 1979 by WH Freeman and Co. Reproduced with permission.)

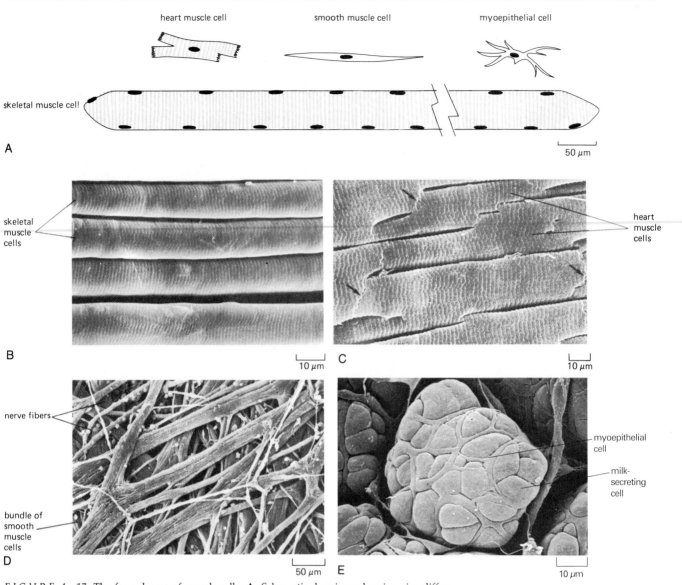

FIGURE 4–17. The four classes of muscle cells. **A**, Schematic drawings showing size differences among muscle types. **B**, Skeletal muscle. **C**, Heart muscle. **D**, Smooth muscle (bladder). **E**, Myoepithelial cells in a mammary gland. (**A**, **B**, and **D** from Alberts B, et al (eds): *Molecular Biology of the Cell*, 2nd ed. New York, Garland Press, 1989, p 984. **B** courtesy of Junzo Deskati. **C** from Fujiwara T: Cardiac muscle, in Canal ED (ed): *Handbook of Microscopic Anatomy*. Berlin, Springer-Verlag, 1986. **D** courtesy of Satoshi Nakasiro. **E** from Nagato T, Yoshida Y, Yoshida A, Uehara Y: *Cell Tissue Res* 1980;209:1–10. Reproduced with permission.)

The structure of smooth muscle differs considerably from that of skeletal and cardiac muscle. The actin and myosin filaments are less organized in smooth muscle, and the muscle does not have striations. Smooth muscle contraction tends to be slower and can be maintained indefinitely. This is critical to the function of blood vessels, which must maintain a degree of contraction or vascular tone to maintain the blood pressure. Smooth muscle differs in the way actin-myosin crossbridges are formed and in the calcium-binding regulatory proteins. When **calmodulin,** the calcium-binding protein in smooth muscle, binds calcium, it stimulates the rate of crossbridge formation by myosin. Smooth muscle contraction is highly de-

pendent on the diffusion of extracellular calcium into the cell through calcium channels in the plasma membrane (sarcolemma). Thus, like cardiac muscle, smooth muscle can also be affected by drugs that alter the calcium channel's ability to conduct calcium. For example, calcium channel–blocking drugs are used to cause the smooth muscle in arterial blood vessels to relax as a treatment for high blood pressure.

Myoepithelial cells represent the fourth class of muscle cells. They are located in the ducts of some glands such as the mammary, sweat, and salivary glands. Unlike all other types of muscle, myoepithelial cells lie in the epithelium and are derived from embryonic ectoderm. Myoepithelial cells contract in response to specific stimuli (e.g., oxytocin in the mammary gland) and serve to expel the contents from the gland.

Nervous Tissue

Nervous tissue is widely distributed throughout the body, providing a rapid communication network between the central nervous system and various body parts. Nerve cells are specialized to generate and transmit electrical impulses very rapidly. Like muscle, nerves are excitable: they respond to stimulation by altering their electrical potentials. This excitability is due to the presence of voltage-sensitive ion channels located in the plasma membrane of the nerve cell. Movement of ions through these channels results in the production and propagation of **action potentials** along the length of the neuron. Neurons communicate their action potentials to other nerve and muscle cells through **synapses.** At the synapse, the presynaptic neuron releases a chemical neurotransmitter into the space between itself and the next neuron, where it diffuses across and interacts with the postsynaptic neuron.

A typical neuron is composed of three parts: a cell body, an axon, and one or more dendrites (Fig. 4–18). The **cell body** contains the nucleus and other cytoplasmic organelles. The **axon** is generally long (as long as 1 meter) and may be encased in a myelin sheath. The axons usually conduct impulses away from the cell body, whereas the **dendritic processes** usually receive information and conduct impulses toward the cell body. Neurons are classified on the basis of the number of projections extending from the cell body. Neurons, like cardiac muscle cells, are permanent and unable to replicate. However, under certain favorable conditions a partially injured neuron may be able to regenerate.

In addition to neurons, nervous tissue contains a variety of supportive cells termed **neuroglia** ("nerve glue") that nourish, protect, insulate, and clean up debris in the central nervous system. These include the astrocytes, oligodendrioglia, ependymal cells, and microglia. (See Chapter 42 for a detailed description of nervous system anatomy and physiology.)

KEY CONCEPTS

- The structure and function of cells are influenced by the genome and environment as well as by developmental history.
- Three important mechanisms of cell development and differentiation are (1) cell-to-cell signals, (2) chemical gradients, and (3) interaction with the extracellular matrix.
- Differentiated cell types have different capacities to divide. Some tissues, such as nerve and cardiac muscle, are terminally differentiated and have limited ability to divide. Other cell types, such as skin and bone marrow, maintain stem cells, which have great capacity to proliferate.
- Different cell types in the adult human are classified into four major categories: epithelium (e.g., skin, glands, endothelium), connective tissue (e.g., bone, cartilage, fat, blood), muscle (e.g., skeletal, cardiac, smooth), and nervous tissue (e.g., neuronal, glial).

Principles of Inheritance

Thus far this chapter has explained how the unique structure of DNA is able to direct the day-to-day activities of a cell and how DNA may be regulated so that the cell can respond to environmental changes and differentiate into specialized cell types within the body. DNA is also the vehicle whereby genes are passed from parent to offspring. In this section the processes of somatic cell division (mitosis) and germ cell division (meiosis) are contrasted and the basic principles of inheritance are reviewed.

Chromosomes

In humans, cellular DNA is organized into 46 different chromosome units that become visible under the microscope only during cell division.[23] During mitosis, chromosomes look like X's of varying sizes and shapes. The chromosome is really made up of two identical linear chromosome units, called **chromatids,** which separate during mitosis. The point at the mid-

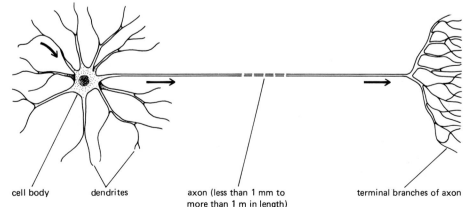

FIGURE 4–18. Diagram of a typical neuron showing the cell body, axon, and dendrites. Neurons have many shapes and sizes. (From Alberts B, et al (eds): *Molecular Biology of the Cell,* 2nd ed. New York, Garland Press, 1989, p 1061. Reproduced with permission.)

cell body   dendrites

axon (less than 1 mm to more than 1 m in length)

terminal branches of axon

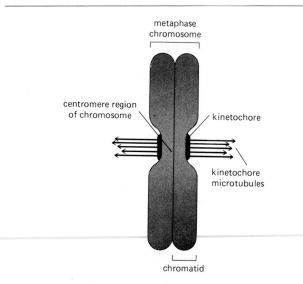

FIGURE 4 – 19. Drawing of a chromosome, showing the two sister chromatids attached at the centromere. The kinetochore microtubules are part of the mitotic apparatus that pulls the chromosome apart during cell division. (From Alberts B, et al (eds): *Molecular Biology of the Cell,* 2nd ed. New York, Garland Press, 1989, p 769. Reproduced with permission.)

dle of the X where the two sister chromatids are joined together is the **centromere** (Fig. 4–19). Human chromosomes are **diploid;** they occur as pairs. One member of the pair comes from the mother and one member comes from the father. Under the microscope the members of a pair appear to be identical (**homologous**) even though they are different in DNA sequence. Chromosomes are characterized based on total size, length of the arms of the X, and their characteristic banding patterns when exposed to certain stains (Fig. 4–20). Of the 23 pairs of chromosomes, 22 are homologous and are called **autosomes.** The remaining pair, the **sex chromosomes,** differs between males and females. Females receive an X chromosome from each parent (homologous), whereas males receive an X chromosome from their mothers and a Y from their fathers (nonhomologous).

Mitosis

The chromosomes of body cells are duplicated and distributed equally to the cell's progeny when it divides in the process called **mitosis,** such that each

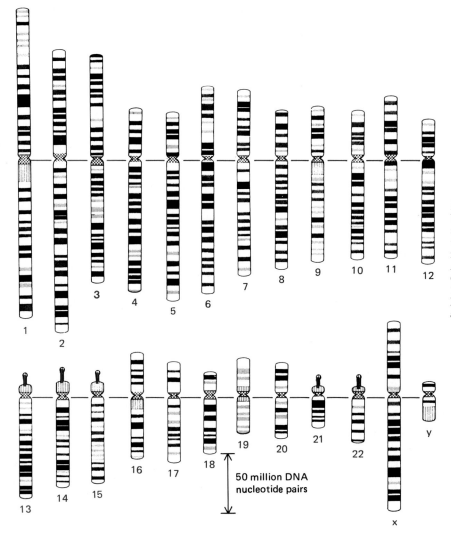

FIGURE 4 – 20. A standard map of the banding pattern of each of the 23 chromosomes of the human. Somatic cells contain two copies of each chromosome. The centromere region is marked by the line. (From Alberts B, et al (eds): *Molecular Biology of the Cell,* 2nd ed. New York, Garland Press, 1989, p 505. Adapted with permission from Franke U: *Cytogenet Cell Genet* 1981;31:24–32 and S. Karger AG, Basel.)

daughter cell receives an identical full set of 46 chromosomes. Mitosis proceeds through six stages, beginning with *prophase,* in which the chromosomes condense and become visible, and ending with *cytokinesis,* when cell division is accomplished. The stages of mitotic cell division are explained in Figure 4–21. Mitosis is responsible for the growth of body cells in which little genetic variation is needed or desired. A more elaborate cell division process occurs in the germ cells where significant chromosomal rearrangements occur.

Meiosis

Although sex is not necessary for reproduction in some organisms (many plants, some worms, and even some species of lizards), it does confer certain benefits to those who utilize it. **Sexual reproduction** allows the mixing of genomes from two different individuals to produce offspring that differ genetically from one another and from their parents. This source of genetic variability is advantageous to the species because it allows for adaptation and evolution in a changing environment. In order for two germ cells (egg and sperm) to combine to form a cell with the normal complement of 46 chromosomes (23 pairs), each germ cell must contribute only half of the total. **Meiosis** refers to this special form of cell division which results in germ cells that are **haploid;** they have half of the normal number of chromosomes. In contrast to mitosis, meiosis involves two divisions of the chromosomal DNA. A comparison of meiotic and mitotic cell division is shown in Figure 4–22.

During the first phase of meiosis, duplicated sister chromatids come in close contact with their homologous pairs. Portions of the homologous chromosomes are exchanged in a process called **crossing over** (Fig. 4–23). This results in a mixing of the maternal and paternal genes of the cell to form a new combination of genes within the chromosomes. **Genetic recombination** is very precise such that genes are exchanged intact and not interrupted in the middle. The first cellular division of meiosis results in two cells, each with 46 chromosomes. These two cells undergo a second division in which the sister chromatids are pulled apart (similar to normal mitosis), resulting in four cells, each having only 23 chromosomes. Each of the germ cells has a different combination of genes that, when passed on through sexual reproduction, will form a new, genetically unique individual.

Genetic Inheritance

"Whom does the baby look like?" is a question frequently asked of new parents. It is common knowledge that **traits** tend to run in families, but Gregor Mendel, a 19th century monk turned geneticist, was the first to notice that traits were transmitted in a predictable way from parent to offspring.[24] Height, weight, skin color, eye color, and hair color are some of the physical traits that characterize an individual. **Phenotype** refers to the physical and biochemical attributes of an individual that are outwardly apparent. These traits are a result of the expression of the individual's unique genetic makeup, or **genotype.** The genotype is a result of the union of 23 maternal and 23 paternal chromosomes at conception. Thus, an individual actually receives two sets of genes, one set from each parent. The genes that code for a particular trait, such as eye color, are located at a particular position (locus) on the chromosome and come in several forms, or **alleles.** In the case of eye color, there are two common alleles, blue and brown. A person actually has two alleles for each gene, one received from each parent. If both alleles for a trait are identical, the individual is **homozygous** for that trait. If two different alleles are present, the individual is **heterozygous** for the trait. Using the eye color example again, if an individual receives a blue eye color allele from each parent, he or she is homozygous for eye color. If a blue eye color allele is received from one parent and a brown eye color allele is received from the other parent, the individual is heterozygous for that trait.

Some traits, like eye color, involve only one gene locus and are called **single-gene** traits. (Variations in shade may be determined by other genes.) The transmission of single-gene traits from parent to offspring follows predictable patterns that can be demonstrated using the Punnett square (Fig. 4–24). In the Punnett square, the alleles for a gene are represented by capital and lowercase letters. The capital letter represents the **dominant** allele and the lowercase letter is the **recessive** allele. As the term implies, the trait of the dominant allele is apparent and will mask the recessive allele. A recessive trait is apparent only if *both* alleles for the trait are recessive (homozygous). The Punnett square is based on the Mendelian principle that all genes are independent and will be inherited in a random manner. Thus, if both parents are heterozygous for a dominant trait (Aa), the offspring will have a 25 percent probability of being AA, a 50 percent probability of being Aa, and a 25 percent probability of being aa. Persons having the AA and Aa genotypes will express the trait in a similar manner. The trait will be absent in the aa genotype. Many genetic diseases are carried in the recessive allele and are manifested only by the aa genotype. Persons who are heterozygous for the disease (Aa) are said to be **carriers** because they are able to pass the defective recessive gene to their offspring even though they do not exhibit the trait.

Some alleles are not clearly dominant or recessive and result in a blending or **intermediate expression** of the trait. Blood type, for example, has three distinct alleles—A, B, and O. A and B may both be expressed together, resulting in the AB blood type. Other traits result from the interaction of several gene loci and are called **polygenic** or multifactorial. Polygenic traits are heritable, but predicting their occurrence is more difficult. Polygenic traits are often affected by environmental factors. As examples, height, weight, and

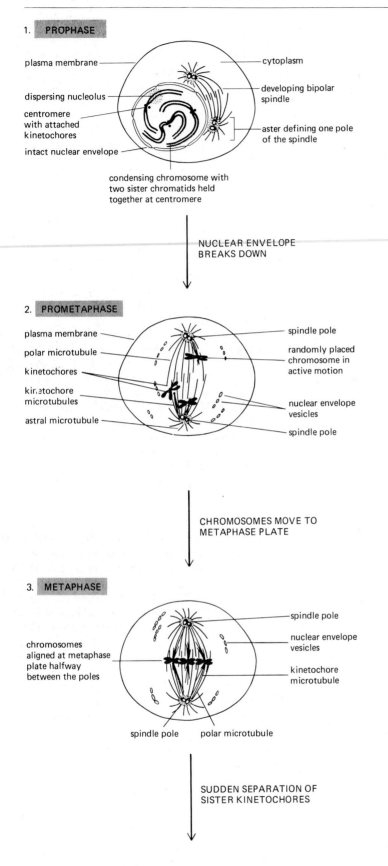

1. PROPHASE

plasma membrane

dispersing nucleolus

centromere with attached kinetochores

intact nuclear envelope

cytoplasm

developing bipolar spindle

aster defining one pole of the spindle

condensing chromosome with two sister chromatids held together at centromere

NUCLEAR ENVELOPE BREAKS DOWN

2. PROMETAPHASE

plasma membrane

polar microtubule

kinetochores

kinetochore microtubules

astral microtubule

spindle pole

randomly placed chromosome in active motion

nuclear envelope vesicles

spindle pole

CHROMOSOMES MOVE TO METAPHASE PLATE

3. METAPHASE

chromosomes aligned at metaphase plate halfway between the poles

spindle pole

nuclear envelope vesicles

kinetochore microtubule

spindle pole   polar microtubule

SUDDEN SEPARATION OF SISTER KINETOCHORES

1   PROPHASE

As viewed in the microscope, the transition from the G_2 phase to the M phase of the cell cycle is not a sharply defined event. The chromatin, which is diffuse in interphase, slowly condenses into well-defined chromosomes, the exact number of which is characteristic of the particular species. Each chromosome has duplicated during the preceding S phase and consists of two sister *chromatids;* each of these contains a specific DNA sequence known as a *centromere,* which is required for proper segregation. Toward the end of prophase, the cytoplasmic microtubules that are part of the interphase cytoskeleton disassemble and the main component of the mitotic apparatus, the *mitotic spindle,* begins to form. This is a bipolar structure composed of microtubules and associated proteins. The spindle assembles initially outside the nucleus.

2   PROMETAPHASE

Prometaphase starts abruptly with disruption of the nuclear envelope, which breaks into membrane vesicles that are indistinguishable from bits of endoplasmic reticulum. These vesicles remain visible around the spindle during mitosis. The spindle microtubules, which have been lying outside the nucleus, can now enter the nuclear region. Specialized protein complexes called *kinetochores* mature on each centromere and attach to some of the spindle microtubules, which are then called *kinetochore microtubules.* The remaining microtubules in the spindle are called *polar microtubules,* while those outside the spindle are called *astral microtubules.* The kinetochore microtubules extend in opposite directions from the two sister chromatids in each chromosome, exerting tension on the chromosomes, which are thereby thrown into agitated motion.

3   METAPHASE

The kinetochore microtubules eventually align the chromosomes in one plane halfway between the spindle poles. Each chromosome is held in tension at this *metaphase plate* by the paired kinetochores and their associated microtubules, which are attached to opposite poles of the spindle.

F I G U R E   4 – 21. The six stages of mitotic cell division. (From Alberts B, et al (eds): *Molecular Biology of the Cell,* 2nd ed. New York, Garland Press, 1989, pp 766–767. Reproduced with permission.)

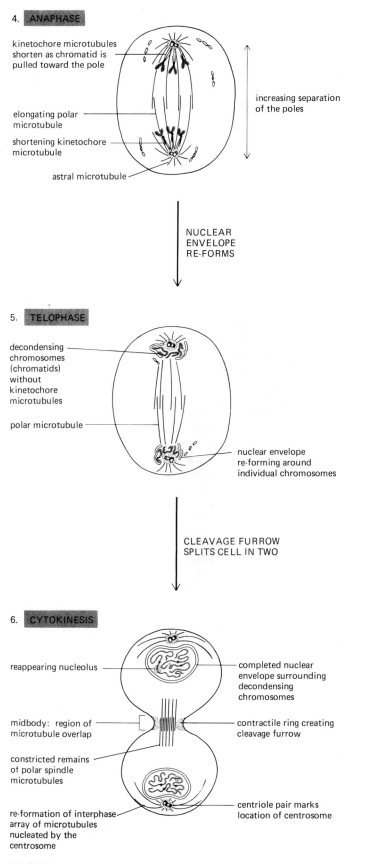

4. **ANAPHASE**

kinetochore microtubules
shorten as chromatid is
pulled toward the pole

increasing separation
of the poles

elongating polar
microtubule

shortening kinetochore
microtubule

astral microtubule

NUCLEAR
ENVELOPE
RE-FORMS

5. **TELOPHASE**

decondensing
chromosomes
(chromatids)
without
kinetochore
microtubules

polar microtubule

nuclear envelope
re-forming around
individual chromosomes

CLEAVAGE FURROW
SPLITS CELL IN TWO

6. **CYTOKINESIS**

reappearing nucleolus

completed nuclear
envelope surrounding
decondensing
chromosomes

midbody: region of
microtubule overlap

contractile ring creating
cleavage furrow

constricted remains
of polar spindle
microtubules

re-formation of interphase
array of microtubules
nucleated by the
centrosome

centriole pair marks
location of centrosome

FIGURE 4–21 Continued

4 ANAPHASE

Triggered by a specific signal, anaphase
begins abruptly as the paired
kinetochores on each chromosome
separate, allowing each chromatid to be
pulled slowly toward the spindle pole it
faces. All chromatids move at the same
speed, typically about 1 μm per minute.
Two categories of movement can be
distinguished. During *anaphase A,*
kinetochore microtubules shorten as the
chromosomes approach the poles.
During *anaphase B,* the polar
microtubules elongate and the two
poles of the spindle move farther apart.
Anaphase typically lasts only a few
minutes.

5 TELOPHASE

In telophase (*telos,* end) the separated
daughter chromatids arrive at the poles
and the kinetochore microtubules
disappear. The polar microtubules
elongate still more, and a new nuclear
envelope re-forms around each group of
daughter chromosomes. The condensed
chromatin expands once more, the
nucleoli—which had disappeared at
prophase—begin to reappear, and
mitosis is at an end.

6 CYTOKINESIS

The cytoplasm divides by a process
known as *cleavage,* which usually starts
sometime during anaphase. The process
is illustrated here as it occurs in animal
cells. The membrane around the middle
of the cell, perpendicular to the spindle
axis and between the daughter nuclei, is
drawn inward to form a *cleavage
furrow,* which gradually deepens until it
encounters the narrow remains of the
mitotic spindle between the two nuclei.
This thin bridge, or *midbody,* may
persist for some time before it narrows
and finally breaks at each end, leaving
two separated daughter cells.

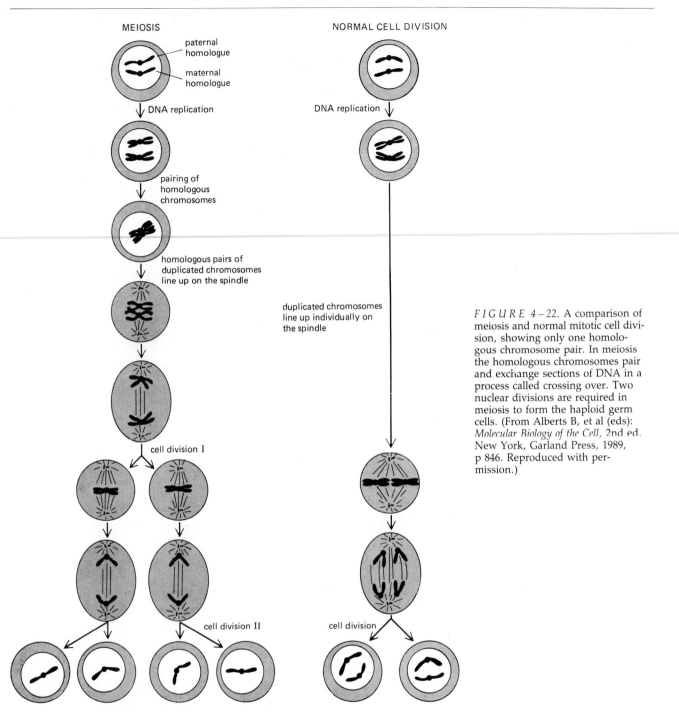

FIGURE 4–22. A comparison of meiosis and normal mitotic cell division, showing only one homologous chromosome pair. In meiosis the homologous chromosomes pair and exchange sections of DNA in a process called crossing over. Two nuclear divisions are required in meiosis to form the haploid germ cells. (From Alberts B, et al (eds): *Molecular Biology of the Cell*, 2nd ed. New York, Garland Press, 1989, p 846. Reproduced with permission.)

FIGURE 4–23. Crossing over during meiotic prophase I results in a reassortment of genes between homologous chromosomes. (From Alberts et al (eds): *Molecular Biology of the Cell*, 2nd ed. New York, Garland Press, 1989, p 847. Reproduced with permission.)

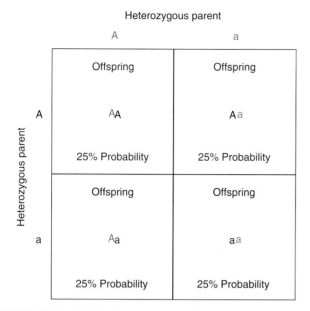

Heterozygous parent

	A	a
A	Offspring AA 25% Probability	Offspring Aa 25% Probability
a	Offspring Aa 25% Probability	Offspring aa 25% Probability

FIGURE 4–24. The Punnett square shows the distribution of parental genes to their offspring. This example shows the mating of two heterozygous individuals. Dominant genes are denoted by the capital A, recessive genes by the lowercase a.

blood pressure are polygenic traits; however, dietary intake will certainly influence the ultimate expression of these genes.

KEY CONCEPTS

- Human DNA is organized into 46 chromosomes (23 pairs). Paired chromosomes look similar under the microscope but differ in DNA sequence. One member of each pair is inherited from the mother, the other from the father.

- Twenty-two pairs of chromosomes are autosomes. The remaining pair, the sex chromosomes, confers maleness (XY) or femaleness (XX).

- During cell division, the chromosomes are distributed to daughter cells. Mitosis results in the equal distribution of chromosomes to both daughter cells (23 pairs each). Meiosis results in four daughter cells, each having one-half the normal number of chromosomes (23). Mitosis occurs in somatic cells and meiosis occurs in germ cells.

- Genes that code for a particular trait come in several forms or alleles. Genotype refers to the particular set of alleles an individual receives. Phenotype refers to an individual's observable attributes. People with different genotypes may have similar phenotypes.

- Some traits involve only one gene locus and are called single-gene traits. The transmission of these traits from parent to offspring follows predictable patterns. The expression of single-gene traits is determined by whether the gene is dominant or recessive. Dominant genes usually code for functional enzymes; recessive genes do not. Traits resulting from the interaction of several genes are polygenic and do not follow predictable patterns of inheritance.

Summary

From the foregoing discussion of genetics and inheritance, it is apparent that, to some extent, all diseases are genetic. Some diseases such as enzyme deficiencies are purely inherited with little environmental influence. At the other end of the spectrum are diseases such as infections which, although environmentally induced, are still influenced by one's genetic susceptibility. In addition to being the elements of heredity, genes also direct the day-to-day activities of the cell. Both of these functions are accomplished by DNA, which provides the template for replication of the genome in preparation for mitosis and meiosis and directs the synthesis of cellular proteins. All the cells of the body possess the same DNA, but through complex processes of differentiation they become specialized to perform particular functions. It is believed that different sets of genes are active in different cell types. The four major classes of differentiated tissues are epithelial, connective, muscle, and nerve. These four tissues interdependently form the functioning systems of the body.

REFERENCES

1. Alberts B, Bray D, Lewis J, Raff M, Roberts K, Watson J: Small molecules, energy, and biosynthesis, in Alberts B, et al (eds): *Molecular Biology of the Cell*, 2nd ed. New York, Garland Press, 1989.
2. Watson JD, Crick FHC: Molecular structure of nucleic acids: A structure for deoxyribose nucleic acid. *Nature* 1953;171:737–738.
3. Kornberg A: *DNA Replication*. San Francisco, WH Freeman & Co, 1980.
4. Fersht AR: Enzymatic editing mechanisms in protein synthesis and DNA replication. *Trends Biochem Sci* 1980;5:262–265.
5. Crick FHC: The genetic code: III. *Sci Am* 1966;215(4):55–62.
6. Cold Spring Harbor: *The Genetic Code. Cold Spring Harbor Symp Quant Biol*, vol 31, 1966.
7. Alberts B, Bray D, Lewis J, Raff M, Roberts K, Watson J: Basic genetic mechanisms, in Alberts B, et al (eds): *Molecular Biology of the Cell*, 2nd ed. New York, Garland Press, 1989.
8. Steitz JA: Snurps. *Sci Am* 1988;258(6):56–63.
9. Spirin AS: *Ribosome Structure and Protein Synthesis*. Menlo Park, CA, Benjamin-Cummings, 1986.
10. Darnell JE Jr: Variety in the level of gene control in eucaryotic cells. *Nature* 1982;297:365–371.
11. McKnight SL: Molecular zippers in gene regulation. *Sci Am* 1991;264(4):54–64.
12. Alberts B, Bray D, Lewis J, Raff M, Roberts K, Watson J: Control of gene expression, in Alberts B, et al (eds): *Molecular Biology of the Cell*, 2nd ed. New York, Garland Press, 1989.
13. Gilbert W, Muller-Hill B: The *lac* operator is DNA. *Proc Natl Acad Sci USA* 1967;58:2415–2421.
14. Gurdon JB: The developmental capacity of nuclei taken from intestinal epithelium cells of feeding tadpoles. *J Embryol Exp Morphol* 1962;10:622–640.
15. Gartler SM, Riggs AD: Mammalian X-chromosome inactivation. *Annu Rev Genet* 1983;17:155–190.
16. Kelly SJ: Studies of the development potential on 4- and 8-cell stage mouse biasomeres. *J Exp Zool* 1977;200:365–376.
17. Wolpert L: Positional information and pattern formation. *Curr Top Dev Biol* 1971;6:183–224.
18. Wylie CC, Stott D, Donovan PJ: Primordial germ cell migration, in Browder LW (ed): *Developmental Biology: A Comprehensive Synthesis*. New York, Plenum Press, 1986, vol 2: *The Cellular Basis of Morphogenesis*.
19. Bereiter-Hahn J, Matolsty AG, Richards KS: In Bereiter-Hahn J, et al (eds): *Biology of the Integument*. New York, Springer, 1986, vol 2: *Vertebrates*.

20. Cormack D: *Ham's Histology*, 9th ed. Philadelphia, JB Lippincott, 1987.
21. Murphy R: Muscle, in Berne RM, Levy MN (eds): *Principles of Physiology*. St. Louis, CV Mosby, 1990, pp 152–185.
22. Alberts B, Bray D, Lewis J, Raff M, Roberts K, Watson J: Differentiated cells and the maintenance of tissues, in Alberts B, et al (eds): *Molecular Biology of the Cell*, 2nd ed. New York, Garland Press, 1989.
23. Alberts B, Bray D, Lewis J, Raff M, Roberts K, Watson J: The cell nucleus, in Alberts B, et al (eds): *Molecular Biology of the Cell*, 2nd ed. New York, Garland Press, 1989.
24. Bateson W: *Mendel's Principles of Heredity*. London, Cambridge University Press, 1902.

BIBLIOGRAPHY

Adolph KW: *Genome Research in Molecular Medicine and Virology*. San Diego, Academic Press, 1993.

Alberts B, et al (eds): *Molecular Biology of the Cell*, 2nd ed. New York, Garland Press, 1989.

Balling R, Ebensperger C, Hoffmann I, Imai K, Koseki H, Mizutani Y, Wallin J: The genetics of skeletal development. *Ann Genet* 1993;36(1):56–62.

Bellairs R, Sanders EJ, Lash JW: *Formation and Differentiation of Early Embryonic Mesoderm*. New York, Plenum Press, 1992.

Browder LW: *Developmental Biology: A Comprehensive Synthesis*. New York, Plenum Press, 1986, vol 2: *The Cellular Basis of Morphogenesis*.

Claassen E, Zegers ND, Laman JD, Boersma WJ: Use of synthetic peptides for the production of site (amino acid) specific polyclonal and monoclonal antibodies. *Year Immunol* 1993;7: 150–161.

Corden JL: RNA polymerase II transcription cycles. *Curr Opin Genet Dev* 1993;3(2): 213–218.

Cormack D: *Ham's Histology*, 9th ed. Philadelphia, JB Lippincott, 1987.

Devlin TM: *Textbook of Biochemistry: With Clinical Correlations*, 3rd ed. New York, Wiley-Liss, 1992.

Doolittle RF: Stein and Moore Award address: Reconstructing history with amino acid sequences. *Protein Sci* 1992;1(2):191–200.

Ebright RH: Transcription activation at Class I CAP-dependent promoters. *Mol Microbiol* 1993;8(5):797–802.

Horwich AL, Willison KR: Protein folding in the cell: Functions of two families of molecular chaperone, hsp 60 and TF55-TCP1. *Philos Trans R Soc Lond Biol* 1993;339(1289):313–325.

Ishihama A: Protein-protein communication within the transcription apparatus. *J Bacteriol* 1993;175(9):2483–2489.

Jonat C, Stein B, Ponta H, Herrlich P, Rahmsdorf HJ: Positive and negative regulation of collagenase gene expression. *Matrix Suppl* 1992;1:145–155.

Lis J, Wu C: Protein traffic on the heat shock promoter: Parking, stalling, and trucking along. *Cell* 1993;74(1):1–4.

Luzio JP, Thompson RJ: *Molecular Medical Biochemistry*. Cambridge, Cambridge University Press, 1990.

McInnes RR, Byers PH: Biochemical genetics: Examples of life after cloning. *Curr Opin Genet Dev* 1993;3(3):475–483.

Mendel G, in Corcos AF, Monaghan FV (eds): *Gregor Mendel's Experiments on Plant Hybrids: A Guided Study*. New Brunswick, Rutgers University Press, 1993.

Newman CM, Magee AI: Posttranslational processing of the *ras* superfamily of small GTP-binding proteins. *Biochim Biophys Acta* 1993;1155(1):79–96.

North AK, Klose KE, Stedman KM, Kustu S: Prokaryotic enhancer-binding proteins reflect eukaryote-like modularity: The puzzle of nitrogen regulatory protein C. *J Bacteriol* 1993;175(14): 4267–4273.

Oh SK, Sarnow P: Gene regulation: Translational initiation by internal ribosome binding. *Curr Opin Genet Dev* 1993;3(3):295–300.

Sachs L, Lotem J: Control of programmed cell death in normal and leukemic cells: New implications for therapy. *Blood* 1993;82(1): 15–21.

Samara G, Sawicki MP, Hurwitz M, Passaro E Jr: Molecular biology and therapy of disease. *Am J Surg* 1993;165(6):720–727.

Sultan C, Lobaccaro JM, Belon C, Terraza A, Lumbroso S: Molecular biology of disorders of sex differentiation. *Horm Res* 1992; 38(3–4):105–113.

Tate PH, Bird AP: Effects of DNA methylation on DNA-binding proteins and gene expression. *Curr Opin Genet Dev* 1993;3(2): 226–231.

Taylor SS, Knighton DR, Zheng J, Sowadski JM, Gibbs CS, Zoller MJ: A template for the protein kinase family. *Trends Biochem Sci* 1993;18(3):84–89.

von Kitzing E: Modeling DNA structures: Molecular mechanics and molecular dynamics. *Methods Enzymol* 1992;211:449–467.

Wilkins AS: *Genetic Analysis of Animal Development*, 2nd ed. New York, Wiley-Liss, 1993.

CHAPTER 5
Genetic and Developmental Disorders

JACQUELYN L. BANASIK

KEY TERMS

aneuploidy: An abnormal number of chromosomes—either too few (hypoploidy) or too many (hyperploidy, polyploidy).

consanguinity: Mating of blood-related individuals.

teratogen: An agent or factor that causes damage or physical defects in a developing embryo.

translocation: The shifting of a segment of one chromosome into another chromosome.

Geneticists and parents alike have marveled at the development of a recognizable human baby, with eyes and ears, toes and fingers, from its simple beginning as a single cell containing one set of genes. Considering the enormous list of potentially disasterous genetic and environmental influences, the birth of a healthy normal child does, indeed, seem something of a miracle. While the risk of bearing a child with mental or physical defects is small for most parents, it is real, and often a source of worry during the prenatal period. It has been estimated that most people harbor between five and eight defective genes that are recessive and therefore of little consequence until they are transmitted to offspring.[1,2] Additionally, there are many known and unknown environmental hazards to which the parent and fetus may be exposed. Structural defects that are due to errors in development and are present at birth are called **congenital malformations.** It is estimated that about 3 percent of newborns have a major malformation of cosmetic or functional significance.[3] Based on the 1990 census,[4] it is estimated that each year in the United States more than 400,000 infants are born with physical or mental damage.

Congenital disorders are generally grouped according to genetic or environmental causes. As many as two thirds of birth malformations have no identifiable cause.[5] In this chapter, the genetic and environmental causes of congenital disorders will be described, as well as the principles of diagnosis, counseling, and gene therapy.

Genetic Disorders

Genetic disorders may be apparent at birth or may not be clinically evident until much later in life. The great majority of genetic disorders are inherited from the affected individual's parents. However, 15 percent to 20 percent represent new mutations that arise during fetal development.[1] The genetic disorders encountered clinically are only a small percentage of those that occur, representing the less extreme aberrations that permit live birth. It has been estimated that about 60 percent of spontaneous abortions have demonstrable chromosomal abnormalities, and many more may have hidden genetic defects.[1,6]

Disorders that are genetic in origin can be divided into three groups: (1) chromosomal aberrations, (2) single-gene or Mendelian disorders, and (3) multifactorial or polygenic disorders.

Chromosomal Abnormalities

Chromosomal defects are generally due to an abnormal number of chromosomes or alterations in the structure of one or more chromosomes. These defects result from errors in the separation or crossing-over of chromosomes during meiosis or mitosis.

Aberrant Number of Chromosomes

The normal human germ cell contains 23 chromosomes. The union of sperm and egg results in a fertilized egg with the full complement of 46 chromosomes—22 autosomes and two sex chromosomes. **Aneuploidy** refers to an abnormal number of chromosomes—either more or less than 46. The usual causes of aneuploidy are nondisjunction and anaphase lag. **Nondisjunction** means that the paired homologous chromosomes fail to separate normally during either the first or second meiotic division (see Chap. 4). The resulting germ cells will then have an abnormal number of chromosomes: one will have 22 chromosomes and one will have 24. When the chromosomes from the abnormal germ cell are combined with a normal germ cell containing 23 chromosomes, the fertilized cell will either be deficient by one chromosome (45) or have an extra chromosome (47) (Fig. 5–1). In **anaphase lag,** one chromosome lags behind and is therefore left out of the newly formed cell nucleus. This results in one daughter cell with the normal number of chromosomes and one with a deficiency of one chromosome, a condition called **monosomy. Polysomy** refers to the condition of too many chromosomes.

The causes of abnormalities in chromosome number are poorly understood. Radiation, viruses, and chemicals have been implicated because they can interfere with mitosis and meiosis in experimental animals. Their role in causing aneuploidy in humans is unproved. Two conditions are known to increase the risk of abnormalities in chromosome number in humans: advanced maternal age and abnormalites in parental chromosome structure.[7,8] There is no precise explanation for the higher risk of nondisjunction with these conditions.

In general, monosomy involving the autosomes is not compatible with life. Autosomal polysomy may result in a viable fetus. The extra autosomal chromosomes are nearly always associated with severely disabled infants.[1] Disorders involving extra or missing sex chromosomes are relatively more common and less debilitating.

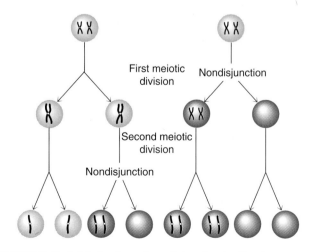

$F I G U R E$ $5-1$. Mechanism of nondisjunction leading to aneuploidy.

Abnormal Chromosome Structure

Alterations in chromosome structure are usually due to breakage and loss or rearrangement of pieces of the chromosomes during meiosis or mitosis.[9] During meiosis, the homologous chromosomes normally pair up and exchange genetic alleles in a process called **crossing-over.** Normal crossing-over involves precise gene exchange between homologues only, with no net gain or loss of DNA. When the normal process of crossing-over goes awry, portions of chromosomes may be lost, attached upside down, or attached to the wrong chromosome. Mitosis also presents opportunities for chromosomal breakage and rearrangement. The severity of the chromosomal rearrangement ranges from insignificant to lethal, depending on the number and importance of the gene loci involved. The common types of chromosomal rearrangements are translocations, inversions, deletions, and duplications (Fig. 5–2).

Chromosomal **translocations** result from the exchange of pieces of DNA between nonhomologous chromosomes. If no genetic material is lost, as in a reciprocal translocation, the individual may have no symptoms of the disorder. However, an individual with a reciprocal translocation is at increased risk of producing abnormal gametes. The exchange of a long chromatid for a short one results in the formation of one very large chromosome and one very small chromosome (see Fig. 5–2). This is called a Robertsonian translocation and is responsible for a rare hereditary form of Down's syndrome discussed later in the chapter.

Inversion refers to the removal and upside-down reinsertion of a section of chromosome (see Fig. 5–2). Like balanced translocations, inversions involve no net loss or gain of genetic material and are often without consequence to the individual. Difficulties result, however, when homologous chromosomes attempt to pair up during meiosis. The chromosome with an inverted section may not pair up properly, resulting in duplications or loss of genes at the time of crossing-over. Thus, the offspring of an individual harboring an inversion may be affected.

Loss of chromosomal material is called **deletion.** Deletions result from a break in the arm of a single chromosome, resulting in a fragment of DNA with no centromere. The piece is then lost at the next cell division. Chromosomal deletions have been associated with some forms of cancer, including retinoblastoma (see Chap. 6).

In contrast to a deletion, where genes are lost, a **duplication** results in extra copies of a portion of DNA. The consequences of duplications are generally less severe than those from loss of genetic material.

Examples of Autosomal Chromosome Disorders

Trisomy 21 (Down's Syndrome). Trisomy 21 is a chromosomal disorder in which individuals have an extra 21st chromosome. It is the most common of the chromosomal disorders and a leading cause of mental retardation, occurring in about 1 in 700 live births.[10] The syndrome, first described by Langdon Down in 1866,[11] includes mental

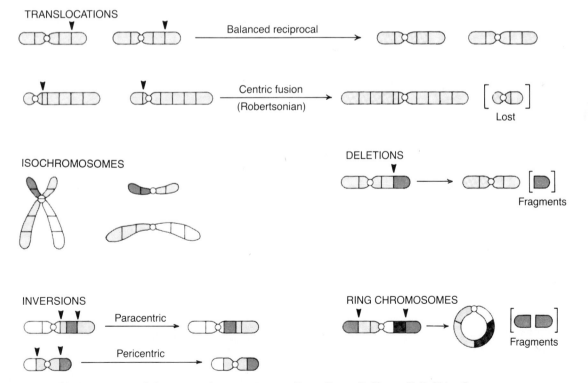

FIGURE 5–2. Types of chromosomal rearrangement. (From Cotran R, Kumar V, Robbins S (eds): *Robbins Pathologic Basis of Disease,* 5th ed. Philadelphia, WB Saunders, 1994. Reproduced with permission.)

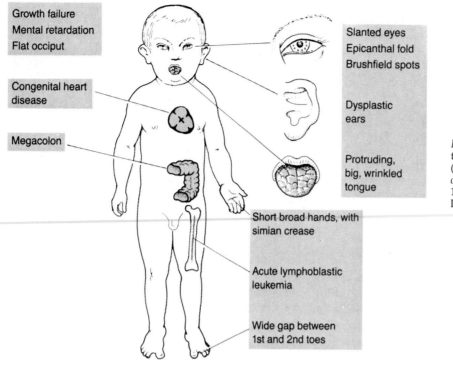

Growth failure
Mental retardation
Flat occiput

Congenital heart
disease

Megacolon

Slanted eyes
Epicanthal fold
Brushfield spots

Dysplastic
ears

Protruding,
big, wrinkled
tongue

Short broad hands, with
simian crease

Acute lymphoblastic
leukemia

Wide gap between
1st and 2nd toes

FIGURE 5–3. Typical clinical manifestations of trisomy 21 (Down's syndrome). (From Rubin E, Farber J: *Essential Pathology*. Philadelphia, JB Lippincott, 1990, p 141. Reproduced with permission. Artist: Dimitri Karetnikov.)

retardation, protruding tongue, low-set ears, epicanthal folds, poor muscle tone, and short stature (Fig. 5–3). Children with Down's syndrome are often afflicted with congenital heart deformities and an increased susceptibility to respiratory infections and leukemia. Three fourths of the fetuses known to have trisomy 21 are stillborn or aborted.[10]

A rare form of Down's syndrome (about 4 percent of cases) is due to a chromosomal translocation of the long arm of chromosome 21 to another chromosome. This form is said to be inherited because the abnormal chromosome is passed on from parent to offspring. In contrast, the etiology of trisomy 21 is not well understood, although it is clearly associated with advanced maternal age.[12] Table 5–1 shows a rise in the incidence

of Down's syndrome from maternal age 20 to 45. The reason for increased susceptibility of the ovum to nondisjunction with age remains unknown.[7] In up to 20 percent of cases, the extra chromosome 21 is thought to be of paternal origin; however, no correlation with paternal age has been found.[8]

Trisomy 18 (Edwards' Syndrome) **and trisomy 13 (Patau's Syndrome).** Trisomy of chromosomes 18 or 13 is much less common than trisomy 21 and more severe. Mental retardation is quite severe, and average life expectancy is only a few weeks beyond birth. Trisomies involving chromosomes 8, 9, and 22 also have been described, but are extremely rare.[10]

Cri du Chat Syndrome. Deletion of the short arm of chromosome 5 results in a syndrome characterized by severe mental retardation, round face, and congenital heart anomalies.[1] The syndrome was so named because of the characteristic cry, which resembles a cat crying. Some children afflicted with this syndrome survive to adulthood, and they generally thrive better than those with the trisomies.

Examples of Sex Chromosome Disorders

Klinefelter's Syndrome. The incidence of Klinefelter's syndrome is about 1 in 850 live births, making it one of the most common genetic diseases of the sex chromosomes.[1] Individuals with Klinefelter's syndrome usually have an extra X chromosome—an XXY genotype. However, individuals with more than one extra X (XXXY and XXXXY) have also been described. The presence of the Y chromosome determines the sex of these individuals to be male; however, the extra

TABLE 5–1. Frequency of Trisomy 21 (Down's Syndrome) in Relation to Maternal Age

Maternal Age	Frequency of Trisomy 21 at Birth
20	1/1,500
25	1/1,350
30	1/900
35	1/380
37	1/240
39	1/150
41	1/85
43	1/50
45	1/28

Adapted with permission from Connor JM, Ferguson-Smith MA (eds): *Essential Medical Genetics*. London, Blackwell Scientific Publications, 1991.

X chromosome(s) result in abnormal sexual development. The condition is rarely diagnosed prior to puberty, when lack of secondary sex characteristics becomes apparent. Associated symptoms reflect a lack of testosterone and include testicular atrophy and infertility, tall stature with long arms and legs, feminine hair distribution, high-pitched voice, and impaired intelligence (Fig. 5–4).

Turner's Syndrome. Also known as monosomy X, Turner's syndrome is associated with the presence of only one normal X chromosome and no Y chromosome. The absence of the Y chromosome results in a female phenotype; however, the ovaries fail to develop, and affected individuals are sterile. In some cases of Turner's syndrome the second X chromosome is not entirely missing but is structurally abnormal. In the great majority of cases, the missing or damaged X chromosome is of

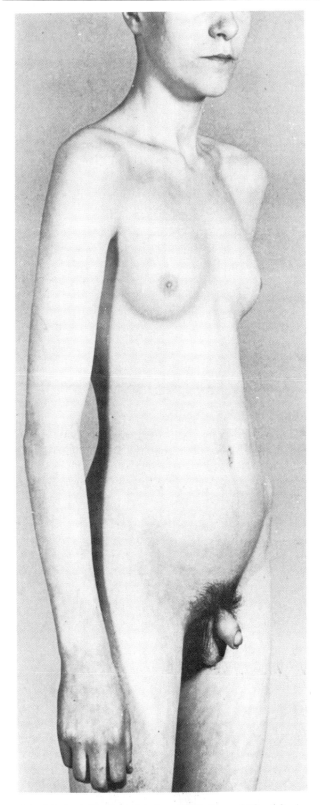

F I G U R E 5 – 4. Typical clinical manifestations of Klinefelter's syndrome. (From Connor JM, Ferguson-Smith MA: *Essential Med ical Genetics,* 3rd ed. London, Blackwell Scientific Publications, 1991, p 136. Reproduced with permission.)

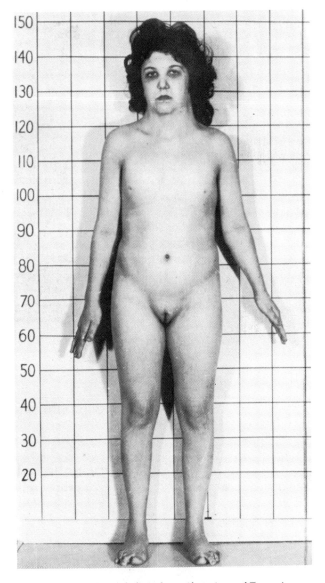

F I G U R E 5 – 5. Typical clinical manifestations of Turner's syndrome. (From Connor JM, Ferguson-Smith MA: *Essential Medical Genetics,* 3rd ed. London, Blackwell Scientific Publications, 1991, p 138. Reproduced with permission.)

paternal origin and may be related to advanced age of the father.[13] Only about 3 percent of infants with monosomy X survive to birth, and there is a high postnatal mortality as well. The incidence is 1 in 5,000 female births.[10] The principal characteristics of Turner's syndrome include short stature, webbing of the neck, fibrous ovaries, sterility, amenorrhea, a wide chest, and congenital heart defects (Fig. 5–5).

Multiple X Females and Double Y Males. A relatively common disorder of the sex chromosomes is the presence of an extra copy of the X chromosome in females (XXX) or of the Y in males (XYY). Most individuals appear normal; however, females may experience menstrual abnormalities, and males will generally be taller than average. A tendency toward mental retardation has been noted in females with more than four X chromosomes.

Mendelian Disorders
(Single-Gene Disorders)

Mendelian disorders result from alterations or **mutations** of single genes. The affected genes may code for abnormal enzymes, structural proteins, or regulatory proteins. An individual has two variants or alleles of each gene, one allele from each parent. A recessive gene is expressed only when the individual is homozygous for the gene—i.e., the individual has two identical copies. Dominant genes require only one allele to be expressed. Mendelian disorders are generally classified according to the *location* of the defective gene (autosomal or sex chromosome) and the *mode of transmission* (dominant or recessive). The great majority of Mendelian disorders are familial (mutant genes inherited from the parents), but 10 percent to 15 per-

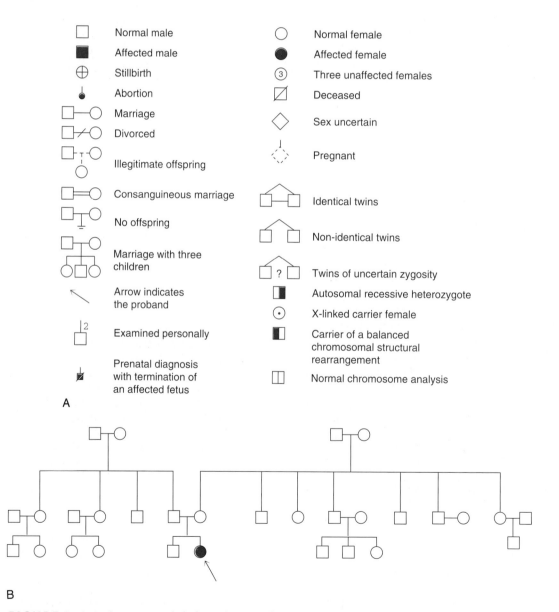

FIGURE 5–6. **A,** Common symbols for pedigree analysis. **B,** Typical family pedigree chart.

cent represent new mutations. In many cases the particular gene responsible for a Mendelian disease has not been identified. A detailed **pedigree** may be used to trace the transmission of the disease through the history of a family. The pedigree chart (Fig. 5–6), showing family relationships and which members have been affected by the disease, is a useful tool in determining the mode of inheritance as recessive, dominant, or sex-linked.

DNA Mutation and Repair

Genetic mutation is a rare event despite the daily exposure of cells to numerous mutagenic influences. Radiation, chemicals, viruses, and even some products of normal cellular metabolism are all potentially mutagenic. In a typical cell, more than 5,000 adenine and guanine DNA bases are lost and over 100 cytosine bases are damaged each day due to thermal disruption.[14] Many other types of DNA damage also occur, but only a few of these changes result in permanent alterations (mutations). The stability of the genes, and thus the low mutation rate, depends on efficient DNA repair mechanisms.

There are a variety of cellular DNA repair mechanisms. All require the presence of a normal complementary DNA template in order to repair the damaged strand of DNA correctly. Single-stranded breaks or loss of bases from only one DNA strand are readily repaired. Double-stranded breaks, involving both strands of complementary DNA, may result in permanent loss of genetic information. Different types of DNA damage are detected and repaired by different enzyme systems. The steps in one type of DNA repair are shown in Figure 5–7.

Genetic mutations are generally of two types: a **point mutation,** which involves a single base pair substitution, or a **frame-shift mutation,** which often changes the genetic code dramatically. Point mutations may go unnoticed or may cause significant genetic diseases. A sequence of three DNA bases (codon) is required to code for each amino acid. A point mutation in the gene may cause the affected codon to signify an abnormal amino acid. The inclusion of the abnormal amino acid in the sequence of the protein may or may not be of clinical significance. A frame-shift mutation is due to the addition or removal of one or more bases, which changes the "reading frame" of the DNA sequence. The DNA sequence is normally "read" in groups of three bases, with no spaces between. All of the codon triplets will be changed in the DNA region downstream from the mutation—resulting in a protein with a greatly altered amino acid sequence (Fig. 5–8).

Autosomal Dominant Disorders

Autosomal dominant disorders are due to a mutation of a dominant gene located on one of the autosomes. Autosomal dominant disorders follow predictable patterns of inheritance (Fig. 5–9), which may be summarized as follows:

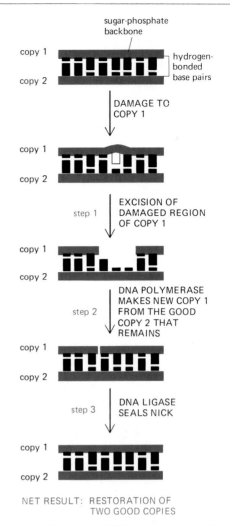

FIGURE 5–7. The steps of DNA repair. In step 1 the damaged section is removed; in steps 2 and 3 the original DNA sequence is restored. (From Alberts B, et al (eds): *Molecular Biology of the Cell,* 2nd ed. New York, Garland Press, 1989, p 223. Reproduced with permission.)

1. Males and females are equally affected.
2. Affected individuals have an affected parent.
3. Unaffected individuals do not transmit the disease.
4. Offspring of an affected individual (with normal mate) have a 50:50 chance of inheriting the disease.
5. The rare mating of two individuals, each carrying one copy of the defective gene (heterozygous), results in a 3 in 4 chance of producing an affected offspring.

The list of known autosomal dominant disorders is long. Many are described in later chapters as they relate to system pathophysiology. A partial list is presented in Table 5–2. In general, autosomal dominant disorders involve key structural proteins or regulatory proteins such as membrane receptors. Marfan's syndrome and Huntington's disease are commonly cited examples of autosomal dominant disorders.

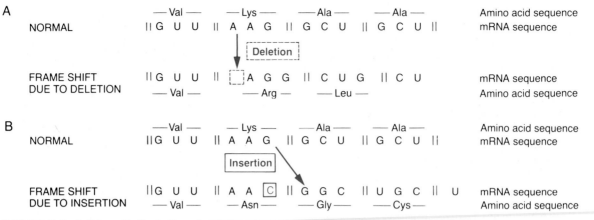

A

| | | —Val— | —Lys— | —Ala— | —Ala— | Amino acid sequence |
NORMAL   ‖G U U ‖A A G ‖G C U ‖G C U ‖   mRNA sequence

Deletion

FRAME SHIFT   ‖G U U ‖ A G G ‖C U G ‖C U   mRNA sequence
DUE TO DELETION   —Val—   —Arg—   —Leu—   Amino acid sequence

B

| | | —Val— | —Lys— | —Ala— | —Ala— | Amino acid sequence |
NORMAL   ‖G U U ‖A A G ‖G C U ‖G C U ‖   mRNA sequence

Insertion

FRAME SHIFT   ‖G U U ‖A A C ‖G G C ‖U G C ‖U   mRNA sequence
DUE TO INSERTION   —Val—   —Asn—   —Gly—   —Cys—   Amino acid sequence

FIGURE 5–8. Schematic illustration of mutations that alter the DNA reading frame by (**A**) deletion of a base or (**B**) insertion of a base. (From Cotran R, Kumar V, Robbins S (eds): *Robbins Pathologic Basis of Disease*, 4th ed. Philadelphia, WB Saunders, 1989, p 126. Reproduced with permission.)

Marfan's Syndrome. Marfan's syndrome is a disorder of the connective tissues of the body. Individuals with Marfan's syndrome are typically tall and slender with long, thin arms and legs (Fig. 5–10). Because of the long, thin fingers, this syndrome has also been called arachnodactyly—"spider fingers." It is commonly suggested that President Abraham Lincoln may have had this disorder. Although skeletal and joint deformities are problematic, the cardiovascular lesions are the most life-threatening. The medial layer of blood vessels, particularly the aorta, tends to be weak and susceptible to dilation and rupture. Dysfunction of the heart valves may occur from poor connective tissue support. The genetic defect responsible for the abnormal connective tissue has not been defin-

itively identified but is thought to be a defect in either elastin or collagen.[15–17]

Huntington's Disease. Huntington's disease is an autosomal dominant disease that primarily affects neurologic function.[13] The symptoms of mental deterioration and involuntary movements of the arms and legs do not appear until approximately age 40. The disease was formerly called Huntington's chorea because of the uncontrolled movements of the limbs (Greek *khoreia* = dance). The delayed onset of symptoms results in the possibility of transmitting the disease to offspring prior to knowing that one carries the defective gene. Pedigree analysis and genetic counseling for patients and families harboring the gene for Huntington's disease is extremely important.

A   PEDIGREE CHART

One affected parent (Aa)   Two affected parents (both Aa)
One normal parent (aa)

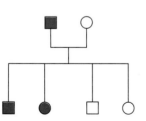

FIGURE 5–9. Typical pattern of inheritance of an autosomal dominant trait. **A,** Pedigree chart. **B,** Punnett square.

B   PUNNETT SQUARE

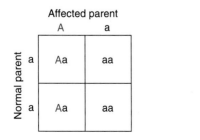

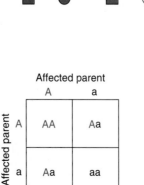

TABLE 5–2. Major Known Autosomal Dominant Disorders

Adult polycystic kidney disease
Familial hypercholesterolemia
Huntington's disease
Marfan's syndrome
Neurofibromatosis (Recklinghausen's disease)
Hereditary spherocytosis
von Willebrand's disease

Data from Cotran R, Kumar V, Robbins S (eds): *Robbins Pathologic Basis of Disease*, 4th ed. Philadelphia, WB Saunders, 1989.

Autosomal Recessive Disorders

Autosomal recessive disorders are due to a mutation of a recessive gene located on one of the autosomes. Autosomal recessive disorders follow predictable patterns of inheritance (Fig. 5–11), which may be summarized as follows:

1. Males and females are equally affected.
2. In most cases the disease is not apparent in the parents or relatives of the affected individual, but both parents are carriers of the mutant recessive gene.
3. Unaffected individuals may transmit the disease to offspring.
4. The mating of two carriers (heterozygous) results in a 1 in 4 chance of producing an affected offspring, and a 2 in 4 chance of producing an offspring who carries the disease.

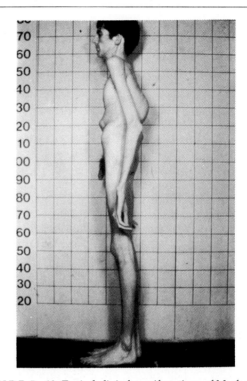

FIGURE 5–10. Typical clinical manifestations of Marfan's syndrome. (From Connor JM, Ferguson-Smith MA: *Essential Medical Genetics*, 3rd ed. London, Blackwell Scientific Publications, 1991. Reproduced with permission.)

A PEDIGREE CHART

One heterozygous carrier parent (Aa)
One affected parent (aa)

Two heterozygous carrier parents (both Aa)

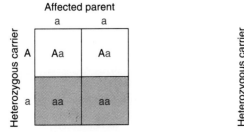
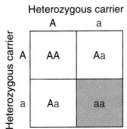

B PUNNETT SQUARE

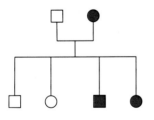

Affected parent

	a	a
A	Aa	Aa
a	aa	aa

Heterozygous carrier

	A	a
A	AA	Aa
a	Aa	aa

FIGURE 5–11. Typical pattern of inheritance of an autosomal recessive trait. **A**, Pedigree chart. **B**, Punnett square.

It is believed that nearly everyone carries one or more mutant recessive genes. Related individuals are more likely to carry the *same* recessive genes. Since recessive diseases are only expressed when both alleles for a particular gene are mutant (homozygous), they are often associated with **consanguinity**—the mating of related individuals.[18] The closer the biological relationship, the greater the proportion of shared genes and the greater the risk of producing affected offspring.

Recessive disorders often involve abnormal enzymatic functions. The gene for a particular enzyme may be absent or in a mutant, and therefore nonfunctional, form. The enzyme deficiency is not apparent in heterozygotes carrying one normal gene and one mutant gene, because the normal gene produces enough of the necessary enzyme. In the homozygous state, neither gene for the enzyme is functional, resulting in an enzyme deficiency. A partial listing of the large number of autosomal recessive disorders that have been identified is given in Table 5–3. Many of these diseases involve inability to metabolize nutrients (inborn errors of metabolism) or to synthesize cellular components because of enzyme deficiencies. Albinism and phenylketonuria are two examples. Other disorders are described in the discussions of system pathophysiology in later chapters.

Albinism. Albinism refers to a lack of pigmentation of the hair, skin, and eye. There are at least six different forms of oculocutaneous albinism, all of which are transmitted as autosomal recessive disorders. Some forms of albinism are associated with organ defects. The defect in one form of albinism has been traced to lack of the enzyme **tyrosinase,** which catalyzes the formation of dopa from tyrosine. Dopa is a precursor of the pigment melanin. Individuals with albinism are at risk for sunburn and skin cancer, and generally exhibit impaired vision and photosensitivity.[1]

Phenylketonuria. Phenylketonuria (PKU) results from an inability to metabolize the amino acid phenylalanine due to lack of the enzyme *phenylalanine hydroxylase.*[13] It is one of several enzyme deficiencies that are often referred to as **inborn errors of metabolism.** The symptoms of the disorder are due to the buildup of dietary phenylalanine in the body, which primarily affects the nervous system. Children with PKU tend to be overly irritable and tremorous and have slowly developing mental retardation. Excess phenylalanine is excreted in the urine in the form of phenylketones—hence the name phenylketonuria. The enzyme deficiency can be detected soon after birth and treated with a low-phenylalanine diet. Because treatment must be instituted very early in order to prevent mental retardation, routine testing for PKU is performed at birth.

Sex-Linked (X-Linked) Disorders

Sex-linked disorders are due to a mutation of the sex chromosomes. Disorders linked to the Y chromosome are extremely rare, and for that reason the terms sex-linked and X-linked are often used interchangeably. Nearly all X-linked disorders are recessive. Females will express the X-linked disease only in the rare instance in which both X chromosomes carry the defective gene. Males, however, do not have the safety margin of two X chromosomes and will express the disease if their one and only X chromosome is abnormal. X-linked disorders follow predictable patterns of inheritance which are dependent on the sex of the offspring and may be summarized as follows:

1. Affected individuals are almost always males.
2. Affected fathers transmit the defective gene to none of their sons but all of their daughters.
3. Unaffected males do not carry the defective gene.
4. A carrier female has a 1 in 2 chance of producing an affected son and a 1 in 2 chance of producing a carrier daughter.
5. Females are affected only in the rare homozygous state which may occur from the mating of an affected or carrier mother and an affected father.

Several X-linked recessive disorders have been identified, as presented in Table 5–4. A well-known example of an X-linked disease is hemophilia A.

Hemophilia A. Hemophilia A is a bleeding disorder associated with a deficiency of Factor VIII, a protein necessary for blood clotting.[19] Individuals afflicted with hemophilia A bleed easily and profusely from seemingly minor injuries. The transmission of hemophilia A in the European royal families constitutes one of the best-known pedigrees available (Fig. 5–12). Queen Victoria of England was the first known carrier of the disease. A number of her male descendants were affected by it.

TABLE 5–3. Major Known Autosomal Recessive Disorders

Albinism
α_1-Antitrypsin deficiency
Cystic fibrosis
Galactosemia
Glycogen storage disease
Lysosomal storage diseases
Phenylketonuria
Severe combined immunodeficiency
Sickle cell anemia

Data from Cotran R, Kumar V, Robbins S (eds): *Robbins Pathologic Basis of Disease*, 4th ed. Philadelphia, WB Saunders, 1989.

TABLE 5–4. Major Known X-Linked (Recessive) Disorders

Hemophilia A
Glucose-6-phosphate dehydrogenase deficiency
Agammaglobulinemia
Muscular dystrophy (certain forms)

Data from Cotran R, Kumar V, Robbins S (eds): *Robbins Pathologic Basis of Disease*, 4th ed. Philadelphia, WB Saunders, 1989.

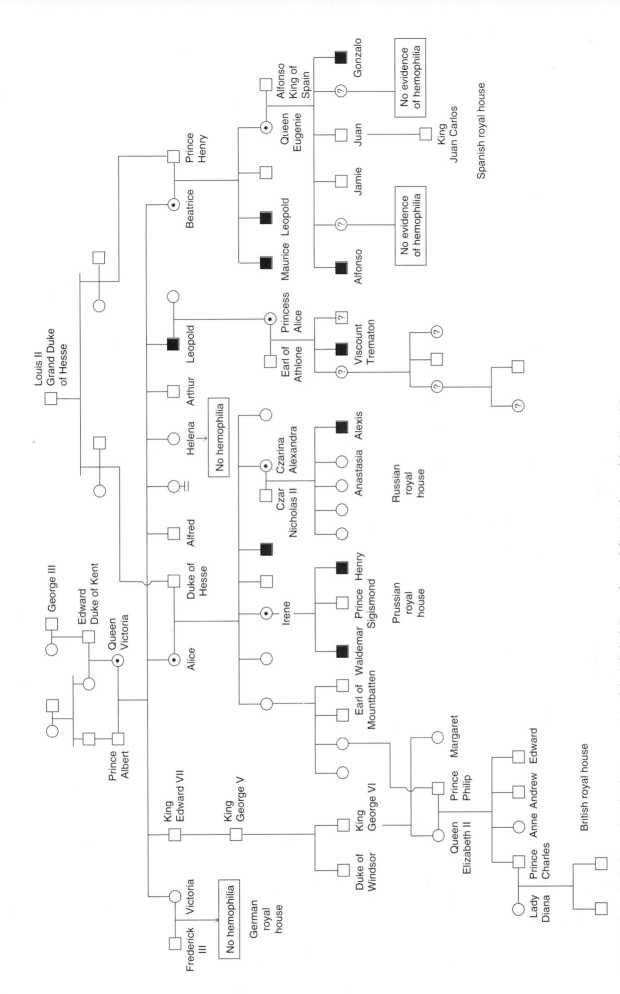

FIGURE 5-12. Pedigree chart for the transmission of the X-linked disease hemophilia A in the royal families of Europe.

Multifactorial (Polygenic) Disorders

Multifactorial disorders are thought to involve two or more mutant genes that act together to produce the trait. Multifactorial disorders are greatly influenced by environmental factors, so that they do not follow clear-cut modes of inheritance but do tend to "run in families." Characteristics that are governed by multifactorial inheritance tend to have a range of expression in the population. For example, height, weight, and intelligence are multifactorial. Most multifactorial disorders also present a range of severity, although a few disorders are either present or not. In the latter case, it may be that a certain threshold number of defective genes must be inherited before the disease is expressed.[1,20]

It is extremely difficult to predict the risk of occurrence of multifactorial disorders based on family history. The risk of recurrence of a typical multifactorial disorder is in the range of 2 percent to 7 percent.[13] Thus, the parents of one affected child have a 2 percent to 7 percent chance of bearing a second affected child. The risk rises to about 9 percent after the birth of a second affected child.[13] The number of genes contributing to the disorder, the degree to which the disease is expressed, and environmental influences (most of which may be undetermined) all affect the true risk of recurrence. It is apparent why multifactorial inheritance has been called "a geneticist's nightmare."

In contrast to single-gene and chromosomal abnormalities, which are rare, multifactorial disorders are very common. High blood pressure, cancer, diabetes mellitus, cleft lip, and several forms of congenital heart defects are governed by multifactorial inheritance. This list is destined to grow as knowledge of the role of genetic mechanisms in cellular function and disease expands.

KEY CONCEPTS

- Genetic disorders are of three general types: chromosomal aberrations, single-gene disorders, and polygenic disorders.
- Chromosome disorders result from an abnormality in number or structure. The presence of one chromosome is termed monosomy (e.g., Turner's syndrome), and the presence of an excessive number of chromosomes is called polysomy (e.g., Down's syndrome). Abnormal rearrangement of portions of the chromosomes (translocation, inversion, deletion, duplication) can result in loss or unusual expression of genes.
- Single-gene disorders result from mutations that alter the nucleotide sequence of one particular gene. Single-gene disorders are transmitted predictably and include autosomal dominant (e.g., Huntington's disease), autosomal recessive (phenylketonuria), and sex-linked (hemophilia) disorders.

- Polygenic disorders are very common and result from the interaction of multiple genes. Disorders such as high blood pressure, cancer, and diabetes are polygenic.

Environmentally Induced Congenital Disorders

Adverse influences during intrauterine life are a significant cause of errors in fetal development that result in congenital malformations. The study of developmental anomalies is called **teratology** (Greek *teraton* = monster). Environmental influences that may adversely affect the developing fetus, such as chemicals, radiation, and viral infections, are called **teratogens**. Many substances are thought to have teratogenic potential, based on experiments in animals, but few are proved in humans. Exposure to a known teratogen may, but need not, result in a congenital malformation. Susceptibility to a teratogen depends on the amount of exposure, the developmental stage of the fetus when exposed, the prior condition of the mother, and the genetic predisposition of the fetus.[5]

Periods of Fetal Vulnerability

The timing of the exposure to a teratogen greatly influences fetal susceptibility and the resulting type of malformation. The intrauterine development of humans can be divided into two stages: (1) the embryonic period, which extends from conception to 9 weeks of development, followed by (2) the fetal period, which continues until birth. Prior to the third week of gestation, exposure to a teratogen generally either damages so few cells that the fetus develops normally, or damages so many cells that the fetus cannot survive and spontaneously aborts. Between the third and ninth week of gestation the fetus is very vulnerable to teratogenesis, with the fourth and fifth weeks the time of peak susceptibility.[5] Organ development (organogenesis) occurs during this period and is very sensitive to injury, regardless of the etiology. Each organ has a critical period during which it is most vulnerable to malformation (Fig. 5–13). The fetal period, from 3 to 9 months, is primarily concerned with further growth and maturation of the organs and is significantly less susceptible to errors of morphogenesis. Fetal insults occurring after the third month are more likely to result in growth retardation or injury to normally formed organs. Unfortunately, an embryo may be exposed to teratogens during the vulnerable period because the mother does not yet realize she is pregnant.

Teratogenic Agents

The teratogenic potential of many agents is unknown. Several chemicals, some infections, and large doses of radiation are definitely associated with a higher risk

Embryonic period (weeks)

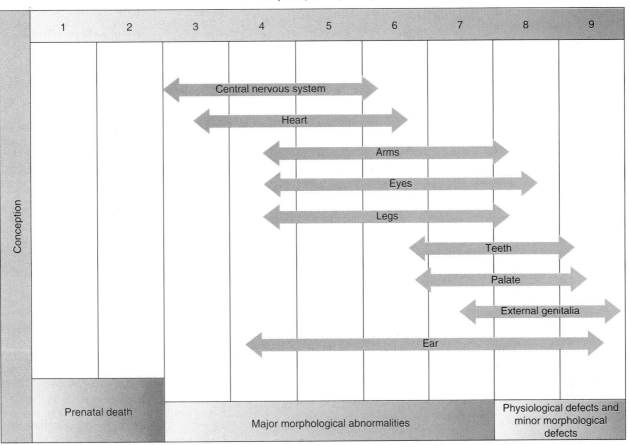

FIGURE 5-13. The vulnerable periods of fetal organ development.

of congenital disorders. In general, teratogens cause errors in morphogenesis by interfering with cell proliferation, migration, or differentiation. The specific mechanisms of action of most teratogens are unknown.

Chemicals and Drugs

The list of proved teratogenic chemicals and drugs includes thalidomide, alcohol, anticonvulsants, warfarin, folate antagonists, androgenic hormones, and organic mercury. Almost no drugs or chemicals are considered to be totally safe, and the current trend is to discourage pregnant women from using *any* drugs or chemicals. Two agents, thalidomide and alcohol, illustrate the teratogenic potential of chemicals.

In the 1960s, a jump in the incidence of congenital limb deformities was traced to maternal use of **thalidomide,** a tranquilizer, between the 28th and 50th day of pregnancy.[5,13] Exposure during the vulnerable period was associated with a very high risk (50 percent–80 percent) of fetal malformation. Typically, the arms were short and flipper-like, although deformities ranged from mild abnormalities of the digits to complete absence of the limbs. Damage to other structures, particularly the ears and heart, also occurred. Thalidomide is one of the most potent teratogens known.

The chronic ingestion of large amounts of alcohol is now known to cause a group of congenital anomalies referred to as **fetal alcohol syndrome.** It is estimated that between 1 and 5 of every 1,000 newborns suffer from alcohol-induced anomalies.[21] Affected infants suffer from growth retardation, neurologic disorders, malformations of the head and face, and atrial septal heart defects. Chronic alcohol intake of six or more hard drinks per day carries a significant risk for causing fetal alcohol syndrome.[22,23] There is insufficient data to determine what, if any, level of alcohol intake during pregnancy is safe. Apart from any direct teratogenic effect, alcohol also causes acute and transient collapse of the umbilical cord, which could damage the fetus by interrupting its oxygen supply.[24] Complete abstinence from alcohol during pregnancy is generally recommended.

Infectious Agents

A number of microorganisms have been implicated in the development of congenital malformations. Certain viral infections appear to carry the greatest threat, although protozoa and bacteria have also been implicated. As with other teratogens, the gestational age of the fetus at the time of infection is critically important. Perhaps the best known viral teratogen is **rubella.** The risk period for rubella infection begins just prior to conception and extends to 20 weeks' gestation, after which the virus rarely crosses the placenta. Rubella-induced defects vary but typically include cataracts, deafness, and heart defects. Several other organisms cause a similar constellation of congenital defects, so the acronym TORCH was developed to alert clinicians to the potential teratogenicity of these infections. TORCH stands for *toxoplasmosis, others, rubella, cytomegalovirus, herpes.* The major features of the TORCH complex are shown in Figure 5–14. The category of "others" includes several less frequently seen causes: hepatitis B, coxsackie virus B, mumps, poliovirus, and others. All microorganisms of the TORCH complex are able to cross the placenta and infect the fetus.

Toxoplasmosis is a protozoal infection that can be contracted from ingestion of raw or undercooked meat and from contact with cat feces. **Cytomegalovirus** and **herpes simplex virus** are generally transmitted to the fetus by chronic carrier mothers. Cytomega-

lovirus and herpes simplex virus often colonize the genital area of the mothers. Infants who escape infection in utero may still acquire the virus as they pass through the birth canal (see Chap. 34).

Radiation

In addition to being mutagenic, radiation is also teratogenic. The teratogenic potential of radiation became apparent from the increased incidence of congenital malformations in children born to women exposed to radiation of the cervix for cancer and in the children of atomic bomb victims in World War II. It is not known if lower levels of radiation, such as those used in diagnostic x-rays, are teratogenic. It is generally recommended that pregnant women avoid diagnostic x-rays or use appropriate lead shielding.

Other Disorders of Infancy

An infant may be afflicted with a variety of problems at birth that do not fall into the category of genetic or developmental malformations. These problems generally arise later in uterine life and often involve mechanical factors or problems with the health of the mother and placenta. For example, babies with low birth weight or immaturity at birth may have difficulty breathing and taking in adequate nutrition. Interruption of the placental oxygen supply due to maternal hemorrhage, sedation, or blood incompatibility may result in fetal brain injury. A difficult labor and delivery may result in a variety of injuries during the birthing process. The details of these diseases of infancy and childhood may be found in specialized texts.

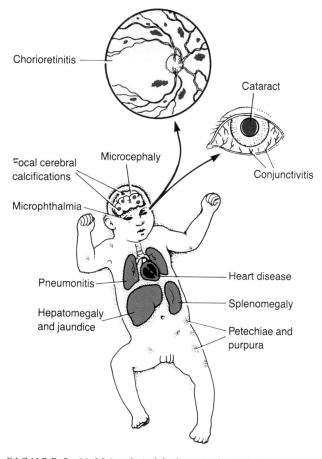

F I G U R E 5 – 14. Major clinical findings in the TORCH complex of infective congenital disorders. (From Rubin E, Farber J: *Essential Pathology.* Philadelphia, JB Lippincott, 1990, p 136. Reproduced with permission. Artist: Dimitri Karetnikov.)

Labels in figure: Chorioretinitis; Cataract; Focal cerebral calcifications; Microcephaly; Conjunctivitis; Microphthalmia; Pneumonitis; Heart disease; Splenomegaly; Hepatomegaly and jaundice; Petechiae and purpura

KEY CONCEPTS

- **Environmental factors that adversely affect the developing fetus are called teratogens. Exposure to teratogens is particularly dangerous during the third to ninth weeks of gestation.**

- **Known teratogens include chemicals and drugs, infections, and radiation. The teratogenic potential of many chemicals and drugs is unknown, so pregnant women are usually advised to avoid all drugs if possible.**

- **Of the infectious agents, viruses are the most teratogenic, particularly organisms of the TORCH variety (toxoplasmosis, rubella, cytomegalovirus, herpesvirus).**

Diagnosis, Counseling, and Gene Therapy

In recent years, the ability to diagnose and treat genetic and developmental disorders has improved dramatically. Although pedigree analysis continues to be an important method for identifying at-risk individuals, for a number of disorders it is now possible to definitely determine whether a particular fetus is afflicted. Unfortunately, individuals at risk for transmitting recessive genetic diseases often are not identified until the birth of an afflicted child. Genetic counseling and prenatal assessment then become extremely important in assisting the family in regard to future pregnancies.

Prenatal Diagnosis and Counseling

A number of conditions are associated with a higher risk of congenital anomalies and are indications for instituting counseling and prenatal diagnostic examination. These conditions include (1) maternal age of 35 or greater, (2) bearing a previous child with a chromosomal disorder (such as trisomy 21), (3) a known family history of X-linked disorders, (4) a family history of inborn errors of metabolism, (5) the occurrence of neural tube anomalies in a previous pregnancy, and (6) known carriers of recessive genetic disorders. As diagnostic methods become more sophisticated, tests for other risk factors may be possible.

At present, ultrasound and amniocentesis are the mainstays of prenatal diagnostic examination. **Ultrasound** is a noninvasive procedure that uses sound waves to produce a reflected image of the fetus. It is commonly used to determine gestational age, fetal position, and placental location. Ultrasound is also useful in detecting visible congenital anomalies such as spina bifida (neural tube defect), heart defects, and malformations of the face, head, body, and limbs. It is useless for determining biochemical or chromosomal alterations. **Amniocentesis** may be performed to determine genetic and developmental disorders not detectable by ultrasound. During amniocentesis, a needle is inserted through the abdomen and into the uterus. A sample of amniotic fluid containing skin cells shed by the fetus is removed for analysis. The amniotic fluid can be analyzed for abnormal levels of certain substances secreted by the fetus, such as α-fetoprotein, which indicates neural tube defects. The live skin cells can be cultured and subjected to biochemical and chromosome analysis. Only certain genetic and developmental disorders can be reliably detected by these procedures, and they may not provide the needed information until relatively late in the pregnancy. Amniocentesis cannot generally be performed prior to the 16th week of gestation, and 2 or 3 more weeks may be required to culture skin cells and subject them to analysis. **Chorionic villus biopsy** involves the removal of a bit of tissue directly from the chorion. It can be performed at 8 weeks' gestation. The early diagnosis of congenital disorders allows a greater number of treatment options. Some disorders can be treated in utero; others may require early delivery, immediate surgery, or cesarean section to minimize fetal trauma. Prior warning of fetal difficulties allows parents time to prepare emotionally for the birth of the child. In some instances, termination of the pregnancy may be the treatment of choice.

Human Genome Project and Gene Therapy

Painstaking pedigree analysis has allowed geneticists to assign a number of genetic traits and diseases to particular locations on the chromosomes. The process of determining the chromosomal location of genes is often called **mapping.** Recent techniques in genetic analysis have radically improved the ability to assign genes to specific chromosomal locations. Two of these techniques, somatic cell hybridization and in situ hybridization, have been particularly fruitful. Not only are the locations of many genes being found, but the entire DNA sequence of many genes is being determined. It has been predicted that the DNA sequence of the entire human genome, containing 3 billion base pairs, will be determined in about 15 years.[25,26] A great deal of money and effort is going into the Human Genome Project in an effort to map and sequence the entire human genome.[27] The maps of the 23 human chromosomes as of 1994 are shown in the appendix.

An exciting outcome of the genome project is the potential for **gene therapy**—the treatment of genetic disease by replacing the defective gene with a normal healthy one. This idea once sounded like science fiction, but clinical trials are already underway to treat children who suffer from a rare condition called severe combined immunodeficiency (SCID) by introducing a functional gene for the enzyme adenosine deaminase. Children who suffer from SCID have severely compromised immune systems and generally die from overwhelming infections.[28,29]

Gene therapy has the potential for alleviating human suffering by curing genetic diseases, but it is accompanied by a number of moral and ethical dilemmas. Tampering with the human gene pool could have serious implications for human evolution. There is also the potential for misusing the technology to create "new and improved" human beings.

KEY CONCEPTS

- Risk factors that indicate the need for prenatal diagnostic examination and counseling include advanced maternal age (over 35 years), a family history of recessive or sex-linked disorders, and the birth of a previous child with chromosomal or neural tube defects.
- Ultrasound, amniocentesis, and chorionic villus biopsy are the mainstays of prenatal assessment for genetic disorders.
- Gene therapy is the treatment of genetic disease by replacing defective genes with normal genes.

Summary

Genetic and developmental disorders are responsible for a number of congenital malformations. Congenital disorders are caused by genetic and environmental factors that disrupt normal fetal development. Genetic disorders are classified as (1) chromosomal alterations, including structural and numerical abnormalities, and (2) Mendelian disorders, including autosomal dominant, autosomal recessive, and X-linked disorders. Known environmental teratogens include radiation, infectious organisms, and a number of chemicals and drugs. The fetus is particularly susceptible to teratogens during the period of organogenesis, which extends from the third to the ninth week of gestation. Pedigree analysis, ultrasound, amniocentesis, and chorionic villus biopsy may provide helpful information regarding genetic risk and the prenatal condition of at-risk infants. The Human Genome Project, which is mapping and sequencing the entire human genome, may allow the development of gene replacement therapy for a variety of genetic diseases in the near future.

REFERENCES

1. Cotran RS, Kumar V, Robbins SL: Genetic disorders, in Cotran RS, Kumar V, Robbins SL (eds): *Robbins Pathologic Basis of Disease*, 4th ed. Philadelphia, WB Saunders, 1989.
2. Erbe RW: Current concepts in genetics: Principles of medical genetics (parts 1 and 2). *N Engl J Med* 1976;294(7):381, 294(9):480–482.
3. Shepard TH: Human teratogenicity. *Adv Pediatr* 1986;33: 225–268.
4. US Bureau of the Census: *Statistical Abstracts of the United States: 1991*, 111th ed. Washington, DC, US Government Printing Office, 1991.
5. Cotran RS, Kumar V, Robbins SL: Diseases of infancy and childhood, in Cotran RS, Kumar V, Robbins SL (eds): *Robbins Pathologic Basis of Disease*, 4th ed. Philadelphia, WB Saunders, 1989.
6. Connor JM, Ferguson-Smith MA: Chromosome aberrations, in Connor JM, Ferguson-Smith MA (eds): *Essential Medical Genetics*. London, Blackwell Scientific Publications, 1991.
7. Hassold TJ, Jacobs PA: Trisomy in man. *Annu Rev Genet* 1984;18:69–97.
8. Juberg RC, Mowrey PN: Origin of nondisjunction in trisomy 21 syndrome: All studies compiled, parental age analysis, and international comparisons. *Am J Med Genet* 1983;16(1):111–116.
9. Ayala FJ, Kiger JA: *Modern Genetics*. Menlo Park, CA, Benjamin/Cummings, 1980.
10. Connor JM, Ferguson-Smith MA: Chromosome disorders, in Connor JM, Ferguson-Smith MA (eds): *Essential Medical Genetics*. London, Blackwell Scientific Publications, 1991.
11. Down JHL: Observations on an ethnic classification of idiots. *Clin Lect Rep London Hosp* 1866;3:259–262.
12. Thompson MW, McInnes RR, Willard HF (eds): *Thompson and Thompson Genetics in Medicine*, 5th ed. Philadelphia, WB Saunders, 1991.
13. Damjanov I: Developmental and genetic diseases, in Rubin E, Farber J (eds): *Essential Pathology*. Philadelphia, JB Lippincott, 1990.
14. Alberts B, Bray D, Lewis J, Raff M, Roberts K, Watson J: Basic genetic mechanisms, in Alberts B, Bray D, Lewis J, Raff M, Roberts K, Watson J (eds): *Molecular Biology of the Cell*, 2nd ed. New York, Garland Press, 1989.
15. Pope FM, Nichols AC, Lewkonia RM, Halme T, Dorrance DE, Pomerance A: Clinical and genetic heterogeneity of the Marphan syndrome. *Curr Probl Dermatol* 1987;17:95–110.
16. Pope FM, Nichols AC: Molecular abnormalities of collagen in human disease. *Arch Dis Child* 1987;62:523–528.
17. Ogilvie DJ, Wordsworth BP, Priestley LM, Dalgleish R, Schmidtke J, Zoll B, Sykes BC: Segregation of all four major fibrillar collagen genes in the Marphan syndrome. *Am J Hum Genet* 1987;41:1071–1082.
18. Connor JM, Ferguson-Smith MA: Population genetics, in Connor JM, Ferguson-Smith MA (eds): *Essential Medical Genetics*. London, Blackwell Scientific Publications, 1991.
19. Connor JM, Ferguson-Smith MA: Single-gene disorders, in Connor JM, Ferguson-Smith MA (eds): *Essential Medical Genetics*. London, Blackwell Scientific Publications, 1991.
20. Connor JM, Ferguson-Smith MA: Multifactorial inheritance, in Connor JM, Ferguson-Smith MA (eds): *Essential Medical Genetics*. London, Blackwell Scientific Publications, 1991.
21. Golbus MS: Teratology for the obstetrician: Current status. *Obstet Gynecol* 1980;55(3):269–277.
22. Beckman DA, Brent RL: Mechanism of known environmental teratogens: Drugs and chemicals. *Clin Perinatol* 1986;13(3): 649–687.
23. Jones KL: The fetal alcohol syndrome. *Growth Genet Horm* 1988;4(1):1–3.
24. Mukherjee AB, Hodgen GD: Maternal alcohol exposure induces transient impairment of umbilical circulation and fetal hypoxia in monkeys. *Science* 1982;218(4573):700–702.
25. Stephens JC, Cavanaugh ML, Gradie MI, Mador ML, Kidd KK: Mapping the human genome: Current status. *Science* 1990;250:237–244.
26. McKusick VA: Presidential Address, Eighth International Congress of Human Genetics: Human genetics: The last 35 years, the present, and the future. *Am J Hum Genet* 1992;50:663–670.
27. The human genome 1993: Human genetic disorders. *J NIH Res* 1993;5(8):123–152.
28. Verma IM: Gene therapy. *Sci Am* 1990;263(5):68–84.
29. Anderson WF: Human gene therapy. *Science* 1992;256:808–813.

BIBLIOGRAPHY

British Medical Association: *Our Genetic Future: The Science and Ethics of Genetic Technology*. Oxford, Oxford University Press, 1992.

Burton BK, Schulz CJ, Burd LI: Limb anomalies associated with chorionic villus sampling. *Obstet Gynecol* 1992;79(5 pt 1): 726–730.

Carey JC, Stevens CA, Haskins R: Craniofacial malformations and their syndromes: An overview for the speech and hearing practitioner. *Clin Commun Disord* 1992;2(4):59–72.

Connor JM, Ferguson-Smith MA: *Essential Medical Genetics*, London, Blackwell Scientific Publications, 1991.

Cotran RS, Kumar V, Robbins SL (eds): *Robbins Pathologic Basis of Disease*, 4th ed. Philadelphia, WB Saunders, 1989.

Holland B, Kyriacou C: *Genetics and Society*. Wokingham, England, Addison-Wesley, 1993.

Hubbard R, Wald E: *Exploding the Gene Myth: How Genetic Information Is Produced and Manipulated by Scientists, Physicians, Employers, Insurance Companies, Educators, and Law Enforcers*. Boston, Beacon Press, 1993.

(The) Human genome 1993: Human genetic disorders. *J NIH Res* 1993;5(8):123–152.

Lindhout D, Omtzigt JG: Pregnancy and the risk of teratogenicity. *Epilepsia* 1992;33(suppl 4):S41–S48.

Los FJ, Hagenaars AM, Marrink J, Cohen-Overbeek TE, Gaillard JL, Brandenburg H: Maternal serum alpha-fetoprotein levels and fetal outcome in early second-trimester oligohydramnios. *Prenat Diagn* 1992;12(4):285–292.

Milunsky A: *Genetic Disorders and the Fetus: Diagnosis, Prevention, and Treatment*, 3rd ed. Baltimore, Johns Hopkins University Press, 1992.

National Down Syndrome Society: *Down Syndrome and Alzheimer Disease: Proceedings of the National Down Syndrome Society Conference on Down Syndrome and Alzheimer Disease*. New York, Wiley-Liss, 1992.

Poole AE, Redford Badwal DA: Structural abnormalities of the craniofacial complex and congenital malformations. *Pediatr Clin North Am* 1991;38(5):1089–1125.

Redline RW, Neish A, Holmes LB, Collins T: Homeobox genes and congenital malformations. *Lab Invest* 1992;66(6):659–670.

Verma IM: Gene therapy. *Sci Am* 1990;263:68–72, 81–84.

White E: *Genes, Brains, and Politics: Self-selection and Social Life*. Westport, CT, Praeger, 1993.

Wilson RD, Chitayat D, McGillivray BC: Fetal ultrasound abnormalities: Correlation with fetal karyotype, autopsy findings, and postnatal outcome. Five-year prospective study. *Am J Med Genet* 1992;44(5):586–590.

CHAPTER 6
Neoplasia

JACQUELYN L. BANASIK

KEY TERMS

anaplasia: A lack of differentiated features in a tumor cell as evidenced by variations in cell size and shape and by abnormal nuclei.

anti-oncogenes: Genes that regulate groups of growth-promoting genes and suppress tumor formation. Also called tumor suppression genes.

autocrine signaling: The secretion of factors that positively feed back onto the cell that secreted them. Usually used in reference to growth factors.

benign tumor: A type of tumor that is strictly local, usually well differentiated, and does not metastasize.

carcinogens: Substances that initiate or promote the development of cancers. Most carcinogens cause cancer by damaging DNA.

grading: Assignment of degree of differentiation of tumor cells by histologic examination. The degree of anaplasia usually correlates with the degree of malignancy.

malignant tumor: A type of tumor that has a tendency to invade local tissues and spread to distant sites (metastasize). Malignant tumors are generally poorly differentiated and associated with a poor prognosis if not promptly treated.

metastasis: Dissemination of cancer cells from the location of origin to other areas in the body.

neoplasia: An abnormal proliferation of cells; may be benign or malignant.

oncogenes: Genes associated with the initiation of cancerous behavior in a cell.

proto-oncogenes: Normal cellular genes that are growth promoting and usually inhibited in nonproliferating cells. When erroneously activated, they become oncogenes and lead to cancer.

staging: The process of determining the extent and location of cancer within an individual.

---

*N*eoplasia means "new growth." In common use, the term implies an *abnormality* of cellular growth and is used interchangeably with the term *tumor*. Neoplasia is associated with uncertain and sometimes life-threatening consequences. It is no surprise that the discovery of a tumor in an individual can evoke feelings of disbelief, anger, and dread. Characterization of the tumor cells is of critical importance to determine if the tumor is benign or malignant (cancerous). The diagnosis of a **benign** growth is received with great relief, as the tumor is generally easily cured. The diagnosis of a **malignant** cancer, on the other hand, heralds months of intensive and often uncomfortable treatment with uncertain outcomes.

The effective treatment and prevention of cancer have been hampered by lack of knowledge of the fundamental causes of cancer. It is increasingly clear that *cancer is due to altered expression of cellular genes.* Unfortunately, identification of the genes involved and their effects on cellular function has been slow to unfold. More than 40 potential cancer-causing genes (oncogenes) have been proposed to date. A unified theory of cancer causation is finally emerging, bringing with it the hope of new methods for cancer therapy.

Benign Versus Malignant Growth

Characteristics of Benign and Malignant Tumors

The terms benign and malignant refer to the overall consequences of a tumor on the host. Generally, malignant tumors have the potential to kill the host if left untreated, whereas benign tumors do not. This difference is not strict, for some benign tumors may be located in critical areas. For example, a benign tumor may be life-threatening if it causes pressure on the brain or blocks an airway or blood vessel. Conversely, a malignant tumor may be so slow-growing and stationary that it poses little threat to the host.

Histologic examination of a tumor is the primary mode for determining its benign or malignant nature. The characterization of a tumor as benign or malignant is based more on experience than on scientific principle. Certain tumor characteristics have historically been shown to indicate malignant potential. Important considerations include localization of the tumor and the differentiation of tumor cells.

Benign tumors do not invade adjacent tissue or spread to distant sites (**metastasize**).[1] Many benign tumors are encapsulated by connective tissue, indicating strictly local growth. Any indication that tumor cells have penetrated local tissues, lymphatics, or blood vessels suggests a malignant nature with potential to spread.

As a general rule, benign cells more closely resemble their tissue type of origin (e.g., skin, liver, and so forth) than malignant cells. The degree of differentiation has traditionally been used to predict malignant potential. A lack of differentiated features in a cancer cell is called **anaplasia.** A greater degree of anaplasia is correlated with a more aggressively malignant tumor.[2] Anaplasia is indicated by variation in cell size and shape within the tumor (Fig. 6–1), enlarged nuclei, abnormal mitoses, and bizarre-looking giant cells. Regardless of appearance, invasion of local tissue or evidence of metastasis confirms the diagnosis of malignancy.

Other differences between benign and malignant tumors have been noted (Table 6–1). Benign tumors generally grow more slowly, have little vascularity, rarely have necrotic areas, and often retain functions similar to those of the tissue of origin. Conversely, malignant tumors often grow rapidly and may initiate vessel growth in the tumor. They frequently have necrotic areas and are dysfunctional.

Tumor Terminology

General rules for the naming of tumors have been developed to indicate the tissue of origin and the benign or malignant nature of the tumor. The suffix -*oma* is used to indicate a benign tumor, whereas *carcinoma* and *sarcoma* are used to indicate malignant tumors. Carcinoma refers to malignant tumors of epithelial origin and sarcoma to malignant tumors of mesenchymal origin. Thus, a benign tumor of glandular tissue would be called an adenoma, but a malig-

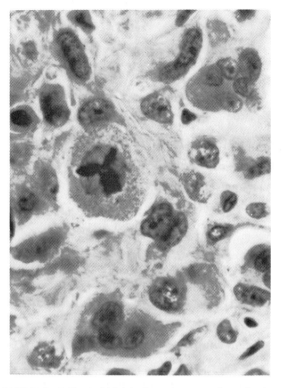

F I G U R E 6 – 1. Typical histologic appearance of anaplastic tumor cells showing variation in cell sizes and shapes. (From Cotran RS, Kumar V, Robbins SL (eds): *Robbins Pathologic Basis of Disease,* 5th ed. Philadelphia, WB Saunders, 1994. Reproduced with permission.)

nant tumor of the same tissue would be called an adenocarcinoma (Table 6–2). There are some notable exceptions to the rules. Lymphomas, hepatomas, and melanomas are all highly malignant, despite their *-oma* suffix. Leukemia refers to a malignant growth of white blood cells.

Metastatic Processes

Loss of Growth Control

Cancer cells are characterized by a lack of normal growth controls, which enables them to break their

TABLE 6–1. General Characteristics of Benign and Malignant Tumors

Characteristic	Benign	Malignant
Histology	Typical of tissue of origin	Anaplastic, with abnormal cell size and shape
	Few mitoses	Many mitoses
Growth rate	Slow	Rapid
Localization/ metastasis	Strictly local, often encapsulated/no metastasis	Infiltrative/frequent metastases
Tumor necrosis	Rare	Common
Recurrence after treatment	Rare	Common
Prognosis	Good	Poor if untreated

attachments, penetrate blood vessels and lymphatics, and invade tissues at distant locations. This process is called **metastasis.** Several abnormal growth properties of cancer cells have been noted in cell culture experiments, including loss of topoinhibition,[3] loss of anchorage dependence,[4] and decreased reliance on growth-promoting factors.[5] An understanding of these properties may help uncover the biological mechanisms of cancer cells.

Cells growing in normal tissues have predictable relationships with neighboring cells. In a particular tissue, the rate of cell growth is precisely matched to the rate of cell death. Normal cells respond to contact with other cells and extracellular matrix molecules by altering their growth rates. Normal cells proliferate only when space is available and the right component of growth-stimulating factors is present. Tumor cells, however, do not obey the rules; they have escaped the normal mechanisms of growth control. Normal cells, when grown in culture, will spread on the bottom of the dish and begin to grow and divide until they make contact with other cells; then they stop. This is called **topoinhibition,** or contact inhibition (see Chap. 2). Cancerous cells do not stop dividing when they contact other cells. They pile up on one another and will continue to divide until they use up the culture medium and die (Fig. 6–2).

The mechanism of topoinhibition is uncertain but is thought to involve changes in cell shape that are transmitted to the cell nucleus by the cytoskeleton.[6] Additionally, cells may signal their neighbors through gap junctions, pores that connect adjacent cells together. Cancer cells in culture have been noted to have reduced numbers of gap junctions[7]; however, the mechanism for loss of topoinhibiton is largely unexplained.

Normal cells in culture must have a solid substance on which to grow. This is termed **anchorage-dependent growth.** Cancer cells have acquired the ability to proliferate in suspension. Apparently, matrix molecules such as fibronectin that stimulate normal cells are not required by cancerous cells.

Tumor cells also have **reduced requirements for growth factors.** Growth factors are locally produced

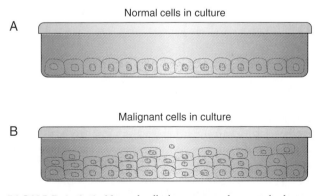

F I G U R E 6 – 2. **A,** Normal cells form a monolayer at the bottom of the culture dish. **B,** Malignant cells continue to divide and pile up on one another. Some malignant cells grow in suspension.

TABLE 6–2. Nomenclature for Neoplastic Diseases

Cell or Tissue of Origin	Benign	Malignant
Tumors of Epithelial Origin		
Squamous cells	Squamous cell papilloma	Squamous cell carcinoma
Basal cells	—	Basal cell carcinoma
Glandular or ductal epithelium	Adenoma	Adenocarcinoma
	Cystadenoma	Cystadenocarcinoma
Transitional cells	Transitional cell papilloma	Transitional cell carcinoma
Bile duct	Bile duct adenoma	Bile duct carcinoma (cholangiocarcinoma)
Liver cells	Hepatocellular adenoma	Hepatocellular carcinoma
Melanocytes	Nevus	Malignant melanoma
Renal epithelium	Renal tubular adenoma	Renal cell carcinoma
Skin adnexal glands		
Sweat glands	Sweat gland adenoma	Sweat gland carcinoma
Sebaceous glands	Sebaceous gland adenoma	Sebaceous gland carcinoma
Germ cells (testis and ovary)	—	Seminoma (dysgerminoma)
		Embryonal carcinoma, yolk sac carcinoma
Tumors of Mesenchymal Origin		
Hematopoietic/lymphoid tissue	—	Leukemia
		Lymphoma
		Hodgkin's disease
		Multiple myeloma
Neural and retinal tissue		
Nerve sheath	Neurilemmoma, neurofibroma	Malignant peripheral nerve sheath tumor
Nerve cells	Ganglioneuroma	Neuroblastoma
Retinal cells (cones)	—	Retinoblastoma
Connective tissue		
Fibrous tissue	Fibromatosis (desmoid)	Fibrosarcoma
Fat	Lipoma	Liposarcoma
Bone	Osteoma	Osteogenic sarcoma
Cartilage	Chondroma	Chondrosarcoma
Muscle		
Smooth muscle	Leiomyoma	Leiomyosarcoma
Striated muscle	Rhabdomyoma	Rhabdomyosarcoma
Endothelial and related tissues		
Blood vessels	Hemangioma	Angiosarcoma
		Kaposi's sarcoma
Lymph vessels	Lymphangioma	Lymphangiosarcoma
Synovium	—	Synovial sarcoma
Mesothelium	—	Malignant mesothelioma
Meninges	Meningioma	Malignant meningioma

From Holleb J, et al (eds): *American Cancer Society Textbook of Clinical Oncology,* 1991, p 8. Reproduced by permission of the American Cancer Society, Atlanta.

(paracrine) peptide hormones that bind to cell surface receptors on target cells. Binding of growth factors initiates a cascade of intracellular responses that leads to cell proliferation. It has recently been proposed that cancer cells may make and respond to their own growth factors, which would remove them from feedback control.[8]

Escape from Tissue of Origin

In order for tumor cells to gain access to the blood or lymphatic circulation, they must first escape the basement membrane of the tissue of origin, move through the extracellular space, and penetrate the basement membrane of the vessel. This process is thought to involve binding to matrix components such as laminin via specific laminin receptors on the tumor cell, followed by release of enzymes such as proteases and collagenases that digest the basement membrane.[9] The cancer cell then squeezes through the rift by ameboid movement. The process is repeated at the vessel basement membrane to access the blood or lymphatic vessel. When the cell reaches the tissue to be colonized, it must again traverse the basement membranes, using similar mechanisms (Fig. 6–3).

Patterns of Spread

The survival of tumor cells in the circulation is not guaranteed. They may be detected by immune cells and destroyed. Only about 0.1 percent of tumor cells survive longer than 24 hours when injected into mice.[10] Some tumor cell types appear to prefer specific target organs. Sometimes the pattern of metastasis is related to the circulatory flow. For example, metastatic tumors from the colon often seed the liver because they travel in the portal vein. The localization of most metastatic tumors is not so easily explained by blood flow patterns, and some tumor cells appear to "home" to specific targets. This homing ability is poorly understood but may involve chemotactic signals from the organ to which the tumor cells respond. Spread via

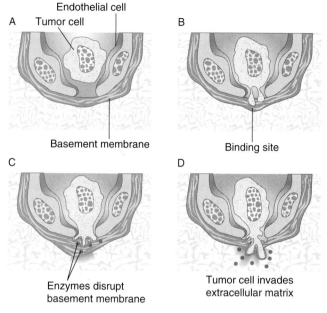

A — Endothelial cell — Tumor cell — Basement membrane

B — Binding site

C — Enzymes disrupt basement membrane

D — Tumor cell invades extracellular matrix

FIGURE 6-3. The mechanisms of tumor invasion and metastasis allow tumor cells to penetrate the basement membrane (BM) and enter tissues. **A,** The tumor cell causes endothelial cells to retract and expose the BM. **B,** Tumor cell attaches to BM via receptors to proteins such as laminin. **C,** Enzymes secreted by tumor cells digest a hole in the BM. **D,** The tumor cell moves through the BM to enter the tissues, secreting enzymes as it goes.

lymphatics is somewhat more predictable than spread by blood flow. Generally the lymph nodes that immediately drain the tissue of cancer origin are colonized first, then the tumor cells tend to spread contiguously from node to node. Hodgkin's disease, a lymphoma, is particularly noted for its orderly spread via the lymphatics.

Tumor Markers

Tumor cells exhibit various degrees of **differentiation,** or resemblance to the parent tissue of origin. Tumor markers are substances associated with tumor cells that may be helpful in identifying the tissue of origin of poorly differentiated metastatic tumors. Identification of the tissue of origin has important implications for prognosis and selection of treatment. Tumor markers rely on the retention of at least some characteristics of the parent tissue type. Enzymes and other proteins that are specific to a particular cell type are commonly used as tumor markers. For example, production of thyroglobulin protein is specific for thyroid tumor cells. Melanoma cells express the antigens HMB-45 and S100, which is helpful in identification as melanocytes. See Table 6–3 for other examples of antigen, hormone, and enzyme markers used to identify tumor cell types.

Grading and Staging of Tumors

Grading and staging of tumors is done to predict the clinical behavior of a malignant tumor and to guide therapy. **Grading** refers to the histologic characterization of tumor cells and is basically a determination of the degree of anaplasia. Most grading systems classify tumors into three or four classes of increasing degrees of malignancy. A greater degree of anaplasia indicates a greater malignant potential. The correlation between the grade of the tumor and its biological behavior is not perfect. Some low-grade tumors have proved to be quite malignant.

The choice of treatment modality is usually influenced more by the stage of the tumor than by its histologic grade. **Staging** describes the location and pattern of spread of a tumor within the host. Factors such as tumor size, extent of local growth, lymph node and organ involvement, and the presence of distant metastases are considered. Several staging systems exist; however, the international TNM (*tumor, node, metastasis*) system is used extensively as a general framework for staging tumors.[11] Particular staging criteria vary with tumors in different organ systems. Examples of staging criteria for breast and colon cancers are shown in Tables 6–4 and 6–5.

Until recently, tumor staging relied primarily on radiography and exploratory surgery. The availability of computed tomography (CT) and magnetic resonance imaging (MRI) as well as other highly sophisticated imaging techniques has revolutionized cancer detection. CT and MRI allow noninvasive exploration of the tissues of the entire body. The computerized images can then be scrutinized for any signs of abnormality which might indicate the presence of hidden tumors. CT and MRI rely primarily on detection of differences in tissue density and therefore are not totally specific for tumors. They can, however, guide the selection of sites for exploration and biopsy and potentially reduce unnecessary surgery.

An exciting new research development in cancer detection is the use of antibodies to track down cancer cells. Antibodies can be raised against specific antigens present on the surface of tumor cells. The antibodies are also bound to a radioactive isotope, such as ^{125}I, which can be detected by imaging. As methods for identifying tumor antigens and raising specific antibodies are improved, this technology may provide the potential for finding very small numbers of tumor cells hidden in the body.

The results of the staging procedure will determine which of the mainstays of cancer treatment—surgery, radiation therapy, or chemotherapy—may be employed, singly or in combination, to destroy the cancer cells. Localized tumors may be treated with surgery and radiation therapy, whereas evidence of metastasis generally necessitates the addition of chemotherapy.

KEY CONCEPTS

- **Malignant tumors will kill the host, benign tumors generally will not. The primary difference between malignant and benign tumors is the propensity of**

T A B L E 6 – 3. Selected Markers Useful for Tumor Identification

Marker	Commonly Associated Tumor
Antigens	
Carcinoembryonic antigen	Adenosarcoma of colon, pancreas, breast, ovary, lung, stomach
Desmin	Myogenic (muscle) sarcoma
CA 125	Genital carcinoma
CA 19-9	GI, pancreatic carcinoma; melanoma
HMB-45	Melanoma
S 100 protein	Melanoma
α-Fetoprotein	Hepatic carcinoma, gonadal tumors
Hormones	
Human chorionic gonadotropin (hCG)	Gonadal tumors
Calcitonin	Medullary thyroid cancer
Thyroglobulin	Thyroid carcinoma
Isoenzymes	
Prostatic acid phosphatase	Prostate adenocarcinoma
Neuron-specific enolase	Small cell carcinoma of lung, neuroblastoma
Immunoglobulins	
Monoclonal Ig	Multiple myeloma

Adapted from Holleb J, et al (eds): *American Cancer Society Textbook of Clinical Oncology*, 1991, pp 16, 22. Reproduced by permission of the American Cancer Society, Atlanta.

malignant tumors to invade adjacent tissues and spread to distant sites (metastasize).

- The suffix *-oma* is used to indicate a benign tumor (e.g., fibroma). *Carcinoma* and *sarcoma* are used to indicate malignancy (e.g., fibrosarcoma). Exceptions include melanomas, lymphomas, hepatomas, and leukemia, all of which are malignant.

- Abnormalities of cancer cells include loss of topoinhibition, loss of anchorage dependence, and decreased reliance on growth-promoting factors. Malignant cells produce specialized laminin receptors and proteolytic enzymes to enable them to escape the tissue of origin and metastasize.

- Grading and staging are done to predict tumor behavior and guide therapy. Grading is the histologic characterization of tumor cells. Staging describes the location and pattern of tumor spread within the host. The TNM staging system describes the *t*umor size, lymph *n*odes affected, and degree of *m*etastasis.

Principles of Cancer Biology

Despite much progress in our understanding of how mechanisms of growth control and cellular differentiation may go awry, there is still no simple answer to the question, "What causes cancer?" It is increasingly evident, however, that cancer is a disorder of DNA. The strongest support for a genetic basis of cancer comes from the observation that cancer often results from agents known to damage DNA. In the 1970s a

T A B L E 6 – 4. TNM Staging Criteria for Breast Cancer

Primary Tumor (T)

Tx	Primary tumor cannot be assessed
T0	No evidence of primary tumor
Tis	Carcinoma in situ. Intraductal carcinoma, lobular carcinoma in situ, or Paget's disease of the nipple with no tumor
T1	Tumor 2 cm or less in greatest dimension
T1a	0.5 cm or less in greatest dimension
T1b	More than 0.5 cm but not more than 1 cm in greatest dimension
T1c	More than 1 cm but not more than 2 cm in greatest dimension
T2	Tumor more than 2 cm but not more than 5 cm in greatest dimension
T3	Tumor more than 5 cm in greatest dimension
T4	Tumor of any size with direct extension to chest wall or skin
T4a	Extension to chest wall
T4b	Edema (including peau d'orange) or ulceration of the skin of breast or satellite nodules confined to same breast
T4c	Both T4a and T4b
T4d	Inflammatory carcinoma

Lymph Node (N)

Nx	Regional lymph nodes cannot be assessed
N0	No regional lymph node metastasis
N1	Metastasis to movable ipsilateral axillary lymph node(s)
N2	Metastasis to ipsilateral axillary lymph node(s) fixed to one another or to other structures.
N3	Metastasis to ipsilateral internal mammary lymph node(s)

Distant Metastasis (M)

Mx	Presence of distant metastasis cannot be assessed
M0	No distant metastasis
M1	Distant metastasis (includes metastasis to ipsilateral supraclavicular lymph nodes)

From Holleb A, et al (eds): *American Cancer Society Textbook of Clinical Oncology*, 1991, p 184. Reproduced by permission of the American Cancer Society, Atlanta.

number of potential cancer-causing agents (**carcinogens**) were identified by demonstrating their mutagenic potential.[12] The suggestion that mutant genes were the basis for cancer launched intense research to identify the cancer-causing gene or genes, or **oncogenes**.

T A B L E 6 – 5. AJC Staging Criteria for Colon Cancer, American Joint Committee on Cancer

Description	Stage
Mucosa or submucosa only	T1
Muscle or serosa	T2
Extension to contiguous structures	T3
No fistula	
With fistula	T4
Extension beyond contiguous structures	T5
No regional node involvement	N0
Regional	N1
Juxtaregional	

Adapted from Holleb J, et al (eds): *American Cancer Society Textbook of Clinical Oncology*, 1991, p 214. Reproduced by permission of the American Cancer Society, Atlanta.

Discovery of Oncogenes

It was known since the early 1960s that certain viruses were associated with cancer in various animal models. Researchers speculated that a virus could introduce a mutant, cancer-causing gene into the host cells. Indeed, malignant cells containing the cancer-causing viruses were shown to have incorporated a small number of viral genes into their cellular DNA.[13] The presence of these oncogenes was required to maintain the malignant state of the cell. It was clear that the viral oncogenes were responsible for initiating tumor formation in the animal cells. A model for the causation of cancer was begining to emerge, but at the time no virally induced *human* cancers were known.

Researchers postulated that human cancers could be associated with mutant cellular oncogenes mediated by factors other than viruses, such as chemicals and radiation. In the early 1980s researchers began to isolate mutant genes from cancerous cells. The cancer-related genes were found to arise from normal cellular genes of very similar structure, sometimes differing by only one base pair.[14] The normal cellular genes are believed to be important for regulation of growth and differentiation. These genes have been called **proto-oncogenes.** In a noncancerous, fully differentiated cell, proto-oncogene expression is tightly controlled. When mutation releases a proto-oncogene from its regulated state, growth control in the cell is deregulated.

Surprisingly, some of the cellular oncogenes were found to be very similar or identical to viral oncogenes from RNA tumor viruses (retroviruses). Retroviruses are composed of RNA and possess a unique enzyme, reverse transcriptase, that directs the synthesis of a DNA copy of the viral RNA. The DNA copy can then be incorporated into the cellular DNA and become part of the host's genome. At some future time the viral DNA may begin actively coding for viral RNA, which can leave the host cell and infect others. Apparently, the tendency of retroviruses to slip in and out of host genomes allows them to pick up some of the host's genes, namely the growth-promoting proto-oncogenes.

Mechanisms of Oncogene Activation

Proto-oncogenes become activated oncogenes when the normal controls that keep them in check are disrupted. Proto-oncogenes and oncogenes do not lead to the cancerous state unless they are actively transcribed within the host cell. Transcription of the oncogene results in the production of abnormal proteins that initiate and/or promote the cancerous state. There are three general ways in which an oncogene can be activated (Fig. 6–4). (1) Oncogenes may be introduced into the host cell by a retrovirus. (2) A proto-oncogene within the cell may suffer a mutagenic event that changes its structure. (3) A gene that normally suppresses the proto-oncogene may be damaged or lost, allowing the proto-oncogene to become abnormally active.

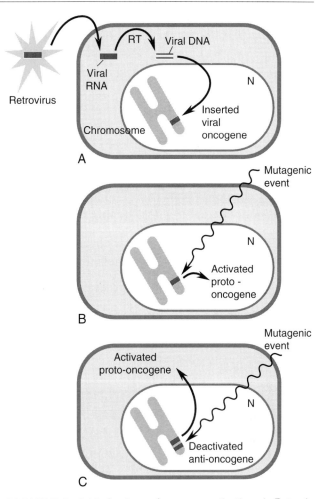

FIGURE 6–4. Mechanisms of oncogene activation. **A,** Retroviral insertion. **B,** Proto-oncogene mutation. **C,** Anti-oncogene mutation. *RT,* reverse transcriptase; *N,* nucleus.

Retroviral Oncogenes

At least three retroviruses are thought to be causative factors in some human cancers. Human immunodeficiency virus (HIV) is associated with Kaposi's sarcoma, Epstein-Barr virus (EBV) with Burkitt's lymphoma, and human T-lymphocyte virus I (HTLV-I) with adult T-cell leukemia-lymphoma. The degree of viral oncogene expression depends on where the oncogene is inserted in the host DNA. Insertion near a promoter sequence may result in continuous transcription of the oncogene. Viral oncogenes are outside of the normal DNA transcription controls and thus are not responsive to growth-suppressing signals.

Proto-oncogene Mutations

Proto-oncogenes are normal growth-promoting genes that are thought to be active when appropriate growth-promoting signals reach the cell. They are especially active during embryogenesis. If a mutation of the proto-oncogene occurs, it may be released from its normal regulation. The mutation may change the sequence of proto-oncogene DNA so that regulatory proteins no longer have the right fit to bind it and keep it inactive. Mutations that cause a large section of DNA to be transposed to another area on the chromosome or to a different chromosome may also remove the proto-oncogene from its repressors.

Anti-oncogene Mutations

Genes that suppress growth-promoting genes and/or promote cellular differentiation have been termed **anti-oncogenes** because of their suspected role in the suppression of tumor formation. Tumor suppression genes are difficult to study because they are noticeable only when they aren't there! The first anti-oncogene to be discovered was the Rb gene, so named because of its role in retinoblastoma, a cancer of the eye.[15] A familial form of retinoblastoma is associated with the transmission of a genetic defect—a portion of chromosome 13 is missing. This is where the Rb anti-oncogene is normally located. An absent Rb anti-oncogene predisposes an individual to cancer, but cancer will not develop unless the other copy of the Rb gene (from the other parent) is also damaged (Fig. 6–5). A number of cancers are suspected to result from the loss of anti-oncogenes at specific chromosome locations (Table 6–6).

Cellular Effects of Oncogene Activation

Maintenance of normal cellular growth and differentiation is dependent on appropriate cell-to-cell interactions and responsiveness to environmental signals. Activation of cellular oncogenes disrupts cellular communication by coding for proteins that are abnormal in structure, function, or quantity. The ways in which these abnormal proteins cause cellular dysfunction

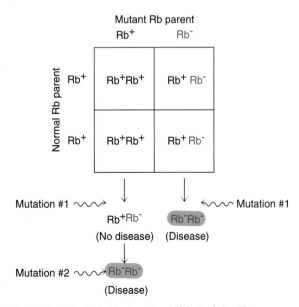

FIGURE 6–5. Both DNA copies (alleles) of the Rb tumor suppression gene must be dysfunctional (Rb⁻Rb⁻) for retinoblastoma to occur. Inheriting a defective Rb gene (Rb⁻) predisposes an individual to the development of cancer.

TABLE 6–6. Cancers Associated With Loss of Anti-oncogenes

Name	Tumor Involvement	Chromosomal Site
	Neuroblastoma	1p
	Small cell lung carcinoma	3p
	Colon carcinoma	5q
	Wilms' tumor	11p
	Bladder carcinoma	11p
	Retinoblastoma, osteosarcoma	13q
	Ductal breast carcinoma	13q
p53	Astrocytoma, colon carcinoma	17p
DCC	Colon carcinoma	18q
	Meningioma, acoustic neuroma	22q

From Holleb J, et al (eds): *American Cancer Society Textbook of Clinical Oncology*, 1991, p 687. Reproduced by permission of the American Cancer Society, Atlanta.

are only partly understood. However, a framework for describing the essential nature of cancer is beginning to unfold. The role of growth factors appears to be of central importance.

Normally, a great deal of intercellular communication is accomplished through the transmission of growth factors. Growth factors are small peptides that are manufactured by cells and secreted into the extracellular space. They diffuse to nearby cells and interact with receptors on the target cell surface. Binding of growth factors to cell surface receptors activates growth-promoting cascades within the cell. Tumor cells are much less dependent on the presence of growth factors than normal cells are. They do not require these growth-promoting signals from the environment in order to grow.

The first clues about how cancer cells may achieve growth factor independence were revealed when oncogenes were discovered. Many oncogenes actually coded for growth factors. This allowed the cancer cell to produce its own growth factor proteins so it was no longer dependent on other cells. Nearly all of the other known oncogenes are suspected to act via the growth factor pathways. There are at least four ways that oncogene expression could affect these pathways (Fig. 6–6). Each mechanism allows the cancerous cell to self-stimulate, thus releasing it from environmental feedback.

Production of Autocrine Growth Factors

In most cases, normally differentiated cells do not produce growth factors to which they can also respond.[16] In order to respond to a particular growth factor, the cell must have the appropriate complementary receptor on its cell surface. So, cells that produce a particular growth factor normally do not have a receptor for that particular growth factor on their cell surface. However, all cells in the body have essentially the same DNA and therefore have the genetic capability of making any of the growth factors. During differentiation into specific cell types, some of these genes get turned off, or repressed. A mutation that causes

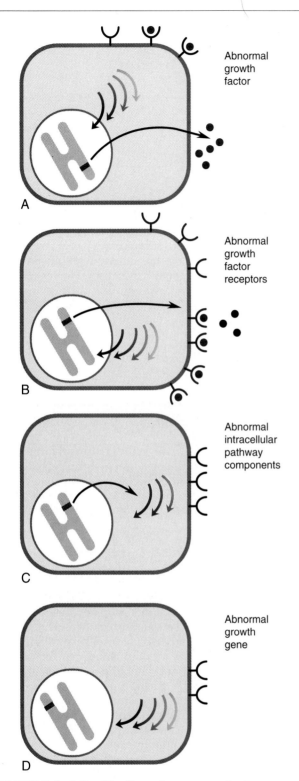

growth factor (PDGF), and transforming growth factor-beta (TGF-β).

Production of Autocrine Growth Factor Receptors

Growth factors cannot penetrate the cell membrane directly, so their presence at the cell surface must be transmitted intracellularly by cell surface receptors. Receptors are transmembrane proteins with the growth factor–binding area on the outside of the cell and an enzyme-activating area on the inside of the cell. These receptors are extremely specific; they will bind with only one particular growth factor. Binding activates a series of reactions within the cell that eventually leads to cell growth.

A mutational event may allow the expression of receptors that should not be present at all, or excessive amounts of normally present receptors; or it may produce receptors with abnormally high affinity. All of these changes result in excessive responsiveness to the growth factors normally present in the cell's environment. Some mutant receptors may even be active in the absence of growth factors. Some cancer cells, particularly breast carcinomas, are known to express huge numbers of abnormal receptors on their cell surface.

Abnormal Intracellular Signaling Pathways

A third way in which oncogenes may allow growth factor independence is by the manufacture of excessive or abnormal components of the intracellular growth-signaling pathways. These pathways involve numerous enzymes and chemicals that are only partly known. They normally function to transmit growth signals from activated receptors at the cell surface to the cell nucleus. These pathways therefore have been called second messenger cascades. An oncogene that codes for excessive or abnormal second messenger components could cause activation of the pathway, even though no signal was received at the cell surface.

Abnormal Nuclear Genes for Growth

The entire growth factor pathway, including the growth factor, the receptor, and the second messenger cascade, ultimately affects transcription of growth genes in the nucleus. It is possible that in some cancers, these genes may become activated in the absence of any message from the growth factor pathway. Very little is known about the genes responsible for prodding the cell out of its dormant state and causing it to proliferate. They are thought to be regulatory genes that control whole groups of other genes. If they become self-activated, the cell could grow despite the absence of growth-promoting signals from the cells environment.

FIGURE 6–6. Possible effects of oncogene activation on growth-signaling pathways. **A,** Production of growth factors. **B,** Production of growth factor receptors. **C,** Intracellular pathway disturbances. **D,** Activation of genes for growth.

production of a growth factor for which the cell also has receptors leads to **autocrine** or self-stimulation of growth. Common growth factors secreted by tumor cells include transforming growth factor-alpha (TGF-α), epidermal growth factor (EGF), platelet-derived

In summary, many known oncogenes appear to act by releasing cancer cell growth from its dependence on growth factors in the environment. This may be accomplished by the production of abnormal growth factors, growth factor receptors, or second messenger components. Additionally, growth factor independence may occur when target genes in the nucleus become self-activated and no longer rely on stimulation from the growth factor pathways.

Multistep Nature of Carcinogenesis

From the above discussion, it would seem that simply introducing an oncogene into a normal cell would be sufficient to transform it into a malignant cell. This has proved not to be the case. Growth regulation of mammalian cells appears to be organized, so that single oncogenes are unable to induce conversion to full malignancy. Different oncogenes work in distinct ways and may affect only a subset of the changes necessary to achieve full malignancy. For example, introduction of the *ras* oncogene into normal cells in culture causes them to show anchorage independence, but they are unable to form tumors when inoculated into an animal. Similarly, the *myc* oncogene allows cells to grow indefinitely in culture, but these immortal cells are still unable to induce tumor formation. However, when both the *ras* and *myc* oncogenes are introduced into normal cells, they become fully malignant (Fig. 6–7).[5]

These culture experiments support the clinical observation that carcinogenesis is a multistep phenomenon.[17] The steps of carcinogenesis have been labeled

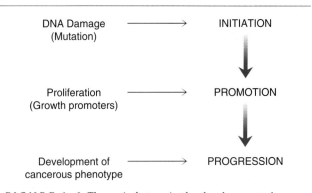

FIGURE 6–8. Theoretical steps in the development of cancer include initiation, promotion, and progression.

initiation, promotion, and progression (Fig. 6–8). The **initiating event** is a genetic mutation. However, the genetic mutation is not evident until the mutant cell proliferates. *Proliferation* is a requirement for cancer development, and nonproliferating cells cannot cause cancer. This is why terminally differentiated cells such as cardiac myocytes or nerve cells do not become cancerous.

Promotion is the stage during which the mutant cell proliferates. The movement from initiation to promotion may involve the activation of another oncogene from another mutational event. The two activated oncogenes may then act synergistically to cause proliferation of the mutant cell. Alternatively, the promoting event may be inactivation of an anti-oncogene that has kept proliferation in check. Because most cells have two DNA copies of each anti-oncogene, a mutation in both copies might be required for tumor promotion. Nonmutating factors may also be important in promoting cellular proliferation. Nutritional factors and infection, for example, may provide a stimulus for cellular proliferation.

Progression is the stage during which the mutant, proliferating cell begins to exhibit malignant behaviors. Generally, the mutation suffered during initiation is not sufficient to cause the biochemical changes necessary for malignant behavior. The proliferating cells are clones of the mutant initiating cell and therefore have the same genotype, but they exhibit a wide variation in phenotype. Phenotype refers to the cell's traits, such as morphology, metabolism, and biochemical makeup. Cells whose phenotype gives them a growth advantage will proliferate more readily. With each cycle of proliferation an opportunity for chance variation arises. In the end, highly evolved tumor cells are generated that differ significantly from their normal ancestors. These cells have developed characteristics, such as laminin receptors, lytic enzymes and anchorage independence, that enable them to behave malignantly.[18]

The fact that conversion from normal cell type to malignant cell type requires multiple steps implies many opportunities to intervene in the process. Prevention of the initiating mutation may be difficult, since carcinogens are ubiquitous; however, therapies

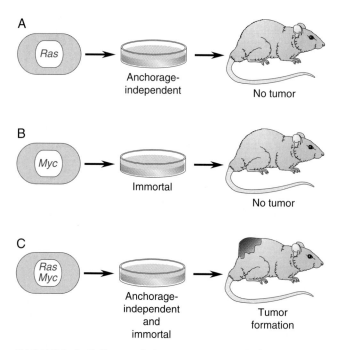

FIGURE 6–7. Synergy between oncogenes may be necessary to initiate malignant growth. **A,** *Ras* gene only. **B,** *Myc* gene only. **C,** Synergy between *ras* and *myc* genes.

to prevent promotion and progression could render the initial mutation harmless. As the biochemical processes governing promotion and progression become clearer, strategies for blocking these stages may be developed.

KEY CONCEPTS

- Cancer results from genetic damage. Genes thought to cause cancer are called oncogenes. Oncogenes may be expressed in a cell by at least three mechanisms: (1) introduction of an oncogene by a virus, (2) mutation of a proto-oncogene, causing it to become an active oncogene, and (3) mutation of an anti-oncogene that eliminates its oncogene-suppressing properties.

- Oncogene activation could cause increased cell growth by at least four mechanisms. These are (1) production of autocrine growth factors, (2) production of abnormal receptors, (3) alterations in intracellular signaling pathways, and (4) direct activation of nuclear genes.

- Full expression of cancer in a host is a multistep process. These steps have been described as initiation, promotion, and progression. The initiating event is thought to be a genetic mutation. Promotion refers to the stage in which the mutant cell is induced to proliferate. Progression is the stage during which the mutant, proliferating cells begin to exhibit malignant behaviors.

Cancer–Host Interactions

Immune Responses to Cancer

It has been suggested that the cancerous transformation of cells may be a relatively common event in life, yet few of these cells survive to give rise to cancer. The immune system is believed to play an important role in the detection and eradication of these cancerous cells. The primary support for this view comes from the observation that people who are immunocompromised have a greater incidence of cancer. In order to rid the body of cancer cells, the immune system must be able to recognize them as such, and then mediate their destruction.

Recognition of Tumor Cells

Recognition of tumor cells as different from their normal counterparts is the basis of tumor immunology. Recognition depends on the expression of abnormal molecules or antigens on the cancer cell surface (Fig. 6–9). Tumor cells may be recognized by cells of the natural or specific immune systems (see Chap. 9). The basis for recognition by nonspecific or natural immune cells is not well understood. The specific immune cells recognize particular antigens on the cell surface called tumor-associated antigens (TAA).[19] A subset of TAA

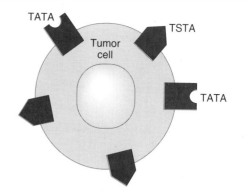

FIGURE 6–9. Cancer cells express abnormal antigens on their cell surface that can activate immune cells. *TSTA,* tumor-specific transplantation antigens; *TATA,* tumor-associated transplantation antigens.

are specific to certain types of tumor cells and have been given the name tumor-specific transplantation antigens (TSTA). TSTA can induce specific resistance to tumor growth in an immunized host. Controversy exists regarding whether all or even most tumors express TSTA. Most experimental cancers induced by viral oncogenes and chemical carcinogens have been shown to possess TSTA; however, some "spontaneous" tumors—those having no known etiology—appear to lack TSTA. It is unclear whether most human tumors possess these specific tumor antigens. A second subset of TAA consists of the tumor-associated transplantation antigens (TATA). These antigens are commonly expressed on a wide variety of different tumor types and sometimes on normal cells. They are less efficient at generating an immune response but are more widely distributed, making them potential targets for immunodetection and immunotherapy.

A number of immune cells work together to rid the body of cancerous cells (Fig. 6–10). Immune cells have been classically categorized into those mediating natural or nonspecific immunity and those mediating acquired or specific immunity. Cancer surveillance is achieved by cells from both categories. Of particular importance are the nonspecific macrophages and natural killer (NK) cells, and the specific B- and T-lymphocytes.

Role of Natural Immunity

Macrophages are believed to be important in the detection of cancer cells and may have some ability to lyse them. A role for macrophages is supported by several circumstantial lines of evidence:

1. Macrophages tend to accumulate in tumors.
2. Macrophages are able to inhibit tumor growth and cause cell lysis in vitro.
3. Factors known to suppress macrophage activity have been associated with increased tumor formation.

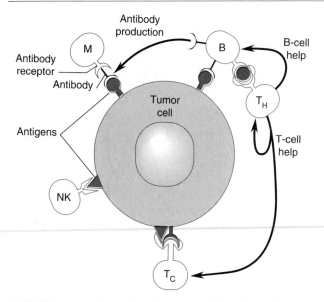

FIGURE 6–10. A number of immune cells work together to kill cancer cells, including macrophages (*M*), natural killer cells (*NK*), B-lymphocytes (*B*), helper T-lymphocytes (*T_H*) and cytotoxic T-lymphocytes (*T_C*).

4. Stimulation of macrophages by immunomodulators has been associated with reduced tumor formation.

The mechanisms by which macrophages are able to locate cancer cells are poorly understood. Macrophages are nonspecific; they can be activated by a number of different aspects of the abnormal cell. Once activated, the macrophage secretes a number of proteins, called cytokines, which boost the response of other immune cells. Macrophages are phagocytic and may achieve some degree of cancer cell lysis through their lysosomal enzymes.

Natural killer cells are a type of lymphocyte, but they do not have the distinctive markers present on B- and T-lymphocytes. Unlike B- and T-lymphocytes, which are specific for a particular antigen, NK cells are nonspecific. They are able to recognize abnormal cells in the same way that macrophages do. NK cells have potent cytotoxic (cell-killing) activity. Like macrophages, NK cells accumulate in tumors and are able to lyse tumor cells in vitro.

Role of Specific Immunity

T- and B-lymphocytes mediate specific immunity in the body. A particular T- or B-cell will become activated by only one particular antigen. Once activated by an antigen, T- and B-cells retain a memory of the antigen and are able to quickly mount an immune response at the next exposure. However, they are useless against antigens of different structure. B- and T-cells are activated by abnormal antigens on the surface of cancer cells. Some antigens are more immuno-

genic than others and elicit a greater B- and T-cell response. Tumor cells that more closely resemble normal cells are less immunogenic.

When B-cells are activated they produce antibodies against the tumor cell. Antibodies are able to bind to the tumor, making it more noticeable to macrophages and NK cells. Antibodies can also cause tumor cell lysis by activating proteins in the blood called complement. Certain complement fragments poke holes in the tumor cell membrane, causing it to rupture and die. B-cell activation is very dependent on growth-promoting signals from T-cells. Certain T-cells, called T-helper cells, produce and release B-cell growth factors (cytokines) that greatly amplify proliferation and antibody secretion of B-cells.

Another type of T-cell, the cytotoxic T-cell, may also be important in tumor cell lysis. Cytotoxic T-cells secrete enzymes that are able to perforate target cell membranes and cause them to rupture. Cytotoxic T-cells also require help from T-helper cells to become optimally activated.

In summary, the immune system has the capacity for recognition and eradication of tumor cells. The efficiency with which the immune system is able to accomplish these goals depends on the ability to recognize cancer cells as being different from self cells. In reality, this may be difficult to achieve, as cancer cells may closely resemble their normal ancestors. In addition, cancer cells appear to have developed means to escape immune system detection, and persons with apparently normal immune systems often die of cancer.

Effects of Cancer on the Immune System

Individuals with cancer often demonstrate deficits in immune system competence.[20] Cancer cells are known to secrete substances that suppress the immune system. Individuals with cancer may have reduced populations of T- and B-cells and may respond poorly to injected antigens. The mechanisms by which cancer cells depress immune responses are not well understood, but the prognosis for cancer recovery is poorer when the immune system is depressed.

In addition to the general immunodepressive effects of cancer, some cancer cells have developed ways to elude immune system detection. For example, cancer cells can internalize their immunoreactive cell surface antigens when antibodies attach to them. A reduction in antigenic sites decreases the likelihood of further stimulation of antibody production. Some tumors escape detection because they are coated with normal extracellular matrix molecules such as glycoproteins. The glycoproteins physically cover up the antigenic tumor markers. Tumor cells that closely resemble normal cells may trigger the production of T-suppressor cells that suppress the activity of other immune cells. T-suppressor cells are a subclass of T-lymphocytes. The conditions that activate them are as yet poorly understood, but they are probably important in keeping the immune system in check so that normal tissues are not attacked. Difficulty differentiating between the tumor cell and a normal cell may result in the production of T-suppressor cells that actually aid tumor cell growth.

Effects of Cancer on the Host

The effects of cancer on the host vary widely, depending on the location of the tumor and the extent and number of metastases. Early-stage cancer may be asymptomatic. As the tumor increases in size and spreads through the body, a number of symptoms become apparent. These include pain, cachexia, bone marrow suppression, and infection. Once treatment has begun, patients may also suffer hair loss and sloughing of mucosal membranes.

Pain is often the most feared complication of the disease process. Pain may be due to invasion of metastatic cells into organs or bone, leading to activation of pain and pressure receptors in the tissues. Tissue destruction and inflammation may contribute to cancer pain. Pain is strongly influenced by fear and fatigue. Cancer treatment may contribute to overall pain because of procedures requiring biopsy and drug administration through veins. Fortunately, pain can usually be well controlled through the use of analgesics. The introduction of patient-controlled analgesia has been effective in reducing patient fears of inadequate therapy for pain.

Cachexia refers to an overall weight loss and generalized weakness (Fig. 6–11). Many factors contribute to cancer cachexia, including loss of appetite (anorexia) and increased metabolic rate. Anorexia accompanies many disease processes and may result from toxins released by the cancer cells or immune cells. Cancer patients may have aversions to specific foods and may feel full after only a few bites. Nausea and vomiting are common complications of cancer therapy and contribute to decreased nutrient intake. Despite the minimal nutrient intake, body metabolism remains high. Cancer cells may compete with normal cells for available nutrients. Nutrients are mobilized from fat and protein stores in the body and consumed by the hypermetabolic cells. Some patients may require nutritional supplementation via enteral or parenteral routes.

Bone marrow suppression contributes to the anemia, leukopenia, and thrombocytopenia that often accompany cancer. Bone marrow suppression may be due to invasion and destruction of blood-forming cells in the bone marrow, poor nutrition, and chemotherapeutic drugs. Anemia refers to a deficiency in circulating red cells. In addition to decreased production of blood cell precursors in the bone marrow, anemia may result from chronic or acute bleeding. Signs and symptoms of anemia are related to a decrease in oxygen-carrying capacity such as fatigue, increased heart rate, and increased respiratory rate.

Leukopenia refers to a decrease in circulating white blood cells (WBCs), or leukocytes. Malignant invasion of the bone marrow is a primary cause of leukopenia. Malnutrition and chemotherapy are contributing factors. A deficiency in WBCs reduces the patient's ability to fight infection. Infection is a major cause of morbidity and mortality in cancer patients. Often the offending organism is *opportunistic*; it is unable to infect an immunocompetent host and becomes virulent only when a person is immunocompromised. Infections are very difficult to treat because the host is unable to mount an effective immune response. Infections are also difficult to prevent, because 80 percent of the infecting organisms are from the patient's own endogenous flora (skin, GI tract). The development of severe leukopenia or infection during treatment may necessitate termination of chemotherapy to allow bone marrow recovery.

Thrombocytopenia is a deficiency in circulating platelets. Platelets are important mediators of blood clotting. Platelet deficiencies predispose to life-threatening hemorrhage. A platelet count of less than $20,000/mm^3$ has been associated with spontaneous hemorrhage.

Anemia, leukopenia, and thrombocytopenia may be treated by administration of blood products containing these elements. In fact, blood replacement therapy is used more often in cancer patients than in any other medical condition. When chemotherapy is terminated, stem cells in the bone marrow generally recover, and the production of blood cells resumes.

Hair loss and the sloughing of mucosal membranes are complications of radiation therapy and chemotherapy. Treatment is designed to kill the rapidly proliferating cancer cells, but normal cells with high growth rates such as mucosal epithelia and hair follicle cells are also damaged. Damaged mucosa is a pri-

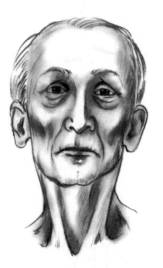

FIGURE 6–11. General emaciated appearance in cancer cachexia. (From Jarvis C. *Physical Examination and Health Assessment.* Philadelphia, WB Saunders, 1992, p 306.)

mary source of cancer pain and anorexia and may provide a portal for the invasion of organisms from the skin or gastrointestinal tract.

If left untreated, cancer has the potential to kill the host. The cause of death is multifactorial. Infection, hemorrhage, and organ failure are the primary causes of cancer death. The failure of cancer-ridden organs such as the liver, kidney, brain, and lung results in the loss of life-sustaining functions. Treatment for cancer can also be detrimental to the host, contributing to immunosuppression and platelet deficiencies. The additive effects of one or more of these factors may lead to cancer death.

KEY CONCEPTS

- In order for the host's immune system to fight cancer, the cancerous cell must be recognized as such. Most tumor cells appear to express unusual antigens on their cell surface, which immune cells may recognize.
- Cancer surveillance is accomplished primarily by macrophages, natural killer cells, and lymphocytes.
- Regardless of the type of malignancy, affected individuals exhibit characteristic signs and symptoms. These include pain, cachexia, bone marrow suppression, and infection. Bone marrow suppression manifests as anemia, leukopenia, and thrombocytopenia.

Cancer Therapy

The overall cure rate for cancer is approximately 51 percent, with some types of cancer having much higher or lower rates of cure.[21] A patient is considered to be cured if there is no evidence of cancer recurrence for 5 years after treatment. Early detection of cancer, while it remains localized in the tissue of origin, is associated with the best prognosis for cure. Patients with metastatic invasion of regional lymph nodes still have a good opportunity for cure with appropriate therapy. Widespread invasion of multiple tissues and organs is associated with a poor prognosis, and therapy is generally aimed at palliation of symptoms rather than cure of the disease. The mainstays of cancer therapy are surgery, radiation therapy, and chemotherapy. Immunotherapy may be the future of cancer therapy, but at present it is still mostly supplementary to the standard treatment methods. The choice of treatment depends largely on the results of the staging procedure. A greater degree of metastasis requires a more aggressive therapeutic approach.

Surgery

More than 60 percent of patients with cancer are treated surgically.[22] Surgery can cure a large proportion of localized cancers. The main benefit of surgery

is removal of a tumor with minimal damage to other body cells. The surgeon generally removes a margin of normal-appearing tissue around the resected tumor to ensure complete tumor removal. Lymph nodes are biopsied and also removed if evidence of metastasis is present. Surgical resection of some tumors can be tricky if vital structures such as neurons or blood vessels are involved. Surgery does involve risks related to anesthesia, infection, and blood loss. The surgical procedure may be disfiguring or may result in loss of function. Surgical resection as the sole treatment of solid tumors is curative in only 30 percent of patients because most patients already have undetectable metastases at the time of diagnosis.[22] Therefore, surgical resection is commonly followed by radiation therapy or chemotherapy. Even one remaining cancer cell could be sufficient to reinitiate tumor formation.

Radiation Therapy

Ionizing radiation is primarily used for two reasons: (1) to kill tumor cells that are not resectable because of location in a vital or inaccessible area, and (2) to kill tumor cells that may have escaped the surgeon's knife and remain undetected in the area. Radiation kills cells by damaging their nuclear DNA. Cells that are rapidly cycling are more susceptible to radiation death because there is little time for DNA repair. The damaged DNA is passed on to daughter cells, causing them to die.

It is difficult to kill all the cells of a large tumor by irradiation because they are heterogeneous; they are in different phases of mitosis and cycling at different rates. A radiation dose large enough to kill all the tumor cells would be sufficient to kill the normal cells as well. Radiation is most effective at eradicating small groups of tumor cells.[23] It is often used in combination with surgery. Radiation is also useful for palliative reductions in tumor size. Pain from bone and brain tumors may be effectively treated by radiation therapy that shrinks the tumor. Tumors with bleeding surfaces may be coagulated with radiation to decrease blood loss.

A certain degree of destruction of normal cells in the irradiated field is expected with radiation therapy. The guiding principle behind radiation therapy is give the maximum dose the normal tissues can tolerate, and hope that it kills the tumor. Radiation is best used when tumor cells are regionally located. Whole-body irradiation to kill tumor cells in distant locations is not recommended because of the likelihood of life-threatening tissue damage.

Chemotherapy

Chemotherapy refers to the systemic administration of anticancer chemicals. Chemotherapy is used to treat cancers that are known or suspected to be disseminated in the body. Unlike surgery or radiation

TABLE 6–7. Standard Chemotherapeutic Agents

Class	Drug	Mechanism of Action
Alkylating agents	Nitrogen mustard Mechlorethamine Melphalan Chlorambucil Cyclophosphamide Ifosfamide	DNA alkylation leading to strand breaks and cross-links that disrupt DNA replication and transcription. Active throughout cell cycle.
Antimetabolites	Methotrexate 5-Fluorouracil (5-FU) Cytosine arabinoside 6-Mercaptopurine 6-Thioguanine	Substitute for or compete with a metabolite, thus interfering with DNA and RNA synthesis. Active mainly during S-phase.
Antitumor antibiotics	Actinomycin D Bleomycin Mitomycin C Doxorubicin Daunorubicin	Various effects on DNA, such as fragmentation, binding, and cross-linking strands. Interfere with transcription.
Plant alkaloids	Vincristine Vinblastine	Bind to mitotic proteins (tubulin) and prevent formation of mitotic spindle. Cells arrest in mitosis.
	Etoposide	Causes DNA strand breaks. Cells arrest in mitosis.
Hormones	Estrogens (DES) Gonadotropin-releasing hormone	Decrease leutinizing hormone secretion and inhibit prostate tumor growth.
	Tamoxifen	Estrodiol antagonist. Inhibits estrogen-dependent tumors (breast).
	Corticosteroids	Bind to and lyse lymphoid cancer cells.
Miscellaneous agents	Cisplatin	Activated platinum causes DNA cross-linking.

Data from Holleb J, et al (eds): *American Cancer Society Textbook of Clinical Oncology*, 1991.

therapy, which are locally or regionally applied, chemotherapeutic drugs can find their cancer cell targets in areas throughout the entire body. The standard chemotherapeutic agents are listed in Table 6–7.

Most chemotherapeutic agents are cytotoxic because they interfere with some aspect of cell division. The more rapidly dividing cells are more susceptible to the killing effects of chemotherapeutic agents. In a large tumor mass, the rates of cell division are very diverse, with many slowly dividing cells. At any one time, only a portion of the tumor cells will be in a cell cycle stage that is susceptible to chemotherapy. Several courses of chemotherapy are generally necessary to ensure that all tumor cells have been killed.[24] It is difficult to kill slowly cycling tumor cells without also killing normal cells that are cycling at approximately the same rate. Small tumors are easier to eradicate because rates of cell division are generally faster. To effect a cure, the "stem" cells that give rise to clones of malignant cells must be destroyed. Unfortunately, stem cells do not divide as rapidly as other tumor cells. Resection or irradiation to reduce tumor size may prompt the stem cells to divide, thus making them more susceptible to chemotherapy.

The chemotherapeutics are not selective for tumor cells, and a certain amount of normal cell death also occurs. Rapidly dividing cells, particularly those of the bone marrow, intestinal epithelia, and hair follicles, are most affected. Bone marrow depression is a most serious side effect as it predisposes the patient to anemia, bleeding, and infection.

Immunotherapy

Harnessing the power of the immune system to fight cancer is a particularly appealing idea because of the potential for *specificity*. Traditional forms of treatment are not selective for cancer cells and result in unavoidable damage to normal tissues. The immune system, on the other hand, is noted for its ability to make subtle distinctions between normal and abnormal or foreign cells. Thus, the immune system could potentially deliver a "silver bullet" directly to tumor cells, leaving normal cells completely unaffected.

Despite much progress in understanding the immune system in the last several years, the hope for effective immunotherapy for cancer has not yet been realized. Current modes of immunomodulation primarily involve the use of interferons, interleukins, and monoclonal antibodies. These therapies are generally used as adjuncts to surgery, radiation, and chemotherapy.

Interferons are glycoproteins produced by immune cells in response to viral infection. Interferons inhibit cell proliferation and are stimulatory to NK cells, T-cells, and macrophages. Interferon-alpha has been successfully used to treat hairy cell leukemia, a rare B-cell malignancy.[25] However, response to interferon therapy in other proliferative disorders has been less impressive. Interferon therapy produces symptoms similar to those of a viral infection: fever, chills, and muscle aches.

Interleukins are peptides produced and secreted by WBCs. They are also called lymphokines or cytokines. Interkeukin-2 (IL-2) is an important cytokine secreted by activated T-helper cells. It stimulates the proliferation of T-cells, NK cells, and macrophages. IL-2 can be used to stimulate the growth of these immune cells in culture. Immune cells taken from a patient's blood can be grown in culture in the presence of IL-2. Then the greatly expanded number of immune cells can be given back to the patient, along with intravenous infusions of IL-2. Such treatment has been associated with regression of some tumors (melanoma, renal cell carcinoma), but the response rate has been lower than anticipated.[26] Because IL-2 toxicity is high, causing severe allergic reactions in many individuals, the future of IL-2 therapy for cancer is unclear.

The use of monoclonal antibodies (antibodies having identical structure) in cancer therapy is currently the subject of intense investigation. Monoclonal antibodies specifically bind with target antigens and therefore could be used in several ways to treat cancer. The use of monoclonal antibodies relies heavily on the ability to identify tumor cell antigens, antigens that are always and only present on tumor cells. This has proved to be a difficult task. If successful, the antibody could be used to deliver a cytotoxic drug directly to the cancer cell, avoiding drug interactions with normal cells. Similarly, antibodies could be used to direct other cytotoxic cells such as macrophages and T-cells to tumor cells lurking in the body. Antibodies could be attached to a radioactive label and injected into a patient to screen for recurrence of tumor growth.

Immunotherapy is still in its infancy, and it is difficult to predict what impact it may ultimately have on cancer detection and therapy. As progress is made in identifying tumor antigens, immunotherapy may become a prominent form of cancer therapy. Even immunization against some forms of cancer is not beyond the realm of probability.

KEY CONCEPTS

- Early detection of cancer while it remains localized is associated with the best prognosis for cure. Cure is defined as no recurrence for 5 years after treatment. The overall cure rate for cancer is about 51 percent.
- The mainstays of cancer therapy are surgery, radiation therapy, and chemotherapy. Surgery and radiation therapy are effective for cancers that are local-

ized. Chemotherapy is the treatment of choice for cancers known or suspected to be disseminated in the body.

- Cells that divide rapidly are the most susceptible to damage from radiation therapy or chemotherapy. In addition to cancer cells, however, rapidly dividing normal cells may be killed. Cells of the bone marrow, hair follicles, and gastrointestinal mucosa are particularly susceptible.

- Immunotherapy is a relatively new form of treatment for cancer that has the potential to specifically target cancer cells. At present, interferon, interleukin-2, and monoclonal antibodies are being used to boost the immune system's ability to locate and destroy cancer cells.

Epidemiology and Cancer Risk Factors

Cancer accounts for approximately 22 percent of all deaths, making it the second leading cause of death in the United States. It is surpassed only by heart diseases, which account for about 36 percent of deaths.[27] Most cancer deaths (66 percent) occur in persons over age 65. The American Cancer Society estimates that 30 percent of persons now living will develop cancer; with today's current cure rates, half will die a cancer-related death.[28] Fortunately, the current view of cancer causation predicts that most cancer is preventable. Indeed, cancer is thought to be a life-style–related disease. The two life-style factors of particular importance are tobacco use and nutrition—factors that are certainly amenable to modification. Despite the common view to the contrary, very few cancers are attributable to environmental carcinogens. Statistics regarding some of the major forms of cancer are shown in Figure 6–12. Further discussions of particular cancers can be found in chapters relating to corresponding body systems.

Tobacco Use

The impact of tobacco use on cancer-related death can be most vividly seen by looking at cancer death rates in the United States from 1930 to 1990 (Fig. 6–13). While all other cancer-related death rates declined or remained relatively stable, the death rate from lung cancer increased dramatically. The increase is attributable almost entirely to smoking. Lung cancer remains the leading cause of cancer death, despite a recent decline in the number of male smokers, from 64 percent in the 1950s to 30 percent in the 1990s.[29] Unfortunately, American women have not followed this trend, and the number of teenage female smokers continues to rise. Lung cancer has one of the worst survival rates of all cancers—only 13 percent.[27] In addition to lung cancer, tobacco use has been linked

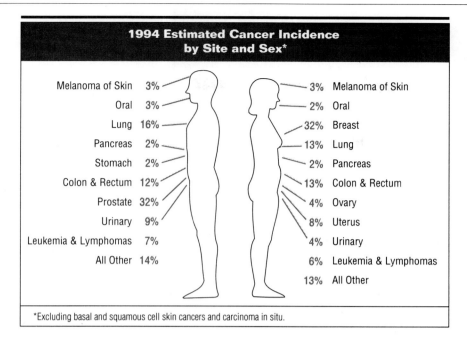

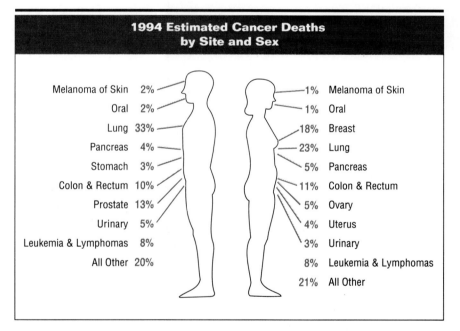

FIGURE 6–12. 1994 estimated cancer incidence and deaths, by site and sex. (From Ca: *A Cancer Journal for Clinicians.* CA 44:7–26, 1994.)

Cancer Death Rates by Site, Males, United States, 1930-90

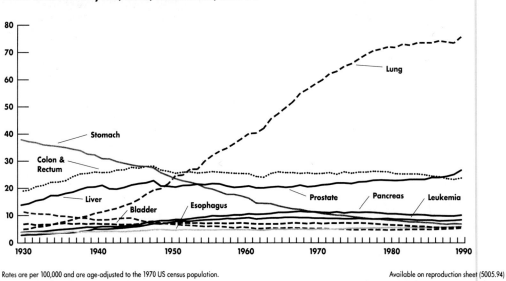

Rates are per 100,000 and are age-adjusted to the 1970 US census population.

Available on reproduction sheet (5005.94)

Cancer Death Rates by Site, Females, United States, 1930-90

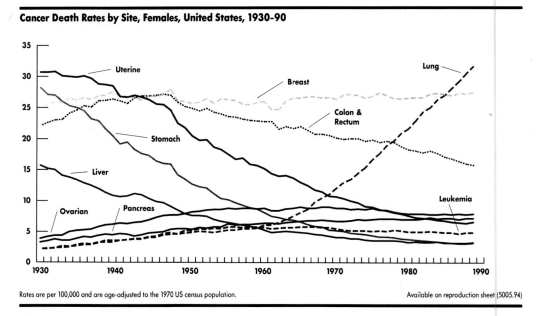

Rates are per 100,000 and are age-adjusted to the 1970 US census population.

Available on reproduction sheet (5005.94)

FIGURE 6–13. The U.S. cancer death rates per 100,000 persons from 1930 to 1990. (From American Cancer Society *Cancer Facts and Figures—1994.* Used by permission © 1994 American Cancer Society, Inc.)

with cancer of the pancreas, bladder, kidney, mouth, and esophagus.

Carcinogens can be grouped into two major types: those that cause genetic damage (initiators), and those that promote growth of the tumor (promoters). Tobacco smoke contains hundreds of compounds, many of which have known genotoxicity (e.g., polycyclic aromatic hydrocarbons, nicotine derivatives) and probably serve as initiators. Tobacco smoke also contains promoters, which spur the mutant cells to proliferate. Promotion appears to be dose dependent, with the risk of cancer increasing sharply as use increases above 20 cigarettes per day.[30] Cessation of smoking results in a decline in cancer risk owing to removal of promoters. Even a moderate decrease in the number of cigarettes smoked could be expected to reduce cancer risk.

Nutrition

The results of studies on the relationship between cancer and nutrition are confusing and contradictory. The general opinion seems to be that diet is associated with cancer risk, but there is little agreement on what that association might be. The two most discussed dietary factors related to cancer are fat and fiber. Despite tremendous advertising by the food industry, there is little scientific basis for recommending changes in dietary intake of fat or fiber for cancer risk reduction.

Fat

Several epidemiologic studies done in the 1970s and early 1980s suggested a relationship between high-fat diets and the development of breast, colon, and prostate cancers. A large number of recent studies have cast doubt on these findings by reporting no correlation between levels of fat intake and cancer development in a variety of populations.[31] In some studies, higher fat intake was found to be protective against some cancers. Further research on the specific type of fat intake and other cofactors is needed to clarify the fat–cancer relationship. One explanation for discrepant results might be that high-fat diets tend to be high-calorie diets. Several studies in animals have shown that regardless of fat intake, tumor growth may be inhibited by caloric restrictions. Thus, caloric rather than fat intake may be the important consideration. Recommendations regarding amount and type of fat intake should be viewed cautiously, as no clear scientific basis for these recommendations is yet available.

Fiber

Fiber is a general term for nondigestable dietary substances that remain in the intestinal lumen, increasing fecal bulk and improving bowel regularity. Fiber includes a diversity of compounds such as cellulose, bran, and pectin. An association between fiber intake and colorectal cancer was proposed in the early 1970s, based on a study comparing the incidence of certain ailments in Americans versus Africans.[32] A number of correlational and comparison studies done since that time have yielded conflicting results. In a 1987 review of the literature, Pilch related the findings of 44 studies (22 correlational studies and 22 case comparison studies).[33] Twenty-three studies reported a protective role for fiber in colon cancer; 14 found no relationship. Seven studies showed that fiber increased the risk of colon cancer. Animal studies do little to clarify the issue. Because fiber is associated with beneficial effects on digestion and elimination, fiber intake in the range of 10 to 13 g per 1,000 calories consumed is generally recommended. However, the effect of fiber on colorectal cancer risk remains unclear.

KEY CONCEPTS

- Cancer is primarily a disease of the elderly (over age 65). It is estimated that 30 percent of persons now living will develop cancer.
- The development of most cancers is related to lifestyle, particularly tobacco use and nutrition. Smoking cessation is considered important in reducing cancer risk. Guidelines regarding nutrition are less clear. Although a low-fat, high-fiber diet is usually recommended, there is, at present, little scientific basis to support these modifications.

Summary

Neoplasia is an abnormal growth of a benign or malignant nature. Benign tumors resemble their parent cells and are strictly local, whereas malignant tumors are anaplastic, invade local tissues, and may spread to distant sites (metastasize). The most important consideration for cancer treatment is the degree of cancer spread in the body, which can be determined by staging procedures. Cancer is treated by surgical removal, radiation therapy, chemotherapy, and sometimes immunotherapy.

Cancer cells have complex relationships with the host. The host immune system is capable of, but not always successful in, recognizing and killing cancer cells. Cancer cells exert immunosuppressive effects on the host as well as leading to pain, cachexia, and bone marrow suppression. If untreated, cancer has the potential to kill the host by multifactorial processes, including infection, hemorrhage, and organ failure. If treated, cancer has an overall cure rate of approximately 51 percent.

The primary cause of cancer is thought to be a carcinogenic life-style, with environmental carcinogens playing a lesser role. Tobacco use and improper nutrition are the two most studied carcinogenic lifestyle traits. The effects of tobacco are clearly carcinogenic through its ability to cause genetic damage as well as to promote the growth of mutant cells. The evidence linking nutritional factors such as fat and fiber intake to cancer risk is less convincing.

Cancer develops when oncogenes or proto-oncogenes become inappropriately activated in the cell. This is usually due to a mutational event in the cell DNA. Inactivation of a tumor suppressor gene, or anti-oncogene, may also contribute to the expression of oncogenes. Oncogenes are thought to disrupt normal intercellular communication, which normally exerts growth-controlling effects on the cell. This is accomplished primarily through the production of abnormal growth factors, growth factor receptors, or second messenger components which allow the cancer cell to manufacture its own growth-promoting signals.

REFERENCES

1. Pfeifer JD, Wick MD: The pathologic evaluation of neoplastic diseases, in Holleb A, Fink DJ, Murphy GP (eds): *American Cancer Society Textbook of Clinical Oncology.* Atlanta, American Cancer Society, 1991, pp 7–24.
2. Rubin E, Farber J: Neoplasia, in Rubin E, Farber J (eds): *Essential Pathology.* Philadelphia, JB Lippincott, 1990, pp 94–131.
3. Temin HM, Rubin H: Characteristics of an assay for Rous sarcoma virus and Rous sarcoma cells in tissue culture. *Virology* 1958;6:669–688.
4. Macpherson I, Montagnier L: Agar suspension culture for the selective assay of cells transformed by polyoma virus. *Virology* 1964;23:291–294.
5. Land H, Parada LF, Weinberg RA: Cellular oncogenes and multistep carcinogenesis. *Science* 1983;222:771–778.
6. Folkman J, Moscona A: Role of cell shape in growth control. *Nature* 1978;273:345–349.
7. Yamaski H, Katoh Y: Further evidence for the involvement of gap junctional intercellular communication in function and maintenance of transformed foci in BALB/c 3T3 cells. *Cancer Res* 1988;48:3490–3495.
8. Sporn MB, Todaro GJ: Autocrine secretion and malignant transformation of cells. *N Engl J Med* 1980;303:878–880.
9. Liotta L: Cancer cell invasion and metastasis. *Sci Am* 1992; 266(2):54–63.
10. Fisher B, Fisher ER: Experimental studies of factors influencing hepatic metastases: I. The effect of number of tumor cells injected and time of growth. *Cancer* 1959;12:926–941.
11. American Joint Committee on Cancer: *Manual for Staging of Cancer,* 3rd ed. Philadelphia, JB Lippincott, 1988.
12. McCann J, Ames BN: Detection of carcinogens as mutagens in the *Salmonella*/microsome test—assay for 300 chemicals: Discussion. *Proc Natl Acad Sci USA* 1976;73:950–955.
13. Dulbecco R: Cell transformation by viruses. *Science* 1969;166:962–968.
14. Shilo BZ, Weinberg RA: DNA sequences homologous to vertebrate oncogenes are conserved in *Drosophila melanogaster. Proc Natl Acad Sci USA* 1981;78:6789–6792.
15. Weinberg RA: Tumor suppressor genes. *Science* 1991;254:1138–1146.
16. Cross M, Dexter M: Growth factors in development, transformation and tumorigenesis. *Cell* 1991;64:271–280.
17. Weinberg RA: Oncogenes, antioncogenes, and the molecular bases of multistep carcinogenesis. *Cancer Res* 1989;49:3713–3721.
18. Templeton DJ, Weinberg RA: Principles of cancer biology, in Holleb A, Fink DJ, Murphy GP (eds): *American Cancer Society Textbook of Clinical Oncology.* Atlanta, American Cancer Society, 1991, pp 678–689.
19. Herberman RB: Principles of tumor immunology, in Holleb A, Fink DJ, Murphy GP (eds): *American Cancer Society Textbook of Clinical Oncology.* Atlanta, American Cancer Society, 1991, pp 69–79.
20. Specter S, Friedman H: Immunosuppressive factors produced by tumors and their effects on the RES, in Herberman RB, Friedman H (eds): *The Reticuloendothelial System: A Comprehensive Treatise.* New York, Plenum Press, 1983, vol 5: *Cancer,* pp 315–326.
21. McKenna RJ: Supportive care and rehabilitation of the cancer patient, in Holleb A, Fink DJ, Murphy GP (eds): *American Cancer Society Textbook of Clinical Oncology.* Atlanta, American Cancer Society, 1991, pp 544–554.
22. Eberlein TJ, Wilson RE: Principles of surgical oncology, in Holleb A, Fink DJ, Murphy GP (eds): *American Cancer Society Textbook of Clinical Oncology.* Atlanta, American Cancer Society, 1991, pp 25–34.
23. Hendrickson FR, Withers HR: Principles of radiation oncology, in Holleb A, Fink DJ, Murphy GP (eds): *American Cancer Society Textbook of Clinical Oncology.* Atlanta, American Cancer Society, 1991, pp 35–46.
24. Cooper MR, Cooper MR: Principles of medical oncology, in Holleb A, Fink DJ, Murphy GP (eds): *American Cancer Society Textbook of Clinical Oncology.* Atlanta, American Cancer Society, 1991, pp 47–68.
25. Golomb HM: The treatment of hairy-cell leukemia. *Blood* 1987;69:979–983.
26. Rosenberg SA, Lotze MT, Muul LM, et al: Observations of the systemic administration of autologous lymphokine activated killer cells and recombinant interleukin-2 to patients with metastatic cancer. *N Engl J Med* 1985;313:1485–1489.
27. Garfinkel L: Cancer statistics and trends, in Holleb A, Fink DJ, Murphy GP (eds): *American Cancer Society Textbook of Clinical Oncology.* Atlanta, American Cancer Society, 1991, pp 1–6.
28. American Cancer Society: *Cancer Facts and Figures—1990.* Atlanta, American Cancer Society, 1990.
29. US Public Health Service, National Cancer Institute, Division of Cancer Prevention and Control: *1987 Annual Cancer Statistics Review.* NIH Publication no 88-2789. Washington, DC, US Government Printing Office, 1988.
30. Weisberger JG, Horn CL: The cause of cancer, in Holleb A, Fink DJ, Murphy GP (eds): *American Cancer Society Textbook of Clinical Oncology.* Atlanta, American Cancer Society, 1991, pp 80–98.
31. Kritchevsky D: Diet and cancer, in Holleb A, Fink DJ, Murphy GP (eds): *American Cancer Society Textbook of Clinical Oncology.* Atlanta, American Cancer Society, 1991, pp 125–132.
32. Burkitt DP, Walker ARP, Painter NS: Dietary fiber and disease. *JAMA* 1974;229:1068–1074.
33. Pilch SM (ed): *Physiological Effects and Health Consequences of Dietary Fiber.* Bethesda, MD, FASEB, 1987.

BIBLIOGRAPHY

American Cancer Society: *Cancer Facts and Figures—1990.* Atlanta, American Cancer Society, 1990.

American Joint Committee on Cancer: *Manual for Staging of Cancer,* 3rd ed. Philadelphia, JB Lippincott, 1988.

Ankathil R, Nair MK: Molecular pathogenesis of chronic myelogenous leukaemia. *Natl Med J India* 1992;5(5):219–222.

Ankathil R, Vijayakumar T, Nair MK: Molecular cytogenetics of human cancer. *Natl Med J India* 1992;5(2):63–68.

Borrow J, Solomon E: Molecular analysis of the t(15;17) translocation in acute promyelocytic leukaemia. *Baillieres Clin Haematol* 1992;5(4):833–856.

Brennan RG: The winged-helix DNA-binding motif: Another helix-turn-helix takeoff. *Cell* 1993;74(5):773–776.

Chemically Induced Cell Proliferation Conference: *Chemically Induced Cell Proliferation: Implications for Risk Assessment.* Proceedings of the Chemically Induced Cell Proliferation Conference held in Austin, Texas, Nov. 29–Dec. 2, 1989. New York, Wiley-Liss, 1991.

Hodgson SV, Maher ER: *A Practical Guide to Human Cancer Genetics.* Cambridge, Cambridge University Press, 1993.

Holleb A, Fink DJ, Murphy GP (eds): *American Cancer Society Textbook of Clinical Oncology.* Atlanta, American Cancer Society, 1991.

Lippman ME, Dickson RB: Growth regulation of cancer-II: *Proceedings of a UCLA Symposium,* held in Keystone, Colorado, January 21–27, 1989. New York, Wiley-Liss, 1990.

Whitfield JF: *Calcium, Cell Cycles, and Cancer.* Boca Raton, CRC Press, 1990.

Yang SS, Warner HR: *The Underlying Molecular, Cellular, and Immunological Factors in Cancer and Aging.* New York, Plenum Press, 1993.

UNIT III
Alterations in Defense

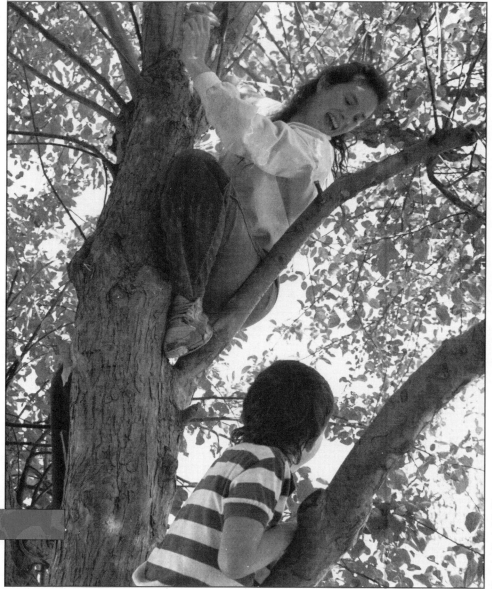

Mother and her child enjoy a playful moment together. Both persons are HIV positive.

Photo by Rachel DeHaan

*I*f nations were defended as effectively as the human body against invasion, there would be far fewer wars. Faced with an epidemic or the onset of seemingly incurable diseases, we may think that we are fragile or vulnerable, when in fact vigilant, powerful bodily defenses protect us continually. Much of our bodily activity is devoted specifically to the detection of threats to our health, to their shrewd assessment by our immune system, and to the mounting of an overwhelming response intended to destroy them. Unseen and unsensed in our daily lives, our defensive systems protect us against the threats around us.

The estimated 400,000 annual American deaths attributed to tobacco smoking remind us that we often subvert our own defenses by persisting in unhealthful habits. We also damage each other, when, for example, we release toxic substances into the environment. But when we give ourselves a chance for good health, we can usually depend on the immune system to provide the alertness, ingenuity, and strong defenses to combat disease.

Today, partly through research into autoimmune diseases and the virus that produces acquired immunodeficiency syndrome (AIDS), both potentially deadly threats to human immunity, we are learning more about how the system works.

Detection of the agents of disease is a key.

The immune responses do their work ingeniously by recognizing the difference between the molecules that are ours (self), that make up ourselves, and those that do not belong. The body employs two lines of defense, the innate, or specific, and the adaptive, or nonspecific, immune systems. The innate system recognizes certain microbes and destroys them; the adaptive system recognizes even infectious organisms it has not seen before by piecing together gene segments, "like a patchwork quilt," one researcher observed, enabling immune cells to respond.

Recent research, much of it intended to discover ways to immunize people against AIDS or cure the diseases associated with the syndrome, reveals in ever greater detail the intricacy and the certainty of the response to pathogens. The immune system detects the seemingly infinite number of viruses, bacteria, and other foreign elements that threaten human health and responds swiftly to suppress them, protecting the body's integrity unless or until it is deceived or overwhelmed.

Scientists, including those who understand the evolution of the immune system most thoroughly, argue that while human immune defenses are evolving rapidly in response to new challenges, a number of factors, aggravated by the environments in which most of us live, threaten to overwhelm them.

The human immune system may be outsmarted by new forms of infection, such as viruses transmitted from another species. But even here the immune system shows its reliability because, supplied from a "storehouse of variability," it is able to respond flexibly to new as well as familiar threats, overcoming even quickly evolving pathogens or viruses,

such as human immunodeficiency virus, that seem to adapt ingeniously to the body's defenses.

But progress and the worldwide increase in population are on the side of the pathogens. Air travel, population growth, and the crowding of people into megacities have vastly increased the ease with which people can become exposed to agents of disease. New microbes emerge, threatening not only the resourcefulness of the immune system but medical science's ability to support it. The recent emer-

FRONTIERS OF RESEARCH
Immune System Responses
Michael J. Kirkhorn

gence of drug-resistant strains of the tuberculosis bacillus provides a reminder that "even old pathogens invent new tricks." Health professionals are alarmed by the emergence of bacteria that are immune to antibiotics. Every disease-causing bacterium now has at least one strain that resists antibiotics, and some resist nearly all of the available medicines.

Autoimmune diseases threaten the body's defenses by turning those defenses against the body. Deceived by viruses or bacteria seeking access to the body by mimicking antibodies that belong to the healthy self, the immune system mobilizes itself for a misguided attack on the tissue it is supposed to protect. Autoimmune diseases include multiple sclerosis, rheumatoid arthritis, juvenile diabetes mellitus, myasthenia gravis, Graves' disease, and systemic lupus erythematosus.

Research intended to relieve the suffering of the victims of these and other autoimmune diseases is proceeding rapidly. Genetic factors are evident in most autoimmune illnesses, and genetic engineering is providing some of the answers.

Autoimmunity is surprisingly widespread. It affects about 5 percent of adults in Europe and North America, two thirds of them women. If it turns out that atherosclerosis, which causes stroke and heart attack, involves an autoimmune response, research into autoimmunity may produce therapies that will control cardiovascular disease, which causes half the deaths in the industrialized world.

Obviously, the immune system needs help. Immunization provides one set of possibilities. Advances in genetic engineering and immunology, which allow ever greater precision in attacks on tumor cells, have renewed interest in vaccines. No longer are cancer vaccines made from whole tumor cells and immune-stimulating chemicals. Genetically engineered vaccines aim for very specific immune reactions.

CHAPTER 7
Stress, Adaptation, and Coping

BILLIE SEVERTSEN and MARYANN F. PRANULIS

KEY TERMS

adaptation: Adjustment to a change in internal or external conditions or circumstances. Adaptation implies changing.

coping: A measure of the individual's resourcefulness and ability to deal with stress and stressors. Coping implies standing firm.

general adaptation syndrome: Described by Hans Selye as the total organism's nonspecific response to stress. The GAS response occurs in the following stages: (1) Alarm reaction, in which the body recognizes the stressor and the pituitary-adrenocortical system responds by producing the hormones essential to either fight or flee. In this stage, heart rate increases, blood sugar is elevated, pupils dilate, and digestion slows. (2) Resistance or adaptive stage, in which the body begins to repair the effect of the arousal. The acute stress symptoms diminish or disappear. If, however, the stress continues, adaptation fails in its attempts to maintain the defense. (3) Exhaustion stage, which occurs when the body can no longer respond to the stress. As a consequence, one or several of a great variety of diseases may develop.

homeostasis: State of equilibrium of the internal environment of the body that is maintained by the dynamic processes of feedback and regulation.

stress: The result produced when an organism is acted upon by forces that disrupt homeostasis.

stressor: An agent or condition capable of producing stress. The term denotes the physical (gravity, mechanical force, pathogen, injury) and psychological (fear, anxiety, crisis, joy) forces that may be experienced by individuals.

*O*ne fundamental principle in the biological sciences is that an organism must be able to adapt to its environment to survive and remain healthy. Numerous clinical specialists are beginning to realize that current health problems are inextricably linked to the way people adapt to their surroundings. Difficulties involved in adapting to the environment constitute an important component of the etiology of many diseases.

Today, individuals suffer from a multitude of environmental stressors: overcrowding, competition, noise, dirt, chemicals, pollution, infectious organisms, and other threats of bodily harm. In their own experiences, most people are familiar with the effects of stress. Everyone experiences some degree of stress most of the time. Stress is not always detrimental. A certain degree of stress is vital and necessary. For example, physical stress associated with activity such as walking or running causes bones to become harder by stimulating osteoblastic activity and calcification. The physical stress of walking also helps to determine the shape of bones. Stress can increase mental and physical alertness and can enhance productivity. Mild, brief stress states can be perceived as pleasant or exciting and can be positive—such as the experience of watching a dramatic movie. Under conditions of stress, important discoveries have been made and works of art have been produced.

Stress is a state that is associated with feelings, but it manifests physiologically as well as in behavioral changes. Psychological and sociocultural stressors produce physiologic changes as well as mental effects, and physiologic stressors can give rise to psychological changes.

This chapter provides a historical perspective on the concept of stress and homeostasis and reviews the neurophysiologic and biochemical events that are set in motion during stressful events.

Stress and Homeostasis

Living organisms survive by maintaining an immensely complex dynamic and harmonious equilibrium called **homeostasis** or **dynamic steady state.** Homeostasis represents an interaction between catabolism and anabolism—a process of constant change in both positive and negative directions. Because organisms are constantly challenged or threatened by intrinsic or extrinsic disturbing forces or stressors, the dynamic steady state required for successful adaptation is maintained by counteracting/reestablishing forces or adaptational responses. These forces consist of a number of physical or mental reactions that attempt to counteract the effects of the stressors.

Stress is defined as a state of tension that can lead to disharmony or threatened homeostasis. The amount of stress a person can tolerate before being overwhelmed depends on the adaptive capacity of that person. Everyone has a different adaptive capacity, and the limits of adaptability may be genetically determined. If adaptation is successful, the dynamic steady state (homeostasis) is maintained or restored. Homeostasis will be disrupted if the adaptive response is insufficient, inappropriate, or excessive. Consistent faulty adaptation will usually result in illness.

Historical Perspectives

Contemporary concepts regarding homeostasis have a long history. In the beginning of the Classical era, Heraclitus was the first to suggest that a static, unchanged state was not the natural condition, but rather that the capacity to undergo constant change was intrinsic to all things.[1] Shortly afterward, Empedocles proposed the corollary that all matter consisted of elements and qualities in dynamic opposition or alliance to one another, and that balance or harmony was a necessary condition for the survival of living organisms.[1] One hundred years later, Hippocrates equated health to a harmonious balance of the elements, and illness and disease to a systematic disharmony of these elements.[1] The terms dyscrasia and idiosyncrasy are derived from the Hippocratic concept of health and disease, meaning, respectively, a defective or peculiar mixing of the elements.[1] Hippocrates also suggested that the disturbing forces that produced the disharmony of disease derived from natural rather than supernatural sources, and that the counterbalancing or adaptive forces were of a natural origin as well. Thus he introduced the concept that "Nature is the healer of disease," a notion later echoed by the Romans when they referred to the counterbalancing forces as *vis medicatrix naturae,* or the healing power of nature.[1]

During Europe's Renaissance, Thomas Sydenham extended the Hippocratic concept of disease as a systematic disharmony brought about by disturbing forces when he suggested that an individual's adaptive response to such forces could itself be capable of producing pathologic changes.[1] Claude Bernard extended the notion of harmony or steady state in the nineteenth century when he introduced the concept of the *milieu interieur,* or the principle of a dynamic internal physiologic equilibrium.[1]

In 1935, Walter B. Cannon published "Stresses and Strains of Homeostasis,"[2] an application of the engineering concept of stress and strain to physiology. Further, Cannon extended the homeostatic concept to emotions as well as physical states. He first described the "fight-or-flight" reaction—the body's increased ability to run or confront due to greater alertness and focused attention and increased oxygen and glucose. Cannon also connected this response to the actions of epinephrine and norepinephrine. These studies further defined Cannon's initial observations that cats exhibiting a rage response to anesthesia had more rapid blood clotting than cats not evincing rage.[3] At about the same time that Cannon was considering these concepts, Hans Selye was also writing about stress.

KEY CONCEPTS

- Stress is defined as a state of disharmony or a threat to homeostasis. If adaptation is successful, the dynamic steady state of homeostasis is maintained or restored.
- Stress evokes the "fight-or-flight" reaction, which confers greater alertness, focused attention, increased energy, and a readiness to run or confront.

Selye's Contributions to Stress Research

Selye was experimenting with hormonal preparations in rats when he serendipitously uncovered a biological basis for stress. Selye was expecting to find different changes in rats injected with different hormonal preparations. But, to his amazement, the same three changes occurred in successive trials. The cortex of the rats' adrenal glands had enlarged, but the lymphatic organs (thymus, spleen, and lymph nodes) had shrunk, and bleeding ulcers of the stomach and duodenum developed in every animal. When Selye experimented with other noxious agents—such as loud noise, extracts from pituitary glands, kidneys, and spleens, and even a poison—the same three changes occurred. The organ changes seemed to occur together and were characteristic not only of one particular kind of injury but of any and all kinds of harmful stimuli. Selye termed the stimuli **stressors** and concluded that the manifestations resulting from the stressors represented a nonspecific response to any noxious stimuli. Because many diverse agents caused the same syndrome, Selye suggested that it be called the **general adaptation syndrome** (**GAS**) and that it include the following three components: *alarm reaction, stage of resistance,* and *stage of exhaustion*.[4] According to Selye's theory, all individuals move through the first two stages innumerable times, becoming adapted or habituated to the stressors encountered during ordinary life.[5] For example, when one first gazes at a bright light, the light acts as a stressor, triggering an *alarm reaction.* As one continues to look at the light, *adaptation* to the stressor occurs, marking a stage of resistance. The stage of *exhaustion* occurs if one continues to look at the bright light—indeed the eye will become permanently damaged if one continues to stare at the light after exhaustion. Observations of this phenomenon have led to the differentiation between focal stimuli and contextual stimuli as described by Hellerman[6] and Roy.[7]

General Adaptation Syndrome

Each component of GAS, the stress syndrome, can be subdivided into several different physiologic responses (Table 7–1). The easiest way to understand the entire response is to examine each component separately.

Alarm Reaction

The alarm reaction has been called the fight-or-flight response because it gives the body a boost of energy to either run or confront. The muscles receive increased blood, enriched with both oxygen and glucose. Respiration is increased, leading to increased oxygen consumption, and the liver gives up its stored glucose, releasing it into the bloodstream.

An alarm reaction begins when the hypothalamus perceives a need to activate the GAS in response to a stressor. The stressor might be an argument with a friend, or an upper respiratory tract infection, or running a marathon, or winning the lottery. The hypothalamus perceives the occurrence as stress and mediates the activation of the sympathetic nervous system, enabling the body to react very quickly to the stressor and coordinate many diffuse responses (Fig. 7–1). The hypothalamus also notifies the pituitary gland. The hypothalamus synthesizes corticotropin-releasing hormone (CRH), which triggers the release of adrenocorticotropic hormone (ACTH) by the anterior pituitary. It also synthesizes antidiuretic hormone (ADH), which is released by the posterior pituitary. The pituitary gland is stimulated to release a variety of hormones (Fig. 7–2). Once the pituitary becomes involved in the response, the alarm reaction cannot be turned off or deactivated. It must run its course, progressing through the stage of resistance.

TABLE 7–1. The Three Stages of the General Adaptation Syndrome

Alarm	Resistance	Exhaustion
Increased secretion of glucocorticoids and resultant changes	Glucocorticoid secretion returns to normal	Increased glucocorticoid secretion but eventually markedly decreased secretion
Increased activity of sympathetic nervous system	Sympathetic activity returns to normal	Stress triad (hypertrophied adrenals, atrophied thymus and lymph nodes, bleeding ulcers in stomach and duodenum)
Increased norepinephrine secretion by adrenal medulla	Norepinephrine secretion returns to normal	
"Fight-or-flight" syndrome of changes	"Fight-or-flight" syndrome disappears	
Low resistance to stressors	High resistance (adaptation) to stressor	Loss of resistance to stressor; may lead to death

From Thibodeau GA, Patton KT: *Anatomy & Physiology,* 2nd ed. St. Louis, Mosby–Year Book, 1993, p 570. Reproduced with permission.

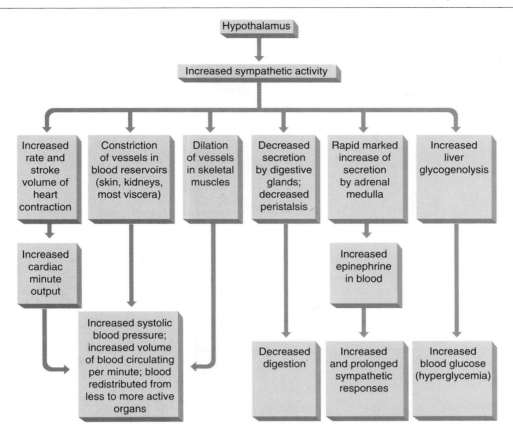

FIGURE 7-1. Alarm reaction responses resulting from increased sympathetic activity. Note that these are the responses commonly referred to as the "fight-or-flight" reaction. (Adapted with permission from Thibodeau GA, Patton KT: *Anatomy and Physiology*, 2nd ed. St. Louis, Mosby–Year Book, 1993, p 570.)

Stage of Resistance

If the physiologic mechanisms described above were to continue unabated, the body would soon suffer undue wear and tear and become permanently damaged. The stage of resistance is the stage in which the body becomes adapted to its previous stressed state and is returned to a state of homeostasis.

As the body moves into the stage of resistance, cortisol and aldosterone are secreted in excess. A principal action of aldosterone is to increase sodium and water retention, thereby contributing to an increase in blood volume. Cortisol is anti-inflammatory in nature and minimizes some symptoms of stress as discussed above.

In the stage of resistance, the body repairs itself as the stressor is addressed and resolved. Homeostasis is restored to the organism.

Selye postulated that adaptation or a return to homeostasis uses energy. Adaptation or habituation to stress refers to either the length of time needed to reach the stage of resistance or the vigor and scope of physiologic responses to the stressor. For example, loud noise is a known stressor. Yet people living near busy airports usually reach a point at which they barely notice the loud noises that frequently occur over their houses. These individuals could be charac-terized as persons who have **habituated** to the stress of loud noises.

Adaptation to a particular stressor comes about in several ways. One important way to habituate is to manipulate or "train" the hypothalamus to react less forcefully to its perceived threat by the stressor. Perception can be altered to resist the negative effects of the stressor; part of the perceptual set regarding loud noise is related to uncertainty about what the noise means. People who live near an airport might well understand why the loud noise occurs (an airplane taking off or landing) and actually may be reassured by the sound. On a conscious level, loud noises from the adjacent airport mean that everything is as it should be.

The hypothalamus can also be trained to pay less attention to some stressors. By ignoring certain stressors, inappropriate triggering of the GAS is avoided. Consequently, more acceptable levels of stress are maintained in the individual. Techniques that accomplish this desensitization of the hypothalamus are ones that change the predominant brain waves of the individual from beta to alpha, which is a slower, normal brain wave.

Examples of therapies that use this principle are biofeedback, visualization, and meditation. Use of these techniques 20 to 30 minutes per day enhances

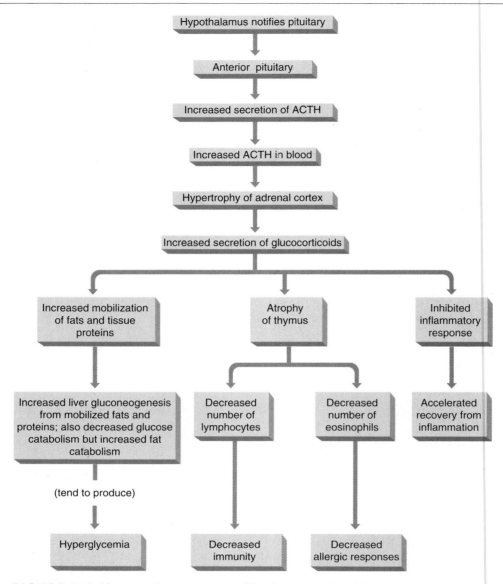

FIGURE 7-2. Alarm reaction responses resulting from activation of the pituitary. (Adapted with permission from Thibodeau GA, Patton KT: *Anatomy and Physiology,* 2nd ed. St. Louis, Mosby–Year Book, 1993, p 569.)

the ability to alter one's perception of stressors and to modulate the stress response. Migraine headache, chronic back pain, and hypertension are examples of conditions that have been successfully treated in this way.

Stage of Exhaustion

Exhaustion occurs as the body is no longer able to bring about a return of homeostasis following the influence of stressors. Instead of going into a stage of resistance, it becomes exhausted and unable to adapt. Selye postulated that when the energy resources of an individual are completely used up, death will occur because the individual is unable to adapt. He speculated that individuals possess both superficial and

deep adaptive energy. Superficial energy can be replaced from the deep adaptive stores. But, when the deep adaptive energy stores are depleted, no other resource exists to help the person recover from stress. This is the point at which people often seek professional health care since they can't seem to adapt to the problem without medical or nursing intervention, or they have developed problems as a result of faulty adaptation.

Local Adaptation Syndrome

A miniature version of the GAS is the local adaptation syndrome (LAS). This phenomenon, initially isolated by Selye, explains the classic inflammatory response. (See Chapters 8 and 9 for a full explanation of infection and inflammation.) Signs of inflammation include redness, swelling or edema, pain, drainage in some instances, and limitation of movement. The nature of an inflammatory reaction is both to separate the inflamed entity from the rest of the body by encapsulation and to destroy the foreign invader by enzyme and inflammatory cell attack. LAS and GAS are compared and contrasted in Table 7–2. Selye's hypotheses about stress are summarized in Figure 7–3.

Although Selye's work has been widely disseminated and used as the theoretical foundation for a considerable volume of research in nursing and other disciplines, his theory has also been widely criticized. The notion that stress is purely a physiologic response has been challenged. It is difficult to know whether the physical stressor itself or one's thoughts and feelings about it actually produce the neuroendocrine response.

Many physiologists resist Selye's concept of nonspecificity. Adaptive bodily responses are selective and are organized to counteract the specific bodily changes that elicit them. It is difficult to explain how any nonspecific physiologic or biochemical response could help the body adapt, for example, to both cold and heat.[8] No single hormone, in fact, responds to all stressful stimuli in the nonspecific fashion implied in Selye's definition of the GAS. Physiologically, the body adapts to cold by conserving heat (peripheral vasoconstriction) and producing more heat (shivering). It adapts to heat by increasing heat loss (peripheral vasodilation and sweating) and decreasing heat production.

Selye's definitions of stress differed from the definitions proposed in physics, where the terms originated. This led to confusion rather than precision. Others criticized Selye's formulations because he was an endocrinologist by specialty and, therefore, not "eminently qualified" to conduct mind-body research or to generate theory about the mind-body interaction. Selye's formulations, however, made sense to the general public and a broad spectrum of professionals in a variety of life sciences. His contributions to knowledge about stress, coping, and adaptation are considered classics which contributed greatly to de-

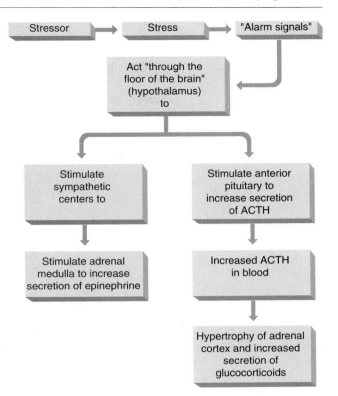

FIGURE 7–3. Selye's hypothesis about activation of the stress response. (Redrawn with permission from Thibodeau GA, Patton KT: *Anatomy and Physiology*, 2nd ed. St. Louis, Mosby–Year Book, 1993, p 571.)

veloping knowledge about neurohormonal transmission.

Subsequently, researchers such as Holmes,[9] Rahe,[10] Mason,[11] and Lazarus[12] further studied the concepts of stress, leading to increased knowledge of adaptation, coping, and the physiologic, biochemical, and psychological responses in stress. Most recently, pioneering research has begun to focus on interactions between the three major integrative systems of the body: the immune, nervous, and endocrine systems.

TABLE 7–2. Comparison of LAS and GAS

Local Adaptation Syndrome	General Adaptation Syndrome
1. Physiologic response is localized; entire body not involved	1. Physiologic response involves entire organism
2. Adaptive response to a stressor	2. Adaptive response to a stressor
3. Short-term response without long-term consequences	3. Long-term response; depletes reservoir of adaptive energy
4. Restorative response—organism returns to homeostasis	4. Restorative response—organism returns to homeostasis (stage of resistance) or deteriorates (stage of exhaustion)

KEY CONCEPTS

- Selye discovered that a number of noxious stimuli or stressors evoked the same type of response in experimental animals. He called this generalized response the general adaptation syndrome. Three common physiologic responses occurred in response to stress: (1) hyperplasia of the adrenal cortex, (2) atrophy of lymphoid tissues, and (3) ulceration of the stomach and duodenum.
- Selye described three phases of the stress response: alarm, resistance, and exhaustion. The alarm reaction is the initial response to stress. The major features of the alarm reaction are attributable to activation of the sympathetic nervous system. During the stage of resistance, sympathetic activity declines while secretion of adrenocortical hormones is high.

If the stressor continues, habituation or adaptation may occur such that the hypothalamus fails to respond with alarm. If the stressor is too great or prolonged, energy reserves may be depleted, leading to the stage of exhaustion.

- Localized inflammatory processes were characterized by Selye as the local adaptation syndrome. Localized inflammation is characterized by redness, swelling, pain, and altered function.

Current Concepts of Stress

With ongoing research, Selye's original view of the stress response has been revised. Current concepts are presented in Figure 7–4. Activation of the stress system leads to changes that improve the organism's ability to regain homeostasis and increase survival chances.

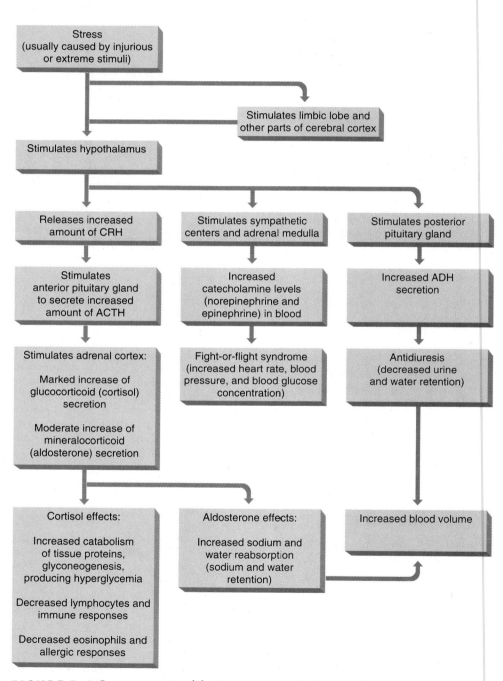

FIGURE 7–4. Current concepts of the stress response. (Redrawn with permission from Thibodeau GA, Patton KT: *Anatomy and Physiology*, 2nd ed. St. Louis, Mosby–Year Book, 1993, p 572.)

Neuroendocrine Interactions

Catecholamine Release ✓

The endocrine system reacts to stress by secreting hormones necessary to alter metabolic processes and restore homeostasis. The reaction of the nervous system involves both the brain and the autonomic nervous systems, primarily the sympathetic nervous system. Neuroendocrine interactions in response to a stressor are summarized in Figure 7–5.

The hypothalamus prompts the release of catecholamines from the sympathetic nervous system, the excitatory portion of the autonomic nervous system. Catecholamines (epinephrine and norepinephrine) are synthesized locally in sympathetic neurons (norepinephrine) and the adrenal medulla (epinephrine and norepinephrine). Catecholamines cannot cross the blood-brain barrier but instead circulate in plasma in a loose association with albumin. Circulating catecholamines have essentially the same effect as direct sympathetic stimulation, causing increased heart rate, increased blood pressure, and increased blood flow to skeletal muscles. Catecholamine response accounts for the increased strength experienced by or witnessed in people during the alarm phase. The effects of norepinephrine and epinephrine are described below.

Norepinephrine. Norepinephrine released from the adrenal medulla goes to the liver and skeletal muscle, but is then rapidly metabolized. Very little adrenal norepinephrine reaches distal tissue.[13] The effects caused by norepinephrine during the stress response are primarily from the sympathetic nervous system.[14] Norepinephrine regulates blood pressure because it is the primary constrictor of smooth muscle in all blood vessels.[15] During stress, norepinephrine raises blood pressure by constricting peripheral vessels. Norepinephrine also reduces gastric secretion. Norepinephrine causes pupils of the eyes to dilate, accounting for the "wide-eyed" appearance of persons experiencing stress.

Epinephrine. Epinephrine causes some of the same effects as norepinephrine, yet it has greater influence on cardiac action.[16] Epinephrine enhances myocardial contractility, increases the heart rate, and increases venous return to the heart, all of which increase cardiac output and blood pressure.[17] Epinephrine also has metabolic effects, increasing glycogenolysis and the release of glucose from the liver.[18] Through the actions of epinephrine, a person has a suddenly increased feeling of muscular strength and aggressiveness.

The metabolic actions of epinephrine aid the metabolic actions of cortisol, which are similar. Brain systems influence and are influenced by both the sympathetic nervous system and the endocrine system responses. In the brain, increased blood flow and increased glucose metabolism lead to increased atten-

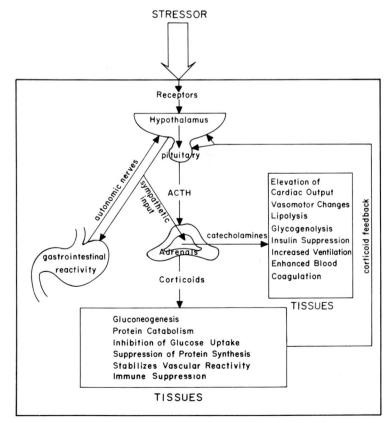

FIGURE 7–5. Neuroendocrine interactions in response to a stressor. Receptors respond to the stressor stimulus and relay the information to the hypothalamus, which controls both the pituitary (adrenal cortex) and the autonomic nervous system (sympathetic pathways). Most of the stress reaction throughout the body is then mediated by secretions of catecholamines and cortical steroids. (From Ramsey JM: *Basic Pathophysiology: Modern Stress and the Disease Process.* Menlo Park, Calif, Addison-Wesley, 1982, p 58. Reproduced with permission.)

tion, vigilance, and alertness. All of these effects prepare the body to take physical action—to "fight or flee."

Table 7–3 summarizes the physiologic effects of epinephrine and norepinephrine.

Hypothalamic, Pituitary, and Adrenal Hormone Release

The endocrine system contributes hypothalamic, pituitary, and adrenal hormones. These hormones include CRH, ACTH, ADH, glucocorticoids (cortisol), and mineralocorticoids (aldosterone)

Aldosterone. At least 95 percent of the mineralocorticoid activity of adrenocortical secretion is due to aldosterone.[19] The primary effect of this steroid is to increase renal tubular resorption of sodium and increase renal excretion of potassium.[20] Through osmotic force, water tends to follow sodium; therefore, excessive resorption of sodium results in an increased extracellular fluid volume, which in turn elevates blood pressure. Aldosterone secretion is normally stimulated by a decreased extracellular fluid volume as well as by the renin-angiotensin mechanism, which responds to diminished blood flow to the kidneys.[21]

Cortisol. About 95 percent of the glucocorticoid activity of adrenocortical secretion is due to cortisol, also known as hydrocortisone.[22] One of the primary effects of cortisol is the stimulation of gluconeogenesis in the liver. Cortisol action may increase the rate of conversion of amino acids to keto acids to glucose by as much as six to ten times.[23] The gluconeogenesis promoted by cortisol ensures an adequate source of glucose (energy) for body tissues in general, and nerve cells in particular. Cortisol also inhibits the uptake and

TABLE 7–3. Physiologic Effects of Adrenal Catecholamines

Effect	Principal Hormone
Vasoconstriction	Norepinephrine
Inhibition of gastrointestinal action	Norepinephrine
Pupil dilation	Norepinephrine
Rate of cardiac contraction	Epinephrine
Force of cardiac contraction	Epinephrine
Stimulates metabolic rate	Epinephrine
Stimulates conversion of glycogen to glucose	Epinephrine
Suppresses secretion of insulin	Epinephrine
Stimulates secretion of glucagon	Epinephrine
Stimulates lipolysis	Epinephrine
Stimulates cholesterol synthesis	Epinephrine
Inhibits cholesterol degradation	Epinephrine
Dilates bronchial airways	Both epinephrine and norepinephrine
Stimulates secretion of ACTH	Norepinephrine
Promotes skeletal muscle contractility	Epinephrine
Increases rate of blood coagulability	Epinephrine
Arouses central nervous system activity	Norepinephrine

From Ramsey JM: *Basic Pathophysiology: Modern Stress and the Disease Process.* Menlo Park, Calif, Addison-Wesley, 1982. p 53, Reproduced with permission.

oxidation of glucose by many body cells, preserving it for nerve cells. The overall action of cortisol on carbohydrate metabolism results in an elevation of blood glucose.

Cortisol enhances the elevation of blood glucose promoted by other hormones, such as epinephrine, glucagon, and somatotropic growth hormone, and this supportive action by cortisol is said to be *permissive* for the actions of other hormones. Because cortisol is necessary for the maintenance of normal blood pressure and cardiac output, it is also permissive for the action of the catecholamines.

Cortisol affects protein metabolism. It has an *anabolic* effect, or increases the rate of synthesis, of proteins and RNA in liver. Cortisol has *catabolic* effects in muscle, lymphoid tissue, adipose tissue, skin, and bone. The overall breakdown effect of proteins results in a negative nitrogen balance and an increase in circulating amino acids. The resultant pooling of amino acids from catabolized proteins may ensure amino acid availability for protein synthesis in certain cells. There is some evidence that cortisol depresses transport of amino acids into muscle cells while enhancing their uptake into the liver, where they are converted to glucose.[24]

In the gastrointestinal tract, cortisol promotes gastric secretion. This is opposite to the effect of norepinephrine, which reduces gastric secretion. Gastric secretion may be stimulated by excessive cortisol, with resultant ulceration of the gastric mucosa—perhaps accounting for the gastrointestinal ulceration observed by Selye.

Cortisol acts as an immunosuppressant by suppressing protein synthesis, including the synthesis of antibodies. Cortisol also reduces populations of eosinophils, lymphocytes, and macrophages.[25] Large doses of cortisol are known to promote atrophy of lymphoid tissue in the thymus, spleen, and lymph nodes. This action of cortisol could account for the lymphoid atrophy observed by Selye.

The ability of cortisol and other glucocorticoids to suppress the inflammatory response provides the basis for the major therapeutic use of these steroids. Glucocorticoids inhibit the accumulation of leukocytes at the site of inflammation and inhibit the release of substances involved in the inflammatory process (e.g., kinins, plasminogen-activating factor, prostaglandins, and histamine) from the leukocytes. However, if glucocorticoids are secreted in excess, the antiinflammatory effects can be detrimental to wound healing. At the site of an inflammatory response, cortisol inhibits fibroblast proliferation and function—accounting for the poor wound healing, increased susceptibility to infection, and decreased inflammatory response that are often seen in individuals with glucocorticoid excess.[26] Table 7–4 summarizes the major physiologic effects of cortisol.

In general, glucocorticoids are believed to facilitate peripheral changes that promote an adaptive redirection of energy. Oxygen and nutrients are directed to the central nervous system and the stressed body site(s). The availability of vital materials is enhanced

TABLE 7–4. Major Physiologic Actions of Cortisol

Carbohydrate and lipid metabolism	Diminishes peripheral uptake and utilization of glucose
	Promotes gluconeogenesis in liver cells
	Enhances the gluconeogenic response to other hormones
	Promotes lipolysis in adipose tissue
Protein metabolism	Stimulates degradation of body protein
	Depresses protein synthesis (including immunoglobulin)
	Increases plasma level of amino acids
	Stimulates deamination in the liver
Membrane permeability	Suppresses membrane permeability of all cells and organelles, but particularly those of lysosomes, and capillary endothelium
	Inhibits the formation and release of histamine and bradykinin
	Permissive for vasoconstrictive action of norepinephrine
Immune reserve	Decreases the tissue mass of all lymphatic tissues
	Promotes rapid decrease in circulating lymphocytes, eosinophils, basophils, and macrophages
Other effects	Promotes gastric secretion
	Enhances urinary excretion
	Decreases proliferation of fibroblasts in connective tissue

From Ramsey JM: *Basic Pathophysiology: Modern Stress and the Disease Process.* Menlo Park, Calif, Addison-Wesley, 1982, p 56. Reproduced with permission.

by increased blood pressure, heart rate, respiratory rate, and glucose. Cortisol also modulates immune responses as described above.

Stress and Other Hormones

Growth Hormone

Growth hormone (somatotropin) is released from the anterior pituitary gland and affects protein, lipid, and carbohydrate metabolism. Growth hormone levels increase in the blood following a variety of *intensely* stressful physical or psychological stimuli, such as strenuous exercise or extreme fear.[27] In most circumstances, the increase in growth hormone occurs only with a parallel rise in cortisol secretion.[28]

Prolactin

Prolactin is released from the anterior pituitary gland and is necessary for lactation and breast development. Prolactin levels in plasma increase from a variety of stressful physical and psychological stimuli.[29] Unlike growth hormone, prolactin levels show little change after exercise. However, like growth hormone, prolactin appears to require more intense stimuli than those leading to increases in catecholamine or cortisol levels.[30] Prolactin levels also increase in the plasma following a variety of sexual stimuli, for example stimulation of the nipple or areola in women.

Testosterone

Testosterone, a hormone secreted by Leydig cells, regulates male secondary sex characteristics and libido. Testosterone levels *decrease* after exposure to physically and psychologically stressful stimuli, as a result of a still unknown mechanism.[31]

Stress and Endorphin Release

Other brain systems involved include the mesocortical and mesolimbic dopamine systems, the amygdala/hippocampus complex, and arcuate pro-opiomelanocortin neurons. These brain systems also facilitate neural pathways mediating arousal, alertness, vigilance, cognition, focused attention, and aggression, and inhibit other pathways, such as feeding and reproduction.[32] Anticipatory and cognitive functions are increased by stimulation of prefrontal cortex neurons in the mesocortical dopamine system.[33] Motivational and reward functions are stimulated by the mesolimbic dopamine system.[34]

The amygdala area of the brain retrieves and analyzes emotional information. This stimulates the GAS in response to an emotional stressor such as fear or generates emotional responses to the stressor. The hippocampus area of the brain counteracts the functions of the amygdala, moderating emotional tone.

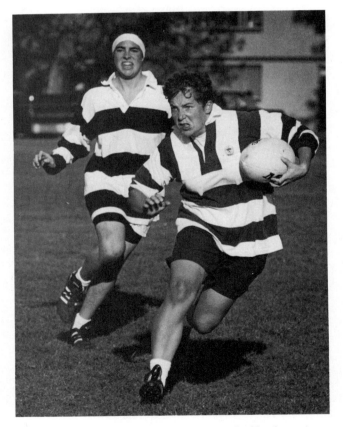

FIGURE 7–6. Growth hormone levels in the blood may increase in response to the stress of rugby. (Photographer: Kathleen Kelly, Spokane, Wash.)

Stimulation of the arcuate pro-opiomelanocortin neurons in the central nervous system may increase self-analgesia due to the generation of β-endorphins.[35] The term *endorphin* was coined by combining the words endogenous and morphine. Like morphine, endorphins raise the pain threshold and produce both sedation and euphoria. As endorphin levels rise, individuals experience these pleasurable sensations. The stress of exercise[36] (Fig. 7–6), the excitement of dance, the anticipation of eating delicious food, or the drama of combat or contact sports can all produce a concomitant increase in endorphin levels.

Neuroendocrine and Immune System Interactions

It is well documented that the endocrine system is inextricably linked to the nervous system and to virtually every other physiologic system. It is also well documented that the autonomic nervous system and the immune system are connected to each other. Principal organs of the immune system are illustrated in Figure 7–7. Sympathetic innervation of both blood vessels supplying immune organs and the parenchyma (the functional parts) of immune organs (fields of lymphocytes) provides the basis for the connection between these two systems. The parenchymal fibers are usually found in areas of T-cells. Precisely how and to what extent this direct autonomic innervation of lymphoid tissues actually regulates immune function is not yet clear.[37] The existence of autonomic innervation of lymphoid tissues and the presence of immune cell receptors for numerous neurochemicals have sparked intense interest in experiments to test directly whether the autonomic nervous system can modulate immune function in intact animals.[38] This hypothesis is illustrated in Figure 7–8.

Although cumulative evidence supports a potentially important role for immunomodulation by the sympathetic nervous system, substantial further work is required to clarify the precise nature and mechanisms of the influence on immune response.

How the neuroendocrine and immune systems are interconnected is another topic of investigation. The endocrine system might well be expected to respond to the intrusion of foreign (nonself) molecules recognized by the immune system. And, there is now considerable evidence that the immune and neuroendocrine systems are thoroughly integrated through the expression of a shared set of hormones and a shared set of receptors for these hormones.[39–41]

An intriguing view, consistent with the above evidence, is that the immune system may serve a sensory function, conveying to the nervous system general signals about the presence of such *noncognitive stimuli* as bacteria or viruses which the nervous system cannot directly detect. These signals would then evoke

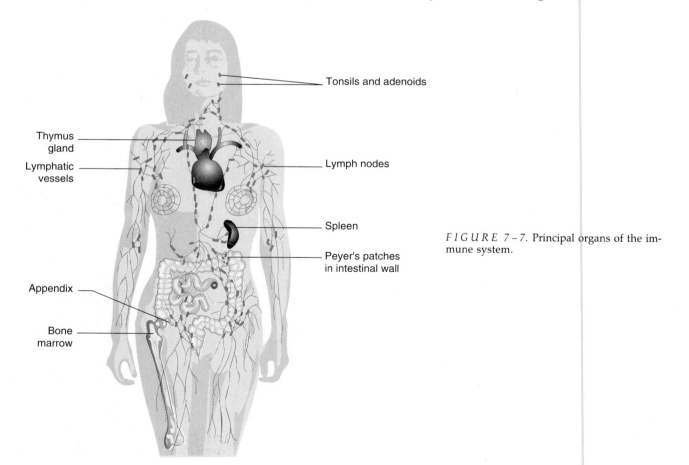

Thymus gland

Lymphatic vessels

Appendix

Bone marrow

Tonsils and adenoids

Lymph nodes

Spleen

Peyer's patches in intestinal wall

FIGURE 7–7. Principal organs of the immune system.

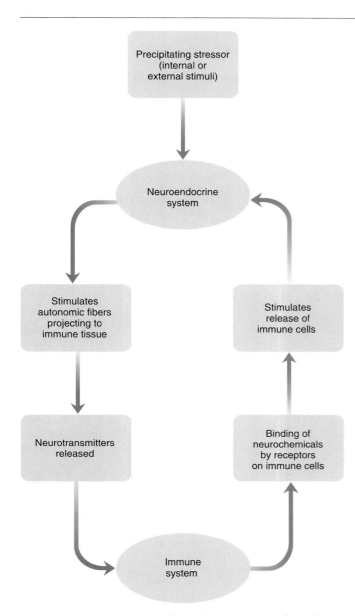

FIGURE 7-8. Model simplifying the complex regulatory loop hypothesized to exist between immune and neuroendocrine systems. Autonomic innervation of lymphoid tissue might thus play a role in directly modulating immune cell function.

neuroendocrine changes that may have physiologic, immunologic, and behavioral consequences. If this pathway is in fact active in vivo, then immune responses can induce hormone release similar to that produced when stressful stimuli are perceived directly by the brain. For example, through immune system signals, bacteria associated with an infection would activate the pituitary-adrenal system, resulting in increased secretions of ACTH and glucocorticoids (Fig. 7–9).

There are at least three extant hypotheses to explain the ways the immune system signals the neuroendocrine system that an immunogenic challenge exists. One hypothesis is that immune cell production

of soluble factors acts on the hypothalamus and influences the hypothalamic-pituitary-adrenal (HPA) axis, raising blood glucocorticoid levels.[42] A second possibility for immune-neuroendocrine signaling is by immune cell production of neuroactive peptides that could act on nearby lymphocytes.[43] A third possibility is through the action of thymosin peptides, which would help stimulate T-cell differentiation and function.[44] Figure 7–10 illustrates a proposed role of thymosins in helping to mediate brain-immune system interactions.

Much evidence supports the existence of brain and immune system responsiveness. Several different stress paradigms have shown that stress can elevate endorphin levels. Stressors varying in seemingly minor detail can result in distinctly different forms of analgesia. Theoretically, these endorphins could exert their effects on immune responses.

In preliminary clinical trials, endorphins have actually been shown to play complex roles in elevating the number of lymphocytes—the number of active T-cells, and the number of cells in several T-cell subsets.[45] It may be that endogenous opioid systems may modulate the immune system and even be shown to influence in vitro and in vivo tumor growth in at least some tumor systems. The resolution of the enhancing and inhibiting effects of opioids on immune responses and a full understanding of the extent to which the immune effects of opioids are causally related to opioid effects on cancer growth require further research. A schematic diagram summarizing neural and neurohumoral mechanisms by which stress and morphine might affect the immune system and tumors is presented in Figure 7–11.

Although the development of the immune and neuroendocrine systems appears to be extensively intertwined, the molecular mechanisms for this developmental interdependency still remain unknown. Recent discovery of a lymphokine product of stimulated lymphocytes, termed neuroleukin, has generated considerable interest.[46] The gene for neuroleukin has now been cloned and sequenced; the protein product is neurotrophic for spinal and sensory neurons and also can support the growth in culture of sensory neurons and some embryonic spinal neurons.[47]

Stress and Disease

Broadly speaking, the stress response depends not only on its capacity to respond quickly to appropriate stimuli, but also on its ability to respond to counterregulatory elements that prevent an over-response. Every aspect of the stress response—including that originating from an inflammatory/immune reaction—must briskly respond to restraining forces. If not kept in check, these responses contribute to the process of pathologic change.

Stress system dysfunction is characterized by sustained hyperactivity or hypoactivity in response to various pathophysiologic states that cut across the traditional boundaries of medical disciplines. These

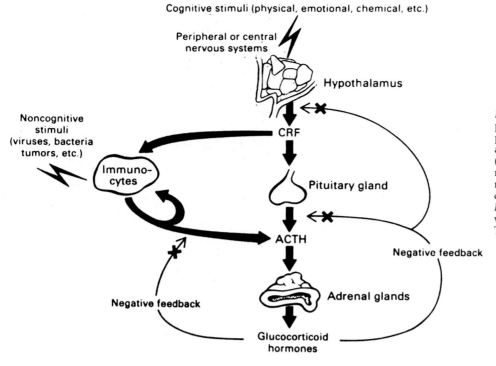

FIGURE 7–9. Illustration of apparent connections between the hypothalamic-pituitary-adrenal axis and cells of the immune system. (From Blalock JE, Harbour-Menamin D, Smith EM: Peptide hormones shared by the neuroendocrine and immunologic systems. *J Immunol* 1985;135:859s. Reproduced with permission. Copyright 1985, The Journal of Immunology.)

include a range of psychiatric, endocrine, and inflammatory disorders, or susceptibility to such disorders.

Hair loss, emotional tension, mouth sores, asthma, heart palpitations, neuromuscular movements (tics), tension headaches, muscle contraction backache, digestive disturbances, and irritable bladder are all common disorders that may be caused or exacerbated by stress. Skin outbreaks such as acne, or reproductive disorders such as menstrual irregularity in women or impotence in men, are also affected by the undesirable effects of too much stress. Table 7–5 summarizes some of the physiologic and psychological effects of too much stress and Figure 7–12 depicts the multiple organs that can be involved in dysregulation of the stress response. The specific stress-

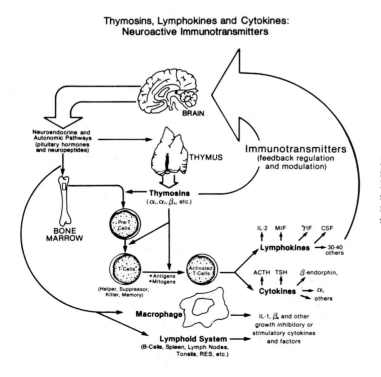

FIGURE 7–10. Illustration of proposed role of thymosins in helping to mediate brain-immune interactions. (From Hall NR, et al: Evidence that thymosins and other biological response modifiers can function as neuroactive immunotransmitters. *J Immunol* 1985;135:807s. Reproduced with permission. Copyright 1985, The Journal of Immunology.)

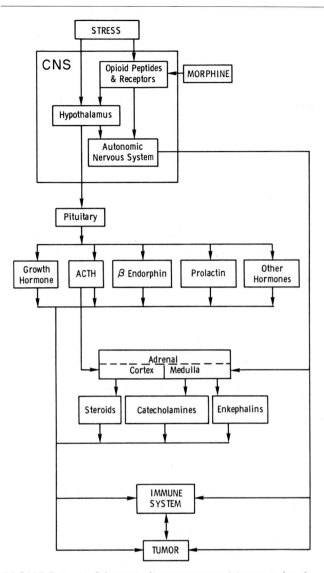

FIGURE 7–11. Schematic diagram summarizing neural and neurohumoral mechanisms by which stress and morphine might affect the immune system and tumors. (From Shavit Y, et al: Stress, opioid peptides, the immune system, and cancer. *J Immunol* 1985;135:836s. Reproduced with permission. Copyright 1985, The Journal of Immunology.)

induced mechanisms causing these disorders are as yet unclear. Research into the interconnections between the immune and neuroendocrine systems may provide answers.

Stress and Aging

Aging itself is a stressful event. Although age-related changes in organs and systems occur slowly, gradually, and almost imperceptibly to the affected individual, the changes have an impact on how individuals are able to tolerate stress. It has been hypothesized that stress and stress-related mechanisms augment age-related changes in the body.[48] Research suggests that stress promotes anatomic and biochemical

changes occurring at the neuromuscular junction to reduce available transmitter chemicals, such as acetylcholine, and decrease communication between nerve and muscle cells.[49] The result is chronic fatigue and reduced physical strength.

In addition to such physiologic factors, social factors such as retirement, loss of income, and the death of friends or family—a general reduction of social support—all contribute to altered ability to manage stress and to cope. Elderly persons are not only at risk for stress-related disorders, they also have diminished immune function to protect themselves. The alterations in immunity associated with aging are described in Chapter 10.

KEY CONCEPTS

- **The stress response involves three major body systems—nervous, endocrine, and immune. These systems work together in a coordinated manner to summon the body's defenses in response to a variety of stressors including psychological, physiologic, and immunologic.**
- **The primary role of the nervous system is appraisal of a stimulus as stressful and activation of the sympathetic nervous system. Norepinephrine released from sympathetic nerve endings increases heart rate and contractility, constricts blood vessels, enhances**

TABLE 7–5. Physical and Behavioral Indicators of Too Much Stress

Physiologic Indicators of High Stress Levels

Elevated blood pressure
Increased muscle tension
Elevated pulse
Increased respiration
Sweaty palms
Cold extremities (hands and feet)
Fatigue
Tension headache
Upset stomach—nausea, vomiting, diarrhea
Change in appetite
Change in weight
Increased blood catecholamine level
Hyperglycemia
Restlessness
Insomnia

Behavioral and Emotional Indicators of High Stress

Anxiety (nonspecific fears)
Depression
Increased use of mind-altering substances (e.g., alcohol, chemical substances)
Change in eating, sleeping, or activity pattern
Mental exhaustion
Feelings of inadequacy; loss of self-esteem
Increased irritability
Loss of motivation
Decreased productivity
Inability to make good judgments
Inability to concentrate
Increased absenteeism and illness
Increased proneness to accidents

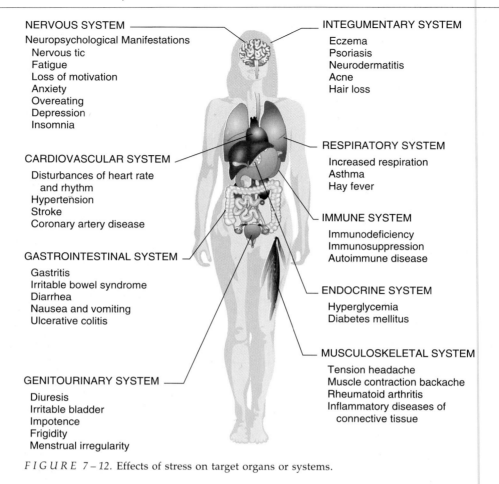

NERVOUS SYSTEM
Neuropsychological Manifestations
Nervous tic
Fatigue
Loss of motivation
Anxiety
Overeating
Depression
Insomnia

CARDIOVASCULAR SYSTEM
Disturbances of heart rate
and rhythm
Hypertension
Stroke
Coronary artery disease

GASTROINTESTINAL SYSTEM
Gastritis
Irritable bowel syndrome
Diarrhea
Nausea and vomiting
Ulcerative colitis

GENITOURINARY SYSTEM
Diuresis
Irritable bladder
Impotence
Frigidity
Menstrual irregularity

INTEGUMENTARY SYSTEM
Eczema
Psoriasis
Neurodermatitis
Acne
Hair loss

RESPIRATORY SYSTEM
Increased respiration
Asthma
Hay fever

IMMUNE SYSTEM
Immunodeficiency
Immunosuppression
Autoimmune disease

ENDOCRINE SYSTEM
Hyperglycemia
Diabetes mellitus

MUSCULOSKELETAL SYSTEM
Tension headache
Muscle contraction backache
Rheumatoid arthritis
Inflammatory diseases of
connective tissue

F I G U R E 7 – 12. Effects of stress on target organs or systems.

blood flow to skeletal muscle, reduces gastrointestinal motility and secretion, and dilates the pupil of the eye.

• Important stress-related endocrine hormones include epinephrine from the adrenal medulla, cortisol from the adrenal cortex, and antidiuretic hormone from the posterior pituitary. Epinephrine's actions are similar to those of norepinephrine and are particularly important for increasing cardiac performance and the release of glucose from the liver. Cortisol has synergistic effects with catecholamines in regulating vascular smooth muscle and is anti-inflammatory. Antidiuretic hormone is important for blood volume regulation.

• Secretion of a number of hormones is altered with stress, but a precise role in the stress response is unknown. Growth hormone may increase or decrease, depending on the stress level. Prolactin increases and testosterone and thyroid-stimulating hormone decrease with stress. Endorphins increase, leading to decreased perception of pain, sedation, and euphoria.

• The role of the immune system in the stress response is less well characterized. Catecholamines and stress hormones affect the activity of immune cells, and immune-released cytokines, such as neuro-active peptides (e.g., neuroleukin), may influence the neuroendocrine system.

• A number of disorders are thought to be related to excessive stress or inappropriate stress responses. These include asthma, palpitations, headaches, menstrual irregularity, skin rashes, and digestive disturbances.

Stress and Stressors

Stressors may impinge on a person from the external environment (e.g., ionizing radiation) or may arise from within the individual (e.g., low blood glucose level, or an imagined or symbolic threat). Stressors may be physical (heat), chemical (drugs or toxins), biological (bacteria), sociocultural (overcrowding, relationships with other people) or psychological (a threat to self-esteem, lack of love).

Stress itself can become a source of new stressors. In other words, an attempt to adapt to one stress may lead to other stresses. For example, in response to stress produced by an infection, a person may take an antibiotic. If the person has an allergic reaction to the antibiotic, additional stress is produced.

Stressors and Circadian Cycles

A person is also subject to many biological rhythms. These rhythms developed during the course of evolution in response to environmental processes and are now inherent in every organism. Although the environmental periodicity no longer causes the biological rhythm, it acts as a synchronizing agent for the self-sustained cycle within the organism. For example, a powerful synchronizing agent is the light-dark (day/night) cycle. Biological cycles may occur over varying lengths of time. Lunar (28 days) and circadian (about 1-day) cycles are very common. For example, the menstrual cycle follows a lunar cycle. Body temperature, many hormone levels, and periods of rest and activity, for example, exhibit circadian rhythms. As a result of circadian cycles, a person is a different physiologic and psychological system at each hour of the day. The phase of the circadian cycles at the time the stressor impinges on the individual, therefore, will partly determine the effects of the stressor. The effects of long-lasting stress may be influenced by the extent to which the stress interferes with the mechanism for synchronizing the innate cycle with the environmental process.

Scope, Intensity, and Duration of Stressors

Stressors also vary in scope, intensity, and duration. The amount of stress humans can withstand varies considerably from person to person and from situation to situation. These contrasting responses are due to varying individual inherent characteristics. During war, individuals exposed to the stress of combat become nonfunctional at different levels for the degree of stress experienced. But, at certain degrees of intensity and duration, *no one* can experience stress and remain functional.

A given stressor can affect the same person in different ways at different times. Throughout life, a person goes through a number of critical stages in development. At certain critical stages, a person may be more vulnerable to a particular stressor than at other times. For example, a high level of bilirubin in the blood can cause brain damage in a newborn because, at this stage of development, the blood-brain barrier is immature and bilirubin can enter the brain. In an adult, however, the blood-brain barrier is impermeable to bilirubin, and a high concentration of bilirubin in the blood usually does not have a neurotoxic effect.

Stressors may be classified as *low* or *high intensity*. A stressor may not be perceived as very intense initially but, over many years, can produce negative effects. For example, living or working for years in a crowded, busy environment may promote physiologic changes that produce hypertensive symptoms. On the other hand, a stressor may be perceived from the outset as having *high intensity*—such as the effect of being involved in a car accident. An example of a *low-intensity* stressor is chapped lips from the effects of a mild windburn.

Stressors may also have a wide or a narrow scope. An individual with a mild, sunburned nose has experienced a *narrow scope* stressor. In this case, the stress of sunburn only affects a small area of the skin briefly. By comparison, a newly divorced single parent with bronchitis, reduced income, and no health care benefits has a *broad scope* stressor—affecting many dimensions.

The amount of stress humans can withstand without having a deleterious response varies from individual to individual and from situation to situation. The magnitude of the human stress response depends on the nature of the stressor, the strength or magnitude of the stressor, and the meaning that the stressor has for the individual. The way a person *perceives* a situation (whether consciously or unconsciously) is also significant. Perception depends on the individual's genetic constitution, earlier conditioning influences, past life experiences, and cultural pressures. An expert golfer, for example, studying the "lie" of a ball near a big sandtrap is not likely to perceive the situation as a stressor. On the other hand, appraisal of the ball's position by an amateur golfer is likely to cause stress—especially during a golf tournament. Besides perception of the stressor, *mediating factors*, such as personal and external resources and coping strategies, affect response.

KEY CONCEPTS

- Response to a stressor depends on its magnitude and the meaning the stressor has for an individual. Stressors may be perceived as more or less stressful. Perception depends on genetic constitution, past experiences and conditioning, and cultural influences. Stressors may be external or from within. They may be physical, chemical, biological, sociocultural, or psychological.
- Stressors may be perceived differently at different times, and individuals may be more vulnerable to effects of stressors at certain times. The stage of development, circadian rhythms, and the effects of other previous or concurrent stressors all contribute to the stress response.

Coping and Adaptation

Coping is a term used in lay as well as professional language. It is common to hear statements like, "He's coping so well with the death of his wife. He arranged the entire funeral and the care of his three children and he returned to work the day after the funeral." Or: "Margie just fell apart after her baby died. She didn't want to see anyone and cried for days. It's a month now and she hasn't returned to work. I think she should see someone who can help her cope better."

While in Western cultures there is a fascination with the bizarre, with natural disasters, and with violence, and an outpouring of generosity and depersonalized caring toward the victims, there is also a general avoidance of painful reality and a reluctance to personally share another person's burden or pain. This reluctance is manifested in statements idealizing nonemotional or highly controlled emotional reactions in behavioral responses to life events and stressful situations. Although the above lay expressions sound suspiciously close to professional psychiatric definitions of *denial*, **coping** is actually the biopsychosocial process of *thinking and functioning appropriately and effectively, as culturally defined, in a stressful situation in order to withstand the stressful situation or the stress generated by the situation.*[50]

In some societies, the display of emotions associated with momentous life events is valued and expected. For example, among orthodox Jews, wailing as an expression of mourning is an appropriate response to the death of a loved one during the first 24 hours after death. In this instance, the outpouring of emotion is an effort to withstand the pain—the internal stress—of the loss. The expression of pain is accepted, and the grieving person is nurtured and protected during this period of time. In Western cultures, coping is often viewed as the ability to carry on with the activities of daily living without a display of emotional reactions during and after stressful life events. Coping implies *standing firm* and is demonstrated in (1) ability to communicate emotions verbally and nonverbally, (2) ability to control emotions, (3) verbal demonstration of ability to perceive reality, (4) verbal demonstration of ability to think logically and to participate in problem-solving activities, and (5) ability to cooperate with others in carrying out desired activities.[51] Figure 7–13 depicts a family coping with the illness of a loved one. Note the controlled emotion and the staunchness expressed by the affected individual.

Coping responses are elicited by internal or external stressors. Lazarus' empirically based, *cognitive appraisal theory* of coping is perhaps the most widely accepted and widely tested of all the coping theories

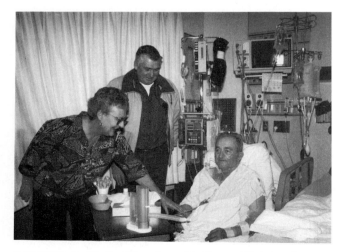

F I G U R E   7 – 13. Family coping with illness. (Photograph courtesy of St. Elizabeth Medical Center, Yakima, WA.)

in the latter half of the twentieth century. Unlike those who acknowledged the importance of threat appraisal but focused on emotion as a driving force, Lazarus focused on the role of cognitive appraisal in the stress-coping-adaptation sequence. Lazarus proposed that an event or potential stressor could be viewed as a challenge, a threat, or a benign (nonchallenging, nonthreatening) event. In his earlier formulations, he proposed that coping responses were provoked only by events perceived to be threatening. He described two types of coping strategies: *problem-focused strategies* and *emotion-focused strategies.* The goal of problem-focused strategies was the resolution of the problem or the stressful situation, whereas the goal of emotion-focused strategies was to reduce the painful emotion associated with the stressful situation. He gave primacy to the importance of problem-focused strategies and suggested that emotion-focused strategies were immature responses at best, and dysfunctional.[12] However, in his more recent theorizing, Lazarus gave increased emphasis to the role of emotions in the stress-coping-adaptation sequence and credited Janis' insightful work as a major contribution to understanding the phenomenon of coping.[52]

The terms "coping" and "adapting" are often used interchangeably. Coping and adaptation are two, almost inseparable processes that are integral parts of life. However, while coping implies standing firm, *adapting* implies changing. **Adapting** is defined as the "biopsychosocial process of changing to become suited to a new or changed situation."[50] Change in itself is potentially stressful and capable of provoking a stress reaction.[53] Proponents of life events theories assert that life events (also referred to as life changes and life crises) are stressful events or stressors provoking a stress reaction.[9] It is proposed that *pleasant* life events such as marriage, the birth of an anticipated child, a desired geographic move, and a job promotion, as well as *unpleasant* events such as the death of a loved one, both require adaptive responses that provoke a stress reaction, regardless of a person's cultural orientation.[10] Adaptation, by definition, is a potentially stressful event. When a person encounters a favorable or an unfavorable life event requiring a personal change or adaptation, the person is confronted by external (situational) and internal (adaptive) changes—both of which may generate a stress reaction.

Sequence of Stress-Adaptation-Coping Events

Coping responses can be elicited by (1) an external life event, (2) internal stress generated by an external event or situation perceived as threatening, or (3) the process of adapting to an external situation requiring change. It thus appears that any event may be perceived as an actual or potential threat or challenge. Mental mechanisms, beliefs, values, and expectations alter a person's perception of the event and provoke a reaction (thoughts and feelings). Typical reactions include feelings of fear-anxiety-anger, helplessness-hopelessness, or optimism. The reaction in turn provokes coping strategies (behavioral responses) aimed at dealing with the event (problem-focused) or dealing with the feelings provoked by the event (emotion-focused). The potential outcomes include (1) resolution of the stressful situation, and (2) continuation or exacerbation of the stressful situation or the stress generated by the situation, culminating, eventually, in death.[12,50–52]

A coping strategy is *functional* if it helps resolve either the situation or the feelings. A coping strategy is *ineffective* or *dysfunctional* if it does not achieve the desired goal. A coping strategy achieving a goal other than the intended goal is also known as *dysfunctional coping*.

KEY CONCEPTS

- **Coping is the biopsychosocial process of thinking and functioning appropriately, as culturally defined, in a stressful situation. In Western cultures, coping is usually viewed as the ability to carry on normal activities without excessive emotional reactions.**
- **Two types of coping strategies are (1) problem-focused strategies, in which the goal is to resolve the problem, and (2) emotion-focused strategies, in which the goal is to reduce emotional pain. A coping strategy is considered functional if it helps resolve the situation or the feelings.**
- **Adapting is the biopsychosocial process of changing to become suited to a new or changed situation. Changing situations or life events are potential stressors that may provoke a stress response. Any event may be an actual or potential stressor.**

Summary

Stress and related concepts can be traced as far back as written science and medicine. Physiologic mechanisms for coping with adversity have not evolved appreciably over the past several thousand years despite increased societal complexity. As living in a society becomes more demanding, the level of stress increases. The *choices* that individuals must make in order to survive in a society are more numerous and more critical.

The physiologic responses to social pressures, information overload, and rapid change resemble those set into motion during physical danger and outright threats to survival. The stress system coordinates the generalized stress response, which takes place when a stressor of any kind exceeds a threshold.

Recent technological advances have permitted understanding of some of the neurophysiologic and biochemical events that promote successful coping and adaptation to stressful situations, as well as identification of illnesses that occur as a result of, or associated with, dysregulation of the stress response. There has been an exponential increase in knowledge regarding the interaction among components of the stress system and between the stress system and other brain elements involved in the coping response regulating emotion, cognitive function, and behavior, as well as between the neuraxes responsible for reproduction, growth, and immunity.

REFERENCES

1. Clendening L: *Sourcebook of Medical History.* New York, Dover Publications, 1942.
2. Cannon WB: Stress and strains of homeostasis. *Am J Med Sci* 1935;189:1–14.
3. Cannon WB: The Influence of Emotional States on the Function of the Alimentary Canal. *Am J Med Sci* 1909;480–487.
4. Selye H: The general adaptation syndrome and the diseases of adaptation. *J Clin Endocrinol* 1946;6:117–230.
5. Selye H: *The Stress of Life,* 2nd ed. New York, McGraw-Hill, 1976.
6. Roy C, Roberts SL: *Theory Construction in Nursing: An Adaptation Model.* Englewood Cliffs, NJ, Prentice-Hall, 1981.
7. Roy C, Andrews HA: *The Roy Adaptation Model: The Definitive Statement.* Norwalk, CT, Appleton & Lange, 1991.
8. Lindsay AM, Carrieri VK: Stress response, in Lindsay AM, Carrieri VK, West CM (eds): *Pathophysiological Phenomena in Nursing: Human Responses to Illness.* Philadelphia, WB Saunders, 1986.
9. Holmes TH, Rahe RH: The social readjustment rating scale. *J Psychosom Res* 1967;11:213–218.
10. Rahe RH: Life-change measurement as a predictor of illness. *Proc R Soc Med* 1968;61:1124–1128.
11. Mason JW: A reevaluation of the concept of non-specificity in stress theory. *J Psychiatr Res* 1971;8:1977–1981.
12. Lazarus RS: Psychological stress and coping in adaptation and illness, in Lipowski ZJ, Lipsih DR, Whybrow PC (eds): *Psychosomatic Medicine: Current Trends and Clinical Applications.* New York, Oxford University Press, 1977.
13. Rose RN: Psychoendocrinology, in Wilson JD, Foster GW (eds): *Williams Textbook of Endocrinology,* 7th ed. Philadelphia, WB Saunders, 1985.
14. Guyton AC: *Textbook of Medical Physiology,* 8th ed. Philadelphia, WB Saunders, 1991.
15. Makara GB, Palkovits M, Szentagothai J: The endocrine hypothalamus and the hormonal response to stress, in Selye H (ed): *Selye's Guide to Stress Research.* New York, Van Nostrand Reinhold Co, 1980, vol 1.
16. Livnat S, Felten SY, Carlson SL, Bellinger DL, Felten DL: Involvement of peripheral and central catecholamine systems in neural-immune interactions. *J Neuroimmunol* 1985;10:5.
17. Williams RH: *Textbook of Endocrinology.* Philadelphia, WB Saunders, 1985.
18. Frederickson R, Hendrie HC, Hingtgen JN, Aprison MH: *Neuroregulation of Autonomic, Endocrine, and Immune Systems.* Boston, Martinus Nijhoff, 1986.
19. Reiser MF: *Mind, Brain, Body.* New York, Basic Books, 1984.
20. Granner DK: Hormones of the adrenal medulla, in Murray RK, et al (eds): *Harper's Biochemistry,* 21st ed. Norwalk, CT, Appleton & Lange, 1988.
21. Lee SW, Tsou A-P, Chan H, Thomas J, Petrie K, Eugui EM, Allison AC: Glucocorticoids selectively inhibit the transcription of the interleukin 1-beta gene and decrease the stability of interleukin 1-beta mRNA. *Proc Natl Acad Sci USA* 1988;85:1204.
22. Fauci AS, Dale DC: The effect of in vitro hydrocortisone on subpopulations of human lymphocytes. *J Clin Invest* 1974;53:240–246.
23. Fauci AS: Corticosteroids and circulating lymphocytes. *Transplant Proc* 1975;7:37–48.
24. Grayson J, Dooley NJ, Koski IR, Blaese RM: Immunoglobulin production induced in vitro by glucocorticoid hormones: T-cell dependent stimulation of immunoglobulin production without B-cell proliferation in cultures of human peripheral lymphocytes. *J Clin Invest* 1981;68:1538–1547.
25. Berne RM, Levy MN: *Physiology,* 2nd ed. St. Louis, CV Mosby, 1988.

26. Thibodeau GA, Patton KT: *Anatomy and Physiology*, 2nd ed. St. Louis, Mosby–Year Book, 1993, pp 571–573.
27. Schalach DS: The influence of physical stress and exercise on growth hormone and insulin secretion in man. *J Clin Endocrinol Metabol* 1967;69:256–269.
28. Vander AJ, Luciano DS: *Human Physiology: The Mechanisms of Body Function*, 5th ed. New York, McGraw-Hill, 1990.
29. Shiu RPC, Friesen HG: Mechanisms of action of prolactin in the control of mammary gland function. *Annu Rev Physiol* 1980;42:83–96.
30. Noel GL, Suih HK, Stone JG, Frantz AG: Human prolactin and growth hormone release during surgery and other conditions of stress. *J Clin Endocrinol Metabol* 1972;35:840–851.
31. Aakvaag A, Bentdal O, Quigstad K, Walstad P, Rohnningen H, Fonnum F: Testosterone and testosterone-binding globulin (TcBG) in young men during prolonged stress. *Int J Androl* 1978;I:22–31.
32. Jungkunz G, Engel RR, King UG, Kuss HJ: Endogenous opiates increase pain tolerance after stress in humans. *Psychiatry Res* 1983;8:13–18.
33. Plotnikoff NP, Faith RE, Murgo AJ, Good RA: *Enkephalins and Endorphins: Stress and the Immune System*. New York, Plenum Press, 1986.
34. Ader R: *Psychoneuroimmunology*. Orlando, Fla, Academic Press, 1981.
35. Cohen MR, Pickar D, Dubois M, Bunney WE Jr: Stress-induced plasma beta-endorphin immunoreactivity may predict postoperative morphine usage. *Psychiatry Res* 1982;6:7–12.
36. Colt EWD, Wardlow SL, Franz AG: The effect of running on plasma beta-endorphin. *Life Sci* 1981;28:1637–1640.
37. Bullock K: Neuroanatomy of lymphoid tissue: A review, in Guillemin R, Cohen M (eds): *Neural Modulation of Immunity*. New York, Raven Press, 1985.
38. Pruett SB, Ensley DK, Crittenen TL: The role of chemical-induced stress responses in immunosuppression: A review of quantitative associations and cause-effect relationships between chemical-induced stress responses and immunosuppression. *J Toxicol Environ Health* 1993;39(2):163–192.
39. Carr DJ, Weigent DA, Blalock JE: Hormones common to the neuroendocrine and immune systems. *Drug Des Deliv* 1989;4(3):187–197.
40. Eskay RL, Grino M, Chen HT: Interleukins, signal transduction, and the immune system-mediated stress response. *Adv Exp Med Biol* 1990;274:332–343.
41. Weigent DA, Carr DJ, Blalock JE: Bidirectional communication between the neuroendocrine and immune systems: Common hormones and hormone receptors. *Ann NY Acad Sci* 1990;579:17–27.
42. Guillemin R, Cohn M, Melnechuk T: *Neural Modulation of Immunity*. New York, Raven Press, 1985.
43. Khansari DN, Murgo AJ, Faith RE: Effect of stress on the immune system. *Immunol Today* 1990;11(5):170–175.
44. Hall NR, McGillis JP: Evidence that thymosins and other biological response modifiers can function as neuroactive immunotransmitters. *J Immunol* 1985;135(2 suppl):806s–811s.
45. Fox BH, Newberry BH: *Impacts of Psychoendocrine Systems in Cancer and Immunity*. Lewiston, NY, CJ Hogrefe, 1984.
46. Bonneau RH, Kiecolt-Glaser JK, Glaser R: Stress-induced modulation of the immune response. *Ann NY Acad Sci* 1990;594:253–269.
47. Biondi M, Kotzalidis GD: Human psychoneuroimmunology today. *J Clin Lab Anal* 1990;4:22–38.
48. Cooper EL: *Stress, Immunity, and Aging*. New York, Marcel Dekker, New York, 1984.
49. Bieliaukas LA: *Stress and Its Relationship to Health and Illness*. Boulder, Colo, Westview Press, 1982.
50. Pranulis MS: Coping with an acute myocardial infarction, in Gentry WD, Williams RB (eds): *Psychological Aspects of Myocardial Infarction and Coronary Care*. St. Louis, CV Mosby, 1975.
51. Folkman S: Personal control and stress and coping processes: A theoretical analysis. *J Pers Soc Psychol* 1984;46:839–852.
52. Lazarus RS, Folkman S: *Stress, Appraisal, and Coping*. New York, Springer, 1984.
53. Aldrich CK, Mendkoff E: Relocation of the aged and disabled: A mortality study. *J Am Geriatr Soc* 1963;II:185–194.

BIBLIOGRAPHY

Antonovsky A: *Health, Stress, and Coping*. San Francisco, Jossey-Bass, 1979.

Biondi M, Kotzalidis GD: Human psychoneuroimmunology today. *J Clin Lab Anal* 1990;4:22–38.

Bonneau RH, Kiecolt-Glaser JK, Glaser R: Stress-induced modulation of the immune response. *Ann NY Acad Sci* 1990;594:253–269.

Cannon WB: *The Wisdom of the Body*. New York, WW Norton, 1963.

French JRP, Rodgers W, Cobb S: Adjustment as person-environment fit, in Coehlo GV, Hamburg DA, Adams JE (eds): *Coping and Adaptation*. New York, Basic Books, 1974.

Krueger E, Krueger GR: How does the subjective experience of stress relate to the breakdown of the human immune system? *In Vivo* 1991;5:207–215.

La Via MF, Workman EA: Psychoneuroimmunology: Where are we, where are we going? *Recent Prog Med* 1991;82:637–641.

Lyon ML: Psychoneuroimmunology: The problem of situatedness of illness and the conceptualization of healing. *Cult Med Psychiatry* 1993;17:77–97.

Mason JW: Organization of psychoendocrine mechanisms: A review and reconsideration of research, in Greenfield NS, Steinbach R (eds): *Handbook of Psychophysiology*. New York, Holt, Rinehart & Winston, 1972, pp 3–91.

Mason JW: Specificity in the organization of neuroendocrine response profiles, in Seeman P, Brown G (eds): *Frontiers in Neurology and Neuroscience Research*. Toronto, University of Toronto Press, 1974.

Mason JW: An historical review of the stress field. *J Hum Stress* 1975;1:6–12.

Mason JW, Brady JV: Plasma 17-hydroxycortico-steroid changes related to reserpine effects on emotional behaviors. *Science* 1956;124:983–984.

Selye H: Perspectives in stress research. *Perspect Biol Med* 1959;2:403–416.

Selye H: Confusion and controversy in the stress field. *J Hum Stress* 1975;1:38–44.

Stein M: Stress, depression, and the immune system. *J Clin Psychiatry* 1989;50:35–40.

Vollhardt LT: Psychoneuroimmunology: A literature review. *Am J Orthopsychiatry* 1991;6:35–47.

Wolf S, Goodell H: *Stress and Disease*. Springfield, Ill, Charles C Thomas, 1956.

CHAPTER 8
Infectious Processes

FAITH YOUNG PETERSON and MARK PUHLMAN

Normal Microbial Flora

Types of Microorganisms
Bacteria
Viruses
Fungi
Parasites

Host–Parasite Relationship
Microorganism Factors
Environmental Factors
Host Defense System
   Mechanical Epithelial Barriers
   Biochemical Epithelial Barriers

Manifestations of Infection
Phagocytosis
Interferons
Fever
Specific Immune Response

Host Factors That Decrease Resistance to Infection
Nutrition
Chronic Illness
Acute Illness
Age
Stress
Immunocompromised Host

Summary

KEY TERMS

bacteria: Tiny, primitive cells that lack nuclei. Bacteria cause infection by parasitizing tissues or otherwise disrupting normal function.

fungi: Simple organisms similar to plants that lack the chlorophyll pigments necessary to make their own food. Fungi become parasites of other tissues, including those of the human body, since they cannot produce their own food.

infection: The state or condition in which the body is invaded by a pathogen that, under favorable conditions, multiplies and produces injurious effects. Localized infection is usually accompanied by inflammation, but inflammation may occur without infection.

infectious disease: Disease caused by a variety of organisms including bacteria, fungi, viruses, and helminths (parasitic worms); transferred by environmental contagion, nosocomial organisms (acquired during hospitalization), and/or endogenous microflora present in the nose and throat, skin, or bowel.

pathogen: An organism capable of causing disease.

protozoa: Protists, or one-celled organisms larger than bacteria, differentiated by DNA organized into a nucleus. Many types of protozoan parasites are found in human tissue.

virus: Intracellular parasite that consists of a DNA or RNA core surrounded by a protein coat and, sometimes, a lipoprotein envelope. Viruses act by invading human cells and causing the production of viral components.

*I*nfection is the cause of death for many people afflicted with a chronic or critical illness. The very young and the very old are particularly susceptible to infections. Infections are caused by microorganisms that gain entry into the body. Once a microorganism adheres to or invades the human body, the signs and symptoms generally associated with infection are generated. The microorganisms that cause infection and disease are called **pathogens.** The major types of microorganisms that can cause infections include bacteria, viruses, fungi, and parasites.

Many hospitalized patients are at risk for the development of **sepsis,** an overwhelming infection that may lead to multiple organ failure, irreversible hypotension, and death.[1] Health care professionals play a vital role in the prevention, early detection, and treatment of infections.

This chapter presents materials on infectious agents, the host–parasite relationship, and the human host's defense system. The factors that may interfere with the body's ability to defend itself from infection and the clinical manifestations of infection will also be discussed, with an emphasis on the identification of risk factors for infection.

Normal Microbial Flora

The interactions between a host, such as a human, and the microorganisms that reside on or in the host are referred to as the **host–parasite relationship.** Large numbers of microorganisms reside on the skin and in the gastrointestinal (GI) tract and vagina of the human host. These microbes normally cause no harm to the host. They are parasites that depend on the host's environment—temperature, moisture, nutrients, and other parasites. They obtain nutrients from the host to grow and reproduce. The host and normal parasite flora usually balance their interactions to the benefit of each in order to grow and survive—a *symbiotic relationship.*

Interestingly, these bacteria have a role in protecting the host from other pathogens by using nutrients and thus preventing other microbial colonization.[2] Normal bacterial flora also participate in metabolic processes such as the synthesis of vitamin K in the colon.[3] Harmless inhabitation of the skin or mucous membranes by these microorganisms is called *colonization.*

Resident flora are usually of a specific type and occupy a certain environment in or on the host. These flora will recolonize quickly if disturbed. For example, normal resident flora of the skin include bacteria such as *Corynebacterium, Staphylococcus epidermidis, Streptococcus viridans,* as well as fungi, yeasts, and even mycobacteria.[4] Transient flora are microorganisms that can be either harmless or potentially harmful. They reside temporarily in or on the host but do not establish permanent residency. For example, antibiotic therapy can disrupt the balance of normal bacterial

flora leading to a secondary infection by a fungus. Antibiotic therapy can also kill vitamin K–producing bacteria in the intestines. This causes a vitamin K deficiency that leads to an increased risk of bleeding.

Normal flora can become pathogenic if they gain entry into the body when the immune system is compromised. These infections are referred to as *opportunistic.* An increased number of people are at risk for opportunistic infections due to diseases of the immune system and therapies that depress the immune system.

When a microorganism is capable of consistently causing disease in all infected hosts, the organism is considered to be *virulent.* As summarized by Bellanti, "Virulence thus represents the interaction between the properties of the host and the pathogen that permits expression of the pathogenic properties of a parasite to the detriment of the host."[5]

KEY CONCEPTS

- A number of microorganisms are considered resident flora because they live on or in the host without causing disease. Resident flora benefit the host by synthesizing molecules and inhibiting the growth of nonresident microorganisms.
- If the host's immune system is compromised, resident flora may become pathogenic, resulting in opportunistic infection.

Types of Microorganisms

Bacteria

Bacteria are single-celled, procaryotic organisms. They live in the intestines of humans and other creatures and are required for digestion. They live in the soil and are responsible for its fertility. They degrade dead tissue, breaking it down for other organisms to use. Among the countless types of bacteria that exist, only a small percentage are known to be harmful to humans.

Bacteria are classified into four major groups based on their cell wall shape and mechanism of movement: *gliding bacteria* (e.g., myxobacteria), *spirochetes* (e.g., *Treponema pallidum*), *mycoplasmas* (e.g., *Mycoplasma pneumoniae*), and *rigid bacteria.* The rigid bacteria are further broken down into actinomycetes (e.g., *Mycobacterium tuberculosis*) and unicellular forms.

The unicellular forms of rigid bacteria include *intracellular obligate parasites* and *free-living bacteria.* The intracellular obligate parasites consist of *rickettsiae* and *chlamydiae.* Intracellular obligate parasites must live within a host cell to survive.

Free-living bacteria are classified into three basic shapes. *Cocci* are round and nonmotile. They may stick together in clumps that look like bunches of grapes (e.g., staphylococcus), in twos (e.g., diplococcus), or in long strands (e.g., streptococcus). *Bacilli,* by comparison, are rod-shaped and may be motile (e.g., *Pseudomonas aeruginosa*). About half of the species are motile and half are nonmotile. The third shape is the *spiral* (e.g., *Spirillum*).

Bacteria are further differentiated by their ability or inability to retain a basic dye after iodine fixation, known as the *Gram stain reaction*. The *Gram stain* separates bacteria into gram-positive organisms, which look dark purple under the microscope, gram-negative organisms, which look pink, or acid-fast organisms, which resist staining but, once stained, resist decoloration.[4] Further differentiation of bacteria is based on nutritional requirements, such as whether or not the organism is aerobic or anaerobic, colony characteristics, and antibiotic resistance.

Pathogenic bacteria owe the ability to infect humans to their structure and proteins. For example, pili enhance certain bacteria's capacity to adhere to the host's surface, improving the bacteria's virulence. Other bacteria have mucopolysaccharide layers or enzymes that facilitate their invasiveness. Figure 8–1 classifies examples of pathogenic bacteria according to the part of the human body that they commonly infect.

EYES
- *Chlamydia trachomatis*
- *Streptococcus pneumoniae*
- *Staphylococcus aureus*
- *Neisseria gonorrhoeae*

THROAT
- *Corynebacterium diptheriae*
- *Streptococcus pyogenes*
- *Bordetella pertussis*

LUNGS
- *Mycoplasma pneumoniae*
- *Legionella pneumophila*
- *Streptococcus pneumoniae*
- *Hemophilus influenzae*
- *Mycobacterium tuberculosis*

LIVER
- *Clostridium*
- *Enterococci*
- Gram-negative *bacilli*

INTESTINES
- *Clostridium difficile*
- *Clostridium perfringens*
- *Salmonella*
- *Shigellae*

VAGINA AND UTERUS
- *Neisseria gonorrhoeae*
- *Chlamydia trachomatis*
- Gram-negative *bacilli*

SKIN
- *Staphylococcus aureus*
- *Streptococcus pyogenes*

BRAIN AND MENINGES
- *Hemophilus influenzae*
- *Neisseria meningitidis*
- *Streptococcus pneumoniae*

EAR
- *Streptococcus pneumoniae*
- *Hemophilus influenzae*
- Gram-negative enteric *bacilli*

HEART
- *Streptococci viridans*
- *Staphylococcus aureus*
- *Enterococci*

KIDNEY
- Gram-negative *bacilli*
- *Escherichia coli*

PROSTATE AND TESTES
- Gram-negative *bacilli*
- *Neisseria gonorrhoeae*

URETHRA
- *Neisseria gonorrhoeae*
- *Chlamydia trachomatis*
- Gram-negative enteric *bacilli*

BONE
- *Staphylococcus aureus*
- Gram-negative enteric *bacilli*
- *Mycobacterium tuberculosis*

JOINTS
- *Staphylococcus aureus*
- *Neisseria gonorrhoeae*
- *Streptococcus pyogenes*

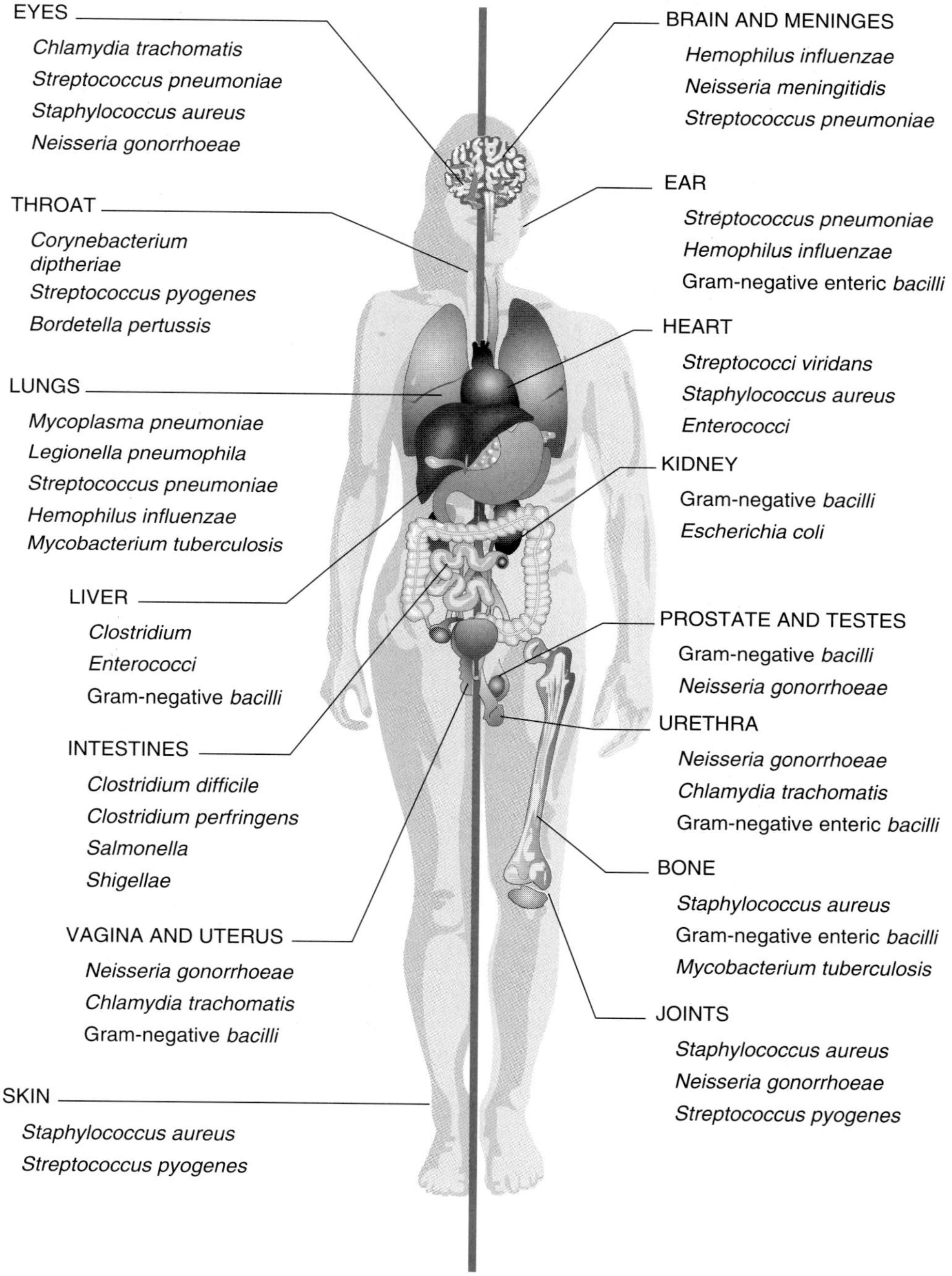

FIGURE 8–1. Examples of pathogenic bacteria classified according to the part of the human body that they commonly infect.

Table 8–1 summarizes primary pathogens associated with specific infections in the human host. Table 8–2 summarizes antimicrobial selection based on the infecting organism.

Viruses

Viruses are tiny genetic parasites, ranging in size from 20 to 300 nanometers (nm).[4] They are composed of genetic DNA or RNA and a capsule surrounding the genetic material. Viruses have only enough genetic information to code for two to 60 proteins. Viruses are totally dependent on the host cell for energy and the "machinery" to replicate themselves. A comparison of viruses and other microorganisms is contained in Table 8–3.

Viruses were once differentiated only by size. With advances in genetic mapping and the use of the electron microscope, viruses can now be classified by the genetic makeup of the organism, the mode of replication, and the structure of the viral capsule, also known as the *capsid*.

All viruses must enter a host cell in order to survive. A virus invades a host cell by several methods. A virus can adhere to the cell membrane, causing phagocytosis. Once inside the host cell, the virus capsule is removed, exposing viral genetic material to the cell's interior. Another way a virus can invade a host cell is by sticking to the surface of the host cell and

TABLE 8–1. Examples of Primary Pathogens Associated With Specific Infections

Burns	Paranasal and Middle Ear	Pleura	Urethra
Staphylococcus aureus *Streptococcus pyogenes* (Group A) *Pseudomonas aeruginosa* Gram-negative bacilli	*Streptococcus pneumoniae* *Streptococcus pyogenes* (Group A) *Hemophilus influenzae* Gram-negative enteric bacilli *Pseudomonas aeruginosa* Anaerobic streptococci *Staphylococcus aureus*	*Staphylococcus aureus* *Streptococcus pneumoniae* *Hemophilus influenzae* Gram-negative bacilli Anaerobic streptococci *Bacteroides* spp. *Fusobacterium* *Streptococcus pyogenes* (Group A) *Mycobacterium tuberculosis*	*Neisseria gonorrhoeae* *Chlamydia trachomatis* *Trichomonas vaginalis* Gram-negative enteric bacilli *Ureaplasma urealyticum*
Skin Infections	**Throat**		**Prostate**
Staphylococcus aureus *Streptococcus pyogenes* (Group A) Gram-negative bacilli *Treponema pallidum*	*Streptococcus pyogenes* (Group A) *Neisseria gonorrhoeae* *Bacteroides* spp. *Fusobacterium* Spirochetes *Corynebacterium diphtheria* *Bordetella pertussis*	**Endocardium** *Viridans* group of streptococci *Staphylococcus aureus* Enterococci Other streptococci *Staphylococcus epidermidis* Gram-negative enteric bacilli *Pseudomonas aeruginosa*	Gram-negative enteric bacilli *Neisseria gonorrhoeae* *Staphylococcus aureus*
Decubitus and Surgical Wounds			**Epididymis and Testes**
Staphylococcus aureus Gram-negative enteric bacilli *Pseudomonas aeruginosa* *Streptococcus pyogenes* (Group A) Anaerobic streptococci *Clostridium* spp. Enterococci *Bacteroides* spp.	**Lungs** *Mycoplasma pneumoniae* *Streptococcus pneumoniae* *Hemophilus influenzae* *Staphylococcus aureus* *Klebsiella* *Pseudomonas aeruginosa* Gram-negative bacilli *Streptococcus pyogenes* (Group A) *Mycobacterium tuberculosis* *Chlamydia psittaci* *Legionella pneumophila* Anaerobic streptococci *Bacteroides* spp. *Coxiella burnetii*	**Peritoneum** *Escherichia coli* Gram-negative bacilli Enterococci *Bacteroides fragilis* Anaerobic streptococci *Clostridium* spp. *Streptococcus pneumoniae* *Streptococcus pyogenes* (Group A) *Neisseria gonorrhoeae* *Mycobacterium tuberculosis*	Gram-negative bacilli *Neisseria gonorrhoeae* *Chlamydia trachomatis* *Mycobacterium tuberculosis*
Meninges			**Bone (Osteomyelitis)** *Staphylococcus aureus* *Salmonella* Gram-negative enteric bacilli *Streptococcus pyogenes* (Group A) *Mycobacterium tuberculosis* Anaerobic streptococci *Pseudomonas aeruginosa*
Neisseria meningitidis *Hemophilus influenzae* *Streptococcus pneumoniae* *Streptococcus* spp. *Escherichia coli* Gram-negative bacilli *Streptococcus pyogenes* (Group A) *Staphylococcus aureus* *Mycobacterium tuberculosis* *Listeria monocytogenes* Enterococci (neonatal period) *Treponema pallidum* *Leptospira*	**Lung Abscess** Anaerobic streptococci *Bacteroides* spp. *Fusobacterium* *Staphylococcus aureus* *Klebsiella* Gram-negative bacilli *Streptococcus pneumoniae* *Enterococcus*	**Biliary Tract** *Escherichia coli* Gram-negative bacilli *Enterococcus* spp. *Staphylococcus aureus* *Clostridium* spp. Streptococci (aerobic and anaerobic)	**Joints** *Staphylococcus aureus* *Neisseria gonorrhoeae* *Streptococcus pyogenes* (Group A) Gram-negative enteric bacilli *Pseudomonas aeruginosa* *Streptococcus pneumoniae* *Neisseria meningitidis* *Hemophilus influenzae* (in children) *Mycobacterium tuberculosis*
Brain Abscess		**Kidney and Bladder**	
Streptococci (aerobic and anaerobic) *Bacteroides* spp. *Staphylococcus aureus*		*Escherichia coli* Gram-negative bacilli *Staphylococcus aureus* *Staphylococcus epidermidis* *Mycobacterium tuberculosis*	

Data from Woodley M, Whelan A: *Manual of Medical Therapeutics*, 27th ed. St. Louis, MO, Department of Medicine, Washington University School of Medicine, 1993.

TABLE 8–2. Antimicrobial Selection Based on Organisms

Organism	Drug of Choice
I. Gram-Positive Cocci	
Staphylococcus aureus	
Non-penicillinase-producing	Penicillin G or V (oral)
	Cephalosporin
Penicillinase-producing	A-penicillinase-resistant penicillin
	Cephalosporin
Methicillin-resistant	Vancomycin
Streptococcus	
Groups A, C, G	Penicillin G or V (oral)
	Cephalosporin
Group B	Penicillin G or ampicillin
	Cephalosporin
Streptococcus viridans	Penicillin G + aminoglycoside
Streptococcus, anaerobic	Penicillin G
	Clindamycin
	Cephalosporin
Enterococcus	Ampicillin, amoxicillin, penicillin G, or vancomycin, + aminoglycoside
Pneumococcus	Penicillin G or V (oral)
II. Gram-Negative Cocci	
Neisseria meningitidis	
Meningitis or bacteremia	Penicillin G
	Chloramphenicol
Neisseria gonorrhoeae	Penicillin G
Genital	Ampicillin
	Tetracycline
III. Gram-Positive Bacilli	
Bacillus anthracis	Penicillin G
	Erythromycin
Listeria monocytogenes	Ampicillin + aminoglycoside
	Tetracycline
Clostridium tetani	Penicillin G
	Cephalosporin
Clostridium perfringens	Penicillin G
	Cephalosporin
Corynebacterium diphtheriae	Erythromycin
	Penicillin G
IV. Gram-Negative Bacilli	
Escherichia coli	Aminoglycoside
	Cephalosporin
Klebsiella pneumoniae	Aminoglycoside
	Cephalosporin
Enterobacter	Aminoglycoside
	Cephalosporin
Legionella pneumophila	Erythromycin
	Tetracycline
	Rifampin
Serratia	Aminoglycoside
	Trimethoprim-sulfamethoxazole (TMP-SMX)
Proteus mirabilis	Ampicillin
	Cephalosporin
	Aminoglycoside
Proteus vulgaris	Aminoglycoside
	Chloramphenicol
Pseudomonas	
aeruginosa	Aminoglycoside + ticarcillin, piperacillin, or aziocillin
pseudomallei	TMP-SMX
cepacia	TMP-SMX
Bacteroides (except *B. fragilis*)	Penicillin
	Chloramphenicol

TABLE 8–2. Antimicrobial Selection Based on Organisms *Continued*

Organism	Drug of Choice
Salmonella	Chloramphenicol
	Ampicillin
	TMP-SMX
Shigella	TMP-SMX
	Chloramphenicol
Hemophilus influenzae	Chloramphenicol
Meningitis, epiglottitis	Ampicillin
Other sites	Ampicillin, TMP-SMX
Bordetella pertussis	Erythromycin
	TMP-SMX
Brucella	Tetracycline + streptomycin
Acinetobacter	Aminoglycoside
	Minocycline
Francisella tularensis	Streptomycin
Yersinia pestis	Streptomycin
Vibrio cholerae	Tetracycline
	TMP-SMX
V. Spirochetes	
Treponema	
pallidum	Penicillin G
	Tetracycline
pertenue	Penicillin G
	Tetracycline
Leptospira	Penicillin G
	Tetracycline
Borrelia recurrentis	Tetracycline
	Penicillin
VI. Acid-Fast Bacilli	
Mycobacterium tuberculosis	Isoniazid (INH) + rifampin, INH + Ethambutol
Mycobacterium leprae	Dapsone + rifampin, clofazimine
VII. *Chlamydia*	
psittaci	Tetracycline
	Erythromycin
trachomatis	Tetracycline
	Erythromycin
VIII. *Mycoplasma pneumoniae*	Tetracycline
	Erythromycin
IX. *Rickettsia*	Tetracycline
	Chloramphenicol

Data from Harvey AM, Johns RJ, McKusick VA et al: *The Principles and Practice of Medicine*, 22nd ed. Norwalk, CT, Appleton & Lange, 1988, and from Jawetz E, Melnick JL, Adelberg EA: *Review of Medical Microbiology*, 17th ed. Norwalk, CT, Appleton & Lange, 1987.

injecting viral genetic material directly into the interior of the host cell.

Some viruses manufacture an *envelope* that surrounds the viral capsid. The envelope is made of host cell proteins. The virus may be released from the host cells by budding from the cell's surface without destroying the host cell (Fig. 8–2).

Viruses that do not manufacture an envelope are usually released by *lysing* the host cell, thus destroying it. The mechanism of lysis seems to be a progressive breakdown of the host cell's maintenance mechanisms with resultant buildup of waste products intracellularly and lack of nutrient transport into the cell. Ultimately the cell wall is disrupted and the cell lyses.

Two major categories of viruses exist: those that contain DNA and those that contain RNA. RNA vi-

TABLE 8–3. A Comparison of Viruses and Other Microorganisms

Organism	Grows in Nonliving Media	Contains Both DNA and RNA	Contains Ribosomes (Energy-Producing Organelles)	Sensitive to Antibiotics
Bacteria	Yes	Yes	Yes	Yes
Mycoplasmas	Yes	Yes	Yes	Yes
Rickettsiae	No	Yes	Yes	Yes
Chlamydiae	No	Yes	Yes	Yes
Viruses	No	No	No	No

ruses are characterized as either *retroviruses* or *straight replicating viruses*. In the following paragraphs, the various categories will be discussed.

The *DNA virus* (e.g., herpes simplex virus) produces its messenger RNA in the host cell's nucleus with the host cell's enzymes. The proteins and the DNA of the virus are thus replicated and assembled in the host cell.

RNA viruses (e.g., influenza virus [Fig. 8–3]), by comparison, replicate their genetic information in one of two ways. *Retroviruses* contain encoding information for the enzyme reverse transcriptase, so that they can create both messenger RNA and DNA from their own genome. The viral DNA is incorporated into the host cell's DNA, and when the host cell replicates, the viral DNA also replicates, thus perpetuating the viral genome as long as the host cell line survives. Viral proteins and RNA are manufactured using the virus' messenger RNA and the host cell's organelles. Human immunodeficiency virus (HIV), the retrovirus that causes acquired immunodeficiency syndrome (AIDS), is an example of a virus that causes permanent change in the human genome and function of the host cell. HIV is a retrovirus.

In contrast to RNA retroviruses, the *straight replicating viruses* reproduce in one of two ways, depending on whether the single-stranded RNA is a positive or negative copy. Viruses in which the RNA is single *positive* copy use the strand as a direct template to replicate RNA polymerase, a protein, and a negative RNA copy. The negative copy gives rise to many positive copies that can either be included in reproduced viruses or used as a template for more proteins. The RNA viruses that possess a *negative* copy replicate in a similar manner, except that the genome must be translated to a positive copy before it can replicate proteins and other viruses.

Fungi

Fungi are nonphotosynthetic, eucaryotic protists that are disseminated through the environment. They can reproduce by simply dividing (asexually) or by combining their genetic information before dividing (sexually). Infections caused by fungi are called *mycotic infections*, or *mycoses*.

Certain fungi live as normal flora (e.g., *Candida*) and become bothersome only when they are not kept in check by other body flora or by the immune system

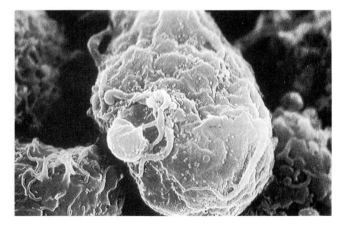

FIGURE 8–2. Scanning electron micrograph of HIV-I–infected T4 lymphocytes. The AIDS virus is budding from the plasma membrane of the lymphocytes. (Courtesy of Centers for Disease Control and Prevention, Atlanta.)

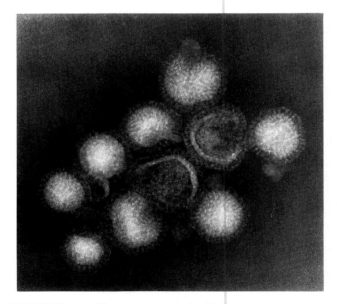

FIGURE 8–3. Electron micrograph of influenza virus, an RNA virus (×150,000). (Courtesy of Dr. F. A. Murphy, Centers for Disease Control and Prevention, Atlanta.)

(*opportunistic fungi*). Examples of opportunistic fungi are *Candida*, Phycomycetes, and *Aspergillus*.

Superficial mycoses, such as that caused by the dermatophytes (e.g., tinea pedis), occur only on superficial, dead, keratinized tissue like hair, epithelium, and nails.[4] In tinea pedis (athlete's foot), infection occurs only in people who wear shoes.

Subcutaneous mycoses occur when fungi are introduced into subcutaneous tissue during trauma. These fungi, when present in the tissues, cause chronic granulomatous disease.[4] An example is *Sporothrix schenckii*. This fungus causes sporotrichosis, which may spread through the lymph system.

Systemic mycoses may occur in both healthy and immunocompromised hosts. Because the fungi causing systemic infections are usually found in the soil, the infections are usually endemic to certain regions where the fungus is found.[4] Infection is caused by inhalation of dust containing the fungus. Because of the endemic nature of these fungi, large segments of the population within the endemic area may have been exposed and infected as children without any symptoms. If symptoms develop, they are usually self-limiting and mild. But for those with altered immune systems, the disease becomes severe and disseminated. Examples of systemic mycoses are histoplasmosis, blastomycosis, and coccidiodomycosis.[4]

To illustrate, *Histoplasma capsulatum* is a fungus that commonly occurs in soils found in the central and eastern United States. *Histoplasma* also occurs in soils rich with chicken feces or bat guano. Humans and animals exposed to dust storms in endemic areas or contaminated with these feces are most likely to be infected. They may also have positive histoplasmin skin tests and may show calcified sites of infection within their lungs.[4]

Conditions that predispose an individual to the potential for an opportunistic fungal infection or to a disseminated pathogenic fungal infection are AIDS, leukemia, cancer chemotherapy, organ transplantation with immune-suppressing therapy, alcoholism, drug abuse, and malnutrition. Opportunistic infections also thrive when the natural flora has been altered with antibiotics or when the environment con-

TABLE 8-4. Fungal Infections

Infection	Distribution	Mode of Transmission	Vector	Symptoms	Primary Site(s)	Secondary Site(s)
Cryptococcosis	Everywhere	Inhalation	Pigeon feces	Fever, cough, weight loss, pleuritic pain, CNS disturbances	Pulmonary system	Meninges, skin, bone
Candidiasis	Normal flora	Ever-present	N/A	Mucocutaneous pain and itching at site of infection	Fungemia, endocarditis	Kidneys, eyes, heart
Phycomycosis (Mucormycosis)	Everywhere	Inhalation, ingestion, wound contamination	Decayed matter, soil	Rhinocerebral mucormycosis: destruction of CN II, IV, V, VI; erosion of carotid artery; meningitis; brain abscess. Pulmonary mucormycosis: dyspnea, chest pain, hemoptysis	Nose, brain, lung	Rare
Histoplasmosis	River valleys (e.g., Mississippi and Ohio) in tropical and temperate zones	Inhalation	Bird and bat feces	Flulike: cough, fever, myalgias, weight loss, anemia, leukopenia, thrombocytopenia, fever, painful oropharyngeal ulcers	Pulmonary system	Bone marrow
Coccidiodomycosis (San Joaquin Valley Fever)	Semi-arid U.S. (e.g., California), southwestern U.S. (Arizona, Nevada)	Inhalation	Dust, dirt	Cough, fever pleuritic chest pain, weight loss, fever, dyspnea, chest pain, CNS disturbances	Pulmonary system	Skin, bone, joints, meninges
Blastomycosis	Southeastern U.S., south central U.S., midwestern U.S., Great Lakes Region	Inhalation	Unknown	Flulike: pleuritic chest pain, arthralgias, erythema nodosum, weight loss, fever, cough, chest pain	Pulmonary system	Skin, bone, joints, male GU tract
Aspergillosis	Everywhere	Inhalation	Decaying vegetation	Dyspnea, chest pain, hemoptysis, wheezing	Pulmonary system	Brain, kidney, liver

tains more nutrients in which the fungi can grow, such as the hyperglycemic bloodstream of a diabetic.

Generally, cultures of fungi are difficult to grow artificially in a laboratory. The most common method of identification is by visualizing their characteristic shapes on a slide of infected tissue.

Drugs used to treat fungal diseases include keto-konazole or amphotericin B. Treatment is usually reversed for disseminated disease, as the local infection is usually self-limited. Treatment is also initiated for those who do not have an intact immune system, such as persons with AIDS. Table 8–4 summarizes important aspects of the most common fungi.

Parasites

Parasites are representatives of four families of the animal kingdom: the Protozoa, or single-celled animals; the Nemathelminthes, or roundworms; the Platyhelminthes, or flatworms; and the Arthropoda, or invertebrate animals with jointed appendages.[4] These parasites live on or in the human body during some part of their life cycle. They depend on their human host for shelter and sustenance. Many parasites have very complicated life cycles that include a larval and adult stage. They rely on particular hosts and vectors to transmit the infection from host to host.

Multiple environmental factors affect the prevalence of parasitic infections: hot and humid climatic conditions; overcrowded living conditions; the presence of insect vectors in bed linen or clothing; improper sewage disposal such as the use of human sewage for fertilizer; the lack of clean water; and the consumption of contaminated raw meat or vegetables. Sexual practices such as unprotected anal intercourse or sexual activity with multiple partners increase the likelihood of transmission of parasites. The nutritional and immune status of the host also have an effect on the symptoms and the aggressiveness of the parasitic infection.

The symptoms of parasitic infection depend on the area in which infestation develops. Protozoan infestation of the GI tract produces cramping, abdominal pain, and bloody diarrhea (amebiasis). Infestation of the blood produces fever, chills, rigor, and later anemia, all of which are associated with malaria (*Plasmodium* infection). Acute pruritus and rash occur in an infection of the skin with *Sarcoptes scabiei* (scabies).

Identification of the infectious agent is usually accomplished by visualizing either the adult parasite or its ova. This can be done by direct observation of the area (inspection of the skin or hair) or by microscopic examination of blood, feces, or tissue samples.

Table 8–5 summarizes various parasitic infections

TABLE 8–5. Parasitic Infections

Parasitic Agent	Common Name of Disease	Location of Infection	Symptoms	Mode of Transmission
Helminths (Worms)				
Nematodes (round-worms)				
Ancylostoma duodenale	Hookworm	Blood vessels of gut	Anemia	Skin penetration
Ascaris lumbricoides	Giant roundworm	Small intestine, lungs	Pneumonitis (rare), intestinal obstruction (rare)	Oral (fecal contamination), auto-infection
Enterobius vermicularis	Pinworm	Cecum	Anal pruritus	Oral
Onchocerca volvulus	River blindness	Skin, eye	Blindness	Insect inoculation
Strongyloides stercoralis	Strongyloidiasis	Small intestine, lungs	Eosinophilia, urticaria, rash, abdominal pain, pneumonitis	Skin penetration, auto-infection
Trichinella spiralis	Trichinosis	Muscles	Muscular pain, eosinophilia, fever, periorbital edema	Oral (infected meat)
Trichuris trichiura	Whipworm	Intestine	Rectal prolapse	Oral (fecal contamination)
Wuchereria bancrofti	Filariasis	Lymphatics	Elephantiasis	Insect (mosquito)
Trematodes				
Clonorchis sinensis	Liver fluke	Liver	Biliary obstruction (rare)	Oral—raw fish
Fasciola hepatica	Liver fluke	Liver	Fever, right upper quadrant abdominal pain, eosinophilia	Oral
Fasciolopsis buski	Intestinal fluke	Liver	Abdominal pain, diarrhea	Oral
Paragonimus westermani	Lung fluke	Lung, intestine	Eosinophilia, cough, chest pain, bronchitis	Oral—poorly cooked freshwater crab or crayfish
Schistosoma haematobium	Blood fluke	Urinary tract	Acute: rash, fever, cough, chills	Skin inoculation
Schistosoma japonicum	Blood fluke	Mesenteric blood vessels	Hepatomegaly, splenomegaly	Skin inoculation
Schistosoma mansoni	Blood fluke	Mesenteric blood vessels	Lymphadenopathy, eosinophilia	Skin inoculation

TABLE 8–5. Parasitic Infections Continued

Parasitic Agent	Common Name of Disease	Location of Infection	Symptoms	Mode of Transmission
Cestodes (tapeworms)				
Diphyllobothrium latum	Fish tapeworm	Intestine	Megaloblastic anemia	Oral—poorly cooked fish
Taenia saginata	Beef tapeworm	Intestine	Mild abdominal pain	Oral—poorly cooked beef
Taenia solium	Pork tapeworm	Intestine	Mild abdominal pain	Oral–poorly cooked pork
Echinococcus granulosus	Hydatid cyst	Lungs, liver	Cholestasis, liver congestion and atrophy, biliary obstruction	Oral—inoculation with sheep, cattle, or dog feces
Protozoa				
Entamoeba histolytica	Amebic dysentery	Intestine	Bloody, mucoid diarrhea; colicky abdominal pain	Contaminated water, raw vegetables
Plamodium spp.	Malaria	Liver, erythrocytes	High fever, chills, rigor, anemia, headache, malaise, chest pain, abdominal pain	Female *Anopheles* mosquito
Leishmania spp.	Kala-azar; cutaneous and mucocutaneous leishmaniasis	Reticuloendothelial cells of the body; disseminates to spleen, liver, bone marrow, lymph glands	Chronic: abdominal discomfort, ascites, fever, weakness, pallor, weight loss, cough / Acute: sudden fever, chills	All transmission accomplished through bite of sandflies after biting specific infected mammals
Trypanosoma spp.		Bloodstream	Local inflammation, lymphadenopathy, muscular necrosis including myocardium (heart failure), esophagus, and colon (dilation); fever, malaise, anorexia, edema of face	Insects—hematophagous (blood-drinking) *Triatoma*
T. cruzi	Chagas' disease			
T. brucei	African sleeping sickness	Bloodstream	Fever, malaise, headache, rash, CNS disturbances	*Glossina* flies (tsetse flies)
Toxoplasma gondii	Toxoplasmosis	Throughout body	Acute: usually asymptomatic / Immunosuppressed: encephalitis, myocarditis, pneumonitis / Newborn: impaired vision, neurologic disorders	Eating raw or undercooked meat, poultry, or dairy foods; oral inoculation with cat feces
Pneumocystis carinii	Pneumonitis	Lungs	Fever, cough, tachypnea, costal retractions, cyanosis	Inhalation
Giardia lamblia	Epidemic diarrhea	Intestine	Acute, self-limited diarrhea; occasionally malabsorption with weight loss	Fecal contamination of water; person-to-person
Trichomonas vaginalis	Trichomoniasis (vaginitis)	Vagina	Irritation, discharge	Venereal
Ectoparasites				
Pediculus humanus var. *corporis*	Body louse	All hair-covered parts of body	Puritus / Nits at base of hair shaft	Person-to-person, via fomites
var. *capitis*	Head louse	Head area		
Pediculus pubis	Pubic louse	Pubic area		
Sarcoptes scabiei var. *hominis*	Scabies	Skin	Puritus, worse at night; linear burrows in folds of fingers, elbows, knees, axillae, pelvic girdle	Person-to-person
Maggots (larvae of dipterous flies	Myiasis	Necrotic tissue	Depends on location of infestation	Dipterous flies
Chiggers (mites)		Skin	Intense puritus, hemorrhagic papules	Inhabit dogs, rabbits, cats, rats; foul cheese, flour, house dust
Ticks		Skin	Can transmit tick paralysis, Lyme disease	Reside in wooded and grassy areas

of humans, including the common name, location, symptoms, and mode of transmission.

KEY CONCEPTS

- Microorganisms responsible for infections in humans include bacteria, viruses, fungi, and parasites.
- Bacteria are characterized according to shape (cocci, rods, spirals), reactions to stains (gram-negative, gram-positive, acid-fast), and oxygen requirements (aerobic, anaerobic).
- Viruses are bits of genetic material (DNA, RNA) with associated proteins and lipids. Viruses are intracellular pathogens that use the host's energy sources and enzymes to replicate. Viral replication may or may not destroy the host cell. DNA viruses may incorporate directly into the host genome. RNA viruses serve as templates for the production of viral RNA and proteins.
- Retroviruses are RNA viruses that contain a special enzyme, called reverse transcriptase, that mediates the synthesis of a DNA copy of the RNA virus. The DNA can then be incorporated into the host genome and passed on to daughter cells when the cell divides.
- Fungal infections can be superficial (e.g., ringworm, athlete's foot), subcutaneous (e.g., sporotrichosis), or systemic (e.g., histoplasmosis). Systemic fungal infections tend to be opportunistic, occurring only when the host's immune system is compromised.
- Parasites include protozoa, helminths (roundworms, flatworms), and arthropods. Manifestations of parasitic infections vary depending on the organism. Common sites of parasitic infestation are the skin and GI tract.

Host–Parasite Relationship

The human body is designed to defend itself against pathogens with its nonspecific and specific immune systems. The first line of defense is the nonspecific immune system, which consists of the skin and mucous membranes. These prevent the entry of microorganisms into the body. If pathogens do enter the body, making it a host, components of the immune system detect their presence and attempt to destroy them. In healthy humans, potentially infectious parasites are usually defeated before the body becomes a host. **Infectious disease** occurs when pathogens enter a host, causing signs and symptoms of illness.

The ability of the human body to resist infection requires an intact host–parasite defense system. Host and environmental factors such as nutrition, age, illness, air quality, sanitation, and stress may alter the host's resistance to infection. In addition, the characteristics of the pathogen such as virulence, toxins, adherence, and invasiveness may allow it to evade the human defense system and colonize. The relationship

between the host, the parasite, and the environment as shown in Figure 8–4 is the framework for understanding infectious processes.

Microorganism Factors

Microorganisms possess certain characteristics that assist in their penetration and survival in the host despite an intact defense system. Virulence, toxin production, microbial adherence, and invasiveness are microorganism factors that influence the development of infection within the host.

Microbial adherence is the ability of the microorganism to latch on to and gain entrance into the host. Without the ability to either directly penetrate a host or stick to the host's tissue surface, pathogens are removed by normal host defenses. Entry into the host can occur directly, as with a surgical wound, arthropod bite, or direct penetration. An infected female *Anopheles* mosquito can inject *Plasmodium vivax* with its bite, causing malaria. *Ancylostoma duodenale* (hookworm) directly penetrates the skin when the skin comes in contact with infected soil.

Entry can also occur through the microorganism's ability to adhere to the host's epithelial cells because of adhesions on the cell surface of certain microorganisms. The type of adhesion varies. For example, the mechanism of adhesion of *Escherichia coli* is protein K88, and Group A streptococci adhesions are lipoteichoic acids.[4] Some bacteria, like *E. coli*, have *pili* or *fimbriae* (hairlike structures) that enable them to attach to glycoproteins containing mannose on their hosts.[6] Microbes are also attracted to and able to attach to certain cell surface proteins such as fibronectin or to the rough surfaces of intravascular or intracavity catheters.

Microbial development of a slime layer also facilitates adherence. The slime layer is the result of extracellular synthesis of a substance, usually a mucopolysaccharide, by enzymes on the surface of the bacteria. The slime layer, called *glycocalyx*, acts as a glue or adhesive that sticks the bacteria to host surfaces. For example, the slime layer produced by *Streptococcus mutans* allows the bacteria to adhere to tooth enamel, forming plaque.[4]

Virulence and invasiveness factors include a variety of mechanisms that microorganisms have evolved to elude and block host defenses or assist in host invasion. These characteristics contribute to the pathogenicity of the microorganism by enabling it to penetrate natural barriers, resist death by phagocytosis, or survive antimicrobial therapy. Examples include bacterial enzymes, encapsulization, mutation, mobility, endospore formation, and resistance to phagocytosis and antimicrobial therapy.

Bacterial enzymes (such as fibrinolysin, coagulase, and hyaluronidase) aid in the microorganism's ability to spread or invade tissues. Most enzymes dissolve or hydrolyze blood, collagen, or connective tissue components. Fibrinolysin, produced by streptococci, dissolves coagulated plasma, which allows local

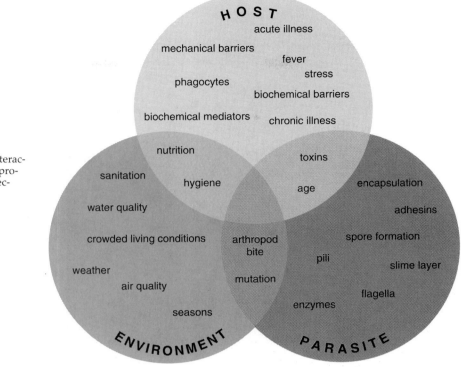

FIGURE 8-4. This depiction of the interactions of host, parasite, and environment provides a framework for understanding infectious processes.

microbial spread into host tissues. Hyaluronidase is secreted by staphylococci, clostridia, streptococci, and others.[4] This enzyme helps local microbial tissue spread by dissolving a connective tissue component called hyaluronic acid.

Encapsulization prevents opsonization (nonself recognition and binding) by antibodies, which stops the microorganism from being phagocytized. For example, *Streptococcus pneumoniae* (pneumococci) diplococci have a polysaccharide capsule that protects them from phagocytosis. The bacterial slime layer also protects the bacteria from phagocytosis.

To illustrate, *Mycobacterium tuberculosis* bacilli are not killed by macrophages. Rather, they are able to reside engulfed in endosomes within macrophages, reticuloendothelial cells, and giant cells. Their invasiveness is related to their ability to form tiny, hard, lipid hydrophobic cell capsules, their ability to form parallel chains (serpentine cords), and their resistance to chemical agents. The *M. tuberculosis* capsules are called tubercles. Within the capsule, the bacilli can reside indefinitely until the host's immune system declines.[7]

Other bacteria are capable of endospore formation. Formation of an endospore allows the microorganism to survive under harsh environmental conditions. The endospore state is specifically triggered by bacterial genes under conditions of decreasing nutrients, such as decreasing nitrogen or carbon in the environment. The endospore, which is capable of regeneration under favorable conditions, is a resting cell

that is released when the microorganism dies. It is highly resistant to heat, lack of moisture, and chemicals. Examples of endospore-forming bacteria include *Clostridium, Bacillus,* and *Coxiella burnetii.*

Microorganisms are also able to mutate in response to changes in the host's environment in order to successfully infect the host. For example, the development of methicillin-resistant *Staphylococcus aureus* is the result of successful mutation of the organism in response to excessive antibody exposure. The ability of *S. aureus* to become antibiotic resistant began with the introduction of penicillin and continues today (Table 8–6).

Other bacteria have *flagella,* motile appendages that allow the bacterium to move or swim toward nutrients in a favorable environment. This movement, called chemotaxis, is usually toward sugar or amino acid concentrations in the environment. Other microorganisms block aspects of the host's immune system, such as by obstructing antigen processing and encouraging the growth of suppressor cells.

Microorganisms may also produce toxins in the host that can affect the host's cells systemically or locally. The toxins are classified as exotoxins or endotoxins. *Exotoxins* are polypeptide toxins that are produced and released by the organism. They are highly antigenic, highly toxic, and unstable when exposed to heat. They cause illness and death by binding to specific receptors in target organs and by interfering with vital metabolic pathways. Some exotoxin-producing bacteria include *Clostridium botulinum, C.*

TABLE 8–6. Historical Progression of Staphylococcus aureus Resistance to Antibiotics

Antibiotic Introduced	Resistance Appeared
Penicillin, 1941	1940s
Streptomycin, 1944	Mid-1940s
Tetracycline, 1948	1950s
Erythromycin, 1952	1950s
Gentamicin, 1964	Mid-1970s
Methicillin, 1959	Late 1960s

From Morita MM: Methicillin-resistant *Staphylococcus aureus:* Past, present and future. *Nurs Clin North Am* 1993;28:625–637. Reproduced with permission.

tetani, Staphylococcus aureus, and *Shigella dysenteriae.*[4] For example, *C. tetani* produces an exotoxin called tetanospasmin that is a powerful neurotoxin. Tetanospasmin interferes with synaptic transmission in the spinal cord and blocks acetylcholine release from nerves at muscle end-plates. This leads to tetany, muscle spasms, characteristic "lockjaw" (trismus), and seizures.

Endotoxins are associated with gram-negative bacteria, Enterobacteriaceae, which are the causative agents of septic shock. Endotoxin is an immunogenic part of the bacterial cell wall (lipopolysaccharide) that triggers a massive immune response when the bacterium lyses. The subsequent immune response leads to shock, vascular collapse, and multiple organ failure. (See Chapter 54 for a further discussion of sepsis.)

Environmental Factors

Environmental factors such as sanitation, air quality, crowded living conditions, and weather also affect the balance between host and parasite. Infections may be transmitted by inhalation of polluted dust or air, by ingestion of contaminated food and water, or by insect or parasite vectors. To illustrate, tuberculosis and poliomyelitis are known to occur in crowded living conditions with poor nutrition and hygiene. Viral hepatitis type A is transmitted by the fecal-oral route, usually by consuming contaminated food or water or by eating sewage-contaminated clams.

Some infections occur only in certain regions or areas. African sleeping sickness, caused by the parasite *Trypanosoma brucei rhodesiense,* occurs only in woodland and savannah areas south and east of Lake Tanganyika. This environmental limitation is related to the environmental range of its vector, the tsetse fly, *Glossina morsitans.*[4]

Many infections are known to have seasonal patterns. For example, poliomyelitis occurs during the summer and fall in temperate zones and year round in the tropics. Aseptic meningitis also tends to occur during the summer and fall. Epidemic typhus caused by *Rickettsia prowazekii* occurs in the winter or in cool climates under conditions of poor sanitation and poor hygiene. It is under these conditions that the human host is most likely to be wearing clothes and can be bitten by the human louse, which is the vector.[4]

Host Defense System

The host defense system is multifaceted, consisting of a *nonspecific* immune response, composed of mechanical and biochemical barriers, phagocytes, and chemical mediators, and a *specific* immune response. (Host immune systems are discussed in greater detail in Chapters 9 and 10.) The body's exterior is an effective mechanical and biochemical barrier to most organisms and infectious agents. The epithelium is difficult for organisms to penetrate because of its structure, pH, continual cell sloughing process, attachment prevention, the passage of secretory IgA through the epithelium from lymphocytes, and the production of biochemical agents.

In the acute care setting, these barriers may be interrupted or destroyed by medical interventions. For instance, endotracheal tubes, urinary catheters, and invasive monitoring catheters interfere with protective epithelial surfaces. Every day, nurses intervene to decrease or ameliorate the damage of these invasive techniques.

Mechanical Epithelial Barriers

The skin is an important mechanical barrier. Intact physical barriers act as blockades to foreign material entering the body. The epithelial cells of the skin provide multilayer protection from the many microorganisms the body comes in contact with. The dry surface of the skin does not promote the growth of organisms, as moisture is preferred. Constant shedding of the epidermis and mucosal membranes aids in the removal of any microorganisms that are attached to their surfaces. For example, an intestinal epithelial cell half-life is 30 hours, which limits the number of bacteria that could attach to the cell. The high fat content of the skin inhibits the growth of bacteria and fungi.[8]

The mucous membrane linings of the GI and genitourinary tracts provide a barrier separating the sterile internal body from the external environment. The lungs are protected with a bilayer mucous lining. The sticky consistency of mucous membranes traps microorganisms, and the cilia sweep the microorganisms away. The mucociliary system and alveolar macrophages are important for ridding the lungs of trapped microorganisms.[2] Mechanisms such as coughing, sneezing, and voiding help remove particles trapped on mucous membranes from the body.

Removal or degradation of the body's mechanical barriers creates a setting in which infection is likely. For example, burn victims who have lost portions of their skin barrier are at high risk for infection. Hospitalized patients who have incisions or intravenous and urinary catheters are at risk for infection because their skin barrier has been breached. The normal action of cilia in the respiratory tract in removing foreign particles is blocked by endotracheal tubes. When a urinary catheter is in place, the flushing of bacteria from the urinary tract opening (meatus) is bypassed (Fig. 8–5).

Biochemical Epithelial Barriers

Chemical barriers enhance the effectiveness of the mechanical barriers.[2] The acid environment of the skin, urine, and vagina inhibits bacterial growth. The secretion of hydrochloric acid with a pH of 1 to 2 by the stomach actually kills microorganisms. Saliva, mucus, tears, and sweat contain antimicrobial chemicals such as lysozyme. Lysozyme is an enzyme that destroys bacterial cell walls and is bactericidal.[2] Lactoferrin is another mucosal protein that keeps bacterial replication low by inhibiting the free iron necessary for bacterial growth. Sebaceous gland secretions act as antifungals. In addition, secretory immunoglobulins (IgA, IgM, IgG) are present in many of the body's secretions, preventing entry of bacteria and viruses through mucous membranes. (See Chapters 9 and 10 for a further discussion of immunoglobulins.)

KEY CONCEPTS

- *Microorganisms possess characteristics that enhance their pathogenic potential. Adherence is improved by the presence of adhesions, slime layers, and pili. Escape from immune detection and destruction is enhanced by encapsulation, spore formation, muta-* tion, flagella, and toxin production. Microorganisms that possess these characteristics are more virulent and likely to cause disease.
- *Environmental factors influence the likelihood of exposure to and infection by microorganisms. Sanitation, air quality, crowded living conditions, and weather are important factors.*
- *The host has several lines of defense to prevent infection and fight microorganisms. The first lines of defense are mechanical and biochemical barriers. Skin and mucous membranes are multilayered and shed continuously, which removes attached microorganisms. The lungs are endowed with cilia that sweep away mucus and trapped debris.*
- *The acidity of urinary, vaginal, skin, and stomach secretions retards microbial growth. Degradative enzymes and secretory immunoglobulins in body secretions help destroy microorganisms before they gain access to the body.*

Manifestations of Infection

The body reacts to invasion by an infectious organism with an inflammatory response. The inflammatory response occurs within seconds. The function of the inflammatory response is to localize and contain microorganisms. The inflammatory response has both nonspecific and specific components.

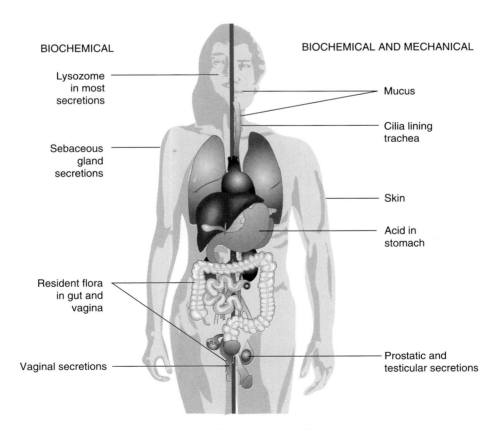

BIOCHEMICAL

Lysozome in most secretions

Sebaceous gland secretions

Resident flora in gut and vagina

Vaginal secretions

BIOCHEMICAL AND MECHANICAL

Mucus

Cilia lining trachea

Skin

Acid in stomach

Prostatic and testicular secretions

FIGURE 8–5. Some of the mechanical and biochemical barriers of the human body.

The clinical manifestations of infection are varied. Symptoms depend on whether the infection is localized or systemic, the location of the infection, the age of the host, and the causative organism. The symptoms most commonly associated with infection are generated from the immune response. If the immune system is depressed, these symptoms may be blunted.

The classic manifestations of infection are fever and leukocytosis. Signs of inflammation that may appear at the site of infection include redness, swelling, heat, tenderness or pain, and loss of function. Systemic symptoms may be nonspecific and vague such as headache, fatigue, lethargy, loss of appetite, and body aches.

The elderly may exhibit either subnormal temperatures or a mild elevation in temperature. Pneumonia in the elderly is likely to manifest with an elevated respiratory rate, loss of appetite, weakness, lethargy, or confusion.[9] A urinary tract infection in the elderly may be asymptomatic. Infants usually have fever, decreased appetite, difficulty with feeding, lethargy, irritability, or a change in the quality of the cry.[10]

Phagocytosis

Phagocytosis is an important component of the nonspecific immune response. *Phagocytosis* is the process of engulfing and destroying microorganisms by granulocytes such as neutrophils and macrophages. Figure 8–6 shows the phagocytic processes of ingestion and intracellular digestion.[5]

The inflammatory response aids in the increased production of phagocytic cells. Chemotaxis attracts the phagocytes to the site of injury.[3] The circulatory system transports the phagocytic cells to the site of injury. Neutrophils are the first cells to arrive and play a vital role in host defense. Inadequate numbers or impaired phagocytic functioning of neutrophils decreases resistance to infection.

Phagocytic cells also release mediators of inflammation such as serotonin, prostaglandins, histamine, lysomal enzymes, clotting factors, kinin, complement fragments, and immune factors. Interleukin-1 (IL-1), released from monocytes and macrophages, helps to mediate the host response. IL-1 is involved in chemotaxis for neutrophils, B-cells, and T-cells; the hepatic synthesis of acute phase proteins; neutrophilia; and lymphocyte stimulation.

Interferons

Interferons make up a group of proteins that are important in defending against viral infections. As cells become infected by virus they produce interferon. Different cell types produce different types of interferon such as interferon-alpha or interferon-beta. Lymphocytes and natural killer cells produce interferon-gamma after activation by antigen. Interferons cause a state of resistance through induction of host cell enzymes that affect transcription and translation of viral genes. They also affect how the host cell will respond to lymphocytes and natural killer (NK) cells. Interferons act to increase viral recognition by the immune system, activate cells to kill viruses such as NK cells and macrophages, and inhibit viral replication.[11] Researchers believe that interferon-induced production of nitric oxide synthetase is one of the ways viral replication is stopped.[12]

Fever

Fever is another nonspecific defense mechanism against invading organisms and is important to the body's response to infection and inflammation. It re-

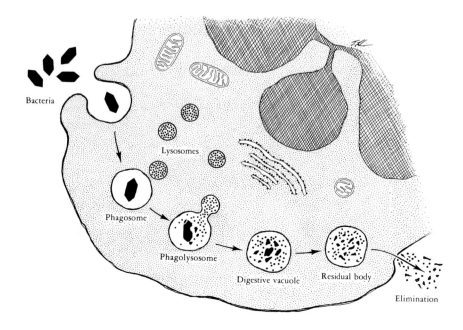

FIGURE 8–6. Schematic representation of phagocytosis showing ingestion process and intracellular digestion. (From Bellanti JA: *Immunology III.* Philadelphia, WB Saunders, 1985, p 18. Reproduced with permission.)

Bacteria

Lysosomes

Phagosome

Phagolysosome

Digestive vacuole

Residual body

Elimination

sults from the release of IL-1 from macrophages. IL-1 is one of the substances known as endogenous pyrogens. Other endogenous pyrogens are interleukin-6 (IL-6) and tumor necrosis factor. *Endogenous pyrogens* are fever-producing substances found in plasma during infection or immune reactions.

Fever is a cardinal sign of infection. Body temperature is regulated in the brain with thermoregulatory mechanisms to raise or lower temperature. Normal temperature is maintained at 37° C (98.6° F) ± 1°. In response to endogenous pyrogens, the brain will reset to a higher temperature, and thermoregulatory mechanisms will cause a rise in temperature until the setpoint is reached. In addition, fever augments host defenses by increasing interferon production and enhancing its effects. Fever may also inhibit bacterial proliferation by interfering with iron metabolism in bacteria.

Although uncomfortable, most fevers are not usually harmful. However, fever can be detrimental in certain clinical situations because it increases the metabolic rate, decreases the seizure threshold, and increases protein catabolism.[3] For example, fever in an individual who has marginal cardiac output will cause the heart to beat faster and may lead to decompensation and congestive heart failure (Fig. 8–7).

Specific Immune Response

The specific immune response includes the humoral and cellular immune response and takes several days to fully develop. The response is triggered through recognition of a specific antigen.[13] (Refer to Chapter 9, Inflammation and Immunity.) Defects in either the humoral or cellular immune system predispose the host to infection. Chronic infections, particularly with opportunistic organisms, are seen when the specific immune response is impaired.

Host Factors That Decrease Resistance to Infection

There are numerous host factors that alter a person's resistance to infection. Prevention and early detection of infection are aided by the identification of high-risk individuals.

Nutrition

Adequate nutrition is necessary to maintain a healthy immune system. It has long been recognized that malnutrition is a risk factor in the development of infections. Protein-energy malnutrition is associated with defects in cell-mediated immunity (specific), impaired intracellular killing by neutrophils, reduced complement activity, and decreased levels of secretory IgA.[14]

Vitamin and trace element deficiencies have been associated with specific defects in the immune system. Severe iron deficiency alters the functioning of some of the cellular components of the immune system and

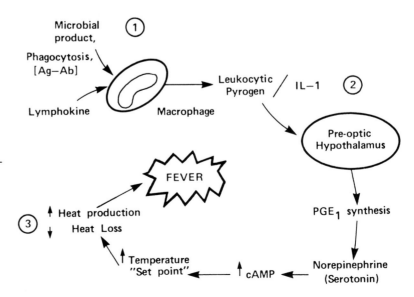

FIGURE 8–7. Pathogenesis of fever. (From Root RK: Infectious diseases: Pathogenic mechanism and host responses, in Smith LH, Thier SO (eds): *Biological Principles of Disease*, 2nd ed. Philadelphia, WB Saunders, 1985, p 163. Modified from Bernheim HA, Block LH, Atkins E: Fever: Pathogenesis, pathophysiology and purpose. *Ann Intern Med* 1979;91:261. Reproduced with permission.)

is believed to increase the susceptibility to infection.[14] Excess amounts of trace elements and fatty acids may also depress the immune system, which emphasizes the need for the intake of optimal amounts of nutrients.

The host responding to an infection will need additional protein and nutrients to fight the microbial invasion. Decreased nutrition during this period of time can lead to a negative nitrogen balance. *Anergy* in the preoperative patient has been a marker for increased postoperative morbidity and sepsis.[15] Anergy, or the failure to mount a localized response to a known antigen when given intradermally, can result from protein-energy malnutrition.

Chronic Illness

Chronic illnesses such as diabetes, cancer, heart disease, and renal failure are associated with increased risk for infection. Deaths in patients with chronic illnesses are frequently directly related to an infectious process. Infections are cited as the leading cause of death in patients with acute renal failure and diabetes.[16,17]

Diabetes alters the host's ability to resist infection. Phagocytosis is impaired with hyperglycemia.[18] Detection of the pain of infection may be delayed due to neuropathies. An increased virulence of some microorganisms is seen when exposed to hyperglycemic environments.[17] With increased glucose levels, *Candida* has been shown to flourish, with increased resistance to phagocytosis.

Circulatory problems associated with cardiac failure or peripheral vascular disease are a risk factor for infection. The cellular components of the immune system are dependent on the circulatory system to deliver them to the site of infection. In addition, antimicrobial agents need to be transported to the site of infection. Many pathogens thrive in areas with poor tissue perfusion.

Acute Illness

Acute illnesses such as trauma or burns alter the body's resistance to infection. Impaired skin integrity allows microorganisms to enter the body. Infections in trauma patients are caused by more virulent, pathogenic organisms and are usually nosocomial (hospital-acquired) infections.[19] Immobility, loss of natural barriers, the dilutional effects on circulating immunocytes, invasive catheters, and antibiotic therapy increase the risk of infection in the trauma patient.

For example, abdominal trauma may result in spleen injury and possible therapeutic splenectomy. Patients with splenectomy are at high risk for developing an overwhelming infection due to *Streptococcus pneumoniae*. The spleen normally facilitates the phagocytosis of encapsulated bacteria. Prevention of life-threatening infections is aided by vaccination of all splenectomy patients with the pneumococcal vaccine.[19]

Age

Age is also a variable in the ability to resist infections. Infants are at an increased risk for infection owing to an immature immune system. The lack of previous exposure to microorganisms makes the immune system naive and less efficient in mounting a defense.[5] A newborn is susceptible to gram-negative bacterial infections and sepsis due to the lack of IgM. Detection of infection in the newborn is based on a high level of suspicion and accurate detection of the subtle signs of lethargy, feeding difficulties, temperature control problems, and changes in vital signs.[20]

The elderly are more susceptible to infection because of declining function of the immune system. Depressed cell-mediated immunity, changes in T-lymphocyte functioning, and atrophy of the thymus gland are some of the factors that may cause decreased immunity.[21] There is greater morbidity and mortality associated with infection in the elderly.[22] Respiratory and urinary tract infections are the most common sites of infection in the elderly. However, the diversity and type of infections in the elderly are greater than in other age groups, leading to higher frequencies of sepsis and bacteremia.[22] Infection may also present atypically, with absence of fever and the sudden onset of confusion. The subtle changes and lack of fever obscure clinical recognition of the presence of an infectious process.[14,22]

Stress

Stress has been implicated in predisposing an individual to an infectious process. An example is the outbreak of a latent herpes simplex infection in response to stress. Stress hormones such as corticosteroids are known for their effects to depress the immune system. Complex interactions exist between the immune system and neuroendocrine system. Hormones such as corticosteroids, endorphins, and lymphokines participate in the regulatory loop between the two systems. (For further discussion, see Chapter 7.)

Immunocompromised Host

Immunosuppression may result from a systemic disease involving the immune system or from the treatment of a disease. Defects may occur in one or more of the limbs of the immune response: phagocytic, complement, cellular, or humoral. A person is considered immunocompromised when such a defect is known to exist. The defect may be caused by a disease such as AIDS, complement deficiencies, or the absence of humoral antibody production. The defect may also be drug-induced. Agents that can cause immunosuppression are antimetabolites, corticosteroids, cyclosporin, and antibiotics.[11] The immunocompromised host is highly susceptible to life-threatening infections. Meticulous care in the prevention of infection is a high priority for this patient.

KEY CONCEPTS

- **Malnutrition may depress immune function because many immune components require adequate proteins, vitamins, and minerals for synthesis. Immunoglobulins, complement factors, and clotting factors require adequate protein metabolism by the liver.**
- **Chronic illnesses such as diabetes and cardiovascular disease predispose to infection because circulation of immune components may be impaired and a high-glucose medium may enhance bacterial growth.**
- **Trauma, burns, invasive instrumentation, antibiotics, and immunosuppressive therapies, which may accompany acute illnesses, predispose to infection by altering the normal host defenses.**
- **The very young and very old are more susceptible to infection because of an immature or degenerating immune function. In the elderly, fever may be absent during infections.**
- **Stress is associated with increased secretion of corticosteroids, which are believed to depress immune function. Exogenous steroids and other immunosuppressive therapies (radiation, antibiotics, anticancer drugs) also increase the risk of infection.**

Summary

Health care professionals play a key role in the prevention and early detection of infectious processes in hospital and community settings. The identification of high-risk individuals who are more susceptible to infection will assist in the earlier detection of the manifestations of infection. Treatment of infections requires optimizing the client's host defense system and is supplemented by pharmacologic and nutritional interventions.

REFERENCES

1. Root RK: Infectious diseases: Pathogenic mechanism and host responses, in Smith LH, Thier SO (eds): *Biological Principles of Disease*, 2nd ed. Philadelphia, WB Saunders, 1985.
2. Vander AJ, Sherman JH, Luciano DS: *Human Physiology: The Mechanisms of Body Function*, 4th ed. New York, McGraw-Hill, 1985.
3. Guyton AC: *Textbook of Medical Physiology*, 8th ed. Philadelphia, WB Saunders, 1991.
4. Jawetz E, et al: *Review of Medical Microbiology*, 17th ed. Norwalk, Conn, Appleton & Lange, 1987.
5. Bellanti JA: *Immunology III*. Philadelphia, WB Saunders, 1985.
6. Sharon N, Lis H: Carbohydrates in cell recognition. *Sci Am* 1993;268(1):82–89.
7. Boutotte J: Tuberculosis: The second time around. *Nursing* 1993;93(5):42–49.
8. Stites DP, Terr AI: *Basic and Clinical Immunology*, 7th ed. Norwalk, Conn, Appleton & Lange, 1991.
9. Golightly MG, Dolan JT: Assessment of immunologic function, in Dolan JT (ed): *Critical Care Nursing: Clinical Management Through the Nursing Process*. Philadelphia, FA Davis, 1991.
10. Karupiah G, Xie QW, Buller RM, et al: Inhibition of viral replication by interferon-γ-induced nitric oxide synthase. *Science* 1993;261:1445–1448.
11. Nossal GJV: Current concepts: Immunology. The basic components of the immune system. *N Eng J Med* 1987;326:1320–1325.
12. Chandra RK: Nutrition, immunity, and infection: Present knowledge and future directions. *Lancet* 1983;1:688–691.
13. Christou NV, Tellado-Rodriguez J, Chartrand L, et al: Estimating mortality risk in preoperative patients using immunologic, nutritional, and acute phase response variables. *Ann Surg* 1989;210:69–77.
14. Stark JL: The renal system, In Alspach JG (ed): *Core Curriculum for Critical Care Nursing*, 4th ed. Philadelphia, WB Saunders, 1991.
15. Hostetter MK: Handicaps to host defense: Effects of hyperglycemia on C3 and *Candida albicans*. *Diabetes* 1990;39:271–275.
16. Rayfield EJ, Ault MJ, Keusch GT, et al: Infection and diabetes: The case for glucose control. *Am J Med* 1982;72:439–450.
17. Hoyt NJ: Host defense mechanisms and compromises in the trauma patient. *Crit Care Nurs Clin North Am* 1989;1:753–765.
18. Miller MK, Pan JS: Life-threatening infections in the newborn, in Shoemaker WC (ed): *Textbook of Critical Care*, 2nd ed. Philadelphia, WB Saunders, 1989.
19. Jeppesen ME: Laboratory values for the elderly, in Carnevale DL, Patrick M (eds): *Nursing Management for the Elderly*, 2nd ed. Philadelphia, JB Lippincott, 1986.
20. Yoshikawa TT, Norman DC: Antibiotic therapy: What to consider when treating geriatric patients. *Hosp Formulary* 1993;28:754–768.
21. Blalock JE, Smith EM: A complete regulatory loop between the immune and neuroendocrine systems. *Fed Proc* 1985;44:108–111.
22. Patrick M: Respiratory problems, in Carnevale DL, Patrick M (eds): *Nursing Management for the Elderly*, 2nd ed. Philadelphia, JB Lippincott, 1986.

BIBLIOGRAPHY

Balows A: *Manual of Clinical Microbiology*, 5th ed. Washington, DC, American Society of Microbiology, 1991.

Boyd R: *Basic Medical Microbiology*. Boston, Little, Brown & Co, 1991.

Cohen FL: Immunologic impairment, infection, and AIDS in the aging patient. *Crit Care Nurs Q* 1989;12:38–45.

Dinarello CA, et al: New concepts on the pathogenesis of fever. *Rev Infect Dis* 1988;10:168–190.

Ganz T: Neutrophil receptors, in Lehrer RI (moderator): Neutrophils and Host Defense. *Ann Intern Med* 1988;109:127–142.

Harvey AM: *Principles and Practices of Medicine*, 22nd ed. Norwalk, Conn, Appleton-Century-Crofts, 1988.

Mandell G: *Principles and Practice of Infectious Diseases*. New York, John Wiley & Sons, 1990.

Morita MM: Methicillin-resistant *Staphylococcus aureus:* Past, present and future. *Nurs Clin North Am* 1993;28:625–637.

Paul WE: Infectious diseases and the immune system. *Sci Am* 1993;269:91–97.

Tellado JM, Giannias B, Kapadia B, et al: Anergic patients before elective surgery have enhanced nonspecific host-defense capacity. *Arch Surg* 1990;125:49–53.

Wertz MJ: Infection, in Patrick ML, et al (eds): *Medical-Surgical Nursing: Pathophysiological Concepts*. Philadelphia, JB Lippincott, 1986.

West JB: *Pulmonary Pathophysiology: The Essentials*. Baltimore, Williams & Wilkins, 1977.

Woodley M, Whelan A: *Manual of Medical Therapeutics*, 27th ed. St. Louis, MO, Department of Medicine, Washington University School of Medicine, 1993.

CHAPTER 9
Inflammation and Immunity

FAITH YOUNG PETERSON, JULIE SYMES, and PAM SPRINGER

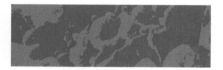

KEY TERMS

antibody: Substance produced by B-cells that destroys or inactivates a specific antigen.

antigen: Macromolecule that provokes an immune system response.

B-cell: Lymphocyte that produces antibodies that attack pathogens or directs other cells to attack them.

basophils: Leukocytes that are functionally and chemically related to the mast cell and have an average diameter of 8 to 10 μ, a kidney-shaped nucleus, and large deep basophilic granules, which contain vasoactive amine and heparin and are important in IgE binding.

complement: Refers to the system that activates immune cytolysis (dissolving of cells) and other biological functions through the use of some 20 distinct serum proteins. Complement activation can occur by the classical or the alternative pathways.

cytokines: Peptide factors released by immune cells when they contact specific antigens. They have signaling, inflammatory, growth, and inhibitory functions.

eosinophils: Leukocytes that are the same size as neutrophils but have a two-lobed nucleus and large, coarse eosinophilic granules that fill the cell; participate in allergic and inflammatory responses.

granulocytes: A leukocyte 8 to 12 μ in diameter with polymorphic nuclei and cytoplasmic granules.

inflammation: The body's protective response at the site of injury or tissue destruction. It is important to recognize that while infectious agents can produce inflammation, infection is not synonymous with inflammation.

macrophage: Mature monocytes that migrate out of the blood vessels to fixed sites in the lymphoid tissues.

major histocompatibility complex: The chromosomal regions that control histocompatibility or transplantation antigens are closely interrelated complexes. Chemical structure, tissue distribution, and function determine placement as Class I antigens (present on virtually all nucleated cells and proteins) or Class II antigens (found mainly on antigen-presenting cells, B-cells, and some activated T-cells).

monocytes and macrophages: Large (14–19 μ), occasionally motile immature macrophages that make up the mononuclear phagocyte system and circulate in the blood for 3 days before maturing.

neutrophils: Highly phagocytic leukocytes containing small lysosomal granules and a segmented nucleus with two to five lobes.

nonspecific immunity: Mechanisms that resist a variety of threatening agents or conditions.

phagocytosis: Ingestion and destruction of pathogens by leukocytes.

specific immunity: Mechanisms that provide protection against specific types of bacteria or toxins.

T-cell: Lymphocyte that provides cellular immunity, has regulatory functions, and attacks antigen in association with other cells.

---

*H*uman host defenses represent a complex system of organs and specialized cells that defend the body against attacks from exogenous (external) invaders as well as endogenous (internal) threats. Components of the *nonspecific* or *innate* and *specific* or *adaptive* immune systems provide for prevention, surveillance, and destruction of threats. Inflammation and immunity include all of the physiologic mechanisms that enable the body to recognize, attack, destroy, and eliminate foreign substances or microorganisms.

Nonspecific defenses are constantly elicited by such events as physical injury and bacterial or viral invasion. *Specific* defenses, by comparison, are engaged in response to a particular bacterium, virus, or molecule and involve specific immune cells. Nonspecific and specific defenses, although discussed separately in this chapter, are complementary and interdependent.

As discussed in Chapter 8, part of the nonspecific immune system involves mechanical and biochemical barriers. The other part of the nonspecific immune system is composed of phagocytes and their chemical mediators and the clotting system. This chapter will further clarify the cellular components of the nonspecific immune system and discuss the components of the specific immune system.

Components of the Immune System

The cells of the immune and inflammatory systems are composed of granulocytes, monocytes, macrophages, and lymphocytes, the last derived from the lymphoid system. The organs of the lymphoid system are the bone marrow, thymus, lymph nodes, spleen, tonsils, adenoids, appendix, and gut-associated lymphoid tissue (GALT), also known as Peyer's patches, in the small and large intestine. The lymphatic vessels and the blood, also part of the lymphoid system organs, carry the lymphocytes to and from places in the body. Lymphoid tissues are stationed throughout the body and are chiefly concerned with the growth, development, and deployment of phagocytic, cellular, and humoral defense.

Bone marrow is contained within all the bones of the body. The primary function of bone marrow is **hematopoiesis,** or the formation of blood cells. There are two kinds of bone marrow, red and yellow. Hematopoiesis is carried out by red (functioning) marrow. By adulthood, red marrow is confined to the pelvis, sternum, ribs, cranium, the ends of the long bones, and the vertebral spine. Yellow or fatty bone marrow is found in the remaining bones. It does not contribute to hematopoiesis.

Cellular Components

Red marrow, the source of all blood cells and platelets, produces an immature, undifferentiated cell called a **stem cell.** This immature stem cell is also referred to as pluripotent, multipotent, totipotent, and omnipotent, indicating the potential of the stem cell to develop along multiple pathways (Fig. 9–1).

When the stem cell is first created in the bone marrow, it is undifferentiated. The cell is not yet committed to a specific type. At this stage the stem cell is flexible and has the potential to become any one of a variety of mature blood cells. The specific cell type of the mature stem cell depends on which maturational pathway it follows.

The selection of or commitment to a maturational pathway appears to be an irreversible event. For instance, if a stem cell is committed to the platelet pathway and becomes a megakaryocyte, it is not able to revert to the pluripotent state and later become a T-lymphocyte. The cell may stop in the maturational process and never completely mature, but once commitment to a specific maturational pathway occurs, the cell continues to follow that path.

The maturational pathway of any stem cell depends, to some extent, on the body's needs at the time, and also on the presence of specific chemicals (termed *factors* or *proteins*) that stimulate specific commitment and induce maturation. For example, erythropoietin is synthesized in the kidney. When immature stem cells are exposed to erythropoietin, the immature stem cells are committed to the erythrocyte maturational pathway and eventually become mature red blood cells.

Normally, blood cells are released into the bloodstream when they reach maturity. On occasion, when the demand for a particular blood cell is high, the bone marrow may respond by releasing the needed blood component while cells are still immature. Figure 9–2 shows the maturational sequence of committed, or differentiated, stem cells.

Granulocytes

Leukocytes, or white blood cells (WBCs), are the primary effector cells of the immune system. Each of the six different types of leukocytes found in blood has a special job to perform. Three of these types are **granulocytes,** called neutrophils, eosinophils, and basophils. The other three WBC types are **monocytes, T-lymphocytes,** and **B-lymphocytes** (plasma cells). All of the leukocytes are a part of the nonspecific defense system except lymphocytes, which are part of the adaptive or specific defense system. Granulocytes, monocytes, and macrophages are the primary leukocytes that protect the body from invading organisms by ingesting or *phagocytizing* them. Table 9–1 describes the roles of the different leukocytes.

Phagocytosis is a process by which material is actually engulfed and ingested by leukocytes. Phagocytosis facilitates clearance of toxic material and the breakdown of dead substances. Phagocytosis involves the following four steps: (1) recognition and adherence to the target, (2) engulfment and ingestion, (3) fusion of the ingested material with the lysosomes of the target, and (4) destruction of the target by lysosomal enzymes.

Any organism that penetrates an epithelial surface will encounter phagocytic cells. Because phagocytes function by engulfing foreign particles and destroying them, they are strategically placed in the body where they will encounter foreigners. Phagocytic cells are found in such places as the liver, as Kupffer cells; in the synovial cavity lining, as A-cells; and in the brain, as microglial cells (Fig. 9–3).

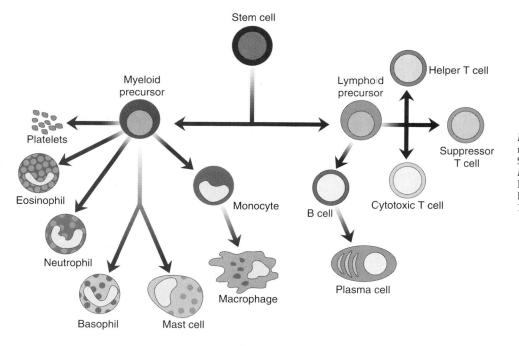

FIGURE 9–1. Cells of the immune system. (Redrawn from Schindler LW: *Understanding the Immune System.* NIH Publication No. 92-529. U.S. Department of Health and Human Services, 1991, p 5.)

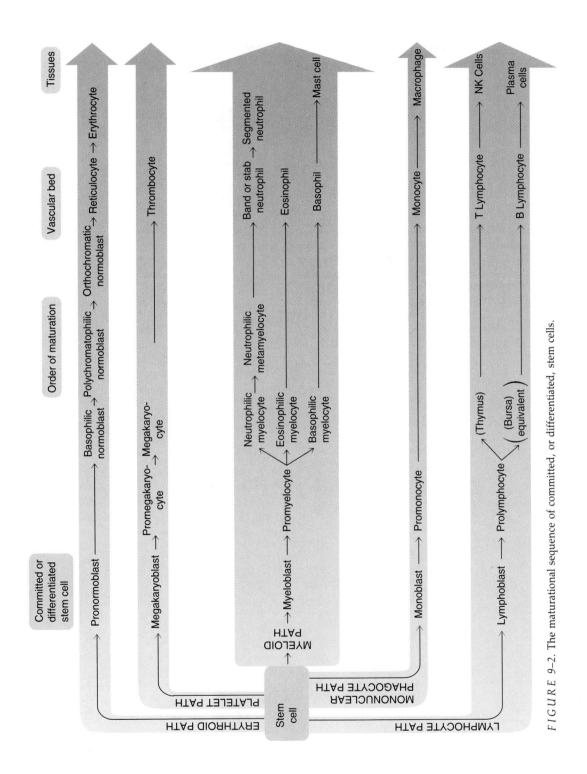

FIGURE 9–2. The maturational sequence of committed, or differentiated, stem cells.

T A B L E 9 – 1. Leukocyte Proportions and Functions

Type	Percentage Present	Role in Inflammation
Neutrophils	60–80	First to appear after injury; phagocytosis
Lymphocytes	20–30	Immune response
Monocytes (macrophages)	3–8	Phagocytosis
Eosinophils	1–6	Allergic reactions, parasite infection
Basophils	0–2	Contain histamine; mediate type I allergic reactions, initiate inflammation

Neutrophils are circulating granulocytes that are also known as polymorphonuclear leukocytes (PMNs). Neutrophils comprise 60 percent to 80 percent of the total WBC count and are the most numerous phagocytes in the blood. Neutrophils normally have 2 to 5 nuclear lobes and coarse, clumped chromatin. Neutrophils arise in the bone marrow from a stem cell and, after a series of divisions, undergo a period of maturation. The stages of maturation, as illustrated

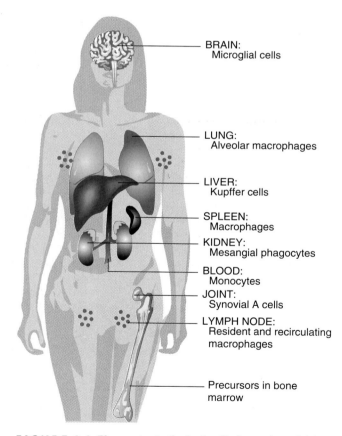

F I G U R E 9–3. Phagocytes in the body. (Redrawn from Schindler LW: *Understanding the Immune System.* NIH Publication No. 92-529. U.S. Department of Health and Human Services, 1991, p 9.)

in Figure 9–2, are: myeloblast → promyelocyte → metamyelocyte → band cell → mature neutrophil.

Neutrophils are stored in the bone marrow, where they number about 10 times the quantity of circulating neutrophils. These stored neutrophils are called as needed into the circulation, where they have a half-life of 4 to 10 hours. Circulating neutrophils have two interchangeable divisions—an *axial pool* and a *marginal pool*.[1] Axial pool neutrophils circulate around in the blood, while those in the marginal pool move slowly along the vascular endothelium, accelerating the neutrophil response to inflammation.[1]

Neutrophils are attracted to areas of inflammation or bacterial proliferation by chemotactic factors such as complement fragment C5a, fibrinopeptides, neutrophilic cationic proteins, lymphokines, certain growth factors such as platelet-derived growth factor and transforming growth factor-beta, and fragments from the breakdown of collagen and fibronectin. Each of these factors may play a role under certain circumstances. For example, lymphokines are almost certainly involved during delayed-hypersensitivity immune reactions (see Chap. 10).

Initially during an acute infection, **neutrophilia**, or an increase in the number of circulating neutrophils, occurs as the bone marrow releases stored neutrophils. As neutrophils are consumed and demand exceeds production, an increase in the immature (band) neutrophils occurs. This increase in band cells is referred to as a "shift to the left" of normal. (See Fig. 9–1.) In general, the greater the shift to the left, the more severe is the infection. A "shift to the right," an increase in mature neutrophils, is associated with pernicious anemia, chronic morphine addiction, or liver disease.

Neutropenia (a neutrophil count $< 1,000/mm^3$) renders a patient very susceptible to overwhelming infections. A person who has a fever and neutropenia can die in 24 hours without antibiotics. Individuals with aplastic anemia or patients receiving chemotherapy or radiation therapy for cancer often have neutropenia. (See Chapter 11 for a further discussion of neutropenia.)

Neutrophils have the capacity to release preformed potent chemical mediators or synthesize other chemical mediators that enable them to digest microorganisms. Over 50 toxins released by neutrophils have been identified—particularly oxidizing agents and powerful enzymes.[2] Because of the mediators and the ability to generate oxidative bursts with release of oxidizing metabolites, neutrophils can cause extensive damage to normal tissue during their inflammatory response.[2] Sometimes the body is ineffective in controlling the neutrophil chemical mediators to prevent extensive normal tissue damage.

Eosinophils are circulating granulocytes that have 2 nuclear lobes and stain brilliant red-orange with eosin. They make up 1 percent to 6 percent of the total WBC count. Eosinophils mature in the bone marrow (3–6 days) and circulate in the blood for about 30 minutes. They have a half-life of 12 days in tissues. Eosinophils arise from a common stem cell and undergo a maturation process similar to that of neutrophils.

Containing chemical granules, eosinophils have receptors for IgE and complement (CR3).[1] They are capable of killing target cells but are not as efficient as neutrophils. Eosinophils are particularly associated with, and increase in number during, allergic reactions and infection with intestinal parasites. Eosinophils may function to help control an inflammatory reaction by releasing enzymes that break down certain chemical mediators such as histamine and leukotrienes.

Basophils are granulocytes characterized by granules that stain blue with basophilic dyes. Basophils account for 0 percent to 2 percent of the total leukocyte count. Both mast cells and basophils arise from the bone marrow. Mature basophils circulate in the vascular system, while mast cells are found in connective tissues, especially around blood vessels and under mucosal surfaces. When stimulated, mature basophils can migrate into connective tissue, but once in the tissue, basophils and mast cells do not reenter the circulation.

The average basophil life span is measured in days, while mast cells can live weeks to months.[3] Although both mast cells and basophils have IgE receptors, they are heterogeneous with varying degrees of responsiveness, reactivity, and mediator content.[3] For example, lung mast cells are different from skin mast cells. Skin mast cells contain more intragranular chymase and are more sensitive to substance P and other neuropeptides. This diversity allows mast cells to respond to changes in their microenvironments.[3]

Both mast cells and basophil granules contain histamine, platelet-activating factor, and other vasoactive amines that are important mediators of immediate hypersensitivity responses. *Degranulation* of mast cells and basophils begins the inflammatory response and is characteristically associated with allergy or type I hypersensitivity reactions. (See Chapter 10 for further information.) However, mast cells and basophils are also involved in wound healing and chronic inflammatory conditions.

Mononuclear Phagocytes—Monocytes and Macrophages

The **mononuclear phagocyte system** (MPS) comprises generalized groups of cells that are widely distributed throughout the body, where they eliminate foreign materials from the blood, lymph, and tissues. The mononuclear phagocytes include both monocytes, composing 3 percent to 8 percent of total circulating leukocytes, and macrophages, found in certain tissues of the body. **Monocytes** from the circulating blood migrate into the various organs and tissues to become macrophages. The term MPS has replaced the term reticuloendothelial system (RES).

Macrophages are found throughout the body's tissues such as alveolar macrophages in the lungs, microglial cells in the brain, and Kupffer cells in the liver. Macrophages can be activated by lymphokines, immune complexes, and complement protein (C3b). Macrophages are powerful phagocytes, each capable of destroying as many as 100 bacteria. They also can engulf and destroy much larger bacteria, and can survive for many months after destroying bacteria. Because of their phagocytic and debridement functions, macrophages are the predominant phagocytic cells in late inflammation.

Macrophages are very versatile and play many parts in the immune response. Not only do they ingest particulate matter, macrophages also present antigens (make foreign material recognizable) to T-cells, initiating the immune response. Macrophages also release chemical mediators that are involved in inflammation and stimulate wound healing. Monocytes and macrophages also have receptors for lymphokines, substances that are secreted by lymphocytes.

Lymphocytes

The adaptive division of the immune system contains two subdivisions called cellular and humoral immunity. **Cellular** or **cell-mediated immunity** is moderated by sensitized or activated *T-lymphocytes*. **T-cells**, or thymus-derived lymphocytes, are responsible for cellular immunity; they have effector and regulatory functions. T-cell regulatory functions mobilize or deactivate the other cells in the immune system. T-cells are important activators of B-cells. T-cell effector functions include the ability to phagocytize or kill foreign invaders. Cellular immunity is effective against viruses, mycobacteria, and fungi and is a component in transplant rejection, delayed hypersensitivity, and tumor destruction.

Humoral-mediated immunity is mediated by *bursa equivalent–derived lymphocytes*, or **B-cells**, and *antibodies*. B-cells enhance the inflammatory response through their differentiation into *plasma cells*, which secrete antibodies. B-cells are important to the immune system because of their specificity and ability to remember antigens, allowing immediate response on subsequent exposure. They are one of the cell types that can process antigens to present to T-cells, causing T-cell activation.

Antigen-antibody complexes function to activate the common or classic pathway of the complement cascade, enhance phagocytosis, activate killer cells, and directly neutralize bacterial toxins and viruses. The humoral system is particularly effective in bacterial phagocytosis and viral neutralization and is involved in anaphylaxis and immune deficiency diseases.

Both T-cells and B-cells derive from a common lymphoid stem cell and are called **lymphocytes.** Together they make up approximately 20 percent of all leukocytes. Their average life span is 4 years, with a range of 3 to 20 years. Their subsequent differentiation and maturation are regulated by separate organs. Morphologically, T-cells and B-cells are small, agranular lymphocytes with more nuclear material than cytoplasm. There are fewer B-cells than T-cells. T-cells compose approximately 80 percent and B-cells 12 percent to 15 percent of all lymphocytes.[4]

Once mature lymphocytes leave their primary lymphoid organs, they travel through the blood to localize in peripheral or secondary lymphoid tissues, including lymph nodes, spleen, tonsils, and Peyer's patches in the intestine. The lymphocytes leave the vascular space through specialized vessels called high endothelial venules[5,6] and locate in these peripheral sites. Within the secondary lymph tissues, the compact lymphocytes move around freely but stay in a resting state until activated. When exposed to antigen, T-cells are activated in the paracortex of lymph nodes while B-cells are activated in the germinal centers of lymph nodes.[5] Once activated they migrate into lymph vessels and travel to the bloodstream, where they are taken to inflammatory sites.

KEY CONCEPTS

- **Major components of the immune system are bone marrow, thymus, lymph nodes, spleen, the mononuclear phagocyte system, and white blood cells. Accessory systems include the complement and clotting cascades and kinins.**
- **Blood cells are produced in the bone marrow in response to specific poietin growth factors. Granulocytes (neutrophils, basophils, eosinophils) and monocytes (macrophages) are nonspecific phagocytic cells. Lymphocytes (B-cells, T-cells) are specific cells that react only to particular antigens. Other blood components produced by bone marrow are erythrocytes and platelets.**
- **Neutrophils are the most numerous WBCs in blood. A large storage pool lies in the bone marrow and can be mobilized in response to antigen. Neutrophils are the predominant WBC type in early infection. They migrate to the area following chemotactic factors and perform phagocytic functions. During infection, larger numbers of immature neutrophils (bands) are released into the blood, termed a "shift to the left."**
- **Eosinophils make up 1 percent to 6 percent of circulating WBCs. They predominate in allergic reactions and parasitic infections. Eosinophils may restrain inflammation by degrading chemical mediators of inflammation.**
- **Basophils compose 0 percent to 2 percent of circulating WBCs. Basophils located in tissues are called mast cells. Basophils and mast cells have IgE receptors on their surfaces and release inflammatory mediators when they are activated by antigen or trauma.**
- **Monocytes compose 3 percent to 8 percent of circulating WBCs. Monocytes located in tissues are called macrophages. Monocytes and macrophages are distributed in strategic locations throughout the body, including the skin, lungs, GI tract, liver, spleen, and lymph. Macrophages are powerful**

phagocytes and are predominant in late inflammation.
- **T-lymphocytes are the major effectors of cell-mediated immunity. T-lymphocytes interact with specific antigens on cell surfaces. They are important in immunity against foreign, infected, or mutant cells. In addition, they secrete cytokines, which boost the immune response of B-cells and other cell types. T-cells make up about 80 percent of total lymphocytes.**
- **B-lymphocytes are the major effectors of antibody-mediated immunity. Activated B-lymphocytes secrete antibodies that protect against soluble antigens as well as cell-associated antigens. B-cells activate T-cells by presenting soluble antigen to them.**

Complement

Complement is an extension and enhancer of both inflammation and immunity. The complement system consists of over 25 chemically and immunologically distinct plasma proteins that interact with antibody, one another, and cell membranes.[7] Most complement proteins are synthesized in the liver, although they can be synthesized by macrophages and other cells. Half of the complement proteins are replaced every 24 hours.[8]

The complement proteins circulate in the blood in an inactive form. Activation of the complement cascade occurs via two different pathways, the classical and the alternative (or properdin) pathways. In both pathways, the inactive complement proteins are converted to their active form in a sequence of reactions. Activation of these pathways eventually leads to lysis of the foreign cell.

The *classical pathway* is primarily triggered by IgG or IgM antibody-antigen complexes, but it can also be triggered by denatured DNA, bacterial cellular membranes, myelin basic proteins, endotoxin, and polyanions.[7] The *alternative pathway* is initiated by aggregated IgA, trypsin-like enzymes, lipopolysaccharide (bacterial cell walls), plant and bacterial polysaccharides, and endotoxin.[7] In the classical pathway, an antibody hooked onto an antigen combines with C1, the first of the complement substances. This sets in motion a domino effect called the complement cascade (Fig. 9–4).

The major actions of complement proteins include cell lysis, facilitation of phagocytosis (opsonization), immune adherence, chemotaxis, and enzyme-like functions that allow cell wall destruction. Complement can also mediate inflammatory processes by acting as an anaphylatoxin. The complement cascade causes the release of inflammatory agents and also interacts with the coagulation and kinin systems.

For example, C3a functions as an anaphylatoxin. The products released from activation of C3a cause stimulation of histamine release from mast cells, contraction of smooth muscle, and endothelial cell rounding up. The complement protein C3b activates phagocytosis by neutrophils and macrophages. This

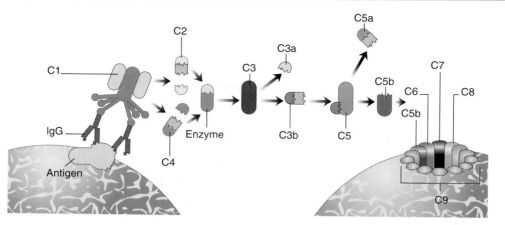

FIGURE 9–4. The complement cascade is activated by the first complement molecule, C1, that identifies an antigen-antibody complex. This event begins a domino effect, with each of the remaining complement proteins performing its part in the attack sequence. The end result is a hole in the membrane of the offending cell and destruction of the cell. (Redrawn from Schindler LW: *Understanding the Immune System.* NIH Publication No. 92-529. U.S. Department of Health and Human Services, 1991, p 11.)

process can enhance the number of bacteria engulfed. Complement protein fragment C5a is both a powerful anaphylatoxin and a potent chemotactic agent. C5a causes chemotaxis so that neutrophils and monocytes will migrate to the inflamed tissue. C5a also activates neutrophils by triggering their oxidative activity and increasing their glucose uptake.

Fragments C5 through C9 form what is called the membrane attack unit. This unit has a direct cytotoxic effect by attacking bacterial cell walls and disrupting the lipid bilayer. This allows free movement of water and sodium into the bacterial cell, causing it to burst. Figure 9–5 shows an overview of the actions of the complement system.

Kinins

Bradykinin and kallidin are two of the many kinins present in the body. Kinins are small polypeptides that cause powerful vasodilation. They are especially active in the inflammatory process. The kinin system is linked to the clotting system via the Hageman factor and is activated with the activation of clotting.[7]

The first step in this process is the conversion of Factor XII to Factor XIIa (Fig. 9–6). Factor XIIa converts a substance known as prekallikrein to kallikrein.[7] Kallikrein converts precursor substances known as kininogens to kinins. The most prevalent is kallidin, which is then converted to bradykinin.[7]

Activated kinins cause increased vascular permeability, vasodilation, and smooth muscle contraction. Allergic rhinitis, viral nasal inflammation, and asthma are conditions affected by the activation of the kinin system.[7] The kinins are also responsible for pain (dolor), which is one of the classic signs of inflammation. For example, the kinin system is thought to cause the severe pain in pancreatitis.[7]

Coagulation Cascade

The blood coagulation cascade's major purpose is to stop bleeding. It is also intimately involved in in-

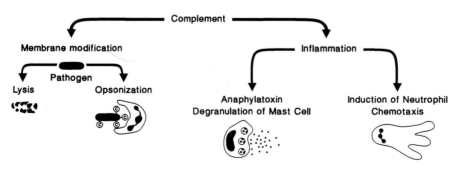

FIGURE 9–5. A diagram of the functions of complement. The primary function of complement is to alter the membranes of pathogens by lysis or opsonization. Additionally, complement components promote inflammation by stimulating histamine release from certain cells and/or by attracting phagocytic cells to an area of inflammation. (From Liszewski MK, Atkinson JP; The Complement System. In Paul WE (ed): *Fundamental Immunology*, 3rd ed. New York, Raven Press, 1993, p 920. Reproduced with permission.)

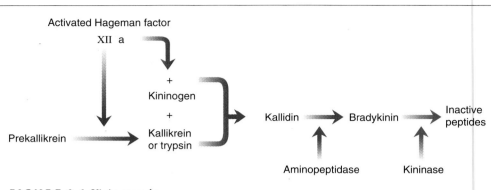

F I G U R E 9–6. Kinin cascade.

flammation and the triggering of the complement and kinin systems. The blood coagulation cascade is comprised of 12 coagulation factors and multiple conversion enzymes. Most of the coagulation factors are synthesized in the liver except for three factors—Factor III comes from any body tissue, Factor VIII is probably produced by vascular endothelial cells, and Factor XIII is most likely secreted by platelets.[7]

The blood coagulation cascade can be initiated by either the intrinsic or extrinsic pathway (see Fig. 13–1). The *intrinsic pathway* is initiated by some internal trauma such as a foreign substance, blood cell damage, or exposure to damaged endothelial cells. This causes activation of Factor XIIa (Hageman factor) and a cascade process that results in Factor X. The *extrinsic pathway* is initiated by blood exposure to injured tissue. Factor III (tissue thromboplastin III), calcium ions, and Factor VII combine to form Factor X.

From Factor X through the development of the fibrin clot, the rest of the blood coagulation pathway is identical. Factor X with calcium ions, phospholipids, and Factor V activates prothrombin to become thrombin. Thrombin with calcium ions activates fibrinogen to become fibrin.

The key linkage between the complement, kinin, and clotting systems is activated Factor XII (Hageman factor). This factor combines with kininogen and prekallikrein to initiate the kinin cascade and joins with

plasminogen to initiate the development of the complement cascade via C1 (Fig. 9–7).

Cytokines

Cytokines are polypeptide signaling molecules that affect the functions of other immune cells by stimulating surface receptors. Cytokines function as immune hormones, communicating when to increase cellular reaction and reproduction and when to suppress reactions in active cells.[9] Cytokines are also called monokines, lymphokines, and interleukins, depending on their cell of origin. Cytokines produced by macrophages and monocytes are called *monokines*. Cytokines produced by lymphocytes are called *lymphokines*. *Interleukins* are produced by a variety of WBC types.

Lymphokines bind to specific receptors on target cells and orchestrate a myriad of other cells and substances, including the elements of the inflammatory response. Lymphokines encourage cell growth, promote cell activation, direct cellular traffic, destroy target cells, and incite macrophages.

Although T-cells are not the only cells that produce cytokines throughout the body, T-cells also produce a number of lymphokines that affect the humoral and cellular immune systems. Lymphokines can act

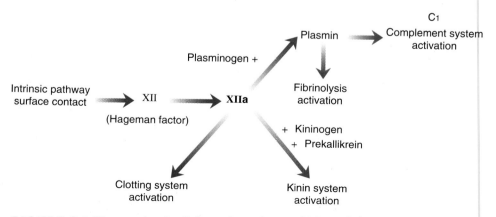

F I G U R E 9–7. Diagram showing linkage of complement, kinin, and clotting systems.

locally or systemically. Some are named for their specific function, such as T-cell growth factor, which increases T-cell production. Other lymphokines can manifest more than one biological property.

Unlike antibodies, lymphokines produced in response to antigens are not specific for that antigen. They amplify the immune system response to the antigen in a nonspecific manner. Lymphokines increase T-cell and B-cell production and maturation and enhance or increase cytolytic, antiviral, and immunologic activities.

One of the first cytokines to be investigated was *interferon*, produced by T-cells, macrophages, and cells outside the immune system. Interferons, a family of proteins, are antiviral in nature. Other cytokines

such as lymphotoxin (from lymphocytes) and tumor necrosis factor (TNF) (from macrophages) kill tumor cells. TNF also inhibits viruses and parasites. Interleukin-1 activates T-cells. Interleukin-2 (IL-2) spurs additional T-cell proliferation and magnifies T-cell response. Other lymphokines are secreted to attract and direct more cells in the response, such as macrophage-activating factor, interleukin-4 (IL-4), and interleukin-6 (IL-6).

Cytokines were initially given descriptive names. These names were later changed as the cytokine's basic structure was identified. This phenomenon of naming and then renaming has caused confusion. Table 9–2 lists the common names and functions of the cytokines.

TABLE 9–2. Cytokines and Their Functions

Immune Modulator	Also Known as	Origin	Function
Interferon-alpha (IFN-α)	Leukocyte Interferon	Secreted by leukocytes and induced by RNA or DNA viruses and by single- or double-stranded polyribonucleotide	Inhibits virus replication; toxic to cancer cells; stimulates leukocytes; facilitates killer cell activity; produces fever; increases B- and T-cell activity
Interferon-beta (IFN-β)	Immune interferon	Secreted by fibroblasts and induced by RNA or DNA viruses and by single- or double-stranded polyribonucleotide	Inhibits virus replication; toxic to cancer cells; facilitates killer cell activity; produces fever
Interferon-gamma (IFN-γ)	Immune interferon	Lymphokine secreted by activated T-cells	Inhibits virus replication; promotes antigen expression; activates macrophages; inhibits cell growth; induces myeloid cell lines
Interleukin-1 (IL-1)	Endogenous pyrogen Lymphocyte-activating factor Leukocyte endogenous mediator Hemopoietin 1	Monokine; mononuclear phagocyte	Stimulates T-cells and macrophages; induces acute phase reaction of inflammation, induces IL-2 secretion, fever production; similar to tumor necrosis factor (TNF) and endogenous pyrogen
Interleukin-2 (IL-2)	T-cell growth factor	Lymphokine secreted mainly by helper T-cells	Promotes the growth of T-cells; enhances function of natural killer (NK) cells; assists T-cell maturation in thymus
Interleukin-3 (IL-3)	Multipotential colony-stimulating factor Mast cell growth factor	Synthesized by T-cells, endothelial cells, fibroblasts, and other cells	Induces proliferation and differentiation of other lymphocytes, pluripotential stem cells, mast cells
Interleukin-4 (IL-4)	B-cell–stimulating factor I (BSF I)	Lymphokine	Promotes T-cell/B-cell interactions; promotes synthesis of IgE by B-cells and T-cell growth; promotes mast cell and hematopoietic cell growth
Interleukin-5 (IL-5)	T-cell replacing factor Eosinophil differentiation factor (BSF II)	Lymphokine secreted by T-cells	Promotes the growth and differentiation of B-cells to secrete IgA; induces differentiation of eosinophils
Interleukin-6 (IL-6)	BSF II Interferon-beta 2 Hepatocyte-stimulating factor (HSF)	Cytokine secreted by mononuclear phagocyte, T-cells, tumors, and nonlymphoid cells (i.e., fibroblasts)	Promotes immunoglobulin secretion by B-cells; induces fever; promotes release of inflammation factors from liver cells; promotes differentiation of hematopoietic stem cells and nerve cells
Lymphotoxin	Cachectin	Protein secreted from T-cells	Kills target cells; 30 percent identical to TNF
Tumor necrosis factor (TNF)	Cachectin	Monokine	Induces leukocytosis, fever, weight loss, inflammation, necrosis of some tumors; stimulates lymphokine synthesis; activates macrophages; toxic to viruses and tumor cells
Macrophage activation factor (MAF)		Leukocytes Fibroblasts	Increases lysomes in macrophages; increases phagocytic activity
Myocardial depressant factor (MDF)		Leukocytes	Decreases cardiac output by decreasing myofibril contractile force

KEY CONCEPTS

- The complement system consists of over 25 plasma proteins that interact in a cascade fashion to produce important mediators of inflammation and immunity. The cascade can be activated by nonspecific antigens (alternative pathway) or by antigen-antibody complexes (classical pathway).

- The most important effector fragments of the complement cascade are C3a, which mediates inflammation; C5a, which is a chemotactic agent; and C6 through C9, the membrane attack complex, which mediates cell lysis.

- Kinins are small peptides that mediate aspects of inflammation, including vasodilation, increased vascular permeability, and pain. Kinin activation is mediated by clotting Factor XIIa.

- The coagulation cascade consists of 12 clotting factors that mediate the formation of fibrin clots. Formation of fibrin clots can be initiated by the intrinsic or extrinsic pathways. Fibrin helps prevent the antigen from disseminating through blood and lymph.

- Cytokines are peptide factors released by immune cells. Cytokines have many functions, including inflammatory mediators, intercellular communication signals, growth factors, and growth inhibitors. Macrophages and lymphocytes are important sources of cytokines.

Nonspecific Immunity and Inflammation

Nonspecific defenses act following external or internal threats such as physical injury or exposure to a foreign material. While they may be selective in differentiating "self" from "nonself," they are not dependent on specific recognition.[2]

Previous exposure to foreign material is not required for the nonspecific defenses to act. The nonspecific defenses include the external barrier of the epithelium; the pH of body fluids, mucus, and bioactive substances; inflammation along with pyrogens and body temperature; phagocytosis; and chemical mediators.

Inflammatory Process

Inflammation is an example of nonspecific defense that occurs in response to tissue injury. Inflammation occurs when cells are injured, regardless of the cause of the injury. It is a protective mechanism that also begins the healing process. The inflammatory response has three purposes: (1) to neutralize and destroy invading and harmful agents, (2) to limit the spread of harmful agents to other tissue, and (3) to prepare any damaged tissue for repair.[10]

Everyone has had the opportunity to become familiar with the inflammatory process on a first-hand basis. Each time you have scratched your arm, cut your finger, or smashed your foot, your body used the inflammatory response to initiate healing. Five cardinal signs of inflammation have been described: (1) redness (rubor), (2) swelling (tumor), (3) heat (calor), (4) pain (dolor), and (5) loss of function (functio laesa). The suffix *-itis* is commonly used to describe conditions that exhibit inflammation. For example, appendicitis, tendinitis, and nephritis refer to inflammation of the appendix, tendon, and kidney, respectively.

There are many causes of inflammation. Any injury to tissue will evoke the inflammatory response. Injury can arise from sources outside the body (exogenous) or from sources inside the body (endogenous).[11] Surgery, trauma, burns, and skin injury from chemicals are all examples of exogenous injuries. Endogenous injuries may result from tissue ischemia such as a myocardial infarction or pulmonary embolism.

Inflammation and infection are commonly confused because they often coexist. Under normal conditions, infection is always accompanied by inflammation; however, not all inflammation involves an infectious agent. For example, inflammation can occur with sprain injuries to joints, myocardial infarction, sterile surgical incisions, thrombophlebitis, and blister formation as a result of either temperature extremes or mechanical trauma. Examples of inflammation that are associated with noninfectious invasion by foreign proteins include allergic rhinitis, some types of contact dermatitis, and other immediate-type allergic reactions. Inflammatory responses that are associated with invasion by pathogens include otitis media, appendicitis, bronchitis, bacterial peritonitis, viral hepatitis, and bacterial myocarditis, among others.

Inflammation may be categorized as either acute or chronic. Acute inflammation is short in duration, lasting less than 2 weeks and involving a discrete set of events. Chronic inflammation tends to be more diffuse, extends over a longer period of time, and may result in the formation of scar tissue and deformity. The inflammatory response is remarkably the same, regardless of the cause. Events in the inflammatory process include (1) chemical responses, (2) vascular responses, and (3) cellular responses (WBC movement and phagocytosis).[12] The inflammatory response is outlined in Figure 9–8.

Chemical Responses

Whenever tissues are injured, chemical mediators are released by activated granulocytes, lymphocytes, and macrophages. These chemicals include histamine, prostaglandins, leukotrienes, cytokines, oxygen radicals, and enzymes. Histamine affects the vascular response by increasing vascular dilation and permeability and allowing fluid to escape from the blood vessels. Prostaglandins are believed to be responsible for the pain associated with inflammation. Cytokines activate and stimulate proliferation of other cells as well as increase lysis of target cells. Enzymes, oxidizing

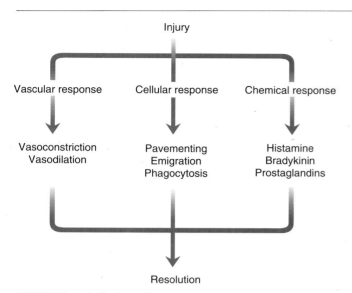

FIGURE 9–8. Outline of the inflammatory response.

agents, and arachidonic acid metabolites attack lipids and proteins, causing cell membrane destruction and digestion of intercellular matrix and protein structures.

Histamine. Histamine is found widely distributed throughout the body. Mast cells and basophils synthesize histamine. During degranulation, large amounts of histamine are released. Histamine is the first chemical mediator in the inflammation response.

Histamine's actions in acute inflammation are mediated by H_1 receptors. Histamine is a potent venous dilator. It also increases the permeability of blood vessel walls by the rounding up of endothelial cells. Histamine allows fluid exudation from the vascular space. Histamine also causes bronchial constriction and mucus production.

Arachidonic Acid Metabolites. Arachidonic acid metabolites include prostaglandins, leukotrienes, thromboxanes, and endogenous pyrogen (EP). Arachidonic acid metabolites are phospholipid compounds metabolized from stored arachidonic acid in the cell membrane.

Prostaglandins arise from the cyclooxygenase pathway.[4] Prostaglandins involved in inflammation contribute to vasodilation, increased permeability, and platelet aggregation. They produce more erythema than histamine.[13] Prostaglandin D_2 also acts as a chemotactic factor and stimulates neutrophil skin infiltration. Prostaglandins also cause pain by enhancing the sensitivity of pain endings.[14]

Five types of leukotrienes are generated from the lipoxygenase pathway: leukotriene A_4 (LTA_4), leukotriene B_4 (LTB_4), leukotriene C_4 (LTC_4), leukotriene D_4 (LTD_4), and leukotriene E_4 (LTE_4). LTA_4, an unstable 5,6-epoxy derivative, is enzymatically converted to LTB_4. LTB_4 is a potent chemotactic agent that causes aggregation of leukocytes; LTC_4, LTD_4, and LTE_4 all cause smooth muscle contractility, bronchospasm, and increased vascular permeability.

Enzymes. Granulocytes and macrophages secrete a wide variety of enzymes that digest protein structures. Some of these enzymes include lysozyme, lactoferrin, cationic proteins, neutral proteases, collagenase, elastase, and acid hydrolases. Neutrophils and macrophages specialize in collagen and intercellular matrix degradation or digestion. Peptide bonds are cleaved in the intercellular matrix by collagenase, elastase, proteinase, and gelatinase.[2]

Oxidizing agents are the most destructive of all cell enzymes or toxins.[2] These oxidizing agents are formed as a result of the NADPH oxidase enzyme system that lies on the plasma membrane of the neutrophil.[2] Neutrophils are capable of synthesizing and assailing microorganisms with these oxidizing agents, which include the following oxygen radicals: superoxide (O_2^-), hydrogen peroxide (H_2O_2), and hydroxyl ions (OH^-). Oxidizing agents directly attack cell membranes, increasing permeability (Fig. 9–9).

Acute Vascular Response

Immediately after injury the precapillary arterioles around the injured area constrict due to tissue damage.[10] This vasoconstriction period lasts from 2 seconds up to 5 or 10 minutes[12,15] and produces tissue hypoxia and acidosis.[14] The amount of vasoconstriction depends on the degree of vascular injury.

Mast cells in the area of injury degranulate with the release of chemical mediators, particularly histamine. One of the early actions of the mediators is to cause endothelial cells to begin contraction and rounding up. Following vasoconstriction, there is a period of arteriolar vasodilation. An increased number of capillaries are involved in carrying blood at this time.[16] Because of the dilated blood vessels and open capillaries, more blood is carried to the injured area, resulting in the redness, pain, and heat of inflammation.

The greater volume of blood increases the amount of pressure within the blood vessels (hydrostatic pressure). The increased pressure actually pushes fluid out of the blood vessels and into the surrounding tissues.

During this period, platelets move into the site and adhere to exposed vascular collagen. The platelets release fibronectin to form a meshwork trap and stimulate the intrinsic clotting cascade to help reduce bleeding. Platelets release a number of peptide growth factors, including platelet-derived growth factor (PDGF), transforming growth factor-beta (TGF-β), epidermal growth factor (EGF), and insulin-like growth factor (IGF-I).[17] PDGF stimulates fibroblastic cell proliferation. IGF-I is a potent vascular endothelial cell chemotactic factor and increases neovascularization.[17] The blood coagulation cascade is also triggered, leading to the formation of a fibrin clot. Usually early clot formation occurs within several minutes.

At the same time, venous capillaries become more permeable due to the chemical mediators released—allowing more fluid to leak into the sur-

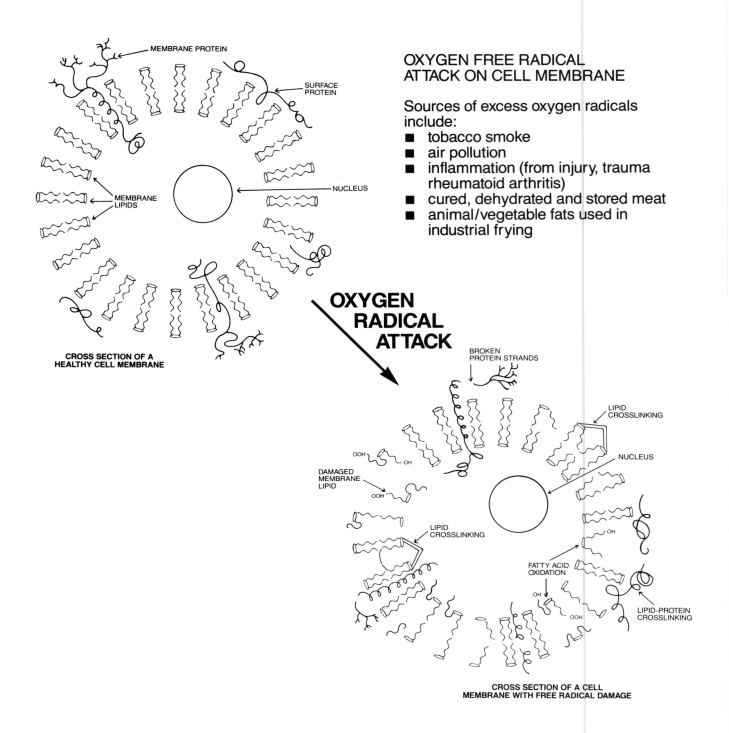

OXYGEN FREE RADICAL
ATTACK ON CELL MEMBRANE

Sources of excess oxygen radicals
include:
- tobacco smoke
- air pollution
- inflammation (from injury, trauma
  rheumatoid arthritis)
- cured, dehydrated and stored meat
- animal/vegetable fats used in
  industrial frying

Oxygen radicals are extremely reactive and short-lived by-products of body metabolism capable of damaging living tissue. Oxygen free radicals can attack cell membranes, causing damage to lipids and proteins. They cause oxidation of lipids (lipid peroxides—fats chemically altered by oxygen radicals that are unable to perform normal cellular functions). This process can impair a cell's ability to function or even destroy it.

FIGURE 9–9. How oxygen radicals cause tissue injury. (Courtesy of the Upjohn Company.)

rounding tissue. In addition to redness and heat, these chemical changes and fluid leakage are responsible for pain and impaired function. During this time, fibrin is also deposited in the lymph system, causing lymphatic blockage.[10] The above changes are responsible for the swelling found with inflammation. This lymphatic blockage "walls off" the area of inflammation from the surrounding tissue and delays the spread of toxins.[8]

The vascular changes that occur soon after injury are beneficial to the injured tissue because irritating or toxic agents are diluted by the fluid that leaks out of the blood vessels into surrounding tissue. Additionally, when the fluid leaves the blood vessels, the remaining blood becomes viscous (thick) and circulation is slowed.

Acute Cellular Response

As the blood flow slows, neutrophils move to the sides of the blood vessels lining the endothelium of the vessels. This process is referred to as *margination* or *pavementing*. By lining the edges of the blood vessels, neutrophils are better able to move out of the vessels and into the tissues.[8,15]

Once margination and the rounding up of endothelial cells have occurred, neutrophils can squeeze out of the blood vessels. The neutrophils are thus free to travel to the inflamed tissue. This process of passing through the blood vessel walls and migrating to the inflamed tissue is referred to as *emigration* or *diapedesis*. Diapedesis begins within a few minutes to hours of injury. Even though the pores lining the vessels are much smaller than the neutrophils, the neutrophils are able to slide through a small portion at a time.[14]

Neutrophils are attracted to the inflamed tissue by a process called **chemotaxis.** Biochemical mediators that attract the neutrophils include bacterial toxins, degenerative products of the inflamed tissue, the C5a complement fragment, and other substances.[14] Neutrophils are thus guided through the tissue to an area of injury by these chemicals. Because neutrophils are highly mobile, they are first on the scene to begin phagocytosis and producing collagenase to break down dead tissue. Neutrophils also liberate endogenous pyrogens, which contributes to the development of fever.

Eosinophils also respond to the site of inflammation. They are especially helpful during parasitic infections. They are rich in chemical mediators such as hydrolases and perioxidases. However, they often act to limit or control the extent of the inflammation.

Chronic Cellular Response

Features that signal the beginning of the chromic cellular response are the dominance of macrophages and the appearance of fibroblasts and lymphocytes. Macrophages are essential for wound healing because of their phagocytosis and debridement functions. Macrophages produce a variety of chemical media-

tors—proteases, interferon, prostaglandins. Proteases help to remove foreign protein from the wound. Macrophages also release tissue thromboplastin to facilitate hemostasis and stimulate fibroblast activity. Macrophages secrete other peptide growth factors, such as angiogenic factor, which encourages neovascularization. This angiogenic factor causes endothelial cells and new vessels to form in the inflamed area.

Lymphocytes also move into the inflamed area to regulate macrophages, and stimulate B-cells should they be necessary. Typically, granulation tissue is formed.[15]

Healing

Inflammatory responses can terminate or be resolved in several ways over time. Usually the reconstructive phase begins 3 to 4 days after injury and persists for 2 weeks. The major cells involved in this phase include fibroblasts, endothelial cells, and myofibroblasts.

Fibroblasts are found all over the body and are thought to originate in mesenchymal primitive tissue. They synthesize connective tissue and are able to migrate. Fibroblasts are stimulated to make collagen, proteoglycans, and fibronectin by lactate, ascorbic acid, low oxygen, and an acid pH (7.2).[15] Macrophages secrete lactate and release growth factors that stimulate fibroblasts. Fibroblasts are subject to contact and density inhibition, allowing for orderly cellular growth. Myofibroblasts develop at the wound edge and provide for wound contraction.

Collagen consists of different types of fibrous glycoproteins and is the most plentiful protein in the body.[18] These differences in glycoprotein give structure to dissimilar tissues. Of all of the types of glycoproteins, four categories have been well defined. Type I collagen comprises 90 percent of body collagen.[18] Type I is associated with collagen fibrils and results in skin, bones, tendons, ligaments, cornea, and internal organs. Type II collagen consists of thinner collagen fibrils and high amounts of carbohydrate and hydroxylysine. It results in cartilage, intervertebral disks, notochord, and the vitreous body of the eye.[18] Type III collagen has fibrils that are associated with skin, blood vessels, and internal organs.[18] Type IV collagen produces a sheetlike meshwork that is associated with basement membranes (basal laminae).[18]

Endothelial cells grow into the connective tissue gel stimulated by angiogenic substance. They usually develop capillary beds from existing vessels. The new capillaries are able to bring in nutrients for tissue repair and wound healing. However, because the new capillaries are leaky, they contribute to continuing edema.

Regeneration of lost tissue into the same tissue type requires survival of the basement membrane and the ability to regenerate. Some cell types regenerate constantly; among these types are the epithelial cells of the skin and mucous membranes, bone marrow cells, and lymphoid cells. Cells of the liver, pancreas, endocrine glands, and renal tubules are also able to regenerate when necessary. However, some permanent cells are unable to regenerate at all, such as neurons and muscle cells.

The maturation phase of wound healing occurs several weeks after the injury and may last for 2 years or more. It is characterized by wound remodeling by fibroblasts, macrophages, neutrophils, and eosinophils. Wound remodeling is the process of collagen deposition and lysis with debridement of the wound edges. During this phase the wound changes color, from bright red to pink to whitish. As long as a wound is pink, the maturation phase is not completed.

Inflammatory Exudates

Exudate is fluid that leaks out of the blood vessels combined with the neutrophils and the debris from phagocytosis. Exudate may vary in composition, but all types have similar functions. These functions include (1) transport of leukocytes and antibodies, (2) dilution of toxins and irritating substances, and (3) the transport of nutrients necessary for tissue repair.

Serous exudate is watery, has a low protein content, and is similar to the fluid that collects under a blister. This type of exudate generally accompanies mild inflammation. With mild inflammation the permeability of the blood vessels is not greatly changed. As a result, only some protein molecules escape from the vessels. Because many molecules do not leave the blood vessels, serous exudate (with low protein content) develops.

With a greater injury, more inflammation occurs, and the blood vessels become more permeable. Because of this increased permeability, more protein is able to pass through the vessel walls. Fibrinogen, a large protein molecule, is able to pass through a highly permeable blood vessel wall. *Fibrinous exudate* is sticky and thick. A fibrinous exudate may need to be removed to allow healing; otherwise scar tissue and adhesions may develop. In some instances, however, fibrinous exudate may be beneficial. In the case of acute appendicitis, fibrinous exudate may actually wall off and localize the infection and prevent its spread.

Purulent exudate is called pus. Purulent exudate generally occurs in severe inflammation accompanied by infection. Purulent exudate is primarily composed of leukocytes (particularly neutrophils), protein, and tissue debris. Purulent exudate generally must be removed or drained for healing to take place.

Hemorrhagic exudate has a large component of red blood cells. This type of exudate is usually present with the severest inflammation. Hemorrhagic exudate occurs when there is severe leakage from blood vessels or when there is necrosis or breakdown of blood vessels.

Systemic Manifestations of Inflammation

Inflammation is associated with both localized and systemic signs and symptoms. The localized symptoms, described previously, occur with both acute and chronic inflammation. Depending on the magnitude of injury and the resistance of the individual, localized inflammation can lead to systemic involvement, which was covered in Chapter 8. They include an elevation in body temperature (fever is almost universal in severe inflammation), leukocytosis, and an elevated erythrocyte sedimentation rate.

KEY CONCEPTS

- Previous exposure to foreign antigens is not required for activation of nonspecific immune defenses. Inflammation is an important part of nonspecific immunity that localizes harmful agents and brings phagocytic cells to the area. Classic manifestations of inflammation are redness, swelling, heat, pain, and loss of function.
- Inflammatory chemicals such as histamine, prostaglandins, and leukotrienes are released primarily from injured tissues, mast cells, macrophages, and neutrophils. These chemicals increase vascular permeability, vasodilate, and attract immune cells to the area (chemotaxis). White cells also release proteolytic enzymes and oxidizing agents to destroy and digest antigens.
- The acute vascular response to injury begins with temporary vasoconstriction, followed by prolonged vasodilation. Vasodilation is accompanied by increased permeability and filtration of fluid into localized tissues. Activation of platelets and fibrin clot formation plugs localized vessels and lymphatics, preventing spread of inflammation.
- During the acute cellular phase of inflammation, leukocytes migrate to the inflamed area, collect at the side of the vessel, and squeeze through into the tissue. Neutrophils arrive in large numbers and begin active phagocytosis. With chronic inflammation, macrophages and lymphocytes predominate.
- Healing is mediated by growth factors released from platelets and immune cells that stimulate fibroblasts to divide and manufacture extracellular matrix proteins. Endothelial cells respond to angiogenic growth factors by forming capillary networks.
- Inflammatory exudates function to transport immune cells, antibodies, and nutrients to the tissue and dilute the offending substances. Serous exudate is watery and low in protein; fibrinous exudate is thick, sticky, and high in protein; purulent exudate contains infective organisms, leukocytes, and cellular debris; and hemorrhagic exudate contains red blood cells.

Specific Immunity

Adaptive resistance (or specific defense) is an essential component in mammal immune systems and is seen only in vertebrates. Therefore, it is a more recent evolutionary immunologic development. **Adaptive resis-**

tance has the characteristics of *specificity, memory, mobility, replicability,* and *cooperativity.*[5] In other words, the adaptive immune system is specific, discriminating, and involves antigen memory. The components of adaptive resistance can distinguish between self and nonself. These components can increase their response to a remembered antigen, but they must be stimulated to become active. However, on first exposure to antigen, the specific defense may take up to 7 days to gear up.

The cellular components of the system can circulate throughout the body and interact with other cells. Sell in 1987 outlined the functional abilities of the adaptive immune system as (1) specific recognition of foreign invaders, (2) rapid synthesis and delivery of immune products to infection sites, (3) differentiation and direction of specific action against nonself foreign invaders, and (4) deactivation mechanisms.[12]

Overview of the Self-Nonself Recognition System

Immune tolerance is the ability of the immune system to recognize a person's own cells ("self") as well as limit lymphocyte response. During maturation, every lymphocyte develops receptors that recognize certain molecular sequences.[19] Immune tolerance relies on cell receptor recognition—the capability of lymphocytes to recognize cell-surface receptors for self.[19-21] Unfortunately, the difference between "self" and "nonself" is not always clear.[19] If antigen-binding receptors interact with self antigens on the host cell, the lymphocyte does not survive. The inability to clearly distinguish self, an autoimmune response, is discussed further in Chapter 10.

There are several theories regarding the development of tolerance. The *clonal deletion* or *suicide theory* was developed by Joshua Lederberg of Rockefeller University in 1959.[22] Lederberg suggested that immature T-cells recognizing antigen might die. He postulated that immature T-cells recognizing self products would die or be destroyed. This theory appears to have the most research support in recent investigations by the National Jewish Center for Immunology and Respiratory Medicine in Denver.

Other theories include the clonal selection theory, clonal anergy or clonal silencing theory, antigen blockade theories, and T-suppressor cell theory. The clonal selection theory was developed in the 1950s by F. M. Burnet at the University of Melbourne.[19] This theory was developed to explain the reason why most people do not exhibit autoimmune diseases. Burnet suggested that antibodies were genetically determined and did not develop in response to a specific antigen presentation.[20] When exposed to an antigen, antibodies are selected that "match" the antigen and are rapidly cloned. He felt that all self antigen clones are destroyed before birth, leaving only foreign-reacting clones.

The clonal anergy or clonal silencing theory was developed by Nossal and others. This theory suggests that antigen contact during T-cell and B-cell differentiation is one of the major causes of immune tolerance.[20,21] Nossal believes that differentiating lymphocytes undergo a tolerance-sensitive phase in which exposure to antigens causes receptor downregulation that produces tolerance and not immunity.[22] These cells are hyporeactive and do not react to the antigen to which they were exposed. Nossal also indicates that premature lymphocytes may be purged through clonal abortion before they become immunocompetent.[21] He suggests that T-suppressor cells may be involved in destroying antiself T-cells that escape the thymus.[21]

The antigen blockade theories submit that B-cell receptors are blocked by specific types of antigens. These antigens patch or cap the receptors so that they are frozen or prevented from functioning normally. The T-suppressor theory states that suppressor T-cells actively work to contain autoimmune responses in the body.[22]

Major Histocompatibility Complex

Recognition of "foreign" or "antigen" mandates that the system also recognize self. This involves genes on chromosome 6 known as the **major histocompatibility complex** (MHC) genes.[11] In humans, the MHC is also known as **human lymphocyte antigen** (HLA) complex. The MHC molecules are the same in all of a person's cells but differ in structure from person to person.[23] Two classes of MHC important in immunology are class I and class II. Class I molecules are glycoproteins found on the surface of all tissue cells. Class II molecules are only found on certain cells, including B-cells, antigen-presenting cells (monocytes and macrophages), and some activated T-cells. Expression of class II molecules on other types of cells may predispose to certain autoimmune diseases.[24]

MHC molecules are also associated with disease states as indicators of disease. As an infected cell degrades bacteria or virus into small protein fragments (peptides), these peptides are linked to recently synthesized class I MHC molecules in the cell's endoplasmic reticulum.[23] These MHC molecules transport the peptides to the cell surface for immune system recognition.[23] In other words, the altered MHC molecules act to signal infection or disease on the cell's surface. In order for cytotoxic, killer T-cells to kill an infected cell, it must be marked with a class I molecule bound with a foreign peptide.[23]

For this reason, MHC class I molecules are important considerations in transplantation. MHC histocompatibility must be present or graft rejection will occur. Therefore, parents and siblings with MHC-identical markers make the best tissue matches.

MHC class II molecules can also display or mark diseased cells, but they do so in a different manner. Class II MHC molecules are found in macrophages and B-cells and do not stimulate killer T-cells.[23] The class II MHC molecules bind to foreign peptides contained in the antigen-presenting cell and move to the surface for recognition by helper T-cells.[23] The helper T-cells then stimulate or activate the presenting cell.

T-Cell Development and Function

T-cell differentiation and maturation are regulated by the thymus. For this reason, T-cells are called thymus-derived lymphocytes. Within the thymus, pre-T-cells become lymphoblasts, which mature into prolymphocytes. Thymic hormones such as thymosin, thymopoietin, thymic humoral factor, and thymulin, secreted by the endocrine epithelial cells in the thymus, are responsible for the development of T-cell subpopulations. Only T-cells with MHC class I or class II receptors on their surface survive to maturity.[6]

T-cells are responsible for cellular immunity with effector and regulatory functions. T-cell subpopulations include memory cells, regulatory cells, and effector cells. *Memory T-cells* remain sensitized to one antigen and circulate in small numbers. With reexposure to their specific antigen, they clone rapidly and circulate in large numbers. They are T-cell memory banks which speed up and enhance the immune response. *Regulatory T-cells* include helper (T4 or CD4) and suppressor (T8) cells. *Effector T-cells* (CD8) include cytoxic T-cells and and killer T-cells. These cells are capable of directly reacting to infected or mutant (neoplastic) cells.

Helper T-Cells

Helper (CD4) T-cells recognize antigens that have been processed and presented to them via antigen-processing cells such as B-cells or macrophages. In response to activation, CD4 cells secrete lymphokines that call B-cells and other inflammatory cells to the sites of infection and stimulate functioning B-cells to manufacture antibodies. Some helper T-cell subgroups have been found to be involved in the infiltration of tumors with antitumor activity.[15] CD4 T-cells have receptors that bind with MHC class II molecules. Without helper (T4) cells, the immune system is not effective.

Suppressor T-Cells

Suppressor cells (T8) inhibit the actions of helper T-cells and B-cells. Suppressor cells help keep the helper T-cells and other immune system cells in check. Suppressor cells may be factors in self-tolerance and acquired immunologic tolerance. It may be the balance between helper and suppressor cells that keeps the immune system functioning normally.

Cytotoxic and Killer T-Cells

Killer T-cells have receptors for MHC class I molecules. Killer cells phagocytize or ingest target cells. Cytotoxic cells lyse or kill target cells. Specifically, cytotoxic cells attach to the foreign cell and directly rupture the cell membrane, improve phagocytic actions (opsonization), and make cells more vulnerable to chemical attack via production of lymphokines.

KEY CONCEPTS

- Specific immunity refers to functions of B- and T-lymphocytes. Each lymphocyte recognizes and reacts to only one particular antigen. On initial exposure to an antigen, lymphocytes undergo clonal expansion so that there are many lymphocytes throughout the body that can recognize and react to that particular antigen. These cells are called memory cells. Subsequent exposure results in a much faster and larger lymphocyte response.

- T- and B-lymphocytes are believed to react only with foreign antigens. Lymphocytes capable of reacting with self tissues are thought to be destroyed or permanently inactivated during fetal development. One theory suggests that lymphocytes must come in contact with all self antigens during fetal development, and those that do not specifically bind self are allowed to survive. MHC proteins on cell surfaces are important markers for self—each person has unique MHC protein structures.

- T-lymphocytes are only able to bind antigens when they are presented on the surface of cells. Cytotoxic T-cells (CD8+) react to cells that express foreign MHC class I proteins on their surface. Helper T-cells (CD4+) bind to cells that express altered MHC class II proteins on their surface. MHC class II proteins are found on antigen-presenting cells (B-cells and macrophages). These cells engulf foreign antigens and combine the antigens with MHC class II proteins on their cell surface. Any helper T-cell having the right receptor to bind the MHC-antigen complex is activated. Activated T-cells proliferate and secrete cytokines.

- T-cells, which mature in the thymus, have subgroups including helper, cytotoxic, and suppressor T-cells. Helper T-cells perform a central role in specific immunity. Activation of helper T-cells results in secretion of cytokines necessary for clonal expansion of T- and B-lymphocytes. Cytotoxic T-cells locate and lyse abnormal cells. Suppressor T-cells are thought to nonspecifically inhibit the immune response.

B-Cell Development and Function

In birds, B-cell differentiation and maturation are regulated by the bursa. Humans have no bursa, so the term *bursa equivalent* is used. The bursa equivalent is not a specific organ in the human body. It is hypothesized to include primarily bone marrow, lymphoid organs, the fetal liver, and/or tissues in the gastrointestinal tract. Within the bursa equivalent, pre-B-cells become lymphoblasts that mature into prolymphocytes. Once B-cells leave the bursa equivalent, they aggregate in lymph nodes and the spleen.

B-cells are responsible for antibody (humoral)-mediated immunity. B-cells have two subpopulations, memory cells and plasma cells. Memory B-cells contain antigen receptors and function like memory T-cells. In other words, memory of the initial antigen is stored in memory B-cells. When exposed to the same type of antigen in the future, these memory B-cells are able to respond with appropriate antibodies.

Plasma cells differentiate from B-cells on antigen stimulation and activation. When foreign antigen is carried to the lymphoid tissues, it causes a clone of antigen-specific B-cells to differentiate into plasma cells. The plasma cells then synthesize and secrete a single antibody or immunoglobulin with one kind of light and heavy chain.[23] These antibodies then bind to the antigen, usually one molecule on the surface of the virus or bacteria. Therefore, each antibody is specific for one antigen.

Antigen Recognition and Presentation

Antigen is a term used to define materials that evoke an immune response. An **antigen** can be a bacterium, a virus, a fungus, a parasite, mutated cells, transplanted tissue, foreign protein, or a part or product of one of these materials.

Immune response specificity occurs because lymphocytes have specific receptors on their cell surfaces that combine with only one particular antigen. An antigen expresses its "foreignness" by characteristic shapes called *epitopes* (parts of molecules that are often unique to that organism), also known as **antigenic determinants,** which protrude from its surface. *Paratopes*, also known as antibody-combining sites, are the parts of antibodies that combine with the epitopes on the identified antigen (Fig. 9–10).

Antigen recognition and processing allow both specificity of response and memory of the antigen. These two components, specificity and memory, are key elements of effective immunity.

Antibodies or Immunoglobulins

Antibodies or immunoglobulins are structurally related glycoproteins that form the basis of humoral-mediated immunity. Antibodies can function in a

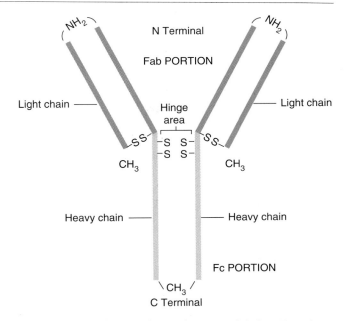

FIGURE 9–11. Structural unit of immunoglobulin. The Fab portion, or the amino ends of the polypeptide chains, binds to antigens specifically. This antigen-binding ability is primarily due to the behavior of the light chains. The hinge area gives the immunoglobulin molecule flexibility. The angle of the arms of the Y can range from 0 to 180 degrees. The Fc portion or carboxy end of the polypeptide chains mediates biological activity by binding to other immune cells, phagocytic cells, platelets, and components of the complement system.

variety of ways. Antibodies can act as antitoxins by neutralizing bacterial toxins. This antitoxin function works by preventing binding of toxins to tissue cells or by capturing the toxin, allowing it to be surrounded by phagocytic cells that provide lysis. Antibodies also function in the neutralization of viruses. In this process, antibodies either prevent the binding of viruses to host tissues or they bind to the antigen, causing an agglutination reaction. Antibodies can unleash the complement cascade, causing cell lysis.

Some antibodies can **opsonize** bacteria. In this situation, antibodies help macrophages recognize bacteria by coating bacterial antigens. Macrophages have receptors for the antibody tails (Fc), which help them attach to the bacteria and improve the efficiency of phagocytosis. The process is called **opsonization,** and the antibodies are called **opsonins.** Antibodies can thus make the inflammatory process more specific.

Immunoglobulin genes possess a high degree of variability necessary for developing a tremendous number of different antibodies with antigen-specific, three-dimensional binding sites. Each immunoglobulin molecule contains two identical light polypeptide chains joined by disulfide bonds to two identical heavy polypeptide chains. The geometry of the relationship between the heavy (H) and light (L) chains forms a Y-like structure. The H chains form the stem of the Y and the L chains are on the outside of the arms of the Y. The H chain structure differs between classes of immunoglobulins and determines their class and subclass. Figure 9–11 shows the basic structural

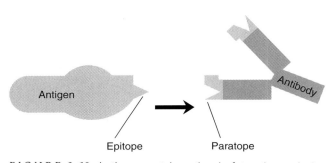

FIGURE 9–10. Antigens contain antigenic determinants (epitopes), and antibodies contain antibody combining sites (paratopes).

TABLE 9–3. Diagram and Properties of Immunoglobulin Classes

Property	IgG1	IgG2	IgG3	IgG4	IgA1	IgA2	sIgA	IgM	IgD	IgE
Half-life (days)	23–25				6			5	3	2.5
Percent total immunoglobulin	80%				13%			6%	0–1%	0.002%
Molecular wt (daltons)	146,000	146,000	170,000	146,000	160,000	160,000	385,000	900,000	184,000	200,000
Complement fixation	++	+	+++	0	–	–	–	+++	–	–
Placental transfer	+++	++	+++	++	–	–	–	–	–	–
Receptor for macrophage	+++	0	+++	0	–	–	–	–	–	–
Reaction with staph protein A	+++	+++	0	+++	–	–	–	–	–	–
Passive cutaneous anaphylaxis	+++	0	+++	+++	–	–	–	–	–	+
Transported across epithelium	–	–	–	–	+	+	+	Occasionally	–	–
Prominent antibody activity	Anti-Rh against infections	Antilevan, antidextran	Anti-Rh	Anti-XIII	Against infections	Against infections	Against infections	ABO isoagglutinins rheumatoid factor	Binds to B-cells in presence of IgM	Mast cell sensitization cytophilic antibody skin sensitizing antibody
Cell binding functions:										
Mononuclear cells	+	–	+	–	–	–	–	–	–	?/+
Neutrophils	+	–	+	+	+	+	+	–	–	–
Mast cells/basophils	–	–	–	?	+	+	+	+	+	+++
T-cells/B-cells	+	+	+	+	–	+	+	+	+	+
Platelets	+	+	+	+	–	–	–	+	–	?

Data from Roitt IM: *Essential Immunology*, 7th ed. Oxford, Blackwell Scientific Publications, 1991; Sell S: *Immunology, Immunopathology and Immunity*, 4th ed. Amsterdam, Elsevier, 1987; Widmann FK: *An Introduction to Clinical Immunology*. Philadelphia, F. A. Davis, 1989 unit of immunoglobulin. This structural geometry allows each end of the molecule to have different functions.

Immunoglobulins are differentiated into five classes: IgG, IgM, IgA, IgD, and IgE. These immunoglobulins differ one from another, even though they have the same basic structural unit. Table 9–3 gives the structure and properties of immunoglobulin classes.

IgG is the most common type of immunoglobulin, accounting for 70 percent to 75 percent of all immunoglobulins. It is found in nearly equal proportions in the intravascular and intercellular compartments and has a long half-life of 23 days. It is composed of four subclasses: IgG1, IgG2, IgG3, and IgG4. The subclasses are differentiated on the basis of the number of interchain disulphide bonds and differing H chains. They have differing biological properties. The basic diagram of IgG is the Y structure.

IgM composes 10 percent of immunoglobulins and is predominantly found in the intravascular pool. Small amounts of IgM are also found in mucosal secretions such as tears, mucus, sputum, and gastrointestinal secretions.[14] It has a half-life of 5 days. IgM is the first immunoglobulin class produced by fetuses.[12] It is also the first immunoglobulin to be produced on exposure to antigens or after immunization. IgM is the major antibody found on B-cell surfaces.[25] IgM is the antibody class that is best in fixing complement, which is important for cytotoxic functions in the immune system.[12] It is important to note that only one molecule of IgM is needed to fix complement, while two molecules of IgG are needed to do the same thing. IgM is a very large molecule with a pentameter geometry.

IgA is the major immunoglobulin found in external or mucous secretions and composes 15 percent to 20 percent of the immunoglobulin pool. It has a short half-life of 5 days. It is primarily found in saliva, tears, tracheobronchial secretions, colostrum, milk, and gastrointestinal and genitourinary secretions.[25] IgA has three identified subclasses: IgA1, IgA2, and secretory IgA (sIgA). SIgA is the type most commonly found in mucous secretions. It is one of the body's first defenders against antigens and is especially important in antiviral protection.[25] IgA has a double Y geometry connected by a J chain, an extra protein called a transport piece or secretory component. This transport piece, produced by glandular or secretory mucosal cells, protects sIgA from proteolysis and facilitates IgA secretion into external fluids.

IgD is only a trace serum immunoglobulin (<1 percent) but is found on the membrane of circulating and/or immature B-cells along with IgM. It has a half-life of 3 days. Little is known about its function. It is thought to be a cellular antigen receptor acting against such antigens as insulin, penicillin, milk proteins, diphtheria toxoid, nuclear antigens, and thyroid antigens.[25] IgD, when bound with antigen, stimulates the B-cell to multiply, differentiate, and secrete other specific immunoglobulins.

IgE is found on the surface membrane of basophils and mast cells. Only trace amounts of IgE are identified in the serum. IgE has a half-life of 2.5 days. It plays a role in immunity against helminthic parasites and is responsible for initiating inflammatory reactions, allergic reactions, and hypersensitivity diseases (i.e., asthma, hay fever). Specifically, IgE causes mast cells to release a variety of active substances, including histamine, serotonin, and leukotrienes (slow-reacting substance of anaphylaxis).

B- and T-Cell Interdependence

When a new antigen is presented to the immune system, it takes the components of the immune system some time to organize a response. First, the antigen enters the body via the blood, skin, mucous membranes, or peritoneum. Then one of two processes can occur: either B-cells and suppressor T-cells are directly activated by antigen, a process called **T-cell-independent activation,** or the antigen is presented by B-cells or macrophages to helper T-cells, which then stimulate B-cell production of antibodies in a process called **T-cell-dependent activation.**[20]

T-cell-independent activation occurs with some soluble antigens. The B-cell response generally is not strong, and immunogenic memory is decreased. An antigen generally associated with T-cell-independent activation is dextran, a polysaccharide polymer.

T-cell-dependent activation involves antigen-presenting macrophages or other antigen-presenting cells such as B-cells. Antigen-presenting macrophages are located in strategic places to interdict antigens: in lymph nodes, spleen, bone marrow, Kupffer cells (liver), pleura, peritoneum, Langerhans cells (skin), and alveoli.

The antigen enters the macrophages via endocytosis and is processed by the macrophage (Fig. 9–12A). After the macrophage takes in the antigen, it digests it and binds a peptide fragment of the antigen to a class II MHC molecule. The MHC class II molecule then moves to the cell surface, where it displays the antigen fragments. Still bound to the antigen fragment is the MHC molecule needed for the T-cell to recognize the antigen. Helper T-cells look for antigen bound to class II MHC molecules. The macrophage places the MHC proteins containing the antigen determinant on its surface. This way, helper T-cells can recognize both self and antigen.

It is important to note that most T-cells must go through this antigen-presenting process in order to effectively respond to the infection. While the antigen presentation is taking place, the macrophage also secretes biologically active molecules that regulate the growth and differentiation of lymphocytes.

Next, helper T-cells combine with the MHC II and "antigen" on the macrophages. The T-helper cells stimulate the formation of T-memory cells and activate specific B-cells. Then, B-cells form plasma cells that secrete antibodies and memory cells that "remember" the antigen, allowing for a quicker response in the future (Fig. 9–12*B*).

Passive and Active Immunity

The immune response is due to specificity and memory by specific defenses. For each individual, immunity may be achieved actively or passively.

Passive Immunity

Passive immunity involves the humoral immune system. It includes the passive transfer of plasma (sera) containing preformed antibodies to a specific antigen from a protected or an immunized person to an unprotected or nonimmunized person. It is indicated in the following situations: (1) B-cell immunodeficiencies, (2) exposure of persons with high susceptibility to a disease without time for active immunization, or (3) when antibody injection may alleviate or suppress the effects of an antigenic toxin.[26]

This passive transfer of antibodies can occur in a variety of ways. In the fetus, IgG1 and IgG3 are the only maternal antibodies that can cross the placental barrier. Most of the time, these antibodies are beneficial and assist the newborn in resisting antigens, based on maternal exposure. However, these antibodies can be damaging to the fetus, as is the case in hemolytic disease of the newborn.

Antibodies, complement, and macrophage functions are deficient at birth. Besides maternal IgG1 and IgG3 received in utero, newborns receive IgA antibodies through breast milk. The infant's immature gastrointestinal tract and low proteolytic enzyme activity do not destroy all protein, which allows some of the IgA antibodies to be absorbed. These antibodies assist the infant in defending against bacterial and viral infections during infancy. It has been hypothesized by some researchers that IgA antibodies in breast milk "modify the ways that proteins cross the infant's highly permeable intestinal mucosa and thereby cause breast-fed infants to have fewer food allergies in later life."[8]

Another method of passive immunity is by direct injection of antibodies into an unprotected person. This is called serotherapy. The unprotected individual can receive a variety of substances, including immune globulin (human) such as IgG; specific immune globulins like hepatitis B immune globulin (human) or rabies immune globulin (human); and human plasma containing all antibodies or animal antibodies such as diphtheria antitoxin, tetanus antitoxin, botulism antitoxin, and antirabies serum.

Human immune globulin contains mostly IgG with traces of IgA and IgM. It is a sterile, concentrated protein solution that contains antibodies from the pooled plasma of many adults. It can be given intramuscularly or intravenously, depending on the product. Although these antibodies contain foreign proteins, they rarely are the cause of an adverse immune response.

Human immune globulins are used as *prophylaxis* against hepatitis A and measles and as *therapy* for the following conditions: antibody deficiency disorders, Kawasaki disease, pediatric AIDS, or hypogammaglo-

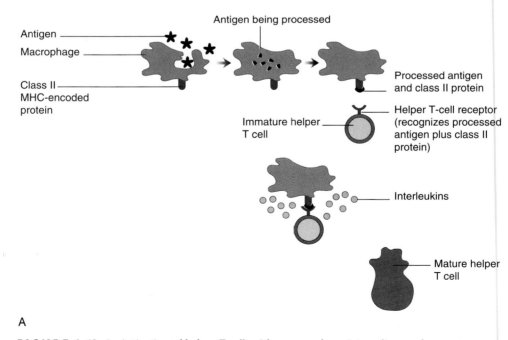

A

FIGURE 9–12. **A,** Activation of helper T-cells. After macrophage internalizes and processes antigen, it presents antigen fragments on its surface. Antigen combined with class II protein attracts helper T-cell; interleukins help T-cell mature.

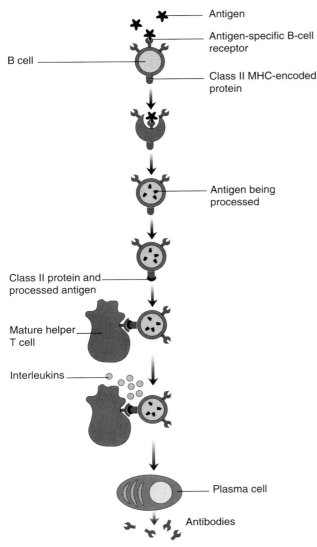

B cell

Antigen

Antigen-specific B-cell receptor

Class II MHC-encoded protein

Antigen being processed

Class II protein and processed antigen

Mature helper T cell

Interleukins

Plasma cell

Antibodies

B

F I G U R E 9–12 Continued **B,** Activation of B-cells to make antibody. B-cell uses receptor to bind matching antigen, which it engulfs and processes. B-cell then presents a piece of antigen, bound to class II protein, on its surface. Complex binds to mature helper T-cell, which releases interleukins that transform B-cell into antibody-secreting plasma cell. (Redrawn from Schindler LW: *Understanding the Immune System.* NIH Publication No. 92–529. U.S. Department of Health and Human Services, 1991, pp 16–17.)

bulinemia in chronic lymphocytic leukemia. Additionally, human immune globulins are used therapeutically for bone marrow transplantation patients and low birth weight infants.

Specific human immune globulins differ from human immune globulins only in the selection of the pooled donors. In other words, only people with high titers of antibodies against the specific antigens needed would be selected for the donor pool. For example, only people with high hepatitis B titers would be used in the pool of donors for hepatitis B immune globulin (HBIG) human.

Animal antibodies are given in specific situations only when necessary because of the significant risks when giving animal sera. Patients who have specific animal allergies or a history of asthma, allergic rhinitis, or other allergies are highly susceptible to developing serum sickness, anaphylaxis, or acute febrile reactions. Animal antibodies are usually given to ameliorate toxins or venoms, including botulism, diphtheria, rabies, tetanus, snakebite, or spider bites. Human plasma is rarely used in infectious disease medicine at this time.

Active Immunity

Active immunity is a protective state caused by the body's immune response as a result of active infection or immunization in which antibodies to a specific antigen are generated to defend against future exposure to the antigen. In other words, the adaptive immune system, after having been exposed to a certain antigen, remembers the antigen and initiates a quick response. This exposure to antigen can be through active infection and antigen processing or through immunization. The adaptive immune system must be exposed to the antigen long enough and in sufficient dose to stimulate an immune response, but not so long as to create overwhelming infection.

The process following exposure or immunization by vaccination involves both cellular and humoral immunity. Upon exposure to the antigen, T-cells, via antigen-presenting cells, stimulate B-cells to replicate, remember, and differentiate into plasma cells. The plasma cells then synthesize and secrete antibodies specific for the antigen. After this initial exposure, both B-cells and T-cells remember the antigen and are capable of both a heightened and rapid response to reexposure to the antigen (Fig. 9–13).

Immunization tricks the immune system into responding to a perceived infection. Vaccines contain altered microorganisms or toxins that retain their ability to stimulate the immune system (antigenic properties) but do not have pathogenic properties. For example, polio vaccine contains live altered bacteria that stimulate the immune system without causing disease. Vaccines can contain live and attenuated (altered) or killed infectious agents.

Vaccines that contain live altered virus or bacteria cause active infection but little injury to the vaccinated individual. These vaccines provide good humoral and cellular immunity with longer lasting memory and often lifetime immunity. An example of long-lasting immunity with a live attenuated vaccine is measles vaccine. Live attenuated vaccines therefore are generally better than those vaccines with inactivated or killed infectious agents. The inactivated or killed vaccines will provide adequate cellular immunity, but humoral immunity, especially IgA, and memory functions may be deficient. An example of shorter lasting immunity with a killed bacteria is pertussis vaccine. Table 9–4 lists all vaccines registered in the United States.

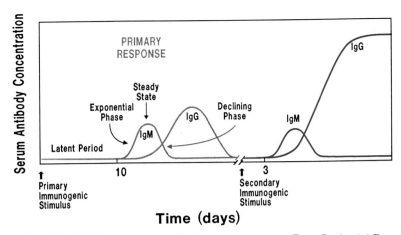

FIGURE 9–13. Time phases in the immune response. (From Benjamini E, Leskowitz S: *Immunology: A Short Course.* New York, Wiley-Liss, Inc., a division of John Wiley & Sons, Inc., page 155. © 1988 Wiley-Liss, Inc. Reprinted by permission of John Wiley & Sons, Inc.

TABLE 9–4. Vaccines Licensed in the United States and Their Routes of Administration

Vaccine*	Type	Route[†]
BCG	Live bacteria	ID (preferred) or SC
Cholera	Inactivated bacteria	SC, IM, or ID[‡]
DTP	Toxoids and inactivated bacteria	IM
Hepatitis B	Inactivated viral antigen: yeast recombinant-derived, plasma-derived	IM; if risk of hemorrhage, SC
Haemophilus b		
Polysaccharide (HBPV)	Polysaccharide	SC or IM
Conjugate (HbCV)	Polysaccharide-protein conjugate	IM
Influenza	Inactivated virus	IM
	Subvirion (split)	IM
Measles	Live virus	SC
Meningococcal	Polysaccharide	SC or IM
MMR	Live viruses	SC
MR	Live viruses	SC
Mumps	Live virus	SC
Plague	Inactivated bacteria	IM
Pneumococcal	Polysaccharide	IM or SC
Poliovirus (trivalent)		
OPV	Live virus	Oral
IPV	Inactivated virus	SC
Rabies	Inactivated virus	IM or ID[‡,§]
Rubella	Live virus	SC
Tetanus and Td, DT (adsorbed)	Toxoids	IM
Tetanus (fluid)	Toxoid	SC
Typhoid		
Parenteral	Inactivated bacteria	SC (boosters may be ID[‡])
Oral	Live attenuated bacteria	Oral
Yellow fever	Live attenuated virus	SC

*BCG = Bacillus of Calmette and Guérin (tuberculosis); DTP = diphtheria and tetanus toxoids and pertussis vaccine adsorbed; HBPV = Haemophilus b polysaccharide vaccine; HbCV = Haemophilus b conjugate vaccine; MMR = measles, mumps, and rubella vaccines; MR = measles and rubella vaccines; OPV = oral poliovirus vaccine; IPV = inactivated poliovirus vaccine; Td = tetanus and diphtheria toxoid (for children ≥ 7 years old and adults); DT = diphtheria and tetanus toxoids (for children < 7 years old).
[†]ID = Intradermal; SC = subcutaneous; IM = intramuscular.
[‡]The intradermal dose is different from the subcutaneous and intramuscular doses.
[§]Used for prophylaxis only.
From Committee on Infectious Diseases, American Academy of Pediatrics: *Report of the Committee on Infectious Diseases,* 22nd ed. Elk Grove Village, Ill, 1991, p 11. Copyright © 1991 American Academy of Pediatrics. Reprinted with permission.

- B-lymphocytes mature in bone marrow and lymph tissue. B-cells have receptors on their surfaces that are able to bind antigens. Each B-cell is able to bind only one particular antigen. Antigen binding causes the B-cell to divide (clonal expansion). Some of the daughter cells become plasma cells, which actively produce and secrete antibodies. Other daughter cells (memory cells) resemble the original cell and distribute in lymph throughout the body. On subsequent exposure to the antigen, antibody production is rapid.

- Antibodies are proteins that are able to specifically bind a particular antigen. Antibodies have several functions. They form complexes with antigens that may neutralize the antigen and remove it from the circulation. Antigen-antibody complexes are a trigger for the complement cascade. Antigens coated with antibody (opsonized) are more easily localized by phagocytic cells.

- The five major antibody classes are IgG, IgM, IgA, IgD, and IgE. Antibody class is determined by the structure of the Fc portion. IgG is the most prevalent antibody class (75 percent). IgM is the first kind to be produced on antigen exposure. IgA is found primarily in body secretions. IgD is present in trace amounts; its function is poorly characterized. IgE binds to basophil and mast cell membranes and mediates inflammation.

- B- and T-cell functions are interdependent. T-cells are unable to respond to soluble antigens. B-cells are able to process free antigen and present it to T-cells. On first exposure, B-cells are minimally activated by antigen unless they are stimulated by cytokines released from T-cells.

- Administration of preformed antibodies confers passive immunity. Passive immunity provides immediate but temporary protection. Active immunity occurs when individuals are exposed to antigen that stimulates their own lymphocytes to produce memory cells. Active immunity confers long-term protection, but may take several weeks to develop.

Integrated Function of Specific and Nonspecific Immunity

The nonspecific and specific cells of the immune system work interdependently to protect the host from foreign antigens. In most cases, an antigen will simultaneously activate both a nonspecific and a specific immune response. Efficient interdependent function depends on a complex communication network that includes a large number of intercellular messengers such as the cytokines. The following paragraphs describe some of the known ways in which cells of specific and nonspecific immunity interact.

Macrophages are nonspecific cells that release mediators important for inflammation and call other WBCs to the area. For example, tissue necrosis factor (TNF) and IL-1 initiate inflammation and also spur other nonspecific cells in the vicinity to produce colony-stimulating factors (CSFs). The CSFs secreted by macrophages and other cells induce the bone marrow to increase production of granulocytes and monocytes. IL-1 enhances the proliferation of specific cells: T-helper cells and B-cells. Macrophages secrete interferon, which inhibits viral replication in infected immune cells. Activated macrophages also secrete IL-6, which is the principal growth factor for B-lymphocytes.

A number of the proteins secreted by macrophages are chemotactic factors that attract other immune cells to the area. In particular, peptides of the IL-8 family are believed to behave as chemotactic factors.

In addition to nonspecific enhancement of other immune cells, macrophages also specifically activate helper T-cells. Macrophages phagocytize and present foreign antigen to helper T-cells. A helper T-cell with the appropriate receptor on its cell surface then binds the presented antigen, causing the helper T-cell to be activated. Activated helper T-cells then secrete a whole group of cytokines that activate other specific and nonspecific immune cells and enhance production of cells in the bone marrow. For example, T-cells release IL-3, which causes generalized multilineage hematopoiesis, and IL-7, which specifically increases the production of B-cells. T-cells also secrete factors that initiate proliferation of already formed B-cells and T-cells (IL-4, IL-5, IL-6).

In addition, activated T-cells secrete a peptide called interferon-gamma that feeds back to macrophages and neutrophils and enhances their phagocytic potential. Cytokines released from both the specific and nonspecific immune cells thus form a complex signaling network that allows the various cells of the immune system to function cooperatively.

Another example of nonspecific and specific immune cell interdependence is evident in the complement system. Complement activation is often triggered by antigen-antibody complexes. Antibody formation is a function of specific immunity (B-cells), yet complement activation is an integral part of the nonspecific system, resulting in the production of chemotactic factors and inflammatory mediators.

Antibodies also enhance the function of nonspecific phagocytic cells by collecting antigen into large complexes that are easier for nonspecific cells to locate and phagocytize. Indeed, the functions of the specific and nonspecific systems are so intertwined that it is misleading to categorize them as separate entities. This is done primarily to simplify the complex immune system to make it easier to study. In reality, the immune system functions as a complex and integrated whole.

- Specific and nonspecific immune cells work together to protect the body from foreign antigens. Macrophages play a central role because they are commonly the first immune cell to encounter the antigen. Macrophages secrete cytokines that stimulate WBC production (IL-1, CSF, IL-6) and help them localize the area (IL-8). Macrophages are antigen-presenting cells that engulf and display antigen on their cell surface in association with MHC class II proteins.

- Helper T-cells are specifically activated by macrophages presenting antigen on their surfaces. Helper T-cells secrete cytokines that stimulate production of WBC in the marrow (IL-3, IL-7) and initiate proliferation of mature B- and T-cells (IL-4, IL-5, IL-6). T-cells secrete interferon-gamma, which stimulates the phagocytic potential of macrophages and neutrophils.

- B-cells secrete antibodies that help phagocytic cells localize and destroy antigens and form complexes that initiate the complement cascade.

Limiting Factors

In order for inflammation to resolve, there must be adequate control of the inflammatory process, basic nutrient availability, and appropriate growth factors. Other systemic factors affecting inflammation resolution include age, the presence of chronic illness, and innervation. Local factors such as blood supply, cell type, control of inflammatory chemical mediators, and cell growth regulation also affect healing.

The potent chemical mediators involved in inflammation can be destructive to normal tissues if not kept in check. The body has a number of mechanisms to prevent excess response and limit inflammation.

Eosinophils can function to control inflammation by releasing enzymes that break down certain chemical mediators such as histamine and leukotrienes. Some histamine (H_2) receptors function to inhibit and control acute cellular inflammation. To control the complement, kinin, and clotting systems, C1 inhibitor, a glycoprotein, inhibits both the Hageman factor and activated portions of C1 (C1r and C1s). Other portions of the complement system are regulated by C4-binding proteins, factor I and factor H, and vitronectin (S protein). Of particular importance is S-protein, which prevents complement membrane attack complex (C6–C9) from attaching to and lysing cell membranes.

To stop the effect of superoxide, there are a number of antioxidants including superoxide dismutases, glutathione peroxidases, and catalases.[27] Vitamin E and beta-carotene are fat-soluble vitamins that react with oxygen radicals and prevent membrane damage.[27] Uric acid and vitamin C neutralize oxidizing agents in the cytoplasm.[27]

External pharmacologic agents such as prostaglandin inhibitors (aspirin and ibuprofen) inhibit prostaglandin synthesis by suppressing enzymes active in the production of prostaglandins and by retarding leukocyte motility. Prostaglandin inhibitors can be used to relieve symptoms resulting from acute or chronic inflammation. Glucocorticoids (discussed in Chap. 7) are also anti-inflammatory agents.

Nutritionally, the body must have adequate amounts of proteins, carbohydrates, lipids, vitamins, and minerals. Proteins for tissue repair as well as transport binding proteins are necessary. Research has demonstrated that malnutrition decreases healing and reduces the strength of the collagen and other proteins in wounds.[28] Impaired intake of nutrients combined with a hypermetabolic state also affects healing. For example, a normally well-nourished, healthy person who experiences multiple trauma in a motor vehicle accident may not heal well if a catabolic, hypermetabolic, negative nitrogen and nutrient state develops.

Oxygenation is critical to resolution of inflammation. Oxygenation at the local level depends on adequate circulatory volume of blood, adequate pumping mechanisms, an intact vascular bed, and neovascularization. Because collagen can only be synthesized in the presence of molecular oxygen, even temporary anoxia changes the strength and quality of collagen fibers.[28] Ischemia associated with inflammation will also increase the chance of infection. Local blood supply also impacts healing. For example, skin tissue heals faster than bone tissue.

Chronic diseases such as diabetes and cardiovascular disease also affect inflammation and healing. In both cases, the microcirculation and systemic circulations are impaired. Diabetics are further affected by deficient collagen and defective granulocyte functions.[28] Persons who take steroids are also at risk of impaired inflammation and healing. They may not have the benefit of a strong inflammatory response when needed. They will also have chronically poor wound healing. Individuals with cancer are affected by competition for nutrients, neutropenia, and the effects of chemotherapy on inflammation and bone marrow cells.

Individuals who develop hypertrophic scars and keloids have overabundant dermal collagen deposition.[28] Research has suggested that keloid and hypertrophic scar development may be linked to IgG antibody-antigen reactions in the skin.[28] Inadequate growth factors such as insulin, thyroid-stimulating factor, growth hormone, epidermal growth factor, and angiogenesis factor may inhibit regeneration and delay healing.

KEY CONCEPTS

- Mechanisms to inhibit and control the immune response include suppressor T-cell function, complement inhibitors, proteolytic degradation of inflammatory mediators by eosinophils, and antioxidants.

- Factors that may adversely suppress immune function include anti-inflammatory drugs, malnutrition, poor circulation, and chronic debilitating diseases.

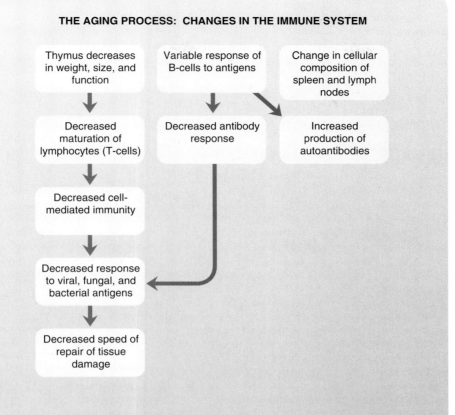

THE AGING PROCESS: CHANGES IN THE IMMUNE SYSTEM

In the elderly, immune system function is altered with a decreased ability to respond to antigenic stimulation. The elderly are able to respond to infections with previously produced "remembered" antibodies. However, they are less able to respond to new antigens. As a result of these changes, there is decreased speed of repair of tissue damage and increased vulnerability to disease.

The cells of the immune system in the elderly are not able to proliferate or reproduce as effectively as in younger persons. Although the total number of T-cells remains the same, T-cell function is decreased. T-cells are less able to proliferate and have decreased cytotoxicity. Antibody production also decreases, especially antibodies such as IgG that are T-cell dependent. There is also a rise in autoantibody production, which may influence the increase in autoimmune disease in the elderly.

Thymus size decreases after puberty, causing a decline in thymic hormone production, decreased T-cell differentiation, and reduced T-cell related B-cell differentiation. Usually thymic hormone secretions stop after age 60. However, the role of thymus involution in elderly immune system changes is currently uncertain.

Summary

The immune system arises from the bone marrow and has two functional divisions—the nonspecific or innate immune system and the specific or adaptive immune system. Both divisions continuously interact to protect the host. They communicate and are activated by each other. Almost all antigens that induce an inflammatory response will also initiate an immune response.

The nonspecific immune system is characterized by phagocytic cells such as neutrophils, the blood coagulation system, chemical mediators, and mechanical and biochemical barriers. This system responds rapidly the same way to every antigen. The specific immune system is characterized by T-cells and B-cells. It has the ability to remember and respond to specific antigens. Together, the parts of the immune system function to protect against external and internal threats.

REFERENCES

1. Broide DH: Inflammatory cells: Structure and function, in Stites DP, Terr AI (eds): *Basic and Clinical Immunology*, 7th ed. Los Altos, Calif, Appleton & Lange, 1991.
2. Weiss SJ: Tissue destruction by neutrophils. *N Engl J Med* 1989;320(6):365–374.
3. Galli SJ: New concepts about the mast cell. *N Engl J Med* 1993;328(4):257–265.
4. Frey AM: The immune system and intravenous administration of immune globulin: Part I. The immune system. *J Intravenous Nurs* 1991;14(5):315–330.
5. Nossal GJV: Life, death and the immune system. *Sci Am* 1993;269(3):53–62.
6. Weissman IL, Cooper MD: How the immune system develops, in Stites DP, Terr AI (eds): *Basic and Clinical Immunology*, 7th eds. Los Altos, Calif, Appleton & Lange, 1991.
7. Frank MM: Complement and kinin, in Stites DP, Terr AI (eds): *Basic and Clinical Immunology*, 7th ed. Los Altos, Calif, Appleton & Lange, 1991.
8. Widmann FK: *An Introduction to Clinical Immunology.* Philadelphia, FA Davis, 1989.
9. Fitzbiggons SJ: Harnessing the immune system. *Technol Rev* 1993;96(6):42–48.
10. Gurka AM: The immune system: Implications for critical care nursing. *Crit Care Nurse* 1990;9(7):24–35.
11. Claman HM: The biology of the immune response. *JAMA* 1992;268(20):2790–2796.
12. Sell S: *Immunology, Immunopathology and Immunity*, 4th ed. Amsterdam, Elsevier, 1987.
13. Wasserman SI: Mediators of inflammation, in Stites DP, Terr AI (eds): *Basic and Clinical Immunology*, 7th ed. Los Altos, Calif, Appleton & Lange, 1991.
14. Ernst PB, Underdown BJ, Bienenstock J: Immunity in mucosal tissues, in Stites DP, Stobo JD, Wells JV (eds): *Basic and Clinical Immunology*, 6th ed. Los Altos, Calif, Appleton & Lange, 1987.
15. Reinhold U, Abken H, Kukel S, et al: Tumor-infiltrating lymphocytes isolated from Ki-1-positive large cell lymphoma of the skin. *Cancer* 1991;68(10):2155–2160.
16. Siskind GW: Aging and the immune system, in Warner HR, et al (eds): *Modern Biological Theories of Aging.* New York, Raven Press, 1987.
17. Bennett NT, Schultz GS: Growth factors and wound healing: Biochemical properties of growth factors and their receptors. *Am J Surg* 1993;165(6):728–737.
18. Alberts S, et al: *Molecular Biology of the Cell*, 2nd ed. New York, Garland Publishing, 1989.
19. Cohen IR: The self, the world and autoimmunity. *Sci Am* 1988;258(4):52–60.
20. Theofilopoulos AN: Autoimmunity, in Stites DP, Stobo JD, Wells JV (eds): *Basic and Clinical Immunology*, 6th ed. Los Altos, Calif, Appleton & Lange, 1987.
21. Nossal GJV: Immunologic tolerance: Collaboration between antigen and lymphokines. *Science* 1989;245:147–153.
22. Marrack P, Kappler JW: How the immune system recognizes the body. *Sci Am* 1993;269(3):81–89.
23. Janeway C: How the immune system recognizes invaders. *Sci Am* 1993;269(3):73–79.
24. Schwartz BD: The human leukocyte antigen complex, in Stein JH (ed): *Internal Medicine.* Boston, Little, Brown & Co, 1990, vol II.
25. Goodman JW: Immunoglobulin structure and function, in Stites DP, Terr AI (eds): *Basic and Clinical Immunology*, 7th ed. Los Altos, Calif, Appleton & Lange, 1991.
26. Committee on Infectious Diseases, American Academy of Pediatrics: *Report of the Committee on Infectious Diseases.* Elk Grove Village, Ill, American Academy of Pediatrics, 1991.
27. Rusting RL: Why do we age? *Sci Am* 1992;267(6):130–141.
28. Carrico TJ, Mehrhof AI, Cohen IK: Biology of wound healing. *Surg Clin North Am* 1984;64(4):721–733.

BIBLIOGRAPHY

Anderson DC, Stiehm R: Immunization. *JAMA* 1987;258(20):3001–3004.

Beal GN: Immunologic aspects of endocrine diseases. *JAMA* 1987;258(20):2952–2956.

Beardsley T: Paradise lost? Microbes mount a comeback as drug resistance spreads. *Sci Am* 1992;267(11):18–20.

Bellanti JA: *Immunology III.* Philadelphia, WB Saunders, 1985.

Benjamini E, Leskowitz S: *Immunology: A Short Course.* New York, Alan R Liss, 1988.

Blackman M, Kappler J, Marrack P: The role of the T cell receptor in positive and negative selection of developing T cells. *Science* 1990;248:1335–1341.

Capron A, Dessaint J: From protective immunity to allergy: The cellular partners of IgE. *Chem Immunol* 1990;49:236–244.

Clowes GHA: *Trauma, Sepsis and Shock: The Physiological Basis.* New York, Marcel Dekker, 1988.

Dinarello CA, Mier JW: Current concepts: Lymphokines. *N Engl J Med* 1987;317(15):940–945.

Dinarello CA, Wolff SM: The role of interleukin-1 in disease. *N Engl J Med* 1993;328(2):106–113.

Dorian B, Garfinkle PR: Stress, immunity, and illness: A review. *Psychol Med* 1987;17:393–407.

Fidler MR: Immunologic anatomy and physiology, in Kinney MR, Packa DR, Dunbar SB (eds): *AACN's Clinical Reference for Critical Care Nursing*, 2nd ed. New York, McGraw-Hill, 1988.

Frey AM: The immune system: Part II. Intravenous administration of immune globulin. *J Intravenous Nurs* 1991;14(6):396–405.

Gardner P, Schaffner W: Immunization of adults. *N Engl J Med* 1993;328(17):1252–1258.

Grawlikowski J: White cells at war. *AJN* 1992;92(3):44–51.

Groenwald S: Physiology of the immune system. *Heart Lung* 1980;9(4):645–650.

Hadden JW: Immunopharmacology: Immunomodulation and immunotherapy. *JAMA* 1987;258(20):3005–3010.

Jackson BS, Jones MB: Hematologic anatomy and physiology, in Kinney MR, Packa DR, Dunbar SB (eds): *AACN's Clinical Reference for Critical Care Nursing*, 2nd ed. New York, McGraw-Hill, 1988.

Jaffe HS, Sherwin SA: Immunomodulators, in Stites DP, Terr AI (eds): *Basic and Clinical Immunology*, 7th ed. Los Altos, Calif, Appleton & Lange, 1991.

Kaliner M: Immediate hypersensitivity. *J Allergy Clin Immunol* 1989;84(6):1028–1031.

Kirkpatrick CH: Transplantation immunology. *JAMA* 1987;258(20):2993–3000.

Kohn RR: Aging and age-related diseases: Normal processes, in Johnson HA (ed): *Relations Between Normal Aging and Disease.* New York, Raven Press, 1985.

Koshland DE: Recognizing self from nonself. *Science* 1990;248:1273.

Lasser A: The mononuclear phagocytic system: A review. *Hum Pathol* 1983;14(2):108–126.

Ledford DK, Espinoza LR: Immunologic aspects of cardiovascular disease. *JAMA* 1987;258(20):2974–2982.

Lenert P, et al: Human CD4 binds immunoglobulins. *Science* 1990;248:1639–1643.

Martin L, Fritzler M: Antibodies, in Stein JH (ed): *Internal Medicine.* Boston, Little, Brown & Co, 1990, vol II.

Meek K: Analysis of junctional diversity during B lymphocyte development. *Science* 1990;250:820–822.

McCord JM: Oxygen-derived radicals: A link between reperfusion injury and inflammation. *Fed Proc* 1987;46(7):2402–2406.

National Institute of Child Health and Human Development Intravenous Immunoglobulin Study Group: Intravenous immune globulin for the prevention of bacterial infections in children with symptomatic human immunodeficiency virus infection. *N Engl J Med* 1991;325(2):73–80.

National Vaccine Advisory Committee: The measles epidemic: The problems, barriers, and recommendations. *JAMA* 1991;266:1547–1552.

Old LJ: Tumor necrosis factor. *Sci Am* 1988;258(5):59–60, 69–75.

Ovary Z: Of immediate hypersensitivity: Remembrances of things past. *Allergy Proc* 1988;9(6):671–675.

Perlmutter RM: Antibodies: Structure and genetics, in Stein JH (ed): *Internal Medicine.* Boston, Little, Brown & Co, 1990, vol II.

Peter G: Childhood immunizations. *N Engl J Med* 1992;327(25):1794–1800.

Ramsdell F, Fowlkes BJ: Clonal deletion versus clonal anergy: The role of the thymus in inducing self tolerance. *Science* 1990;248:1342–1348.

Richardson S: Human Physiological Defenses (computer program). Salt Lake City, University of Utah, 1988.

Roitt I: *Essential Immunology.* Boston, Blackwell Scientific Publications, 1991.

Russell RL: Evidence for and against the theory of developmentally programmed aging, in Warner HR, et al (eds): *Modern Biological Theories of Aging.* New York, Raven Press, 1987.

Saul RL, Gee P, Ames BN: Free radicals, DNA damage, and aging, in Warner HR, et al (eds): *Modern Biological Theories of Aging.* New York, Raven Press, 1987.

Schmid-Schonbein GW: Capillary plugging by granulocytes and the no-reflow phenomenon in the microcirculation. *Fed Proc* 1987;46(7):2397–2401.

Schwartz RH: A cell culture model for T lymphocyte clonal anergy. *Science* 1990;248:1349–1356.

Sprent J, Gao EK, Webb SR: T cell reactivity to MHC molecules: Immunity versus tolerance. *Science* 1990;248:1357–1363.

Steinberg AD: Tolerance and autoimmunity, in Stein JH (ed): *Internal Medicine.* Boston, Little, Brown & Co, 1990, vol II.

Steinman L: Autoimmune disease. *Sci Am* 1993;9(3):107–114.

Stites DP, Terr AI: *Basic and Clinical Immunology,* 7th ed. Los Altos, Calif, Appleton & Lange, 1991.

Stobo JD: The human immune response, in Stein JH (ed): *Internal Medicine.* Boston, Little, Brown & Co, 1990, vol II.

Strober W, James SP: The immunopathogenesis of gastrointestinal and hepatobiliary diseases. *JAMA* 1987;258(20):2962–2969.

Trentham DE, Dynesius-Trentham RA, Orav EJ, et al: Effects of oral administration of type II collagen on rheumatoid arthritis. *Science* 1993;261:1727–1730.

Vander AJ, Sherman JH, Luciano DS: *Human Physiology: The Mechanisms of Body Function,* 4th ed. New York, McGraw-Hill, 1985.

Virella G, Patrick CC, Goust J: Diagnostic evaluation of cell-mediated immunity. *Immunol Series* 1990;50:303–321.

Von Boehmer H, Kisielow P: Self-nonself discrimination by T cells. *Science* 1990;248:1369–1373.

Ware JA, Heistad DD: Platelet-endothelium interactions. *N Engl J Med* 1993;328(9):628–635.

Wayne SJ, Rhyne RL, Garry PJ, et al: Cell-mediated immunity as a predictor of morbidity and mortality in subjects over 60. *J Gerontol* 1990;45(2):M45–48.

Wilson CB: Immune aspects of renal diseases. *JAMA* 1987;258(20):2957–2961.

Young JD, Cohn ZA: How killer cells kill. *Sci Am* 1988;258(1):38–44.

Zweiman B, Arnason BG: Immunologic aspects of neurological and neuromuscular diseases. *JAMA* 1987;258(20):2970–2973.

CHAPTER 10
Alterations in Immune Function

FAITH YOUNG PETERSON

KEY TERMS

acquired or secondary immunodeficiency: An immunodeficiency that develops after birth and is the result of an illness rather than a genetic defect. Examples include impaired immune function secondary to poor nutrition or a medication. This type of immunodeficiency may be reversible.

acquired immunodeficiency syndrome (AIDS): A syndrome caused by the human immunodeficiency virus (HIV).

allergy: Type I hypersensitivity of the immune system to relatively harmless environmental agents. Antigens that trigger an allergic response are often called allergens.

autoimmunity: An inappropriate and excessive response to self antigens. Disorders that result from an autoimmune response are called autoimmune diseases.

congenital immunodeficiency: A rare condition that results from improper development of immune system components before birth.

human immunodeficiency virus: An RNA-containing virus (retrovirus) that appears to infect T-cells.

hypersensitivity: A type of inappropriate or excessive response of the immune system.

immunodeficiency: Failure of immune system mechanisms to defend against pathogens. There are two broad categories of immune deficiencies, based on the mechanism of lymphocyte dysfunction—primary and acquired.

The purposes of the immune system are to defend the body against invasion or infection by foreign substances called antigens, assist the body to maintain a steady state, and patrol for and destroy cells that are abnormal or damaged. Antigens or immunogens are foreign substances, cells, toxins, or proteins that cause the components of the immune system to react and respond. The ability to stimulate an immune response is called **immunogenicity.**

In some disease states, proteins or cells within the body can be recognized as "foreign," also bringing on an immune response. This response is called autoimmunity. In other disease states, the person is unable to defend adequately against pathogens. The person is then said to have an immunodeficiency. Immunodeficiency diseases are caused by a defect in one or more immune system components. These diseases range from severe to mild depending on the immune system component affected. Immunodeficiencies can also be either primary or secondary (acquired). The person with hypersensitivity has an excessive immune response.

This chapter addresses alterations in immune function. It will focus upon changes that cause inappropriate immune responses, excessive immune reactions, and failures of the immune system to respond to pathogens.

Autoimmunity

Autoimmunity occurs when the immune system fails to recognize a person's own cells ("self") for some reason. Autoimmune diseases are the direct result of the reaction between self antigens and the immune system. Autoimmune diseases can be either *organ-nonspecific and generalized* or *organ-specific and localized.* An example of an organ-nonspecific autoimmune disease is systemic lupus erythematosus (SLE). Examples of organ-specific autoimmune diseases are myasthenia gravis and Graves' disease. No one theory can explain the loss of tolerance for all autoimmune diseases. A number of factors interacting together most probably contribute to the development of autoimmunity. For this reason, autoimmune diseases are said to be multifactorial and may be polygenic.

Many immunologic factors can lead to the development of autoimmunity. The theory of antigenic mimicry emphasizes the similarities between molecular segments or epitopes of foreign antigens and the person's own cells.[1] The basis of this theory is that the basic components of self and foreign cells are the same. For example, all cells, whether self or foreign, are made up of proteins, carbohydrates, nucleic acids, and lipids. Cells with the same or similar molecular segments as foreign epitopes can "fit" lymphocyte receptors. Therefore, these self antigens can be attacked as foreign under certain circumstances when the normal cell has been altered, for example, by a viral infection that stimulates the immune response.

The theory proposing a release of sequestered antigens suggests that certain self antigens are isolated from the immune system within an organ during the neonatal period.[2] When the organ is damaged later in life, these antigens are exposed to the immune system, which does not recognize them as self. Therefore, the damaged cells are attacked and destroyed further.

There are a number of T-cell theories. These include thymus gland defects, decreased T-suppressor cell function, and altered T-helper cell function. The theory attributing autoimmunity to thymus gland defects states that the maturation and differentiation of T-cells are affected by decreased hormone secretion.[2] This is thought to be a major factor in the development of generalized autoimmune diseases such as SLE. The theory attributing autoimmunity to decreased T-suppressor cell activity states that decreased numbers of T-suppressor cells fail to repress immunoglobulin activity.[2] However, this theory does not adequately explain tissue- or organ-specific autoimmune damage. The altered T-helper cell function theory asserts that changed T-helper cells lose their self tolerance through a variety of mechanisms.

There are also a number of B-cell theories of autoimmunity. The theory attributing autoimmunity to escape of B-cell tolerance proposes that certain B-cells lose their responsiveness to T-suppressor cell messages.[2] The B-cell activation theories, which are well supported clinically and experimentally, suggest that extrinsic factors or intrinsic, genetic B-cell defects cause autoantibody production and an increase in the number and activity of B-cells.[2,3] A number of extrinsic factors, including viruses, bacteria, antibiotics, proteolytic enzymes, and lipopolysaccharides, have been found to be B-cell–activating factors that could trigger autoantibody production.

Research into genetic defects in the major histocompatibility complex (MHC), defects in macrophage function, defects in bone marrow stem cells, and defects in tolerance induction suggests that abnormal functioning in any of these systems could contribute to autoimmunity.[2] Sex hormones and sex-linked genes are thought to influence the expression of autoimmune diseases. The exact mechanisms of this interaction have not been established. The relationship between the development of autoimmune disease and sex is significant. For example, women are nine times more likely to develop SLE than men.[2]

Certain MHC genes appear to increase the risk of developing autoimmune disease. The strongest correlation of MHC molecules with autoimmune disease is the linkage between MHC or the HLA-B27 phenotype and ankylosing spondylitis. In this case, 95 percent of all people with ankylosing spondylitis have a positive B27 phenotype. However, not everyone with a positive B27 phenotype develops ankylosing spondylitis, owing to differences in the way antigen is presented to the immune system. Other diseases are associated with different MHC phenotypes, but the correlation between risk for disease and the disease marker is much lower. For example, Addison's disease is associated with the DR3 phenotype, but it has only a 6 percent risk correlation.

Viral infections may be associated with the development of autoimmunity. Viruses can activate B-cells, decrease the function of T-cells, contribute to the development of antigenic mimicry, or insert viral components on cell surfaces, triggering immune reactions.[2] For example, Epstein-Barr virus (EBV) has been frequently cited as a cause of autoimmune disease. Other factors that may contribute to autoimmunity include environmental triggers leading to inflammation or lymphokine release that activates antiself T-cells.[4]

KEY CONCEPTS

- Autoimmune disorders occur when the immune system erroneously reacts with "self" tissues. These disorders are thought to be polygenic and multifactorial; however, the exact etiology is unknown.
- The antigenic mimicry theory proposes that since self and foreign antigens are composed of the same basic building blocks—proteins, carbohydrates, nucleic acids, and lipids—small alterations in self tissue may lead to immunogenic attack.
- Release of sequestered antigens theory suggests that self antigens that do not come in direct contact with lymphocytes during fetal development may cause autoimmune reactions if they are subsequently released from sequestration.
- Abnormal production of subclasses of T-lymphocytes, particularly T-suppressor cells, has been proposed as a reason for the development of autoimmunity as well as the development of abnormal B-cells that do not respond to T-suppressor cell signals.
- A genetic component is likely since certain autoimmune disorders are more commonly associated with particular major histocompatibility complex types and female gender.
- Viruses may also be causative in the development of autoimmune disorders. Viruses may alter self cells, thus precipitating an immune attack. Formed antibodies may then cross-react with similar but uninfected cells.

Alterations in Immune Function: Hyperfunction

Hypersensitivity is a disorder that results from a specific antigen-antibody reaction or a specific antigen-lymphocyte interaction. The immune response in hypersensitivity reactions is often inappropriate or excessive. There are four classes or types of hypersensitivity. Each type is characterized by a specific cellular or antibody response. Although the diseases or syndromes associated with each type differ in their clinical signs and symptoms, the underlying pathophysiology is similar within each type. Table 10–1 differentiates each of the four major types of hypersensitivity.

Allergy and Hypersensitivity

Type I Hypersensitivity

Type I hypersensitivity is also known as *atopic hypersensitivity* or *anaphylactic allergic reaction*. Type I hypersensitivity is a sensitization reaction characterized by signs and symptoms of an allergic reaction immediately following contact with an antigen (allergen). The reaction occurs within 15 to 30 minutes after exposure to the allergen. Immunoglobulin E (IgE) is the principal antibody mediating this reaction. Mast cells are the principal effector cells, with support from other IgE-stimulated effector cells, including eosinophils and macrophages.[5] Examples of this type of hypersensitivity reaction include anaphylaxis to a bee sting, asthma, seasonal allergic rhinitis, allergies, and eczema. Common allergenic medications, insects, and foods that can trigger type I hypersensitivity are listed in Table 10–2.

Mast cells, found throughout the body in all loose connective tissue, are covered with IgE receptors—up to 500,000 on their cell surface.[6] This makes them particularly responsive to antigens. The initial incident during a type I hypersensitivity response is the cross-linking of two IgE receptors to one antigen on the mast cell at the site of the allergen's entry into the body (Fig. 10–1). Cross-linking of IgE and the allergen causes a series of actions that results in immediate, massive, local mast cell degranulation of preformed and newly formed mediators and the release of mediators by other IgE-triggered effector cells.[5] The release of mediators causes an inflammatory cell response.

Mast cells, basophils, and other effector cells release many mediators. Some of the mediators are preformed, such as histamine, heparin, kininogenase and tryptase (proteolytic enzymes), and chemotactic factors (eosinophilic chemotactic factor of anaphylaxis, ECF-A; platelet-activating factor, PAF; and chemotactic factor leukotriene B4, LIB4). Other mediators are formed during the degranulation process. Examples of newly formed mediators include superoxide, prostaglandins, thromboxanes, leukotrienes (slow-reacting substance of anaphylaxis, SRS-A), bradykinin, PAF, and interleukins (IL-3, IL-4, IL-5, IL-6).[6]

Histamine binds to both H_1 and H_2 receptors. (The H stands for histamine.) The histamine that binds to H_1 receptors is responsible for increased vascular permeability, vasodilation, urticaria formation, bronchial constriction with wheezing and coughing, and increased gut permeability. The histamine that binds to H_2 receptors counteracts the actions of the H_1 receptors by decreasing overall degranulation, increasing lymphocyte activation, and decreasing neutrophil chemotaxis and enzyme release. The proteolytic enzymes, kininogenase and tryptase, activate the kinin pathway and C3, which triggers the complement cascade. Heparin decreases clot formation. The chemotactic factors call or activate other inflammatory and immune cells. Leukotrienes (SRS-A) cause smooth muscle contraction and increase vascular permeability.

TABLE 10–1. The Four Types of Hypersensitivity

	Type I: Atopic, Anaphylactic	Type II: Cytotoxic, Cytolytic	Type III: Immune Complex (Arthus)	Type IV: Delayed Hypersensitivity
Mediated by	Immunoglobin IgE	Immunoglobin IgM or IgG	Immunoglobin IgG	Td Lymphocytes
Complement activation	No	Yes	Yes	No
Immune response	Ag plus IgE, leading to mast cell degranulation	Surface Ag and Ab, leading to killer cell cytotoxic action or complement-mediated lysis	Ag-Ab complex in tissues; complement activated and PMNs attracted	Ag-sensitized T-cells release lymphokines, leading to inflammatory reactions, and attract macrophages which release mediator
Peak action	15–30 min	15–30 min	6 hr	24–48 hr
Serum transferability	Yes	Yes	Yes	No
Cell transferability	No	No	No	Yes (T-cells)
Genetic mechanisms	Familial High IgE level HLA-linked Ir genes General hyperresponsiveness	None	Familial (autoimmune) HLA specificities	None
Causes of reaction (allergy)	T-cell deficiency Abnormal mediator feedback Environmental factors and Ag	Exposure to Ag on foreign tissue, cells, or graft	Persistent infection—microbe Ag Extrinsic environmental Ag Autoimmunity—self Ag	Intradermal Ag Epidermal Ag Dermal Ag
Manifestation (examples)	Anaphylaxis, asthma, rhinitis eczema	ABO transfusions, hemolytic disease of newborn, myasthenia gravis	Glomerulonephritis, systemic lupus, farmer's lung, arthritis, vasculitis	Guillain-Barré disease, tuberculin test, contact dermatitis, tissue graft rejection, multiple sclerosis

Data from Sell S: *Immunology, Immunopathology and Immunity,* 4th ed. Amsterdam, Elsevier, 1987, chap 13; and Roitt I: *Essential Immunology,* 7th ed. Oxford, Blackwell Scientific Publications, 1991, chaps 19–23.
Abbreviations: Ag, antigen; Ab, antibody; PMN, polymorphonuclear leukocyte.

Treatment for type I hypersensitivity primarily involves pharmacologic management using antihistamines, β-adrenergics, theophyllines, cromolyn sodium, corticosteroids, and/or anticholinergics. Anti-

TABLE 10–2. Possible Causes of Human Anaphylaxis

Medications
  Penicillin, penicillin analogues, and other antibiotics
  Radiographic contrast media
  Aspirin, indomethacin, and other analgesics
  Allergenic extracts
  Biologicals
    Serum proteins, including gamma globulin
    Insulin and other hormones
    Vaccines
    Enzymes such as penicillinase
  Local anesthetics
Hymenoptera (stinging) insects
  Polistes wasps
  Honeybees
  Fire ants
  Hornets and yellow jackets
Foods
  Nuts
  Seafoods, especially shellfish
  Eggs
  Fruit, especially citrus and strawberries
  Tartrazine, yellow dye no. 5

histamines such as Benedryl are used to moderate the effect of vasoactive mediators such as histamine. This action decreases vascular permeability and bronchoconstriction. β-Adrenergic sympathomimetics and theophyllines are used to decrease bronchoconstriction and bronchospasm. Available orally, parenterally, and via inhalers, these medications have a rapid onset. β-adrenergics that can be given include metaproterenol, terbutaline, albuterol, and epinephrine. Theophyllines given include aminophylline, theophylline, and oxtriphylline. Cromolyn sodium stabilizes mast cell membranes. Corticosteroids are used to decrease the inflammatory response. Anticholinergics are used to block the parasympathetic system, allowing greater sympathetic activity. This indirectly causes bronchodilation.

There is increasing evidence that genetic mechanisms influence type I hypersensitivity, with a strong hereditary linkage regarding IgE response to antigens (allergens).[6] This genetic component involves both the ability to respond to an allergen and the general ability to produce an IgE antibody response. For example, children born to two allergic parents have a 50 percent chance of being allergic. Children born to one normal and one allergic parent have a 30 percent chance of being allergic (Fig. 10–2).

Researchers are currently exploring two genetic avenues that influence hyperresponsiveness and al-

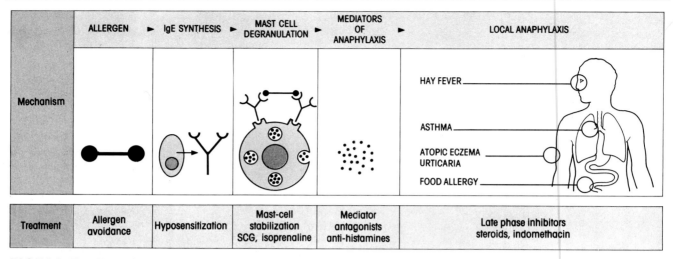

FIGURE 10–1. Type I hypersensitivity response. (From Roitt I: *Essential Immunology*, 7th ed. Oxford, Blackwell Scientific Publications, 1991, p 256. Reproduced with permission.)

lergies. These include research on IgE levels and T-suppressor cell function. High IgE levels have been found in some hypersensitive people. It has also been found that low levels of T-suppressor cells are associated with high IgE levels and the MHC genes HLA-B8 and HLA-Dw3. HLA-B8 may be linked to T-suppressor cell control of immune responses. These findings suggest that there is T-cell control of IgE production. However, not all allergic people have high IgE levels.

Recent research has shown that there are two T-helper cell types, called Th1 and Th2, in allergic reac-

tions.[8] Of these two cell types, Th2 is more prevalent. The Th2 cells release IL-4 and IL-5. IL-4 stimulates B-cell IgE production contributing to high levels of IgE.[8] The Th1 cells secrete interferon-gamma and IL-2. Interferon-gamma secretion hampers B-cell IgE antibody stimulation.[8] This research implies that an individual's mix of Th1 and Th2 cells may contribute to allergic reactivity.

There are several other hypotheses regarding the causes of allergic, type I hypersensitivity reactions. It is hypothesized that there is a T-suppressor cell deficiency or abnormal mediator feedback that in-

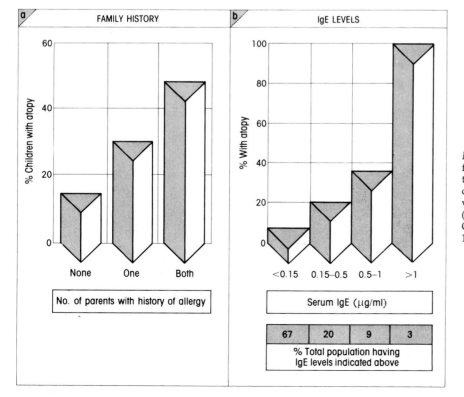

FIGURE 10–2. Genetic mechanisms that influence type I hypersensitivity: **a**, family history; **b**, IgE levels—the higher the serum IgE concentration, the greater the chance of developing allergy (type I hypersensitivity). (From Roitt I: *Essential Immunology*, 7th ed. Oxford, Blackwell Scientific Publications, 1991, p 257. Reproduced with permission.)

creases mast cell degranulation and the inflammatory response. Environmental pollutants may increase mucosal permeability and enhance antigen (allergen) entry into the body. This increased entry would subsequently increase IgE responsiveness.

There is also the allergic breakthrough hypothesis. This hypothesis suggests that in both high IgE and low IgE responders, the overt expression of clinical symptoms is seen only when some allergic breakthrough level is exceeded. Exceeding this hypothesized level may depend on the presence of concomitant factors such as viral infections of the upper respiratory tract, transient IgA deficiency, or decreased T-suppressor cell activity.

Research has shown that protective, proactive actions taken during pregnancy can decrease the likelihood that the child will develop type I hypersensitivity. These actions include avoiding foods to which the mother is allergic, limiting excesses of one type of food during the last trimester of pregnancy, avoiding whole eggs during the last month before delivery and while breast-feeding, and limiting cow's milk to two glasses per day.[9] Other actions to be taken during the child's infancy include avoiding exposure to environmental pollution, breast-feeding for a minimum of 6 months, supplementation with non-cow's milk products such as soy milk, giving solid foods only after the infant is 6 months old, keeping the infant's room as free of dust and molds as possible, and keeping pets (dogs, cats, birds) out of the home.[9,10]

Another avenue of preventing type I hypersensitivity reactions involves the use of desensitization therapy (immunotherapy) or cromolyn sodium. Cromolyn sodium (Intal) stabilizes mast cells and inhibits mast cell degranulation, which decreases the release of the vasoactive mediators.[6] This medication is used primarily for patients with asthma.

Desensitization therapy or immunotherapy is more successful in patients with hay fever than in patients with other types of allergies.[11] It involves both environmental control of external allergens and titrated pharmacologic exposure to allergens. Environmental control involves a systematic plan to decrease exposure to house dust, molds, and animal dander. Pets are kept out of the house. The person must avoid food allergens, wool carpets, goosedown or feather pillows, dried plants, and exposure to other animal and vegetable products.[11] The person is urged to use air conditioning and electronic air filters.[11]

Pharmacologic desensitization involves injecting a person with a sufficient amount of antigen (allergen) on a regular basis over a course of months or years, followed by periodic maintenance or booster therapy.[12] Progressively over time, the dose is increased until the person can tolerate the allergen without a type I hypersensitivity reaction.[11] The goal of this therapy is a change in immunoglobulins so that there is an increase in IgG and IgA blocking antibodies, no increase in IgE during allergy season, decreased basophil reactivity, and a decreased lymphocyte reactivity to allergens.[12]

Type II Hypersensitivity

Type II hypersensitivity is also known as *cytotoxic* or *cytolytic hypersensitivity*. Type II hypersensitivity is characterized by antibodies that attack antigens on the surface of specific cells or tissues. This reaction is immediate, occurring within 15 to 30 minutes after exposure to the antigen. It is mediated by the complement system and a variety of principal effector cells, including tissue macrophages, platelets, killer cells, neutrophils, and eosinophils. IgG and IgM are the principal antibodies. Examples of this type of hypersensitivity reaction include ABO transfusion reactions, hemolytic disease of the newborn, myasthenia gravis, thyroiditis, hyperacute graft rejections, and autoimmune hemolytic anemias.

The initial incident during a type II hypersensitivity response is the exposure to antigen on the surface of foreign cells. The Fab portion of the IgG or IgM antibodies binds to the antigens on the target foreign cell, forming an antigen-antibody complex. (Refer also to Chapter 9 for a discussion of IgG and IgM antibodies.) The Fc region of the IgG or IgM antibodies sticks out away from the cell membrane surface. The Fc region then acts as a bridge between the antigen and complement or the effector cells.[7] This antigen-antibody complex formation with Fc bridging specifically precipitates a cytotoxic reaction by effector cells or complement-mediated lysis (Fig. 10–3).

Complement-mediated lysis occurs through the classical pathway activation of complement. Activated complement component, C3b, is bound to the target cell by the Fc region of IgG or IgM. C3b increases opsonization, which in turn increases the capacity of the system to allow lysis by other effector cells or by complement itself. Lysis of the foreign cell is by complement via the C5–C9 membrane attack complex (Fig. 10–4).

Effector cells in cytotoxic reactions link to exposed Fc and C3 receptors. Once this bridging occurs, the foreign cell is phagocytized and destroyed by lyso-

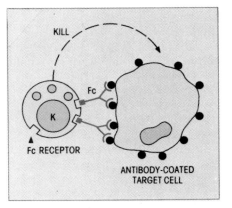

FIGURE 10–3. Cell death of antibody-coated target by killer T-cells. The surface receptors on the killer T-cells bind to the antibody-coated target cell, causing cell destruction. (From Roitt I: *Essential Immunology*, 7th ed. Oxford, Blackwell Scientific Publications, 1991, p 261. Reproduced with permission.)

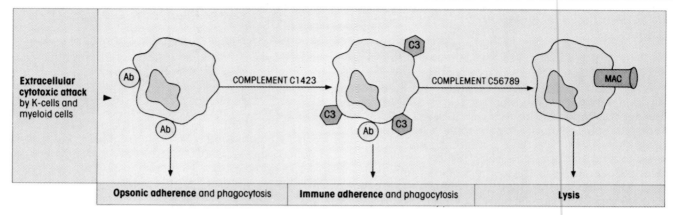

FIGURE 10–4. Type II hypersensitivity response. Antibodies directed against cell surface antigens cause cell death not only by complement-mediated lysis but also by adherence reactions leading to phagocytosis, or through nonphagocytic extracellular killing. (From Roitt I: *Essential Immunology*, 7th ed. Oxford, Blackwell Scientific Publications, 1991, p 261. Reproduced with permission.)

somes within the effector cell. In hypersensitivity reactions that involve large areas, effector cells such as neutrophils are unable to surround or engulf the area. Therefore, the neutrophils release their lysosomes outside their membrane in order to destroy the involved cells.[7]

For example, a major blood group transfusion reaction is a type II hypersensitivity reaction. It occurs when a person receives blood from someone with a different blood group type (Table 10–3). If a person with type A blood having type A antigens and anti-B antibodies incorrectly receives type B blood with B antigens and anti-A antibodies, the anti-B antibodies will attach to the surface of the infused B red blood cells (RBCs) and the anti-A antibodies in the infusion will attach to the surface of the circulating A RBCs. This will stimulate antigen-antibody complex formation and the destruction of large numbers of RBCs. The resulting signs and symptoms of this major blood group reaction include fever, chills, flushing, tachycardia, hypotension, low back pain, pleuritic chest pain, nausea, vomiting, restlessness, anxiety, oliguria, and headache. This may progress to anaphylaxis, shock, and death.

Hemolytic disease of the newborn (HDNB) or erythroblastosis fetalis is another example of type II hypersensitivity. This occurs during pregnancy when an RhG negative mother is sensitized to her fetus's Rh+ red cell group antigens due to exposure during a previous pregnancy. The mother's IgG Rh-positive antibodies cross the placental barrier and attack the fetus's RBCs. The mother's prior exposure usually occurs during birth or miscarriage of a previous Rh-positive child, when there is mixing of fetal and maternal blood. After this exposure, the mother develops Rh-positive antibodies that affect her subsequent children. Usually the first Rh-positive child is not affected unless there is placental tearing or leakage into the mother's circulation.

Myasthenia gravis is another example of type II hypersensitivity. In this case, there are antibodies to the acetylcholine receptor on muscle membrane surfaces, primarily the motor end-plate. With the antigen-antibody formation at the receptor site, complement attacks the receptor. Effector cells are not thought to be involved in this type II hypersensitivity reaction.[7] The loss of acetylcholine stimulation at the motor end-plate causes the extreme muscular weakness associated with myasthenia gravis. Other autoantibodies associated with type II hypersensitivity are listed in Table 10–4.

Hyperacute graft rejection is a type II hypersensitivity reaction that affects transplanted tissues, particularly the kidney. It occurs when the transplanted donor tissue has an antigen to which the recipient has preformed antibodies. For example, when a tissue from a blood type A or B donor is transplanted into a blood type O recipient, the recipient has anti-A and anti-B antibodies. These antibodies will immediately attack the foreign transplanted tissue.

As in other type II hypersensitivity reactions, onset begins immediately after revascularization in the transplant procedure. This antigen-antibody complex formation with Fc bridging triggers effector cell infiltration and complement-mediated lysis of the donor tissues, inflammation, vascular thrombosis, and hemorrhage. The reaction happens so quickly that the tissue is not even vascularized. Within 48 hours after transplantation, the graft tissue is ravaged and no longer functioning.

TABLE 10–3. ABO Blood Groups

Blood Group (Phenotype)	Antigens	Antibodies to ABO in serum
A	A	Anti-B
B	B	Anti-A
AB	A and B	None
O	H	Anti-A, anti-B

TABLE 10–4. Diseases and Autoantibodies Associated with Type II Hypersensitivity

Disease	Antigen/Autoantibody
Type I diabetes	Islet cells
Insulin-resistant diabetic states	Insulin receptor
Myasthenia gravis	Acetylcholine receptor
Addison's disease	Adrenal epithelial cells
Autoimmune hemolytic anemia	Red cell membrane
Immune thrombocytopenic purpura	Platelet membrane
Autoimmune neutropenia	Neutrophil antigens
Pernicious anemia	Intrinsic factor, gastric parietal cells
Lymphocytic thyroiditis	Thyroglobulin
Graves' disease	Receptor for thyroid-stimulating hormone
Pemphigus vulgaris	Desmosomes
Hyperacute graft rejection	Donor antigens

Adapted with permission from Widmann FK: *An Introduction to Clinical Immunology.* Philadelphia, FA Davis, 1989, p 247.

Type III Hypersensitivity ✓

Type III hypersensitivity is also known as *immune complex* or *arthus's reaction.* Type III hypersensitivity is characterized by antigen-antibody complex deposition into tissues, causing an inflammatory reaction. This reaction peaks 6 hours after exposure to the antigen. IgG is the principal antibody. The principal effector cells are neutrophils and mast cells. Examples of this type of hypersensitivity reaction include serum sickness, glomerulonephritis, SLE, arthritis, and vasculitis. Table 10–5 lists the diseases associated with type III hypersensitivity.

Type III hypersensitivity reactions involve a sequential process that begins with an interaction between a circulating soluble antigen and soluble antibody or between an insoluble antigen and a soluble antibody.[13] Depending on the concentration of anti-

TABLE 10–5. Diseases Associated with Type III Hypersensitivity

Immune complex glomerulonephritis
Systemic lupus erythematosus (SLE)
SLE-associated glomerulonephritis
Acute allergic alveolitis
Farmer's lung disease
Pigeon fancier's disease
Postinfectious arthritis
Drug-sensitivity arthritis
Rheumatoid arthritis
Serum sickness
Henoch-Schönlein purpura
Drug-induced vasculitis
Polyarteritis nodosa
Wegener's granulomatosis
Goodpasture's syndrome

Adapted with permission from Widmann FK: *An Introduction to Clinical Immunology.* Philadelphia, FA Davis, 1989, pp 252–253.

gen and antibody, multiple cross-linking of antigen and antibody occurs.

This complex is unlike smaller complexes, which can remain suspended and be removed via the urine. It is also unlike the very large-sized complexes, which can be more easily phagocytized because they are more easily marked or fixed by complement. Large complexes are phagocytized by the reticuloendothelial system—particularly the Kupffer cells in the liver.[7,14] When both antigen and antibody are soluble, the complex precipitates out of the body fluid and is deposited into tissues. When only the antibody is soluble, the antibody reacts with the fixed antigen in the tissues. Then, the antibody within the complex links with the complement system via its Fc receptors.

The activation of the classical complement cascade releases C3a and C5a as well as the membrane attack complex. C3a, with its anaphylatoxin function, stimulates release of histamine from mast cells, indirectly increasing vascular permeability and vasodilation. This causes bronchial smooth muscle contraction, which causes bronchial constriction, wheezing, and coughing. C3a also causes the rounding up of endothelial cells, thereby increasing vascular permeability. The increased vascular permeability leads to edema formation, which allows cellular inflammatory components to move around easier. It also dilutes and limits the duration of action of mediators. C5a is an even more powerful component than C3a. It is a powerful anaphylatoxin with actions the same as those of C3a. It is also a powerful chemotactic agent for neutrophils. C5a also causes a respiratory burst within neutrophils, causing an increase in oxygen consumption 50 times normal, increased glucose uptake and procoagulant activity.

As a result of the activation of complement, neutrophils, macrophages, and mast cells are attracted to the area and are activated. These cells begin lysis and destruction of the tissues via the release of cytokines and the inflammatory response. The inflammation causes tissue destruction, scarring, and further reaction of the immune system against the damaged tissue (Fig. 10–5).[14]

Antigen-antibody complex deposition in tissues is affected by a number of factors. Increased vascular permeability as a result of histamine or other vasoactive mediator release is hypothesized to be an important factor in tissue deposition.[7,13] Researchers have found that even small immune complexes can be deposited in tissues treated with vasoactive mediators.[7] Sites of increased turbulence and blood pressure tend to have increased immune complex deposition.[7] These sites include the glomerular capillaries, choroid plexus, ciliary body, and vessel curves or bifurcations.

Intermediate-sized immune complexes tend to be deposited because they do not fix complement well, do not bind with RBCs well, and are not removed by the reticuloendothelial system well. Occasionally even small immune complexes can be deposited if they are so numerous that the phagocytic cells are overwhelmed. The deposition of immune complexes also depends on their immunoglobulin class and the

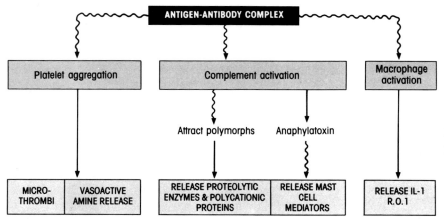

FIGURE 10–5. Type III immune complex–mediated hypersensitivity. (From Roitt I: *Essential Immunology*, 7th ed. Oxford, Blackwell Scientific Publications, 1991, p 265. Reproduced with permission.)

affinity between the antigen and antibody.[7,13] Lastly, deposition may be affected by the type of antigen or by the relationship between the immune complex and the sites with increased collagen.[7] Because there is a strong affinity between DNA and collagen, there may be increased deposition of DNA–anti-DNA immune complexes in collagen membranes such as in the kidney.[7]

There are three possible scenerios that can precipitate type III hypersensitivity. First, a *persistent low-grade infection* due to a microbial or viral agent can stimulate a weak antibody response. The continuing nature of persistent infection and antibody response leads to chronic immune complex production.[7] Second, an extrinsic environmental antigen from molds, plants, or animals can be inhaled into the lung. This *inhalation of antigen* causes antigen-antibody complex formation in alveoli. Third, an autoimmune process can develop in which *autoantibodies attack self antigens*. In this case, the body forms antibodies to some of its own cells. Because the cells persist over time, there is chronic immune complex production and deposition in tissues.

Immune complex glomerulonephritis is an example of a type III hypersensitivity reaction due to persistent low-grade infection. It involves the interaction of soluble exogenous antigen with soluble antibody. It is the cause of most glomerulonephritis cases. Glomerulonephritis typically occurs 10 days to 2 weeks following an infection with a *Streptococcus* bacterial strain. The immune complex is deposited in the glomerular capillary wall and the mesangium.[13] This deposition causes proteinuria, hematuria, hypertension, oliguria, and red cell casts in the urine. In some types of glomerulonephritis, the patient may have edema, nephrotic syndrome, and acute renal failure that may progress to chronic renal failure.

The treatment of glomerulonephritis involves the use of corticosteroids to decrease inflammation.[13] In certain situations, cyclophosphamide and azathioprine may be used as immunosuppressives. Antihistamines and antiserotonins have been tried in order to decrease vasoactive mediators and vascular permeability. Anticoagulants and antiplatelet medications

such as aspirin as well as plasmapheresis are currently being studied. In plasmapheresis, plasma is removed from the blood and type-specific fresh frozen plasma or albumin is used to replace the withdrawn plasma.

✓ Systemic lupus erythematosus (SLE) is another example of type III hypersensitivity reaction due to autoantibody production. SLE is a member of the group of diseases variably called autoimmune, connective tissue, collagen-vascular, or inflammatory disorders. SLE tends to occur more frequently in women than in men, with an incidence of 7.6 per 100,000.[15] It is primarily characterized by the development of antibodies against nuclear antigens such as DNA, deoxyribonucleohistone, and RNA.[15,16] Production of autoantibodies to the RBCs, neutrophils, platelets, lymphocytes, and other organs or tissues may also occur.[16] SLE is associated with decreased serum complement levels.

Antinuclear and anti-DNA autoantibodies attack and deposit on collagen-rich tissues, including the glomerular basement membrane and the dermal-epidermal junction.[16] However, autoantibodies can react with DNA anywhere in the body. The immune complex deposition and resulting inflammatory response cause the signs and symptoms of SLE.

The disorder has a variety of signs and symptoms because any organ system can be involved in SLE. Kidney involvement leads to nephritis and glomerulonephritis. Skin symptoms include an erythmatous rash on exposed skin, purpura, alopecia, mucosal ulcerations, subcutaneous nodules, and splinter hemorrhages.[16] The patient may have symptoms of arthritis or polyarthralgia, pleurisy, pericarditis, restrictive pulmonary disease, retinal changes, thrombocytopenia, anemia, and gastrointestinal (GI) ulceration.[15] Central nervous system (CNS) involvement includes neuritis, seizures, depression, or psychosis.[15]

The treatment of SLE ranges from giving nonsteroidal anti-inflammatory agents such as aspirin to systemic corticosteroids. Corticosteroids decrease inflammation and provide immunosuppression, which can decrease symptoms and add to the patient's quality of life. Antimalarials such as hydroxychloroquine or chloroquine are occasionally used in cases with skin involvement because they bind and alter DNA.[15] If the patient does not respond to corticosteroids, immunosuppressives such as cyclophosphamide, chlorambucil, or azathioprine can be used.

Type IV Hypersensitivity ✓

Type IV hypersensitivity is also known as *delayed hypersensitivity*. Delayed hypersensitivity is characterized by tissue damage that results from a delayed cellular reaction to an antigenic challenge. Unlike other hypersensitivity reactions, there is no primary antibody involvement.[14] Rather, antigen-sensitized cytotoxic T-cells mediate the reaction by releasing lymphokines (cytokines). The principal effector cells are lymphocytes and macrophages, with mast cells involved in the early phases. This reaction peaks 24 hours to 14 days after exposure to the antigen.[7,17]

In general, type IV hypersensitivity reactions involve a series of events that evolves over time. Recent studies indicate that mast cell degranulation occurs early in the evolution of a delayed hypersensitivity reaction, followed by lymphocyte and macrophage invasion.[18] Unlike what occurs in type I hypersensitivity reactions, the mast cell degranulation is a local event with limited response of target cells, inhibiting cytokines, and selected release of cytokines by mast cells. The reaction is also limited by the action of T-suppressor cells, which inhibit other T-cell actions. The combined actions of T-cell and mast cell mediators call macrophages to the site.

There are several types of delayed hypersensitivity reactions. These include contact hypersensitivity, cutaneous basophil hypersensitivity (Jones-Mote), tuberculin-type hypersensitivity, granulomatous hypersensitivity, and transplant rejection.

Contact hypersensitivity is the most familiar type IV hypersensitivity. It is an allergic response to a wide variety of plant oils, chemicals, ointments, clothing, cosmetics, dyes, and adhesives. Contact hypersensitivity is an epidermal phenomenon. As a delayed reaction, it peaks in 48 to 72 hours. The reaction is slow because the skin-penetrating antigen is very small and in an incomplete form. This incomplete, lipid-soluble antigen is called a *hapten*. The hapten must first penetrate the epidermis, where it links with a normal body protein in the epidermis called a *carrier*. Only after the hapten combines with the carrier is it a complete antigen. The now complete antigen can then be presented to T-cells via epidermal macrophages called Langerhan's cells located in the suprabasal epidermis. Then, the antigen-sensitized T-cells release lymphokines, which initiate an inflammatory response and attract other effector cells. Effector cells in contact hypersensitivity include macrophages but not neutrophils.[7]

After primary exposure or immunization, there is a cellular reaction at each subsequent exposure site.[14] Cross-reactivity with related substances also occurs with contact hypersensitivity. For example, a person with contact dermatitis to nickel will react when exposed to a variety of nickel alloys, including the metals in earrings, zippers, and belt buckles.[14] The skin symptoms resulting from contact dermatitis include redness, edema, itching, and blisters. People with sensitivities may also experience respiratory symptoms if exposed to aerosolized hapten.[14] This could occur when a person is downwind from burning poison ivy or burning tires.

Cutaneous basophil hypersensitivity (Jones-Mote) is a lymphocyte-mediated basophil reaction. This reaction is produced by soluble antigen that triggers T-cell activation. The T-cells then release cytokines and activate basophils, which infiltrate the area. It is a delayed reaction that peaks in 24 hours and can last 7 to 10 days.[7] The reaction will disappear when antibody to the antigen arrives. An example of this type of hypersensitivity is skin graft reactions and rejection.

Tuberculin-type hypersensitivity occurs when someone who has tuberculosis or antibodies to it is exposed to tuberculin in a tuberculin test. It is a dermal phenomenon that peaks in 48 to 72 hours.[7] The person will experience redness, induration, and inflammation at the site of the subcutaneous injection. Because the injected amount is so small, the reaction will disappear when the antigen is degraded.[14] However, people with severe reactions may experience tissue necrosis at the site.

Granulomatous hypersensitivity reactions are a primary defense against intracellular infections and represent a chronic type IV hypersensitivity reaction.[17] It is a protective, defense reaction that eventually causes tissue destruction because of the persistence of the antigen. In this type of hypersensitivity, antigen is not destroyed within the macrophages. This is either due to failure of lysozyme-phagocyte fusion, as in tuberculosis and leprosy, or to material resistance to internal lysozymes, as in retained suture material. In an effort to protect the host, lymphocytes and macrophages actually cause the tissue damage by releasing cytokines and stimulating an inflammatory response (Fig. 10–6).

After the bacteria or sutures are ingested, the host walls off the area using a variety of inflammatory cells including macrophages, lymphocytes, tissue histiocytes, eosinophils, plasma cells, giant, and epithelioid cells.[17] This collection of inflammatory cells form a ball-like mass called a granuloma. The predominant cell in the granuloma is the macrophage.[17] Macrophages and macrophage-derived epithelioid cells make up the core of the granuloma. Epithelioid cells come from macrophages and are large, flat cells with lots of endoplasmic reticulum. When epithelioid cells fuse, they form multinucleated giant cells.[17,19] This core is surrounded by lymphocytes. Over time, fibroblastic activity and increased collagen synthesis cause the granuloma to become fibrotic with scar formation. Often there is central necrosis within the granuloma, called caseous or cheesy necrosis. Patient's with granulomatous diseases present with a variety of symptoms. Table 10–6 lists the granulomatous diseases.

Chronic transplant rejection is another type IV

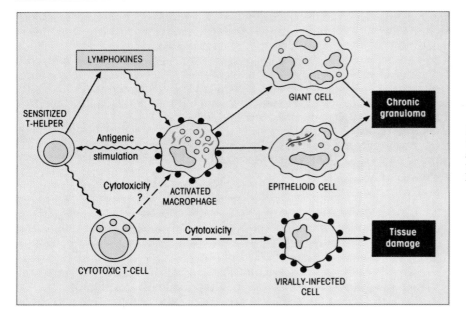

FIGURE 10–6. The cellular basis of type IV hypersensitivity. (From Roitt I: *Essential Immunology,* 7th ed. Oxford, Blackwell Scientific Publications, 1991, p 271. Reproduced with permission.)

hypersensitivity reaction. In this type of rejection, sensitized T-lymphocyte and macrophage infiltration of the donor tissues is seen. Helper T-cells and cytotoxic T-cells work together in graft rejection. Specifically, helper T-cells release lymphokines that stimulate and activate cytotoxic T-cells.[20] The resulting inflammation and release of cytokines cause tissue edema and vascular impairment, leading to necrosis, fibrosis, scarring, and decreased function. As in other delayed hypersensitivity reactions, chronic transplant rejection occurs months to years after transplantation. It can occur with kidney, heart, liver, pancreas, and bone transplants. In each case, symptoms may include delayed healing, poor vascularization, and decreasing function. Treatment includes the use of corticosteroids, cyclosporine, azathioprine, and antilymphocyte globulin (ALG).[21] Cyclosporine is used because of its inhibition of helper T-cells; ALG is used because of its cytolytic effect on lymphocytes.[21] Azathioprine inhibits T-cell function and mediated responses.[22]

Graft-versus-host disease (GvHD) is another type IV hypersensitivity reaction, but with a twist. This disease involves a host and donor that are not HLA identical or histocompatible. The host tissue HLA antigens differ from the donated tissue HLA antigens. In GvHD, the host is immunosuppressed with deficient cellular immunity, but the donor tissue is fully immunocompetent. For example, this type of disease can occur during bone marrow transplantation where the host is without immunity but the transplanted tissue is fully functional. The donor tissue lymphocytes are able to recognize the host tissues as foreign. Because the host is not able to seek out and destroy the donor's lymphocytes, the host is overwhelmed and attacked by the donor lymphocytes.

GvHD can occur in patients undergoing any type of tissue transplantation or as a consequence of blood transfusions.[23] GvHD can be acute, occurring within 10 to 70 days, or chronic, developing after 180 days. The skin, liver, and GI systems are primarily affected, with associated symptoms including skin rashes, severe diarrhea, hepatomegaly, and jaundice.[24,25]

Prevention of GvHD includes a number of approaches. First, patients at high risk for transfusion-associated GvHD should receive gamma-irradiated blood products. Patients at high risk include premature newborns and patients who have undergone bone marrow and organ transplantations, those with congenital immunodeficiency syndromes, patients with Hodgkin's disease, patients with solid tumors, and people with AIDS.[23] Second, prevention of GvHD in patients can include a 3- to 12-month course of immunosuppression with methotrexate, cyclophosphamide, or cyclosporine after transplantation.[24] Third, prevention can involve limiting transplantation to HLA genotypical identical siblings.[25] Fourth, in bone marrow transplantation, it can involve transplanting T-cell–depleted bone marrow.[25]

Treatment of GvHD is difficult. It involves the use of anti-human thymocyte globulin (ATG), prednisone, cyclosporine, methotrexate, and monoclonal antibodies.[24] Combination protocols of these agents

TABLE 10–6. Granulomatous Diseases Associated With Type IV Hypersensitivity

Disease	Bacterium
Tuberculosis	*Mycoplasma tuberculosis*
Leprosy	*Mycoplasma leprae*
Histoplasmosis	*Histoplasma capsulatum*
Coccidioidomycosis	*Coccidioides immitis*
Brucellosis	*Brucella abortus*
	Brucella suis (less common)
	Brucella melitensis (less common)
Tularemia	*Francisella (Pasteurella) tularensis*

are common and tend to be more effective than single-agent therapy.[25]

- Type I hypersensitivity is an immediate allergic or anaphylactic type reaction mediated primarily by sensitized mast cells. The reaction is initiated when IgE antibodies located on the mast cell membrane are bound by antigen, leading to cross-linking of IgE receptors. Mast cell degranulation releases chemicals that mediate the signs and symptoms of anaphylaxis. Released histamine, kinins, prostaglandins, interleukins, and leukotrienes result in increased vascular permeability, vasodilation, hypotension, urticaria, and bronchoconstriction. Examples of type I reactions include drug reactions, bee sting reactions, and asthma.

- Type II hypersensitivity occurs when antibodies are formed against antigens on cell surfaces, resulting in lysis of target cells. Cell lysis may be mediated by activated complement fragments (membrane attack complex) or by phagocytic cells that are attracted to target cells by the attached antibodies. Examples include transfusion reactions, erythroblastosis fetalis, and myasthenia gravis.

- Type III hypersensitivity reactions occur when antigen-antibody complexes are deposited in tissues, resulting in tissue inflammation and destruction. Antigen-antibody complexes activate the complement cascade and subsequently attract phagocytic cells to the tissue. Persistent low-grade infections, the inhalation of antigens into alveoli, and autoimmune system production of antibodies may result in chronic production of antigen-antibody complexes. Examples include glomerulonephritis and systemic lupus erythematosus.

- Type IV hypersensitivity reactions are T-cell mediated and do not require antibody production, in contrast to types I, II, and III. Sensitized T-cells react with altered or foreign cells and initiate inflammation. Contact dermatitis, tuberculin reactions, transplant rejection, and graft-versus-host disease are examples.

Alterations in Immune Function: Hypofunction

Primary Immunodeficiency Disorders

Primary immunodeficiency disorders result from a functional decrease in one or more components of the immune system. These disorders can affect lymphocytes, antibodies, phagocytes, and complement proteins.[26] The most common disorders are listed in Table 10–7. They are congenital disorders, often genetically sex-linked. The first clinical indicators of immunodeficiency disorders are the signs and symptoms of infection, and the disorders are often first suspected when an infant has severe recurrent or untreatable infections.

B-Cell and T-Cell Combined Disorders

Severe combined immunodeficiency disorders (SCID) are due to embryonic defects that wipe out stem cells in the bone marrow. They include a group of disorders that are characterized by severe immune system dysfunction and a variety of clinical features. The most common SCIDs are autosomal recessive (or Swiss type), autosomal recessive with enzyme adenosine deaminase (ADA) deficiency, X-linked recessive, defective expression of MHC antigens, and SCID with leukopenia or reticular dysgenesis.

Infants with SCID due to autosomal recessive or X-linked recessive disease lack T-cell, B-cell, and natural killer cell functions. Antibody titers are decreased, with lack of antibody formation after immunization. T-cells are low in number or absent, but the ratio of helper to suppressor cells is not inverted, as in acquired immunodeficiency syndrome (AIDS). Some infants have increased numbers of B-cells but they are unable to function.[14,26] Generally, most patients have small, hypoplastic thymuses.[26] Infants with SCID due to defective expression of MHC antigens have poor antibody production with decreased IgG, IgM, and IgA. Lymphocyte numbers are normal to slightly decreased. T-cell function is decreased. Infants with reticular dysgenesis have failure of both lymphocytes and granulocytes. Although the fetus grows normally, the infant is severely affected, with deceased numbers of lymphocytes, decreased antibodies, and decreased phagocytic cells.[14]

Infants with these syndromes develop infections such as otitis, pneumonia, and diarrhea shortly after birth. They are prone to develop sepsis, opportunistic infections with such pathogens as *Candida albicans* or *Pneumocystis carinii*, infections with such viruses as cytomegalovirus or herpes, and common childhood diseases such as varicella and measles.[26] Because of the severity of the infections, most affected infants do not grow normally once an infection develops. Treatment includes bone marrow transplantation. However, these infants are at high risk for developing GvHD. Infants with reticular dysgenesis usually die within the first few months of life.[14]

Wiskott-Aldrich syndrome is an X-linked immunodeficiency disorder that affects both T-cells and B-cells.[14] It is characterized by the presence of eczema, thrombocytopenic purpura, and infection. In this syndrome, antibody concentrations are variable, with IgE and IgA usually elevated, IgG normal to low, and IgM usually decreased. This antibody variability is due to increased antibody catabolism. There is also associated platelet deficiency. T-cells are present but function deficiently.[14] Affected infants have particular difficulty mounting immune responses to polysaccharide antigens which include bacterial cell walls.[26] For this reason, they are prone to pneumococcal infections, including pneumonia, meningitis, otitis media, and sepsis. They are also subject to renal disease and ma-

TABLE 10–7. Primary Immunodeficiency Disorders

Disorder	Functional Deficiency
Bruton's X-linked agammaglobulinemia	Antibody
Common variable (acquired) hypogammaglobulinemia	Antibody
Selective IgA deficiency	IgA antibody
Secretory component deficiency—chronic mucocutaneous candidiasis	Secretory IgA
Selective IgM deficiency	IgM antibody
Selective deficiency of IgG subclasses	IgG antibody subclass
Immunodeficiency with elevated IgM	IgG and IgA antibodies
Transient hypogammaglobulinemia of infancy	Low antibodies
Antibody deficiency with near-normal immunoglobulins	Antibody
Duncan's X-linked lymphoproliferative disease	Anti-Epstein-Barr virus–linked antigen antibody
DiGeorge's syndrome (congenital thymic hypoplasia or aplasia)	Primarily T-cells
Nezelof's syndrome	T-cells, antibodies, neutropenia
Autosomal recessive severe combined immunodeficiency syndrome (SCID)	T-cells, antibodies
Autosomal recessive SCID with ADA deficiency	T-cells, antibodies
X-linked recessive SCID	T-cells, antibodies
Defective expression of major histocompatibility complex (MHC) antigens	T-cells, antibodies
SCID with leukopenia (reticular dysgenesis)	T-cells, antibodies, granulocytes
Wiskott-Aldrich syndrome (immunodeficiency with eczema and thrombocytopenia)	Antibody, T-cells
Ataxia, telangiectasia	Antibody, T-cells
Cartilage-hair hypoplasia	T-cells
Immunodeficiency with thymoma	T-cells, antibody
Hyperimmunoglobulinemia E	Excessive IgE
Lymphocyte function antigen 1 deficiency	Cytotoxic cells, phagocytic cells
Chediak-Higashi-Steinbrink syndrome	Natural killer cells, phagocytic cells
Chronic granulomatous disease of childhood	Phagocytic cells
Acquired immunodeficiency syndrome	T-cells, CD4 cells

Adapted with permission from Widmann FK: *An Introduction to Clinical Immunology.* Philadelphia, FA Davis, 1989, p 194. Data from Buckley RH: Immunodeficiency diseases. *JAMA* 1992;268(20):2797–2806.

lignancies. The average age at death of these infants is 3.5 years[27]; survival beyond adolescence is rare.[26]

Infants with the Wiskott-Aldrich syndrome are often treated with splenectomy, antibody replacement therapy, and antibiotic therapy. Bone marrow transplantation is an option that shows some promise in this disorder.

T-Cell Disorders

DiGeorge's syndrome or *thymic hypoplasia* is a developmental T-cell disorder associated with total or partial loss of thymus gland function.[14] The aplastic or hypoplastic thymus is unable to assist in the maturation of T-cells. Therefore, there is a deficiency of T-cells. B-cells are normal. Because it is a developmental disorder, this syndrome is often associated with other congenital problems such as cardiac and great vessel anomalies, hypoparathyroidism with hypocalcemia, esophageal atresia, and unusual facial features including mandibular hypoplasia and low-set ears.[14,26] Infants with partial loss of thymus function may not have trouble with infections. However, infants with total loss of thymus function resemble children with SCID and rarely live to age 6 years.[27]

Chronic mucocutaneous candidiasis is an autosomal recessive T-cell disorder characterized by severe skin and mucous membrane infection with *Candida albicans.*[14] B-cell and T-cell functions are usually normal except for the inability of the T-cells to respond to the *Candida.*[14,26] Occasionally, IgA levels may be affected. This disorder is associated with high endocrine gland autoantibodies and hypoactivity. Affected patients often develop autoimmune endocrine deficiences.

There is no known cure for this disorder. The goal of treatment is to reduce the severity of skin and mucous membrane infection and to decrease disfigurement from infection and scarring.

B-Cell Disorders

✓The most common immunodeficiency disorder is *selective IgA deficiency.* This disorder affects 1 in 400 persons. It is a B-cell disorder characterized by failure of IgA-bearing lymphocytes to become plasma cells, with resulting lack of serum and secretory IgA.[14,26,27] Genetically, it can be an autosomal recessive or autosomal dominant disease.[14] People with this disorder are prone to respiratory, GI, and genitourinary (GU) tract infections. They tend to have many autoantibodies (including anti-IgA antibodies) with a high incidence of vascular and collagen autoimmune diseases. They often react to cow's milk and can develop sprue-like conditions. Because they have severe allergic reactions to blood or blood products containing IgA, exogenous IgA replacement is contraindicated. Treatment includes prevention of infection and treatment of infection with appropriate antibiotics.

Bruton's X-linked agammaglobulinemia or *congenital hypogammaglobulinemia* is a B-cell disorder due to dysplastic B-cell tissue (bursa equivalent). In 1952, it was the first immunodeficiency disorder identified.[27] In this case, alteration in the function of the bursa equivalent results in B-cell deficiency with decreased serum concentrations of IgG, IgA, and IgM.[14] T-cell numbers are increased and the thymus is normal. Male infants are affected but are not usually diagnosed with this disorder until they are 6 to 9 months old because of passive maternal IgG protection.[14,26] Frequent infections occur in these infants, including pneumonia, otitis, meningitis, sinusitis, and septicemia.[26] Despite the infections, these infants can grow normally if treated with antibiotics and recurrent administration of human gamma-globulin. However, passive immunotherapy is not always effective. If the child survives to adulthood, life expectancy is decreased and rheumatoid arthritis is common.[14]

Transient hypogammaglobulinemia of infancy is a self-limiting condition in which the infant is slow to develop normal immunoglobulin levels.[14] The infant experiences a lengthened period of low IgG levels after birth.[7] Affected infants are able to develop normal immunoglobulin levels and immune system functions by approximately age 4. During the period of low antibody levels, they are more susceptible to infections, particularly respiratory tract infections.

KEY CONCEPTS

- Primary deficiencies in immune function may be congenital, genetic, or acquired. Secondary deficiencies are conditions that impair immune function secondarily to other processes such as poor nutrition, stress, or drugs.
- Absence of stem cells in the marrow results in severe combined immunodeficiency disorder (SCID). Functional B- and T-lymphocytes are lacking, and infants with SCID easily succumb to sepsis and opportunistic infections. Other types of primary immunodeficiency disorders affect a particular cell type: DiGeorge's syndrome occurs with T-cell agenesis related to lack of thymus function, chronic mucocutaneous candidiasis is due to abnormal T-cells that cannot respond to *Candida,* and Selective IgA deficiency is due to B-cell abnormality.

Human Immunodeficiency Virus and Acquired Immunodeficiency Syndrome

Acquired immunodeficiency syndrome is a primary immunodeficiency disease caused by one of two retroviruses, **human immunodeficiency virus** (HIV) type I and HIV type II. HIV's emergence worldwide has triggered major research efforts to better understand and combat its lethal effects on the immune system.

Retroviruses were one of the first viruses discovered at the turn of the century as the cause of cancers in chickens.[28] Originally, they were identified only in nonhuman species, where their presence was generally harmless or occasionally associated with tumors and slowly progressive cardiovascular, pulmonary, or neurologic diseases. Retroviruses have subsequently been identified in most animal species.[29]

HIV is very closely related to primate retroviruses, particularly the green monkey virus and macaque monkey virus called simian immunodeficiency virus STLV-III or SIV.[30,31] This primate retrovirus does not cause disease in monkeys. It is hypothesized that a virus similar to STLV-III may have crossed species into humans, initiating a series of mutations that became HIV.[31,32]

In 1980, the first human retroviruses were found to affect T-cells. The human T-lymphocyte virus HTLV-I was found to infect T-cells, causing adult T-cell leukemia.[30] HTLV-II was subsequently discovered and found to be associated with the development of hairy cell leukemias and T-cell leukemias.[30] HTLV-IV is associated with patients who have chronic lymphomas, but this relationship is not well established.[29] These are transforming, cancer-causing viruses that were originally thought to be closely linked to HIV. This has proved not to be correct.[31] However, their discovery enlightened Gallo, Essex, and Montagnier, who were able to narrow their search for the cause of AIDS.[31]

In 1981 the first descriptions of immunodeficiency disease in previously healthy persons appeared in the medical literature.[33] But the specific retrovirus causing HIV infection and AIDS was not isolated until 1983 (Montagnier) and 1984 (Gallo). HIV is a type of retrovirus from a subfamily called lentiviruses (Lentivirinae). This subfamily is so named from the Latin (*Lentus,* slow) because infection occurs slowly over time.[31] It was originally labeled human T-lymphotropic virus III (HTLV-III) and was renamed human immunodeficiency virus (HIV). HIV type 2, a related but distinct retrovirus, was later identified in 1986 and is most closely related to simian immunodeficiency virus.[31]

Although the syndrome was not reported until 1981, isolated cases of HIV or HIV-like infections had been reported beginning in the 1950s and 1960s. Positive tests on serum for HIV antibodies were found in samples taken from a small region in Central Africa in the 1950s. This infection appears to have remained localized before spreading to the rest of Central Africa during the late 1960s and early 1970s. It is commonly thought that HIV reached Haiti in the late 1970s and may have reached Europe and the Americas from there.[34]

HIV is nondiscriminatory. It infects people worldwide without regard for age, race, sex, or social class. Currently, there are an estimated 19.5 million adults infected with HIV worldwide.[35] This figure is expected

HIV also known as HTLV

to increase to 40 million people by the year 2000.[36] In the United States, approximately 1 million people are infected with HIV.[37,38] To date, there have been 195,000 cases of AIDS, with a 65 percent mortality rate.[39] Between 1991 and 1993, 165,000 to 215,000 people will die of AIDS.[38] It is estimated that 5,000 people a day worldwide are infected with HIV.[36]

Both HIV 1 and HIV 2 are found worldwide. They are similar in structure and function. They are differentiated by their point of origin. HIV 1 is thought to have originated in Central Africa, and HIV 2 was originally isolated in West Africa.[30] HIV type 1 is the causative organism for most AIDS cases found in the United States.[26]

Transmission ✓

HIV 1 and 2 can infect people through several known routes of transmission. HIV is known to be transmitted in blood, semen, vaginal, and cervical secretions, amniotic fluids, and breast milk. HIV is known to be present in but not believed to be transmitted in urine, saliva, tears, cerebrospinal fluid, and possibly feces.

Because of these known routes of transmission, those at highest risk of developing HIV infection include IV drug users who share needles, unprotected sexual partners of IV drug users, unprotected male or female sexual partners of homosexual or bisexual men, recipients of HIV-contaminated blood or blood products, and people who have multiple sexual partners, who have unprotected sex with a partner of unknown HIV status, or who have unprotected sex outside of a monogamous relationship.

Heterosexual intercourse with infected partners is the major route of transmission of HIV, with 56.8 percent of the cases due to sexual intercourse with an IV drug user.[40,41] Because of this, women are the fastest growing risk group with a larger proportionate infection rate increase than men (Fig. 10–7).[41–43] AIDS is currently the leading cause of death in 20 to 40-year-old women in New York City and is predicted to become one of the leading causes of death in all women between the ages of 20 and 45 years.[42] The World Health Organization (WHO) states that more than 3 million women are infected worldwide.[44] Black and Hispanic women had the highest infection rate increases.[41] Because child-bearing women are at risk, pregnant HIV-infected women also risk transmitting HIV to their fetus. This risk is 20 percent to 50 percent for each pregnancy, with increasing risk in subsequent pregnancies for each HIV-positive fetus born.[45] Women who are diagnosed with AIDS die more quickly than their male counterparts.[42]

Routine social contact with people who are HIV positive does not increase one's risk of getting HIV. For example, using public restrooms, swimming in public swimming pools, touching or hugging someone who is HIV positive, or eating with community utensils or in restaurants are safe practices. One cannot get HIV infection from insects like mosquitoes.

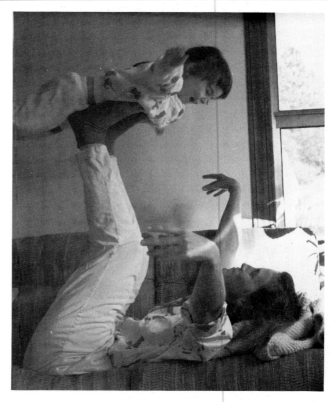

F I G U R E 10–7. Mother and child, both HIV positive. AIDS will be a leading cause of death in all women by the year 2000. (Photographer: Rachel DeHaan, Spokane, WA.)

Prevention is essential. Safe sex practices include abstinence, use of a condom (barrier protection) during sexual intercourse, avoiding multiple sexual partners, and knowing the HIV status of all sexual partners.[46] Spermicides may inactivate HIV and other sexually transmitted diseases but must be used with a male or female condom.[47] HIV infection in drug users can be prevented by using sterile needles and avoiding dirty or shared needles. HIV infection in infants can be prevented by avoiding pregnancy when engaging in high-risk behaviors.

Medical and health care personnel are at risk through occupational exposure to blood and bodily fluids. Self-protection though the use of universal precautions can decrease risk by reducing exposure.[48] Health care providers should carefully wash their hands before and immediately after patient contact. It is essential to wear disposable gloves for any actual or potential contact with blood or body secretions, when handling items contaminated with blood or body fluids, when performing finger or heel sticks, or when the health care provider has scratches or cuts on the hand.

Gowns or plastic aprons, masks, goggles, or face shields should be worn to protect face and clothing when there is risk of airborne droplets of blood or body fluids. Protective gear should be changed between patients. Needles and sharps should be disposed of in rigid, puncture-proof containers. They should not be bent, broken, or recapped prior to disposal. Resuscitation bags and masks should be available to minimize the need for mouth-to-mouth procedures.

Hallmarks of HIV Infection

The hallmark of HIV infection is the decrease in CD4 or T-helper/inducer lymphocytes. CD4 or T-helper cells are necessary for appropriate immune responsiveness because they are the cells that mediate between the antigen-presenting cells and other immune cells such as B-cells and other T-cells. The CD4 lymphocytes are characterized by the presence of the CD4 receptor (Fig. 10–8).

In addition to these cellular immune system abnormalities, there are accompanying humoral immune dysfunctions. B-cell numbers remain normal.[49] IgG levels are elevated, with hypergammaglobulinemia; IgM levels are elevated in early infection; and IgA levels are elevated in late infection. Despite these elevations, there is decreased responsiveness to polysaccharide (bacterial cell wall) antigens. Immune complexes are increased and B-cell differentiation and responses to antigens are decreased.[50,51] Macrophage numbers remain normal, but their functions are generally decreased.[49]

In order to diagnose HIV infection, laboratory tests such as enzyme-linked immunosorbent assay test (ELISA) and the Western blot test are used to detect the presence of HIV antibodies, which in infected persons are in measurable quantities. The ELISA test is positive for HIV antibodies if the blood of an infected person reacts with the surface antigen of a killed HIV virus. When the ELISA test is positive, a second test, the Western blot test, is used to confirm the presence of HIV antibodies. The Western blot test uses an expensive process called electrophoresis, so it is usually used only as a confirmatory test.

There are other laboratory and diagnostic tests that assist in the identification of persons infected with HIV, including a complete blood cell count and a chemistry panel or screen. A specific indicator of disease progression is a blood serum laboratory test for T-helper and T-suppressor cell ratio. Diagnostic tests such as chest x-rays are helpful in determining the presence of secondary infections such as pneumonia or *Pneumocystis carinii* infection. Table 10–8 lists helpful diagnostic and laboratory tests used to diagnose or predict the course of HIV infection.

Etiology

HIV is an RNA virus that causes a defect in cell-mediated immunity. HIV is a retrovirus; the viral RNA must be converted into DNA before the viral genes can be expressed. Like other retroviruses, HIV differs from DNA viruses because the RNA genome cannot replicate without undergoing transformation into DNA. (See also Chapter 8 for a discussion of retroviruses.)

HIV consists of a core or *capsid* of two strands or chains of RNA, protein and enzymes surrounded by a spherical viral envelope one ten-thousandth of a millimeter across.[35] The viral envelope consists of a cell membrane derived from the host cell from which protrude viral glycoprotein studs. The outside of the viral envelope looks like a studded ball (Fig. 10–9). *Glycoprotein 120* (gp120) and *glycoprotein 41* (gp41) are the two HIV envelope proteins that cover the viral particle surface. Gp120 is the most external and distal part of each "stud," while gp41 is the bridge that holds it onto the virion surface. Although the viral particle (virion) is roughly spherical, there is great diversity

TABLE 10–8. Tests Used to Diagnose HIV Infection

Complete blood cell count
  White blood cell count normal to decreased
  Lymphopenia (<30 percent of WBCs)
  Thrombocytopenia (decreased platelet count)
Lymphocyte screen
  Reduced helper/suppressor T-cell ratio
  T4 (helper) lymphocytes decreased
  T8 (suppressor) lymphocytes increased
Quantitative immunoglobulin
  IgG increased
  IgA frequently increased
Chemistry panel
  Lactic dehydrogenase (LDH) increased (all fractions)
  Serum albumin decreased
  Total protein increased
  Cholesterol decreased
  SGOT and SGPT elevated
Anergy panel
  Nonreactive (anergic) or poorly reactive to infectious agents or environmental materials, i.e., pokeweed, phytohemagglutinin mitogens and antigens, mumps, candidin
Hepatitis B surface antigen
  To detect presence of hepatitis B/C
Blood cultures
  To detect septicemia
Chest x-ray
  To detect *Pneumocystis carinii* or tuberculosis

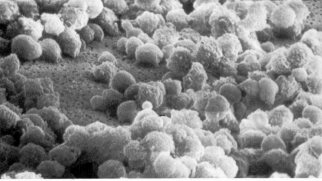

FIGURE 10–8. Scanning electron micrograph (low magnification) of population of AIDS-infected lymphocytes. (Courtesy of Centers for Disease Control and Prevention, Atlanta.)

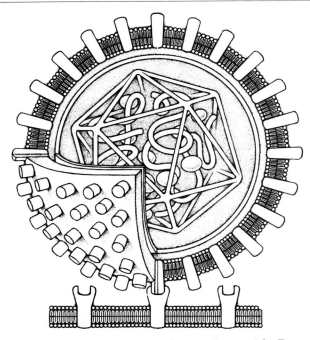

F I G U R E 10–9. Schematic view of a retrovirus particle. Two identical single strands of viral RNA are within the viral core. The core is surrounded by an envelope that is derived from host membranes enriched with viral glycoprotein. Interaction of the envelope glycoprotein with a host-encoded cell surface receptor (CD4) is shown at the bottom. (From Varmus H: Retroviruses. *Science* 1988;240:1427–1435. Copyright 1988 by the AAAS. As adapted from Varmus H: *Advances in Oncology* 1987; copyright 1987 *Advances in Oncology*.)

in size and shape—such as comet-shaped virion and virion with tails.[31]

The core is protected by the viral envelope. Between the envelope and core is a protein layer called p17.[35] The capsid itself is composed of a protein called p24.[35] Within the capsid, the two strands of RNA compose the viral genome (Fig. 10–10).

This genome contains all of the information regulating the virus's structural format and growth during its life cycle. The enzymes within the core are also very important because they facilitate the conversion of RNA into DNA. This conversion is the means of information transfer with this virus. The enzymes include *reverse transcriptase, integrase,* and *protease. Reverse transcriptase* is composed of two associated enzymes called *polymerase* and *ribonuclease.*

Once inside the body, HIV particles are attracted to cells with receptors on their surface, called CD4. The HIV envelope protein, gp120, specifically binds to the CD4 receptor. Once the HIV particle is bound to the CD4 receptor on the host cell, gp41 implants itself in the cell membrane. This sequence of events causes the viral particle and the cell to fuse. The core of the virus is then injected into the cytoplasm of the host cell, producing infection (Fig. 10–11).

Once in the cytoplasm, a single-strand DNA copy is made by reverse transcriptase from the viral RNA.

Using the single-strand DNA as a template, DNA *polymerase* copies it to make a second DNA strand and destroys the original RNA strands. The accuracy of the DNA transcription is poor, with frequent mutations.[35] This ability to mutate makes HIV easily resistant to antiviral medications.

Once formed, the new viral DNA, containing at least nine genes, migrates to the cell nucleus. Inside the nucleus, *integrase* splices the viral DNA, called *provirus,* into the host cell's DNA. Once in the host cell's DNA, the viral DNA (provirus) will be replicated together with the host cell's DNA during every cell division. Now the infection is permanent. The viral DNA is permanently part of the host cell's DNA.

Pathogenesis

The production of new virus is variable and dependent on the host's cellular activity as well as the interaction between HIV regulatory genes (gene names: *tat, nef, rev*).[35] In some cells, such as T-cells, HIV can lie dormant until activated; in other cells, such as macrophages and monocytes, RNA copies of HIV are consistently being made and released without destroying the host cell. Other host cellular factors that influence viral production of HIV include lack of proteins, inhibition by other proteins, or low concentrations of initiation factors.

The process of building new virus particles begins within the host cell's DNA. Segments at the end of the viral genome tell the host cell to make RNA copies of the viral DNA. Some of the genes direct the host cell to manufacture viral envelope proteins (gene name: *env*) and enzymes (gene name: *pol*), while other RNA strands become future genetic material (gene name: *gag*).

The assembly of new virus particles, called *virions,* occurs at the cell membrane. Three produced proteins migrate to the cell periphery and attach to the cell membrane, causing the viral material to bud out from the membrane. The protein-cutting enzyme, protease, separates the envelope proteins from enzymes and RNA genetic material and binds the viral core. Therefore, the completed virion has a host cell membrane from which the envelope proteins gp120 and gp41 stick out like spikes (Fig. 10–12).

During early infection, HIV is widespread throughout the body, with detectable viremia and viral seeding of lymph tissues.[52] This progresses to an asymptomatic phase of infection with little detectable virus in the blood. However, during this period, seeded HIV replicates in the lymph nodes, gradually destroying the lymph tissue during the infection.[35] This is associated with chronic lymphadenopathy and a persistent, gradual decline in CD4 T-cell numbers. Pantaleo et al. have hypothesized that the lymphadenopathy is caused by a vigorous intralymphoid immune response against HIV infection.[52] At the end of the infection, viremia again occurs. It is hypothesized that the destroyed lymph nodes are no longer capable of removing or holding virus, allowing viral escape into the bloodstream (Fig. 10–13).[35,52]

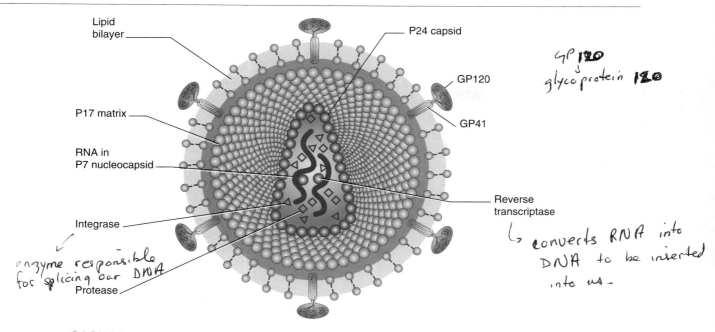

FIGURE 10–10. HIV retrovirus particle.

Once viral production starts, host cell death can occur. Cells may die due to the accumulation of intracellular viral DNA or the loss of normal cellular protein synthesis due to the infection.[52]

Most methods of host cell death involve the envelope protein gp120 or immune processes. Cross-linking of CD4 and gp120 can trigger automatic preprogrammed T-cell death, called *apoptosis*.[52] CD4 and gp120 cross-linking can also cause the cell to stop dividing and decreases the cell's ability to fight infection. This is called *anergy*.[35,52] Profuse viral production with multiple CD4 receptors in close proximity can also cause host cell death. Multiple virion buds with

gp120 on their surfaces attach to the surrounding host cell membrane CD4 receptors. This causes tearing of the host cell membrane with subsequent cellular edema and death.

Another process of cell death occurs when multiple uninfected cells become fused together with infected cells by the virus. This mass of cells is called a *syncytium formation*.[31] It can lead to a large number of cell deaths from a single event.

Cell death can occur when the immune system makes antibodies to the viral envelope protein. When gp120 is shed, it binds to uninfected CD4 receptors. Then the immune system attacks the uninfected but

FIGURE 10–11. Sequence of HIV infection and replication in CD4 cells. (Redrawn with permission from Schecter J: The frustrating fight against AIDS. *Technol Rev* 1987;90:65.)

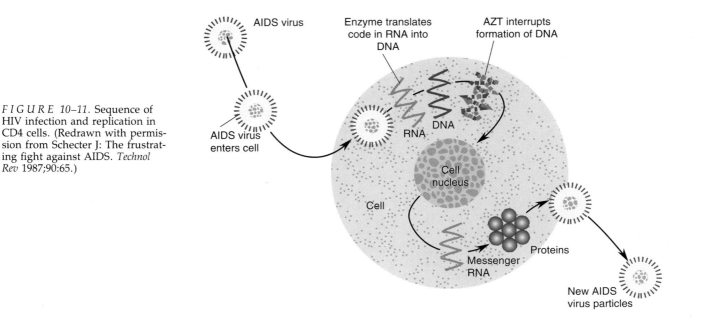

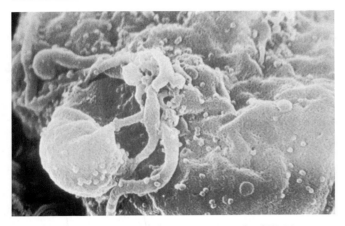

FIGURE 10–12. Scanning electron micrograph of HIV-I–infected T4 lymphocytes showing virus budding from the plasma membrane of the lymphocytes. (Courtesy of Centers for Disease Control and Prevention, Atlanta.)

antibody-coated cells with the complement system or killer T-cells, killing the uninfected host cells.[31,35] This can be antibody-dependent cellular cytotoxicity or natural killer cell cytotoxicity.[53]

Cell death can happen secondary to a type III hypersensitivity reaction. GP120 and gp41 have characteristics similar to MHC class antigens. In this case, the body may fail to recognize the difference between gp120 and "self MHC markers" and attack normal cells as nonself.[35] This causes destruction of large numbers of T-cells.[31,53] Cells may also be affected by

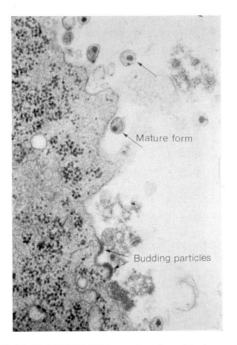

Mature form

Budding particles

FIGURE 10–13. HIV-I/LAV-type virus found in hemophiliac patient who developed AIDS. Magnification of virus particles ranges in size from 90 to 120 nm. (Courtesy of Centers for Disease Control and Prevention, Atlanta.)

T-cell–mediated cytotoxicity or by cytokines and inflammation resulting from infection.[31,53]

Staging and Symptoms

HIV infection is a syndrome and not a disease. This means that the virus can express itself in many ways. The CD4 receptor is found on most cells infected by HIV, including T-cells, microglial cells, lymph nodes, alveolar macrophages, thymus gland, bone marrow, and Langerhans cells in the skin. Other cells infected by HIV include glial cells in the brain, endothelial cells, cervical cells, retinal cells, transformed B-cells and bone marrow–derived circulating dendritic cells, and enterochromaffin cells in the colon, duodenum, and rectum.[53] As a result of this widespread involvement, the signs and symptoms of HIV infection are widespread and diverse.

No one symptom typifies HIV infection. However, groups of signs and symptoms are useful in staging the progress of the infection. There are a number of different classification systems that categorize groups of symptoms into stages. Each of the proposed systems utilize different approaches to describe the maturation of HIV from asymptomatic infection until the development of AIDS. The three major systems include the ARC-AIDS system, the Centers for Disease Control (CDC) system, and the Walter Reed classification systems.

A simple three-stage evolution of HIV infection from AIDS-related complex (ARC) to AIDS highlights the first classification system. The first stage involves the initial infection with HIV and seropositive conversion. This stage is associated with no symptoms except for an initial flulike syndrome.

The second stage is known as AIDS-related complex, or ARC. Persons with ARC have a positive HIV antibody titer and changes in other immune system functions. The person with symptoms of ARC must also have two or more of the following symptoms: weight loss, fever, night sweats, chronic diarrhea, lymphadenopathy (swollen nodes), or yeast infections.

The third stage is AIDS, the syndrome. The person has a positive HIV antibody titer, an altered T4:T8 cell ratio, and severe symptoms. In this case, the number of T4 cells is uncharacteristically lower than the number of T8 cells. The person has opportunistic infections or secondary tumor development.

The Walter Reed (WR) classification system is a more detailed categorization of HIV that uses laboratory testing as criteria for staging. In Stage 0, there is exposure to the virus. It appears in the CSF and blood but is not detected on laboratory tests because there are no antibodies yet. There are usually no symptoms. It is a time of rapid virus replication. The person is infectious but does not know it.

Stage 1 (WR-1) is marked by seroconversion. The T4-cell (CD4 cell) count remains greater than 400. The seroconversion process generally takes 3 weeks to 6 months after exposure, but may take as little as 2 weeks or as long as 14 months. At the time of sero-conversion, the person experiences flulike or mono-nucleosis-like symptoms. These symptoms include fever, chills, headaches, nausea, vomiting, fatigue, weakness, arthralgias, sore throat, stiff neck, photophobia, irritability, and rash. The rash is not the same in everyone and may be maculopapular, vesicular, or urticarial. The person may even develop encephalopathy. During WR-1, the numbers of white cells, including lymphocytes, are decreased except for an increased number of T8 suppressor cells. Platelets are also decreased. The person has an elevated erythrocyte sedimentation rate. Then, after the first few weeks, the symptoms disappear. However, HIV is still present, and the person continues to be infectious throughout the rest of the course of the infection.

Stage 2 can last 3 to 5 years. It is a latency period in which the virus stays in check. Production of virus occurs only sporadically and in certain cells. The person feels well but may experience some chronic lymphadenopathy. The T4 cell count is greater than 400.

Stage 3 is characterized by rapid virus production that occurs for up to 18 months after the latency period. There is a persistent and continuous drop in the T4 count to below 400.

In Stage 4, T4 cell counts continue to remain below 400. The person only partially responds to skin tests (partial anergy). In other words, there is limited reaction to a tuberculin test or other type IV (delayed) hypersensitivity test.

Stage 5 is characterized by a T4 count below 200. There is total absence of type IV hypersensitivity reactions (complete anergy). Severe viral or fungal infections of the skin and mucous membranes develop. Oral and/or genital herpes simplex and candidiasis usually develop, as well as fuzzy white patches on the tongue called oral hairy leukoplakia. The person has cytomegalovirus and/or Epstein-Barr virus infection as well as other opportunistic infections.

Stage 6 is also known as opportunistic infection–defined AIDS. The T4 count is less than 100. The person typically has one or more opportunistic infections, including *Pneumocystis carinii* pneumonia, *Toxoplasma gondii* (neural toxoplasmosis), cryptosporidiosis (gastroenteritis) and *Mycobacterium avium-tuberculosis*. The person usually has one or more tumors or cancers, including Kaposi's sarcoma (a connective tissue skin cancer), lymphomas, or cancer of the rectum and tongue (Fig. 10–14).

The CDC system is a simple matrix classification system for adults and children. In this system, T-cell counts are linked with clinical symptomatology.[54] The CDC has defined three T-cell categories and three clinical categories that are mutually exclusive. The T-cell categories define three T-cell ranges. In category 1, the T-cell count is greater than or equal to 500/μL; in category 2, T-cell counts range from 200 to 499/μL; and in category 3, the T-cell count is less than 200/μL.[54]

The clinical categories are labeled A through C. Category A includes a variety of clinical conditions including asymptomatic, persistent generalized

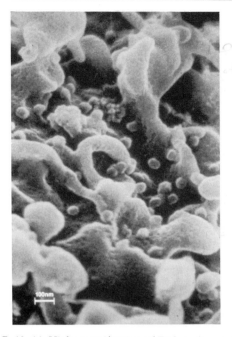

F I G U R E 10–14. High magnification of T4 lymphocyte infected with HIV-I. (Courtesy of Centers for Disease Control and Prevention, Atlanta.)

lymphadenopathy and a current or history of acute HIV infection with accompanying illness.[54] Category B includes conditions that are secondary to impaired cell-mediated immunity such as candidiasis (oral or vaginal), fever, persistent diarrhea, oral hairy leukoplakia, shingles, idiopathic thrombocytopenic purpura, pelvic inflammatory disease, listeriosis, and peripheral neuropathy.[54] Category C includes conditions that are listed in the AIDS surveillance case definition.[54] An individual in category C will remain in this category. The CDC classification matrix is given in Table 10–9.

Clinical Manifestations and Treatment

HIV affects all body systems but chiefly the cutaneous, pulmonary, GI, neurologic, and optic systems. Nearly

TABLE 10–9. CDC HIV/AIDS Classification Matrix

CD4 T-Cell Categories	Clinical Categories		
	A *Asymptomatic, acute HIV*	*B* *Symptomatic not (A) or (C)*	*C* *AIDS indicator*
1 ≥500/μL	A1	B1	C1
2 200–499/μL	A2	B2	C2
3 <200/μL AIDS indicator T-cell count	A3	B3	C3

From 1993 revised classification system for HIV infection and expanded surveillance case definition for AIDS among adolescents and adults. *MMWR* 41 (RR-17):1–6.

all persons with HIV develop GI manifestations. Approximately 50 percent of all persons with HIV develop pulmonary and cutaneous indications, and 50 percent to 60 percent develop neurologic symptoms.[33,55] Table 10–10 outlines the common agents of infection in patients with AIDS.

Gastrointestinal manifestations are nearly universal in persons with HIV. In fact, the GI tract may be the major target organ in HIV infection.[30] The GI complications are usually due to the multiple opportunistic infectious agents that have been identified, although tumors may also occur in the GI tract. HIV may or may not be a significant direct pathogen.[30] Some of the most significant infectious agents are viruses such as cytomegalovirus and herpes simplex; fungi such as *Candida*; bacteria such as *Salmonella*, *Shigella*, *Clostridium difficile*, *Chlamydia trachomatis*, and *Campylobacter*; and parasites such as *Giardia*, *Isospora*, *Entamoeba histolytica*, and *Cryptosporidium*.[56]

GI symptoms include chronic diarrhea, oral candidiasis, anorexia, nausea, vomiting, mucous membrane ulcers, retrosternal pain on swallowing, abdominal pain, and low serum vitamin B_{12}. The diarrhea is often watery or bloody, causing malabsorption that results in severe weight loss. Ulcerations may occur secondary to the inflammation. Treatment involves the use of antibiotics such as vancomycin (Vancocin), amikacin (Amikin) ampicillin, ciprofloxacin (Cipro), erythromycin, trimethoprim-sulfamethoxazole (Bactrim), metronidazole (Flagyl), clotrimazole troches (Mycelex), ganciclovir (Cytovene), spiramycin (Rovamycine), and eflornithin (Ornidyl).

Pulmonary manifestations are a major source of morbidity and mortality in AIDS patients. These complications include opportunistic pneumonias such as *Pneumocystis carinii*, cytomegalovirus, *Mycobacterium avium-tuberculosis*, *Histoplasma*, or *Staphylococcus* and parenchymal lung diseases including Kaposi's sarcoma, lymphoma, nonspecific pneumonitis, and ARDS. *Pneumocystis carinii* is the most common presenting opportunistic infection in AIDS.[33]

Pneumocystis carinii pneumonia (PCP) is caused by a protozoon that prefers alveolar environments. It infects most people during early childhood but does not cause disease in immunocompetent persons. However, with immunodeficiency and T4 cell counts below 200, *Pneumocystis* becomes activated. The symptoms of PCP infection are similar to those of adult respiratory distress syndrome (ARDS) (Fig. 10–15). These symptoms include decreased phospholipid (surfactant) production, dry cough, dyspnea, tachypnea, chest discomfort, and marked pallor and cyanosis. Treatment includes the use of trimethoprim-sulfamethoxazole (Bactrim, Septra), dapsone-trimethoprim), and parenteral and aerosolized pentamidine (NebuPent, Pentam 300). Experimental treatments include the use of dapsone-pyrimethamine,[57] clindamycin-primaquine, eflornithine, and trimetrexate-leucovorin.[58] Survival rates are 57 percent to 59 percent with the first infection and 25 percent with a second infection.

Cutaneous manifestations occur both early and late in the course of HIV infection. The origin of these manifestations may be allergic, infectious, or neoplastic. Symptoms of the cutaneous manifestations depend on the cause. Allergic causes may be due to drug reactions or the development of seborrheic dermatitis or skin-colored papular eruptions. Viral causes include herpes simplex, varicella zoster, Epstein-Barr virus, and human papillomavirus. The development of genital warts from human papillomavirus is an early symptom of HIV disease in women. For mucocutaneous viral infections, acyclovir (Zovirax) or vidarabine are the recommended antiviral agents.

Oral hairy leukoplakia is an example of an oral mucous membrane viral infection thought to be due to Epstein-Barr virus or human papillomavirus. Oral hairy leukoplakia is characterized by white to gray, raised "hairy" lesions that form on the tongue and buccal mucosa. These lesions cannot be removed or scraped off using a tongue blade, which differentiates this infection from oral candida or thrush (Fig. 10–16, Color Plate I).

Other infectious causes of cutaneous manifestations can be bacterial, such as *Mycobacterium avium* or *Staphylococcus aureus*; fungal, including *Candida*, *Cryptococcus*, or *Histoplasma*; or the mites that cause scabies. Vaginal candidiasis is the most common early skin symptom in HIV-positive women.[59] Neoplasms can also occur, including Kaposi's sarcoma, squamous cell carcinoma, basal cell carcinoma, or cutaneous lymphomas. Up to 83 percent of persons with AIDS get seborrheic dermatitis and 20 percent get papular eruptions.[33]

Kaposi's sarcoma is an AIDS-related malignancy that affects the skin and mucous membranes, lymphatics, and other internal organs. It is one of the few

T A B L E 10–10. Common Agents of Infection in Patients With AIDS

Viruses	Fungi
Herpes simplex 1 and 2	*Candida albicans*
Herpes zoster	*Cryptococcus neoformans*
Cytomegalovirus	*Histoplasma capsulatum*
JC virus	*Coccidioides immitis*
Epstein-Barr virus	*Nocardia*
Human papillomavirus	
Varicella	
Adenovirus	
Bacteria	**Protozoa**
Campylobacter spp.	*Pneumocystis carinii*
Shigella spp.	*Toxoplasma gondii*
Neisseria spp.	*Isospora belli*
Salmonella spp.	*Cryptosporidium*
Chlamydia spp.	*Giardia lamblia*
Staphylococcus spp.	*Entamoeba histolytica*
H. influenzae	
Legionella spp.	
Treponema spp.	
Mycobacteria spp.	

Data from Stites DP, Terr AI: *Basic and Clinical Immunology*, 7th ed. Los Altos, Calif., Appleton & Lange, 1991; Ungvarski PJ, Schmidt J: AIDS patients under attack. *RN* 1992;55(11):35–44; Anastasi JK, Rivera JL: Identify the skin manifestations of H.I.V. *Nursing* 1992;92(11):58–61.

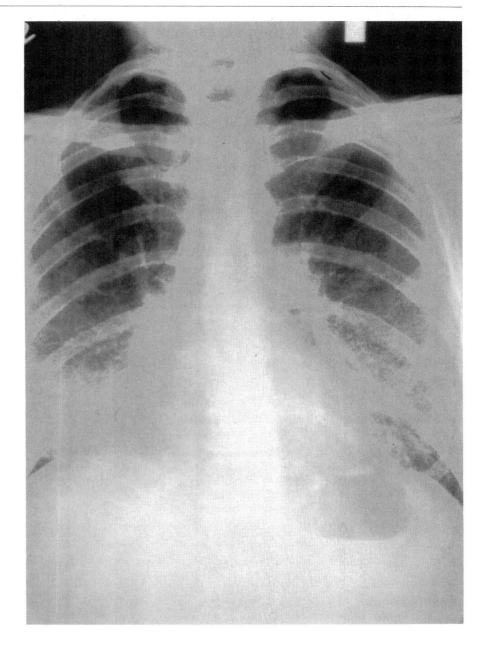

FIGURE 10–15. Pneumocystis carinii. Chest radiograph showing bilateral lower lobar interstitial infiltrates. (From Friedman-Kien AE: *Color Atlas of AIDS.* Philadelphia, WB Saunders, 1989. Reproduced with permission.)

neoplasms indicative of immune system dysfunction. Before 1981, it was rarely found in the United States except in elderly men of Mediterranean or Eastern European Jewish ancestry.[60] With the AIDS epidemic, it is now found in young, formerly healthy persons who live in the United States, are homosexual or bisexual, and who develop AIDS. It rarely occurs in other high-risk groups or in women in the United States. It is the most common tumor found in HIV-infected homosexual men.[61]

The skin lesions of Kaposi's sarcoma are individual tumors that begin as flat or macular subcutaneous patches. The patches initially range in color from light pink to deep purple and are painless and nonpruritic (Fig. 10–17, Color Plate I). The lesions evolve from the patches into thickened plaques or large nodules that can change to a brown color over time especially in darkly pigmented persons (Fig. 10–18, Color Plate I). They may occur anywhere on the body, although they usually begin on the face, scalp, or in the mouth. They range in size from a few millimeters to coalesced lesions covering large areas of the body. The lesions are highly vascular but do not bleed excessively.[60,61]

Kaposi's sarcoma is often treated with radiation therapy and chemotherapy. Surgery is rarely indicated except to remove large, uncomfortable lesions. Radiation therapy is used primarily for oral or cutaneous lesions. Vinblastine, vincristine, etoposide (VP-16-213), doxorubicin, and interferon-alpha have been useful chemotherapeutic agents in the treatment of

Kaposi's sarcoma.[61,62] Persons with the best prognosis with Kaposi's tend to have limited disease with no other opportunistic infections and no weight loss, fevers, or night sweats.[62]

Neurologic manifestations are often the reason that people with HIV seek treatment. HIV invades the neurologic system early in the course of infection. It infects glial cells, endothelial cells, and brain macrophages. Central and peripheral nervous system manifestations may be due to HIV infection directly or may be due to infectious agents or neoplasms.[33] Opportunistic infectious agents that can affect the neurologic system include *Toxoplasma* and *Cryptococcus*. A variety of peripheral neuropathies can result from HIV infection directly, although some may be due to herpes zoster infection.

HIV encephalopathy (AIDS dementia complex, subacute or AIDS encephalopathy) is the most common neurologic manifestation. The cause of HIV encephalopathy is due directly or indirectly to HIV infection or viral products, cytokine-related cellular damage, and the competition or interference between gp120 and neuroleukin, a nerve growth factor.[33,63] This disorder can affect both adults and children.

HIV encephalopathy is a syndrome characterized by progressive cognitive impairment or dementia like that seen in Huntington's disease or Parkinson's disease. The neurologic symptoms include confusion, forgetfulness, loss of concentration, handwriting changes, slower verbal and motor responses, headache, apathy, and focal motor deficits such as clumsiness, weakness, loss of balance, and slurred speech.[33,55,63] Associated generalized symptoms consist of fever and mild metabolic acidosis. Behavioral symptoms include personality changes, social withdrawal, depression, and less commonly anxiety and hyperactivity. In children, the head circumference does not increase with age.[55] Computed tomography shows diffuse atrophy and ventricular enlargement in most cases.[55] CSF analysis shows elevated protein and abnormal IgG levels.

As the disorder progresses, the neurologic symptoms become more severe. Ataxia, hypertonia, tremors, and incontinence appear. The person may be alert but cognitively impaired, mute, and paraplegic. The person may also develop hemianopsia (partial blindness), myoclonus, and seizures. The person may become comatose and lethargic with other systemic dysfunctions.

Renal impairment can also occur with HIV infection. HIV can affect the kidneys, causing AIDS-associated nephropathy (AIDS-related glomerulopathy) and drug-induced ischemia and renal failure. *Hematologically*, people with HIV have anemia, thrombocytopenia, and granulocytopenia.

Ocular manifestations of HIV infection may be of infectious or noninfectious origin. Noninfectious causes of ocular problems include HIV retinopathy and malignancy. Infectious causes consist of bacteria such as syphilis and *Staphylococcus*; fungi including *Candida*, *Cryptococcus*, and *Histoplasma*; protozoa such as *Pneumocystis* and *Toxoplasma*; and viruses such as herpes simplex and cytomegalovirus.

The most severe type of ocular infection is *cytomegalovirus retinitis*. After an insidious onset, ocular CMV precipitates hemorrhages, exudates, and vasculitis in the retina. The CMV retinal infection leads to destruction and necrosis of the retina, with resulting blindness.[64] CMV retinitis affects 10 percent to 15 percent of all people with AIDS.[65] Treatment for CMV retinitis includes ganciclovir (Cytovene) and trisodium phosphonoformate (Foscavir, Foscarnet).[65] HIV-associated retinopathy causes the development of cotton wool spots and microvascular retinal changes, including retinal hemorrhages.[64] These changes are usually not as severe as CMV retinitis.

HIV-related endocrine dysfunction is usually associated with changes in hormone secretion secondary to the stress response; destruction of endocrine tissue due to infection, cancer, or inflammation; or the use of pharmacologic agents.[66] Adrenal secretion of cortisol is elevated at the expense of other hormones. Most endocrine dysfunction is subtle, with few overt manifestations.

The treatment of HIV infection involves the use of several medications. The first and most widely used is 3'-azido-3'-deoxythymidine (AZT, Zidovudine, Retrovir). AZT is used because it effectively inhibits reverse transcriptase. It is rapidly absorbed when taken orally and can penetrate the blood-brain barrier. However, recent studies have shown that the early use of AZT does not delay the onset of HIV or prolong life.[67] Granulocyte colony-stimulating factor filgrastim (G-CSF Neupogen) is also being used to increase nonspecific immunity by increasing neutrophils in those persons with neutropenia. Recent research on the use of IV immunoglobulin in HIV-infected children with T-cell counts above 200/mm^3 showed a decrease in serious bacterial, minor bacterial, viral, and opportunistic infections.[68]

Prevention of HIV infection by active immunity via vaccine is the ultimate goal of current research. At this time, several experimental vaccines are being tested. The HGP-30 vaccine contains a synthetic copy of p17, a core HIV protein.[67] GP160 vaccine is a genetically engineered form of gp160, an HIV envelope protein.[69,70] An inactivated HIV vaccine, GP120, has had its envelope removed and its immunogenic proteins enhanced.[69,70] Ongoing research is quantifying the ability of these vaccines to stimulate both cellular and humoral responses to HIV.

Secondary Immunodeficiency Disorders

A number of physical, psychosocial, nutritional, environmental, and pharmacologic factors can, singly or in combination, lead to the development of **secondary immunodeficiency disorders**. Many of these linkages were discussed in Chapter 8.

Studies of physical and psychosocial stress, decreased social support, depression, and bereavement have shown that changes occur, especially decreases in immune functioning.[71] T-cells and B-cells decrease after surgery.[72] And a number of pharmaceuticals affect the immune system. For example, cancer pharmacotherapeutic drugs often lead to a decline in immune function. Anesthetics (halothane, cyclopropane, nitrous oxide, ether), alcohol, antibiotics, and steroids decrease cellular and/or humoral immunity.[72]

A number of studies have linked immune system competency and nutritional status. Malnutritional states can lead to protein depletion as well as iron, carbohydrate, and lipid deficiencies.[72,73] Overnutrition, especially hyperlipidemia, can lead to lymphocyte and granulocyte dysfunctions.[73] Kinsella in 1990 stated that deficiencies, imbalances, or excess nutritional factors may impair the development of all stem cells, alter the recognition and processing of antigens, hurt immune cell proliferation, reduce phagocytic and cytolytic capacity, and harm cooperative interactions between cells in the immune system.[73]

KEY CONCEPTS

- Acquired Immunodeficiency Syndrome (AIDS) is a primary disorder caused by viral infection of white blood cells. It is a major health concern because it carries a very poor prognosis.

  Etiology: Human immunodeficiency virus types 1 and 2 are retroviruses that primarily infect CD4+ lymphocytes and macrophages and lead to AIDS. Sexual intercourse and the shared use of contaminated needles to inject drugs intravenously are the most common routes of transmission.

  Epidemiology and prevention: High-risk populations include IV drug users, sexual partners of IV drug users, and bisexual or homosexual men. Use of condoms and sterile needles decreases risk of infection. Exposure to blood and body fluids of infected individuals through skin, mucous membranes, and accidental needle sticks is the primary risk factor for health care workers. The universal use of body substance isolation decreases risk of infection.

  Pathophysiology: The hallmark of AIDS is a decrease in CD4+ (T-helper) lymphocytes. B-cell responsiveness is decreased because of dependence on T-helper cell cytokines. Macrophages also have CD4+ receptors and are targets for HIV infection. HIV gains access to CD4+ cells by attaching to the CD4+ receptor on the cell surface. Attachment is mediated by viral envelope protein gp120. Once inside the cell, reverse transcriptase directs the synthesis of DNA using the viral RNA template. Viral DNA may then be integrated into the host genome. Viral DNA may lie dormant in T-cells for years until it is stimulated to begin active transcription. Dysfunction of T-cells occurs via several mechanisms: Cross-linking of CD4+ receptors by viruses may result in T-cell death or anergy; viruses may cause several T-cells to be linked together, followed by cell fusion and death; B-cells may form antibodies against infected T-cells; viral budding may cause excessive loss of cell membrane.

  Staging and classification: HIV infection is a progressive disease characterized by different clinical manifestations at each stage. Individuals move through the stages at different rates. The early stage of viral seeding is characterized by flulike symptoms and the formation of anti-HIV antibodies (seroconversion). Next, symptoms of early immune dysfunction are present, including lymphadenopathy, fever, and night sweats. This stage is followed by a surge in viral production and a drop in the CD4+ lymphocyte count. In the later stages, CD4+ counts continue to fall and the person is subject to a number of opportunistic infections and tumor formation.

  Clinical manifestations: AIDS, the end stage of HIV infection, is characterized by opportunistic infection and tumor formation. Most body systems are affected. GI symptoms include diarrhea, ulceration, anorexia, and candidiasis. Pulmonary symptoms include pneumonia, particularly *Pneumocystis carinii*, and ARDS. Skin symptoms include *Candida*, herpes, HPV, and EBV infections and Kaposi's sarcoma. Neurologic manifestations include peripheral neuropathy, encephalopathy with dementia, headache, apathy, and focal deficits.

  Treatment: Effective treatment for HIV and AIDS has been elusive. Antivirals such as AZT, which inhibits reverse transcriptase, have not been very effective. Efforts to stimulate immune function with peptide growth factors are under investigation. Aggressive treatment of opportunistic infections with appropriate antibiotics and antivirals is a large part of the treatment regimen.

Summary

Humans live in an environment teeming with substances capable of producing immunologic responses. Contact with antigen leads not only to induction of a protective immune response, but also to reactions that can be damaging to tissues. This chapter highlighted some of the recent advances in basic immunology and general disorders of the immune system. Some specific immunologic diseases and age-related considerations have also been presented.

REFERENCES

1. Cohen IR: The self, the world and autoimmunity. *Sci Am* 1988;258(4):52–60.
2. Theofilopoulos AN: Autoimmunity, in Stites DP, Stobo JD, Wells JV (eds): *Basic and Clinical Immunology*, 6th ed. Los Altos, Calif, Appleton & Lange, 1987.
3. Marrack P, Kappler JW: How the immune system recognizes the body. *Sci Am* 1993;269(3):81–89.
4. Sinha A, Lopez MT, McDevitt HO: Autoimmune diseases: The failure of self tolerance. *Science* 1990;248:1380–1388.
5. Capron A, Dessaint J: From protective immunity to allergy: The cellular partners of IgE. *Chem Immunol* 1990;49:236–244.

6. Kaliner M, Lemanske R: Rhinitis and asthma. *JAMA* 1992;268(20):2807–2829.
7. Roitt I: *Essential Immunology.* Oxford, England, Blackwell Scientific Publications, 1991.
8. Lichtenstein LM: Allergy and the immune system. *Sci Am* 1993;269(3):117–123.
9. Dewey J: Stopping allergies before they start. *Nursing 84* (September 1984), p 19.
10. Gergen PJ, Weiss KB: Changing patterns of asthma hospitalization among children: 1979 to 1987. *JAMA* 1988;264(13):1688–1692.
11. Long BC, Phipps WJ: *Medical-Surgical Nursing: A Nursing Process Approach.* St. Louis, CV Mosby, 1989.
12. Creticos PS: Immunotherapy with allergens. *JAMA* 1992;268(20):2834–2839.
13. Wilson CB, Yamamoto T, Ward DM: Renal diseases, in Stites DP, Stobo JD, Wells JV (eds): *Basic and Clinical Immunology,* 6th ed. Los Altos, Calif, Appleton & Lange, 1987.
14. Widmann FK: *An Introduction to Clinical Immunology.* Philadelphia, FA Davis, 1989.
15. Condemi JJ: The autoimmune diseases. *JAMA* 1992;268(20):2882–2892.
16. Fye KH, Sack KE: Rheumatic diseases, in Stites DP, Stobo JD, Wells JV (eds): *Basic and Clinical Immunology,* 6th ed. Los Altos, Calif, Appleton & Lange, 1987.
17. Geppert TD, Lipsky PE: Cellular immunity, in Stein JH (ed): *Internal Medicine.* Boston, Little, Brown & Co, 1990, vol II.
18. Waldorf HA, Walsh LJ, Schechter NM, Murphy GF: Early cellular events in evolving cutaneous delayed hypersensitivity in humans. *Am J Pathol* 1991;138(2):477–486.
19. Lasser A: The mononuclear phagocytic system: A review. *Hum Pathol* 1983;14(2):108–126.
20. Bach FH, Sachs DH: Current concepts: Transplant immunology. *N Engl J Med* 1987;317(8):489–492.
21. Krull K, Hatswell E: Single-lung allograft: A nursing perspective. *Crit Care Nurse* 1989;8(6):35–56.
22. Hadden JW, Smith DL: Immunopharmacology: Immunomodulation and immunotherapy. *JAMA* 1992;268(20):2964–2969.
23. Anderson KC, Goodnough LT, Sayers PN, Pisciotto PT, Kurtz SR, Lane TA, Anderson CS, Silberstein E: Variation in blood component irradiation practice: Implications for prevention of transfusion-associated graft-versus-host disease. *Blood* 1991;77(5):2096–2102.
24. Garovoy MR, Melzer JS, Gibbs VC, Bozdech M: Clinical transplantation, in Stites DP, Stobo JD, Wells JV (eds): *Basic and Clinical Immunology,* 6th ed. Los Altos, Calif, Appleton & Lange, 1987.
25. Caudell KA: Graft-versus-host disease, in Whedon MB: *Bone Marrow Transplantation: Principles, Practice, and Nursing Insights.* Boston, Jones and Bartlett, 1991.
26. Buckley RH: Immunodeficiency diseases. *JAMA* 1992;268(20):2797–2806.
27. Frey AM: The immune system and intravenous administration of immune globulin: Part I. The immune system. *J Intravenous Nurs* 1991;14(5):315–330.
28. Varmus H: Retroviruses. *Science* 1988;240:1427–1435.
29. Gold JWM: HIV-1 infection. *Med Clin North Am* 1992;76(1):1–18.
30. Gallo RC, Montagnier L: The AIDS epidemic, in *The Science of AIDS.* Salt Lake City, Freeman Press, 1989.
31. Haase AT: Biology of human immunodeficiency virus and related viruses, in Holmes KK, Cates W Jr, Lemon SM, Stamm WE (eds): *Sexually Transmitted Diseases,* 2nd ed. New York, McGraw-Hill, 1990, pp 305–315.
32. Osborn JE: The AIDS epidemic: An overview of the science. *Issues Sci Technol* 1986;II(2):40–55.
33. Hirsch MS: Clinical manifestations of HIV infection in adults in industrialized countries, in Holmes KK, Cates W Jr, Lemon SM, Stamm WE (eds): *Sexually Transmitted Diseases,* 2nd ed. New York, McGraw-Hill, 1990, pp 331–342.
34. Gallo RC: The AIDS virus. *Sci Am* 1987;256(1):47–56.
35. Greene WC: AIDS and the immune system. *Sci Am* 1993;269(3):99–105.
36. Centers for Disease Control: World AIDS Day—December 1, 1993. *MMWR* 1993;42(45):1.
37. Beneson AS: *Control of Communicable Diseases in Man,* 15th ed. Washington, DC, American Public Health Association, 1990.
38. Mortality attributable to HIV infection/AIDS—United States, 1981–1990. *MMWR* 1991;40(3):41–44.
39. Leerhsen C, Foot D, Gordon G, et al: Magic's message. *Newsweek* 1991;118(21):58–62.
40. Hankins CA: Women and HIV infection and AIDS in Canada: Should we worry? *Can Med Assoc J* 1990;143:1171–1173.
41. Update: Acquired immunodeficiency syndrome—United States: 1992. *MMWR* 1993;42(28):547–551.
42. Smeltzer SC, Whipple B: Women and HIV infection. *Image J Nurs Scholarship* 1991;23(4):249–256.
43. Guinan ME: HIV, heterosexual transmission, and women. *JAMA* 1992;268(4):520–521.
44. Hankins CA, Handley MA: HIV disease and AIDS in women: Current knowledge and a research agenda. *J AIDS* 1992; 5:957–979.
45. Minkoff HL, McCalla S, Delke I, Stevens R, Salwen M, Feldman J: The relationship of cocaine use to syphilis and human immunodeficiency virus infections among inner city parturient women. *Am J Obstet Gynecol* 1990;163(2):521–526.
46. Williams AB: Women at risk: An AIDS educational needs assessment. *Image J Nurs Scholarship* 1991;23(4):208–213.
47. Centers for Disease Control: Update: Barrier protection against HIV infection and other sexually transmitted diseases. *MMWR* 1993;42(30):589–591.
48. U.S. Department of Health and Human Services: Recommendations for prevention of HIV transmission in health-care settings. *MMWR* 1987;36(2S):2S–18S.
49. Flaskerud JH: *AIDS/HIV Infection: A Reference Guide for Nursing Professionals.* Philadelphia, WB Saunders, 1989.
50. Fling JA, Fischer JR Jr, Boswell RN, Reid MJ: The relationship of serum IgA concentration to human immunodeficiency virus (HIV) infection: A cross-sectional study of HIV-seropositive individuals detected by screening in the United States Air Force. *J Allergy Clin Immunol* 1988;82(6):965–970.
51. Cohn DL: Bacterial pneumonia in the HIV-infected patient. *Infect Dis Clin North Am* 1991;5(3):485–507.
52. Pantaleo G, Graziosi C, Fauci AS: The immunopathogenesis of human immunodeficiency virus infection. *N Engl J Med* 1993;328(5):327–335.
53. Koenig S, Fauci AS: Immunology of HIV infection, in Holmes KK, et al (eds): *Sexually Transmitted Diseases.* New York, McGraw-Hill, 1990, pp 317–330.
54. 1993 Revised classification system for HIV infection and expanded surveillance case definition for AIDS among adolescents and adults. *MMWR* 1992;41(RR-17):1–6.
55. McArthur JH, Palenick JG, Bowersox LL: Human immunodeficiency virus and the nervous system. *Nurs Clin North Am* 1988;23(4):823–841.
56. Tanowitz HB, Simon D, Wittner M: Gastrointestinal manifestations. *Med Clin North Am* 1992;76(1):45–62.
57. Girard PM, Landman R, Gaudebout C, et al: Dapsone-pyrimethamine compared with aerosolized pentamidine as primary prophylaxis against *Pneumocystis carinii* pneumonia and toxoplasmosis in HIV infection. *N Engl J Med* 1993;328(21):1514–1520.
58. Bernard EM, Sepkowitz KA, Telzak EE, Armstrong D: Pneumocystosis. *Med Clin North Am* 1992;76(1):107–119.
59. Kelly PJ, Holman S: The new face of AIDS. *Am J Nurs* 1993;93(3):26–34.
60. Friedman-Kien AE, Ostreicher R, Saltzman B: Clinical manifestations of classical, endemic African, and epidemic AIDS-associated Kaposi's sarcoma, in Friedman-Kien AE (ed): *Color Atlas of AIDS.* Philadelphia, WB Saunders, 1989.
61. Krown SE, Myskowski PL, Paredes J: Kaposi's sarcoma. *Med Clin North Am* 1992;76(1):235–252.
62. Volberding PA: AIDS-related malignancies, in Holmes KK, Cates W Jr, Lemon SM, Stamm WE (eds): *Sexually Transmitted Diseases,* 2nd ed. New York, McGraw-Hill, 1990, pp 685–690.
63. Brew BJ: Central and peripheral nervous system abnormalities. *Med Clin North Am* 1992;76(1):63–81.
64. deSmet MC, Nussenbatt RB: Ocular manifestations of AIDS. *JAMA* 1991;266(21):3019–3022.
65. Plona RP, Schremp PS: Nursing care of patients with ocular manifestations of human immunodeficiency virus infection. *Nurs Clin North Am* 1992;27(3):793–805.

66. Grinspoon SK, Bilezikian JP: HIV disease and the endocrine system. *N Engl J Med* 1992;327(19):1360–1365.
67. Broader use for rifabutin, vaccine research progress and other news from the AIDS front. *Hosp Formul* 1993;28:827–828.
68. Mofenson LM, Moye J Jr, Bethel, et al: Prophylactic intravenous immunoglobulin in HIV-infected children with CD4+ counts of 0.20 × 10⁹/1 or more. *JAMA* 1992;268(4):483–488.
69. AIDS vaccine research: Two different approaches show promise. *Hosp Formul* 1992;27(10):976–977.
70. Weinstein SM: AIDS—Pharmacologic update. *J Intravenous Nurs* 1992;15(4):220–229.
71. Hillhouse J, Adler C: Stress, health, and immunity: A review of the literature and implications for the nursing profession. *Holistic Nurs Pract* 1991;5(4):22–31.
72. Gurka AM: The immune system: Implications for critical care nursing. *Crit Care Nurse* 1990;9(7):24–35.
73. Kinsella JE, Lokesh B: Dietary lipids, eicosanoids, and the immune system. *Crit Care Med* 1990;18(2):S94–S113.

BIBLIOGRAPHY

Allen JR, Setlow VP: Heterosexual transmission of HIV. *JAMA* 1991;266(12):1695–1696.

Anastasi JK, Rivera JL: DDI and DDC. *RN* 1991;54(11):41–43.

Anastasi JK, Rivera JL: Identify the skin manifestations of H.I.V. *Nursing* 1992;92(11):58–61.

Arico M, Caselli D, D'Argenio P, et al: Malignancies in children with human immunodeficiency virus type 1 infection. *Cancer* 1991;68(11):2473–2477.

Barnes DM: Solo actions of AIDS virus coat. *Science* 1987;237:971–973.

Blackman M, Kappler J, Marrack P: The role of the T cell receptor in positive and negative selection of developing T cells. *Science* 1990;248:1335–1341.

Bozzette SA, Larsen RA, Chiu J, et al: A placebo-controlled trial of maintenance therapy with fluconazole after treatment of cryptococcal meningitis in the acquired immunodeficiency syndrome. *N Engl J Med* 1991;324:580–584.

Claman HM: The biology of the immune response. *JAMA* 1992;268(20):2790–2796.

Connolly KJ, Allan JD, Fitch H, et al: Phase I study of 2'-3'-dideoxyinosine administered orally twice daily to patients with AIDS or AIDS-related complex and hematologic intolerance to zidovudine. *Am J Med* 1991;91:471–478.

Daar ES, Meyer RD: Bacterial and fungal infections. *Med Clin North Am* 1992;76(1):173–204.

Denning DW, Armstrong RW, Lewis BH, Stevens DA: Elevated cerebrospinal fluid pressures in patients with cryptococcal meningitis and acquired immunodeficiency syndrome. *Am J Med* 1991;91(3):267–272.

DeVita VT, Hellman S, Rosenberg SA: *AIDS: Etiology, Diagnosis, Treatment, and Prevention*, 2nd ed. Philadelphia, JB Lippincott, 1988.

Dinarello CA, Mier JW: Current concepts: Lymphokines. *N Engl J Med* 1987;317(15):940–945.

Easterbrook PJ, Keruly JC, Creagh-Kirk T, Richmon DD, Chaisson RE, Moore RD: Racial and ethnic differences in outcome in zidovudine-treated patients with advanced HIV disease. *JAMA* 1991;266(19):2713–2718.

Farizo KM, Buehler JW, Chamberland ME, et al: Spectrum of disease in persons with human immunodeficiency virus infection in the United States. *JAMA* 1992;267(13):1778–1805.

Flaskerud JH, Thompson J: Beliefs about AIDS, health, and illness in low-income white women. *Nurs Res* 1991;40(5):266–271.

Frey AM: The immune system: Part II. Intravenous administration of immune globulin. *J Intravenous Nurs* 1991;14(6):396–405.

Gellin BG, Soave R: Coccidian infections in AIDS: Toxoplasmosis, cryptosporidiosis, and isosporiasis. *Med Clin North Am* 1992;76(1):205–234.

Gerbert B: Primary care physicians and AIDS: Attitudinal and structural barriers to care. *JAMA* 1991;266(20):2837–2842.

Guarner J, de Rio C, Carr D, et al: Non-Hodgkin's lymphomas in patients with human immunodeficiency virus infection. *Cancer* 1991;68(11):2460–2465.

Hadden JW: Immunopharmacology: Immunomodulation and immunotherapy. *JAMA* 1987;258(20):3005–3010.

Haseltine WA, Wong-Staal F: The molecular biology of the AIDS virus, in *The Science of AIDS*. Salt Lake City, Freeman Press, 1989.

Heinemann MH: Ophthalmic problems. *Med Clin North Am* 1992;76(1):83–98.

Heyward WL, Curran JW: The epidemiology of AIDS in the U.S., in *The Science of AIDS*. Salt Lake City, Freeman Press, 1989.

Higgins DL, Galavotti C, O'Reilly KR, et al: Evidence for the effects of HIV antibody counseling and testing on risk behaviors. *JAMA* 1991;266(17):2419–2429.

Houldin AD, Lev E, Prystowsky MB, Redei E, Lowery BJ: Psychoneuroimmunology: A review of literature. *Holistic Nurs Pract* 1991;5(4):10–21.

Hu WS, Temin HM: Retroviral recombination and reverse transcription. *Science* 1990;250:1227–1232.

Jacobsberg LB, Perry S: Psychiatric disturbances. *Med Clin North Am* 1992;76(1):99–106.

Janeway CA: How the immune system recognizes invaders. *Sci Am* 1993;269(3):73–79.

Kaliner M: Immediate hypersensitivity. *J Allergy Clin Immunol* 1989;84(6):1028–1031.

Koshland DE: Recognizing self from nonself. *Science* 1990;248(4961):1273.

Lagakos S: Effects of zidovudine therapy in minority and other subpopulations with early HIV infection. *JAMA* 1991;266(19):2709–2712.

Lenert P, Kroon D, Spiegelberg H, Golub ES, Zeneth M: Human CD4 binds immunoglobulins. *Science* 1990;248(4963):1639–1643.

Levine AM: AIDS-associated malignant lymphoma. *Med Clin North Am* 1992;76(1):253–268.

Levine AM, Sullivan-Halley J, Pike MC, et al: Human immunodeficiency virus–related lymphoma: Prognostic factors predictive of survival. *Cancer* 1991;68(11):2466–2472.

Lucente FE: Otolaryngologic aspects of acquired immunodeficiency syndrome. *Med Clin North Am* 1991;75(6):1389–1398.

Martin L, Fritzler M: Autoantibodies, in Stein JH (ed): *Internal Medicine*. Boston, Little, Brown & Co, 1990, vol II.

Mitsuya H, Yarchoan R, Broder S: Molecular targets for AIDS therapy. *Science* 1990;249:1533–1544.

Moore JP, McKeating JA, Weiss RA, Satlentau QJ: Dissociation of gp120 from HIV-1 virions induced by soluble CD4. *Science* 1990;250:1139–1142.

Moss GB, Kreiss JK: The interrelationship between human immunodeficiency virus infection and other sexually transmitted diseases. *Med Clin North Am* 1990;74(6):1647–1660.

National Vaccine Advisory Committee: The measles epidemic: The problems, barriers, and recommendations. *JAMA* 1991;266(11):1547–1552.

O'Connor PG, Molde S, Henry S, Shockcor WT, Schottenfeld RS: Human immunodeficiency virus infection in intravenous drug users: A model for primary care. *Am J Med* 1992;93(10):382–386.

Padian NS, Shiboski SC, Jewell NP: Female-to-male transmission of human immunodeficiency virus. *JAMA* 1991;266(12):1664–1667.

Pan American Health Organization: *AIDS: Profile of an Epidemic*. Washington, DC, Pan American Health Organization and World Health Organization, 1989.

Pearlstein G: Renal system complications in HIV infection. *Crit Care Nurs Clin North Am* 1990;2(1):79–87.

Perlmutter RM: Antibodies: Structure and genetics, in Stein JH (ed): *Internal Medicine*. Boston, Little, Brown & Co, 1990, vol II.

Phillips TP, Bloch D: *Nursing and the HIV Epidemic: A National Action Agenda*. Washington, DC, U.S. Department of Health and Human Services, Public Health Service, 1989.

Phillips AN, Elford J, Sabin C, Bofill M, Janossy G, Lee CA: Immunodeficiency and the risk of death in HIV infection. *JAMA* 1992;268(19):2662–2666.

Pitchenik AE, Fertel D: Tuberculosis and nontuberculous mycobacterial disease. *Med Clin North Am* 1992;76(1):121–172.

Porter SB, Sande MA: Toxoplasmosis of the central nervous system in the acquired immunodeficiency syndrome. *N Engl J Med* 327(23):1643–1648.

Ramsdell F, Fowlkes BJ: Clonal deletion versus clonal anergy: The role of the thymus in inducing self tolerance. *Science* 1990;248(4961):1342–1348.

Redfield RR, Burke DS: HIV infection: The clinical picture, in *The Science of AIDS*. Salt Lake City, Freeman Press, 1989.

St. Louis ME, Conway GA, Hayman CR, et al: Human immunodeficiency virus infection in disadvantaged adolescents. *JAMA* 1991;266(17):2387–2391.

Sasaki T, Muryoi T, Hatakeyama A, et al: Circulating anti-DNA immune complexes in active lupus nephritis. *Am J Med* 1991;91:355–362.

Saul RL, Gee P, Ames BN: Free radicals, DNA damage, and aging, in Warner HR, et al (eds): *Modern Biological Theories of Aging*. New York, Raven Press, 1987.

Scherer P: How AIDS attacks the brain. *Am J Nurs* 1990;90:44–52.

Schwartz RH: A cell culture model for T lymphocyte clonal anergy. *Science* 1990;248:1349–1356.

Sell S: *Immunology, Immunopathology and Immunity,* 4th ed. Amsterdam, Elsevier, 1987.

Selwyn PA, Sckell BM, Alcabes P, Friedland GH, Klein RS, Schoenbaum EE: High risk of active tuberculosis in HIV-infected drug users with cutaneous anergy. *JAMA* 1992;268(4):504–509.

Sloand EM, et al: HIV testing: State of the art. *JAMA* 1991;266(20):2861–2866.

Sprent J, Gao EK, Webb SR: T cell reactivity to MHC molecules: Immunity versus tolerance. *Science* 1990;248:1357–1363.

Stein M, Mayer K: Drug therapy of major opportunistic infections in HIV-infected patients. *Hosp Formul* 1991;26(9):706–713.

Steinberg AD: Tolerance and autoimmunity, in Stein JH (ed): *Internal Medicine*. Boston, Little, Brown & Co, 1990, vol II.

Steinman L: Autoimmune disease. *Sci Am* 1993;269(3):107–114.

Stites DP, Terr AI: *Basic and Clinical Immunology,* 7th ed. Los Altos, Calif, Appleton & Lange, 1991.

Stobo JD: The human immune response, in Stein JH (ed): *Internal Medicine*. Boston, Little, Brown & Co, 1990, vol II.

Strohl RA: Progress in HIV disease. *Nurs Acumen* 1991;3(1):1.

Tharp MD: IgE and immediate hypersensitivity. *Dermatol Clin* 1990;8(4):619–631.

Ungvarski PJ, Schmidt J: AIDS patients under attack. *RN* 1992;55(11):35–44.

Virella G, Patrick CC, Goust J: Diagnostic evaluation of cell-mediated immunity. *Immunol Series* 1990;50:303–321.

Von Boehmer H, Kisielow P: Self-nonself discrimination by T cells. *Science* 1990;248:1369–1373.

Wasserman SI: Immediate hypersensitivity, in Stein JH (ed): *Internal Medicine*. Boston, Little, Brown & Co, 1990, vol II.

Wayne SJ, Rhyne RL, Garry PJ, Goodwin JS: Cell-mediated immunity as a predictor of morbidity and mortality in subjects over 60. *J Gerontol* 1990;45(2):M45–M48.

Weber JN, Weiss RA: HIV infection: The cellular picture, in *The Science of AIDS*. Salt Lake City, Freeman Press, 1989.

White DA, Zaman MK: Pulmonary disease. *Med Clin North Am* 1992;76(1):19–44.

Whitley RJ, Gnann JW: Acyclovir: A decade later. *N Engl J Med* 1992;327(11):782–789.

Wormser GP: *AIDS and Other Manifestations of HIV Infection*. Park Ridge, NJ, Noyes Publications, 1987.

Wright K: Mycoplasmas in the AIDS spotlight. *Science* 1990;248:682–683.

Young JD, Cohn ZA: How killer cells kill. *Sci Am* 1988;258(1):38–44.

COLOR PLATE I

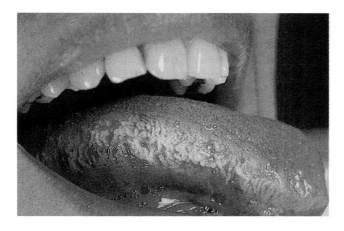

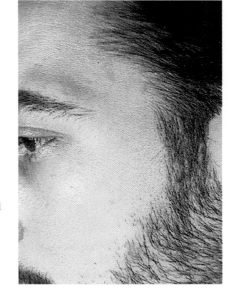

FIGURE 10–16. Hairy leukoplakia. (From Friedman-Kien AE: *Color Atlas of AIDS.* Philadelphia, WB Saunders, 1989. Reproduced with permission.)

FIGURE 10–17. Epidemic Kaposi's sarcoma, patch stage. Note multiple patch-stage lesions on the temple and bearded areas of the face. The lesions are slightly irregular in shape and widely dispersed over the rest of the body. (From Friedman-Kien AE: *Color Atlas of AIDS.* Philadelphia, WB Saunders, 1989. Reproduced with permission.)

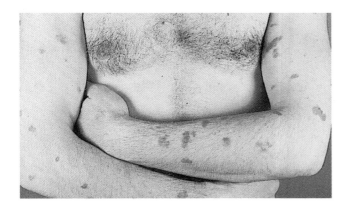

FIGURE 10–18. Epidemic Kaposi's sarcoma, plaque stage. Note multiple elongated and irregularly shaped violet to brown plaque lesions of Kaposi's sarcoma on the upper extremities. (From Friedman-Kien AE: *Color Atlas of AIDS.* Philadelphia, WB Saunders, 1989. Reproduced with permission.)

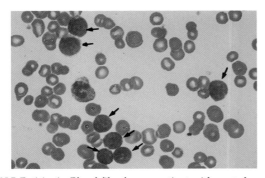

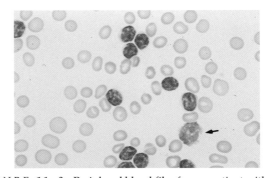

FIGURE 11–1. Blood film from a patient with acute lymphocytic leukemia showing blast forms with somewhat clumped, dense nuclear chromatin. (Courtesy of Pamela G. Kidd, M.D., Department of Laboratory Medicine, University of Washington, Seattle.)

FIGURE 11–2. Peripheral blood film from a patient with chronic lymphocytic leukemia showing small lymphocytes with dense, clumped nuclear chromatin and light blue cytoplasm. *Arrow* points to a smudged cell—an artifact arising from slide preparation. (Courtesy of Pamela G. Kidd, M.D., Department of Laboratory Medicine, University of Washington, Seattle.)

COLOR PLATE II

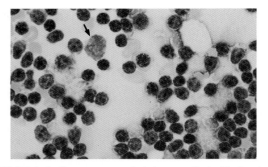

FIGURE 11–3. Bone marrow aspirate from a patient with chronic lymphocytic leukemia showing a monotonous presentation of small lymphoid cells with coarse nuclear chromatin and light blue cytoplasm. There is one larger monocytoid cell (*arrow*). (Courtesy of Pamela G. Kidd, M.D., Department of Laboratory Medicine, University of Washington, Seattle.)

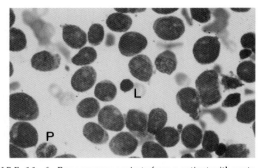

FIGURE 11–6. Bone marrow aspirate from a patient with acute myelogenous leukemia showing myeloblasts with loose nuclear chromatin, nucleoli, and moderate cytoplasm. Note the lymphocyte (L) and the polymorphonuclear leukocyte (P) for size comparison. (Coutesy of Pamela G. Kidd, M.D., Department of Laboratory Medicine, University of Washington, Seattle.)

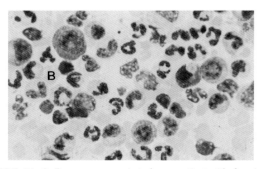

FIGURE 11–8. Bone marrow aspirate from a patient with chronic myelogenous leukemia showing abundance of polymorphonuclear leukocytes (PMNs) with immature granulocytes and a single basophil (B). (Courtesy of Pamela G. Kidd, M.D., Department of Laboratory Medicine, University of Washington, Seattle.)

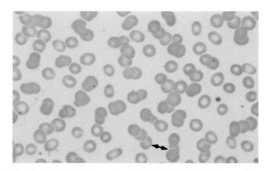

FIGURE 11–15. Multiple myeloma blood film illustrating rouleaux formation—a linear clumping of RBCs produced by an abnormal protein (globulin). (Courtesy of Pamela G. Kidd, M.D., Department of Laboratory Medicine, University of Washington, Seattle.)

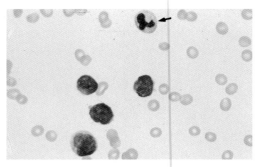

FIGURE 11–5. Blood film from a patient with acute myelogenous leukemia showing four myeloblasts and one polymorphonuclear leukocyte (*arrow*). Note scanty cytoplasm of blast cells and absence of platelets. (Courtesy of Pamela G. Kidd, M.D., Department of Laboratory Medicine, University of Washington, Seattle.)

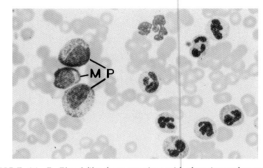

FIGURE 11–7. Blood film from a patient with chronic myelogenous leukemia showing mature granulocytes. Note three immature cells: one myelocyte (M) and two promyelocytes (P). (Courtesy of Pamela G. Kidd, M.D., Department of Laboratory Medicine, University of Washington, Seattle.)

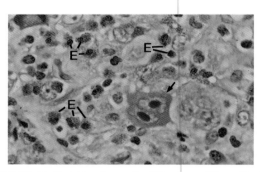

FIGURE 11–11. Hodgkins disease. Reed-Sternberg cell (*arrow*) is a large cell with an opaque cytoplasm, clear nuclear chromatin, and larger dense nucleoli. In close proximity is a larger histiocytic cell with a lobulated nucleus, nonprominent nucleoli, and pink cytoplasm. Note also abundant eosinophils (E). (Courtesy of Pamela G. Kidd, M.D., Department of Laboratory Medicine, University of Washington, Seattle.)

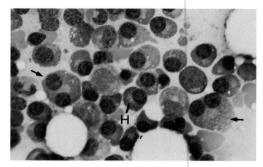

FIGURE 11–16. Multiple myeloma bone marrow aspirate. Plasma cell proliferation illustrated by moderate-sized cells with eccentric nuclei and an opaque blue cytoplasm with a clear paranuclear zone. The clear paranuclear zone is called a höf (H). Also present are two binucleated plasma cells (*arrows*). (Courtesy of Pamela G. Kidd, M.D., Department of Laboratory Medicine, University of Washington, Seattle.)

CHAPTER 11
Lymphoproliferative Disorders

LINDA BELSKY-LOHR and LEE-ELLEN C. COPSTEAD

KEY TERMS

Hodgkin's disease or Hodgkin's lymphoma: A progressive abnormal neoplasm of the primary lymph nodes characterized by painless enlargement of the lymph nodes, spleen, and lymphoid tissues.

leukemia: A malignant disease of the blood and blood-forming organs, with abnormal development of leukocytes and their precursors in the blood and bone marrow. The clinical classification of leukemia depends on the type of cells involved—myeloid (myelogenous), lymphoid (lymphogenous), or monocytic; its duration; and its acute or chronic progression.

leukocytes or white blood cells: Cells that protect the body from disease by phagocytosis of microorganisms and other debris and participate in the immune system.

lymphopoiesis: The developmental process from pluripotential stem cells to mature differentiated lymphocytes.

lymphoproliferation: A proliferation of cells of the lymphoreticular and myeloproliferative systems. Lymphoproliferative disorders are malignant diseases that include lymphocytic, histiocytic, and monocytic leukemias, multiple myeloma, and Hodgkin's disease.

multiple myeloma or plasma cell myeloma: A malignant abnormal growth of plasma cells characterized by widespread osteolytic lesions and originating in multiple bone marrow tumors.

myeloproliferation: The abnormal production of bone marrow components, including erythroblasts, granulocytes, and megakaryocytes.

non-Hodgkin's lymphomas: A group of malignant solid lymphoid tumors that are clinically similar to Hodgkin's disease, although the giant Reed-Sternberg cells are absent and metastasis is faster. The disease begins in the lymphoid components of the immune system.

---

*W*hite **blood cells** (WBCs) or **leukocytes** function by a variety of mechanisms to provide the individual with protection from invading nonself cells (viruses, bacteria, molds, spores, pollens, protozoa, helminths, proteins, and cells from other living organisms) and from self cells that are no longer normal (see Chap. 8). These protective functions are generally dependent on maintaining normal numbers and ratios of many specific mature circulating leukocytes. When any one type of WBC is present in either abnormally high or abnormally low amounts, hematopoietic function and immune function may be altered to some degree, causing the individual to be at risk for specific complications. This chapter discusses the pathologic changes and implications for treatment for persons with disorders characterized by malignant overgrowth of specific cell forms of the lymphoproliferative and myeloproliferative hematopoietic systems: the leukemias, lymphomas, and multiple myeloma.

Signs and symptoms of neoplasias of the blood and blood-forming tissues are dependent on the type of malignancy that exists. The leukemias may be conceptualized as *liquid* tumors, primarily involving the bone marrow. Therefore, pallor, fatigue, fever, recurrent infections, petechiae, purpura, and gross bleeding may be present at the time of diagnosis. Such disorders render the individual susceptible to invasion and attack by infectious agents, prone to life-threatening bleeding episodes, and unable to tolerate the usual routine of daily activities. *Solid* tumors of the blood and blood-forming tissues, such as the lymphomas or multiple myeloma, may present initially with an enlarged lymph node (lymphoma) or small tumors scattered haphazardly through the skeletal system, causing bone pain (multiple myeloma).

A complete data base should focus on skin color, petechiae, bruising, or occult or gross bleeding; liver, splenic, lymph node, or joint enlargement; vital signs; and any complaints of shortness of breath or bone pain.

Depending on the diagnosis, interventions may be implemented that attempt to alter the patient's adaptations to the disease. Additionally, the patient with a malignancy needs emotional support. Fears and uncertainty about all matters of everyday life may abound. An intense course of chemotherapy means time spent hospitalized with low blood counts, the need for blood product and antibiotic support, possible hair loss, pain, nausea, vomiting, and fertility concerns. Furthermore, the family unit and significant others may be profoundly affected by the diagnosis of a malignancy. The nurse is in a prime position to offer and facilitate emotional support. National coping and support groups with local affiliations are available to provide the cancer patient with the reassurance that the cancer experience need not be endured alone. Once the diagnosis has been established and therapy has begun, the goal for the patient is to try to maintain as normal a life as is possible. Patient teaching promotes independence and gives the person a feeling of control.

Leukemias

The **leukemias** are a group of malignant disorders involving abnormal overproduction of a specific cell type, usually at an immature stage, in the bone marrow. Leukemic cells are initially confined to the bone marrow; however, subsequent invasion extends to other organs and tissues of the body as well as the peripheral blood. Accumulation of the leukemic cell in the bone marrow prevents the occurrence of normal **lymphopoiesis** (lymphocyte production), **leukopoiesis** (granulocyte and monocyte production), **erythropoiesis** (RBC production), and **megakaryopoiesis** (platelet production). The end result for the patient diagnosed with leukemia is a functionally incompetent bone marrow.

Leukemia may be acute in onset and short in duration or may have an insidious onset and persist as a chronic disorder. The types of leukemia are further categorized by the specific maturational pathway from which the abnormal cells arise. Leukemias in which the abnormal cells arise from within the committed lymphoid maturational pathways are categorized as **lymphocytic** or **lymphoblastic** (see Fig. 11–9). Leukemias in which the abnormal cells arise within the committed myeloid maturational pathways are categorized as **myelocytic** or **myelogenous** (see Fig. 11–4). Several subtypes exist for each of these and are categorized by the degree of maturity of the abnormal cell and the specific cell type involved. Table 11–1 pre-

TABLE 11-1. French-American-British (FAB) Classification of the Leukemias

Acute Lymphoblastic Leukemia (ALL)

L1 Lymphoblastic leukemia
  Predominance of small lymphoblasts
  Childhood type
L2 Lymphoblastic leukemia
  Predominance of large lymphoblasts
  Heterogeneous type
L3 Predominance of large, more primitive lymphoblasts
  Lymphoma type

Acute Nonlymphoblastic Leukemia (ANLL)

M0 Acute undifferentiated leukemia
  Not classifiable
M1 Acute myeloblastic leukemia (AML)
  Without maturation—most common
  Less than 3 percent promyelocytes
M2 Acute myeloblastic leukemia (AML)
  Some maturation
  More than 3 percent promyelocytes
M3 Acute promyelocytic leukemia (APML)
  More than 30 percent promyelocytes
M4 Acute myelomonocytic leukemia (AMML)
  Minor component—myelocyte or monocyte—is more
  than 20 percent in peripheral blood and/or BM
M5a Acute monocytic leukemia (AMOL)
  Poorly differentiated
M5b Acute monocytic leukemia (AMOL)
  Differentiated
M6 Erythroleukemia

From Bennett JM, Catovsky D, Daniel MT, et al: Proposals for the classification of the acute leukemias. *Br J Haematol* 1976;33:451–458. Reproduced with permission of Blackwell Scientific Publications, Ltd.

sents the French-American-British (FAB) classification of the leukemias.[1]

This chapter will focus on the four most common types of leukemia: acute lymphocytic leukemia, chronic lymphocytic leukemia, acute myelogenous leukemia (also commonly called acute nonlymphocytic leukemia), and chronic myelogenous leukemia, or chronic nonlymphocytic leukemia. Certainly there are less common forms of leukemia. The student is referred to a hematology textbook for those varieties.

Acute Lymphocytic Leukemia

Acute lymphocytic leukemia (ALL) is a malignant disorder involving the lymphocytic lineage. In ALL, the abnormal leukemic cell resembles an immature lymphocyte or lymphoblast. The leukemic blast cell is morphologically similar to the normal blast cell. Figure 11–1 (Color Plate I) shows the blood film from a person with ALL, illustrating blast forms. Unlike the normal blast cell, however, the leukemic blast cell does not mature and is also incompetent, which means that it has incomplete functionality. Leukemic lymphoblasts accumulate in the bone marrow, crushing out precursors for normal lymphopoiesis, erythropoiesis, and megakaryopoiesis.

Acute lymphocytic leukemia is predominantly a disorder of children. It is the most common malig-

nancy in childhood and ranks as the second leading cause of death in that age group. The peak incidence occurs between the ages of 2 and 10 years. A second rise in incidence occurs during middle and older adulthood. With treatment, the survival rate for children is 93 percent, but the prognosis for adults is poorer.[2]

Chronic Lymphocytic Leukemia

Chronic lymphocytic leukemia (CLL), the rarest of the major leukemia groups, is defined as a proliferative disorder of lymphoid tissues. In CLL, abnormal and incompetent lymphocytes initially involve the lymph nodes, but the disease progresses until further involvement of the reticuloendothelial system (liver, spleen) and invasion of the bone marrow ensue. Eventually, the lining of the respiratory and gastrointestinal tracts and the skin exhibit evidence of infiltration by leukemic cells. As the disease process continues, normal bone marrow elements are replaced by abnormal lymphocytes. This replacement interferes with normal hematopoiesis. Figures 11–2 (Color Plate I) and 11–3 (Color Plate II) show the typical small, abnormal lymphocytes in peripheral blood and bone marrow aspirates.

The lymphocytes in chronic lymphocytic leukemia are also immunologically incompetent. Hypogammaglobulinemia is a characteristic of late-stage disease. The defect seems to involve immunoglobulin-producing B-lymphocytes.

Chronic lymphocytic leukemia has an insidious onset. Usually it is found by accident on routine blood count examinations. CLL is most prevalent in the Western hemisphere. It primarily affects individuals older than age 50 and has a possible genetic predisposition. The prognosis, even with treatment, is poor.[3]

Acute Myelogenous Leukemia

Acute myelogenous leukemia (AML), also known as acute nonlymphocytic leukemia (ANLL), is defined as a malignant disorder involving the pluripotent myelocytic stem cell of the bone marrow. (The hematopoietic cascade is reviewed in Figure 11–4.) Most frequently the granulocytic lineage is involved; however, other marrow elements can be affected. The terminology used to define and describe the different varieties of AML tends to be confusing at best. However, the descriptors used identify the cell precursor most prominent in the bone marrow. Examples of different varieties or types of AML include acute granulocytic leukemia, acute promyelocytic leukemia, acute myelomonocytic leukemia, and erythroleukemia. Acute granulocytic leukemia, myelomonocytic leukemia, and erythroleukemia differ morphologically, but clinically they are similar. Acute promyelocytic leukemia is a rare leukemia and tends to be accompanied by the development of disseminated intravascular coagulation (DIC) during relapse. However, when controlled by chemotherapeutic agents, it resembles the most common varieties.

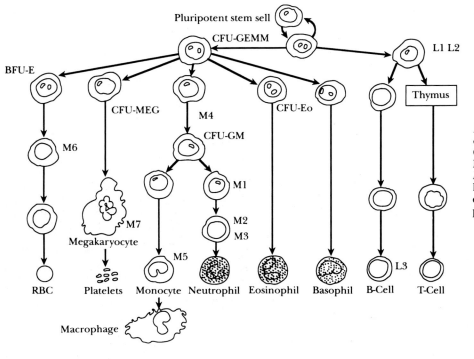

Pluripotent stem sell

CFU-GEMM

L1 L2

BFU-E

Thymus

CFU-MEG

M4

CFU-Eo

M6

CFU-GM

M1

M7

M2

Megakaryocyte

M3

M5

L3

RBC   Platelets   Monocyte   Neutrophil   Eosinophil   Basophil   B-Cell   T-Cell

Macrophage

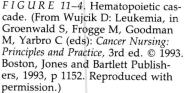

F I G U R E 11–4. Hematopoietic cascade. (From Wujcik D: Leukemia, in Groenwald S, Frogge M, Goodman M, Yarbro C (eds): *Cancer Nursing: Principles and Practice,* 3rd ed. © 1993. Boston, Jones and Bartlett Publishers, 1993, p 1152. Reproduced with permission.)

Acute granulocytic leukemia is the most common of the acute myelogenous leukemias and will be discussed as a prototype. Often the terms acute myelogenous leukemia and acute granulocytic leukemia are used interchangeably.

Acute granulocytic leukemia involves abnormal proliferation and accumulation of immature granulocytes (myeloblasts) (Figs. 11–5, 11–6, Color Plate II). Proliferation of the immature granulocyte may be either slower or faster than normal granulocytes. Regardless of the speed of cell division, the abnormal leukemia cells eventually crowd out normal cells in the bone marrow.[4]

Acute granulocytic leukemia is rare in adolescents, but the majority of acute nonlymphocytic leukemias diagnosed during the neonatal period and early infancy are acute granulocytic leukemia. There is a rising incidence in middle age, peaking in the eighth and ninth decades of life.[5]

Chronic Myelogenous Leukemia

Chronic myelogenous leukemia (CML), also known as chronic nonlymphocytic leukemia (CNLL), is defined as a malignant disorder characterized by abnormal and excessive accumulation and overgrowth of granulocytes in the bone marrow (Figs. 11–7, 11–8, Color Plate II). These granulocytes are associated with a unique chromosomal abnormality, the Ph[1] (Philadelphia) chromosome. Additionally, they seem to have a lengthened life span and retain their ability to fight infection through phagocytosis.[6]

The onset and progression of CML are insidious. Remission of CML may be successful for as long as 4 years. However, almost 70 percent of patients with

CML will undergo an acute transformation, or *blast crisis.*[7] During blast crisis, the leukemia resembles acute granulocytic leukemia, but unlike the latter, acute transformation is not amenable to chemotherapy, and death usually occurs within months.[8]

CML represents approximately 20 percent of all leukemias in the Western hemisphere.[7] It does occur in adolescents, but the peak incidence occurs between the age of 25 and 60 years. CML in the neonate tends to have a rapid progression of infiltration and invasion.[7]

Etiology

The exact cause of any of the leukemias is not known. It seems clear, however, that the pathogenesis is multifactorial. Review of the literature reveals possible chemical, viral, radiation, and genetic stimuli preceding the development of leukemia.[6,9] However, it is nearly impossible to identify the causative factor(s) in individual cases of leukemia. The basic mechanism appears to involve gene damage of cells, leading to transformation of those cells from the normal state to a malignant state. The processes appear to be the same as for the development of solid tumors (see Chap. 6).

The following conditions and factors constitute possible risk factors for the development of leukemia: ionizing radiation, chemicals and drugs, marrow hypoplasia, environmental interactions, genetic factors, viral factors, immunologic factors, and interactive factors. Exposure to large quantities of ionizing radiation appears to be a major risk factor in the development of leukemia. Exposures ranging from therapeutic irradiation for diseases such as ankylosing spondylitis and Hodgkin's disease to irradiation from the atomic bomb at Hiroshima or the Chernobyl accident are associated with leukemia.

Many different chemicals and drugs have been linked to the development of leukemia. Of these chemicals, benzene is the most closely associated with the development of leukemia. Phenylbutazone, arsenic, and chloramphenicol also appear to be related to the later development of leukemia. Unfortunately, antineoplastic drugs, especially alkylating agents, used as treatment for other malignant conditions are also linked to leukemia development.[2]

Marrow hypoplasia can also increase the risk of leukemia. A reduction or alteration in production of hematopoietic cells may predispose individuals to leukemia. Examples of conditions associated with the later development of leukemia include Fanconi's anemia, paroxysmal nocturnal hemoglobinurias during the aplastic phase, and myelodysplastic syndromes.[10] Environmental factors that predispose to leukemia are difficult to identify, as they can be multiple and interactive. Such exposures include in utero irradiation, maternal irradiation, and early childhood viral disease.

An increase in the frequency of leukemia among the following populations suggests possible genetic involvement: identical twins of persons with leukemia and individuals with Down's syndrome, Bloom's syndrome, Fanconi's anemia, and Klinefelter's syndrome. Chromosomal aberration may be an important factor in the development of leukemia in these syndromes.[6]

The ribonucleic acid (RNA) viruses have been implicated in the causation of leukemia. Retroviruses that carry the gene for reverse transcriptase are also suspected of producing leukemia.[11]

A deficiency in the immune system may favor the development of leukemia. It has not yet been determined whether leukemia among immunodeficient individuals is a result of immunosurveillance failure or if the pathologic mechanisms that cause the immune deficiency also trigger malignant transformation of leukopoietic cells.[12,13]

The interaction of multiple host and environmental factors may result in leukemia. The interaction of these factors is tolerated differently by each person, frequently making it difficult to determine the etiology of any specific leukemia.

Pathogenesis

The basic pathologic defect in leukemia is a malignant transformation of the stem cells of early committed precursor leukocyte cells, producing an abnormal proliferation of a specific type of leukocyte. The immature leukocytes, which are functionally abnormal, are produced in excessive quantities in the bone marrow, essentially shutting down normal bone marrow production of erythrocytes, platelets, and functionally mature leukocytes. This situation leads to anemia, thrombocytopenia, and leukopenia of normal WBC types, even though the affected individual has a greatly elevated number of abnormal circulating WBCs. Death usually results from infection or hemorrhage unless treatment is instituted. For the acute leukemias, these pathologic changes occur rapidly and progress quickly to death without intervention. Chronic leukemia may be present for many years before overt pathologic changes related to the illness are manifested. Usually, chronic leukemia progresses to a blast crisis stage, in which the leukemia becomes an acute illness closely resembling acute leukemia.

Clinical Manifestations

Clinical manifestations are related to the lack of normal hematopoiesis in the bone marrow. Bone marrow dysfunction results in varying degrees of leukopenia, anemia, and thrombocytopenia. It is these three deficiencies that cause the most common clinical manifestations in the leukemic patient, regardless of the type of leukemia present. Tables 11–2 and 11–3 list the primary and secondary manifestations of the leukemias and summarize their features at presentation.

Anemia, with a hematocrit of 25 percent to 30 percent or hemoglobin levels of 8–10 g/dL, may manifest with pallor, fatigue, malaise, shortness of breath, dyspnea, or decreased activity tolerance.[14] These symptoms occur based on the rate of red cell decrease as much as on the absolute values present. Chronically low hemoglobin and hematocrit may be tolerated better than a drastic drop in one or both values. Transfusion may be warranted when the hematocrit approaches 30 percent. Thrombocytopenia with a platelet count below 20,000/mm^3 manifests as petechiae, easy bruising, bleeding gums, occult hematuria, or retinal hemorrhages. There is an inverse relationship between the number of thrombocytes and the incidence of severe bleeding episodes. Leukopenia, when present, leaves the patient at risk for developing infection. Infection may be caused by bacterial, viral, fungal, or protozoal organisms. There is also an inverse relationship between the number of leukocytes, particularly granulocytes, and the incidence of infection. Infection is suspected in the presence of fever (temperature > 38.5° C) and is treated aggressively with broad-spectrum bactericidal agents. Infection in the neutropenic patient may quickly evolve into life-threatening sepsis.

Other manifestations of leukemia include lymphadenopathy, joint swelling and pain, weight loss, anorexia, and varying degrees of hepatosplenomegaly. Sternal tenderness is frequently present in CML. Gingival hyperplasia frequently accompanies acute granulocytic leukemia. Meningeal involvement is more common in children than adults and is more frequently encountered in children with ALL. However, it should be remembered that central nervous system (CNS) involvement is possible in any of the leukemias. Meningeal or CNS involvement is also related to the poor ability of chemotherapeutic agents to cross the blood-brain barrier. Meningeal involvement presents as an increase in intracranial pressure. Signs and

TABLE 11-2. Manifestations of Leukemia

	Organ	Manifestations
Primary Manifestations		
Result from the proliferation of leukocytes within blood-forming organs	Bone marrow	Hyperplasia of abnormal cells Hypoplasia of all normal cellular components Thrombocytopenia leads to bleeding Erythrocytopenia leads to anemia Granulocytopenia leads to infection
	Spleen and liver	Hepatosplenomegaly Changed consistency: Acute leukemia—soft Chronic leukemia—hard Infarction causes pain Hypersplenism leads to pancytopenia
	Lymph nodes	Lymphadenopathy May be painful Obstruction of adjacent organs or structures
Secondary Manifestations		
Result from the infiltration of leukemic cells into body tissues *or* consequences of bone marrow suppression	Liver	Hepatomegaly May be painful or tender
	Bones, joints, and muscle	Enlargement of the cortex of the long bones in children with acute lymphoblastic leukemia Osteolytic lesions Goutlike symptoms Pain Swelling
	Central nervous system	Thrombosis } Hemorrhage } paralysis Increased intracranial pressure Headache Vomiting
	Skin	Purpura Petechiae Ecchymoses Infection
	Gastrointestinal system	Ulceration Hemorrhage Infection
	Mouth, throat, and nose	Bleeding gums Epistaxis Ulceration Necrosis Infection
	Lungs	Infarction Infection Pleural effusion
	Eyes	Retinal hemorrhage Subconjunctival hemorrhage Papilledema Visual disturbances
	Kidneys	Bilateral asymmetric enlargement Hyperuricemia Rare pyelonephritis leads to renal failure

From Wujcik D: Leukemia, in Groenwald S, Frogge M, Goodman M, Yarbro C (eds): *Cancer Nursing: Principles and Practice*, 3rd ed. © 1993. Boston, Jones and Bartlett Publishers, 1993, p 1153. Reproduced with permission.

TABLE 11–3. Comparative Features of the Leukemias at Presentation

Description	Median Age	Initial Remission Rate	Median Survival With Treatment	Splenomegaly	Infection	Adenopathy	Hemoglobin	White Blood Cell Count	Platelets
Acute myelogenous leukemia	50–60	60 percent–70 percent	10–15 mo	No	Yes	No	Low	Variable	Low
Acute lymphoblastic leukemia	4	Adult 70 percent; children 90 percent	Adult 2 yr; children 5 yr	Yes	Yes	Yes	Low	Variable	Low
Chronic myelogenous leukemia	49	90 percent	3 yr	Yes	No	No	Low	100,000–300,000 granulocytes	Normal or low
Chronic lymphocytic leukemia	60	90 percent	4–6 yr	Yes	Yes	Yes	Low	20,000 lymphocytes	Low

From Wujcik D: Leukemia, in Groenwald S, Frogge M, Goodman M, Yarbro C (eds): *Cancer Nursing: Principles and Practice*, 3rd ed. © 1993. Boston, Jones and Bartlett Publishers, 1993, p 1154. Reproduced with permission.

symptoms of increased intracranial pressure include nausea and vomiting, headaches, blurred vision, and cranial nerve dysfunction. Papilledema may be visualized on funduscopic examination.

Treatment

In general, the leukemic patient and family need an extensive teaching program. Teaching should include information about the leukemia disease process, the procedures used during the diagnostic and maintenance phases of treatment, radiation therapy, antineoplastic drug therapy prescribed, signs and symptoms warranting medical intervention, precautionary measures needed for home care, and over-the-counter medications that should be avoided. From this long list of teaching needs, it is easy to see that the person with leukemia may feel overwhelmed. Therefore, teaching must be a carefully planned endeavor. Coordination of the teaching between the acute care setting and ambulatory care setting is most important.

The remainder of this section focuses on three specific management areas: pharmacologic management, nutritional management, and the treatment of complications.

Pharmacologic Management

The goal of therapy is remission—the absence of any detectable leukemic cells in the bone marrow. Antineoplastic drug therapy varies with the morphologic type of leukemia and the stage of treatment. Basically, drug treatment for the acute leukemias has three phases: *remission-induction phase, remission-consolidation phase,* and *remission-maintenance phase.*

Once the diagnosis is established, remission-induction phase treatment begins. The aim of treatment in this phase is to destroy as many leukemic cells as possible and return the bone marrow to a functionally "normal" state. At the time of diagnosis, it is estimated that the number of leukemic cells is between 1×10^{12} and 1×10^{14}. These leukemic cells are found predominantly in the bone marrow.

Remission-induction phase treatment cannot destroy all leukemic cells present at the time of diagnosis. The inability to achieve complete leukemic cell destruction during the remission-induction phase is because some leukemic cells grow slowly and do not respond to chemotherapy. Actively dividing leukemic cells (approximately $1 \times 10^{3-4}$ cells) are found in the bone marrow, in tissues and organs, and in the peripheral blood. The second pool of quiescent leukemic cells is much larger ($1 \times 10^{8-9}$ cells) and is primarily present in the bone marrow. Because these cells are not actively replicating, they are difficult to kill with chemotherapeutic drugs. It is hoped that over a 2- to 3-year period, these cells will become active and therefore amenable to treatment.

Drugs are used in combination during remission-induction phase treatment for ALL and AML. Single-agent drug therapy has been found to be less effective than combinations of antineoplastic agents. Vincristine and prednisone are most commonly used in ALL. Often a third drug, such as L-asparaginase or daunorubicin, is added to treatment. Complete remission for adults and children with ALL is possible. Complete remission rates for adults are approximately 75 percent; in children, complete remission is accomplished in 80 percent to 90 percent of all cases.[15]

A second phase of antineoplastic drug therapy, called remission-consolidation phase, is sometimes employed. The goal of remission-consolidation phase treatment is to further reduce the leukemic cell population. Remission-consolidation phase treatment is usually short, averaging about 3 or 4 days. Drugs commonly used for this phase of treatment in the acute leukemias are methotrexate, cyclophosphamide, hydrocortisone, cytosine arabinoside (Cytarabine), L-asparaginase, and 6-thioguanine.

Remission-maintenance phase treatment occurs once remission is established. The goal of remission-maintenance phase treatment is to further destroy the leukemic cell population. This phase is continued for 2 to 3 years postdiagnosis. Research evidence strongly suggests that continuing chemotherapy beyond a 2- to 3-year period does not alter the relapse rate. Drugs used most commonly in the acute leukemias include 6-mercaptopurine, 6-thioguanine, cyclophosphamide, vincristine, methotrexate, cytosine arabinoside, and hydroxyurea. In ALL, it appears that methotrexate and 6-mercaptopurine are the most important drugs to maintain remission.[16]

Acute myelogenous leukemia has not been as amenable to remission-induction phase treatment as acute lymphocytic leukemia. Currently, combinations of chemotherapy are used. Drugs such as vincristine, prednisone, cytosine arabinoside, cyclophosphamide, and 6-thioguanine are often used in various combinations. With the establishment of more aggressive chemotherapeutic protocols, such as daunorubicin and cytosine arabinoside, the remission rate approaches 75 percent.[5]

The chronic leukemias require a somewhat different pharmacologic approach. Remission is never completely established. Instead, the chronic leukemias are, more or less, controlled for as long as possible. The drugs of choice for CLL are chlorambucil and cyclophosphamide. A new agent, fludarabine phosphate (Fludara), may be useful in controlling CLL that is refractory to chlorambucil and cyclophosphamide.[17] Phase III clinical trials are underway comparing Fludara alone versus chlorambucil and cyclophosphamide given together versus chlorambucil, cyclophosamide, and Fludara. Because studies are ongoing, results are not yet known.

In CML, interferon-alpha, busulfan, melphalan, and uracil mustard are used. Blood counts, especially quantitative leukocyte determinations, are carefully monitored and medication doses are adjusted accordingly. Drug therapy for the chronic leukemias may be administered intermittently or continuously. In children and adults, the CNS acts as a sanctuary for leukemic cells. Once abnormal cells invade the CNS, conventional routes of chemotherapy are unsuccessful, related to the poor ability of chemotherapeutic agents to cross the blood-brain barrier. Therefore, CNS involvement is treated via the intrathecal route. Intrathecal administration necessitates performing a lumbar puncture. The antineoplastic agent is then diluted with cerebrospinal fluid and a minimum volume of nonpreservative diluents to minimize fluid volume shifts from the CNS. Finally, the medication is instilled. Intrathecal instillation of chemotherapeutic agents is not without risk. Neurologic abnormalities, either transient or permanent, have occurred. The following drugs are used for the CNS treatment of leukemia: methotrexate, cytosine arabinoside, aminopterin, and hydrocortisone. Because vincristine sulfate is extremely neurotoxic, it is *never* given intrathecally.

Some treatment protocols combine intrathecal medication with cranial irradiation; other treatment programs use intrathecal medication only. Regardless of the treatment protocol, the purpose remains the same: to eradicate leukemic cells from the sanctuary of the CNS.

Aspirin or aspirin-containing products and medications containing guaifenesin should not be administered to the patient with leukemia. Aspirin and guaifenesin interfere with adequate platelet function. Aspirin is found in many over-the-counter cold and flu medications; guaifenesin is contained in over-the-counter cough suppressants. Patients should be taught to read all medication labels before taking the medication. It is wise to encourage patients to seek medical attention before self-medicating.

Nutritional Management

Patients with leukemia may experience anorexia, weight loss, nausea, vomiting, and stomatitis. Children and adolescents on chemotherapy may experience a slowing of growth. These adaptations may be related to the disease process of leukemia or to the treatment protocols. Weight losses, weight gains (fluid retention while taking corticosteroids), or slowing of linear growth should be noted and acted upon quickly. In the presence of delayed growth or weight loss, a diet high in proteins and calories is needed. Supplemental feedings of high protein and high caloric content may need to be added to the patient's 24-hour regimen. Fluid retention caused by corticosteroids can be reduced by placing the patient on a reduced sodium diet.

Complications

Infection

Infections can be fatal for the leukemic patient. During the remission-induction phase, the most common infections are caused by bacterial and fungal organisms. The mortality from either fungal or bacterial infection is high. The most common infection during the remission-maintenance phase is viral. Infection is related to the degree of leukopenia present. As the neutrophil count decreases, the infection rate increases. Isolation of the neutropenic patient is usually instituted. Some institutions have laminar air flow units available, in which special filters purify the air the patient breathes. Some institutions use protective isolation or reverse isolation techniques. Regardless of the isolation technique used, the purpose remains the same: to protect the patient against the occurrence of infection. It is important to avoid large crowds and prevent contact with contagious individuals when blood counts are low.

Rectal temperatures, enemas, and suppositories are avoided in order to prevent infection by damaging the rectal mucosa. Intramuscular injections are avoided because they break the skin integrity and create a portal for bacterial invasion and abscess formation.

Patients may have an altered inflammatory response and may not exhibit the usual signs of inflammation and infection, such as purulent discharge. An elevated temperature signals a potential problem of infection. Whenever infection is suspected in a leukopenic patient, cultures are taken of blood, urine, throat, etc., in an attempt to identify the location of infection and the causative organism. Broad-spectrum antibiotics are started initially until the organism is identified.

Recently a group of drugs has been added to the oncologist's arsenal against neutropenia associated with chemotherapy. Colony-stimulating factors, as they are called, stimulate and direct development of specific cell lines within the patient's bone marrow. There are colony-stimulating factors for the red cell line and the white cell line. Our discussion will be limited to the most commonly used white cell stimulating factor, granulocyte-CSF, or G-CSF.

As discussed in Chapters 8 and 9, neutrophils are granulocytes (white blood cells) responsible for body defense against infectious organisms. When the neutrophil count falls, the risk for infection climbs. Additionally, the longer a patient is neutropenic, the more likely is the development of a life-threatening infection.

Research[18] has demonstrated that the administration of G-CSF can reduce the length of neutropenic episodes. The most common use of G-CSF is during anticipated periods of neutropenia, thus reducing the risk of infection. Such clinical applications include administration after bone marrow transplantation to speed up bone marrow recovery time, and administration to augment high-dose chemotherapy protocols, allowing the oncologist to maximize the benefit of chemotherapy while reducing the risk of deleterious side effects.

Anemia

Anemia is a common complication of leukemia. Causes of anemia are abnormal bone marrow replacement by leukemic cells and bone marrow suppression by chemotherapeutic agents. The leukemic patient may demonstrate pallor, shortness of breath, tachycardia, and limited activity tolerance in response to anemia. These patients frequently need replacement transfusion therapy in the form of packed RBCs.

Bleeding

Thrombocytopenia with resultant hemorrhage can be life-threatening. Care is focused on preventing major hemorrhagic episodes. Assessment for signs or symptoms of hemorrhage includes monitoring changes in level of consciousness (intracranial bleeding). Hematemesis and epistaxis may be provoked with or without injury.

Not all bleeding is apparent and life-threatening. Frequently the leukemic patient experiences occult bleeding. Gingival oozing may occur after brushing teeth or eating. Occult hematuria is common. Assessment includes testing stools, emesis, and urine for occult blood. Rectal temperatures, enemas, rectal suppositories, and intramuscular injections are avoided as these may lead to severe hemorrhagic episodes.

Pain

The leukemic patient may have pain. Pain most commonly involves the bones and joints and is due to pressure caused by infiltration and accumulation of leukemic cells in the bone marrow. Hemarthrosis may also occur and can be painful. Narcotics may be given in an attempt to control the pain, or chemotherapy may be administered when the pain is thought to be caused by leukemic infiltration.

Alopecia

Body image changes caused by chemotherapy or radiation therapy interfere with the individual's ability to cope with the disease process. *Alopecia* (hair loss) creates a common body image change. However, alopecia is only a temporary consequence of treatment. Until the hair grows back, wigs, toupées, decorative scarfs, or caps may help promote a more positive body image.

KEY CONCEPTS

- Leukemias are malignant disorders characterized by overproduction of abnormal WBCs (leukocytes) in the marrow. Accumulation of abnormal cells interferes with the production of other normal marrow cells, including platelets, RBCs, and WBCs. Risk factors for the development of leukemia include exposure to chemical, viral, and radiation mutagens and immunodeficiency disorders.

- The classification of leukemia is based on the cell type involved (lymphocytes or nonlymphocytes) and the rapidity of disease progression (acute or chronic). Acute lymphocytic leukemia affects children primarily, has an acute onset, responds well to treatment, and has a relatively good prognosis. Chronic lymphocytic leukemia affects adults primarily, has an insidious onset, responds less well to treatment, and has a poorer prognosis than acute lymphocytic leukemia. Acute nonlymphocytic leukemia affects adults primarily, has an acute onset, and responds relatively well to treatment. Chronic nonlymphocytic leukemia affects adults primarily, has an insidious onset, and responds poorly to treatment. Both acute and chronic nonlymphocytic leukemia may be associated with abnormal proliferation of any of the myelogenous cells (platelets, RBCs, granulocytes and monocytes).

- Manifestations of leukemia are due to insufficient quantities of normal marrow cells as evidenced by anemia, thrombocytopenia, and leukopenia of normal cells. Anemia manifests with pallor, fatigue, dyspnea, and decreased activity tolerance. Thrombocytopenia manifests with petechiae, bleeding gums, hematuria, and prolonged bleeding time. Leukopenia manifests with frequent, recurrent infections. Symptoms due to malignant overproliferation of leukemic cells include lymphadenopathy, weight loss, sternal tenderness, and bone pain. Infiltration of leukemic cells into the brain may manifests as increased intracranial pressure.

- Chemotherapy is the mainstay of treatment. Several courses may be needed to kill leukemic cells which replicate slowly. Chemotherapy is more effective in acute leukemias because cells are more rapidly dividing. Chronic leukemias have populations of slowly dividing cells that are difficult to eradicate with chemotherapy. Remission is not completely achieved, but cell growth is kept in check.

- Treatment for leukemia is associated with a number of potential complications requiring monitoring and treatment. Chemotherapy destroys rapidly growing normal cells as well as leukemic cells. This leads to further anemia, leukopenia, and thrombocytopenia. Rapidly dividing hair and mucous membrane cells are also affected, leading to alopecia and stomatitis. Transfusions of blood products may be needed. Stimulation of WBC production by administration of colony-stimulating factors may be indicated.

Hodgkin's Disease

Unlike the leukemias, malignant lymphomas differ in the degree of differentiation of the affected cells and the location of production of these cells. **Lymphomas** are malignancies characterized by a proliferation of **committed lymphocytes** rather than the stem cell precursors, as in leukemia. (Figure 11–9 shows the maturation sequence of the lymphocyte.) Note that the malignant proliferation does not occur in the bone marrow, but rather in the other lymphoid tissues scattered throughout the body, especially the lymph nodes and the spleen. As such, lymphomas are actually solid-tissue masses rather than cellular suspensions within the blood and the bone marrow.

Hodgkin's disease is a malignant disorder of the lymph nodes characterized by the presence of Reed-Sternberg cells on histopathologic examination. Hodgkin's disease metastasizes predominantly via the lymphatics along predictable, contiguous pathways and represents 40 percent of all malignant lymphomas.[19] Figure 11–10 shows the orderly pattern of contiguous lymphoid spread in Hodgkin's disease.

Hodgkin's disease occurs across the age continuum, with half of the cases occurring between the ages of 20 and 40. Less than 10 percent of all cases occur before 10 years of age.[20] The overall incidence

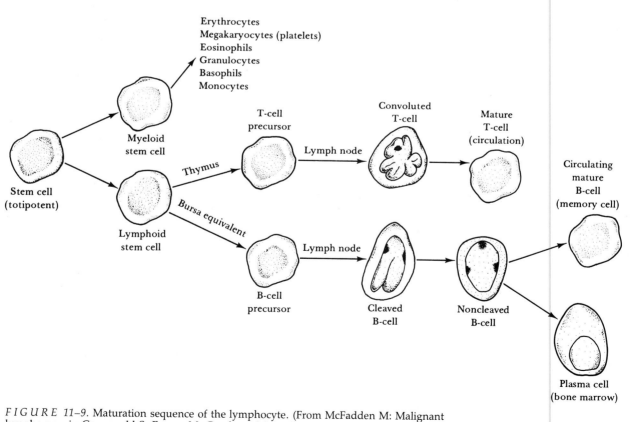

FIGURE 11–9. Maturation sequence of the lymphocyte. (From McFadden M: Malignant lymphomas, in Groenwald S, Frogge M, Goodman M, Yarbro C (eds): *Cancer Nursing: Principles and Practice*, 3rd ed. © 1993. Boston, Jones and Bartlett Publishers, 1993, p 1204. Reproduced with permission. Illustrator: J. Thommen.)

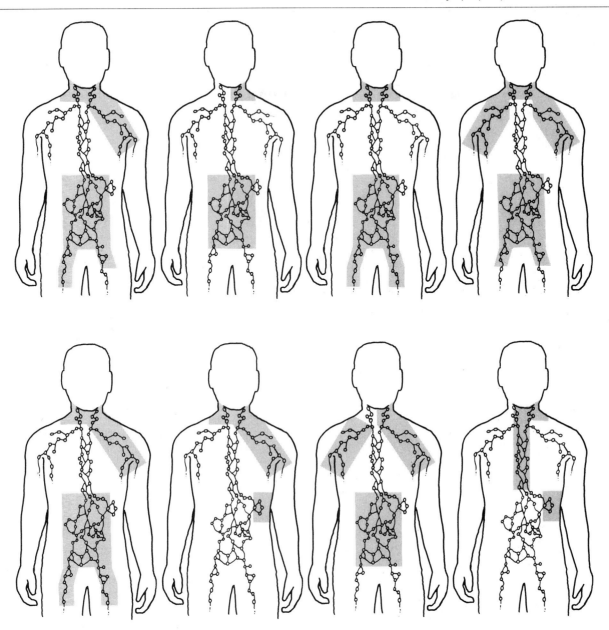

FIGURE 11–10. Orderly pattern of contiguous lymphoid spread in Hodgkin's disease. (From Rosenberg SA: Hodgkin's disease: No stage beyond cure. *Hosp Pract* 1986;21(8):97. Reproduced with permission. Illustration by Bunji Tagawa.)

of Hodgkin's disease is higher in the male population, and disease in males carries a poorer prognosis than disease in females.[20]

Etiology and Pathogenesis

The exact etiology is unknown. But, many believe there are predisposing genetic and environmental factors that cause Hodgkin's disease among family members. Factors implicated as possible causes include viral infections and previous exposure to alkylating chemical agents. Hodgkin's disease usually originates in a single lymph node or a single chain of nodes. The lymphoid tissues within the node undergo malignant transformation and usually initiate some inflammatory processes at the same time. These nodes contain the Reed-Sternberg cell, which is a characteristic marker of Hodgkin's disease (Fig. 11–11, Color Plate II). This initially localized disease first metastasizes to other lymphoid structures and eventually invades nonlymphoid tissues.[21]

Clinical Manifestations

The usual clinical presentation includes painless lymph node enlargement that may be accompanied by fever, night sweats, pruritus, weight loss, and malaise.

Usually, lymph node enlargement occurs in nodes above the diaphragm, the cervical nodes being the most commonly involved. Other supradiaphragmatic nodes that may be involved are the axillary and mediastinal nodes. Signs and symptoms associated with axillary and mediastinal lymphadenopathy include cough, dyspnea, and superior vena cava obstruction.[21] Less commonly, subdiaphragmatic lymphadenopathy is present. If lymph nodes below the diaphragm are involved, most likely they are inguinal nodes. Mesenteric nodes are rarely involved.[21,22]

Other clinical manifestations may include retroperitoneal lymph node enlargement, hepatosplenomegaly, and bone involvement. These manifestations usually occur later as the disease becomes more disseminated. However, a small number of patients may present with disseminated disease at the time of diagnosis.

Hodgkin's disease has been divided into four subgroups, based on the histopathologic findings at the time of lymph node biopsy.[23] These subgroups are (1) lymphocyte predominance, (2) nodular sclerosis, (3) mixed cellularity, and (4) lymphocyte depletion. Table 11–4 summarizes the major histologic findings of each type.

The lymphocyte predominance type carries the best prognosis, with a 90 percent 5-year disease-free survival rate. Lymphocyte predominance represents approximately 16 percent of all cases of Hodgkin's disease. The nodular sclerosing type has a 70 percent 5-year survival rate.[24] It represents approximately 35 percent of all cases of Hodgkin's disease.[25] The mixed cellularity type represents approximately one third of all Hodgkin's disease and has a 4 percent 5-year disease-free survival rate.[22] The lymphocyte depletion type represents approximately 16 percent of all Hodgkin's disease cases.[26] Lymphocyte depletion is usually associated with extensive disease at the time of diagnosis and carries an overall poor prognosis.

Not only is Hodgkin's disease classified according to the histopathologic findings, it is also staged. A staging workup is performed to detect the extent of malignancy at the time of diagnosis. Clinical staging dictates the treatment modality best suited to provide the patient with the greatest chance for long-term survival and cure.

Historically, there has been controversy regarding which clinical staging protocol to use. The staging protocol used today was first introduced in 1971 at the Ann Arbor symposium on staging in Hodgkin's disease.[27] This staging protocol relies on clinical signs and symptoms and tissue sampling usually performed during laparotomy. The stages are described in Table 11–5. Each stage is further classified into an A or a B category. The A category designates that the patient is without certain symptoms or is symptom free. The B category denotes that the patient does have certain symptoms. These symptoms include weight loss of greater than 10 percent of body weight 6 months prior to diagnosis, unexplained fever greater than 38° C, and night sweats.[22] Figure 11–12 illustrates the staging system.

In order to properly diagnose and stage Hodgkin's disease, a large suite of tests is performed. The purpose of the staging workup is to detect the extent of the disease process, thereby identifying the clinical stage. The clinical stage in turn dictates the treatment modalities utilized. Therefore, to provide patients with the best chance for cure, it is important that they complete the staging tests. Some of the tests may be quite uncomfortable, and the rationale for performing the staging workup may seem elusive. Clinical and pathologic staging procedures are summarized in Table 11–6.

Patients undergoing a staging workup for Hodgkin's disease are subjected to invasion of many body parts. These patients will need a lot of emotional support and education. It is useful to note that because of improvements in therapy over the past 10 years, Stage A disease is potentially curable.

TABLE 11–4. Classification of Hodgkin's Disease Based on Histopathologic Findings on Lymph Node Biopsy

Subgroup	Major Histologic Features	Approximate Frequency (%)
Lymphocyte predominance	Abundant normal-appearing lymphocytes with or without benign histiocytes; occasionally nodular, rare Reed-Sternberg cells	2–10
Nodular sclerosis	Nodules of lymphoid tissue separated by bands of collagen; numerous variants of Reed-Sternberg cells	40–80
Mixed cellularity	Pleomorphic infiltrate of eosinophils, plasma cells, histiocytes, and lymphocytes, with numerous Reed-Sternberg cells	20–40
Lymphocyte depletion	Paucity of lymphocytes with numerous Reed-Sternberg cells, diffuse fibrosis, and necrosis	2–15

From Carson C, Callaghan ME: Hematopoietic and immunologic cancers, in Baird SB, McCorkle R, Grant M (Eds): *Cancer Nursing: A Comprehensive Textbook*. Philadelphia, WB Saunders, 1991, p 552. Originally adapted from Rosenberg SA: Hodgkin's disease: No stage beyond cure. *Hosp Pract* 1986;21(8):92. Reproduced with permission.

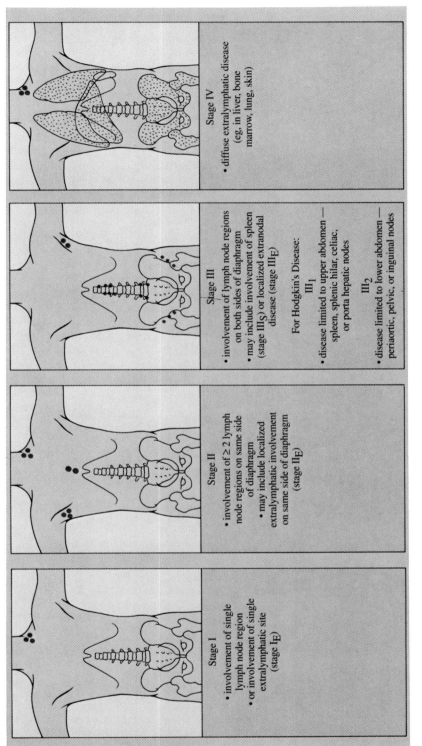

FIGURE 11–12. Ann Arbor staging system for Hodgkin's disease and non-Hodgkin's lymphoma. (From *Atlas of Diagnostic Oncology,* by Arthur T. Skarin, M.D., Gower Medical Publishing an imprint of Times Mirror International Publishers, Ltd., 1991, p 12.6. Reproduced with permission.)

TABLE 11–5. Ann Arbor Staging System for Hodgkin's Disease and Non-Hodgkin's Lymphoma

Stage	Definition
I	Involvement of a single lymph node region (I) or of a single extralymphatic organ or site (I_E).
II	Involvement of two or more lymph node regions on the same side of the diaphragm (II) or involvement of an extralymphatic organ or site and one or more lymph node regions on the same side of the diaphragm (II_E).
III	Involvement of lymph nodes on both sides of the diaphragm (III), which may also be accompanied by localized involvement of extralymphatic organs or sites (III_E) or involvement of the spleen (III_S), or both (III_SE).
IV	Diffuse or disseminated involvement of one or more extralymphatic* organs or tissues, with or without associated lymph node involvement.

Each stage is subclassified by the presence (B) or absence (A) of one or more of the following unexplained symptoms:
Weight loss >10 percent over 6 months
Fever >38° C
Night sweats

*Extralymphatic may include the following sites: lung, bone, bone marrow, liver, or brain.
From Carson C, Callaghan ME: Hematopoietic and immunologic cancers, in Baird SB, McCorkle R, Grant M (eds): *Cancer Nursing: A Comprehensive Textbook.* Philadelphia, WB Saunders, 1991, p 552. Reproduced with permission.

Another diagnostic procedure that is of utmost importance is the lymph node biopsy. This single procedure establishes the diagnosis of Hodgkin's disease from the presence of Reed-Sternberg cells. In addition, lymph node biopsy enables the pathologist to classify Hodgkin's disease as either lymphocyte predominant, modular sclerosis, mixed cellularity, or lymphocyte depletion Hodgkin's disease.

Laboratory findings are not unique to Hodgkin's disease, but certain characteristic patterns have been established. Neutrophilic leukocytosis may be present, as well as a mild normocytic, normochromic anemia and eosinophilia. Both Coombs-positive and Coombs-negative hemolytic anemia may be present. An elevated leukocyte alkaline phosphatase level, elevated serum copper level, and elevated erythrocyte sedimentation rate are often associated with exacerbations. An elevation in serum alkaline phosphatase may signal liver and bone metastasis. Hypergammaglobulinemia is common, while hypogammaglobulinemia may occur with advanced disease.

Treatment

Radiation and Pharmacologic Management

Radiation therapy is the primary treatment of Hodgkin's disease Stages I, II, and IIIA.[24] Figure 11–13 illustrates the radiation fields used in treating lymph nodes both above and below the diaphragm. Subtotal nodal irradiation includes fields I and II and is the most commonly used radiation treatment for Stages IA and IIA laparotomy-negative patients.

Although radiation therapy is the primary treatment modality used in Stages I, II, and IIIA Hodgkin's disease, chemotherapy has found a place in the management of more disseminated disease, i.e., Stages IIIB and IV. Even patients with widespread disease at the time of diagnosis and patients who have shown evidence of cross-resistance to one chemotherapeutic protocol still have a chance for long-term survival.

Two major chemotherapeutic protocols are used in the management of Hodgkin's disease. All three protocols use combinations of antineoplastic drugs. The most common protocol used today is the MOPP regimen. It was first developed in the 1960s by DeVita and co-workers[28] at the National Cancer Institute. It includes the drugs nitrogen mustard (Mustargen), vincristine (Oncovin), procarbazine, and prednisone.

The complete remission rate with the MOPP regimen is 80 percent.[28] Some patients do not achieve a complete remission or become refractory to the MOPP protocol. For these patients, hope still exists with another protocol. The ABVD protocol has been found effective for those patients not attaining a complete

TABLE 11–6. Staging Procedures for Hodgkin's Disease

Clinical Staging (CS)

Adequate surgical biopsy reviewed by an experienced hemopathologist. In primary extranodal lymphomas, biopsy should also include a lymph node when palpable.
Detailed history with special attention to the presence or absence of systemic symptoms.
Careful physical examination, emphasizing node chains, size of liver and spleen, Waldeyer's ring inspection, and bony tenderness.
Routine laboratory tests: complete blood count, erythrosedimentation rate, liver function tests, serum uric acid, serum copper.
Chest roentgenogram (posteroanterior and lateral) with measurement of mass/thoracic ratio.
Bilateral lower extremity lymphogram.
Chest and abdominal computed CT scan or MRI.
Radioisotopic evaluation with gallium 67 when the results of other conventional diagnostic procedures are inconclusive.

Pathologic Staging (PS)

Core needle biopsy of bone marrow from posterior iliac crest. Biopsy should be bilateral, especially in the presence of CS III and in patients with systemic symptoms.
Needle or surgical biopsy of any suspicious extranodal (e.g., hepatic, splenic, osseous, pulmonary, cutaneous) lesion(s).
Cytologic examination of any effusion.
Staging laparotomy with splenectomy, needle and wedge biopsy of liver, and biopsies of para-aortic, mesenteric, portal, and splenic hilar lymph node remains indicated after negative bone marrow biopsy in initial stages (CS I to II) only if therapeutic decisions will depend on the identification of occult abdominal involvement.

From Bonadonna G, Wiernik PH, Santoro A: Clinical treatment of Hodgkin's disease, in Wiernik PH, Canellos GP, Kyle RA, Schiffer CA (eds): *Neoplastic Diseases of the Blood*, 2nd ed. New York, Churchill Livingstone, 1991. Reproduced with permission.

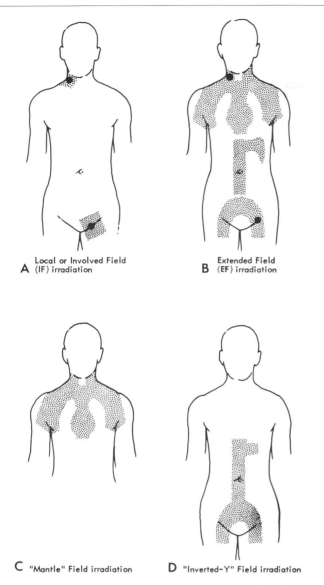

A Local or Involved Field (IF) irradiation

B Extended Field (EF) irradiation

C "Mantle" Field irradiation

D "Inverted-Y" Field irradiation

FIGURE 11–13. Radiation fields in the treatment of Hodgkin's disease. (From Haskell CM, Parker RG: Hodgkin's disease, in Haskell C (ed): *Cancer Treatment*, 2nd ed. Philadelphia, WB Saunders, 1985, pp 758–788. Reproduced with permission.)

remission or relapsing while on the MOPP protocol. The ABVD regimen includes Adriamycin (doxorubicin), bleomycin, vincristine, and DTIC (imidazole carboxamide or dacarbazine).[29] Additionally, radiation therapy and chemotherapy can be combined to give the patient the best chance for long-term sustained remission. Maintenance-phase chemotherapy has not been found useful.

Nutritional Management

The patient may have experienced a weight loss of greater than 10 percent of body weight prior to diagnosis. Serum protein studies may be indicated, and if total serum protein and albumin levels are found low,

a diet high in protein and carbohydrates is needed. Nutritional supplements may be administered.

Complications

Bone marrow suppression can lead to leukopenia, anemia, and thrombocytopenia. Thus, the patient is prone to infection, anemia, and major as well as minor bleeding episodes. Refer to the section on complications of leukemia for further discussion.

KEY CONCEPTS

- Hodgkin's disease is characterized by malignant transformation of lymph node cells called Reed-Sternberg cells. Spread of malignant cells occurs along predictable, contiguous pathways. Most commonly a single cervical lymph node is involved initially, with slow progression to nearby nodes.
- Manifestations of Hodgkin's disease include painless lymph node enlargement, fever, night sweats, and weight loss.
- Staging is done to determine the degree of dissemination. When affected lymph nodes are localized to one area (Stage I) or one side of the diaphragm (Stage II), the prognosis for cure is very good. Dissemination to lymph nodes above and below the diaphragm (Stage III) or to extralymphatic organs or tissues (Stage IV) carries a poorer prognosis, but cure is still possible.
- Radiation is the primary therapy for early-stage Hodgkin's disease. More disseminated disease may be treated with chemotherapeutic protocols (i.e., MOPP or ABVD regimens). Treatment may lead to bone marrow suppression and predispose to anemia, thrombocytopenia, and leukopenia.

Non-Hodgkin's Lymphoma

The malignancies included in the classification **non-Hodgkin's lymphoma** (NHL) are all of those malignant lymphomas that do not fit into the schema of Hodgkin's disease. The majority of non-Hodgkin's lymphomas arise from lymph nodes, but these lymphomas can originate in virtually any tissue or organ. With the exception of a few subtypes, most non-Hodgkin's lymphomas occur in older adults. Males are at slightly higher risk than females.

The classification of non-Hodgkin's lymphoma includes a wide variety of malignant lymphomas. These lymphomas differ histologically one from another. This group of disorders is subdivided into two main classes, lymphocyte malignancies and histiocyte malignancies (Fig. 11–14). The lymphocytic lymphomas include (1) malignant lymphoma, well-differentiated lymphocytic, (2) malignant lymphoma, poorly differentiated lymphocytic, (3) undifferentiated lymphoma, monomorphic, (4) undifferentiated lymphoma, pleomorphic, (5) histiocytic lymphoma (B lymphocytes),

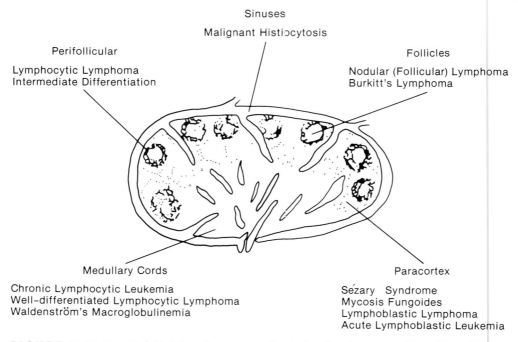

Sinuses
Malignant Histiocytosis

Perifollicular
Lymphocytic Lymphoma
Intermediate Differentiation

Follicles
Nodular (Follicular) Lymphoma
Burkitt's Lymphoma

Medullary Cords
Chronic Lymphocytic Leukemia
Well-differentiated Lymphocytic Lymphoma
Waldenström's Macroglobulinemia

Paracortex
Sézary Syndrome
Mycosis Fungoides
Lymphoblastic Lymphoma
Acute Lymphoblastic Leukemia

FIGURE 11–14. Non-Hodgkin's lymphomas according to functional anatomy. (From Mann RB, Jaffe ES, Bernard CW: Malignant lymphomas: A conceptual understanding of morphological diversity. *Am J Pathol* 1972;94:103–191. Reproduced with permission.)

and (6) mixed lymphoma (lymphocytic-histiocytic). The histiocytic type includes only one variety: histiocytic lymphoma. In this chapter, the non-Hodgkin's lymphomas will be considered collectively.

In non-Hodgkin's lymphoma, extranodal involvement, unpredictable metastasis, and wide dissemination of malignancy are present early in the disease process and usually are encountered at the time of diagnosis.

Etiology and Pathogenesis

The exact etiology is unknown, but factors such as viral infection, exposure to ionizing radiation, and exposure to toxic chemicals have been implicated. Theories of causality currently focus on virology and immune suppression.

Clinical Manifestations

The clinical manifestations of non-Hodgkin's lymphoma are similar to those of Hodgkin's disease. They include painless lymph node enlargement with or without fever, sweating, weight loss, malaise, and pruritus.

Differences between non-Hodgkin's lymphoma and Hodgkin's disease do exist, however, and clinical differences are summarized in Table 11–7. Hodgkin's disease is more easily treated to achieve complete remission. Extranodal involvement occurs early in the course of non-Hodgkin's lymphoma; it is frequently present on diagnosis. Manifestations of extranodal disease may include involvement of the skin, gastroin-

testinal tract, bone, and bone marrow. The systemic manifestations of non-Hodgkin's lymphoma are listed in Table 11–8.

Transformation to leukemia occurs in approximately 13 percent of lymphoma cases with high pe-

TABLE 11–7. Clinical Differences in Hodgkin's Disease and Non-Hodgkin's Lymphoma

Characteristic	Hodgkin's Disease	Non-Hodgkin's Lymphoma
Nodal disease	Contiguous spread	Noncontiguous
Extranodal disease	Uncommon	More common involvement of gastrointestinal tract, testes, bone marrow
Site of disease	Mediastinal involvement common in 50 percent of patients	Mediastinal involvement less common (20 percent)
	Bone marrow involvement uncommon	Bone marrow involvement common
	Liver involvement uncommon	Liver involvement common
Extent of disease	Often localized	Rarely localized (10 percent)
B symptoms	Common (40 percent)	Uncommon (20 percent)

From Carson C, Callaghan ME: Hematopoietic and immunologic cancers, in Baird SB, McCorkle R, Grant M (eds): *Cancer Nursing: A Comprehensive Textbook.* Philadelphia, WB Saunders, 1991, p 558. Originally adapted from DeVita VT Jr, Hellman S, Rosenberg SA (eds): *Cancer: Principles and Practice of Oncology,* 4th ed. Philadelphia, JB Lippincott, 1993, p 1883. Reproduced with permission.

TABLE 11-8. Systemic Alterations in Non-Hodgkin's Lymphoma

System	Manifestations
Lymphoid system	Lymphadenopathy—peripheral or central Hepatosplenomegaly Thymic (anterior superior mediastinal) mass Waldeyer's ring involvement Bone marrow involvement
Gastrointestinal system	Abdominal or pelvic mass Upper or lower gastrointestinal bleeding Malabsorption Intussusception Perforation Fistula Biliary obstruction Pancreatic mass Ascites Salivary gland swelling
Genitourinary system	Renal mass, ureteric obstruction Testicular mass Ovarian mass Vaginal bleeding
Nervous system	Meningeal involvement Cranial nerve palsies Intracranial mass (extradural or intra-cerebral) Paraspinal mass Intraorbital, periorbital, or ocular mass Peripheral neuropathy Progressive multifocal leukoencephalopathy
Endocrine system	Thyroid mass Adrenal mass
Other	Bone involvement Paranasal sinus involvement Jaw involvement Skin infiltration Venous or (rarely) arterial obstruction Pericardial effusion Pulmonary infiltration
General	Pyrexia/night sweats Weight loss Lethargy

From Magrath IT, Wilson W, Horvath K, et al: Clinical features and staging, in Magrath IT (ed): *The Non-Hodgkin's Lymphomas*. Baltimore, Williams & Wilkins, 1990. Reproduced with permission.

ripheral lymphocyte counts.[28] The staging of non-Hodgkin's lymphoma is identical to that used in Hodgkin's disease. Diagnostic procedures and the staging workup are similar to those used in Hodgkin's disease. As with all malignancies, diagnosis of cell type is based on histopathologic tissue sampling.

Treatment

The prognosis for the patient with non-Hodgkin's lymphoma is variable. Favorable outcomes are being realized with increasing frequency in localized disease (Stages I and II). For those patients experiencing disseminated disease (Stages III and IV), long-term periods free of disease are becoming more common. The future development of less toxic, more effective che-

motherapeutic treatment protocols holds great promise for these patients.

Pharmacologic Management

As with Hodgkin's disease, collaboration among the hematologist-oncologist, radiation oncologist, and surgical oncologist is needed to develop the best treatment plan for the individual patient. Therapeutic management is predicted by the clinical stage, histologic type, age of the patient, and bone marrow integrity at the time of diagnosis.

The primary purpose of surgery in the treatment of non-Hodgkin's lymphoma is in diagnosis and clinical staging of the disorder. Radiation therapy as the primary treatment modality is employed in localized disease (Stages I and II). In advanced, disseminated disease, radiation therapy is used in combination with adjuvant chemotherapy.

For advanced lymphoma (Stages III and IV), chemotherapy is prescribed. Multi-agent protocols give the best chance for long-term disease-free survival. Combinations of cyclophosphamide (Cytoxan), vincristine, prednisone, procarbazine, doxorubicin (Adriamycin), and bleomycin are used for disease control.[30] Single-agent treatment programs were used in the past; however, remissions with single-agent therapy were short-lived.

Nutritional Management

Nutritional management of the patient with non-Hodgkin's lymphoma is similar to that for the patient with Hodgkin's disease.

Complications
Oncologic Emergencies

Oncologic emergencies occur more frequently in non-Hodgkin's lymphoma than in Hodgkin's disease. Superior vena cava obstruction and spinal cord compression are two of the most common oncologic emergencies occurring with non-Hodgkin's lymphoma. Other complications include CNS involvement. Infections secondary to primary malignancies, bone involvement, and joint effusions are also complications.

KEY CONCEPTS

- Non-Hodgkin's lymphomas are a diverse group of malignant diseases of lymphoid tissue. The characteristic Reed-Sternberg cell is not present. Non-Hodgkin's lymphomas do not spread in a predictable manner and often are disseminated at diagnosis.
- The clinical manifestations are similar to those of Hodgkin's disease and include painless lymph node enlargement, fever, night sweats, and weight loss.

- The prognosis varies, depending on the stage of dissemination at diagnosis and the malignant characteristics of the involved cell type. Radiation therapy and chemotherapy are the usual therapies.

Multiple Myeloma

Multiple myeloma, also known as **plasma cell myeloma,** is a malignant disorder characterized by proliferation of abnormal plasma cells (mature B-cells) in the bone marrow (Figs. 11–15, 11–16, Color Plate II). Single or multiple tumors containing abnormal plasma cells are found throughout the marrow. Additionally, immunoglobulin synthesis is disturbed. Infiltration of abnormal plasma cells is not limited to the bone. Multiple myeloma disseminates throughout the body, ultimately involving the lymph nodes, liver, spleen, and kidneys.

Multiple myeloma occurs exclusively in the adult population, usually affecting individuals over 40 years of age. The peak incidence is in the sixth decade of life.[31] The male-female ratio is 2 : 1.[32]

Etiology and Pathogenesis

The exact etiology is unknown, but genetic predisposition, oncogenic viruses, inflammatory stimuli, and chronic antigenic stimulation are all theoretical possibilities.[33] Essentially, an excess number of abnormal plasma cells infiltrate the bone marrow and develop into tumors and ultimately destroy bone; they then invade lymph nodes, liver, spleen, and kidneys. These plasma cells produce an abnormal immunoglobulin which is often referred to as a myeloma protein (Bence Jones protein). Multiple myeloma occurs in middle-aged and elderly clients, and in males more often than females.

Clinical Manifestations

The onset of multiple myeloma is generally slow and insidious, and most affected individuals remain asymptomatic until the disease is somewhat advanced. The patient may experience a presymptomatic phase lasting from 5 to 20 years. During this time, the person's only complaint may be that of frequent episodes of infection, particularly pneumonia. Some patients without symptoms are diagnosed from the presence of Bence Jones proteinuria and an elevated total serum protein level.

The earliest and most frequent complaint is bone pain. Spontaneous pathologic fractures may also occur. Skeletal changes are caused by loss of calcium from bone tissue, resulting in hypercalcemia, and by invasion of the bone marrow by abnormal plasma cells. Anemia, fatigue, repeated infection and bleeding tendencies (such as purpura and epistaxis) represent dysfunction or impairment of function of the bone marrow. Anorexia, nausea, vomiting, and weight loss, as well as confusion, may also be presenting signs and symptoms.

Renal insufficiency is a complication experienced by approximately one half of these patients. Impairment of renal function is due to hypercalcemia, hyperviscosity of the blood caused by proteinemia, and hyperuricemia. Most commonly the renal tubule is affected, resulting in proteinuria. The Bence Jones protein, a light chain protein by-product of antibody breakdown, may be excreted in the urine.

The diagnosis is made using multiple testing procedures. A complete history and physical examination are performed. Complete blood cell counts with quantitative platelet determinations may demonstrate granulocytopenia, anemia, and thrombocytopenia. Serum studies show hypercalcemia, hyperuricemia, and proteinuria. Prothrombin times and partial thromboplastin times may be altered. The erythrocyte sedimentation rate is elevated. Quantitative immunoglobulin assays indicate monoclonal immunoglobulin abnormalities. Monoclonal immunoglobulin abnormalities or plasma cell dyscrasias indicate an expansion of a single clone of immunoglobulin-secreting cells and a resultant increase in serum levels of a single homogeneous immunoglobin or its fragments. Radiologic studies of the ribs, spine, skull, and pelvis show a characteristic "punched-out" or "honeycombed" appearance. Twenty-four-hour urinalysis may demonstrate the presence of Bence Jones protein. The diagnosis is confirmed by bone marrow biopsy. Normally, the plasma cell concentration in the bone marrow is approximately 5 percent.[34] In multiple myeloma, abnormal plasma cell proliferation may range between 30 percent and 95 percent.[35]

Treatment

Pharmacologic Management

Antineoplastic agents are used to induce and maintain a remission. The alkylating agents melphalan (Alkeran) and cyclophosphamide (Cytoxan) are most commonly used. Additionally, prednisone may be added to the patient's chemotherapeutic program. Remission induction rates currently approach 60 percent.[36] Survival after this protocol is approximately 2 to 5 years.

If these agents should fail, more aggressive therapy can be employed. More recently, a 4-day continuous infusion of vincristine sulfate and Adriamycin has been used in combination with oral dexamethasone for those patients in whom first-line therapy fails.[36]

Supportive pharmacologic management may be employed in an attempt to enhance renal function and promote an optimum level of comfort for these patients. Diuretics, particularly furosemide (Lasix), may be ordered to prevent complications, such as congestive heart failure secondary to impaired renal function. Additionally, Lasix enhances the excretion of calcium ions and therefore is useful in controlling or reducing hypercalcemia. Oral phosphate drugs can also assist in promoting calcium ion excretion by binding with free calcium ions and aiding excretion via the kidneys. However, oral phosphate agents must be used with caution in patients already having renal impairment. Allopurinol (Zyloprim) reduces the uric acid formation caused by rapid cell destruction by inhibiting xanthine oxidase formation. This agent, which is also used in leukemias for the same reason, is important in preventing uric acid nephropathy caused by the hyperuricemia. Narcotic analgesics used in conjunction with muscle relaxants are used to control the pain associated with malignant invasion of the bone marrow by plasma cells.

Nutritional Management

Patients with multiple myeloma can experience severe anorexia, weight loss, nausea, vomiting, diarrhea, or constipation related to the disease process itself, the effects of chemotherapy and radiation therapy, or as complications of immobility, an increased need for fluids, and the increased use of pain medications. A diet high in proteins, vitamins, minerals, and carbohydrates should be offered. Small, frequent (six) meals a day may be more easily managed and tolerated by the patient. Pretreatment with antiemetics may be indicated.

Complications

Dehydration

Dehydration can become a life-threatening complication by causing renal shutdown. Acute renal failure can be precipitated by the accompanying hyperuricemia, proteinemia, hypercalcemia, and increased viscosity of the blood. Patients with multiple myeloma have a fluid need requirement above that of maintenance. Fluid requirements should be encouraged to 1½ to 2 times normal (approximately 4–5 L/day). These patients should never suffer a sustained period of no fluid intake. If an NPO status must be assumed by the patient for diagnostic procedures, an intravenous route with an appropriate rate of flow is warranted. In this case, renal disease is easier to prevent than treat. If renal shutdown does occur, hemodialysis may need to be instituted.

KEY CONCEPTS

- **Multiple myeloma is due to malignant transformation of antibody-secreting B-lymphocytes (plasma cells). It primarily affects adults over 40 years of age. Malignant plasma cells infiltrate bone marrow, lymph nodes, liver, spleen, and kidney.**
- **The onset of clinical symptoms is insidious. Bone pain, pathologic bone fractures, anemia, thrombocytopenia, leukopenia, and renal insufficiency may occur.**
- **Malignant cells represent a single clone of transformed B-cells that all secrete the same (monoclonal) antibody. Detection of excessive monoclonal**

- **antibody and characteristic monoclonal antibody degradation products (Bence Jones proteins) in the urine aids in diagnosis.**
- **Infiltration and breakdown of bones result in spinal compression, fractures, and hypercalcemia. Large amounts of Bence Jones protein may impair renal tubular function, leading to renal failure. Diuretics and high fluid intake may reduce the risk of renal impairment. Chemotherapy is the mainstay of treatment.**

Summary

Multiple myeloma is basically a multifocal **plasma cell cancer** of the osseous system that in the course of its dissemination may involve many extraosseous sites. Most patients are symptomatic when diagnosed. Clinical manifestations stem from the effects of (1) infiltration of organs, particularly the bones, by tumorous masses of plasma cells and (2) the abnormal immunoglobulins secreted by the tumor cells.

In 99 percent of patients with multiple myeloma, electrophoretic analysis will disclose increased levels of one of the immunoglobulin classes in the blood or light chains in the urine (Bence Jones protein). Identification of these proteins in the blood and urine is one of the most important diagnostic features of the disease.

By comparison, the **leukemias** are malignant neoplasms of **hematopoietic stem cells** that are characterized by diffuse replacement of the bone marrow by neoplastic cells. In most cases the leukemic cells spill over into the blood, where they may be seen in large numbers. These cells may also infiltrate the liver, spleen, lymph nodes, and other tissues throughout the body. Although the presence of excessive numbers of abnormal cells in the peripheral blood is the most dramatic manifestation of leukemia, note that the leukemias are primary disorders of the *bone marrow*.

Malignant lymphomas, on the other hand, are characterized by the proliferation of cells native to the **lymphoid tissues,** i.e., lymphocytes, histiocytes, and their precursors and derivatives. Within the broad group of malignant lymphomas, **Hodgkin's disease** is segregated from all other forms, which constitute the non-Hodgkin's lymphomas. Although both have their origin in the lymphoid tissues, Hodgkin's disease is set apart by the presence of a distinctive unifying morphologic feature, the Reed-Sternberg giant cell.

For all persons suffering from these lymphoproliferative disorders, the *diagnostic period* may be especially long. Consequently, patients must be provided with explanations of the need for multiple examinations. Emotional support during this period is especially important.

Nursing's role in the management of patients with neoplastic disorders of the blood and blood-forming tissues includes education of the patient and family regarding the disease process and the medical treatments prescribed. Patients and family members need education with continued reinforcement of material, owing both to their lack of medical knowledge and to the emotional impact of the diagnosis, which makes learning difficult, especially in the early stages of diagnosis.

REFERENCES

1. Bennett JM, Catovsky D, Daniel MT, et al: Proposals for the classification of the acute leukemias. *Br J Haematol* 1976; 33:451–458.
2. Henderson ES, Han T: Current therapy of acute and chronic leukemia in adults. *CA* 1986;36:322–350.
3. Foon KA, Gale RP: Chronic lymphocytic leukemia, in Gale RP (ed): *Leukemia Therapy.* Boston, Blackwell Scientific Publications, 1986, p 165.
4. Zigelboim J, Foon K, Gale R: Acute myelogenous leukemia, in Haskell C (ed): *Cancer Treatment,* 2nd ed. Philadelphia, WB Saunders, 1985, pp 694–706.
5. Gale RP, Foon KA: Therapy of acute myelogenous leukemia. *Semin Hematol* 1987;24:40–54.
6. Lichtman MA: Chronic myelogenous leukemia and related disorders, in Williams WJ, Beutler E, Erslev AJ, Lichtman MA (eds): *Hematology,* 4th ed. New York, McGraw-Hill, 1990, pp 202–212.
7. Champlin RE: Chronic myelogenous leukemia in leukemia therapy, in Gale RP (ed): *Leukemia Therapy.* Boston, Blackwell Scientific Publications, 1986, p 148.
8. Cunningham I, Gee T, Dowling M, et al: Results of treatment of Ph1 + chronic myelogenous leukemia with an intensive treatment regimen (L-5 protocol). *Blood* 1979;53:375–393.
9. Berenson J, Zigelboim J, Gale R: Acute lymphoblastic leukemia, in Haskell C (ed): *Cancer Treatment,* 2nd ed. Philadelphia, WB Saunders, 1985, pp 706–721.
10. Bakemeier RF, Zagers G, Cooper FA, Rubin P: The malignant lymphomas: Hodgkin's disease and non-Hodgkin's lymphoma, multiple myeloma, and macroglobulinemia, in Bakemeier RF (ed): *Clinical Oncology for Medical Students and Physicians.* Rochester, NY, American Cancer Society, 1983, pp 346–369.
11. Jacobs AD, Gale RP: Acute lymphoblastic leukemia in adults, in Gale RP (ed): *Leukemia Therapy.* Boston, Blackwell Scientific Publications, 1986, pp 71–98.
12. Blayney DW, Jaffe ES, Blatner WA, et al: The human T-cell leukemia/lymphoma virus associated with American adult T-cell leukemia/lymphoma. *Blood* 1983;62(2):401–405.
13. Bloomfield CD, Rowley JD, Goldman AI, Lawler SD, Walker LM, Mitelman F: For the Third International Workshop on chromosomal abnormalities and their clinical significance in acute lymphoblastic leukemia. *Cancer Res* 1983;43:868–873.
14. Henderson ES: Acute leukemia: General considerations, in Williams WJ, Beutler E, Erslev AJ, Lichtman MA (eds): *Hematology,* 4th ed. New York, McGraw-Hill, 1990, pp 236–251.
15. Champlin RE, Gale RP: Bone marrow transplantation for acute leukemia: Recent advances and comparison with alternative therapies. *Semin Hematol* 1987;24:55–67.
16. Hoelzer D, Gale RO: Acute lymphoblastic leukemia in adults: Recent progress, future progress, future direction. *Semin Hematol* 1987;24:27–34.
17. Keating MJ, Kantarjian H, Talpaz M, et al: Fludarabine: A new agent with major activity against chronic lymphocytic leukemia. *Blood* 1989;74:19–25.
18. Advani R, Chao NJ, Horning SJ, et al: GM-CSF as adjunct to autologous hemopoietic stem transplantation for lymphoma. *Ann Intern Med* 1992;116(3):183–189.
19. DeVita VT Jr, Hellman S, Rosenberg SA: *Cancer: Principles and Practice of Oncology,* 2nd ed. Philadelphia, JB Lippincott, 1985.
20. American Cancer Society: *Cancer Facts and Figures—1993.* Atlanta, American Cancer Society, 1993, pp 7–26.
21. Kaplan HS: Hodgkin's disease: Biology, treatment, prognosis. *Blood* 1981;57:813–822.
22. Rosenberg SA: Hodgkin's disease: No stage beyond cure. *Hosp Pract* 1986;21(8):91–98, 101–108.
23. Carson C, Callaghan ME: Hematopoietic and immunologic cancers, in Baird SB, McCorkle R, Grant M (eds): *Cancer Nursing: A Comprehensive Textbook.* Philadelphia, WB Saunders, 1991, p 552.
24. Haskell CM, Parker RG: Hodgkin's disease, in Haskell C (ed): *Cancer Treatment,* 2nd ed. Philadelphia, WB Saunders, 1985, pp 758–788.
25. Lacher MJ: Hodgkin's disease: Historical perspective, current status and future directions. *CA* 1985;35:88–94.
26. Rapaport SI: *Introduction to Hematology.* Philadelphia, JB Lippincott, 1987.
27. Skarin AT: *Dana Farber Cancer Institute Atlas of Diagnostic Oncology.* Philadelphia, JB Lippincott, 1991.
28. DeVita VT Jr, Hubbard S, Young R, Longo D: The role of chemotherapy in diffuse aggressive lymphoma. *Semin Hematol* 1988;25:2–10.
29. Bentino JR: Clinical pharmacology and toxicity of antineoplastic drugs, in Williams WJ, Beutler E, Erslev AJ, Lichtman MA (eds): *Hematology,* 4th ed. New York, McGraw-Hill, 1990, pp 279–288.
30. Connors JM, Fisher RI, Armitage JO: Decision making in the treatment of malignant lymphoma. American Society of Hematology educational session, Atlanta, American Society of Hematology, December 1989.
31. Anderson MG: The lymphomas and multiple myeloma, in Baird SB, Donhower MG, Stalsbrohen VL, Ades PB (eds): *A Cancer Source Book for Nurses,* 6th ed. Atlanta, American Cancer Society, 1991, pp 286–295.
32. Sheridan C: Multiple myeloma, in Groenwald SL, Frogge MH, Goodman M, Yarbo CH (eds): *Cancer Nursing: Principles and Practice,* 2nd ed. Boston, Jones and Bartlett, 1990, pp 991–998.
33. Bubley GJ, Schnipper LE: Multiple myeloma, in Holleb AI (ed): *American Cancer Society Textbook of Clinical Oncology.* Atlanta, American Cancer Society, 1991, pp 397–409.
34. Cherng NC, Asal NR, Kuebler JP, et al: Prognostic factors in multiple myeloma. *Cancer* 1991;67(12):3150–3156.
35. Duffy TP: The many pitfalls of diagnosis of myeloma. *N Engl J Med* 1992;326(6):394–396.
36. Boccadoro M, Marmont F, Tribalto M, et al: Multiple myeloma: VMCP/VBAP alternating combination chemotherapy is not superior to melphalan and prednisone even in high-risk patients. *J Clin Oncol* 1991;9(3):444–448.

BIBLIOGRAPHY

Aisenberg AC: A historical overview of malignant lymphomas, in Wiernik PH, Canellos GP, Kyle RA, Schiffer CA (eds): *Neoplastic Diseases of the Blood,* 2nd ed. New York, Churchill Livingstone, 1991, pp 597–607.

Alexanian RJ, Barlogie B, Dixon D: Renal failure in multiple myeloma: Pathogenesis and prognostic implications. *Arch Intern Med* 1990;150(8):1693–1695.

Appelbaum JW: The role of the oncogene in the pathogenesis of cancer. *Semin Oncol Nurs* 1992;8:51–62.

Bonadonna G, Wiernik PH, Santoro A: Clinical treatment of Hodgkin's disease, in Wiernik PH, Canellos GP, Kyle RA, Schiffer CA (eds): *Neoplastic Diseases of the Blood,* 2nd ed. New York, Churchill Livingstone, 1991, pp 701–727.

Boring CC, Squires TS, Tong T: Cancer statistics. *CA* 1993;43:7–26.

Canellos GP: Can MOPP be replaced in the treatment of advanced Hodgkin's disease? *Semin Oncol* 1990;17(2 suppl):2–6.

Cheson BD: New modalities of therapy in chronic lymphocytic leukemia. *Crit Rev Oncol Hematol* 1991;11:167–177.

Eyre HJ, Farver ML: Hodgkin's disease and non-Hodgkin's lymphoma, in Holleb AI, Fink DJ, Murphy GP (eds): *Textbook of Clinical Oncology.* Atlanta, American Cancer Society, 1991, pp 377–396.

Gail, MH, Pluda JM, Rabkin CS, et al: Projections of the incidence of non-Hodgkin's lymphoma related to acquired immunodeficiency syndrome. *JNCI* 1991;83:695–701.

Gaynor ER, Fisher RI: Diffuse aggressive lymphomas in adults, in Magrath IT (ed): *The Non-Hodgkin's Lymphomas.* Baltimore, Williams & Wilkins, 1990, pp 317–329.

Gianni AM, Bregni M, Siena S, et al: Recombinant human granulocyte-macrophage colony-stimulating factor reduces hematologic toxicity and widens clinical applicability of high-dose cyclophosphamide treatment in breast cancer and non-Hodgkin's lymphoma. *J Clin Oncol* 1990;8:368–378.

Haluska FG, Tsujimoto Y, Croce CM: The molecular genetics of non-Hodgkin's lymphomas, in Magrath IT (ed): *The Non-Hodgkin's Lymphomas.* Baltimore, Williams & Wilkins, 1990, pp 96–108.

Hardy R, Horning SJ: Molecular studies in the clinical evaluation of non-Hodgkin's lymphoma. *Hematol Oncol Clin North Am* 1991;5:891–900.

Jacobson DR, Zolla-Pazner S: Immunosuppression and infection in multiple myeloma, in Wiernik PH (ed): *Neoplastic Diseases of the Blood.* New York, Churchill Livingstone, 1991, pp 415–426.

Keegan P, Ozer H: Immunology of the lymphomas, in Wiernik PH, Canellos GP, Kyle RA, Schiffer CA (eds): *Neoplastic Diseases of the Blood,* 2nd ed. New York, Churchill Livingstone, 1991, pp 663–688.

Lester EP, Ultmann JE: Lymphoma, in Williams WJ, Beutler E, Ersley AJ, Lichtman MA (eds): *Hematology,* 4th ed. New York, McGraw-Hill, 1990, pp 1067–1087.

Levine EG, Bloomfield CD: Leukemias and myelodysplastic syndromes secondary to drug, radiation, and environmental exposure. *Semin Oncol* 1992;19:47–84.

Magrath IT: Lymphocyte ontogeny: A conceptual basis for understanding neoplasia of the immune system, in Magrath IT (ed): *The Non-Hodgkin's Lymphomas.* Baltimore, Williams & Wilkins, 1990, pp 29–48.

Magrath IT: The non-Hodgkin's lymphomas: An introduction, in Magrath IT (ed): *The Non-Hodgkin's Lymphomas.* Baltimore, Williams & Wilkins, 1990, pp 1–14.

Magrath IT, Wilson W, Horvath K, et al: Clinical features and staging, in Magrath IT (ed): *The Non-Hodgkin's Lymphomas.* Baltimore, Williams & Wilkins, 1990, pp 180–199.

McNally JC, Stair J: Potential for infection, in McNally JC, Somerville ET, Miaskowski C, Rostad M (eds): *Guidelines for Oncology Nursing Practice.* Philadelphia, WB Saunders, 1991, pp 191–202.

Medeiros LJ, Jaffe ES: Pathology of malignant lymphomas, in Wiernik PH, Canellos GP, Kyle RA, Schimpff CA (eds): *Neoplastic Diseases of the Blood,* 2nd ed. New York, Churchill Livingstone, 1991, pp 631–661.

Ohno R, Tomonoage M, Kobayaski T, et al: Effect of granulocyte colony stimulating factor after intensive induction therapy in relapsed or refractory acute leukemia. *N Engl J Med* 1990; 323:871–877.

Oniboni AC: Infection in the neutropenic patient. *Semin Oncol Nurs* 1990;6:50–60.

Parker BA, Green MR: Hodgkin's disease, in Moosa AR, Schimpff SC, Robson MC (eds): *Comprehensive Textbook of Oncology,* 2nd ed. Baltimore, Williams & Wilkins, 1991, vol 2, pp 1257–1267.

Parker JW, Lukes RJ: Neoplasms of the immune system, in Stites DP, Terr AI (eds): *Basic and Clinical Immunology,* 7th ed. Norwalk, Conn, Appleton & Lange, 1991, pp 599–631.

Purtilo DR, Stevenson M: Lymphotropic viruses as etiologic agents of lymphoma. *Hematol Oncol Clin North Am* 1991;5:901–923.

Rahr VA, Tucker R: Non-Hodgkin's lymphoma: Understanding the disease. *Cancer Nurs* 1990;13:56–91.

Riedel DA: Epidemiology of multiple myeloma, in Wiernik PH (ed): *Neoplastic Diseases of the Blood.* New York, Churchill Livingstone, 1991, pp 347–372.

Rostad M: Potential for injury related to anemia, in McNally JC, Somerville ET, Miaskowski C, Rostad M (eds): *Guidance for Oncology Nursing Practice.* Philadelphia, WB Saunders, 1991, pp 208–215.

Sandlund J, Magrath IT: Lymphoblastic lymphomas, in Magrath IT (ed): *The Non-Hodgkin's Lymphomas.* Baltimore, Williams & Wilkins, 1990, pp 240–255.

Stevenson MA, Stanton SC, Cossman J: Involvement of the bell-2 gene in Hodgkin's disease. *JNCI* 1990;82:855–858.

Urba WJ, Longo DK: Burkitt's lymphoma, in Moosa AR, Schimpff SC, Robson MC (eds): *Comprehensive Textbook of Oncology,* 2nd ed. Baltimore, Williams & Wilkins, 1991, vol 2, pp 1296–1301.

Urba WJ, Longo DL: Lymphocytic lymphomas: Clinical course and management, in Moosa AR, Schimpff SC, Robson MC (eds): *Comprehensive Textbook of Oncology,* 2nd ed. Baltimore, Williams & Wilkins, 1991, vol 2, pp 1277–1295.

Urba WJ, Longo DL: Lymphocytic lymphomas: Epidemiology, etiology, pathology, and staging, in Moosa AR, Schimpff SC, Robson MC (eds): *Comprehensive Textbook of Oncology,* 2nd ed. Baltimore, Williams & Wilkins, 1991, vol 2, pp 1268–1276.

Vose JM, Bierman PJ, Armitage JO: Non-Hodgkin's lymphoma, in Wiernik PH, Canellos GP, Kyle RA, Schiffer CA (eds): *Neoplastic Diseases of the Blood,* 2nd ed. New York, Churchill Livingstone, 1991, pp 739–751.

Wright DH: Pathogenesis of non-Hodgkin's lymphoma: Clues from geography, in Magrath IT (ed): *The Non-Hodgkin's Lymphomas.* Baltimore, Williams & Wilkins, 1990, pp 122–134.

Yarbro CH: Lymphomas, in Groenwald SL, Frogge MH, Goodman M, Yarbro CH (eds): *Cancer Nursing: Principles and Practice,* 2nd ed. Boston, Jones and Bartlett, 1990, pp 974–989.

UNIT IV

Alterations in Oxygen Transport, Blood Coagulation, Blood Flow, and Blood Pressure

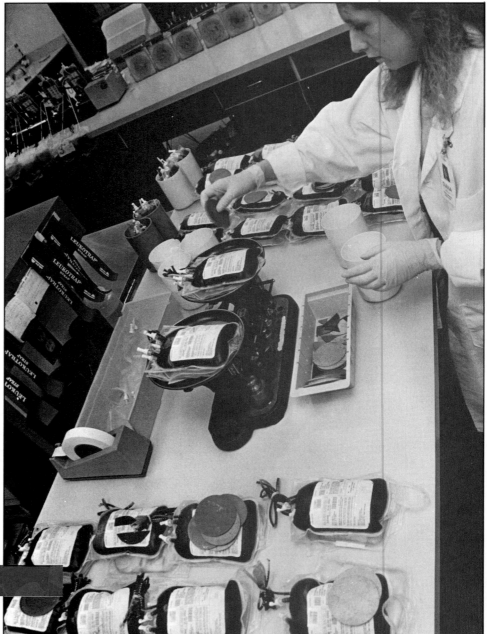

Packed red cells are weighed at a blood bank.

Photo by Kathleen Kelly

*V*oluntary blood donors are among the heroines and heroes of our time. They provide the precious fluid that allows the survival of accident victims and surgical patients. But there are times when voluntarism is not enough. When blood replacement supplies run low, an additional concern is added to the multitude of worries that attend therapy and healing, reviving one of the dreams of medicine, which is to find ways to bypass the donor. Gene therapy may eventually produce the means for the therapeutic production of blood cells.

Donors donate, but the producers of blood cells are hormones—specifically, hematopoietic hormones, or hemopoietins. They provide the variety of blood cell types the body requires.

All of the many types of blood cells develop from a single type that originates in the blood marrow, stem cells, which have been called the most primitive cells known to exist in the body. The stem cells reside in the bone marrow—in adults, principally the marrow of membranous bones. The supply of red blood cells (RBCs) issuing from the marrow is regulated by a feedback cycle that ensures an adequate supply of cells for tissue oxygenation. When oxygen carried to the tissues decreases, the bone marrow immediately begins to produce more RBCs, as it does in response to various forms of anemia. White blood cells, or leukocytes, indispensable to the immune system's ability to resist disease, are formed in the bone marrow and in lymph tissue.

By influencing the development of stem cells, hemopoietins promote the production of particular kinds of blood cells and prepare them for their work in the body. Several years ago the genes for some of these hormones were cloned, which meant that quantities of them could be made. This opened up the possibility for the production of specific blood cells for use in therapy, perhaps eventually obviating transfusion.

Because the blood is contained in a dynamic system, and because that system is influenced by the ordinary details of daily life—what we eat and how much, whether we exercise, the state of our emotions—healthy blood flow also is a frontier of research.

Nowhere is the frontier more evident than in our increasing understanding of the serious health consequences of high blood pressure and the simple daily choices that can prevent illness.

The human body is a container of carefully balanced pressures. The flow of blood is monitored by the body. When pressures exceed the limits tolerated by monitoring systems, intervention sometimes is required. Blood flow to each tissue is monitored by microvessels, which measure what each tissue needs, thus controlling local blood flow. Nervous control of circulation also helps control tissue blood flow.

The heart pays attention to the demands of the tissues, responding to the return of blood through the veins and to nerve signals that make it pump the required amounts of blood. The arterial pressure itself is carefully regulated; if it falls below its normal mean level, immediate circulatory changes—increased heart pumping, contraction of venous reservoirs, constriction of arterioles—provide more blood for the arteriolar tree. Kidneys play their part by secreting pressure-controlling hormones and by regulating blood volume.

Hypertension, or high blood pressure, is a concern to medical professionals because it influences a number of disorders, including strokes, coronary artery disease, and renal disease. Current estimates indicate that about 50 mil-

FRONTIERS OF RESEARCH
Blood and Circulatory Disturbances
Michael J. Kirkhorn

lion Americans, a little less than 20 percent of the population, suffer from high blood pressure.

Findings from the Treatment of Mild Hypertension Study reported in 1993 have contributed to understanding of the effects of life-style modifications, including weight reduction, restriction of sodium consumption, aerobic exercise, and reduction of alcohol drinking, in subjects with only marginally high blood pressure.

An article in the *Journal of the American Medical Association* suggested that the results of this long-term study—a significant reduction of blood pressure and no additional treatment required for 59 percent of the volunteer subjects—indicate that "life-style modification be used as definitive or adjunctive therapy in all hypertensive patients." Citing another current study by the Veterans Administration Cooperative Study Group on Antihypertensive Agents, the *JAMA* article points out that the life-style study showed results equaling those achieved with diltiazem hydrochloride, which the VA study showed was the drug most successful in lowering diastolic blood pressure.

The emphasis on life-style—our daily habits, guided or unguided by prudence—is substantiated in other recent findings. A report on the Framingham Study, in which a group of men and women with no initial signs of hypertension were followed for 18 to 20 years to determine whether anxiety and anger influenced the onset of hypertension, showed that "feelings of anxiety or tension may increase the risk of hypertension among middle-aged men." In this study, no relationship between anxiety and hypertension was found in middle-aged women. The researchers recommended consideration of "behavioral treatment for hypertension . . . as part of a nonpharmacologic treatment program among anxious middle-aged men with mild to moderate hypertension" and as an adjunct to treatment with antihypertensive drugs.

CHAPTER 12
Alterations in Oxygen Transport

MARIE KOTTER and SUSAN OSGUTHORPE

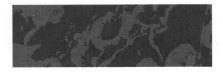

KEY TERMS

anemia: A deficiency of red blood cells.

erythroblastosis: Presence of erythroblasts in the blood due to failure of their maturation in the bone marrow.

erythromelalgia: Painful erythema (redness of the skin) of the palms and soles due to congestion of the capillaries.

erythropoiesis: Process producing red blood cells.

hematopoiesis: Process of development from pluripotential stem cells to mature, differentiated red cells, neutrophils, eosinophils, basophils, monocytes, and platelets.

hemoglobin: Oxygen-carrying protein in the red blood cells.

hemolysis: Separation of hemoglobin from red blood cells and its appearance in the fluid in which the corpuscles are suspended.

hyperplasia: Abnormal multiplication or increase in the number of normal cells in normal arrangement in a tissue.

megaloblastic dysplasia: Abnormal development of large red cells and non-lymphocytic bone marrow cells.

megaloblasts: Large abnormal hemopoietic bone marrow cells.

pancytopenia: Decreased production of red cells, white cells, and platelets.

panmyelosis: Overproduction of normal red cells, white cells, and platelets.

platelets: Circulating cytoplasmic fragments of megakaryocytes that are essential in the formation of blood clots and in the control of bleeding.

polycythemia: An excess of circulating red blood cells.

red blood cells or erythrocytes: Cells responsible for transporting oxygen to the tissues, removing carbon dioxide from the tissues, and buffering blood pH.

relative anemia: "Anemia" characterized by normal total red cell mass with disturbances in the regulation of plasma volume.

relative polycythemia: "Polycythemia" characterized by normal total red cell mass with disturbances in the regulation of plasma volume.

reticulocytosis: Increase in the number of circulating reticulocytes.

spherocyte: An abnormal, biconvex, spherical erythrocyte that is less biconvex than a normal erythrocyte.

thrombocytopenia: A decrease in circulating blood platelets.

---

*B*lood is a critical body fluid composed of formed elements and cells suspended in plasma, circulating through the cardiovascular system. As the transport system of the body, it is involved in the physiologic and pathologic activities of all organs. The **red blood cell** (RBC), or **erythrocyte,** is essential to oxygen transport within the circulatory system. Red cells bind to hemoglobin molecules, which are designed to move oxygen efficiently from the lungs to other body tissues. Hemoglobin also aids in acid-base balance. Additionally, RBCs interact with water to carry carbon dioxide away from the cells and back to the lungs for expiration.

Composition of Blood

The total blood volume averages 75.5 mL/kg in men and 66.5 mL/kg in women, which is 5 to 6 liters or 7 percent to 8 percent of body weight. The blood cells make up 45 percent and blood plasma 55 percent of the blood volume. Blood plasma is composed of about 92 percent water and 7 percent plasma proteins (Fig. 12–1). The arterial pH of normal blood is 7.35 to 7.45.[1]

Organic and Inorganic Components

The plasma proteins are formed mainly in the liver. They are nondiffusible and important in regulating blood volume and the body's fluid balance. Plasma proteins contribute to blood viscosity, which is important in maintaining blood pressure. There are three general types of plasma proteins. The first is serum albumin, which is an important factor in maintaining blood volume and pressure. The second type of plasma protein is serum globulin, which is composed of three general fractions. The alpha fraction is associated with the transport of bilirubin, lipids, and steroids; the beta fraction is associated with the transport of iron and copper in plasma; and the gamma fraction contains the antibody molecules. Fibrinogen is the third type of plasma protein. It is the precursor of fibrin, which forms the framework of blood clots. Regulatory proteins such as hormones and enzymes are also present in the plasma. Diffusible anabolic substances such as sodium chloride, calcium, potassium, carbonic acid, iodine, and iron are used by body cells and make up 0.9 percent of plasma. Also included in this category are nutritive organic materials such as amino acids, glucose, fats, and cholesterol, which are foodstuffs in solution absorbed from the gastrointestinal (GI) tract. They are transported to other body tissues for utilization and storage. Diffusible catabolic constituents such as urea, uric acid, xanthine, creatine, creatinine, and ammonia are products of tissue activity that are transported from the tissues to the kidneys and skin for excretion (Table 12–1).[1]

Cellular Components

Erythrocytes

Of the cellular elements of blood (Fig. 12–2), **red cells** or **erythrocytes** are the most numerous, with normal concentrations ranging from 4.2 to 6.2 million cells/mm^3. Red cells are responsible for transporting oxygen to the tissues, removing carbon dioxide from the tissues, and buffering blood pH. Erythrocytes have no cytoplasmic organelles, nucleus, mitochondria, or ribosomes. They live for 80 to 120 days in the circula-

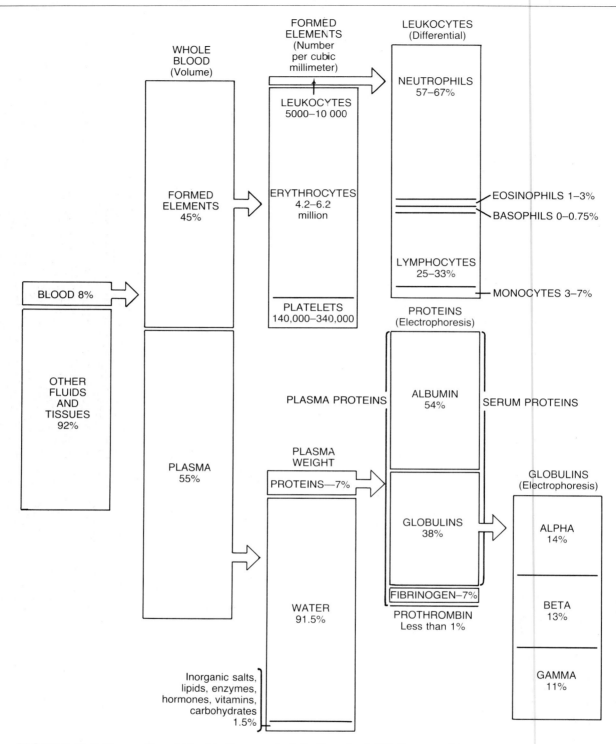

F I G U R E 12–1. Composition of blood in the normal adult. (From Jacob SW, Francone CA: *Elements of Anatomy and Physiology*, 2nd ed. Philadelphia, WB Saunders, 1989, p 164.)

TABLE 12–1. Organic and Inorganic Components of Blood

Constituent	Amount/Concentration	Major Functions
Water	92 percent of plasma weight	Medium for carrying all other constituents
Electrolytes	Total <1 percent of plasma weight	Keep H_2O in extracellular compartment; act as buffers; function in membrane excitability
NA^+	136–145 mEq/L (142 mM)	
K^+	3.5–5 mEq/L (4 mM)	
Ca^{++}	4.5–5.5 mEq/L (2.5 mM)	
Mg^{++}	1.5–2.5 mEq/L (1.5 mM)	
CL^-	100–106 mEq/L (103 mM)	
HCO_3^-	27 mEq/L (27 mM)	
Phosphate (mostly HPO_4^{2-})	3–4.5 mEq/L (1 mM)	
SO_4^{2-}	.5–1.5 mEq/L (0.5 mM)	
Proteins	6–8 g/dL (2.5 mM)	Provide colloid osmotic pressure of plasma; act as buffers; bind other plasma constituents (lipids, hormones, vitamins, metals, etc); clotting factors; enzymes; enzyme precursors; antibodies (immune globulins); hormones
Albumins	3.5–5.5 g/dL	
Globulins	1.5–.3 g/dL	
Fibrinogen	.2–.4 g/dL	
Gases—arterial plasma		By-product of oxygenation; most CO_2 content is from HCO_3 and acts as a buffer
CO_2 content	22–20 mmol/L plasma	
		Oxygenation
O_2	Pao_2 80 mm Hg or greater (arterial); $P\bar{v}o_2$ 30–40 mm Hg (venous)	
		By-product of protein catabolism
N_2	0.9 mL/dL	
		Provide nutrition and substances for tissue repair
Nutrients		
Glucose and other carbohydrates	70–105 mg/dL (5.6 mM)	
Total amino acids	40 mg/dL (2 mM)	
Total lipids	450 mg/dL (7.5 mM)	
Cholesterol	150–250 mg/dL (4–7 mM)	
Individual vitamins	0.0001–2.5 mg/dL	
Individual trace elements	0.001–0.3 mg/dL	
Waste products		
Urea (BUN)	10–20 mg/dL (5.7 mM)	End product of protein catabolism
Creatinine	.7–1.5 mg/dL (0.09 mM)	End product from energy metabolism
Uric acid	2.5–8 mg/dL (0.3 mM)	End product of protein metabolism
Bilirubin	.3–1.1 mg/dL (0.003–0.018 mM)	End product of red blood cell destruction
Individual hormones	0.000001–0.05 mg/dL	Functions specific to target tissue

Adapted with permission from Vander AJ, Sherman JH, Luciano DS: *Human Physiology: The Mechanisms of Body Functions,* 5th ed. New York, McGraw-Hill, 1990.

tion, die, and are replaced. Hemoglobin is the main functional constituent of the red cell. It is a protein that enables the blood to transport 100 times more oxygen than could be transported in plasma alone. An intraerythrocytic enzyme, carbonic anhydrase, is responsible for the buffering mechanism of red cells.[1]

The erythrocyte's size and shape also contribute to its function as a gas carrier (Fig. 12–3). It is a small, biconcave disk about 7.2 μ in diameter that must circulate through splenic sinusoids and capillaries, which are only 2 μ in diameter. This remarkable feat is accomplished through a property called reversible deformability, which allows the RBC to assume a torpedo-like conformation and then return to a biconcave disk shape.[2]

Leukocytes

Leukocytes, or **white blood cells,** protect the body from disease by phagocytosis of microorganisms and other debris and participate in immune antibody formation. Leukocytes act primarily in the tissues but are also transported in the circulatory and lymphatic systems. The average adult has approximately 5,000–10,000 leukocytes/mm³ of blood. Leukocytes are further divided into categories according to structure and function.[1]

Granulocytes are motile cells 8 μ to 12 μ in diameter with polymorphic nuclei and cytoplasmic granules. These granules contain digestive enzymes and biochemical mediators that kill or break down microorganisms and other phagocytic debris. Granulocytes use ameboid movement to migrate through vessel walls to tissue in response to chemotactic factors.[1]

Granulocytes are divided into three categories. **Neutrophilic granulocytes,** which compose 57 percent to 67 percent of leukocytes, contain small lysosomal granules and a segmented nucleus with two to five lobes. Immature neutrophils, which lack a segmented nucleus, are called bands. Neutrophils are the chief phagocytes in the early phase of inflammation. They ingest and destroy microorganisms and debris and then die. Upon death and lysis of these cells, digestive enzymes are released that dissolve debris

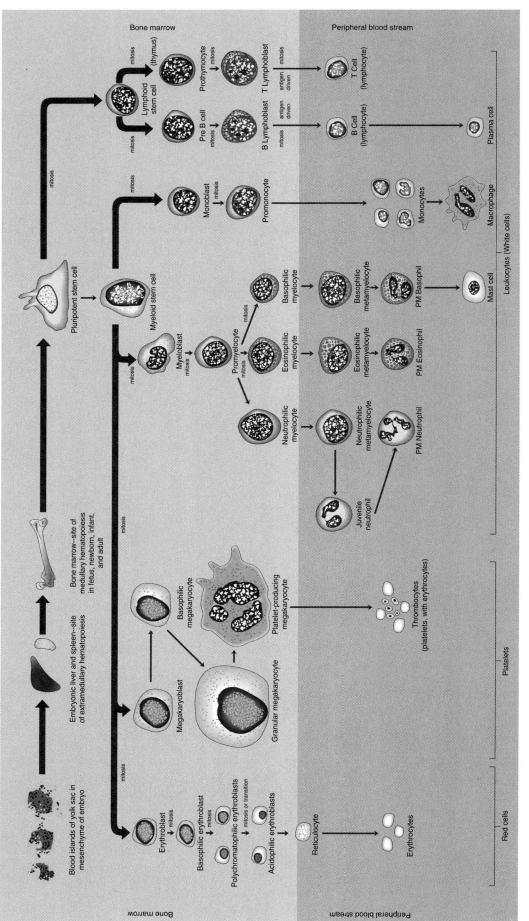

FIGURE 12–2. Maturation of human blood cells. Probable pathways of blood cell differentiation from the pluripotent stem cell to mature leukocytes, erythrocytes, and platelets. Production of cells begins in embryo blood islands of the yolk sac. As the embryo matures, production shifts to the liver and spleen (extramedullary hematopoiesis) and progresses to bone marrow (medullary hematopoiesis). In an adult, all production is in the bone marrow. Current thinking is that all cell production begins with a pluripotent stem cell which differentiates into either a myeloid stem cell or a lymphoid stem cell, which then differentiates into specific blast cells. For example, red cell differentiation begins with the proerythroblast, which matures into a basophilic erythroblast, to a polychromatophilic erythroblast, and to an acidophilic erythroblast, all of which are found in the bone marrow. Red cell differentiation concludes with production of reticulocytes and mature red cells (erythrocytes), which normally are found only in the peripheral blood.

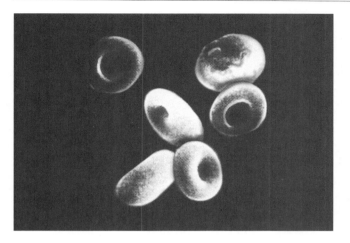

FIGURE 12–3. Mature erythrocytes, redrawn from a scanning electron micrograph.

and prepare the site for healing. Neutrophils live about 4 days if they have not participated in an inflammatory process.[1]

Eosinophilic granulocytes are the same size as neutrophils and have a two-lobed nucleus. They contain large, coarse, eosinophilic granules that fill the cell. Eosinophils, which compose only 1 percent to 4 percent of the normal leukocyte count in adults, ingest antigen-antibody complexes induced by IgE-mediated reactions to attack parasites. They also help control inflammatory processes and may participate in hypersensitivity reactions to other allergens. High eosinophil counts are often found in people experiencing type I allergic reactions such as asthma or hay fever (Table 12–2).[3]

Basophilic granulocytes are functionally and chemically related to the mast cell and have an average diameter of 8 μ to 10 μ. They have a kidney-shaped nucleus and large, deep basophilic granules in the cytoplasm. The granules contain the vasoactive amines histamine, bradykinin, and serotonin, and the anticoagulant heparin. Basophils compose less than 1 percent of the circulating leukocytes, and some researchers suggest their primary function is to release vasoactive amines and heparin. All of the body's blood histamine is thought to be in basophils and mast cells and is released when multivalent antigens (from allergens) bind to and cross-link the IgE molecules that are bound to the mast cells.[4]

Monocytes and macrophages are large (14–19 μ), occasionally motile leukocytes that make up the mononuclear phagocyte system. Monocytes are immature macrophages that circulate in the blood for 3 days before maturing into macrophages that migrate out of the blood vessels to fixed sites in the lymphoid tissues. Macrophages may be active for months or years before they migrate to an inflammatory site in the body where they ingest microorganisms, debris, or dead host cells such as red cells. They compose 3 percent to 7 percent of the circulating leukocytes.[5]

TABLE 12–2. Blood Cells

Cell	Structural Characteristics	Normal Amounts in Circulating Blood*	Function	Life Span
Erythrocyte (red blood cell)	Nonnucleated bi-concave disk containing hemoglobin	Male: 4.7–6.1 $\times$ 10^{12}/L Female: 4.2–5.4 $\times$ 10^{12}/L	Gas transport to and from tissue cells and lungs	80–120 days
Leukocyte (white blood cell)	Nucleated cell	4.8–10.8 $\times$ 10^9/L	Body defense mechanisms	See below
Lymphocyte	Mononuclear immunocyte	1.2–3.4 $\times$ 10^9/L, 20–44% leukocyte differential	Humoral and cell-mediated immunity	Days or years, depending on type
Neutrophil	Segmented polymorphonuclear granulocyte with neutrophilic granules	1.4–6.5 $\times$ 10^9/L, 50%–70% leukocyte differential	Phagocytosis, particularly during early phase of inflammation	5 days
Eosinophil	Segmented polymorphonuclear granulocyte with cosinophilic granules	0–0.7 $\times$ 10^9/L, 0%–4% leukocyte differential	Phagocytosis, antibody-mediated defense against parasites, participate in mucosal immune response	Unknown
Basophil	Segmented polymorphonuclear granulocyte with barophilic granules	0–0.2 $\times$ 10^9/L 0%–2% leukocyte differential	Transport and release heparin and histamine, involved in immune and inflammatory responses	Unknown
Monocyte-macrophage	Large mononuclear phagocyte	0.11–0.59 $\times$ 10^9/L, 2%–9% leukocyte differential	Phagocytosis; process and present antigens	Months or years
Platelet	Diskoid cytoplasmic fragment derived from megakarocytes	130–400 $\times$ 10^9/L	Hemostasis following vascular injury; form hemostatic plug, provide cofactors, maintain vascular endothelium	8–12 days

*In system of international units.

Lymphocytes are the primary cells in the immune response. They compose 25 percent to 33 percent of the circulating leukocytes. There are two basic types of lymphocytes: T-cells, which are involved in cell-mediated immunity, and B-cells, which are involved in humoral immunity. Detailed information on immune mechanisms is provided in Chapter 10.[5]

Platelets

Platelets, which are essential in the formation of blood clots and in the control of bleeding, are circulating cytoplasmic fragments of megakaryocytes. They contain cytoplasmic granules that release biochemical mediators involved in the hemostatic process. Normally, 150,000–400,000 platelets/mm[3] circulate freely in the blood. An additional one third of the body's platelets are in a reserve pool in the spleen. When a vessel is damaged, collagen is exposed; circulating platelets adhere to this "foreign" surface, aggregate, degranulate, and release a variety of biochemicals. Finally, they form a platelet plug with fibrin strands to seal the injury.

The amounts of the different cellular components in the blood vary with age. Table 12–3 gives normal values from birth to 21 years.[5]

KEY CONCEPTS

- Of the 4 to 6 liters of blood in the circulatory system, approximately 45 percent is composed of blood cells and 55 percent is plasma. The plasma fraction contains dissolved substances, including nutrients, ions, plasma proteins, metabolic wastes, hormones, and enzymes.
- Red cells function to carry oxygen and carbon dioxide in the blood. They have a limited life span of 80 to 120 days because they contain no cytoplasmic organelles and thus are unable to replace lost or damaged cellular components. The normal red cell concentration is 4.2–6.2 million/mm[3].
- Leukocytes, or white blood cells, are the other cell type present in blood. Leukocytes circulate in much lower numbers than red cells (5,000–10,000/mm[3]). Leukocytes are of three major kinds: granulocytes, monocytes (macrophages), and lymphocytes.
- Platelets are small, cellular fragments of megakaryocytes. The normal platelet count is 150,000–450,000/mm[3].

Structure and Function of Red Blood Cells

The cellular components of blood originate in the yolk sac mesenchyme, move to the liver and spleen during fetal life, and finally are limited to the marrow of the body skeleton (Fig. 12–4). Bone marrow provides a special environment for hematopoietic cell proliferation and maturation. Developing cells are held in a fine reticulin mesh that provides free access to plasma nutrients but retains developing cells until their maturity allows penetration of the endothelial barrier. In times of need, immature cells are released early into the circulation, where their presence is a sign of hematopoietic system stress or disease.[5]

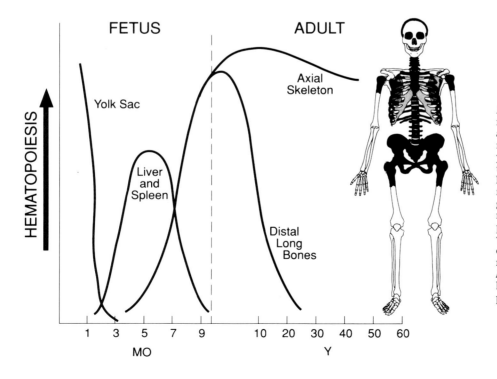

FIGURE 12–4. Location of active marrow growth in the fetus and adult. During fetal development, hemopoiesis is first established in the yolk sac mesenchyme, later moves to the liver and spleen, and finally is limited to the bony skeleton. From infancy to adulthood, there is a progressive restriction of productive marrow to the axial skeleton and proximal ends of the long bones, which appear as shaded areas on the drawing of the skeleton. (From Hillman RS, Finch CA (eds): *Red Cell Manual*, 6th ed. Philadelphia, FA Davis, 1992, p 2. Reproduced with permission.)

TABLE 12–3. *Development of Hematologic Values*

Age	Hemoglobin (g)	Hematocrit (%)	RBC Count (million per mm³)	Platelets (thousand per mm³)	Reticulocytes (%)	WBC Count (per mm³)	PMN Count, Adult	Band Forms (%)	Eosinophils (%)	Basophils (%)	Lymphocytes (%)	Monocytes (%)
Birth	17.6	55	5.5	350.0	5.0	9,000–30,000 (av., 18,000)	9,400 (52%)	9.1	2.2	0.6	31	5.8
24 hr	18.0	56	5.3	400.0	5.2	9,400–34,000 (av., 19,045)	9,800 (52%)	9.2	2.4	0.5	31	5.8
1 wk	17.0	54	5.0	300.0	1.0	5,000–21,000 (av., 12,279)	4,700 (39%)	6.8	4.1	0.4	41	9.1
2 mo	12.4	30	4.3	260.0	0.5	5,500–18,000 (av., 11,000)	3,300 (30%)	4.4	2.7	0.5	57	5.9
6 mo	11.5	34	4.6	250.0	0.8	6,000–17,500 (av., 11,900)	3,300 (28%)	3.8	2.5	0.4	61	4.8
2 yr	12.9	40	4.8	250.0	1.0	6,000–17,000 (av., 10,680)	3,200 (30%)	3.0	2.6	0.5	59	5.0
6 yr	14.1	42	4.8	250.0	1.0	5,000–14,500 (av., 8,500)	4,000 (48%)	3.0	2.7	0.6	42	4.7
14 yr	15.0	45(♂) 42(♀)	5.1	250.0	1.0	4,500–13,000 (av., 7,900)	4,200 (53%)	3.0	2.5	0.5	37	4.7
21 yr	15.0	45(♂) 42(♀)	5.1	250.0	1.0	4,500–11,000 (av., 7,400)	4,200 (56%)	3.0	2.7	0.5	34	4.0

From Platt W: *Color Atlas and Textbook of Hematology*, 2nd ed. Philadelphia, JB Lippincott, 1979, p 4. Reproduced by permission of William R. Platt, M.D.

Hematopoiesis

Hematopoiesis is the developmental process from pluripotential stem cells to mature, differentiated red cells, neutrophils, eosinophils, basophils, monocytes, and platelets. **Lymphopoiesis** describes this process for lymphocytes. Both hematopoietic and lymphopoietic stem cells probably derive from a single totipotent stem cell pool in fetal development, but it is uncertain if this is the functioning stem cell after birth (Fig. 12–5). Research suggests that a pluripotent stem cell that is stimulated by erythropoietin and other poietins to cause further differentiation into separate cell lines may be the primary stem cell in adults.[6]

Hematopoiesis is a two-stage process that involves mitotic division or proliferation and maturation or differentiation. Each type of blood cell has stem cells that undergo mitosis when stimulated by a specific biochemical signal indicating that the number of circulating cells has decreased. Medullary or bone marrow hematopoiesis continues throughout life and can be accelerated by several mechanisms, including (1) an increase in differentiation of daughter cells, (2) an increase in number of stem cells, and (3) conversion of yellow (fatty) bone marrow (which does not produce cells) to red marrow (which does produce cells). Marrow conversion is stimulated by erythropoietin, which is the hormone that stimulates erythrocyte production. In adults, extramedullary hemopoiesis, when blood cells are produced in tissues other than bone, is usually a disease symptom.[7]

Erythrocyte development is shown in detail in Figure 12–2. During this process, the cell changes from a large nucleated cell, rich in ribosomes, to a reticulocyte, a small disk that has lost its nucleus. The reticulocyte leaves the marrow, enters the bloodstream, and matures into an erythrocyte in 24 to 48

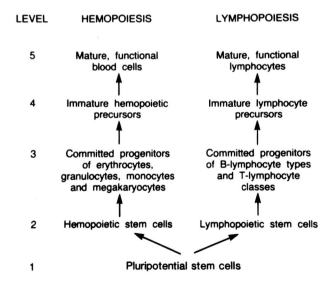

FIGURE 12–5. Stem cells and normal hemopoiesis. (From Williams WJ, et al (eds): *Hematology*, 4th ed. New York, McGraw-Hill, 1990, p 152. Reproduced by permission of McGraw-Hill, Inc.)

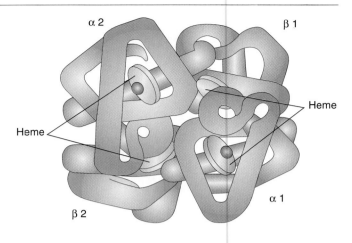

FIGURE 12–6. Molecular structure of hemoglobin. The molecule is a spherical tetramer weighing approximately 64,500 daltons. It contains two α and two β polypeptide chains and four heme groups.

hours. During this period, mitochondria and ribosomes disappear, and the cell can no longer synthesize hemoglobin or metabolize. The normal reticulocyte count is 1 percent of the total RBC count. This makes it a useful test to determine erythropoietic activity.[7]

Hemoglobin Synthesis

The immature red cell can be viewed as a factory for hemoglobin synthesis. In a mature red cell, **hemoglobin,** the oxygen-carrying protein, composes about 90 percent of the cell's dry weight in the form of approximately 300 hemoglobin molecules. Hemoglobin is composed of two pairs of polypeptide chains, the globins, each having an attached heme molecule that is composed of iron plus a protoporphyrin molecule (Fig. 12–6).[8]

After dietary iron is absorbed in the duodenum and proximal jejunum, it is transported through the plasma by the protein transferrin to transferrin iron receptors on the red cell membrane. The transferrin-receptor complex is engulfed by the cell into an invagination of the cell surface. The invagination becomes sealed off and forms an intracytoplasmic vacuole. Iron is then released and either stored as ferritin or used to synthesize heme (Fig. 12–7).[5]

About 67 percent of total body iron is bound to heme in erythrocytes and muscle cells and 30 percent is stored bound to ferritin or hemosiderin-containing macrophages and hepatic parenchymal cells. The remaining 3 percent is lost daily in urine, sweat, bile, and epithelial cells shed in the intestines.

The mitochondria are responsible for the synthesis of protoporphyrin. The final heme molecule consists of four porphyrin moieties assembled in a ring structure around a central iron molecule (Fig. 12–8).[5]

Globin is assembled from two pairs of polypeptide chains produced on specific ribosomes. The protein chain produced in fetal life is altered after birth by

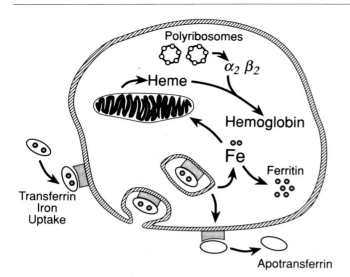

FIGURE 12-7. Intracellular pathways for iron uptake and incorporation into hemoglobin. The iron-transferrin complex is picked up by a membrane-associated receptor and brought into the cell by invagination and formation of an intracytoplasmic vacuole. The iron is then released and stored as intracytoplasmic ferritin or used to synthesize heme, the precursor of hemoglobin. The transferrin receptor complex is returned to the cell membrane, where the apotransferrin is expelled back into circulation. (From Hillman RS, Finch CA (eds): *Red Cell Manual*, 6th ed. Philadelphia, FA Davis, 1992, p 8. Reproduced with permission.)

sequential gene suppression and activation. At birth, red cells contain mainly fetal hemoglobin, hemoglobin F, which is composed of two α-chains and two γ-chains. Hemoglobin F is a more efficient gas carrier under decreased oxygen tension than hemoglobin A and releases CO_2 more readily. Within a few months, fetal hemoglobin disappears and is replaced by adult hemoglobin, hemoglobin A (Fig. 12–9). Hemoglobin A is composed of two α-chains and two β-chains and makes up 97 percent of the hemoglobin found in adults.[9] Folates and vitamin B_{12} are absorbed from

food by the ileal mucosa. Vitamin B_{12} requires intrinsic factor in the gastric juice for absorption. Intrinsic factor is secreted by the stomach parietal cells and binds to vitamin B_{12}. The complex then moves down the GI tract to the ileum, where it attaches to specific receptor sites on the ileum mucosal cell. It is absorbed into the cell, released, and transported in the blood to the tissues and liver (Fig. 12–10).[10]

Several hundred abnormal hemoglobins have been described. Most are characterized by the substitution of only one amino acid and are classified by the polypeptide chain in which the substitution occurs.[11]

Nutritional Requirements for Erythropoiesis

In addition to iron, which is required for hemoglobin synthesis, the normal development of erythrocytes requires adequate supplies of protein, vitamins, and minerals. Erythropoiesis cannot proceed in the absence of vitamins, especially B_{12}, folate, B_6, riboflavin, pantothenic acid, niacin, ascorbic acid, and vitamin E. Folate deficiencies or vitamin B_{12} deficiencies lead to impaired DNA synthesis in erythroid cells because the vitamins are coenzymes in a large number of key reactions in cellular metabolism.

Energy and Maintenance of Erythrocytes

For the red cell to perform efficiently and survive in the circulation for the full 120-day life span, it must have a source of energy. Without an energy source, the red cell becomes sodium logged and potassium depleted. The shape changes from a biconcave disk to a sphere, and it is quickly removed from the circulation by the filtering action of the spleen and the reticuloendothelial system. The chief metabolic pathway, accounting for about 90 percent of the glucose used, is the anaerobic or Embden-Meyerhof pathway.

FIGURE 12-8. Heme formation. The mitochondrion is responsible for the synthesis of protoporphyrin, a stepwise process beginning with the formation of δ-aminolevulinic acid from glycine and succinyl-CoA, with pyridoxal-5-phosphate (PLP) as an essential cofactor. The sequence of porphobilinogen, uroporphyrin, and coproporphyrin formation then occurs in the cytoplasm, followed by an intramitochondrial assembly of protoporphyrin and iron to form heme. The structure of the final product, the heme molecule, is shown. It consists of four porphyrin moieties assembled in a ring structure around a central iron molecule. (From Hillman RS, Finch CA (eds): *Red Cell Manual*, 6th ed. Philadelphia, FA Davis, 1992, p 9. Reproduced with permission.)

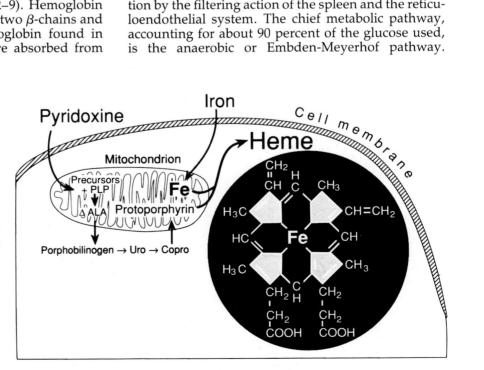

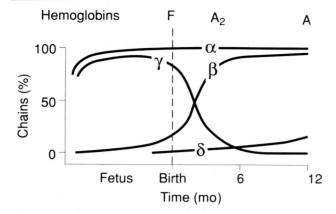

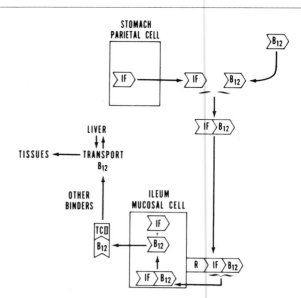

FIGURE 12–9. Changes in hemoglobin with development. Sequential suppression and activation of individual globin genes in the immediate postnatal period result in a switch from fetal hemoglobin (hemoglobin F: two α-chains and two γ-chains) to adult hemoglobin (hemoglobin A: two α-chains and two β-chains). A small amount of hemoglobin A$_2$ (two α-chains and two δ-chains) is also present in the adult. (Adapted with permission from Hillman RS, Finch CA (eds): *Red Cell Manual*, 6th ed. Philadelphia, FA Davis, 1992, p 9.)

FIGURE 12–10. Absorption, transport, and storage of vitamin B$_{12}$. IF, intrinsic factor; R, tissue binders; TC II, transcobalamin II. (From Miale J (ed): *Laboratory Medicine Hematology*, 6th ed. St. Louis, CV Mosby, 1982, p 425. Reproduced with permission.)

About 10 percent of the glucose undergoes aerobic glycolysis in the hexose monophosphate shunt. Deficiencies of enzymes that regulate these pathways can be due to natural causes, such as the normal aging process, or to an inherited deficiency of an enzyme.[12]

Cell membrane structures are matrices formed from a double layer of phospholipids. In the red cell membrane, the globular proteins floating on the "sea of lipids" are formed to a protein network on the cytoplasmic surface of the membrane. One half of the mass of the membrane is lipid, which is partially responsible for many of its physical characteristics. Both passive cation permeability and mechanical flexibility can be significantly influenced by changing the lipid composition of the membrane. Maintaining and renewing membrane lipids are important in well-developed normal cells, and problems in these pathways produce premature cell death.[13]

Red Cell Production

When blood is described as a single body system, it is called the **erythron** (Fig. 12–11). The erythron includes the blood cells and their bone marrow precursors, so that it is much larger than the liver. The size of the erythron increases or decreases based on the erythropoietic process and the pathologic changes in red cells seen in anemias.[14] Erythropoiesis is controlled by a system sensitive to alterations in the concentration of hemoglobin in the blood. A decrease in hemoglobin decreases the tissue oxygen tension in the kidney. In response to this hypoxia, the kidney secretes a hormone, erythropoietin, that stimulates primitive stem cells in the bone marrow to differenti-

ate into proerythroblasts, thereby increasing the erythron (Fig. 12–12).[15] Other types of hypoxia can also initiate this response.

Red Cell Destruction

As the red cell ages, the various enzyme activities decrease, membrane lipids decrease, hemoglobin A$_3$ and methemoglobin increase, and there are changes in cell size. The cell loses its ability to deform and becomes increasingly fragile. These aging red cells are then removed by the mononuclear phagocytic system. The red cells are digested by proteolytic and lipolytic enzymes in phagolysosomes of macrophages. Some 80 percent to 90 percent of this process occurs in macrophages of the spleen and liver. Only 10 percent to 20 percent of normal destruction occurs intravascularly.[16]

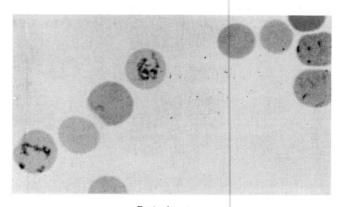

Reticulocytes

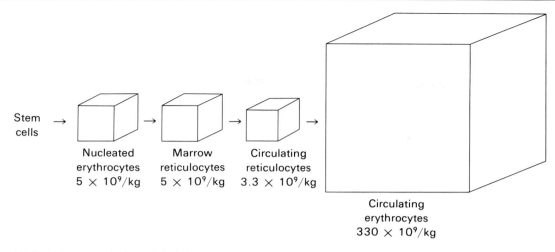

FIGURE 12–11. Scale model of the erythron, showing the relative proportions of each of the components. The numbers below each box indicate the average number of cells per kilogram of body weight. (From Wintrobe M, et al (eds): *Clinical Hematology*, 8th ed. Philadelphia, Lea & Febiger, 1981, p 109. Reproduced with permission.)

Globin is broken down into amino acids and the iron is recycled. Porphyrin is reduced to bilirubin, which is transported to the liver and conjugated by glucuronyl transferase. Finally, conjugated bilirubin is excreted in the bile as glucuronide. Bacteria in the intestine convert conjugated bilirubin into urobilinogen, which is excreted primarily in the stool but also in the urine. Any condition causing increased red cell destruction increases the load of bilirubin to be cleared, which leads to increased serum levels of unconjugated bilirubin and increased excretion of urobilinogen (Fig. 12–13).[16]

KEY CONCEPTS

- **Red cell development from pluripotent stem cells in the bone marrow is stimulated by a growth factor called erythropoietin. Erythropoietin is secreted into the bloodstream by kidney cells in response to low oxygen tension in the blood.**

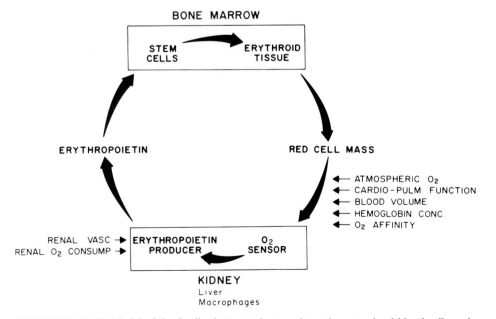

FIGURE 12–12. Model of the feedback circuit that regulates the rate of red blood cell production to the need for oxygen in the peripheral tissues. (From Williams WJ, et al (eds): *Hematology*, 3rd ed. New York, McGraw-Hill, 1983, p 373. Reproduced by permission of McGraw-Hill, Inc.)

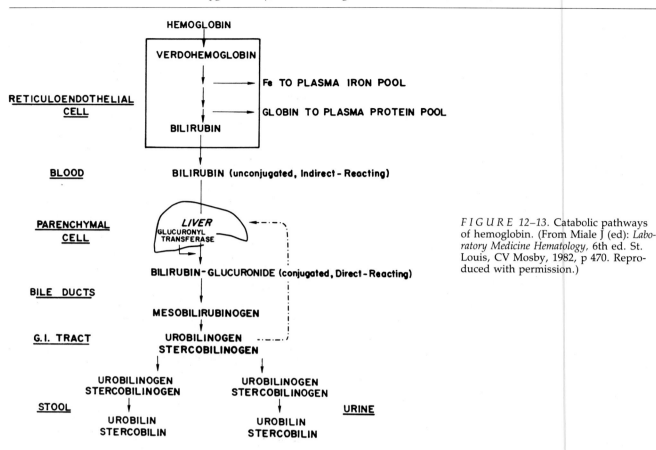

FIGURE 12–13. Catabolic pathways of hemoglobin. (From Miale J (ed): *Laboratory Medicine Hematology*, 6th ed. St. Louis, CV Mosby, 1982, p 470. Reproduced with permission.)

- During development, red cells lose their nuclei and other cytoplasmic organelles. A reticulocyte is an immature red cell that still retains some cellular organelles. An increased blood reticulocyte count is a useful indicator of increased red cell production.

- Hemoglobin is the major component of red cells. It is composed of two pairs of polypeptide chains, each of which has a heme molecule attached. Oxygen can bind reversibly to an iron molecule at the center of each heme. When fully saturated, a hemoglobin molecule carries four oxygen molecules, or 1.34 mL of oxygen per gram of hemoglobin.

- Red cell production requires adequate amounts of several nutrients, particularly iron, vitamin B_{12}, and folate. Lack of intrinsic factor inhibits absorption of B_{12} from the small intestine and is a risk factor for anemia.

- Red cells rely on glycolysis for energy production because they do not contain mitochondria. As energy production declines due to red cell aging and loss of essential glycolytic enzymes, the cell swells, gets trapped in the spleen, and is removed from the circulation. Red cell degradation releases bilirubin, a toxic substance that is conjugated in the liver and excreted in urine and bile.

Gas Transport and Acid-Base Balance

RBCs have many important functions in the body related to gas transport and acid-base balance.[17,18] RBCs contain hemoglobin, which is responsible for oxygen transport to the body tissues.[17] Oxygen combines with the heme portion of hemoglobin in a loose and reversible bond in the pulmonary capillary with a high Po_2 and is carried to the tissues with a low Po_2, where it is released.[18] Large quantities of carbonic anhydrase in RBCs catalyze the reaction between carbon dioxide and water produced by cellular metabolism in the tissues to form carbonic acid and subsequently hydrogen and bicarbonate for elimination by the lungs and kidneys.[17] Finally, the hemoglobin protein directly binds with carbon dioxide to form carbaminohemoglobin for carbon dioxide transport, which is an acid-base buffer responsible for as much as 50 percent of the whole blood buffering power.

Oxygen Transport

The transport of oxygen to the body tissues and the removal of carbon dioxide is a complex process involving external respiration, hemoglobin concentration, hemoglobin-oxygen affinity, arterial oxygen saturation, cardiac output, blood viscosity, internal respiration, and changes in oxygen supply and demand (Fig. 12–14).

External respiration includes the following processes: (1) ventilation or movement of air between the atmosphere and the alveoli, (2) distribution of air within the lungs to maintain appropriate oxygen and carbon dioxide concentrations in the alveoli, (3) diffusion or movement of oxygen and carbon dioxide across the alveolar membrane, and (4) perfusion of the pulmonary capillary bed.[19]

Approximately 97 percent of oxygen is transported in the blood loosely and reversibly combined with hemoglobin (oxyhemoglobin) in the red cells, and 3 percent is dissolved in plasma.[18, 19] Each hemoglobin molecule can bind four atoms of oxygen. Despite a combining potential of 1.39 mL of oxygen per gram of hemoglobin in pure hemoglobin, a maximum of about 1.34 mL of oxygen per gram of hemoglobin is available, owing to a reduction of about 4 percent by impurities such as methemoglobin.[18] The blood of a normal person contains approximately 15 grams of hemoglobin per 100 mL of blood.[18] Therefore, in the average person, the hemoglobin in 100 mL of blood can combine with almost 20 mL of oxygen if the hemoglobin is 100 percent saturated. This value is expressed as 20 volumes percent (vol percent).[18]

The partial pressure of oxygen (Po_2) reflects the pressure or tension that oxygen exerts when it is dissolved in blood. Partial pressure is measured in millimeters of mercury (mm Hg).[20] In the pulmonary capillaries, where Po_2 is high, oxygen binds easily with

hemoglobin, but in the tissue capillaries, where Po_2 is low, oxygen is released from hemoglobin.[18] The partial pressure affects the ability of oxygen to associate with hemoglobin-binding sites in the lungs and the ability of oxygen to be released or dissociated from these sites at the tissue level.[20] The partial pressure of oxygen in arterial blood (Pao_2) is usually 80 to 100 mm Hg, whereas the partial pressure of oxygen in venous blood ($P\bar{v}o_2$) is usually 35 to 40 mm Hg.[20] The amount of hemoglobin bound to oxygen relative to the total amount of hemoglobin, both reduced and oxygenated, is expressed as the oxygen saturation, in a percentage.[20,21] Arterial blood (Sao_2) is normally saturated with oxygen at 95 percent to 100 percent, whereas venous blood ($S\bar{v}o_2$) is saturated at 60 percent to 80 percent.[18–20]

The oxygen-hemoglobin dissociation curve (Fig. 12–15) demonstrates the relationship between Po_2 and So_2. The upper part of the curve represents oxygen uptake in the lungs, and demonstrates that significant changes in Po_2 result in only small changes in So_2 to help ensure adequate oxygen delivery to the tissues.[19,20] On the steep lower portion of the curve, reflecting the venous blood, small changes in venous Po_2 result in large changes in $S\bar{v}o_2$.[20] Therefore, the tissues are protected with an available oxygen reserve as large quantities of oxygen are released from the blood for relatively small decreases in Po_2 to a critical $P\bar{v}o_2$ level of approximately 30 mm Hg, at which point the oxygen reserve is quickly depleted.[20] Normally, tissue Po_2 does not rise above 40 mm Hg to enhance diffusion of oxygen from the blood to the tissues, and venous blood has a $P\bar{v}o_2$ of 40 mm Hg with a satura-

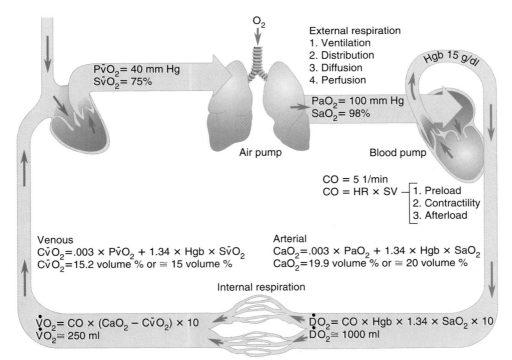

Figure 12.14
Copstead/Perspectives on Pathophysiology

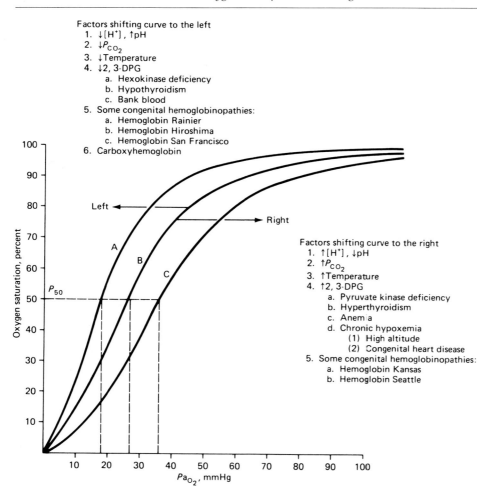

Factors shifting curve to the left
1. $\downarrow[H^+]$, $\uparrow$pH
2. $\downarrow P_{CO_2}$
3. $\downarrow$Temperature
4. $\downarrow$2, 3-DPG
    a. Hexokinase deficiency
    b. Hypothyroidism
    c. Bank blood
5. Some congenital hemoglobinopathies:
    a. Hemoglobin Rainier
    b. Hemoglobin Hiroshima
    c. Hemoglobin San Francisco
6. Carboxyhemoglobin

Factors shifting curve to the right
1. $\uparrow[H^+]$, $\downarrow$pH
2. $\uparrow P_{CO_2}$
3. $\uparrow$Temperature
4. $\uparrow$2, 3-DPG
    a. Pyruvate kinase deficiency
    b. Hyperthyroidism
    c. Anemia
    d. Chronic hypoxemia
      (1) High altitude
      (2) Congenital heart disease
5. Some congenital hemoglobinopathies:
    a. Hemoglobin Kansas
    b. Hemoglobin Seattle

FIGURE 12–15. Oxygen-hemoglobin dissociation curve. Factors affecting hemoglobin's affinity for oxygen. Curve *B* is the standard oxyhemoglobin dissociation curve. Factors that shift the curve to the left are represented in curve *A*; factors that shift the curve to the right are represented in curve *C*. (From Gottlieb JE: Breathing and gas exchange, in Kinney MR, Packa DR, Dunbar SB (eds): *AACN's Clinical Reference for Critical Care Nursing*, 3rd ed. New York, McGraw-Hill, 1993, p 672. Reproduced by permission.)

tion of 75 percent, compared to a Pao_2 of 95 mm Hg with a saturation of 97 percent in the arterial blood.[18]

The ability of oxygen to combine with hemoglobin and the strength of this bond, independent of Po_2, is known as the oxygen-hemoglobin affinity. The number of hemoglobin-binding sites occupied by oxygen (saturation) increases with the affinity of hemoglobin for oxygen; and as the affinity of hemoglobin for oxygen decreases, the saturation decreases and oxygen is released to the cells.[20] The ability of hemoglobin to release oxygen to the tissues is commonly assessed at point P_{50} on the oxygen-hemoglobin dissociation curve.[19] The affinity of hemoglobin for oxygen at point P_{50} on the oxyhemoglobin dissociation curve is where 50 percent of the hemoglobin is saturated at 27 mm Hg in a healthy person at 37° C, an arterial pH of 7.40, a Pco_2 of 40 mm Hg, and normal 2,3-DPG and hemoglobin levels.[19] A decrease in oxygen affinity (shift to the right on the oxyhemoglobin dissociation curve) or an increase in oxygen affinity (shift to the left) can be caused by the conditions listed in Figure 12–15.

A shift of the oxyhemoglobin dissociation curve to the right enhances oxygen release to the cell (see Fig. 12–15).[18,21] The shift provides the increase in oxygen delivery that is needed during exercise and other types of stress, as well as in chronic disease states.[18]

A shift of the oxyhemoglobin dissociation curve to the left is seen with a decrease in H^+ ion concentration, a decrease in Pco_2, an increase in pH, a decrease in temperature, a decrease in 2,3-DPG, some congenital hemoglobinopathies, and carboxyhemoglobin.[18]

Arterial blood oxygen content (Cao_2) and venous blood oxygen content ($C\bar{v}o_2$) can be calculated by considering the oxygen capacity of hemoglobin, the oxygen combined with hemoglobin, and the oxygen dissolved in plasma.

Oxygen capacity of Hb (vol %)
$$= Hb \text{ (g/100 mL)} \times 1.34 \text{ (mL O}_2\text{/g Hb)}$$
$$15 \times 1.34 = 20.1 \text{ vol \%}$$

Oxygen combined with Hb (vol %)
$$= Hb \text{ (g/100 mL)} \times 1.34 \text{ (mL O}_2\text{/g Hb)} \times \text{saturation (\%)}$$
$$15 \times 1.34 \times 97.5\% = 19.6 \text{ vol \% in arterial blood}$$
$$15 \times 1.34 \times 75\% = 15.1 \text{ vol \% in venous blood}$$

Oxygen dissolved in plasma (vol %)
$$= Po_2 \text{ (mm Hg)} \times 0.003 \text{ (vol \%/mm Hg)}$$
$$100 \times 0.003 = .3 \text{ vol \% in arterial blood}$$
$$75 \times 0.003 = .2 \text{ vol \% in venous blood}$$

Therefore,

Total oxygen content = oxygen combined with Hb
+ oxygen dissolved in plasma in arterial blood

$$19.6 \text{ vol } \% + 0.3 \text{ vol } \% = 19.9 \text{ vol } \% \text{ } Cao_2$$

Oxygen combined with Hb
+ oxygen dissolved in plasma in venous blood

$$15.1 \text{ vol } \% + 0.2 \text{ vol } \% = 15.3 \text{ vol } \% \text{ } C\bar{v}o_2$$

Oxygen delivery, or $\dot{D}o_2$, is the amount of oxygen (in mL) delivered per minute to the tissues.[19] It is calculated by multiplying the arterial oxygen content (Cao_2) by the cardiac output. Cardiac output depends on heart rate, preload, stroke volume, and afterload (see Chap. 16) and is usually between 4 and 8 L/min. Therefore, oxygen delivery is approximately 1,000 mL/min.

Oxygen delivery (mL/min)
= cardiac output (L/min) $\times$ Cao_2 $\times$ 10

$$995 \text{ mL/min} = 5 \text{ L/min} \times 19.9 \text{ vol } \% \times 10$$

Cardiac output (CO) and blood viscosity both determine blood flow.[22] Blood viscosity is a function of the hematocrit, flow rate, vessel size, red cell shape or deformity, plasma viscosity, and erythrocyte aggregation produced by the interaction of plasma proteins with RBCs.[22]

Oxygen consumption ($\dot{V}o_2$) is the amount of oxygen consumed by the tissues, and it is measured in milliliters of oxygen per minute. Once the oxygen reaches the tissues, oxygen consumption is controlled by the rate of energy expenditure within the cells or the rate at which adenosine diphosphate (ADP) is formed from adenosine triphosphate (ATP) to provide energy.[18] The increasing concentration of ADP enhances the metabolic utilization of oxygen and nutrients, which releases energy.[18] Oxygen consumption can be determined by subtracting the oxygen remaining in the venous blood (venous transport) from the oxygen delivered to the tissues by the arteries (arterial transport), and is known as the Fick equation.[21]

Oxygen consumption = arterial oxygen transport
− venous oxygen transport

$$\dot{V}o_2 = CO \times (Cao_2 - C\bar{v}o_2) \times 10$$

$$225 \text{ mL} = 5 \text{ L/min} \times (19.6 \text{ vol } \% - 15.2 \text{ vol } \%) \times 10$$

Gas values (pressure and content) relative to the oxygenation of blood are detailed in Table 12–4.

Carbon Dioxide Transport

RBCs are important in the transport of carbon dioxide in the blood. Carbon dioxide, a by-product of cellular metabolism, is transported in three forms in the blood: (1) as dissolved gas, (2) as bicarbonate ion (HCO_3^-), and (3) in association with hemoglobin (Fig. 12–16).[18] Dissolved carbon dioxide combines slowly with water in the plasma to form carbonic acid (H_2CO_3), but in the red cell, the presence of carbonic anhydrase as a catalyst significantly accelerates this reaction.[18,21] Carbonic acid rapidly dissociates into hydrogen ions (H^+) and bicarbonate ions (HCO_3^-).[18,21] As the concentration of HCO_3^- in the red cell increases, it diffuses into the plasma, whereas the H^+ remains, causing chloride to diffuse from the plasma into the red cell to maintain

TABLE 12–4. Gas Values Significant to the Oxygenation of Blood

Cao_2	The arterial blood oxygen content is the amount of oxygen carried in the arterial blood and is the sum of oxyhemoglobin plus the amount of oxygen dissolved in the plasma. It is measured in milliliters of oxygen per deciliter of blood (mL/dL), or volume percent. Normal Cao_2 is approximately 20 vol percent.
$C\bar{v}o_2$	The venous blood oxygen content is the amount of oxygen carried in the venous blood and is the sum of oxyghemoglobin plus the amount of oxygen dissolved in the plasma. It is measured in milliliters of oxygen per deciliter of blood (mL/dL), or volume percent. Normal $C\bar{v}o_2$ is approximately 15 vol percent.
$\dot{D}o_2$	Oxygen delivery or transport is the amount of oxygen delivered to the tissues. It is measured in milliliters of oxygen per minute (mL/min). Normal arterial $\dot{D}o_2$ is approximately 1,000 mL O_2/min. Normal venous $\dot{D}o_2$ is approximately 750 mL O_2/min.
Pao_2	The partial pressure of oxygen in arterial blood, measured in millimeters of mercury (mm Hg). It reflects the tension or pressure that is exerted by oxygen when it is dissolved in plasma. Normal Pao_2 is 80 to 100 mm Hg.
$Paco_2$	The partial pressure of carbon dioxide in arterial blood, measured in millimeters of mercury (mm Hg). It reflects the tension or pressure that is exerted by carbon dioxide when it is dissolved in plasma. Normal $Paco_2$ is 35 to 45 mm Hg.
$P\bar{v}o_2$	The partial pressure of oxygen in venous blood, measured in millimeters of mercury (mm Hg). It reflects the tension or pressure that is exerted by oxygen when it is dissolved in plasma. Normal $P\bar{v}o_2$ is 35 to 40 mm Hg.
$P\bar{v}co_2$	The partial pressure of carbon dioxide in venous blood, measured in millimeters of mercury (mm Hg). It reflects the tension or pressure that is exerted by carbon dioxide when it is dissolved in plasma. Normal $P\bar{v}co_2$ is 41 to 51 mm Hg.
Sao_2	The amount of hemoglobin bound to oxygen relative to the total amount of hemoglobin, both reduced and bound, in arterial blood and expressed as a percentage. Normal Sao_2 is 95 percent to 100 percent.
$S\bar{v}o_2$	The amount of hemoglobin bound to oxygen relative to the total amount of hemoglobin, both reduced and bound, in venous blood and expressed as a percentage. Normal $S\bar{v}o_2$ is 60 percent to 80 percent.
$\dot{V}o_2$	Oxygen consumption is the amount of oxygen consumed by the tissues. It is measured in milliliters of oxygen per minute (mL/min). Oxygen consumption is derived from the difference between arterial oxygen transport and venous oxygen transport. Normal $\dot{V}o_2$ is 200 to 250 mL O_2/min.

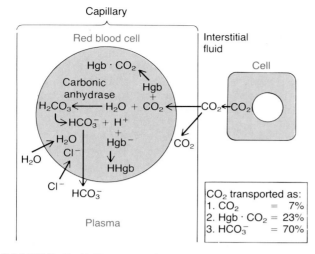

FIGURE 12–16. Transport of carbon dioxide in the blood. (From Guyton AC: Transport of oxygen and carbon dioxide in the blood and body fluids, in Guyton AC: *Textbook of Medical Physiology*, 8th ed. Philadelphia, WB Saunders, 1991, p 440. Reproduced with permission.)

electrical neutrality. This is referred to as the **chloride shift.**[19]

Hemoglobin provides an excellent acid-base buffer by reacting with the free hydrogen ions and directly with carbon dioxide to form carbaminohemoglobin (Hb-CO$_2$), which is easily dissociated in the lungs as carbon dioxide for exhalation.[18] Unloading of oxygen at the tissues facilitates the loading of carbon dioxide and is referred to as the Haldane effect.[18,19]

Alterations in Oxygen Transport

There must be sufficient circulating hemoglobin mass to meet the metabolic needs of the body. A feedback mechanism ensures that when there is a decrease in the oxygen reaching the tissues, there is a compensatory increase in the production of red cells.[22] The feedback mechanism regulating RBC production is under the control of erythropoietin.[5,22] As stem cells differentiate into the erythroid committed line, the most primitive stem cell is referred to as the erythroid burst-forming unit (BFU-E), which is controlled by growth factors derived from T-lymphocytes and macrophages and to a lesser degree by erythropoietin.[5,22] The BFU-E further differentiates into colony-forming units (CFU-E) more responsive to erythropoietin, and subsequently into normoblasts and mature RBCs.[5,22] The majority of erythropoietin is actively secreted by the kidney. Ten percent of erythropoietin is formed elsewhere in the body.[5,22–24]

Factors that decrease hemoglobin mass such as anemia or decreased arterial saturation (such as hypoxia from either cardiac or pulmonary conditions) impair oxygen delivery to the body tissues.[22] This stimulates an increased release of erythropoietin and the production of RBCs.[22] Figure 12–17 illustrates normal

regulation of erythropoiesis and the compensatory regulation of erythropoiesis that is seen in hypoxia, anemia, and polycythemia vera.[22]

KEY CONCEPTS

- Nearly all (97 percent) of the oxygen transported in blood is bound to hemoglobin within the red cells. Only 3 percent is dissolved in plasma. At a normal Pao$_2$, hemoglobin is 95 percent to 100 percent saturated with oxygen. About one fourth of the bound oxygen is unloaded to the tissues, resulting in a venous hemoglobin saturation of about 75 percent.

- The oxyhemoglobin saturation curve describes the relationship between the partial pressure of oxygen and hemoglobin saturation. In the lung, where Po$_2$ is high (100 mm Hg), oxygen is loaded onto hemoglobin. In the tissues, where Po$_2$ is low (40 mm Hg), oxygen is unloaded from hemoglobin to tissues.

- The affinity of hemoglobin for oxygen is affected by temperature, acid-base status, 2,3-DPG levels, and carbon dioxide. Affinity decreases at the tissue level due to increased acid, 2,3-DPG, and carbon dioxide. This shift to the right of the oxyhemoglobin dissociation curve enhances unloading of oxygen to the tissue. A shift to the left occurs at the lung, where blood is more alkalotic and carbon dioxide levels are lower. The increased affinity of hemoglobin for oxygen at the lung facilitates oxygen binding.

- The oxygen content of arterial blood is calculated by adding the amount bound to hemoglobin (Hb) plus the amount dissolved in plasma: Cao$_2$ = (Hb × 1.34 × Sao$_2$) + (Pao$_2$ × .003). Oxygen delivery to the body tissues is calculated by multiplying Cao$_2$ times cardiac output (CO): Do$_2$ = Cao$_2$ × CO × 10.

- The consumption of oxygen by tissues can be estimated using the Fick equation: V̇o$_2$ = CO × (Cao$_2$ − C̄v̄o$_2$) × 10. Oxygen consumption increases with increased tissue metabolism.

- Hemoglobin is an important factor in carbon dioxide transport in the blood. At the tissue, hemoglobin binds carbon dioxide to form carbaminohemoglobin, which then releases carbon dioxide at the lung. Red cells contain the enzyme carbonic anhydrase, which greatly increases conversion of carbon dioxide and water into HCO$_3^-$ and H$^+$ at the tissue level. At the lung, the reaction proceeds in reverse, producing carbon dioxide, which is eliminated by the lungs.

Anemias

Erythrocyte disorders are divided into two groups (Table 12–5): (1) **anemia,** defined as a deficit of red cells, and (2) **polycythemia,** defined as an excess of red cells. In discussing the various erythrocyte disorders in terms of the classification system given in Table 12–6, it is possible to review the more common anemias without the comprehensive review detailed in hematology reference books. An anemic patient has tissue hypoxia due to the low oxygen-carrying capacity of the blood. In contrast, a polycythemic patient has increased whole blood viscosity and blood volume due to the increase in number of RBCs.

Relative anemia and **relative polycythemia** are characterized by normal total red cell mass with disturbances in the regulation of plasma volume. In pregnancy, the average plasma volume is 43 percent greater than in nonpregnant women, which causes a "dilutional anemia."

Absolute anemias are those anemias with an actual decrease in numbers of red cells. This can be caused by decreased production of red cells or increased destruction of red cells.[25]

General Effects of Anemia

The clinical manifestations of anemia include a reduction in oxygen-carrying capacity, tissue hypoxia, and compensatory mechanisms to restore tissue oxygenation.[26] Increased pulmonary and cardiac function increases the oxygen consumption, and an increase in oxygen extraction occurs to protect tissues. Selective tissue perfusion provides shunting to vital organs in short-term compensation, and increased erythropoi-

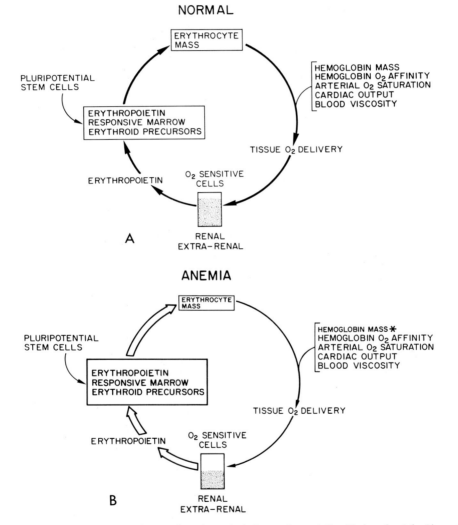

FIGURE 12–17. Regulation of erythropoiesis by erythropoietin. Under physiologic conditions, erythropoietin secretion is low. Any factor decreasing oxygen delivery to the oxygen-sensitive cells results in increased secretion of erythropoietin and a compensatory increase in erythrocyte production as illustrated in **B** for anemia, with a decrease in erythrocyte mass, and in **C** for hypoxia, with a decrease in arterial oxygen saturation. A decrease in oxygen requirements produces a relative oxygen surfeit, resulting in decreased erythropoietin secretion and a compensatory decrease in erythrocyte production, as illustrated in **C** for polycythemia vera: as autonomous production of red cells increases, tissue oxygen delivery increases, resulting in a decreased erythropoietin release. (From Wheby MS: Differentiation, biochemistry and physiology of the erythrocyte, in Thorup OA (ed): *Leavell and Thorup's Fundamentals of Clinical Hematology*, 5th ed. Philadelphia, WB Saunders, 1987, pp 68–69. Reproduced with permission.)

Illustration continued on following page

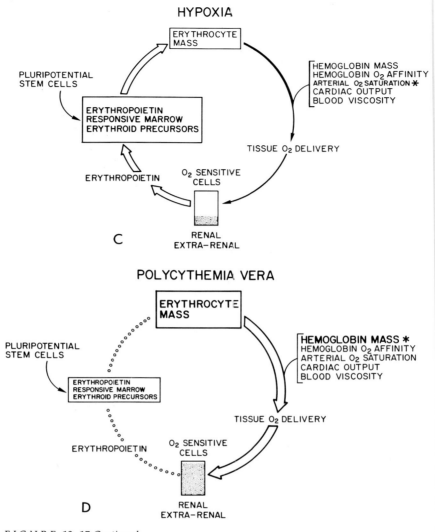

F I G U R E 12–17 Continued

etic activity is stimulated to provide long-term compensation.[26] Specific symptoms related to these causes are vasoconstriction, pallor, tachypnea, dyspnea, tachycardia, angina pectoris, high-output failure, intermittent claudication, night cramps in muscles, headache, light-headedness, tinnitus, roaring in the ears, faintness, and GI and genitourinary (GU) symptoms.[26]

Anemias Related to Decreased Red Cell Production

Aplastic Anemia

Etiology and Pathogenesis. Aplastic anemia is an example of a stem cell disorder which is characterized by a reduction of hematopoietic tissue in the bone marrow, fatty marrow replacement, and pancytopenia. The decrease in functional bone marrow mass is usually caused by toxic, radiant, or immunologic injury to the bone marrow stem cells, which causes a

decrease in red cells, white cells, and platelets, or **pancytopenia.**[27]

Chloramphenicol and benzene are two chemical substances that have a significant history of causing aplastic anemia. Exposure to lethal or sublethal amounts of whole-body irradiation results in extensive cell death in the bone marrow and intestines. The biological effect of radiation depends on the amount of radiant energy absorbed by the tissues.[27]

Laboratory Features. **Pancytopenia** in aplastic anemia is characterized by low red cell, white cell, and platelet counts. The magnitude of the **granulocytopenia** is very important for the immediate prognosis. An absolute granulocyte count of less than 200/mm³ results in immediate susceptibility to infectious complications. Coagulation tests are generally normal except for the bleeding time, which reflects the low platelet count.[27]

Clinical Manifestations. In aplastic anemia, the decreased bone marrow function results in pancytopenia or anemia, leukopenia, and **thrombocytopenia.**[27–30] The onset is usually insidious, and patients often pre-

TABLE 12–5. Classification of Erythrocyte Disorders

Anemia

Relative
1. Macroglobulinemia
2. Pregnancy
3. Nutritional deficiency
4. Splenomegaly

Absolute
1. Anemia predominantly caused by decreased red cell production
   a. Disturbance of proliferation and differentiation of hemopoietic stem cells
      (1) Aplastic anemia
      (2) Dyshemopoietic anemia
   b. Disturbance of proliferation and differentiation of erythroid progenitor or precursor cells
      (1) Pure red cell aplasia
      (2) Anemia of chronic renal failure
      (3) Anemia of endocrine disorders
      (4) Congenital dyserythropoietic anemia
   c. Disturbance of DNA synthesis (megaloblastic anemia)
      (1) Vitamin B_{12} deficiency
      (2) Folic acid deficiency
      (3) Acquired and congenital defects in purine and pyrimidine metabolism
   d. Disturbance of hemoglobin synthesis (hypochromic anemia)
      (1) Iron deficiency
      (2) Congenital atransferrinemia and idiopathic pulmonary hemosiderosis
      (3) Thalassemia
   e. Unknown or multiple mechanisms
      (1) Anemia of chronic disorders
      (2) Anemia associated with marrow infiltration
      (3) Anemia associated with nutritional deficiencies
      (4) Sideroblastic anemia
2. Anemia caused predominantly by increased erythrocyte destruction or loss
   a. Intrinsic abnormality
      (1) Membrane defect
         (a) Hereditary spherocytosis
         (b) Hereditary elliptocytosis
         (c) Hereditary stomatocytosis
         (d) Acanthocytosis
      (2) Enzyme deficiency
         (a) Glucose-6-phosphate dehydrogenase deficiency
         (b) Pyruvate kinase (PK) and other enzyme deficiencies
         (c) Porphyria

      (3) Globin abnormality (hemoglobinopathy)
         (a) Sickle cell disease and related disorders
         (b) Unstable hemoglobins
         (c) Low-oxygen-affinity hemoglobinopathies
      (4) Paroxysmal nocturnal hemoglobinuria
   b. Extrinsic abnormality
      (1) Mechanical
         (a) March hemoglobinuria
         (b) Traumatic cardiac hemolytic anemia
         (c) Microangiopathic hemolytic anemia
      (2) Chemical or physical
         (a) Hemolytic anemia due to chemical or physical agents
      (3) Infectious
         (a) Hemolytic anemia due to infection with microorganisms
      (4) Antibody-mediated
         (a) Acquired hemolytic anemia due to warm-reacting autoantibodies
         (b) Cryopathic hemolytic syndrome
         (c) Drug reaction involving antibodies reacting with erythrocytes
         (d) Alloimmune hemolytic disease of the newborn
      (5) Hyperactivity of the monocyte-macrophage system
         (a) Hypersplenism
      (6) Blood loss
         (a) Acute blood loss anemia

Polycythemia (Erythrocytosis)

Relative
1. Dehydration
2. Spurious (stress or smokers) erythrocytosis

Absolute
1. Primary
   a. Polycythemia vera
   b. Erythremia
2. Secondary
   a. Appropriate
      (1) Altitude
      (2) Cardiopulmonary disorder
      (3) Increased affinity of hemoglobin for oxygen
   b. Inappropriate
      (1) Renal tumor and cyst
      (2) Hepatoma
      (3) Cerebellar hemangioblastoma

From Williams WJ, et al (eds): *Hematology*, 3rd ed. New York, McGraw-Hill, 1983, p 407. Reproduced by permission of McGraw-Hill, Inc.

sent only after the late manifestations of pancytopenia are evident. These include weakness, fatigue, lethargy, pallor, dyspnea, palpitations, and the tachycardia of anemia; fever and bacterial or fungal infections (particularly in the mouth or perirectal area) secondary to neutropenia; and petechiae, bruising, nosebleeds, retinal hemorrhage, and increased menstrual flow from thrombocytopenia.[27,29,30] Grayish brown skin pigmentation, testicular atrophy, and enlargement of the spleen, liver, and lymph nodes are seen in

patients under observation and treatment for aplastic anemia. These clinical features are thought to be related to blood transfusions.[30]

Treatment. Treatment for aplastic anemia is directed at withdrawal of causative factors, supportive care, and therapy to restore normal hematopoiesis.[27–30] Removing the identified causative factor usually has no effect on the overall clinical course.[29] Transfusion therapy to provide an adequate number of erythrocytes and platelets has been effective, particu-

TABLE 12–6. Replacement Therapy for Vitamin B₁₂ and Folic Acid Deficiency Anemia

	Vitamin B$_{12}$ Deficiency	Folate Deficiency
Vitamin form	Cyanocobalamin or hydroxocobalamin	Folic acid
Route	Intramuscular	Oral
Dose		
Initial	Cyanocobalamin: 1,000 μg daily while in hospital; then weekly × 6 Hydroxocobalamin: 1,000 μg × 6 over 2–3 weeks	1 mg daily or twice a day for 1–4 months
Maintenance	Cyanocobalamin: 100–1,000 μg per month Hydroxocobalamin: 1,000 μg every 3 months	Depends on disease—may be needed for sprue, hemolytic anemias, renal dialysis
Prophylaxis	Total gastrectomy Ileal resection Gastric bypass (?)	Pregnancy Prematurity Dialysis

From Eichner EH: Megaloblastic anemias, in Stein JH, et al (eds): *Internal Medicine*, 3rd ed. Boston, Little, Brown & Co, 1990, p 1088. Reproduced with permission; © 1990, Little, Brown and Company.

larly when the platelets have been matched for HLA antigens to prevent sensitization in long-term patients.[27,29,30] Aggressive treatment of infections when fever or localized signs appear is indicated, as is providing protective environments (reverse isolation, laminar flow rooms, and "life islands") when granulocyte counts fall below 200/μL.[27,29,30] Stimulation of the bone marrow (myelostimulatory therapy) with androgens, etiocholanolone, lithium, and ceruloplasmin has been effective.[27,29,30] Antilymphocyte globulin (ALG) and antithymocyte globulin (ATG) are used in conjunction with granulocyte-macrophage colony-stimulating factor (GM-CSF) and bone marrow transplantation, depending on the age of the patient and the response to therapy.[27–30] Splenectomy affords an increase in the effective life span of the available circulating blood cells; however, there is no evidence to support improved bone marrow function after splenectomy, and patients do not experience remission.[27,30]

Course and Prognosis. The overall mortality in adults with aplastic anemia is 65 percent to 75 percent, with a median survival time of about 3 months.[31–33] Children with acquired aplastic anemia have a 50 percent survival rate whether they are treated with supportive care or myelostimulatory agents.[34–36] Patients who have undergone bone marrow transplantation from an HLA-identical sibling have survival rates of 70 percent in young patients or those who have not received blood products.[29] In general, the prognosis is best when the causative agent can be identified and eliminated so that the bone marrow can recover. The outlook is better for patients with erythrocyte hypoplasia than for those with pancytopenia. Patients with severe pancytopenic aplastic anemia have the worst prognosis.[30]

Anemia of Chronic Renal Failure

Etiology and Pathogenesis. The anemia of chronic renal failure occurs from (1) failure of the renal excretory function, leading to hemolysis, bone marrow cell depression, and blood loss, and (2) failure of the renal endocrine function, which causes impaired erythropoietin production and bone marrow compensation.[37]

Laboratory Features. This anemia is characterized by a decreased red cell count and low hemoglobin and hematocrit values. Some red cells appear grossly deformed with a few large spicules. The total and differential leukocyte counts and the platelet count are usually normal.[37]

Clinical Manifestations. Any of the clinical manifestations described above (see General Effects of Anemia) may be evident in chronic renal failure. The anemia of chronic renal failure is due to a decrease in or absence of erythropoietin. The hematocrit falls in proportion to the degree of renal insufficiency, and uremia occurs as the glomerular filtration rate falls below 40 mL/min.[38] Signs and symptoms usually manifest when the hematocrit falls to 20 percent or below and include those listed under General Effects of Anemia. Due to increased utilization of immunosuppressive therapy in chronic renal failure, thrombocytopenia and neutropenia also develop, and many patients present with purpura and GI and gynecologic bleeding.[39–41] Patients treated with androgen therapy

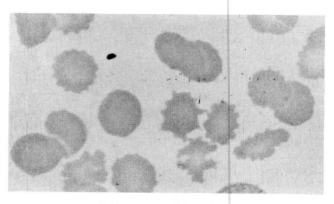

Schistocytes and Burr Cells

often present with fluid retention, hirsutism, skin infections, cholestasis, acne, virilization in women, pain at the injection site, and hematomas.[37,42]

Treatment. Therapy consists of providing the elements necessary for red cell production in the form of adequate nutritional intake, multivitamins with folic acid, and iron therapy in those patients with documented iron deficiency.[37,38,42,43] Transfusion with packed cells or intravenous (IV) synthetic erythropoietin is used to increase the oxygen-carrying capacity; androgen therapy to stimulate erythropoietin production is also used.[37,38,42,43]

Course and Prognosis. Chronic renal insufficiency is a progressive disease. When compromised kidney function causes dangerous or irreversible clinical consequences, renal substitution therapy with hemodialysis, hemofiltration, or peritoneal dialysis is usually required.[43,44] Renal transplantation is justified only when the relative risk of surgery is outweighed by the prospects for successful allograft function.[45] One-year patient survival rates are 95 percent to 97 percent following transplantation.[45]

Anemias of Vitamin B₁₂ or Folate Deficiency

Etiology and Pathogenesis. The anemia resulting from a deficiency of either vitamin B_{12} or folic acid is caused by a disruption in DNA synthesis of the blast cells in the bone marrow. This disruption produces very large abnormal bone marrow cells called **megaloblasts.** In the peripheral blood the red cells are larger than normal and macrocytic, the granulocytes are hypersegmented, and the numbers of red cells, white cells, and platelets are decreased.

The classic anemia in this classification is pernicious anemia. The fundamental defect causing pernicious anemia is the lack of intrinsic factor. Without it, vitamin B_{12} cannot be absorbed, thus leading to vitamin B_{12} deficiency. This deficiency results in disordered nucleic acid metabolism, which causes **megaloblastic dysplasia,** a condition involving abnormal production and maturation of red cell, white cell, and platelet systems. There is strong evidence that pernicious anemia develops as a result of genetically determined autoimmune disease which is manifested by serum and gastric juice antibodies against intrinsic factor and parietal cells.[46] The biochemical basis of the neurologic lesions in pernicious anemia is not known. There can be peripheral nerve degeneration, degeneration of the posterior columns of the spinal cord, or both together. There is some evidence of abnormal fatty acid metabolism in the peripheral nerves and degeneration of the white matter in the spinal cord in animals.[47]

Laboratory Features. The peripheral blood shows low RBC counts of 500,000–750,000/mm³, low WBC counts of 4,000–5,000/mm³, and low platelet counts of 50,000/mm³. These counts are usually not as low as those seen in aplastic anemia. The bone marrow shows megaloblastic dysplasia, which results in a pe-

ripheral blood picture of macrocytosis and hypersegmented neutrophils. The Schilling test, which measures excretion of radioactive B_{12}, is low and the serum level of vitamin B_{12} is low. Gastric analysis reveals a lack of free hydrochloric acid in the gastric juice (achlorhydria).[47]

Folate deficiencies resemble vitamin B_{12} deficiencies except for the neurologic disease, which is more characteristic of vitamin B_{12} deficiency. Folate deficiencies are usually the result of dietary deficiencies, alcoholism and cirrhosis, pregnancy, or infancy.

Clinical Manifestations. The clinical features of vitamin B_{12} deficiency include nonspecific manifestations of megaloblastic anemia or nonspecific glossitis, elevated serum lactic dehydrogenase levels, weight loss, neurologic abnormalities, decreased serum B_{12} levels, methylmalonic acidemia, and response to vitamin B_{12} therapy with lack of response to folic acid therapy.[47] The neurologic abnormalities include symmetric paresthesias of the feet and hands with vibratory sense and proprioception disturbances. The paresthesias progress to spastic ataxia owing to degenerative changes of the dorsal and lateral columns of the spinal cord. Cerebral signs include irritability, somnolence, memory impairment, and perversion of taste, smell, and vision, as well as psychological and mental derangement often referred to as "megaloblastic madness."[47–49] Folate deficiency manifestations include those of nonspecific megaloblastic anemia as well as a history of circumstances likely to result in folic acid deficiency such as a poor or fad diet, frank malabsorption, or alcoholism. In folate deficiency, cerebral symptoms such as irritability, memory loss, and personality changes are seen.[47–49]

Treatment. Replacement of vitamin B_{12} and folic acid is indicated in vitamin B_{12} and folic acid deficiency anemias, respectively (see Table 12–6). Transfusion therapy may be indicated in elderly or critically ill patients.[47–49] Serum hypokalemia should be treated with potassium supplements to prevent sudden death, reportedly associated with a sharp drop in serum potassium seen in vitamin B_{12} therapy.[50]

Course and Prognosis. The majority of patients respond well to replacement therapy; however, continued assessment and monitoring of these patients are essential to prevent hematologic or neurologic relapse secondary to inadequate therapy.[51] Prophylactic vitamin B_{12} is indicated in patients who have undergone total gastrectomy, ileal resection, and gastric bypass. Prophylactic folic acid is useful during pregnancy, in premature infants, and for patients on dialysis therapy.[48]

Iron Deficiency Anemia

Etiology and Pathogenesis. Iron deficiency, the most common nutritional deficiency in the world, is the most common cause of anemia. Iron deficiency results in the unavailability of iron for hemoglobin synthesis. This may be due to low intake, diminished absorption, physiologically increased requirements such as pregnancy, excessive iron loss such as chronic hemorrhage, or inadequate utilization of iron such as anemia of chronic disorders. Iron is one of the most carefully conserved body substances, and under normal conditions very little is lost except as a result of bleeding. Normal dietary requirements, if 10 percent is absorbed, are as follows: adult men, 10 mg/day; adult women, 20 mg/day; and pregnant women, 35 mg/day. A normal diet supplies the adult with about 10–15 mg/day.[52]

Laboratory Features. In latent iron deficiency there may be no anemia, but after receiving iron, these patients respond with a significant increase in blood hemoglobin. In a typical case caused by chronic bleeding, the reduction in hemoglobin concentration is proportionately greater than the reduction in the red cell count. The red cells are smaller and paler than normal cells due to the decreased amount of hemoglobin and are described as hypochromic, microcytic red cells. The white cells are usually normal. The platelet count varies, depending on the cause of the deficiency. In severely anemic children and infants, thrombocytopenia may be present. In patients who are bleeding, thrombocytosis may be present. Serum ferritin is decreased, serum iron is decreased, iron binding capacity is increased, and tissue iron stores are decreased.[52]

Clinical Manifestations. The majority of patients are asymptomatic; however, patients may experience general symptoms of anemia such as weakness, fatigue, dyspnea, palpitations, irritability, headaches, light-headedness, and pica (craving for nonfood substances, particularly ice).[53–56] In severe cases, GI symptoms are seen, such as glossitis and stomatitis, esophageal webbing, and atrophic gastritis, as well as changes in the fingernails, conjunctival pallor, and splenomegaly.[53–56]

Treatment. Iron deficiency anemia is treated with oral administration of ferrous sulfate (300 mg one to three times daily) between meals or ferrous gluconate until hematologic normality is reached. Thereafter it is important to continue the treatment for 4 to 6 months to build iron stores to approximately 500 mg.[56] Urgent treatment may be accomplished with iron-dextran infusions or intramuscular injections of 200 or

500 mg.[53,55,56] Nutritional therapy alone is not therapeutic but rather is an adjunct to care.[55] Although iron therapy will remediate the iron deficiency anemia, the underlying cause must be sought and corrected.[56]

Course and Prognosis. The symptoms may be alleviated in the first few days of treatment. The reticulocyte count usually reaches maximum levels in 7 to 12 days, and the hemoglobin is usually normal by 2 months.[55] The prognosis is excellent if the underlying cause is benign; however, even in patients with incurable disease states, treatment of iron deficiency anemia with iron therapy can increase the comfort of the patient.[55]

Anemias Related to Inherited Disorders of the Red Cell

Thalassemia

Anemia can also be caused by increased destruction or hemolysis of red cells. Hemolytic anemias are characterized by decreased red cell survival rates. The thalassemias are examples of an anemia caused by decreased red cell survival rates.[57] The red cells produced are abnormal and prone to destruction. This destruction is based on an intrinsic defect in the red cells.

Etiology and Pathogenesis. The thalassemias are a group of diseases associated with the presence of mutant genes that suppress the rate of synthesis of globin chains. Thalassemias are classified according to the polypeptide chain or chains with deficient synthesis, such as α-thalassemia or β-thalassemia.[57]

A deficiency in one or more polypeptide chains causes decreased hemoglobin synthesis and an imbalance between α- and non-α-chain production. Because of the lack of hemoglobin, the anemia is severe and the peripheral cells are microcytic and hypochromic. The disruption of the globin balance causes the normal chains to build up and precipitate within the cytoplasm. This damages the cell membranes, which leads to premature cell destruction. For example, in homozygous β-thalassemia, the deficiency of β-chain synthesis results in the accumulation of α-chains, which aggregate to form insoluble inclusions in bone marrow erythroid precursors. These inclusions cause early destruction of 70 percent to 85 percent of marrow normoblasts. In response to this massive destruction, erythroid cell proliferation in homozygous β-thalassemia is significant.[57]

Laboratory Features. Laboratory values vary, depending on the severity of the imbalance, which is determined by the genetic pattern. Due to the decrease in hemoglobin, the red cells are hypochromic and microcytic. Many target cells are present. In homozygous or major syndromes the hemoglobin is often less than 7 gm/dL, and there are nucleated red cells in the peripheral blood. The leukocyte number is usually increased, but platelet number is normal. The bone marrow is hypercellular with profound normoblastic hyperplasia. There is evidence of hemolysis

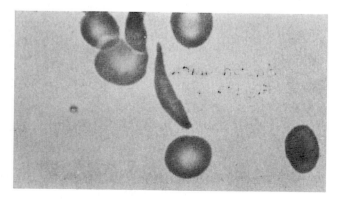

Sickle Cell

with increased unconjugated bilirubin levels and increased excretion of urobilin and urobilinogen.[57]

Clinical Manifestations. Patients may have any of the clinical manifestations described earlier (see General Effects of Anemia). The clinical findings are the result of α- or β-globin production in α-thalassemias and α-globin chain excess and persistent hemoglobin F production in the β-thalassemias.[57–60]

α-Thalassemias are found primarily in Asian individuals; however, they have also been increasingly documented in individuals of Mediterranean or African descent.[59] Usually patients with α-thalassemia minor are silent carriers or present with mild to moderate anemia. They are identified during familial studies following the identification of a family member with Bart's hemoglobin, hydrops fetalis, or hemoglobin H disease (α-thalassemia major).[57,59] Infants with hemoglobin Bart's fetalis syndrome are pale, edematous, and have hepatomegaly, splenomegaly, and ascites.[57,59] Individuals with hemoglobin H disease have typical facies and bone changes seen in β-thalassemia, splenomegaly, and hepatomegaly.[57,59]

β-Thalassemia occurs mainly in individuals of Mediterranean descent and presents as thalassemia major, intermedia, or minor.[59] Patients with thalassemia major have skull bone deformities from intra- and extramedullary bone marrow expansion, mongoloid facies, bowing and rarefaction of long bones, extension of bone marrow into paraspinal or intraabdominal tumors, hepatomegaly, splenomegaly, and cardiac failure or endocrinopathies such as diabetes mellitus and hypogonadism from excessive intestinal iron absorption.[58] Patients with thalassemia intermedia show fewer effects of iron overload, growth retardation, marrow expansion, and splenomegaly; however, deforming bone and joint disease, chronic leg ulceration, and infection are common in this form of thalassemia.[57,58] Thalassemia minor is usually relatively asymptomatic.[59]

Treatment. Children with thalassemia are treated with blood transfusion therapy to maintain a hemoglobin level of 10–14 g/dL to ensure normal growth and development and to avoid skeletal deformities. Subcutaneous infusion with desferrioxamine, an iron-chelating agent, 8 to 12 hours daily for 5 to 6 days a week at doses of 2–6 g/day is required to manage iron overload from transfusion therapy.[57–59] Splenectomy is indicated in cases with hypersplenism, but it requires aggressive management of infection following the procedure.[58] Bone marrow transplantation has been used in severe β-thalassemia. The best candidates are younger children, as older children have a high rejection and mortality rate.[58] Folic acid administration is used. As this is a genetically transmitted disease, it is important for patients and parents to receive appropriate genetic counseling.[58]

Course and Prognosis. Infants with hemoglobin Bart's hydrops fetalis are usually stillborn or die within hours to days of birth. Some patients with hemoglobin H disease live a full life.[59] Patients with β-thalassemia intermedia can expect to live until middle age; however, iron loading and crippling bone disease occur in the third and fourth decades.[61,62] Individuals with β-thalassemia major who are transfusion dependent rarely live past 25 years of age, and the death rate increases markedly after age 15.[63]

Sickle Cell Anemia

Etiology and Pathogenesis. Sickle cell anemia is caused by hemoglobin S, which is a substitution of valine for glutamic acid in the sixth position of the β-chain. This disease is the most common heritable hematologic disease in the world.[10] This apparently minor change in the molecular structure causes profound changes in hemoglobin stability and solubility. Hemoglobin S, under decreased oxygen tension, undergoes polymerization, which caused the red cell to assume a sickled shape. Patients who are homozygous produce only hemoglobin S.[64] No Hb A is synthesized, since all the β-chains are S chains which combine with normal α-chains to form Hb S. In heterozygous patients with sickle cell trait, both normal and S chains are formed[65]. Since fewer abnormal chains are produced than normal ones, the amount of Hb A usually exceeds that of Hb S. It has been suggested that preferential sickling of cells with malarial parasites reduces the number of parasites and allows children with sickle cell trait who are infected with these parasites to reach reproductive age. This may have provided a selective advantage to the Hb S trait, thereby preventing S from being genetically eliminated.[10]

The pathogenetic signs and symptoms of sickle cell disease all relate to the red cell sickling. Sickled red cells have a decreased survival time, which causes anemia. Sickled cells cause vascular occlusion, which results in capillary stasis, venous thrombosis, and arterial emboli. The most dangerous feature of sickle cell anemia is the occurrence of acute episodes of "crisis," which can be hemolytic or vascular (Fig. 12–18).[10,64,65]

Laboratory Features. The laboratory features in sickle cell anemia are distinctive. The anemia is usually severe, with hypochromic red cells of different shapes and sizes. Target red cells are present, and occasionally sickled cells can be seen on smears. Red cell breakdown products are increased, which increases serum bilirubin, urobilinogen, and urobilin levels. Acute hemolytic crisis is characterized by hemoglobinuria, leukocytosis, and normoblastosis; diffuse intravascular coagulation may develop.[10,64,65]

Clinical Manifestations. Sickle cell anemia and sickle cell trait are found almost entirely in the black race.[59] Hemolysis of the sickle cells occurs in the spleen or vascular space, and vaso-occlusive events occur in the small capillaries and venules caused by sickle cells.[58,60] The red cell life span is already shortened by the sickling and may precipitate a hemolytic crisis with jaundice.[64] Sudden massive pooling of red cells, particularly in the spleen, can create a sequestration crisis, which is thought to result in the deaths that occur in the first years of life.[64] Infarctive crises or painful episodes are a result of obstruction of blood

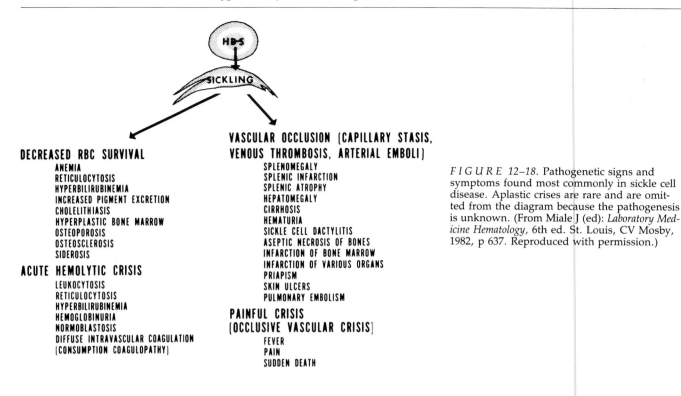

DECREASED RBC SURVIVAL
ANEMIA
RETICULOCYTOSIS
HYPERBILIRUBINEMIA
INCREASED PIGMENT EXCRETION
CHOLELITHIASIS
HYPERPLASTIC BONE MARROW
OSTEOPOROSIS
OSTEOSCLEROSIS
SIDEROSIS

ACUTE HEMOLYTIC CRISIS
LEUKOCYTOSIS
RETICULOCYTOSIS
HYPERBILIRUBINEMIA
HEMOGLOBINURIA
NORMOBLASTOSIS
DIFFUSE INTRAVASCULAR COAGULATION
(CONSUMPTION COAGULOPATHY)

VASCULAR OCCLUSION (CAPILLARY STASIS, VENOUS THROMBOSIS, ARTERIAL EMBOLI)
SPLENOMEGALY
SPLENIC INFARCTION
SPLENIC ATROPHY
HEPATOMEGALY
CIRRHOSIS
HEMATURIA
SICKLE CELL DACTYLITIS
ASEPTIC NECROSIS OF BONES
INFARCTION OF BONE MARROW
INFARCTION OF VARIOUS ORGANS
PRIAPISM
SKIN ULCERS
PULMONARY EMBOLISM

PAINFUL CRISIS (OCCLUSIVE VASCULAR CRISIS)
FEVER
PAIN
SUDDEN DEATH

FIGURE 12–18. Pathogenetic signs and symptoms found most commonly in sickle cell disease. Aplastic crises are rare and are omitted from the diagram because the pathogenesis is unknown. (From Miale J (ed): *Laboratory Medicine Hematology,* 6th ed. St. Louis, CV Mosby, 1982, p 637. Reproduced with permission.)

vessels, tissue hypoxia, and tissue death, and may occur throughout the body.[58,59,64] Vaso-occlusive events are described in Table 12–7. Children with sickle cell anemia are shorter and experience delayed puberty, but attain normal height with late adolescent growth.[64] Bony abnormalities, "hand-foot" syndrome with periostitis of the metacarpal and metatarsal bones, splenomegaly, inability to concentrate urine, priapism with subsequent impotence, underdeveloped genitalia and hypogonadism, hepatomegaly, jaundice, gallstones, tachycardia, acute chest syndrome (fever, chest pain, increasing white cell count, and pulmonary infiltrates), retinal vessel obstruction, cerebrovascular accidents, and leg ulcers are all seen in sickle cell disease patients.[64] Pregnant women exhibit signs of pyelonephritis, pulmonary infarction, pneumonia, antepartum hemorrhage, premature fetal delivery, and fetal death.[64]

TABLE 12–7. Vaso-Occlusive Consequences of Sickle Cell Disease

Event	Incidence	Features
Acute		
Painful episodes	>50% of patients with Hb SS and Hb S β-thalassemia	Mild to severe pain, one or several areas
Chest syndrome	10%–20% of adults	Difficult to distinguish from pneumonia; may involve entire lung
Priapism	10%–40% of males	Can have a more chronic form; causes impotence
Cerebrovascular accidents	5%–10% of children	Usually subarachnoid bleeding in adults
Hepatopathy	<2% of adults	Bilirubin may reach >80 mg/dL
Chronic		
Aseptic bone necrosis	10%–25% of adults	Hips and shoulders, common in Hb SC
Proliferative retinopathy	50% of adults with Hb SC, <5% Hb SS	Can lead to retinal detachment
Leg ulcers	10%–20%	Can be severe and disabling
Functional asplenia and autosplenectomy	Starts in infancy; >90% of adults with Hb SS	Predisposes to sepsis
Nephropathy	Renal failure in older patients	Nephrotic syndrome, renal failure

From Sternberg MH: Hemoglobinopathies and thalassemias, in Stein JH, et al (eds): *Internal Medicine,* 3rd ed. Boston, Little, Brown & Co, 1990, p 1095. Reproduced with permission; © 1990, Little, Brown and Company.

Treatment. Currently there are no safe effective antisickling agents, and treatment is primarily supportive in vaso-occlusive crisis with hydration, analgesics, hypnotics, a search for infection, and subsequent appropriate antibiotic therapy.[59] Transfusions are used to restore normal hematocrit levels, and splenectomy is performed in children with sequestration syndrome.[58,59,64] During pregnancy, folic acid should be given, along with iron supplements if iron deficiency is present; however, transfusion should be given only when clinical and hematologic indicators are present.[58]

Course and Prognosis. Sickle cell anemia is a serious disorder, and many patients die in childhood, especially in sequestration crisis.[59] Functional hyposplenia predisposes individuals to infections such as pneumonia and chronic pyelonephritis with renal failure.[59] Heart failure, bone marrow and fat emboli, shock, and organ failure are frequent causes of death. In developed countries, patients may survive into the third and fourth decades, whereas survival past childhood in underdeveloped countries is unusual.[58]

Hereditary Spherocytosis

Etiology and Pathogenesis. In hereditary spherocytosis, the red cells have abnormal membranes, which cause them to have a decreased survival time. The disease is inherited as an autosomal dominant trait and is characterized by red cells that are fragile microspherocytes. In addition, there is increased destruction of **spherocytes** (abnormal spherical erythrocytes) in the spleen. Patients have anemia, intermittent jaundice, splenomegaly, and uniform responsiveness to splenectomy. Current research suggests that the intrinsic defect is in the protein portion of the membrane.[66]

Laboratory Features. The concentration of hemoglobin within the red cells is increased. Reticulocytosis is present, and microspherocytes are seen on the blood smear. Osmotic fragility is increased, and serum unconjugated bilirubin is increased. Following splenectomy, the hemoglobin is in the high normal range.[65]

Clinical Manifestations. Hereditary spherocytosis is the most common hereditary hemolytic anemia and is most common in people with a northern European background.[59,66,67] The major clinical manifestations are anemia, jaundice, splenomegaly, bile pigment gallstones, and chronic leg ulcers.[59,66] The anemia is usually mild due to compensation by the erythropoietic bone marrow cells. Aplastic crisis precipitated by an infection may be seen with associated fever, abdominal discomfort, nausea, vomiting, rapidly increasing weakness, pallor, tachycardia, low blood pressure, and shock.[59,66]

Treatment. Treatment usually consists of splenectomy, which may be performed in infancy in severe cases but more commonly is done in late childhood. Transfusion is usually indicated only in aplastic crisis.[59,66,68]

Course and Prognosis. Most patients have no or mild anemia, fluctuating degrees of jaundice, and episodes of aplastic or hemolytic anemia.[66] Splenectomy is usually curative; however, the subsequent risk of acquiring a serious infection is significant.[66]

Glucose-6-Phosphate Dehydrogenase Deficiency

Etiology and Pathogenesis. The energy required for membrane function and cellular integrity is derived from the anaerobic and aerobic metabolism of glucose. Traditionally, hemolytic anemias caused by enzyme deficiencies are called nonspherocytic, to distinguish them from classic hereditary spherocytosis. When black soldiers receiving the antimalarial drug Primaquine began suffering hemolytic episodes, a type of hemolytic anemia caused by a deficiency of glucose-6-phosphate dehydrogenase (G-6-PD, an enzyme in the red cell glycolitic pathway) was discovered.[69] When G-6-PD–deficient RBCs are challenged by one of several drugs, glutathione is depleted, Heinz bodies form, and glucose use is inhibited. These three events cause membrane damage, which results in removal of the damaged cells by reticuloendothelial cells. Except in rare instances, G-6-PD–deficient persons do not have hemolytic anemia unless challenged by drugs.[69]

Laboratory Features. Usually this anemia is first recognized during or following an infectious illness or following exposure to a suspect drug or chemical. The hematologic tests reflect the severity of the hemolytic episode. The diagnosis is made using a specific test which measures G-6-PD activity.[69]

Clinical Manifestations. Most individuals have no clinical manifestations of this disease.[59,70] When they occur, hemolytic anemia is triggered by drug administration, infection, diabetic acidosis, the newborn period, and, in one subset, exposure to fava beans.[59,70]

Treatment. Treatment is usually preventative through avoidance of drugs that trigger hemolytic episodes, and aggressive infection management.[70] Some patients may require transfusion therapy.[70]

Course and Prognosis. The prognosis is usually good as the episodes of hemolytic crisis are usually self-limiting except in fava bean–susceptible individuals, in whom shock may develop in a short period of time.[70]

Anemias Related to Extrinsic Red Cell Destruction or Loss

The final categories in absolute anemias are caused by extrinsic abnormalities. The most important of these categories are the immune hemolytic anemias caused by antibodies to red cells. These anemias are subdivided into those caused by isoantibodies, which are the result of accidental immunization of individuals, such as hemolytic disease of the newborn, and those caused by autoantibodies, where individuals make antibodies against their own red cells.

Hemolytic Disease of the Newborn

Etiology and Pathogenesis. When fetal red cells cross the placenta, they may stimulate the production of maternal antibodies against antigens on the fetal red cell not inherited from the mother. These maternal antibodies cross into the fetal circulation and cause destruction of fetal cells. Fetal-maternal ABO incompatibility is the most common cause of hemolytic disease of the newborn (HDNB), but Rh incompatibility is clinically more important because of the severity of the hemolytic disease in the fetus.[71] With the introduction of Rh treatment, the total incidence of HDNB in Rh-negative women has been greatly reduced.[72]

Laboratory Features. Anemia, **reticulocytosis** (an increased number of circulating reticulocytes), and nucleated red cells are seen in the peripheral blood. There is a rough correlation between the hemoglobin levels and the severity of the disease.[71] Untreated infants may experience a rapid fall in hemoglobin levels after birth.[72] **Leukocytosis** is present, but platelet counts are usually normal. Infants with severe disease may have thrombocytopenia. Serum bilirubin, a hemolytic breakdown product, is readily transferred across the placenta. At birth, the baby's bilirubin level reflects both the severity of the **hemolytic** process and the ability of the baby's liver enzyme system to conjugate and excrete bilirubin. Cord blood red cells show a characteristic positive direct antiglobulin test, reflecting the maternal antibodies attached to the infant's red cells.[71,72]

During pregnancy, laboratory tests of amniotic fluid for bilirubin and antibodies and test of the mother's peripheral blood for maternal sensitization are useful in predicting whether infants will be affected by HDNB.[71,72]

Clinical Manifestations. The clinical manifestations of this disease are hemolytic anemia, extramedullary erythropoiesis, and hyperbilirubinemia.[72] Jaundice, petechial hemorrhages, hepatomegaly, splenomegaly, heart failure (with pulmonary edema, pleural effusions, ascites, and edema), kernicterus (a condition in the newborn marked by severe neural symptoms, associated with high levels of bilirubin in the blood), and diffuse intravascular coagulation are seen in these infants. Many infants die in utero.[59,72]

Treatment. Amniocentesis, in utero transfusion, and early delivery have been performed on fetuses with severe **erythroblastosis.**[59,72] Exchange transfusion lowers the serum bilirubin and the antibody content of the neonatal blood and removes cells susceptible to hemolysis.[59] Phototherapy and phenobarbital are used to lower the bilirubin. Albumin has been used to increase the albumin-binding capacity and reduce the risk of kernicterus and the need for exchange transfusion.[59,72]

Course and Prognosis. Many infants appear normal at birth, only to develop jaundice within 2 to 3 hours. Petechial hemorrhages develop soon after birth, and kernicterus is usually seen late in the second day of significant jaundice.[59] Successful Rho-gam administration prevention programs have reduced the perinatal mortality to about 1 percent to 2 percent.[72]

Antibody-Mediated Drug Reactions

Etiology and Pathogenesis. Drug-induced immune hemolytic anemias are examples of diseases where exposure to a drug causes destruction and lysis of the allergic or sensitized person's own red cells. Drugs can lead to red cell hemolysis by four different immune mechanisms (Table 12–8).[73]

Hapten Mechanisms. In this mechanism, exemplified by penicillin, the drug combines with a component of the RBC membrane. An antibody is developed against the drug. When the drug is given again, it coats the red cells, and the antibody attaches to the drug–red cell complex.[73] The antigen-antibody complex then causes hemolysis.

Immune Complex Formation. In this situation, the drug alone induces an antibody response. Subsequent administration of the drug causes formation of drug-antibody complexes which bind complement and attach to the RBC. The RBC is an "innocent bystander" and is hemolyzed. The immune complex can also bind to platelet and leukocyte membranes, causing anemia,

TABLE 12–8. Types of Drug-Induced Hemolytic Anemia

Type	Role of Drug	Type of Attachment to RBC	Mechanism of Cell Destruction	Direct Antiglobulin Test Positive With	Example
Hapten	Combines with RBC membrane	Antibody attached to drug-RBC complex	Agglutination, extravascular	Anti-IgG	Penicillin
Immune complex formation	Induces antibody to drug	Drug-antibody complex attached to RBC membrane	Lysis, intravascular	Anticomplement	Stibophen Quinidine
Autoantibody	Induces antibody to RBC	Antibody to RBC membrane Rh antigens	Agglutination, extravascular	Anti-IgG	α-Methyldopa
Nonspecific	Alters RBC membrane protein	Plasma proteins attach to altered RBC protein	Unknown	Anti-IgG, anticomplement, other antibodies	Cephalosporins

From Williams WJ, et al (eds): *Hematology*, 3rd ed. New York, McGraw-Hill, 1983, p 607. Reproduced by permission of McGraw-Hill, Inc.

leukopenia, and thrombocytopenia. Quinidine is a common drug causing this type of reaction.[73]

Autoantibody Induction. This mechanism was first studied in cases of hemolytic anemia with patients taking the antihypertensive agent β-methyldopa (Aldomet 1). The drug appears to induce antibody formation to red cell membrane Rh antigens.[73] About one fourth of the patients receiving this drug develop a positive antiglobulin test.

Nonspecific. In the final mechanism, seen in cephalosporin sensitivity, the drug alters the RBC membrane protein. Plasma proteins attach to the altered RBC protein and cause a positive serologic test but no cell hemolysis.[73]

Laboratory Features. The laboratory features for all four mechanisms are nonspecific and show increased red cell turnover and anemia if hemolysis becomes decompensated. Serologic tests such as the direct antiglobulin test will be positive. Leukopenia and thrombocytopenia are sometimes seen when there is drug-induced platelet or leukocyte destruction.[73]

Clinical Manifestations. Immune drug-induced hemolytic anemias vary in symptomatology and severity, depending on the mechanism involved.[59,74–76] Hapten (e.g., penicillin) and autoimmune (e.g., methyldopa) drug-induced hemolytic anemias have an insidious onset of symptoms over a period of weeks; however, immune complex hemolysis (e.g., quinine or quinidine) may have sudden, severe hemolysis with hemoglobinuria and result in acute renal failure.[75]

Treatment. Recognition and discontinuing the responsible drug are usually the only treatment necessary.[75]

Course and Prognosis. Immune hemolytic anemia due to drugs is usually mild and the prognosis is good; however, with severe hemolysis, death can occur.[75]

Acute Blood Loss

Etiology and Pathogenesis. Acute blood loss anemia may present after trauma or secondary to a disease process.[77] Acute blood loss anemia decreases the overall blood volume and impairs oxygen delivery.[77]

Laboratory Features. There is a decrease in both the hematocrit and hemoglobin due to blood loss. The hematocrit is less than 40 percent in men and 37 percent in women. The hemoglobin concentration is less than 14 g/dL in men and 12 g/dL in women.[77]

Clinical Manifestations. In a normal 70-kg person with a 5,000 mL total blood volume, 10 percent loss of blood (500 mL) rarely causes any clinical signs except occasional vasovagal syncope. A 20 percent loss (1,000 mL) usually causes no clinical symptoms at rest, but tachycardia is seen with exercise and a slight postural drop in blood pressure occurs.[77–82] A person with a 30 percent loss (1,500 mL) usually presents with flat neck veins when supine, postural hypotension, and exercise tachycardia. A 40 percent loss (2,000 mL) causes the patient's central venous pressure, cardiac output, and arterial blood pressure to fall below normal while supine and at rest, with associated air hunger, tachycardia, and cold, clammy skin.[77–82] A 50 percent loss of total blood volume (2,500 mL) often causes shock and death.[77–82]

Treatment. Blood volume replacement therapy with crystalloid solutions, colloid solutions (plasma protein, albumin, or dextran), and fresh whole blood is essential in the early management of acute hemorrhage to restore blood volume and to prevent shock.[77] Complete reliance on fresh whole blood for treating acute blood loss is contraindicated and should be reserved for patients with a low red cell mass, where tissue hypoxia is a threat.[77] Replacement of red cell mass by increased red cell production is a gradual process occurring over 2 to 5 days as the marrow stem cells proliferate and mature. Maximum red cell production is seen by the 10th day post hemorrhage.[77]

Course and Prognosis. With adequate replacement therapy, the prognosis is excellent; however, the underlying cause must be identified and treated.

Other Extrinsic Abnormalities

Other agents such as mechanical heart valves or open heart bypass machines may cause physical damage to the red cells, resulting in hemolysis. Drugs and chemicals, physical agents such as burns, or infectious agents such as malaria may result in anemia. Finally, hypersplenism and splenomegaly can cause anemia, leukopenia, or thrombocytopenia severe enough to require splenectomy.[83]

Transfusion Therapy

Medical indications for transfusion therapy are restoration or maintenance of oxygen-carrying capacity, blood volume, hemostasis, and leukocyte function.[84,85] A summary of blood components, indications, actions, contraindications, precautions, and hazards is presented in Table 12–9. Types of transfusion reactions, signs and symptoms, usual causes, treatment, and precautions are summarized in Table 12–10.

KEY CONCEPTS

- **The general effects of anemia are due to tissue hypoxia and efforts to compensate for low oxygen-carrying capacity. Vasoconstriction, pallor, tachypnea, dyspnea, tachycardia, ischemic pain, lethargy, and light-headedness may be present. In addition, signs and symptoms relating to the specific cause of the anemia may be present. These accompanying manifestations are helpful in determining the cause of the anemia.**

- **Anemia may be due to abnormally low production of red cells and/or excessive loss or destruction. A decreased production of red cells may be due to stem cell failure (aplastic anemia), lack of erythropoietin (renal disease), or nutritional deficiencies of iron, vitamin B_{12}, or folate. Excessive red cell loss**

TABLE 12–9. Summary of Blood Components

Component	Major Indications	Action	Not Indicated for	Special Precautions	Hazards	Rate of Infusion
Whole blood	Symptomatic anemia with large volume deficit	Restoration of oxygen-carrying capacity, restoration of blood volume	Condition responsive to specific component	Must be ABO-identical; labile coagulation factors deteriorate within 24 hr after collection	Infectious diseases; septic/toxic, allergic, febrile reactions; circulatory overload	For massive loss, as fast as patient can tolerate
Red blood cells	Symptomatic anemia	Restoration of oxygen-carrying capacity	Pharmacologically treatable anemia, coagulation deficiency	Must be ABO-compatible	Infectious diseases; septic/toxic, allergic, febrile reactions	As patient can tolerate but less than 4 hr
Red blood cells, leukocytes removed	Symptomatic anemia, febrile reactions from leukocyte antibodies	Restoration of oxygen-carrying capacity	Pharmacologically treatable anemia, coagulation deficiency	Must be ABO-compatible	Infectious diseases; septic/toxic allergic reaction (unless plasma also removed, e.g., by washing)	As patient can tolerate but less than 4 hr
Red blood cells, adenine-saline added	Symptomatic anemia with volume deficit	Restoration of oxygen-carrying capacity	Pharmacologically treatable anemia, coagulation deficiency	Must be ABO-compatible	Infectious diseases; septic/toxic, allergic, febrile reactions; circulatory overload	As patient can tolerate but less than 4 hr
Fresh frozen plasma	Deficit of labile and stable plasma coagulation factors and TTP	Source of labile and nonlabile plasma factors	Condition responsive to volume replacement	Should be ABO-compatible	Infectious diseases, allergic reactions, circulatory overload	Less than 4 hr
Liquid plasma and plasma	Deficit of stable coagulation factors	Source of nonlabile factors	Deficit of labile coagulation factors or volume replacement	Should be ABO-compatible	Infectious diseases, allergic reactions	Less than 4 hr
Cryoprecipitated AHF	Hemophilia A, von Willebrand's disease hypofibrinogenemia Factor XIII deficiency	Provides Factor VIII, fibrinogen, VWF, Factor XIII	Conditions not deficient in contained factors	Frequent repeat doses may be necessary	Infectious diseases, allergic reactions	Less than 4 hr
Platelets; platelets, pheresis	Bleeding from thrombocytopenia or platelet function abnormality	Improves hemostasis	Plasma coagulation deficits and some conditions with rapid platelet destruction (e.g., ITP)	Should not use some microaggregate filters (check manufacturer's instructions)	Infectious diseases; septic/toxic, allergic, febrile reactions	Less than 4 hr
Granulocytes	Neutropenia with infection	Provides granulocytes	Infection responsive to antibiotics	Must be ABO-compatible; do not use depth-type microaggregate filters	Infectious diseases, allergic reactions, febrile reactions	One pheresis unit over 2–4 hr period; closely observe for reactions

Adapted with permission from Summary Chart of Blood Components, *Circular of Information for the Use of Human Blood and Blood Components*. American Red Cross, Council of Community Blood Centers, and American Association of Blood Banks, 1991, pp 14–15.

may be due to hemolysis (ABO and Rh incompatibility, drugs) or bleeding (surgery, trauma). Inherited disorders of red cells often impair production and increase destruction of red cells.

- Determining the etiology of anemia is based on the history, differential signs and symptoms, and laboratory studies. The important differentiating features of the major anemias are as follows:

  Aplastic anemia: History of toxic or radiation injury to bone marrow. Accompanying leukopenia and thrombocytopenia. Red cells are normocytic, normochromic.

  Chronic renal failure: History of renal disease. Decreased erythropoietin (EPO) level and EPO responsiveness. Red cells are normocytic, normochromic.

  B_{12} and folate deficiency: History of poor intake or GI disease. Accompanying neurologic dysfunction. Red cells are megaloblastic (macrocytic).

  Iron deficiency: History of poor intake or chronic blood loss. Decreased serum ferritin and iron levels. Red cells are microcytic, hypochromic.

  Hemolytic: History of ABO or Rh incompatibility, or drug exposure. Increased bilirubin, jaundice, positive direct antiglobulin. Red cells are normocytic, normochromic.

  Acute blood loss: History of trauma, surgery, or known bleeding. Accompanying manifestations of volume depletion. Red cells are normal. Anemia may not be apparent until fluid loss is replaced.

- Inherited disorders of the red cell (thalassemia, sickle cell anemia, spherocytosis, G-6-PD deficiency) predispose red cells to early destruction because of abnormalities in hemoglobin structure, cell shape, membrane structure, or energy production. Manifestations of hemolysis (e.g., bilirubin, jaundice) are often present.

- The general treatment of anemias is aimed at removing the cause, if possible; restoring oxygen-carrying capacity with blood transfusion when necessary; and preventing the complications of ischemia (e.g., with rest, oxygen therapy) and hemolysis (increased fluid intake, treatment of high bilirubin levels).

Polycythemia

In polycythemias, red cells are present in excess, which increases the whole blood viscosity, which in turn causes the clinical manifestations such as hypertension.

Polycythemia Vera

Etiology and Pathogenesis. Polycythemia vera is a chronic **panmyelosis** and is part of the spectrum of myeloproliferative disorders. There is overproduction of normal red cells, white cells, and platelets. The cause is unknown. Some researchers have postulated that it is the result of damage to the undifferentiated stem cell by a virus or other agents.[86]

Laboratory Features. The diagnosis depends primarily on laboratory studies, which show an absolute increase in red cell mass and leukocytosis and thrombocytosis. The bone marrow shows **hyperplasia** of red cell, white cell, and platelet series and extension of active hematopoietic marrow into bones of the extremities. Uric acid is increased due to excessive cell proliferation, which results in an increased number of cells being destroyed. Arterial oxygen saturation is normal, which differentiates polycythemia vera from secondary (hypoxemic) erythrocytosis. Secondary findings include elevated serum vitamin B_{12} and elevated leukocyte alkaline phosphatase levels (Table 12–11).[83]

Clinical Manifestations. Common clinical manifestations include occlusive vascular lesions, mucosal hemorrhage, and hypertension, but each phase of the disease presents somewhat differently. Most of the clinical symptoms of polycythemia vera are related to the increased red cell mass, which gives rise to an increased blood viscosity.[86–89] The onset is insidious with variable manifestations in virtually any organ system.[86,87] Clinical symptoms appear between 50 and 75 years of age, and they appear more often in males and blacks.[87] In the pre-erythrocytic or developmental phase, splenomegaly, night sweats, and postbathing pruritus are common.[88] Other patients experience mild thrombohemorrhagic symptoms or **erythromelalgia** (painful erythematous palms and soles from an increased number of circulating platelets).[88]

In the erythrocytic phase, occlusive vascular lesions such as transient ischemic attacks, cerebrovascular accidents, myocardial ischemia or infarctions, portal venous obstruction, or superficial venous thrombosis occur and may be the first indication of the presence of the disease.[87,88] The hyperviscosity produces symptoms of reduced cerebral blood flow such as headaches, dizziness, and visual disturbances.[88]

Mucosal hemorrhage manifestations including epistaxis, ecchymosis, and GI and GU bleeding occur. Progressive splenomegaly, intermittent claudication, peptic ulcers, hyperuricemia, and gout are often seen.[87,88] The most striking feature is a ruddy or florid

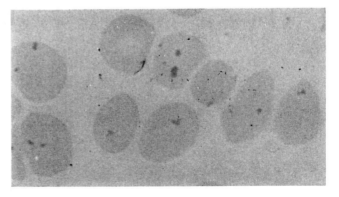

Heinz Bodies

TABLE 12-10. Transfusion Reactions

Type	Signs and Symptoms	Usual Cause	Treatment	Precautions
Acute intravascular hemolytic (immune)	Hemoglobinemia and hemoglobinuria, fever, chills, anxiety, shock, disseminated intravascular coagulation, dyspnea, chest pain, flank pain, nausea/vomiting, headache, pain at needle site and along venous tract	Incompatibility due to clerical errors; involves ABO (primarily) or other erythrocyte antigen-antibody incompatibility	Stop transfusion; hydrate, support blood pressure and respiration; induce diuresis; treat shock and DIC	Positively identify donor and recipient blood types and groups before transfusion is begun; verify with one other nurse or physician Transfuse blood slowly for first 15–20 min and/or initial one-fifth volume of blood; remain with patient In event of signs or symptoms, stop transfusion immediately, maintain patient intravenous line, and notify physician Save donor blood to re-crossmatch with patient's blood Monitor blood pressure for shock Insert urinary catheter and monitor hourly outputs Send sample of patient's blood and urine to laboratory for presence of hemoglobin (indicates intravascular hemolysis) Observe for signs of hemorrhage resulting from DIC Support medical therapies to reverse shock
Delayed extravascular hemolytic (immune)	Fever, malaise, indirect hyperbilirubinemia, increased urine urobilinogen, falling hematocrit	Destruction of RBCs; usually involves non-ABO Ag-Ab incompatibility occurring 3–10 days post transfusion	Monitor hematocrit, renal function, coagulation profile; no acute treatment generally required	Observe for posttransfusion anemia and decreasing benefit from successive transfusion
Febrile	Fever, chills, rarely hypotension	Antibodies to leukocytes or plasma proteins	Stop transfusion; give antipyretics; acetaminophen (or aspirin if not thrombocytopenic)	Use of leukocyte-poor RBCs is less likely to cause reaction
Allergic	Urticaria (hives), flushing, wheezing, laryngeal edema, rarely hypotension or anaphylaxis	Antibodies to plasma proteins	Stop transfusion; give antihistamine; if severe, epinephrine and/or steroids	Pretransfusion antihistamine; use of washed RBC components
Hypervolemic	Dyspnea, rales, hypertension, pulmonary edema, cardiac arrhythmias, precordial pain, cyanosis, dry cough, distended neck veins	Too rapid or excessive blood transfusion	Induce diuresis; phlebotomy; support cardiorespiratory system as needed	Transfuse blood slowly Prevent overload by using packed RBCs or administering divided amounts of blood Use infusion pump to regulate and maintain flow rate If signs of overload, stop transfusion immediately Place patient in semi-Fowler position to increase venous resistance

Reaction	Signs and Symptoms	Blood Factors	Nursing Responsibilities	Prevention
Noncardiogenic pulmonary edema	Dyspnea, pulmonary edema, normal cardiac pressures	Anti-HLA or antileukocyte antibodies	Support blood pressure and respiration (may require intubation)	Use washed RBCs; avoid unnecessary transfusion
Hypothermia	Chills, low temperature, irregular heart rate, possible cardiac arrest	Rapid infusion of cold blood products	Monitor temperature; if markedly subnormal, stop transfusion	Allow blood to warm at room temperature (<1 hr); Use an electric warming coil to rapidly warm blood
Electrolyte disturbances, hyperkalemia	Nausea, diarrhea, muscular weakness, flaccid paralysis, paresthesia of extremities, bradycardia, apprehension, cardiac arrest	Massive transfusions or in patients with renal problems	Kayexalate enemas if potassium >5.0 mEq/L	Use washed RBCs or fresh blood if patient at risk
Citrate intoxication (hypocalcemia)	Tingling in fingers, tetany, muscular cramps, carpopedal spasm, hyperactive reflexes, convulsions, laryngeal spasm, respiratory arrest	Massive transfusion of blood	Stop transfusion, administer calcium IV if severe	Infuse blood slowly (citrate reaction less likely to occur); If signs of tetany occur, clamp tubing immediately, maintain patient intravenous line, and notify physician
Air emboli	Sudden difficulty in breathing, sharp pain in chest, apprehension, respiratory or cardiac arrest	Air emboli from blood administered under pressure	Stop transfusion, turn patient on left side, aspirate right atrial/ventricular air emboli	When infusing blood under pressure before container is empty, if air is observed in tubing, clamp tubing immediately below air bubble, clear tubing of air by aspirating air with syringe or disconnecting tubing and allowing blood to flow until air has escaped
Bacterial sepsis	Shock, chills, fever	Contaminated blood component	Stop transfusion; support blood pressure; give antibiotics	Care in blood collection and storage
Delayed reactions, transmission of infection	Signs of infection after transfusion; e.g., jaundice from hepatitis, bacterial or toxin contamination—high fever, severe headache or substernal pain, hypotension, intense flushing, vomiting/diarrhea	Hepatitis, AIDS, malaria, syphilis, bacteria, viruses, other	Stop transfusion, send culture; sensitivity tests, treat specific infection	Blood is tested for HBsAg (hepatitis B), syphilis, and in most centers HTLV-III (AIDS); positive units are destroyed; Individuals at risk for carrying certain viruses are deterred from donation; Observe for signs of infection

Adapted with permission from Whaley LR, Wong L (eds): *Nursing Care of Infants and Children*, 4th ed. St. Louis, CV Mosby, 1991; and Pisciotto PT, Civarella D, Kurtz SR, Lane TA, Moroff G, Morrison FS, Roberts SC (eds): *Blood Transfusion Therapy: A Physician's Handbook*, 3rd ed. Arlington, Va, American Association of Blood Banks, 1989.

TABLE 12–11. Differential Diagnosis of Polycythemia Vera From Secondary Polycythemia and Spurious Erythrocytosis

Findings	Polycythemia Vera	Secondary Polycythemia	Spurious Erythrocytosis
Splenomegaly	Present	Absent	Absent
Arterial oxygen saturation	Normal	Decreased or normal	Normal
Thrombocytosis	Present	Absent	Absent
Blood histamine	Increased	Normal	Normal
Serum VB$_{12}$BC	Increased	Normal	Normal
Serum vitamin B$_{12}$	Increased	Normal	Normal
Leukocyte alkaline phosphatase	Increased	Normal	Normal
Bone marrow	Panmyelosis	Erythroid hyperplasia	Normal
Basophil count	Increased	Normal	Normal
Leukocytosis	Present	Absent	Absent
Erythropoietin	Decreased	Increased	Normal
Serum iron concentration	Decreased	Normal	Normal

From Williams WJ, et al (eds): *Hematology*, 3rd ed. New York, McGraw-Hill, 1983, p 630. Reproduced by permission of McGraw-Hill, Inc.

face, telangiectasis of the cheeks and nose, and purplish cyanosis of the lips and ears.[86–89] Hypertension is seen in about half of the patients. Distension of the retinal veins with a dark purple coloring is another important clinical finding.[87] As the disease develops into the spent or postpolycythemia myeloid metaplasia phase, many patients complain only of asthenia; however, progressive splenomegaly, severe anemia, hemorrhage (particularly cutaneous), hepatomegaly, weight loss, and wasting often occur.[87,88]

Treatment. There is no cure. Treatment is directed at reducing the increased blood volume, blood viscosity, red cell mass, and platelet counts by phlebotomy, radioactive phosphorus, and chemotherapeutic agents.[86–89] Phlebotomy of 350 to 500 mL every other day until a normal hematocrit is reached alleviates many symptoms for most patients. Phlebotomy of only 200 to 300 mL should be considered for elderly patients or those with cardiovascular disease.[86,87] In the past, a hematocrit of 50 percent was used as the upper limit of hematocrit tolerated before phlebotomy was used. Recently, studies have found that increased vascular complications, decreased cerebral blood flow, and decreased mental alertness occurred when hematocrits began to exceed 46 percent.[90–92] Phlebotomy is effective in controlling red cell mass, but myelosuppressive therapy is needed to control hepatosplenomegaly and thrombocytosis.[93,94] This is accomplished with radioactive phosphorus (2.3 mCi/m^2) given IV following an initial series of phlebotomies, and may require a follow-up dose in 12 to 16 weeks to bring the disease under control.[86] It is effective in 75 percent to 80 percent of cases, and remissions lasting 6 to 24 months often occur.[95–97] Chemotherapy with the alkylating agents of busulfan and pipobroman are recommended as they do not increase the risk of acute leukemia seen with chlorambucil.[98,99]

Course and Prognosis. Untreated polycythemia vera has a poor prognosis, with a survival of less than 2 years.[100,101] The development of thrombosis, hemorrhage, and myeloproliferative syndromes is common.[87] Treated patients have a median survival of 7 to 15 years, with the most common causes of death being thrombosis, hemorrhage, leukemia, and other myeloproliferative conditions.[86,87]

Secondary Polycythemia

Etiology and Pathogenesis. Secondary polycythemia is an absolute erythrocytosis caused by an increased stimulation of RBC production, usually in response to tissue hypoxia. There are inappropriate secondary polycythemias which are caused by renal or other organ tumors which cause an increase in erythropoietin production.

As this type of polycythemia demonstrates an increase in red cell mass with no involvement of other marrow elements, it is most commonly seen with a known hypoxic stimulus, inappropriate erythropoietin, or excess adrenocortical steroids or androgens.[87]

Laboratory Features. The laboratory findings confirm increased red cell production with no increase in white cells or platelets. Erythropoietin is increased.[102]

Clinical Manifestations. The symptoms are those of the underlying disease state such as cardiovascular disease with right-to-left shunt, chronic lung disease or alveolar hypoventilation, low barometric pressure, or abnormal hemoglobin concentration.[87,89]

Treatment. As this is a physiologic compensation, the clinical treatment is directed at identifying and treating the underlying cause.[87,103] Phlebotomy has been used to reduce cardiovascular work and appears to be helpful in both the cardiovascular and chronic obstructive pulmonary disease patient.[103]

Course and Prognosis. The course and prognosis are influenced by the underlying disease process.

Relative Polycythemia

Etiology and Pathogenesis. Relative (spurious) polycythemia is characterized by an increased hematocrit in the presence of normal or decreased total RBC mass. There are two types of patients showing this characteristic. The first group has this laboratory value secondary to an obvious disturbance in fluid balance, such as is seen in severe dehydration or endocrinologic disorders. The other group, often described as having stress polycythemia, has hypertension, increased hematocrits, and no increase in total RBC mass or obvious fluid loss. Research is continuing on the etiology and pathogenesis of the phenomena.[103]

Laboratory Features. All hematologic tests are normal except for elevated hematocrit, hemoglobin, and red cell counts. The red cell volume is normal. Increased cholesterol and uric acid values are common.[103]

Clinical Manifestations. The manifestations depend on the underlying cause. In dehydration, the patient will have flat neck veins, skin turgor, thirst, tachycardia, and, in severe cases, low cardiac output and blood pressure. If the underlying condition is stress related, the symptoms are those of a catecholamine stress response. These patients are usually white middle-aged men.[104] In patients with spurious polycythemia due to smoking, the problem is usually chronic and the symptoms due to hyperviscosity described for polycythemia vera are often found.[87,104]

Treatment. As this is a spurious polycythemia, it is important to recognize and treat the underlying cause. Fluid administration and management will resolve dehydration; however, spurious polycythemia is likely to be associated with a long-term condition that will require concurrent medical management. When the condition is a result of stress, identification of the stressors and stress management are indicated, with long-term follow-up.[87,104] In spurious polycythemia due to smoking, the patient must stop smoking for the condition to resolve.[87,104]

Course and Prognosis. The long-term prognosis is excellent if the underlying condition is identified and resolved, but patients with chronic anxiety or an inability to quit smoking may experience the same complications related to erythrocytosis as are seen in polycythemia vera.[87,104]

KEY CONCEPTS

- **Three types of polycythemia have been identified, according to etiology. Polycythemia vera is associated with malignant transformation of bone marrow stem cells. Secondary polycythemia is due to chronic hypoxemia, with a resultant increase in erythropoietin production. Relative polycythemia is due to dehydration, which causes a spurious increase in RBC count.**

- **Differential diagnosis of the type of polycythemia is based on the history and accompanying manifestations.**

  Polycythemia vera: Absence of hypoxemia and dehydration. Accompanying leukocytosis and thrombocytosis.

  Secondary polycythemia: History of lung disease or living at high altitude. Hypoxemia evident on blood gas evaluation.

  Relative polycythemia: History of fluid loss or poor intake. Accompanying manifestations of dehydration.

- **Treatment of polycythemia is aimed at removing the cause if possible. Phlebotomy and bone marrow–suppressing agents may be used for polycythemia vera. Major complications of polycythemia are increased blood viscosity and the risk of thrombi.**

Summary

The ultimate purpose of the erythron is to ensure that there is adequate oxygen delivery with respect to oxygen demand. This is enhanced by the unique ability of hemoglobin in RBCs to carry and release oxygen at a suitable tension to support energy-generating systems in the body tissues. Anemia, as a deficit in RBCs, poses a serious threat to oxygen transport and to the ability of the body to receive adequate oxygenation. Intense research in RBC physiology and pathophysiology continually yields new information for a better understanding of erythrocyte disorders, improved treatment modalities, and improved prognoses.

REFERENCES

1. Platt W: Introduction to hematology, in Platt W (ed): *Color Atlas and Textbook of Hematology.* Philadelphia, JB Lippincott, 1974, pp 1–6.
2. Branemark PI, Lindstrom J: Shape of circulating blood corpuscles. *Biorheology* 1963;1:139.
3. Connell JT: Morphological changes in eosinophils in allergic disease. *J Allergy Clin Immunol* 1968;41:1–9.
4. Stallman PJ, Aalberse RC: Quantitation of basophil-bound IgE in atopic and nonatopic subjects. *Int Arch Allergy Appl Immunol* 1977;54:114–120.
5. Hillman RS, Finch CA: General characteristics of the erythron, in Hillman RS, Finch CA (eds): *Red Cell Manual,* 5th ed. Philadelphia, FA Davis, 1985, pp 1–32.
6. Erslev AJ: Production of erythrocytes, in Williams WJ, et al (eds): *Hematology,* 3rd ed. New York, McGraw-Hill, 1983, pp 365–376.
7. Diggs L, Sturm D, Bell A: *The Morphology of Human Blood Cells.* Abbott Park, Ill, Abbott Laboratories, 1985, pp 1–86.
8. Hoffbrand AV, Pettit JE: Blood cell formation, in *Essential Haematology.* Oxford, Blackwell Scientific Publications, 1980, pp 1–27.
9. Wintrobe M, et al: The mature erythrocyte, in Wintrobe M, et al (eds): *Clinical Hematology,* 8th ed. Philadelphia, Lea & Febiger, 1981, pp 89–104.
10. Miale J: Folic acid, vitamin B$_{12}$, and macrocytic anemia, in Miale J (ed): *Laboratory Medicine Hematology,* 6th ed. St. Louis, CV Mosby, 1982, pp 416–444.
11. Miale J: Anemia due to decreased erythrocyte survival—the hemoglobinopathies, in Miale J (ed): *Laboratory Medicine Hematology,* 6th ed. St. Louis, CV Mosby, 1982, pp 602–657.
12. Beutler E: Energy metabolism and maintenance of erythrocytes, in Williams WJ, et al (eds): *Hematology,* 3rd ed. New York, McGraw-Hill, 1983, pp 331–345.
13. Shohet S: Red cell membrane lipids: renewal and metabolism,

in Williams WJ, et al (eds): *Hematology*, 3rd ed. New York, McGraw-Hill, 1983, pp 345–353.

14. Wintrobe M, et al: Erythropoiesis, in Wintrobe M, et al (eds): *Clinical Hematology*, 8th ed. Philadelphia, Lea & Febiger, 1981, pp 108–135.

15. Erslev AJ: Production of erythrocytes, in Williams WJ, et al (eds): *Hematology*, 3rd ed. New York, McGraw-Hill, 1983, pp 365–376.

16. Miale J: The erythrocyte: Porphyrin and hemoglobin metabolism, in Miale J (ed): *Laboratory Medicine Hematology*, 6th ed. St. Louis, CV Mosby, 1982, pp 445–474.

17. Guyton AC: Red blood cells, anemia, polycythemia, in Guyton AC (ed): *Textbook of Medical Physiology*, 8th ed. Philadelphia, WB Saunders, 1991, pp 356–364.

18. Guyton AC: Transport of oxygen and carbon dioxide in the blood and body fluids, in Guyton AC: *Textbook of Medical Physiology*, 8th ed. Philadelphia, WB Saunders, 1991, pp 433–443.

19. Williams SM: The pulmonary system, in Alspach JG, Williams SM (eds): *Core Curriculum for Critical Care Nursing*, 3rd ed. Philadelphia, WB Saunders, 1985, pp 2–97.

20. American Edwards Laboratories: *Continuous S$\bar{v}$O$_2$ Monitoring: Theory and Applications*. Irvine, Calif, American Edwards Laboratories, nd.

21. Gottlieb JE: Breathing and gas exchange, in Kinney MR, Packa DR, Dunbar SB (eds): *AACN's Clinical Reference for Critical-Care Nursing*, 2nd ed. New York, McGraw-Hill, 1988, pp 160–192.

22. Wheby MS: Differentiation, biochemistry and physiology of the erythrocyte, in Thorup OA (ed): *Leavell and Thorup's Fundamentals of Clinical Hematology*, 5th ed. Philadelphia, WB Saunders, 1987, pp 64–89.

23. Jackson LO: Sites of formation of erythropoietin, in Jacobson LO, Doyle MA (eds): *Erythropoiesis*. New York, Grune & Stratton, 1962.

24. Jacobson LO, Goldwasser E, Pried W, Plzak L: The role of the kidney in erythropoiesis. *Nature* 1957;179:633–634.

25. Erslev AJ: Classification of erythrocyte disorders, in Williams WJ, et al (eds): *Hematology*, 3rd ed. New York, McGraw-Hill, 1983, pp 406–409.

26. Erslev AJ: Erythrocyte disorders—general considerations, in Williams WJ, et al (eds): *Hematology*, 2nd ed. New York, McGraw-Hill, 1977, pp 249–255.

27. Erslev AJ: Aplastic anemia, in Williams WJ, et al (eds): *Hematology*, 3rd ed. New York, McGraw-Hill, 1983, pp 151–170.

28. Deisseroth AB, Wallerstein RO: Bone marrow failure: Aplastic anemia, myelodysplastic syndrome, myelophthisic syndrome, agnogenic myeloid metaplasia and pure red-cell aplasia, in Kelley WN, et al (eds): *Textbook of Internal Medicine*. Philadelphia, JB Lippincott, 1989, pp 1202–1206.

29. Gale RP: Bone marrow failure, in Stein JH, et al (eds): *Internal Medicine*, 3rd ed. Boston, Little, Brown & Co, 1990, pp 1109–1114.

30. Quesenberry PJ: Bone marrow failure, in Thorup OA (ed): *Leavell and Thorup's Fundamentals of Clinical Hematology*, 5th ed. Philadelphia, WB Saunders, 1987, pp 349–372.

31. Vincent PC, DeGruchy GC: Complications and treatment of acquired aplastic anemia. *Br J Med Haematol* 1967;13:977–999.

32. Lewis SM: Course and prognosis in aplastic anemia. *Br Med J* 1965;1:1027–1031.

33. Lynch RE, Williams DM, Reading JC, Cartwright GE: The prognosis in aplastic anemia. *Blood* 1975;45:517–528.

34. Heyn RM, Ertel IJ, Tubergen DG: Course of acquired aplastic anemia in children treated with supportive care. *JAMA* 1969;208:1372–1378.

35. Li FP, Alter BP, Nathan DG: The mortality of acquired aplastic anemia in children. *Blood* 1972;40:153–162.

36. Deposito P, Akatsuka J, Thatcher LG, Smith NJ: Bone marrow failure in pediatric patients. *J Pediatr* 1964;64:683–696.

37. Erslev AJ: Anemia of chronic renal failure, in Williams WJ, et al (eds): *Hematology*, 3rd ed. New York, McGraw-Hill, 1983, pp 417–425.

38. Luke RG, Strom TB: Chronic renal failure, in Stein JH, et al (eds): *Internal Medicine*, 3rd ed. Boston, Little, Brown & Co, 1990, pp 801–821.

39. Castaldi PA, Rozenberg MC, Stewart JH: The bleeding disorder of uremia: A qualitative platelet defect. *Lancet* 1966; 2:66–69.

40. Rabiner SF, Drake RF: Platelet function as an indicator of adequate dialysis. *Kidney Int* 1975;2(suppl):144–146.

41. Rabiner SF: Uremic bleeding, in Spaet TH (ed): *Progress in Hemostasis and Thrombosis*. New York, Grune & Stratton, 1972, pp 233–250.

42. Williams ME, Wheby MS: Anemia associated with other conditions, in Thorup OA (ed): *Leavell and Thorup's Fundamentals of Clinical Hematology*, 5th ed. Philadelphia, WB Saunders, 1987, pp 373–393.

43. Ziyadeh FN, Agus ZS: Approach to the patient with chronic renal failure, in Kelley WN, et al (eds): *Textbook of Internal Medicine*. Philadelphia, JB Lippincott, 1989, pp 883–890.

44. Swartz RD: Clinical approach to renal substitution therapy: Dialysis and hemofiltration, in Kelley WN, et al (eds): *Textbook of Internal Medicine*. Philadelphia, JB Lippincott, 1989, pp 890–896.

45. Rocher LL: Approach to the patient with renal transplant, in Kelley WN, et al (eds): *Textbook of Internal Medicine*. Philadelphia, JB Lippincott, 1989, pp 896–900.

46. Chanarin I, James D: Humoral and cell-mediated intrinsic factor antibody in pernicious anemia. *Lancet* 1974;1:1078–1080.

47. Beck WS: The megaloblastic anemia, in Williams WJ, et al (eds): *Hematology*, 3rd ed. New York, McGraw-Hill, 1983, pp 434–465.

48. Eichner EH: Megaloblastic anemias, in Stein JH, et al (eds): *Internal Medicine*, 3rd ed. Boston, Little, Brown & Co, 1990, pp 1082–1088.

49. Carmel R: Nutritional biochemistry of megaloblastic anemias, in Kelley WN, et al (eds): *Textbook of Internal Medicine*. Philadelphia, JB Lippincott, 1989, pp 1388–1391.

50. Lawson DH, Murray RM, Parker JLW: Early mortality in megaloblastic anemias. *Q J Med* 1972;41:1–14.

51. Colon-Otero G, Wheby MS: Disorders of cobalamin and folate metabolism, in Thorup OA (ed): *Leavell and Thorup's Fundamentals of Clinical Hematology*, 5th ed. Philadelphia, WB Saunders, 1987, pp 185–211.

52. Wintrobe M, et al: Iron deficiency and iron-deficiency anemia, in Wintrobe M, et al (eds): *Clinical Hematology*, 8th ed. Philadelphia, Lea & Febiger, 1981, pp 617–645.

53. Lipschitz DA: Disorders of iron metabolism, in Stein JH, et al (eds): *Internal Medicine*, 3rd ed. Boston, Little, Brown & Co, 1990, pp 1074–1082.

54. Cook JD: Blood loss, iron deficiency, and iron-lending anemias, in Kelley WN, et al (eds): *Textbook of Internal Medicine*. Philadelphia, JB Lippincott, 1989, pp 1432–1436.

55. Fairbanks VF, Beutler E: *Iron Deficiency*, 3rd ed. New York, McGraw-Hill, 1983, pp 466–489.

56. Wheby MS: Disorders of iron metabolism, in Thorup OA (ed): *Leavell and Thorup's Fundamentals of Clinical Hematology*, 5th ed. Philadelphia, WB Saunders, 1987, pp 212–250.

57. Weatherall DJ: The thalassemias, in Williams WJ, et al (eds): *Hematology*, 3rd ed. New York, McGraw-Hill, 1983, pp 493–521.

58. Steinberg MH: Hemoglobinopathies and thalassemias, in Stein JH, et al (eds): *Internal Medicine*, 3rd ed. Boston, Little, Brown & Co, 1990, pp 1089–1098.

59. Mohler DN, Thorup OA: Hemolytic anemia, in Thorup OA (ed): *Leavell and Thorup's Fundamentals of Clinical Hematology*, 5th ed. Philadelphia, WB Saunders, 1987, pp 251–348.

60. Benz BJ: The hemoglobinopathies, in Kelley WN, et al (eds): *Textbook of Internal Medicine*. Philadelphia, JB Lippincott, 1989, pp 1423–1432.

61. Weatherall DJ, Clegg JB: *The Thalassemia Syndromes*, 3rd ed. Oxford, Blackwell Scientific Publications, 1981.

62. Weatherall DJ: The iron loading anemias, in Martell AE, Anderson WF, Badman DG (eds): *Development of Iron Chelators for Clinical Use*. New York, Elsevier, 1981, p 3.

63. Modell B, Letski EA, Flynn DM, Peto R, Weatherall DJ: Survival and desferrioxamine in thalassemia major. *Br Med J* 1982;284:1081–1084.

64. Beutler E: Erythrocyte disorders—anemias related to abnormal globin, in Williams WJ, et al (eds): *Hematology*, 3rd ed. New York, McGraw-Hill, 1983, pp 583–609.

65. Wintrobe M, et al: Hemoglobinopathies S, C, D, E, and O and associated diseases, in Wintrobe M, et al (eds): *Clinical Hematology*, 8th ed. Philadelphia, Lea & Febiger, 1981, pp 835–836.

66. Jandl JH, Cooper RA: Erythrocyte disorders—anemias due to increased destruction of erythrocytes with abnormal shape and normal hemoglobin (membrane defects?), in Williams WJ, et al (eds): *Hematology*, 3rd ed. New York, McGraw-Hill, 1983, pp 547–553.

67. Lessin LS: Hemolytic anemias due to intracorpuscular abnormalities, in Kelley WN, et al (eds): *Textbook of Internal Medicine*. Philadelphia, JB Lippincott, 1989, pp 1441–1446.

68. Parker JC: Hereditary red cell enzymopathies and membrane defects, in Stein JH, et al (eds): *Internal Medicine*, 3rd ed. Boston, Little, Brown & Co, 1990, pp 1098–1102.

69. Miale J: Anemia due to decreased erythrocyte survival—congenital and acquired hemolytic anemias, in Miale J (ed): *Laboratory Medicine Hematology*, 6th ed. St. Louis, CV Mosby, 1982, pp 550–601.

70. Beutler E: Erythrocyte disorders—anemias due to increased destruction of erythrocytes with enzyme deficiencies, in Williams WJ, et al (eds): *Hematology*, 3rd ed. New York, McGraw-Hill, 1983, pp 561–574.

71. Wintrobe M, et al: Hemolytic disease of the newborn (HDN), in Wintrobe M, et al (eds): *Clinical Hematology*, 8th ed. Philadelphia, Lea & Febiger, 1981, pp 909–920.

72. Bowman JM: Alloimmune hemolytic disease of the newborn, in Williams WJ, et al (eds): *Hematology*, 3rd ed. New York, McGraw-Hill, 1983, pp 653–659.

73. Swisher SN, Burka ER: Drug reactions involving antibodies reacting with erythrocytes, in Williams WJ, et al (eds): *Hematology*, 2nd ed. New York, McGraw-Hill, 1977, pp 605–610.

74. Petz LD: Hemolytic anemias due to acquired abnormalities of the red blood cell membrane, in Kelley WN, et al (eds): *Textbook of Internal Medicine*. Philadelphia, JB Lippincott, 1989, pp 1446–1450.

75. Packman CH, Leddy JP: Drug-related immunologic injury of erythrocytes, in Williams WJ, et al (eds): *Hematology*, 3rd ed. New York, McGraw-Hill, 1983, pp 647–653.

76. LoBuglio AF: Acquired hemolytic anemias, in Stein JH, et al (eds): *Internal Medicine*, 3rd ed. Boston, Little, Brown & Co, 1990, pp 1102–1109.

77. Hillman RS: Erythrocyte disorders—anemias due to acute blood loss, in Williams WJ, et al (eds): *Hematology*, 3rd ed. New York, McGraw-Hill, 1983, pp 667–672.

78. Finch CA, Lenfant C: Oxygen transport in man. *N Engl J Med* 1972;286:407–415.

79. Ebert RV, Stead EA, Gibson JG: Response of normal subjects to acute blood loss. *Arch Intern Med* 1941;68:578–590.

80. Theyl RA, Tuohy GF: Hemodynamics and blood volume during operation with ether anesthesia and unreplaced blood loss. *Anesthesiology* 1964;25:6–14.

81. Howarth S, Sharpey-Schafer EP: Low blood pressure phases following hemorrhage. *Lancet* 1947;1:18–20.

82. Tovey GH, Lennon GG: Blood volume studies in accidental hemorrhage. *J Obstet Gynaecol Br Commonw* 1962;5:749–752.

83. Beutler E: Hemolytic anemia due to chemical and physical agents, in Williams W, et al (eds): *Hematology*, 3rd ed. New York, McGraw-Hill, 1983, pp 625–628.

84. Kasprisin CA: Recipient considerations, in Reynolds AW, Steckler D (eds): *Practical Aspects of Blood Administration*. Arlington, Va, American Association of Blood Banks, 1986, pp 1–21.

85. American Association of Blood Banks: Blood transfusion practice, in Walker RH, et al (eds): *Technical Manual*, 10th ed. Arlington, Va, American Association of Blood Banks, 1990, pp 341–375.

86. Murphy S: Hemopoietic stem cell disorders—myeloproliferative disorders, in Williams WJ, et al (eds): *Hematology*, 3rd ed. New York, McGraw-Hill, 1983, pp 185–196.

87. Niskanen E: Polycythemia, in Thorup OA (ed): *Leavell and Thorup's Fundamentals of Clinical Hematology*, 5th ed. Philadelphia, WB Saunders, 1987, pp 409–423.

88. Frenkel EP: Polycythemia vera, in Kelley WN, et al (eds): *Textbook of Internal Medicine*. Philadelphia, JB Lippincott, 1989, pp 1181–1184.

89. Krantz SB: Polycythemia, in Stein JH, et al (eds): *Internal Medicine*, 3rd ed. Boston, Little, Brown & Co, 1990, pp 1119–1124.

90. Humphrey PR, et al: Cerebral blood-flow and viscosity in relative polycythemia. *Lancet* 1979;2:873–877.

91. Willison JR, et al: Effect of high hematocrit on alertness. *Lancet* 1980;1:846–848.

92. Pearson TC, Wetherley-Mein G: Vascular occlusive episodes and venous hematocrit in primary proliferative polycythemia. *Lancet* 1978;2:1219–1222.

93. Wasserman JD: Influence of therapy on causes of death in polycythemia vera. *Clin Res* 1981;29:573A.

94. Modan B, Lilienfeld AM: Polycythemia vera and leukemia—the role of radiation treatment. A study of 1222 patients. *Medicine* 1965;44:305–344.

95. Lawrence JH: *Polycythemia: Physiology, Diagnosis and Treatment Based on 303 Cases*. Modern Medical Monographs, no. 13. New York, Grune & Stratton, 1955.

96. Perkins J, Israels MCG, Wilkinson JF: Polycythemia vera: Clinical studies on a series of 127 patients managed without radiation therapy. *Q J Med* 1964;33:499–518.

97. Wasserman LR: Polycythemia vera—its course and treatment. Relation to myeloid metaplasia and leukemia. *Bull NY Acad Med* 1954;5:343–375.

98. Haanen C, Mathe G, Hayat M: Treatment of polycythemia vera by radiophosphorus or busulfan: A randomized trial. *Br J Cancer* 1981;44:75–80.

99. Najman A, et al: Pipobroman therapy of polycythemia vera. *Blood* 1982;59:890–894.

100. Chievitz E, Thiede T: Complications and causes of death in polycythemia vera. *Acta Med Scand* 1962;172:513–523.

101. Videbaeck A: Polycythemia vera: Course and prognosis. *Acta Med Scand* 1950;138:179–187.

102. Erslev AJ: Secondary polycythemia, in Williams WJ, et al (eds): *Hematology*, 3rd ed. New York, McGraw-Hill, 1983, pp 673–684.

103. Frenkel EP: Approach to the management of polycythemia, in Kelley WN, et al (eds): *Textbook of Internal Medicine*. Philadelphia, JB Lippincott, 1989, pp 1331–1337.

104. Erslev AJ: Relative polycythemia, in Williams WJ, et al (eds): *Hematology*, 3rd ed. New York, McGraw-Hill, 1983, pp 684–686.

BIBLIOGRAPHY

American Association of Critical Care Nurses, Alspach JG: *Core Curriculum for Critical Care Nursing*, 4th ed. Philadelphia, WB Saunders, 1991.

American Edwards Laboratories: *Continuous S$\bar{v}$O$_2$ Monitoring: Theory and Applications*. Irvine, Calif, American Edwards Laboratories, nd.

Guyton AC: *Textbook of Medical Physiology*, 8th ed. Philadelphia, WB Saunders, 1991.

Harmening D (ed): *Clinical Hematology and Fundamentals of Hemostasis*, 2nd ed. Philadelphia, FA Davis, 1992.

Hillman RS, Finch CA (eds): *Red Cell Manual*, 5th ed. Philadelphia, FA Davis, 1985.

Hoffbrand AV, Pettit JE (eds): *Essential Haematology*. Oxford, Blackwell Scientific Publications, 1980.

Kelley WN, et al (eds): *Textbook of Internal Medicine*. Philadelphia, JB Lippincott, 1989.

Kinney MR, Packa DR, Dunbar SB (eds): *AACN's Clinical Reference for Critical-Care Nursing*, 2nd ed. New York, McGraw-Hill, 1988.

Miale J (ed): *Laboratory Medicine Hematology*, 6th ed. St. Louis, CV Mosby, 1982.

Platt W (ed): *Color Atlas and Textbook of Hematology*. Philadelphia, JB Lippincott, 1974.

Reynolds AW, Steckler D (eds): *Practical Aspects of Blood Administration*. Arlington, Va, American Association of Blood Banks, 1986.

Stein JH, et al (eds): *Internal Medicine*, 3rd ed. Boston, Little, Brown & Co, 1990.

Thorup OA Jr (ed): *Leavell and Thorup's Fundamentals of Clinical Hematology*, 5th ed. Philadelphia, WB Saunders, 1987.

Walker RH, et al (eds): *Technical Manual*, 10th ed. Arlington, Va, American Association of Blood Banks, 1990.

Williams WJ, et al (eds): *Hematology*, 3rd ed. New York, McGraw-Hill, 1983.

Wintrobe M, et al (eds): *Clinical Hematology*, 8th ed. Philadelphia, Lea & Febiger, 1981.

CHAPTER 13
Alterations in Hemostasis and Blood Coagulation

EDITH RANDALL

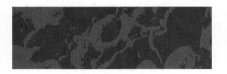

KEY TERMS

coagulation: The process of blood clot formation.

coagulopathy: An abnormality in blood clot formation resulting in bleeding.

ecchymosis: Discoloration of the skin (bruise) caused by escape of blood into the tissues.

fibrinolysis: Dissolution or breakup of a fibrin clot.

hemarthrosis: Blood in a joint cavity.

hematoma: A mass caused by collection of blood that has extravasated into a tissue or cavity.

hemostasis: Arrest of bleeding; prevention of blood loss.

petechiae: Nonblanching, pinpoint red or purple spots caused by capillary hemorrhages.

purpura: Hemorrhagic lesions 2–4 mm in diameter; petechiae that occur in groups or patches.

thrombocytopenia: Deficiency in the number of circulating platelets in the blood.

The term **hemostasis** means arrest of bleeding or prevention of blood loss after a blood vessel is injured. Hemostasis is accomplished via a complex interaction involving the vessel wall, circulating platelets, and plasma coagulation proteins. If hemostasis is inadequate, bleeding results; if hemostasis is excessive, inappropriate clotting or thrombosis results.

This chapter reviews the process of hemostasis and how that process is evaluated by means of clinical assessment and laboratory tests. The focus of the chapter is on disorders of hemostasis and coagulation that result in bleeding. Disorders that result in thrombosis are discussed in Chapter 14, Alterations in Blood Flow.

The Process of Hemostasis

Stages of Hemostasis

Primary hemostasis, the initial response to injury, involves the interaction between platelets and the injured blood vessel. The immediate response of the vessel to trauma is vasoconstriction to reduce blood loss. Although nervous reflex may play a part, this vasoconstriction results primarily from local myogenic spasm that may last from minutes to hours. The degree of vascular spasm is greater with a blunt or crushing injury (resulting in less bleeding) than with a sharp cut to a vessel.[1]

A second component of primary hemostasis is formation of a platelet plug. Platelets not only adhere to endothelial collagen exposed by injury, they also aggregate (clump together) at the site of vessel injury. The formation of this platelet plug is usually completed within 3 to 7 minutes.

Secondary hemostasis involves the formation of a fibrin clot, or **coagulation,** at the site of injury to maintain hemostasis already initiated. Clotting factors are activated and participate in a series of events that catalyzes or facilitates the conversion of fibrinogen to fibrin. This process takes an average of 3 to 10 minutes.

Clot retraction, the final stage of clot formation, is the process in which the components of the fibrin clot—the platelet plug, fibrin strands, and trapped red blood cells—are compressed or contracted to form a firm clot. This stage takes approximately 1 hour.

Platelets

Platelets play an integral role in hemostasis; thus, it is important to review their nature and function. A normal platelet count is between 150,000 and 350,000 per cubic millimeter (mm^3).[2] Platelets, the smallest of the formed elements in the blood, are produced from megakaryocytes in the bone marrow. Approximately 70 percent of platelets are found in the circulation and 30 percent in the spleen.[3] Factors such as the stress response, epinephrine, and exercise may stimulate platelet production.[4] The average life span of a platelet

is 10 days. On completion of its life span, a platelet is eliminated from the circulation by the tissue macrophage system.[1]

Platelets play a complex role in the process of hemostasis. Initially, platelets adhere to subendothelial collagen exposed by trauma. After adhesion, the platelets become activated and release substances such as thromboxane A_2, adenosine diphosphate (ADP), serotonin, growth factor, von Willebrand factor, and calcium. These substances enhance vasoconstriction, facilitate platelet aggregation, and promote vessel repair and healing.[3–5]

In addition to the major role of platelets in primary hemostasis, they are also involved in secondary hemostasis. Platelets catalyze interactions between activated coagulation factors and thus accelerate the conversion of prothrombin to thrombin. Platelets also play a role in clot retraction.

Blood Coagulation Factors

Blood coagulation factors, with the exception of tissue factor (Factor III, tissue thromboplastin) and calcium, are plasma proteins that circulate in the bloodstream in an inactive state. These factors are listed in Table 13–1 according to the internationally standardized nomenclature. The factors are numbered in the order of their discovery, not the order in which they participate in the clotting cascade. Some factors have both active and inactive forms; the letter "a" after the Roman numeral designates the active form.

The liver is responsible for the synthesis of coagulation factors, with the exception of part of Factor VIII. Factors II, VII, IX, and X are dependent on vitamin K for synthesis and normal activity. Some of the coagulation proteins can also be synthesized by other cells such as megakaryocytes and endothelial cells.[6]

Fibrin Clot

In normal hemostasis, activation of the intrinsic and extrinsic pathways and, in turn, the common final pathway produces the fibrin clot. Effective hemostasis is the result of interactions between all of these pathways (Fig. 13–1).

The intrinsic pathway of coagulation begins when blood comes into contact with altered vascular endothelium or another negatively charged surface such as glass. This contact phase of coagulation involves four factors: prekallikrein, high molecular weight kininogen (HMWK), Factor XI, and Factor XII. These four factors form a complex, and a series of events occurs. Factor XII is activated to Factor XIIa, which in turn activates XI to XIa and prekallikrein to its active form, kallikrein. Kallikrein liberates bradykinin from HMWK. The release of bradykinin produces an initial vasodilation followed by release of angiotensin II and vasoconstriction. The major role of Factor XIa is activation of Factor IX to Factor IXa in the presence of calcium. Factor IXa then activates Factor X to Factor Xa in the presence of Factor VIII, calcium, and phospho-

T A B L E   13 – 1. Blood Coagulation Factors

Factors	Other Designations
I	Fibrinogen
II	Prothrombin
III	Tissue factor; tissue thromboplastin
IV	Calcium
V	Proaccelerin; labile factor
VI	This factor is no longer considered a distinct part of coagulation
VII	Stable factor; serum prothrombin conversion accelerator
VIII	Antihemophilic globulin; antihemophilic factor
IX	Christmas factor
X	Stuart factor; Stuart-Prower factor
XI	Plasma thromboplastin antecedent (PTA)
XII	Hageman factor
XIII	Fibrin stabilizing factor
Prekallikrein	Fletcher factor
High molecular weight kininogen	Contact activation cofactor

lipid. This activation usually takes place on the membrane of stimulated platelets. The common final pathway is initiated by Factor Xa.

The extrinsic pathway of coagulation begins when tissue factor from injured tissue activates Factor VII. Factor VIIa activates Factor X to Xa, which in turn initiates the common final pathway. Factor VIIa also activates Factor IX in the intrinsic system.

The common final pathway of coagulation is initiated by Factor X, which is activated by both the intrinsic and extrinsic pathways. Factor Xa, in the presence of Factor V, calcium, and phospholipid, converts prothrombin (Factor II) to thrombin. This conversion is facilitated by the presence of activated platelets. Thrombin then cleaves fibrinogen to form an insoluble fibrin clot. Thrombin also activates Factor XIII, which promotes fibrin stabilization. The clot is further stabilized by clot retraction. Thrombin also helps to perpetuate the clotting cascade by activating Factors V and VIII.

Fibrinolysis

At the same time the fibrin clot is forming, the process of **fibrinolysis** or clot dissolution is initiated (Fig. 13–2). Factor XII, HMWK, kallikrein, and thrombin are involved in the release of plasminogen activators. The plasminogen activators cleave plasminogen, a plasma protein that has been incorporated into the fibrin clot, to its active form, plasmin. Plasmin digests fibrinogen and fibrin and inactivates blood coagulation Factors V and VIII. Fibrin degradation products, or fibrin split products, result from the dissolution of the fibrin clot.

The entire process of hemostasis is complex. In addition to the events already discussed, natural anticoagulants such as antithrombin III, protein C, and protein S exist to inhibit inappropriate clot formation. The Kupffer cells of the liver and the macrophages of the spleen and bone marrow clear the circulation of activated clotting factors and fibrin degradation prod-

ucts. Antiplasmins that inhibit plasmin exist to prevent inappropriate fibrinolysis. All of these factors and mechanisms are present to create a balance between clot production and clot dissolution. The optimal goal is that normal hemostasis is achieved and maintained.

KEY CONCEPTS

- Hemostasis involves several critical steps. These include vasospasm, formation of a platelet plug, and activation of the clotting cascade to form a fibrin clot.
- Factors released from platelets contribute to hemostasis by enhancing vasoconstriction, platelet aggregation, and vessel repair.
- Fibrin clot formation can be initiated by the intrinsic or extrinsic pathway. Each pathway requires the sequential activation of specific clotting factors, ultimately resulting in enzymatic cleavage of fibrinogen to form an insoluble fibrin clot.
- Initiation of fibrinolysis occurs simultaneously with clot formation to prevent excessive clotting and vessel occlusion.

Evaluation of Hemostasis and Coagulation

Data obtained from clinical assessment and laboratory tests facilitate the identification and evaluation of a hemostatic abnormality. Evaluation of a patient for a bleeding tendency is indicated in the following circumstances: when there is a history of bleeding, during active bleeding unresponsive to standard interventions, and as part of screening prior to surgery. A bleeding tendency may be inherited or acquired and may result from defects in blood vessels, platelets, or coagulation factors. The goal of the evaluation process is to identify if a problem exists and to determine

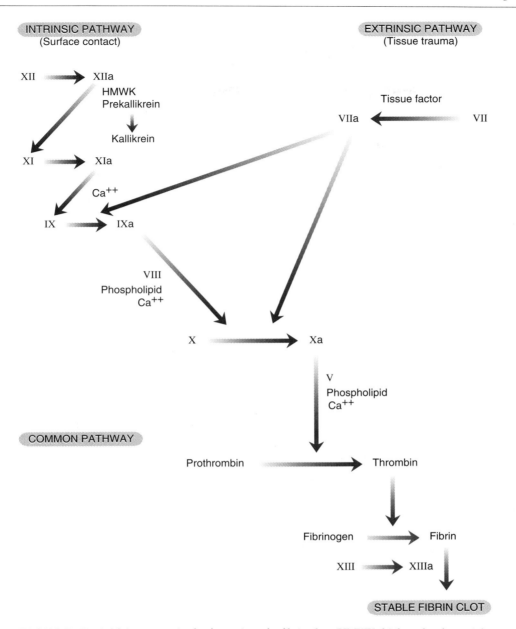

FIGURE 13–1. Major events in the formation of a fibrin clot. (HMWK, high molecular weight kininogen; Ca^{++}, calcium.)

the underlying cause so that appropriate management can be initiated.

Clinical Assessment

Both the family history and the personal history are important in evaluating a bleeding problem (Table 13–2). A family history of bleeding in males is often linked to one of the hemophilias, which account for the majority of serious inherited coagulation problems.[7] The location, severity, duration, and setting in which bleeding occurs are also important clues to the type of defect present. Bleeding associated with vascular and platelet defects usually occurs immediately

after trauma (e.g., dental extraction), involves skin or mucous membranes, and is brief in duration. Delayed bleeding or bleeding into muscles or joints is typical of coagulation defects.[8]

Systemic disease such as uremia, liver disease, systemic lupus erythematosus, and malignancies may be associated with a bleeding problem. Medication history, including use of over-the-counter products, is another important aspect in the evaluation of a hemostatic defect. A common cause of acquired bleeding problems is drug ingestion. Specific drugs that alter hemostasis include aspirin and aspirin-containing preparations, nonsteroidal anti-inflammatory agents, antibiotics, anticoagulants, alcohol, and chemotherapeutic agents.

Plasminogen

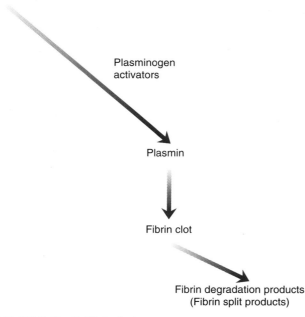

F I G U R E 13 – 2. Fibrinolysis.

As the history is obtained, the physical examination can begin. Many of the physical findings of bleeding are manifested in the skin and mucous membranes. The individual may appear pale or jaundiced. Pallor is associated with a marked decrease in hemoglobin; jaundice is associated with liver disease and perhaps associated coagulation disorders.

Petechiae are flat, pinpoint, nonblanching red or purple spots caused by capillary hemorrhages within the skin and mucous membranes. Petechiae are commonly seen with vascular and platelet disorders. They are usually present on dependent areas of the body, such as the legs, or on areas constricted by clothing such as tight stockings. Not all petechiae indicate a bleeding problem. Petechiae found on other body areas not constricted by tight clothing, such as the abdomen or thorax, may be associated with infectious disease. Petechiae may be seen in the newborn as a result of the trauma of delivery, not due to a bleeding problem.

When petechiae occur in groups or patches, the term **purpura** is used. Purpuric lesions are often pruritic (itchy). Fever and malaise may be present, as may effusions into joints or viscera, manifested by joint or abdominal pain.

Ecchymosis occurs when blood escapes into the tissues, producing a bruise. If the area is raised, it is called a **hematoma. Hemarthrosis,** manifested by swelling and pain, is bleeding into a joint. Large ecchymoses, hematomas, and hemarthroses are seen in coagulation disorders.

A telangiectasia is a lesion created by dilation of capillaries and small arteries, typically on the lips, tongue, tips of the fingers and toes, and sometimes in visceral vessels. These thin, dilated, tortuous vessels are red to violet in color, blanch with pressure, and tend to bleed with minimal trauma. Spider telangiectasias branch into the subcutaneous and dermal layers of the skin and are often associated with liver disease.

Other significant findings of a bleeding disorder on physical examination include blood (bright red, rusty, black) in drainage or excreta such as feces, urine, emesis, or gastric drainage. Acute abdominal or flank pain may indicate internal bleeding. Hypovolemia from bleeding may present as hypotension, tachycardia, pallor, altered mentation, or decreased urine output. Two of the most life-threatening sites of bleeding are the oropharynx (resulting in airway compromise) and within the head. "Intracerebral hemorrhage is one of the leading causes of death in patients with severe coagulation disorders."[5]

Laboratory Tests

Many laboratory tests are available to aid in the diagnosis of hemostasis problems (Table 13–3). Basic screening includes a complete blood cell (CBC) count, including a platelet count and peripheral smear, bleeding time, prothrombin time, activated partial thromboplastin time, and thrombin time.[8] These screening tests evaluate both primary and secondary hemostasis. The CBC determines if anemia is present,

T A B L E 13 – 2. Historical Clues to Bleeding Disorders

History	Possible Disorder/Cause
Family history of bleeding in males	Hemophilia A or B
Family history of bleeding in both males and females	Von Willebrand's disease
Acquired bruising tendency	Aspirin (or other drug) ingestion; thrombocytopenia
Bruising or bleeding associated with another illness	Drug ingestion; thrombocytopenia; anticoagulant therapy
Inappropriate bleeding during/following surgery	Mild coagulation factor deficiency; von Willebrand's disease; thrombocytopenia; aspirin ingestion; anticoagulant therapy
Delayed bleeding after trauma/surgery	Factor XIII deficiency

Adapted with permission from Andreoli TE, et al: *Cecil Essentials of Medicine,* 3rd ed. Philadelphia, WB Saunders, 1993, p 401.

the platelet count determines the number of platelets, and the peripheral smear indicates the number and gross morphology of platelets. The bleeding time evaluates vascular status and platelet function. The prothrombin time assesses the extrinsic pathway of coagulation, and the activated partial thromboplastin time assesses the intrinsic pathway. Thrombin time measures the time needed to convert fibrinogen to fibrin; this reflects the quantity and quality of fibrinogen as well as the influence of any inhibitors.

Further laboratory investigation is necessary if abnormalities are identified on the screening tests, or if, despite normal screening tests, there is obviously a bleeding problem. Specific tests are available to assess abnormal platelet function, the presence of circulating anticoagulants, and levels of individual coagulation factors.

KEY CONCEPTS

- Bleeding tendencies may be inherited or acquired. A history of abnormal bleeding, liver disease, or anticoagulant drug use may be important risk factors. Physical findings of petechiae, purpura, ecchymosis, telangiectasias, and occult or frank bleeding are indicative.
- Usual laboratory tests include platelet count, bleeding time, prothrombin time (extrinsic pathway), activated thromboplastin time (intrinsic pathway), thrombin time, and fibrin split products.

Disorders of Hemostasis and Coagulation

Vascular Disorders

Vascular disorders of hemostasis and coagulation are those in which the primary cause of bleeding is a problem with the vascular component of primary hemostasis. The vascular defect may be acquired (e.g., related to ingestion of a specific drug) or inherited.

Vascular Purpura

Etiology. Vascular purpura is a disorder in which purpura—patches of petechiae, or pinpoint hemorrhages, on the skin—is present; the primary cause of the purpura, or more extensive bleeding in some cases, is an abnormality of the vessels or the tissues that support them.

Allergic purpura (anaphylactoid purpura, Henoch-Schönlein purpura) is most often seen in children between the ages of 4 and 7.[9,10] Drug-induced purpura may result from many drugs, including atropine, chloral hydrate, and other sedatives; sulfa drugs; procaine penicillin; and coumarin. Purpura and perhaps severe hemorrhage are components of the Ehlers-Danlos syndrome and osteogenesis imperfecta, both inherited disorders of connective tissue. Acquired disorders of connective tissue such as scurvy (vitamin C

deficiency), senile purpura (seen in the elderly), and corticosteroid purpura (associated with steroid drug therapy) may also result in purpuric lesions.

Pathogenesis. The allergic purpuras are thought to result from an autoimmune process that produces inflammation or vasculitis of small vessels. As a result, there is perivascular infiltration and serosanguinous effusions into surrounding tissues, producing the characteristic purpura.

The pathophysiology of drug-induced purpura is not well understood. An autoimmune process like that described in the preceding paragraph has been proposed.

Structural abnormalities of vessels and perivascular supportive tissue provide the mechanism for bleeding in many of the vascular purpuras. These abnormalities may be inherited or acquired. In Ehlers-Danlos syndrome and osteogenesis imperfecta, the vascular abnormality is thought to result from decreased or poor-quality collagen and elastin; both are necessary for perivascular support. Vitamin C deficiency, seen in scurvy, results in defective collagen synthesis. The lack of proper collagen support for the vessels leads to bleeding. In the elderly (senile purpura), there is loss of subcutaneous fat and changes in connective tissue which allow for more mobility of the skin. The resulting shearing force causes rupture of small vessels.[11] Steroids appear to induce catabolism of proteins in supportive tissues decreasing the mechanical strength of the microvasculature.

Clinical Manifestations. Purpura and other evidence of bleeding, in some instances, is characteristic of the vascular purpuras. The purpuric lesions characteristically appear and fade or disappear in groups, are not elevated, and do not blanch with pressure.

With the allergic purpuras, the lesions tend to be palpable and are found on the proximal extremities, especially on the legs and buttocks; they may be accompanied by fever, itching, arthralgia, and paresthesia. Bleeding from the lesions themselves and generalized bleeding are uncommon. Usually an allergic purpura is a self-limited disorder and the prognosis is good.

Generalized purpura is characteristic of drug-induced vascular purpura. The purpura quickly subsides when the drug is discontinued. Other bleeding manifestations are uncommon.

The purpura associated with inherited connective tissue disorders, such as Ehlers-Danlos syndrome, often is accompanied by large ecchymoses and hematomas.

The purpura seen with scurvy typically occurs around hair follicles and on the medial surfaces of the thighs and buttocks. Ecchymoses and large hematomas may also occur.

Senile purpura and corticosteroid purpura generally occur on the dorsum of the hands and forearms and are aggravated by trauma. Other bleeding is uncommon.

Diagnosis. The diagnosis of a vascular purpura is one of exclusion after platelet disorders and coagula-

TABLE 13–3. Select Laboratory Tests Used to Assess Bleeding

Test	Normal Value*	Purpose or Significance
Platelet count	150,000–350,000/mm^3	Determines number of platelets; decr. in ITP, anemias, DIC, infection, chemotherapy; incr. in leukemia, cancer, splenectomy
Bleeding time	3–10 min	Assesses platelet and vascular response; incr. in thrombocytopenia, vascular defects, severe liver disease, DIC, von Willebrand's disease, aspirin ingestion
Prothrombin time (PT)	10–14 sec; 100%	Evaluates the extrinsic pathway of coagulation; incr. in vitamin K deficiency, hemorrhagic disease of the newborn, liver disease, DIC, anticoagulant therapy
Activated partial thromboplastin time (APTT)	33–45 sec	Evaluates the intrinsic pathway of coagulation; incr. in hemophilia, vitamin K deficiency, liver disease, DIC, circulating anticoagulants, heparin therapy
Thrombin time (TT)	15 sec, or control + 5 sec	Measures conversion of fibrinogen to fibrin; incr. in DIC, liver disease, low fibrinogen
Fibrinogen†	200–400 mg/dL	Measures fibrinogen level; decr. in liver disease, DIC
Fibrin split products (FSP) or fibrin degradation products (FDP)†	<3 µg/mL	Measures by-products from breakdown of fibrin clot; incr. in DIC, hypoxia, leukemia, thromboembolic disorders
Clot retraction†	1 hr: evidence of shrinking and incr. firmness 24 hr: 50% of volume is clot, 50% is serum	Rough measure of platelet function; decr. in thrombocytopenia, von Willebrand's disease
Platelet aggregation†	Visible aggregates form in <5 min	Measures rate and percentage of aggregation; decr. in mononucleosis, ITP, von Willebrand's disease, leukemia, aspirin ingestion, thrombasthenia, Bernard-Soulier syndrome
Tourniquet test (Rumpel-Leede test, capillary fragility test)†	No petechiae or occasional petechiae	Evaluates vascular fragility and platelet function; positive test in thrombocytopenia, vascular purpuras, thrombasthenia
Euglobin lysis time†	No lysis of fibrin clot at 37°C for 3 hr; clot is observed for 24 hr	Assesses fibrinolysis; incr. lysis in DIC, incompatible blood transfusion, cirrhosis, cancer, obstetric complications

*Value may vary, depending on source.
†Tests not included in a routine coagulation screen.
Abbreviations: ITP, idiopathic thrombocytopenic purpura; DIC, disseminated intravascular coagulation; incr., increased; decr., decreased.

tion disorders have been ruled out. An abnormal tourniquet test (positive Rumpel-Leede test) in the setting of a normal or increased bleeding time, normal platelet count, and normal coagulation studies suggests a problem with the vascular component of hemostasis.

Treatment. Treatment for a vascular purpura includes removal or avoidance of the causative agent if one is identified (e.g., penicillin) and intervention to relieve symptoms such as itching. If more extensive bleeding accompanies the purpura, identification of the cause as well as intervention to control the bleeding is necessary.

Hereditary Hemorrhagic Telangiectasia

Etiology. A telangiectasia is a dilated and/or tortuous small blood vessel, found in the skin or mucous membranes, that has a tendency to bleed spontaneously or following minor trauma. Hereditary hemorrhagic telangiectasia (Osler-Weber-Rendu disease) is transmitted as an autosomal dominant trait; the vascular abnormalities can be seen in children but become more prominent after puberty, peaking between the fourth and fifth decades. As the telangiectases—the skin spots resulting from the vascular lesion—become more prominent, the frequency and severity of the bleeding increase. Bleeding tends to be less severe in females than males.[12] The prognosis is good with this vascular disorder.

Pathogenesis. The telangiectases result from an abnormality in vascular development. The vessel wall is composed of a single layer of endothelium; thus, support and contractile properties are deficient, leading to spontaneous bleeding or bleeding with only minor trauma. Any mucosal surface—e.g., respiratory, gastrointestinal, and genitourinary tracts—may be involved. Vascular malformations in the lung, pulmonary arteriovenous fistulas, occur in 15 percent to 20 percent of patients.[12]

Clinical Manifestations. Bright red or purple lesions, ranging from pinpoint to 3 mm in diameter, can be found on the nasal mucous membranes, lips, palate, tongue, face, trunk, palms of the hands, and the soles of the feet. Typically the lesions are flat and blanch with pressure.

The most common clinical problem is mucous membrane bleeding, especially epistaxis. Bleeding, however, may occur from telangiectases in any area. Frequent bleeding episodes may result in anemia.

Diagnosis. The diagnosis is confirmed from the presence of multiple telangiectases, repeated episodes of bleeding, or a family history of bleeding in both sexes. If telangiectases are not easily visible, the diagnosis is more difficult to make.

Treatment. Treatment is primarily supportive and includes use of topical hemostatic agents or cauterization if the bleeding site is accessible; nasal tamponade; and iron replacement. Blood transfusions and surgical intervention for uncontrolled bleeding or removal of an arteriovenous fistula may be considered in select cases.

Platelet Disorders

Platelet disorders of hemostasis and coagulation are those in which the primary cause of bleeding is an abnormality in the quantity or the quality of platelets.

Thrombocytopenia

Etiology. **Thrombocytopenia** is a common cause of generalized bleeding. Thrombocytopenia is present when the platelet count falls below 150,000/mm³; however, bleeding does not typically occur at this level.[13] Platelet counts of 50,000/mm³ may result in bleeding following minor trauma; at 20,000/mm³, a hematologic emergency exists because spontaneous bleeding may occur.[5,13] Some of the many causes of thrombocytopenia are listed in Table 13–4.

Idiopathic thrombocytopenic purpura (ITP) is a thrombocytopenia that occurs in the absence of toxic or drug exposure or a disease associated with decreased platelets. Acute ITP occurs most frequently in young children of either sex following an acute viral infection.[14,15] Resolution is usually spontaneous, and the prognosis is good. Chronic ITP is more common in adults. The onset is insidious, and women are affected more often than men. If a woman with ITP is pregnant, she can deliver a thrombocytopenic infant because the antiplatelet antibody crosses the placenta. Adult ITP may precede or occur in association with diseases of altered immunity such as systemic lupus erythematosus, lymphoproliferative disease, or acquired immunodeficiency syndrome (AIDS).

Pathogenesis. Four mechanisms are responsible for thrombocytopenia: decreased platelet production, decreased platelet survival, splenic sequestration (pooling), and intravascular dilution of circulating platelets (see Table 13–4). Regardless of the mechanism responsible for thrombocytopenia, there are fewer platelets available and inadequate hemostasis is the potential result.

Platelets are produced by bone marrow megakaryocytes. Platelet production falls when the number of megakaryocytes is reduced or when the process of platelet production (thrombocytopoiesis) is ineffective. Although numerous causes of decreased platelet production are listed in Table 13–4, drugs are often responsible. Bone marrow suppression from chemotherapy and alcohol ingestion are common reasons for decreased platelets.[13,16] In the elderly, thiazide diuretics are the most likely drugs to cause thrombocytopenia.[17]

The average life span of a platelet is 10 days. Decreased platelet survival may be the result of an antibody-mediated immune mechanism that destroys platelets (e.g., ITP, heparin) or the result of increased consumption of platelets, as seen in disseminated intravascular coagulation. Direct trauma to platelets from vascular or valvular prostheses may also be responsible for decreased platelet survival.

Normally, 30 percent of total platelets can be found in the spleen; the remaining 70 percent are circulating. When the spleen is enlarged (splenomegaly), as many as 90 percent of the platelets may be pooled or sequestered in the spleen; thus the circulat-

TABLE 13–4. Some Causes of Thrombocytopenia

Cause	Mechanism
Folate/B₁₂ deficiency, radiation therapy, chemotherapy, drugs (alcohol, anticonvulsants, thiazide diuretics), aplastic/hypoplastic anemias, leukemia, lymphoma, viral infections	Decr. platelet production: decr. megakaryocytes, ineffective production
Viral infections, drugs (digitalis, quinidine, penicillins, heparin), vascular/valvular prostheses, DIC, AIDS, sepsis, ITP	Decr. platelet survival: incr. destruction, incr. consumption
Hypersplenism (secondary to portal hypertension in hepatic disease, leukemia, lymphoma)	Splenic pooling of platelets
Massive blood transfusion	Dilution of platelets

Abbreviations: DIC, disseminated intravascular coagulation; AIDS, acquired immune deficiency syndrome; ITP, idiopathic thrombocytopenic purpura; incr., increased; decr., decreased.

ing number of platelets is markedly decreased.[18] If the spleen cannot be felt on physical examination, platelet sequestration can be ruled out as the primary mechanism of the thrombocytopenia.

The final mechanism responsible for thrombocytopenia is dilution of circulating platelets by administration of massive transfusions. Platelets degenerate in stored blood; thus, when a large amount of blood deficient in platelets is transfused, thrombocytopenia results.

Clinical Manifestations. Clinical manifestations of thrombocytopenia are generally absent until the platelet count falls below 100,000/mm³. Increased bruising and prolonged bleeding following minor trauma may be seen with a platelet count of 50,000/mm³. Petechiae and purpura are prominent with platelet counts below 50,000/mm³. Spontaneous mucosal, deep tissue, and intracranial bleeding may be seen with platelet counts below 20,000/mm³.

Diagnosis. Thrombocytopenia is diagnosed by the presence of a low platelet count. The bleeding time is prolonged and clot retraction is poor to absent. Prothrombin time, partial thromboplastin time, and other coagulation studies are normal. The CBC count will indicate if the thrombocytopenia is isolated or if there is an associated problem such as anemia. Gross morphology of platelets, evaluated from the peripheral blood smear, and bone marrow examination provide additional information regarding the mechanism for the thrombocytopenia. Because many drugs are associated with thrombocytopenia, careful review of all medications the patient is taking is also necessary in the search for the cause of the thrombocytopenia.

Treatment. The treatment of thrombocytopenia is based on the identified cause or mechanism and may include any of the following: discontinuation of any suspected drug; avoidance of aspirin and aspirin-like drugs that alter normal platelet function; administration of corticosteroids to increase platelet production and to decrease splenic sequestration of platelets; platelet transfusions; plasma exchange transfusions; or splenectomy. Splenectomy results in removal of a major site of platelet destruction and also eliminates a source for production of antiplatelet antibodies.

Thrombocytosis

Etiology. Thrombocytosis is generally defined as a platelet count above 400,000/mm³. Transitory thrombocytosis is seen following stress or physical exercise. Secondary or reactive thrombocytosis occurs as a response to hemorrhage, inflammatory diseases, malignancy, infection, hemolysis, or splenectomy. Primary thrombocytosis or thrombocythemia is seen with polycythemia vera and chronic granulocytic leukemia.

Pathogenesis. In all types of thrombocytosis, the number of platelets is increased, but the mechanism of the increase varies. Transitory thrombocytosis results from release of preformed platelets, not increased production. As the name implies, the elevation in platelet count is transient. Secondary thrombocytosis results

from an actual increase in platelet production via an unknown mechanism. With primary thrombocytosis, there is abnormal proliferation of megakaryocytes in the bone marrow, resulting in as much as a 15-fold increase in platelet production.[19] The pathophysiologic basis for the excessive bleeding or thrombosis that may result is not well understood.

Clinical Manifestations. In general, transitory and secondary thrombocytosis do not result in hemorrhage or thrombotic complications. Hemorrhage into the skin and mucous membrane, as well as gastrointestinal bleeding, may be seen with primary thrombocytosis. Thrombosis resulting in peripheral vascular ischemia or pulmonary embolism may further complicate the clinical picture. Thromboembolic events are the most common cause of death. However, the course of the disease is benign in most patients.

Diagnosis. The diagnosis is made on the basis of a high platelet count. Bleeding time may be normal or prolonged, and platelet aggregation is normal or impaired. The history and clinical presentation, as well as additional laboratory tests such as bone marrow examination, aid in determining the type of thrombocytosis.

Treatment. No treatment is necessary with transitory and secondary thrombocytosis. Reducing platelet production with the use of cytotoxic agents such as hydroxyurea is one approach to treating primary thrombocytosis. Antiplatelet therapy (e.g., aspirin or dipyridamole) with its risk of bleeding may also be employed. In the presence of acute bleeding or thrombosis, platelet pheresis may be used to temporarily control the platelet count.

Qualitative Platelet Disorders

Etiology. Although the number of platelets may be normal, the ability of the platelets to function in the hemostatic process may be abnormal; thus a qualitative platelet disorder is present. Inherited defects in platelet function such as Bernard-Soulier syndrome (giant platelet syndrome), von Willebrand's disease, and thrombasthenia (Glanzman's disease) are rare. In contrast, acquired disorders of platelet function are common; they are often associated with drugs, especially aspirin; with uremia; or with another hematologic disease such as leukemia.

Pathogenesis. Whether the qualitative platelet disorder is inherited or acquired, at least one of the aspects of platelet function (adhesion, aggregation, or release reaction) is abnormal; a bleeding tendency results. In both Bernard-Soulier syndrome and von Willebrand's disease, platelet adhesion is abnormal. Platelet aggregation is the problem in thrombasthenia. Aspirin and other nonsteroidal anti-inflammatory agents inhibit production of thromboxane A_2 and thus impair both platelet aggregation and the platelet release reaction.

Clinical Manifestations. The clinical presentation of a qualitative platelet disorder is some form of bleeding tendency, such as petechiae and purpura on skin and mucous membranes, epistaxis, gastrointestinal bleeding, or menorrhagia. Acquired platelet function defects may also result in excessive bleeding during and following surgical procedures.

Diagnosis. With qualitative platelet defects, the bleeding time is prolonged but the platelet count and other routine coagulation screening tests are normal. Although a bleeding time greater than 10 minutes is associated with a slight increase in bleeding tendency, the risk is not significantly increased until the bleeding time exceeds 15 or 20 minutes.[5]

Special laboratory tests that more specifically evaluate platelet function, such as platelet aggregation studies, are necessary to determine the exact cause of bleeding.[8] Other coexisting hematologic defects may make diagnosis of a platelet defect difficult.

Treatment. If the platelet disorder is drug induced, the offending drug is discontinued. Transfusion with normal platelets is the usual intervention if treatment is necessary because of bleeding. Administration of desmopressin or cryoprecipitate is the treatment of choice when von Willebrand's disease is the underlying cause of bleeding.[5] The treatment for von Willebrand's disease is described in the following section.

KEY CONCEPTS

- Disorders of the vasculature that result in altered hemostasis include inflammation (allergic purpura), structural abnormalities (collagen diseases), and weakened vessel walls (telangiectasia).
- An insufficient quantity of platelets ($<50,000/mm^3$) results from decreased production, sequestration, increased destruction, and dilution. Important causes of thrombocytopenia include autoimmune destruction (ITP), disseminated intravascular coagulation (DIC), and mechanical destruction (artificial valves).
- Excessive quantity of platelets ($>400,000/mm^3$) results from excessive production (cancerous proliferation of bone marrow cells). Thrombocythemia may result in excessive coagulation with thrombosis or excessive bleeding.
- A normal platelet count does not ensure adequate platelet function. Platelet adhesion, aggregation, and degranulation may be abnormal, resulting in a prolonged bleeding time. The usual cause is drug related (e.g., aspirin), but, rarely, the platelet defect is inherited (e.g., von Willebrand's disease).

Coagulation Disorders

Coagulation disorders or **coagulopathies** are those defects of hemostasis and coagulation in which the primary cause of bleeding is a problem with the formation, stabilization, or lysis of the fibrin clot.

Hemophilia

Etiology. Hemophilia is rare in the general population, but it is the most common severe inherited coagulation disorder. Although bleeding may be apparent in infancy (e.g., intracranial bleeding, bleeding after circumcision), usually the disorder is diagnosed in early childhood once the child becomes active.

Hemophilia A, the classic form of the disease, accounts for approximately 85 percent of cases of clinical hemophilia. Hemophilia A is due to Factor VIII deficiency.[20] The majority of patients inherit this X-linked recessive disorder; hemophilia is transmitted by an asymptomatic carrier female to an affected son. Approximately 20 percent of patients with hemophilia A will have a negative family history because of a spontaneous mutation of the hemophilic gene.

Less common than hemophilia A is hemophilia B, also known as Christmas disease. Factor IX is deficient in this form of hemophilia.

The hemophilias are often classified according to the extent to which the specific coagulation factor (Factor VIII or Factor IX) is deficient. Patients with severe hemophilia have less than 1 percent normal coagulation factor activity, patients with moderate hemophilia have 1 percent to 5 percent normal coagulation factor activity, and patients with mild hemophilia have 5 percent to 25 percent normal coagulation factor activity.[21]

Of critical concern in the hemophilic patient is intracranial hemorrhage and other serious bleeding episodes. Because of advances in treatment, however, a normal life span is possible for many.

Pathogenesis. Hemophilia A results from the lack of Factor VIII or the abnormal function of Factor VIII. Hemophilia B results from the lack of Factor IX or the abnormal function of Factor IX. A deficiency or malfunction in either factor interferes with the normal sequence of events in the intrinsic pathway of coagulation and, in turn, the eventual production of fibrin clot. Inability to form a fibrin clot results in bleeding.

Clinical Manifestations. Once clinical evidence of bleeding is present, hemophilia A and B are indistinguishable. Patients with mild hemophilia may actually be asymptomatic until stressed by surgery or trauma. Prolonged bleeding from relatively minor trauma and occasionally spontaneous bleeding are characteristic of moderate hemophilia. With severe hemophilia, frequent episodes of spontaneous bleeding are likely.

Any of the following clinical manifestations may occur: easy bruising, prolonged bleeding from the nasal or oral mucosa, deep tissue hematomas, hemarthrosis, spontaneous hematuria, gastrointestinal bleeding, and intracranial bleeding. The hallmark of hemophilia is hemarthrosis. Repeated episodes of hemarthroses may result in joint deformity.

Major long-term complications of hemophilia include progressive joint deformity due to repeated hemarthroses; and hepatitis, cirrhosis, and AIDS related to repeated transfusions.

Diagnosis. Hemophilia is considered as the cause of bleeding when the family history is positive for bleeding in males, there is a history of joint bleeding and hematomas, and joint deformity is present on the physical examination. Laboratory tests consistent with hemophilia include a normal or slightly prolonged bleeding time, a normal prothrombin time, and a prolonged activated partial thromboplastin time. Factor assay verifies a deficiency in either Factor VIII or Factor IX. Early in pregnancy, chorionic villus biopsy or amniocentesis may be done to identify factor deficiency; thus, prenatal diagnosis of hemophilia is possible.[22]

Treatment. The patient and family must learn about hemophilia, including how to recognize and appropriately respond to bleeding episodes, what lifestyle changes will be necessary, and how the disease is transmitted. Prevention of injury and avoidance of aspirin and aspirin-like drugs, which alter platelet function in achieving and maintaining hemostasis, are important parts of treatment. Joint bleeding is managed by immobilization of the limb and application of ice.

With dental procedures requiring local anesthesia, prophylactic administration of Factor VIII should be considered in the patient with hemophilia A. Bleeding episodes due to hemophilia A are managed primarily by the administration of cryoprecipitate or other preparations of Factor VIII concentrate. The goal of therapy is to obtain a Factor VIII level at least 30 percent of normal.[23-25] Up to 20 percent of patients with severe hemophilia develop Factor VIII inhibitor, an antibody that rapidly inactivates transfused Factor VIII.[21,22] Plasmapheresis and immunosuppressive therapy are sometimes necessary to maintain adequate Factor VIII levels in these patients.

Mild to moderate bleeding due to hemophilia B is managed with the administration of fresh or fresh frozen plasma or cryoprecipitate. Konyne or Proplex, a concentrate containing Factors II, VII, IX, and X, is another therapeutic option; these concentrates are associated with a high risk of hepatitis.

Von Willebrand's Disease

Etiology. Von Willebrand's disease is inherited as an autosomal dominant disorder of Factor VIII carrier protein and platelet dysfunction. In rare cases, von Willebrand's disease is an autosomal recessive disorder.[7] Several less common subtypes of the disease have been identified, but all have some defect in von Willebrand factor, a plasma protein. Von Willebrand's disease occurs in both females and males. Bleeding manifestations of the disease tend to become more severe with age.

Pathogenesis. Von Willebrand factor and Factor VIII normally circulate in plasma as a complex. Von Willebrand factor is necessary for stabilization of Factor VIII in the circulation and for normal adherence of platelets to damaged vascular endothelium.[23,26] In von Willebrand's disease, the level of von Willebrand factor is decreased or absent; Factor VIII may be mildly to severely depressed. Absence of platelet adhesion at the site of vascular injury, plus deficient Factor VIII activity in the intrinsic coagulation pathway, both contribute to the bleeding seen in von Willebrand's disease.

Clinical Manifestations. Epistaxis, mucosal bleeding, ecchymoses, gastrointestinal bleeding, and menorrhagia are common clinical manifestations of von Willebrand's disease. Once hemostasis is achieved, it can usually be maintained. Hemarthrosis is rare. Although not common, von Willebrand's disease should be considered as a possible cause of excessive surgical bleeding. Bleeding manifestations may decrease during pregnancy because levels of von Willebrand factor and Factor VIII rise during this time.[7]

Diagnosis. The history and clinical presentation initially suggest the possibility of von Willebrand's disease as the cause of bleeding. Laboratory tests consistent with the disease include an increased bleeding time, prolonged activated partial thromboplastin time, normal platelet count, and normal prothrombin time. More specialized testing will verify that plasma von Willebrand factor is decreased and Factor VIII activity is reduced.

Treatment. Mild forms of classic von Willebrand's disease can be treated with desmopressin (DDAVP), which causes release of von Willebrand factor and Factor VIII from vascular endothelial cells.[21] Excessive menstrual bleeding can be managed with hormonal suppression. Severe bleeding is treated with cryoprecipitate that contains both Factor VIII and von Willebrand factor. Aspirin and aspirin-containing drugs, which inhibit normal platelet function in hemostasis, should be avoided in patients with von Willebrand's disease.

Complications of therapy for severe von Willebrand's disease include hepatitis and AIDS related to transfusions with blood products. Antibodies that inhibit the activity of von Willebrand factor may develop, but this is rare.

Hemorrhagic Disease of the Newborn

Etiology. As the name implies, this coagulation disorder is seen in the newborn, typically 48 to 72 hours after birth. Hemorrhagic disease of the newborn is more common in breast-fed babies (who do not receive vitamin K supplement) than in formula-fed babies. It is rare in Western countries because of routine administration of vitamin K to newborns.

Pathogenesis. This bleeding disorder results from a deficiency of the vitamin K–dependent coagulation factors, Factors II, VII, IX, and X. The levels of these factors are approximately 50 percent of normal in umbilical cord blood; the levels decline rapidly after birth, hitting their lowest at 48 to 72 hours. In a small number of infants the decline is so significant that severe bleeding results. After 72 hours, the levels of these coagulation factors gradually increase over the course of several weeks. This increase is primarily due to absorption of vitamin K from the diet. Cow's milk has a significantly higher content of vitamin K than breast milk; thus, breast-fed babies need vitamin K supplementation.

Hepatic immaturity may also contribute to hemorrhagic disease of the newborn. The liver may be unable to initially produce adequate levels of the vitamin K–dependent coagulation factors.

Clinical Manifestations. Evidence of bleeding, such as melena, bleeding from the umbilicus, and hematuria, appears on the second or third day of life. Life-threatening complications include intracranial hemorrhage and hypovolemic shock.

Diagnosis. The diagnosis is primarily based on the clinical presentation, particularly the timing of the onset of bleeding. The prothrombin time is prolonged; vitamin K–dependent clotting factors are decreased.

Treatment. Administration of vitamin K prophylactically to the newborn prevents the severe decline of the vitamin K–dependent coagulation factors and for the most part eliminates this coagulation disorder.

If evidence of hemorrhage is present, vitamin K should be administered. For severe hemorrhage, fresh plasma will replenish the deficient coagulation factors and stop the bleeding. Fresh whole blood will correct severe anemia and shock.

Premature infants may experience bleeding due to platelet abnormalities and a deficiency in several coagulation factors. Because of hepatic immaturity, vitamin K is ineffective therapy in these infants. Fresh plasma is the treatment of choice for the premature infant with bleeding complications.

Disseminated Intravascular Coagulation

Etiology. Disseminated intravascular coagulation (DIC) is an acquired hemorrhagic syndrome in which both clotting and bleeding occur simultaneously. Widespread clotting in small vessels leads to consumption of the clotting factors and platelets, which in turn leads to bleeding. DIC occurs secondary to a variety of factors, including malignancy, sepsis, snakebite, abruptio placentae, trauma and crushing injuries, transfusions of incompatible blood, burns, shock, and severe liver disease.[6,14,27]

Pathogenesis. DIC represents a paradox of both thrombosis and hemorrhage. Accelerated intravascular clotting in small vessels is initiated by contact of the blood with damaged vascular endothelium (sepsis, burns), release of procoagulant substances into the blood (snake venom, malignancy), generation of procoagulants in the blood (incompatible blood transfusion), or stagnant blood flow (shock). Coagulation factors, especially prothrombin, platelets, Factor V, and Factor VIII, are rapidly consumed. At the same time, the fibrinolytic system is activated to break down the clots. The fibrin degradation products that result act as circulating anticoagulants. The combination of coagulation, anticoagulation, and fibrinolysis ultimately leads to hemorrhage.[27]

Clinical Manifestations. Although both bleeding and clotting are part of the syndrome, initially bleeding is more apparent clinically. Petechiae and ecchymoses on skin and mucous membranes, as well as bleeding from orifices and any site of injury, such as venipuncture and injection sites, may be present. Acrocyanosis (cold, mottled fingers and toes) may also be apparent. Thrombi in the pulmonary microcirculation (small vessels) may result in dyspnea, hemoptysis, crackles. Patients with DIC are also predisposed to acute renal failure due to microthrombi in the renal microvasculature.

Diagnosis. The diagnosis of DIC is based on a high index of suspicion. The typical clinical picture described above, plus the presence of a predisposing cause, should make DIC a consideration. Abnormal coagulation studies that help confirm the diagnosis include increases in the bleeding time, prothrombin time, activated partial thromboplastin time, fibrin split products (FSP), and thrombin time; the fibrinogen level and platelet count are decreased. A newer test, D-dimer, is being used to confirm fibrin split products. An elevated FSP plus elevated D-dimer is highly predictive of DIC.[8,27]

Treatment. The cornerstone of treatment for DIC is removal or correction of the underlying cause and support of major organ systems. Replacement of depleted clotting factors with fresh frozen plasma, packed red blood cells, platelets, or cryoprecipitate may be necessary. Although controversial, heparin may be utilized to minimize further consumption of clotting factors in the microcirculation and also to deactivate the fibrinolytic system.[6,8,27]

Acquired Vitamin K Deficiency

Etiology. Acquired vitamin K deficiency may result in bleeding due to a coagulation defect. Vitamin K, a fat-soluble vitamin, is obtained via the diet and intestinal flora. Vitamin K is then absorbed by the intestine and stored in the liver. Normal absorption is dependent on bile acids and adequate mucosal function in the intestine. Vitamin K is necessary for normal synthesis and function of coagulation proteins (Factors II, VII, IX, and X) as well as coagulation inhibitors (proteins C and S).

Vitamin K deficiency with its associated risk for bleeding may occur with the following: malnutrition, malabsorption (including biliary disease), chronic hepatic disease, antibiotic therapy, and oral anticoagulation therapy. As many as 25 percent of patients treated with oral anticoagulants will develop bleeding complications.[28]

Pathogenesis. One of the many functions of the liver is the synthesis and transport of bile, which is necessary for fat digestion and normal absorption in the small intestine. Vitamin K is a fat-soluble vitamin; if fat malabsorption occurs due to a lack of bile, vitamin K is not absorbed, resulting in a vitamin K deficiency. In the newborn, especially the premature infant, vitamin K deficiency may be related to liver immaturity and the lack of vitamin K synthesis by the intestine until the gut is colonized with the flora that produce vitamin K. Coumarin-type drugs are vitamin

K antagonists that inhibit the normal role of vitamin K in the synthesis of clotting factors. The net effect is decreased clotting factor activity.

Although vitamin K is deficient, the liver continues to synthesize the vitamin K–dependent coagulation factors. The coagulation activity of these factors, however, is impaired, resulting in bleeding.[23]

Clinical Manifestations. Evidence of bleeding may present in a variety of ways, including mucosal and gastrointestinal bleeding, ecchymoses, menorrhagia, and hematuria. Surgical bleeding may be a significant problem in the patient with a vitamin K deficiency.

Diagnosis. Vitamin K deficiency should be considered as the cause for bleeding when the prothrombin time is increased but other coagulation studies are normal.[8] Of the vitamin K–dependent clotting factors, Factor VII (extrinsic pathway) has the shortest half-life; thus, the prothrombin time prolongs first. Ultimately, the activated partial thromboplastin time will also be prolonged as clotting factors in the intrinsic pathway become deficient.

Treatment. Parenteral administration of vitamin K rapidly restores levels in the liver with normal production of coagulation factors in 8 to 16 hours.[22,28] Fresh frozen plasma, with an immediate supply of clotting factors, is the treatment of choice for severe hemorrhage. Correction or removal of the cause for vitamin K deficiency is also an important part of therapy.

Hepatic Disease

Etiology. A common complication of many hepatic disorders is abnormal hemostasis. With the exception of part of the antihemophilic factor, all plasma protein clotting factors, fibrinolytic factors, and their inhibitors are synthesized totally or predominantly by the liver.[29,30] If liver function is altered by disease, bleeding is one manifestation. Often patients initially bleed because of an anatomic defect such as esophageal varices; however, the bleeding is exacerbated by abnormal hemostasis.

Pathogenesis. Several factors may contribute to the abnormal hemostasis seen in liver disease. Liver disease alters the synthesis and transport of bile, which is necessary for normal fat digestion and absorption. Impaired absorption and metabolism of vitamin K, which is fat soluble, result in decreased hepatic synthesis of coagulation Factors II, VII, IX, and X. Altered liver function also results in decreased synthesis of fibrinogen and Factors V and XI.[30] A deficiency in any of the coagulation factors can interrupt the normal process of fibrin clot formation. In addition to synthesis of coagulation factors, the liver also plays a role in removing activated coagulation proteins and activated fibrinolytic proteins from the circulation. Failure to adequately filter these proteins may result in an imbalance between clot formation and clot dissolution (fibrinolysis), manifesting clinically as DIC.[30] Liver disease may also alter normal production of inhibitors of coagulation (antithrombin III, proteins C and S);

this contributes to the hypercoaguable component of DIC.[23,30]

Another factor contributing to the bleeding associated with liver disease is thrombocytopenia. A low platelet count is common in liver disease. The exact mechanism is unknown but may relate to splenomegaly associated with portal hypertension.[6,13,30] Sequestration of platelets in the enlarged spleen depletes the number circulating and available for normal hemostasis.

Clinical Manifestations. Patients with chronic, rather than acute, liver disease are more likely to have clinical evidence of a bleeding problem. Typical clinical features may include any of the following: petechiae, ecchymoses, spider telangiectases, bleeding from venipuncture sites or esophageal varices, and gastrointestinal bleeding. DIC may complicate the clinical presentation. Bleeding may not be a problem until the patient has surgery or a biopsy.

Diagnosis. The patient with liver disease and associated bleeding will commonly have a decreased platelet count, normal or decreased fibrinogen levels, and prolonged prothrombin and activated partial thromboplastin times. More specific coagulation studies may be indicated in some situations.

Treatment. Treatment may be instituted prophylactically prior to surgery or biopsy, or it may be mandated by a bleeding episode. The degree of abnormality on coagulation tests or the severity of the bleeding will influence the aggressiveness of therapy. Because of the high likelihood of vitamin K deficiency, administration of vitamin K may be the initial intervention. Platelet infusions are appropriate if significant thrombocytopenia is present. Fresh frozen plasma is the primary replacement product utilized to supply coagulation factors. Administration of large quantities of plasma carries the risk of precipitating hepatic encephalopathy and fluid overload.

KEY CONCEPTS

- Coagulation disorders result from defects in the clotting cascade or fibrinolytic process. These disorders may be inherited or acquired.

- The hemophilias are inherited bleeding disorders due to deficient clotting factor production. The most common are hemophilia A (Factor VIII) and hemophilia B (Factor IX).

- Von Willebrand's disease is an inherited bleeding disorder due to abnormal Factor VIII carrier protein production. The disease results in deficient Factor VIII in the circulation and decreased platelet function.

- Vitamin K deficiency is associated with several coagulation disorders, including hemorrhagic disease of the newborn and bleeding related to malnutrition and liver disease. Vitamin K is a necessary cofactor for liver production of Factors II, VII, IX, and X.

- Disseminated intravascular coagulation (DIC) is an acquired bleeding syndrome associated with a number of etiologic factors including trauma, malignancy, burns, shock, and abruptio placentae. DIC is characterized by widespread clot formation in small vessels. Clotting factors and platelets are consumed, leaving the patient with deficient resources for appropriate clot formation. The platelet count and fibrinogen levels are typically decreased and prothrombin time, partial thromboplastin time, thrombin time, bleeding time, and fibrin split products are elevated.

Summary

The presence of unexpected overt or covert bleeding may signal an acquired or inherited problem with hemostasis. A review of normal hemostasis, as well as information on select disorders of hemostasis and coagulation, has been presented in this chapter. With a sound knowledge base, the health care professional is in a position to play a key role in the recognition, diagnosis, and treatment of a bleeding problem.

REFERENCES

1. Guyton A: *Textbook of Medical Physiology*, 8th ed. Philadelphia, WB Saunders, 1991, pp 390–399.
2. George J: Evaluation of hemostasis and thrombosis, in Stein J (ed): *Internal Medicine*. Boston, Little, Brown & Co, 1990, pp 992–996.
3. Jennings B: The hematologic system, in Alspach J (ed): *Core Curriculum for Critical Care Nursing*. Philadelphia, WB Saunders, 1991, pp 675–689.
4. Diethorn M, Weld L: Physiologic mechanisms of hemostasis and fibrinolysis. *J Cardiovasc Nurs* 1989;4(1):1–10.
5. Handin R: Bleeding and thrombosis, in Wilson J, et al (eds): *Harrison's Principles of Internal Medicine*. New York, McGraw-Hill, 1991, pp 348–353.
6. Dolan J: *Critical Care Nursing: Clinical Management Through the Nursing Process*. Philadelphia, FA Davis, 1991, pp 1271–1311.
7. Perry E, Hall M: Hereditary bleeding, in Reisdorff E, Roberts MR, Wiegenstein JG (eds): *Pediatric Emergency Medicine*. Philadelphia, WB Saunders, 1993, pp 476–484.
8. Wallerstein R: Laboratory evaluation of a bleeding patient. *West J Med* 1989;150(1):51–58.
9. Swerlick R, Lawley T: Cutaneous vasculitis: Its relationship to systemic disease. *Med Clin North Am* 1989;73(5):1221–1235.
10. Champoux A: Henoch-Schönlein purpura, in Reisdorff E, Roberts MR, Wiegenstein JG (eds): *Pediatric Emergency Medicine*. Philadelphia, WB Saunders, 1993, pp 405–408.
11. Gottlieb A: Nonallergic purpura, in Williams W (ed): *Hematology*. New York, McGraw-Hill, 1990, pp 1434–1441.
12. Gottlieb A: Hereditary hemorrhagic telangiectasia, in Williams W (ed): *Hematology*. New York, McGraw-Hill, 1990, pp 1449–1452.
13. Schneiderman E: Thrombocytopenia in the critically ill patient. *Crit Care Nurs Q* 1990;13(2):1–6.
14. Swearingen P, Keen J: *Manual of Critical Care*. St. Louis, CV Mosby, 1991, pp 427–440.
15. Gordon J, et al: Hematologic disorders in the pediatric intensive care unit, in Rogers M (ed): *Textbook of Pediatric Intensive Care*. Baltimore, Williams & Wilkins, 1992, pp 1357–1402.
16. Nugent D, Tarantino M: Hematology-oncology problems in the intensive care unit, in Fuhrman B, Zimmerman J: *Pediatric Critical Care*. St. Louis, CV Mosby, 1992, pp 815–827.
17. Fox F, Auestad A: Geriatric emergency clinical pharmacology. *Emerg Clin North Am* 1990;8(2):221–239.
18. Aster R, George J: Thrombocytopenia due to sequestration of platelets, in Williams W (ed): *Hematology*. New York, McGraw-Hill, 1990, pp 1398–1400.
19. Williams W: Thrombocytosis, in Williams W (ed): *Hematology*. New York, McGraw-Hill, 1990, pp 1403–1406.
20. Guyton A: *Human Physiology and Mechanisms of Disease*, 5th ed. Philadelphia, WB Saunders, 1992, pp 272–279.
21. Goldsmith J: Plasma component therapy: II. Hemostatic defects and their therapy, in Lubin N (ed): *Transfusion Therapy in Infants and Children*. Baltimore, Johns Hopkins University Press, 1991, pp 152–174.
22. Handin R: Disorders of coagulation and thrombosis, in Wilson J, et al (eds): *Harrison's Principles of Internal Medicine*. New York, McGraw-Hill, 1991, pp 1505–1511.
23. White G II: Disorders of blood coagulation, in Stein J (ed): *Internal Medicine*. Boston, Little, Brown & Co, 1990, pp 1048–1062.
24. Rick M, Gralnick H: Inherited disorders of blood coagulation, in Kelley W (ed): *Textbook of Internal Medicine*. Philadelphia, JB Lippincott, 1992, pp 1262–1267.
25. Levine P: The congenital coagulopathies, in Rippe J, et al (eds): *Intensive Care Medicine*. Boston, Little, Brown & Co, 1991, pp 1023–1031.
26. Gralnick H: Von Willebrand's disease, in Kelley W (ed): *Textbook of Internal Medicine*. Philadelphia, JB Lippincott, 1992, pp 1493–1509.
27. Epstein C, Bakanauskas A: Clinical management of DIC: early nursing interventions. *Crit Care Nurs* 1991;11(10):42–53.
28. Bang N: Diagnosis and management of bleeding disorders, in Shoemaker W, et al (eds): *Textbook of Critical Care*. Philadelphia, WB Saunders, 1989, pp 869–886.
29. Ansell J: Acquired bleeding disorders, in Rippe J, et al (eds): *Intensive Care Medicine*. Boston, Little, Brown & Co, 1991, pp 1013–1023.
30. Gralnick H: Acquired disorders of coagulation, in Kelley W (ed): *Textbook of Internal Medicine*. Philadelphia, JB Lippincott, 1992, pp 1267–1271.

BIBLIOGRAPHY

Acevedo M: Blood dyscrasias: Polycythemia, idiopathic thrombocytopenic purpura, and thrombotic thrombocytopenic purpura. *J Intravenous Nurs* 1992;15(1):52–57.
Aledort LM: New approaches to management of bleeding disorders. *Hosp Pract* 1989;24(2):207.
Bailes BK: Disseminated intravascular coagulation: Principles, treatment, nursing management. *AORN J* 1992;55(2):515.
Berg DE: Components and defects of the coagulation system. *Nurse Practitioner Forum* 1992;3(2):62–71.
Burns ER: When to suspect a bleeding disorder. *Emerg Med* 1990;22(11):67.
Ellison N: Perioperative disorders of hemostasis. *Current Rev Post Anesth Care Nurses* 1989;11(19):150–156.
Gobel BH: Plasma and plasma derivative therapy for coagulation disorders. *Semin Oncol Nurs* 1990;6(2):129–135.
Harmening DM: *Clinical Hematology and Fundamentals of Hemostasis*. Philadelphia, FA Davis, 1992.
Heimbach LJ, Newman JG: Shock lung and DIC. *Emergency* 1992;24(12):48.
Kesteven P, Saunders P: Disseminated intravascular coagulation. *Care Crit Ill* 1993;9(1):22.
Kimble C: Neonatal petechiae: Strategies for nursing interventions. *Pediatr Nurs* 1992;18(3):208.
Lee GR, et al: *Wintrobe's Clinical Hematology*. Philadelphia, Lea & Febiger, 1993.
Litwack K: Bleeding and coagulation in the PACU. *Crit Care Nurs Clin North Am* 1991;3(1):121–127.
Lynch M, Potter M: Henoch-Schönlein purpura: A case study. *Pediatr Nurs* 1990;16(6):561–566.
Mills D: When blood won't clot—hemophilia. *RN* 1992;55(11):28–33.
Mills DA: Hemophilia, in Thomas D (ed): *Quick Reference to Pediatric Emergency Nursing*. Gaithersburg, Md, Aspen Publishers, 1991.

Nathan DG, Oski FA: *Hematology of Infancy and Childhood*. Philadelphia, WB Saunders, 1993.

Peric-Knowlton W: Thromboembolic disorders: Current practice issues. *Nurse Practitioner Forum* 1992;3(2):60–61.

Ratnoff OD, Forbes CD: *Disorders of Hemostasis*. Philadelphia, WB Saunders, 1991.

Scott RB: Common blood disorders: A primary care approach. *Geriatrics* 1993;48(4):72.

Sedlak SK, Mace D: Hidden problems with bleeding in trauma patients. *J Emerg Nurs* 1989; 15(5):422–429.

Spivak JL, Eichner ER: *The Fundamentals of Clinical Hematology*. Baltimore, Johns Hopkins University Press, 1993.

Volker DL: Challenge of disseminated intravascular coagulation. *Dimensions Oncol Nurs* 1991;5(2):26–31.

Vosburgh E: Rational intervention in von Willebrand's disease. *Hosp Pract* 1993;28(3A):31.

Waldrop G, et al: Heparin-induced thrombocytopenia and thrombosis. *Dimensions Crit Care Nurs* 1991;10(6):330–344.

CHAPTER 14
Alterations in Blood Flow

ROBERTA EMERSON

KEY TERMS

aneurysm: Local dilation of arterial wall.

arteriosclerosis: Generalized term for pathologic conditions resulting in decreased distensibility of arteries.

arteriovenous fistula: Abnormal communication between an artery and a vein.

arteriovenous malformation: A type of arteriovenous fistula resulting in a tangle of vessels within the vasculature of the brain.

atherosclerosis: A type of arteriosclerosis characterized by proliferation of smooth muscle cells and lipid collection within the walls of arteries, resulting in narrowed lumina and impaired ability to dilate.

chronic venous insufficiency: Varicosity of the deep veins.

edema: Excessive amount of fluid in the interstitial space.

embolus: A collection of material (thrombus, air, fat, tumor cells, bacteria, amniotic fluid) propelled by blood flow to another site where it lodges and results in obstruction of flow.

hemodynamics: Principles of blood flow.

ischemia: Alteration in flow through the arterial system, producing tissue hypoxia.

phlebitis: Inflammation of a vein.

thrombophlebitis: Inflammation of a vein accompanied by the formation of a clot.

thrombus: Stationary blood clot formed within a vessel.

varicose veins: Incompetency of the superficial veins of the extremities, producing engorgement.

vasculitis: Inflammation of the lining (intima) of an artery.

vasospasm: Sudden, involuntary constriction of an artery, producing obstruction of flow.

---

*T*he primary functions of the circulatory system are the transportation of oxygen and nutrients and the removal of metabolic waste products within the body. In order to perform these functions, a complex circuitry of vessels traverses the body (Fig. 14–1), powered by the pumping action of the heart. Movement of blood through the lungs is provided by the right side of the heart. Systemic blood flow is supplied by the left side of the heart.

Nutrients are absorbed into the blood it moves through the gastrointestinal tract via the splanchnic circulation. Oxygen uptake and the release of carbon dioxide occur in the specialized vascular bed of the pulmonary circulation. Additional metabolic by-products are carried by the blood to the kidneys for elimination. Effective transportation of oxygen and nutrients and the removal of waste materials depend on proper functioning of the circulatory system.

Organization of the Circulatory and Lymphatic Systems

After passing through the pulmonary circulatory system and leaving the left side of the heart, blood flows through a graduated series of tubes to all of the cells of the body before returning to the right side of the heart. The powerful left ventricle propels the blood into the aorta, arteries, arterioles, and finally to the capillary bed. Here the proximity of capillary endothelium to the other cells of the body facilitates the movement of nutrients and oxygen into the cells and the removal of cellular metabolic wastes. Capillary blood is then collected by venules which flow into veins, returning blood to the vena cava and the right side of the heart (Fig. 14–2). The entire process, moving 5 liters of blood through the entire circuit, takes only about a minute.

The lymphatic system is a specialized scheme of channels and tissues (nodes). It is not arranged in a circuit as is the circulatory system. Instead, the lymphatic vessels begin blindly deep in the body's connective tissue. One of the functions of the lymphatic system is to reabsorb fluid that leaks out of the vascular network into the interstitium during movement through the capillary network and return it to the general circulation. During the process of exchange that occurs at a cellular level within the capillary bed, some fluid moves into the interstitium and fails to return. This lost fluid can amount to as much as 2–4 L/day. At this microcirculatory level, lymphatic vessels lie in close proximity to the capillary vasculature. The fluid is absorbed by the lymphatics, renamed "lymph," and returned to the venous circulation by way of the thoracic duct and the right lymphatic duct (Fig. 14–3). (See Chapter 9 for a discussion of the role of the lymphatics in the immune response.)

Vessel Structure

In order to carry out their specialized functions, the circulatory vessels and lymphatic vessels are markedly different structurally. A knowledge of the morphology of these vessels enhances an understanding of the alterations in function produced by disease.

Blood Vessel Structure

Structurally, arteries, capillaries, and veins have significant variation. The primary differences between the smaller arterial and venous vessels occur in the quantities of muscle and connective tissue present. In arterioles, the principal tissue is muscle, whereas in venules muscle is scarce and connective tissue predominates. Larger arteries and veins vary in the composition of the walls and in the size and shape of the vessels. Capillary walls are composed of a single layer of endothelial cells. These extremely simple structures carry out extraordinarily complex functions.

Anatomy of Arteries and Veins. The walls of both arteries and veins are composed of three microscopically distinct layers, or **tunicas: the intima,** the **media,** and the **adventitia.** The histologic components of these coats are similar in arteries and veins (Fig. 14–4). Generally, the walls of veins are not as thick as the walls of arteries, but the lumina are larger.

The **intima** consists of a layer of endothelial cells that is in direct contact with the blood as it flows through the vessel. The intimal layer of veins protrudes into the lumen, creating the valves that prevent the backflow of blood. Arterial intima is characterized by an inner elastic membrane next to the endothelial cells. This elastic membrane is thickest in the aorta and decreases in density until only scattered elastic fibers can be identified in the smallest of arterioles. With increasing age, the intimal wall of arteries becomes thicker and less elastic. This interferes with diffusion of nutrients into the wall, causing the internal elastic membrane to degenerate and calcify.[1]

The **media,** or middle layer, exhibits the greatest

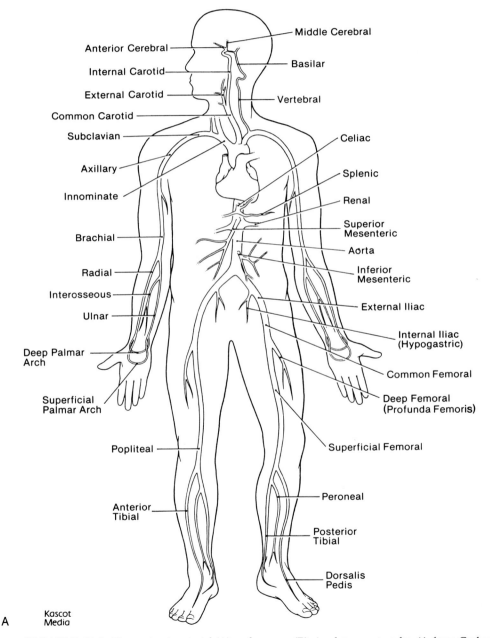

A   Kascot
Media

FIGURE 14–1. The systemic arterial (**A**) and venous (**B**) circulatory networks. (**A** from Graham LM, O'Keefe MF: Arterial disease, in Fahey VA (ed): *Vascular Nursing.* Philadelphia, WB Saunders, 1993, p 5. **B** from Rohrer MJ: The venous system: Basic considerations, *op cit,* p 23. Reproduced with permission.)

Figure continued on following page

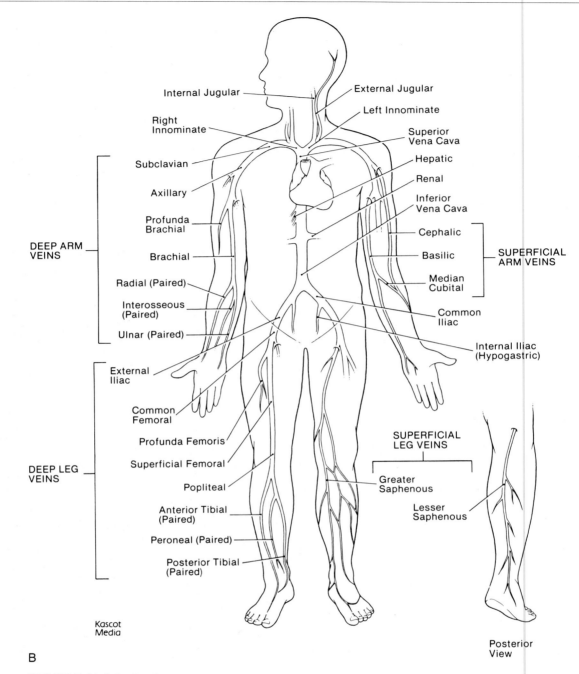

Internal Jugular

External Jugular

Right Innominate

Left Innominate

Superior Vena Cava

Subclavian

Hepatic

Axillary

Renal

Inferior Vena Cava

Profunda Brachial

Cephalic

DEEP ARM VEINS

Brachial

Basilic

SUPERFICIAL ARM VEINS

Radial (Paired)

Median Cubital

Interosseous (Paired)

Ulnar (Paired)

Common Iliac

Internal Iliac (Hypogastric)

External Iliac

Common Femoral

Profunda Femoris

SUPERFICIAL LEG VEINS

Superficial Femoral

DEEP LEG VEINS

Popliteal

Greater Saphenous

Anterior Tibial (Paired)

Lesser Saphenous

Peroneal (Paired)

Posterior Tibial (Paired)

Kascot Media

B

Posterior View

F I G U R E   14–1 Continued

differences between arteries and veins. In all arteries the media is the thickest of the tunicas. Large arteries have smooth muscle fibers arranged in a circular pattern and interspersed with elastic fibers. Moving to ever-smaller arterioles, the smooth muscle remains but the elastic tissue disappears. This thick, smooth muscle layer is responsible for the firmness and limited distensibility of arteries. With advancing age, changes in the intima result in decreased nutrition to the media, causing degeneration of this smooth muscle tissue.[1] In veins, the media also has smooth muscle, usually arranged in a circular pat-

tern with some longitudinal strands. The quantity of smooth muscle decreases as the veins become larger. Venous media also contains collagenous connective tissue, but elastic tissue is rare except in the largest veins.

In veins, the **adventitia** is the thickest layer. It is composed of collagenous connective tissue and longitudinal smooth muscle. In larger arteries there is a discernible external elastic membrane in the adventitia. This membrane is eliminated as the arteries become smaller. Arterial adventitia consists predominantly of collagenous connective tissue. Some larger

PULMONIC
CIRCULATION

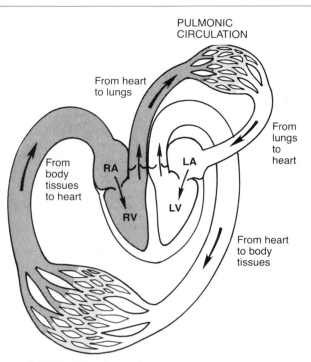

SYSTEMIC CIRCULATION

F I G U R E 14–2. The circulatory system. Oxygenated blood leaves the pulmonic circulation and returns to the heart via the left atrium (LA) and left ventricle (LV). From the left side of the heart, the oxygenated blood enters the systemic circulation, where gas and metabolic exchange occurs. Blood returns to the right side of the heart, through the right atria (RA) and right ventricle (RV), which propels it back into the lungs. (From Black JM, Matassarin-Jacobs E: *Luckmann and Sorensen's Medical-surgical Nursing: A Psychophysiologic Approach*, 4th ed. Philadelphia, WB Saunders, 1993, p 1092. Reproduced with permission.)

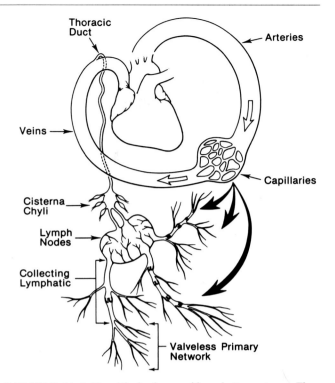

F I G U R E 14–3. Simplified scheme of lymphatic anatomy. The lymphatic capillaries collect vascular capillary excess fluid and return it to the venous circulation. (From Dixon MB, Bergan JJ: Lymphedema, in Fahey VA (ed): *Vascular Nursing*. Philadelphia, WB Saunders, 1993, p 34. Reproduced with permission.)

vessels also contain isolated, longitudinally arranged fibers of smooth muscle.

Anatomy of Capillaries. Capillaries are composed of a single thickness of endothelium. Moving from the end of an arteriole to the beginning of a venule, capillaries narrow to a diameter barely sufficient for a single red blood cell (RBC) to pass through. In some tissues, one or two smooth muscle cells form a precapillary sphincter that controls flow through the vessel (Fig. 14–5).

There are spaces between the endothelial cells that vary in size from organ system to organ system. These spaces, or **pores,** permit certain constituents to pass out of the capillaries. For example, capillary beds in the brain have very small spaces and permit only very small molecules to pass through. The space between endothelial cells of the brain is so small that it is referred to as the **blood-brain barrier.** In parts of the kidneys, however, capillaries are more porous, allowing much larger molecules to enter or exit the circulation. This is the process of **ultrafiltration.** The size of the spaces between the endothelial cells of capillary walls determines the **capillary permeability** of a specific capillary bed.

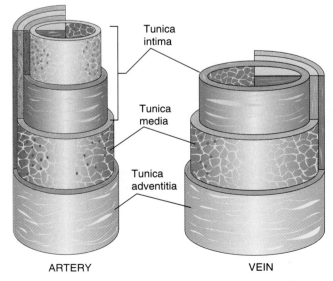

ARTERY   VEIN

F I G U R E 14–4. Tunicas of arteries and veins, showing the thicker walls of the arteries.

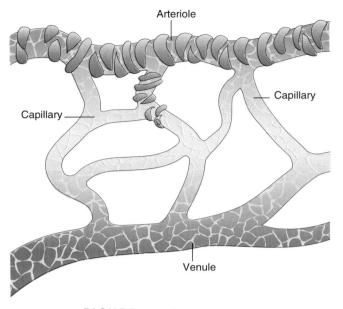

F I G U R E 14–5. Capillary network.

Lymphatic Structure

Lymphatic vessels are thin-walled and most resemble veins in appearance. Like their counterparts in the circulatory system, they range in size from lymphatic capillaries to vessels of increasing diameter. Like veins, lymphatics have valves composed of folds of their inner layer that extend into the lumen of the channels (Fig. 14–6). The walls of lymphatic capillaries contain contractile fibers that are stimulated when stretched, causing the vessels to contract.

KEY CONCEPTS

- Arteries and veins have three distinct layers. The intima, the innermost layer, is composed of a single layer of endothelial cells. The media, or middle layer, is composed of smooth muscle and elastin.

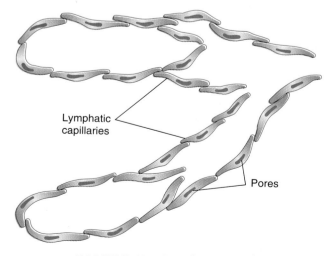

F I G U R E 14–6. Lymphatic network.

Media is thicker in arteries than in veins. The adventitia, the outermost layer, is composed of supporting connective tissue.

- Capillaries have only a single layer of endothelial cells. The permeability of capillaries is determined by how tightly the endothelial cells join together.

Principles of Flow

Hemodynamics of the Circulatory System

The principles of blood flow are known as circulatory **hemodynamics.** These principles govern the quantity of blood passing by a given point in a specific period of time. Therefore, blood flow may be recorded as a given number of liters, milliliters, or cubic centimeters per second, minute, or hour. A discussion of the hemodynamics of the circulatory system includes the attributes of pressure, resistance, velocity, laminar and turbulent flows, wall tension, and compliance.

Blood Flow, Pressure, and Resistance

Blood flow is accomplished by movement along a **pressure gradient** within the vascular bed. This means that blood moves from an area of higher pressure to an area of lower pressure. The arterial walls with their thick muscular media coat provide the high-pressure end of the gradient. Seeking a lower pressure, blood moves into the venous system. The thinner, more pliable walls of the venous vascular bed furnish the low-pressure portion of the pressure gradient. The greater the pressure difference, the faster is the blood flow.

The movement of blood through the vascular system is opposed by the force of **resistance.** The relationship between blood flow and resistance is an inverse one: as resistance increases, blood flow decreases. This force has several determinants, each of which can change resistance considerably.

Two of the determinants of resistance are *vessel length* and *vessel radius*. Resistance increases with the length of the vessel. As illustrated in Figure 14–7, given three vessels of the same radius, doubling the length reduces the flow by 50 percent. Reducing the vessel length by half increases the flow by 100 percent. These changes in flow occur when the pressure gradient remains constant and are due solely to variations in vessel length. Resistance decreases as the radius of a vessel increases. Resistance is inversely related to the fourth power of the vessel's radius, or r^4. Therefore, increasing the radius of the vessel produces an exponential increase in blood flow. Figure 14–8 demonstrates the effect of doubling the radius of a vessel on the flow of blood, if all other factors related to flow are held constant. The resulting flow of blood is 16 times greater in the greater-diameter vessel.

Although there is variability in the length of vessels throughout the circulatory system, vessels are

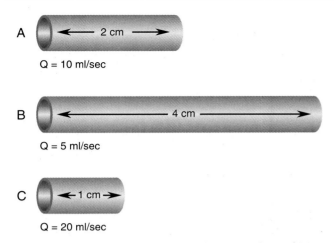

FIGURE 14-7. Relationship of vessel length to blood flow.

incapable of altering their own length. There is, however, considerable ability to change the diameter of vessel walls in normal physiology, and many disease processes are associated with changes in the size of the vessel lumen. Even minor changes will produce major alterations in resistance and hence blood flow. This makes changes in diameter the most important determinant of resistance.

The third determinant of resistance is the *viscosity* of the blood itself. Viscosity denotes the thickness of a fluid. When the blood is more viscous, the friction between the cells and the liquid increases, and resistance to flow increases. Blood is composed of a suspension of cellular material and plasma. Roughly 99 percent of the cellular constituents of the blood are RBCs. Increasing the relative concentration of RBCs or decreasing the plasma component results in more viscous blood, hence more resistance and slower blood flow. This is what occurs in dehydration, when the plasma component is relatively decreased, or in polycythemia, when the number of RBCs increases.

The relationship between the variables of pressure difference and resistance and their effect on blood flow is expressed by **Ohm's law,** as follows:

$$Q = P/R,$$

where Q is the blood flow, P is the pressure difference between two points, and R is resistance. Altering any one of the determinants of resistance will produce a change in flow. Likewise, if the pressure difference within the circulatory system is changed, it will result in a change in the flow of blood. This is best visualized in the arterioles, the major site of resistance in the vascular system (Fig. 14-9).

Total peripheral resistance refers to the resistance throughout the entire vascular system. It can be calculated based upon the pressure difference between the arteries and the veins. The resulting peripheral resistance units (PRU) are expressed as mm Hg/mL/sec and are known as hybrid units with little clinical value. Clinically, **systemic vascular resistance** (SVR) is used to denote resistance peripheral to the heart and lungs. SVR converts PRU to metric units and is measured in dynes/sec/cm^5, which is more useful in the clinical setting. SVR is calculated based on the following formula:

$$SVR = \frac{MAP - CVP}{CO} \times 80,$$

where the mean arterial pressure (MAP) is 70–105 mm Hg, the central venous pressure (CVP) is 0–8 mm Hg, and cardiac output (CO) is 4–8 L/min. The resulting range for SVR is 700–1,600 dynes/sec/cm^5. Since the primary determinant of SVR is the resistance vessels, or the arterial bed, diseases and drug therapies that affect the arterial bed have the most profound impact on the SVR.

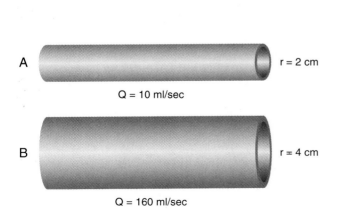

FIGURE 14-8. Relationship of vessel radius to blood flow.

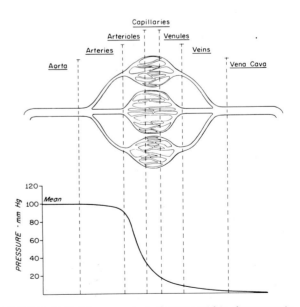

FIGURE 14-9. Mean pressure changes within the systemic vasculature. A significant decrease in pressure occurs as blood flows through the arterioles into the capillaries. The figure illustrates the role of the arterioles in the determination of vascular resistance. Because of the large number of capillaries, total resistance is not increased with the decreased radius of the capillaries. (From Patton HD, et al (eds): *Textbook of Physiology,* 21st ed. Philadelphia, WB Saunders, 1989, p 778. Reproduced with permission.)

Velocity and Laminar and Turbulent Flow

Blood flow is defined as the volume of blood that passes a given point in a given unit of time and is measured in milliliters or liters per second. **Velocity** is a measure of the distance traveled in a given interval of time and is usually expressed in centimeters per second. Velocity is governed by the total cross-sectional area and varies inversely with it. An increase in the total cross-sectional area will produce a decrease in velocity, a decrease in the total cross-sectional area will produce an increase in velocity. The total cross-sectional area of the arterial bed is the smallest of any vessel in the circulatory system. Next smallest in total cross-sectional area is the venous bed. The capillary beds of the body combine to produce the greatest total cross-sectional area. The dividing and subdividing of vessels within the circulatory system results in greater velocity in the arterial and venous beds than in the capillary bed (Fig. 14–10). An understanding of the concept of velocity enhances discussion of laminar and turbulent flow.

When blood flows through a long, smooth-walled vessel, it does so in layers. The velocity of the layers varies, with blood in the center moving much faster than blood in the outer layers. The blood in the center layer moves fastest because it is in contact with blood only. The outermost layer is in contact with the vessel wall, which exerts friction against the cellular components in the blood. Many of the cells stick to the intima. This layer may flow only minimally, if at all.

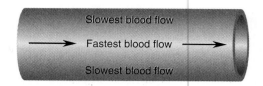

FIGURE 14–11. Parabolic profile of laminar blood flow.

Layers of blood between this outer layer and the central core of blood slide over one another with increasing velocity. This is referred to as the parabolic profile of **laminar flow** and is illustrated in Figure 14–11.

The streamlined nature of laminar flow is disrupted by normal anatomy and by pathologic processes creating turbulent flow. **Turbulent flow** is an interruption in the forward current of blood flow by crosswise flow. The same process can be seen in a river, where boulders interrupting the flow produce whirlpools and the characteristic roar of rapids. In the human body, turbulent flow through blood vessels can be auscultated as a *bruit.* Sometimes it can be palpated as well, and then it is called a *thrill.* This turbulence may be due to blood moving through branching vessels at a sharp angle, blood flowing around an obstruction in the vessel, or blood flowing over a roughened intimal surface. Turbulent flow alters the parabolic profile seen with laminar flow, slowing velocity around the source of the turbulence.[2] Slowing of flow can cause cellular components of the blood to adhere to one another, the turbulent focus, and the intimal wall, promoting the formation of clots.

Wall Tension and Compliance

The relationship between distending pressure and wall tension is expressed by the **law of Laplace** and is illustrated in Figure 14–12. This physical principle has broad applications in physiology; however, the present discussion focuses on its implications for blood vessels. The **distending pressure** (*P*) is the **transmural pressure,** or pressure on one side of the

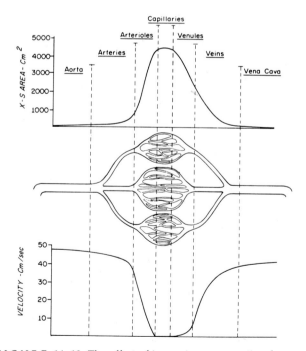

FIGURE 14–10. The effect of increasing cross-sectional area on the velocity of blood flow. Increased cross-sectional area in the capillary bed results in a significant decrease in velocity when compared to the arterial and venous networks. (From Patton HD, et al (eds): *Textbook of Physiology,* 21st ed. Philadelphia, WB Saunders, 1989, p 777.)

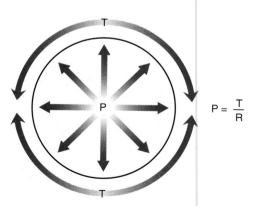

$$P = \frac{T}{R}$$

FIGURE 14–12. Law of Laplace as applied to a blood vessel. Distending pressure (*P*) is the difference between the pressures on either side of the vessel and is equal to the wall tension (*T*) divided by the radius of the blood vessel (*r*).

vessel wall minus the pressure on the other side of the blood vessel. This distending pressure (*P*) is equal to the wall tension (*T*) divided by the radius of the blood vessel (*r*). An increase in radius or distending pressure results in increased wall tension.

When the pressure of the blood in the vessel begins to fall, wall tension forces exceed distending forces, the radius decreases, flow declines, and resistance increases. The distending pressure may reach a point at which it is no longer possible to hold the blood vessel open. If the pressure reaches 20 mm Hg, a point called the *critical closing pressure,* blood flow will cease entirely.[3]

The smaller the radius of the blood vessel, as in a capillary compared to an artery or vein, the less tension is needed in the wall to balance out the distending pressure. Wall tensions fall rapidly from 170,000 dynes/cm in the aorta to 16 dynes/cm in the capillaries, rising to 21,000 dynes/cm in the vena cava.[4]

Wall tension is a product of the elasticity of the vessel and is a force that opposes the distending pressure. How wall tension in a given vessel responds to changes in distending pressures is based on its compliance. **Compliance** reflects the distensibility of a blood vessel—its ability to accept an increased volume of blood. The large quantity of muscle tissue in much of the arterial system limits its distensibility. Veins, however, are highly distensible and compliant, capable of holding a large quantity of blood at a low pressure. Because of this quality, veins are referred to as *capacitance vessels.* When the body is at rest, 75 percent of the total blood volume is found in the systemic venous system. When a patient is given a transfusion of blood, the vast majority of it will remain in the systemic veins, right atria and ventricle, and the pulmonary circulation. Less than 1 percent of the transfused blood moves into the arterial system.[4]

Dynamics in the Microcirculation and Lymphatics

The capillary bed is referred to as the **microcirculation.** Its primary function is the essence of the circulatory system as a whole: the exchange of gases and nutrients. Blood flow in the capillary bed is largely laminar, with minimal turbulence at bifurcations. Variations in smooth muscle tone (vasomotion) in the capillaries are responsible for producing changes in the velocity of flow. Blood flow at this level is directly related to the difference between the arterial and venous pressures and inversely related to SVR. When a patient's arterial pressure falls and he becomes hypotensive, the body attempts to maintain flow in the microcirculation by increasing SVR.

The exchange of materials across the capillary endothelium through the interstitial space, to or from the cells, occurs as a continuous process. Substances pass between cells and capillaries by moving along a concentration gradient (*diffusion*), while fluid moves according to a pressure gradient (*osmosis*).

As fluid moves through the interstitial space, most of it returns to the capillary bed. Normally, approximately 10 percent of the fluid remains in the interstitium and is picked up by the adjacent lymphatic system to be returned to the general circulation. Alteration in the pressure gradient responsible for filtration can allow an excessive amount of fluid to escape into the interstitial space. Increased fluid accumulation in the interstitial space can also occur when the lymphatic flow is impaired or when capillaries become more permeable and "leak" fluid. These are the mechanisms that result in **edema.**

The pressure gradient between the capillary and the interstitium is produced and maintained in accord with the balance of four distinct forces or pressures: capillary pressure, interstitial fluid colloid osmotic pressure, plasma colloid osmotic pressure, and interstitial fluid pressure (Fig. 14–13). This delicate balance of forces is summarized by **Starling's hypothesis,** which states that the net filtration is equal to the combined forces fostering filtration minus the combined forces opposing filtration:

Net filtration pressure (+0.3 mm Hg)
 = (capillary pressure (17 mm Hg)
 + interstitial fluid colloid osmotic pressure
 (5.0 mm Hg))
 − (plasma colloid osmotic pressure (28 mm Hg)
 + interstitial fluid pressure (−6.3 mm Hg))

0.3 mm Hg = ((17 mm Hg + 5 mm Hg)
 − (−6.3 mm Hg + 28 mm Hg))

Clinically, capillary fluid pressure and plasma colloid osmotic pressure are most important to a discussion of pathophysiology. **Capillary fluid pressure** is the blood pressure within the capillary. It is the force pushing fluid from the capillary into the interstitium and is often called the filtration pressure. The strength of this force depends on the blood pressure and resistance within the arterial and venous systems. Patho-

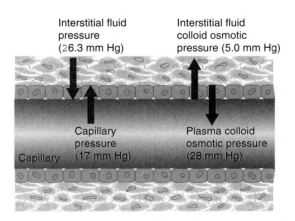

FIGURE 14–13. Components of the capillary pressure gradient. Ultrafiltration reflects the difference between the combined forces forcing fluid out of the capillary (capillary pressure and interstitial fluid colloid osmotic pressure) and those forces attempting to hold fluid in the capillary (plasma colloid osmotic pressure and interstitial fluid pressure).

logic conditions resulting in a change in either the blood pressure or the resistance to flow can alter this force, most frequently increasing it and propelling more fluid into the interstitial space.

Plasma proteins are responsible for the primary force resulting in fluid remaining in the capillary, **plasma colloid osmotic pressure.** Most plasma proteins remain in the capillaries because they are such large molecules that they are not able to move through the capillary walls easily. The vast majority of plasma protein, by weight, is albumin. Although globulins and fibrinogen have greater molecular weight, albumin is present in plasma in greater quantity. The number of dissolved molecules within the plasma determines the plasma colloid osmotic pressure. In the interstitial space, the number of dissolved molecules establishes the interstitial fluid pressure. Albumin, as the smallest of the plasma proteins, will move with some difficulty through the capillary walls and into the interstitium. The plasma has nearly four times the concentration of proteins as the interstitium. For that reason, plasma colloid osmotic pressure normally exceeds that in the interstitium, favoring fluid remaining in the capillaries.[2]

Applying the Starling hypothesis to the net filtration pressure results in a total pressure favoring filtration of 0.3 mm Hg. This pressure difference is responsible for producing the fluid excess, which is then normally picked up by the lymphatic system for eventual return to the circulation. If the pressures alter, resulting in an even greater pressure gradient, more fluid moves from the capillaries into the interstitial space. Likewise, a change in the permeability of the capillary wall allowing plasma protein leakage or a reduction in lymphatic flow will allow fluid to collect in the interstitium. In each case, the result is **edema** (see Chap. 28). When fluid collection in the interstitial space is limited to the extremities, due to impaired flow, the result is **lymphedema.**

Once absorbed into the lymphatic system, interstitial fluid is referred to as **lymph.** It is similar in composition to interstitial fluid, but with a lower concentration of protein. Molecules of fat and bacteria are also found in lymph. Lymph circulates throughout the body at a rate of approximately 3 L/day. Lymphatic flow can be increased by increasing the capillary pressure, decreasing the plasma colloid osmotic pressure, increasing the interstitial fluid colloid osmotic pressure, or increasing the permeability of the capillaries. The interstitial fluid hydrostatic pressure increases (becomes less negative) when any of these factors change, and the lymphatic flow increases.[3]

KEY CONCEPTS

- Physical laws govern the flow of blood through the circulatory system. Predictions regarding blood flow, blood pressure, and resistance to flow can be made using these laws. The important relationships may be summarized as follows:
  1. Flow = Pressure/Resistance
  2. Blood pressure = Flow (CO) × Resistance
  3. Resistance = Pressure/Flow
- The main factors affecting resistance to flow are radius and length of the vessels, and blood viscosity and turbulence. Usually, radius of the vessel is the most important determinant of resistance. Radius affects resistance inversely and to the fourth power $(1/r^4)$. A small decrease in radius results in a large increase in resistance.
- The velocity of blood flow varies inversely with the total cross-sectional area of the vascular bed. The capillaries have the greatest total cross-sectional area and therefore the slowest flow.
- Laplace's law describes the relationships among wall tension, distending pressure, and vessel radius $(P = T/r; T = P \times r)$. An increase in radius or distending pressure will result in increased wall tension.
- The transcapillary exchange of fluid and nutrients is accomplished by the processes of diffusion and filtration. Diffusion refers to movement of solute and is determined by capillary permeability and the size of the concentration gradient. Filtration refers to movement of fluid and is affected in the following way:
  1. Increased capillary hydrostatic pressure and interstitial oncotic pressure enhance filtration.
  2. Increased interstitial hydrostatic pressure and capillary oncotic pressure oppose filtration.
  3. Increased permeability (K) enhances filtration.

Control of Flow

Blood flow throughout the periphery is controlled by extrinsic mechanisms mediated by the autonomic nervous system, the venous and thoracic pumps, and intrinsic autoregulatory mechanisms. Lymphatic flow is controlled by increasing interstitial fluid hydrostatic pressure and by the lymphatic pumps. In health, these mechanisms of control respond to changes in the internal and external environment and compensate rapidly and efficiently. However, in illness these mechanisms may be inadequate to compensate for alterations in flow.

Control of Blood Flow

Extrinsic Mechanisms

The autonomic nervous system provides the primary extrinsic control of blood flow through the sympathetic nervous system (SNS). Although parasympathetic nervous system (PSNS) innervation is important to the regulation of the heart, it is not important to the regulation of peripheral blood flow. Within the medulla, groups of neurons form the **vasomotor center.** This area plays a major role in the maintenance of blood pressure. The vasomotor center responds to direct stimulation and afferent stimuli of both an excitatory and inhibitory nature (see Chap. 15, Alterations in Blood Pressure). A basal rate of discharge from the vasomotor center results in a continuous minimal level of contraction of vascular smooth muscle, referred to as **vasomotor tone.**

All blood vessels except the small venules and capillaries contain smooth muscle that is innervated by adrenergic fibers from the SNS. Because arteries have the most smooth muscle, they are most affected by SNS stimulation. Veins, by contrast, have little neural innervation, and venoconstriction, if it occurs, plays a minimal role in controlling blood flow except in the skin and the splanchnic circulation of the gut. In general, the release of norepinephrine, the SNS postganglionic neurotransmitter, results in arterial vasoconstriction via the α_1 receptors located on the vascular smooth muscle walls. Likewise, drugs that mimic the α_1 response (α agonists such as phenylephrine) produce vasoconstriction, increasing vasomotor tone and diastolic blood pressure. An α antagonist such as prazosin will result in the blockade of α receptors and vasodilation of the arterial bed.

Although there are β_2-adrenergic receptors located on blood vessels found in skeletal muscle which produce vasodilation when stimulated, they are only minimally affected by endogenous norepinephrine from the SNS. Epinephrine, the endogenous catecholamine released by the adrenal medulla, or its exogenous pharmacologic equivalent (Adrenalin) does stimulate these receptors, producing vasodilation.[5] Therefore, their major role is not so much to maintain vasomotor tone but to increase nutrient and oxygen supplies to skeletal muscles during periods of stress.

Blood flow through the venous system is maintained by the pressure gradient from the veins to the right side of the heart, and the venous and thoracic pumps. Blood is propelled through the circuit, pushed by the force of left ventricular contraction and moving forward toward the low-pressure side of the pump on the right side of the heart. In the peripheral veins, the venous pump is activated by skeletal muscle activity. Folds in the intimal wall of the veins form valves. Contraction of the skeletal muscles bordering veins compresses them, forcing the valves open and propelling venous blood back toward the heart. This **venous pump** significantly facilitates venous return. Patients who are immobilized by bed rest lose this valuable mechanism, which results in a decrease in cardiac preload and increased work of the heart in order to maintain the cardiac output. The thoracic pump acts to increase venous return to the heart as intrathoracic pressure changes with breathing. This process, like the venous pump, enhances venous return to the heart (preload) (see Chap. 16).

Intrinsic Mechanisms

Autoregulation refers to the ability of organs to maintain a relatively constant blood flow, regardless of changes in arterial pressure. This flow is *relatively* constant because it has limits; there is a range within which it is maintained. There are a number of theories as to how autoregulation works to meet the needs of individual organs within the body. The *myogenic hypothesis* is based on the observation that as vascular smooth muscle is stretched, it contracts. Therefore, as arterial pressure rises and arterial walls stretch, contraction is stimulated, producing vasoconstriction. The myogenic hypothesis also suggests that resistance to flow is increased with stretch by early closing of precapillary sphincters. The *metabolic hypothesis* proposes that metabolic by-products (metabolites) or substrates exert a direct vasodilatory effect, increasing blood flow to the area. Metabolites might include carbon dioxide or lactic acid. Histamine and prostaglandins are examples of metabolic substrates. A local increase in blood flow is referred to as **hyperemia.** The increase in local blood flow in response to increased metabolic demand is called **active** or **functional hyperemia. Reactive hyperemia** occurs when a temporary reduction in blood flow is interrupted. The body responds by briefly increasing circulation to the area, resulting in the characteristic flushing seen, for instance, when a tourniquet is removed. The *tissue pressure hypothesis* of autoregulation postulates that an acute increase in the pressure within the arterial system will result in an increase in interstitial volume and pressure. This increased tissue pressure, external to the vasculature, results in compression of small vessels which increases resistance and reduces flow.[2]

Control of Lymphatic Flow

The movement of lymph is expedited by **lymphatic pumps.** This is a general term and includes the pumping action of the lymphatics themselves and the pumping effect on the lymphatic vessels produced by activity external to them. Like veins, lymphatic vessels have valves on their intimal surface that allow forward movement of fluid toward the heart and systemic circulation. Compression of lymphatic channels by adjacent skeletal muscles, the smooth muscle of organs, and the pulsatile movement of arteries forces lymph toward the heart. Intrathoracic pressure changes related to breathing increase lymphatic return as well as venous return. Lymphatic flow is therefore enhanced by increased physical activity, increased blood pressure, or increased respiratory rate. Lymphatic contractions are thought to be the primary factor in lymphatic flow. Lymphatic capillaries contract when stretched, propelling lymph forward. The rate of contractions increases as the volume of lymph increases.[4]

KEY CONCEPTS

- The blood flow through a particular vascular bed is regulated centrally by the autonomic nervous system and locally by the organ or tissue.

- In most vascular beds, the sympathetic nervous system (SNS) causes constriction, which increases resistance and reduces flow. Smooth muscle cells in these vascular beds have α_2 receptors that bind the

SNS neurotransmitter norepinephrine, causing contraction. There is no significant parasympathetic innervation of systemic vessels.

- Autoregulation refers to a tissue's ability to regulate its own flow. Autoregulation allows a tissue to maintain optimal flow despite changes in blood pressure or metabolic demands. In instances of high blood pressure or decreased metabolic demand, the arterioles and precapillary sphincters that control flow to the tissue constrict, reducing flow. In instances of low blood pressure or high demand, vessels dilate, increasing flow.

- Lymphatic vessels maintain flow by contracting when stretched with lymph. Intraluminal valves prevent backflow. External compression by contracting muscles enhances lymph flow.

General Mechanisms Resulting in Altered Flow

A reduction in flow through the systemic vasculature results in impaired ability to transport gases and nutrients to and from body tissues. Cells of the body vary in their oxygen demands. **Hypoxia,** an insufficient supply of oxygen, can occur for a multiplicity of reasons, such as a decrease in hemoglobin formation or diminished oxygen transport in the lungs (see Chap. 12). When flow through the arterial system is altered, the cause of hypoxia is **ischemia.** Impairment in flow through the venous system interferes with the removal of metabolic waste products and causes fluid to back up in the system, a condition known as **venous engorgement** or **venous obstruction.** When the lymphatic circulation is altered, the resulting fluid and pressure changes may be visible locally or systemically.

Lymphatic Vessels

The lymphatic circulatory system may be overwhelmed when there are changes in hydrostatic or oncotic pressures or when the movement of fluid at the capillary bed is impaired. The result is **edema,** an excessive amount of fluid in the interstitial spaces. A wide variety of conditions is capable of producing edema. Edema may be local or systemic. (Systemic edema is discussed in detail in Chapter 28.)

When lymphatic flow is altered due to impairment in the circulation of lymph itself, the condition is called **lymphedema.** The result is similarly an excessive quantity of fluid in the interstitium, but the underlying pathology is an obstruction to flow.

Blood Vessels: Obstructions

Pathologies affecting blood flow may involve impedance of the arterial or venous system. Some obstructions to flow are specific to either the arterial or venous portion of the system, but most can occur in some form on both sides. Obstructions to flow that may interfere with either arterial or venous flow are presented in detail in the following discussion. Those that are specifically arterial or venous in nature are detailed more fully later in the chapter.

Thrombosis

A **thrombus** is a stationary blood clot formed within a vessel. **Thrombosis** refers to the formation of clots within vessels, to differentiate it from the clotting process that takes place as a homeostatic mechanism. Thrombi may develop in either the arterial or venous circulatory system. Activation of the clotting or coagulation cascade within the vessel results in thrombosis (see Chap. 13).

Thrombosis is initiated by a change within the blood vessel resulting in localized reduction in flow. Inflammation of blood vessels may be the stimulus for thrombosis in either arteries or veins. When inflammation occurs in a vein (**phlebitis**) and is accompanied by the formation of a thrombus, it is called **thrombophlebitis.** The most common cause of thrombophlebitis is the inflammation produced by the placement of a needle or catheter for intravenous therapy. Thrombosis may also be initiated by a generalized reduction in flow and the release of vasoactive substances that occur in shock states (see Chap. 54). Systemic derangement in coagulation takes place in disseminated intravascular coagulation (DIC), resulting in thrombosis in the microcirculation throughout the body (see Chap. 13). Thrombi may form in veins when blood flow is slowed by an assortment of factors. They may also form in arteries when the surface has been roughened or narrowed by another pathologic process such as arteriosclerosis. Risk factors associated with thrombosis are listed in Table 14–1.

Interventions in the treatment of thrombus formation may be medical or surgical. Ideally, thrombosis

TABLE 14–1. Risk Factors Commonly Associated With Thrombosis

General (arterial and venous)
  Hypercoagulable conditions
    Polycythemia
    Dehydration
    Platelet aggregation
  Pump failure
    Congestive heart failure
    Shock
  Dysrhythmias
  Aging
  Trauma, including surgery
  Drugs
    Anesthetic agents
    Oral contraceptives
    Tobacco
Arterial
  Arteriosclerosis/atherosclerosis
Venous
  Immobilization

is prevented in high-risk individuals through pharmacologic or other medical approaches. The prophylactic (preventative) injection of low doses of heparin (5,000 units subcutaneously every 8 to 12 hours), which inhibits activation of Factor X, the rate-limiting step in the clotting cascade, is effective and commonly used for hospitalized patients. Warfarin sodium (Coumadin) may also be given prophylactically. It is an oral anticoagulant that depresses synthesis by the liver of vitamin K–dependent clotting factors (II, VII, IX, and X). Aspirin in low doses (325 mg every 2 days) inhibits platelet aggregation and may be an important preventive measure in certain thrombotic conditions such as cerebral vascular accidents. Once a thrombus has formed, anticoagulant therapy is continued to prevent the formation of further thrombi, but it is not effective in dissolving an existing clot. Therapeutic doses of subcutaneous or intravenous heparin may be instituted. At these higher dosages, heparin inhibits the synthesis of thrombin and prevents the formation of a stable fibrin clot by blocking the conversion of fibrinogen to fibrin and impairing the activation of fibrin-stabilizing factor (Factor XIII). **Thrombolytic agents** such as streptokinase, urokinase, and alteplase are intravenous drugs that are capable of dissolving clots. Their current use is limited to patients with thrombi in the coronary or pulmonary vasculature. Their use must be closely supervised; patients receiving thrombolytic therapy are usually in critical care settings.[6] Additional medical prophylactic interventions include the use of antiembolic stockings or sequential compression devices for immobilized patients, and initiation of ambulation as soon as possible.

Because thrombi partially or completely occlude flow through the involved vessel, they can produce ischemia distal to that point in an artery or congestion behind the obstruction in a vein. A thrombus that only partially occludes a vessel continues to be affected by the force of blood flow. Eventually, it may break free from the vessel wall and become an embolus.

Embolus Formation

An **embolus** is a collection of material that forms a clot within the bloodstream. This traveling clot is propelled by blood flow to a distant point, where it lodges to produce a new site of obstruction.

An embolus may be a **thromboembolus,** having begun as a thrombus that was subsequently dislodged from the vessel intima. Most thromboemboli in the venous system originate in the deep veins of the pelvis and lower extremities. They traverse the venous circulation and return to the right side of the heart, eventually lodging in the arterial side of the pulmonary vasculature and resulting in a **pulmonary embolism.** Thromboemboli from the venous circulation are the most frequent cause of pulmonary emboli, but the etiology may be nonthrombotic, as is the case for tumor, fat, air, amniotic, or bacterial emboli (see Chap. 22). **Embolectomy** is the surgical removal of an embolus and is usually confined to thromboemboli. The use of this surgical technique is dependent on the location of the embolus. In patients who experience repeated emboli, usually originating from the peripheral venous system, a filter may be surgically implanted in the inferior aorta. As the blood passes through the filter, emboli are trapped and cannot progress into the pulmonary circulation.

Various other materials, some totally foreign to the bloodstream, if present in sufficient quantity can also form emboli. **Fat emboli** are aggregates of fat molecules released into the blood after trauma or surgery involving bones. Most frequently the long bones of the legs are the source of these emboli. Pressure changes are generated within the traumatized bone, forcing molecules of fat into the bloodstream. Malignancy produces metastasis by various means, one of which is via the blood as **tumor emboli.** Collections of bacteria and exudate may break free from a source within the circulation such as the leaflets of the valves of the heart in bacterial endocarditis. Once in the bloodstream, the **bacterial emboli** travel on, eventually occluding circulation and becoming a new site of infection. Air from the external environment is a foreign material when found in the bloodstream as **air emboli.** Bubbles of air, having most likely entered the blood through an intravenous line, come to rest in small blood vessels. It is difficult to identify the specific volume of air that can sufficiently obstruct flow to result in deleterious effects. In animal research, the quantity of air necessary to produce death varies, partially affected by the speed with which it is injected. Under some circumstances, a 5-cc injection of air will result in death of animal models. At other times, a 100-cc bolus of air will not produce adverse effects.[4]

Pressure changes in the abdomen during labor and delivery may force amniotic fluid into the bloodstream as **amniotic fluid emboli.** Here the emboli cause a different set of problems. Amniotic fluid cannot perform the functions of the blood in carrying gases and nutrients, but as a fluid it does not produce obstruction to flow. Instead, the proteins and cells in amniotic fluid act as antigens, initiating an immune response (see Chap. 9).

Vasospasm

Vasospasm is a sudden, involuntary constriction of an artery that results in obstruction to flow. It may be mediated by environmental factors such as exposure to cold or emotional stress, producing a localized response.

Inflammation

Vasculitis is inflammation of the intima of an artery. Inflammation of the lining of a vein is called **phlebitis.** If superficial, these inflammations may be visible as reddened, tender streaks on the skin. Of more significance is their ability to serve as foci for the thrombotic process.

Arteritis (angiitis) is a specific term that identifies an inflammatory process of autoimmune origin in arteries. The initiating stimulus for this autoimmune disease is frequently an infectious process, viral or bacterial (especially streptococcal), or an adverse response to drugs such as sulfonamides or phenothiazines.

Mechanical Compression

A variety of forces external to the vascular system may result in partial or complete obstruction of blood flow. Trauma may produce direct pressure on a blood vessel, resulting in occlusion. This same effect may result from constriction due to casts or tight dressings. Swelling secondary to bleeding or edema within a fascial compartment will eventually compromise the circulation in vessels that pass through the compartment, producing **compartment syndrome.** Prolonged occlusion produces neurovascular alterations that can be assessed before the ischemia is irreversible.

Blood Vessels: Structural Alterations

An assortment of pathologies in blood vessel structure will produce alterations in blood flow. The structure of arteries or veins may be changed secondary to congenital anomalies or pathologic processes triggered later in life.

Valvular Incompetence

The intimal folds of veins that form the valves can be damaged, interfering with the effective flow of blood through a portion of the venous system (**valvular incompetence**). The susequent pathologies may affect superficial veins (**varicose veins**) to deep veins (**chronic venous insufficiency**), resulting in severe tissue hypoxia and **venous stasis ulcers.**

Arteriosclerosis/Atherosclerosis

Arteriosclerosis is a complex condition that produces structural changes within arteries. **Atherosclerosis,** a specific type of arteriosclerosis, produces an increase in the number of smooth muscle cells and a collection of lipids within the intima of medium- and large-sized arteries. This process eventually narrows the lumina and decreases their ability to dilate. Atherosclerotic changes are responsible for or contribute to many diseases throughout the body such as hypertension, renal failure, coronary artery disease, and cerebral vascular disease.

Aneurysms

Aneurysms are localized dilations of arterial walls. They vary in the severity of their consequences, depending on their size, type, and location. All aneurysms produce an alteration in flow due to the changes in vessel diameter. But more significant is the fact that the aneurysm represents a weakened area in the artery that may eventually rupture.

Arteriovenous Fistulas

Arteriovenous (AV) **fistulas** are abnormal communications between arteries and veins. They are usually congenital in origin but may result from traumatic injury. Symptoms depend on the size and location of the fistula. Because AV fistulas provide a shortcut between the two vascular systems, they can result in alterations in oxygenation to the involved tissues and systemic hemodynamic changes. One of the most common and serious types of AV fistulas is the **arteriovenous malformation** (AVM). An AVM is a tangled knot of arteries and veins found within the brain vasculature. It may be responsible for such signs and symptoms as headaches, cerebral vascular accident, (stroke due to bleeding), dementia, or seizures (see Chaps. 43–44). If the AV fistula is sufficient to cause hemodynamic changes, surgery is performed to ligate all of the branches of the fistula and isolate it from the general circulation.

KEY CONCEPTS

- Altered blood flow results from obstructive processes. Obstruction results in reduced flow beyond the obstruction and increased pressure before the obstruction (upstream). In the arterial system, obstruction manifests primarily as distal ischemia. In the venous system, obstruction manifests as edema.
- The causes of vessel obstructions include thrombi, emboli, vasospasm, external compression (e.g., compartment syndrome), and structural alterations (e.g., atherosclerotic plaques, aneurysms).

Alterations in Arterial Flow

Alterations in arterial flow result from obstruction (arteriosclerosis, atherosclerosis, arteritis, vasospasm, thrombi, emboli and acute occlusion) or mechanical alterations (AV fistulas and aneurysms).

Arteriosclerosis/Atherosclerosis

Arteriosclerosis is a generic term meaning "hardening of the arteries" and broadly includes three pathologic processes: Monckeberg's sclerosis, or medial calcific sclerosis, arteriolar sclerosis, and atherosclerosis. Monckeberg's sclerosis is characterized by calcium deposition in the tunica media of intermediate-sized arteries. The result is thickening and increased rigidity of the vessel wall, but no reduction in flow. Arteriolar sclerosis is characterized by thickening and luminal narrowing of the small arteries that occur in association with hypertension. **Atherosclerosis,** the most common arteriosclerotic process, affects intermediate-sized and large arteries. Smooth muscle cells and lipids collect along the intimal surface, producing a narrowing of the luminal diameter and a reduction in flow (Fig. 14–14).[7]

Atherosclerosis is the pathologic origin for the vast majority of arterial disease and is the cause of nearly half of deaths in the United States and Western Europe. Atherosclerosis tends to develop in large and medium-sized arteries, most frequently the coronary, cerebral, and femoral arteries and the aorta. Over 60 percent of the mortality associated with atherosclerosis is due to occlusion of coronary arteries (coronary artery disease, CAD), producing myocardial ischemia and infarction. The remainder of the deaths due to atherosclerosis are secondary to thrombotic or hemorrhagic processes in such organ systems as the brain, kidneys, liver, gastrointestinal tract, and the extremities.[3] When the peripheral vascular system is affected, it is most often the lower extremities, and the disease process is called **arteriosclerosis** or **atherosclerosis obliterans** (Fig. 14–15). Research results from the Framingham Study identified the development of lower extremity arterial disease in 5 percent of the subjects over the course of the 24-year data collection interval.[8]

The precise pathologic mechanism of atherosclerosis is unknown; it is most likely a combination of factors. The insidiousness of the disease process has affected the speed and specificity of research. The three primary pathologic processes currently appear to be (1) a response to serum lipid levels, (2) reaction to injury of the vessel wall, and (3) cellular transformation. Each hypothesis has spawned considerable research attention.

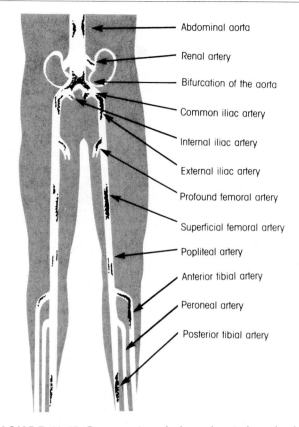

- Abdominal aorta
- Renal artery
- Bifurcation of the aorta
- Common iliac artery
- Internal iliac artery
- External iliac artery
- Profound femoral artery
- Superficial femoral artery
- Popliteal artery
- Anterior tibial artery
- Peroneal artery
- Posterior tibial artery

FIGURE 14–15. Common sites of atherosclerosis from the descending aorta distal to the lower extremities. (From Wagner MM: Pathophysiology related to peripheral vascular disease. *Nurs Clin North Am* 1986;21(2):196. Reproduced with permission.)

Pathogenesis

Lipid insudation is currently held to be the most important factor in the pathogenesis of atherosclerosis. According to the theory, high concentrations of cholesterol in the serum in the form of low-density lipoproteins (LDLs) are transported into the muscle tissues of the artery, where they produce irritation and proliferation of muscle cells.[7]

Cholesterol is a necessary component of cellular membranes and is used in the manufacture of steroids within the body. Cholesterol itself is highly insoluble and is transported throughout the body in the form of **lipoproteins,** cholesterol cores with protein shells. Although there are several forms of lipoproteins, LDLs and high-density lipoproteins (HDLs) are most important to the discussion of atherosclerosis. Receptors on the surface of the LDL molecule bind with receptors on cell membranes, allowing it to be absorbed into the cell. These receptors abound in the muscle cells of arteries. The protein coat is dissolved and the cholesterol is used to meet the cellular needs. The excess cholesterol that is not removed is stored and acts as a cellular irritant; the precise mechanism is unclear. But the correlation between high levels of serum LDLs and cholesterol is clearly significant in

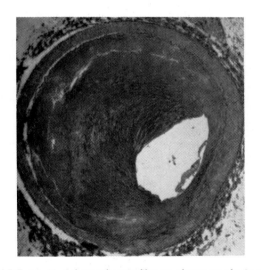

FIGURE 14–14. Atherosclerotic fibrous plaque producing a significant reduction in the lumen of a coronary artery. (From Robbins SL, Cotran RS, Kumar V: *Pathologic Basis of Disease,* 3rd ed. Philadelphia, WB Saunders, 1984, p 511. Reproduced with permission.)

the development of atherosclerosis. HDL seems to serve as a protective mechanism in the formation of atherosclerosis. It is postulated that HDL is able to remove cholesterol from formations in the arterial walls and transport it back to the liver.[3] Consequently, cholesterol levels and lipoprotein profiles are closely supervised. An acceptable total cholesterol level for an adult is less than 280 mg/dL. Levels of LDL are felt to be detrimental if greater than 160 mg/dL. Protective levels of HDL are those greater than 35 mg/dL.[7] A major preventive intervention related to atherosclerosis is encouraging the consumption of a low-fat diet, with those fats being primarily polyunsaturated (from vegetable sources as opposed to animal).

The **reaction to injury** hypothesis is grounded in nonspecific damage to the endothelial surface of the arterial intima, producing an alteration in wall permeability. The normal barrier is lost, and serum constituents such as platelets and large quantities of lipoproteins enter the intimal lining. Platelets aggregate and some are damaged, releasing platelet-derived growth factor (PDGF), which stimulates growth of smooth muscle cells. Media smooth muscle cells, normally protected by an intact intima, are drawn toward the intima and proliferate. The essence of this hypothesis is chronicity of irritation, in contrast to mild intermittent irritation, which is reversible. Chronic irritation may be due to smoking, hypercholesterolemia, and such hemodynamic stressors as hypertension, diabetes mellitus, and high levels of circulating catecholamines, angiotensin, or hormones.[9]

The **cellular transformation** or **monoclonal hypothesis** theorizes that the origin of each single atherosclerotic plaque is a single muscle cell that mutates into a benign tumor. Seminal work on this theory was done by Benditt.[10] The supporting histologic evidence is the large percentage of atherosclerotic plaques in humans that appear to be monoclonal, originating in a single cell. Mutagenic factors such as smoking, viruses, and cellular injury have been postulated.[7,10]

Process

Regardless of the specific mechanism, the arterial wall undergoes a series of morphologic changes that result in structural alterations. Initial changes involve only the intimal wall, but secondary alterations occur within the media. Atherosclerotic lesions are generally divided into three types, indicative of advancing pathology.

The earliest anomaly, the **fatty streak,** is a yellowish smooth muscle cell filled with lipids. Although it protrudes into the intimal lumen slightly, it results in no significant alteration in flow and no signs or symptoms. Fatty streaks have been found at autopsy of very young children.[11]

Fibrous plaques (atheromas) are the lesions most characteristic of atherosclerosis. They appear as a yellow-gray or whitish colored elevation, extruding from the intima and producing varying degrees of alteration in blood flow. Histologically, the lesions are lipid-filled smooth muscle cells encased in collagen fibers and additional lipids. As the lesion grows, it invades the tunica media on one side and traps blood constituents on the other.

The **complicated lesion** represents the most advanced form of the disease. Deep within the lesion, necrosis occurs owing to lack of blood supply, and dead tissue accumulates. Cellular debris, hemorrhage and thrombus formation, and lipid calcification all contribute to the increasing rigidity of the lesion. The vessel wall may be destroyed as the lesion grows and calcifies. Before signs or symptoms appear, the blood flow to a given organ or tissue normally must be diminished by more than 50 percent to 75 percent. Since the process is so slow, collateral circulation may have time to develop, further postponing the development of clinically recognizable disease.

Risk Factors

Historically, health care has focus on preventing atherosclerosis by manipulation of predisposing factors. These risk factors are categorized as modifiable or nonmodifiable, according to the individual's degree of control over them (Table 14–2). It is often difficult to isolate the effect of a single risk factor since they most frequently occur in combination with one another.

The most frequently cited prospective research into atherosclerotic risk factors began in 1948 in Framingham, Massachusetts.[8] Initially, 5,209 men and women between the ages of 30 and 59 volunteered to be subjects in the study. The purpose of the study was to identify factors associated with the development of atherosclerosis over a long period of time. The Framingham study is ongoing, with researchers now studying the children of the original participants. Much of the available information regarding atherosclerotic risk factors is based on the results of this research.

The precise mechanisms associated with smoking and atherogenesis have not been clearly elucidated. Certain constituents of cigarette smoke, in addition to being carcinogenic, have been found to stimulate

TABLE 14–2. Risk Factors Associated with Atherosclerosis

Modifiable risk factors
    Smoking
    Elevated blood pressure
    Glucose intolerance
    Elevated cholesterol and low-density lipoproteins
    Decreased physical activity
    Obesity
    Weight fluctuations
    Stress management
Nonmodifiable risk factors
    Age
    Sex
    Race
    Heredity

the release of catecholamines, increasing blood pressure, heart rate, and oxygen consumption and resulting in increased work for the heart. The release of catecholamines also enhances the release of free fatty acids and glucose. Nicotine has a direct vasospastic effect on blood vessels and increases platelet aggregation.[12] Statistics support the increased incidence of atherosclerosis, especially CAD, among smokers.[13] The risk increases with an increase in the amount of smoking and the length of time the individual has smoked. Stopping smoking results in a reduction of the risk. Death from myocardial infarction is also more common among smokers.[11]

Increases in both systolic and diastolic blood pressure are associated with an increased incidence of atherosclerosis. Diastolic blood pressure elevations are probably more significant, for they represent the status of the cardiovascular system when it is at rest. The risk diminishes with interventions directed toward lowering the blood pressure.[11] Hypertension is often found in the presence of other risk factors. (See Chapter 15 for a discussion of hypertension.)

Elevated serum cholesterol and LDL levels were discussed in the previous section as significant contributors to the development of atherosclerosis. In addition to dietary fat intake, smoking and diabetes mellitus have been found to be associated with elevations in LDL and reduced levels of HDL.[7]

Glucose intolerance is affiliated with diabetes mellitus, a disease in which an absolute lack of or a decreased response to insulin produces a derangement in metabolism (see Chap. 41). Atherosclerosis is highly correlated with glucose intolerance, probably because of the alterations in carbohydrate and fat metabolism and the direct damage to vessel basement membrane with elevated blood sugar levels. The incidence of atherosclerotic diseases is much higher among those with diabetes mellitus than in the general population, but it does not appear to be related to the degree of hyperglycemia.[11] Individuals with diabetes mellitus are also more likely to have other risk factors such as obesity, hypertension, and elevated serum lipids.

Obesity, defined as a body weight 30 percent or greater than the ideal, is thought to be a contributing risk factor for atherosclerosis, in that it may accelerate the process. Abdominally distributed obesity seems to be most highly correlated with atherosclerosis.[11] Weight gain is associated with increasing serum cholesterol and LDL levels, increasing systolic blood pressure, glucose intolerance, and a sedentary life-style.

Physical activity has been found to increase HDL levels, the collateral circulation, and vessel size, and to decrease total cholesterol levels, glucose intolerance, body weight, and blood pressure. Clearly, all of these events can retard the development and mitigate the severity of atherosclerosis. Research likewise substantiates physical inactivity as a risk factor for cardiovascular disease.[7,11]

Stress and personality factors have received considerable attention as risk factors for atherosclerosis over the past 10 to 20 years. It is extremely difficult to isolate these facets and examine them quantitatively and qualitatively. Objectively, stress results in the release of endogenous catecholamines that contribute to the work of the cardiovascular system. Subjectively, the rushed, stressed person is less inclined to exercise and eat wisely and more inclined to smoke and be hypertensive.

Certain risk factors are not modifiable and hence not manipulable for prevention purposes. As an individual ages, changes occur in the proliferation of smooth muscle of blood vessels. Stem cells in the media—cells that result in differentiated cells—decline in their speed of replication. Thus, **clonal senescence** is hypothesized to be a risk factor for the eventual morphologic changes found with atherosclerosis. This particular risk factor correlates well with the monoclonal hypothesis of atherogenesis.

Sex is another nonmodifiable risk factor. Men have a higher incidence of atherosclerosis earlier in life than women, apparently owing to the protective aspects of estrogen. After menopause, this advantage is lost. It may be lost earlier if women smoke, have hypertension, have increased serum cholesterol, or take oral contraceptives. Postmenopausal hormone replacement seems to reduce the incidence of CAD and provide a degree of protection.[14]

A strong family history, especially of CAD is an important predictor of its occurrence and subsequent prognosis. The specific mechanism is uncertain, but most likely it is a combination of genetic and environmental factors. Certain of the modifiable risk factors are also known to have a genetic component.

Studies of ethnicity as a nonmodifiable risk factor associated with atherosclerosis have predominantly focused on the increased incidence of CAD and hypertension among black Americans compared with white Americans.[15] Research among Hispanic Americans indicates a lower incidence of CAD and subsequent mortality than in non-Hispanic Americans.[16] In both cases, the overlap of genetic and environmental factors makes ethnicity as an isolated independent variable difficult to evaluate.

Clinical Manifestations, Diagnosis, and Treatment

Disease manifestations vary with the tissues involved and the severity of altered flow. Atherosclerosis is an underlying pathology for much of the hypertension, renal disease, cardiac disease, peripheral arterial disease, and stroke seen in health care practice. Decreased organ or tissue function occurs, and diagnosis and treatment approaches vary. Patient history and physical assessment provide significant information. Noninvasive tests such as Doppler flow studies may identify areas of occlusion or diminished flow. **Plethysmography** may be used to measure changes in the relative size of extremities associated with blood flow. **Ankle pressures** are obtained with a blood pressure cuff and Doppler ultrasonography and compared with brachial blood pressures in the *ankle-brachial in-*

dex. A normal A:B index is 1.0; an index less than 1.0 is indicative of diminished arterial flow. Exercise or stress testing may be performed to evaluate the pain of arterial occlusive disease (intermittent claudication). Angiography—radiologic studies of blood flow—is the most frequently employed diagnostic examination.[17] (See Chapter 17 for a discussion of coronary artery disease, Chapter 15 for a discussion of hypertension, Chapter 28 for a discussion of renal failure, and Chapter 43 for a discussion of cerebral vascular accidents.)

Identification of and interventions directed toward modifiable risk factors are the major thrusts of treatment, regardless of the organs or tissues affected.[12,18] Drugs to reduce cholesterol and LDL levels are usually prescribed sparingly, and only if diet and exercise have been ineffective. **Balloon angioplasty,** the surgical radiologic fragmentation of atherosclerotic plaques by inflating a specially equipped catheter, is commonly performed on both coronary and peripheral arteries. **Laser angioplasty** is being combined with balloon angioplasty to create an opening in significantly obstructed peripheral vessels before the balloon is inflated. Laser angioplasty is being investigated as a potential intervention for atherosclerotic coronary arteries. Currently, when balloon angioplasty of the coronary arteries is unacceptable or fails to result in satisfactory improvement, **coronary artery bypass surgery** is performed. Autologous donor grafts, either from the saphenous veins or from the internal mammary arteries, are used. Peripheral arterial bypass grafts are named for their sites or origin and termination (e.g., aortofemoral, femoropopliteal). Synthetic graft material is more common for peripheral vascular bypass surgery.[19]

Arteritis: Thromboangiitis Obliterans

Thromboangiitis obliterans (Buerger's disease) is a rather rare inflammatory condition affecting small and

TABLE 14–3. Defining Characteristics of Arteriosclerosis Obliterans

Skin assessment
- Cool or cold to touch
- Decreased or absent hair growth
- Dry, thin, glossy appearance
- Thickened nails
- Pallor when elevated, rubor when dependent
- Diminished or absent pulses

Pain assessment
- Sharp and stabbing
- Intensified with activity
- Relieved by rest or dependency

Ulcer assessment
- Severely painful
- Pale, gray base
- Well-defined edges
- Located on heels, lateral malleolus, between distal portions of phalanges, pretibial area

medium-sized arteries of the upper and lower extremities and producing varying degrees of obstruction. The inflammation is accompanied by thrombosis, fibrosis, and scarring that may extend to neighboring nerves. It is associated with cigarette smoking and found most frequently in young men under the age of 40.[20]

Veins may also be affected, but the signs and symptoms relate to obstruction of arterial flow (Table 14–3). Patients complain of pain with activity (**intermittent claudication;** Fig. 14–16) and sensitivity to cold. Peripheral pulses are diminished. Ulceration may occur. Patients are encouraged to cease smoking. Bypass surgery is rarely an option because the involved vessels are too distal.[21]

Raynaud's Syndrome

An extreme vasoconstrictive response of the arteries in the hands and fingers produces the characteristic

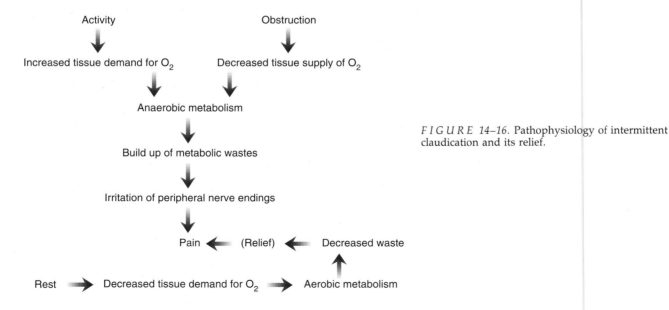

FIGURE 14–16. Pathophysiology of intermittent claudication and its relief.

Deep vein thrombosis is treated aggressively. Deep vein thrombosis of the lower extremities and pelvic veins is the most frequent source of pulmonary emboli. Patients are hospitalized, and intravenous anticoagulation therapy may be initiated. Occasionally, patients are treated on an outpatient basis with oral anticoagulants (Coumadin). Patients who have previously developed deep vein thromboses are at risk for further hypercoagulation and may be prophylactically anticoagulated with antiplatelet therapy (low-dose aspirin). With subsequent hospitalization, these patients frequently are begun on low-dose heparin therapy prophylactically.[6]

KEY CONCEPTS

- **Common causes of venous obstruction are incompetent valves (as may occur with obesity, pregnancy, right heart failure, prolonged standing), varicose veins, and deep vein thrombosis.**
- **Edema, stasis ulcers, and pain usually accompany chronic venous obstruction.**
- **Deep vein thrombosis is potentially life-threatening because of the likelihood of embolization to the pulmonary circulation. It is aggressively treated with immobilization of the extremity and the administrations of anticoagulants.**

Alterations in Lymphatic Flow

Lymphedema

Lymphedema occurs when the normal flow of lymph is obstructed or altered in some fashion (Fig. 14–20). It is often differentiated as primary or secondary. Primary lymphedema is related to a congenital absence or decreased numbers of lymphatics or obstruction of the thoracic duct or the cisterna chyli. Secondary lymphedema is most frequently due to the surgical removal of lymph nodes or destruction of the lymphatics by radiation therapy in the treatment of malignancies.

Patients may present with bilateral or unilateral edema, usually beginning in the feet or hands and progressing centrally. This form of edema is not associated with the skin changes (pigmentation, ulceration) seen with edema originating from the systemic venous system. Chronic congestion produces subcutaneous fibrosis, resulting in thick, rough skin.[28]

Medical treatment includes external pneumatic compression devices, elastic stockings, and diuretics. Surgical removal of skin and subcutaneous tissue followed by split-thickness skin grafts over the muscle may be helpful but produces physically unattractive results. Reconstructive surgery may be done to create lymphovenous bypasses, but these often result in thrombosis. Other surgical interventions have been attempted, depending on the location of the problem, with varying degrees of success.[28]

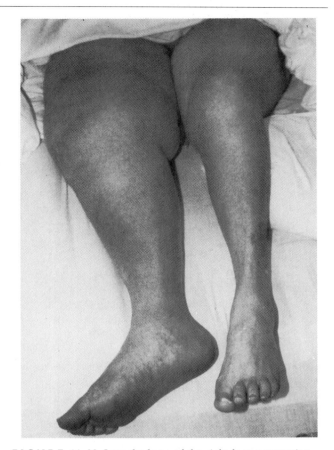

FIGURE 14–20. Lymphedema of the right lower extremity due to removal of iliofemoral nodes and radiation therapy for rectal cancer. (From Dixon MB, Bergan JJ: Lymphedema, in Fahey VA (ed): *Vascular Nursing*. Philadelphia, WB Saunders, 1988, p 37. Reproduced with permission.)

KEY CONCEPTS

- **Obstruction to lymph flow is most commonly due to surgical removal of or radiation damage to lymphatic vessels during treatment of cancer.**
- **Manifestations of lymphatic obstruction include regional edema and thickened subcutaneous tissue.**

Summary

The circulatory system is organized to facilitate its dual role of oxygen and nutrient transport and removal of metabolic waste products. The arrangement and unique structure of the circulatory vessels permit the system to carry out these roles.

An understanding of the principles and control of flow aids in the comprehension of the pathologies resulting in alterations in flow. Principles of flow, or the hemodynamics of the circulation, include concepts and physical laws relating to relationships of flow, pressure and resistance, velocity, and laminar and turbulent flow, and wall tension and compliance. Control of blood flow is through both extrinsic and intrinsic mechanisms. Lymphatic flow is controlled through the lymphatic pump system, governed by skeletal muscle, and the smooth muscle of organs and arteries.

Pathophysiologic changes that result in alterations in blood flow can be classified as either due to obstruction (thrombosis, emboli, vasospasm, inflammation, mechanical compression) or to structural alterations (valvular incompetence, arteriosclerosis/atherosclerosis, aneurysms, arteriovenous fistulas). Conditions that produce alterations in arterial or venous flow are due to one of these primary processes. Pathologic conditions of the lymphatic system are essentially due to disruption of the normal pressure relationships or an obstruction within the circulatory system, for proper functioning of the lymphatic system depends on the appropriate functioning of the vascular system.

REFERENCES

1. Johnson WTM, et al: Arterial intimal embrittlement: A possible factor in atherogenesis. *Atherosclerosis* 1986;59:161–171.
2. Guzzetta CS, Dossey BM: *Cardiovascular Nursing: Bodymind Tapestry.* St. Louis, CV Mosby, 1984.
3. Guyton A: *Textbook of Medical Physiology,* 8th ed. Philadelphia, WB Saunders, 1991.
4. Ganong WF: *Review of Medical Physiology,* 13th ed. Norwalk Conn, Appleton & Lange, 1987.
5. Patton HD, Fuchs AF, Hille B, Scher AM, Steiner R: *Textbook of Physiology,* 21st ed. Philadelphia, WB Saunders, 1989.
6. Malseed RT, Harrigan GS: *Textbook of Pharmacology and Nursing Care.* Philadelphia, JB Lippincott, 1989.
7. Underhill SL, et al: *Cardiac Nursing,* 2nd ed. Philadelphia, JB Lippincott, 1989.
8. Dawber TR: *The Framingham Study: The Epidemiology of Atherosclerotic Disease.* Cambridge, Harvard University Press, 1980.
9. Ross R: The pathogenesis of atherosclerosis: An update. *N Engl J Med* 1986;314:488–498.
10. Benditt EP: Implications of the monoclonal character of human atherosclerotic plaques. *Am J Pathol* 1977;86(3):693.
11. Wilson JD, et al: *Harrison's Principles of Internal Medicine,* 12th ed. New York, McGraw-Hill, 1991.
12. Doyle EJ: Treatment modalities in peripheral vascular disease. *Nurs Clin North Am* 1986;21(2):241–253.
13. Bondy B: An overview of arterial disease. *J Cardiovasc Nurs* 1987;1(2):1–11.
14. Murdaugh C: Coronary artery disease in women. *J Cardiovasc Nurs* 1990;4(4):35–50.
15. Keller C: Coronary artery disease in blacks. *J Cardiovasc Nurs* 1990;4(4):1–12.
16. Derenowski J: Coronary artery disease in Hispanics. *J Cardiovasc Nurs* 1990;4(4):13–21.
17. Massey JA: Diagnostic testing for peripheral vascular disease. *Nurs Clin North Am* 1986;21(2):207–218.
18. Turner J: Nursing intervention in patients with peripheral vascular disease. *Nurs Clin North Am* 1986;21(2):233–240.
19. Dixon MB, Nunnelee J: Arterial reconstruction for atherosclerotic occlusive disease. *J Cardiovasc Nurs* 1987;1(2):36–49.
20. Juergens JL: Thromboangiitis obliterans, in Rutherford RB (ed): *Vascular Surgery,* 2nd ed. Philadelphia, WB Saunders, 1984.
21. Graham LM, O'Keefe MF: Arterial disease, in Fahey VA (ed): *Vascular Nursing.* Philadelphia, WB Saunders, 1988.
22. Porter JM: Raynaud's syndrome and associated vasospastic conditions of the extremities, in Rutherford RB (ed): *Vascular Surgery,* 2nd ed. Philadelphia, WB Saunders, 1984.
23. Wagner MM: Pathophysiology related to peripheral vascular disease. *Nurs Clin North Am* 1986;21(2):195–218.
24. Crawford ES, Snyder DM: Thoracoabdominal aortic aneurysms, in Rutherford RB (ed): *Vascular Surgery,* 2nd ed. Philadelphia, WB Saunders, 1984.
25. Gordon RD, Fogarty TJ: Peripheral arterial embolism, in Rutherford RB (ed): *Vascular Surgery,* 2nd ed. Philadelphia, WB Saunders, 1984.
26. Hobbs JT: The treatment of varicose veins by sclerosing therapy, in Rutherford RB (ed): *Vascular Surgery,* 2nd ed. Philadelphia, WB Saunders, 1984.
27. Burnham SJ: Operative treatment of varicose veins, in Rutherford RB (ed): *Vascular Surgery,* 2nd ed. Philadelphia, WB Saunders, 1984.
28. Dixon MB, Bergan JJ: Lymphedema, in Fahey VA (ed): *Vascular Nursing.* Philadelphia, WB Saunders, 1988.

BIBLIOGRAPHY

Anidjar S, Kieffer E: Pathogenesis of acquired aneurysms of the abdominal aorta. *Ann Vasc Surg* 1992;6:298–305.

Bacharach JM, Colville DS, Lie JT: Accelerated atherosclerosis, aneurysmal disease, and aortitis: Possible pathogenetic association with cocaine abuse. *Int Angiol* 1992;11:83–86.

Campisi C: A rational approach to the management of lymphedema. *Lymphology* 1991;24:48–53.

Casley-Smith JR: The pathophysiology of lymphedema and the action of benzopyrones in reducing it. *Lymphology* 1988;21:190–194.

Crotty TP: The origin and the progression of varicose veins. *Med Hypotheses* 1992;37:198–204.

Glagov S, Zaring C, Ku DN: Hemodynamics and atherosclerosis: Insights and perspectives gained from studies of human arteries. *Arch Pathol Lab Med* 1988;112:1018–1031.

Haft JI, al-Zarka AM: Comparison of the natural history of irregular and smooth coronary lesions: Insights into the pathogenesis, progression and prognosis of coronary atherosclerosis. *Am Heart J* 1993;126:551–561.

Kuhn FE, Mohler ER, Rackley CE: Cholesterol and lipoproteins: Beyond atherogenesis. *Clin Cardiol* 1992;12:883–890.

Novo S, et al: Prevalence of risk factors in patients with peripheral arterial disease: A clinical and epidemiological evaluation. *Int Angiol* 1992;11:218–229.

Raines EW, Ross R: Smooth muscle cells and the pathogenesis of the lesions of atherosclerosis. *Br Heart J* 1993;69:930–937.

Resin E: Sodium and obesity in the pathogenesis of hypertension. *Am J Hypertens* 1990;3:164–167.

Ross R: The pathogenesis of atherosclerosis: A perspective for the 1990's. *Nature* 1993;362:801–809.

Ruderman NB, Schneider SH: Diabetes, exercise and atherosclerosis. *Diabetes Care* 1992;15:1787–1793.

Schwartz CJ, Valente AJ, Sprague EA: A modern view of atherogenesis. *Am J Cardiol* 1993;71:98–148.

Young JR: The swollen leg: Clinical significance and differential diagnosis. *Cardiol Clin* 1991;9:443–456.

CHAPTER 15
Alterations in Blood Pressure

CHRISTINE HENSHAW

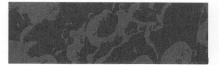

KEY TERMS

accelerated (malignant) high blood pressure: Rapidly progressing, potentially fatal form of hypertension in which diastolic blood pressure exceeds 120 mm Hg.

cardiac output: The amount of blood pumped by the heart each minute.

diastolic blood pressure: The minimum pressure in the arteries just prior to the next ventricular ejection.

high blood pressure/hypertension: Elevation of blood pressure above 140 mm Hg systolic and/or 90 mm Hg diastolic.

isolated systolic hypertension: An elevation in systolic blood pressure above 140 mm Hg, without an increase in diastolic blood pressure. Most commonly occurs in the elderly.

Korotkoff sounds: Sounds heard when auscultating arterial blood pressure. As the pressure in the blood pressure cuff is released, blood begins to flow turbulently through the artery, producing noises.

mean arterial pressure: The average pressure in the arterial system through the cardiac cycle; estimated clinically as diastolic pressure plus one third of the pulse pressure.

orthostatic (postural) hypotension: Increase in heart rate of more than 15 percent and decrease in either systolic blood pressure, by more than 15 mm Hg, or diastolic blood pressure, by more than 10 mm Hg.

pheochromocytoma: Tumors of the adrenal gland that secrete catecholamines, resulting in elevated blood pressure. An example of a condition that causes secondary high blood pressure.

pregnancy-induced hypertension: Elevated blood pressure that occurs during pregnancy. Blood pressure returns to normal after delivery.

primary (idiopathic, essential) hypertension: High blood pressure of unidentified etiology. Accounts for 90 percent of cases of high blood pressure.

pulse pressure: The difference between the systolic and diastolic blood pressures.

secondary hypertension: High blood pressure in which the cause can be identified.

systolic blood pressure: The maximum pressure in the aorta and major arteries during ventricular ejection of blood.

total peripheral resistance: The impedance to blood flow exerted by the arterioles; determined primarily by vascular diameter. Total peripheral resistance is composed of systemic vascular resistance and pulmonary vascular resistance.

white coat phenomenon: Elevated blood pressure readings when measured by a physician.

A complex array of mechanisms work together with the actions of other systems to perfuse body tissues. Chapter 14 presented mechanisms that control blood flow. For the human body to function effectively, blood flow must be accompanied by an adequate perfusion pressure.

Arterial blood pressure is the driving force that propels fluids throughout the body. Although blood pressure fluctuates, it is perhaps the most closely regulated physiological parameter in the circulatory system. The present chapter describes factors affecting blood pressure, measurement of blood pressure, and alterations in blood pressure.

Function of the Arterial and Pulmonary Systems

Arterial blood pressure is the pressure generated by the heart as it contracts and ejects blood into the systemic arterial vascular system. As blood travels through the vascular system, the pressure decreases: rapidly as the blood passes through the arterioles, then more slowly as the blood passes through the capillaries and the venous system (Fig. 15–1). By the time the blood has returned to the right atrium, the pressure is almost entirely dissipated. This decrease in pressure is due to the resistance to flow offered by the vascular system; the arterioles offer the most resistance. Because fluid moves from an area of high pressure to an area of low pressure, the pressure difference between the aorta and the right atrium is the force that propels blood through the vasculature. Arterial blood pressure is recorded as a systolic and a diastolic value, for example, 120/80, with 120 being the systolic value and 80 being the diastolic value, and is measured in millimeters of mercury (mm Hg) or torr.[1,2]

Systolic blood pressure reflects the maximum pressure in the aorta and major arteries during ventricular ejection of blood and averages 120 mm Hg in the normal, healthy adult. Ventricular contraction forces blood into the distensible aorta where much of the stroke volume of that contraction is retained (Fig. 15–2). The volume in the aorta and the large arteries exerts pressure on arterial walls; this pressure is the systolic arterial pressure. An increase or decrease in volume can produce a corresponding elevation or reduction in systolic blood pressure, assuming no other changes in the system.

During diastole, passive elastic recoil of the arterial walls ejects blood out of the aorta and into the peripheral arteries. **Diastolic pressure** reflects the minimum pressure in these vessels during the pre-ejection rest period, just prior to the subsequent ventricular contraction. Because the next contraction occurs before all the blood is ejected, the pressure never falls to zero. The minimum pressure (diastolic pressure) is determined in part by the diameter of the arterioles, which is also the major determinant of systemic vascular resistance (SVR). Therefore the diastolic blood pressure reading provides an estimate of SVR. Vasoconstriction, a narrowing of vessel diameter, increases SVR and diastolic blood pressure; vasodilation reduces SVR and diastolic blood pressure. The average diastolic blood pressure in the healthy adult is 80 mm Hg.[1,2]

Arterial Pressure Pulses

The contour of the arterial pressure wave can be approximated by palpating the arterial pulse. At the carotid artery, the information obtained most closely reflects central hemodynamics and cardiac events. As one moves to more peripheral sites, the arterial pressures dissipate and the similarity to central hemodynamics diminishes.[3]

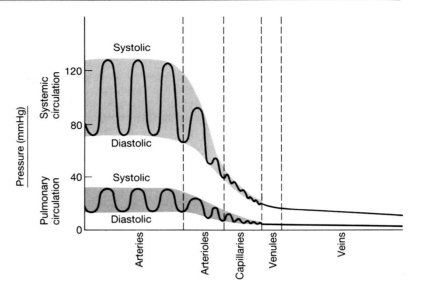

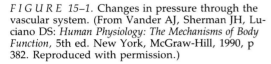

FIGURE 15–1. Changes in pressure through the vascular system. (From Vander AJ, Sherman JH, Luciano DS: *Human Physiology: The Mechanisms of Body Function*, 5th ed. New York, McGraw-Hill, 1990, p 382. Reproduced with permission.)

The difference between the systolic and diastolic blood pressures is termed the **arterial pulse pressure. Pulse pressure** is determined by stroke volume (the amount of blood ejected with each heart beat), the speed at which the stroke volume is ejected, and arterial distensibility.[2]

Mean arterial pressure (MAP) is the average pressure in the system throughout the cardiac cycle. Because more time is spent in diastole than in systole at normal heart rates, MAP is not the arithmetic average of the diastolic and systolic pressures, but rather reflects the relative time spent in each portion of the cardiac cycle. MAP is derived most accurately by using intra-arterial blood pressure measurement, dividing the area under the arterial pressure curve by the time of one cardiac cycle. Clinically, the formula used to estimate MAP is diastolic pressure plus one third of the pulse pressure.[1,2]

Determinants of Blood Pressure

The relation between pressure, flow, and resistance in a system is defined by the formula: Flow is equal

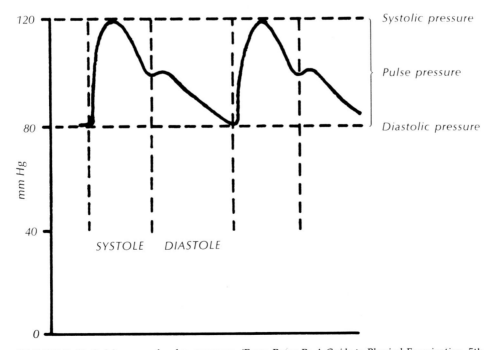

FIGURE 15–2. Measure of pulse pressure. (From Bates B: *A Guide to Physical Examination*, 5th ed. Philadelphia, JB Lippincott, 1991, p 274. Reproduced with permission.)

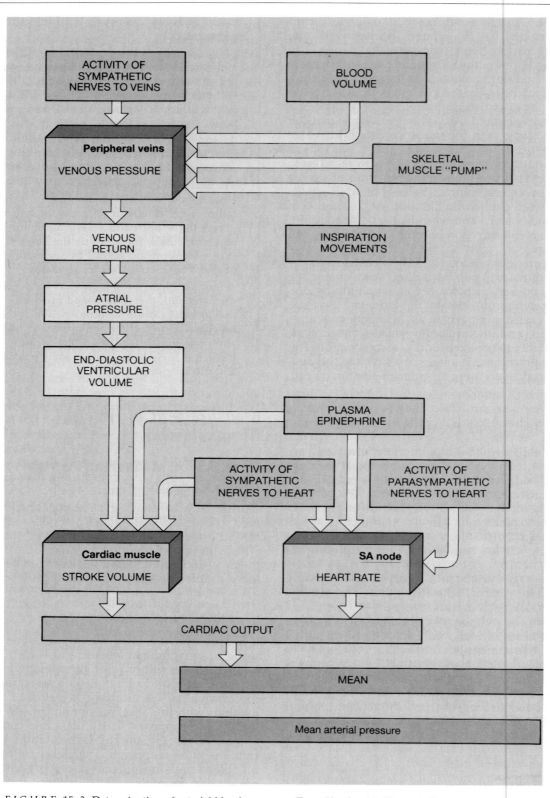

FIGURE 15–3. Determination of arterial blood pressure. (From Vander AJ, Sherman JH, Luciano DS: *Human Physiology: The Mechanisms of Body Function,* 5th ed. New York, McGraw-Hill, 1990, pp 404–405. Reproduced with permission.)

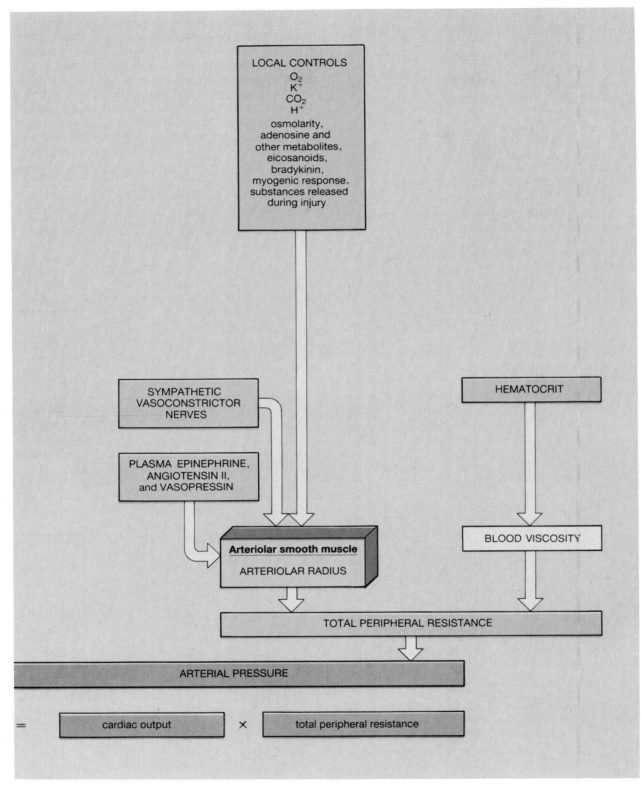

FIGURE 15–3 Continued

placed over the brachial artery. The return of blood flow through the artery is signaled by the **Korotkoff sounds,** named after the Russian physician who first described them. The sounds are due to turbulent flow through the partially occluded artery (Table 15–1). Phase I is associated with the onset of tapping sounds heard through the stethoscope and is recorded as the systolic blood pressure. Phase IV is signaled by an abrupt muffling of sound and is recorded as the diastolic blood pressure in children. In adults, the disappearance of sounds, phase V, signals diastolic blood pressure.[10]

Palpation should be used prior to obtaining an auscultated blood pressure to avoid missing the auscultatory gap. The **auscultatory gap** is that time during cuff deflation after the systolic blood pressure when the Korotkoff sounds disappear (Fig. 15–4). The sounds reappear at the beginning of phase III. If the cuff initially was not inflated high enough, the resumption of Korotkoff sounds during phase III may be mistaken for the onset of sounds in phase I. The auscultatory gap happens most frequently in persons with hypertension; if the auscultatory gap is missed, the blood pressure recorded will be too low. Once the blood pressure is known and an auscultatory gap is ruled out, it is not necessary to estimate blood pressure by palpating the pulse prior to auscultation. The palpatory method also is useful when auscultatory blood pressures are difficult to obtain, for example, in persons with low blood pressure, as in shock.[10,11]

Another indirect method combines the Doppler technique with the use of a sphygmomanometer. Ultrasonic impulses are transmitted from a transducer placed over an artery to the blood cells flowing through the artery. The impulses are reflected back to the transducer, which translates the impulses into audible sound. As the blood pressure cuff is deflated, the transducer is placed over an artery. The onset of sounds from the Doppler instrument is equivalent to phase I of the Korotkoff sounds and signals systolic blood pressure. It is recorded as a Doppler pressure, for example, 120/D. As with palpated pressures, no diastolic measurement is obtained. This technique, as with palpated measurement, is useful in persons in whom blood pressure is difficult to measure by auscultation, for example, persons with low blood pressure.

Direct Methods

Direct measurement of arterial blood pressure also is possible. A catheter is introduced into a peripheral artery, such as the radial, brachial, or femoral artery, and is connected to a pressure transducer. Pressure from the artery is transmitted to and exerts pressure on the diaphragm at the air–fluid interface in a dome attached to the transducer. The transducer converts the pressure on the diaphragm to electrical signals. The electrical signals are amplified, filtered, and displayed on a monitor in waveforms. Digital readings often are displayed.[12]

Factors That Affect Blood Pressure Measurement

A number of factors can affect blood pressure measurements. These factors are of two types: technical factors and factors involving the subjective influences of the observer (Table 15–2).

Technical aspects include such things as body positioning and size of the cuff used. If the arm used for blood pressure measurement is positioned above the level of the heart, the blood pressure may be artificially lowered; if the arm is below the heart, blood pressure may be artificially raised. If the arm is unsupported, isometric activity by the patient in an effort to keep the arm elevated may result in falsely high readings.[10] The American Heart Association recommends use of a cuff with a bladder width that is 40 percent of the circumference of the midpoint of the limb.[10] Cuffs with bladders that are too narrow will result in falsely elevated blood pressure readings; bladders that are too wide result in erroneously low readings.

The second type of factor that can affect blood pressure measurement is the subjective influence of the observer. Observer bias is the phenomenon that occurs when the person measuring blood pressure unconsciously "hears" a lower blood pressure in a healthy young adult and a higher pressure in, for example, an obese person.[10]

Terminal digit preference is the unconscious preference to end a blood pressure reading in a certain

T A B L E 15 – 1. Phases and Descriptions of Korotkoff Sounds

Phase	Sound	Indication
I	First appearance of faint, clear tapping sounds	Systolic pressure
II	Sounds developing a murmuring or swishing quality	—
III	Sounds become crisper and increase in intensity	—
IV	Distinct, abrupt muffling of sounds	Diastolic (children)
V	Sounds disappear	Diastolic (adults)

Developed from information on Frolich ED, Grim C, Labarthe DR, Maxwell MH, Perloff D, Weidman WH: *Recommendations for Human Blood Pressure Determination by Sphygmomanometers.* Dallas, American Heart Association, 1987.

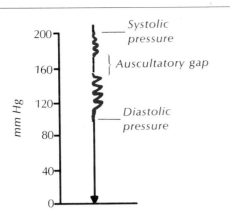

FIGURE 15-4. Auscultatory gap. (From Bates B: *A Guide to Physical Examination*, 5th ed. Philadelphia, JB Lippincott, 1991, p 283. Reproduced with permission.)

number, for example 90 mm Hg rather than 88 mm Hg. The digits 0 and 5 are recorded most frequently.[13] When blood pressure readings are near critical diagnostic thresholds, for example 90 mm Hg diastolic, there is a tendency to record lower rather than higher readings.[14] The reader is referred to Frolich et al[10] for a detailed discussion of factors that interfere with accurate blood pressure measurement.

KEY CONCEPTS

- Erroneous blood pressure measurements may be due to a missed auscultatory gap, hydrostatic pressure changes with changes in arm position, inappropriate cuff size, or observer bias.

Hypertension

Definition

High blood pressure is defined as blood pressure persistently elevated above 140 mm Hg systolic and/or 90 mm Hg diastolic. In the United States, more than 50 million people have or are being treated for high blood pressure.[15] A classification scheme for blood pressure has been developed based on the knowledge that as blood pressure, both systolic and diastolic, increases, so does the risk of cardiovascular complications (Table 15-3).

Risk Factors

Age

Blood pressure rises consistently with age, beginning at levels as low as 50/40 mm Hg in newborns and increasing to over 200 mm Hg in some elderly subjects.[5] High blood pressure in children is classified as "significant" when it is greater than or equal to the 95th percentile for age, and "severe" when it is greater than or equal to the 99th percentile for age (Table 15-4). High blood pressure occurs in about 5 percent of children in the United States, but more than 50 percent of people over 55 years of age have high blood pressure.[15-17] High blood pressure in childhood is a predictor of hypertension in adult life, especially in association with obesity.[18]

The increase in blood pressure with age is primarily attributable to arteriosclerosis. This mainly affects

TABLE 15-2. Technical, Subjective, and Other Factors That Influence Blood Pressure Readings

Factor	Effect on Blood Pressure (BP)
Technical Factors	
Cuff	
Too wide, too long	BP decreased
Too narrow, too short	BP increased
Arm position	
Above heart	BP decreased
Below heart	BP increased
Unsupported	BP increased
Excessive pressure on head of stethoscope	Diastolic progressively decreased with increasing pressure
<1 min between readings	BP increased
Respiration	BP increased during inspiration
Subjective Factors	
Terminal digit preference	Tendency to end BP in zero
Observer bias	Record BP higher or lower, depending on recorder's biases
Poor hearing	Altered reading
Other Factors	
"White coat" phenomenon	Higher BP reading when measured by a physician
Eating, smoking, taking caffeine, exercising within 30 min of BP	Increased BP
Speaking while BP measured	Increased BP

TABLE 15–3. Classification of Blood Pressure (BP) for Adults Aged 18 Years and Older

Category	Systolic (mm Hg)	Diastolic (mm Hg)
Normal	<130	<85
High normal	130–139	85–89
Isolated systolic hypertension	140+	<90
Hypertension		
Stage 1 (mild)	140–159	90–99
Stage 2 (moderate)	160–179	100–109
Stage 3 (severe)	180–209	110–119
Stage 4 (very severe)	≥210	≥120

Adapted with permission from The Fifth Report of the Joint National Committee on Detection, Evaluation, and Treatment of High Blood Pressure. *Arch Intern Med* 1993;153(2):161.

the systolic blood pressure and accounts for the isolated systolic high blood pressure seen most often in the elderly.[5]

Race

High blood pressure occurs two to three times more frequently in African-Americans than in whites, especially at diastolic levels above 105 mm Hg.[15,19–21] Elevated blood pressures appear earlier in African-Americans, and target organ damage is more severe than in Americans of European, Hispanic, or Native American descent.[15,18–20] The reason for this difference in African-Americans is not known, although African-Americans with high blood pressure have lower renin levels than do other Americans with high blood pres-

sure.[22] Possibly because of these lower renin levels, antihypertensive drugs that work primarily through altering the renin mechanisms, such as β-adrenergic-blocking agents and ACE inhibitors, when used alone, are less effective in this population. When used in combination therapy, these drugs are equally effective across ethnic groups.[15,23] Recent studies suggest that an enhanced sensitivity to vasopressin in African-Americans may account for some of the blood pressure variation seen in this population.[23]

Obesity

Excess weight is associated with elevated levels of blood pressure.[24] In the 20- to 39-year-old age group, high blood pressure occurs twice as often in overweight as in normal weight persons.[25] The mechanism by which excess weight contributes to high blood pressure is not known; however, weight reduction in overweight individuals is known to reduce blood pressure.[26] Obesity in childhood is a predictor of high blood pressure in adulthood.[17,18]

Excess Sodium Intake

Epidemiologic studies indicate that in members of cultures with high sodium intake, arterial blood pressures are higher than in individuals from cultures with low sodium intake (Fig. 15–5). Excess sodium intake has been associated with elevated levels of blood pressure in some persons, labeled "sodium responders." This association has not, however, revealed the cause of the high blood pressure; the blood pressure of sodium nonresponders is not increased when sodium intake is increased, nor is it reduced when sodium intake is restricted.[5]

TABLE 15–4. Classification of Hypertension in the Young

Age Group	≥95th Percentile (Significant)	≥99th Percentile (Severe)
Newborns, d		
7 (SBP)	> 95	>105
8–30 (SBP)	>103	>109
Infants <2 yr		
SBP	>111	>117
DBP	> 73	> 81
Children, yr		
3–5		
SBP	>115	>123
DBP	> 75	> 83
6–9		
SBP	>121	>129
DBP	> 77	> 85
10–12		
SBP	>125	>133
DBP	> 81	> 89
13–15		
SBP	>135	>143
DBP	> 85	> 91
Adolescents, 16–18 yr		
SBP	>141	>149
DBP	> 91	> 97

Adapted with permission from The 1988 Report of the Joint National Committee on Detection, Evaluation, and Treatment of High Blood Pressure. *Arch Intern Med* 1988;148:1023.

Classification of High Blood Pressure

Primary High Blood Pressure

In at least 90 percent of people with high blood pressure, no cause can be identified. These cases are described as **primary** or **idiopathic** or **essential high**

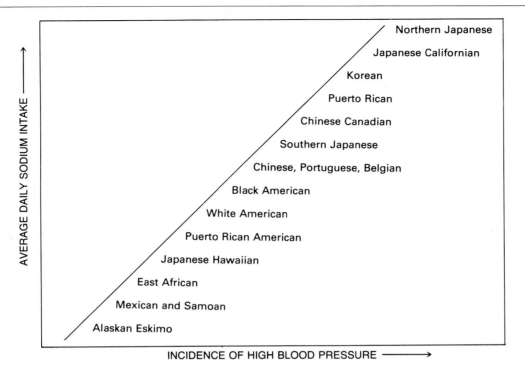

FIGURE 15–5. Cultural differences in blood pressure as related to sodium intake. (From Sollek MV, Lee KA: High blood pressure, in Underhill SL, et al (eds): *Cardiac Nursing*, 2nd ed. Philadelphia, JB Lippincott, 1989, p 817. Originally adapted from Meneely GR, Battarbee HD: High sodium–low potassium environment and hypertension. *Am J Cardiol* 1976;38(6):776; Meneely GR, Dahl LK: Electrolytes in hypertension: The effects of sodium chloride. *Med Clin North Am* 1961;45(2):280. Reproduced with permission.)

blood pressure. Studies of twins living apart show a high correlation in blood pressure, suggesting a genetic component to high blood pressure.[27] The risk factors listed previously play a contributing but not necessarily causative role in the development of high blood pressure. Other environmental factors such as stress have also been identified as contributing to high blood pressure.

Alterations in a variety of physiologic mechanisms currently are being investigated for their role in high blood pressure. The renin-angiotensin-aldosterone system and the mechanisms controlling sodium excretion are of interest. The renin-angiotensin-aldosterone system usually is activated in response to low renal perfusion. This results in renal retention of sodium and water, which increases vascular volume, renal perfusion, and blood pressure. Fifteen percent of people with high blood pressure are found to have high levels of renin activity. In situations of low circulating fluid volume and sodium deficiency, renin activity is stimulated, producing sodium and water retention and vasoconstriction.[16]

On the other hand, 30 percent of people with high blood pressure, including African-Americans, have been found to have low renin activity.[16] This is linked to sodium excess, which reduces renin activity; however, the effect is the same as in high renin activity: increased vascular volume and elevated blood pressure. Most people with high blood pressure have normal renin activity levels.[16]

Stimulation of the renin-angiotensin-aldosterone system results in the release of aldosterone. In response to aldosterone, the kidneys retain the positively charged sodium ion and in exchange excrete the cation potassium. In examining the influence of sodium intake on blood pressure, it becomes apparent that potassium levels also must be evaluated. The possibility of reducing blood pressure by increasing potassium intake rather than by restricting sodium intake is being investigated.[16]

The vascular endothelium is now believed to be a hormone-producing endocrine gland in its own right. Endothelial cells produce a number of vasoactive substances; an excess of those that produce vasoconstriction or a deficit in substances that produce vasodilation may result in high blood pressure.[28]

Recent studies have examined the role of vasopressin in the development of primary hypertension. Enhanced sensitivity to vasopressin has been identified in African-Americans with high blood pressure; this may explain some of the ethnic variability in blood pressure.[29]

Non-insulin-dependent diabetes mellitus (NIDDM) has been identified as a risk factor for essential hypertension. The prevalence of hypertension in subjects with NIDDM is up to 50 percent.[30,31] Obesity in patients with NIDDM explains some of this increased risk of hypertension. Obesity, NIDDM, and hypertension all may be accompanied by insulin resistance and hyperinsulinemia. The hypertensive mechanisms of insulin are not yet known; hypotheses include increased norepinephrine release, sodium retention, and increased vascular tone by affecting the sodium transport mechanisms in blood vessels. Insulin also is associated with an accelerated rate of atherosclerosis development.[30] Hyperinsulinism and insulin resistance have been noted in nonobese normotensive individuals with a family history of hypertension.[32] Blood pressure has been found to decline in African-American diabetic hypertensives as blood sugar is reduced, independent of a change in antihypertensive medications.[33] Secondary hypertension has not been associated with insulin resistance.[34]

Other areas of inquiry into the etiology of essential hypertension include increased sensitivity to angiotensin II[35] and the role of electrolytes in the development of hypertension.

Secondary High Blood Pressure

Of the 5 percent of children with high blood pressure, 80 percent of cases are attributable to some identifiable cause. Less than 10 percent of adult high blood pressure is of the secondary type.[15,16] A variety of health problems can lead to high blood pressure.

Renal Disorders. Renal disease is the most frequent cause of secondary high blood pressure, accounting for about 5 percent of all cases and 70 to 95 percent of high blood pressure in children.[16,19] Conditions that produce excess secretion of renin may result in high blood pressure. Renal artery stenosis, for example, may reduce renal perfusion and stimulate activation of the renin-angiotensin-aldosterone system, resulting in increased renin. Subsequent retention of sodium and water, along with vasoconstriction, results in elevated blood pressure.[16,36] Wilms' tumor is a renin-secreting tumor that produces increased blood pressure, activating the renin-angiotensin-aldosterone system, with resultant sodium and water retention and vasoconstriction. Any form of renal failure that results in retention of sodium and water may produce hypertension. Hypertension also may cause renal failure by damaging the arterioles that supply the kidneys. Reduction in blood flow to the kidneys stimulates the renin-angiotensin-aldosterone system, producing sodium and water retention and vasoconstriction that reduces blood flow further. This vicious cycle continues, aggravating the renal failure and the hypertension.[16,36]

Endocrine Disorders. Elevated levels of adrenal cortical hormones can result in high blood pressure. Both the glucocorticoids (cortisol) and mineralocorticoids (aldosterone) promote sodium and water retention by the kidneys, resulting in elevated blood pressure. Examples of conditions that produce excesses of these hormones are primary aldosteronism, Cushing's syndrome, and exogenous administration of glucocorticoids.[16,36]

Pheochromocytomas, tumors of chromaffin tissue seen most commonly in the adrenal medullae, secrete catecholamines, producing sympathetic nervous system stimulation resulting in vasoconstriction, increased heart rate and increased cardiac output. This excess secretion of catecholamines dramatically elevates blood pressures and may result in death within 6 months if not treated.[5,16]

Other endocrine disorders that may result in high blood pressure include acromegaly, which is associated with increased aldosterone levels (producing sodium and water retention) and hypo- or hyperthyroidism. Hypothyroidism reduces cardiac output; this is balanced by an increase in SVR, producing elevated diastolic blood pressure readings. Thyroid hormone enhances the effects of the sympathetic nervous system (faster heart rate, strengthened contractility and vasoconstriction); hyperthyroidism, therefore, may also produce high blood pressure.[16] Hyperparathyroidism may result in blood pressure by unknown mechanisms.[36]

Vascular Disorders. Arteriosclerosis raises SVR and therefore increases blood pressure, particularly diastolic blood pressure. In addition, arteriosclerosis may narrow renal arteries, resulting in stimulation of the renin-angiotensin-aldosterone system. Paradoxically, high blood pressure accelerates atherosclerosis, producing a self-perpetuating cycle.[5,16]

Coarctation of the aorta may produce high blood pressure in children and adults. Ejection of blood into the narrowed aorta results in an elevated systolic blood pressure in the arms. An identifying feature of high blood pressure due to coarctation of the aorta is the presence of normal or lower blood pressure in the legs, compared to the arms.[15,16]

Neurologic Disorders. Problems that cause elevated intracranial pressure, such as intracerebral hemorrhage and subdural hematoma, may result in elevated blood pressure. Pressure on the posterior hypothalamus, the medulla, or on nerve pathways (for example, from tumors) may produce excessive catecholamine stimulation and increased blood pressure. Benign or malignant tumors of the sympathetic nervous system may produce hypertension.[16]

Spinal cord injuries may produce hypertension in response to stimuli such as a full bladder, a phenomenon called autonomic hyperreflexia or dysreflexia (see Chap. 44).[16]

Exogenous Compounds. Many prescription and over-the-counter medications can cause elevations in blood pressure. Sympathomimetics (drugs that mimic the sympathetic nervous system), amphetamines, tricyclic antidepressants, corticosteroids, and oral contraceptives are some of the drugs known to produce high blood pressure. Caffeine and nicotine, by producing vasoconstriction, also can increase blood pressure (Table 15–5). So-called recreational drugs, particularly cocaine, may also have significant cardiovascular effects, including hypertension.

Isolated Systolic Hypertension

Estimates of the prevalence of high blood pressure in the elderly (both systolic and diastolic) range from 44 to 75 percent. Isolated systolic high blood pressure, defined as systolic blood pressure greater than or

TABLE 15–5. Exogenous Compounds That Cause High Blood Pressure

Sympathomimetic agents	Tryptophan- and Tyramine-containing foods
Amphetamine	Chicken liver
Caffeine	Pickled herring
Adrenalin	Yeast extract
Dopamine	Broad beans
Nicotine	Matured cheeses (especially cheddar)
Methyldopa	Beer
Tyramine	Wines (especially Chianti)
Tricyclic antidepressants	Oral contraceptives
Phenacetin-containing analgesics	Trace metals, minerals, and electrolytes
Licorice	Cadmium
Chewing tobacco	Lead
Steroid therapy	Mercury
Monoamine oxidase inhibitors	Magnesium
Isocarboxazid (Marplan)	Sodium
Isoniazid	Zinc
Nialamide (Niamid)	Selenium
Pargyline (Eutonyl)	Calcium
Phenelzine (Nardil)	Potassium
Procarbazine	
Tranylcypromine (Parnate)	

Adapted with permission from Sollek MV, Lee KA: High blood pressure, in Underhill SL, Woods SL, Froelicher ESS, Halpenny CJ (eds): *Cardiac Nursing*, 2nd ed. Philadelphia, JB Lippincott, 1989.

equal to 140 mm Hg with diastolic blood pressure less than 90 mm Hg, occurs in approximately 10 percent of persons 65 to 74 years of age[5,15] and in 24 percent of those 80 years old or older.[37] Decreased distensibility of the aorta and large arteries in the elderly occurs as arteriosclerosis progresses with age. This reduced distensibility produces an elevation in systolic blood pressure without an increase in diastolic blood pressure.[5,15,38]

Isolated systolic hypertension is associated with higher risk of stroke, other cardiovascular diseases, and death.[38,39] Treatment guidelines for isolated systolic hypertension are the same as those for combined systolic and diastolic high blood pressure,[15] and treatment has been shown to be effective in reducing the risks listed above.[39,40]

Pregnancy-Induced Hypertension

Blood pressure normally decreases during the first two trimesters of pregnancy, then gradually returns to normal levels during the third trimester. The initial decrease in blood pressure apparently is due to a decrease in TPR, as CO is increased 40 to 60 percent during pregnancy. As TPR returns to normal levels, blood pressure rises. During pregnancy, there also is an increase in levels of angiotensin II and aldosterone, promoting vasoconstriction and sodium and water retention.[15,16]

Because of the cardiovascular changes that occur with pregnancy, the usual criteria for adult high blood pressure do not apply. The American College of Obstetricians and Gynecologists suggests the following criteria to aid in the diagnosis of high blood pressure during pregnancy: (1) blood pressure greater than 140/90 mm Hg, (2) an increase in systolic blood pressure of 30 mm Hg, or (3) an increase in diastolic blood pressure of 15 mm Hg.[41]

Pregnancy-induced hypertension (PIH), or **preeclampsia,** is characterized by elevated blood pressure, proteinuria, and edema. Several proposed mechanisms are under investigation. An increased sensitivity to angiotensin II, hormonal changes that increase vasoconstriction, and a tendency toward a reduced calcium intake during pregnancy may combine to produce elevated blood pressure.[36] Systemic vasospasm, possibly due to an imbalance in the production of thromboxane, a vasoconstricting substance, and prostacyclin, a vasodilator, may produce high blood pressure.[42]

Usually developing after the 20th week of gestation, PIH may occur earlier in the pregnancy. Onset during the second trimester is associated with increased maternal and fetal risk.[42] The condition occurs during first and subsequent pregnancies, and blood pressure returns to normal between pregnancies. Treatment with aspirin during pregnancy may prevent PIH.[42,43]

Chronic hypertension is high blood pressure unrelated to the pregnancy. Blood pressure fluctuations resemble those in normal pregnant women; that is, blood pressure decreases early in the pregnancy and increases during the last 3 months. These changes in blood pressure may be mistaken for PIH in women with previously undiagnosed chronic hypertension. Unlike women with PIH, however, women with chronic high blood pressure will remain hypertensive after delivery. Chronic high blood pressure increases the risk of PIH.

Transient or late high blood pressure occurs during the last trimester of pregnancy or in the early postdelivery period. Blood pressure returns to normal levels within 10 days after delivery.[16]

Accelerated High Blood Pressure

Accelerated (malignant) high blood pressure is a rapidly progressing, potentially fatal form of hypertension in which diastolic blood pressure exceeds 120 mm Hg. Although only about 1 percent of all hypertensive persons develop accelerated hypertension, the 1-year mortality rate if untreated approaches 90 percent. African-Americans, males, and middle-aged people are most likely to develop this form of high blood pressure. Severe emotional stress, excessive salt intake, and abrupt discontinuation of antihypertensive medication without tapering are examples of situations that may trigger a hypertensive crisis; any disease that produces high blood pressure can result in the accelerated form.[16] The most common mechanism of malignant hypertension is bilateral renal artery stenosis.[36]

In addition to extremely high blood pressures, evidence of target organ damage is present. Any organ may be damaged, but the kidneys are most commonly involved. Damage to the afferent arterioles produces stiff, thickened arterioles that are less responsive to changes in perfusion. Renal failure may ensue. Other potential problems resulting from arterial damage include encephalopathy, cardiac failure, dissecting aortic aneurysm, and severe retinopathy in the form of papilledema.[16]

Effects of High Blood Pressure

Cardiac

Elevated systemic blood pressure requires that the left ventricle work harder to overcome the resistance to ejection of blood. In response, the left ventricular muscle hypertrophies, which increases myocardial oxygen demand. The work load of the left ventricle increases as blood pressure increases. When the myocardial oxygen demand exceeds the supply, heart failure develops (see Chap. 18).[5,16]

Vascular

Sustained high blood pressure causes changes in the walls of arteries and arterioles. High blood pressure accelerates the development of atherosclerosis in the aorta and in the medium- to large-sized arteries, resulting in isolated systolic high blood pressure in the elderly. Atherosclerosis also contributes to cerebral infarction.[16]

Arteriosclerosis in the smaller arteries and arterioles contributes to cerebrovascular disease and peripheral vascular disease. Fibrinoid necrosis occurs in the small arterioles and produces lesions in the kidneys and in the retina of the eyes.[16]

Signs and Symptoms

The phrase "silent killer" is aptly applied to high blood pressure and summarizes the fact that few signs and symptoms of high blood pressure exist. When signs and symptoms do occur, they may signify advanced high blood pressure and represent damage to target organs. The degree and duration of elevated blood pressure determine the severity of target organ damage and signs and symptoms.[5,16]

High blood pressure increases myocardial work load and produces left ventricular hypertrophy (LVH). When myocardial oxygen demand exceeds supply, heart failure occurs. Signs and symptoms of left ventricular failure include crackles in the lungs, dyspnea, and fatigue. LVH may be seen on chest radiographs and produces characteristic changes on the electrocardiogram, consisting of increased voltage and repolarization abnormalities. LVH is a serious consequence of hypertension associated with a 21 to 33 percent mortality within 5 years of diagnosis.[17,22,44]

Acceleration of atherosclerosis along with hypertrophy and edema of vessel walls produces coronary artery narrowing and further myocardial ischemia. This may lead to angina pectoris and myocardial infarction.[16]

Other cardiovascular outcomes of high blood pressure include the development and rupture of aortic aneurysms and the development of peripheral arterial disease with intermittent claudication. Cerebrovascular accidents (strokes) are a major complication of high blood pressure. Signs and symptoms depend on the location of the infarct and range from transient symptoms to aphasia and hemiplegia. Nonspecific signs and symptoms of cerebrovascular diseases due to high blood pressure may include headache, irritability, fatigue, seizures, and coma.[16]

In the retina of the eye, arterioles and arteries may be examined using noninvasive techniques. Hypertensive retinopathy is graded on a scale of I to IV, with grade I changes signifying recent onset of high blood pressure or mild levels of high blood pressure. Grade IV changes (papilledema) indicate severe, accelerated high blood pressure. Hypertensive retinopathy may produce visual changes ranging from blurred vision to blindness.[16]

Arteriolar changes associated with high blood pressure cause serious problems in the kidneys. Renal artery obstruction, decreased renal perfusion, and altered nephron function result in renal failure. Proteinuria, nocturia, and azotemia may occur.[16]

Diagnosis

A diagnosis of high blood pressure is made after a minimum of two blood pressure measurements on separate occasions reveal elevated readings. All the guidelines of the American Heart Association for blood measurement detection should be followed.[8] The **"white coat" phenomenon**—elevated blood pressure readings when measured by a physician—must be taken into account, and home blood pressure monitoring may aid in making the diagnosis.[45]

The medical history is focused on risk factors for high blood pressure, including family history, and the presence of other cardiovascular risk factors. Careful determination of the use of prescription and over-the-counter medications as well as recreational drugs should be made (see Table 15–5).

In addition to blood pressure determination, the physical examination includes assessment for target organ damage (for example, funduscopic examination of the eyes), assessment of arteries for the presence of bruits, and neurologic evaluation. Useful diagnostic tests include an electrocardiogram, assessment of serum lipids, assessment of renal function, and assessment of serum electrolytes.[15]

Treatment

Several clinical trials have demonstrated a decrease in mortality and morbidity with blood pressure reduction.[46–49] The goal of therapy is to achieve and maintain a blood pressure less than 140/90 mm Hg. Decisions about initiation of and type of therapy depend on the severity of blood pressure, the presence of target organ damage, and the presence of other cardiovascular risk factors. Therapies and goals for isolated systolic hypertension are the same as for systodiastolic hypertension.[37]

The most recent set of hypertension treatment guidelines was published in the Fifth Report of the Joint National Committee on Detection, Evaluation, and Treatment of High Blood Pressure. This report outlined a new classification system of hypertension that substituted the use of Stages 1, 2, 3, and 4 for the terms "mild," "moderate," and "severe." This change was prompted by the erroneous assumption that mild hypertension was not a serious condition requiring medical attention.[15]

Other changes from previous guidelines included an emphasis on life-style modifications in the treatment of hypertension, and a new treatment algorithm (Fig. 15–6) that replaced the "stepped-care" approach first described in the 1970s.[15]

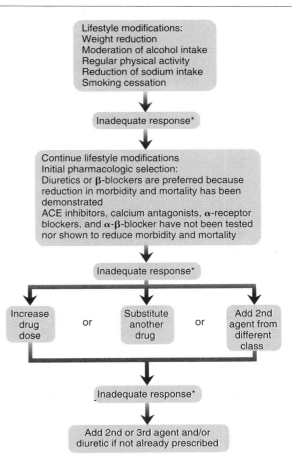

FIGURE 15–6. Treatment algorithm. Asterisk indicates that response means the patient achieved goal blood pressure or is making considerable progress toward this goal. ACE, angiotensin-converting enzyme. (Redrawn from Fifth Report of the Joint National Committee on Detection, Evaluation, and Treatment of High Blood Pressure. *Arch Intern Med* 1993;153:161. Reproduced with permission.)

Life-Style Modifications

In persons with Stage 1 and Stage 2 hypertension, and in those without evidence of target organ damage, life-style modifications may be instituted initially without concomitant pharmacologic therapy, both to lower blood pressure and to reduce the effects of other cardiovascular risk factors. In Stages 3 and 4 hypertension, life-style modifications should be instituted along with pharmacologic treatment.[15]

Weight reduction in overweight persons may lower blood pressure, often enough to achieve normal blood pressure levels. The blood pressure–lowering effects of antihypertensive medications are enhanced by weight reduction.[15,50]

Excess alcohol intake contributes to high blood pressure and should be restricted to 1 ounce of ethanol per day (two ounces of 100 proof whiskey, 8 ounces of wine, or 24 ounces of beer).[15,51]

Moderate sodium restriction of 1.5 to 2.5 grams per day will reduce blood pressure in "sodium-sensitive" individuals.[15,51] Sodium-sensitive individuals tend to be older, obese, black, and to have higher initial blood pressures. Salt sensitivity also is associated with low plasma renin activity.[52]

Sodium-restricted diets potentiate the effects of some antihypertensive medications. Excess dietary salt intake promotes excretion of calcium and potassium in the urine, possibly promoting vasoconstriction and increased blood pressure.[52] Conversely, extreme sodium restriction may elevate blood pressure in some individuals and has been associated with increased norepinephrine, renin, and cholesterol levels.[52]

High potassium and calcium intake may reduce or suppress the increase in blood pressure that occurs after salt loading.[52] Potassium supplementation has been found to reduce blood pressure.[50,51] Increased calcium intake has been shown to reduce blood pressure in pregnant women.[53]

Nicotine is not associated with the long-term development of high blood pressure but, because of its vasoconstrictive properties, does cause acute elevations to occur. For this reason, and because of the role of nicotine in other cardiovascular disease and in pulmonary disease, smoking cessation is encouraged.[15,16,50]

Some individuals successfully lower blood pressure using biofeedback and relaxation techniques.[15,50,51] Regular aerobic exercise reduces blood pressure, independent of weight loss.[15,51] Reduction of dietary fat intake reduces serum cholesterol levels, facilitates weight loss, and possibly reduces blood pressure directly.[15,50]

Pharmacologic Therapy

In persons with diastolic blood pressures above 95 mm Hg, drug therapy has been shown to reduce cardiovascular morbidity and mortality. When diastolic blood pressure is 90 to 94 mm Hg and other cardiovascular risk factors are present, use of drug therapy still is warranted. If there are no other cardiovascular risk factors and diastolic blood pressure is less than 95 mm Hg, nonpharmacologic methods to reduce blood pressure should be instituted[15]; preliminary evidence suggests pharmacologic treatment may be effective with acceptable risk.[48]

Following a vigorous 6-month trial of life-style modifications, drug therapy may be instituted in persons with Stage 1 or Stage 2 hypertension whose blood pressure remains greater than 140/90 mm Hg. Pharmacologic therapy may be instituted immediately, along with life-style modifications, in persons with Stage 3 or 4 hypertension.

Initial drug therapy should begin with diuretics or β blockers (Table 15–6). Drugs from other classifications, for example calcium antagonists and ACE inhibitors, while effective in reducing blood pressure, have not been demonstrated to be effective in reducing morbidity and mortality. For this reason, they should not be used for initial monotherapy except in special situations.

Other considerations in the choice of initial therapy include demographic considerations, concomitant diseases, and quality of life issues. Although age and gender have not been found to determine drug responsiveness, African-Americans generally are more responsive to diuretics and calcium antagonists than to β blockers or ACE inhibitors.

Although some antihypertensive drugs worsen some diseases, other diseases may be ameliorated. For example, β blockers may worsen asthma but may improve angina pectoris. Use of an antihypertensive drug that also treats a concomitant disease may simplify the medication regimen and reduce costs.

Many of the antihypertensive agents have undesirable side effects. Compliance with the medication plan may be significantly influenced by drugs that impair sexual function, impair mental acuity, or reduce exercise tolerance. The cost of the therapy must be considered when selecting antihypertensive ther-

TABLE 15–6. Classification of Antihypertensive Medications

Diuretics	Centrally acting alpha blockers
Thiazides and related sulfonamide diuretics	Clonidine
Chlorothiazide	Guanabenz
Chlorthalidone	Guanfacine
Hydrochlorothiazide	Methyldopa
Indapamide	Peripheral acting adrenergic antagonists
Metolazone	Guanadrel
Polythiazide	Guanethidine
Loop diuretics	Rauwolfia
Bumetanide	Reserpine
Ethacrynic acid	Angiotensin-converting enzyme inhibitors
Furosemide	Benzapril
Potassium-sparing agents	Captopril
Amiloride	Cilazapril
Spironolactone	Enalapril
Triamterene	Fosinopril
Adrenergic inhibitors	Lisinopril
β-adrenergic blockers	Perindopril
Acebutolol	Quinapril
Atenolol	Ramipril
Metoprolol	Sdpirapril
Nadolol	Calcium antagonists
Pindolol	Amlodipine
Propanolol	Diltiazem
Timolol	Felodipine
Combined α, β-adrenergic blocker	Isradipine
Labetalol	Nicardipine
α₁-adrenergic blockers	Nifedipine
Doxazosin	Verapamil
Prazosin	Vasodilators
Terazosin	Hydralazine
	Minoxidil

Adapted with permission from The Fifth Report of the Joint National Committee on Detection, Evaluation, and Treatment of High Blood Pressure. *Arch Intern Med* 1993;153:165.

apy. Inability to pay for the medication may be a hidden reason for failure of drug therapy.[15]

If adequate blood pressure control is not achieved after 1 to 3 months of therapy, the dose is increased, a drug of a different class is substituted, or a drug of a different class is added. Addition of a drug with a different mode of action from the first often will allow smaller doses of drugs to be used, thereby reducing the incidence of side effects. Once adequate blood pressure control has been achieved, combination drugs may be used to simplify the medication regimen and reduce costs.[15]

After blood pressure control has been achieved and maintained for at least 1 year, pharmacologic therapy may be gradually and slowly reduced. This is most often effective in clients who also are using non-pharmacologic adjuncts in blood pressure control. Tapering or elimination of blood pressure medication requires careful monitoring to avoid return of blood pressure to previously elevated levels.[15]

Hypertensive Crisis

In some instances, urgent lowering of blood pressure may be necessary to avoid serious organ damage or death. Severe perioperative hypertension, accelerated hypertension, intracranial hemorrhage, and dissecting aortic aneurysms are examples of situations requiring rapid reduction of blood pressure. Intravenous (IV) agents are used in these situations and require monitoring in intensive care units. Examples of IV agents include sodium nitroprusside, nitroglycerin, hydralazine, labetalol, and methyldopa.[15]

KEY CONCEPTS

- High blood pressure is arbitrarily defined as a blood pressure above 140 mm Hg systolic and/or 90 mm Hg diastolic. Chronic high blood pressure is associated with an increased risk of left ventricular hypertrophy, left heart failure, and atherosclerosis.
- Several risk factors for development of hypertension have been proposed: age, ethnicity and family history, obesity, and high sodium intake.
- Persons who develop primary hypertension have a genetic predisposition (polygenic) which can be influenced by environmental factors such as life-style and diet. An imbalance of endothelium-derived mediators may be important in development of hypertension. The endothelium secretes and processes a number of vascular constricting and relaxing factors.
- Secondary hypertension is rare and refers to high blood pressure of known etiology, such as renal artery stenosis, renal failure, hypersecretion of aldosterone or catecholamines, hyperthyroidism, increased intracranial pressure, and drugs.
- Hypertension is associated with headache, retinopathy, seizures, and coma; however, there may be no symptoms. The diagnosis is made after at least two elevated blood pressure readings on separate occasions.

- Treatment centers on measures to decrease vascular resistance and/or blood volume. Weight reduction, moderation of alcohol intake, sodium and fat restriction, and relaxation may be recommended. Drugs may be used to decrease vascular resistance (ACE inhibitors, adrenergic inhibitors, calcium antagonists, direct vasodilators) and reduce blood volume (diuretics).

Orthostatic Hypotension

Successful change of position from supine to upright requires an intact cardiovascular system and adequate fluid volume. When the upright position is assumed, blood volume transiently shifts to the lower extremities. The baroreceptors in the carotid arteries and in the arch of the aorta sense a decrease in circulating volume and trigger the responses outlined in Figure 15–3. These mechanisms result in peripheral vasoconstriction and increased heart rate in an attempt to restore MAP. During change from a supine to an upright position, the normal postural vital sign response includes an increase in heart rate up to 15 percent above resting, a decrease of up to 15 mm Hg in systolic blood pressure, and a change in diastolic blood pressure ranging from a 5 mm Hg reduction to a 10 mm Hg increase.[5,11]

Two types of problems alter the normal response to postural change. Saline depletion results in an exaggerated pulse increase (greater than 15 percent), and a decrease in either systolic (greater than 15 mm Hg) or diastolic (greater than 10 mm Hg) blood pressure. The cardiovascular responses to a reduction in MAP are intact, but a lack of fluid volume prevents a rapid return to normal vital signs with positional change. As a result, positional change may be accompanied by dizziness, light-headedness, or syncope as cerebral blood flow is reduced.[11]

Impaired cardiovascular response constitutes the other type of problem that produces an altered vital sign response to postural change. One of two mechanisms is involved: inadequate peripheral vasoconstriction or inadequate heart rate increase. The vital sign response to inadequate peripheral vasoconstriction mimics that of saline depletion (heart rate increased more than 15 percent and either a reduction in systolic blood pressure of more than 15 mm Hg or a reduction in diastolic blood pressure of more than 10 mm Hg), and differentiation between the two is based on client history. Peripheral neuropathy, as occurs in diabetics, may limit peripheral vasoconstriction; a history of saline loss, as occurs with diuretic therapy, suggests fluid volume deficit. It is important to remember that the two mechanisms could occur simultaneously.[11]

The second cardiovascular mechanism of abnormal vital sign response to positional change is autonomic insufficiency. In this case, the anticipated increase in heart rate in response to low MAP is blunted. This may represent primary dysfunction of the cardiovascular reflex mechanisms but more commonly is the result of drug therapy with agents that prevent an increase in heart rate, for example, the β-adrenergic blocking agents.[11]

Management of orthostatic hypotension depends on the etiology. Orthostatic hypotension due to fluid volume deficit is treated by restoring fluid volume. Unless due to pharmacologic therapy, persons with orthostatic hypotension due to impaired cardiovascular responses must be taught to minimize the blood pressure changes that result from position change. This is accomplished by teaching the person to make position changes slowly to allow gradual compensation to the upright position. The same instructions should be given to the person with orthostatic hypotension due to pharmacologic therapy, if the medication cannot be discontinued.

KEY CONCEPTS

- Orthostatic hypotension is due to a drop in cardiac output when the upright position is assumed. Activation of the baroreceptors usually minimizes the drop in blood pressure by increasing heart rate and vascular resistance. An increase in heart rate of 15 percent or more above supine or a fall in systolic (>15 mm Hg) or diastolic (>10 mm Hg) blood pressure is defined as orthostatic hypotension.

- The usual cause of orthostatic hypotension is intravascular volume depletion.

- An impaired baroreceptor reflex may also result in orthostatic hypotension. Adrenergic blocking drugs, peripheral neuropathy, and spinal cord injury can interrupt the normal baroreceptor reflex pathway.

Summary

Arterial blood pressure, specifically, mean arterial pressure, is a closely regulated physiologic parameter. A variety of mechanisms interact to maintain the blood pressure necessary to perfuse body tissues.

Mechanisms that elevate blood pressure may be stimulated in response to such situations as hemorrhage or low renal perfusion, as occurs in heart failure or shock, or those mechanisms may be activated in the absence of identifiable stimuli, as in primary hypertension. Primary hypertension is a significant public health problem, affecting millions of Americans. Reduction of elevated blood pressure is vital in preventing damage to body organs and may be achieved by life-style modification or pharmacologic methods.

Intact cardiovascular reflexes and sufficient fluid volume both are necessary for the maintenance of adequate blood pressure with positional change. Alterations in volume status, peripheral vasoconstriction, or in heart rate response can interfere with the ability to successfully assume an upright posture.

REFERENCES

1. Vander AJ, Sherman JH, Luciano DS: *Human Physiology: The Mechanisms of Body Function*, 5th ed. New York, McGraw-Hill, 1990.
2. Halpenny CJ: The systemic circulation, in Underhill SL, et al (eds): *Cardiac Nursing*, 2nd ed. Philadelphia, JB Lippincott, 1989.
3. Bates B: *A Guide to Physical Examination*, 5th ed. Philadelphia, JB Lippincott, 1991.
4. Halpenny CJ: Regulation of cardiac output and blood pressure, in Underhill SL, et al (eds): *Cardiac Nursing*, 2nd ed. Philadelphia, JB Lippincott, 1989.
5. Guyton AC: *Textbook of Medical Physiology*, 8th ed. Philadelphia, WB Saunders, 1991.
6. Green JF: *Mechanical Concepts in Cardiovascular and Pulmonary Physiology*. Philadelphia, Lea & Febiger, 1977.
7. Tulassay T: Physiology of blood pressure. *Child Nephrol Urol* 1992;12(2–3):70–77.
8. Hollister AS, Inagami T: Atrial natriuretic factor and hypertension. *Am J Hypertens* 1991;4(10 pt 1):850–865.
9. O'Brien ET, O'Malley K: *Essentials of Blood Pressure Measurement*. Edinburgh, Churchill Livingstone, 1981.
10. Frolich ED, Grim C, Labarthe DR, Maxwell MH, Perloff D, Weidman WH: *Recommendations for Human Blood Pressure Determination by Sphygmomanometers*. Dallas, American Heart Association, 1987.
11. Underhill SL: History taking and physical examination, in Underhill SL, et al (eds): *Cardiac Nursing*, 2nd ed. Philadelphia, JB Lippincott, 1989.
12. Gardner PE, Woods SL: Hemodynamic monitoring, in Underhill SL, et al (eds): *Cardiac Nursing*, 2nd ed. Philadelphia, JB Lippincott, 1989.
13. Hessel PA: Terminal digit preference in blood pressure measurements: Effects on epidemiological associations. *Int J Epidemiol* 1986;15(1):122–125.
14. Patterson JR: Sources of error in recording the blood pressure of patients with hypertension in general practice. *Br Med J (Clin Res)* 1984;289:1661–1664.
15. Fifth report of the Joint National Committee on Detection, Evaluation, and Treatment of High Blood Pressure. *Arch Intern Med* 1993;153(2):154.
16. Sollek MV, Lee KA: High blood pressure, in Underhill SL, et al (eds): *Cardiac Nursing*, 2nd ed. Philadelphia, JB Lippincott, 1989.
17. Mahoney LT, Clarke WR, Burns TL, Lauer RM: Childhood predictors of high blood pressure. *Am J Hypertens* 1991;4(suppl 11):608S–610S.
18. Jamerson K, Julius S: Predictors of blood pressure and hypertension. *Am J Hypertens* 1991;4(suppl 11):598S–602S.
19. American Heart Association: *1993 Heart and Stroke Facts*. Dallas, American Heart Association, 1993.
20. Stamler J, Stamler R, Liu K: High blood pressure, in Connor WE, Bristow JD: *Coronary Heart Disease: Prevention, Complications, and Treatment*. Philadelphia, JB Lippincott, 1985.
21. Leong GM, Kainer G: Diet, salt, anthropologic and hereditary factors in hypertension. *Child Nephrol Urol* 1992;12(2–3):96–105.
22. Saunders E: Hypertension in blacks. *Med Clin North Am* 1987;71(5):1013–1029.
23. Saunders E: Stepped care and profiled care in the treatment of hypertension: Considerations for black Americans. *Am J Med* 1986;81(6C):39–44.
24. Aristimuno GG, Foster TA, Voors AW, et al: Influence of persistent obesity in children on cardiovascular risk factors: The Bogalusa heart study. *Circulation* 1984;69(5):895–904.
25. Stamler R, Stamler J, Riedlinger WF: Weight and blood pressure. *JAMA* 1978;240(15):1607–1610.
26. Reisin E, Abel R, Modan M, et al: Effects of weight loss without salt restriction on the reduction of blood pressure in overweight hypertensive patients. *N Engl J Med* 1978;298(1):1–6.
27. Miall WE: Genetic considerations concerning hypertension. *Ann NY Acad Sci* 1978;304:18–27.
28. Panza JA, Quyyumi AA, Brush JE, Epstein SE: Abnormal endothelium-dependent vascular relaxation in patients with essential hypertension. *N Engl J Med* 1990;323(1):22–27.
29. Goldsmith MF: African lineage, hypertension linked. *JAMA* 1991;266(15):2049.
30. Tuck M: Glucose, insulin, and insulin resistance as biochemical predictors of hypertension. *Am J Hypertens* 1991;4(suppl 11):638S–641S.

31. Lindholm LH: Cardiovascular risk factors and their interactions in hypertensives. *J Hypertens* 1991;9(suppl 3):S3–S6.
32. Facchini F, Chen YDI, Clinkingbeard C, Jeppesen J, Reaven GM: Insulin resistance, hyperinsulinemia, and dyslipidemia in nonobese individuals with a family history of hypertension. *Am J Hypertens* 1992;5(10):694–699.
33. Jaber LA, Melchior WR, Rutledge DR: Possible correlation between glycemia and blood pressure in black, diabetic, hypertensive patients. *Ann Pharmacother* 1992;26(7–8):882–886.
34. Shamiss A, Carroll J, Rosenthal T: Insulin resistance in secondary hypertension. *Am J Hypertens* 1992;5(1):26–28.
35. Widgren BR, Herlitz H, Aurell M, Berglund G, Wikstrand J, Andersson OK: Increased systemic and renal vascular sensitivity to angiotensin II in normotensive men with positive family histories of hypertension. *Am J Hypertens* 1992;5(3):167–174.
36. Streeten DHP, Anderson GH: Secondary hypertension: An overview of its causes and management. *Drugs* 1992;43(6): 805–819.
37. Hall WD: Treatment of systolic hypertension. *Heart Dis Stroke* 1992;1(5):271–273.
38. Nichols WW, Nicolini FA, Pepine CJ: Determinants of isolated systolic hypertension in the elderly. *J Hypertens* 1992;10 (suppl 6):S73–S77.
39. SHEP Cooperative Research Group: Prevention of stroke by antihypertensive drug treatment in older persons with isolated systolic hypertension. *JAMA* 1991;265(24):3255–3264.
40. Menard J, Day M, Chatellier G, Laragh JH: Some lessons from Systolic Hypertension in the Elderly Program (SHEP). *Am J Hypertens* 1992;5(5 pt 1):325–330.
41. Maikranz P, Lindheimer MD: Hypertension in pregnancy. *Med Clin North Am* 1987;71(5):1031–1049.
42. Davies NJ: Hypertensive disorders of pregnancy for the trainee. *Br J Hosp Med* 1992;47(8):613–619.
43. Uzan S, Beaufils M, Breart G, Bazin B, Capitant C, Paris J: Prevention of pre-eclampsia with low-dose aspirin: Results of the apreda trial. *Eur J Obstet Gynecol Reprod Biol* 1992;44:12.
44. Kannel WB: Left ventricular hypertrophy as a risk factor: The Framingham experience. *J Hypertens* 1991;9(suppl 2):S3–S9.
45. Mancia G, et al: Effects of blood-pressure measurement by the doctor on patient's blood pressure and heart rate. *Lancet* 1983;2:695–698.
46. Hypertension Detection and Follow-up Program Cooperative Group: Five-year findings of the Hypertension Detection and Follow-up Program. *JAMA* 1979;242(23):2562–2571.
47. Multiple Risk Factor Intervention Trial Research Group: Multiple Risk Factor Intervention Trial. *JAMA* 1982;248(12): 1465–1477.
48. Luque-Otero M, Fernandez-Pinilla C: The J-curve: the importance of gradual reduction of blood pressure. *Drugs* 1992;44(suppl 1):56–60.
49. Walker WG, Neaton JD, Cutler JA, Neuwirth R, Cohen JD: Renal function change in hypertensive members of the Multiple Risk Factor Intervention Trial. *JAMA* 1992;268(21):3085–3091.
50. Silverberg DS: Non-pharmacological treatment of hypertension. *J Hypertens* 1990;(suppl 4):S21–S26.
51. Fotherby BMD, Potter JF: Potassium supplementation reduces clinic and ambulatory blood pressure in elderly hypertensive patients. *J Hypertens* 1992;10(11):1403–1408.
52. Muntzel M, Drueke T: A comprehensive review of the salt and blood pressure relationship. *Am J Hypertens* 1992;5(suppl 4):1S–42S.
53. Knight KB, Keith RE: Calcium supplementation in normotensive and hypertensive pregnant women. *Am J Clin Nutr* 1992;55(4):891–895.

BIBLIOGRAPHY

Blaufox MD, Lee HB, Davis B, Oberman A, Wassertheil-Smoller S, Langford H: Renin predicts diastolic blood pressure response to nonpharmacologic and pharmacologic therapy. *JAMA* 1992;267(9):1221–1225.

Calhoun DA, Oparial S: Treatment of hypertensive crisis. *N Engl J Med* 1990;323(17):1177–1183.

Hollister AS, Inagami T: Atrial natriuretic factor and hypertension. *Am J Hypertens* 1991;4(10 pt 1):850–859.

Lind L, Lithell H, Gustafsson IB, Pollare T, Ljunghall S: Metabolic cardiovascular risk factors and sodium sensitivity in hypertensive subjects. *Am J Hypertens* 1992;4(8):502–505.

Mangino MW: Hypertension in elders: Clinical diagnosis and treatment considerations. *J Gerontol Nurs* 1991;17(12):14–22.

National High Blood Pressure Education Program Working Groups: National High Blood Pressure Education Program Working Group report on primary prevention of hypertension. *Arch Intern Med* 1993;153(2):186–208.

Rich GM, McCullough M, Olmedo A, Malarick C, Moor TJ: Blood pressure and renal blood flow responses to dietary calcium and sodium intake in humans. *Am J Hypertens* 1991;4(suppl 11):642S–645S.

Silverberg DS: Non-pharmacological treatment of hypertension. *J Hypertens* 1990;8(suppl 4):S21–S26.

Stamler J, Stamler R, Neaton JC: Blood pressure, systolic and diastolic, and cardiovascular risks. *Arch Intern Med* 1993; 153(5):598–615.

Trials of Hypertension Prevention Collaborative Research Group: The effects of nonpharmacologic interventions on blood pressure of persons with high normal levels. *JAMA* 1992; 167(9):1213–1220.

Van Hooft IMS, Grobbee DE, Derkx FHM, de Leeuw PE, Schalekamp MADH, Hofman A: Renal hemodynamics and the renin-angiotensin-aldosterone system in normotensive subjects with hypertensive and normotensive parents. *N Engl J Med* 1991;324(19):1305–1311.

Vane JR, Anggard EE, Botting RM: Regulatory functions of the vascular endothelium. *N Engl J Med* 1990;323(1):27–36.

Wassertheil-Smoller S, Oberman A, Blaufox MD, Davis B, Langford H: The Trial of Antihypertensive Interventions and Management (TAIM) study. *Am J Hypertens* 1992;5(1):37–44.

U N I T V
Alterations in Cardiac Function

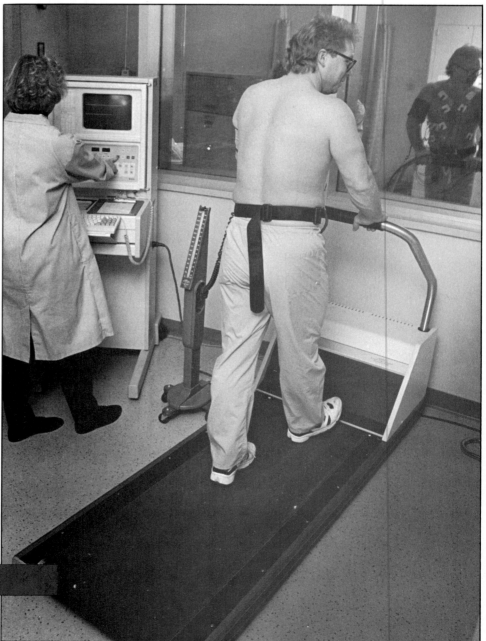

Cardiac rhythm and blood pressure are monitored in response to the stress of exercise.

We carry with us a crude geography of the body, empirically unreliable, or at least limited in accuracy. But it serves its purposes, and sometimes it turns out to be partly helpful. We assume that the brain contains conscious processes and we oppose its stringencies to the language of the heart, which throbs with emotion.

In fact the heart does respond to emotional stress. When we say that under some forms of stimulation—romance, surprise, fear, or other excitement—our hearts go "pitter-pat," we are actually describing a quickened cardiac cycle in which the interval shrinks between the period of relaxation, called *diastole,* and the contraction in which the blood is pumped from the heart, called *systole.*

To the trained ear the heart valves make a *lub dub lub dub* sound. But whatever the sound the heart makes, and however well we understand its essential function as a blood pump, we also know with increasing certainty that concern with the heart's proper functioning—its health—involves attention to the patient's emotional state, diet, and daily habits, as well as to the heart's medical condition when trouble arises.

Medical professionals are continually reminded not to underestimate the influence of psychosocial factors in coronary heart disease. New findings revealing that emotionally depressed myocardial infarction survivors may have five times the mortality rate of others suggest, according to the *Journal of the American Medical Association,* that "it is now time to develop and evaluate interventions aimed at ameliorating the harmful effects of these risk factors."

Current research reminds health care professionals that some primary factors in most cardiac disease are habits which, if they are changed, provide preventive care for the heart, forestalling disease and even in some cases reversing its effects.

High cholesterol levels, strongly influenced by diet, remain a foremost cardiovascular villain.

Health care professionals screen cardiovascular patients for high blood cholesterol values. Recently, researchers have been asking which categories of the population would benefit most from cholesterol testing. The National Cholesterol Education Program recommended that all Americans 20 years old or older should be tested and treated if necessary, another of those indications, found in many fields of specialization, that testing, observation, and early diagnosis are keys to the prevention of disease. The alternatives—therapy and surgery after disease has progressed—are far more expensive and costly in human terms.

That study assumed that a cholesterol-lowering diet would be helpful, but other research suggests that lipid-lowering drugs will be required in many cases. Assuming a possible need for lifelong treatment, this is an expensive therapy. Therefore it is all the more important that the target populations for screening and treatment be exactly specified. Another study recommends that screening and treatment in young adults be limited to those with known coronary heart disease or other short-term risk factors.

Health care professionals from different backgrounds often are in a position to influence patients, or prospective patients, to change their habits in ways that will help them avoid treatment, including surgery, which they may require if they pay no attention to cholesterol levels, diet, exercise, or emotional stress. But the effectiveness of treatment is an important consideration not only for cardiologist and patient but for all professionals who offer advice on health matters.

For heart surgeons, the relative value of current directions of treatment remains undecided. Many new options have been devised and offered, but as medical professionals evaluate new therapies, they still find themselves in disagreement on established treatments. One yet to be deter-

FRONTIERS OF RESEARCH
Heart Disease, Heart Attacks, and Health Habits
Michael J. Kirkhorn

mined balance is found in the uncertainty about the relative value of angioplasty and bypass surgery. The number of patients undergoing percutaneous transluminal coronary angioplasty is approaching the number who have undergone coronary artery bypass graft surgery.

Recent studies indicated that patients with acute myocardial infarction benefited from prompt and skillful percutaneous transluminal coronary angioplasty, which shortened hospital stays, lowered ensuing costs, and produced fewer readmissions than thrombolytic therapy without angioplasty.

An Emory University study found that for patients with two-vessel coronary artery disease, complete revascularization was more often achieved with surgery. Five-year survival was 93 percent for angioplasty patients and 89 percent for surgical patients, who tended to be older, with more concomitant illnesses. Angioplasty patients required much more frequent additional revascularization treatment, 43 percent at five years, as opposed to 7 percent for surgical patients.

Other research shows that while mortality from coronary heart disease is decreasing, the rate of decline is half as steep for women as for men. Men and women die in roughly equal proportions from myocardial infarction.

Most studies of myocardial infarction have emphasized disease among men. As a result, surgical equipment for common therapies such as coronary artery bypass graft surgery and percutaneous transluminal coronary angioplasty were initially developed for men, as were the first artificial hearts.

Once again, the threat to health is the result of a combination of inherent susceptibilities and bad habits. Hypertension contributes greatly to the possibility of coronary heart disease among women as well as men. Women who smoke more than 24 cigarettes a day increase their risk of myocardial infarction by 10 times, and oral contraceptive users who smoke increase their risk by 20 times over nonusers who do not smoke.

CHAPTER 16
Cardiac Function

JACQUELYN L. BANASIK

KEY TERMS

afterload: The impedance that must be overcome in order to eject blood from the cardiac chamber.

autoregulation: The intrinsic tendency of an organ or tissue to maintain adequate blood flow despite changes in metabolism or blood pressure.

cardiac output: A measure of the amount of blood pumped by the heart in 1 minute, usually expressed in liters per minute.

creatine kinase: An enzyme that catalyzes the transfer of a phosphate group between ATP and creatine. The isoenzyme found in cardiac muscle is called CK-MB.

crossbridge: The interaction between thick and thin filaments of the contractile apparatus when myosin heads bind to actin.

ejection fraction: Stroke volume divided by end-diastolic volume; indicates pumping efficiency of the ventricle.

Frank-Starling law of the heart: Describes the relationship between diastolic stretch and subsequent increased strength of contraction. Also called the length-tension relationship.

preload: The volume of blood in the cardiac chamber just prior to systole (end-diastolic volume).

rhythmicity: The ability to beat rhythmically without external stimuli. Also called *automaticity.*

stroke volume: The volume of blood ejected from the ventricle in one systole (end-diastolic volume minus end-systolic volume).

---

*T*he primary function of the heart is to produce the driving force that propels blood through the vessels of the circulatory system. Along with the lungs, the heart works to distribute oxygenated blood and nutrients to tissues and organs of the body. The heart's functional capabilities are directly related to its anatomic characteristics.

Functional Anatomy of the Heart

The heart is located in the **mediastinum,** suspended between the lungs, behind the sternum, and in front of the vertebral column, thoracic aorta, and esophagus (Fig. 16–1).[1] When viewed from the front, the heart appears rotated to the left so that the right atrium and right ventricle are most anterior. The **base** of the heart occupies the right chest and is relatively fixed in place by its attachments to the great vessels. The **apex** of the heart lies primarily in the left chest and is directed forward toward the anterior chest wall. With each heartbeat, a characteristic thrust or point of maximal impulse (PMI) is generally palpable where the apex strikes against the chest. The PMI is normally located on the left chest where the fifth intercostal space and midclavicular line intersect. Variations in heart size and position within the chest may be related to age, body size, shape, weight, or pathologic conditions of the heart and other nearby structures.

Functionally important cardiac tissues include connective tissues, which form the fibrous skeleton and valves; cardiac muscle, which produces the contractile force; and epithelial tissue, which lines the cardiac chambers and covers the outer surfaces of the heart. The **fibrous skeleton** consists of four rings that provide a firm scaffold for attachment of cardiac muscle and the cardiac valves. Four cardiac valves control the direction of blood flow through the heart (Fig. 16–2). The **mitral atrioventricular valve** (bicuspid) directs blood flow from the left atrium to the left ventricle while the **tricuspid atrioventricular valve** directs blood from the right atrium to the right ventricle. Edges of the AV valves are attached to valvular rings formed by the fibrous skeleton. Valve leaflets are tethered to papillary muscles of the ventricular chambers by connective tissues called **chordae tendineae. Papil-**lary muscles attach to ventricular walls and help prevent the valve leaflets from bending backward into the atria during ventricular contraction (Fig. 16–3). The AV valves open passively during diastole when the pressure of blood in the atria exceeds that in the ventricles. Ventricular contraction reverses the pressure gradient and causes AV valves to snap shut, preventing blood from flowing backward into the atria.

Two **semilunar valves** are located in the ventricular outflow tracts. The **pulmonic valve** lies between the right ventricle and pulmonary artery and the **aortic valve** lies between the left ventricle and aortic artery. Compared to the AV valves, the semilunar valves are thicker and are not supported by fibrous cords. They open and close passively according to pressure gradients, just as the AV valves do. When intraventricular pressures exceed pulmonary and aortic artery pressures, the semilunar valves remain open and then close when ventricular pressures fall below aortic and pulmonary artery pressures.

The cardiac muscle layer (**myocardium**) produces the contractile force that pushes blood through the circulatory system. Heart muscle is organized into four separate chambers of varying muscular wall thickness, reflecting the degree of pressure work required from each chamber. Atria serve primarily as conduits and have a thinner layer of muscle than the ventricles. The left ventricle is two to three times as thick as the right ventricle because higher pressures are required to eject blood into the systemic circulation than into the pulmonic system. Layers of cardiac muscle are arranged in spirals so that contraction results in a squeezing force that generates pressure within the chambers (Fig. 16–4). Normal chamber pressures are given in Table 16–1. Alterations in chamber pressures may reflect pathologic cardiovascular changes such as valvular disorders, blood volume abnormalities, and heart failure (see Chaps. 17 and 18).

Cardiac chambers and valves are lined by a layer of squamous epithelial cells called **endocardium.** The endocardial layer provides a smooth surface on which blood can slide and thus prevents it from clotting and minimizes trauma to red cells. The endocardium is continuous with endothelium of the vascular system. Outer surfaces of the heart are also covered by a layer of epithelial cells, called **epicardium,** which is part

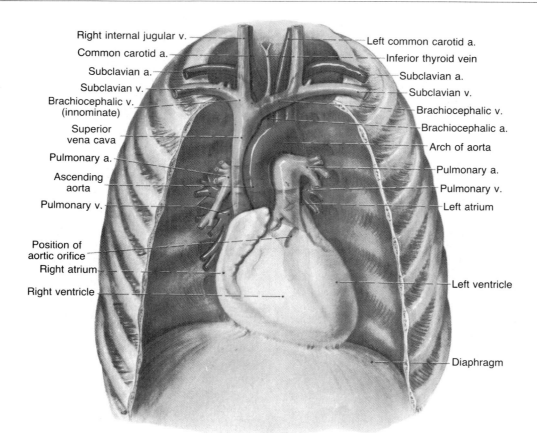

Right internal jugular v.
Common carotid a.
Subclavian a.
Subclavian v.
Brachiocephalic v. (innominate)
Superior vena cava
Pulmonary a.
Ascending aorta
Pulmonary v.
Position of aortic orifice
Right atrium
Right ventricle

Left common carotid a.
Inferior thyroid vein
Subclavian a.
Subclavian v.
Brachiocephalic v.
Brachiocephalic a.
Arch of aorta
Pulmonary a.
Pulmonary v.
Left atrium
Left ventricle
Diaphragm

F I G U R E 16–1. Position of the heart in the chest cavity. (From Jacob SW, Francone CA, Lossow WJ: *Structure and Function in Man,* 5th ed. Philadelphia, WB Saunders, 1982. Reproduced with permission.)

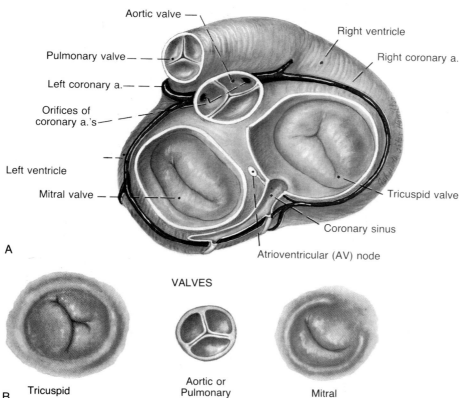

Aortic valve
Pulmonary valve
Left coronary a.
Orifices of coronary a.'s
Left ventricle
Mitral valve

Right ventricle
Right coronary a.
Tricuspid valve
Coronary sinus
Atrioventricular (AV) node

A

VALVES

Tricuspid

Aortic or Pulmonary

Mitral

B

F I G U R E 16–2. **A,** Position of the heart valves as viewed from above. **B,** Configuration of the heart valves showing the two cusps of the mitral valve and the three cusps of the tricuspid valve. The pulmonary and aortic valves have three leaflets. (**A** from Jacob SW, Francone CA: *Elements of Anatomy and Physiology,* 2nd ed. Philadelphia, WB Saunders, 1989, p 179. **B** from Jacob SW, Francone CA, Lossow WJ: *Structure and Function in Man,* 5th ed. Philadelphia, WB Saunders, 1982. Reproduced with permission.)

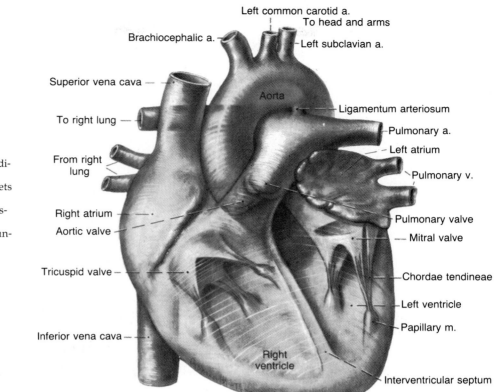

Left common carotid a.

To head and arms

Brachiocephalic a.

Left subclavian a.

Superior vena cava

Aorta

Ligamentum arteriosum

To right lung

Pulmonary a.

Left atrium

From right lung

Pulmonary v.

Right atrium

Pulmonary valve

Aortic valve

Mitral valve

Tricuspid valve

Chordae tendineae

Left ventricle

Papillary m.

Inferior vena cava

Right ventricle

Interventricular septum

FIGURE 16–3. The chordae tendineae and papillary muscles attach the mitral and tricuspid valve leaflets to the ventricular myocardium. (From Jacob SW, Francone CA, Lossow WJ: *Structure and Function in Man*, 5th ed. Philadelphia, WB Saunders, 1982. Reproduced with permission.)

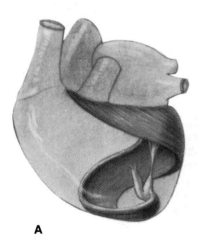

A

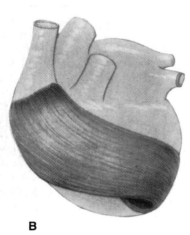

B

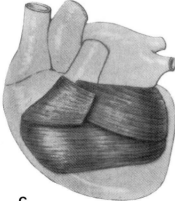

C

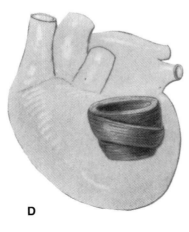

D

FIGURE 16–4. Ventricular muscle is arranged in spiral layers. *A* through *D* depict progressively deeper layers of cardiac muscle. (From Jacob SW, Francone CA, Lossow WJ: *Structure and Function in Man*, 5th ed. Philadelphia, WB Saunders, 1982, p 369. Reproduced with permission.)

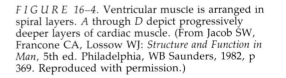

T A B L E 16 – 1. Normal Pressures in the Heart

Location	Pressure (mm Hg)*
Right atrium	0–8
Right ventricle	15–28 / 0–8
Pulmonary artery	15–28 / 4–12
Left atrium	4–12
Left ventricle	100–120 / 4–12
Aorta	100–120 / 60–80

*Right and left atrial pressures listed as means; other pressures written as systolic/diastolic.

of a protective covering called the pericardium. The **pericardium** is actually composed of two layers that envelop the heart like a sac (Fig. 16–5). The inner layer (**visceral pericardium**) is attached directly to the heart's outer surface, while an outer layer (**parietal pericardium**) forms a sac around the heart. Visceral and parietal pericardial layers are separated by a thin, fluid-filled space (**pericardial space**) that usually contains 10 to 30 mL of serous fluid. This fluid lubricates pericardial surfaces and reduces friction as layers slide against one another during cardiac contraction.

KEY CONCEPTS

> • Blood flows from the right atria to the right ventricle through the tricuspid valve. The pulmonic valve lies between the right ventricle and the pulmonary artery. Blood flows from the left atria to the left ven-

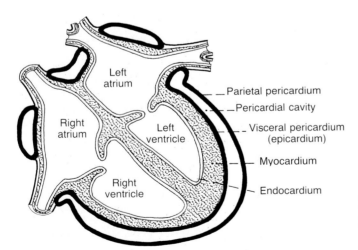

F I G U R E 16–5. The pericardial sac is composed of two layers separated by a narrow fluid-filled space. The visceral pericardium (epicardium) is attached directly to the heart's surface, while the parietal pericardium forms the outer layer of the sac. (From Jacob SW, Francone CA: *Elements of Anatomy and Physiology*, 2nd ed. Philadelphia, WB Saunders, 1989, p 177. Reproduced with permission.)

tricle through the mitral valve. The aortic valve lies between the left ventricle and the aorta.

> • Heart muscle (myocardium) is lined with endothelium on the inner surface and covered with epicardium on the outer surface.

> • The pericardial sac envelops and protects the heart from friction.

Circulatory System

The circulatory systems of the lungs and body can be viewed as two separate but dependent systems. The left heart chambers produce the force to propel blood through the vessels of the systemic (body) circulation. The left atrium receives oxygenated blood from the lungs by way of the pulmonary veins and delivers it to the left ventricle. This oxygenated blood is pumped by the left ventricle into the aorta, which supplies the arteries of the systemic circulation. Venous blood is collected from capillary networks of the body and returned to the right atrium by way of the venae cavae. Blood from the head returns to the right atrium through the superior vena cava, and blood from the body returns via the inferior vena cava.

The right heart receives deoxygenated blood from the systemic circulation and pumps it through the lungs by way of the pulmonary artery. The pulmonary artery divides into left and right branches, which subdivide to supply blood to pulmonary capillary beds. Exchange of respiratory gases occurs at the pulmonary capillaries so that the blood delivered to the left atrium by pulmonary veins is well oxygenated.

Left and right heart circulations are connected in series such that the output of one becomes the input of the other. Thus, the functions of the right and left heart are interdependent. Failure of one side of the heart to pump efficiently will soon lead to dysfunction of the other side.

KEY CONCEPTS

> • The right heart chambers pump deoxygenated (venous) blood through the lungs. The left heart chambers pump oxygenated blood through the systemic circulation.

Cardiac Cycle

Each heartbeat is composed of a period of contraction (**systole**) followed by a period of relaxation (**diastole**). The interval from one heartbeat to the next is called a **cardiac cycle** and includes ventricular, atrial, and aortic (or pulmonic) events.[2] Each of these events is associated with characteristic pressure changes within the cardiac chambers. Pressure changes result in valvular opening and closing and unidirectional movement of blood through the heart. The various events of the cardiac cycle are illustrated in Figure 16–6.

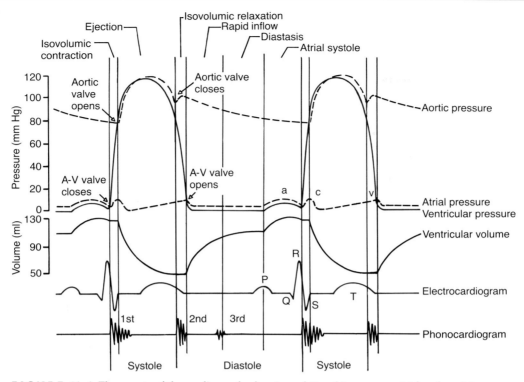

FIGURE 16–6. The events of the cardiac cycle showing relationships among atrial and ventricular pressures, ventricular volume, and aortic pressure. (From Guyton AC: *Textbook of Medical Physiology*, 8th ed. Philadelphia, WB Saunders, 1991, p 102. Reproduced with permission.)

The cardiac cycle can be described sequentially beginning with ventricular filling. During diastole the ventricles are relaxed and blood flows in from the atria through open AV valves. Initially ventricular filling occurs passively because of a pressure gradient between the atria and ventricles. Toward the end of ventricular diastole, the atria contract, squeezing more blood through the AV valves into the ventricles. Atrial contraction increases the ventricular blood volume by 20 to 30 percent.

Isovolumic Contraction

Immediately following atrial systole the ventricles begin to contract, causing intraventricular pressure to rise and the AV valves to close. AV valve closure produces a sound that can be heard at the chest wall and is termed S_1. Ventricular pressure rises rapidly during isovolumic contraction because all four cardiac valves are closed and the volume of blood within the ventricular chamber is forcefully compressed by the powerful ventricular myocardium.

Ventricular Ejection

Ventricular contraction results in a rapid rise in ventricular pressure. As ventricular pressure exceeds aortic pressure, the aortic valve is forced open and a period of rapid ejection of blood from the ventricle follows. The rapid ejection phase is followed by a period of reduced ejection as aortic pressure rises and ventricular pressures and volumes fall. These events occur on the right side of the heart in a similar manner, although pressure gradients are lower.

Isovolumic Relaxation

The isovolumic relaxation phase begins with semilunar valve closure in response to falling ventricular pressures and ends when the AV valves open to allow ventricular filling. Ventricular blood volume remains constant during this period because all four cardiac valves remain closed. Closure of the semilunar valves causes the second heart sound, S_2. Opening of the AV valves signals the beginning of rapid ventricular filling and the start of another cardiac cycle.

Atrial Events

Atrial pressure waves have three characteristic curves, the **a**, **c**, and **v** waves (see Fig. 16–6). The a wave corresponds to atrial contraction which immediately precedes AV valve closure. The c wave occurs early in ventricular systole and is thought to represent bulging of AV valves into the atrial chambers. The v waves have a gradual incline representing filling of the atrium as blood returns from the circulation. The v wave drops rapidly as atrial pressure is relieved by AV valve opening. A large v wave is often associated with inadequate closure of the AV valve, resulting in regurgitation of ventricular blood back into the atrium during ventricular systole.

Aortic and Pulmonary Artery Events

Aortic and pulmonary artery pressures rise and fall in relation to the cardiac cycle. Arterial pressures fall to their lowest value just prior to semilunar valve opening. This lowest pressure is called **diastolic blood pressure.** Arterial pressure reaches its maximum during ventricular ejection and is called **systolic blood pressure.** A characteristic notch (*dicrotic notch*) in the arterial pressure curve may be seen as the semilunar valves close.

The difference in aortic pressure between systole and diastole is partly dependent on the aorta's elastic characteristics. During systole, the aorta stretches to accommodate blood ejected by the ventricle. The stretched aorta has "stored" or potential energy that is released during diastole to maintain driving pressure and keep blood continuously flowing through the circulation. Aortic stiffening, as occurs with aging or arteriosclerosis, may result in higher systolic and lower diastolic blood pressures due to loss of aortic elastic properties.[2]

KEY CONCEPTS

- Characteristic pressure wave changes that occur during the cardiac cycle may be useful in diagnosing cardiac disease and identifying heart catheter location.
- The atria have three characteristic waves, a, c, and v. The a wave corresponds to atrial contraction, the c wave corresponds to ventricular contraction, and the v wave corresponds to atrial filling.
- The ventricles have four important phases, isovolumic contraction, ejection, isovolumic relaxation, and diastolic filling. The rate and amplitude of these pressures reflect chamber volume, contractility, and valvular function.
- Pressure changes in the aorta during a cardiac cycle are partly dependent on the elasticity of the aorta. Differences between systolic and diastolic pressures are less with a compliant aorta. Aortic stiffness results in higher systolic and lower diastolic pressures.

Coronary Circulation

Anatomy of the Coronary Vessels

The blood supply to the heart muscle is provided by the coronary arteries (Fig. 16–7). Right and left coronary artery openings are located within the sinuses of Valsalva, in the aortic root, just beyond the aortic valve.[3] The **right coronary artery** (RCA) originates in the sinus of Valsalva near the aortic valve's anterior cusp and passes diagonally toward the right

ventricle in the AV groove. In approximately 80 percent of the population, the RCA gives rise to a posterior descending vessel that supplies blood to the heart's posterior aspect. The **left main coronary artery** arises near the aortic posterior cusp and travels a short distance anteriorly before dividing into the **anterior descending** and **circumflex** branches. The anterior descending branch supplies septal, anterior, and apical areas of the left ventricle while the circumflex artery supplies lateral and posterior left ventricle. The three major coronary arteries give rise to a number of smaller branches that penetrate the myocardium and branch into small arterioles and capillaries. Areas supplied by divisions of the coronary arteries are listed in Table 16–2. Most of the heart's capillary beds drain into the coronary veins, which then empty into the right atrium through the coronary sinus (Fig. 16–8).

Regulation of Coronary Blood Flow

Blood flow through coronary vessels is determined by the same physical principles that govern flow through other vessels of the body, namely driving pressure and vascular resistance to flow.[4] **Driving pressure** through the coronary arteries is determined by aortic blood pressure and right atrial pressure. This relationship may be expressed as: coronary driving pressure = aortic pressure − right atrial pressure. Thus, an increase in aortic pressure enhances coronary blood flow, whereas an increase in right atrial pressure opposes coronary flow.

Coronary **vascular resistance** has two major determinants: (1) coronary artery diameter and (2) the degree of external compression due to myocardial contraction. Coronary artery diameter is continuously adjusted to maintain blood flow at a level adequate for myocardial demands. **Autoregulation** is the term used to describe the intrinsic ability of the arteries to adjust blood flow according to tissue needs. Vessel dilation (*vasodilation*) occurs in response to increased tissue metabolism, while decreased metabolic activity

T A B L E 16 – 2. Areas Supplied by the Coronary Arteries

Artery	Area Supplied
Right coronary	Right atrium (55 percent of persons) Right ventricle Intraventricular septum Sinus node (55 percent of persons) AV node Bundle of His
Left anterior descending	Right atrium (45 percent of persons) Right ventricle (minor) Left ventricle (anterior, apex) Anterior papillary muscles Right and left bundle branches Intraventricular septum
Left circumflex	Left atrium Left ventricle (posterior, anterior) Sinus node (45 percent of persons)

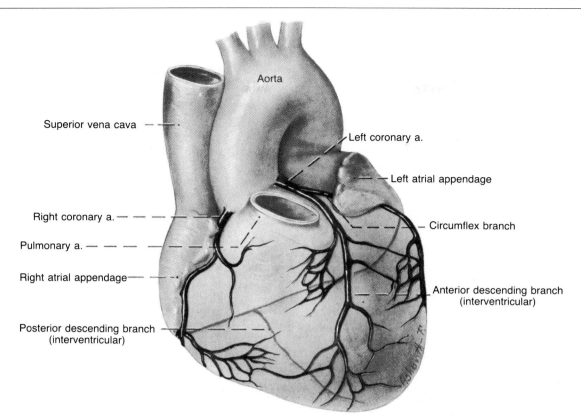

FIGURE 16–7. Coronary arteries supplying the heart. (From Jacob SW, Francone CA, Lossow WJ: *Structure and Function in Man*, 5th ed. Philadelphia, WB Saunders, 1982. Reproduced with permission.)

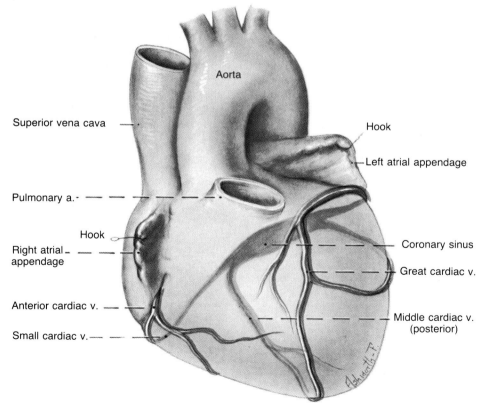

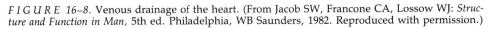

FIGURE 16–8. Venous drainage of the heart. (From Jacob SW, Francone CA, Lossow WJ: *Structure and Function in Man*, 5th ed. Philadelphia, WB Saunders, 1982. Reproduced with permission.)

results in a decreased vessel diameter (*vasoconstriction*). The mechanism of autoregulation is best explained by the **metabolic hypothesis,** which says that increased metabolism results in a buildup of vasodilatory chemicals in the vessel. Smooth muscle encircling the vessel relaxes in response to the chemicals, increasing vessel diameter. Several vasodilating substances have been proposed, including potassium ions, hydrogen ions, carbon dioxide, prostaglandins, and adenosine. The endothelial cells that line vessels are known to secrete a variety of relaxing and constricting factors, most of which have not yet been well characterized. An increase in the level of adenosine (derived from adenosine triphosphate [ATP]) is currently believed to be the chief vasodilatory chemical. A low level of oxygen in the blood (*hypoxemia*) also may cause vasodilation. Whatever their identity, the vasodilatory substances are washed away as blood flow increases in response to increased vessel diameter. A declining level of vasodilatory chemicals results in vasoconstriction. Thus, vessel diameter is continuously adjusted according to concentrations of vasodilatory chemicals, which are directly related to the tissue's metabolic activity.

Vessel diameter is also regulated by the autonomic nervous system. The coronary arteries are primarily innervated by sympathetic nerves, but they also receive a small amount of parasympathetic innervation. Sympathetic nervous activity results in vasoconstriction; parasympathetic activity results in vasodilation. Vessel diameter is therefore an interplay between nervous system and autoregulatory influences.

In addition to vessel diameter, coronary resistance is affected by myocardial contraction. During systole, cardiac muscle compression creates a marked rise in coronary resistance that reduces coronary blood flow (perfusion). Blood flow to the left ventricle is greatly decreased during systole because of the pressures generated by the thick muscular layer. Blood vessels that penetrate the myocardium to supply the innermost endocardial areas are more compromised during contraction than are outer epicardial vessels. Even though coronary artery driving pressure is greatest during ventricular systole, little blood flow reaches the ventricles because of the high external pressure applied to the coronary vessels as the myocardium contracts. Therefore, most myocardial blood flow occurs during the diastolic interval between ventricular contractions. The time the heart spends in diastole is directly related to heart rate. Faster heart rates reduce diastolic time and decrease coronary artery blood flow.

Cardiac muscle needs a continuous supply of oxygen and nutrients in order to perform its pumping functions. A disruption in cardiac blood flow (*ischemia*) generally results in some degree of pump failure and damage to cardiac tissues. Myocardial ischemia may be caused by conditions that reduce coronary blood flow or increase myocardial demands for oxygen. These include (1) a reduced driving pressure (low aortic blood pressure or high right atrial pressure), (2) a reduced vessel diameter (hypertrophy, arteriosclerosis, thrombosis, vasoconstricting chemicals), (3) reduced perfusion time (high heart rates, some dysrhythmias), and (4) increased metabolic demands (fever, sepsis, anemia).

KEY CONCEPTS

- The right and left coronary arteries originate from the aortic root, within the sinuses of Valsalva. In most people the right coronary artery perfuses the right ventricle, atrioventricular node, sinoatrial node, and right atrium.
- The left coronary artery divides into the left circumflex artery and left anterior descending artery, which perfuse the left atrium and ventricle.
- Coronary blood flow is regulated centrally by the autonomic nervous system and locally by autoregulation. The amount of coronary flow depends on driving pressure and coronary resistance. Coronary resistance is dependent mostly on vessel diameter.
- Although driving pressure is highest during systole, there is little coronary flow because of vessel compression by the contracting myocardium. Most blood flow occurs during diastole.

Microanatomy of Cardiac Myocytes

Cardiac muscle cells are divided into two general types: working cells, which have primarily mechanical pumping functions, and electrical cells, which primarily transmit electrical impulses. Both types are *excitable:* they are able to produce and transmit action potentials. Working myocardial cells are packed with contractile filaments and make up the bulk of the atrial and ventricular muscle. Electrical cells function to initiate and coordinate contraction of the working cells.

Myocyte Structure

Typical myocardial cells (myocytes) are illustrated in Figure 16–9. Cardiac myocytes are described as muscle "fibers" because of their long narrow shape. The plasma membrane (**sarcolemma**) of one cardiac cell is joined to other nearby cells by junctions called **intercalated discs,** which allow the rapid passage of electrical impulses from one cell to the next. The intercalated discs permit the many separate cells of the myocardium to function together in a coordinated manner. This arrangement is called a **functional syncytium.** The sarcolemma also forms membrane-lined channels that penetrate the cell and become the **transverse tubules** (t-tubules) (Fig. 16–10). T-tubules permit extracellular fluid and ions to diffuse near intracellular structures. Movement of ions across the sarcolemma is an essential part of cellular excitation and the subsequent contraction of intracellular elements. Cellular contractile elements are simultaneously activated because signals at the cell surface are rapidly transmitted internally by the t-tubules.[5]

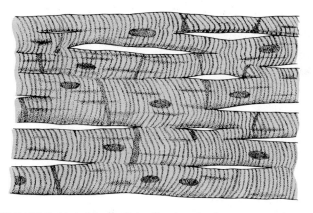

FIGURE 16-9. Myocardial cells, showing long narrow shape and interconnecting junctions, forming a functional syncytium. (From Guyton AC: *Textbook of Medical Physiology*, 8th ed. Philadelphia, WB Saunders, 1991, p 99. Reproduced with permission.)

The **sarcoplasmic reticulum** (SR) is an extensive labyrinth of hollow membrane that stores significant amounts of intracellular calcium. It contains voltage-sensitive channels that open briefly during depolarization and allow calcium ions to flow into the cytoplasm.

The SR also contains powerful calcium pumps which recover calcium ions from the cytoplasm and return them to the SR.

Cardiac muscle cells are packed with large numbers of **mitochondria** that are strategically positioned along the contractile fibers of the cell. The heart is also endowed with an extensive capillary network, approximately one capillary per muscle cell. The large numbers of mitochondria and abundant oxygen supply are necessary to keep pace with the high ATP requirements of the contractile elements.

Structure of the Contractile Apparatus

Microscopic inspection of the cardiac myocyte reveals a typical pattern of banding called *striation*.[6] This striated appearance is due to an organized structure of the proteins (myofibrils) of the contractile apparatus (Fig. 16-11). The contractile proteins, actin and myosin, are called filaments because they are long and narrow. **Myosin** filaments are larger and referred to as **thick filaments. Thin filaments** are actually composed of three different types of proteins bundled together. **Actin** is the primary constituent of thin fil-

FIGURE 16-10. A schematic diagram of a portion of a cardiac myocyte showing the transverse tubules which extend horizontally from the plasma membrane into the cell interior. (From Fawcett DW: *Bloom and Fawcett: A Textbook of Histology.* Philadelphia, WB Saunders Company, 1986. Copyright Chapman & Hall, New York. Modified after Essner E, Novikoff AB, Quintana N: *J Cell Biol* 1965;25:209 by copyright permission of the Rockefeller University Press. Artist: Sylvia Colard Keene. Reproduced with permission.)

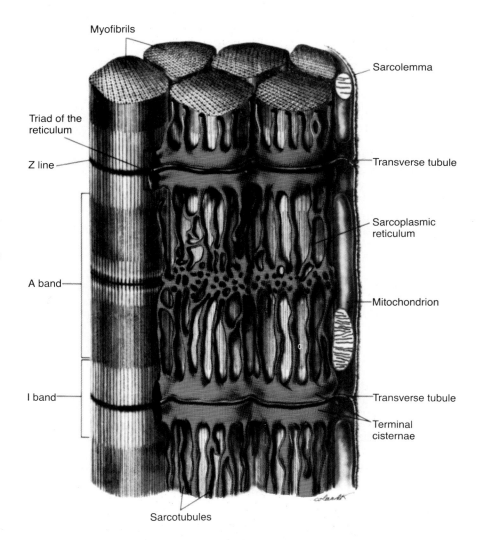

Myofibrils

Sarcolemma

Triad of the reticulum

Z line

Transverse tubule

Sarcoplasmic reticulum

A band

Mitochondrion

I band

Transverse tubule

Terminal cisternae

Sarcotubules

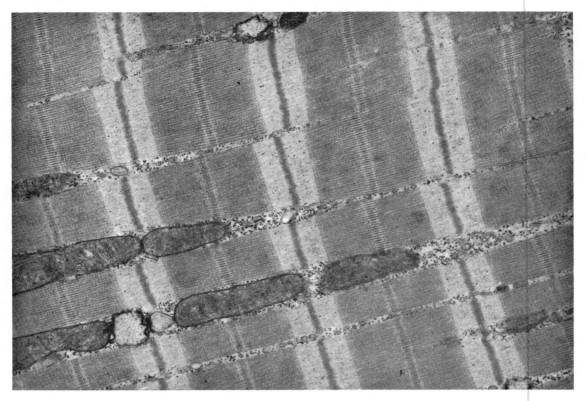

F I G U R E 16–11. Electron micrograph of muscle fibrils showing characteristic banding pattern. (From Fawcett DW: *The Cell.* Philadelphia, WB Saunders, 1981. Reproduced with permission.)

aments, with smaller amounts of the proteins **tropomyosin** and **troponin** bound to it.

The thick and thin filaments are specifically arranged in contractile units called **sarcomeres** (Fig. 16–12). Sarcomeres are defined by dark bands called **Z lines,** which lie perpendicular to actin and myosin filaments. A sarcomere extends from one Z line to the next. Thin actin filaments are attached to Z lines and extend from them. The **I bands** (isotropic) are light in color and correspond to the position of thin actin filaments extending in both directions from the Z line. Thick myosin filaments lie parallel to and in between the thin filaments. Each myosin filament is actually surrounded by six thin filaments (Fig. 16–13). The dark **A band** corresponds to an area where the actin and myosin filaments overlap. An **M line** marks the center of the A band and the midpoint of the myosin filaments. One other zone, the **H zone,** corresponds to a region occupied solely by myosin filaments with no actin filament overlap. An efficient, synchronized contraction is enhanced by this precise arrangement of contractile elements.

Characteristics of Contractile Filaments

Myosin molecules are composed of six polypeptide chains, two heavy (H) chains and four light (L) chains. These light and heavy chains are organized into a tail region and two globular "head" areas. The myosin heads interact with actin filaments to produce muscle contraction. Thick filaments are made up of many myosin molecules with tail regions bundled together and heads sticking out at intervals along the bundle. The head regions are flexible and can bend and pull as needed during muscle contraction. Myosin head groups are oriented in opposite directions on either

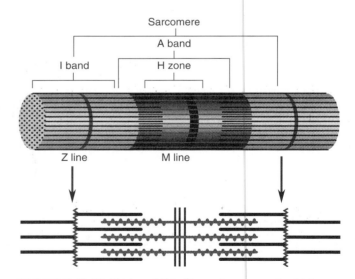

F I G U R E 16–12. Thick and thin filaments are organized into contractile units called sarcomeres. A sarcomere extends from one Z line to the next and represents the fundamental unit of muscle contraction. See text for description of bands, zones, and lines.

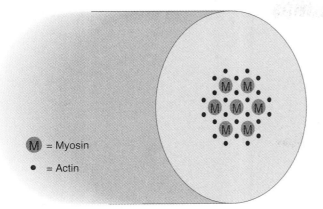

FIGURE 16–13. Each myosin filament is surrounded by six actin filaments, with which it binds.

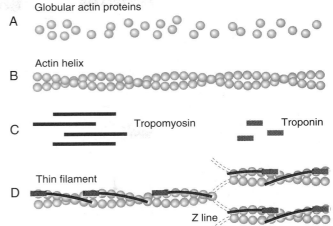

Globular actin proteins

A

Actin helix

B

C   Tropomyosin   Troponin

Thin filament

D

Z line

FIGURE 16–15. Schematic of the proteins which make up the thin filament. **A**, Globular actin proteins combine to form long double-helix filaments. **B** and **C**, the proteins troponin and tropomyosin combine with the actin helix to form the thin filament (**D**).

side of the center tail region (Fig. 16–14). Myosin head groups, which have enzymatic properties, are able to cleave ATP and release energy necessary for muscle contraction.

As previously mentioned, thin filaments are composed of three different proteins: actin, tropomyosin, and troponin. Actin filaments are actually polymers of many globular actin proteins attached end to end like two strings of beads and then twisted together, forming a helix (Fig. 16–15). Each of the actin beads has a site that can bind with myosin heads. Tropomyosins are long, slender proteins that bind to a string of seven actin beads. When myocardial muscle is relaxed, tropomyosin molecules cover the myosin-binding sites on the actin beads. A third protein, troponin, is attached to each tropomyosin molecule and is also bound to the actin filament. Each troponin is able to bind four molecules of calcium ion. As described below, tropomyosin and troponin are important regulatory proteins that control the activities of actin and myosin filaments.

KEY CONCEPTS

- **The myocardial cells of the heart behave as a syncytium because they are joined by gap junctions (intercalated discs) that permit the flow of ions from one cell to the next.**

- **Myocytes are packed with actin and myosin proteins which form the contractile apparatus. The thick filaments are composed of myosin proteins. Myosin has enzymatic activity and splits ATP, releasing energy needed for movement of the filaments.**

- **The thin filament is composed of actin and two regulatory proteins, troponin and tropomyosin. At rest, tropomyosin covers myosin-binding sites on actin. The position of tropomyosin is regulated by the calcium-binding protein, troponin.**

Molecular Basis of Contraction

Overview of Contraction

The heart's pumping action is accomplished by the additive contractions of the many myocytes that form the cardiac chambers. Because each myocyte contributes only a small amount to overall muscle shortening, all cells of the chamber must shorten simultaneously to produce a forceful contraction. The specialized cells of the conduction system function to stimulate myocardial contraction in a coordinated way. An action potential traveling down the conduction system is the usual trigger for contraction. Cardiac myocyte depolarization causes ion channels in the plasma membrane and t-tubules to open, permitting sodium and calcium entry and release of calcium from sarcoplasmic reticulum. The presence of free cal-

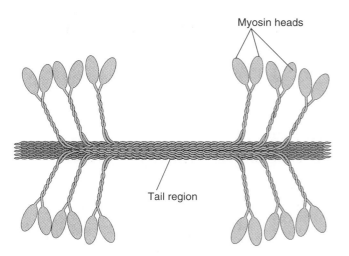

Myosin heads

Tail region

FIGURE 16–14. Myosin head groups are oriented in opposite directions on either side of the center tail region.

cium in the sarcoplasm (muscle cytoplasm) results in contraction. These events describe the process of excitation-contraction coupling.

Sliding Filament/Crossbridge Theory of Muscle Contraction

The sliding filament or crossbridge theory of muscle contraction is suggested by the anatomical configuration of the sarcomere described earlier. Muscle shortening is accomplished by increasing the amount of overlap of actin and myosin filaments. The Z lines at the ends of the sarcomere move closer together as interdigitating actin and myosin filaments slide past one another. Myosin head groups grip binding sites on the actin beads and pull the thin filaments toward the sarcomere's center. Each time a myosin head binds an actin bead it forms a **crossbridge.** Flexible myosin heads move in a ratchet-like manner to tug on the actin filaments (Fig. 16–16). Each ratcheting motion moves actin filaments only minutely, and many sequential crossbridge formations are required to shorten the sarcomere. Thus, myosin heads bend back and forth, binding and pulling on the actin filaments in a steplike fashion. Actin filaments are prevented from slipping back to their original position because some myosin-actin bonds are forming while others are releasing. The making and the subsequent breaking of each actin-myosin crossbridge requires one molecule of ATP. Consequently, tremendous quantities of ATP are hydrolyzed with each cardiac contraction.

ATP hydrolysis, which occurs at the myosin head region, provides the energy for contraction and also affects the ability of myosin to bind actin. Myosin has two functional states or conformations: (1) a low-affinity state in which it does not bind actin, and (2) a high-affinity state in which it avidly binds actin. The affinity of the myosin head for actin depends on whether ATP is present (low affinity) or adenosine diphosphate (ADP) and inorganic phosphate (Pi) are present (high affinity). A proposed sequence of crossbridge formation (Fig. 16–17) is as follows: (1) Free myosin heads bind ATP and hydrolyze it to ADP and Pi, which remain on the myosin. (2) Myosin heads now have a high affinity for actin and stretch out to bind it. (3) If binding sites on actin are accessible,

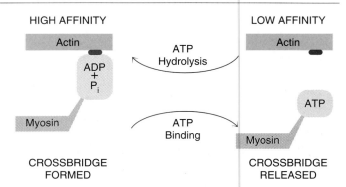

FIGURE 16–17. The affinity of the myosin for actin binding sites depends on whether ATP is bound to myosin (low affinity) or ADP + Pi are bound (high affinity).

myosin binds to the actin, resulting in a ratchet movement of the myosin (power stroke) and release of ADP and Pi. (4) With loss of ADP and Pi, myosin is able to bind another molecule of ATP. (5) The myosin heads with ATP bound have a low affinity for actin and let go. (6) ATP is again hydrolyzed to ADP and Pi, and another crossbridge cycle is initiated. Continued crossbridge cycling is dependent on the availability of ATP. Lack of ATP results in fewer crossbridge cycles and inability of the muscle to shorten normally.

Role of Calcium in Muscle Contraction

Muscle contraction is dependent on an adequate amount of calcium ion in the cytoplasm. In the absence of free intracellular calcium, no muscle contraction will take place, even though myosin head groups have high affinity for actin binding sites. This phenomenon can be explained in the following way. Myosin heads are prevented from binding to actin by tropomyosin proteins, which lie on top of actin binding sites. The position of tropomyosin protein is controlled by troponin. When calcium is absent, troponin induces tropomyosin to cover the actin binding sites. When calcium is present, troponin allows tropomyosin to move over and uncover the binding sites (Fig. 16–18). Crossbridge formation immediately ensues because myosin heads have high affinity for these sites in the relaxed state.

Energy of Muscle Relaxation

Although muscle relaxation is generally viewed as a passive phenomenon, it actually requires energy. Muscle relaxation is accomplished by removing calcium ions from the sarcoplasm. As calcium levels fall, calcium diffuses away from the troponin molecules and tropomyosin is induced to cover the actin binding sites. With actin binding sites covered, myosin heads are unable to initiate crossbridge formation, and thick and thin filaments slide back to their resting position. Removal of calcium ions is an energy-requiring pro-

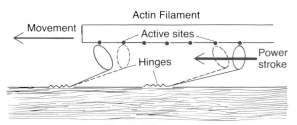

FIGURE 16–16. Flexible myosin heads bind and tug on the thin filaments in a ratchet-like manner. (From Guyton AC: *Textbook of Medical Physiology,* 8th ed. Philadelphia, WB Saunders, 1991, p 72. Reproduced with permission.)

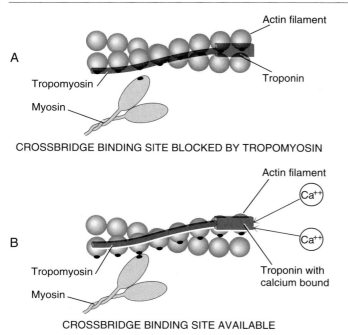

A

Actin filament

Tropomyosin

Troponin

Myosin

CROSSBRIDGE BINDING SITE BLOCKED BY TROPOMYOSIN

B

Actin filament

Ca^{++}

Ca^{++}

Tropomyosin

Troponin with calcium bound

Myosin

CROSSBRIDGE BINDING SITE AVAILABLE

F I G U R E 16–18. Troponin and tropomyosin are proteins that regulate the ability of actin and myosin to form crossbridges. **A**, In the absence of calcium, tropomyosin covers the binding sites on actin and inhibits crossbridge formation. **B**, In the presence of calcium, troponin induces the tropomyosin to "uncover" the actin binding sites and allows crossbridge formation.

cess. Membrane pumps located in the sarcolemma and sarcoplasmic reticulum actively move calcium out of the sarcoplasm against a concentration gradient (Fig. 16–19). The sarcolemma contains two different calcium pumps: one that requires ATP and one that uses the potential energy of the sodium gradient to remove calcium from the cell. Calcium pumps on the sarcoplasmic reticulum require ATP.

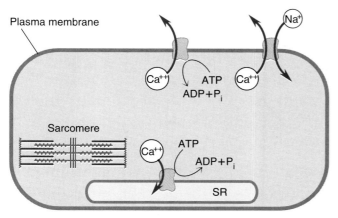

Plasma membrane

Na^+

Sarcomere

Ca^{++} ATP ADP+P_i Ca^{++}

Ca^{++} ATP ADP+P_i

SR

Cardiac muscle cell

F I G U R E 16–19. Calcium ions are removed from the cardiac muscle cell cytoplasm by energy-dependent protein transporters in the plasma membrane and sarcoplasmic reticulum (SR) membrane.

KEY CONCEPTS

- Contraction of cardiac muscle is accomplished by shortening of individual sarcomeres. This is due to increased overlap of actin and myosin filaments. Myosin heads bind to specific sites on actin and pull the thin filaments toward the center.
- ATP hydrolysis provides the energy for crossbridging and also affects the affinity of myosin for actin. Myosin has high affinity for actin when ADP and P_i are bound, and low affinity when ATP is bound. Myosin cycles between high- and low-affinity states, making and breaking crossbridges with the actin filament.
- The presence of intracellular free calcium ion (Ca^{++}) is necessary for muscle contraction to occur. When Ca^{++} is absent, actin binding sites are covered and not accessible for crossbridging. Binding of Ca^{++} to troponin induces the movement of tropomyosin to uncover actin binding sites.
- Muscle relaxation is due to removal of Ca^{++} from the cytoplasm. This is an energy-requiring process.

Cardiac Energy Metabolism

The heart, like other tissues in the body, utilizes energy from ATP hydrolysis to drive its energy-requiring functions. Synthesis of ATP in cardiac muscle cells is accomplished by the same glycolytic and oxidative reactions described in detail in Chapter 2.

Oxygen Utilization

Recall that oxidative phosphorylation is much more efficient than glycolysis, producing a total of 34 to 36 ATP molecules per glucose molecule compared to only two ATP molecules produced from glycolysis. Because the heart is continuously active, its energy requirements are considerable. Very little ATP is stored in myocardial cells so a continuous supply of oxygen and nutrients is necessary to support ongoing ATP synthesis. Even under normal resting conditions, the heart extracts a large portion of oxygen from the blood perfusing it. Conditions of increased oxygen demand, therefore, must be met by increasing the rate of coronary blood flow. When oxygen delivery is insufficient to meet requirements for oxidative phosphorylation, the cell must rely on ATP produced by glycolysis. Unfortunately, glycolysis produces only enough ATP to maintain the cell for a few minutes. In addition, anaerobic glycolysis results in local buildup of lactic acid, which may further impair cardiac performance.

Under conditions of relative ATP excess, myocardial cells are able to transfer energy to a storage form called creatine phosphate (CP). This transfer is accomplished by the enzyme, **creatine kinase** (CK), in the following reaction: ATP + creatine ↔ ADP + CP. Although amounts of cellular CP are limited, they provide an immediate source of energy when cellular ATP levels are low. Under conditions of ischemia, the enzymatic reaction would proceed in reverse, utilizing CP and ADP to produce ATP.

The enzyme creatine kinase is also useful in the diagnosis of myocardial cell damage. Damaged cells leak their enzymes into extracellular fluid and eventually into the bloodstream. Elevated levels of blood CK are indicative of cell membrane damage. Different types of tissue contain different forms of CK (isoenzymes). The MB form of creatine kinase is found in cardiac muscle, and elevated serum levels of this enzyme are indicative of myocardial infarction.[7]

Substrate Utilization

The primary foodstuffs that fuel energy-producing enzymatic processes in cardiac muscle are glucose and fatty acids.[8] Amino acids are less important metabolic substrates for cardiac muscle except during states of starvation. The relative amounts of fatty acids and glucose used by the heart muscle depend on their concentration in blood. Fatty acids are the preferred fuel, particularly in a fasting state, when glucose levels are lower. Under fasting conditions, fatty acids account for approximately 85 percent of myocardial fuel and glucose contributes only 15 percent. After eating, when blood sugar levels rise, glucose utilization may increase to about 50 percent. Fatty acid metabolism requires oxygen and is therefore not useful under conditions of ischemia.

KEY CONCEPTS

- **Creatine phosphate is an immediately available storage form of energy. In conditions of low ATP availability, creatine phosphate is converted to ATP by the enzyme creatine kinase.**
- **The primary energy substrates for the heart are fatty acids and glucose.**

Cardiac Electrophysiology

The plasma membranes of cardiac cells are endowed with special ion channels that make the cells excitable. Excitable tissues are able to generate and conduct action potentials. The heart is rhythmically activated by action potentials, which are generated and transmitted by a specialized conduction system. Spread of an action potential over cardiac muscle cell surfaces results in myocardial contraction. An understanding of the electrophysiologic properties of the heart is important because many cardiac disorders include disturbances in electrical function.

Cardiac Resting Potential

Like other cells, resting cardiac cells are negatively charged on the inside with respect to the outside (see Chap. 2). Differences in potassium ion concentration

across the cell membrane determine the resting membrane potential. Cardiac muscle cells generally have a resting membrane potential of -85 to -95 millivolts (mV). An increase in extracellular potassium ion tends to depolarize the cell (make it less negative), and a lower than normal extracellular potassium tends to hyperpolarize the cell (make it more negative). The degree of polarization is an important determinant of the ease with which an action potential can be initiated. It is easier to reach threshold and initiate an action potential when the membrane is already partially depolarized.

Cardiac Action Potentials

Depolarization of cardiac cells to a threshold point results in activation of voltage-sensitive ion channels in the membrane. A myocardial action potential (Fig. 16–20) results from movement of ions through these open voltage-gated channels. The action potential in ventricular cells has five characteristic phases, which can be measured by a voltmeter connected to a microelectrode inserted into the cell.

Phase 0. Phase 0 begins when the membrane potential approaches threshold and voltage-gated "fast" sodium channels open momentarily. Due to a steep electrochemical gradient for sodium entry, rapid influx of sodium ions occurs. Sodium entry depolarizes

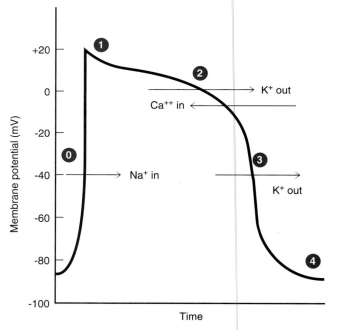

F I G U R E 16–20. The cardiac myocardial action potential has five characteristic phases, representing changes in ion movement through the plasma membrane. Phase 0: rapid upstroke due to sodium influx. Phase 1: slight repolarization due to closure of sodium channels and beginning potassium efflux. Phase 2: plateau due to offsetting influx of calcium and efflux of potassium. Phase 3: rapid repolarization due to closure of calcium channels and continued potassium efflux. Phase 4: resting membrane potential reestablished due to closure of all voltage-sensitive channels.

the cell by neutralizing the difference in charge (polarity) across the membrane. A steep depolarizing deflection is shown on the voltmeter.

Phase 1. Phase 1 is identified on the voltmeter as a small repolarizing deflection that corresponds to closure of the "fast" sodium channels and beginning efflux of potassium from the cell. The interior of the cell is now more positively charged, which induces potassium ions to leave the cell.

Phase 2. Phase 2 is also called the *plateau phase* because little change in membrane potential occurs during this time, even though ions continue to move across the membrane. Phase 2 is primarily associated with an influx of calcium ions, which is offset by an efflux of potassium ions. Calcium channels open and close slowly in comparison to fast sodium channels and are thus referred to as slow channels.

Phase 3. Phase 3 is characterized by a rapid return to the resting membrane potential. This is accomplished by closure of the slow calcium channels and continued and even more rapid efflux of potassium ions from the cell. Sodium channels remain absolutely refractory during phases 1, 2, and early 3. The latter part of phase 3 represents a **relative refractory period,** when sodium channels may be induced to open but a larger than normal depolarizing stimulus is required.

Phase 4. Phase 4 corresponds to the period of time between action potentials when no changes in membrane voltage are evident and the resting membrane potential is present. The Na^+/K^+ pump and Ca^{2+} pumps work continuously throughout the phases to maintain the internal and external concentrations of sodium, potassium, and calcium ions.

Rhythmicity of Myocardial Cells

Rhythmicity (**automaticity**) refers to intermittent, spontaneous generation of action potentials. A requirement for rhythmicity is that the cell membrane have sufficient "leak" channels for cation entry. Leak channels in automatic cells allow influx of sodium ions independent of any particular stimulus. Over time, the flow of positive ions into a cell will depolarize the membrane and result in generation of an action potential. Although automatic cells possess fast sodium channels, they are perpetually inactivated (refractory) because the resting membrane potential remains above −55 mV. Action potentials are achieved by opening of the voltage-gated slow calcium channels, making the rate of membrane depolarization and repolarization slower than in ventricular muscle cells. Repolarization is achieved in large part by exodus of potassium ions from the cell. Rhythmic cells have a recognizable action potential that is characterized by a sloping phase 4 (Fig. 16–21), in contrast to the flat phase 4 of ventricular muscle cells.

The rate of rhythmic discharge is determined in part by rates of cation entry through leak channels. In a normal heart, a cell with the fastest rate of spontaneous depolarization becomes the pacemaker for the rest of the heart. Cells in the sinoatrial (SA) node,

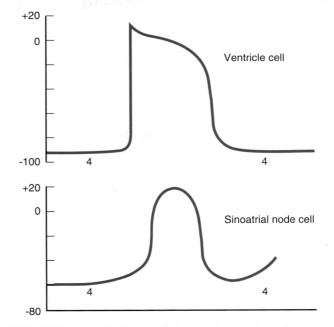

FIGURE 16–21. Rhythmic cells have a sloping phase 4, in contrast to the flat phase 4 of the ventricular muscle cell.

located in the right atrium, generally function as the heart's pacemaker because they have the fastest rate of spontaneous depolarization. However, other myocardial cells are also capable of spontaneous depolarization and may initiate an action potential in certain circumstances.

The steepness of the slope of phase 4 depolarization determines the rate of action potential generation. Several factors determine the steepness of the slope, including membrane permeability to sodium, calcium, and potassium. For example, a reduction in potassium ions leaving the cell would enhance depolarization and result in a faster rate. Rhythmicity may be influenced by the autonomic nervous system, drugs, and electrolyte balance.

Specialized Conduction System of the Heart

Some myocardial cells are specialized to conduct action potentials throughout the heart in an organized and rapid manner. These cells make up the conduction system of the heart shown in Figure 16–22. Normal excitation of the heart follows a pathway beginning with the SA node, atrial internodal pathways, AV node, ventricular bundle branches, and finally Purkinje fibers.

The **SA node** is located in the right atrium near the superior vena cava inlet. It receives innervation from sympathetic and parasympathetic branches of the autonomic nervous system. The SA node generally serves as a pacemaker for the heart, generating about 75 action potentials per minute in a resting adult. SA action potentials are spread contiguously to adjacent atrial cells at a rate of about 0.3 m/sec. A

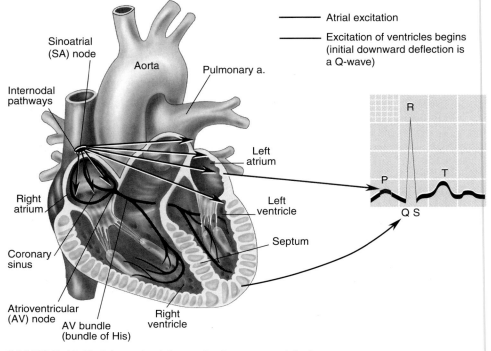

FIGURE 16–22. Schematic of the conducting system of the heart.

fibrous skeleton separates atria from ventricles and prevents spread of impulses from atrial cells to ventricular cells. There are several small bundles of atrial muscle cells that conduct impulses slightly faster (1.0 m/sec) than the usual atrial cell. One such bundle, the anterior interatrial band (Bachmann's bundle), conducts impulses from the SA node to the left atrium. The existence of three other bundles that conduct impulses from the SA node to the AV node has been suggested[2,5] but still remains controversial. Atrial depolarization results in atrial contraction, which increases the volume delivered to the still relaxed ventricular chambers.

After traversing the atria, the impulse initiated at the SA node arrives at the **AV node** located in the posterior septal wall of the right atrium just behind the tricuspid valve. There is a characteristic slowing of impulse conduction through the AV node, which allows for completion of atrial contraction prior to beginning ventricular systole. The AV node is actually composed of several different types of fibers that have somewhat different action potential conduction times. Overall, it normally takes about 0.13 second for an impulse to pass through the AV node. The slowness of conduction through AV fibers is related to two factors: (1) cells in the AV region have less negative resting membrane potentials and therefore a slower phase 0, and (2) there are few gap junctions between AV nodal cells so that cell-to-cell conduction of action potentials is more difficult due to high resistance. The AV node is richly innervated by the autonomic nervous system. The AV node spontaneously depolarizes at a rate of 40 to 60 times per minute and will become the heart's pacemaker if the SA node fails.

Purkinje cells, which lead from the AV node to ventricular myocardium, are vastly different from AV nodal cells. They are large and well structured to conduct impulses very rapidly. After penetrating the AV fibrous barrier, the bundle of Purkinje fibers travels 5 to 15 mm down the intraventricular septum toward the apex. The **main bundle** then divides into **left** and **right bundle branches,** which travel down the left and right sides of the intraventricular septum. Successive branches of Purkinje fibers penetrate the ventricular muscle mass from the endocardial side. Intraventricular septal areas are depolarized first, followed by apical muscle, and finally the lateral walls (Fig. 16–23). The total time elapsed between main bundle branch and terminal Purkinje fiber depolarization is only 0.03 second. Therefore, the entire ventricular endocardium is activated almost simultaneously. Purkinje fibers are capable of spontaneous depolarization at a rate of 15 to 40 times per minute and may become pacemakers for the heart if impulses from the SA and AV nodes are interrupted.

Action potentials are rapidly transmitted from the terminal Purkinje fibers to **cardiac muscle fibers** and then spread contiguously from cell to cell through the ventricular muscle. Approximately 0.03 second is required for the impulse to be transmitted through the ventricular myocardium. Impulses normally travel from the terminations of Purkinje fibers at endocardial surfaces toward the epicardial surfaces. Depolarization of the ventricular myocardium is followed by contraction and ejection of blood from the ventricles.

The ability of faster pacemakers to suppress the automatic discharge of slower pacemakers is called **overdrive suppression.** A slower pacemaker may be

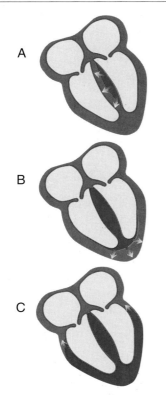

FIGURE 16-23. Sequence of ventricular depolarization showing septal depolarization in a left to right direction (**A**), followed by apical depolarization in an endocardial to epicardial direction (**B**) and finally depolarization of the lateral walls (**C**).

revealed if the normal pacemaker is suddenly interrupted. Sometimes it takes a period of time for the slower pacemaker to "kick in" and begin pacing at its intrinsic rate. A previously rapid rate of depolarizations apparently enhances the activity of membrane Na$^+$/K$^+$ pumps, resulting in a period of hyperpolarization (more negative resting potential) when the faster pacemaker suddenly stops. Thus, it takes a bit longer to reach threshold and initiate the first action potential.

Autonomic Regulation of Rhythmicity

Both sympathetic and parasympathetic nerves supply the heart. Sympathetic innervation is widespread to all areas, including the ventricular myocardium. Parasympathetic innervation, by way of the vagus nerves, is localized primarily in SA and AV nodal areas. The autonomic nervous system exerts control over heart rate and velocity of impulse conduction. In general, **sympathetic activation** increases heart rate (*chronotropic effect*) and increases speed of conduction (*dromotropic effect*) as well as inducing heart muscle to contract more forcefully (*inotropic effect*). These effects are achieved by release of the neurotransmitter norepinephrine (NE) from sympathetic nerve endings. Binding of NE to receptors on heart muscle cell membranes results in opening of membrane channels, which allows more rapid sodium and calcium ion entry.

Parasympathetic activation primarily results in a reduction in heart rate and speed of action potential conduction. Acetylcholine is the neurotransmitter released by parasympathetic nerve endings. Acetylcholine binding by receptors on heart cells increases membrane permeability to potassium ion, allowing it to leak from the cell. The resulting hyperpolarization makes it more difficult to reach threshold and initiate an action potential. The resting heart is normally under a degree of parasympathetic influence, which results in an SA discharge rate of about 75 beats per minute. If parasympathetic activity is blocked, the spontaneous discharge rate of SA nodal cells increases to about 100.

KEY CONCEPTS

- The cardiac resting membrane potential is about −90 mV. The resting membrane potential is determined by the ratio of intracellular to extracellular K$^+$.
- The five phases of the cardiac action potential are due to changes in ion conductance through the plasma membrane. The main changes in ion conductance result from opening of the fast Na$^+$ channels (phase 0), slow Ca^{++} channels (plateau), and K$^+$ channels (repolarization) in the plasma membrane.
- Spontaneous generation of action potentials in automatic cells is due to progressive leak of Na$^+$ and Ca^{++} into the cell via "leak" channels. The rate of leak determines the rate of pacemaker discharge. Parasympathetic influence increases K$^+$ efflux and slows the rate. Sympathetic influence increases influx of Na$^+$ and Ca^{++} and increases the rate.
- The usual conduction pathway for depolarization of the heart begins at the SA node, progresses through the atria, enters the AV node, and activates the His-Purkinje fibers. Purkinje fibers leave the AV node and divide into left and right branches that innervate the endocardial surface of the ventricular myocardium.

Electrocardiography

As action potentials spread from cell to cell throughout the myocardium, an electrical current is transmitted to the body surface and can be detected by electrodes placed on the skin.[9] A recording of these electrical currents is called an **electrocardiogram** (ECG). The ECG is a useful indicator of abnormalities of the heart's conduction system. Irregularities in initiation of impulses, conduction rates, and conduction pathways can be identified. The ECG looks different from the cardiac action potential described previously because it registers depolarizing and repolarizing currents in the whole heart rather than the activity of individual myocytes (Fig. 16–24).

Electrical currents traveling through the heart have both direction and magnitude and are often described as **vectors.** At any instant in time, electrical

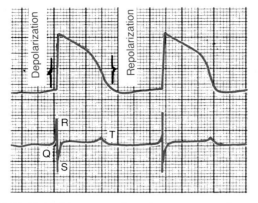

FIGURE 16–24. Upper recording, action potential from a single ventricular muscle cell, showing rapid depolarization and prolonged repolarization phases. Lower recording, electrocardiogram of potentials from the heart as a whole recorded simultaneously. (From Guyton AC: *Textbook of Medical Physiology*, 8th ed. Philadelphia, WB Saunders, 1991, p 119. Reproduced with permission.)

currents are moving in various directions through different regions of the heart. Waveforms recorded at the ECG electrodes are algebraic sums of all of these vectors. Patterns of electrical activity recorded by the ECG vary according to the placement of electrodes on the body. In general, a wave of depolarization moving toward a positive electrode will register as an upward deflection on the ECG. A wave of repolarization moving away from a positive electrode also will register as an upward deflection on the ECG. A downward deflection results from a wave of depolarization moving away from a positive electrode (Fig. 16–25). Placement of a positive electrode on the lower left extremity (lead II) results in the typical ECG pattern shown in Figure 16–26. A description of the usual electrode placements is included in the section on diagnostic tests at the end of this chapter.

Each deflection on the ECG has a normal characteristic shape and time interval (see Fig. 16–25). The three major wave complexes are the **P wave,** which corresponds to atrial depolarization, the **QRS complex,** which represents ventricular depolarization, and the **T wave,** which reflects ventricular repolarization. The **P-R interval,** between the beginning of the P wave and the beginning of the QRS complex, includes atrial, AV node, and His-Purkinje fiber depolarization. The normal sequence of ventricular depolarization begins with the septum, followed by the apex, and finally the base of the ventricular walls. Septal depolarization begins on the left septal surface and then travels toward the right, resulting in a negative deflection, the **Q wave** in lead II (Fig. 16–27). A large upright **R wave** corresponds to a wave of depolarization traveling down the ventricles toward the apex. Depolarization of the ventricular base, since it moves in a direction away from the lower limb electrode, is recorded as a negative **S wave.** The **S-T interval,** between the S wave and the beginning of the T wave, is isoelectric (flat), as the entire ventricle is depolarized

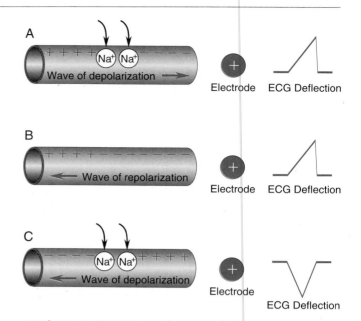

FIGURE 16–25. ECG waveforms may be positive (upward) or negative (downward) depending on the location of electrodes on the chest. **A,** A wave of depolarization moving toward a positive electrode results in a positive deflection. **B,** A wave of repolarization moving away from a positive electrode results in a positive deflection. **C,** A wave of depolarization moving away from a positive electrode results in a negative deflection.

and no detectable current is flowing. The Q-T interval, from the beginning of the QRS complex to the end of the T wave, is commonly measured as an indicator of ventricular systole. The T wave is normally upright in lead II, representing a wave of repolarization moving away from a positive electrode. Abnormalities in any time intervals may indicate abnormal conduction pathways and enhanced or slowed conduction times. Rhythm disturbances are discussed in detail in Chapter 18.

KEY CONCEPTS

- The ECG represents an algebraic sum of all depolarizing and repolarizing currents occurring in the heart. ECGs are useful for detecting conduction and rhythm disturbances.
- The major deflections of the ECG are:
  P wave: atrial depolarization
  P-R interval: atrial, AV node, and Purkinje depolarization
  Q wave: septal depolarization
  R wave: apical depolarization
  S wave: depolarization of lateral walls (base)
  T wave: ventricular repolarization

Determinants of Cardiac Output

Cardiac output is a measure of the amount of blood pumped out of the heart each minute. Since the heart's primary function is to pump enough blood

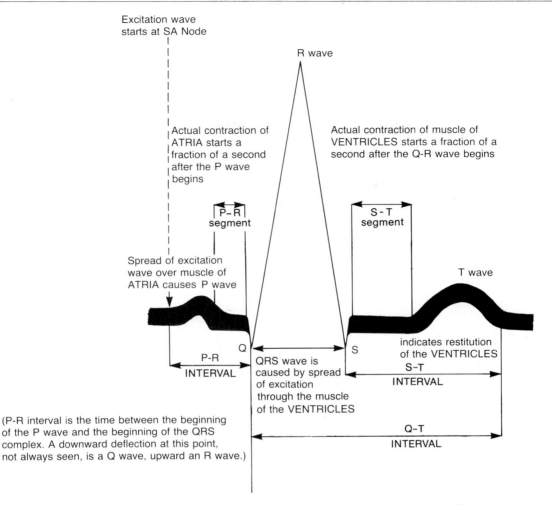

Excitation wave
starts at SA Node

R wave

Actual contraction of
ATRIA starts a
fraction of a second
after the P wave
begins

Actual contraction of muscle of
VENTRICLES starts a fraction of a
second after the Q-R wave begins

P–R
segment

S-T
segment

Spread of excitation
wave over muscle of
ATRIA causes P wave

T wave

Q

P-R
INTERVAL

S

QRS wave is
caused by spread
of excitation
through the muscle
of the VENTRICLES

indicates restitution
of the VENTRICLES

S-T
INTERVAL

(P-R interval is the time between the beginning
of the P wave and the beginning of the QRS
complex. A downward deflection at this point,
not always seen, is a Q wave, upward an R wave.)

Q-T
INTERVAL

FIGURE 16–26. Usual ECG pattern recorded from lead II, showing characteristic waves and intervals. (From Jacob SW, Francone CA: *Elements of Anatomy and Physiology*, 2nd ed. Philadelphia, WB Saunders, 1989, p 182. Reproduced with permission.)

to circulate oxygen and nutrients to tissues, cardiac output is an extremely important indicator of cardiovascular health. The normal resting cardiac output is approximately 5 to 6 L/min but varies with body size and age. Cardiac output is often indexed to body surface area in an attempt to adjust for these differences (cardiac index = cardiac output ÷ body surface area). A normal cardiac index ranges from 2.8 to 3.3 L/min/m². Regardless of the actual liters pumped per minute, the adequacy of tissue perfusion is ultimately important.

Cardiac output is a product of heart rate and stroke volume (CO = HR × SV). **Stroke volume** refers to the amount of blood ejected from the ventricle with each contraction. An increase in heart rate (to a point) and/or an increase in stroke volume will result in a greater cardiac output. Conversely, a low heart rate and/or a decreased stroke volume will cause cardiac output to fall. To a certain extent, a change in one factor can be compensated for by a change in the other, thus maintaining cardiac output at a constant level. For example, it is common for an individual with limited stroke volume due to cardiac disease to have a high resting heart rate. Any physiologic, pharmacologic, or pathologic process that alters heart rate or stroke volume may affect cardiac output and therefore tissue perfusion.

Determinants of Heart Rate

Heart rate is primarily determined by influences of the autonomic nervous system. Release of norepinephrine by **sympathetic nerve** endings in the heart results in increased heart rate. A similar effect results from circulating norepinephrine and epinephrine released from the adrenal gland during sympathetic stimulation. Sympathetic activation of the heart is regulated by several reflex pathways that constantly monitor blood pressure and metabolic activity in the body. In general, detection of inadequate blood pressure, a lack of oxygen, or a buildup of metabolic end products results in activation of the sympathetic nervous system. Specialized sensory nerve endings,

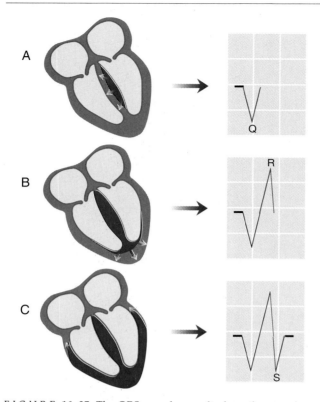

FIGURE 16–27. The QRS complex results from the sequence of ventricular depolarization. **A**, In lead II, septal depolarization is in a direction away from the positive electrode, resulting in a negative Q wave. **B**, Depolarization of the apex of the heart is in a direction toward the positive electrode, resulting in a large positive R wave. **C**, Depolarization of the lateral walls and base of the ventricles is in a direction away from the positive electrode, resulting in a negative S wave.

called **baroreceptors,** located in the aortic arch and carotid arteries respond to changes in blood pressure and transmit this information to the central nervous system (CNS). A fall in blood pressure causes parasympathetic system inhibition and cardiac sympathetic nerve activation, resulting in a rise in heart rate. Conversely, a rise in blood pressure causes heart rate to fall because of parasympathetic activation and sympathetic inhibition. Under normal resting conditions, the heart rate is under parasympathetic influence, with a usual rate of 60 to 80 beats per minute.

Because blood pressure is influenced by arteriolar resistance, it is not always a good indicator of cardiac output, so other monitoring systems are utilized. **Chemoreceptors** provide additional information to the CNS about the adequacy of cardiac output (and lung function). Chemoreceptors located in the carotid arteries, aortic arch, and hypothalamus respond to the levels of oxygen, carbon dioxide, and pH of the blood. Detection of inadequate oxygen or excessive carbon dioxide and H^+ results in sympathetic activation and an increase in heart rate. A reduction in carbon dioxide or alkalemia results in parasympathetic activation and decreased heart rate.

In addition to baroreceptors and chemoreceptors, other sensory fibers that detect pressure are located within the cardiac chambers. These sensory receptors respond to changes in intrachamber pressure, which reflect the volume of blood in the chamber. Atrial or ventricular overdistention activates the sympathetic system and increases heart rate. Heart rate may also be influenced by higher CNS activities that do not involve reflex pathways. Anxiety, fear, and excitement may activate the sympathetic system, for example. A variety of drugs can mimic or block the effects of both sympathetic and parasympathetic systems and therefore influence heart rate (see Chap. 17).

In general, an increase in heart rate will result in an increase in cardiac output; however, at very high heart rates, cardiac output may actually fall. At high heart rates, the time for diastolic ventricular filling is significantly reduced, resulting in a low stroke volume. The benefit of increased heart rate is therefore undermined by impaired pumping efficiency.

Determinants of Stroke Volume

Three major factors influence stroke volume: (1) the volume of blood in the heart, (2) the contractile capabilities of heart muscle, and (3) impedance opposing ejection of blood from the ventricle. Each of these factors is in turn influenced by many other physiologic, pharmacologic, and sometimes pathologic variables.

Volume of Blood in the Heart. The heart can only pump as much blood as is delivered to it by the circulatory system. Blood returning to the heart from the circulation is often called **venous return.** Normally, venous return is equal to cardiac output because the circulatory system is just that—a circuit. However, there may be inequalities over several heartbeats when changes in blood volume or blood distribution occur. The heart is well suited to adjust to these beat-to-beat changes in venous return, such that the healthy heart pumps essentially whatever amount is delivered to it.

The amount of blood present in the ventricles just prior to contraction (end-diastolic volume) is an important determinant of stroke volume. The relationship between diastolic volume and the force of myocardial contraction is known as the **Frank-Starling law of the heart.**[2,10] In essence, this law states that an increase in resting muscle fiber length will result in a greater development of muscle tension. Ventricular muscle fiber length is determined by the volume of blood it contains, commonly called the **preload.** An increase in preload results in a greater force of contraction and therefore a larger stroke volume. In this way, the ventricle is able to adjust its stroke volume, beat by beat, according to the amount of blood to be pumped.

The Frank-Starling law of the heart may be understood by recalling the molecular structure of contractile units of heart muscle. For contraction to occur, the actin and myosin filaments that make up the sarcomere must form crossbridges and slide together. Stretching the muscle prior to contraction would allow greater numbers of crossbridges to form, resulting in a more forceful contraction (Fig. 16–28). Overstretch, however, would disengage the actin and myosin filaments and disrupt crossbridge formation. On the other hand, if sarcomere length is already short prior to contraction, little contraction is possible because actin filaments begin to overlap and interfere with each other.

The cardiac function curve describes the effects of preload on ventricular stroke volume (Fig. 16–29). In practice, stroke volume and ventricular end-diastolic volume are difficult to measure, and other indicators, such as ventricular pressure and cardiac output, may be used. Cardiac function curves can be measured in persons with poorly functioning hearts to determine the best filling volume (preload) for optimizing cardiac output. Often, the failing heart requires a higher than normal preload in order to maintain a normal cardiac output.

Contractile Capabilities of the Heart. Heart muscle contractility depends on several factors, including: (1) the amount of contractile proteins in the muscle cells, (2) the availability of ATP and calcium ions, and (3) the degree of sympathetic or pharmacologic stimulation. Contractility is, by definition, independent of fiber end-diastolic length and is therefore not affected by preload. Given an adequate ATP supply, the contractile state of the normal myocardium is primarily determined by factors that increase or prolong the presence of free calcium ions within the myocardial cell. In general, an increased intracellular free calcium level can be accomplished by enhanced release from internal stores, enhanced entry from extracellular fluid, and reduced extrusion/sequestration.

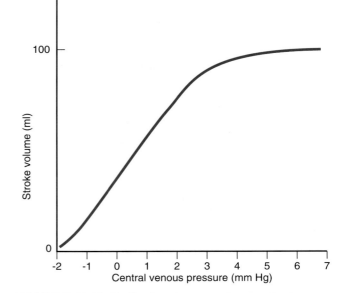

FIGURE 16–29. Cardiac function curve showing the dependence of ventricular stroke volume on preload.

A variety of agents, called positive inotropes, are associated with increased intracellular calcium levels in the heart. These include the sympathetic neurotransmitters norepinephrine and epinephrine, thyroid hormone, caffeine, digitalis, and many others. Agents that depress contractility, called negative inotropes, achieve their effects by reducing intracellular calcium levels. These agents include calcium channel blockers, parasympathomimetics, and sympathetic blocking drugs. The baroreceptor reflex, described previously in relation to heart rate, is also an important regulator of stroke volume through its effects on contractility.

Cardiac disease may adversely affect contractility because of an inadequate oxygen supply or because of actual myocardial cell death. These disorders are discussed in Chapter 17.

Impedance to Ejection from the Ventricle. The third major determinant of stroke volume is **afterload,** which refers to the impedance that must be overcome in order to eject blood from the chamber. Left ventricular afterload is determined primarily by aortic pressure. Normally the aortic valve offers little impedance to flow; however, aortic valve narrowing may significantly increase afterload. An increase in afterload will result in a decrease in stroke volume unless contractility or preload (or both) is adjusted to compensate. Conversely, a decrease in afterload will allow a larger than normal volume of blood to be ejected from the heart, requiring less myocardial work.

The ventricles normally eject only about 60 to 70 percent of their end-diastolic volume during contraction; the remaining 30 to 40 percent remains in the ventricle. **Ejection fraction** is influenced by afterload as well as preload and contractile state. A reduced ejection fraction is a common finding in persons suffering from myocardial infarction.

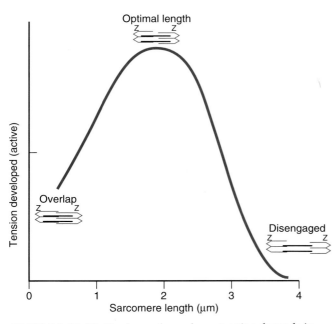

FIGURE 16–28. The force of muscle contraction depends in part on its resting length prior to activation. At short lengths, filaments may overlap and interfere with crossbridge formation. At optimal length, the greatest tension is developed and crossbridge formation is enhanced. With excessive stretch the filaments may disengage and no longer form crossbridges, resulting in inability to contract.

Cardiac Work

The work done by the heart can be described as the amount of energy (ATP) exerted to perform its pumping function. The four determinants of cardiac output described in the previous section—heart rate, preload, contractility, and afterload—are also the major determinants of cardiac energy requirements. An increase in any of these four factors will increase ATP requirements and therefore cardiac cell oxygen requirements. High afterload is most detrimental, as it greatly increases cardiac work without producing a higher cardiac output.

KEY CONCEPTS

- Cardiac output is the product of the heart rate times the stroke volume (CO = HR × SV). An increase in heart rate or stroke volume will increase cardiac output. An increase in heart rate can compensate for a decrease in stroke volume.

- Heart rate is controlled primarily by the autonomic nervous system. Factors that increase heart rate include low blood pressure (baroreceptors), acidemia (chemoreceptors), atrial and ventricular overdistention (stretch receptors), and emotions. Activation of the vagus nerve will decrease heart rate.

- Stroke volume is influenced by preload. According to the Frank-Starling law, increased preload stretches the sarcomere, resulting in more forceful contraction.

- Increased contractility increases stroke volume by causing a greater percentage of the ventricular volume to be ejected. Any factor that enhances the concentration of intracellular Ca^{++} will increase contractility.

- Increased afterload will decrease stroke volume. Afterload is determined primarily by the resistance of the arterial system. Vasoconstriction and high aortic pressure increase afterload.

- Any factor that increases heart rate, preload, contractility, or afterload will increase the work load of the heart.

Endocrine Function of the Heart

In addition to its pumping function, the heart also has an endocrine function: secretion of atrial natriuretic peptide (ANP).[11] ANP is synthesized by myocytes in the atria and released in response to atrial stretch. Increased atrial stretch occurs when blood volume becomes excessive. ANP causes enhanced excretion of sodium and water by the kidney. In general, the effects of ANP are antagonistic to those of the renin-angiotensin-aldosterone system (see Chap. 26).

Tests of Cardiac Function

In addition to history, laboratory, and physical assessment, a number of diagnostic tests may be employed to evaluate cardiac function.[3] The **electrocardiogram** is routinely obtained and provides information about the heart's conduction patterns. **Echocardiography, phonocardiography,** and **nuclear cardiography** are tests that use various modes to image the heart. A more direct assessment of cardiac function can be obtained by **cardiac catheterization.** Each of these studies is briefly described in this section.

Electrocardiography

The **electrocardiograph** (ECG) graphically records electrical currents generated by cardiac cells. The current is registered by skin electrodes placed in particular positions on the body. The standard ECG has 12 different leads that are obtained through ten skin electrodes: three standard bipolar limb leads, three aug-

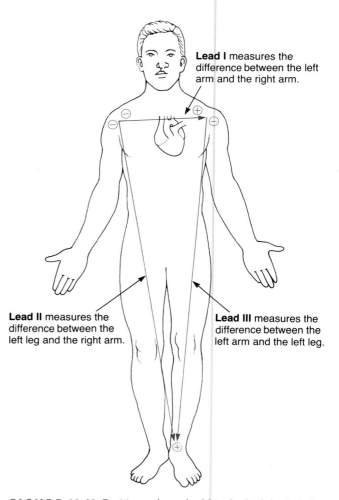

FIGURE 16–30. Positions of standard bipolar limb leads I, II, and III. (From Ignatavicius DD, Bayne MV: *Medical-Surgical Nursing: A Nursing Process Approach.* Philadelphia, WB Saunders, 1991, p 2103. Reproduced with permission.)

mented unipolar limb leads, and six unipolar chest leads. Bipolar leads represent a difference in electrical potential between two electrodes, one positive and one negative. Augmented unipolar limb leads represent a difference in potential between one electrode and the average of the other two limb electrodes. Unipolar chest leads represent a difference in potential between the chest electrode and a location at the center of the heart. Each lead provides a different ECG recording because of its particular "view" of current flow through the heart.

The three standard bipolar limb leads are lead I, lead II, and lead III (Fig. 16–30): Lead I measures the current between the right arm and left arm, lead II measures the current between the right arm and left leg, and lead III measures the current between the left arm and left leg. A normal ECG from leads I, II, and III is illustrated in Figure 16–31.

Electrode placement for the augmented unipolar limb leads is illustrated in Figure 16–32. Unipolar limb lead electrodes provide the positive pole: lead aVR is recorded from the right arm, lead aVL is recorded from the left arm, and lead aVF is recorded from the left leg. In these leads, *a* stands for augmented, *V* stands for voltage, and *R, L,* and *F* indicate the location of the unipolar lead; *right* arm, *left* arm, and *foot* (left). A normal ECG from these leads is illustrated in Figure 16–33.

Precordial unipolar chest leads are obtained from electrodes placed in six positions over the heart on the anterior chest (Fig. 16–34). Chest leads are designated as V_1, V_2, V_3, V_4, V_5, and V_6. The normal ECG from the chest leads is illustrated in Figure 16–35. The chest leads provide a horizontal view of the heart, whereas the limb leads provide a view of the frontal plane.

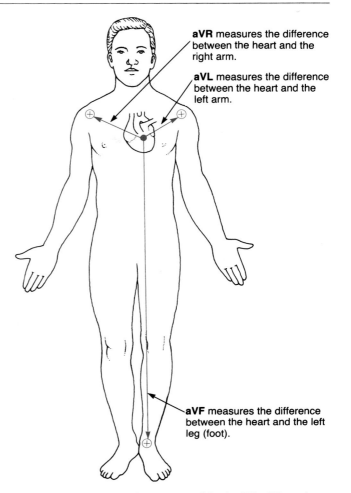

aVR measures the difference between the heart and the right arm.

aVL measures the difference between the heart and the left arm.

aVF measures the difference between the heart and the left leg (foot).

FIGURE 16–32. Unipolar augmented leads aVR, aVL, and aVF. (From Ignatavicius DD, Bayne MV: *Medical-Surgical Nursing: A Nursing Process Approach.* Philadelphia, WB Saunders, 1991, p 2104. Reproduced with permission.)

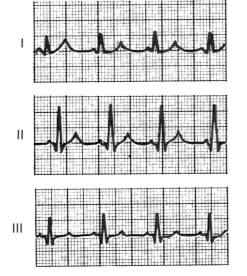

FIGURE 16–31. Normal ECG recorded from the three standard bipolar limb leads. (From Guyton AC: *Textbook of Medical Physiology,* 8th ed. Philadelphia, WB Saunders, 1991, p 122. Reproduced with permission.)

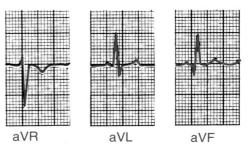

aVR   aVL   aVF

FIGURE 16–33. Normal ECG recorded from the three unipolar augmented leads. (From Guyton AC: *Textbook of Medical Physiology,* 8th ed. Philadelphia, WB Saunders, 1991, p 122. Reproduced with permission.)

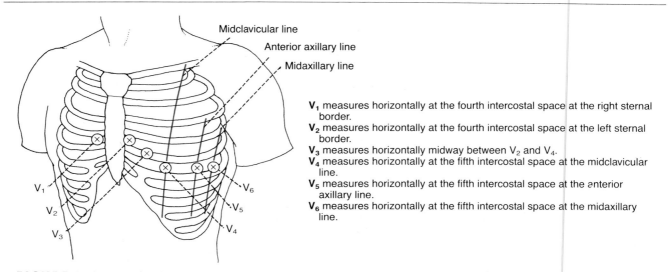

Midclavicular line

Anterior axillary line

Midaxillary line

V₁ measures horizontally at the fourth intercostal space at the right sternal border.
V₂ measures horizontally at the fourth intercostal space at the left sternal border.
V₃ measures horizontally midway between V₂ and V₄.
V₄ measures horizontally at the fifth intercostal space at the midclavicular line.
V₅ measures horizontally at the fifth intercostal space at the anterior axillary line.
V₆ measures horizontally at the fifth intercostal space at the midaxillary line.

F I G U R E   16–34. Unipolar chest (precordial) leads V_1 through V_6. (From Ignatavicius DD, Bayne MV: *Medical-Surgical Nursing: A Nursing Process Approach.* Philadelphia, WB Saunders, 1991, p 2104. Reproduced with permission.)

ECGs are usually recorded for a short period of time when the subject is resting. Sequential ECGs are useful for determining changes over time. In some cases it is necessary to monitor the ECG for an extended period of time to capture rhythm problems that occur infrequently or with particular activities. This is accomplished by continuous ambulatory monitoring (e.g., Holter monitoring) over a 24- to 48-hour period. An ECG can also be recorded during exercise to monitor the effects of exercise stress on cardiovascular function. An exercise test (stress test) is usually performed while the subject progressively increases his effort on a treadmill or stationary bicycle. The exercise ECG is particularly useful for assessing the adequacy of coronary circulation when myocardial work load is increased.

The **vectorcardiogram** is a special kind of electrocardiogram which differs substantially from the standard 12-lead ECG. The vectorcardiogram detects heart depolarization in two planes simultaneously and displays it as two-dimensional vector loops. Seven electrodes are placed on the body surface, including five chest positions, one left leg position, and one forehead or neck position. Depolarizations are measured in each of three planes of the body: horizontal plane, frontal plane, and sagittal plane. Thus, a vectorcardiogram provides a three-dimensional view of the heart, whereas a standard ECG provides only a two-dimensional view. The vectorcardiogram may be more sensitive than the standard 12-lead ECG in picking up changes due to myocardial infarction.

Echocardiography

Echocardiography uses reflected sound waves (ultrasound) to provide an image of cardiac structure and motion within the chest. The cardiac echo is obtained by placing a blunt probe on the chest surface that transmits and receives high-frequency sound waves. Sound waves traveling through chest and heart structures are reflected back to the receiving probe. The time between sound wave emission and detection of reflected waves is used to calculate distances between the probe and reflecting tissue. The sound waves are not heard or felt by the subject and have no known detrimental effects on tissues. The probe is moved across the chest to assess cardiac structures of interest, and recordings are videotaped for later viewing. Echocardiograms are particularly useful for diagnosis of heart enlargement, valvular disorders, collections of fluid in the pericardial space, cardiac tumors, and abnormalities in left ventricular motion. An echocardiogram is shown in Figure 16–36.

Phonocardiography

Phonocardiography is a graphic representation of heart sounds obtained by auscultation with special microphones placed on the chest wall. Sound waves produced by various cardiac events are transduced into a visual recording. Phonocardiography may be useful for characterizing abnormal heart sounds produced by insufficient or stenosed valves, stiffened

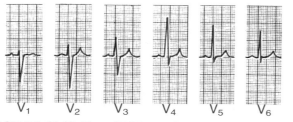

V₁   V₂   V₃   V₄   V₅   V₆

F I G U R E   16–35. Normal ECG recorded from the six unipolar chest leads, V_1 through V_6. (From Guyton AC: *Textbook of Medical Physiology,* 8th ed. Philadelphia, WB Saunders, 1991, p 122. Reproduced with permission.)

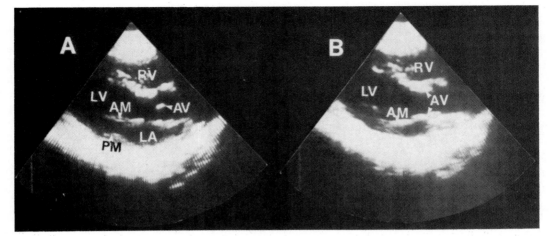

FIGURE 16–36. Long-axis cross-sectional echocardiograph of the left ventricle (LV), right ventricle (RV), mitral valve, aortic valve, and left atrium (LA) during diastole (**A**) and systole (**B**). During diastole the anterior (AM) and posterior (PM) mitral leaflets are apart and the aortic valve leaflets (AV) come together. In systole the mitral leaflets come together and the aortic leaflets separate. (From Braunwald E (ed): *Heart Disease: A Textbook of Cardiovascular Medicine*, 4th ed. Philadelphia, WB Saunders, 1992, p 67. Reproduced with permission.)

cardiac chambers, congenital defects, and excessive cardiac volumes. A phonocardiogram is shown in Figure 16–37.

Nuclear Cardiography

Radioactive substances injected into the bloodstream can be used to trace the patterns of blood flow in the heart. Radiation exposure is minimal, as very small amounts of radioactive substances are used. The most common nuclear imaging tests are technetium pyro-phosphate scanning, thallium imaging, and gated blood pool scanning.

Technetium scanning is used to visualize infarcted areas of cardiac muscle that accumulate the radioisotope. The radioactive technetium is injected into the bloodstream and then allowed to clear from the system for 2 hours. Infarcted cardiac tissues appear as "hot spots" when scanned with a gamma scintillation camera, which measures radioactive disintegrations of the ^{99m}Tc radioisotope.

Thallium imaging is used to assess the adequacy of blood flow to cardiac tissues. After injection of radioactive thallium (^{201}Tl), the heart is quickly scanned to visualize the amount of radioactivity taken up by cardiac tissues. Healthy cardiac tissues that receive adequate blood supply actively accumulate the isotope. Areas of inadequate blood flow or infarcted tissue do not accumulate isotope and appear as "cold spots" on the scan.

Gated pool scanning is used primarily to assess left ventricular motion and ejection fraction. Before it is injected intravenously, radioactive technetium is attached to albumin or red cells, and therefore remains in the bloodstream and is not taken up by cells. Computer imaging is used to analyze blood flow through the chambers of the heart over many cardiac cycles. The dynamics of ventricular motion, such as hypercontractility or hypocontractility, may be visualized.

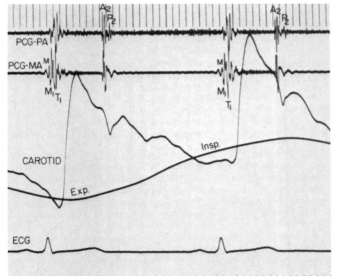

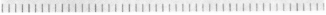

FIGURE 16–37. The normal phonocardiogram showing the first heart sound, PCG-MA, and the second heart sound, A_2-P_2. (From Braunwald E (ed): *Heart Disease: A Textbook of Cardiovascular Medicine*, 3rd ed. Philadelphia, WB Saunders, 1988, p 44. Reproduced with permission.)

Cardiac Catheterization/ Coronary Angiography

Of the many available diagnostic tools for cardiac evaluation, cardiac catheterization/coronary angiography provides the most definitive information. Cardiac catheterization/coronary angiography may be used to determine important structural and hemodynamic characteristics, for it affords direct measurement of pressures within cardiac chambers; visualization of chamber size, shape, and movement; sampling for blood oxygen content in various heart regions; measurement of cardiac output and ejection fraction; and visualization and treatment of coronary artery obstructions.

Cardiac catheterization angiography is associated with several serious risks, including bleeding, dysrhythmias, heart perforation, and coronary ischemia. However, the value of information supplied is generally believed to far outweigh the risks. Catheterization is frequently used to evaluate suspected or confirmed coronary artery disease, valvular dysfunction, congenital defects, left ventricular dysfunction, and coronary bypass graft patency.

Assessment of the left side of the heart, including the coronary arteries, is achieved by passing a catheter through a femoral or brachial artery into the aorta. The catheter is then manipulated into the left ventricle or left atrium to assess chamber pressures, and a ventriculogram is obtained. Contrast dye injected into the ventricular chamber is monitored by fluoroscopy to assess ventricular function. The catheter is usually pulled back into the aorta and then advanced into one or more of the coronary ostia. The patency of the coronary arteries can be visualized by injecting contrast dye into them and monitoring by fluoroscopy (Fig. 16–38). When contrast dye is in the coronary artery, a period of cardiac ischemia is produced during which the patient may experience angina, dysrhythmias, and coronary spasms.

Right heart catheterization is done to evaluate

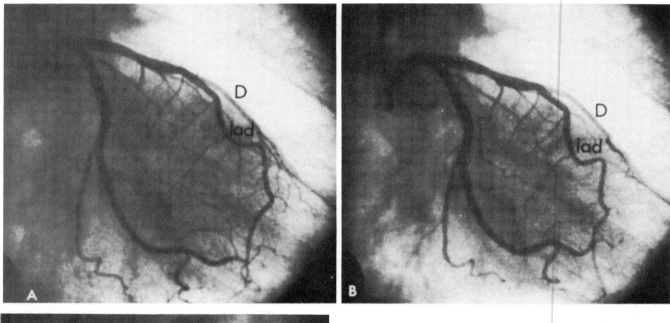

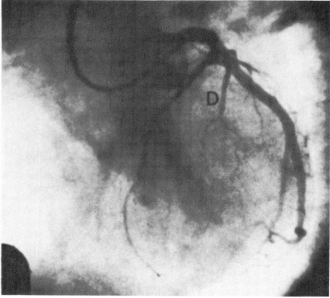

FIGURE 16–38. Coronary artery angiography. **A,** Right anterior oblique view during diastole. **B,** Right anterior oblique view during systole. **C,** Left anterior oblique view. D = diagonal branch; lad, left anterior descending coronary artery. (From Braunwald E (ed): *Heart Disease: A Textbook of Cardiovascular Medicine,* 2nd ed. Philadelphia, WB Saunders, 1984, p 327. Reproduced with permission.)

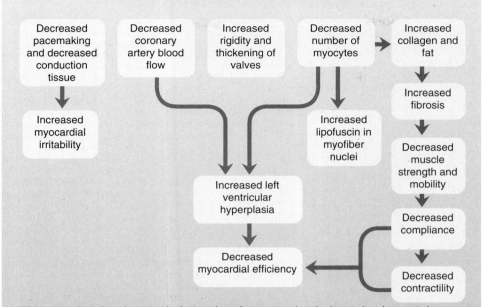

THE AGING PROCESS: CHANGES IN THE HEART

With aging, there is a decrease in the number of myocytes, but the heart size does not change appreciably. With the loss of overall cardiac muscle tissue, there is a corresponding expansion in myocardial collagen and fat. The left ventricular muscle wall becomes thicker, with a resulting increase in oxygen demand. The endocardium becomes fibrotic and sclerosed. Cross-linking of the collagen tissue within the heart muscle increases myocardial stiffening, which causes decreased compliance. The decrease in compliance produces a decline in cardiac contractility, which reduces the heart's pumping ability. The rate of ventricular relaxation decreases.

Fibrotic changes in cardiac valves result from a combination of hemodynamic stress and generalized thickening. There is also a decrease in coronary artery blood flow to the myocardium, which affects myocardial oxygen and nutrient supply. The myocardial cells increase in size, with increased lipofuscin pigment and lipid deposition.

Within the specialized electrical conduction tissue, there is loss of myocytes in and fibrosis of conduction pathways, especially in the sinoatrial (SA) node, atrioventricular (AV) node, and bundle of His. There is a decreased number of pacemaker cells in the SA node resulting in less responsiveness of the SA node to adrenergic stimulation. Myocardial cell irritability increases. On the electrocardiogram, the P wave may be notched or slurred. The PR interval is longer, and the QRS amplitude decreases. The axis may shift left due to left ventricular muscle thickening (hypertrophy). The T wave may be notched, and the amplitude may decrease.

The changes previously noted affect cardiac function. The resting heart rate in the elderly is unchanged. During stress or exercise, the aging heart is unable to respond quickly with an elevated rate, and the maximum heart rate elevation is reduced. Once the heart rate is elevated, it takes a much longer time for the heart rate to return to its resting rate. The cardiac stroke volume and cardiac output generally decrease with stress. Oxygen consumption in the myocardium is reduced, resulting in less efficient function when stressed and an overall decreased cardiac reserve.

right heart structures. The catheter is introduced into a vein, usually femoral or antecubital, then threaded through the inferior vena cava and into the heart. Pressures and blood samples are obtained as the catheter is advanced into the right atrium, ventricle, and pulmonary artery. Right heart catheterization is useful in assessing tricuspid and pulmonary valve disorders, pulmonary hypertension, septal defects, and right ventricular function.

In the last 15 years, coronary angiography has moved from a method of assessment only to a method of treatment for coronary occlusion. The coronary catheter can be used to direct thrombolytic agents to the site of coronary thrombosis and rapidly restore blood flow to ischemic areas. Laser therapy and coronary balloon angioplasty can also be performed during coronary angiography. These methods clear the coronary obstruction through thermal and mechanical means. The success of these approaches to treatment of coronary obstruction depends largely on how soon after an ischemic event they are done.

Summary

The heart's primary function is to pump sufficient blood to deliver oxygen and nutrients to the body. The heart may be viewed as two separate pumps: a right heart that perfuses the lungs and a left heart that perfuses the systemic circulation. The left ventricle must generate higher pressures and therefore has a thicker myocardial mass and higher energy requirements. Because little ATP storage in cardiac cells is possible, the coronary arteries must deliver a steady supply of oxygen and nutrients. Cardiac contraction can be described by the sliding filament/crossbridge theory and occurs only in the presence of ATP and free calcium ions. Any factor that enhances intracellular calcium ion concentration will result in generation of a greater contractile force.

A coordinated cardiac contraction is possible because the heart's conduction system activates the chambers in a sequential manner. The sinoatrial node is the usual pacemaker because it has the highest intrinsic rate of diastolic depolarization. Diastolic depolarization rate is strongly influenced by the autonomic nervous system. The ECG records electrical activity of the heart and is a useful indicator of cardiac conduction abnormalities.

The ultimate indicator of cardiac function is the cardiac output, which is the product of heart rate and stroke volume. The autonomic nervous system is the main regulator of heart rate, while stroke volume is influenced by preload, afterload, and contractility.

These factors are also the primary determinants of myocardial work and energy expenditure.

REFERENCES

1. Warwick R, Williams PL (eds): *Grays Anatomy*, 35th ed. Philadelphia, WB Saunders, 1980.
2. Guyton AC: Unit III—The heart, in: *Textbook of Medical Physiology*, 8th ed. Philadelphia, WB Saunders, 1991, pp 97–123.
3. Braunwald E (ed): *Heart Disease: A Textbook of Cardiovascular Medicine*, 4th ed. Philadelphia, WB Saunders, 1992.
4. Factor S, Kirk E: Pathophysiology of myocardial ischemia, in Hurst JW, et al (eds): *The Heart*, 6th ed. New York, McGraw-Hill, 1986, p 857.
5. Berne RM, Levy MN: The cardiac pump, in Berne RM, Levy MN (eds): *Principles of Physiology*. St. Louis, CV Mosby, 1990.
6. Alberts B, Bray D, Lewis J, Raff M, Roberts K, Watson J: The cytoskeleton, in Alberts B, et al (eds): *Molecular Biology of the Cell*, 2nd ed. New York, Garland Publishing, 1989.
7. DeWood M, et al: Clinical laboratory measurement in cardiac disease, in Halstead J, Halstead C (eds): *The Laboratory in Clinical Medicine*, 2nd ed. Philadelphia, WB Saunders, 1981.
8. Morgan H, Neely J: Metabolic regulation and myocardial function, in Hurst JW, et al (eds): *The Heart*, 6th ed. New York, McGraw-Hill, 1986.
9. Conover MB: *Understanding Electrocardiography: Arrhythmias and 12-Lead ECG*, 5th ed. St. Louis, CV Mosby, 1988.
10. Starling EH: *The Linacre Lecture on the Law of the Heart*. London, Longmans Green & Co, 1918.
11. Cantin M, Genest J: The heart as an endocrine gland. *Sci Am* 1986;2:76–81.

BIBLIOGRAPHY

Berne RM, Levy MN (eds): *Principles of Physiology*. St. Louis, CV Mosby, 1990.
Dzau VJ: Local contractile and growth modulators in the myocardium. *Clin Cardiol* 1993;16(5 suppl 2):115–119.
Edvinsson L, Uddman R (eds): *Vascular Innervation and Receptor Mechanisms: New Perspectives*. San Diego, Academic Press, 1993.
Ferrari AU: Modulation of parasympathetic and baroreceptor control of heart rate. *Cardioscience* 1993;4(1):9–13.
Glitsch HG, Tappe A: The Na^+/K^+ pump of cardiac Purkinje cells is preferentially fuelled by glycolytic ATP production. *Pflugers Arch* 1993;422(4):380–385.
Guyton AC: *Textbook of Medical Physiology*, 8th ed. Philadelphia, WB Saunders, 1991.
Hille B: *Ionic Channels of Excitable Membranes*, 2nd ed. Sunderland, Mass, Sinauer Associates, 1992.
Johnson MD, Friedman E: G proteins in cardiovascular function and dysfunction. *Biochem Pharmacol* 1993;45(12):2365–2372.
Katz AM: *Physiology of the Heart*, 2nd ed. New York, Raven Press, 1992.
Kern MJ: Perspective: The cellular influences of calcium antagonists on systemic and coronary hemodynamics. *Am J Cardiol* 1992;69(7):3B–7B.
Moffett D, Moffett S, Schauf C: *Human Physiology: Foundations and Frontiers*, 2nd ed. St. Louis, CV Mosby, 1993.
Rowell LB: *Human Cardiovascular Control*. New York, Oxford University Press, 1993.
Ruegg JC: *Calcium in Muscle Contraction: Cellular and Molecular Physiology*, 2nd ed. Berlin, Springer-Verlag, 1992.
Xiao RP, Lakatta EG: Deterioration of beta-adrenergic modulation of cardiovascular function with aging. *Ann NY Acad Sci* 1992;673:293–310.

CHAPTER 17
Alterations in Cardiac Function

JACQUELYN L. BANASIK

KEY TERMS

angina pectoris: A paroxysmal chest pain most often due to cardiac ischemia associated with atherosclerotic coronary artery disease.

cardiac tamponade: Abnormal external pressure on the heart resulting in poor cardiac filling and decreased cardiac output.

cardiomyopathy: Diseases that primarily affect myocardial cells, often of unknown etiology.

myocardial infarction: Localized area of cardiac necrosis most often associated with ischemic heart disease.

regurgitation (valvular): Retrograde blood flow through a cardiac valve when the valve is supposed to be closed.

shunt (cardiac): An abnormal route of blood flow through the heart.

stenosis (valvular): Obstruction to blood flow through open cardiac valves.

subendocardium: The part of the myocardium lying in proximity to the endocardial surface.

sudden cardiac death: Death due to cardiac causes within 24 hours of onset of symptoms.

transmural: Denotes entire thickness of the myocardial wall. A transmural myocardial infarction extends through the entire cardiac muscle layer.

---

*T*he incidence of heart disease has increased rapidly during the 1900s and now claims the lives of approximately 750,000 persons annually in the United States.[1] Heart disease is the predominant cause of death and disability in the industrialized world. Nearly twice as many people die from cardiac disorders as from all types of cancers combined. Since the late 1960s, however, a substantial decline in cardiac mortality has been achieved in the United States due to improvements in treatment and prevention. Great progress has been made in the treatment of ischemic heart disease, which accounts for about 80 percent of all heart diseases.[2] Other forms of cardiac disease, including endocardial and valvular disease, myocardial disease, pericardial disease, and congenital heart defects, account for the remaining 20 percent of cases. Common sequelae of many of these disorders are heart failure and rhythm disturbances, which are covered in Chapter 18.

Ischemic Heart Disease

The category of ischemic heart disease (IHD) includes several related disorders that are characterized by an imbalance between the supply and demand of the heart for oxygenated blood. In a great majority of cases, the cause of insufficient myocardial oxygen supply is a reduction in blood flow through the coronary arteries. Because the coronary arteries are most often narrowed or obstructed by plaques, IHD has commonly been called coronary artery disease (CAD). In more than 90 percent of cases of IHD, the coronary arteries suffer reduced blood flow due to obstructive atherosclerotic narrowings, vasospasm, or blood clot.[3,4] In addition to reduced coronary blood flow, IHD may result from a great increase in demand for oxygen, as occurs during strenuous exercise or with a fall in the blood oxygen content. Coronary obstruction is much more frequently the cause of cardiac ischemia then either high oxygen demand or low blood oxygen content.

Pathogenesis

Ischemia of cardiac cells occurs when the oxygen supply is insufficient to meet metabolic demands. Myocardial cells are unable to store much adenosine triphosphate (ATP) and therefore must continually receive a supply of oxygen for aerobic synthesis of ATP. ATP is essential to power myocardial contraction as well as for cell maintenance. Because the heart is unable to stop and rest when ATP supplies dwindle, it is essential that a steady flow of oxygen be provided.

Any factor that decreases myocardial oxygen supply or increases myocardial oxygen demand can upset the balance and result in cellular ischemia. The critical factor in meeting cellular demands for oxygen is adequate coronary perfusion. Even conditions resulting in very high myocardial oxygen consumption will seldom lead to ischemia unless there is some element of CAD. Therefore, the pathophysiology of IHD primarily has to do with derangements of coronary perfusion. Five pathophysiologic mechanisms may affect coronary perfusion: (1) coronary atherosclerosis, (2) platelet aggregation and thrombus formation, (3) coronary vasospasm, (4) nonatherosclerotic coronary disease, and (5) hemodynamic alterations.

Coronary Atherosclerosis

Atherosclerosis of the coronary arteries is present in over 90 percent of persons with IHD.[5] The development of stenotic atherosclerotic lesions in the coronary arteries is similar to that described for peripheral vessels. Although several hypotheses have been put forth to explain the pathogenesis of atherosclerosis, none has been proved. These hypotheses are summarized in Table 17–1 and discussed in Chapter 14.

Since the late 1960s attention has focused on an apparent association of certain traits and habits with the development of coronary atherosclerosis and IHD. These so-called "risk factors" for coronary atherosclerosis include innate factors such as age, sex, and family history and several modifiable factors including hyperlipidemia, diabetes, hypertension, smoking, and a sedentary life-style. These risk factors are described in detail in Chapter 14, and only hyperlipidemia, a factor of particular relevance to coronary atherosclerosis, is described here.

The observation that atherosclerotic plaques are composed primarily of lipid prompted the idea that abnormal lipid metabolism was a likely culprit in the development of IHD. A great deal of evidence has accumulated to indicate that hyperlipidemia is indeed a major risk factor for atherosclerotic heart disease. This evidence is summarized in Table 17–2. There appears to be no critical plasma lipid level that would

TABLE 17–1. Summary of Theories of Atherosclerosis

Hypothesis	Major Features
Response to injury	Injurious agents (shear force, chemicals, infection, or other trauma) cause a loss of endothelial cell membrane integrity. Platelets stick to the surface and release growth factors for smooth muscle cells (PDGF).
Monoclonal	Many plaques are known to be derived from one precursor smooth muscle cell (monoclonal). Some unknown factors, perhaps viruses or carcinogens, are thought to cause transformation of the muscle cell such that it reproduces excessively.
Lipid insudation (infiltration)	Endothelial cells exposed to high levels of blood lipids may take up excessive amounts by endocytosis, which results in cellular dysfunction. Macrophages are currently believed to play a role by engulfing excess lipids and transporting them into the arterial wall as they migrate into the tissue.
Intimal cell mass	Intimal cell masses are focal accumulations of smooth muscle cells located in the intima of the arteries at branch points and areas of high shear forces. Intimal masses are present in infants and are more pronounced in males. These may be the precursors of atherosclerotic lesions later in life due to chronic mechanical or biochemical injury.

identify those at risk. Rather, the risk of IHD increases proportionately as the lipid level increases. Lipids are transported through the bloodstream in combination with proteins. Certain lipid-protein molecules (lipoproteins) are associated with a greater risk of atherosclerosis. The five major kinds of lipoproteins are shown in Figure 17–1. High levels of low-density lipoproteins (LDLs), which are high in cholesterol, have been associated with the highest risk. Very-low-density lipoproteins (VLDLs), which have large amounts of triglycerides, also appear to increase risk. High-density lipoproteins (HDLs), on the other hand, have been correlated with a decreased risk of atherosclerosis.[6]

The mechanisms whereby LDL and VLDL cause, and HDL prevents, atherosclerosis are unknown. HDLs may transport cholesterol from the vessel back to the liver for excretion, thus clearing away atheromatous plaque. The role of LDL and indirectly VLDL is to bring cholesterol to the peripheral tissues. Cholesterol uptake by peripheral cells is mediated by receptors (LDL receptors) on cell surfaces that bind and promote endocytosis of cholesterol. Extreme cases of hyperlip-idemia result in individuals who lack functional LDL receptors. These disorders run in families and are associated with genetically linked defects in the LDL receptor.

Atherosclerotic lesions generally increase in size over many years and progressively occlude the lumen of vessels. A significant reduction in blood flow results when a plaque occupies 75 percent of the arterial lumen. Clinically significant atherosclerotic plaques may be located anywhere within the three major coronary arteries or major secondary branches. All three coronary arteries are often simultaneously affected although some individuals have only one or two diseased vessels. Surprisingly, the extent and severity of the atherosclerotic lesions are not a good predictor of the severity of IHD.

Platelet Aggregation and Thrombus Formation

The sudden obstruction of coronary blood flow that results in acute myocardial ischemia is usually associ-

TABLE 17–2. Evidence Implicating Hyperlipidemia in Atherosclerotic Heart Disease

1. Atherosclerotic plaques are rich in cholesterol, which is derived primarily from serum lipoproteins.
2. Atherosclerosis can be produced in experimental animals by feeding diets that increase plasma cholesterol levels.
3. Genetic disorders causing severe hypercholesterolemia lead to early, severe atherosclerosis.
4. Acquired diseases such as hypothyroidism and nephrotic syndrome which cause hyperlipidemia are associated with an increased incidence of ischemic heart disease.
5. Populations having higher blood cholesterol levels have a higher mortality from ischemic heart disease.
6. Recent prospective studies have shown that treatment with diet modification and cholesterol-lowering drugs reduces cardiovascular mortality in selected patients with hypercholesterolemia.

Data from Cotran RS, Kumar V, Robbins SL (eds): *Robbins Pathologic Basis of Disease*, 4th ed. Philadelphia, WB Saunders, 1989.

	MAJOR LIPIDS	MAJOR APOPROTEIN(S)
Chylomicron 80–500 nm	80–95% TG (dietary)	C proteins, AI, AII, B48
VLDL 30–80 nm	45–65% TG (endogenous) 25% cholesterol	C proteins, B48, E
IDL 30 nm	45% cholesterol	B100, E
LDL 15–25 nm	70% cholesterol	B100
HDL 5–12 nm	<25% cholesterol	AI, AII

F I G U R E 17–1. The five major kinds of lipoproteins. (From Cotran RS, Kumar V, Robbins SL (eds): *Robbins Pathologic Basis of Disease,* 4th ed. Philadelphia, WB Saunders, 1989, p 560. Reproduced with permission.)

ated with the formation of a clot in the coronary artery. Clots generally form at the sites of preexisting atherosclerotic plaques. Rupture of the plaque exposes a rough area composed of collagen and other molecules which are thrombogenic—they induce clot formation. Clot formation begins with adherence of platelets to the ruptured plaque. The platelets that initially attach release chemicals that attract more platelets, resulting in aggregation and plug formation. The coagulation cascade may also be initiated, resulting in formation of a platelet-fibrin clot that may occlude the vessel or may break loose and travel farther along the vessel. Chemicals released by activated platelets include several vasoactive products (histamine, serotonin, thromboxane) that may contribute to spasm of the coronary vessel, further reducing blood flow. Realization of the role that platelets play in the progression of coronary obstruction has resulted in the prophylactic use of anticoagulants such as aspirin to prevent thrombus formation. Preliminary results of the long-term use of small doses of aspirin suggest a reduction in IHD mortality.[7]

Coronary Vasospasm

Vasospasm of atherosclerotic coronary arteries has been documented in some patients with IHD. Very rarely, acute vasospasm has been associated with myocardial damage in patients with no preexisting atherosclerotic lesions. Spasm of the coronary artery in a stenotic area could lead to disruption or rupture of the plaque and cause platelet aggregation. Conversely, platelet activation with release of vasoactive chemicals could contribute to vasospasm.

Nonatherosclerotic Coronary Disease

Several nonatherosclerotic disorders are associated with alterations in coronary perfusion. These include diseases that result in coronary inflammation such as lupus erythematosus, Kawasaki syndrome, and polyarteritis nodosa. Traumatic injury to the coronary arteries and cocaine-induced vasospasm are examples of other nonatherosclerotic processes that may result in coronary obstruction.

Hemodynamic Alterations

Recall from Chapter 16 that coronary blood flow depends on driving pressure and coronary resistance. A fall in driving pressure may significantly reduce coronary perfusion, particularly in vessels having high resistance to flow due to atherosclerotic narrowing. Conditions such as shock, hemorrhage, or anesthesia may be associated with a fall in blood pressure, which decreases driving pressure and coronary perfusion, resulting in myocardial ischemia.

One or a combination of these five mechanisms is thought to be responsible for the development of the ischemic heart diseases discussed in the next section.

KEY CONCEPTS

- Cardiac ischemia occurs when the heart's demand for oxygenated blood exceeds its supply. In most cases ischemia is a result of insufficient blood flow through the coronary arteries.
- Ischemic heart disease (IHD) is most often associated with coronary atherosclerosis. Risk factors for IHD are the same as for atherosclerosis of other arteries: advancing age, male gender, family history, hyperlipidemia, diabetes, smoking, hypertension, and a sedentary life-style.
- Acute occlusion of a coronary vessel is usually due to thrombus formation at the site of an atherosclerotic plaque. Prophylactic use of anticoagulants may decrease mortality from IHD.
- IHD may uncommonly be caused by coronary vasospasm, inflammation and trauma of the coronaries, or a low perfusion pressure due to volume depletion or shock.

Ischemic Syndromes

Four ischemic syndromes have been identified, according to the severity and onset of cardiac ischemia: (1) angina pectoris, (2) myocardial infarction, (3) chronic IHD, and (4) sudden cardiac death, which may occur in association with any of the other three syndromes. The four syndromes of IHD are late manifestations of slowly progressing coronary atherosclerosis over a span of several decades.

Angina Pectoris

Angina pectoris is characterized by chest pain associated with intermittent myocardial ischemia. The length and the severity of the myocardial ischemia are insufficient to result in death of cells. Bouts of chest pain and associated symptoms are generally recurrent and may be precipitated by conditions that increase myocardial oxygen demand, such as exercise, stress, sympathetic nervous system activation, and increased preload, afterload, heart rate, or muscle mass. Ischemic pain receptors from the myocardium travel to the central nervous system (CNS) with the eighth cervical and first through fourth thoracic dorsal root ganglia. Sensory neurons from the jaw, neck, and arm also travel in these nerve trunks, so that heart pain may be perceived as emanating from these body parts. This is called *referred pain. Anginal pain* may be described as burning, crushing, squeezing, or choking. Pain is sometimes represented by expressions such as "an elephant is sitting on my chest," or by the patient placing a tight fist on the chest. Anginal pain may be mistakenly attributed to indigestion.

Anginal ischemia, although temporary, may result in inefficient cardiac pumping with resultant pulmonary congestion and shortness of breath. Three patterns of angina pectoris have been described: stable or typical angina, Prinzmetal's or variant angina, and unstable or crescendo angina. All of these patterns are associated with underlying coronary vessel disease and may be exhibited in a particular individual at different times and under different conditions.

Stable angina is the most common form and is therefore called classic or typical angina. Stable angina is characterized by stenotic atherosclerotic coronary vessels that reduce coronary blood flow to a critical level. The stenosed arteries dilate poorly in response to increased myocardial oxygen requirements. Under conditions of increased myocardial work load, such as during physical exertion or emotional strain, coronary perfusion is inadequate and ischemia results. The onset of anginal pain is generally predictable and elicited by similar stimuli each time. Stable angina is generally relieved by rest and nitroglycerin, a drug that causes peripheral vasodilation and reduces myocardial work load.

Prinzmetal's variant angina is characterized by unpredictable attacks of anginal pain. Although most individuals with Prinzmetal's angina have significant coronary atherosclerosis, the onset of ischemic symptoms is unrelated to physical or emotional exertion, heart rate, or other obvious causes of increased myocardial oxygen demand. Vasospasm has been identified as the probable mechanism leading to variant angina, although the cause of the vasospasm is unknown. Proposed mechanisms include atherosclerosis-induced hypercontractility, abnormal secretion of vasospastic chemicals by local mast cells, and abnormal calcium flux across the vascular smooth muscle. Variant angina responds well to treatment with calcium channel blocking drugs, which inhibit vascular smooth muscle contraction.

Unstable angina is characterized by a pattern of anginal attacks that occur with increasing frequency and severity over time. Unstable angina may represent a degree of ischemia that comes precariously close to causing actual death of cardiac tissue. Unstable angina is thought to progress to actual infarction of cardiac tissue in some cases and is therefore carefully evaluated and actively treated. In most patients, rupture of an atherosclerotic lesion with superimposed thrombus formation is present. However, collateral vessels provide enough perfusion to prevent actual cellular death. Vasospasm may also be involved. Unstable angina may be viewed as lying in between the reversible ischemia of classic angina on one end of the spectrum and the irreversible condition of myocardial infarction at the other end.

Myocardial Infarction

Myocardial infarction (MI) results from prolonged or total disruption of blood flow to the myocardium, causing irreversible cellular death. Acute MI is the most important form of IHD, resulting in about 500,000 deaths annually in the United States.[2] It is estimated that an American male has greater than a one in five chance of sustaining an MI or fatal ischemic event before the age of 65. An MI may occur at any age, but the frequency rises with advancing age. Females under 45 have a sixfold lesser risk of MI than men of the same age. After menopause the rate of MI in women approaches that of their male counterparts and becomes essentially equal by age 80.[8]

Precipitating Factors. Coronary atherosclerosis is the dominant pathogenetic mechanism for MI, just as it is for other forms of IHD. There is some controversy regarding the sequence of events that tips the scales from reversible ischemia to irreversible MI. Two types of MI have been described, each having different morphology and clinical significance. The **transmural infarct** involves the entire thickness of the ventricular wall and is the more serious of the two types. It is also the more common. A **subendocardial infarct,** in contrast, involves only the inner one third to one half of the ventricular wall (Fig. 17–2) and is generally associated with less severe symptoms. These lesions are not exclusive: the subendocardial MI can extend across the ventricular wall to become a transmural MI under certain circumstances. It is believed by some investigators that the pathophysiology of these two types of MI are somewhat different.

In about 90 percent of transmural MIs, the initiating event is believed to be development of a thrombus on top of an ulcerated or cracked atherosclerotic plaque.[9] The initiating event is a sudden change in structure of the plaque—cracking, hemorrhaging, or

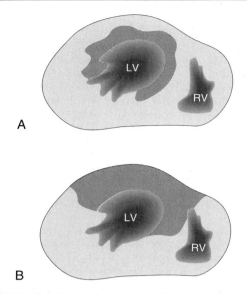

F I G U R E   17–2. Comparison of subendocardial infarct (**A**) and transmural infarct (**B**). RV, right ventricle; LV, left ventricle.

ulceration. The involved atheromatous plaque is usually already large enough to cause at least a 75 percent reduction in blood flow prior to the MI. The cause of plaque rupture remains uncertain but may involve local vasospasm with resulting trauma. Platelets passing by the surface of the ruptured plaque adhere to it, initiate formation of a platelet plug, and activate the clotting cascade. The resultant thrombus grows in size until it occludes the vessel and triggers the transmural MI. The thrombus theory of acute transmural MI was controversial for many years because only 50 percent of persons dying from transmural MI had demonstrable thrombus at autopsy. Then DeWood and co-workers[10] demonstrated that about 90 percent of persons with acute MI had an intracoronary thrombus within 4 hours of onset of symptoms, but only 60 percent had thrombi 12 to 24 hours later. This suggested that the thrombus was quickly dissolved by natural mechanisms after the occlusive event. Further support for the thrombus theory comes from the effectiveness of thrombolytic therapy, which successfully restores flow through obstructed coronary vessels in 75 to 95 percent of cases.[11]

The mechanism of transmural MI in the remaining 10 percent of cases having no thrombus formation remains speculative. In some instances no significant underlying atherosclerosis is present. Persistent vasospasm may be the culprit.

The pathophysiology of the subendocardial type of MI is less well established. The subendocardial surfaces of the heart are most vulnerable to any reduction in blood flow. The coronary arteries enter the myocardium at the outer epicardial surface and traverse thick ventricular walls before finally delivering blood to the endocardial areas. Factors such as an increased demand for oxygen in the setting of generalized atherosclerosis may be involved, although a role for thrombus has also been proposed. There is almost always underlying atherosclerotic coronary disease, but often no critical stenosis resulting in greater than 75 percent occlusion.

Cellular Pathophysiology. The cellular consequences of an acute interruption of blood flow to the myocardium do not occur instantaneously or uniformly. Acute occlusion causes a range of cellular events, depending on the availability and adequacy of collateral blood flow, the relative work load, and the length of time that flow is interrupted. A typical transmural infarct has several zones composed of cells in various stages of ischemia and death.

Experiments in animal models indicate that complete occlusion of a coronary vessel results in a predictable pattern of cellular dysfunction and death.[1] Depletion of ATP in acutely ischemic cells begins immediately, followed within 1 to 2 minutes by impaired ability to contract. Within 10 minutes, cellular concentrations of ATP fall to one-half normal, and irreversible cell injury occurs after 20 to 40 minutes of complete occlusion (Table 17–3). Ischemic necrosis begins in the subendocardial zone and spreads across the ventricular wall toward epicardial surfaces. Epicardial areas are spared for longer periods of time because they enjoy the greatest collateral network of arterial vessels. The ultimate size of the infarcted tissue depends on the extent, duration, and severity of ischemia. Areas of necrosis may be intermixed with or surrounded by zones of reversibly injured cells that are marginally perfused by collaterals. "Rescue" of these potentially salvageable cells is the focus of most treatment.

Morphology. Nearly all transmural infarcts are located in the left ventricular (LV) walls.[1] Isolated right ventricular (RV) infarction occurs in only 1 to 3 percent of MIs. Occlusion of the left anterior descending artery causes 40 to 50 percent of acute MIs, the right coronary artery contributes another 30 to 40 percent, and the left circumflex another 15 to 20 percent. The locations of the resulting infarcts are shown in Table 17–4. It is common for an individual with IHD to suffer from more than one MI during his lifetime.

The area of necrosis resulting from MI undergoes a series of morphologic changes as the infarct ages. These morphologic changes generally cannot be detected on gross examination until 6 to 12 hours post infarct. After 18 to 24 hours the area of infarct becomes paler than surrounding tissues. Thereafter the area of infarct becomes obvious as it turns yellowish and soft with a rim of red vascular connective tissue. At 1 to 2 weeks the necrotic tissue is progressively degraded and cleared away. Infarcted myocardium is particularly weakened and susceptible to rupture at this time. By 6 weeks the necrotic tissue has been replaced by tough fibrous scar tissue.

Clinical Course and Symptoms. The diagnosis of MI is based on three primary indicators: (1) symptoms, (2) electrocardiographic (ECG) changes, and (3) elevations of specific enzymes in the blood. Other diagnostic examinations such as cardiac catheterization, echocardiography, and radionuclide scintigraphy may also be done to provide additional information.

TABLE 17–3. Cellular Events Following Myocardial Infarction

Time	Electron Microscope	Histochemistry	Light Microscope	Gross Changes
0–½ hr	*Reversible injury* Mitochondrial swelling; distortion of cristae; matrix densities; relaxation of myofibrils	↓ Dehydrogenases ↓ Oxidases ↓ Phosphorylases ↓ Glycogen ↓ K and ↑ Na$^+$ and Ca^{++}	?Waviness of fibers at border	
1–2 hr	*Irreversible injury* Sarcolemmal disruption: mitochondrial amorphous densities			
4–12 hr	Margination of nuclear chromatin		Beginning coagulation necrosis; edema hemorrhage; beginning neutrophilic infiltrate	
18–24 hr			Continuing coagulation necrosis; pallor (pyknosis of nuclei, shrunken eosinophilic cytoplasm), marginal contraction band necrosis	Pallor
24–72 hr			Total coagulative necrosis with loss of nuclei and striations; heavy interstitial infiltrate of neutrophils	Pallor, sometimes hyperemia
3–7 d			Beginning disintegration of dead myofibers and resorption of sarcoplasm by macrophages; onset of marginal fibrovascular response	Hyperemic border, central yellow-brown softening
10 d			Well-developed necrotic changes; prominent fibrovascular reaction in margins	Maximally yellow and soft vascularized margins, redbrown and depressed
7th wk				Scarring complete

From Cotran RS, Kumar V, Robbins SL (eds): *Robbins Pathologic Basis of Disease*, 4th ed. Philadelphia, WB Saunders, 1989, p 611. Reproduced with permission.

Symptoms. Severe crushing, excruciating chest pain that may radiate to the arm, shoulder, or jaw is the harbinger of acute MI. Pain is commonly accompanied by nausea, vomiting, sweating, and shortness of breath. In contrast to anginal pain, infarction pain generally lasts more than 15 minutes and is not relieved by rest or nitroglycerin. In some instances, however, the MI is entirely asymptomatic and may elude detection. Asymptomatic MI has been called "silent MI" and may be detected only serendipitously at a later date. Pain may be difficult to assess in individuals with a tendency to ignore or deny their symptoms. Thus, although pain is an important indicator of ischemia, other clinical information is often needed to correctly distinguish between angina, infarction, and noncardiac sources.

Electrocardiographic Changes. Myocardial ischemia and infarction often result in characteristic changes on ECG waveforms. Infarction is typified by the appearance of abnormally deep or wide Q waves and inverted T waves (Fig. 17–3). These changes are very specific for MI and when present are diagnostic. However, specific Q and T wave changes may be absent in 20 to 30 percent of patients suffering MIs.

Dysrhythmias and the characteristic S-T segment changes that accompany MI are attributed to injured and ischemic cells that have not yet become necrotic. Reversibly injured cells have limited ATP supplies to power membrane pumps and are predisposed to leakage of ions across their cell membranes. Abnormal ion flux may result in continuous current flow even

TABLE 17–4. Location of Myocardial Infarction According to Coronary Artery Affected

Arterial Obstruction	Location of Infarct
Left anterior descending (40–50% of infarcts)	Anterior wall of LV near apex Anterior 2/3 of interventricular septum
Right coronary (30–40% of infarcts)	Posterior wall of LV Posterior 1/3 of interventricular septum
Left circumflex (15–20% of infarcts)	Lateral wall of LV

Data from Cotran RS, Kumar V, Robbins SL (eds): *Robbins Pathologic Basis of Disease*, 4th ed. Philadelphia, WB Saunders, 1989.

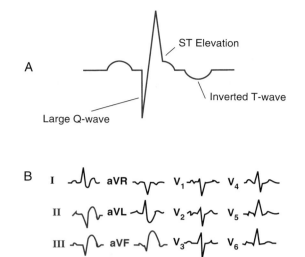

FIGURE 17–3. **A,** Typical ECG infarction pattern showing abnormally large Q wave and inverted T wave. **B,** Typical ECG in inferior myocardial infarction. Note leads II, III, aVF.

when the heart is at rest. This current leak may be detected by the ECG as S-T segment elevation.

The 12-lead ECG is used to localize the injured region of the LV. Various leads of the 12-lead ECG "look at" different regions of the heart. Abnormalities such as Q waves and S-T segment elevation in a particular lead or leads indicates that the damage is localized to the part of the LV "seen" by that lead. MIs may thus be described as anterior, lateral, posterior, septal, inferior, or any combination of these areas. (The 12-lead ECG is described in Chapter 16.)

Serum Enzymes. The appearance of certain intracellular enzymes in the blood after myocardial cell death is a very sensitive and reliable indicator of MI. Myocardial cell death leads to elevated serum levels of glutamic oxaloacetic transaminase (GOT, SGOT, AST), lactate dehydrogenase (LDH), and creatine kinase (CK). An increase in these enzymes suggests leakage from fatally damaged cells that have lost plasma membrane integrity. Cardiac cells contain particular forms of LDH and CK called isoenzymes. Cardiac isoenzymes have a slightly different amino acid sequence than other cell types. In particular, myocytes contain the isoenzymes MB-CK and LDH-1 and LDH-2. There is normally a small amount of LDH-1 in the blood and a slightly greater amount of LDH-2. After MI, the MB-CK and LDH levels rise in the blood. The ratio of LDH-1 to LDH-2 reverses from the normal pattern

as more LDH-1 isoenzyme is present than LDH-2. This is called a *flipped LDH* enzyme pattern. An elevated level of serum MB-CK is considered to be the best indicator of acute MI. Enzymes are elevated for a short time only and return to normal within several days (Table 17–5). Therefore, enzyme elevations are useful diagnostically only during the acute period of the MI.

In addition to chest pain, ECG abnormalities, and serum enzyme elevations, the person experiencing an MI may exhibit signs of cardiac inflammation, including fever, leukocytosis, and an elevated sedimentation rate. Symptoms of circulatory inadequacy including fatigue, restlessness, anxiety, and weakness may be present. Insufficient myocardial contraction after MI may result in low cardiac output. Several compensatory mechanisms are evoked in response to the inadequate cardiac output. In particular, the sympathetic nervous system is activated, thus increasing heart rate, contractility, and blood pressure. Unfortunately, the body's attempts to improve cardiac output cause the already damaged heart to work even harder. The events following MI are summarized in Figure 17–4. Compensatory mechanisms are shown in Figure 17–5.

Prognosis and Treatment. It is difficult to determine a prognosis for acute MI because many variables affect the outcome, including the extent and location of the infarct, previous cardiovascular health, age, and the presence of other disease processes. Of particular importance is the rapidity with which treatment is sought. Most deaths from MI occur before the victim reaches the hospital. Overall mortality within 1 year of MI is about 35 percent.[1] In approximately 10 to 20 percent of cases an MI is not accompanied by any complications (*uncomplicated MI*) and the patient recovers rapidly. However, the remaining 80 to 90 percent of MIs are followed by one or more complications.[1] Potential complications include cardiac dysrhythmias, congestive heart failure, cardiogenic shock, ventricular rupture, and thromboembolism.

Treatment of MI is directed at decreasing myocardial oxygen demand and increasing myocardial oxygen supply, while monitoring for and treating complications as they arise. Measures to reduce myocardial work load frequently include preload and afterload reduction, heart rate control, pain relief, and activity restriction. Sympathetic antagonists, nitrates, and morphine sulfate are the mainstays of drug therapy. Measures to increase oxygen delivery to the ischemic areas include thrombolytic drugs, coronary bypass

TABLE 17–5. Time Course of Enzyme Elevations After Myocardial Infarction

Enzyme	Initial Rise	Peak	Return to Normal
Creatine kinase	4–6 hr	24 hr	2–4 d
Glutamine oxaloacetic transaminase	8–12 hr	24–48 hr	4–6 d
Lactate dehydrogenase	12–24 hr	3–6 d	8–14 d

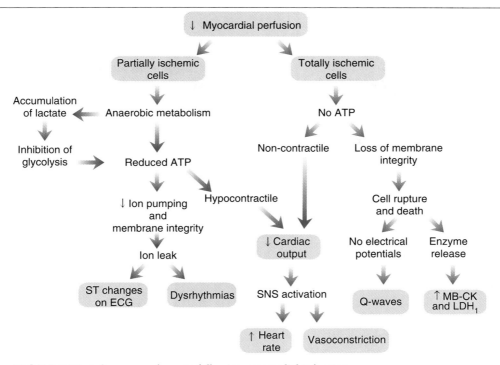

FIGURE 17-4. Summary of events following myocardial infarction.

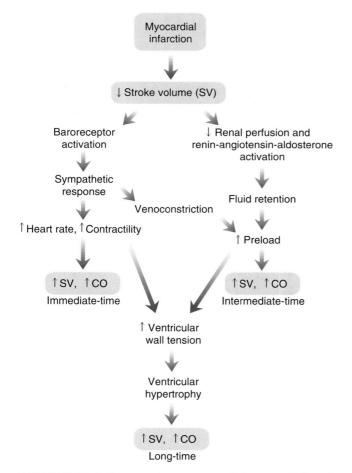

FIGURE 17-5. Compensatory responses to increase stroke volume (SV) and maintain cardiac output (CO) following myocardial infarction.

grafting, and balloon angioplasty. Thrombolytic agents can be administered systemically or directly into the blocked coronary artery. Common thrombolytics include streptokinase and tissue plasminogen activator (tPA). Coronary bypass grafting may be done to treat MI or to prevent it. This procedure uses an alternative vessel (mammary artery or saphenous leg vein) to circumvent the blocked portion of the coronary artery and reestablish flow downstream from an occlusion. A balloon-tipped catheter may be inserted into a blocked coronary to reopen it. This procedure is called percutaneous transluminal coronary angioplasty (PTCA). When the balloon is correctly positioned at the site of stenosis, it is inflated to crush the stenotic area and increase vessel diameter.

Early detection and treatment of dysrhythmias and conduction disorders are an important part of the immediate care of an MI patient. Many dysrhythmias are life-threatening and, at the very least, lead to decreased cardiac output or increased myocardial work load. Continuous ECG monitoring is generally the standard of care because of the high incidence of electrical disturbances following MI. Common dysrhythmias and conduction disorders are described in Chapter 18.

Chronic Ischemic Heart Disease

Chronic IHD has been designated to classify patients in whom heart failure develops insidiously as a consequence of progressive ischemic myocardial damage. In most cases there is a history of angina or MI, often many years prior to the onset of heart failure. Heart failure appears to be a consequence of slow, progressive atrophy of myocytes due to chronic ischemia. The disease is usually found in elderly individuals. Atrophic and dead cells are scattered throughout the myocardium rather than being localized, as occurs with MI. The prognosis for chronic IHD is quite poor, with death from congestive heart failure the common outcome. Heart failure is further discussed in Chapter 18.

Sudden Cardiac Death

Sudden cardiac death (SCD) is usually defined as unexpected death from cardiac causes within 1 hour of the onset of symptoms. Ischemic heart disease is at the root of a vast majority of cases of SCD. Rarely, SCD may be a complication of hereditary or acquired structural or electrical abnormalities. It is estimated that 300,000 to 400,000 individuals die each year in the United States from SCD.[12] SCD is most often associated with coronary atherosclerosis, although MI is found in only 25 percent of cases.[13] It appears that a lethal dysrhythmia such as asystole or ventricular fibrillation is the primary cause of death. Ischemia, diffuse myocardial atrophy, scarring and fibrosis of old MI tissue, and electrolyte imbalances are factors that may predispose the heart to the electrical abnormalities that lead to SCD.

KEY CONCEPTS

- The four ischemic heart disease syndromes are angina pectoris, myocardial infarction (MI), chronic ischemic heart disease, and sudden cardiac death. These are all due to progressive coronary atherosclerosis.

- Angina is characterized by intermittent bouts of chest pain brought on by exertion and generally relieved by rest. No permanent myocardial damage occurs.

- Prolonged or severe ischemia results in MI that is characterized by severe, unrelieved chest pain, nausea and vomiting, diaphoresis, shortness of breath, and inflammation (fever, increased WBC count, increased sedimentation rate).

- Enzyme elevations and ECG changes are diagnostic of MI. The enzyme changes are increased serum MB-CK fraction and flipped LDH enzymes (LDH-1 > LDH-2). ECG changes include large Q waves and inverted T waves.

- A drop in cardiac output due to MI triggers a number of compensatory responses, including sympathetic activation. The sympathetic nervous system increases heart rate, contractility, and blood pressure, all of which increase myocardial work load. Treatment usually includes efforts to decrease sympathetic nervous system activation of the heart (e.g., rest, heart rate control, pain relief, and afterload reduction).

Endocardial and Valvular Diseases

Endocardial and valvular structures may be damaged by inflammation and scarring, calcification, or congenital malformations. These processes interfere with the normal valvular properties of unimpeded flow and unidirectional flow. Although congenital malformations may affect any valve, acquired valvular disorders generally involve the mitral or aortic valves. Abnormalities of valvular function cause altered hemodynamics in the heart and generally result in an increased myocardial work load. Ultimately, heart failure may result from significant valvular dysfunction.

Normally, heart valves open completely, so that little or no pressure difference can be measured on either side of the valve. Failure of a valve to open completely is termed **stenosis**. Significant hemodynamic consequences generally occur when the valve opening is reduced to one half of normal. The degree of stenosis can be estimated by development of an abnormal pressure gradient across the valve. Stenosis results in extra pressure work for the heart, as blood must be forced through the high resistance of a narrow valve opening. Stenosis generally progresses slowly over years to decades, allowing time for affected heart chambers to compensate through dilation and hypertrophy.

Regurgitation or **insufficiency** refers to inability of a valve to close completely, thereby allowing blood to flow in a reverse direction. Regurgitation may develop suddenly due to valvular infection or rupture of a supporting papillary muscle. Sudden regurgitation is poorly tolerated, as little compensation is possible. Regurgitation results in extra volume work for the heart as more blood must be pumped to maintain adequate forward flow.

Diseased valves may exhibit elements of both stenosis and regurgitation, although one problem usually predominates. Postinflammatory scarring due to rheumatic heart disease and valvular calcification with aging are the primary causes of stenosis. A wide variety of diseases of the endocardium may lead to valvular regurgitation. These include rheumatic heart disease and infective endocarditis, which are discussed later in this chapter. Damaged valves are susceptible to infection, and antibiotic prophylaxis is therefore indicated for surgical and diagnostic procedures. The common causes of acquired mitral and aortic valvular diseases are listed in Table 17–6.

Disorders of the Mitral Valve

Three important disorders of the mitral valve are stenosis, regurgitation, and mitral valve prolapse. In **mitral stenosis** the flow of blood from the left atrium (LA) into the LV is impaired. Mitral stenosis is characterized by an abnormal LA/LV pressure gradient during ventricular diastole (Fig. 17–6). Normally the pressures in the atrium and ventricle are nearly equal

TABLE 17–6. Major Causes of Acquired Valvular Heart Disease

Mitral Valve Disease	Aortic Valve Disease
Mitral Stenosis	*Aortic Stenosis*
Postinflammatory scarring (rheumatic heart disease)	Postinflammatory scarring (rheumatic heart disease)
	Senile calcific aortic stenosis
	Calcification of congenitally deformed valve
Mitral Regurgitation	*Aortic Regurgitation*
Abnormalities of leaflets and commissures	Intrinsic valvular disease
Postinflammatory scarring	Postinflammatory scarring (rheumatic heart disease)
Infective endocarditis	Infective endocarditis
Floppy mitral valve	Aortic disease
Abnormalities of tensor apparatus	Syphilitic aortitis
Rupture of papillary muscle	Ankylosing spondylitis
Papillary muscle dysfunction (fibrosis)	Rheumatoid arthritis
Rupture of chordae tendineae	Marfan's syndrome
Abnormalities of left ventricular cavity and/or anulus	
LV enlargement (myocarditis, congestive cardiomyopathy)	
Calcification of mitral ring	

From Schoen FJ Jr: Symposium on cardiovascular pathology, part II. Surgical pathology of removed natural and prosthetic valves. *Hum Pathol* 1987;18:558. Reproduced with permission.

during ventricular diastole when the mitral valve is open. Figure 17–6 shows that with mitral valve stenosis, the atrial pressure remains higher than ventricular pressure throughout diastole. As stenosis worsens, the pressure gradient often increases. Increased pressure work of the LA leads to atrial chamber enlargement and hypertrophy. Progressive narrowing of the mitral valve may lead to markedly elevated LA pressures and increased pulmonary vascular pressure. If uncorrected, mitral stenosis may result in chronic pulmonary hypertension, RV hypertrophy, and right-sided heart failure.

Signs and symptoms of mitral stenosis are due to backup of volume and pressure in the LA and pulmonary circulation as well as decreased stroke volume of the LV due to deficient filling. Symptoms are exacerbated by conditions that further decrease LV filling, such as increased heart rate or other tachydysrhythmias. Atrial dysrhythmias, such as atrial fibrillation, are common due to excessive atrial volume. Atrial enlargement and fibrillation also predispose to the development of atrial clots, which may dislodge and result in systemic embolization. Signs and symptoms of mitral stenosis from pulmonary congestion may include orthopnea, cough, dyspnea on exertion, paroxysmal nocturnal dyspnea, abnormal breath sounds, and poor arterial oxygenation. Reduced LV stroke volume may be apparent as fatigue, poor activity tolerance, and weakness. Blood rushing through the narrowed mitral valve during ventricular diastole may be heard as a diastolic murmur at the heart's apex. In many cases, an abnormal heart sound, an opening snap, may also be heard.

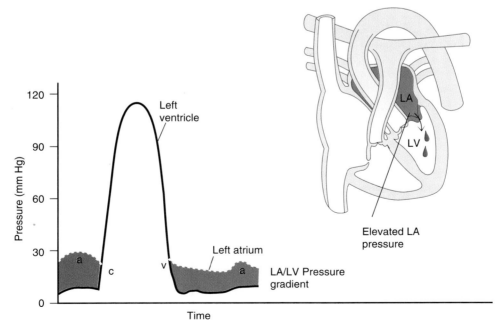

FIGURE 17–6. Mitral stenosis is characterized by an abnormal left atrial to left ventricular pressure gradient (*shaded area*).

In **mitral regurgitation** there is a backflow of blood from the LV into the LA during ventricular systole. Regurgitant flow elevates LA volume and pressure, leading to characteristic giant v waves on the atrial pressure monitor (Fig. 17–7). The severity of mitral insufficiency is related to the amount of LV stroke volume which is regurgitant. The LV must pump a greater volume to maintain an effective stroke volume. Both the LA and LV generally dilate and hypertrophy to compensate for the extra volume they are required to pump. Mitral regurgitation may lead to left heart failure if severe and uncorrected. Signs and symptoms of mitral regurgitation are similar to those described for mitral stenosis and result from pulmonary congestion and poor cardiac output. The murmur of mitral regurgitation occurs throughout ventricular systole (pansystolic).

As many as 7 percent of persons in the United States have mitral valves that balloon up into the LA during ventricular systole.[14] This condition is called **mitral valve prolapse** (Fig. 17–8). Women between the ages of 20 to 40 years are most often affected. In a great majority of cases the disorder is asymptomatic and is diagnosed only incidentally on routine physical examination. In some cases the prolapse is sufficient to cause a degree of mitral regurgitation. The cause of this valvular abnormality is uncertain, although it is commonly associated with other connective tissue disorders such as Marfan's syndrome or scoliosis.

Mitral valve prolapse may be detected by a midsystolic click or systolic murmur. Symptomatic individuals may experience palpitations, rhythm abnormalities, dizziness, fatigue, dyspnea, chest pain, or psychiatric manifestations such as depression and anxiety. The large majority have no untoward effects and are usually unaware of their condition. However, there are four serious, although rare, complications of mitral valve prolapse: (1) Infective endocarditis is more frequent and may warrant prophylactic antibiotics for invasive procedures. (2) A slow, insidious onset of mitral regurgitation may necessitate treatment. (3) Dysrhythmias may develop. (4) Sudden death may occur in association with fatal ventricular dysrhythmias, although it is considered a remote risk unless other cardiac pathology also is present.

Surgical repair for mitral prolapse is rarely indicated.

Disorders of the Aortic Valve

The primary disorders of the aortic valve are stenosis and regurgitation. With the decline in incidence of rheumatic fever, the predominant cause of aortic stenosis is age-related calcification. The hallmark of this disorder is calcium deposits piled up on the aortic cusps (Fig. 17–9). These aortic calcifications build up over several decades and generally become clinically apparent after age 70 to 90 years. Rheumatic heart disease, on the other hand, occurs primarily in children and young adults and now accounts for only about 10 percent of cases of acquired aortic stenosis. Causes of aortic regurgitation are similar to those of mitral regurgitation (see Table 17–6).

Aortic stenosis results in obstruction to aortic outflow from the LV during systole. This is characterized by a LV/Ao pressure gradient during ventricular ejection (Fig. 17–10). The LV develops high systolic pressures to overcome resistance of the stenotic aortic valve. The slow development of aortic stenosis allows

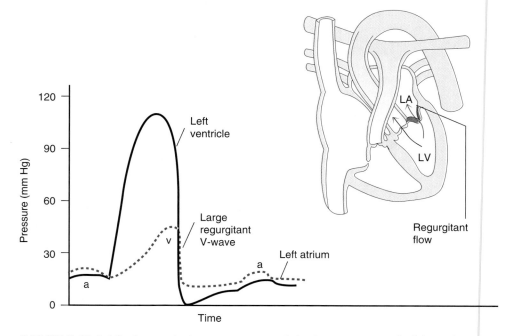

F I G U R E 17–7. Mitral regurgitation causes characteristic giant v waves on the left atrial pressure monitor.

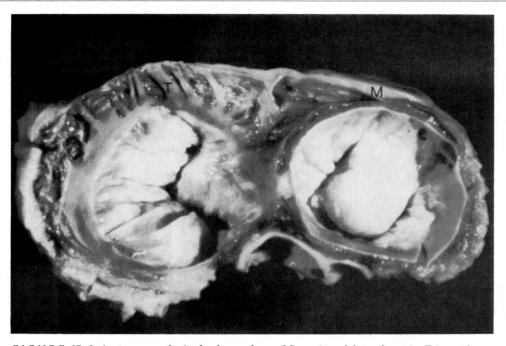

FIGURE 17–8. Appearance of mitral valve prolapse (M) as viewed from the atria. Tricuspid prolapse (T) is also present. (From Cotran RS, Kumar V, Robbins SL (eds): *Robbins Pathologic Basis of Disease*, 4th ed. Philadelphia, WB Saunders, 1989, p 629. Courtesy of L Riddick, MD, medical examiner, Alabama Institute of Forensic Sciences, and W Roberts, MD, National Institutes of Health, Bethesda, Md. Reproduced with permission.)

FIGURE 17–9. Appearance of calcium deposits on valvular cusps. (From Cotran RS, Kumar V, Robbins SL (eds): *Robbins Pathologic Basis of Disease*, 4th ed. Philadelphia, WB Saunders, 1989, p 627. Reproduced with permission.)

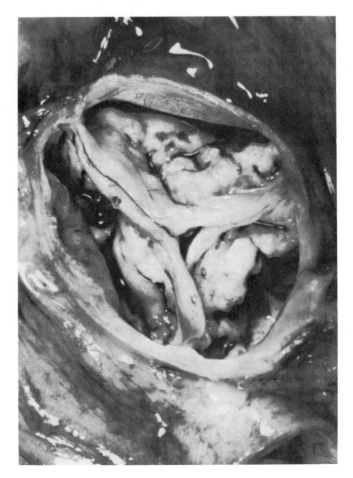

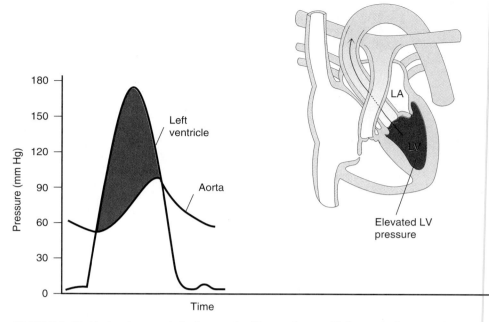

F I G U R E 17–10. Aortic stenosis is characterized by an abnormal left ventricular to aortic pressure gradient (*shaded area*).

the heart to maintain stroke volume by compensatory LV hypertrophy. The combination of high LV pressure and hypertrophy predisposes the heart to ischemia and attacks of anginal pain. Continued high LV afterload from a stenotic aortic valve may lead to left heart failure. Symptoms of aortic stenosis are due to diminished cardiac output, with pulmonary complications occurring later as the LV fails. Syncope, fatigue, low systolic blood pressure, and faint pulses are common signs and symptoms. A characteristic murmur occurs during ventricular systole and varies in intensity, getting progressively louder and then diminishing (crescendo-decrescendo). The heart rate is generally slow, allowing for a necessarily long ejection phase. Surgical correction is indicated for symptomatic aortic stenosis.

Aortic regurgitation results from an incompetent aortic valve that allows blood to leak back from the aorta into the LV during diastole. The LV becomes volume overloaded because it contains its usual preload, received from the atrium, plus regurgitant blood from the aorta. The LV compensates for this extra volume work with hypertrophy and dilation. A larger than normal stroke volume is thus achieved, resulting in a high systolic blood pressure. Diastolic blood pressure is generally lower than normal due to rapid runoff of blood into the ventricle. The large stroke volume and rapid decline in diastolic blood pressure result in a bounding peripheral pulsation (Fig. 17–11). Aortic insufficiency is characterized by a high-pitched blowing murmur during ventricular diastole. Patients may complain of palpitations and a throbbing or pounding heart due to the large ventricular stroke volume. The major complication of aortic regurgitation is left heart failure due to the high ventricular work load.

Rheumatic Heart Disease

Rheumatic heart disease is an uncommon but serious consequence of rheumatic fever. The incidence of rheumatic fever has steadily declined in the United States, but the disease still affects an estimated 15 to 20 million people a year worldwide.[15] Rheumatic fever is an acute inflammatory disease that follows infection with Group A β-hemolytic streptococci. Damage to tissues (principally joints, the heart, and the kidneys) is due to immune attack on the individual's own tissues. Antibodies against the streptococcal antigens are directed against self tissues. This may be an autoimmune phenomenon or a cross-reactivity between

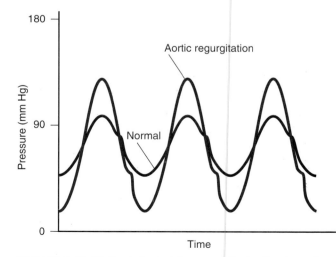

F I G U R E 17–11. Typical arterial pressure fluctuation in aortic regurgitation.

streptococcal antigens and certain tissue molecules. It is unknown why some individuals experience progressive tissue damage while others suffer no lasting consequences. A genetic predisposition to heightened immune responsiveness has been suggested.

The acute infection occurs primarily in children and is accompanied by fever and a sore throat. Only 3 percent of children with pharyngeal streptococcal infection go on to develop rheumatic fever.[1] Prompt initiation of antibiotic therapy is often effective in preventing rheumatic fever. Rheumatic fever diffusely affects connective tissue in joints, the heart, and the skin. The CNS and kidney are also frequently involved. Fifty to 75 percent of children and 35 percent of adults with rheumatic fever develop rheumatic heart disease.[16] Inflammation of the heart can include all layers, resulting in carditis. Endocardial inflammation results in valvular swelling, erosions, and clumping of platelets and fibrin on valve leaflets. Scarring and shortening of valvular structures may occur and become progressively more severe. The myocardium and pericardium may show signs of rheumatic inflammation. Other hallmarks of rheumatic fever include joint inflammation, involuntary movements (Sydenham's chorea), and a distinctive truncal rash. An elevated antibody titer against streptococcal products (streptolysin O) may help confirm the diagnosis. Unfortunately, individuals who experience rheumatic fever have a 50 percent chance of recurrence if they have another pharyngeal streptococcal infection.

Infective Endocarditis

Infective endocarditis is due to invasion and colonization of endocardial structures by microorganisms, with resulting inflammation. A variety of organisms are known to have an affinity for the endocardium, and for the cardiac valves in particular. Valvular lesions include growths of microorganisms enmeshed in fibrin deposits. These growths are called **vegetations** and may become quite large, interfering with valvular function and predisposing to embolus formation. The most common bacterial culprits are several strains of streptococci and *Staphylococcus aureus*. A requisite for infective endocarditis is invasion of the bloodstream by infective organisms. The portal of entry may be obvious, as with an overt infection, intravenous (IV) drug addiction, or invasive surgical or dental procedures. Sometimes the source may be less obvious, such as the gastrointestinal tract or oral cavity. Once the organism enters the circulation, several factors influence its ability to attack the endocardial structures and cause disease.

Acute infective endocarditis may theoretically develop in any individual if host resistance is low, the organism is highly virulent, and the bacterial invasion is sufficiently large. Acute infective endocarditis usually affects individuals with previously normal valves and leads to death in 50 to 60 percent of victims.[17] Intravenous drug abusers are particularly susceptible to acute infective endocarditis.

Subacute infective endocarditis has a more insidious onset and generally affects individuals with some preexisting propensity for valvular colonization. The offending organisms are less virulent. Rheumatic heart disease, congenital heart abnormalities, mitral valve prolapse, calcified valves, and artificial valves are important predisposing factors. Immunosuppression and persistent inoculation through IV drug abuse are other predisposing influences. *Staphylococcus aureus*, *S. epidermidis*, and *Candida*, which colonize the skin, are common offenders in IV drug users. The valves on the right side of the heart are usually infected in this population.

Organisms associated with subacute infective endocarditis are not virulent enough to attack normal healthy endocardium and are able to gain a foothold only in hearts having some underlying predisposition. Preexisting cardiac disease may allow the formation of platelet-fibrin deposits on the valves due to abnormal or stagnant blood flow patterns. These deposits become the site of organism attachment. Antibodies against the invader may further assist attachment by causing clumping together of organisms.

The diagnostic findings in both acute and subacute infective endocarditis are much the same. Large, bulky, bacteria-laden vegetations hang from the heart valves and adjacent endocardial surfaces. In addition to the risk of embolization, vegetations may cause erosion or perforation of the underlying valve leaflet. In acute forms, adjacent myocardium may be eroded and abscessed. With time, valvular vegetations become fibrotic and calcified. Unfortunately, the clinical presentation of subacute infective endocarditis is quite nonspecific, with low-grade fever the most consistent sign. Nonspecific fatigue, weight loss, and flulike symptoms may be the only clues. Positive blood cultures may help confirm the diagnosis.

Acute infective endocarditis has a more obvious onset with fever, chills, malaise, and frequently a heart murmur. Complications such as valvular insufficiency, embolization, and renal disease generally occur early in the course of the disease. The treatment for acute and subacute types centers on antibiotic therapy, with surgical replacement of valves when indicated. Prevention through prophylactic antibiotic therapy in individuals at risk is an important consideration.

The endocardium is prey to many other disorders such as systemic lupus erythematosus (an immunologic disease), calcium deposition secondary to renal disease, and nonbacterial thrombotic endocarditis secondary to hypercoagulable states associated with cancer.

KEY CONCEPTS

- **Valvular disorders are of two types. Stenotic valves fail to open properly, causing an abnormal pressure gradient across the valve and increasing the pressure work of the heart. Regurgitant valves allow blood to flow backward across the valve, resulting in extra volume work for the heart.**

- Mitral stenosis is characterized by a large left atrial to left ventricular gradient during ventricular diastole. Mitral stenosis leads to left atrial and pulmonary congestion.
- Mitral regurgitation is characterized by large v waves in the left atrial pressure tracing. Mitral regurgitation increases the work of the left atrium and ventricle and can lead to left heart failure.
- Aortic stenosis results in obstruction to outflow of blood from the left ventricle. It is characterized by a large left ventricular to aortic pressure gradient during systole. The extra pressure work can lead to left ventricular hypertrophy and failure.
- Aortic regurgitation is characterized by a high systolic and low diastolic blood pressure and a bounding pulse. Left ventricular failure may result, owing to high volume work.
- Rheumatic heart disease results from immune-mediated damage to the endocardium following Group A β-hemolytic infection.
- Acute and subacute infective endocarditis result in growth of bacteria-laden vegetations on heart valves. In addition to valvular erosion and scarring, embolization may occur.

Myocardial Diseases

In addition to the diseases already discussed, which secondarily affect the myocardium as a consequence of inadequate blood supply or endocardial infections, there are two additional categories of diseases of heart muscle, myocarditis and cardiomyopathy. Myocarditis is an inflammatory disorder of the heart muscle characterized by necrosis and degeneration of heart muscle cells. Cardiomyopathy includes several disorders of the heart muscle that may be genetic or acquired but are noninflammatory. The division of these categories is somewhat arbitrary; however, the clinical course of myocarditis is generally acute and stormy, with recovery or death from cardiac failure occurring weeks to months after the onset of symptoms. In contrast, the cardiomyopathies generally evolve more insidiously over years, with few symptoms until the heart slips into failure.

Myocarditis

Myocarditis is characterized by inflammation, leukocyte infiltration, and necrosis of cardiac muscle cells. Causes of myocarditis are innumerable but include all microbial agents, several forms of immune-mediated diseases, and several physical agents. Table 17–7 lists the more common causes of myocarditis. The true incidence of myocarditis is unknown because the diagnosis relies largely on circumstantial evidence.

Most cases of myocarditis are associated with viral infections. Immunosuppressed individuals and infants are particularly vulnerable. Cardiac involvement

TABLE 17–7. Major Causes of Myocarditis

Viruses	Metazoa
Coxsackie A and B virus	Echinococcus
ECHO virus, types 6, 7, 19, 22	Trichinella
Influenza virus	
Poliomyelitis virus	***Immune-Mediated Reactions***
Human immunodeficiency virus	Poststreptococcal (rheumatic fever)
Hepatitis virus	Systemic lupus erythematosus
Epstein-Barr virus (infectious mononucleosis)	Systemic sclerosis
Cytomegalovirus	Methyldopa
	Sulfonamides
Chlamydia	Penicillin
	Para-aminosalicylic acid
C. psittaci	Streptomycin
	Transplant rejection
Rickettsia	
	Physical Agents
R. typhi (typhus fever)	
R. tsutsugamushi (scrub typhus)	Radiation
	Heat stroke
Bacteria	
	Unknown
Corynebacterium (diphtheria)	
Salmonella	Sarcoidosis
Mycobacterium (tuberculosis)	Giant cell (Fiedler's) myocarditis
Streptococcus (β-hemolytic)	Kawasaki's disease
Neisseria (meningococcus)	
Leptospira (Weil's disease)	
Borrelia (relapsing fever)	
Fungi and Protozoa	
Trypanosoma (Chagas' disease)	
Aspergillus	
Blastomyces	
Cryptococcus	
Candida	
Coccidioidomyces	

From Cotran RS, Kumar V, Robbins SL (eds): *Robbins Pathologic Basis of Disease*, 4th ed. Philadelphia, WB Saunders, 1989, p 641. Reproduced with permission.

generally appears days or weeks after a viral infection elsewhere in the body. Documenting a viral cause is often impossible, but a rising antibody titer supports the diagnosis. The mechanism of viral myocarditis is uncertain. Direct viral cytotoxicity may occur, or the virus may evoke an immune response directed against the heart. Most investigators currently believe the second mechanism to be most likely. In countries other than the United States, nonviral organisms are more commonly associated with myocarditis. For example, *Trypanosoma crusi* is endemic in areas of South America, affecting about half the population. Of these, myocarditis occurs in about 80 percent of cases, causing death in a large proportion.[18]

In some cases of myocarditis, the individual's immune system appears to be the causative agent. Antibodies or activated lymphocytes are formed against heart tissues. Several drugs, including penicillin, have a propensity to evoke a hyperactive immune response in some individuals and may cause an allergic-type reaction that affects the myocardium. Regardless of the specific cause, there is a characteristic inflammation of cardiac muscle.

Acute myocarditis is most often characterized by general dilation of all four heart chambers. The ventricular myocardium is "flabby" with patchy or diffuse necrotic lesions. The heart muscle appears inflamed and edematous with white blood cell (WBC) infiltrates. Endocardial structures are usually normal. The clinical course of acute myocarditis varies in severity from asymptomatic to rapidly evolving heart failure. Generalized symptoms related to the inflammatory process may be present, as well as ECG changes due to myocardial cell death. Many persons recover completely, while others have progressive disease that manifests years later as "dilated cardiomyopathy." Thus, there is overlap and difficulty separating the myocarditis and cardiomyopathic forms of myocardial disease.

Cardiomyopathy

Cardiomyopathy is variously defined by different groups. The World Health Organization restricts the term to "noninflammatory heart muscle disease of unknown cause."[19] Others have adopted the terms **primary cardiomyopathy** for the unknown etiology category and **secondary cardiomyopathy** for myocardial dysfunction of known etiology. Both categories exclude hypertensive, congenital, valvular, ischemic, pericardial, and inflammatory myocardial disorders.

Primary Cardiomyopathy

The primary cardiomyopathies are, by definition, of unknown etiology. However, there are strong correlations with genetic and environmental causes for some types. Three types of primary cardiomyopathy can be identified, based on morphology and pathophysiology: dilated, hypertrophic, and restrictive.

Dilated or **congestive cardiomyopathy** is characterized by cardiac failure associated with dilation of all four heart chambers. Four factors are suspected in the initiation of dilated cardiomyopathy: (1) alcohol toxicity, (2) genetic abnormality, (3) pregnancy, and (4) postviral myocarditis. Alcohol and its metabolites are toxic to heart muscle cells and are associated with thiamine and other nutritional deficiencies. However, the exact mechanism of alcohol-associated cardiomyopathy remains unclear, justifying its continued inclusion in the category of primary cardiomyopathy. *Peripartum cardiomyopathy* is the term applied to cases of dilated cardiomyopathy discovered just before or just after delivery. A nutritional deficiency is suspected because, in most instances, it occurs in poor women having frequent pregnancies. In rare cases, dilated cardiomyopathy runs in families and has a presumed genetic basis. The nature of the genetic link has not been identified. Postviral myocarditis is an attractive pathogenetic mechanism for dilated cardiomyopathy, as previously discussed. Myocardial biopsies often reveal signs of inflammatory injury; however, progression from acute myocarditis to dilated cardiomyopathy has rarely been documented. A variety of other causes have been proposed as well. In fact, dilated cardiomyopathy is a bit of a catch-all term invoked to cover cases of dilated congestive failure having no well-defined origin.

Histologic examination of hearts with dilated cardiomyopathy reveals vague, nonspecific changes, or even no changes at all, in up to 25 percent of cases.[20] An occasional hypertrophied or atrophied myocyte may be apparent, along with mild fibrosis. The clinical presentation is one of slowly progressing biventricular heart failure. The diagnosis is based on exclusion of other causes. Cardiac transplantation is the only definitive treatment.

In contrast to dilated cardiomyopathy, **hypertrophic cardiomyopathy** is characterized by a thickened, hypercontracting heart. The hypertrophy is often not uniform throughout the heart and may primarily affect the septum, leading to the term *idiopathic hypertrophic subaortic stenosis* (IHSS). The LV is usually more involved than the RV. There is substantial evidence that this form of cardiomyopathy is transmitted genetically in an autosomal dominant pattern in half of the cases. The nature of the genetic defect is unknown. Abnormalities of cardiac myosin proteins have been suggested.[21]

Hypertrophic cardiomyopathy may be asymptomatic or may manifest with symptoms of ventricular outflow obstruction. Outflow obstruction is particularly problematic when the myocardial hypertrophy is localized in the subaortic septal region. Strenuous activity may precipitate profound outflow obstruction, negligible stroke volume, and sudden death. Other factors contributing to reduced stroke volume are a smaller intraventricular chamber size and a noncompliant ventricle. Microscopically, the hypertrophied muscle cells appear disorganized and haphazardly oriented. These changes may be a result of the high intraventricular pressures generated or the impaired blood supply, rather than themselves be causative factors.

The clinical course of hypertrophic cardiomyopathy is variable, with most patients experiencing little change in cardiac function over many years. In some patients congestive failure develops, which may actually improve the situation because reduced systolic contraction results in less outflow obstruction. Surgery to thin the septal thickening is rarely performed any longer, as it has been superseded by drug therapy. In general, drugs that increase myocardial contractility or heart rate are avoided because they further impair diastolic filling and worsen aortic outflow obstruction. β-Adrenergic antagonists and calcium channel blocking drugs may be used to dampen the hypercontractility. Long-term survival is possible.

Restrictive cardiomyopathy is the rarest form and is characterized by a stiff, fibrotic ventricle with impaired diastolic filling. The proposed mechanisms for development of ventricular fibrosis remain speculative and include amyloidosis, genetic inheritance, postviral syndrome, malnutrition, autoimmune disease, and even heavy consumption of bananas (rich in serotonin).[1] Regardless of the specific cause, the myocardium becomes fibrosed, rigid, and noncompliant. The major difficulty is restricted diastolic filling with resultant low stroke volume and congestive heart failure. Calcium channel blocking drugs may be instituted to enhance diastolic relaxation.

Secondary Cardiomyopathy

Cardiomyopathies of presumed known origin compose the category of secondary cardiomyopathy. Typical features are patchy necrosis, swelling, and fatty changes in the myocardium. Table 17–8 lists causative agents associated with secondary cardiomyopathy. Symptoms are generally similar to those described for dilated cardiomyopathy and are due to poor stroke volume and pulmonary congestion.

KEY CONCEPTS

- Myocarditis is an inflammatory disorder characterized by scattered necrotic and dead heart muscle cells. Most cases are associated with viral infections. The major complication of myocarditis is dilation of the four heart chambers, with reduced contractility.
- Cardiomyopathies encompass a number of disorders of heart muscle that may be genetic or acquired but are not inflammatory. In most cases the exact cause is unknown.
- Dilated cardiomyopathy is characterized by enlargement of all four chambers and reduced contractility.
- Hypertrophic cardiomyopathy affects primarily the left ventricle and ventricular septum. Conditions that increase contractility of the heart (exercise,

TABLE 17–8. Major Associations of Secondary Cardiomyopathy

Toxic	Neuromuscular Disease
Alcohol	Friedreich's ataxia
Cobalt	Muscular dystrophy
Catecholamines	Congenital atrophies
Carbon monoxide	
Lithium	*Storage Disorders*
Hydrocarbons	
Arsenic	Hunter-Hurler syndrome
Cyclophosphamide	Glycogen storage disease
Doxorubicin (Adriamycin)	Fabry's disease
Daunorubicin	Sandhoff's disease
Metabolic Disease	*Infiltrative*
	Leukemia
Hyperthyroidism	Carcinomatosis
Hypothyroidism	Sarcoidosis
Hypokalemia	
Hyperkalemia	*Immunologic*
Nutritional deficiency—thiamine, protein, other avitaminoses	Post transplant
Hemochromatosis	

From Cotran RS, Kumar V, Robbins SL (eds): *Robbins Pathologic Basis of Disease*, 4th ed. Philadelphia, WB Saunders, 1989, p 648. Reproduced with permission.

drugs) can result in obstruction of ventricular outflow and reduced cardiac output.
- Restrictive cardiomyopathy is characterized by a stiff, fibrotic left ventricle that resists diastolic filling. Decreased cardiac output and left-sided congestive failure can result.

Pericardial Diseases

Pericardial disorders are rarely isolated processes of primary etiology; rather, they are sequelae of other disorders such as systemic infection, trauma, metabolic derangement, or neoplasia. Despite the diversity of causative factors, pericardial involvement generally presents as an accumulation of fluid in the pericardial sac or inflammation of pericardial structures.

Pericardial Effusion

An accumulation of noninflammatory fluid in the pericardial sac is called *pericardial effusion*. Normally the pericardial space contains only 30 to 50 mL of thin, clear fluid. Under pathologic conditions, as much as 500 mL may accumulate. The composition of the usual types of effusions are:

1. *Serous*—a transudate secondary to congestive failure or hypoproteinemia.
2. *Serosanguinous*—a mixture of serous fluid and blood that may follow blunt chest trauma or cardiopulmonary resuscitation.
3. *Chylous*—a collection of lymph due to obstruction of lymphatic drainage.
4. *Blood*—hemopericardium usually resulting from penetrating trauma to the heart.

The accumulation of pericardial fluid is generally without clinical significance except as an indicator of underlying disease processes. However, if the fluid accumulation is large or occurs suddenly, the life-threatening condition of **cardiac tamponade** may ensue. Tamponade refers to external compression of the heart chambers such that filling is impaired. Signs and symptoms of cardiac tamponade include reduced stroke volume and compensatory increases in heart rate. Systemic venous congestion occurs as blood is prevented from entering the compressed heart by way of the superior and inferior venae cavae. Venous congestion may be apparent as distended neck veins. Changes in intrathoracic pressure during respiration may have exaggerated effects on cardiac filling. The waxing and waning of blood pressure in synchrony with respiration is called **pulsus paradoxus.** Significant pulsus paradoxus is usually defined as a difference of 10 mm Hg or more in systolic blood pressure between inspiration and expiration. Other manifestations of tamponade include rising filling pressures in the heart chambers, muffled heart sounds, dull chest pain, diminished ECG amplitude, and a compressed cardiac silhouette on x-ray. Treatment of tamponade is aimed at relieving the pericardial pressure by aspi-

TABLE 17–9. Causes of Pericarditis

Infectious Agents	Miscellaneous
Viral	Myocardial infarction
Pyogenic bacteria	Uremia
Tuberculous	Postcardiac surgery
Fungal	Neoplasia
Other parasites	Trauma
	Radiation
Presumably Immunologically Mediated	
Rheumatic fever	
Systemic lupus erythematosus	
Scleroderma	
Postcardiotomy	
Postmyocardial infarction	
Drug-hypersensitivity reaction	

From Cotran RS, Kumar V, Robbins SL (eds): *Robbins Pathologic Basis of Disease*, 4th ed. Philadelphia, WB Saunders, 1989, p 649. Reproduced with permission.

rating the offending fluid. Failure to treat tamponade may result in drastically reduced diastolic filling, cardiovascular collapse, and death.

Nonsymptomatic pericardial effusions may be aspirated (*pericardiocentesis*) or merely monitored and allowed to resolve spontaneously. Treatment is directed at the underlying cause of the effusion.

Pericarditis

Inflammation of the pericardium originates from a variety of causes (Table 17–9). Rarely is the pericardium the primary site of disease. Pericarditis is often categorized into acute and chronic forms; however, these are morphologically and etiologically similar. Chronic pericarditis refers to a healed stage of the acute form that results in chronic pericardial dysfunction.

Acute Pericarditis

Acute pericarditis can be categorized according to the character of the inflammatory exudate—serous, fibrinous, purulent, hemorrhagic, or caseous. The usual etiologic agents and major morphologic findings in each form are summarized in Table 17–10. The symptoms of acute pericarditis are due to the systemic effects of inflammation and pericardial damage and include fever, leukocytosis, malaise, and tachycardia. Sticking and rubbing of the visceral and parietal pericardial layers cause pain, which may radiate to the back and be associated with esophageal discomfort and dysphagia (difficulty swallowing). Acute pericarditis may be confused with anginal pain. Rubbing of the pericardial layers may be heard as a friction rub. The rub can be transient and intermittent and may sound squeaky or like scratchy sandpaper. Epicardial injury due to pericarditis may be apparent on the ECG as S-T segment elevation. Treatment is generally symptomatic and includes measures to relieve pain and minimize inflammation.

Chronic Pericarditis

Healing of an acute form of pericardial inflammation may result in **chronic (healed) pericardial dysfunction** of two principal kinds, adhesive mediastinopericarditis and constrictive pericarditis. **Adhesive media-**

TABLE 17–10. Etiology and Morphology of Types of Pericarditis

Type of Pericarditis	Etiology	Morphology
Serous	Nonbacterial Rheumatic fever Tumors Uremia Viral (coxsackie A, B; adenovirus; influenza virus; mumps)	Epicardial and pericardial inflammation with few WBCs. Volume of fluid is moderate (50–200 mL). Rarely progresses to fibrous adhesions.
Fibrinous and sero-fibrinous	Myocardial infarct Uremia Irradiation Lupus erythematosus Trauma Bacterial infection Viral infection	Inflammation with large amounts of plasma protein including fibrin. Fibrin may cause loose adherence of the pericardial layers. Friction rub is common.
Purulent or suppurative	Bacterial Mycotic Parasitic	Exudate is creamy pus composed of large amounts of protein and WBCs. Large amount of fluid is common (400–500 mL). Progresses to chronic restrictive pericarditis.
Hemorrhagic	Tuberculosis Malignant neoplasm Surgical trauma	Composed of blood mixed with a fibrinous or purulent exudate.
Caseous	Tuberculosis	Cottage cheese-like exudate. Often progresses to chronic restrictive pericarditis.

Data from Cotran RS, Kumar V, Robbins SL (eds): *Robbins Pathologic Basis of Disease*, 4th ed. Philadelphia, WB Saunders, 1989.

stinopericarditis is usually a consequence of suppurative or caseous pericarditis or a complication of previous cardiac surgery. It may also follow significant irradiation of the chest. The pericardial sac is destroyed and the external aspect of the heart adheres to surrounding mediastinal structures. The work load of the heart increases significantly as contraction is opposed by the attached surrounding structures.

Constrictive pericarditis may be a result of previous suppurative or caseous pericarditis, commonly due to tuberculosis. However, in many cases the cause of pericardial dysfunction is unknown. The pericardial sac becomes dense, nonelastic, fibrous, and scarred. It encases the heart like a stiff cage, impairing diastolic filling. The constrictive process generally occurs slowly and may be quite advanced by the time symptoms occur. Symptoms may include exercise intolerance, weakness, fatigue, and systemic venous congestion. Treatment is aimed at relieving the constriction by removal of pericardium (*pericardectomy*) and measures to improve cardiac contractility.

KEY CONCEPTS

- Large accumulations of pericardial fluid can result in cardiac tamponade. External compression of the heart chambers impairs diastolic filling and results in decreased stroke volume. Distended neck veins, pulsus paradoxus, elevated and equalized intrachamber pressures, and muffled heart sounds are indicative.
- Acute pericarditis causes sticking and rubbing of the visceral and parietal pericardial layers. A friction rub, pain radiating to the back, esophageal discomfort, and generalized signs of inflammation are usually present.
- Chronic pericarditis can lead to destruction of the pericardial sac with adhesion of the heart to surrounding mediastinal structures. Cardiac contraction may be impaired.
- Constrictive pericarditis results in a fibrous, scarred pericardium that restricts cardiac filling.

Congenital Heart Diseases

Congenital heart disease is an abnormality of the heart that is present from birth. A wide variety of defects have been described, and only the pathophysiology of the most common defects will be included. A brief description of fetal cardiac development is a necessary prelude to a discussion of the congenital heart diseases.

Embryologic Development

The development of the heart involves a complex orchestration of formation and resorption of structures. A necessarily simplified version of cardiac embryology is presented here. For a thorough treatment of cardiac embryology, the reader is referred to other sources.[22] Abnormalities in the development of four

important heart structures are at the root of most of the common heart defects. These are (1) development of the atrial septum, (2) development of the ventricular septum, (3) division of the main outflow tract (truncus arteriosus) into the pulmonary and aortic arteries, and (4) development of the valves. Each of these is briefly reviewed.

The primitive heart begins as an enlarged tube, much like a blood vessel. The tube has three layers. The inner luminal layer is thin and composed of endothelial cells. This layer will eventually line the inner chambers of the heart and valves. The outermost layer is also thin and is called the myoepicardial mantle. The outer mantle will form the epicardial and muscular structures of the heart. In between these two thin layers of cells is a thick layer of gelatinous substance called cardiac jelly. Cardiac jelly is the precursor to endocardial cushion tissue, which is important in formation of membranes in the heart, including the septa that separate the four chambers of the heart.

By day 23, the heart tube begins to beat. The tube folds upon itself to form an asymmetric loop structure (Fig. 17–12). One bulge of the loop forms a primitive single atrium, another forms the future LV, and a third forms the future RV and common ventricular outflow tract (truncus arteriosus). The common atrium is divided into right and left atria by growth of the interatrial septum. Atrial septation occurs in several steps. First, the *septum primum* is formed passively in the superior surface by an indentation caused by the overlying truncus arteriosus (Fig. 17–13). Next, the superior and inferior endocardial cushions grow and extend toward each other (see Fig. 17–13). These flaps of tissue overlap but do not fuse, so that blood is able to pass through from the right atrium to the left atrium. A reverse in the direction of flow, as occurs

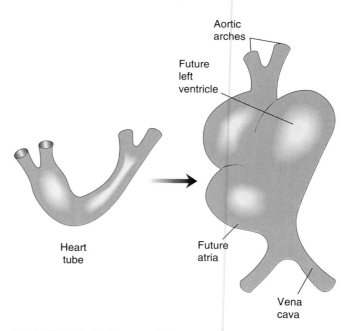

FIGURE 17–12. Asymmetric loop structure in early embryonic development of the heart.

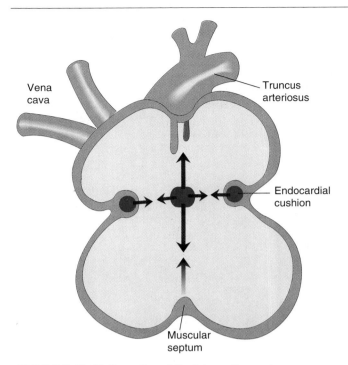

FIGURE 17–13. Formation of the intracardiac septa.

at birth, would push the flap shut and close the hole. This flaplike opening, called the *ostium secundum*, remains open throughout fetal life and is later called the *foramen ovale*.

Septal formation between the ventricles follows a similar pattern. The lower portion of the interventricular septum is formed by circular growth and fusing of the muscular ventricular walls. Then the muscular septum proliferates upward toward the atria. The inferior endocardial cushion tissue also grows downward to meet the uplifting muscular septum (see Fig. 17–13).

At about the same time that the atrial and ventricular septal structures are being elaborated, the common ventricular outflow tract, the truncus arteriosus, is divided into the pulmonary and aortic channels. This is accomplished by growth and eventual fusion of mounds of endocardial cushions located in the wall of the truncus arteriosus. The truncal endocardial cushions go on to form the semilunar valves as well (Fig. 17–14).

The atrioventricular septum and valves are similarly formed by the growth and fusion of the right and left lateral cushions. Superior and inferior cushions also contribute to formation of the septum between atria and ventricles. Leaflets of the valves are initially formed by lumps of cushion material, which are replaced by muscle tissue from the ventricular wall. The muscle tissue also forms the chordae tendineae and papillary muscle structures. Eventually the muscle cells of the leaflets and chordae tendineae are replaced by tough fibrous connective tissue.

When the embryonic heart is fully developed, there remain two important passageways that permit blood flow to bypass the lungs (Fig. 17–15). The foramen ovale lies between the left and right atria and allows blood to bypass the RV. Blood flows right to left through the atrial opening because the pressure in the left atrium is low. High resistance of the deflated lungs also causes RV pressure to be high, which impedes RV filling. The other important structure is the ductus arteriosus, a channel that connects the pulmonary artery and the aorta. Blood flows from the pulmonary artery into the aorta during fetal life because of high vascular resistance in the collapsed lungs. Both of these communications generally close after birth when the lungs inflate and the resistances on the right side of the heart fall. Clamping the umbilical cord also serves to increase systemic vascular resistance, which further augments the reverse in pressure gradient, with left heart pressures now exceeding the right.

Etiology and Incidence

Congenital heart disease is the most common heart disorder among children, with an overall incidence of 0.5 to 1 percent of all live births.[23] Ten of the most common heart defects are listed in Table 17–11, with approximate frequencies of occurrence. In over 90 percent of cases the cause of the heart defect is unknown. Multifactorial inheritance with both genetic and environmental influences is probable. Very few cases of congenital malformations can be clearly attributed to environmental factors. Maternal rubella during the first trimester of pregnancy is the best-documented environmental cause of heart defects. A large number of cardiac teratogens are suspected, based on animal

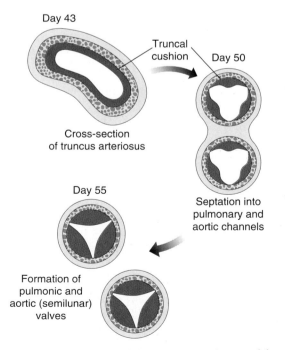

FIGURE 17–14. Septation of the truncus arteriosus and formation of the semilunar valves.

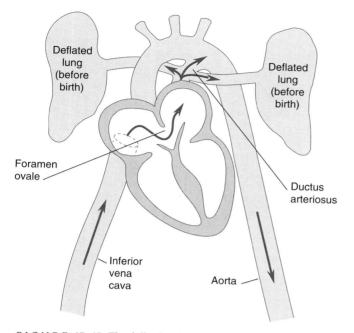

F I G U R E 17–15. The fully developed embryonic heart showing the foramen ovale and ductus arteriosus.

Pathophysiology

The many forms of congenital heart anomalies result in two primary pathologies, shunts or obstructions. A **shunt** denotes an abnormal path of blood flow through the heart or great vessels. The shunt may be further characterized as right to left or left to right, indicating the direction of abnormal blood flow. Right-to-left shunts allow unoxygenated blood from the right heart to enter the left heart and systemic circulation without first passing through the lungs. Infants with right-to-left shunting of blood generally have some degree of cyanosis due to the decreased oxygen content of the arterial blood (cyanotic defect). Conversely, a left-to-right shunt occurs when oxygenated blood from the left heart or aorta flows back into the right heart to be recirculated through the lungs. The blood reaching the systemic circulation is normally oxygenated and the infant is not cyanotic (acyanotic defect). However, the right heart has an increased work load due to the extra shunt blood. In time, the overload of the right heart can result in RV hypertrophy and high right heart pressures. A left-to-right shunt may then progress to a more dangerous right-to-left shunt when right heart pressures exceed pressures in the left heart. Congenital disorders causing abnormal blood flow through the heart include atrial septal defect, ventricular septal defect, patent ductus arteriosus, tetralogy of Fallot, transposition of the great arteries, truncus arteriosus, and tricuspid atresia.

Some heart anomalies produce **obstructions** to blood flow because of abnormal narrowings. Stenosis or atresia (failure to develop) of valves and coarctation of the aorta are the most common obstructive defects. Obstructions do not result in cyanosis but generally increase the work load of the affected chamber. In addition to being classified according to pathology as obstructions or shunts, heart defects are also classified according to the clinical manifestation of cyanosis. The acyanotic disorders include the obstructive disorders and left-to-right shunts. The cyanotic category in-

studies. These include hypoxia, ionizing radiation, and heavy alcohol consumption.

There are several indications that genetic influence is important in cardiac malformation. There is a two- to tenfold increase in the incidence of congenital heart defects among siblings. Several heart defects also occur more frequently in males. However, twin studies show that only in 10 percent of cases does a heart defect (ventricular septal defect) afflict both infants, even though their genotype is identical.[24] Thus, there is a complex interplay between genetic and environmental influences that is as yet poorly understood.

T A B L E 17–11. Approximate Frequencies of Cardiac Malformations

Malformation	Percentage of Congenital Heart Disease	Male-Female Ratio
Ventricular septal defect (VSD)	30	1:1
Patent ductus arteriosus (PDA)	10	1:2.5
Atrial septal defect (ASD)	10	1:3
Pulmonic stenosis	7	1:1
Coarctation of aorta	7	3–4:1
Aortic stenosis	6	3–5:1
Tetralogy of Fallot	6	1:1
Transposition of great arteries	4	3:1
Persistent truncus arteriosus	2	1:1
Triscuspid atresia	1.5	1:1

From Cotran RS, Kumar V, Robbins SL (eds): *Robbins Pathologic Basis of Disease,* 4th ed. Philadelphia, WB Saunders, 1989, p 619. Reproduced with permission.

cludes abnormalities causing right-to-left shunts. Specific heart defects are described further using this categorization.

Acyanotic Congenital Defects

Atrial Septal Defect

During the third to fifth week of fetal development, the left and right atria are separated by flaps of tissue that become the atrial septum. A flaplike opening in the septum, called the foramen ovale, remains patent during intrauterine life such that blood may pass from the right to the left atrium and bypass the uninflated and nonfunctional lungs (Fig. 17–16). The foramen ovale normally remains open in utero because the pressure on the right side of the heart is higher than on the left. With birth, however, the pressure gradient reverses as the lungs inflate and greatly reduce the pulmonary vascular resistance. The higher left-sided pressure forces the flap shut, and fusion of the foramen ovale membrane normally occurs. Ninety percent of **atrial septal defects** (ASDs) occur at the location of the foramen ovale (Table 17–12). The abnormal septal opening may be of variable size. Small defects (<1 cm) are well tolerated. Even larger ASDs may be asymptomatic for many years as long as the shunt flow is left to right and therefore acyanotic. The long-term increase in pulmonary blood flow may eventually lead to pulmonary hypertension, RV hypertrophy, and a reversal of the shunt to a right-to-left pattern. Cyanosis, respiratory difficulty, and right heart failure may then ensue. Large or symptomatic ASDs are commonly repaired surgically early in life, before pulmonary complications occur.

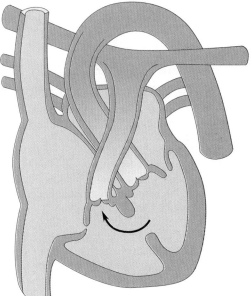

FIGURE 17–17. Ventricular septal defect.

Ventricular Septal Defect

Ventricular septal defect (VSD) is the most common congenital cardiac anomaly. It is frequently associated with other cardiac defects such as tetralogy of Fallot, transposition of the great arteries, and ASDs. The ventricular septum develops between the fifth and sixth weeks of fetal life as the membrane derived from endocardial cushion fuses with the muscular septum (Fig. 17–17). Ninety percent of VSDs are located within the membranous septum, very close to the bundle of His. As with ASD, the functional significance depends largely on the size of the defect. The shunt is initially left to right, as left heart pressures are highest. With the increase in pulmonary blood flow, pulmonary hypertension and RV hypertrophy may result, causing a reversal of the shunt. Large VSDs may be apparent at birth because of rapidly developing right heart failure and a loud systolic murmur. Large, symptomatic defects in infants or moderate defects in older children are repaired surgically to avoid progression to pulmonary vascular disease.

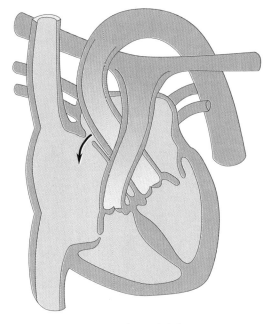

FIGURE 17–16. Atrial septal defect.

TABLE 17–12. Anatomic Locations of Atrial Septal Defects

Type	Location	Frequency
Ostium secundum	Midseptal wall at foramen ovale	90% of cases
Ostium primum	Low in atrial septal wall near AV valves	5% of cases
Sinus venosus	High in atrial septal wall near entrance of superior vena cava	5% of cases

Small VSDs in infants are generally not immediately repaired because of the tendency to close spontaneously.

Patent Ductus Arteriosus

The ductus arteriosus is a normal channel between the pulmonary artery and the aorta that remains open during intrauterine life (Fig. 17–18). Within 1 to 2 days after birth, the ductus arteriosus closes functionally, and within a few weeks it closes permanently. The ductus arteriosus allows blood to flow from the pulmonary artery into the aorta, thus bypassing the lungs. Low oxygen tension and local production of prostaglandins appear to be important in maintaining patency of the channel during fetal life. After birth the flow through the ductus arteriosus is left to right, due to the higher pressure in the aorta. This brings oxygenated blood through the ductus arteriosus and stimulates it to close. In many cases the reason for abnormal continued patency of the ductus arteriosus after birth is not well understood. Conditions that cause low blood oxygen tension may contribute to continued patency. Most often a **patent ductus arteriosus** (PDA) has no clinical significance early in life because the shunt is left to right and no cyanosis is evident. Surgical treatment is usually not immediately undertaken because these defects tend to close spontaneously. Prostaglandin inhibitors may be given to induce closure of the defect. Continued patency of the ductus arteriosus is usually obvious because of a harsh, grinding systolic murmur and often a systolic thrill (vibration). Surgical closure of the PDA is done as soon as it becomes evident that spontaneous closure is unlikely. As with other left-to-right shunt disorders, uncorrected PDA results in pulmonary hyper-

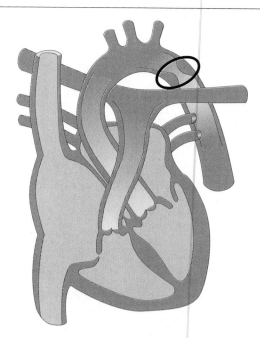

F I G U R E 17–19. Coarctation of the aorta.

tension complicated by respiratory and right heart failure. Eventual reversal of the shunt to a right-to-left pattern results in cyanosis. Because the ductus is usually located distal to the origin of the subclavian artery, the lower extremities may show cyanosis, whereas the upper extremities remain pink.

Coarctation of the Aorta

Coarctation refers to a narrowing or stricture that may impede blood flow. **Coarctation of the aorta** is a common heart defect that affects males three to four times more frequently than females. Narrowing of the aorta may occur anywhere along its length; however, in most cases the coarctation is located just before or just after the ductus arteriosus (Fig. 17–19). Preductal coarctation is usually more severe and often associated with other anomalies. In some instances the aortic stricture is so severe that blood flow to the lower body must be maintained solely through flow through the ductus arteriosus. This results in a very high work load for the right heart and may lead to congestive failure in the early neonatal period. Blood supply to the arms and head is unaffected, as these arteries arise proximal to the stricture. Postductal coarctation is generally less severe and may go unrecognized until adulthood. There is typically an elevated blood pressure in the upper extremities, with weak pulses and low blood pressure in the lower extremities. All types of coarctation are usually accompanied by systolic murmurs and ventricular hypertrophy. The stricture can be repaired surgically by resection of the narrowed region. If left untreated, significant coarctation may lead to congestive heart failure, intracranial hemorrhage, or aortic rupture.

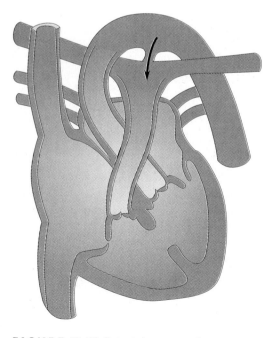

F I G U R E 17–18. Patent ductus arteriosus.

Pulmonary Stenosis or Atresia

Isolated pulmonary stenosis and atresia are included in the category of acyanotic defects because they do not themselves result in cyanosis. However, they often occur in conjunction with other anomalies that allow survival into the neonatal period. The other defects may allow shunting of blood and result in cyanosis. In **pulmonary atresia** there is no communication between the RV and the lungs, so that blood must enter the lungs by first traveling through a septal opening and then through a PDA. The RV is typically underdeveloped (hypoplasia) and the ASD is large. **Pulmonary stenosis** can be mild to severe, depending on the extent of narrowing of the pulmonic valve. Pulmonary stenosis is usually due to abnormal fusion of the valvular cusps. RV hypertrophy occurs secondary to the high ventricular afterload caused by the narrowed outflow opening. Isolated pulmonary stenosis is easily corrected by surgery; however, the prognosis depends in large part on the health of the RV.

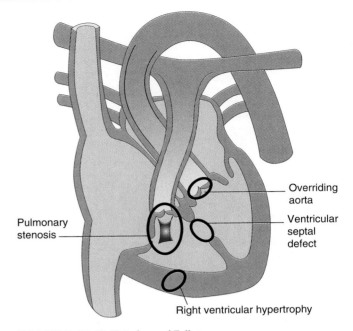

FIGURE 17–20. Tetralogy of Fallot.

Aortic Stenosis or Atresia

Congenital **aortic atresia** is rare and not compatible with survival. Depending on severity, **aortic stenosis** is correctable and associated with a good prognosis. Aortic stenosis may involve the valvular cusps or the subvalvular fibrous ring just below the cusps. The narrowed aortic outflow tract results in a high LV afterload, which causes the LV to hypertrophy. A prominent systolic murmur is usually apparent. Surgical replacement is the definitive treatment if the stenosis is severe, progresses, or becomes symptomatic.

Transposition of the Great Arteries

In the most common form of **transposition of the great arteries,** the aorta arises from the RV and the pulmonary artery arises from the LV (Fig. 17–21). This anomaly results in formation of two separate, noncommunicating circulations. The right heart receives blood from the systemic circulation and recirculates it through the body by way of the aorta. Blood reaching the body has not passed through the lungs and is therefore poorly oxygenated. The left heart receives

Cyanotic Congenital Defects

Tetralogy of Fallot

The four defining features of **tetralogy of Fallot** are (1) a VSD, (2) an aorta positioned above the ventricular septal opening (overriding aorta), (3) pulmonary stenosis that obstructs RV outflow, and (4) RV hypertrophy (Fig. 17–20). The severity of the symptoms is related primarily to the degree of pulmonary stenosis. The heart is generally enlarged due to the extensive RV hypertrophy. Even if the condition is untreated, individuals with tetralogy may live into adulthood. The defect often results in cyanosis because the overriding aorta receives unoxygenated blood from the right heart as well as oxygenated blood from the left heart. The degree of cyanosis depends on the amount of blood received from the right heart, which in turn depends on the degree of pulmonic obstruction. Surgical correction is usually recommended because prolonged palliation carries the risk of infective endocarditis and secondary polycythemia.

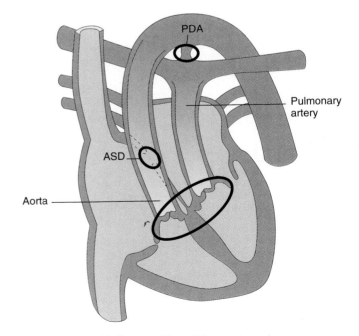

FIGURE 17–21. Transposition of the great arteries.

oxygenated blood from the lungs and then recirculates it through the lungs again, by way of the pulmonary artery. Unless there is some mixing of these separate circulations through other heart defects, such as septal defects, transposition is not compatible with life. Nearly all infants who survive the neonatal period have an interatrial opening, and most also have a PDA. A good deal of mixing must be maintained after birth for the infant to survive. Surgery may be directed at improving the mixing of systemic and pulmonary blood by enlarging or creating openings in the heart. An artificial conduit may also be placed that directs blood from the right atrium into the LV and from the left atrium into the RV. The RV is then able to pump oxygenated blood into the systemic circulation. Long-term survival depends, in part, on the ability of the RV to sustain the increased work load imposed by the high systemic vascular resistance.

Truncus Arteriosus

Truncus arteriosus is a congenital malformation in which the pulmonary artery and aorta fail to separate, resulting in the formation of one large vessel that receives blood from both the right and left ventricles (Fig. 17–22). There is a large VSD and a single valvular structure leading to the single large artery. Mixing of blood from the right and left hearts results in systemic cyanosis. The amount of blood entering the systemic versus the pulmonary circulation depends on the degree of vascular resistance in the two systems. Abnormally high pulmonary blood flow may progress to pulmonary hypertension and RV hypertrophy. Increased pulmonary resistance causes cyanosis to become more severe as more blood enters the systemic circulation. Surgical correction is required for survival.

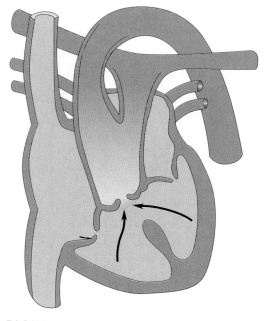

F I G U R E 17–22. Truncus arteriosus.

Tricuspid Atresia

Absence of the tricuspid valve is almost always associated with underdevelopment of the RV and an ASD. Circulation is maintained by the ASD, which allows blood to bypass the RV. A PDA is required in order to perfuse the lungs. In some cases a concomitant VSD is present that may allow some blood to pass into the RV and enter the pulmonary circulation. Cyanosis is present from birth, and there is a high mortality rate. Surgical correction is required for survival.

KEY CONCEPTS

- All the congenital heart anomalies result in two primary pathologies: (1) shunting of blood through abnormal pathways in the heart or great vessels, and (2) obstruction to blood flow due to abnormal narrowings.
- Disorders that result in right-to-left shunting of blood result in cyanosis. These include tetralogy of Fallot, transposition of the great arteries, truncus arteriosus, and tricuspid atresia.
- Disorders that result in left-to-right shunting of blood or obstruction to flow are generally acyanotic. These include atrial septal defect, ventricular septal defect, patent ductus arteriosus, coarctation of the aorta, and pulmonary and aortic stenosis and atresia.

Summary

A variety of disease processes may interfere with the heart's ability to provide the body with oxygenated blood. Among these processes are ischemic heart disease, valvular and endocardial diseases, myocardial diseases, pericardial diseases, and congenital heart defects. The most important forms of ischemic heart disease are angina pectoris and myocardial infarction, both of which usually result from coronary atherosclerosis. Stenotic coronary lesions obstruct blood flow to the myocardium, resulting in ischemia. The distinction between angina and myocardial infarction relies primarily on the presence of myocardial enzymes in the blood. Angina is ischemia without cellular death and therefore does not result in enzyme elevation. Myocardial infarction, on the other hand, is associated with the death of myocardial cells and the subsequent release of intracellular enzymes. Myocardial infarction may be complicated by dysrhythmias and failure of the heart to pump efficiently.

Valvular disorders are of two types: those that impede flow because of stenosis and those that allow regurgitation because of failure to close completely. The general consequence of valvular disorders is an increased myocardial work load due to high afterload (stenosis) or high preload (regurgitation). The heart may eventually decompensate and proceed to congestive heart failure. The endocardial diseases, rheumatic heart disease and infective endocarditis, also primarily affect the heart valves, creating stenosis and regurgitation.

Disorders of the myocardium include myocarditis, which is an inflammatory process, and cardiomyopathy, which is a noninflammatory process, usually of unknown etiology. Most cases of myocarditis are viral; however, it is the immune system's response to the virus that appears to cause myocardial damage. Myocarditis results in a dilated, flabby heart with decreased pumping efficiency. The cardiomyopathies are a diverse group of disorders that may be classified as primary (having unknown etiology) and secondary (due to some known disease process). Primary cardiomyopathies include a dilated form, a hypertrophic form, and a restrictive form. The primary problem in the dilated form is poor contractility of all heart chambers. The hypertrophic form may cause left ventricular outflow obstruction which interferes with cardiac output and increases left ventricular strain. Difficulty in the restrictive form is because of poor diastolic filling due to a stiff, fibrosed ventricular chamber.

Pericardial disorders include accumulations of fluid in the pericardial sac and acute and chronic forms of pericarditis. Pericardial fluid may be serous, serosanguinous, chylous, or frank blood. Pericardial accumulations are usually of little consequence except as indicators of underlying pathophysiology. However, if the accumulation is large or rapid, it may compress the heart and interfere with diastolic filling—a process called cardiac tamponade. Pericarditis refers to inflammation of the pericardium. It is usually secondary to other disease processes. Pericardial inflammation generally causes pain and may be associated with a friction rub. Chronic pericarditis can cause erosion of the pericardial sac such that the epicardial layer of the heart may become fused to other mediastinal structures. Alternatively, chronic pericarditis may cause the pericardial sac to become fibrotic and noncompliant such that it restricts expansion of the heart during diastolic filling.

A number of heart disorders may be present at birth. These can be categorized as obstructions or shunts and as cyanotic or acyanotic. In general, disorders that allow unoxygenated blood from the right heart to enter the systemic circulation (right-to-left shunt) will cause cyanosis. Examples of cyanotic defects include tetralogy of Fallot, transposition of the great arteries, truncus arteriosus, and tricuspid atresia. Examples of acyanotic defects are coarctation of the aorta, atrial and ventricular septal defects, and patent ductus arteriosus.

All heart diseases discussed in this chapter may be complicated by heart failure. Heart failure occurs when the pumping efficiency of the heart is decreased such that cardiac output is subnormal. It is often accompanied by congestion of the lungs or the systemic venous system. Heart failure is discussed in Chapter 18.

REFERENCES

1. Cotran RS, Kumar V, Robbins SL: *Robbins Pathologic Basis of Disease*, 4th ed. Philadelphia, WB Saunders, 1989.
2. American Heart Association: *1988 Heart Facts*. Dallas, American Heart Association National Center, 1988.
3. Reimer K, Jennings R: Myocardial ischemia, hypoxia, and infarction, in Fozzard HA, Haber E, Jennings RB, Katz AM (eds): *The Heart and Cardiovascular System*. New York, Raven Press, 1988.
4. Brown BG: Coronary vasospasm: Observations linking the clinical spectrum of ischemic heart disease to the dynamic pathology of coronary atherosclerosis. *Arch Intern Med* 1988; 141(6):716–722.
5. Roberts WC: The coronary arteries in ischemic heart disease: Facts and fancies. *Triangle* 1977;16(2):77–90.
6. Eder HA, Gidez LI: The clinical significance of the plasma high density lipoproteins. *Med Clin North Am* 1982;66(2):431–440.
7. Steering Committee of the Physicians Health Study Research Group Preliminary Report: Finding from the aspirin component of the ongoing physicians' health study. *N Engl J Med* 1988;318:261–264.
8. Lerner DJ, Kannel WB: Patterns of coronary heart disease, morbidity, and mortality in the sexes: A 26-year follow-up of the Framingham population. *Am Heart J* 1986;111(2):383–390.
9. Willerson JT, Campbell WB, Winniford MD, et al: Conversion from chronic to acute coronary artery disease: Speculation regarding mechanisms. *Am J Cardiol* 1984;54(10):1349–1354.
10. DeWood MA, Spores J, Notsker R, et al: Prevalence of total coronary occlusion during the early hours of transmural myocardial infarction. *N Engl J Med* 1980;303:897–902.
11. Marder V, Sherry S: Thrombolytic therapy: Current status. *N Engl J Med* 1988;318:1512–1520.
12. Myerberg R: Sudden cardiac death: Epidemiology, causes, and mechanisms. *Cardiology* 1987;74(suppl 2):2–9.
13. Cobb LA, Nerner JA, Trobaugh GB: Sudden cardiac death: II. Outcome of resuscitation, management, and future directions. *Mod Concepts Cardiovasc Dis* 1980;49:37–42.
14. Dean G: Mitral valve prolapse. *Hosp Pract* 1985;20:75–81.
15. Gillum R: Trends in acute rheumatic fever and chronic rheumatic heart disease: A national perspective. *Am Heart J* 1986;111(2):430–432.
16. Chen SC, Donahoe JL, Fagan LF: Rheumatic fever in children: A follow-up study with emphasis on cardiac sequelae. *Jpn Heart J* 1981;22:167–172.
17. Durack D, Beeson R: Pathogenesis of infective endocarditis, in Rahimtoola S (ed): *Infective Endocarditis*. New York, Grune & Stratton, 1978, p 1.
18. Fejfar Z: Cardiomyopathies: An international problem. *Cardiology* 1968;52(1):9–19.
19. Report of the WHO/ISFC Task Force on the Definition and Classification of Cardiomyopathies. *Br Heart J* 1980;44:672–673.
20. Olsen EG: Special investigations of COCM: Endomyocardial biopsies (morphological analysis). *Postgrad Med* 1978; 54(633):486–493.
21. Geisterfer-Lowrance AA, Kass S, Tanigawa G, et al: A molecular basis for familial hypertrophic cardiomyopathy: A β cardiac myosin heavy chain gene missense mutation. *Cell* 1990; 62:999–1006.
22. Giuliani ER, Fuster V, Gersh BJ, McGoon MD, McGoon DC (eds): *Cardiology Fundamentals and Practice*, 2nd ed. St. Louis, Mosby–Year Book, 1991, pp 47–110.
23. Hackel D, Jennings R: The heart, in Rubin E, Farber J (ed): *Essential Pathology*. Philadelphia, JB Lippincott, 1990.
24. Newman TB: Etiology of ventricular septal defects: An epidemiologic approach. *Pediatrics* 1985;76:741–749.

BIBLIOGRAPHY

Alpert MA, Hashimi MW: Obesity and the heart. *Am J Med Sci* 1993;306(2):117–123.
Anderson HV, King SB 3rd: Modern approaches to the diagnosis of coronary artery disease. *Am Heart J* 1992;123(5):1312–1323.

Braunwald E (ed): *Heart Disease: A Textbook of Cardiovascular Medicine,* 4th ed. Philadelphia, WB Saunders, 1992.

Brutsaert DL, Sys SU, Gillebert TC: Diastolic failure: Pathophysiology and therapeutic implications. *J Am Coll Cardiol* 1993; 22(1):318–325.

Cannon LA, Marshall JM: Cardiac disease in the elderly population. *Clin Geriatr Med* 1993;9(3):499–525.

Chatterjee K: Complications of acute myocardial infarction. *Curr Probl Cardiol* 1993;18(1):1–79.

Clark LT: Atherogenesis and thrombosis: Mechanisms, pathogenesis, and therapeutic implications. *Am Heart J* 1992;123 (4 pt 2):1106–1109.

de Divitiis O, Celentano A, De Simone G, et al: Management of the patient with left ventricular hypertrophy. *Eur Heart J* 1993;14(suppl D):22–32.

Eng C, Zhao M, Factor SM, Sonnenblick EH: Post-ischaemic cardiac dilatation and remodeling: Reperfusion injury of the interstitium. *Eur Heart J* 1993;14(suppl A):27–32.

Ertl G, Gaudron P, Hu K: Ventricular remodeling after myocardial infarction: Experimental and clinical studies. *Basic Res Cardiol* 1993;88(suppl 1):125–137.

Hurwitz JL, Josephson ME: Sudden cardiac death in patients with chronic coronary heart disease. *Circulation* 1992;85(1 suppl): 143–149.

Juggi JS, Koenig Bernard E, Van Gilst WH: Cardioprotection by angiotensin-converting enzyme (ACE) inhibitors. *Can J Cardiol* 1993;9(4):336–352.

King KB, Clark PC, Norsen LH, Hicks GL Jr: Coronary artery bypass graft surgery in older women and men. *Am J Crit Care* 1992;1(2):28–35.

Lim MC, Tan TZ, Choo M, Lim YT, Soo CS, Ling LH: Review of patients with infective endocarditis of native valves over a five-year period. *Ann Acad Med Singapore* 1993;22(3):296–299.

Limacher MC: Clinical features of coronary heart disease in the elderly. *Cardiovasc Clin* 1992;22(2):63–73.

Marian AJ, Roberts R: Molecular genetics of cardiomyopathies. *Herz* 1993;18(4):230–237.

Messerli FH, Ketelhut R: Left ventricular hypertrophy: An independent risk factor. *J Cardiovasc Pharmacol* 1991;17(suppl 4):S59–S66; discussion, S66–S67.

Nademanee K, Singh BN, Stevenson WG, Weiss JN: Amiodarone and post-MI patients. *Circulation* 1993;88(2):764–774.

Natsume T: Therapeutic advances in the treatment of left ventricular hypertrophy. *Eur Heart J* 1993;14(suppl D):33–37.

Raspa RF, Wilson CC: Calcium channel blockers in the treatment of hypertension. *Am Fam Physician* 1993;48(3):461–470.

Royster RL: Myocardial dysfunction following cardiopulmonary bypass: Recovery patterns, predictors of inotropic need, theoretical concepts of inotropic administration. *J Cardiothorac Vasc Anesth* 1993;7(4 suppl 2):19–25.

Russo AM, O'Connor WH, Waxman HL: Atypical presentations and echocardiographic findings in patients with cardiac tamponade occurring early and late after cardiac surgery. *Chest* 1993;104(1):71–78.

Schultz HS: Experimental studies on the pathogenesis of damage in the heart. *Rec Results Cancer Res* 1993;130:145–156.

Vogt M, Motz WH, Schwartzkopf B, Strauer BD: Pathophysiology and clinical aspects of hypertensive hypertrophy. *Eur Heart J* 1993;14(suppl D):2–7.

Vogt M, Motz W, Strauer BE: ACE-inhibitors in coronary artery disease? *Basic Res Cardiol* 1993;88(suppl 1):43–64.

CHAPTER 18
Heart Failure and Dysrhythmias: Common Sequelae of Cardiac Diseases

JACQUELYN L. BANASIK

KEY TERMS

congestive heart failure: Dysfunctional cardiac pumping that results in congestion of blood behind the dysfunctional cardiac pump. Right heart failure is associated with systemic venous congestion. Left heart failure is associated with pulmonary congestion.

contractility: The ability of cardiac muscle to shorten in response to stimuli that increase cytoplasmic free calcium ion levels.

dysrhythmia: An abnormality of heart rhythm, including altered rates or sites of impulse initiation and abnormal conduction pathways.

ectopy: A cardiac impulse initiated at a site other than the sinoatrial node.

fibrillation: Cardiac dysrhythmia characterized by rapid, random myocardial contractions and discoordinated pumping action.

inotropy: The force or energy of cardiac contraction.

lusitropy: The energy of cardiac relaxation.

orthopnea: Difficult breathing that is relieved by upright position.

reentry: The proposed mechanism for many dysrhythmias, including premature complexes and fibrillation. Reentry occurs when an impulse is able to activate the cardiac muscle more than once due to abnormalities in conduction through a portion of the heart.

*H*eart failure and electrocardiographic dysrhythmias may occur in association with cardiac diseases from a number of different causes. **Heart failure** refers to inability of the heart to maintain sufficient cardiac output to optimally meet metabolic demands of tissues and organs of the body. Heart failure is the potential end point of all serious forms of heart disease. Disturbances in electrical activity of the heart may signify underlying pathophysiologic processes and may also lead to insufficient cardiac output. Neither heart failure nor dysrhythmia is a primary medical diagnosis, and underlying pathophysiologic processes must also be investigated.

Heart Failure

Heart failure is defined as insufficient cardiac output due to cardiac causes. Regardless of specific cause, the pathophysiologic state of heart failure results either from impaired ability of myocardial fibers to contract and relax or from an excessive cardiac work load. Sluggishness of the cardiac pump results in congestion of blood flow through the circulatory systems, leading to **congestive heart failure** (CHF). Most instances of heart failure are due to deterioration of the contractile ability of the heart muscle. Several of the heart diseases discussed in Chapter 17 may lead to impaired **contractility,** including the ischemic syndromes, myocarditis, and dilated cardiomyopathy. Disorders that may impose excessive pressure or volume work on the heart include several congenital heart defects, valvular disorders, high blood pressure, respiratory diseases, anemia, and hyperthyroidism. Fortunately for the student, all of these diverse causes of heart failure result in common pathophysiologic processes and similar signs and symptoms.

Etiology

Diminished Myocardial Contractility

Although diminished myocardial contraction is frequently cited as a basis for heart failure, little is known about the biochemical nature of the dysfunction. Several mechanisms have been proposed to explain elements of the contractile failure, but no clear understanding has yet emerged. In some instances, the failing heart has one or more of the following alterations: a reduced number of beta receptors,[1] an abnormal form of myosin having a reduced ability to utilize adenosine triphosphate (ATP), dysfunctional mitochondria, or altered myocardial calcium metabolism.[2]

A growing body of evidence indicates that a significant reduction in beta$_1$ receptors is often present in failing hearts.[3,4] This has been termed beta receptor downregulation and is thought to result from overexcitation of cardiac beta receptors by sympathetic neurotransmitters as the body's compensatory mechanisms attempt to restore cardiac output. A reduction in the number of beta receptors results in a myocar-

dium that is less responsive to sympathetic stimulation and adrenergic drug therapy.

Recently, it has been recognized that failing hearts often have abnormalities in relaxation (**lusitropy**) as well as contractile function (**inotropy**). The rate and efficiency of relaxation depend in part on the ability of cellular calcium pumps to remove calcium ions from the cytosol. Calcium pumps are energy dependent and regulated, in part, by beta receptors on the cardiac cell membrane.[5] Reduced ATP production and beta receptor downregulation may lead to insufficient diastolic relaxation. Diastolic dysfunction can increase myocardial work load, hamper ventricular filling, and contribute to poor cardiac output.

Impaired contractility due to significant loss of myocardial tissue is a frequent cause of heart failure. Myocardial infarction, with cell death and loss of contractile elements, reduces the heart's contractile force. The degree of pump failure is related to the amount of heart muscle lost.

The severity of decreased contractility may be estimated by measuring the amount of blood that the ventricle is able to eject into the arterial system. A reduced stroke volume, reduced cardiac output, and lowered ejection fraction are associated with heart failure. Ejection fraction is the portion of preload that is ejected with cardiac contraction. A normal heart ejects approximately two thirds of the end-diastolic volume (preload) of the ventricle with each contraction.[6] In heart failure, the ejection fraction is reduced and may fall to 15 or 20 percent in severe cases.

Increased Myocardial Work Load

Myocardial work load has three primary determinants: heart rate, preload (volume work), and afterload (pressure work). A number of heart diseases are associated with excessive volume and pressure work. Valvular and congenital disorders that result in regurgitant or shunt flow increase volume work, whereas the stenotic or obstructive disorders increase pressure work. In addition to these diseases, systemic and pulmonary hypertension increase the pressure work of the left and right ventricles respectively and may lead to heart failure.

KEY CONCEPTS

- Heart failure is a potential consequence of most cardiac disorders. Heart failure occurs when the heart is unable to provide sufficient cardiac output to maintain function of the body.

- Impaired contractility is frequently associated with heart failure. The biochemical basis of impaired contractility is mostly unknown; however, beta receptor downregulation and reduced ATP production are likely etiologic factors.

- In some cases, such as valvular and congenital defects, heart failure is due to excessive work load.

Compensatory Mechanisms

The ability of the healthy heart to improve cardiac output by increasing heart rate, stroke volume, or both is called **cardiac reserve.** With strenuous activity a healthy heart can triple its resting cardiac output by increasing both heart rate and stroke volume. The failing heart, on the other hand, has very limited ability to increase stroke volume on demand, and even mild activity may be poorly tolerated. In severe heart failure, cardiac output at rest may be insufficient to meet metabolic demands, and the condition of *cardiogenic shock* may result (see Chap. 54). Three primary compensatory mechanisms are activated in heart failure to maintain cardiac output: sympathetic nervous system stimulation, increased preload, and myocardial hypertrophy (Fig. 18–1).

Sympathetic Nervous System

Sympathetic activation of the heart is primarily a result of baroreceptor reflex stimulation. The baroreceptors (pressoreceptors) located in the aorta and carotid arteries detect a fall in pressure due to diminished stroke volume and transmit this information to the central nervous system (CNS) (see Chap. 16). The CNS increases activity in the sympathetic nerves to the heart, resulting in increased heart rate and contractility. The failing heart may have reduced responsiveness to sympathetic activation, however, because of impaired contractile ability. Sympathetic activation also causes venoconstriction, which redistributes blood and increases cardiac preload. Sympathetic constriction of arterioles helps to maintain blood pressure

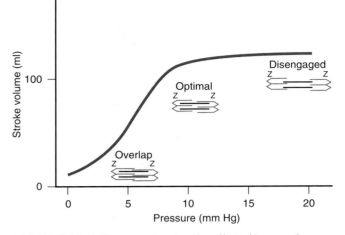

FIGURE 18–2. Diagram showing the effect of increased preload on sarcomere length and stroke volume.

when cardiac output is reduced. Sympathetic activation is an early and immediate compensatory response to insufficient cardiac output.

Increased Preload

Increased **preload** in the cardiac chambers is a consequence of reduced ejection fraction with a resulting increase in residual end-systolic volume. The affected chamber(s) enlarge to accommodate excessive blood volume (cardiac dilation). Decreased cardiac output to the kidney reduces glomerular filtration, resulting in fluid conservation. In addition, the renin-angiotensin-aldosterone cascade may be activated because of reduced cardiac output to the kidney. Angiotensin II and aldosterone enhance sodium and water reabsorption by the kidney, contributing to an elevated blood volume. Increased preload is a compensatory mechanism that enhances the ability of the myocardium to contract forcefully.[6] An enlarged chamber volume causes the myocardial fibers to lengthen during diastole, which results in greater fiber shortening during contraction. This mechanism is attributed to the Frank-Starling law of the heart, which states that diastolic stretch (preload) of myocardial fibers increases the force of contraction.[7] The diastolic length of the muscle fibers is thought to determine the number of effective crossbridge cycles that can be accomplished during systole.[6,8] At short diastolic lengths, fewer crossbridge cycles can be completed before thin filaments begin to overlap and interfere with further shortening. With increasing diastolic length, a greater number of crossbridge cycles is possible before the filaments overlap, and a greater degree of shortening is accomplished. Thus, up to a point, an increase in the volume or preload of the heart will result in a greater force of contraction (Fig. 18–2). If, however, muscle fibers are excessively stretched, thick and thin filaments may be disengaged and therefore unable to

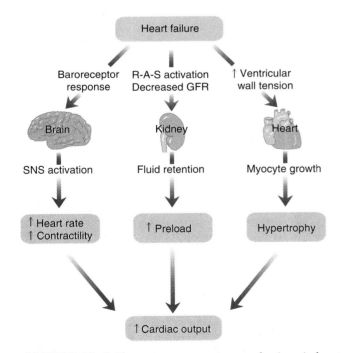

FIGURE 18–1. The major compensatory mechanisms in heart failure that act to restore cardiac output.

effectively make crossbridges. There appears to be an upper limit of effective stretch, beyond which contraction deteriorates and the heart may decompensate. Compensation through enhancement of blood volume takes days to weeks—much longer than sympathetic activation.

Myocardial Hypertrophy

Hypertrophy of cardiac muscle cells is the third mechanism of compensation and generally takes much longer to occur than dilation or sympathetic activation. Hypertrophy appears to result from a chronic elevation of myocardial wall tension.[9] Wall tension may be high as a result of dilation and increased diastolic blood volume or as a consequence of high systolic pressures generated in the chamber. The relationship between myocardial wall tension and intrachamber pressure and diameter is described by the law of Laplace: Tension = transmural pressure × radius/wall thickness. When the ventricular chamber enlarges and pressures increase, more tension is created in the ventricular muscle wall. The development of high systolic pressures in the ventricle may be necessary to overcome a high afterload such as occurs with arterial hypertension and aortic valve stenosis. The hypertrophy of contractile elements in the myocardium boosts the heart's pumping force.

Enhanced preload and cardiac hypertrophy may allow a heart to compensate for increased myocardial work for an extended period of time. At some point, however, the ability to compensate is exceeded, contractility becomes impaired, and decompensation ensues. The factors that determine the end of compensation and the beginning of decompensation are poorly understood. Morphologically, it is not yet possible to differentiate the compensated from the decompensated heart.[2] Neither the amount of dilation and hypertrophy nor the extent of the primary cardiac disease indicates whether the heart is in a compensated or decompensated state. The severity of the cardiac failure may be primarily evident in the hypoxic and congestive dysfunction of other tissues and organs rather than in the heart itself.

Unfortunately, the three compensatory mechanisms of sympathetic activation, increased preload, and hypertrophy, which serve to restore cardiac output to the tissues, also result in an increase in myocardial work and oxygen requirements. A delicate balance must be maintained between the necessity for adequate cardiac output to tissues and the need to minimize cardiac work. Decompensation may occur when the primary disease plus the superimposed burdens of compensation overwhelm the heart's ability to generate adequate contractile force. The focus of therapy for congestive heart failure is to maintain a state of compensation by minimizing cardiac work while optimizing cardiac output—a difficult goal to achieve.

KEY CONCEPTS

- Three compensatory mechanisms are activated in heart failure in an attempt to improve cardiac output. Unfortunately, these responses also increase myocardial work load and may perpetuate the heart failure.

- Sympathetic activation is an early response to reduced cardiac output. Sympathetic nervous system activation increases heart rate, contractility, and arterial vasoconstriction. The failing heart generally has reduced responsiveness to sympathetic nervous system neurotransmittors due to beta receptor downregulation.

- Decreased cardiac output reduces kidney perfusion and leads to volume retention. Extra blood volume increases cardiac preload. Higher preload results in more forceful ejection of blood from the heart (Frank-Starling law) and improves cardiac output.

- Cardiac hypertrophy is stimulated by elevated myocardial wall tension. Hypertrophy adds contractile filaments and improves contractile force.

Pathophysiology

The pathophysiology of heart failure is commonly described according to the side of the heart that has a depressed pumping capability. The etiology, clinical manifestations, and treatment of right and left heart failure differ substantially and the two sides are best considered separately, even though dysfunction of one side of the heart often will eventually affect function of the other side. Recall that the right side of the heart receives blood from the systemic venous circulation and pumps it into the pulmonary system and the left heart receives blood from the pulmonary circulation and delivers it to the systemic arterial system (Fig. 18–3). Insufficient cardiac pumping is manifested by poor cardiac output, called forward failure, and by congestion of blood behind the pump, called backward failure. The clinical manifestations of forward and backward failure differ according to the side of the heart that is dysfunctional.

Left-Sided Heart Failure

Left heart failure is most often associated with left ventricular infarction, cardiomyopathy, aortic and mitral valvular disease, and systemic hypertension.[2] Myocardial infarction and cardiomyopathy are generally associated with impaired myocardial contractility, whereas the valvular diseases and hypertension cause excessive myocardial work. The **forward effects** of left-sided heart failure are due to insufficient cardiac output with diminished delivery of oxygen and nutrients to peripheral tissues and organs (Fig. 18–4). Inadequate perfusion of the brain may lead to symptoms of restlessness, mental fatigue, confusion, anxiety, and impaired memory. Generalized fatigue, activity intolerance, and lethargy may be present (Fig. 18–5).

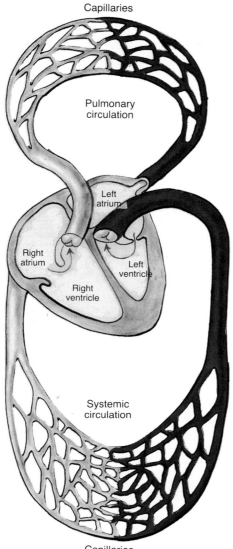

Capillaries

Pulmonary
circulation

Left
atrium

Right
atrium

Left
ventricle

Right
ventricle

Systemic
circulation

Capillaries

FIGURE 18–3. The systemic and pulmonary circulations viewed as separate but interdependent systems. (From Jacob SW, Francone CA: *Essentials of Anatomy and Physiology,* 2nd ed. Philadelphia, WB Saunders, 1989, p 197. Reproduced with permission.)

Reduced perfusion of the kidney results in a decline in urine output with subsequent fluid retention. Activation of the renin-angiotensin-aldosterone cascade contributes to conservation of sodium and water by the kidney and may also cause vascular constriction. Vascular constriction may serve to maintain blood pressure and redistribute reduced cardiac output to vital organs; however, it also increases the afterload against which the damaged left ventricle must pump. If renal blood flow becomes severely limited, the patient with left heart failure may develop kidney failure.

Forward failure also results in activation of the sympathetic nervous system because of the baroreceptor reflex. Sympathetic activation contributes to vascu-

lar constriction and helps maintain blood pressure in the face of reduced cardiac output; however, as with angiotensin II, it increases left ventricular afterload. Sympathetic activation results in a compensatory increase in heart rate that may augment cardiac output to some extent but, again, raises myocardial energy consumption.

The **backward effects** of left heart failure produce dramatic clinical symptoms due to pulmonary dysfunction (see Fig. 18–4). The sluggish pumping of the left heart results in an accumulation of blood within the pulmonary circulation. As blood pressure (hydrostatic) builds within the pulmonary veins and capillaries, fluid is forced from the capillaries into interstitial and alveolar spaces, causing edema. Pulmonary congestion and edema are associated with a number of clinical findings (see Fig. 18–5). **Dyspnea** or breathlessness occurs early in the progression of left heart failure and may be considered the cardinal symptom. Difficulty breathing may be exacerbated by activity (dyspnea on exertion), lying down (orthopnea and paroxysmal nocturnal dyspnea), and blood volume expansion. **Orthopnea** and **paroxysmal nocturnal dyspnea** are due in part to a redistribution of blood volume from the periphery to the heart when the individual lies down. The failing left heart is unable to effectively pump extra volume, and pulmonary congestion is worsened. The severity of orthopnea may be quantified by the degree of head elevation (e.g., number of pillows) used to relieve dyspnea. Paroxysmal nocturnal dyspnea refers to intermittent attacks of severe dyspnea during the night and is a most distressing form of orthopnea. The individual experiences a feeling of suffocation and panic at not being able to overcome the dyspnea.

Clinical signs of pulmonary congestion include cough, respiratory crackles (rales), hypoxemia, high left atrial pressure, and typical findings on x-ray. Cough results from bronchial irritation associated with congestion. In severe cases, sputum may be blood-tinged from breakage of fragile capillaries, and frothy due to fluid buildup in the alveoli. The severity of pulmonary edema can be estimated from the location of crackles within the lung fields. Crackles are abnormal sounds caused by the movement of air through partially fluid-filled alveoli. Edema fluid collects in dependent lung fields because of gravity and progressively moves up the lung as more edema fluid accumulates. For example, in mild pulmonary edema, crackles might be heard only at the base of the upright lung, but with increasing severity they become apparent in the lower one third to one half of the lung. Fluid in the alveoli and interstitial spaces also interferes with alveolar-capillary gas exchange and results in some degree of hypoxemia. Hypoxemia may be detected by arterial blood gas analysis and may be apparent clinically as cyanosis. **Cyanosis** refers to a blue coloration of the skin and results from significant amounts of desaturated hemoglobin in the blood. Cyanosis is a late sign and is clinically evident only when a large amount (about 5 g/dL) of hemoglobin is deoxygenated (normal hemoglobin 15 g/dL).[10]

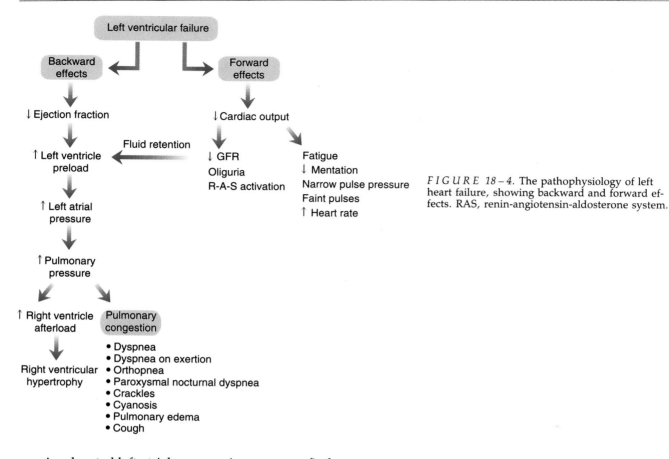

FIGURE 18–4. The pathophysiology of left heart failure, showing backward and forward effects. RAS, renin-angiotensin-aldosterone system.

An elevated left atrial pressure is a common finding in left heart failure due to excessive blood volume and the compensatory responses of atrial dilation and hypertrophy. Atrial pressure can be estimated by inserting a balloon-tipped catheter (Swan-Ganz) into the pulmonary artery. When left atrial pressure reaches 16 to 18 mm Hg, pulmonary edema generally occurs. Typical x-ray findings include an enlarged heart and engorged pulmonary capillaries and lymphatics (Kerley B lines).

Acute cardiogenic pulmonary edema is a life-threatening condition that severely impairs gas exchange, producing dramatic signs and symptoms. The patient exhibits severe dyspnea and anxiety, and a bolt-upright posture is usually assumed to maximize respiratory effort. Bubbly crackles may be heard all the way up the lung from the bases to the apices, and pink frothy sputum may be expectorated or may well up from the trachea. Anxiety and hypoxemia contribute to tachycardia, which may worsen the pumping efficiency of the failing heart. Cyanosis and symptoms of tissue hypoxia are usually apparent. The immediate treatment is aimed at reducing the fluid volume in the lungs and supporting oxygenation.

Right-Sided Heart Failure

Because the right and left hearts are in series, left heart failure eventually increases the burden on the right heart and may cause it to fail as well. The causes

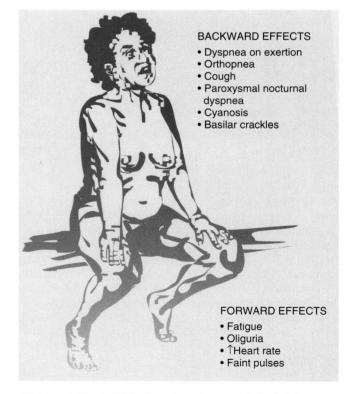

FIGURE 18–5. Clinical manifestations of left heart failure.

of right heart failure must therefore include all the causes of left heart failure. Pure right heart failure is rare and is usually a consequence of right ventricular infarction or pulmonary disease. Only 3 percent of myocardial infarctions occur in the right ventricle; however, right ventricular infarcts are often poorly tolerated and difficult to treat.[11] Pulmonary disorders that result in increased pulmonary vascular resistance impose a high afterload against which the right ventricle must pump. The resultant right ventricular hypertrophy, called **cor pulmonale,** may progress to right ventricular failure as the lung disease worsens.

Any lung disorder that decreases the total cross-sectional area of the lung vasculature can increase pulmonary vascular resistance and produce right ventricular strain. Hypoxemia, for example, causes the pulmonary arterioles to constrict, which increases pulmonary resistance. Destruction or blockage of the vascular bed, such as occurs with emphysema or pulmonary embolus, will similarly reduce the cross-sectional area of the pulmonary vasculature and lead to increased pulmonary resistance. If the increase in pulmonary resistance and right ventricular work load occurs gradually, the right ventricle can compensate by increasing preload and hypertrophy. However, the thin musculature of the right ventricle has limited ability to adjust to acute changes in work load as would occur with a right ventricular infarct or large pulmonary embolus.

The **forward effect**s of right heart failure are very similar to those described for the left heart (Fig. 18–6). If the right heart fails to deliver an adequate amount of blood to the left heart, then systemic cardiac output

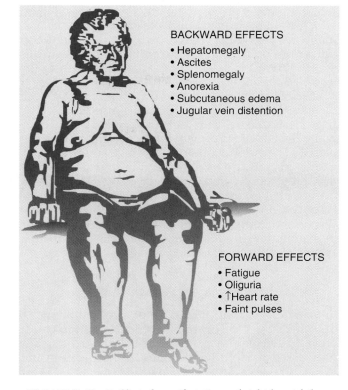

FORWARD EFFECTS
- Fatigue
- Oliguria
- ↑Heart rate
- Faint pulses

BACKWARD EFFECTS
- Hepatomegaly
- Ascites
- Splenomegaly
- Anorexia
- Subcutaneous edema
- Jugular vein distention

FIGURE 18–7. Clinical manifestations of right heart failure.

will be reduced, even though the left ventricle is functioning properly. The forward effects of failure include sympathetic nervous system activation, stimulation of renin release from the kidney with resultant volume expansion, and activity intolerance. There is no direct impairment of pulmonary function due to right heart failure; however, peripheral tissues may suffer from hypoxia due to reduced perfusion.

As with left heart failure, there is congestion of blood behind the failing ventricle due to sluggishness of the pump. The **backward effects** of right heart failure are due to congestion in the systemic venous system (see Fig. 18–6). Systemic venous congestion results in impaired function of the liver, portal system, spleen, kidneys, peripheral subcutaneous tissues, and brain (Fig. 18–7).

The liver is usually somewhat increased in size and weight, but individual hepatocytes may show signs of atrophy and necrosis due to chronic passive congestion.[2] Impedance to blood flow through the liver may cause hydrostatic pressure in the portal system to build, leading to edema formation in the peritoneal cavity (ascites). Increased pressure in the portal system is reflected back to the spleen and gastrointestinal tract. The spleen is generally enlarged (congestive splenomegaly), and gastrointestinal symptoms such as anorexia and abdominal discomfort may be present.

Increased systemic venous pressure causes congestion of the kidneys, which contributes to the decreased glomerular filtration and fluid retention. Fluid

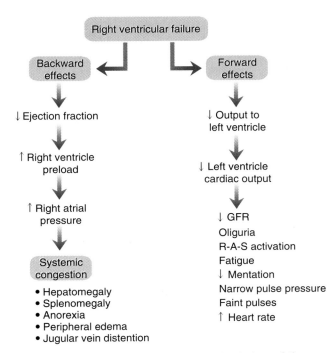

FIGURE 18–6. The pathophysiology of right heart failure, showing backward and forward effects. RAS, renin-angiotensin-aldosterone system.

retention may be perpetuated by the congested liver, which is unable to metabolize plasma aldosterone normally.[2] Excess fluid volume and venous congestion caused by right heart failure result in subcutaneous edema. Edema is usually particularly apparent in the lower extremities.

Drainage of venous blood from the head and neck by way of the superior vena cava is also impeded by right heart failure. The jugular veins may be abnormally distended, and mental functioning may be impaired. The hepatojugular reflux test can be done to assess the severity of right heart failure. The liver is manually compressed, causing a sudden increase in venous blood returning to the right heart, while jugular neck veins are observed for sudden distention. In the absence of right heart failure, the sudden increase in venous return would enter the heart unimpeded and no neck vein distention would be apparent.

Biventricular Heart Failure

In many cases, heart failure is not localized to one or the other side of the heart. Biventricular failure is most often a result of primary left ventricular failure that has progressed to right heart failure. With biventricular failure, there is pulmonary congestion due to left heart failure as well as systemic venous congestion due to right heart failure. The location of the congestive symptoms is a primary clue in determining the type of heart failure present. With pure left heart failure, the lungs are congested but the systemic venous system is not. With pure right heart failure, the systemic system is congested but the pulmonary system is not. In biventricular failure, both pulmonary congestion and systemic venous congestion are present.

KEY CONCEPTS

- **The pathophysiology of heart failure is characterized by the effects of forward failure (reduced cardiac output) and backward failure (congestion behind the pump).**
- **Left-sided heart failure is characterized by pulmonary congestion, which may manifest with dyspnea, orthopnea, crackles, cough, pulmonary edema, and hypoxemia.**
- **Right-sided heart failure is characterized by systemic venous congestion, which may manifest with jugular vein distention, hepatomegaly, splenomegaly, and peripheral edema.**

Treatment

Therapy for congestive heart failure is aimed at improving cardiac output while minimizing congestive symptoms and cardiac work load. These objectives are obtained by manipulating preload, afterload, and contractility. When possible, specific treatment is undertaken to correct the underlying cause of the heart failure. Some pharmacologic agents commonly used in the treatment of heart failure are listed in Table 18–1.

Management of Preload

Congestive heart failure is generally associated with an elevated preload due to an expanded intravascular volume and a reduced ejection fraction. According to the Frank-Starling law of the heart, an elevated preload is desirable because it will enhance systolic shortening and improve cardiac output. Unfortunately, high preload exacerbates congestive symptoms and adds to the work of an already damaged heart. The

T A B L E 18–1. Drugs Commonly Used in the Treatment of Heart Failure

Category of Action	Examples
Preload-Reducing Drugs	
Diuretics	
Loop diuretics	Furosemide (Lasix)
	Ethacrynic acid (Edecrine)
	Bumetanide (Bumex)
Thiazide and thiazide-like	Chlorothiazide (Diuril)
	Hydrochlorothiazide (HCTZ)
	Metolazone (Diulo)
	Chlorthalidone (Hygroton)
	Indapamide (Lozol)
Osmotic diuretic	Mannitol (Osmitrol)
Venodilators	
Narcotic	Morphine
Nitrates	Erythrityl trinitrate
	Isosorbide dinitrate (Isordil)
	Nitroglycerin (Nitrobid)
Angiotensin-converting enzyme inhibitors	Captopril (Capoten)
	Enalapril (Vasotec)
	Lisinopril (Zestril)
Afterload-Reducing Drugs	
Angiotensin-converting enzyme inhibitors	As above
Calcium channel blockers	Diltiazem (Cardizem)
	Nicardipine (Cardene)
	Nifedipine (Procardia)
	Verapamil (Calan)
Centrally acting antiadrenergics	Clonidine (Catapress)
	Quanabenz (Wytensin)
	Methyldopa (Aldomet)
Peripherally acting antiadrenergics	Guanethedine
	Reserpine
Direct vasodilators	Hydralazine (Apresoline)
	Nitroprusside (Nipride)
	Prazosin (Minipress)
	Minoxidil (Rogaine)
Inotropic Drugs (Increase Contractility)	
Cardiac glycosides	Digitoxin
	Digoxin (Lanoxin)
	Deslanoside
Beta adrenergics	Dobutamine (Dobutrex)
	Dopamine (Inotropin)
	Isoproterenol (Isuprel)
Phosphodiesterase inhibitors	Amrinone (Inocor)

aim of therapy, then, is to optimize preload such that congestive symptoms are minimized but cardiac output is not compromised. The right ventricle is particularly sensitive to reductions in preload, and care must be taken to avoid a significant drop in right ventricular output when intravascular volume is decreased.

Several drugs may be administered to reduce intravascular volume, including diuretics and angiotensin-converting enzyme (ACE) inhibitors. Patients may be instructed to modify salt and fluid intake as well. Diuretics promote the excretion of fluid by increasing renal blood flow, blocking sodium and chloride reabsorption, or both. Drugs that inhibit enzymes that convert angiotensin I (inactive) to angiotensin II (active) are called ACE inhibitors. Even though the kidney may continue to produce renin, it has little effect, because angiotensin II and aldosterone production is blocked. Preload may also be reduced by redistribution of blood volume within the vascular system. Drugs that cause venous dilation and peripheral pooling of blood can effectively reduce preload. In acute congestive syndromes, such as pulmonary edema, phlebotomy may also be performed.

Management of Afterload

Afterload represents the resistance against which the ventricle must pump and is an important determinant of myocardial energy consumption. Afterload may be inappropriately high in heart failure because of primary hypertension or sympathetic nervous system activation. As mentioned previously, diminished stroke volume is detected by the aortic and carotid baroreceptors, which results in sympathetic activation. Sympathetic stimulation of the arterioles causes them to constrict, thus increasing vascular resistance, arterial blood pressure, and ventricular afterload. Drugs that cause arteriolar dilation may be used to decrease ventricular afterload. Arteriolar dilation is accomplished by inducing vascular smooth muscle cells to relax by decreasing calcium ions in their cytosol. Calcium entry into the cells can be blocked by calcium channel–blocking drugs or by inhibition of vasoconstrictive neurotransmitters and peptides. Some of these agents have additional effects on venous smooth muscle and cardiac muscle and may reduce preload and myocardial contractility. Careful assessment is required to optimally reduce afterload yet avoid excessive reductions in preload or contractility.

In addition to drug therapy, afterload can be reduced mechanically with the intra-aortic balloon pump (IABP) (Fig. 18–8).[12] This treatment is invasive, associated with several potential complications, and generally reserved for severe cases of left heart failure. A catheter with a balloon at the end is inserted, usually through the femoral artery, into the descending aorta. A machine outside the body intermittently inflates and deflates the balloon in time with cardiac contractions. During ventricular systole, the balloon is quickly deflated, which creates a vacuum effect in the aorta, reduces ventricular afterload, and promotes

ventricular emptying. In addition to improving cardiac output by reducing afterload, the IABP also decreases myocardial strain and improves perfusion of the coronary arteries. Coronary blood flow is enhanced during diastole when the balloon is quickly inflated, raising the driving pressure for flow through the coronary arteries. In some cases, increased coronary blood flow may improve the availability of myocardial ATP and increase contractility.

Management of Contractility

Improvements in contractility are achieved primarily through drug therapy and efforts to optimize oxygen and nutrient delivery to compromised myocardial cells. **Contractility** refers to the rate and extent of force generated by the ventricle during systole and is not dependent on preload.[6] Contractility is enhanced by measures that increase the availability of ATP and intracellular calcium during systole. The synthesis of sufficient ATP depends primarily on the adequacy of myocardial perfusion and oxygenation. Oxygen administration and evaluation of the hemoglobin level may be employed to support oxygen delivery.

The availability of intracellular calcium ions can be enhanced through drugs, including sympathomimetics, digitalis, and other direct positive inotropic agents. Drugs that mimic sympathetic nervous system effects, such as norepinephrine, isoproterenol, and dopamine, may be used in acute situations to improve cardiac output but generally are not suitable for long-term use because of the potential for imposing excessive afterload and dramatically increasing myocardial oxygen consumption.

Digitalis or a related cardiac glycoside is the usual treatment of choice for the long-term management of heart failure. Cardiac glycosides directly inhibit the sodium-potassium pump present in the cell membranes of all cells. This results in an increase in intracellular sodium accumulation and a decreased gradient for sodium entry into the cell (Fig. 18–9). A diminished sodium gradient slows the sodium-dependent calcium pump that normally removes intracellular calcium. This allows more calcium to remain in the cell, thus strengthening myocardial contraction. Digitalis also slows the heart rate through several mechanisms and promotes sodium and water excretion through improved cardiac output to the kidney. Dangerous side effects from digitalis toxicity may occur because inhibition of sodium-potassium pumps in cells throughout the body may disrupt ion balance, cellular volume control, and nerve and muscle transmission. Depletion of serum potassium (hypokalemia) may also slow sodium-potassium pumps and potentiate digitalis toxicity.

Recently, measures to increase the number of functional cardiac beta receptors in failing hearts have been tried, with apparent success. Studies using beta blocking drugs and partial beta agonists have demonstrated improvement in contractile (inotropic) and diastolic (lusitropic) function.[13,14] Presently, beta blocking

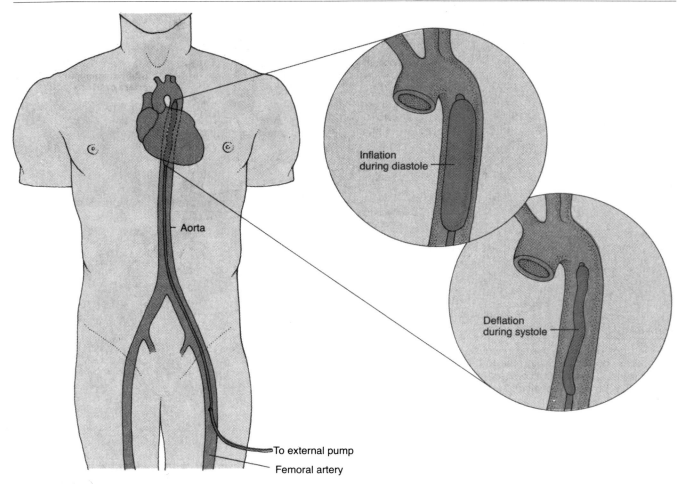

FIGURE 18 – 8. Schematic of an intra-aortic balloon pump (IABP) positioned in the aorta. The balloon deflates during ventricular systole to aid left ventricular emptying by reducing afterload. The balloon inflates during ventricular diastole to increase aortic diastolic pressure and improve coronary artery perfusion. (From Ignatavicius DD, Bayne MV: *Medical-Surgical Nursing: A Nursing Process Approach.* Philadelphia, WB Saunders, 1991, p 2157. Reproduced with permission.)

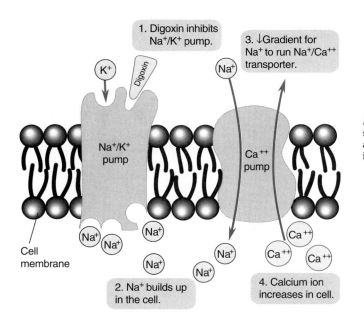

FIGURE 18 – 9. A section of cardiac muscle cell membrane showing the effects of digoxin on the Na^+/K^+ pump resulting in accumulation of intracellular sodium and less efficient calcium ion extrusion.

drugs are generally thought to be contraindicated in heart failure because of their tendency to reduce contractility. However, these new studies suggest that partial beta blockade in selected patients may enhance the number or function of beta receptors in the heart and actually may improve systolic and diastolic function.

KEY CONCEPTS

- The primary aims of treatment are to improve cardiac output and minimize congestive symptoms. These aims are accomplished through the pharmacologic management of preload, afterload, and contractility.
- Diuretics and venodilators are used to alleviate congestion by reducing preload. Preload reduction must be approached cautiously to avoid a reduction in cardiac output.
- Sympathetic antagonists, calcium channel blockers, and direct vasodilators are used to decrease cardiac work load by reducing afterload. Excessive reductions in blood pressure must be avoided.
- Myocardial contractility may be improved by measures that increase oxygen delivery to the heart. In addition, positive inotropic drugs such as digitalis and beta agonists or beta partial agonists may be used to improve contractility.

Cardiac Dysrhythmias

Dysrhythmia refers to an abnormality of the heartbeat. A normal heartbeat is initiated in the sinoatrial (SA) node and follows a consistent pathway of depolarization through the atria, atrioventricular (AV) node, His-Purkinje system, and finally the ventricular myocardium. Electrical depolarization of the heart is normally followed by atrial and then ventricular muscular contraction. A number of factors may lead to disturbances in heartbeat, including hypoxia, electrolyte imbalance, trauma, inflammation, and drugs. Dysrhythmias are significant for two reasons: (1) they indicate an underlying pathophysiologic disorder, and (2) they can disrupt normal cardiac output. Dysrhythmias can be categorized into three major types: abnormal rates of sinus rhythm, abnormal sites (ectopic) of impulse initiation, or disturbances in conduction pathways.

Dysrhythmia Analysis

Electrocardiographic (ECG) recording paper is specifically designed to allow easy measurement of waveform amplitude and duration (Fig. 18–10). Each small box on the ECG paper represents an amplitude of 0.1 millivolt (mV) and a duration of 0.04 second. Larger boxes are also marked on the paper and correspond to 0.5 mV in amplitude (five small boxes) and 0.2 second in duration (five small boxes). These markings allow measurement of waveform amplitude, duration, and heart rate. Rhythm strips presented in this chapter are from a single lead only (usually lead II), but it should be emphasized that thorough ECG interpretation often requires several leads to provide different views of electrical conduction through the heart. (Lead placement is discussed in Chapter 16.)

Normal Sinus Rhythm

Before we proceed to the interpretation of dysrhythmias, the features of normal sinus rhythm must be understood. Normal sinus rhythm is generally defined as an impulse rate between 60 and 100 per minute that begins in the sinus node and follows the normal conduction pathway. Characteristics of normal sinus rhythm are listed in Table 18–2. The rhythm shown in Figure 18–11 is regular. There is a P wave for every QRS, the P-R, QRS, and Q-T intervals are

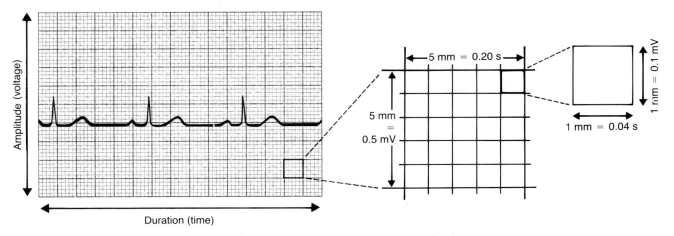

F I G U R E 18–10. Electrocardiographic strip showing the markings for measuring amplitude and duration of waveforms. (From Ignatavicius DD, Bayne MV: *Medical-Surgical Nursing: A Nursing Process Approach.* Philadelphia, WB Saunders, 1991, p 2117. Reproduced with permission.)

TABLE 18–2. Electrocardiographic Characteristics of Normal Sinus Rhythm

Rhythm:	Regular. P-P intervals and R-R intervals may vary as much as 3 mm and still be considered regular.
Rate:	60–100 beats/min.
P waves:	One P wave preceding each QRS.
PR interval:	0.12–0.20 sec, constant.
QRS duration:	0.04–0.10 sec, constant.
QT interval:	<0.40 sec.

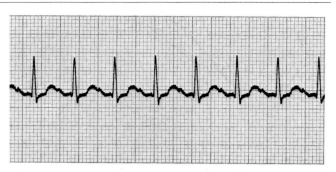

FIGURE 18–12. Sinus tachycardia.

of normal duration, and there are no "funny-looking" beats.

There are several methods for figuring heart rate using the rhythm strip. The easiest but least accurate method is to count the number of QRS complexes within 6 seconds and multiply by ten. ECG paper has 3-second marks along the top that can be used to determine a 6-second interval. A more accurate method for determining heart rate is to count the number of small boxes between complexes. The number of boxes is divided by 1,500 to determine heart rate because there are 1,500 small boxes per minute (1,500 × 0.04 sec = 60 sec). Neither of these methods is accurate with irregular rhythms, so heart rate must be calculated for a longer time interval, usually 1 minute. With this understanding of rate calculation and methods to measure the duration and amplitude of waveforms, one can analyze dysrhythmias.

KEY CONCEPTS

- Measurement of ECG waveform amplitude, duration, and frequency is necessary to analyze cardiac rhythms. ECG paper is marked in small boxes representing 1 mV amplitude and 0.04 second duration.
- Normal sinus rhythm is characterized by regular P-P and R-R intervals, a rate of 60 to 100 beats/min, and normal P-R (0.12–0.20 sec) and QRS (0.04–0.10 sec) intervals.

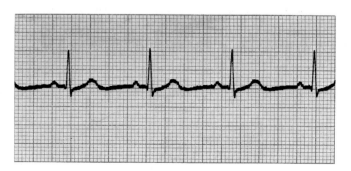

FIGURE 18–11. Normal sinus rhythm.

Abnormal Rates of Sinus Rhythm

Sinus Tachycardia

Sinus tachycardia is an abnormally fast heart rate of greater than 100 beats/min (Fig. 18–12). A number of factors, including sympathetic activation, pain, increased metabolism, low blood pressure, and hypoxia, can lead to sinus tachycardia, making it a very common dysrhythmia. Sinus tachycardia often is a compensatory response to increased demand for cardiac output or reduced stroke volume. Treatment is aimed at correcting the underlying cause. In some instances, however, the rate can become so high that ventricular filling is impaired and cardiac output is compromised. Sympatholytics or calcium channel–blocking agents may then be indicated.

Sinus Bradycardia

A heart rate of less than 60 beats/min is called **bradycardia.** Sinus bradycardia results from slowed impulse generation by the sinus node in response to parasympathetic activity, drugs, or increased stroke volume. Important features of sinus bradycardia are shown in Figure 18–13. Sinus bradycardia may be a normal finding in well-conditioned individuals who have large resting stroke volumes. Abnormal parasympathetic activation can result from pain (vasovagal), carotid sinus massage, endotracheal suctioning, and the Valsalva maneuver (bearing down). Slow heart rates may be well tolerated by some individuals and not require treatment. If the slow heart rate precipitates low cardiac output, it is usually treated with sympathomimetic or parasympatholytic drugs.

Sinus Arrhythmia

A degree of variability in the heart rate, or **sinus arrhythmia,** is a normal finding associated with fluctuations in autonomic influences and respiratory dynamics. Sinus arrhythmia can be particularly pronounced in children. Sinus arrhythmia must be differentiated from a sinus node irregularity called **sick sinus syndrome,** in which alternating periods of sinus bradycardia and tachycardia occur (Fig. 18–14). Sick sinus syn-

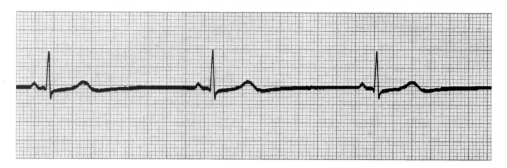

F I G U R E 18 – 13. Sinus bradycardia.

drome may necessitate implantation of a permanent pacemaker. Sinus arrhythmia is a normal finding and thus requires no treatment.

Asystole

The absence of impulse initiation in the heart is called **asystole.** It is characterized by a flat ECG recording lacking recognizable waveforms (Fig. 18–15). Electrical asystole results in mechanical asystole and zero cardiac output. Asystole is a fatal condition if not immediately treated with cardiopulmonary resuscitation. Cardiac pacing may successfully restore an electrical rhythm in some cases. Asystole may result from myocardial infarction, electrical shock, electrolyte disturbances, acidosis, and extreme parasympathetic activity.

KEY CONCEPTS

- **Sinus tachycardia (>100 beats/min) usually occurs from sympathetic activation of the heart. Sympathetic nervous system activation may be compensatory (e.g., occurring in the setting of low blood pressure, low cardiac output, or hypoxemia) or may be due to pain and anxiety.**
- **Sinus bradycardia (<60 beats/min) usually occurs in response to parasympathetic activity. Bradycardia is treated if the slow heart rate precipitates inadequate cardiac output.**
- **Sinus arrhythmia is usually normal and more pronounced in young persons than in older adults.**
- **Asystole (absence of heartbeat) is fatal if not rapidly treated with cardiopulmonary resuscitation or effective pacing.**

Abnormal Site of Impulse Initiation

Initiation of a cardiac impulse at a site other than the SA node occurs primarily for two reasons. First, SA node failure may allow a slower pacemaker to take over. Takeover by a slower pacemaker is called an **escape rhythm.** Second, enhanced excitability of a cardiac cell may cause it to depolarize prematurely, thus overriding the SA node and causing an early beat. Premature beats are initiated outside the SA node and are called **ectopic beats** or ectopy.

F I G U R E 18 – 14. **A,** Sinus arrhythmia is a normal finding that may be particularly pronounced in children. **B,** Sick sinus syndrome. Strips show alternating periods of tachycardia and bradycardia.

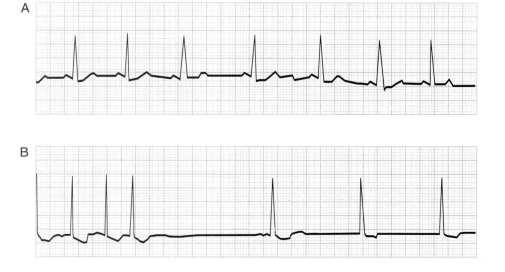

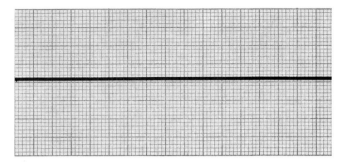

FIGURE 18–15. Asystole.

Escape Rhythms

Escape beats can originate in the AV nodal region or in the ventricular Purkinje fibers. A **junctional escape rhythm** originates in the AV node, has a rate of 40 to 60 per minute, and has a normal QRS configuration (Fig. 18–16). A **ventricular escape rhythm** originates in the Purkinje fibers, has a rate of 15 to 40, and is characterized by an abnormally wide QRS complex on the ECG (Fig. 18–17). An important clue to identifying escape rhythms is the absence of normal P waves and P-R intervals. After the impulse is generated in the Purkinje or nodal cell, it can be conducted backward to the atria. Thus a P wave, if present, may be inverted and located before, during, or after the QRS. Escape rhythms are usually poorly tolerated because they are slow and associated with decreased cardiac output. Failure of the sinus node can be treated with a pacemaker.

Premature Beats and Ectopic Rhythms

Premature atrial complexes (PACs) originate in the atria but not at the SA node. The PAC occurs earlier than normal, is preceded by a P wave, and has a normal QRS configuration (Fig. 18–18). Isolated or rare PACs are not clinically significant. However, frequent PACs may indicate underlying pathophysiology and may be precursors to more serious dysrhythmias.

Paroxysmal atrial tachycardia (PAT) is a burst of atrial complexes resembling several PACs in a row (Fig. 18–19). The rhythm is regular at a rate of 160 to 220 beats/min. It may be difficult to distinguish this rhythm from sinus tachycardia; however, differences in P wave configuration are usually apparent. The period of atrial tachycardia may last for minutes, hours, or days and can result in ischemia. PAT can occur in persons with no underlying heart disease in response to emotional stress or drugs. An episode of PAT may start as a PAC that has an abnormally slow conduction time through the atria and AV node. This is thought to allow the wave of depolarization to reexcite previously depolarized cells, resulting in reentry and perpetuation of the abnormal rhythm.

Reentry is a process in which a cardiac depolarization continues to proceed in a part of the heart after the main impulse has finished its path and the majority of the fibers have repolarized. If the errant impulse proceeds slowly enough, it may eventually meet with nonrefractory cells and initiate an extra, ectopic cardiac depolarization. Reentry processes are produced when electrical conduction in a portion of the heart is abnormally slowed or has an unusually long pathway.

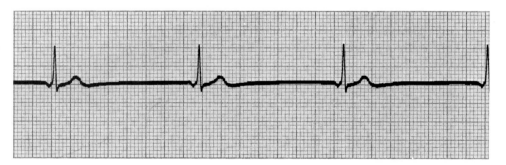

FIGURE 18–16. Junctional escape rhythm.

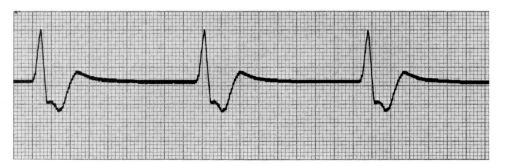

FIGURE 18–17. Ventricular escape rhythm.

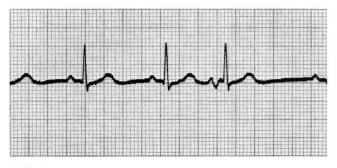

FIGURE 18–18. Premature atrial complex.

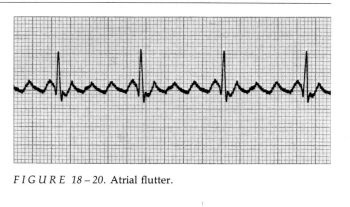

FIGURE 18–20. Atrial flutter.

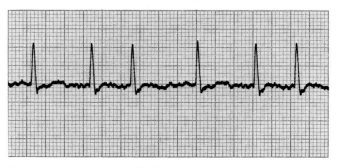

FIGURE 18–21. Atrial fibrillation.

Reentry is the probable culprit in many ectopic dysrhythmias.

Atrial flutter is manifested by a rapid atrial rate of 220 to 350 beats/min and a characteristic sawtoothed pattern of atrial depolarizations (Fig. 18–20). Atrial flutter and PAT are similar except for the more rapid atrial rate, which produces the sawtoothed pattern. The QRS configuration is normal; however, some of the atrial depolarizations may not conduct through the AV node, resulting in a slower ventricular rate. The ventricular rate may be irregular if there is a variable block or may be regular if there is a uniform block such as 2 : 1 or 3 : 1. Reentry is the probable mechanism for atrial flutter. Persons exhibiting atrial flutter usually have underlying heart disease, fluid overload, or atrial ischemia.

Atrial fibrillation is a completely disorganized and irregular atrial rhythm accompanied by an irregular ventricular rhythm of variable rate (Fig. 18–21). The atrial impulses appear as small squiggly waves of various sizes and shapes. Atrial cells cannot respond in an organized manner to depolarizing stimuli at rates faster than about 350. At rates above 350, a chaotic rhythm with asynchronous atrial contractions results. The majority of atrial depolarizations are blocked at the AV node, with few reaching the ventricles and initiating ventricular contraction. Atrial fibrillation causes the atria to quiver rather than contract forcefully. This allows blood to become stagnant in the atria and may lead to formation of thrombi. Additionally, the usual "atrial kick" that normally adds 30 percent more blood to the ventricle prior to systole is lost, and cardiac output may be reduced. Digitalis may be used to treat atrial fibrillation.

Premature junctional complexes can be initiated in two junctional zones: in the area just prior to the AV node, where atrial fibers enter, or in the area just after the AV node, where nodal fibers enter the bundle of His. The impulse spreads upward into the atrium, causing a P wave, and downward into the ventricle, causing a normally configured QRS. The P wave may precede, follow, or be buried in the QRS. Premature junctional beats have the same clinical significance as PACs and are generally well tolerated.

Junctional tachycardia is a rapid junctional discharge in the range of 120 to 200 beats/min (Fig. 18–22). The rhythm resembles a series of junctional premature beats, with P waves preceding, following, or buried in the QRS complexes. Differentiation of the ECG pattern produced by junctional tachycardia from that produced by atrial tachycardia is often difficult, and the term "supraventricular tachycardia" may be used for both.

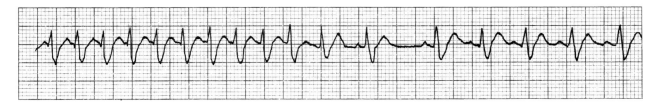

FIGURE 18–19. Paroxysmal atrial tachycardia. (From Ignatavicius DD, Bayne MV: *Medical-Surgical Nursing: A Nursing Process Approach.* Philadelphia, WB Saunders, 1991, p 2122. Reproduced with permission.)

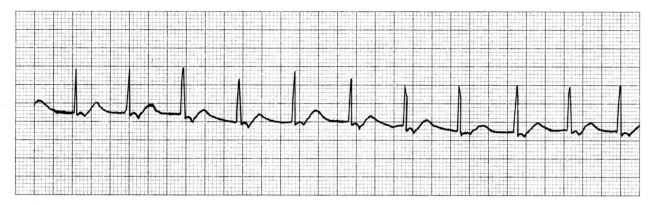

FIGURE 18–22. Junctional tachycardia. (From Ignatavicius DD, Bayne MV: *Medical-Surgical Nursing: A Nursing Process Approach.* Philadelphia, WB Saunders, 1991, p 2122. Reproduced with permission.)

Premature ventricular complexes (PVCs) arise from cells located in the ventricular myocardium. The impulse from this ectopic focus will depolarize the ventricles but doesn't activate the atria or depolarize the sinus node. Thus, the normal rhythm of sinus discharge is not disturbed. The normal sinus impulse is generally buried within the bizzare-looking QRS from the premature ventricular beat. It does not result in a QRS because the ventricles are refractory from the premature depolarization. The next sinus beat occurs just when it normally would have if no premature beat had occurred. Thus, the interval between the sinus beat preceding and the sinus beat following the premature beat is twice the regular interval (Fig. 18–23). This is known as a "compensatory pause" and helps confirm the diagnosis of PVCs. The QRS of the premature complex is prolonged (>0.10 sec) and bizarre in appearance. The T wave is usually in a direction opposite to the main QRS deflection. Premature ventricular beats are commonly associated with coronary artery disease, drug overdose, and electrolyte disturbances. The clinical significance depends in part on the frequency of the premature beats. With high frequency, cardiac output may be compromised. Frequent PVCs may be treated with antiarrhythmic drugs.

Ventricular tachycardia consists of three or more ventricular complexes at a rate greater than 100 per minute (Fig. 18–24). The rhythm is fairly regular and the complexes generally have the same configuration (monomorphic). With rapid rates, it may be difficult to distinguish the QRS complexes from the S-T segments and T waves, and the ECG appears as a series of large, wide, undulating waves. The sinus node usually continues to discharge independently of the ventricular rhythm, and P waves, if seen, are not associated with the QRS.

Reentry is the probable mechanism of ventricular tachycardia in most cases. Ventricular tachycardia is often associated with myocardial ischemia and infarction. Damage to the myocardium results in altered conduction times and conduction pathways, which set the stage for reentry loops. High catecholamine levels and an abnormal electrolyte balance may contribute to the dysrhythmogenesis.

Ventricular tachycardia is a serious dysrhythmia that is nearly always indicative of significant heart disease. It may be fatal unless it is successfully and rapidly treated. Ventricular tachycardia may compromise cardiac output, resulting in loss of consciousness. Treatment consists of rapid administration of antidysrhythmic drugs and, if necessary, cardiopulmonary resuscitation and administration of 10 to 100 joules of electrical current to the chest (cardioversion).

Ventricular fibrillation is a rapid, uncoordinated cardiac rhythm that results in myocardial quivering and lack of effective contraction. The rhythm is generally easily identified, particularly when assessment

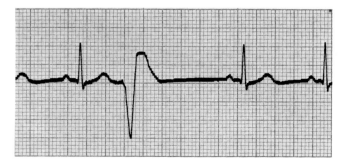

FIGURE 18–23. Premature ventricular complex.

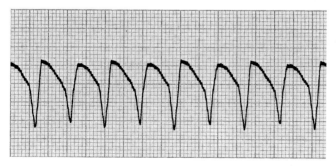

FIGURE 18–24. Ventricular tachycardia.

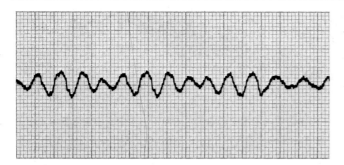

FIGURE 18–25. Ventricular fibrillation.

of the patient indicates absence of pulse and loss of consciousness. The ECG tracing is rapid and erratic, with no identifiable QRS complexes (Fig. 18–25). Ventricular fibrillation results in death if not reversed within minutes.

The same conditions that result in ventricular tachycardia may cause ventricular fibrillation. A critically timed premature beat or accelerating ventricular tachycardia may be the precursor to ventricular fibrillation. The ventricular depolarization is thought to be fractionated into a number of localized reentrant currents within the myocardial mass. The discoordinated depolarizations are sustained because of variability in conduction velocities and refractory periods.

Ventricular fibrillation must be rapidly identified and treated with cardiopulmonary resuscitation and defibrillation with electrical current. Defibrillation differs from cardioversion in that the administration of current is not synchronized with the R wave and the amount of energy delivered is greater (200–350 J). The earlier the patient is defibrillated, the better is the chance for success. In some instances, the ventricular fibrillation pattern is very fine and similar to the tracing seen in asystole. Defibrillation is still indicated. Defibrillation and cardiopulmonary resuscitation are usually followed by administration of antidysrhythmic drugs.

KEY CONCEPTS

- Failure of the SA node to generate impulses may result in a junctional or ventricular escape rhythm. These rhythms are slow and may be poorly tolerated. Absence of P waves is important to determination of escape rhythms.
- In most cases premature beats and ectopic rhythms are attributed to reentry mechanisms. Reentry circuits may be established when portions of the heart have abnormal conduction rates or pathways. Enhanced automaticity has been proposed as an alternate mechanism for generation of ectopic complexes.
- Ventricular tachycardia and ventricular fibrillation are associated with a significant fall in cardiac output and must be rapidly diagnosed and treated.

Conduction Pathway Disturbances

Disturbances of Atrioventricular Conduction

A disturbance in conduction between the sinus impulse and its associated ventricular response has been called **atrioventricular block.** The conduction may be abnormally slowed or completely blocked. The AV block results from a functional or pathologic defect in the AV node, bundle of His, or bundle branches. Three categories of AV block have traditionally been described: first-degree block, second-degree block (which includes type I and type II), and third-degree (complete) block. These AV conduction disorders are associated with different pathologies and clinical implications.

First-degree block is generally identified by a prolonged P-R interval (>0.20 sec) on the ECG (Fig. 18–26). The rhythm remains regular, and each P wave is associated with a QRS. First-degree block is a common finding during infection and may occur in the absence of organic heart disease. Drugs and organic heart disorders, such as myocardial ischemia and congenital heart defects, may cause first-degree block. First-degree block is generally monitored but is not actively treated except to alleviate the underlying cause if possible.

Second-degree block is diagnosed when some of the atrial impulses are not conducted to the ventricles. Two types of second-degree block are identified by the pattern of nonconducted impulses. Type I (Mobitz type I, Wenckebach) is associated with progressively lengthening P-R intervals until one P wave is not conducted (dropped beat). The pattern repeats, causing the QRS complexes to occur in groups. The P-P intervals are constant, whereas the R-R intervals vary (Fig. 18–27). Type I second-degree block is usually due to reversible ischemia of the AV node, often associated with acute myocardial infarction. The ischemic node is slow to recover after each depolarization, resulting in a longer and longer nodal delay until one impulse is not conducted. This gives the AV node time to recover, and the next atrial impulse is conducted more quickly with a nearly normal P-R interval, beginning the cycle again. Treatment is rarely required. If the block progresses to a type II block, a pacemaker may be required.

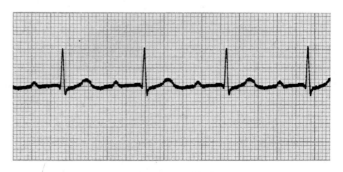

FIGURE 18–26. First-degree AV block.

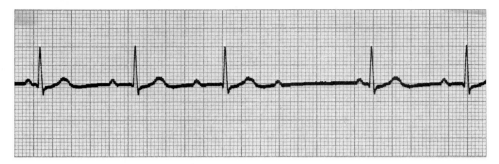

F I G U R E 18 – 27. Second-degree AV block, type I (Wenckebach, Mobitz type I).

Type II second-degree block is identified by the presence of nonconducted P waves (dropped beats) with a consistent P-R interval (Fig. 18–28). The QRS is usually wide (0.12 sec or greater). Type II block is generally associated with pathology of the bundle of His and/or right bundle branch. It is the bundle-branch block that causes the QRS complexes to be abnormally wide. Type II second-degree block is less common than type I but is more serious. It is usually associated with anterior septal myocardial infarction or fibrosis of the conduction system. Type II block may progress to complete heart block with slow ventricular escape rhythm and poor cardiac output. Type II block may also result in severe bradycardia due to the number of dropped beats. Symptomatic type II block may require treatment with a pacemaker.

Third-degree block may occur due to pathology of the AV node, bundle of His, or bundle branches. No impulses are conducted from the atria to the ven-

tricles, and a junctional or ventricular escape rhythm is evident. The ECG shows regularly occurring P waves that are totally independent of the ventricular rhythm (Fig. 18–29). If the QRS complex is narrow, the block is most likely in the AV node, proximal to the bundle of His. A prolonged QRS (>0.12 sec) indicates pathology distal to the bundle of His, within the bundle branches. The severity of symptoms is determined primarily by the heart rate, with slower rhythms being more serious. A pacemaker is generally required.

Abnormal Conduction Pathways

Some individuals have congenital abnormalities of the cardiac conduction system called *accessory pathways.* These extra conduction tracts provide alternate pathways for depolarization of the heart, resulting in ab-

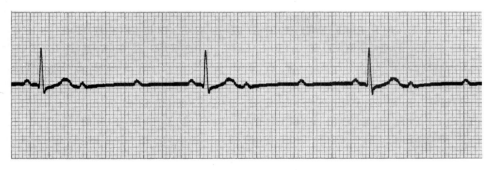

F I G U R E 18 – 28. Second-degree AV block, type II (Mobitz type II).

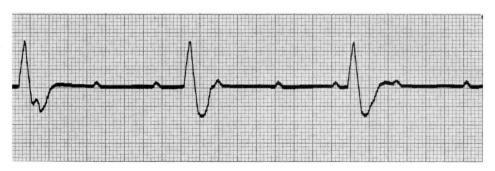

F I G U R E 18 – 29. Third-degree AV block, complete.

normally early ventricular depolarizations following atrial depolarizations. Three types of abnormal conduction pathways (preexcitation syndromes) have been identified.

1. Wolf-Parkinson-White syndrome is caused by accessory pathways that originate in the atria, bypass the AV node, and enter a site in the ventricular myocardium. This results in more rapid activation of the ventricle with a short P-R interval, initial slurring of the QRS (delta wave), and a wide QRS (Fig. 18–30). The accessory pathway may provide a mechanism for reentry and the development of supraventricular tachycardia.

2. Lown-Ganong-Levine syndrome results from accessory connections from the atria to the bundle of His. These connections bypass the AV node but permit normal intraventricular conduction. Thus the ECG shows early depolarization of the ventricles and a short P-R interval, but the QRS is normally configured (Fig. 18–31).

3. Mahaim pathways are accessory tracts that originate in the distal region of the AV node or bundle of His and end in a portion of the ventricular myocardium. The P-R interval is not usually shortened because of normal AV nodal delay; however, a portion of the ventricle may be prematurely depolarized, resulting in a "fusion" beat in which the normal and premature depolarizations occur simultaneously.

Identification and treatment of individuals with preexcitation syndromes is desirable to prevent symptoms of supraventricular tachycardia and to reduce the possibility of deterioration of the rhythm to atrial or ventricular fibrillation. Antidysrhythmic agents and measures to interrupt the pathway, such as vagal stimulation, may be used.

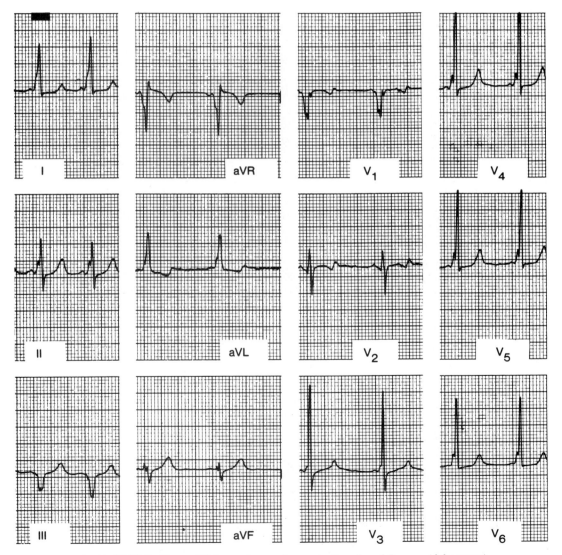

FIGURE 18–30. Wolff-Parkinson-White syndrome demonstrating sloped R wave (delta wave). (Reprinted from *Clinical Electrocardiography for Nurses* by H. M. Sweetwood, p 177, with permission of Aspen Publishers, Inc., © 1983.)

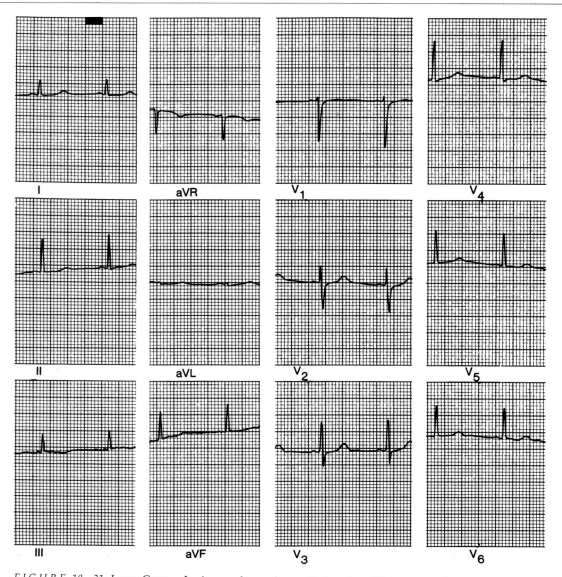

F I G U R E 18 – 31. Lown-Ganong-Levine syndrome demonstrating short PR interval and normal QRS. (Reprinted from *Clinical Electrocardiography for Nurses* by H. M. Sweetwood, p 185, with permission of Aspen Publishers, Inc., © 1983.)

Intraventricular Conduction Defects

Abnormal conduction of impulses through the intraventricular bundle branches is called *bundle-branch block*. The two primary bundles are the right bundle branch, which supplies the right ventricle, and the left bundle branch, which supplies the left ventricle. The left bundle branch is further divided into three fascicles, the anterior fascicle, the posterior fascicle, and the septal fascicle. These supply the anterior, posterior, and septal portions of the left ventricle respectively. Slowed or obstructed conduction occurring in one or more of these bundles results in abnormal ventricular depolarization and wide, bizzare-appearing QRS complexes. Bundle-branch blocks are best detected with ECG leads V_1 and V_6.

Right bundle-branch block may be present in almost any form of heart disease. It is occasionally found in individuals having no clinical evidence of heart disease. Right bundle-branch block can progress to complete heart block in some cases. The ECG pattern is indicative of blocked conduction to the right ventricle such that the left ventricle depolarizes first, then spreads to the right ventricle. Right bundle-branch block is classically associated with a late R wave in lead V_1 and an S wave in V_6. These changes are compared with the normal V_1 and V_6 in Figure 18–32.

Left bundle-branch block causes a delay in left ventricular depolarization. The right ventricle is activated first through the right bundle branch, followed by right-to-left activation of the septum, and finally left ventricular activation. The QRS is abnormally wide (>0.12 sec) but has a nearly normal deflection pattern in V_1 and V_6. In V_1 the small r wave normally associated with septal depolarization is absent, and V_6 consists of a wide R wave (Fig. 18–33). Leads V_4

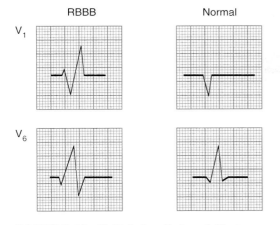

FIGURE 18 – 32. Right bundle-branch block pattern.

through V_6 show a wide, slurred, or notched (rabbit ear) R wave.

Left anterior hemiblock is due to a block in the anterior fascicle of the left bundle which causes the posterior aspect of the left ventricle to be activated first, followed by spread through the left ventricular myocardium in an upward and leftward direction. The ECG pattern shows small initial r waves followed by large S waves in leads II and III. The duration of the QRS is within normal limits.

Left posterior hemiblock is due to a block in the posterior fascicle of the left bundle which causes the anterior left ventricle to be activated first, followed by spread in a downward and rightward direction. The ECG findings include q wave in leads II, III, and aVF and R wave in leads I and aVL. These ECG findings may mimic ventricular hypertrophy or inferolateral myocardial infarction, making recognition difficult.

Combination blocks—Slowed or obstructed conduction may occur simultaneously in more than one bundle or fascicle, leading to the terms *bifascicular block*

and *trifascicular block.* For example, a right bundle-branch block occurring in conjunction with a left posterior hemiblock is called a bilateral or bifascicular block. Trifascicular block refers to a bifascicular bundle block (most commonly right bundle-branch block with left anterior hemiblock) in addition to a first-degree block (prolonged P-R interval). The prolonged P-R interval is usually due to incomplete block in the left posterior fascicle. Complete trifascicular block would make it impossible for a supraventricular depolarization to activate the ventricles, i.e., complete heart block.

KEY CONCEPTS

- Disturbances of AV conduction are generally referred to as AV blocks. First-degree block is characterized by a prolonged P-R interval and usually requires no treatment.

- Two types of second-degree block have been identified. Type I (Wenckebach) is characterized by a progressive prolongation of the P-R interval until one P wave is not conducted. Type I block is associated with AV nodal ischemia. Type II second-degree block is identified by a rhythm showing a consistent P-R interval with some nonconducted P waves. This block is more serious because it has a tendency to progress to complete AV block (third-degree block).

- Third-degree or complete heart block is diagnosed when there is no apparent association between atrial and ventricular conduction. This rhythm is serious, as it is typically associated with slow ventricular rhythm and poor cardiac output.

- Accessory conduction pathways are suspected in persons exhibiting preexcitation syndromes. Severe tachycardias and other reentrant rhythms may occur.

- Disturbances of intraventricular conduction (bundle-branch blocks) are characterized by wide,

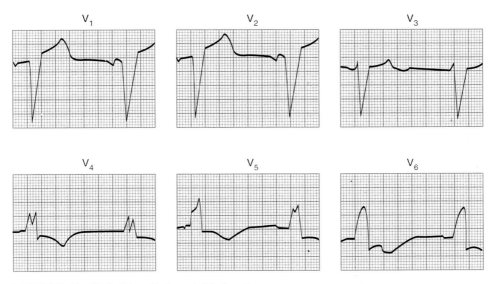

FIGURE 18 – 33. Left bundle-branch block pattern.

TABLE 18-3. Major Electrophysiologic Classes of Antiarrhythmic Compounds

Fast Sodium Channel Blockers	Repolarization Prolonging
Disopyramide	Amiodarone
Procainamide	Bretylium
Quinidine	Sotalol
Lidocaine	
Mexiletine	*Calcium Channel Blockers*
Phenytoin	
Tocainide	Diltiazem
	Nifedapine
Encainide	Verapamil
Flecainide	
Indecainide	*Potassium Channel Openers*
Propafenone	
	Adenosine
Beta Blockers	Adenosine triphosphate
Acebutolol	
Alprenolol	
Atenolol	
Labetolol	
Metoprolol	
Nadolol	
Oxprenol	
Propranolol	
Sotalol	
Timolol	

bizzare-looking QRS complexes. Any of the three ventricular fascicles may be affected (right bundle, left anterior fascicle, left posterior fascicle).

Treatment

Dysrhythmias are generally treated if they cause the patient to experience symptoms or if they are expected to progress to a more serious rhythm. A number of antidysrhythmic drugs (antiarrhythmics) have proved effective in treating many dysrhythmias. These drugs alter the properties of ion movement across cardiac membranes and affect the rate and duration of depolarization and repolarization. The major electrophysiologic classes of antiarrhythmic compounds are summarized in Table 18-3. Treatment may also include measures to improve cardiac output, including pacemakers and drugs to improve contractility and blood pressure. Dysrhythmias causing severely reduced cardiac output, such as severe bradycardia, asystole, ventricular tachycardia, and ventricular fibrillation, require cardiopulmonary resuscitation until an effective cardiac rhythm is established.

Summary

Heart failure may result from a number of cardiac and noncardiac disorders that diminish myocardial contractility or impose an excessive work load on the heart. The consequences of heart failure can be categorized as "forward" effects and "backward" effects. Forward effects are due to decreased cardiac output to the tissues and include decreased renal blood flow, fluid retention, activity intolerance, and mental fatigue. Backward effects are due to congestion of blood behind the sluggishly pumping ventricle. With left heart failure, the congestion is located in the lungs and produces a number of signs and symptoms, including dyspnea, orthopnea, hypoxemia, crackles, and frank pulmonary edema. Right heart failure causes congestion in the systemic venous system leading to congestion and dysfunction of the liver, spleen, and kidney, as well as peripheral subcutaneous edema and distended neck veins. The location of congestive signs and symptoms is the primary clue in differentiating right- and left-sided heart failure.

Three major compensatory mechanisms operate to maintain cardiac output in the failing heart. These are sympathetic activation, increased preload, and cardiac muscle cell hypertrophy. Unfortunately, these mechanisms also increase myocardial work load and oxygen requirements and may overwhelm the heart, causing decompensation. The primary aims of therapy are to improve cardiac output and minimize congestive symptoms and cardiac work load. These aims are achieved through management of preload, afterload, and contractility.

Dysrhythmia refers to an abnormality of the heartbeat. ECG dysrhythmias may occur in association with a number of cardiac and noncardiac disorders. Disturbances in electrical activity of the heart can indicate underlying pathophysiologic processes but are not themselves primary medical diagnoses. Dysrhythmias are significant because they can signal underlying pathophysiologic disorders and can disrupt normal cardiac output. Dysrhythmias can be categorized into three major types including, abnormal rates of sinus rhythm, abnormal site (ectopic) of impulse initiation, and disturbances in conduction pathways. Treatment of dysrhythmias centers on maintaining adequate cardiac output, providing antiarrhythmic drugs as needed, and diagnosing and treating the underlying pathology.

REFERENCES

1. Bristow MR, Ginsburg R, Minobe N, et al: Decreased catecholamine sensitivity and beta-adrenergic receptor density in failing human hearts. *N Engl J Med* 1982;307:205–211.
2. Cotran RS, Kumar V, Robbins SL: *Robbins Pathologic Basis of Disease*, 4th ed. Philadelphia, WB Saunders, 1989.
3. Bristow MR, Ginsburg R, Umans V, et al: β_1 and β_2-adrenergic-receptor subpopulations in nonfailing and failing human ventricular myocardium: Coupling of both receptor subtypes to muscle contraction and selective β_1-receptor downregulation in heart failure. *Circ Res* 1986;59:297–309.
4. Murphee S, Saffitz J: Distribution of β-adrenergic receptors in failing human myocardium. *Circulation* 1989;79:1214–1225.
5. Katz AM: Inotropic and lusitropic abnormalities in heart failure. *Eur Heart J* 1990;11(suppl A):27–31.
6. Guyton AC: *Textbook of Medical Physiology*, 8th ed. Philadelphia, WB Saunders, 1991.
7. Starling EH: *The Linacre Lecture on the Law of the Heart*. London, Longmans Green & Co, 1918.
8. Berne RM, Levy MN: The cardiac pump, in Berne RM, Levy MN (eds): *Principles of Physiology*. St. Louis, CV Mosby, 1990.

9. Schlant RC, Sonneblick EH: Pathophysiology of heart failure, in Hurst JW, et al (eds): *The Heart*, 6th ed. New York, McGraw-Hill, 1986, p. 327.

10. Gold WM: Cyanosis, in Blacklow RS (ed): *MacBryde's Signs and Symptoms*, 6th ed. Philadelphia, JB Lippincott, 1983.

11. Alpert JS, Braunwald E: Acute myocardial infarction: Pathological, pathophysiological, and clinical manifestations, in Braunwald E (ed): *Heart Disease: A Textbook of Cardiovascular Medicine*, 2nd ed. Philadelphia, WB Saunders, 1984.

12. Circulatory assist, in Daily E, Schroeder J: *Techniques in Bedside Hemodynamics Monitoring*, 3rd ed. St. Louis, CV Mosby, 1985.

13. Heilbrunn SM, Shah P, Bristow MR, Valantine HA, Ginsburg R, Fowler MB: Increased β-receptor density and improved hemodynamic response to catecholamine stimulation during long-term metoprolol therapy in heart failure from dilated cardiomyopathy. *Circulation* 1989;79(3):483–490.

14. Heng MK: Beta, partial agonists to treat heart failure: Effects of Xamoterol upon cardiac functions and clinical status. *Clin Cardiol* 1990;13:171–176.

BIBLIOGRAPHY

Arnold JM: The role of phosphodiesterase inhibitors in heart failure. *Pharmacol Ther* 1993;57(2–3):161–170.

Banach K, Bunemann M, Huser J, Pott L: Serum contains a potent factor that decreases beta-adrenergic receptor-stimulated L-type Ca^{2+} current in cardiac myocytes. *Pflugers Arch* 1993;423(3–4):245–250.

Bonow RO, Udelson JE: Left ventricular diastolic dysfunction as a cause of congestive heart failure: Mechanisms and management. *Ann Intern Med* 1992;117(6):502–510.

Brandt RR, Wright RS, Redfield MM, Burnett JC Jr: Atrial natriuretic peptide in heart failure. *J Am Coll Cardiol* 1993;22(4 suppl A):86A–92A.

Bristow MR: Changes in myocardial and vascular receptors in heart failure. *J Am Coll Cardiol* 1993;22(4 suppl A):61A–71A.

Coats AJ: Exercise rehabilitation in chronic heart failure. *J Am Coll Cardiol* 1993;22(4 suppl A):172A–177A.

Cody RJ: Clinical trials of diuretic therapy in heart failure: Research directions and clinical considerations. *J Am Coll Cardiol* 1993;22(4 suppl A):165A–171A.

Cody RJ: Physiological changes due to age: Implications for drug therapy of congestive heart failure. *Drugs Aging* 1993; 3(4):320–334.

Cohn JN: Efficacy of vasodilators in the treatment of heart failure. *J Am Coll Cardiol* 1993;22(4 suppl A):135A–138A.

Cohn JN: Nitrates versus angiotensin-converting enzyme inhibitors for congestive heart failure. *Am J Cardiol* 1993;72(8):21C–24C; discussion, pp 24C–26C.

Davies RH, Sheridan DJ: The treatment of heart failure—what next? *Br J Clin Pharmacol* 1993;35(6):557–563.

Drexler H, Hayoz D, Munzel T, Just H, Zelis R, Brunner HR: Endothelial function in congestive heart failure. *Am Heart J* 1993;126(3 pt 2):761–764.

Elkayam U, Shotan A, Mehra A, Ostrzega E: Calcium channel blockers in heart failure. *J Am Coll Cardiol* 1993;22(4 suppl A):139A–144A.

Ertl G, Gaudron P, Neubauer S, et al: Cardiac dysfunction and development of heart failure. *Eur Heart J* 1993;14 suppl A:33–37.

Fischer TA, Erbel R, Treese N: Current status of phosphodiesterase inhibitors in the treatment of congestive heart failure. *Drugs* 1992;44(6):928–945.

Floras JS: Clinical aspects of sympathetic activation and parasympathetic withdrawal in heart failure. *J Am Coll Cardiol* 1993;22(4 suppl A):72A–84A.

Furukawa T, Myerburg RJ: Mechanisms of arrhythmias in chronic ischemic heart disease. *Cardiovasc Clin* 1992;22(1):19–43.

Garg R, Yusuf S: Current and ongoing randomized trials in heart failure and left ventricular dysfunction. *J Am Coll Cardiol* 1993;22(4 suppl A):194A–197A.

Guyatt GH: Measurement of health-related quality of life in heart failure. *J Am Coll Cardiol* 1993;22(4 suppl A):185A–191A.

Holtz J: Pathophysiology of heart failure and the renin-angiotensin-system. *Basic Res Cardiol* 1993;88(suppl 1):183–201.

Hood WB Jr: Role of converting enzyme inhibitors in the treatment of heart failure. *J Am Coll Cardiol* 1993;22(4 suppl A):154A–157A.

Johnston CI, Fabris B, Yoshida K: The cardiac renin-angiotensin system in heart failure. *Am Heart J* 1993;126(3 pt 2):756–760.

Kelly RA, Smith TW: Digoxin in heart failure: Implications of recent trials. *J Am Coll Cardiol* 1993;22(4 suppl A):107A–112A.

Little WC, Applegate RJ: Congestive heart failure: Systolic and diastolic function. *J Cardiothorac Vasc Anesth* 1993;7(4 suppl 2):2–5.

Litwin SE, Grossman W: Diastolic dysfunction as a cause of heart failure. *J Am Coll Cardiol* 1993;22(4 suppl A):49A–55A.

Morgan HE: Cellular aspects of cardiac failure. *Circulation* 1993;87(5 suppl):IV4–IV6.

Om A, Hess ML: Inotropic therapy of the failing myocardium. *Clin Cardiol* 1993;16(1):5–14.

Packer M: The development of positive inotropic agents for chronic heart failure: How have we gone astray? *J Am Coll Cardiol* 1993;22(4 suppl A):119A–126A.

Parameshwar J, Poole-Wilson PA: The role of calcium antagonists in the treatment of chronic heart failure. *Eur Heart J* 1993;14 suppl A:38–44.

Pfeffer MA: Angiotensin-converting enzyme inhibition in congestive heart failure: Benefit and perspective. *Am Heart J* 1993;126(3 pt 2):789–793.

Pogwizd SM, Corr B: The contribution of nonreentrant mechanisms to malignant ventricular arrhythmias. *Basic Res Cardiol* 1992;87(suppl 2):115–129.

Poole-Wilson PA: Relation of pathophysiologic mechanisms to outcome in heart failure. *J Am Coll Cardiol* 1993;22(4 suppl A):22A–29A.

Rahimtoola SH: The hibernating myocardium in ischaemia and congestive heart failure. *Eur Heart J* 1993;14 suppl A:22–26.

Schwartz K, Chassagne C, Boheler KR: The molecular biology of heart failure. *J Am Coll Cardiol* 1993;22(4 suppl A):30A–33A.

Shah PM, Pai RG: Diastolic heart failure. *Curr Probl Cardiol* 1992;17(12):781–868.

Sneddon JF, Camm AJ: Sinus node disease: Current concepts in diagnosis and therapy. *Drugs* 1992;44(5):728–737.

Thames MD, Kinugawa T, Smith ML, Dibner-Dunlap ME: Abnormalities of baroreflex control in heart failure. *J Am Coll Cardiol* 1993;22(4 suppl A):56A–60A.

Treasure CB, Alexander RW: The dysfunctional endothelium in heart failure. *J Am Coll Cardiol* 1993;22(4 suppl A):129A–134A.

Waldo AL, Biblo LA, Carlson MD: Ventricular arrhythmias in perspective: A current view. *Am Heart J* 1992;123(4 pt 2):1140–1147.

Walker JE: Congestive heart failure in the elderly. *Conn Med* 1993;57(5):293–298.

Weintraub NL, Chaitman BR: Newer concepts in the medical management of patients with congestive heart failure. *Clin Cardiol* 1993;16(5):380–390.

Wilson JR, Mancini DM: Factors contributing to the exercise limitations of heart failure. *J Am Coll Cardiol* 1993;22(4 suppl A):93A–98A.

Young JB: Heart failure, ventricular remodelling and the renin-angiotensin system: Insights from recently completed clinical trials. *Eur Heart J* 1993;14 suppl C:14–17.

UNIT VI
Alterations in Respiratory Function

Breathing and lung function are affected by smoking.

Photo by Kathleen Kelly

Inhale. Exhale.
Hold your breath.
Gasp in surprise or fright.
Catch your breath.
Sigh in relief.
Breathe easier.

*O*ur breathing reveals us. We can conceal a moment of strong emotion by deliberately changing our breathing patterns—by taking some deep breaths, for example, or stifling a reaction to a moment of anxiety. But the need for conscious control only proves how richly meaningful breathing is. Our breathing is us. It even reveals the content of our collaboration with others: To conspire is to breathe together, or, as the dictionary says, to blow or sound together, to plot. Anyone who inspires you is infusing or enkindling you, as though responsive breathing could fill or fire a spirit.

Of course, this giveaway also is life-giving. Breathing, which may reveal us in unguarded moments, also sustains life. But it often is expected to do its work, rhymically inflating the lungs, despite efforts we make to impair our own or other peoples' breathing by contaminating the air the respiratory system requires.

No bodily system is more vulnerable to contamination by outside agents. Each year thousands of smokers die from lung cancer and emphysema. Others suffer lifelong illness from exposure to uranium dust, coal dust, asbestos, and other contaminants encountered either at work or at large in the environment.

The nose does its complicated work, warming, humidifying, and filtering the air we breathe, but this efficient appendage cannot save those who subject themselves, or are subjected, to lethal contamination. Particles too small to be filtered by the nose settle into small bronchioles. This is a cause of lung disease among miners. Tiny particles of cigarette smoke also escape the body's filters, causing lung disease or lung cancer.

Often we inflict these diseases on one another, or allow our habits to aggravate allergies or illnesses among otherwise healthy people.

A young man who has recently taken a job as a newspaper editor begins to experience breathing problems at work. He has a history of asthma but has not been troubled by it recently. His workplace is one that is becoming increasingly rare: A number of other employees are heavy smokers, and there are no rules against smoking in the room where he works.

One morning he is rushed by his wife to an emergency room, suffering from an asthmatic attack. He can inhale, but has the asthmatic's problem exhaling because the bronchial smooth muscle, excited by a reaction set off by some antigen, contracts spastically, increasing resistance in the airway. As an asthmatic, he is hypersensitive to foreign substances in the air. In his case, as his health care provider tells him, he is being injured by tobacco smoke. He chooses to find another job.

But diseases caused or aggravated by outside contaminants are only some of those found in the respiratory system. For others, gene therapy research is revealing new avenues of hope. An article in the *Journal of the American Medical Association* suggests that cystic fibrosis, an intractable respiratory disease normally treated by clearing the airway of secretions, treating infections, and replacing pancreatic enzymes, might now be treated through gene therapy. The disease-related gene has been identified. Cystic fibrosis gene

FRONTIERS OF RESEARCH
Advances in Treatment of Respiratory Disorders
Michael J. Kirkhorn

therapy has been effective in animal models, suggesting that similar therapy could be helpful to human sufferers.

Other respiratory disorders are becoming less ominous through improvements in monitoring, treatment, and care, though they remain dangerous and troubling for the health professionals who diagnose and treat them.

Health professionals have learned to watch alertly for signs of acute respiratory distress syndrome (ARDS), which can develop slowly or suddenly, often with devastating results. Twenty years ago, nine ARDS patients in ten died. The mortality is still above 50 percent, but a medical response can offer the patient a good possibility for recovery.

This life-threatening syndrome has recently been seen by researchers as part of a combination or sequence of disorders associated with systemic inflammatory response (SIRS) and multiple organ dysfunction syndrome (MODS), common critical care conditions characterized by progressive organ failure and, often, by death.

Researchers report that acute lung injury (ALI) and ARDS "play pivotal roles" in most occurrences of SIRS and MODS. Understanding the pathophysiology of the lung disorders has guided researchers in their approach to the often fatal system failures. MODS, organ collapse, is the most common cause of death among ARDS patients.

ARDS also is called high-permeability pulmonary edema. When the endothelial lining of the alveolar capillary membrane is damaged, fluid molecules that would normally remain inside the capillaries leak into surrounding tissues. The result is edema.

This disrupts normal gas exchange. Blood passes through saturated and collapsed alveoli without receiving oxygen. Supplemental oxygen can't reach the damaged alveoli. Heart rate and blood pressure decrease.

ARDS is another of those disorders that present a combination of crucial and exacting responsibilities for the health care professional. The ARDS patient requires careful detection of changes in respiratory status, gas exchange, and oxygen absorption, as well as nourishment adequate to allow the affected individual enough strength to eventually leave the ventilator.

CHAPTER 19
Respiratory Function

LORNA SCHUMANN

KEY TERMS

atresia: Closure of a normally open passage.

carina: A ridgelike structure at the base of the trachea that projects from the area that separates the left and right bronchi.

cilia: Hairlike processes on the surface of some cells.

colloid osmotic pressure: Passage of fluid from an area of less concentration to an area of higher concentration of colloids (large molecules).

compliance: A measure of the ease of elastic distensibility of a hollow organ.

diffusion coefficient: A constant that depends on the properties of the tissue and the gas; the rate of movement of a gas is proportional to the diffusion coefficient.

fistula: An abnormal opening between two organs or between an internal organ and the body surface.

hydrostatic pressure: Pressure exerted by a liquid.

shunt: Movement of blood into the arterial system without passing through areas of the lung.

The primary function of the lungs is gas exchange. Oxygen is transported to the body tissues, and carbon dioxide, a waste product, is transported out of the body. The exchange of these gases takes place at the alveolar-capillary membrane. Because health care professionals play a key role in prevention, treatment, and patient/family education in cases of respiratory disease, knowledge of lung structure and functions is essential.

Structural Organization of the Respiratory System

Embryology

On or about day 26 of embryonic development, formation of the lower respiratory system begins. This early formation consists of a laryngotracheal groove that arises from the wall of the pharynx and gives rise to the epithelium and glands of the larynx, trachea, bronchi, and pulmonary lining. The groove continues to deepen and forms a diverticulum (pouch) that develops into the laryngotracheal tube and bronchial buds.

Initially, the laryngotracheal diverticulum includes the esophagus and the trachea as a single tube. Then longitudinal ridges begin to develop along the tubular wall and form a septum (wall), which separates the esophagus from the trachea. Failure of this septum to develop leads to a **fistula** (abnormal opening), leaving a communication between the esophagus and the trachea. This abnormality occurs about once in every 2,500 births. Congenital malformations of the lower respiratory tract that require medical-surgical intervention are fairly rare. Figure 19–1 shows the four primary types of tracheoesophageal fistulas. Approximately 90 percent of the cases of esophageal **atresia** (blind pouch) are of the type seen in Figure 19–1A. Figures 19–1B, C, and D show variations of tracheoesophageal fistulas.[1]

As the laryngotracheal tube continues to elongate, the lung bud divides into two bronchial buds, which become the bronchi and the right and left lung. It is during this growth period that the right bronchus becomes larger than the left. The right mainstem bronchus is normally more vertical than the left because it is the main continuation of the laryngotracheal tube and branches off the trachea at a 20-degree angle. The left bronchus branches off the trachea in a more horizontal direction at an angle of 40 to 60 degrees. This normal anatomic development increases the chances that a foreign body will lodge in (or that an endotracheal tube will enter) the right mainstem bronchus rather than the left.

Fetal lung development can be divided into four periods. These are described below.

Pseudoglandular Period

The **pseudoglandular period** (5–17 weeks) represents the period of development when the lung resembles a gland. The bronchial divisions are differentiated, and the major elements of lung tissue are present except for those involved in gas exchange: the respiratory bronchioles and alveoli.

Canalicular Period

The **canalicular period** (16–25 weeks) is a period of growth when the bronchi and bronchioles enlarge and vascularization of lung tissue takes place. At the end of this period, respiration is possible because of the

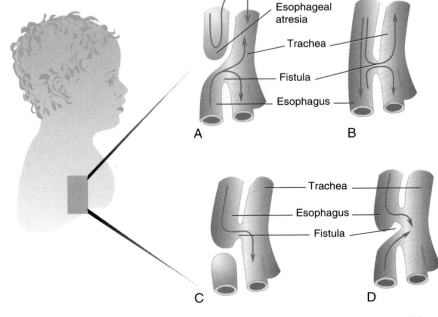

FIGURE 19–1. The four primary types of tracheoesophageal fistulas. **A**, The most common type, with complete atresia (blind pouch) of the esophagus. **B**, A common opening between the trachea and esophagus. **C**, An opening from an esophageal pouch into the trachea. **D**, A double opening from two unconnected ends of the esophagus. *Arrows* indicate flow of fluid from the esophagus to the trachea.

development of respiratory bronchiole and primitive alveoli. Alveoli are grapelike sacs where gas exchange occurs. Type II pneumocytes (epithelial cells that are on the internal surface of alveoli) begin to secrete surfactant at the end of this period. Surfactant is a phospholipid essential for maintaining alveolar patency.

Terminal Sac Period

The **terminal sac period** (24 weeks to birth) is so named because of the development of terminal sacs (future alveoli). As the period progresses, the sacs become thinner and thinner, thus preparing the lung tissue for gas exchange. Proliferation of pulmonary capillaries is also prominent during this period. Infants born prematurely in the early weeks of this period (25–28 weeks) are susceptible to the development of respiratory distress syndrome (RDS) (see Chap. 22).

Alveolar Period

The **alveolar period** (late fetal life to 8 years) is the final period of lung development. During this stage, alveolar ducts form from terminal sacs and alveoli mature by increasing in size and in number. Approximately one eighth to one sixth of the adult number of alveoli are present at birth.[1] During this growth period, there is a lack of structural collateral pathways necessary for maintaining open airways. This may make the individual more susceptible to atelectasis (incomplete expansion) and obstruction. Lung damage during this period may cause permanent defects in lung development.[1,2]

KEY CONCEPTS

- Respiratory system development begins at about day 26 of gestation. Abnormal development of the septum during this time can lead to tracheoesophageal fistula.
- Normal development of the bronchi results in a straighter route from the trachea to the right mainstem bronchus than to the left. Foreign objects are more likely to enter the right bronchus.
- At 25 weeks' gestation, the fetal lung has developed sufficiently to allow respiration. Alveolar development and surfactant production are just beginning.

Anatomy and Physiology

The anatomic arrangement of the respiratory system facilitates humidification, warming, filtering, and conduction of gas. The vast expanse of the alveolar-capillary membrane is more than adequate for normal gas exchange. Anatomically the respiratory system can be divided into two major areas: the upper airway and the lower airway. The upper airway consists of the nasopharyngeal cavity (nasopharynx, oropharynx, laryngopharynx) (Fig. 19–2). The lower airway contains the larynx, trachea, bronchi, bronchopulmonary segments, terminal bronchioles, and the acinus (the alveolar region supplied by one terminal bronchiole, which includes numerous alveoli).

Upper Airway and Nasal Cavity

The **nasal cavity** conducts gases to and from the lungs, and filters, warms, and humidifies the air. It is a rigid box composed of two thirds cartilage and one third bone, which prevents collapse of the area during movement of air. The convoluted turbinates (cone-shaped bones) of the nasal cavity are highly vascular with delicately tuned blood flow to form an efficient heat exchanger. Evaporation of water from the turbinate surface and from the mucus secreted by mucosal

PHARYNX

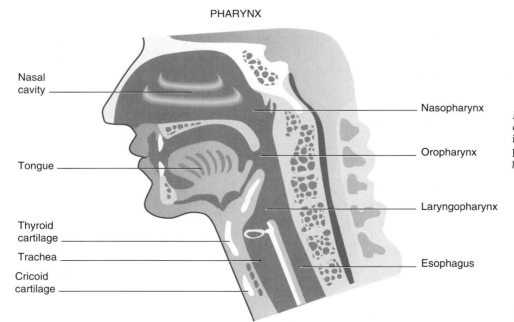

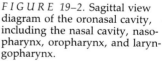

FIGURE 19–2. Sagittal view diagram of the oronasal cavity, including the nasal cavity, nasopharynx, oropharynx, and laryngopharynx.

glands raises the water vapor of the inspired air to normal saturation. Therefore, air is warmed to body temperature and humidified to approximately 80 percent saturation.

Air is filtered by the large hairs (*vibrissae*) of the nasal cavity and **cilia** that line the nasal cavity. The cilia sweep foreign particles trapped by mucus into the nasopharynx, where they are swallowed or expectorated. An electron micrograph of the tracheobronchial lining is shown in Figure 19–3. Pseudostratified ciliated columnar epithelium lines the trachea and bronchi. Goblet cells and mucus-producing glands are contained in this area and are responsible for producing the approximate 100 mL of mucus that is produced daily in the adult. The composition of mucus is 95 percent water plus mucopolysaccharides, mucoproteins, and lipids. Maintenance of water content and fluid balance is important to the mobilization of secretions. A child has more mucus-producing glands and therefore produces more mucus than adults. In the disease state of a child, an overproduction of mucus in combination with small airway size may precipitate tracheobronchial obstruction.[3]

Cilia

Cilia (Fig. 19–4) beat in a sweeping motion like oars rowing a boat at approximately 1,000 to 1,500 strokes per minute.[4,5] Mucociliary transport (movement of mucus upward) is a primary defense mechanism of the tracheobronchial tree. Inhaled particles, bacteria, and macrophages are removed from the respiratory tract by ciliary clearance and cough reflex. Ciliary function is impaired by smoking, alcohol, hypothermia, hyperthermia, cold air, low humidity, starvation, anesthetics, corticosteroids, noxious gases, a cold, and increased mucus.[4,5]

Paranasal Sinuses

The four **paranasal sinuses** are air-containing spaces adjacent to the nasal passages that provide speech resonance and increase the heat and water vapor exchange surfaces. The sinuses are swept clean by mucociliary action when the communicating passages that connect them with the nasal passages remain open.

Eustachian Tube

The **eustachian tube** runs the short distance from the middle ear to the posterior nasopharynx in order to maintain the air in the middle ear at atmospheric pressure. To prevent secretions or food from entering the middle ear during swallowing, the pharyngeal muscles close the eustachian tube briefly. The nasal end of the eustachian tube is surrounded by flexible cartilage arranged in a spiral configuration. The muscles surrounding the eustachian cartilages close the opening

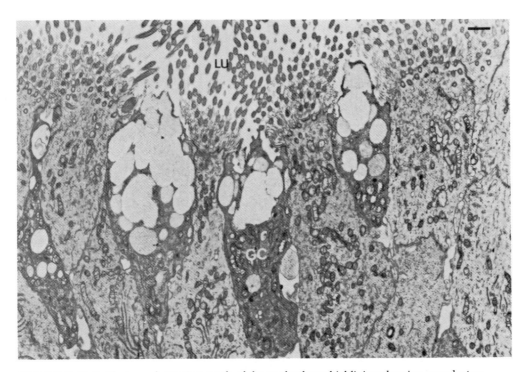

F I G U R E 19–3. Electron photomicrograph of the tracheobronchial lining showing pseudostratified columnar epithelium with goblet cells (*GC*) and mucous glands. *LU,* lumen of the airway; horizontal bar = 1 µm (×6,000). (From Murray JF: *The Normal Lung,* 2nd ed. Philadelphia, WB Saunders, 1986, p 27. Courtesy of Donald McKay, M.D. Reproduced with permission.)

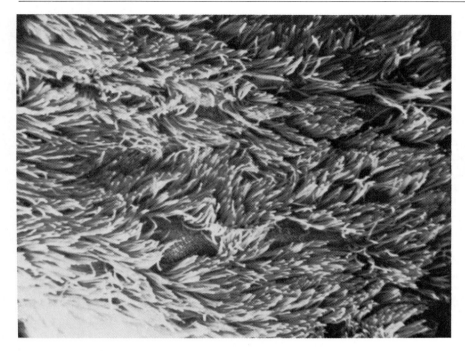

F I G U R E 19–4. Photomicrograph depicting the ciliary lining of a bronchiole in a healthy adult (×2,000). (From Ebert RV, Terracio MJ: *Am Rev Respir Dis* 1975;111:4. Reproduced with permission.)

by pulling the cartilage tighter. Because the tube is shorter in children, the potential for *otitis media* is increased.

Lower Airway

The lower respiratory airway contains the larynx, trachea, bronchi, bronchopulmonary segments, terminal bronchioles, and acinus. The acinus (Fig. 19–5) is composed of bronchioles, alveolar ducts, and alveoli. Air

passes through the nasal cavity or oral cavity into the pharynx, where it is filtered, warmed, and humidified. It then passes from the pharynx to the larynx and finally into the tracheobronchial region.

Larynx

The **larynx** is the transition area between the upper and lower airways. Anatomically it is considered part of the lower airway, but functionally it is similar to

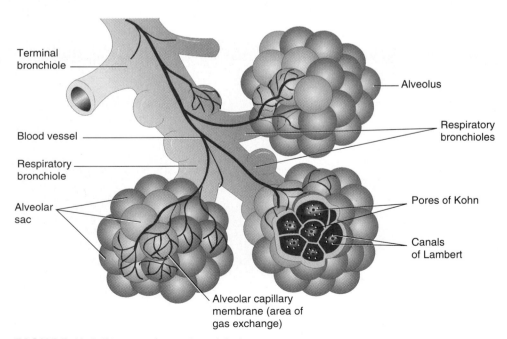

F I G U R E 19–5. Diagram of a portion of the lower respiratory tract, including a terminal bronchiole, respiratory bronchioles, and alveoli, where interchange of O_2 and CO_2 occurs between the thin walls of the alveoli and the capillary membrane.

the upper airway. The larynx contains the epiglottis, vocal cords, and cartilages. The anatomic arrangement of the larynx functions to prevent aspiration during swallowing and to assist in phonation and coughing. The larynx has been named the "voice box" because it contains the vocal cords. Each vocal cord is attached anteriorly to the thyroid cartilage and posteriorly to the arytenoid cartilage. Vibration of the cords leads to phonation.

The major cartilages of the larynx are the thyroid, cricoid, and artenoid. The thyroid cartilage is a large shield-shaped cartilage often referred to as the "Adam's apple." Immediately below the thyroid cartilage, is the site for emergency opening (*cricothyroidotomy*) of the tracheal passageway. The cricoid cartilage lies below the thyroid cartilage and is the narrowest point in the airway of a child. It is the only complete tracheal ring and because of its narrowness in the small child's airway, an endotracheal tube cuff is unnecessary for required intubation of the airway.

Functionally, the larynx provides two important defense functions for the respiratory system. It prevents aspiration of foreign matter during swallowing and provides a mechanism for giving a forceful cough. Food is prevented from entering the trachea during swallowing by closure of the epiglottis. If food or fluid should bypass the epiglottis and enter the tracheobronchial tree, the cough reflex is initiated. A cough reflex is produced when the epiglottis and vocal cords close tightly against air entrapped in the lungs. When the expiratory muscles contract forcefully against the closed epiglottis and vocal cords, a pressure of approximately 100 mm Hg is created. When the cords and epiglottis suddenly open, the high-pressure buildup is allowed to escape. This reflex rapidly removes foreign matter from the tracheobronchial tree.[4,5]

Trachea, Bronchi, and Bronchioles

The **trachea, bronchi,** and **bronchioles** make up the conducting airways that allow passage of gases to and from the gas exchange units. These conducting airways make up a proportionately larger amount of the total airway system in the infant and child than in the adult. The trachea (Fig. 19–6) contains incomplete cartilaginous rings and is approximately 11 to 13 cm long and lies between the cricoid cartilage and the **carina** (ridge located at the lower end of the trachea). Individual variations in tracheal shape include circular, D, C, elliptical, triangular, and U (Fig. 19–7). Of 111 adult tracheas studied, the incidence of shapes was 48.6 percent C, 27 percent U, 12.6 percent D, 8.2 percent elliptical, 1.8 percent circular, and 1.8 percent triangular.[6] These tracheal variations may affect ventilation of patients who have endotracheal tubes in their airways and require mechanical ventilation.

The majority of cough receptors lie at the carina. At the **carina,** the trachea divides into two mainstem (primary) bronchi which contain cartilage and smooth muscle. Viewing the body anteriorly, the carina is located at the angle of Louis, between the sternum and manubrium at the second intercostal space.

Anatomically, the right mainstem bronchus (see Fig. 19–6) is shorter, wider, and more in line with the trachea. For this reason, aspirated materials and endotracheal tubes tend to pass through the right passageway. This is also true for all ages. The small size of the conducting airway in the infant and child makes even a small decrease in the size of the lumen from an obstruction, critical to airway conduction.[3,7] Primary bronchi further divide into five (secondary) lobar branches, three to the right lung and two to the left lung. Each lobar branch enters a lobe of the lung and further divides into bronchopulmonary segments (ten segments in the right lung, nine segments in the left lung) (Fig. 19–8).[4,5] Each bronchopulmonary segment is composed of 50 or more terminal bronchioles (conducting airways) that branch into respiratory bronchioles where gas exchange begins.

Nervous system control over the bronchi and bronchioles is mediated by the autonomic nervous system. Stimulation of the parasympathetic nervous system innervating the bronchial smooth muscle leads to bronchoconstriction. When receptors are stimulated, impulses are carried to the brain by the vagus nerve. Efferent impulses returning from the brain initiate bronchoconstriction. Stimulation of the sympathetic nervous system leads to relaxation of bronchial smooth muscle. Sympathetic stimulation is mediated by β_2-adrenergic receptors, which are under the control of circulating catecholamines. Few, if any, sympathetic nerve fibers exist in the human airway.[8] (Refer to the discussion under Control of Respiration later in this chapter for further information.)

Terminal bronchioles, which include the conducting airways, further subdivide into two or more respiratory bronchioles (16 divisions or generations) where gas exchange begins. The respiratory bronchioles divide into two or more alveolar ducts, which in turn supply several alveoli.

Alveoli

The lung is fully developed by the 8th year of life.[1,2] The large alveolar surface area in conjunction with pulmonary surfactant, a phospholipid produced by type II alveolar cells, lowers surface tension and facilitates gas exchange. In addition to the type II cells found in alveoli, two other types of cells are also found: type I alveolar cells, the basic structural cells of the alveoli; and alveolar macrophages, which act as a defense mechanism by phagocytizing particles in the alveoli. Alveolar macrophages can be damaged by smoking and by inhalation of silica (SiO_2).

Adult lungs contain approximately 300 million **alveoli,** and the newborn lung contains one-eighth to one-sixth the adult number.[1,3–5] An elderly person may also have a reduction in the number of alveoli as part of the normal aging process, but many elderly people retain the same number of alveoli that they had as a younger adult.

Gas exchange occurs in the alveolar units (see Fig. 19–5) where oxygen (O_2) and carbon dioxide (CO_2) transfer across the alveolar capillary membrane. Col-

Structure of Trachea and Major Bronchi

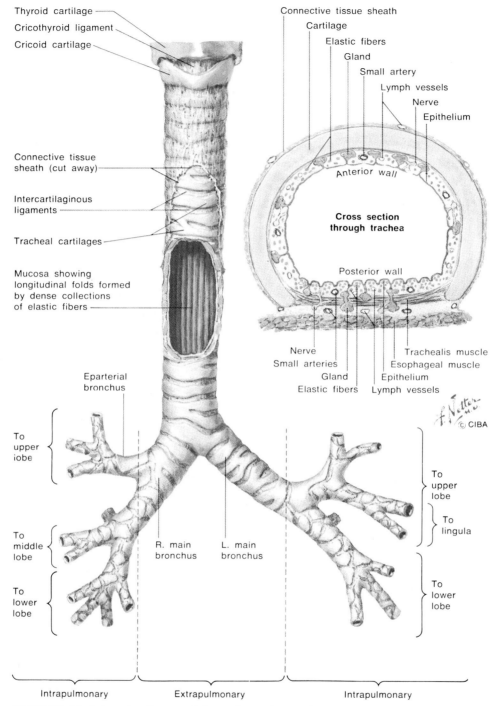

Thyroid cartilage
Cricothyroid ligament
Cricoid cartilage

Connective tissue sheath (cut away)

Intercartilaginous ligaments

Tracheal cartilages

Mucosa showing longitudinal folds formed by dense collections of elastic fibers

Connective tissue sheath
Cartilage
Elastic fibers
Gland
Small artery
Lymph vessels
Nerve
Epithelium

Anterior wall

Cross section through trachea

Posterior wall

Nerve
Small arteries
Gland
Elastic fibers
Trachealis muscle
Esophageal muscle
Epithelium
Lymph vessels

© CIBA

Eparterial bronchus

To upper lobe

To middle lobe

To lower lobe

R. main bronchus
L. main bronchus

To upper lobe

To lingula

To lower lobe

Intrapulmonary   Extrapulmonary   Intrapulmonary

F I G U R E   19–6. Anterior diagram of the trachea and major bronchi. (From Netter FH: *Respiratory System*, Vol. 7. Summit, NJ, CIBA Pharmaceutical Co, 1979, p 23. Reproduced with permission.)

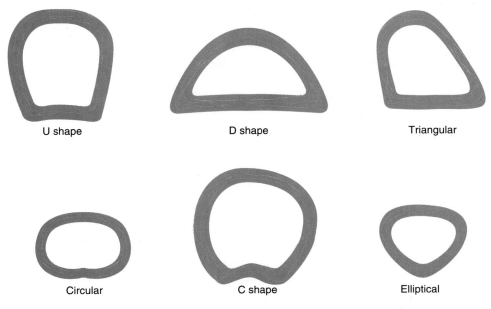

U shape   D shape   Triangular

Circular   C shape   Elliptical

FIGURE 19–7. Examples of variation in tracheal shape.

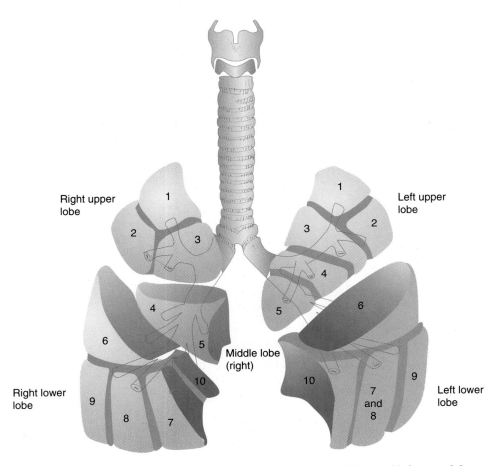

Right upper lobe

Left upper lobe

Right lower lobe

Middle lobe (right)

Left lower lobe

FIGURE 19–8. Bronchopulmonary segments of the human lung. **Right and left upper lobes:** *1* = apical segment, *2* = posterior segment, *3* = anterior segment; **left upper lobe:** *4* = superior segment, *5* = inferior segment; **middle lobe (right):** *4* = lateral segment, *5* = medial segment; **right and left lower lobes:** *6* = superior (apical) segment, *7* = medial basal segment, *8* = anterior basal segment (on left, *7* and *8* combine to form the anterior-medial basal segment), *9* = lateral basal segment, *10* = posterior basal segment.

lateral alveolar ventilation can also occur through holes in the alveolar walls called the pores of Kohn or canals of Lambert. The alveolar membrane is thicker in the neonate and reaches the adult thinness of 0.5 μm by the age of 8.[1,3] In addition, the small child has less collateral ventilation because of fewer pores of Kohn.[3,9] The membrane of an elderly person is even thinner than that of the adult.[4,10–12] This thinner membrane may allow increased transfer of O_2. The healthy older adult has very thin-walled, enlarged air sacs compared to those of a young person. In addition to the thin alveolar wall, there is also a decrease in the number of capillaries present.[4,11,12]

KEY CONCEPTS

- The upper airway includes the nasopharynx, oropharynx, and laryngopharynx. The primary functions of the upper airway are to warm, filter, and humidify inspired air.
- Eustachian tubes connect the middle ear to the nasopharynx. When patent, they function to prevent changes in pressure in the ear. Children are prone to inflammation and closure of the tubes, resulting in otitis media.
- The upper and lower airways are lined with cilia, which move rhythmically to transport mucus and trapped debris out of the respiratory tree. Ciliary function is impaired by a number of factors, among them smoking, alcohol, low humidity, and anesthesia.
- The lower airway includes the structures below the larynx—the trachea, bronchi, bronchioles, and alveoli. The larynx functions to prevent aspiration during swallowing and is the location of the vocal cords.
- The trachea, bronchi, and bronchioles serve as conducting passageways for air. They do not engage in gas exchange. Sympathetic influence on these airways causes relaxation (by means of β_2-adrenergic receptors) and parasympathetic influence causes constriction (by means of acetylcholine receptors).
- Exchange of respiratory gases occurs in the alveoli. The epithelial cells that make up the alveoli are called type I cells (type I pneumocytes). Type II pneumocytes produce surfactant in the alveoli. The grapelike structure of the alveoli provides a huge surface area for gas exchange.

Age-Related Variations

Structural and physiologic variations occur at each end of the age continuum. A summary of anatomic and physiologic respiratory variations by age group is presented in Table 19–1. The data will assist the reader in determining variations in patient care data pertinent to each age group that may vary from standard adult values.

TABLE 19–1. Variations in Anatomy and Physiology of the Respiratory System by Age Grouping

Age Group	P_AO_2 (*mm Hg*)	P_ACO_2 (*mm Hg*)	Ph	Bicarb mEq/L	Anatomic Dead Space	Percent of Alveoli
Young newborns	60–70	45–50	7.3–7.4 (depends on Apgar score)	20–26	Proportionately for size	12.5 to 16.5 adult number
Children	90–100	35–45	7.35–7.45	22–28	Proportionately for size	Adult number by 8 yr old
Adult	90–100	35–45	7.35–7.45	24–30	Approximately 150 cc	300,000/lungs
Elderly after age 60	70–80	35–45	7.30–7.45 (depends on oxygenation)	24–30	Approximately 150–200 cc	≤300,000/lungs

Age Group	Thickness of Alveolar Membrane	No. of Capillaries	Vital Capacity	Tidal Volume	Compliance	Airway Resistance
Young newborns	Thicker than adult	Less than adult	Proportionately less than adult	Proportional to size	More compliant than adult	Greater than adult
Children	Adult by 8 yr old	Adult by 8 yr old	Proportional to size	Proportional to size	Similar to adult	Greater than adult
Adult	Less than 0.5 μ	Adult	4.7 L	500 cc	Static compliant 90–100 mL/ cm H_2O	1.0–1.5 cm H_2O/L/sec
Elderly after age 60	Thinner than adult	Less than adult	Less than adult	Less than adult values (30 percent less by age 80)	Less compliant	Adult level or less

Pulmonary Circulation

Sources of Blood Supply

Blood supply to the lungs comes from two sources: the bronchial artery system, which supplies a small amount of oxygenated blood to the pleura and lung tissues, and the pulmonary artery system, which provides a vast capillary network for O_2 and CO_2 exchange. The capillary networks of the neonate, young child, and elderly person are less than those in the average healthy adult. Oxygen-depleted blood leaves the right ventricle by way of the pulmonary artery trunk, which branches into the right and left pulmonary arteries. The pulmonary arteries further divide into smaller arteries and arterioles that feed into the capillary network where gas exchange occurs from the alveolar capillary membrane.

Factors Influencing Pulmonary Circulation

The capillary network is a low-pressure system that is able to expand two to three times normal size before a significant increase in pulmonary capillary pressures is detectable. The normal pulmonary arterial pressure in a healthy adult is about 22 to 25/8 mm Hg. The mean pulmonary artery pressure is approximately 15 mm Hg. This compares with the high pressure of the systemic circulation which is normally considered to be 120/80 mm Hg, with a mean arterial pressure of 96 mm Hg. Under normal resting conditions, only about 25 percent of pulmonary capillaries are perfused (filled with blood).

The pulmonary circulation has two mechanisms for lowering pulmonary vascular resistance when vascular pressures are increased because of increased blood flow (Fig. 19–9).[4,5,7] The first mechanism is recruitment, which allows opening of previously closed capillary vessels. The second mechanism is distention, which allows for widening of capillary vessels.

Another factor influencing pulmonary circulation is the water balance of the lung tissues. Water balance is regulated by the **hydrostatic pressure, colloid osmotic pressure,** and **capillary permeability.** When capillary hydrostatic pressure exceeds colloid osmotic pressure, fluid moves from the capillary into the interstitium. If the fluid shift is not controlled, the fluid volume will continue to increase until fluid is moved into the alveoli. Alveolar edema is more serious than intestitial edema (fluid in the interstitial space) because of its effect on gas exchange owing to fluid in the alveoli.[4,7] Pulmonary interstitial and alveolar edema is common in disease processes such as congestive heart failure and infectious diseases of the lung. Other disease processes that also increase capillary permeability are adult respiratory distress syndrome (ARDS) and infant respiratory distress syndrome. (See Chapter 22 for further discussion.)

KEY CONCEPTS

- The lungs are perfused by two sources: bronchial arteries bring a small amount of oxygenated blood to nourish lung tissues; pulmonary arteries bring the

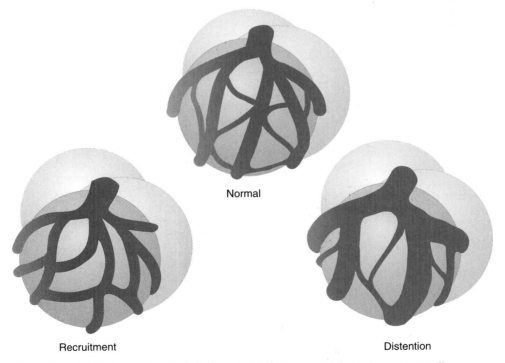

Normal

Recruitment

Distention

FIGURE 19–9. Two mechanisms for lowering pulmonary vascular resistance in capillary vessels. *Recruitment* allows for opening of previously closed capillaries. *Distention* allows for widening of capillary vessels.

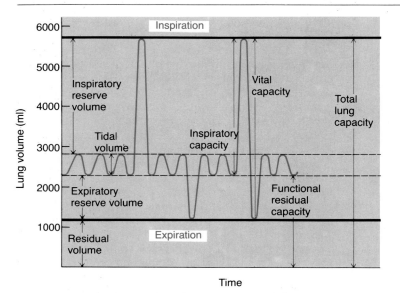

FIGURE 19–10. Schematic representation of the various lung volumes and capacities for a healthy adult. (From Guyton AC: *Textbook of Medical Physiology,* 8th ed. Philadelphia, WB Saunders, 1991, p 407. Reproduced with permission.) (See also Table 19–2.)

entire cardiac output of the right ventricle to the alveoli for gas exchange.

- The lung has a large reserve capacity for gas exchange. At rest only about 25 percent of the pulmonary capillaries are perfused. During periods of high lung blood flow (such as, high cardiac output during exercise), previously unperfused capillaries are recruited, and already perfused capillaries become distended.

- Filtration of fluid through pulmonary capillaries is influenced by hydrostatic pressure and colloid osmotic pressure in the same way as other capillaries. Excessive filtration can lead to pulmonary edema, which interferes with normal gas exchange.

Ventilation, Perfusion, Gas Exchange, and Transport

Respiratory Cycle

The respiratory cycle consists of three processes: ventilation, diffusion, and perfusion. Ventilation is discussed in this section; diffusion and perfusion are discussed under Exchange and Transport of Gases in the Body. The overall effectiveness of the transfer of O_2 and CO_2 between the alveoli and the pulmonary circulation requires a matched distribution of ventilation and perfusion.

Ventilation

Ventilation is the process of moving air into the lungs (alveoli) and distributing air within the lungs to gas exchange units for maintenance of oxygenation and removal of CO_2.[7] Measures of ventilation (amount of air moved) include four lung volumes and four lung capacities. Figure 19–10 schematically presents the various lung volumes and capacities; Table 19–2 defines each term and provides further details.

Lung volumes and capacities vary with individual body size, age (decreased in the neonate, young child, and the elderly)[11–13] and the individual's body position (supine vs. upright). Testing of pulmonary function to measure these volumes and capacities is covered under Obstructive Pulmonary Disease in Chapter 20.

Dead Space

Other concepts important to ventilation are dead space, minute ventilation, and alveolar ventilation. **Dead space** includes three dimensions: anatomic dead space, alveolar dead space, and physiologic dead space. Anatomic dead space includes the volume of nonusable gas (not used in gas exchange) in the conducting airways from the nose down to the respiratory[7,10] bronchioles. The area between the nasal cavity and the terminal bronchioles is considered to be anatomic dead space because gas exchange does not occur in these areas. Generally in the adult this area is equal to 1 mL per pound of ideal body weight, or approximately 150 mL. In the newborn and young child, the anatomic dead space is proportionately larger for its size.[3,9] The anatomic dead space of the elderly person may increase slightly over that of the healthy young adult because of the loss of alveolar sacs, but it typically remains the same. Alveolar dead space is composed of the ventilated but unperfused or underperfused areas of the lung and is often referred to as wasted ventilation.[7] Alveolar dead space increases with the development of pulmonary emboli owing to decreased perfusion. Physiologic dead space (functional dead space) is the sum of the anatomic dead space and alveolar dead space.[10,11] Approximately one third of each breath is wasted as dead space.

Minute Ventilation

Minute ventilation or expired volume ($\dot{V}E$) is the product of tidal volume times respiratory rate per

TABLE 19–2. Human Lung Volumes and Capacities

Lung Volumes

Tidal volume	A normal breath (approximately 500 mL) or the amount of gas entering or leaving the lung during normal breathing
Inspiratory reserve volume	The amount of gas a person is able to inspire above a normal breath (e.g., maximum deep breath, approximately 3 L)
Expiratory reserve volume	The amount of gas expired beyond tidal volume (approximately 1.2 L)
Residual volume	The volume of gas left in the lungs at the end of a maximum expiration (approximately 1.2 L)

Lung Capacities

Vital capacity	The total volume of gas that can be exhaled during maximum expiration (approximately 4.8 L)
Inspiratory capacity	Amount of gas that can be inspired from a resting expiration (approximately 3.5 L)
Functional residual capacity	The amount of gas left in the lungs at the end of a normal expiration (approximately 2.4 L)
Total lung capacity	The amount of gas contained in the lungs at maximum inspiration (approximately 6.0 L)

minute. For example, a person with a tidal volume (milliliters of air inhaled with each breath) of 500 mL, breathing at a rate of 15 breaths/min, has a minute ventilation of 7,500 mL. (Refer to Table 19–2 for typical volumes.)

Alveolar Ventilation

By comparison, **alveolar ventilation** ($\dot{V}A$) equals the difference between tidal volume (V_T) and anatomic dead space volume (V_D) multiplied by the respiratory rate (RR) per minute[10]:

$$(V_T - V_D) \times RR = \text{Alveolar ventilation } (\dot{V}A).$$

Because alveolar ventilation is affected by both anatomic dead space and the respiratory rate, slow deep breathing yields a greater alveolar ventilation than rapid shallow respiration. The patient breathing 25 times/min at a low tidal volume of 200 mL would have an alveolar ventilation of (200 mL − 150 mL) times 25 breaths/min, which equals 1,250 mL. A patient breathing 10 times/min at a tidal volume of 600 mL would have an alveolar ventilation of (600 mL − 150 mL) times 10, or 4,500 mL.

KEY CONCEPTS

- Approximately one third of each breath occupies areas of the lung that do not engage in gas exchange. Total (physiologic) dead space includes the anatomic dead space of the bronchial tree and the dead space of unperfused alveoli.
- Alveolar ventilation may be severely compromised in persons with small tidal volumes or increased dead space. When tidal volume is not significantly greater than dead space, increased respiratory rate is not effective in restoring minute ventilation.

Exchange and Transport of Gases in the Body

Diffusion

The second process in the respiratory cycle is **diffusion**. Diffusion is the movement of gas from a high concentration area to a low concentration area. The alveolar-capillary membrane through which O_2 and CO_2 must diffuse consists of six barriers (Fig. 19–11). For O_2 to reach the hemoglobin molecule, it must pass through surfactant, the alveolar membrane, interstitial fluid, the capillary membrane, plasma, and the red blood cell membrane. The rate of diffusion of a gas is proportional to the tissue area and the difference in gas partial pressure between the two sides of alveoli, and inversely proportional to the tissue thickness that the gas must move through. Oxygen diffuses into the blood from the alveoli, and CO_2 diffuses out of the blood into the alveoli. Under normal conditions, O_2 and CO_2 move across the alveolar-capillary membrane in only 0.25 second. The red blood cell spends about 0.75 second within the pulmonary capillary system surrounding the alveoli, thus allowing an extra 0.50 second of exchange time. Even with mild disease processes, O_2 and CO_2 have adequate time for transfer.

Under abnormal conditions, such as thickening of the alveolar-capillary membrane (pneumonia, pulmonary edema, and interstitial lung disease) and decreased available surface area (emphysema), the diffusion capacity of the lung tissue is impaired. Diffusion capacity may be further impaired by increased physical activity because of the decreased time spent by the red blood cells in the pulmonary capillary system. Thickening of the alveolar-capillary membrane also occurs with aging.

Carbon dioxide is 20 times more diffusible than O_2 because of its greater solubility. Factors that determine the ability and the speed of a gas to

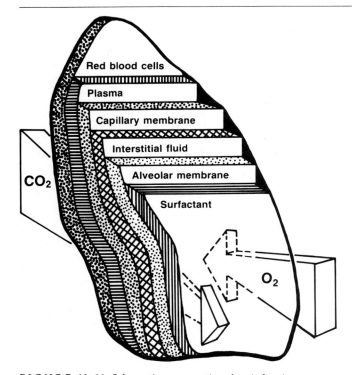

F I G U R E 19–11. Schematic representing the six barriers through which O_2 and CO_2 must diffuse for gas exchange to occur.

diffuse include the available surface area of alveoli and capillaries, the integrity of the capillary and alveolar membranes, the availability of hemoglobin to transport oxygen, the solubility of the gas, the **diffusion coefficient** of the gas, and the differences in partial pressure of the gases on each side of the alveolar membrane. For example, because CO_2 is 24 times more soluble than O_2, it diffuses more rapidly and requires a lower partial pressure.

Conditions that increase the partial pressure contribute to what is termed ventilation-perfusion ($\dot{V}A/\dot{Q}$, where $\dot{V}A$ = alveolar ventilation and $\dot{Q}$ = blood flow) mismatch. These include areas of **shunt** (unoxygenated blood), which have adequate pulmonary capillary blood flow but no ventilation, and areas of mismatched gas distribution (ventilation) to blood distribution (perfusion). The decreased diffusing capacity seen in the aged person is further compromised by a decrease in the number of pulmonary capillaries and decreased lung volume and capacities. The end result is decreased partial pressure of arterial O_2 (PaO_2) and increased $\dot{V}A/\dot{Q}$ mismatch. The PaO_2 drops about 3 to 5 mm Hg for each decade after age 30. Therefore, an 80-year-old individual could be expected to have a PaO_2 of 75 mm Hg. Diffusion is also decreased in the newborn because of the thickness of the alveolar membrane.[3] In a healthy adult, the PaO_2 value would be 90 to 100 mm Hg. (Refer to Table 19–1 for variations in respiratory anatomy/physiology by age grouping.)

The difference between alveolar (PAO_2) and arterial (PaO_2) oxygen tension is a good indicator of diffusion and $\dot{V}A/\dot{Q}$ matching. Alveolar oxygen (PAO_2) is estimated by using the following equation:

$$PAO_2 = FIO_2 (PB - 47) - (PaCO_2 \div 0.8)$$

where FIO_2 = fraction of inspired oxygen, PB = barometric pressure, 47 = constant for water vapor pressure (mm Hg), 0.8 = respiratory quotient, and $PaCO_2$ = laboratory measurement of arterial CO_2 (mm Hg).

The value for PAO_2 is normally very close to that for PaO_2. The difference between alveolar and arterial oxygen tensions is called $A - aDO_2$. A large $A - aDO_2$ indicates poor $\dot{V}A/\dot{Q}$ matching. For example, to calculate $A - aDO_2$ for a person at sea level (PB = 760 mm Hg) breathing room air (FIO_2 = 0.21) with PaO_2 = 75 mm Hg, and $PaCO_2$ = 40 mm Hg:

$$PAO_2 = 0.21 (760 - 47)$$
$$- (40 \div 0.8) \approx 150 - 50 = 100.$$

So, using the arterial blood gas value obtained for the PaO_2:

$$A - aDO_2 = 100 - 75 = 25 \text{ mm Hg.}$$

Perfusion and Oxygen Transport

Perfusion (blood flow) is the third process of the respiratory cycle. The pulmonary circulation is a low-pressure system (25/8 mm Hg). Blood from the right ventricle is pumped into the main pulmonary artery and then into its branches, which go into capillary beds throughout lung tissue. The capillary beds surround the alveoli and allow for easy exchange of O_2 and CO_2.

Oxygen is transported to the tissues by two mechanisms: in the dissolved form in plasma, and in the bound state attached to the hemoglobin molecule. Only about 0.3 mL O_2/100 mL is carried dissolved in the plasma.[7] The remaining O_2 is transported on the hemoglobin molecule. A high concentration (partial pressure) of O_2 in the pulmonary capillaries causes O_2 to bind to the hemoglobin molecule. Heme is an iron-porphyrin compound that joins with the four polypeptide chains of the protein globin. Oxygen binds to each of the four heme sites to form oxyhemoglobin. At the tissue level where the partial pressure of O_2 is low, O_2 is released from the hemoglobin molecule. Dependent on tissue needs, one fourth is normally unloaded at the tissues in a resting individual which results in venous blood being 75 percent saturated.

Fully bound O_2 is considered to be 100 percent saturated and yields a PaO_2 of 95 to 100 mm Hg. Increasing alveolar O_2 above this level will have no further effect on increasing the amount of O_2 carried on the hemoglobin molecule. Oxygen binds to the hemoglobins molecule in the lungs and is delivered to tissues. Oxygen binds when there is a high affinity of oxygen to hemoglobin (at the lungs) and releases when the affinity is decreased at the tissue level to maintain adequate metabolic processes. Below a PaO_2 of 60 mm Hg (90 percent saturation) hemoglobin saturation falls steeply (see Fig. 12–15). The oxyhemoglobin dissociation curve schematic shows the effects of increases and decreases in O_2 affinity at any Pao_2. Decreased O_2 affinity, also termed a "shift to the right," aids in the release of O_2 from the hemoglobin molecule, thus facilitating movement of O_2 from the blood into the tissues.

Increased O_2 affinity, termed a "shift to the left" represents an increased binding of O_2 to the hemoglobin molecule, thus decreasing its delivery to the tissues. Although an increased affinity for O_2 reflects a higher percentage of saturated hemoglobin, its ineffective release in the tissues may be profound. Factors that affect hemoglobin affinity and shift the curve to the left (increased affinity) include alkalosis, hypothermia, decreased $Paco_2$, and decreased 2,3-diphosphoglycerate (2,3-DPG, an end product of red blood cell metabolism). Factors that shift the curve to the right (decreased affinity) include acidosis, hyperthermia, increased $Paco_2$, and increased 2,3-DPG. The availability of O_2 is also decreased by decreased cardiac output and anemia.

Carbon Dioxide Transport

Carbon dioxide, a by-product of cell metabolism, is transported in the blood in four ways: dissolved in plasma (5 to 10 percent of the total CO_2 transport); in carbonic acid in the plasma (insignificant amount); as bicarbonate (60 to 70 percent); and as carbamino compounds on the hemoglobin molecule (20 to 30 percent). The greatest bulk of CO_2 transport is in the bicarbonate form. In the presence of the plasma enzyme, carbonic anhydrase, CO_2 combines with water to form carbonic acid, which in turn almost instantaneously breaks down into bicarbonate ions and hydrogen ions. The released hydrogen ions attach to the hemoglobin molecule, while the bicarbonate ion diffuses into the plasma and combines with sodium. Chloride ions in the surrounding plasma shift into the red blood cell (chloride shift). This chemical process is reversed when the venous blood reaches the lungs, so that CO_2 can diffuse across the alveolar membrane to be exhaled.

Hypoxemia and Hypoxia

Two terms frequently used in discussing decreased Pao_2 are hypoxemia and hypoxia. **Hypoxemia** refers to deficient blood oxygen as measured by low arterial O_2 and low hemoglobin saturation as measured by arterial blood gases. **Hypoxia** refers to a decrease in tissue oxygenation.

The end result of ineffective gas exchange is hypoxia, which is manifested by hypoxemia (decreased Pao_2). Resultant types of hypoxia can be classified into four categories: hypoxic hypoxia, anemic hypoxia, circulatory hypoxia, and histotoxic hypoxia. Hypoxic hypoxia occurs when the Pao_2 is decreased despite normal O_2-carrying capacity. Causes include high altitude, hypoventilation, and airway obstruc-

tion. Oxygen therapy usually provides adequate therapy.

Anemic hypoxia results from a decrease in O_2 carrying capacity. Causes of anemic hypoxia include sickle cell anemia, carbon monoxide poisoning, and other anemias.

Circulatory hypoxia results in a low cardiac output state where the O_2-carrying capacity is normal but blood flow is reduced. Examples of circulatory hypoxia include shock, cardiac arrest, severe blood loss, thyrotoxicosis, and congestive heart failure.

The final classification is histotoxic hypoxia, which occurs when interference of a toxic substance leads to inability of tissues to utilize available oxygen. Cyanide poisoning is an example of this hypoxic classification.

Ventilation-Perfusion Ratios

A factor important to the concepts of ventilation and perfusion is the matching of an adequate volume of air in the alveoli to adequate pulmonary blood flow. In the ideal state, 4 L/min of alveolar ventilation is matched to 5 L/min of capillary blood flow in the lungs, creating a normal $\dot{V}a/\dot{Q}$ ratio of 0.8. Two major factors impacting this normal $\dot{V}a/\dot{Q}$ ratio are right-to-left shunt and regional ventilation and perfusion changes. (Refer to the discussion under Distribution of Ventilation Through the Lung.) Other factors influencing the ratio are position changes, exercise, bed rest, and disease conditions of the lung.

Two concepts essential to a discussion of $\dot{V}a/\dot{Q}$ ratios include distribution of blood flow (perfusion) through the lung, and distribution of ventilation throughout the lung.

Distribution of Blood Flow Through the Lung

Distribution of blood flow (perfusion) is uneven and is affected by body position and exercise. When a person is upright, blood flow is much less in the upper regions of the lungs (apices) than in the lower regions (bases). When a person assumes the supine position, blood flow to the posterior dependent portion of the lung is higher. Blood flow to the anterior nondependent portions is lower, although the redistribution of blood flow is less dramatic than that seen in the upright lung.

The effects of gravity on the lung has led to the concept of three[3] or four[7] lung zones. Figure 19–12 depicts three lung zones. Zone one reflects blood flow in the apices of the lung. Blood flow is minimal because the enlarged alveolar sacs create an alveolar pressure that is higher than capillary pressure, leading to pulmonary capillary collapse. Zone two, the middle region of the lung, has a pulmonary artery pressure greater than the pressure inside the alveoli. This alveolar pressure is greater than pulmonary venous pressure, which results in decreased blood flow to this region. Physiologically the region is marked by inter-

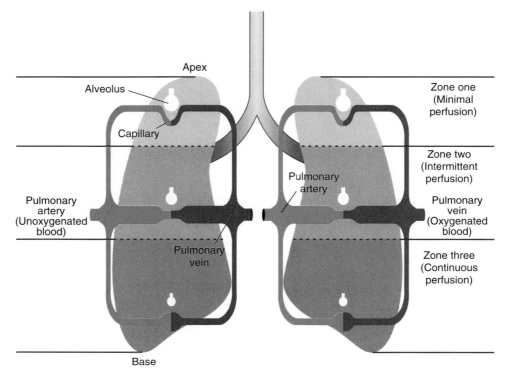

F I G U R E 19–12. Schematic representation of the three lung zones in which different hemodynamic conditions govern blood flow. (See text for discussion.)

mittent perfusion, which increases as one progresses from the upper region of the zone to the lower region of the zone in the upright position.

Zone three represents the ideal state, which is marked by continuous perfusion of lung tissue throughout the entire cardiac cycle. Pulmonary artery pressure is greater than pulmonary venous pressure, which in turn is greater than alveolar pressure. In this zone capillary vessels are distended, and vascular resistance is low.[7,9]

Distribution of Ventilation Through the Lung

Distribution of ventilation is also affected by body position. In the upright individual, the alveoli at the apices of the lung are much larger than those at the base. Figure 19–13 shows the variation in structural size of alveoli at the apex as compared to that at the base. In the normal upright individual, the bases of the lung are better ventilated than the apices. Ventilation per unit volume is greatest near the bottom of the lung and decreases toward the apices.[7] These regional differences are less in a supine person. The greater lung expansion at the bases results from a greater expansion of the ribs at the bases and the downward displacement of the diaphragm, which expands the lower lobes more than the upper lobes. When an individual is in the supine and lateral position, ventilation is best in the dependent lung, but the difference is not as great as that seen in the upright lung. In the

abnormal (diseased) state in which the individual is breathing at low lung volumes, ventilation is best in the nondependent (upper) areas of the lung. With rapid, shallow breathing, air goes to the apices.

Normally, 2 to 3 percent of the total pulmonary capillary blood flow bypasses (right-to-left shunt) alveolar ventilation, creating a decrease in arterial oxygen by 3 to 5 mm Hg. The base of the lung has the greatest blood flow and ventilation. Overall, in the upright lung, the best $\dot{V}A/\dot{Q}$ exchange takes place at the base of the lung. In the elderly adult, there is a decrease in the matching of ventilation to perfusion because of early airway closure in the lower zones (bases) of the lungs with the person upright.[10,12,13]

The discussion on ventilation and perfusion indicates that the best overall ventilation and perfusion occurs in the dependent lung fields (bases) in the upright lung. Factors that interfere with ventilation and perfusion lead to a classification of respiratory disorders according to broad categories of mechanisms of dysfunction such as O_2 failure and ventilatory failure. These factors are discussed in the last section of this chapter.

KEY CONCEPTS

• Oxygen and CO_2 diffuse quickly across alveolar capillary membranes. Complete equilibration of gases occurs in the first third of the capillary under normal conditions. Diffusion may be incomplete when

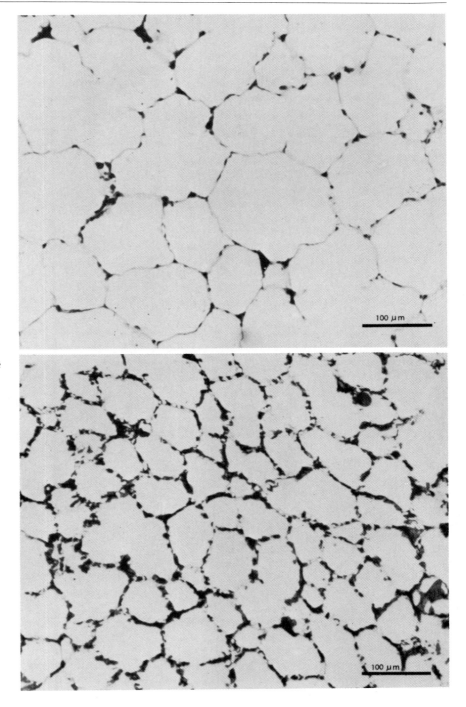

FIGURE 19–13. Sections of lung from the apex (*upper panel*) and 20 cm below the apex (*lower panel*) obtained from a greyhound dog frozen in the vertical position. The upper picture shows what alveoli in the apex (*zone one*) of the lung looks like in the upright position: the air sacs are large and blood flow is diminished. The lower picture represents the base of the lung zone with optimal ventilation and perfusion (×188). (From Murray JF: *The Normal Lung,* 2nd ed. Philadelphia, WB Saunders, 1986, p 110. Courtesy of Jon B. Glazier, M.D. Reproduced with permission.)

the alveolar capillary membrane is abnormally thickened or capillary blood flow is extremely rapid.

- Carbon dioxide is more soluble and diffuses more quickly than O_2. Disorders of diffusion often affect O_2 transfer earlier and more significantly than CO_2 transfer.

- Oxygen is carried in the blood in two forms: dissolved in solution ($PaO_2 \times 0.003$); and bound to hemoglobin ($Hb \times$ saturation $\times 1.34$). Significantly more O_2 is bound than dissolved. Low hemoglobin

and low hemoglobin saturation profoundly affect the O_2 content in the blood.

- The oxyhemoglobin saturation curve describes the relationship between PaO_2 and hemoglobin saturation. At a PaO_2 of 90 to 100 mm Hg, hemoglobin is fully saturated. An increase in PaO_2 above this level does not significantly improve O_2 content.

- The affinity of hemoglobin for O_2 is affected by temperature, acid-base status, 2,3-DPG levels, and CO_2. Affinity decreases at the tissue level because of increased acid, 2,3-DPG, and CO$_2$. This "shift to the right" enhances the unloading of O$_2$ at the tissue. A "shift to the left" occurs at the lung, where the blood is more alkalotic and CO$_2$ levels are lower. Increased affinity of hemoglobin in the lung enhances oxygen binding.

- A general deficiency of O$_2$ in the blood (hypoxemia) results from poor diffusion at the alveoli (hypoxic hypoxia) or anemia (anemic hypoxia). Tissue hypoxia may be due to general hypoxemia or poor perfusion (circulatory hypoxia) or poor uptake of O$_2$ by the tissue (histotoxic hypoxia).

- In order for optimal alveolar-capillary gas exchange to occur, alveoli must be both ventilated and perfused. Ventilation and perfusion are gravity dependent, such that the greatest ventilation and perfusion occur in dependent lung areas. Mismatching of ventilation and perfusion leads to decreased diffusion of gases. The difference between alveolar and arterial oxygen tension (A $-$ aDo$_2$) provides a good index of the adequacy of ventilation-perfusion matching.

- Carbon dioxide is transported in the blood in three major forms: dissolved, as carboxyhemoglobin, and as the bicarbonate ion. The most important of these is bicarbonate ion, which is formed from the combination of CO$_2$ and H$_2$O, forming carbonic acid (H$_2$CO$_3$). Carbonic acid breaks into HCO$_3^-$ and H$^+$. At the lung, the reaction proceeds in the reverse to form CO$_2$, which diffuses into the alveoli.

Control of Respiration

Control of respiration is influenced by a number of factors. These include neural control, chemoreceptors, lung receptors, proprioceptors, and pressure receptors. The factors that regulate respiration are reviewed in this section.

Neural Control

Neural control of the respiratory system is located in the medulla oblongata and the pons, which is commonly referred to as the respiratory center. Nerve impulses travel from the brain stem by way of the phrenic nerve to the diaphragm to stimulate muscular contractions for inspiration. Environmental factors may override the neural control center, but in the normal state they do not exert major control over respiration.

The **medullary respiratory center** within the brain stem consists of two groups of widely dispersed neurons that function as a unit to regulate breathing. The dorsal respiratory group of neurons sends out impulses that stimulate inspiratory muscles (in the intercostals and diaphram). The impulses are released in increasing fashion, termed a "ramp" signal. Impulses begin slowly and increase steadily for about 2 seconds. Abrupt cessation of signals for 3 seconds allows for expiration, then the cycle begins again.[4,5,7] This system establishes the basic respiratory rhythm. Figure 19–14 provides a schematic diagram of these

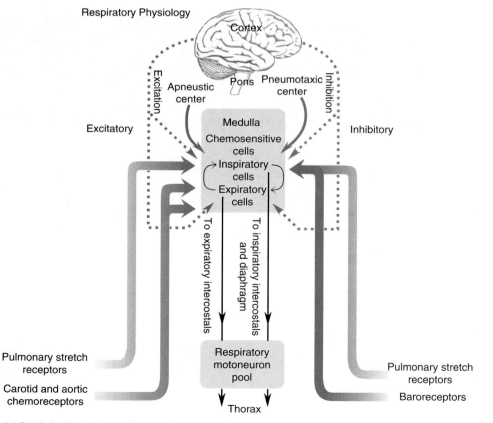

F I G U R E 19–14. Interactive mechanisms influencing control of respiration.

interactive mechanisms on respiratory control. These elements of respiration are described in the following sections.

The **pneumotaxic center of the upper pons** (see Fig. 19–14) appears to influence the rate of respiration and ends inspiration by inhibition of an inspiratory "ramp." In addition, input from the spinal cord, cortex, and midbrain contribute to the normal smooth pattern of respiration.

The **apneustic center of the lower pons** (demonstrated to exist in dogs) influences the pattern of respiration and probably prevents the "switch off" of the inspiratory "ramp." It may function to provide an extra driving force for the inspiratory neurons, thus prolonging inspiration.

Other Centers of Control

Other respiratory control centers include central chemoreceptors, peripheral chemoreceptors, Hering-Breuer reflex, proprioceptors, and pressoreceptors.

The **central chemoreceptors** within the medullary center respond to changes in CO_2 and pH. A small increase in $Paco_2$ leads to stimulation of respiration. Alveolar ventilation can increase tenfold with an acute rise in $Paco_2$. Acidosis or a decrease in pH can also increase alveolar ventilation.

The **peripheral chemoreceptors** located in the aortic arch and carotid bodies respond to decreases in arterial O_2 and pH and increases in arterial $Paco_2$. A severe decrease in Pao_2 (30–60 mm Hg range) leads to stimulation of respiration. Increases in the hydrogen ion concentration (decreased pH) or the $Paco_2$ indirectly increase respiratory activity. However, these effects are not prominent because of the overriding effects of the central chemoreceptors.

The **Hering-Breuer reflex** consists of stretch receptors located in the alveolar septa, bronchi, and bronchioles. Inflation of the lung initiates the response that sends neuronal impulses up the vagus nerve to the medulla to cause inhibition of inspiration. Therefore, the rate and duration of inspiration are effected. This reflex, seen primarily in neonates and at high tidal volumes (greater than 1,500 cc), prevents overdistention of the lung.[4,5,7]

Proprioceptors located in the muscles and tendons of movable joints respond to body movement (exercise). The stimulus of body movement leads to stimulation of respiration (rate and depth) in order to maintain oxygen levels during exercise.[5]

Pressoreceptors (baroreceptors) located in the aortic arch and carotid bodies respond to changes in blood pressure. The aortic arch transmits impulses through the vagus nerve, and the carotid bodies transmit impulses through the glossopharyngeal nerve. An increase in arterial blood pressure leads to increased blood flow with a resultant increase in O_2 to tissue and inhibition of respiration. A decrease in arterial blood pressure below a mean arterial pressure of 80 mm Hg leads to stimulation of respiration.

Environmental Factors

Environmental factors also influence respiration. Individuals demonstrate changes in respiration related to such factors as a cold shower, pin prick, fever, and stress, as well as to airway irritation from air pollution, infection, and smoking.

KEY CONCEPTS

- The medulla oblongata and pons contain the neurons that integrate information regarding the ventilatory status of the body. These respiratory center neurons generate the nervous impulses that stimulate respiratory muscle contraction.
- Respiratory neurons in the medulla create cyclic neuronal firing, which initiates inspiration and establishes the basic inspiratory-expiratory pattern. Pneumotaxic center neurons in the pons primarily influence the rate and depth of respiration.
- Information about the body's respiratory status is provided to brain stem respiratory centers by chemoreceptors, baroreceptors, proprioceptors, and pulmonary stretch receptors.
- Central chemoreceptors located within the medulla detect changes in pH and CO_2. Peripheral chemoreceptors are located in the aorta and carotids and detect changes in arterial pH, CO_2 and Po_2. An increase in CO_2 or a decrease in pH or Po_2 stimulates ventilation.

Mechanics of Breathing

The mechanics of breathing include such concepts as airway resistance, lung compliance, and opposing lung forces (elastic recoil vs. chest wall expansion) of the lung. These factors affect the overall performance of gas exchange.

Airway Resistance

Airway resistance is determined by the relationship between pressure and air flow. It is influenced by airway radius and the pattern of gas flow. Resistance increases as the radius of the airway tube decreases. Resistance is calculated by the following formula:

$$\text{Resistance} = \frac{\text{Pressure difference}}{\text{Rate of air flow}}.$$

The radius of the airway decreases from the trachea to the terminal bronchioles. As mucus builds up in the airway the passage is narrowed, and resistance to air flow increases. Other factors affecting airway resistance include stress, pulmonary conditioning, and age.

The trachea and bronchi contain cartilage and small amounts of muscle. The cartilage assists in maintaining airway passage stability, thus preventing airway collapse. The bronchioles and terminal bronchioles do not contain cartilage, but have increased amounts of smooth muscle that are innervated by the autonomic nervous system. Stimulation of cholinergic fibers leads to bronchoconstriction. Stimulation of the β_2-adrenergic receptors leads to bronchodilation. It appears that the function of the bronchial muscles help to maintain an even distribution of ventilation. A circadian rhythm is associated with bronchial tone, with maximal bronchodilation occurring at about 6:00 P.M. and maximal bronchoconstriction occurring at 6:00 A.M.[4]

Airway resistance is also affected by the pattern of gas flow (Fig. 19–15). Air movement from the nasal cavity through the large bronchi occurs by *turbulent flow*, which creates friction and increases resistance. Bronchospasm in the smaller airways and high gas flow also create turbulent flow. *Laminar flow* occurs in the small airways of the lung and creates minimal resistance to air flow. *Transitional flow* (mixed pattern of flow) occurs in the larger airways, especially at bifurcations. The highest airway resistance is at the nose because of turbulent flow with high velocities of air flow. The lowest airway resistance is in the small bronchioles where turbulent flow is low. Airway resistance is even higher in the newborn than the adult, and continues to be greater than that of the adult up to the age of 5. It changes very little in the elderly lung.[3,9,14]

Lung Compliance

Lung compliance is another factor that influences the work of breathing. Compliance represents lung expansibility and the ease of lung inflation. It is a measure of the relationship between pressure and volume. It is represented by the following formula:

$$Compliance = \frac{\text{Change in volume}}{\text{Change in pressure}}.$$

It is best illustrated by the effort required to blow up a new balloon as compared to blowing up a balloon that has been inflated many times before. Two factors associated with compliance are chest wall expansibility (not usually measured) and lung expansibility. Lung compliance can be measured in the static (motionless) state or dynamic state. **Effective static compliance** is determined by dividing the pressure required to deliver a volume of gas by the tidal volume as delivered by a ventilator. A more accurate measure-ment of compliance requires the insertion of an esophageal balloon. Normal static compliance in a healthy young adult would be 90 to 100 mL/cm H_2O.

Compliance provides an estimate of airway resistance and elasticity. Compliance is a measure of the volume above which an increase in pressure will not increase the volume of gas (normal, 40–50 mL/cm H_2O). Lung compliance is increased in the neonate and young child under the age of $3\frac{1}{2}$ because of their increased chest wall flexibility.[3] Lung compliance may decrease in the elderly because of increasing chest wall rigidity from calcification of costal cartilages, reduced mobility of ribs, and partial contraction of inspiratory muscles.[14] Compliance may be further compromised by loss in the elastic fibers of the lung that occur with age.[14] (There appears to be a reduction in number and thickness of elastic fibers with advancing age.) Changes in the thoracic vertebrae and intervertebral disks also lead to decreased expansion of the chest wall in the elderly.[11,12] Disease processes that make the lung stiffer and decrease respiratory function include pneumonia, pulmonary edema, atelectasis, ARDS, and pulmonary fibrosis. Other factors that decrease compliance by decreasing chest wall distensibility are obesity, abdominal distention, kyphoscoliosis, and abdominal surgery (due to decreased respiratory effort from surgical pain). Lung compliance is increased in patients with emphysema because there is loss of alveoli and elastic tissue.

Opposing Lung Forces

Another factor in the work of breathing is the effect of **opposing lung forces.** The lungs have a natural recoil tendency, whereas the chest wall favors the expanded state. During inspiration the chest wall muscles (external intercostals) contract, elevating the ribs as the diaphragm moves downward. These two actions create a negative intrapleural pressure that causes the lung to expand. During expiration the lung deflates passively because of the elastic recoil (elastic fibers in the lung tissue), relaxation of the diaphragm, and the surface tension of the alveoli. In the normal resting individual, expiration is accomplished almost entirely by relaxation of the diaphragm.[7]

KEY CONCEPTS

- To move air into the lungs, the respiratory muscles generate a negative intrapleural pressure that causes air inflow, owing to the pressure gradient between the atmospheric pressure at the mouth (zero pressure) and the alveolar pressure (negative pressure).

- Airways and tissues of the lung resist inflation. Resistance is provided by the airways, elastic fibers in the lung, and surface tension in the alveoli. The degree of resistance can be estimated by measuring overall lung compliance. A compliant lung requires minimal pressure to accomplish a large increase in

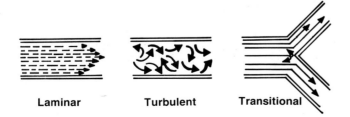

Laminar   **Turbulent**   **Transitional**

FIGURE 19–15. Patterns of gas flow through various sized airways.

volume; a noncompliant (stiff) lung requires the generation of high pressure to inflate the lung.

- Airway resistance is primarily determined by the diameter of the airways. Airway constriction greatly increases airway resistance. Parasympathetic stimulation of the airways results in constriction; sympathetic (β_2) stimulation results in dilation.
- Elastic fibers in the lung are stretched during inspiration, then recoil passively to achieve expiration. Destruction of elastic fibers increases lung compliance; excessive fiber production (fibrosis) decreases lung compliance.
- High surface tension in an alveoli causes the surfaces to stick together, making inflation more difficult. Surfactant functions to reduce surface tension. A lack of surfactant makes the lungs more difficult to inflate (decreased compliance).

Classification of Respiratory Disorders

Respiratory disorders can be classified according to broad categories of mechanisms of dysfunction, such as **ventilatory failure or oxygenation failure.** Additionally, respiratory disorders may also be classified according to categories of lung disease, encompassing changes in structure and function. Changes in structure and function include restrictive disorders, obstructive disorders, vascular disorders, respiratory failure, neoplasms, and infectious processes. The broad classifications of ventilatory failure and oxygen failure are considered briefly in this section, and in later chapters of this unit (Chaps. 20–23), followed by the classifications according to structure and function in the chapters on pathophysiologic diseases.

Ventilatory Failure

Ineffective gas exchange from **ventilatory failure** occurs when an adequate volume of gas is maldistributed, minute ventilation is decreased, and/or alveolar hypoventilation occurs. Maldistribution of gas occurs in patients with emphysema where gas exchange occurs only in some alveolar units.[14] In the healthy lung, some maldistribution of gas occurs because of gravitational forces on the lung. When a person is standing upright, the air spaces at the apex of the lung are more expanded than those at the base of the lung.[2] In addition to the gravitational forces, airway resistance affects distribution of gases. In obstructive pulmonary diseases the increased airway resistance develops in localized regions because of (1) plugging of airways from increased sputum production, (2) mucosal hypertrophy and edema, (3) loss of structural integrity of the airway, and (4) airway narrowing from bronchial smooth muscle contraction when there is hyperactivity of the airways.[14] During expiration, air leaves the areas of least resistance first, thus creating areas of maldistribution of gas. Alveolar hypoventilation leads to increased $Paco_2$ retention and decreased Pao_2. This occurs in patients with peri-

ods of apnea, Pickwickian syndrome, myasthenia gravis, and those under sedation. In patients with pulmonary disease, a greater amount of the tidal volume is wasted, and the compensatory mechanism of increasing the respiratory rate is insufficient to provide adequate alveolar ventilation. Therefore, CO_2 levels become elevated, and O_2 levels drop.

Oxygenation Failure

Ineffective gas exchange related to oxygen failure occurs when ventilation and perfusion are mismatched, when diffusion abnormalities exist, and when right-to-left shunt exists. Abnormal $\dot{V}A/\dot{Q}$ ratios exist when ventilation and perfusion are mismatched in some lung areas. During periods of normal perfusion not all capillaries are open, but the capillary system has the ability to recruit (open up) more capillaries and to distend (expand) capillaries now in use (see Fig. 19–9) to increase alveolar blood flow when necessary as a compensatory mechanism. In addition, 2 to 3 percent of the total blood flow in the lung is not oxygenated because the thesbian, pleural, and bronchial veins drain unoxygenated blood into the left side of the heart and into the pulmonary veins. Ventilation-perfusion equations in Table 19–3 show normal function, low $\dot{V}A/\dot{Q}$, and high $\dot{V}A/\dot{Q}$. The equations reflect the relationship between blood flow and gas distribution.

Areas of low $\dot{V}A/\dot{Q}$ may have normal perfusion, but receive inadequate alveolar ventilation (Fig. 19–16). This effect is similar to shunting of pulmonary artery blood through totally unventilated units. Areas of high $\dot{V}A/\dot{Q}$ (Fig. 19–17) may have adequate ventilation but have areas of decreased perfusion. This effect is similar to having increased dead space, clinically represented by areas of ventilation without blood flow, as seen in the patient with a pulmonary emboli. Although it is difficult clinically to differentiate diffusion defects from shunt effect, abnormalities occur in patients with thickening of the alveolar capillary membrane. Examples of diseases with thickened membranes include Goodpasture's syndrome, systemic lupus erythematosus, sarcoidosis, diffuse interstitial fibrosis, and alveolar cell carcinoma.[3]

Ineffective gas exchange is also seen in patients with pulmonary shunt (Fig. 19–18). A **shunt effect** results from blood passing from the right-to-left heart

TABLE 19–3. Ventilation-Perfusion ($\dot{V}A/\dot{Q}$) Equations*

Low $\dot{V}A/\dot{Q}$ (underventilated):	$\dfrac{2\,\text{L/min alveolar ventilation}}{5\,\text{L/min blood flow}}$
Normal $\dot{V}A/\dot{Q}$:	$\dfrac{4\,\text{L/min alveolar ventilation}}{5\,\text{L/min blood flow}}$
High $\dot{V}A/\dot{Q}$ (underperfused):	$\dfrac{4\,\text{L/min alveolar ventilation}}{2\,\text{L/min blood flow}}$

*$\dot{V}A/\dot{Q}$, where $\dot{V}A$ = alveolar ventilation and $\dot{Q}$ = blood flow.

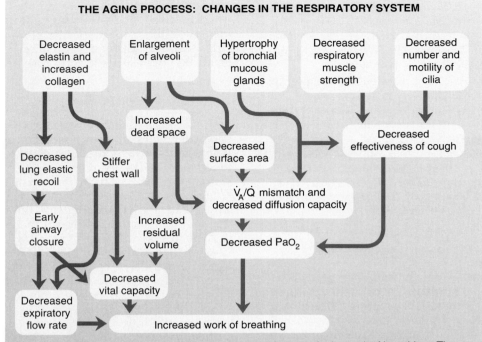

THE AGING PROCESS: CHANGES IN THE RESPIRATORY SYSTEM

With aging, the result of all pulmonary changes is an increase in the work of breathing. The lungs show a reduction in elastin and a rise in collagen, leading to decreased elastic recoil and increased compliance. These changes give rise to increased residual volume and early airway closure. The chest wall becomes stiffer or more rigid due to rib and cartilaginous calcification. The strength of the diaphragm, intercostal muscles, and accessory muscles declines. The stiff chest wall and diminished respiratory muscle strength cause other functional changes, including an increase in dead space and decreased expiratory flow rates and vital capacity.

There is a reduction in the number and motility of cilia resulting in a decrease in respiratory epithelium. There is an increase in and hypertrophy of bronchial mucous glands. The decreased respiratory muscle strength, increased mucus, chest wall stiffness, and cilia loss together reduce cough effectiveness.

Within the lungs, there is enlargement of alveoli and respiratory bronchioles with subsequent decreased surface area. The arterial blood flow through the pulmonary vessels decreases proportionally with changes in cardiac output. The loss of elastic recoil causes the enlarged respiratory bronchioles to collapse or close before the alveoli empty. Alveoli enlargement, along with reduced pulmonary artery blood flow and early airway closure, lowers diffusion capacity and the amount of gas exchange.   It also increases air trapping and residual volume.

Owing to chest wall stiffness and lung rigidity, apical ventilation increases in the elderly whereas basilar ventilation decreases. Ventilation-perfusion ($\dot{V}_A/\dot{Q}$) mismatch occurs as a result of increasing apical ventilation with poor apical capillary blood flow. The result of these changes leads to reduced arterial oxygen pressure (PaO_2). The PaO_2 may decrease when the elderly individual reclines, because of increased $\dot{V}_A/\dot{Q}$ mismatch.

Faith Young Peterson

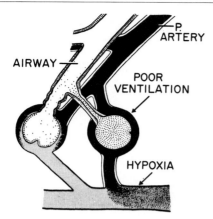

FIGURE 19–16. Schematic diagram of poor ventilation with good perfusion. Low $\dot{V}A/\dot{Q}$ areas contribute poorly oxygenated blood to the systemic circulation, an affect similar to that resulting from venous admixture (shunt effect). (From Cherniack RM, Cherniack L: *Respiration in Health and Disease,* 3rd ed. Philadelphia, WB Saunders, 1983, p 68. Reproduced with permission.)

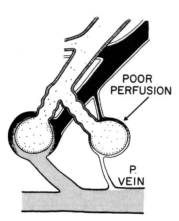

FIGURE 19–17. Schematic diagram of poor perfusion with good ventilation. High $\dot{V}A/\dot{Q}$ areas contribute gas to the mixed expired air, which is high in O_2 and low in CO_2, resulting in increased dead space. (From Cherniack RM, Cherniack L: *Respiration in Health and Disease,* 3rd ed. Philadelphia, WB Saunders, 1983, p 68. Reproduced with permission.)

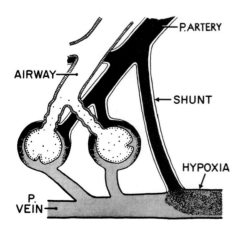

FIGURE 19–18. Hypoxia resulting from true venous admixture (shunt). (From Cherniack RM, Cherniack L: *Respiration in Health and Disease,* 3rd ed. Philadelphia, WB Saunders, 1983, p 70. Reproduced by permission.)

without passing through ventilated areas of the lung. **Shunts** occur in patients with ventricular septal defects, atrial septal defects, patent ductus arteriosus, localized pneumonia, and ARDS. Localized pneumonia and ARDS also have the added effect of $\dot{V}A/\dot{Q}$-mismatch.

Partial pressures of arterial O_2 in the newborn (60–70 mm Hg) and elderly (70–80 mm Hg) are less than that of the adult. The lower O_2 pressure is well tolerated in the newborn because of the presence of fetal hemoglobin, which has the ability to carry 20 to 30 percent more O_2 than adult hemoglobin. The newborn also has a higher hemoglobin concentration (20–21 g/dL) for the first few weeks after birth. Therefore, oxygenation is not normally a problem. The lower Po_2 of the newborn is also associated with an increased Pco_2. Other blood gas values (see Table 19–1) show little difference from those of adults unless there is an oxygenation problem, such as infant respiratory distress syndrome or congenital heart disease.

KEY CONCEPTS

- **Ventilatory failure occurs when alveolar ventilation is insufficient to accomplish adequate gas exchange. Ventilatory failure may result from decreased respiratory rate, decreased tidal volume, or increased dead space. Arterial blood gases demonstrate hypercarbia and hypoxemia.**

- **Oxygenation failure occurs when diffusion of gases across the alveolar capillary interface is impaired. Oxygenation failure may be due to $\dot{V}A/\dot{Q}$ mismatching, right-to-left shunt, or excessive barriers to diffusion. Arterial blood gases demonstrate hypoxemia, but not necessarily hypercarbia.**

Summary

The primary function of the respiratory system is oxygenation of the tissues. This function is accomplished by the movement of O_2 from the atmosphere through the airways to alveolar sacs. The inhaled air is warmed, humidified, and filtered in the upper airway on its way to the alveoli. Once in the alveoli, O_2 is exchanged for CO_2, a gaseous waste product, and is transported by means of hemoglobin molecules to the tissues. The respiratory system has numerous control mechanisms that influence its function. For example, the respiratory control centers may be inhibited when a person has a brain injury, thus leading to inadequate respiration. The health or disease of a patient's cardiovascular, renal, and hematologic systems also affect the functioning of the respiratory system. Health care professionals play a key role in the prevention and treatment of respiratory disease and in patient/family education.

REFERENCES

1. Moore KL, Persaud TVN: *The Developing Human: Clinically Oriented Embryology*, 5th ed. Philadelphia, WB Saunders, 1993.
2. Emery J (ed): *The Anatomy of the Developing Lung*. London, William Heinemann Ltd, 1969.
3. Oakes AR (ed): *Critical Care Nursing of Children and Adolescents*. Philadelphia, WB Saunders, 1981.
4. Ganong WF: *Review of Medical Physiology*, 16th ed. Los Altos, Lange Medical Publications, 1993.
5. Guyton AC: *Textbook of Medical Physiology*, 8th ed. Philadelphia, WB Saunders, 1991.
6. Mackenzie CF: Compromises in the choice of orotracheal or nasotracheal intubation and tracheostomy. *Heart Lung* 1983; 12:485–492.
7. West JB: *Respiratory Physiology: The Essentials*, 4th ed. Baltimore, Williams & Wilkins, 1990.
8. Cherniack NS, Altose MG, Kelsen SG: The respiratory system, in Berne RM, Levy MN (eds): *Physiology*, 3rd ed. St. Louis, CV Mosby, 1993.
9. Behrman RE (ed): *Nelson Textbook of Pediatrics*, 14th ed. Philadelphia, WB Saunders, 1992.
10. Slonim NB, Hamilton LH: *Respiratory Physiology*, 5th ed. St. Louis, CV Mosby, 1988.
11. Cotran RS, Kumar V, Robbins SL: *Robbins Pathologic Basis of Disease*, 5th ed. Philadelphia, WB Saunders, 1994.
12. Robertson D: Physiologic changes and clinical manifestations of aging, in Pagliaro LA, Pagliaro AM (eds): *Pharmacologic Aspects of Aging*. St. Louis, CV Mosby, 1983.
13. Allen SC: The respiratory system, in Brocklehurst JC (ed): *Textbook of Geriatric Medicine and Gerontology*, 4th ed. New York, Churchill Livingstone, 1992.
14. Lareau SC: Respiratory problems, in Carnevali DL, Patrick M (eds): *Nursing Management for the Elderly*, 3rd ed. Philadelphia, JB Lippincott, 1993.
15. Fretwell MD: Aging changes in structure and function, in Carnevali DL, Patrick M (eds): *Nursing Management for the Elderly*, 3rd ed. Philadelphia, JB Lippincott, 1993.

BIBLIOGRAPHY

Barnes PJ: Airway neuropeptides: Roles in fine tuning and in disease? *News Physiol Sci* 1989;4:116–120.
Bartsch P, Maggionni M, Ritter M, Nob C, Vock P, Oetz O: Prevention of high-altitude pulmonary edema by nifedipine. *N Engl J Med* 1991;325:1284–1289.
Baum GL, Wolinsky E: *Textbook of Pulmonary Diseases*, 4th ed. Boston, Little, Brown & Co, 1989.
Biscoe TJ, Duchem MR: Monitoring PO_2 by the carotid chemoreceptor. *News Physiol Sci* 1990;5:229–233.
Chang HK, Paiva M: *Respiratory Physiology: Lung Biology in Health and Disease*. New York, Marcel Dekker, 1989, vol 40.
Crystal RG, West JB (eds): *The Lung: Scientific Foundations*. 2 vols. New York, Raven Press, 1991.
Fels AOS, Cohn ZA: The alveolar macrophage. *J Appl Physiol* 1986;60:353–369.
Gross I: Regulation of fetal lung maturation. *Am J Physiol* 1990; 259:L337–L344.
Hall JB, Schmidt GA, Wood LDH: *Principles of Critical Care*. New York, McGraw-Hill, 1992.
Hawgood S: Pulmonary surfactant apoproteins: Review of protein and genomic structure. *Am J Physiol* 1989;257:L13–L22.
Higenbottam T, Otulana BA, Wallwork J: The physiology of heart-lung transplantation in humans. *News Physiol Sci* 1990;5:71–74.
Kryger MH (ed): *Introduction to Respiratory Medicine*, 2nd ed. New York, Churchill Livingstone, 1990.
Light RW: *Pleural Diseases*, 2nd ed. Malvern, Pa, Lea & Febiger, 1990.
Macklem, PT: The act of breathing. *News Physiol Sci* 1990;5:233–237.
Melamed Y, Shupak A, Bitterman H: Medical problems associated with underwater diving. *N Engl J Med* 1992;326(1):30–35.
Murray JF: *The Normal Lung: The Basis for Diagnosis and Treatment of Pulmonary Disease*, 2nd ed. Philadelphia, WB Saunders, 1986.
Murray JF, Nadel J: *Respiratory Medicine*. Philadelphia, WB Saunders, 1991.
Parillo JE: *Current Therapy in Critical Care Medicine*, 2nd ed. St. Louis, BC Dekker, 1991.
Reynolds HY: Immunologic system in the respiratory tract. *Physiol Rev* 1991;71(4):1117–1133.
Rippe JM, Irwin RS, Alpert JS, Fink MP (eds): *Intensive Care Medicine*, 3rd ed. Boston, Little, Brown & Co, 1991.
Taylor AE, Rehder K, Hyatt RE, Parker JC: *Clinical Respiratory Physiology*. Philadelphia, WB Saunders, 1989.
Ward MP, Milledge JS, West JB: *High Altitude Medicine and Physiology*. Philadelphia, University of Pennsylvania Press, 1989.
West JB: *Physiology: The Essentials*, 4th ed. Baltimore, Williams & Wilkins, 1991.
Wright JR, Dobbs LG: Regulation of pulmonary surfactant secretion and clearance. *Annu Rev Physiol* 1991;53:395–414.

CHAPTER 20
Obstructive Pulmonary Disorders

LORNA SCHUMANN

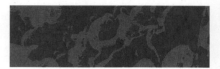

KEY TERMS

bronchiectasis: Abnormal, irreversible dilation of the bronchial walls.

bronchiolitis: Inflammation of small bronchi.

bronchospasm: Narrowing of the bronchi because of an abnormal contraction of the smooth muscles of the bronchi.

chest physiotherapy: Use of percussion and postural drainage to mobilize secretions from specific segments of the lungs.

Heimlich maneuver: An emergency procedure for dislodging an obstruction from the trachea. It requires grasping the choking person from behind by placing your hands around the victim's waist just below the sternum in a fist and pulling inward and upward with force to dislodge the obstruction.

hyposensitization: Reduction in sensitivity to allergens by administering low doses of the allergen, which binds with immunoglobulin G.

metaplasia: Transformation of one kind of tissue to another fully differentiated tissue.

rhinorrhea: Drainage of a watery fluid from the nasal mucosa.

steatorrhea: Passage of high fat content in the feces; seen in malabsorption diseases where there is lack of pancreatic enzymes.

suppurative disease: A disease that produces purulent material (pus).

*T*wenty percent of Americans have experienced some form of respiratory disease, ranging from the common cold to chronic obstructive pulmonary disease. Cancer of the lung accounts for more than 200,000 deaths per year in the United States.[1] Adult respiratory distress syndrome is responsible for 75,000 deaths a year.[1] Chronic obstructive pulmonary disease (COPD) is the fifth leading cause of death in the United States.[2] Health care professionals play a key role in the treatment of these respiratory disorders both in the community and in the hospital setting.

This chapter presents materials related to respiratory diseases covered under the classification of obstructive pulmonary diseases. It includes obstruction of the airway lumen, obstruction from conditions in the wall of the tracheobronchial lumen, and obstruction resulting from increased pressure around the outside of the airway lumen as seen in emphysema secondary to loss of lung elasticity.

Respiratory disorders can be classified according to broad categories of mechanisms for dysfunction, such as ventilatory failure or oxygenation failure, as presented in Chapter 19, or as categories of lung disease encompassing changes in structure and function. Structural and functional disorders include obstructive diseases, restrictive diseases, vascular diseases, respiratory failure, neoplasms, and infectious processes. This chapter and subsequent chapters present respiratory diseases according to disorders of structure and function.

Obstructive Lung Diseases

Obstructive lung diseases are those respiratory disorders that present with increasing resistance to air flow. They are generally caused by conditions that obstruct the inside of the lumen, constrict the wall of the airway, and/or cause increasing pressure around the outside of the airway during exhalation (peribronchial occlusion).

Obstructive diseases of the lung can be classified into those involving (1) obstruction of the airway lumen (foreign body, increased secretions, or aspiration of fluids), (2) obstruction from conditions in the wall of the lumen (asthma, bronchitis), and (3) obstruction resulting from increasing pressure around the outside of the airway lumen (emphysema secondary to loss of lung tissue and elasticity, enlarged lymph node, or tumor).[3] These divisions are mainly terms of convenience, because many disease processes involve several areas of the pulmonary system.

Involvement of the airways produces narrowing of the passages so that obstruction to air flow occurs. The major obstructive airway diseases are bronchitis, emphysema, and asthma. Characteristic pathologic and clinical findings are described for each of these classifications. Clinically, pure forms of emphysema and bronchitis are rare, and most patients present a combination of several or all of these obstructive processes. An explanation of diagnostic tests for the various obstructive diseases is presented at the end of this section.

Obstruction of the Airway Lumen

Bronchiectasis

Etiology. **Bronchiectasis** is either an acquired or congenital disorder and is classified both as an **obstructive** and as a **suppurative** (pus-forming) disorder. Acquired bronchiectasis is now rare in the United States because of early treatment with antibiotics for bronchopulmonary infections. Cystic fibrosis accounts for approximately 50 percent of the cases of bronchiectasis. Children are at higher risk for development of bronchiectasis because of anatomic factors such as small, soft, elastic bronchi. Bronchi in children are easily damaged by overinflation and distention from inflammation and infection.

Bronchiectasis can be classified into two basic anatomic categories according to bronchial shape: saccular, with cavity-like dilations; and cylindrical, with widening of the bronchial walls. A fusiform shape is a combination of saccular and cylindrical changes. These anatomic changes are shown in Figure 20–1.

Pathogenesis. This disorder is characterized by recurrent infection and inflammation of bronchial walls, which leads to persistent dilation of the medium-sized bronchi and bronchioles. Inflammation of bronchi and bronchioles results in destruction of the walls of central bronchi and obliteration of peripheral bronchi and bronchioles.[1] The inflammatory infections are most frequently caused by gram-negative bacteria. The destructive process leads to loss of ciliated epithelium, squamous **metaplasia** (abnormal transformation of normal tissue to abnormal tissue), and pus formation, which in turn leads to obstruction of air flow. The lung tissue of a patient with cystic fibrosis complicated by varicose bronchiectasis is shown in Figure 20–2. The bronchial lumen resembles varicose veins.[1]

Clinical Manifestations. Signs and symptoms frequently seen during the inflammatory phase of the disease include chronic productive cough with copious amounts of purulent, foul-smelling, green, or yellow sputum. The sputum has the characteristic of separating into three layers in a sputum cup.[4] Other clinical features are hemoptysis, crackles, rhonchi, halitosis, and digitial clubbing. Clubbing is caused by decreased oxygenation, which leads to fibrous tissue hyperplasia in the area between the nail and phalanx. It is associated with lymphocytic extravasation, increased vascularity, and edema. The severity of clubbing parallels the severity of pulmonary disease.[5] Digital clubbing can be identified by two methods, as seen in Figure 20–3. Hypoxemia is seen in severe cases. Complications of bronchiectasis are malnutrition, recurrent pneumonia, right ventricular failure, and secondary visceral abscesses.[4]

Diagnosis. Generally, the diagnosis of bronchiectasis is based on a history of chronic productive cough. The patient complains of producing copious amounts of foul-smelling sputum. The chest radiograph may

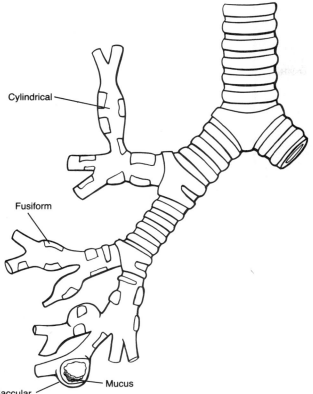

Cylindrical

Fusiform

Saccular — Mucus

FIGURE 20-1. Various types of bronchiectasis. The morphology varies. (From Monahan FD, Drake T, Neighbors M: *Nursing Care of Adults.* Philadelphia, WB Saunders, 1994, p 557. Reproduced with permission.)

reveal small cysts, thickening of bronchial walls, and increased bronchial markings (areas of intensity showing bronchi which are usually not distinct). Pulmonary function tests show decreased air flow and vital capacity in advanced cases. Arterial blood gases reveal hypoxemia (decreased partial pressure of oxygen Pao_2) and hypercapnia (increased partial pressure of carbon dioxide, $Paco_2$) from obstruction to air flow. In advanced cases computed tomography assists in providing a definitive diagnosis of bronchiectasis.[6]

Treatment. Lifelong, daily chest physiotherapy with vigorous chest percussion and postural drainage and inhaled bronchodilators is the mainstay of therapy. This regimen is supplemented with antibiotic therapy selected on the basis of sputum culture results and Gram staining during periodic infections. Proper hydration and nutrition are important in promoting liquefaction of secretions and preventing increased susceptibility to infection resulting from malnutrition. Maintaining adequate nutrition is a problem because patients find that it requires increased energy and effort to eat. Breathing and coughing require increased energy also. Many patients complain of constant fatigue. (Refer to the following section on cystic fibrosis for further discussion on treatment.) In severe cases, when other measures fail, bronchoscopy with bronchial lavage may be necessary to remove thick, purulent secretions. Patient education materials can

be obtained from the Cystic Fibrosis Foundation, 6000 Executive Blvd., Suite 510, Rockville, MD 20852.

Bronchiolitis

Etiology. **Bronchiolitis** is characterized by widespread inflammation of bronchioles because of infectious agents such as respiratory syncytial virus, influenza (type A, B, or C), bacteria (*Hemophilus influenzae,* pneumococci, or hemolytic streptococci), and occasionally by allergic reactions. Respiratory syncytial virus is the cause of bronchiolitis in 75 percent of hospitalized infants.[7] The disease is generally seen in the winter months and usually occurs in children under the age of 2 years. It may also affect adults as a result of toxic fumes or viral infections, or in association with rheumatoid arthritis.[1,4] In adults, bronchiolitis is commonly associated with smoking.[1]

McConnochie and Roghmann,[8] using a case-control method, studied risk factors associated with bronchiolitis. Fifty-three children with bronchiolitis were matched with two control children without bronchiolitis. Multivariate analysis showed that children at high risk for developing bronchiolitis are those with a family history of asthma, presence of "passive smoking" (inhaling smoke from others' cigarettes), and presence of older siblings. The risk of bronchiolitis associated with the presence of older siblings increased linearly with the number and age of older siblings. The authors recommend instructing parents of high-risk infants in reduction of smoking and eliminating contact between infants and older siblings during periods when respiratory virus infection is prevalent.[8]

Carlsen et al[9] also studied risk factors associated with bronchiolitis in 51 hospitalized infants and 24 control children. They found that children born between April and September had an increased incidence of bronchilitis. Other risk factors were increased number of siblings who attended school or nursery school, and shorter periods of breast-feeding.

Pathogenesis. Once initiated by the causal agent, the pathophysiologic mechanisms of bronchiolitis lead to inflammation of the bronchioles. Inflammation leads to an increased number of lymphocytes and exudate. Three possible mechanisms of airway obstruction may occur after the initiation of the inflammatory process. They include the following: (1) inflammatory exudate, which may displace surfactant, leading to airway obstruction; (2) the release of chemical mediators, which may produce bronchiolar constriction; and (3) inflammation, which may induce fibrosis and narrowing of the airway.[1,7] In addition to these changes, goblet cell metaplasia and increased bronchial muscle mass may also occur, resulting in further airway narrowing. Production of thick, tenacious mucus leads to airway obstruction, atelectasis, and hyperinflation.

Clinical Manifestations. The severity and course of the disease are variable, ranging from mild to fatal. Common clinical features include wheezing due to

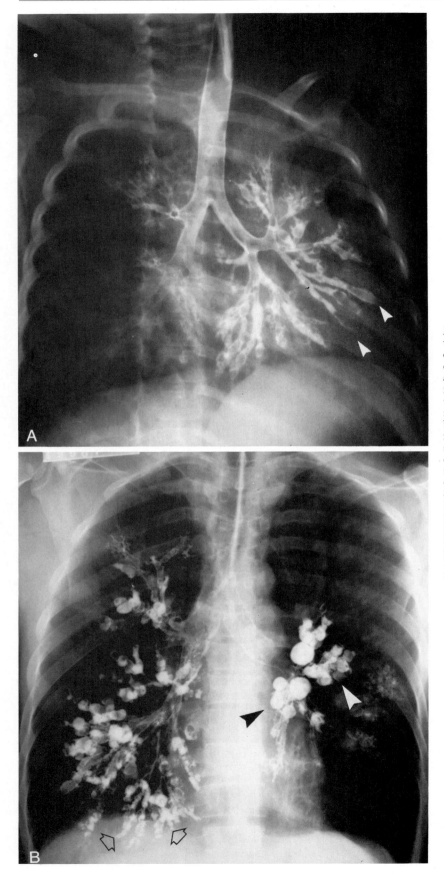

F I G U R E 20 – 2. Bronchographic features of varicose and cystic bronchiectasis. A left tracheobronchogram in a shallow posterior oblique projection (**A**) reveals mildly dilated and slightly irregular bronchi that terminate four to six generations of branchings from the trachea in a squared or bulbous appearance (*arrowheads*). The findings are those of varicose bronchiectasis. A bilateral tracheobronchogram in the anteroposterior projection (**B**) demonstrates a multitude of contrast material-filled cystic spaces resembling a cluster of grapes (*arrowheads*), a characteristic feature of cystic bronchiectasis. Note that the cystic spaces appear after only two to three bronchial generations. Less severe bronchiectasis of varicose type is present in the right lower lobe (*open arrows*). (From Fraser RG, Pare JAP, Pare PD, Fraser RS, Genereux GP: *Diagnosis of Diseases of the Chest.* 3rd ed. Philadelphia, WB Saunders, 1990, vol 3, p 2199. Reproduced with permission.)

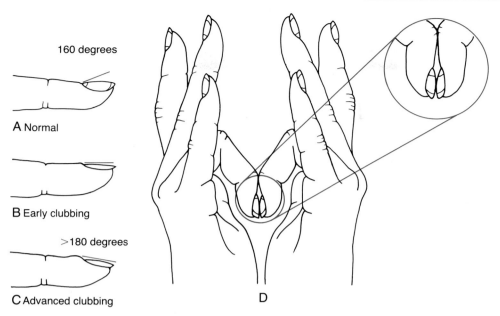

160 degrees

A Normal

B Early clubbing

>180 degrees

C Advanced clubbing

D

FIGURE 20–3. Clubbing. **A**, Normal digit with angle of 160 degrees. **B**, Flattened angle between nail and skin exceeds 180 degrees. **C**, Advanced clubbing with rounded nail. **D**, Clubbing is assessed by the Schamroth technique: the nurse instructs the client to place the nails of the fourth (ring) fingers together while extending the other fingers, and to hold the hands up. A diamond-shaped space between the nails is a normal finding, that is, clubbing is absent. (From Black JM, Matassarin-Jacobs E (eds): *Luckmann and Sorensen's Medical-Surgical Nursing*, 4th ed. Philadelphia, WB Saunders, 1993, p 920. Reproduced with permission.)

bronchospasm, crackles, decreased breath sounds, retractions, increased sputum, dyspnea, and rapid, shallow respirations.

Diagnosis. Patients commonly have an elevated white blood cell count. The chest radiograph may show enlarged air sacs, interstitial infiltrates, atelectasis, or severe hyperinflation. Pulmonary function tests reveal severe obstruction to air flow.

Treatment. Therapy is aimed at maintaining adequate oxygenation by providing humidified oxygen, monitoring blood gases or oxygen saturation, and providing oral or intravenous bronchodilator agents. Table 20–1 provides general information on pharmacologic agents commonly used in the treatment of various respiratory disorders. Use of these agents depends on the severity of the diagnosis and physician preference.

The use of inhaled bronchodilators for the treatment of bronchiolitis remains controversial. Hughes et al[10] tested the efficacy of salbutamol on respiratory mechanics in bronchiolitis. The results showed that salbutamol did not improve the basic respiratory function but rather had the detrimental effect of increasing airway collapse on forced expiration.

Aerosolized ribavirin has been effective in treating patients positive for respiratory syncytial virus (RSV).[11,12] Researchers have found statistically significant improvement in oxygen saturation in patients receiving aerosolized ribavirin over the control groups.

Other therapies include sedation for anxiety, fluid therapy, and the administration of broad-spectrum antibiotics based on culture and sensitivity results. Patients are encouraged to stop smoking and to avoid passive smoke. The use of steroids is controversial, but may be effective in some patients in decreasing inflammation.[4,7]

The use of eye-nose goggles by health care workers is recommended to control the spread of RSV. The virus is spread through the air or by contact with secretions from the eye, nose, or mouth and may not be prevented by the routine use of gowns and masks. Gala et al[13] reported that 34 percent of hospital personnel who did not use goggles and 43 percent of susceptible infants became infected. The use of a mask and goggles lowered the percentages of infection to 5 percent for hospital personnel and 6 percent for susceptible infants.

Agah et al[14] verified these findings and determined that the clinical illness rate was 11 percent in the mask-and-goggle group and 62 percent in the no mask-and-goggle group. They also found that wearing a mask and goggles reduced the infection rate in health care workers from 61 percent to 5 percent.[14]

Cystic Fibrosis

Etiology. Cystic fibrosis (mucoviscidosis) is an autosomal recessive disorder of the exocrine glands. It is the most common chronic lung disease in white children and young adults. The prevalence in white births is 1 in 2,500,[4] which accounts for 95 percent of all cases in the United States. One in 25 caucasians

TABLE 20–1. Common Therapeutic Agents Used in the Treatment of Respiratory Diseases

Classification/Agent	Dosage Forms*	Action
Methylxanthines		
Theophylline, aminophylline	Oral, IV	Bronchodilation
β-Adrenergic Receptor Agonists		
Catecholamines		Bronchodilation
Epinephrine	IV, inhaled	
Isoproterenol	IV, inhaled	
Isoetharine	Inhaled	
Bitolterol	Inhaled	
Resorcinols		
Metaproterenol	Oral, inhaled	
Terbutaline	Oral, IV	
Fenoterol	Inhaled	
Saligen		
Albuterol	Oral, inhaled	
Newer Agents		
Pirbuterol	Inhaled	
Salmeterol xinafoate	Inhaled	
Anticholinergics		
Atropine sulfate	Oral, inhaled	Blocks action of acetycholine and increases intracellular cyclic monophosphate, which lead to bronchodilation
Glycopyrrolate	IV, IM, SC, inhaled	
Ipratropium bromide	Inhaled	
Glucocorticoids		
Beclomethasone	Oral, inhaled	Suppresses inflammation and may potentiate B₂-adrenergic agents
Dexamethasone	Inhaled	
Triamcinolone	IM, inhaled	
Flunisolide	Inhaled	
Methylprednisolone	IV	
Prednisone	Oral	
Mast Cell Stabilizer		
Cromolyn sodium	Inhaled	Stabilizes mast cell membranes
Nedocromil sodium		

*IV, intravenous; IM, intramuscular; SC, subcutaneous.

are heterozygous carriers of the cystic fibrosis gene.[4,15] The incidence in American blacks is rare (1 in 17,000 live births), and it is almost never seen in the Oriental population.[1,15,16] About one third of the 30,000 cases of cystic fibrosis in the United States are in adults.[4,15,17] It can be classified either as an obstructive disorder or as a suppurative (pus-forming) disorder.[17] Hypersecretion of abnormal, thick mucus that obstructs exocrine glands and ducts is a characteristic finding of the disease. The diagnosis is usually made in childhood or early adulthood. Survival past the age of 30 is unusual,[16] and 50 percent of children with cystic fibrosis die before the age of 20.[4,7,18]

With advances in antibiotic therapy, early recogni-

tion, and treatment of complications, patients with cystic fibrosis are living longer into adulthood. Some patients are now having families. Cystic fibrosis is classified as an autosomal recessive disorder. The genetic defect associated with cystic fibrosis involves deletion of three base pairs that code for phenylalanine on chromosome 7. With the loss of these three base pairs, the cystic fibrosis transmembrane regulator is missing.[4,15] The most common genetic deletion, known as ΔF508, occurs in 68 percent of cystic fibrosis patients tested.[15] Research is now under way to further our ability to treat and perhaps cure the disease.

Pathogenesis. Cystic fibrosis primarily affects the pancreas and lungs. The mucus-producing glands of both organs hypertrophy and produce excessive secretions that are thick mucoproteins. The thick eosinophilic mucous secretions plug the glands and ducts of the pancreatic acini, intestinal glands, intrahepatic bile ducts, and the gallbladder, causing dilation and fibrosis.[15] These changes result in decreased production of pancreatic enzymes necessary for digestion of fats, carbohydrates, and proteins, thus leading to increased fat and protein in the stool.[15,19]

The pulmonary bronchial system is also affected by the thick, tenacious mucus that results from failure of chloride channels in the apical membranes of mucosal cells to open. Decreased flow of ions and water results in viscid mucus.[15] The thick mucus causes airway obstruction, atelectasis, and hyperinflation. The thick mucus also decreases ciliary action, thus contributing to mucus stasis, which provides a medium for pulmonary infection. Sweat glands, salivary glands, and lacrimal glands are also affected, leading to high secretions of sodium and chloride.[15]

Clinical Manifestations. Typical findings include a history of cough in a young adult or child; thick, tenacious sputum; recurrent pulmonary infections (commonly *Pseudomonas aeruginosa*); and recurrent episodes of bronchitis. These processes ultimately progress to pneumonia and bronchiectasis; cor pulmonale; exercise intolerance; and steatorrhea (fat in the stool).

Physical examination may reveal digital clubbing, dyspnea, tachypnea, sternal retractions, unequal breath sounds, moist basilar crackles and rhonchi, and a barrel chest that is hyperresonant to percussion.[4] Other findings that vary in the cystic fibrosis population are the following: pancreatic insufficiency, 85 percent; cirrhosis of the liver, 5 to 20 percent; diabetes mellitus, 1 to 10 percent; gallstones, 30 to 35 percent; and nasal polyps, 15 percent.[3,4,15,16,20–22] Infants frequently present with a history of multiple respiratory infections, meconium ileus, failure to thrive, jaundice, salt depletion, and edema.[22]

Huang et al[21] reviewed data on 142 cystic fibrosis subjects ranging in age from 18 to 42 years to determine common clinical features, survival rates, and prognostic factors in survival. Poor prognosis was evidenced by individuals who had low clinical scores as measured by the Scwachman and Kulczycki scoring system. According to Scwachman and Kulczycki, poor prognostic factors for cystic fibrosis included low-weight percentile and *Pseudomonas cepacia* colonization of the lower respiratory tract by the age of 18.[21]

Nutritional assessment reveals depleted fat stores, steatorrhea, anorexia, decreased growth rate in children (weight, height, head circumference), and decreased midarm indices.[22]

Diagnosis. The diagnosis of cystic fibrosis is based on clinical and laboratory findings. Diagnostic studies routinely done include arterial blood gas measurements, pulmonary function tests, and chest radiographs. Specific diagnostic tests for cystic fibrosis include stool examination for fat, sweat electrolyte tests, and genetic testing. A three-way stool collection combined with the dietary history during that time is used to determine fat absorption. A coefficient of fat absorption of less than 93 percent (<85 percent in infants) can be used to define **steatorrhea**.[22] Arterial blood gases commonly show hypoxemia and hypercapnia because of airway obstruction. Pulmonary function tests reveal decreased vital capacity, decreased air flow rates, increased airway resistance, increased functional residual capacity (FRC), and decreased tidal volume. Chest radiographs show evidence of patchy atelectasis, bronchiectasis, obstructive emphysema, cystic lung fields, and peribronchial thickening.[3,4,15,16,20,23] Elevated sedimentation rates are seen in acute exacerbation, owing to increased inflammation of tissue.[18,24]

Sweat electrolyte testing reveals elevated sodium and chloride levels, with over 98 percent of patients having levels above 60 mEq/L.[17,18,22] Most cystic fibrosis patients have levels above 100 mEq/L.[22]

Treatment. Management of the patient with cystic fibrosis involves an interdisciplinary approach utilizing medicine, nursing, occupational therapy, physical therapy, dietary, and psychosocial support.

Because pulmonary disease accounts for the majority of morbidity and mortality associated with cystic fibrosis, treatment is aimed at *aggressive* pharmacologic management of pulmonary infection based on sputum culture and sensitivity results. Treatment of the respiratory system includes the use of conventional bronchodilators, such as theophylline products, and inhaled sympathomimetic medications, such as albuterol or metaproterenol. Mobilization of the thick mucus is a priority. Postural drainage and **chest physiotherapy** help in loosening and draining the sputum. Alternative methods include the forced expiratory technique, which involves coughing (huffing) with an open glottis.[22]

High-dose antibiotic therapy is used for exacerbations of respiratory infections and during periodic hospitalizations for intensive therapy lasting up to 3 to 4 weeks to decrease bacterial growth in the lungs. The period of hospitalization is diminished in some patients and they are discharged as soon as it is seen that the infective organism responds to therapy. Patients are taught to administer intravenous infusions at home. This period of intense high-dose antibiotic therapy is often termed the "clean-out" regimen. "Clean-out" requires initial hospitalization for intravenous infusion of antibiotics such as gentamicin, to-bramycin, ceftazidime, vancomycin, and carbenicillin.[4,16,22] Hypochloremic alkalosis is associated with high-dose carbenicillin therapy. Hypocalcemia and hypomagnesmia may occur in patients receiving gentamicin.[16] For the outpatient, oral cephalosporin (cephalexin, cefaclor, or cefuroxime), trimethoprim-sulfamethoxazole (Septra or Bactrim) or a tetracycline compound may be used.[8,18,22]

Other antibiotics such as dicloxacillin, imipenem, aztreonam, erythromycin, clindamycin, and chloramphenicol may also be given. Antipseudomonal antibiotics such as azlocillin are beneficial for the treatment of acute exacerbations.[24] Aerosolized antibiotics (tobramycin, gentamicin) are effective on a short-term basis for improving pulmonary function tests and reducing hospitalizations.[22] Oxygen has been shown to improve long-term survival.

Nutritional therapy includes low-fat, high-protein diet, and vitamin supplements (especially the fat-soluble vitamins A, D, E, and K). Other pharmacologic therapy related to nutrition is aimed at replacement of pancreatic enzymes (Viokase, Cotazym, Creon, Zymase, Pancrease). Maintenance of weight in children with cystic fibrosis often requires an intake of 150 percent of the calories recommended for healthy children. Emphasis on a low-fat diet has diminished with modern pancreatic enzyme replacement.[15,22] In some cases, enteral feedings or intravenous nutrition may be necessary on a short-term basis. Nutritional management of the adolescent presents a challenge. Salt supplementation may be necessary in hot weather.

A yearly influenza vaccine is recommended for cystic fibrosis patients because of the increased risk of complications associated with infection.[18]

Heart-lung or lung transplantation is currently the only definitive treatment. Results show improved quality of life.[4] Over 200 cystic fibrosis patients worldwide have undergone transplantation, with a 1-year survival of 70 percent.[15] Caine et al[25] compared survival, morbidity, quality of life, and resources in patients who received a heart-lung transplant and those who did not. Patients receiving transplants showed marked improvement in mobility, energy, and quality of life. Survival at 1 year for transplants was almost twice that for nontransplants.[25]

Recent identification of the disease-related gene, the cystic fibrosis transmembrane conductance regulator (CFTR),[26–28] has advanced prospects for corrective gene therapy[29] (Fig. 20–4). Gene therapy has been attempted in rat and mouse models with some success, suggesting that analogous therapy in humans afflicted with the disease will be beneficial. Approval has already been given to several centers in the United States for Phase I human trials using the CFTR adenoviral vector.

CFTR works by encoding a chloride channel and is expressed in the sweat glands, the lungs, and the pancreas. Gene therapy targets the lung epithelial cell through tracheal instillation of a recombinant, replication-defective adenovirus encoding human CFTR. One limiting factor is that the gene has a short-term

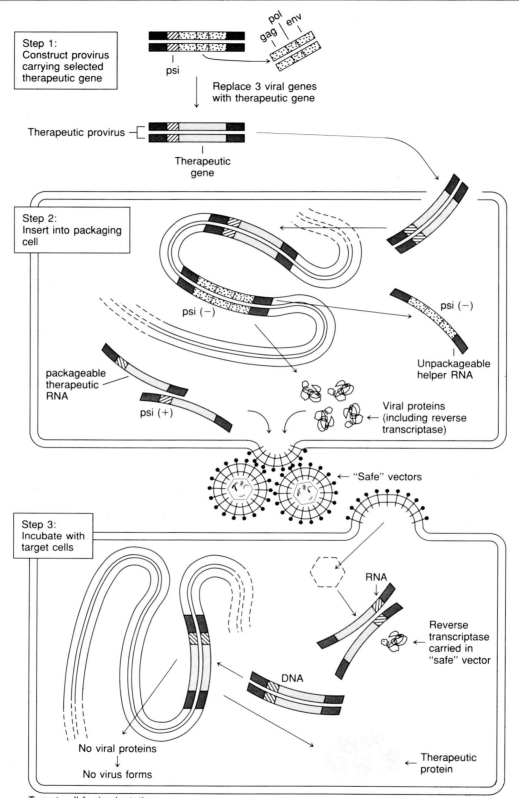

Step 1:
Construct provirus
carrying selected
therapeutic gene

pol
gag | env

psi

Replace 3 viral genes
with therapeutic gene

Therapeutic provirus

Therapeutic
gene

Step 2:
Insert into packaging
cell

psi (−)

psi (−)

Unpackageable
helper RNA

packageable
therapeutic
RNA

psi (+)

Viral proteins
(including reverse
transcriptase)

"Safe" vectors

Step 3:
Incubate with
target cells

RNA

Reverse
transcriptase
carried in
"safe" vector

DNA

No viral proteins

No virus forms

Therapeutic
protein

Target cell for implantation

FIGURE 20–4. See legend on opposite page

expression. In the experiments conducted on rats, expression persisted only 42 days.[30]

Another protocol that relies on gene transfer of a DNA-liposome complex has been approved in England. Further study will be required to determine whether an adenoviral vector can create sufficient cell types without toxicity to produce a long-term therapeutic effect in humans. An additional consideration, due to the vector's short-term expression, is the nature of the host immune response to a highly antigenic adenovirus following repetitive administration. Deoxyribonucleic acid liposome delivery (such as that approved in England) may address these limitations.

Tracheal/Bronchial Obstruction

Etiology. Tracheobronchial obstruction is an acute problem requiring immediate treatment. Causes frequently seen include aspiration of a foreign body (such as a piece of meat, peanut, coin, or so forth), malpositioned endotracheal tube, laryngospasm, epiglottitis, trauma, swelling from smoke inhalation, postsurgical blood clot, and compression of the bronchus or trachea by tumors or enlarged lymph nodes. With inhaled foreign bodies the right lung is affected more often than the left because of the anatomic extension of the right mainstem bronchus from the trachea.[9,31]

Pathogenesis. Obstruction by one of the etiologic agents listed earlier can be partial or complete. The health care worker must be prepared to assess the situation rapidly and immediately progress toward relieving the obstruction.

Clinical Manifestations. With complete obstruction, no movement of air will be heard on auscultation, but the patient may still be making inspiratory chest movements. Other clinical features of complete obstruction include inability to talk, tachycardia, cyanosis, and rapid progression to unconsciousness unless the problem is quickly reversed.

With partial obstruction of the airway, the patient usually presents with stridor, sternal and intercostal retractions, wheezing, nasal flaring, tachypnea, dyspnea, tachycardia, and use of accessory muscles to breathe. Cyanosis is a late sign that usually indicates exhaustion or complete obstruction.

Diagnosis. The diagnosis is based on clinical features and arterial blood gases (ABGs). The ABG values frequently show, hypoxemia and hypercarbia re-

sulting from the airway obstruction. Chest radiographs may reveal the location of the obstruction.

Treatment. Treatment involves opening the obstructed airway as quickly as possible. Blows to the patient's back or use of the **Heimlich maneuver** may be necessary for the foreign body to be expelled. Aspirated contents occluding the airway are suctioned to relieve obstruction. If these methods are unsuccessful, an emergency tracheostomy should be performed in the case of a suspected upper airway obstruction in the subglottic region or above. If emergency treatment has not removed the cause of the obstruction, further intervention must be done, as in the case of tumors. Laser bronchoscopy to remove tracheal and endobronchial lesions has proved very effective. The procedure can be done under local anesthesia.[32]

A tracheal stent (device used to maintain an orifice) can be used to maintain an open airway in patients with stenosis due to caustic aspiration, endotracheal intubation, recurrent infection, or other types of occlusion resulting from surgery or manipulation of the trachea.[33,34] Self-expanding metal stents are currently being used in lung and heart-lung transplant patients who have developed tracheal stenosis.[34]

KEY CONCEPTS

- Obstructive disorders are associated with increased resistance to air flow. Generally, the airways are more narrowed on expiration than inspiration, so that "getting the air out" is most difficult.

- Bronchiectasis is associated with recurrent inflammation of the bronchial walls, chronic cough, and aneurysm-like dilations of the bronchioles. These bronchiolar dilations serve as pockets of infection, producing purulent, foul-smelling sputum. Treatment centers on antibiotic therapy and removal of secretions.

- Bronchiolitis refers to widespread bronchiolar inflammation, often associated with smoking and a number of infectious agents. Inflammation results in mucosal swelling, excessive mucus production, and bronchial muscle constriction—all of which narrow the airway lumen and may lead to wheezing and dyspnea. Treatment centers on bronchodilating agents and treatment of the underlying cause.

- Cystic fibrosis is an autosomal recessive disorder of exocrine glands and mucous cells. Secretions are excessively thick because of insufficient chloride and

---

FIGURE 20–4. Gene therapy may use retroviral vectors to deliver therapeutic genes. In such cases, viruses are made in which viral genes (*gag, pol,* and *env* specifying, respectively, proteins of the viral core, the enzyme reverse transcriptase, and constituents of the coat) are removed and a therapeutic gene substituted. The virus is then inserted into a packaging cell. Here, the defective "therapeutic virus" is helped to replicate and repackage with the aid of a "helper" virus, which "lends" the missing viral protein products to the therapeutic virus. The helper virus, however, is also defective because the *psi* region is deleted (necessary for inclusion of RNA into viral particles). This assumes that the helper virus will not leave the cell. The particles that escape the cell, then, carry therapeutic RNA and no viral genes. They can enter other cells and splice the therapeutic gene in the cellular DNA, but they cannot reproduce. (From Walsh PC, Retik AB, Stamey TA, Vaughan ED (eds): *Campbell's Urology,* 6th ed. Philadelphia, WB Saunders, 1992, p 300. Used with permission.)

water transport. Thick secretions cause airway obstruction, atelectasis, and air trapping. Associated symptoms resulting from dysfunction of the exocrine pancreas are apparent. Treatment centers on removal of secretions and providing antibiotic therapy for complicating respiratory infections.

- Obstruction of the trachea or large bronchi may occur acutely, requiring immediate treatment. Usual causes include foreign body aspiration, trauma, and inflammation. With complete obstruction, no movement of air occurs, even though inspiratory efforts may be observed. Partial airway obstruction is associated with wheezing, retractions, and stridor. Treatment centers on removing the obstruction if possible, or creating a patent airway by a tracheostomy.

Obstruction From Conditions in the Wall of the Lumen

Asthma

Etiology. Asthma is defined **symptomatically** by recurring paroxysms of diffuse wheezing, dyspnea, and cough resulting from spasmodic contractions of the bronchi. Asthma is believed to arise from contraction of airway smooth muscle and from airway inflammation. A key point to the disease is its reversibility. With proper treatment most asthmatics can control the disease and prevent it from developing into emphysema or bronchitis. Asthma occurs in about 2 to 10 percent[4,6,35] of the population and is common among children and adults alike. The overall death rate among asthmatics for 1988 was 0.1 percent.[8]

Although the exact pathogenesis of the disease is not well understood, various etiologic categories or syndromes of asthma have been defined. They include extrinsic asthma, intrinsic asthma, exercise-induced asthma, occupational-induced asthma, drug-induced asthma, cardiac asthma, and triad asthma.

Extrinsic and intrinsic asthma are the two most common forms covered in the literature. The clinical features of all forms are similar, but the cause of asthma varies. **Extrinsic asthma** makes up approximately one third to one half of all cases.[4,6,8] Extrinsic asthma, also called allergic asthma, commonly affects children and young adults. It is commonly associated with a history of hay fever or eczema (atopy), a positive family history of the disease, and positive skin test reactions. Attacks are related to specific antigens and are immunoglobulin E (IgE)-mediated. Pharmacologic therapy, hyposensitization, and environmental control are usually beneficial.[4,36]

In contrast to extrinsic asthma, **intrinsic asthma** frequently develops in middle age and has a less favorable prognosis. Respiratory infections appear to be causative, whereas antigen-antibody reactions appear to have minimal role in the disease process.[36] Attacks are often severe, and patients have a variable response to medical therapy. Hyposensitization therapy and environmental control measures are *not* usually helpful.

Intrinsic asthma is not IgE mediated and occurs in adults. The diagnosis is based on the lack of an allergic reaction. Psychological stress factors, pulmonary irritants, and exercise may precipitate an asthma attack.[1,3] Airways are hyperreactive, and patients may present with extreme dyspnea, orthopnea, and agitation. The prognosis is poorer than with extrinsic asthma.

Exercise-induced asthma is common, especially in children, and often, but not always, is associated with other types of asthma. **Bronchospasm** often occurs 5 to 10 minutes after the exercise period begins. The increased rate and depth of respiration during exercise, especially in cold air, lead to cooling and dehydration of the lower airways. Symptoms occur more rapidly in cold weather. Heat loss, water loss, and increased osmolarity of the lower respiratory mucosa are believed to stimulate mediator release from basophils and tissue mast cells. This mediator release is then thought to produce airway smooth muscle contraction. Running, jogging, and tennis are the most common instigators of exercise-induced asthma. Bicycling and swimming are much less prone to induce symptoms.

Occupational asthma resembles allergic asthma and may be accompanied by positive skin test reactions to protein allergens in the work environment. Occupational exposures to allergens such as fumes from plastic, formaldehyde, isocyanates, some metals, textiles, engine exhaust, sulfur dioxide, fluoride, and western red cedar dust *do not* provoke skin reactions. To prove hypersensitivity, it may be necessary to challenge the patient by inhalation of the suspected dust or fumes in a controlled environment. The individual affected by occupational asthma tends to have progressively more severe attacks with subsequent exposures. Symptoms may clear over a weekend or vacation and recur when the individual is back at work. This repeated history often is sufficient to establish the diagnosis. Hyposensitization in most cases of occupational asthma is ineffective because of lack of an IgE antibody reaction and because the chemicals that cause symptoms usually are toxic when injected.[1,16]

Drug-induced asthma can produce a serious reaction in the asthmatic patient. Symptoms range from mild **rhinorrhea** to respiratory arrest requiring mechanical ventilation.

In patients with nasal polyps, sinusitis, and asthma, ingestion of aspirin may induce severe or occasionally fatal asthmatic attacks. Sometimes anaphylactoid reactions cause a decrease in blood pressure, itching, **rhinorrhea**, or a rash after aspirin ingestion. Aspirin intolerance with asthma usually occurs in adults and may occur severely without previous warning symptoms. Attacks may occur within minutes of ingestion or may be delayed up to 12 hours. Nonsteroidal anti-inflammatory drugs such as indomethacin, ibuprofen, and related drugs may also induce asthma in the aspirin-intolerant patient. Other salicylate products and acetaminophen do not induce asthma in aspirin-intolerant patients.

Aspirin reactions are not immunologically mediated. Therefore, skin testing is not useful for diagnosing aspirin intolerance. Because aspirin and nonsteroidal anti-inflammatory drugs inhibit the conversion of arachidonic acid to prostaglandins, it may be that aspirin shunts arachidonic acid breakdown to the leukotriene system. Leukotrienes are slow-reacting substances of anaphylaxis with powerful bronchoconstriction activity. Leukotrienes are chemicals that are released from mast cells in tracheal and bronchial tissue. (Refer to Figure 20–6 later in this chapter, which shows the chemicals contained in mast cells.) If the history is nondiagnostic, patients may be challenged with small but increasing doses of aspirin. Reactions to aspirin can be severe and prolonged, so that challenge should be performed in the hospital or in the doctor's office with appropriate measures available to treat severe reactions. Avoidance is the most practical approach to this problem because testing can be dangerous.

Asthma can occur from ingestion of food additives. Tartrazine (yellow dye no. 5), which is used to color pharmaceuticals, hair products, and food products, may also produce severe asthma in susceptible people. A complete list of drugs containing tartrazine can be obtained from the Food and Drug Administration.

Monosodium glutamate, used as a flavor enhancer in foods, can produce faintness, nausea, sweating, a fall in blood pressure, and occasionally asthma. Sodium or potassium metabisulfite, used to preserve fruits, vegetables, and meats, can cause anaphylactoid reactions. A challenge with the chemical may be necessary to establish a diagnosis, as metabisulfites are ubiquitous in our society.

Hops in beer have also been implicated in causing severe bronchospasm. Skin reactivity does not occur, and the mechanism of the problem is not IgE mediated. The diagnosis involves a history of exposure followed by symptoms.

Triad asthma is a subcategory of drug-induced asthma representing a combination of intrinsic asthma, aspirin sensitivity, and nasal polyposis.[4,8] **Cardiac asthma** results from bronchospasm precipitated by congestive heart failure.

Pathogenesis. Bronchial asthma is characterized by obstruction and narrowing of airways as a result of **bronchospasm,** increased mucus secretion, and mucosal edema. When smooth muscle spasm is the primary cause, the severity of symptoms may change rapidly. If mucosal edema or mucus secretion resulting from airway inflammation is the major cause, the progression and regression of obstruction occur more slowly. Thickening of the smooth muscle, muscle spasm, and development of mucous plugs in the smaller airways all increase airway obstruction (Fig. 20–5).

With extrinsic asthma, an IgE-mediated response is common and is often associated with the atopic state, manifested by elevated IgE levels, allergic rhinitis, eczema, a family history of allergy, and attacks associated with seasonal, environmental, or occupational exposure. The mechanism of action is initiated by exposure to a specific antigen that has previously been sensitized by mast cells in pulmonary mucosa. When the antigen reacts with the antibody on the surface of the mast cell, packets of chemical mediator substances stored in the cell are released. The chemical mediators that are released include histamine, slow-reacting substances of anaphylaxis (leukotrienes), prostaglandins, bradykinins, eosinophilic chemotactic factor, serotonin, and others.[3,36,37] Research is continuing to determine other factors that trigger bronchospasm and airway inflammation. Figure 20–6 depicts common chemicals that are released by the mast cell and the physiologic effect of these chemicals. Histologic changes in the epithelial basement membrane occur over time. The basement membrane is a complex structure that separates endothelial cells from underlying stroma. The membrane provides tensile strength and physical support to surrounding structures.[1] It also functions as a filter and as a site for cell attachment. The width of basement membrane thickens in asthmatics over time. The width seen in asthmatics is 17.5 μ, while that seen in healthy subjects is 7 μ.[38] Figure 20–6 depicts the pathogenesis of asthma in relation to mast cell release and parasympathetic stimulation by way of the vagus nerve. Vagal stimulation leads to edema, mucus hypersecretion, and bronchoconstriction.

The association of attacks with extrinsic allergens may be obscure. Many allergic asthmatics have immediate, rapidly reversible bronchospasm within an hour of exposure. Most patients will have a second, gradual onset of obstructive symptoms starting within 4 to 12 hours and becoming more severe than the

F I G U R E 20 – 5. The bronchial wall in asthma. Note the hypertrophied, contracted smooth muscle; edema; mucous gland hypertrophy; and secretion in the lumen. (From West JB: *Pulmonary Pathophysiology: The Essentials,* 3rd ed. Baltimore, Williams & Wilkins, 1987, p 81. Reproduced with permission.)

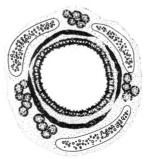

NORMAL

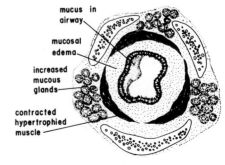

mucus in airway

mucosal edema

increased mucous glands

contracted hypertrophied muscle

ASTHMA

ALLERGIC ASTHMA

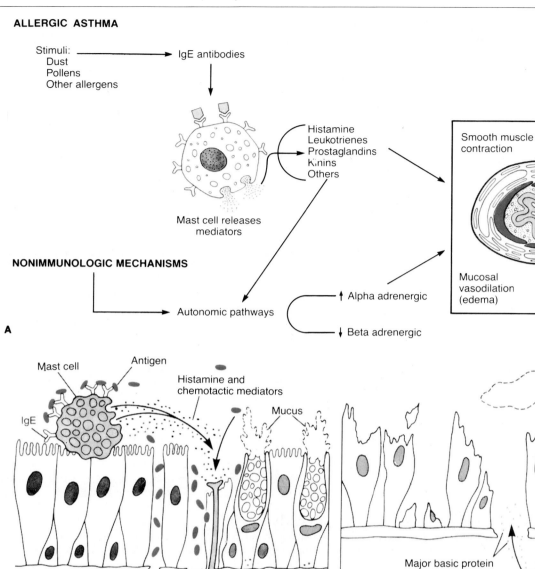

NONIMMUNOLOGIC MECHANISMS

A

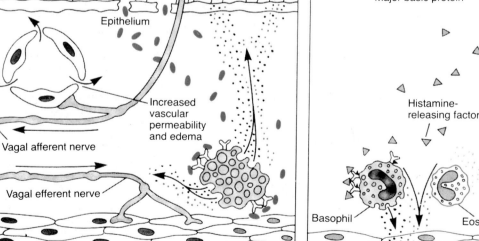

B

F I G U R E   20 – 6. See legend on opposite page

immediate reaction, then subsiding more slowly. This late reaction is more resistant to treatment, and ventilatory changes may persist. Some patients have little or no immediate obstructive response but a severe late response. In such cases the causative exposure may not be obvious.

Clinical Manifestations. Common symptoms are wheezing, feelings of tightness of the chest, dyspnea, and productive cough. Wheezing is caused by vibration in narrowed airways, which act like the uncoupled, vibrating reed of a wind instrument, yielding a musical sound.[39] Sputum is often thick, tenacious, scant, and viscid (sticky). Physical findings vary with the severity of the attack. A mild attack may be associated with a random monophonic expiratory wheezing, tachycardia, and tachypnea. Random monophonic wheezes are located throughout the chest and come and go on examination. The area where they are heard best is indicative of the area of obstruction (for example, if they are heard best at the mouth, this is indicative of large airway obstruction).[39] Tachycardia is an early sign of hypoxemia. A more severe attack requiring medical assistance may be accompanied by the use of accessory muscles of respiration, intercostal retractions, distant breath sounds, orthopnea, agitation, tachypnea, and tachycardia. In the severe state, the patient may appear cyanotic, agitated, restless, and confused. The degree of wheezing is *not* a good indicator of the severity of an asthma attack. The intensity of wheezing is *not* a reliable indicator of blockage of air flow. The measurement of peak expiratory flow rate (PEFR) is the best indicator of reduction in air flow (see discussion under Diagnosis). A PEFR of less than 100 L/min indicates severe obstruction.[4,40] When obstruction is the tightest, the patient cannot move enough air with enough velocity to make wheezing sounds. A patient with severe respiratory distress, prolonged expiration (indicating that the person is having difficulty moving air out of the lungs), neck and intercostal retractions, and minimal air sounds is critically ill and requires emergency intervention.

Diagnosis. The diagnosis of asthma is based on physical findings, sputum examination, pulmonary function tests, blood gases, and chest radiography demonstrating hyperinflation. Abnormal physical findings include presence of a productive cough, wheezing (most often on expiration, although inspiratory wheezing may be present), a hyperinflated chest,

and decreased breath sounds. Sputum samples reveal Charcot-Leyden crystals, eosinophils, and Curschmann's spirals.

Forced expiratory volumes decrease during asthma attacks. PEFR is measured to determine the index of airway function. The PEFR is the maximum flow of expired air attained during a forced vital capacity procedure.[40]

Blood gas values may be normal during a mild attack, but as the bronchospasm increases in intensity, respiratory alkalosis and hypoxemia become prominent findings. Elevation of $Paco_2$ in these patients is a poor prognostic sign, indicating that the patient's ability to continue breathing at a rapid rate has diminished and that exhaustion is imminent.

Determination of allergen(s) is done by skin testing or inhalation of suspected allergens. Skin testing is usually more helpful in young patients who have extrinsic asthma. Bronchial provocation testing with histamine or methacholine may be useful in confirming the diagnosis of asthma in certain cases.

A complete blood cell count can show an elevated number of white blood cells with increased eosinophils. Eosinophils are prominent in the cellular infiltrate of the bronchioles, the sputum, and the peripheral blood. A fall in the total eosinophil count is a valuable measure of effectiveness of corticosteroid treatment. With effective treatment, the total eosinophil count is depressed below $10/mm^3$.[3,4]

Respiratory failure may be evidenced by severe respiratory distress in a patient who shows no radiographic evidence of pneumothorax. As the patient improves, the wheezing becomes louder. When wheezing is no longer heard after an asthma attack, pulmonary function tests may continue to show obstructive changes for several weeks. Some patients will have a slight wheeze continuously between asthma bouts and still be comfortable and functional.

Treatment. Therapy for asthma is first of all aimed at prevention. The patient needs to be taught to avoid those things in the environment that trigger asthma attacks. Environmental control includes dust control; removal of allergens such as feathers, molds, and animal danders; and in some cases, removal of rugs and carpets. Other environmental control factors that help some patients with extrinsic asthma include the use of air purifiers and air conditioners. The patient should also be taught preventive therapy in regard to

---

FIGURE 20-6. **A,** Allergic and nonimmunologic mechanisms in asthma. **B,** Immediate (*left*) and late-phase (*right*) responses in allergic mucosal reactions. The immediate reaction is triggered by binding of antigen to IgE on the surface of superficial mast cells, which release histamine and other mediators. The latter open tight junctions between epithelial cells, allowing antigen to reach mast cells. Mediators increase vascular permeability and mucus production. Histamine and other mediators also interact with afferent nerves to initiate reflex responses. Mast cells also generate chemotactic factors and an influx of basophils, neutrophils, and eosinophils, which signals onset of the late-phase response (*right panel*). Histamine-releasing factors derived from a variety of cells act on basophils. Histamine and other mediators induce the late response. Major basic protein from eosinophils causes most of the epithelial damage. (From Cotran RS, Kumar V, Robbins SL: *Robbins Pathologic Basis of Disease*, 4th ed. Philadelphia, WB Saunders, 1989, p 775. Originally adapted from Lichtenstein L: The nasal late-phase response—an in-vivo model. *Hosp Pract* 1988;23(1):121. Illustration by Ilil Arbel. Reproduced with permission.)

smoking cessation, avoidance of passive smoking, and avoidance of aerosols and odors. Patients should seek early treatment of respiratory infections.

Chemotherapy for all three major obstructive disorders is similar. Refer to Table 20–1 (page 456) for a list of common respiratory drugs used in the treatment of various types of obstructive disorders.

Figure 20–7 shows the site of action of drugs used in the treatment of asthma. For the ambulatory patient with infrequent attacks, inhaled bronchodilators such as albuterol, metaproterenol, and others may provide adequate control.[8] For people with exercise-induced asthma or children with extrinsic asthma, cromolyn sodium or nedocromil sodium and inhaled bronchodilators prior to exercise are helpful. Cromolyn sodium or nedocromil sodium may be equally effective in intrinsic asthma when used prior to an attack. Patients with more frequent attacks require maintenance bronchodilators with inhaled corticosteroids.[8] Theophylline, previously used as first-line therapy for the treatment of asthma, has fallen into disfavor because of its numerous side effects and the availability of inhaled sympathomimetics and corticosteroids. In addition, many clinicians favor inhaled corticosteroids as first-line therapy.[4]

β_2-Adrenergic bronchodilator drugs such as meta-

TABLE 20–2. Patient's Instructions for Use of Inhalation Aerosol

1. **Shake the inhaler well** immediately before each use. Remove the cap from the mouthpiece. Inspect the mouthpiece for the presence of foreign objects before each use.
2. **Breathe out fully through the mouth.** Place the mouthpiece slightly away from the mouth, holding the inhaler in its upright position.
3. Take in a slow, deep breath while depressing the top of the canister.
4. **Hold your breath** for 10 seconds.
5. Wait 1 minute and repeat the procedure.
6. **Cleanse the inhaler thoroughly and frequently.**

proterenol, albuterol, and terbutaline are effective in promoting bronchodilation. Metaproterenol and albuterol come in oral (syrup, tablets) and inhaled (solution or aerosol container) dosages. Terbutaline is available in oral, inhaled, and parenteral dosage forms. Proper administration of inhaled agents is essential for optimum therapy. The recommended method for using metered-dose nebulizers is described in Table 20–2.

Carpentiere et al[41] studied the effects of fenoterol (a bronchodilator) metered-dose aerosol treatment on

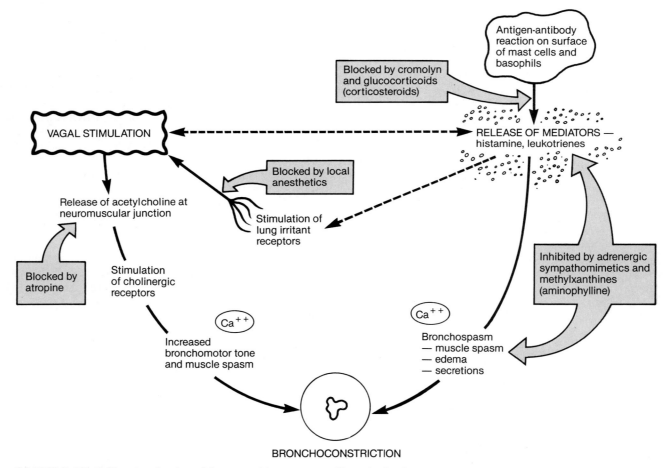

FIGURE 20–7. The site of action of drugs used in treatment of bronchial asthma. *Broken lines* indicate interactions that are not well established. (From Kersten LD: *Comprehensive Respiratory Nursing.* Philadelphia, WB Saunders, 1989, p 104. Reproduced with permission.)

the circadian rhythm of expiratory flow in allergic bronchial asthma. They found statistically significant circadian rhythms of forced expiratory volume in 1 second (FEV_1) in the eight patients studied. The greatest FEV_1 values were found at 10:48 A.M. Others have recorded the lowest FEV_1 values during the early morning hours around 2 A.M. to 6 A.M.[42,43] The use of Fenoterol over a 3-day period diminished the statistical significance of the circadian rhythm. The authors stated that treatment with bronchodilators should be scheduled at periods that reflect the most need in relation to circadian rhythms. Several explanations exist for the increased bronchospasm seen in asthmatics in the early morning hours. They include gastroesophageal reflux resulting from acid entering the trachea,[44] allergic and hormonal factors, rapid-eye-movement sleep,[45] and low levels of cyclic adenosine monophosphate.

Inhaled corticosteroid therapy (beclomethasone, flunisolide, or triamcinolone) is effective in most patients and is available in low and high doses. Because airway inflammation is a key component of asthma treatment, these drugs are effective. It does not have the major side effects of oral steroids but is effective in decreasing the bronchial inflammatory response seen in asthmatics. Oral candidiasis can be a side effect of aerosol steroid therapy; it can be avoided by rinsing the mouth after each use. Inhaled sympathomimetics may be given 15 to 20 minutes prior to inhalation of corticosteroids to enhance delivery of the medication in the airways.[4] Inhaled corticosteroids are useful as prophylaxis but are not administered during an acute asthma episode.

Corticosteroids are used for their anti-inflammatory and immunosuppressant action. Oral doses are useful for short-term use. Long-term use should be avoided if possible because of the side effects of adrenal suppression and multiple adverse effects. If long-term use is necessary, an alternate-day morning dosing schedule is effective in minimizing side effects. When discontinuing oral steroid therapy, it is important to taper the dosage over a 7- to 10-day period. Methotrexate has been tried in patients with chronic asthma who are corticosteroid dependent. Results have not been consistently positive.[4] Other therapies used in more severe asthmatics include use of home oxygen therapy and home administration of small volume nebulizer treatments via intermittent positive pressure ventilation.

Charlton et al evaluated the use of peak-flowmeters in home use as part of a self-management health program. Patients were randomly assigned to a control group or an experimental group (home use of peak-flowmeters). The control group received an intense education course on asthma and received a self-management treatment plan based on symptom treatment.[40] The peak-flowmeter group received an education course and instruction on home use of peak-flowmeters. In the group using home peak-flow metering, the use of oral steroids from 73 percent to 47 percent and the rate of medical consultation decreased from 98 percent to 66 percent. Similar findings were noted in the control group.[40]

Hyposensitization may be used as an adjunct to other therapies. The allergen is first identified by testing with purified allergens using the scratch, prick, or intradermal method. A positive reaction is shown by a flare or wheal occurring at the site in 15 to 20 minutes.

Acute attack or **status asthmaticus** (severe attacks unresponsive to routine therapy) requires more rapid and intense therapy, which includes epinephrine (young patients) or terbutaline given subcutaneously; aminophylline, a loading dose followed by continuous infusion to achieve a therapeutic serum level of 10 to 20 g/mL. In patients requiring high dose aminophylline to obtain a therapeutic level, cimetidine may be added to the regimen to decrease metabolism of drug by the liver. Once air flow has improved, aerosol inhalers (isoproterenol, isoethrane, atropine, ipratropium bromide). Intravenous corticosteroids are the mainstay of therapy. Oxygen therapy with or without mechanical ventilation may be necessary in severe cases.

Epinephrine has been the standard emergency therapy for many years.[35] But many emergency rooms are now initiating therapy with inhaled β-adrenergic aerosolized drugs. Ruddy et al[47] found that metaproterenol, a β-adrenergic aerosolized drug, had fewer side effects, a longer duration of action, and was followed by fewer recurrences of asthma than epinephrine treatment. Shapiro et al[48] recommend the use of aerosolized metaproterenol in children, based on their findings in a prerandomized, double-blind study of 100 children 6 to 12 years old with acute asthma. A dose of 5 mg of metaproterenol provided optimal bronchodilation with only minimal side effects. They also found aerosolized treatments less traumatic to the child than injections. The aerosolized β-adrenergic drugs have a wide margin of safety, and dosages can be individualized to the patient.[35]

The more that patients understand about asthma, the better they are at self-management of the symptoms. Educational materials are available from the American Lung Association, the Asthma and Allergy Foundation of America, and the National Institute of Allergy and Infectious Diseases.

KEY CONCEPTS

- Asthma is characterized by acute, reversible episodes of airway obstruction. Bronchospasm, excessive mucus production, and swelling of the bronchial mucosa lead to the obstructive episode. Wheezing, dyspnea, hyperinflation, and productive cough are common features.

- The severity of an asthma episode may vary from mild to life-threatening, depending on the degree of airway obstruction. With intense narrowing of the bronchi, severe hypoxemia may result.

- Several types of asthma have been identified. Intrinsic asthma is precipitated by exercise, stress, and exposure to pulmonary irritants, but no allergen can be identified. Drugs such as aspirin and exposure to occupational allergens have also been identified as etiologic agents.

- Extrinsic asthma is mediated by IgE, which is produced in response to specific antigens. The IgE binds to mast cells and causes them to release inflammatory chemicals when re-exposed to the antigen. Skin testing may be helpful in identifying suspected allergens.

- Prevention of asthma attacks is an important part of therapy. Avoidance of precipitating factors and prophylactic drug therapy are recommended. Bronchodilators, corticosteroids, and oxygen therapy are mainstays of treatment for an acute attack.

Chronic Bronchitis

Etiology. The major causes of chronic bronchitis are smoking, repeated viral or bacterial respiratory infections, predisposition due to genetic makeup, and inhalation of physical or chemical irritants. To a certain extent, chronic bronchitis is part of the normal aging process. The normal aging process leads to a loss of alveoli, an increase in the size of alveolar ducts, a loss of gas-exchanging surface area, and a decrease in bronchiolar musculature.[1] There is a high prevalence of chronic bronchitis in the British Isles because of environmental conditions, pollution, and socioeconomic factors.[1]

Chronic bronchitis (also referred to as type B chronic obstructive pulmonary disease, COPD) is defined **symptomatically** by hypersecretion of bronchial mucosa and a chronic or recurrent productive cough of more than 3 months' duration and occurring each year for 2 successive years in patients in whom other causes have been excluded.[4] For patients with chronic bronchitis and emphysema, airway obstruction is persistent and nonreversible.

The majority of patients smoke cigarettes and are frequently exposed to other irritants as well. Mortality rates from asthma, bronchitis, and emphysema are higher during times of serious air pollution with sulfur dioxide.[49] Barker and Osmond[50] determined a causal link between acute lower respiratory tract infection in early childhood and chronic bronchitis in adult life.

Pathogenesis. Pathologic changes in the airway include chronic inflammation and swelling of the bronchial mucosa resulting in scarring, increased fibrosis of the mucous membrane, increased numbers (hyperplasia) of bronchial mucous glands and goblet cells, hypertrophy of bronchial glands and goblet cells, and increased bronchial wall thickness, which potentiates obstruction to air flow. Figures 20–8 and 20–9 show the histologic changes seen in chronic bronchitis. Hypertrophy of mucosal glands and goblet cells leads to increased mucus production, which combines with purulent exudate to form bronchial plugs. The mucociliary clearing action is impaired or lost, and some areas of ciliated epithelium are replaced by squamous cells **metaplasia**.[1,4,50] In addition, ciliary function is diminished because of decreased numbers of cilia and decreased action of available cilia.

Often the inflammatory and fibrotic changes may extend into the surrounding alveoli. The narrowed airways and the mucous plugs prevent proper oxygenation and potentiate airway obstruction. High air flow resistance increases the work of breathing, thus leading to increased oxygen demands. In areas of greater obstruction to air flow, alveoli empty and fill more slowly, leading to ventilation-perfusion ($\dot{V}A/\dot{Q}$) mismatch, thus lowering arterial oxygenation. An old clinical term rarely used today, "blue bloater," reflects the pathophysiologic process of oxygen desaturation (cyanosis) and edema associated with heart failure.

Involvement of small pulmonary arteries related to inflammation in the bronchial walls and the compensatory spasm of pulmonary blood vessels from hypoxia produce pulmonary hypertension. As the process of pulmonary hypertension continues, right ventricular end-diastolic pressures increase, leading to right ventricular dilation and right-sided heart failure. Heart failure resulting from lung disease is called **cor pulmonale.** Heart failure results in increased venous pressure, liver engorgement, and dependent edema. Manifestations of heart failure may occur during exacerbations of bronchitis and subside with appropriate treatment.

After severe streptococcal or staphylococcal pneumonia, repeated bouts of bronchitis, infection with

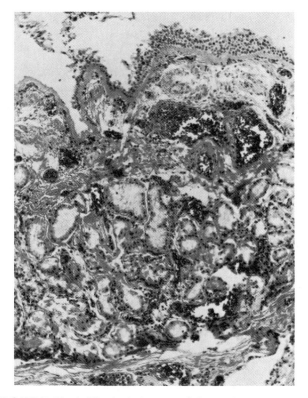

FIGURE 20–8. Histologic features of chronic bronchitis. (Lumen of bronchus is above.) Note slight desquamation of mucosal epithelial cells and marked thickening (approximately twice normal thickness) of mucous gland layer. Vascular congestion is evident. (From Cotran RS, Kumar V, Robbins SL: *Robbins Pathologic Basis of Disease,* 4th ed. Philadelphia, WB Saunders, 1989, p 773. Reproduced with permission.)

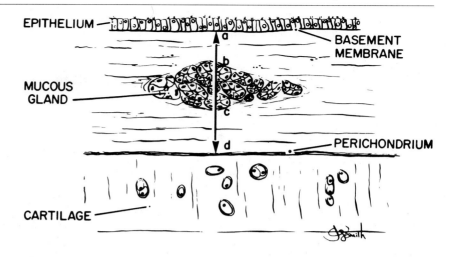

EPITHELIUM

BASEMENT MEMBRANE

MUCOUS GLAND

PERICHONDRIUM

CARTILAGE

FIGURE 20–9. Structure of a normal bronchial wall. In chronic bronchitis the thickness of the mucous glands increases and can be expressed as the Reid index, given by formula $(b - c)/(a - d)$. The ratio is normally less than 0.4. A ratio of 0.7 indicates severe bronchitis. (From Thurlbeck WM: *Chronic Airflow Obstruction in Lung Disease.* Philadelphia, WB Saunders, 1976, p 33. Reproduced with permission.)

the mold *Aspergillus fumigatus,* mucous plugs, foreign bodies, or immunologic deficiencies, destruction of bronchial walls may occur, leaving dilated sacs of purulent material. This is termed **bronchiectasis.** (Refer to the section on bronchiectasis earlier in this chapter for a more detailed description of this disease process.) These dilated sacs contain pools of infected secretion which do not clear themselves and serve as sources of further infection that can spread to adjacent lung fields, or can spread by the lymphatics or venous drainage to other areas of the body, commonly the brain. If bronchiectatic lesions are localized, surgical resection of the affected portions of lung may be helpful. The narrowing of the airways of bronchitis and the turbulent air flow from mucus obstruction produce wheezing resembling asthma.

Clinical Manifestations. The typical clinical presentation is an overweight male of age 40 or more who presents with shortness of breath on exertion, excessive amounts of sputum, chronic cough, evidence of excess body fluids (edema, hypervolemia), and a history of smoking. In addition, the patient often complains of chills, malaise, muscle aches, fatigue, loss of libido, and insomnia. Although the typical patient is a man in his early 40s, the prevalence in women who smoke cigarettes is steadily rising.

Sputum production may be variable and worsens with respiratory infection. Cough and sputum production are most severe in the mornings. Gradually patients develop progressive shortness of breath on exertion. Most patients do not seek help until dyspnea becomes troublesome.

In the end-stage disease process, the patient has severe exertional dyspnea, cyanosis, and dependent edema. Hypoxemia or decreased arterial oxygen leads to pulmonary hypertension, progressing to cor pulmonale.

Diagnosis. Measures used to confirm the diagnosis include chest radiography, which may show congested lung fields, an enlarged horizontal cardiac silhouette, and evidence of previous pulmonary infection; pulmonary function tests showing normal total lung capacity, increased residual volume, and decreased FEV_1; and arterial blood gas evaluation, which

often shows elevated $Paco_2$ and decreased Pao_2 (often below 65 mm Hg). The electrocardiogram may show atrial arrhythmias and evidence of right ventricular hypertrophy. The hematocrit may reveal polycythemia (increased numbers of red blood cells) related to continuous or nocturnal hypoxemia.[4,7] Nocturnal hypoxemia leads to a compensatory production of red blood cells in an attempt to carry more oxygen to the body tissues.

Depending on the severity of the disease, the physical examination may reveal scattered crackles, rhonchi and wheezes, use of accessory muscles to breathe, jugular vein distention, and pedal and ankle edema. Table 20–3 lists the distinguishing features of both chronic bronchitis and emphysema.

Treatment. The treatment for bronchitis and emphysema is similar. Because bronchitis and emphysema are most frequently seen in combination, the therapies covered in this section are for the combined disorder. The overall goals are to (1) block the progression of the disease, (2) return the patient to optimal respiratory function, and (3) return the patient to usual activities of daily living.

Pharmacologic treatment involves the use of bronchodilators (theophylline, terbutaline); cough suppressants, when necessary; and anti-infective agents for infections. Corticosteroids may also be used in the treatment of some patients who have airway inflammation and a component of asthma. (See the Treatment section on asthma in this chapter for an expanded discussion of pharmacologic therapy.)

Low-dose oxygen therapy is recommended for patients with Pao_2 levels less than 55 mm Hg.[43] Oxygen can be delivered through a nasal cannula (0.5–3 L/min) or Venturi mask (28–40 percent) at flow rates sufficient to keep the oxygen saturation above 90 percent. Mechanical ventilation may become necessary for some patients to get them over crisis periods of acute exacerbations.

Oxygen saturation can be measured by routine testing for blood gas values or by the use of noninvasive oxygen saturation monitors. Patients with hypercapnia (high levels of carbon dioxide in the blood) are sensitive to increased levels of oxygen, such as levels

TABLE 20–3. Common Distinguishing Features of Emphysema and Chronic Bronchitis*

Patient Data	Emphysema	Bronchitis
History		
Life-style	Smoker	Smoker
Weight	Weight loss	Overweight
Onset of symptoms	Usually after age 50	Usually after age 40
Sputum	Mild, mucoid	Excessive purulent
Cough	Minimal or absent	Chronic; more severe in mornings
Dyspnea	Progressive exertional dyspnea	Mild to moderate, but may gradually progress to severe exertional dyspnea
Patient Complaints	Shortness of breath on exertion; fatigue, insomnia	Chills, malaise, muscle aches, fatigue, insomnia, loss of libido
Physical Signs		
Edema	Absent	Present
Central cyanosis	Absent	Present in advanced disease
Use of accessory muscles to breathe	Present	Absent until end stage
Body build	Thin, wasted	Stocky, overweight
Anterior-posterior (AP) chest diameter	"Barrel chest," 1:1 ratio AP diameter	Normal
Auscultation of chest	Decreased breath sounds, decreased heart sounds, prolonged expiration	Wheezes, crackles, rhonchi depending on the severity of disease
Percussion	Hyperresonant	Normal
Jugular vein distention	Absent	Present
Other	Pursed-lip breathing	Evidence of right-sided heart failure (cor pulmonale)
General Diagnostic Tests		
Chest radiograph	Narrowed mediastinum; normal or small vertical heart; hyperinflation; low, flat diaphragm; presence of blebs or bullae	Congested lung fields, enlarged horizontal heart
Arterial blood gases	Decreased Pao_2 (60–80 mm Hg); normal or increased $Paco_2$ (increases with advancing disease)	Decreased Pao_2 (60 mm Hg); increased $Paco_2$
Electrocardiogram	Normal or tall symmetric P waves; tachycardia, if hypoxic	Right axis deviation, right ventricular hypertrophy, atrial arrhythmias
Hematocrit	Normal	Polycythemia
Pulmonary Function Tests		
Functional residual volume	Increased	Normal or slight increase
Residual volume	Increased	Increased
Total lung capacity	Increased	Normal
Forced expiratory volume	Decreased	Decreased
Vital capacity	Decreased	Normal or slight decrease
Static lung compliance	Increased	Normal

*Clinically, features of bronchitis and emphysema are not always clear-cut because many of the patients have a combined disease process.

above 3 L/min. With oxygen therapy, carbon dioxide levels tend to be even higher.

Although traditionally the mechanism of carbon dioxide retention with oxygen therapy had been related to a diminished ventilatory drive, current research suggests that oxygen therapy may instead cause increased $\dot{V}A/\dot{Q}$ imbalance, precipitating a rise in carbon dioxide. It is important to remember that all patients with a history of COPD are not carbon dioxide retainers.

Patients with end-stage emphysema or oxygen levels less than 55 mm Hg[51] are frequently placed on low-level oxygen therapy at home. Home oxygen therapy has been demonstrated to retard the development of pulmonary hypertension and cor pulmonale.[50] Portable oxygen saturation monitors for evaluating the effectiveness of oxygen administration at home may also be used.

Supportive therapies include adequate rest, proper hydration (8 to 12 glasses of water per day unless the patient has congestive heart failure), percussion and postural drainage, and physical reconditioning programs using a treadmill or stationary bicycle. Low-tension, high-repetition muscle contractions provide endurance conditioning. High-tension, low-repetition muscle contractions provide strength conditioning. Alternating rest and exercise improves results on pulmonary function tests.[52] Some patients have benefited from the use of inspiratory muscle trainers. These devices cause the user to increase respiratory muscle strength and endurance by increasing the resistance to air flow on inspiration.[53]

Support groups such as the American Lung Association and local Better Breathers organizations are available in many communities. Support groups are helpful in addressing prevention strategies and coping mechanisms. Hospitals also have special organized classes for individuals with emphysema. Special exercise courses designed for respiratory disease patients are also available in some communities. Instructional materials for patients can be obtained from the American Lung Association.

Acute Bronchitis

Etiology. Acute inflammation of the tracheobronchial tree is produced by a variety of viruses such as influenza virus, A or B, parainfluenza, respiratory syncytial virus coronavirus, coxsackie virus, and adenovirus. Nonviral causes include *Mycoplasma* and *Chlamydia*, numerous bacteria, heat or smoke inhalation, inhalation of irritant chemicals such as sulfur dioxide and chlorine, bromine, or fluorine gases, and allergic reactions. Seasonal patterns of acute bronchitis are common. January and February are peak months, and August has the lowest rate. Highest rates are noted in early childhood and old age.[54] The swelling of bronchial mucosa in children leading to obstruction and respiratory distress with wheezing is known as asthmatic bronchitis.

Pathogenesis. The airways become inflamed and narrowed from capillary dilation, swelling from exudation of fluid, infiltration with inflammatory cells, increased mucus production, loss of ciliary function, and loss of portions of the ciliated epithelium. Many viruses and mycoplasmas inhibit macrophages and lymphocytes, temporarily promoting secondary bacterial invasion. Microorganisms may also induce long-lasting hyperirritability of the respiratory tract with associated episodes of bronchospasm.

Clinical Manifestations. Most of these infections are mild and self-limited, requiring only supportive treatment. In children, the smaller airways are most easily obstructed by inflammation, so that severe obstruction may occur. The smaller airways in proportion to body size are due to a smaller size lumen in relation to the vessel wall. Associated inflammation of the larynx and trachea produces croup. Acute inflammation of the epiglottis may rapidly produce severe toxicity and dangerous respiratory obstruction. Epiglottitis should be suspected in children and even adults with fever, severe sore throat, cough, and rapidly developing obstructive dyspnea with stridorous breath sounds and an audible inspiratory wheeze. A lateral radiograph of the pharynx using air as a contrast medium demonstrates glottic swelling. The patient needs immediate antibiotic treatment with amoxicillin and may need emergency endotracheal intubation or tracheostomy to ensure an adequate airway.

The dangers of acute bronchitis include the potential for bacterial invasion, which can worsen symptoms in patients with chronic obstructive pulmonary disease and precipitate serious infections in the aged or those with debilitating disease.

Diagnosis and Treatment. The diagnosis of acute bronchitis is similar to that of chronic bronchitis. Treatment entails identifying the infectious agent and providing appropriate antibiotics.

KEY CONCEPTS

- Chronic bronchitis is an inflammatory disorder of the airways that most commonly results from long-term cigarette smoking. It is defined as a productive cough lasting more than 3 months per year for 2 or more consecutive years. Resultant airway damage is not reversible.

- Chronic bronchitis is associated with persistently narrowed airways because of chronic inflammation, scarring, and excessive mucus production. Airway obstruction leads to poor ventilation of alveoli and impaired exchange of oxygen and carbon dioxide. Blood gases are characterized by low Pao_2, and high $Paco_2$. Persistent hypoxemia causes a compensatory increased in red blood cell production (polycythemia). Cyanosis is usually evident.

- Alveolar hypoxia leads to generalized pulmonary vasoconstriction, pulmonary hypertension, and right ventricular hypertrophy (cor pulmonale) in the person with chronic bronchitis. Right-sided heart failure may occur because of the high pulmonary resistance.

- The treatment of chronic bronchitis centers on removing the etiologic factors (for example, cigarette smoke) providing bronchodilator therapy, removing secretions, preventing respiratory muscle fatigue, and providing low-dose supplemental oxygen. High-dose oxygen is contraindicated because it increases $Paco_2$ levels.

- Acute bronchitis results from temporary inflammation of the tracheobronchial tree. Inflammation may be due to viral, bacterial, fungal, or chemical causes. Symptoms are due to narrowing of inflamed airways and increased mucus production. Dyspnea and cough are common.

- Epiglottitis, or inflammation of the epiglottis, can progress to complete airway obstruction requiring emergency treatment. Epiglottitis is suspected when wheezing and severe dyspnea are found in association with fever, sore throat, and cough.

Obstruction Related to Loss of Lung Parenchyma

Emphysema

Etiology. **Emphysema** (also referred to as type A COPD) is defined **pathologically** by destructive changes of the alveolar walls without fibrosis and abnormal enlargement of the distal air sacs.[1,4] Emphysema is frequently associated with chronic bronchitis. According to the American Lung Association, 14 million Americans have COPD—12 million have bronchitis and 2 million have emphysema.

The causes of emphysema are not fully understood, but emphysema is associated with cigarette smoking, air pollution, and certain occupations such as welding, mining, and working with asbestos. It tends to develop over a long period of time and thus is seen more frequently in the elderly. It is a common disease seen in almost 50 percent of autopsies.[1] A prospective, matched, controlled study of COPD patients showed a higher incidence of lung cancer (8.8 percent) than in the control group (2 percent).[55]

The normal aging process, starting at about age 30, reflects changes similar to those seen in emphysema. These changes include a loss of alveoli, an increase in the size of alveolar ducts, a loss of gas-exchanging surface area (4 percent per decade), and a decrease in bronchiolar musculature.[1]

When emphysema occurs in young to middle-aged adults, it is often associated with a deficiency of α_1-antitrypsin activity in the lung. Garver et al[56] determined that 2 percent of the cases of emphysema in the United States and Europe are associated with a hereditary deficiency of α_1-antitrypsin. Human alpha proteinase inhibitor is used as replacement therapy for these patients.

Emphysema may follow bacterial lung infections such as by staphylococci, which secrete proteases that destroy the elastin proteins responsible for the normal elasticity of the lung tissue. Bacterial infections block mechanisms that normally inhibit the release of proteolytic enzymes from degenerating neutrophilic granulocytes.

Pathogenesis. The pathologic changes leading to alveolar destruction are associated with the release of proteolytic enzymes from inflammatory cells such as neutrophils and macrophages. Smoking is commonly associated with emphysema. Smoking causes alveolar damage in two ways: (1) it leads to inflammation in the lung tissue (parenchyma), thus initiating a chain of events leading to the release of proteolytic enzymes that directly damages alveolar tissue; and (2) it inactivates α_1-antitrypsin, which normally acts to protect the lung parenchyma. Figure 20–10 illustrates the pathogenesis of emphysema.

With the loss of alveolar walls, there is also a marked reduction in the pulmonary capillary bed, which is essential for exchange of oxygen and carbon dioxide between the alveolar air and capillary blood. There is also a loss of elastic tissue in the lung, which leads to a decrease in the size of the smaller bronchioles. The loss of lung tissue leads to a loss of radial traction and increasing pressure around the outside of the airway lumen, which in turn increases airway resistance and decreases air flow. Figure 20–11 shows the effect of decreased radial traction on the size of small bronchioles. Air then becomes trapped in distal alveoli, leading to distended air sacs, which adds to the collapsing pressure on more proximal bronchi and increases airway obstruction. Loss of alveolar walls and air trapping lead to the formation of **bullae,** large, thin-walled cysts in the lung, that further rob the lung of its gas transport function. The appearance of the lung and lung tissue from typical emphysematous patients is shown in Figures 20–12 and 20–13.

Three major classifications of emphysema exist: (1) centriacinar (also called centrilobular), which is associated with both smoking and chronic bronchitis and destroys the respiratory bronchioles; (2) panacinar (also called parlobular), which destroys the alveoli; and (3) paraseptal, which affects the peripheral lobules. Some of the classifications of emphysema and the topographic distribution of emphysema in lung tissue are shown in Figure 20–14.

Clinical Manifestations. Patients with emphysema commonly seek help because of progressive exertional dyspnea. The typical patient is a thin man in his middle 50s who has had increasing shortness of breath for the past 3 to 4 years. The difficulty in breathing is evidenced by the use of accessory muscles to breathe, progressive dyspnea, and the use of pursed-lip breathing in an effort to get more air out over a longer period of time before the small airways collapse. Cough may be minimal or absent. Decreased arterial oxygen saturation remains minor until late in the course of the disease. Late in the disease process the major symptom is dyspnea on exertion. These patients used to be referred to as the "pink puffers," a term related to the physiologic matching of ventilation and perfusion. They tend to have more areas of high ventilation in relation to perfusion; thus maintaining near normal arterial oxygen levels. Ventilation-perfusion matching and a sustained high respiratory rate

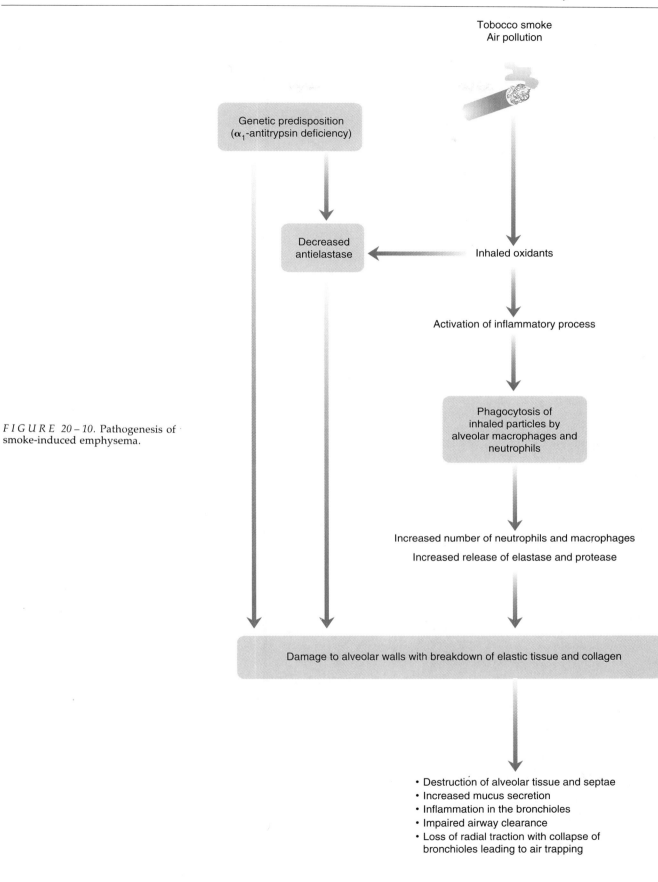

FIGURE 20–10. Pathogenesis of smoke-induced emphysema.

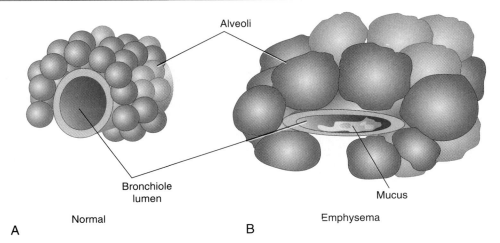

Alveoli

Bronchiole
lumen

Mucus

A   Normal   B   Emphysema

F I G U R E 20 – 11. Loss of radial traction in emphysema leads to airway collapse. **A**, Terminal bronchiole in cross-section. **B**, Terminal bronchiole with narrowed lumen resulting from loss of surrounding alveoli, leading to decreased radial traction and airway collapse.

produce a relatively normal arterial oxygen level until late stages of the disease.[1] As with bronchitis, the incidence is increasing in women who smoke.

Diagnosis. The diagnosis of emphysema is based on the patient's history and physical findings, pulmonary function tests, chest radiographs, arterial blood gases, and electrocardiogram. Changes seen in pulmonary function tests include an increased functional residual capacity, increased residual volume, increased total lung capacity, decreased forced expiratory volume in one second (FEV_1) and decreased vital capacity. Chest radiographs show hyperinflation; a low, flat diaphragm; the presence of blebs or bullae; a narrow mediastinum; and a normal or small vertical heart. Electrocardiographic findings may be

normal or show tall P waves. Tachycardia may be the first sign of decreased oxygenation. Arterial blood gas values typically reveal a mild decrease in Pao_2 (55–80 mm Hg) and a normal (or in late stages, elevated) $Paco_2$ (50–60 mm Hg).

Physical examination reveals a thin, wasted individual who is using accessory muscles to breathe and sits slightly hunched forward in an effort to breathe better. Auscultation and percussion of the lung fields reveal decreased breath sounds, decreased heart sounds, prolonged expiration, decreased diaphragmatic excursion, and a hyperresonant chest. Pursed-lip breathing, chronic morning cough because of mucus buildup at night, and an increased anteroposterior chest diameter (barrel chest) are also frequent

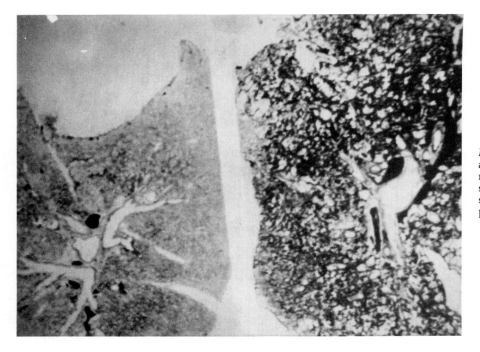

F I G U R E 20 – 12. Gross appearance of emphysematous lung. *Left,* normal lung tissue from a nonsmoker. *Right,* lung tissue from a smoker who has developed emphysema.

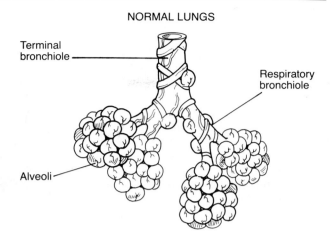

NORMAL LUNGS

Terminal bronchiole

Respiratory bronchiole

Alveoli

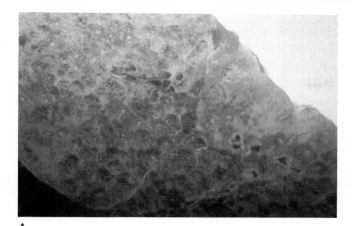

A

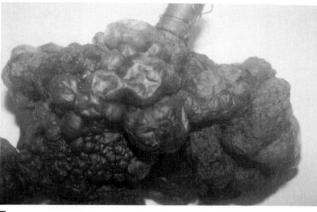

B

FIGURE 20–13. Appearance of slices of emphysematous lung. **A,** Centriacinar (centrilobular) emphysema. **B,** Panacinar (panlobular) emphysema.

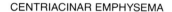

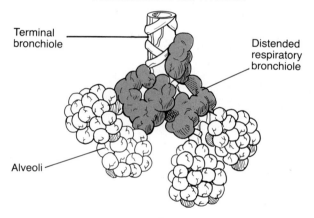

CENTRIACINAR EMPHYSEMA

Terminal bronchiole

Distended respiratory bronchiole

Alveoli

findings. Weight loss occurs because of anorexia and lack of energy to eat.

Treatment. Refer to the Treatment section under chronic bronchitis earlier in this chapter for detailed treatment modalities common to both obstructive lung diseases. Major treatment modalities include:

1. Use of bronchodilators, with inhaled sympathomimetics and ipratropium bromide being preferred
2. Bronchial hygiene to mobilize secretions
3. Cessation of smoking
4. Graded aerobic exercise
5. Abdominal diaphragmatic breathing exercises with pursed-lip breathing to improve muscle conditioning for breathing and exhale more air from the lungs
6. Avoidance of pollution and irritants
7. Home oxygen therapy for continuous use or only during the night and during exercise

An excellent patient teaching manual called *Better Breathing—A Self-Teaching Manual* is available from PAL Medical, Inc., Maitland, Florida. Poor prognosis is associated with weight loss, so treatment is focused on maintaining proper nutrition.

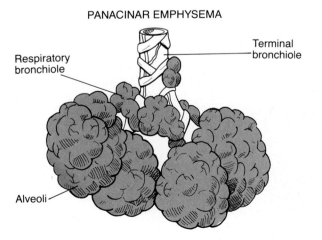

PANACINAR EMPHYSEMA

Respiratory bronchiole

Terminal bronchiole

Alveoli

FIGURE 20–14. Types of emphysema. (From Black JM, Matassarin-Jacobs E (eds): *Luckmann and Sorensen's Medical-Surgical Nursing,* 4th ed. Philadelphia, WB Saunders, 1993, p 1027. Reproduced with permission.)

KEY CONCEPTS

- Emphysema is an obstructive airway disorder that results from destruction of alveoli and small airways. Emphysema occurs primarily in cigarette smokers and is often seen in association with chronic bronchitis.
- Alveolar destruction is due to release of inflammatory proteolytic enzymes that degrade lung proteins. Smoking also inhibits a protective enzyme (α_1-antitrypsin) that normally keeps the proteolytic enzymes in check. Genetic deficiency of α_1-antitrypsin is an uncommon cause of emphysema.
- Emphysema causes two major problems with respiration; (1) a decrease in surface area for gas exchange, and (2) airway collapse from loss of radial traction. Airway collapse is greater on expiration, resulting in air trapping and hyperinflation.
- Emphysema is characterized by dyspnea, weight loss, use of accessory muscles to breathe, a flat diaphragm, and barrel chest. Cyanosis is not present until late stages of the disease. By sustaining high ventilatory effort, a patient can have blood oxygen levels that are generally maintained near normal. Carbon dioxide levels may be low due to hyperventilation.
- Therapy for emphysema is similar to that for chronic bronchitis. Cessation of smoking is necessary to prevent progression of the disease. Present damage is irreversible. Oxygen therapy improves activity tolerance and does not cause elevations in Pa_{CO_2} in people with emphysematous COPD.

Diagnostic Tests

Pulmonary Function Testing

The primary criteria in diagnosing COPD include the demonstration of obstruction to air flow in the lungs. This may be determined in a number of ways, but the most common method is spirometry. Table 20–4 lists common ventilatory parameters referred to in the measurement of spirometry.

Spirometry is performed by asking the patient to inhale deeply and then to exhale, as fast as possible until maximum air is exhaled. The total volume of air exhaled is known as the forced vital capacity (FVC). In order to determine flow, the time required for exhaling the air is also determined. The volume exhaled in the first second is a reliable and reproducible index of obstructive airway disease. This value is known as the forced expiratory volume in 1 second (FEV_1). Figure 20–15 presents spirogram examples of normal, obstructive, and restrictive graphs for forced expiratory volume and forced vital capacity. For all spirometric studies, normal values are based on large population studies of healthy volunteers and are adjusted for height, weight, age and sex data that are available for comparison.

A simple formula has been developed to define and quantify air flow obstruction. If the quotient of

*TABLE 20–4. Common Ventilatory Parameters Used in the Measurement of Obstructive Lung Disease**

Tidal volume	Volume of air inspired and expired with a normal breath (400–500 cc or 5 cc/kg body weight)
Residual volume	Volume of gas left in lung after maximal expiration; stabilizes alveoli
Vital capacity or forced vital capacity	Maximal amount of air that can be expired after a maximal inspiratory effort; includes inspiratory reserve volume, tidal volume, and expiratory reserve volume
Functional residual capacity	Volume of air left in lungs after a normal expiration; includes expiratory reserve volume and reserve volume
Forced expiratory flow rate (FEF_{25}, FEF_{50}, FEF_{75})	Volume of air forcibly exhaled per second or minute at 25 percent, 50 percent, and 75 percent of the FVC
Peak expiratory flow rate	Highest rate of flow sustained for 10 msec or more at which air can be expelled from the lungs

*Refer also to Figure 19–10 in Chapter 19.

the FEV_1 ratio divided by the FVC ratio is 75 percent or greater, no obstruction of airflow is present. If the value obtained is between 60 percent to 70 percent, then mild obstruction of air flow is present. Moderate obstruction is defined as a value of 50 to 60 percent; and severe obstruction is present when the FEV_1/FVC ratio is less than 50 percent. Therefore, using a spirometer and measuring both volume and time, the diagnosis of chronic obstructive pulmonary disease can be made and the severity quantified.

From the spirometric ventilatory measurements (see Table 20–4), other determinations of air flow can be made during the mid to later parts of the vital capacity. These measures are helpful in determining the presence of small airway disease. Some investigators believe that small airway disease may be a precursor to the development of chronic bronchitis and emphysema.[1,3,56]

Frequently, an inhaled bronchodilator, such as isoetharine, albuterol, or metaproterenol, may be given, with repeated testing in 15 to 20 minutes. If the FEV_1 improves by 15 percent or more, the patient is considered to have a positive bronchodilator response indicative of partially reversible bronchospasm of the smooth muscles of the airways. This is most often the case with asthma or asthmatic bronchitis.

A second pulmonary function test known as the diffusion capacity measures the ability of the alveolar air to diffuse into the capillary blood. The technical details of this test are beyond the scope of this book, but it is a valuable test in determining either thickening (fibrosis) of the alveolar-capillary membrane or destruction (emphysema) of the membrane.

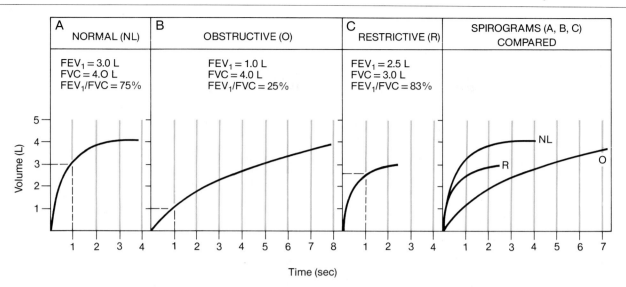

FIGURE 20–15. Distinguishing restrictive from obstructive lung disease. (FEV₁, forced expiratory volume in 1 second; FVC, forced vital capacity; NL, normal lungs; R, restrictive disease; O, obstructive disease. (From Kersten LD: *Comprehensive Respiratory Nursing.* Philadelphia, WB Saunders, 1989, p 376. Reproduced with permission.)

By breathing mixtures of an inert gas, such as helium, the total lung capacity (TLC) can be determined. This volume is composed of the vital capacity (VC) and the residual volume (RV). The residual volume is that volume of air that remains in the lung after a person has voluntarily exhaled all of the air from the lungs. (Refer to Figure 19–10 in Chapter 19.) The ratio of the residual volume to the total lung capacity (RV/TLC) is normally 30 to 35 percent. In some patients with air flow obstruction, air tends to "trap" in the lungs, thereby increasing the residual volume and resulting in overinflation of lung tissue.

Arterial blood gases are also useful as a pulmonary function measurement. Using these values, a careful assessment of both the oxygenation of the patient, as well as the acid-base status can be determined. The normal pH is 7.40, the normal $Paco_2$ is 40 mm Hg, and the normal Pao_2, at sea level, is 80 to 100 mm Hg. In COPD, especially in the severe stage, Pao_2 falls $Paco_2$ rises. Table 20–5 lists normal arterial blood gas values for various individuals.

Bronchial Provocation Tests

The controlled induction of bronchospasm by inhalation of various agents is occasionally used to identify patients with hyperreactive airways and to prove whether certain inhaled substances can produce bronchospasm. Usually a series of inhalations is administered, followed by a series of ventilation measurements. Generally the test is stopped when the FEV₁ falls 20 percent or more compared to the control measurement. Bronchoprovocation is contraindicated if the patient is already exhibiting symptoms or requires continual asthma medication. Allergens can be administered as solutions, dusts, or fumes. The amount administered should be no more than the patient would normally encounter in the environment. If symptoms occur, they can be readily reversed by two to four inhalations of albuterol or metaproterenol.

General hyperreactivity of the bronchi can be detected by having the patient inhale histamine phosphate solutions or methacholine (mecholyl, related to

TABLE 20–5. Normal Arterial Blood Gas Values

Parameter	Adult	Pregnancy	Newborn	COPD (Late findings)
Pao_2	80–100	75–100	60–70	Decreased
$Paco_2$ (mm Hg)	35–45	30–37	35–45	Increased
pH	7.35–7.45	7.35–7.45	7.30–7.40	Decreased
HCO_3 (mEq/L)	24–30	20–26	20–26	Increased
Base excess (mEq/L)	±2	—	—	
O_2 saturation	96%–100%	95%–100%	90%–100%	Decreased

T A B L E 20 – 6. Research Findings in Obstructive Lung Diseases

Authors, Study	Findings
Agah et al[14]	This study evaluated the clinical illness rate in an experimental study that compared a mask-and-goggle group to a no mask-and-goggle control group. The infection rate in the mask-and-goggle group was 11 percent; the control group has a 62 percent infection rate.
Carlsen et al[9]	A comparative study of risk factors associated with bronchiolitis in infants and children was done. Data showed that risk factors were increased number of school age siblings, shorter period of breast feeding, and the season between April and September.
Gala et al[13]	The effect of the use of eye-nose goggles was studied to determine their effectiveness. Data revealed that 34 percent of the hospital personnel without goggles and 43 percent of susceptible infants become infected. The use of goggles lowered the percentages of infection to 5 percent for hospital personnel and 6 percent of susceptible infants. The efficacy of syncytial on respiratory mechanism was tested in patients with bronchiolitis. The results showed that syncytial did not improve basic respiratory function.
McConnochie et al[8]	A cross-control method was used to study risk factors associated with bronchiolitis. Data showed that children at high risk for developing bronchiolitis are with a positive family history of asthma, passive smoking, and presence of older siblings.
Meyers et al[57]	The authors reviewed the records of 100 episodes of bloodstream infections in patients over the age of 65. Survival was 60 percent with these patients having the poorest survival rates.
Cook et al[58]	The peak expiratory flow rates (PEFR) of 3,812 persons age 65 to 105 years, with a median age of 72, were measured. Other variables measured were physical function, cardiovascular measures, and cognitive function. The PEFR was significantly related to age, sex, smoking, and years smoked. Low PEFR was associated with chronic respiratory symptoms.
Philips et al[59]	Forty-eight healthy volunteers with a mean age of 69 years were studied in a clinical sleep laboratory. They underwent spirometry evaluation after spending a night in the sleep role. The findings showed that there was a significant correlation between poor sleep quality and poor performance on pulmonary function tests.
Buist et al[60]	Official statement of the American Thoracic Society, adopted in June 1989. These guidelines were developed to aid practitioners in decision making regarding who should be treated with the experimental and unproved AAT replacement therapy. The article describes appropriate diagnosis and treatment as well as supportive and augmentation therapy.
Haluszka et al[61]	Pulmonary flow resistance, dynamic lung compliance, breathing pattern, arterial blood gases, and intrinsic PEEP were measured in 96 stable COPD patients with varying degrees of airway obstruction. Intrinsic PEEP was correlated with FEV_1, pulmonary flow resistance, and $Paco_2$. These data suggest that PEEP and its concomitant dynamic hyperinflation are increased with increased severity of lung obstruction.
Whitelaw[62]	Despite improvements in drug therapy and disease management plans, asthma deaths are increasing. The author suggests that reliance on bronchodilators and antiasthma medications may make patients complacent. They may spend more time in allergen-containing environments and delay treatment during acute attacks. The treatments that make them feel good may alter their behavior in ways that actually increase their risk of death.
Barnes[63]	The author describes the pathophysiology of asthma as an inflammatory disease, including a discussion on the neurogenic mechanisms and the role of inflammation mediators. The mechanisms of actions of bronchodilators, β-agonists, anticholinergics, anti-inflammatory drugs, and other medications used in asthma treatment are described. The author proposes what he calls a "logical approach to therapy," including the risks and benefits of various treatments, and their long-term consequences.
Salvaterra et al[64]	Pulmonary hypertension is a serious complication of COPD that results in severe disability and contributes to mortality. This article reviews the current methods of diagnosis and treatment of pulmonary hypertension.

acetylcholine) or nebulized distilled water. A fall of over 20 percent in the FEV_1 will identify hyperreactivity.

KEY CONCEPTS

- Obstructive disorders are associated with characteristic abnormalities of pulmonary function tests. These include:

  1. Decreased forced expiratory volume in 1 second (FEV_1)

  2. A low FEV_1/forced vital capacity ratio (< 70 percent)

  3. Improvement in FEV_1 after bronchodilator

  4. Increased residual volume

  5. Increased functional residual capacity

Summary

Health care professionals play a key role in the treatment of respiratory disorders in the hospital and community setting. Obstructive pulmonary diseases have been presented in this chapter. Table 20–6 lists some current research on obstructive airway diseases.

REFERENCES

1. Thurlbeck WM, Miller RR: The respiratory system, in Rubin E, Farber JL (eds): *Pathology*. Philadelphia, JB Lippincott, 1993, pp 542–627.

2. Kuhn C, Askin F: Lungs and mediastinum, in Kissane JM (ed): *Anderson's Pathology*, 9th ed. St. Louis, CV Mosby, 1989.

3. West JB: *Pulmonary Pathophysiology: The Essentials*, 4th ed. Baltimore, Williams & Wilkins, 1992.

4. Stauffer JL: Pulmonary diseases, in Tierney LM, McPhee SJ, Papdakis MA (eds): *Current Medical Diagnosis and Treatment*. Norwalk, Conn, Appleton & Lange, 1994, pp 207–279.

5. Weiss EB: Clubbing, in Greene HC, Glassock RJ, Kelley MS (eds): *Introduction to Clinical Medicine*. Philadelphia, BC Decker, 1991, pp 474–477.

6. Dantzker DD, Tobin MJ, Whatley RE: Respiratory diseases, in Andreoli TE, Carpenter C, Plum F, Smith LH (eds): *Cecil Essentials of Medicine*, 3rd ed. Philadelphia, WB Saunders, 1993, pp 125–180.

7. Heiser MS, Downes JJ: Acute respiratory failure in infants and children due to lower respiratory tract obstructive disorders, in Shoemaker WC, Ayres S, Grenvik A, Holbrook PR, Thompson WL (eds): *Textbook of Critical Care*, 2nd ed. Philadelphia, WB Saunders, 1989, pp 538–547.

8. McConnochie KM, Roghmann KJ: Parental smoking, presence of older siblings, and family history of asthma increase risk of bronchiolitis. *Am J Dis Child* 1986;140:806–812.

9. Carlsen K, Larsen S, Bjerve O, Leegaard J: Acute bronchiolitis: Predisposing factors and characterization of infants at risk. *Pediatr Pulmonol* 1987;3:153–160.

10. Hughes DM, Lesouef PN, Landau LI: Effect of salbutamol on respiratory mechanics in bronchiolitis. *Pediatr Res* 1987;22:83–86.

11. Conrad DA, Christenson JC, Waner JL, Marks MI: Aerosolized ribavirin treatment of respiratory syncytial virus infection in infants hospitalized during an epidemic. *Pediatr Infect Dis J* 1987;6:152–158.

12. Rodriguez WJ, Kim HW, Brandt CD, et al: Aerosolized ribavirin in the treatment of patients with respiratory syncytial virus disease. *Pediatr Infect Dis J* 1987;6:159–163.

13. Gala CL, Hall CB, Schnabel KC, et al: The use of eye-nose goggles to control nosocomial respiratory syncytial virus infection. *JAMA* 1986;256:2706–2708.

14. Agah R, Cherry JD, Garakian AJ, Chapin M: Respiratory syncytial virus (RSV) infection rate in personnel caring for children with RSV infections: Routine isolation procedures versus routine procedures supplemented by use of masks and goggles. *Am J Dis Child* 1987;141:695–697.

15. Light MJ, Harwood IA: Cystic fibrosis. *Hosp Med* 1991;27(4):37.

16. Snyder JD: Gastroenterology, in Graef JW (ed): *Manual of Pediatric Therapeutics*, 4th ed. Boston, Little, Brown & Co, 1988, pp 253–284.

17. Davis PB, di Sant'Agnese PA: Diagnosis and treatment of cystic fibrosis: An update. *Chest* 1984;85(6):802–809.

18. Liss HP: Cystic fibrosis, in Barnes HV (ed): *Clinical Medicine: Selected Problems with Pathophysiologic Correlations*. Chicago, Year Book Medical Publishers, 1988, pp 199–203.

19. *An Introduction to Cystic Fibrosis*. Bethesda, Md, Cystic Fibrosis Foundation, 1987.

20. Thompson JM: Respiratory system, in Thompson JM, McFarland GK, Hirsch JE, Tucker SM, Bowers AC (eds): *Mosby's Manual of Clinical Nursing*. St. Louis, CV Mosby, 1989.

21. Huang NN, Schidlow DV, Szatrowski TH, et al: Clinical features, survival rate, and prognostic factors in young adults with cystic fibrosis. *Am J Med* 1987;82:871–879.

22. Ramsey BW, Farrell PM, Penchaoz P, the Consensus Committee: Nutritional assessment and management in cystic fibrosis: A consensual report. *Am J Clin Nutr* 1992;55:108–116.

23. Umetsu DT: Allergic disorders and immunodeficiency, in Graef JW (ed): *Manual of Pediatric Therapeutics*, 4th ed. Boston, Little, Brown & Co, 1988, pp 463–479.

24. Smith AL: Antibiotic therapy in cystic fibrosis evaluation of clinical trials. *J Pediatr* 1986;108(2):866–870.

25. Caine N, Sharples LD, Smith R, et al: Survival and quality of life of cystic fibrosis patients before and after heart-lung transplantation. *Transplant Proc* 1991;23:1203–1204.

26. Collins FS: Cystic fibrosis: Molecular biology and therapeutic implications. *Science* 1992;256:774–779.

27. Rommens JM, Iannuzzi MC, Kerem BS, et al: Identification of the cystic fibrosis gene: Chromosome walking and jumping. *Science* 1989;245:1059–1065.

28. Riordan JR, Rommens JM, Kerem BS, et al: Identification of the cystic fibrosis gene: Cloning and characterization of complementary DNA. *Science* 1989;245:1066–1073.

29. Kerem BS, Rommens JM, Buchanan JA, et al: Identification of the cystic fibrosis gene: Genetic analysis. *Science* 1989;245:1072–1080.

30. Rosenfeld MA, Yoshimura K, Trapnell BC, et al: In vivo gene transfer of the human cystic fibrosis transmembrane conductance regulator gene to the airway epithelium. *Cell* 1992;68:143–155.

31. Respiratory emergencies, in Potter DO (editorial director), *Emergencies* (Nurse's Reference Library). Springhouse, Pa, Springhouse Corp, 1986, Chap. 4.

32. Lo TC, Beamis JF, Weinstein RS, et al: Intraluminal low-dose rate bracytherapy for malignant endobronchial obstruction. *Radiother Oncol* 1992;23(11):16–20.

33. Tsang V, Williams AM, Goldstrow P: Sequential Silastic and expandable metal stenting for tracheobronchial strictures. *Ann Thorac Surg* 1992;53(5):856–860.

34. Spatenka J, Khaghani A, Irving JD, Theodoropoulos S, Slavik Z, Yacoub MH: Gianturco self-expanding metallic stents in the treatment of tracheobronchial stenosis after single lung and heart/lung transplantation. *Eur J Cardiothorac Surg* 1992;5(12):648–652.

35. Botte RG: Nebulized beta-adrenergic agents in the treatment of acute pediatric asthma. *Pediatr Emerg Care* 1986;2:250–253.

36. Netter FH: *Respiratory system*. Summit, NJ, Ciba-Geigy Corp, 1979.

37. Matus VW, Glennon SA: Respiratory disorders, in Kinney MR, Packa DR, Dunbar SB (eds): *AACN's Clinical Reference for Critical-Care Nursing*, 2nd ed. New York, McGraw-Hill, 1993, pp 774–827.

38. Hogg JC: The pathophysiology of asthma. *Chest* 1982;82:8s–11s.

39. Corwin RW: Wheezing, in Greene HL, Glassock RJ, Kelley MA (eds): *Introduction to Clinical Medicine*. Philadelphia, BC Decker, 1991, pp 488–490.

40. Charlton I, Charlton G, Broomfield J, Mullee MA: Evaluation

of peak flow and symptoms only self management plans for control of asthma in general practice. *Br Med J.* 1990;301: 1355–1359.

41. Carpentiere G, Marino S, Castello F: Effects of inhaled fenoterol on the circadian rhythm of expiratory flow in allergic bronchial asthma. *Chest* 1983;83:211–214.
42. Hetzel MR: The pulmonary clock. *Thorax* 1981;36:481–486.
43. Fairfax AJ, McNabb WR, Davis HJ, Spiro SG: Slow-release oral salbutamol and aminophylline in nocturnal asthma: Relation of overnight changes in lung function and plasma drug levels. *Thorax* 1980;35:526–530.
44. Orringer MB: Respiratory symptoms and oesophageal reflux. *Chest* 1979;76:618–619.
45. Thomas E: Asthma at night [letter]. *Lancet* 1983;1:650–651.
46. Diez Jarilla JL, De Castro Del Pozo S: Asthma [letter]. *Lancet* 1983;1:650–651.
47. Ruddy RM, Kolski G, Scarpa N, Wilmott R: Aerosolized metaproterenol compared to subcutaneous epinephrine in emergency treatment of acute childhood asthma. *Pediatr Pulmonol* 1986;2:230–234.
48. Shaprio GG, Furukama CT, Pierson WE, Chapko MK, Sharpe M, Bierman CW: Double-blind, dose-response study of metaproterenol inhalant solution in children with acute asthma. *J Allergy Clin Immunol* 1987;79:378–386.
49. Imai M, Yosida K, Kitcibatake M: Mortality from asthma and bronchitis associated with changes in sulfur oxides air pollution. *Arch Environ Health* 1986;41:29–35.
50. Barker DP, Osmond C: Childhood respiratory infection and adult chronic bronchitis in England and Wales. *Br Med J* 1986;293:1271–1275.
51. Payne CB: Chronic airflow obstruction, in Barnes HV (ed): *Clinical Medicine: Selected Problems with Pathophysiologic Correlations.* Chicago, Year Book Medical Publishers, 1988, pp 199–203.
52. Braun NMT, Faulkner J, Hughes RL, Roussos C, Sahgal V: Why should respiratory muscles be exercised? *Chest* 1983;84:76–83.
53. Newman LS, Tate RM: Chronic obstructive pulmonary disease and bronchiectasis, in Rakel RE (ed): *Conn's Current Therapy.* Philadelphia, WB Saunders, 1993.
54. Ayres JG: Seasonal patterns of acute bronchitis in general practice in the United Kingdom: 1976–1983. *Thorax* 1986;41:106–110.
55. Skillrud DM, Offord KP, Miller RD: Higher risk of lung cancer in chronic obstructive pulmonary disease: A prospective, matched controlled study. *Ann Intern Med* 1986;105:503–507.
56. Garver RI, Mornex JF, Nukiwa T, et al: Alpha$_1$ antitrypsin deficiency and emphysema caused by homozygous inheritance of non-expressing alpha$_1$-antitrypsin genes. *N Engl J Med* 1986;314:762–766.
57. Meyers BR et al: Bloodstream infections in the elderly. *Am J Med* 1989;86:379–384.
58. Cook NR, et al: Peak expiratory flow rate in an elderly population. *Am J Epidemiol* 1989;130:66–78.
59. Philips B, et al: Sleep quality and pulmonary function in healthy elderly. *Chest* 1989;95:60–64.
60. Boist AS, et al: Guidelines for the approach to the patient with severe hereditary alpha$_1$-antitrypsin deficiency. *Am Rev Respir Dis* 1989;140:1494–1497.
61. Haluszka J, et al: Intrinsic PEEP and arterial Pco$_2$ in stable patients with chronic obstructive pulmonary disease. *Am Rev Respir Dis* 1990;141:1194–1197.
62. Whitelaw WA: Asthma deaths. *Chest* 1991;99:1507–1510.
63. Barnes PJ: A new approach to the treatment of asthma. *N Engl J Med* 1989;321:1517–1527.
64. Salvaterra CG, Rubin LJ: Investigation and management of pulmonary hypertension in chronic obstructive pulmonary disease. *Am Rev Respir Dis* 1993;148:1414–1417.

BIBLIOGRAPHY

American Thoracic Society: Guidelines for the approach to the patient with severe hereditary alpha-1-antitrypsin deficiency. *Am Rev Respir Dis* 1989;140(5):1494–1496.

American Thoracic Society: Lung function testing: Selection of reference values and interpretative strategies. *Am Rev Respir Dis* 1991;144(5):1202–1218.

American Thoracic Society: Standards for the diagnosis and care

of patients with chronic obstructive pulmonary disease (COPD) and asthma. *Am Rev Respir Dis* 1987;136(1):225–244.

Barker AF, Bardana EJ Jr: Bronchiectasis: Update of an orphan disease. *Am Rev Respir Dis* 1988;137:969–978.

Bosco KA, Gerstman BB, Tomita DK: Variations in the use of medication for the treatment of childhood asthma in the Michigan Medicaid population, 1980–1986. *Chest* 1993;104(6):1727–1732.

Collins FS: Cystic fibrosis—molecular biology and implications. *Science* 1992;256(5058):774–779.

Cullen MR, Cherniack MG, Rosenstock L: Occupational medicine (parts 1 and 2). *N Engl J Med.* 1990;322(9):594–601; 322 (10):675–683.

Davis PB: Cystic fibrosis from bench to bedside. *N Engl J Med* 1991;325(8):575–576. Editorial.

Drugs for ambulatory asthma. *Med Lett Drugs Ther* 1991;33:9–12.

Eschenbacher WL, Mannina A: An algorithm for the interpretation of cardiopulmonary exercise tests. *Chest* 1990;97(2):263–267.

Ferguson GT: Corticosteroids and respiratory muscles; Does it matter? *Chest* 1993;104(6):1649–1650.

Fick RB Jr, Stillwell PC: Controversies in the management of pulmonary disease due to cystic fibrosis. *Chest* 1989;95(6):1319–1327.

Filippell MB, Rearick T: Respiratory syncytial virus. *Nurs Clin North Am* 1993;28(3):651–671.

Fitzgerald JM, Hargreave FE: The assessment and management of acute life-threatening asthma. *Chest* 1989;95(4):888–894.

Gardner RM: Standardization of spirometry: A summary of recommendations from the American Thoracic Society. The 1987 update. *Ann Intern Med* 1988;108:217–220.

Hodgkin JE: Prognosis in chronic obstructive pulmonary disease. *Clin Chest Med* 1990;11(3):555–569.

Kelly HW: Correct aerosol medications use and the health professions: Who will teach the teachers? *Chest* 1993; 104(6):1648–1649.

Kokkarinen JI, Tukiainen HO, Terho EO: Effect of corticosteroid treatment on the recovery of pulmonary function in farmer's lung. *Am Rev Respir Dis* 1992;145(1):3–5.

Lindgren C: Respiratory syncytial virus and the sudden infant death syndrome. *Acta Paediatr Suppl* 1993;82:67–69.

LoRusso TJ, Belman MJ, Flashoff JD, Koerner SK: Prediction of maximal exercise capacity in obstructive and restrictive pulmonary disease. *Chest* 1993;194(5):1748–1765.

Lugo RA, Nahata MC: Pathogenesis and treatment of bronchiolitis. *Clin Pharm* 1993;12(2):95–116.

National Asthma Education Program, National Heart, Lung, and Blood Institute: Executive summary: *Guidelines for the Diagnosis and Management of Asthma.* Publication No.91-3042A. Bethesda, Md, *National Institutes of Health,* June 1991.

Neeld DA, Goodman LR, Gurney JW, Greenberger PA, Fink JN: Computerized tomography in the evaluation of allergic bronchopulmonary aspergillosis. *Am Rev Respir Dis* 1990; 142(5):1200–1205.

Petty TL: The National Mucolytic Study: Results of a randomized, double-blind, placebo-controlled study of iodinated glycerol in chronic obstructive bronchitis. *Chest* 1990;97(1):75–83.

Rodrigo G, Rodrigo C: Assessment of the patient with acute asthma in the emergency room: A factor analytic study. *Chest* 1993;104(5):1325–1328.

Rom WN, Travis WD, Brody AR: Cellular and molecular basis of the asbestos-related diseases. *Am Rev Respir Dis* 1991; 143(2):408–422.

Sferlazza SJ, Beckett WS: The respiratory health of welders. *Am Rev Respir Dis* 1991;143(5):1134–1148.

Sharma SK, Pande JN, Verma K: Effect of prednisolone treatment in chronic silicosis. *Am Rev Respir Dis* 1991;143(4):814–821.

Smith L: Childhood asthma: Diagnosis and treatment. *Curr Probl Pediatr* 1993;23(7):271–298.

Spitzer SA, Fink G, Mittleman M: External high-frequency ventilation in severe chronic obstructive pulmonary disease. *Chest* 1993;104(6):1698–1701.

Spitzer WO, Fuissa S, Ernst P, et al: The use of beta-agonists and the risk of death and near death from asthma. *N Engl J Med* 1992;326(8):501–506.

Zagelbaum GL, Welch MA Jr, Doyle PR: *Basic Arterial Blood Gas Interpretation.* Little, Brown & Co, 1988.

Zibrak JB, O'Donnell CR, Morton K: Indications for pulmonary function testing. *Ann Intern Med* 1990;112(10):763–771.

CHAPTER 21
Restrictive Pulmonary Disorders

LORNA SCHUMANN

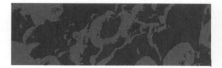

KEY TERMS

effusion: Movement of fluid from blood vessels or lymphatics into a body cavity or tissues.

exudates: Fluid of high protein content that moves into tissues or cavities as part of a reaction to inflammation or injury.

fibrosis: The formation of fibrous connective tissue in place of normal tissue.

granulomas: Tissue that forms into a nodular mass because of inflammation, infection, or injury.

hypersensitivity: An abnormal excessive response to a sensitizing antigen.

hypoventilation: Decreased exchange of air in the alveoli in relation to oxygen consumption, influenced by a decreased rate and depth of respiration.

infiltrates: Fluid or material that has moved into tissues.

interstitial: The space between tissues.

pleurodesis: Installation of a chemically irritating drug (tetracycline, sterile talc, Bleomycin, doxycycline, etc.) into the pleural space.

thoracentesis: Removal of fluid from the chest cavity through a trocar or cannula.

thoracotomy: Surgically opening the chest wall.

transudates: Fluid of low protein content that passes through membranes because of a difference in hydrostatic pressure.

Restrictive pulmonary diseases are the result of decreased expansion of the lungs because of alterations in the lung parenchyma, pleura, chest wall, or neuromuscular apparatus. These disorders may be classified as pulmonary or extrapulmonary and represent acute or chronic patterns of lung dysfunction rather than a single clinical disease. Table 21–1 lists the various disease processes that can be classified as restrictive. These diseases are characterized by a decrease in total lung capacity, vital capacity, functional residual capacity, and residual volume. The greater the decrease in lung volume, the greater the severity of the disease.

This chapter presents information related to restrictive pulmonary diseases that are characterized as **extrapulmonary** in nature, such as chest wall disease, neuromuscular disease, or pleural disease. **Granulomas, fibrosis,** and collagen diseases, characterized as **pulmonary** in nature, are also discussed. Table 21–2 presents data related to variations in respiratory parameters that are affected by restrictive lung disease in infant and elderly populations.

Adult respiratory distress syndrome, ventilatory failure, infant respiratory distress syndrome (hyaline membrane disease), and atelectasis are **intrapulmonary** restrictive diseases, which are discussed in Chapter 22. Respiratory infections, pulmonary vascular disorders, neoplasms, and occupational diseases are also presented in Chapter 22.

TABLE 21–1. Restrictive Pulmonary Disorders

Pulmonary—Diseases of the Lung Parenchyma

Neoplastic diseases	—
Pneumonia	Pneumonias (viral, bacterial, fungal), hypersensitivity pneumonitis
Granulomatous diseases	Sarcoidosis, tuberculosis, coccidiodomycosis, blastomycosis
Pneumoconiosis	Occupational lung diseases
Diffuse interstitial fibrosis	—
Collagen diseases	Rheumatoid arthritis, scleroderma, systemic lupus erythematosus
Atelectasis	—
Pulmonary resection	—
Vascular diseases	Pulmonary edema, pulmonary embolism
Adult respiratory distress syndrome	—

Extrapulmonary Restriction

Chest wall disease	Kyphoscoliosis, ankylosing spondylitis, obesity
Neuromuscular disease	Quadriplegia, hemiplegia, Guillain-Barré, myasthenia gravis, amyotrophic lateral sclerosis, muscular dystrophy
Pleural disease	Pleural effusion, emphysema, hemo/pneumo/chylothorax
Other	Abdominal distention/surgery, pregnancy

Pulmonary Restriction

Diffuse Interstitial Pulmonary Fibrosis

Etiology

Diffuse interstitial pulmonary **fibrosis** is the name typically used for restrictive diseases characterized by thickening of the alveolar interstitium.[1] Controversy surrounds the name of the disease because several terms may be used to describe various aspects or stages of the same disease process. Synonyms frequently presented in the literature include **interstitial pneumonia,** Hamman-Rich syndrome, intrinsic fibrosing alveolitis, cryptogenic fibrosing alveolitis, and idiopathic pulmonary fibrosis. The pathogenesis of the disease is not well understood but may be related to an immune reaction.[1,2] The average survival time after disease onset is 4 years.[3]

Pathogenesis

Pathophysiologic changes include **interstitial** and **alveolar** wall thickening and increased collagen bundles in the interstitium. Lung tissue becomes infiltrated by lymphocytes, macrophages, and plasma cells. Alveolar sacs become scarred and destroyed. These changes in turn lead to large air-filled sacs (cysts) accompanied by dilated terminal and respiratory bronchioles.

Clinical Manifestations

Clinical features include rapid, shallow breathing; dyspnea; irritating, nonproductive cough; clubbing; inspiratory crackles (rales); and marked dyspnea with exercise. Cyanosis is a late finding. Anorexia and weight loss are also noted on physical assessment. As the disease progresses, patients exhibit inability to increase cardiac output with exercise. Arterial oxygen desaturation also occurs with exercise.

Diagnosis

The chest radiograph shows a honeycomb appearance with ground-glass haziness indicative of infiltrates. Transbronchial biopsy, lung scanning, and bronchoalveolar lavage may be used for diagnostic evaluation of the patient. Pulmonary function tests reveal marked reduction in ventilatory capacity because of decreased lung volume and a decreased diffusion capacity of carbon monoxide (used only in test situations). Oxygen levels are also decreased. Increased stimulation of stretch receptors and peripheral chemoreceptors is believed to occur in interstitial lung disease.[3]

Treatment

Primary therapy consists of administration of 40 to 80 mg of corticosteroids per day. Cyclophosphamide and azathioprine have questionable benefit, with only 20 percent of the sample population showing improve-

TABLE 21–2. Respiratory Parameters Impacted by Restrictive Lung Disease

Anatomic Site	Impact on Restrictive Disease
Infant	
Sternum and ribs are cartilaginous with soft chest wall	Diminishes effect of restrictive disease in infants
Ribs are horizontally oriented so that ribs move in and out easily	Diminishes effect of restrictive disease in infants
Accessory muscles of respiration are poorly developed	Majority of respiratory movement relies on diaphragm. Restrictive diseases that compromise diaphragmatic excursion affect respiratory status. For example, thoracic or abdominal surgery, paralysis, and abdominal masses all affect diaphragmatic excursion
Diaphragm rests horizontally and draws lower ribs inward in the supine position so that diaphragmatic excursion is decreased	Leads to compromised effort of breathing
Cartilage of infant larynx is soft, so the airway is compressed when the neck is flexed or hyperextended	Increases airway resistance
During the 1st month of life the neonate is an obligatory nose breather	Nasal obstruction may lead to respiratory distress from decreased air flow
Small diameter of airway leads to increased resistance to air flow	Mucus or edema in the airway may lead to a significant increase in resistance and a decrease in airway diameter
Fewer alveoli than in adults, leading to decreased radial traction applied to the airways	Increased tendency of airways to collapse
Pores of Kohn and channels of Lambert are underdeveloped, leading to fewer collateral ventilation pathways	May lead to respiratory compromise, reducing ventilatory support with restrictive diseases
Elderly	
Decreased ciliary activity	Increased incidence of infection; decreased mucus clearance in all types of respiratory disorders
Decreased chest wall compliance and decreased lung elasticity in some areas of the lung	Leads to a reduction in lung volume; leads to decreased expansion of the lungs and to decreased matching of ventilation and perfusion
Decreased stress tolerance	Increased incidence of disease and trauma with age
Decreased muscle tone	Decreased physical conditioning
Impaired immunity as evidenced by decreased T-cell function; increased autoantibodies	Decreased resistance to infection
Decreased oxygen uptake	Decreased oxygen level in the blood
Decreased vital capacity	Decreased alveolar expansion
Decreased cough reflex	Impaired ability to clear secretions and inhaled particulate matter

ment.[4] However, these drugs have been useful in reducing the dosage of corticosteroids. Lung transplantation has been used successfully in selected patients.[4]

KEY CONCEPTS

- Diffuse interstitial pulmonary fibrosis is a restrictive disorder characterized by thickening of the alveolar interstitium. The disorder is immune mediated, but the etiology remains undetermined.
- Lung tissues are characteristically infiltrated by immune cells (macrophages and lymphocytes). Excess fibrin deposition results in stiff, noncompliant lungs. Vital capacity, tidal volume, functional residual capacity, and diffusion capacity are generally reduced. Respiratory rate increases to compensate for the small tidal volume.
- Treatment centers on drugs to depress immune system activity, such as corticosteroids.

Sarcoidosis

Etiology

Sarcoidosis is categorized as an acute or chronic systemic disease of unknown cause. The acute process occurs more commonly in women in the second or third decades of life.[3,4] The chronic form is seen more commonly in older individuals. The disease usually occurs in the third to fourth decades of life, with the highest incidence seen in North American blacks, Scandinavians, and inhabitants of England.[2,4,5]

Pathogenesis

The disease is characterized by the development of multiple, uniform, noncaseating **granulomas** that affect multiple organ systems, most commonly the lymph nodes and lung tissue. Abnormal T-cell function is also noted with this disease.[5] Other systems frequently involved are the skin, spleen, liver, kidney, and bone marrow. The noncaseating granulomas that form are fibrotic and are surrounded by large histocytes.[4,5] Sarcoid granulomas may also occur in the bronchial airways.

Clinical Manifestations

Sarcoidosis is characterized by malaise, fever, dyspnea of insidious onset, skin rashes, erythema nodosum (lesions marked by the formation of painful nodes on the lower extremities), hepatosplenomegaly, and lymphadenopathy. Patients with the acute disease usually present with enlarged lymph nodes and arthritis, although some patients are asymptomatic.[2] Skin lesions and lacrimal and parotid gland involvement are also noted in the acute process.[4] Iriditis and uveitis may develop. The chronic disease is manifested by pulmonary **infiltration** and **fibrosis**.[6]

Diagnosis

Common laboratory findings in patients with sarcoidosis include leukopenia, increased eosinophil count, elevated sedimentation rate, and increased calcium levels (seen in 15 percent of patients).[6] Approximately 70 percent of patients exhibit anergy (decreased sensitivity to specific antigens). Active cases also demonstrate elevated levels of angiotensin-converting enzyme. A positive Kveim skin test (seen in 75 percent of cases) assists in diagnosis of the disease. A positive Kveim test is indicated by typical tubercles and giant cell formation at the site of interdermal injection of 0.1 cc of Kveim antigen, an extract of spleen from a patient with sarcoidosis.[4] The test requires biopsy samples to be taken at the injection site 3 weeks and 6 weeks following injection. The use of the Kveim test is controversial because of the hazard of injecting human material (antigens) into others.[4,5]

Pulmonary function tests reveal decreased lung volumes, decreased lung compliance, and decreased diffusing capacity. Blood gases show decreased arterial partial pressure of oxygen (Pao_2) and normal or decreased arterial partial pressure of carbon dioxide ($Paco_2$). Transbronchial lung biopsy demonstrates noncaseating **granulomas,** thus providing a definitive diagnosis. Bronchoalveolar lavage may be used to monitor cell content in patients with sarcoidosis.[4]

Chest radiographs allow one to differentiate stages of the disease process, namely: stage 0, normal chest study; stage I, hilar adenopathy alone; stage II, hilar adenopathy and parenchymal involvement; and stage III, parenchymal involvement alone. Pleural effusion is noted in 10 percent of the cases with sarcoidosis.[4]

Treatment

Primary treatment for patients whose disease process does not resolve spontaneously and who develop progressive lung disease or evidence of extrapulmonary sarcoidosis consists of corticosteroids and treatment of symptoms. The prognosis is best for patients with stage I disease.

KEY CONCEPTS

- Sarcoidosis is a restrictive disorder associated with abnormal protein deposits (granulomas) within the lung. Granulomas are fibrotic and are associated with immune cells (histocytes). The cause is unknown.
- Symptoms include progressive dyspnea, fever, enlarged lymph nodes, and generalized symptoms of inflammation. Pulmonary lymph nodes may be primarily affected, with progression to parenchymal involvement. Pulmonary function test results are consistent with a restrictive disorder, demonstrating reduced lung volumes and increased respiratory rate.
- Treatment is symptomatic. Corticosteroids may be used to reduce inflammation.

Hypersensitivity Pneumonitis

Etiology

Hypersensitivity pneumonitis is classified as both a restrictive disease and an occupational disease. It may also be called *extrinsic allergic alveolitis*. Numerous inhaled organic dusts are responsible for the disease process. Table 21–3 lists various sources (allergens) related to the disease. Many people are exposed to these antigens, but only a few people develop a disease process.

Pathogenesis

The causative dust is suspected from the patient's history and confirmed by demonstrating precipitating antibodies in the serum directed toward the causative antigen. The causative antigen combines with the serum antibody in the alveolar walls, leading to a type III **hypersensitivity** reaction. Type III hypersensitivity diseases are caused by the formation of antigen-antibody complexes. (See Chapter 9, Inflammation and Immunity, for further discussion.) These antigen-antibody complexes then elicit the granulomatous inflammation. This in turn leads to lung tissue injury, as evidenced by thickened alveolar walls, formation of **exudate** in the bronchiolar lumen, and infiltration by lymphocytes, plasma cells, and eosinophils.[5]

TABLE 21–3. Causes of Hypersensitivity Pneumonitis

Disease	Antigen	Source
Farmer's lung	*Thermophilia, Actinomyces*	Moldy hay, silage
Bird breeder's lung	Parakeet, pigeon, chicken	Bird excreta, feathers and animal protein
Bagassosis	Thermophilic bacteria	Moldy sugar cane pulp
Mushroom, cork, maple bark, malt, cheesemaker's, redwood lung	Various fungi	Handling moldy products
Granary lung	Wheat weevil	Insect-infected grain
Pituitary extract	Heterologous pituitary and serum proteins	—
Fish meal worker's lung	Protein, fungi	Animal food
Humidifier lung	Thermophilic bacteria, amoebae, and fungi	Humidifiers and evaporative air coolers

Many individuals develop precipitating antibodies (precipitin) from organic dust exposure, but only a few develop pneumonitis.[5] Experiments in animals show that a delayed hypersensitivity (type IV) reaction to the antigen is also required before pneumonitis occurs.[5]

Clinical Manifestations

In the acute disease, symptoms start 4 to 6 hours after exposure. General symptoms may include chills, fever, sweating, shivering, achiness, nausea, lethargy, headache, and malaise.[3,4] Respiratory symptoms may include dyspnea, dry cough, tachypnea, and chest discomfort. Physical findings may include cyanosis (a late sign) and crackles (rales) in the lung bases.[3]

In the chronic form, progressive diffuse pulmonary **fibrosis** develops in the upper lobes—the hallmark of the disease. In the intermediate form, the disease may manifest with acute febrile episodes and progressive fibrosis with cough, dyspnea, fatigue, and eventual cor pulmonale (right-sided heart failure due to lung disorders).

Diagnosis

During the acute phase, transient pulmonary **infiltrates** or increased bronchial markings may be found on chest radiographs, which also show small nodular densities.

Skin testing may produce a red, indurated, hemorrhagic reaction 4 to 12 hours after injection that lasts several days. This reaction suggests precipitin-mediated sensitivity. Skin testing for most precipitating antigens is impractical because most produce irritating reactions before the precipitin reaction occurs, and many individuals without the disease have precipitating antibodies.

Pulmonary function tests show decreased lung volumes and diminished compliance. A decreased diffusing capacity is also noted. Common laboratory findings include an increased white blood cell count and a decreased Pao_2. Hypoxemia worsens with exercise.

Treatment

The goal of therapy is to identify the offending agent and prevent further exposure. This may require a change in environment or occupation. Oral corticosteroids may be used to decrease the inflammatory process.

KEY CONCEPTS

- **Hypersensitivity pneumonitis includes a group of inflammatory lung disorders associated with inhalation of organic particles. Antibodies are produced in response to the inhaled particles, then antigen-antibody complexes deposit in the lung and initiate inflammation and granuloma production.**
- **Hypersensitivity pneumonitis is characterized by general symptoms of inflammation (fever, chills, malaise), dyspnea, dry cough, and tachypnea. Chronic exposure leads to progressive fibrosis and pulmonary dysfunction characteristic of restrictive parenchymal disease.**

Atelectasis

Atelectasis is covered in detail in Chapter 21 in relation to its effect in adult respiratory distress syndrome. Obstruction of the conducting airways into the alveoli leads to collapse of lung tissue in the involved area. It is seen as a postoperative complication in patients who have undergone chest or abdominal surgery. Common causes are mucous obstruction or decreased respiratory expansion because of surgical pain. Common clinical features include dyspnea, tachycardia, decreased chest wall expansion, and, if severe, hypoxemia.

Extrapulmonary Restriction

Diseases of the Pleura

Pneumothorax

Etiology

Pneumothorax is characterized by the accumulation of air in the pleural space. A *primary pneumothorax* is classified as (1) spontaneous, occurring mainly in tall, thin men between 20 and 40 years of age, or (2) secondary, occurring as a result of complications from pulmonary disease (such as asthma, emphysema, cystic fibrosis, or tuberculosis). A specific category of secondary pneumothorax associated with menstruation is called catamenial pneumothorax. A third classification (*tension pneumothorax*) is traumatic, resulting from penetrating or nonpenetrating trauma.

Pathogenesis

Spontaneous pneumothorax results from rupture of subpleural blebs in the apices. The subpleural blebs are believed to occur in the apices as a result of negative mechanical pressures in the upper third of the upright lung field. **Secondary pneumothorax** occurs as a result of asthma, emphysema, cystic fibrosis, or tuberculosis due to rupture of a bleb (large air sac).

    Tension pneumothorax (Fig. 21–1) results from air building up under pressure in the pleural space. The lung on the ipsilateral (same) side collapses and forces the mediastinum toward the contralateral (opposite) side, thus decreasing venous return and cardiac output. With an open, "sucking" chest wall wound, air enters during inspiration but cannot escape during expiration, thus leading to mediastinal (contents of the septum between the two lungs) and tracheal shift.

Clinical Manifestations

The clinical features of pneumothorax include tachycardia, decreased or absent breath sounds, hyperresonance, chest pain on the affected side, and dyspnea. Tension pneumothorax and a large spontaneous

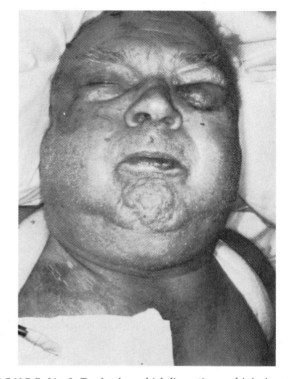

FIGURE 21–2. Tracheobronchial disruption and injuries of the esophagus. (From *Blunt Chest Trauma: General Principles and Management*, Kirsh MM, Sloan H, p 109. Copyright 1977. Published by Little, Brown and Company. Reproduced with permission.)

pneumothorax are emergency situations, with patients presenting with severe tachycardia, hypotension, a tracheal shift to the contralateral side, neck vein distention, hyperresonance, and subcutaneous emphysema (Fig. 21–2).

Diagnosis

Arterial blood gas analysis shows a decreased Pao_2. The chest radiograph shows depression of the hemidiaphragm on the side of the pneumothorax. The diagnosis is usually based on clinical features without

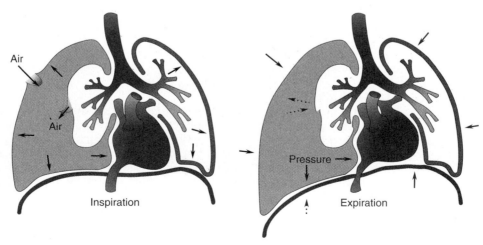

FIGURE 21–1. Tension pneumothorax.

radiographic confirmation. A chest radiograph in tension pneumothorax shows a mediastinal shift (Fig. 21–3).

Treatment

The treatment of pneumothorax depends on the severity of the problem and the cause of the air leak. If the collapse is less than 15 percent, the patient is hospitalized, placed on bed rest, and treated symptomatically.[6] If the collapse is greater than 15 percent, chest tube placement with water seal and suction is necessary.[4] Asymptomatic patients with greater than 15 percent pneumothorax may also be treated conservatively.[6] The amount of suction for the chest tube is prescribed by the physician. Frequently used parameters for chest tube drainage are 2 cm water seal and 20 cm water suction.

Chemical **pleurodesis** may be indicated for patients with spontaneous pneumothorax. Instillation of tetracycline, sterile talc, Bleomycin, doxycycline, etc., into the chest wall cavity promotes adhesion of the visceral pleura to the parietal pleura in an attempt to prevent further ruptures. Patients with a previous pneumothorax should be warned about exposure to high altitude, scuba diving, and smoking. A **thoracotomy** may be performed in patients in whom further spontaneous pneumothoraces and blebs develop.

Pleural Effusion

Etiology

Pleural effusion is not a disease but rather a collection of fluid in the pleural cavity as a result of a disease process. Normally, 15 to 25 mL of serous fluid is contained in the pleural space. The five major types of pleural effusion are transudates, exudates, empyema, hemothorax or hemorrhagic pleural effusions, and chylothorax.[4]

Transudates are low in protein and are frequently associated with severe heart failure or other edematous states such as cirrhosis with ascites, nephrotic syndrome, and myxedema. **Exudates** are high in protein with a ratio of pleural fluid protein to serum protein greater than 0.5.[4] Common causes of exudates are malignancies, infections (especially pneumonia), pulmonary embolism, sarcoidosis, post-myocardial infarction syndrome, and pancreatic disease. Empyema is a high-protein effusion resulting from infection in the pleural space. Hemothorax, the presence of blood in the pleural space, is often the result of chest trauma. Hemorrhagic pleural effusion contains a mixture of blood and pleural fluid. If the hematocrit of the fluid is greater than 50 percent of the hematocrit of peripheral blood, the fluid correction is called a **hemothorax.**[4] Chylothorax or chylous pleural effusion develops from trauma as a result of either leakage of

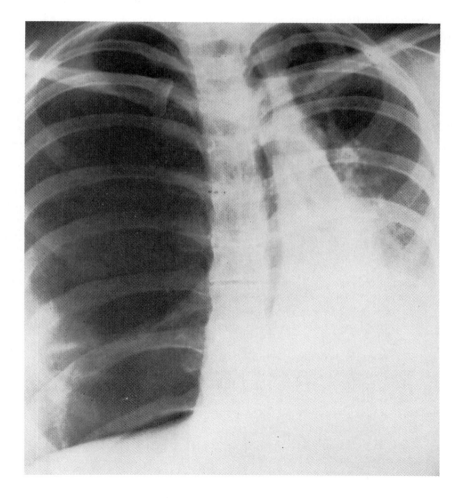

FIGURE 21–3. Upright posteroanterior chest radiograph showing a right-sided tension pneumothorax. Note marked deviation of trachea and cardiac silhouette into the left side of the chest. There is also depression of the right hemidiaphragm. (From *Blunt Chest Trauma: General Principles and Management*, Kirsh MM, Sloan H, p 62. Copyright 1977. Published by Little, Brown and Company. Reproduced with permission.)

chyle (lymph fluid) from the thoracic duct, rheumatoid pleural effusion, or tuberculous pleuritis.[4]

Pathogenesis
Pathophysiologic changes associated with the various types of effusions relate to changes in pleural capillary hydrostatic pressure, colloid oncotic pressure, or intrapleural pressure. The imbalance in these pressures is associated with fluid formation exceeding fluid removal.

Clinical Manifestations
Clinical features vary depending on the cause of the effusion. Small effusions may be asymptomatic (which is common) in patients with less than 300 mL of fluid in the pleural cavity. General features include dyspnea, pleuritic pain, dry cough, decreased chest wall movement, absence of breath sounds over the affected area, dullness to percussion, and decreased tactile fremitus. A massive pleural effusion may lead to a contralateral tracheal shift.

Diagnosis
The composition of **transudate** fluid is diagnostic: low protein, low lactic dehydrogenase (LDH), increased glucose, and a white blood cell (WBC) count of less than 1,000 cells/mm³. **Exudate** findings are variable and depend on the cause of the effusion. General findings of exudates are increased WBCs, increased LDH, and increased protein. **Thoracentesis** should be done to analyze the fluid and to reduce the amount of fluid in the pleural cavity.

Analysis of pleural fluid for pH is helpful in diagnosing the cause of effusion. A pH less than 7.3 indicates cancer or effusion caused by pneumonia, empyema, lupus, rheumatoid arthritis, or tuberculosis.[4,5]

Treatment
Treatment is directed at the underlying cause of the effusion and relieving symptoms. Closed chest tube drainage or **thoracentesis** is indicated if the effusion is large. A **thoracotomy** to control bleeding may be required in patients with excessive bleeding.

KEY CONCEPTS

- **The pleural space is usually a potential space, containing only a tiny amount of fluid for lubrication. Accumulations of air (pneumothorax), pus (empyema), blood (hemothorax), lymph (chylothorax), or transudate in the pleural space can restrict lung expansion.**
- **Tension pneumothorax occurs when pleural air progressively accumulates and develops a positive pressure in the pleura. The ipsilateral lung collapses, and mediastinal structures (trachea, heart) are shifted toward the opposite side. Breath sounds are diminished or absent on the affected side.**
- **Tension pneumothorax and a large, simple (spontaneous) pneumothorax are medical emergencies requiring treatment to remove pleural air and re-**

expand the lung. This usually requires insertion of a chest tube. Chemical pleurodesis may be done in persons prone to spontaneous pneumothorax.
- **A number of disease processes may result in accumulation of fluid in the pleural space. Analysis of the type of fluid (e.g., transudate, blood, pus) is indicative of the underlying disease process. General manifestations include pleuritic pain, diminished breath sounds over the effusion, and dullness to percussion.**

Diseases of the Chest Wall
Kyphoscoliosis

Etiology
Kyphoscoliosis may develop from an unknown cause (idiopathic) or may be related to congenital disease (Pott's disease) or neuromuscular disease (muscular dystrophy, Marfan's syndrome, neurofibromatosis, or Friedreich's ataxia, following poliomyelitis).

Pathogenesis
Commonly, a bony deformity of the chest wall as a result of kyphosis (hunchback appearance; posterior curvature deformity) and scoliosis (lateral curvature deformity) is found (Fig. 21–4). The higher the deformity in the vertebral column, the greater the compromise of respiratory status.[3] Lung volumes are compressed, leading to atelectasis, ventilation-perfusion ($\dot{V}_A/\dot{Q}$) mismatch, and hypoxemia.

Clinical Manifestations
Common clinical features include dyspnea on exertion; rapid, shallow breathing; and chest wall deformity as evidenced by ribs protruding backward with flared ribs on the convex side and crowded ribs on the concave side.

Diagnosis
Diagnostic findings include hypercapnia, hypoxemia (due to $\dot{V}_A/\dot{Q}$ mismatch), and decreased lung volumes and lung capacities as evidenced by decreased values on pulmonary function tests. Also noted are increased pulmonary artery pressures because of the associated arterial hypoxemia. Radiographs show accentuated bony curves.

Treatment
Treatment depends on the severity of the deformity. Screening for scoliosis and kyphoscoliosis in school-children has proved to be an excellent method of early diagnosis. A postural exercise program for mild scoliosis and external braces for moderate scoliosis are recommended. For more advanced cases with curvatures greater than 40 degrees, electrical stimulation of the paraspinal muscles, spinal fusion, and spinal instrument (Harrington rod) placement for surgical stabilization are recommended treatments.

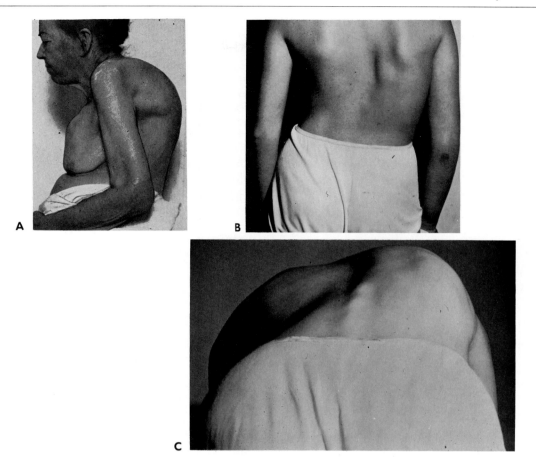

FIGURE 21–4. Kyphosis (**A**) and scoliosis (**B** and **C**) are structural deformities that can interfere with ventilation. (From Delp MH, Manning RT: *Major's Physical Diagnosis*, 9th ed. Philadelphia, WB Saunders Co, 1981. Reproduced with permission.)

Ankylosing Spondylitis

Etiology

Ankylosing spondylitis occurs equally in both sexes and is commonly seen in the second or third decades of life.[4,5] It is characterized by chronic inflammation at the site of ligamentous insertion into the spine or sacroiliac joints. The precise cause is unknown, but persons with the disease have a higher than normal titer of HLA-B27 antigen.[5,7] The respiratory system is affected by limited chest expansion and by the formation of pulmonary fibrosis in the upper lobes, which later develops into bronchiectasis and cavitation.[7]

Pathogenesis

Ankylosing spondylitis is a progressive inflammatory disease leading to immobility of the vertebral joints and fixation of the ribs. The inflammatory process affects the articular processes, costovertebral joints, and sacroiliac joints by inducing a fibrotic response leading to joint calcification, ossification of ligaments, and skeletal immobility.

Clinical Manifestations

Initial symptoms include low- to midback pain and stiffness that is more severe after prolonged rest. With exercise, the pain and stiffness decrease. As the disease process advances, rib cage movement is greatly reduced, leading to restrictive lung dysfunction.

Chest wall muscular atrophy is common and leads to further restriction of rib cage expansion. Breathing is largely accomplished by excursion of the diaphragm as the rib cage becomes immobilized. Associated problems seen with the disease include arthritis, uveitis, spondylitic heart disease, pulmonary fibrosis, and polyarteritis.

Diagnosis

Pulmonary function tests show decreased vital capacity, decreased total lung capacity, and decreased compliance of the respiratory system, mainly the chest wall. Radiographs show destruction of cartilage, erosion of bone, calcification, and bony bridging of joint margins.

Laboratory findings, although not diagnostic of the disease, include an elevated sedimentation rate in 85 percent of cases as well as a decreased RBC count and an increased WBC count. HLA-B27 antigen is seen in 90 percent of cases,[4,7,8] indicative of an immune response.

Treatment

General therapy includes development of an exercise program that includes breathing exercises and mobility exercises. Pharmacologic management with nonsteroidal anti-inflammatory agents provides symptomatic relief of pain and stiffness and promotes function. Indomethacin appears to be the most effective therapy.[4] Pain medications may also be used in these patients.

Obesity

Etiology

Obesity is defined as excessive body fat, with a body weight greater than 120 percent of normal for age, sex, and height.[2] In most cases, obesity results from excessive caloric intake or reduced caloric expenditure. Obese patients are at risk for a variety of disorders, the most common of which are diabetes mellitus, coronary artery disease, degenerative joint disease, gallstones, certain cancers, and pulmonary impairment. Patients with morbid obesity (weight more than twice normal weight) have a tenfold increase in death rate.[4]

Pathogenesis

Endocrine causes of obesity are rare.[4–6] Hypothyroidism, the use of corticosteroids, and hypothalamic lesions can all lead to weight gain; however, the major cause of obesity is excess caloric intake. If obesity is defined as increased adipose tissue (20 percent above normal), then 20 percent of middle-aged American men and 40 percent of middle-aged American women are obese.[5]

TABLE 21-4. Neuromuscular Disorders Affecting the Respiratory System

Disease	Pathogenesis	Pathophysiology	Clinical Features
Poliomyelitis (myelitis is inflammation of the spinal cord)	Develops from an enteral virus acquired by ingestion or respiratory droplet	After a 1- to 3-wk incubation period, the virus invades the intestinal blood supply. Once in the circulation the virus invades all areas of the body. Invasion of the central nervous system leads to neural damage and initiation of an inflammatory reaction.	General symptoms are tremors, muscle weakness. Bulbar poliomyelitis affects the respiratory muscle nerves, leading to respiratory paralysis. Patients usually exhibit shoulder girdle paralysis first, followed by intercostal and diaphragm muscle paralysis. Paralysis may be rapid or slowly progressive. Also seen are diplopia, facial weakness, dysphagia, difficulty chewing, nasal voice, and loss of gag reflex.
Amyotrophic lateral sclerosis	Cause unknown; current theories are autoimmune disease or a slow virus	Affects the anterior horn cells of both upper and lower motor neurons.	Progressive weakness affecting distal more than proximal muscles. Atrophy, fasciculations, and spasticity are noted. Involvement of the respiratory muscles leads to respiratory dysfunction requiring mechanical ventilation.
Muscular dystrophies (most common is Duchenne type)	Hereditary disease (X-linked recessive) passed from mothers to sons	Progressive muscular weakness noted initially in lower extremity muscles. In later years (20s–30s) respiratory muscles become involved. Patients are at risk for respiratory infections.	Progressive muscular weakness and wasting. Skeletal deformities are also common. Involvement of the respiratory muscles (diaphragm, intercostals, and accessory muscles) leads to hypoxia and hypercapnia.
Guillain-Barré (acute idiopathic polyneuropathy)	Exact cause unknown, but thought to be an autoimmune disease triggered by a viral infection	The disease usually follows an infection or inoculation. Peripheral nerves are affected, leading to neural inflammation, demyelination, and axon destruction.	Progressive weakness and loss of motor function beginning in the feet and legs and ascending upward. Sensory loss may also be noted but is not as dramatic as motor loss. Loss of respiratory muscles leads to respiratory failure, which frequently requires mechanical ventilation. Autonomic nervous system symptoms may also be noted (tachycardia, arrhythmias, hypo- or hypertension, loss of sweating).
Myasthenia gravis	Considered an autoimmune disease with both humoral (B-cell) and cell-mediated (T-cell) components	Auto-antibodies and T-cells bind to and damage AChR, leading to decreased functioning of receptors.	Common symptoms are diplopia, ptosis, difficulty swallowing, increased weakness with activity, nasal voice, slurred speech, and weakness of proximal extremities. As the disease progresses, respiratory muscles become involved, leading to respiratory failure. Pneumonia may result from respiratory failure and immobility.

Obesity may be associated with **hypoventilation.** The mechanisms of obesity hypoventilation are reduced ventilatory drive and increased work of breathing. In addition, the increased abdominal size can force the thoracic contents upward into the chest cavity, thus decreasing lung expansion and diaphragmatic shortening. Obesity hypoventilation, also called Pickwickian syndrome, was named for the Charles Dickens character. Pickwickian syndrome is associated with hyperventilation and airway obstruction.

Clinical Manifestations

Obesity hypoventilation is characterized by hypoventilation, somnolence, severe hypoxemia, polycythemia, and cor pulmonale. Patients complain of daytime somnolence, impotence, shortness of breath, headache, and enuresis.

Diagnosis

Arterial blood gases may reveal hypoxemia and hypercapnia. Chest wall compliance, vital capacity, total lung capacity, and expiratory reserve volume are all decreased. Patients may also have an increased RBC count and show signs and symptoms of cor pulmonale and pulmonary hypertension.

Treatment

Primary treatment of obesity consists of weight loss. A weight loss program that includes the family members should be developed. Oxygen delivery through a nasal cannula or mechanical ventilation may be necessary for morbid obesity. Medroxyprogesterone acetate, 10 to 20 mg every 8 hours, may be given. Surgical intervention with gastric stapling or gastric bypass has proved successful in some patients.[2] These operations are intended to permanently curtail food intake.

Neuromuscular Diseases

Neuromuscular diseases that affect the respiratory muscles or their nervous system innervation can lead to respiratory failure. This group of diseases is presented in detail in Table 21–4.

KEY CONCEPTS

- Kyphoscoliosis is a deformity of the bony structure of the chest wall characterized by hunchback and lateral curvature of the spine. The abnormal shape of the chest interferes with the normal mechanics of breathing, resulting in small lung volumes, compression atelectasis, and hypoxemia. Compensatory tachypnea is usually present.
- Ankylosing spondylitis is a progressive inflammatory disease affecting vertebrae and ribs. Chronic inflammation leads to chest wall fibrosis and immobility. Chest wall muscle atrophy and rib cage stiffening result in pulmonary dysfunction characteristic of restrictive disorders.
- Extreme obesity may interfere with the normal mechanics of breathing because of excessive chest weight and abdominal impingement on the chest cavity. Pickwickian syndrome is a disorder of obesity associated with hypoventilation and airway obstruction.

Summary

Restrictive pulmonary diseases have been reviewed. Table 21–5 presents an overview of current research regarding restrictive pulmonary diseases. The primary dysfunctions seen with restrictive diseases are

TABLE 21–5. Summary of Research Findings Related to Restrictive Lung Disease

Authors/Study	Findings
Mabie et al[9]	Four obese (110.7–145.5 kg) antepartum hypertensive women with pulmonary edema were studied. Physiologic results indicated decreased osmotic pressure, increased pulmonary artery pressures, high cardiac output, normal systemic and pulmonary vascular resistance, and increased left ventricular wall thickness. The authors indicated that the pulmonary congestion was due to fluid overload from salt and water retention.
Levy et al[10]	Because differentiation between TB and sarcoidosis is difficult, the researchers attempted to determine if an ELISA could distinguish between the two diseases. The sample consisted of 11 patients with sarcoidosis, 7 with active TB, and 10 healthy volunteers. ELISA differentiated between sarcoidosis and TB with a high degree of reliability.
Trentin et al[11]	This study was done to clarify the natural history of hypersensitivity pneumonitis in 18 nonsmokers. The group that continued to be exposed to the antigen causing the pneumonitis had persistently increased lymphocytes and increased suppressor T-lymphocytes. The unexposed group had a decrease in suppressor T-lymphocytes.
White et al[12]	Six patients with methotrexate pneumonitis (MP) were compared with 7 healthy persons, 7 patients with malignancies not taking methotrexate, and 3 patients with breast cancer taking methotrexate. The MP group showed a significant increase in lymphocytes and a decrease in the percentage of macrophages in comparison to the other groups. The MP group also had a sig-

Table continued on following page

TABLE 21–5. Summary of Research Findings Related to Restrictive Lung Disease Continued

Authors/Study	Findings
	nificant increase in helper T-cells and a decrease in suppressor T-cells compared to the other groups.
Spiteri et al[13]	Ten patients with untreated symptomatic sarcoidosis received 800 μg of budesonide twice daily for 16 wk in pressurized metered doses. Five matched sarcoidosis patients and 10 healthy volunteers received placebo. The 10 budesonide patients noted symptomatic relief and no adverse effects. No significant pulmonary function test improvement was noted in any of the patients. A marked decrease in the bronchoalveolar lavage lymphocytosis was seen in the budesonide group.
Chang et al[14]	One hundred forty adults with pleural effusions were evaluated by thoracentesis, closed pleural biopsy, and fiber-optic bronchoscopy. Thirty-nine had nonneoplastic diseases, 95 had a malignancy, and for 6 patients no diagnosis could be made. Fiber-optic bronchoscopy was more successful in making a diagnosis with patients presenting with hemoptysis or pulmonary lesions on x-ray. Thoracentesis with closed pleural biopsy was more predictive in the absence of x-ray findings of hemoptysis.
Morel et al[15]	The study was conducted to determine the role of anti-acetylcholine receptor (AChR) antibodies in neonatal myasthenia gravis (MG) by AChR antibody titers, toxin-binding blocking antibody, and IgG subclasses. Thirty children of myasthenic mothers were studied. Fourteen infants were symptomatic; 16 were asymptomatic. All infants had circulating anti-AChR antibodies, but levels were significantly higher in symptomatic infants. The best predictor of neonatal MG was a high maternal level of anti-AChR. Eight of 9 affected infants were born to mothers with levels greater than 60 nm.
McKhann et al[16]	Two hundred forty-five patients with Guillain-Barré disease were randomized into control and plasmapheresis groups. Four factors that correlated with poorer outcomes were mean amplitude of compound muscle action potential 20% of normal, older age, time from onset of disease of 7 days or less, and need for ventilatory support. The patient group that progressed the best was the continuous flow pheresis group, with a 0.95 probability of walking at 3 months. The intermittent flow pheresis group had a probability of 0.87, followed by the pheresis group with a probability of 0.73.
Segall[17]	Two patients with Duchenne muscular dystrophy (DMD) were treated with intermittent positive pressure ventilation by nasal mask during sleep. Transcutaneous CO_2 and O_2 readings and ear oximetry measurements were done. In one patient $tcCO_2$ dropped from 72 to 43 mm Hg and tcO_2 increased from 38 to 62 mm Hg. The second patient had smaller changes. Prolonged treatment during sleep resulted in clinical improvement for more than 18 months.
Lorch et al[18]	Five patients with recurrent symptomatic pleural effusion were studied to see if patient rotation during tetracycline administration enhanced contact. Gamma camera images were obtained during instillation of labeled tetracycline. Results indicated that rotation of the patient was not necessary because tetracycline dispersed rapidly and completely without rotation. In one patient, rotation was helpful because the lung was substantially separated from the chest wall.
Midgren et al[19]	Six patients with idiopathic scoliosis and 7 with paralytic scoliosis secondary to polio were tested for pulmonary function during daytime wakefulness. During sleep, So_2 and $tcCO_2$ were measured. Eight of the 13 patients had hypoxemia during sleep. All 8 were hypercapnic during daytime wakefulness. These patients demonstrated hypoventilation during sleep.
Rello et al[20]	The authors compiled statistics from 58 patients with severe community-acquired pneumonia. The most common pathogens causing the disease were *Streptococcus pneumoniae* (37.1%), *Legionella pneumophilia* (22.8%), gram-negative bacilli (11.4%), *Mycobacterium tuberculosis* (11.4%), and *Pneumocystis carinii* (8.5%). The overall death rate in these patients was 22.4%, with 50% of the deaths occurring within 5 days of admission. These early deaths were caused by septic shock, hemoptysis (in the case of TB) or hypoxia. Hypoxia was the major complication in all cases of late deaths. This study is important in planning preventative measures and in the implementation of treatments.
Stein et al[21]	Data from two separate groups of clinical investigators were combined to assess the efficacy of different approaches to the diagnosis and management of patients with acute PE. The practical algorithm derived from this data base suggests that a thorough clinical evaluation, including a $\dot{V}/\dot{Q}$ scan and evaluation for deep venous thrombosis, would decrease the need for pulmonary angiography. Under current diagnostic guidelines, 72% of the patients would undergo pulmonary angiography, versus 33% under the algorithm proposed in this study.

TABLE 21–5. Summary of Research Findings Related to Restrictive Lung Disease Continued

Authors/Study	Findings
Alfageme et al[22]	The authors reported findings in the treatment of 82 episodes of empyema over a 6-year period. Most cases (82%) had some underlying disease such as alcoholism, malignancy, or diabetes. In 73% empyema developed secondary to bronchopulmonary infection. The authors compare the results of treatment with antibiotics only, thoracentesis, chest tube drainage, major surgery, and streptokinase treatments.
Kondoh et al[23]	Idiopathic pulmonary fibrosis is a chronic and fatal disease. Some individuals experience an acute exacerbation, which leads rapidly to severe lung injury. Appropriate therapy for this abrupt worsening has not been established. The authors reported favorable results of corticosteroid therapy in 3 patients. The results are tentative but point to the need for further study.
Frieden et al[24]	Information is compiled on 466 patients who tested positive for *M. tuberculosis* in New York City in April 1991. One third had cultures that included isolates resistant to antituberculosis drugs, including rifampin and isoniazid. This represented a dramatic increase in the incidence of drug-resistant forms of *M. tuberculosis*. The incidence of resistant forms was highest in patients with a history of antituberculosis therapy. The authors urged increased efforts to control and prevent drug-resistant TB.
Gable et al[25]	A retrospective study of the patient records of 171 individuals with lung disease cause by drug-resistant *M. tuberculosis*. Forms of the disease caused by bacilli resistant to both rifampin and isoniazid are very difficult to treat. Despite the use of a variety of chemotherapeutic agents, only about half of the patients had a negative sputum culture. The ramifications of these drug-resistant forms for public health are discussed.

decreased total lung capacity and vital capacity. Patients experience difficulty getting air into their lungs as a common feature.

REFERENCES

1. Bitterman PB: Familial idiopathic pulmonary fibrosis: Evidence of lung inflammation in unaffected family members. *N Engl J Med* 1986;314(21):1343–1347.
2. Felig P, Hanel RJ, Smith LH: Metabolism, in Smith LH, Thier SO (eds): *Pathophysiology: The Biological Principles of Disease*, 2nd ed. Philadelphia, WB Saunders, 1985, pp 321–439.
3. Kersten LD: *Comprehensive Respiratory Nursing: A Decision Making Approach*. Philadelphia, WB Saunders, 1989.
4. Stauffer JL: Pulmonary diseases, in Schroeder SA, Tierney LM, McPhee SI, Papadakis MA, Krupp MA: *Current Medical Diagnosis and Treatment*. Norwalk, Conn, Appleton & Lange, 1993, pp 177–256.
5. Thurlbeck WM, Miller RR: The respiratory system, in Rubin E, Farber JO (eds): *Pathology*. Philadelphia, JB Lippincott, 1993.
6. Way K: Thoracic wall, pleura, mediastinum and lung, in Way LW (ed): *Current Surgical Diagnosis and Treatment*. Norwalk, Conn, Appleton & Lange, 1991, pp 307–348.
7. Hellmann DB: Arthritis and musculoskeletal disorders, in Schroeder SA, Tierney LM, McPhee SI, Papadakis MA, Krupp MA (eds): *Current Medical Diagnosis and Treatment*. Norwalk, Conn, Appleton & Lange, 1992, pp 631–667.
8. West JB: *Pulmonary Pathophysiology—The Essentials*, 4th ed. Baltimore, Williams & Wilkins, 1992.
9. Mabie WC, et al: Circulatory congestion in obese hypertensive women: A subset of pulmonary edema in pregnancy. *Obstet Gynecol* 1988;72:553–558.
10. Levy H, et al: Differentiation of sarcoidosis from tuberculosis using an enzyme-linked immunosorbent assay for the detection of antibodies against *Mycobacterium tuberculosis*. *Chest* 1988;94:1254–1255.
11. Trentin L, et al: Longitudinal study of alucolitis in hypersensitivity pneumonitis patients: An immunologic evaluation. *J Allergy Clin Immunol* 1988;82:577–585.
12. White DA, et al: Methotrexate pneumonitis: Bronchoalveolar lavage findings suggest an immunologic disorder. *Am Rev Respir Dis* 1989;139:19–21.
13. Spiteri MA, et al: Inhaled corticosteroids can modulate the immunopathogenesis of pulmonary sarcoidosis. *Eur Respir J* 1989;2:218–224.
14. Chang SC, et al: The role of fiberoptic bronchoscopy in evaluating the causes of pleural effusions. *Arch Intern Med* 1989;149:855–857.
15. Morel E, Eymard B, Vernet-der Garabedian B, et al: Neonatal myasthenia gravis: A new clinical and immunologic appraisal on 30 cases. *Neurology* 1988;38:138–142.
16. McKhann GM, Griffin JW, Cornblath DR, et al: Plasmapheresis and Guillain-Barré syndrome: Analysis of prognostic factors and the effects of plasmapheresis. *Ann Neurol* 1988;23;347–353.
17. Segall D: Noninvasive nasal mask-assisted ventilation in respiratory failure of Duchenne muscular dystrophy. *Chest* 1988; 93;1298–1300.
18. Lorch DG, Gordon L, Wooten S, et al: Effect of patient positioning on distribution of tetracycline in the pleural space during pleurodesis. *Chest* 1988;93:527–529.
19. Midgren B, Petersson K, Hansson L, et al: Nocturnal hypoxaemia in severe scoliosis. *Br J Dis Chest* 1988;82:226–236.
20. Rello J, Quintana E, Net A, et al: A three-year study of severe community-acquired pneumonia with emphasis on outcome. *Chest* 1993;103:232–235.
21. Stein PD, Hull RD, Saltzman HA, et al: Strategy for diagnosis of patients with suspected acute pulmonary embolism. *Chest* 1993;103:1553–1559.
22. Alfageme I, Munoz F, Pena N: Empyema of the thorax in adults: Etiology, microbiologic findings, and management. *Chest* 1993;103:830–843.
23. Kondoh Y, Taniguchi H, Kawabata T, et al: Acute exacerbation in idiopathic pulmonary fibrosis: Analysis of clinical and pathologic findings in three cases. *Chest* 1993;103:1808–1812.
24. Frieden TR, Sterling T, Pablos-Mendez A, et al: The emergence of drug-resistant tuberculosis in New York City. *N Engl J Med* 1993;328:521–526.
25. Gable M, Iseman MD, Madsen LA, et al: Treatment of 171 patients with primary tuberculosis resistant to isoniazid and rifampin. *N Engl J Med* 1993;328:527–532.

BIBLIOGRAPHY

Casella FJ, Allon M: The kidney in sarcoidosis. *J Am Soc Nephrol* 1993;3(9):1555–1562.

Davidson DL, O'Sullivan AF, Morley KD: HLA antigens in familial Guillain-Barré syndrome. *J Neurol Neurosurg Psychiatry* 1992; 55(6):508–509.

Dryzer SR, Allen ML, Strange C, Sahn SA: A comparison of rotation and nonrotation in tetracycline pleurodesis. *Chest* 1993: 104(6):1763–1766.

Forst LS, Abraham J: Hypersensitivity pneumonitis presenting as sarcoidosis. *Br J Ind Med* 1993;50(6):497–500.

Grassi V, Tantucci C: Respiratory prognosis in chest wall diseases. *Arch Chest Dis* 1993;48(2):183–187.

Heath M: Management of obstructive sleep apnea. *Br J Nurs* 1993;2(16):802–804.

Inselma LS, Millanese A, Deuroloo A: Effect of obesity on pulmonary function in children. *Pediatr Pulmonol* 1993;16(2):130–137.

Marel M, Zrustova M, Stasny B, Light RW: Incidence of pleural effusion in a well-defined region: Epidemiologic study in central Bohemia. *Chest* 1993;104(5):1486–1489.

Murauama J, Yoshizawa Y, Ohtsuka M, Hasegawa S: Lung fibrosis in hypersensitivity pneumonitis. Association with CD4+ but not CD8+ cell dominant alveolitis and insidious onset. *Chest* 1993;104(1):38–43.

Nishimura K, Itoh H, Kitaichi M, Nagai S, Izumi T: Pulmonary sarcoidosis: Correlation of CT and histopathologic findings. *Radiology* 1993;189(1):105–109.

Ogilvie JW: Adult scoliosis: Evaluation and nonsurgical treatment. *Instr Course Lect* 1992;41:251–255.

Pi-Sunyer FS: Medical hazards of obesity. *Ann Intern Med* 1993;119(7 pt 2):655–660.

Pollack CV, Jorden RC: Recognition and management of sarcoidosis in the emergency department. *J Emerg Med* 1993;11(3):297–301.

Remy JM, Remy J, Wallaert B, Muller NL: Subacute and chronic bird breeder hypersensitivity pneumonitis: Sequential evaluation with CT and correlation with lung function tests and bronchoalveolar lavage. *Radiology* 1993;189(1):111–118.

Romero S, Candela A, Martin C, Hernandez L, Trigo C, Gil J: Evaluation of different criteria for the separation of pleural transudates from exudates. *Chest* 1993;104(2):399–404.

Schlock W: Current issues in the assessment of interstitial lung disease. *Arch Chest Dis* 1993;48(3):237–244.

Shammas RL, Movahed A: Sarcoidosis of the heart. *Clin Cardiol* 1993;16(6):462–472.

Sharma OP: Pulmonary sarcoidosis and corticosteroids. *Am Rev Respir Dis* 1993;147(6 pt 1):1598–1600.

Spillane RM, Shepard JA, DeLuca SA: High resolution CT of the lungs. *Am Fam Physician* 1993;48(3):493–498.

Winterbauer RH, Lammert J, Sellard MA, Wu R, Corley D, Springmeyer SC: Bronchoalveolar lavage cell populations in the diagnosis of sarcoidosis. *Chest* 1993;104(2):352–361.

Winterbauer RH, Wu R, Springmeyer SC: Fractional analysis of the 120 ml bronchoalveolar lavage: Determination of the best specimen for diagnosis of sarcoidosis. *Chest* 1993;104(2): 344–351.

Zaccaria S, Zaccaria E, Zanabini S, Patessio A, Braghiroli A, Spada EL, Donner CF: Home mechanical ventilation of kyphoscoliosis. *Arch Chest Dis* 1993;48(2):161–164.

CHAPTER 22
Ventilation and Respiratory Failure

LORNA SCHUMANN

KEY TERMS

atelectasis: Collapse of alveoli.

closing volume: Lung volume at which the lower lung zones collapse and ventilation ceases.

hyaline membranes: Appearance of membranes in alveolar tissue that looks like glass. The alveoli are filled with proteinaceous fluid and epithelial cells.

hypercapnia: An abnormally high amount of carbon dioxide in the blood.

hypoxemia: An abnormally low amount of oxygen in the blood.

positive end-expiratory pressure: A method utilizing a ventilator to maintain positive airway pressure at the end of expiration which results in increased functional residual capacity and decreased shunt.

surfactant: A surface tension–reducing agent produced by type II pneumocytes in the lung.

Acute respiratory failure (ARF) is defined as a state of disturbed gas exchange resulting in abnormal arterial blood gases. The abnormality in arterial blood gases is considered to be an arterial partial pressure of oxygen (Pao_2) of less than 60 mm Hg (hypoxemia) and a partial pressure of carbon dioxide ($Paco_2$) of greater than 50 mm Hg (hypercapnia) with a pH of less than 7.30 when the patient is breathing room air.[1] Patients with respiratory failure can be divided into three categories: (1) failure of respiration or oxygenation leading to hypoxemia and normal or low carbon dioxide levels; (2) failure of ventilation leading to hypercapnia; and (3) a combination of respiratory and ventilatory failure. Chapter 19 provides further discussion of these three categories.

Injury to the lung depends on the nature of the illness, the site of damage, and the severity of injury. Injury to the alveolar-capillary membrane results in increased permeability of the endothelium and epithelium, which in turn can lead to interstitial and alveolar edema. When the injury is severe, hypoxemia increases despite the increased inspired oxygen. Ventilator support with **positive end-expiratory pressure** (PEEP) is used to relieve hypoxemia and reduce intrapulmonary shunting.

This chapter presents information related to ARF and subcategories of adult respiratory distress syndrome (ARDS) and infant respiratory distress syndrome (IRDS), also called hyaline membrane disease. Successful treatment of these diseases requires a highly technical team approach in an intensive care setting.

Acute Respiratory Failure

Acute respiratory failure is a broad term for a variety of disorders that culminate in a deterioration of lung function. The diagnostic features are a rising concentration of carbon dioxide ($Paco_2$) and a falling concentration of oxygen (Pao_2) in the arterial blood. A normal range for $Paco_2$ is 35 to 45 mm Hg, and a normal range for Pao_2 (at sea level) is 80 to 100 mm Hg. A $Paco_2$ greater than 50 mm Hg and a Pao_2 less than 60 mm Hg for a patient breathing room air would arbitrarily define the parameters of acute respiratory failure.[1] However, in clinical practice, the significance of Pao_2 and $Paco_2$ depends on the disease process rather than the specific values.[1]

A number of conditions may cause respiratory failure (Table 22–1), including disorders of the neuromuscular chest apparatus (e.g., poliomyelitis, Guillain-Barré syndrome, quadriplegia, hemiplegia), disorders affecting the chest skeletal system (kyphoscoliosis), and chest trauma (rib and sternal fractures) (see Table 21–4 for discussion of these diseases). Shock, pulmonary emboli, and pulmonary edema may also lead to respiratory failure. Extreme obesity may lead to alveolar hypoventilation, resulting in respiratory failure. The most common primary lung diseases causing ARF are advanced emphysema, pneumonia, asthma, and ARDS.

Etiology

The precise pathophysiologic mechanism of ARF depends on the cause or causes of the disease process. In general, the development of **hypoxemia** is related to poor matching of ventilation and perfusion. The development of **hypercapnea** is related to reduced alveolar ventilation in relation to production of carbon dioxide.

Another mechanism of respiratory failure may be stimulation of the sympathetic nervous system, which leads to selective pulmonary vasoconstriction, increased pulmonary vascular resistance, and tachycardia.[1] Hypercapnia leads to decreased tissue and cellular function, which in turn leads to metabolic and respiratory acidosis, cerebral depression, hypotension, and circulatory failure.[2] In addition, hypercapnia also leads to stimulation of the sympathetic nervous system, which leads to tachycardia and increased cardiac output. If the disease process is chronic, compensation for hypercapnia and acidosis occurs in the renal system by retention of bicarbonate ions and excretion of hydrogen ions. If the process is acute, the patient remains acidotic due to lack of time for renal compensation.

TABLE 22–1. Causes of Acute Respiratory Failure

Central Nervous System

Drug overdose
Cerebral vascular accident (stroke)
Hypothyroidism
Quadriplegia
Hemiplegia

Neuromuscular Diseases

Guillain-Barré
Myasthenia gravis
Tetanus
Amyotrophic lateral sclerosis

Chest Wall and Diaphragm

Trauma (thoracic/abdominal)
Kyphoscoliosis
Upper abdominal or thoracic surgery
Pleural effusion
Hemo/pneumo/chylo thorax

Airways

Laryngospasm
Foreign body aspiration
Asthma
Chronic bronchitis

Pulmonary Parenchyma Diseases

Emphysema
Pulmonary fibrosis
Adult respiratory distress syndrome
Infant respiratory distress syndrome

Vascular Diseases

Pulmonary emboli (blood, fat, air)
Cardiac and noncardiac pulmonary edema
Shock

Clinical Manifestations

Clinical features of ARF vary with the cause. The individual chapters on primary disease processes give precise signs and symptoms. General features include **hypoxia** and **hypercapnia,** which lead to headache, confusion, decreased level of consciousness, dizziness, tremors, and initial hypertension followed by hypotension and tachycardia. Early signs include rapid, shallow breathing with increased inspiratory muscle movement. Late findings include cyanosis, nasal flaring, and sternal and intercostal retractions.[1-3] However, when consciousness is depressed, the latter signs may disappear. The patient is then nearing respiratory arrest.

Diagnosis

Diagnostic tests include measurement of arterial blood gases (ABGs) and chest radiography. A Pa_{O_2} of less than 50 mm Hg and a Pa_{CO_2} of greater than 50 mm Hg are common on room air. Chest radiographic findings depend on the disease process. Other supporting tests include an electrolyte panel with evidence of electrolyte imbalance and a complete blood cell (CBC) count with evidence of infection or anemia. Depending on the severity of respiratory failure, the patient may need monitoring in an intensive care unit.

Treatment

Treatment of ARF depends on the underlying cause. If there is a neuromuscular problem or skeletal weakness, assisted ventilation with a positive-pressure volume ventilator is indicated to maintain airway patency and ensure adequate alveolar ventilation. Intermittent negative-pressure ventilation may be an alternative approach for patients with chronic respiratory failure due to neuromuscular diseases. Braun et al.[4] used negative-pressure ventilation in three men with amyotrophic lateral sclerosis and two men with Duchenne's muscular dystrophy. Results showed stabilization or improvement in vital capacity and reduction in carbon dioxide blood levels after 5 to 11 weeks of therapy.[4]

The primary goal of therapy is to provide adequate oxygenation at the cellular level by maintaining a Pa_{O_2} greater than 60 mm Hg (oxygen saturation > 90 percent). If acute respiratory failure is caused by chronic obstructive pulmonary disease, then vigorous treatment of bronchospasm, infection, and heart failure is required using a combination of methylxanthines, β_2-agonists, corticosteroids, (controversial), antibiotics, and diuretics. Hypotension should be treated promptly with volume replacement and/or vasopressors. The use of corticosteroids in high doses (e.g., methylprednisolone, 25–30 mg/kg body weight) for the first 24 to 48 hours of the disease process is controversial because there is no conclusive evidence of efficacy.[1-3]

General supportive care consists in providing adequate nutrition, maintaining fluid and electrolyte balance, providing pain management, and preventing complications of gastrointestinal stress and bed rest. High-calorie, high-protein, low-carbohydrate nutritional support is recommended. A diet high in carbohydrates should be avoided because of its tendency to increase carbon dioxide production.[5]

KEY CONCEPTS

- Acute respiratory failure is generally diagnosed from arterial blood gas disturbances. The usual defining values are a Pa_{O_2} less than 60 mm Hg and a Pa_{CO_2} greater than 50 mm Hg when the subject is breathing room air.
- Conditions that predispose an individual to hypoventilation, ventilation-perfusion mismatching, or right-to-left shunt may lead to respiratory failure (e.g., drugs, neuromuscular weakness, chest wall deformities or trauma, and parenchymal lung diseases.)
- Manifestations of respiratory failure are due to tissue hypoxia and compensatory responses and include confusion, tremors, hypotension, depressed consciousness, tachypnea, and tachycardia.
- The goal of therapy is to reduce tissue hypoxia by maintaining Pa_{O_2} above 60 mm Hg. Depending on the underlying disease process, this may require mechanical ventilation, supplemental oxygen, nutritional supplementation, bronchodilators, and antibiotics.

Adult Respiratory Distress Syndrome

Etiology

Adult respiratory distress syndrome is a disease characterized by damage to the alveolar-capillary membrane. Clinically, ARDS is recognizable by a decline in the Pa_{O_2} that is refractory (does not respond) to treatment, widespread alveolar infiltrates on the chest radiographs, and severe dyspnea. Mortality statistics range from 43 percent to 63 percent.[1-3,5-11] Patients who recover from the acute injury can expect to return to relatively normal lung function.[11] Follow-up studies (9 months to 4 years) in ARDS survivors show a mild restrictive pulmonary function.[11-13] This syndrome has been reported as having many causes, including severe trauma, sepsis, aspiration of gastric acid, fat emboli syndrome, and shock. Table 22–2 lists the major disorders associated with ARDS.

The precise mechanism of lung injury is not known, but the common denominator appears to be increased permeability of the pulmonary vasculature and alveolar epithelium. Older names used for the syndrome include shock lung, stiff lung, white lung, wet lung, Da Nang lung, postperfusion lung, adult hyaline membrane disease, and pump lung.[3]

T A B L E 22 – 2. Major Disorders Associated With ARDS

Shock (any process leading to a low blood flow state)
Infectious causes
  Sepsis (primarily from gram-negative bacteria)
  Pneumonia (viral, bacterial, fungal)
  Miliary tuberculosis
Trauma-Lung contusion
Embolism
  Fat emboli
  Air emboli
  Thrombus formation
  Amniotic fluid embolism
  Head injury (increased intracranial pressure)
Aspiration
  Gastric contents
  Drowning
Drug overdose
  Heroin
  Methodone
  Darvon
  Barbiturates
Inhaled toxins
  Smoke inhalation
  High concentrations of oxygen (iatrogenic)
  Corrosive chemicals (ammonia, sulfur dioxide, chlorine, and
    others)
High altitude
Radiation
Hematologic disorders
  Disseminated intravascular coagulation
  Massive blood transfusions
  Postcardiopulmonary bypass
  Thrombotic thrombocytopenic purpura
Metabolic disorders
  Pancreatitis
  Uremia
  Paraquat ingestion
Burns
Cancer
Anaphylaxis
Eclampsia

The pathogenetic sequence of events in ARDS is shown in Figure 22–1. The initial injury to the alveolar-capillary membrane may be caused by direct damage, as seen in aspiration of acidic gastric contents, or by indirect damage, as occurs in shock. Therapeutic interventions (shown in the center boxes of Fig. 22–1) may act to compound the effects of the initial lung injury. The resulting injury leads to an increase in permeability, which results in interstitial and alveolar edema.

Pathogenesis

The characteristic pathophysiologic abnormalities of ARDS involve injury to the alveolar-capillary membrane from a wide variety of disorders. Common findings in this type of injury include (1) severe hypoxemia caused by intrapulmonary shunting of blood, (2) a decrease in lung compliance, (3) a decrease in functional residual capacity (FRC), (4) diffuse, fluffy alveolar infiltrates on the chest radiograph, and (5) absence of evidence of cardiogenic pulmonary edema.[2,3,10,14,15]

The mechanism by which the FRC is decreased remains controversial, but three possible explanations exist: (1) fluid-filled alveoli do not function to exchange gas, which leads to loss of lung volume; (2) congestion of the lung decreases compliance; and (3) increased interstitial fluid leads to increased interstitial space pressure and a decreased transmural pressure gradient, which normally functions to keep the small airways open. Early closure and continued closure lead to atelectasis and loss of lung volume.[14]

The decrease in lung compliance, often severe in ARDS, is reflected in the high ventilatory pressures required to deliver an adequate volume of gas. It is thought that this decrease in lung compliance is due to loss or inactivation of **surfactant** with subsequent increased recoil pressure of the lungs.[3,14] In addition, fluid fills the alveoli and impairs ventilation.

The decrease in Pao_2 is a result of normal perfusion of large numbers of alveoli that are poorly ventilated (areas of low ventilation-perfusion) or not ventilated (areas of shunt). Fluid replacement must be closely monitored to prevent overload. The most valid measure of pulmonary vascular fluid status is pulmonary artery capillary pressures (or wedge pressures).

The routine effects of mechanical ventilation with tidal volumes of 10 to 12 mL/kg body weight[1] and PEEP have been well documented.[8,11,16] The large tidal volumes are often effective in preventing or reversing atelectasis. Use of PEEP produces a positive distending pressure across the alveoli and the airways, which maintains patency and increases FRC. With this recruitment of alveoli, Pao_2 increases and the shunt decreases.[14] Another possible effect of PEEP is that it may act to conserve surfactant.[14]

Pathogenesis of Atelectasis Associated With ARDS

Atelectasis is a term derived from the Greek words *ateles,* meaning imperfect, and *ektasis,* meaning expansion. In medical terminology, it refers to the collapse of the gas-exchanging units (alveoli). The most common cause of atelectasis in the hospitalized patient is retained secretions.[17]

Other causes of atelectasis include central nervous system depression, neuromuscular diseases, chest wall and diaphragmatic diseases, airway obstruction, and diseases of the pulmonary parenchyma.

Three factors that are associated with the pathogenesis of atelectasis and that influence the ability of an alveolus to maintain its expiratory volume above the critical volume are (1) closing volume, (2) surfactant, and (3) gas volume denitrogenation.

Closing volume. **Closing volume** refers to the point at which the small airways in the lung bases close.[2,17,18] Under normal conditions, there is a tendency for the small airways to collapse during expiration. When a healthy adult fully expires to residual volume (RV), airways in the dependent lung regions tend to close

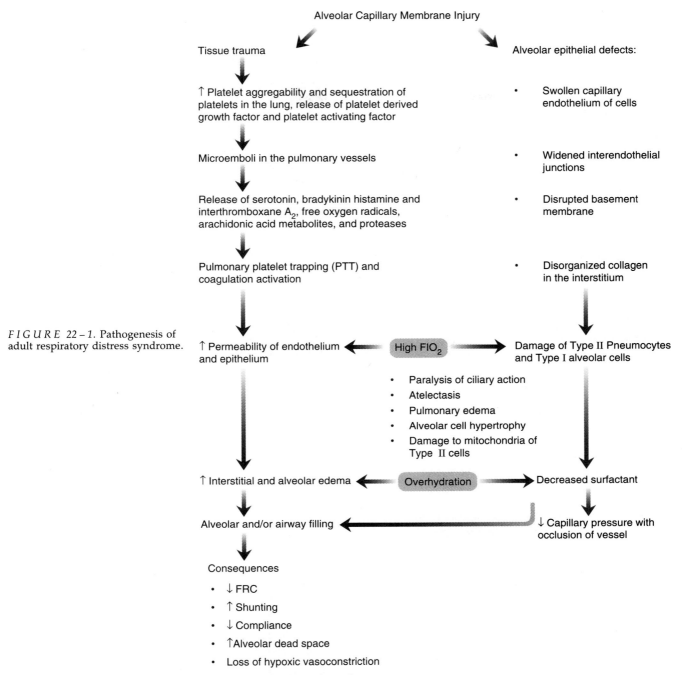

FIGURE 22–1. Pathogenesis of adult respiratory distress syndrome.

because of the more positive intrapleural pressure.[19] Gravitational forces and the weight of the lung in a standing man cause a higher transmural pressure at the apices than the bases. This widens airways at the apices relative to the bases and, in an upright person, can lead to closure of airways at the bases while they are still open at the apices.[2,17–19] The large airways in the upper lobes remain open because intrapleural pressure is approximately 7.5 cm H_2O more negative there. At end-expiration (FRC) in upright man, pleural pressures at the apex and base are −10 and −2.5 cm H_2O, respectively. At low lung volumes (after an exhalation below FRC), the pleural pressures at the apex and base are −4 and +3.5 cm H_2O, respectively.[19]

In diseased lungs, by comparison, loss of elastic recoil and structural supporting tissue and the resultant airway narrowing promote widespread airway collapse and air trapping at or above FRC. If the closing volume is greater than the patient's FRC, the bronchioles will close earlier during expiration.[17] The airway closure results in air "trapping" of the remaining alveolar gas. This trapping may act to ensure that the small alveoli remain above their critical volumes and do not collapse; however, if the closing volume is greater than FRC, the bronchioles will close during expiration and decrease adequate alveolar ventilation, because they may be poorly ventilated during respiration.[20]

Surfactant. **Surfactant** is a phospholipid material secreted by the type II cells of the alveolar lining that acts to lower surface tension and decrease the tendency of the alveoli to collapse at a minimal volume (end of expiration).[18-21] In pathologic states, with the loss of surfactant activity, surface tension remains high at low alveolar volumes. This leads to collapse of alveoli, requiring high pressures to reopen the alveoli. When a patient is placed on positive end-expiratory pressure (PEEP), the alveoli are prevented from collapse during expiration.[22]

Denitrogenation. The volume of gas within a collapsible container is important for maintaining the container in the expanded state. Therefore, the volume of gas remaining in the alveoli at the end of expiration is a key factor in maintaining the alveolus above its critical volume.[17] When a patient is suddenly removed from PEEP for central venous pressure determinations or suctioning, the alveolar units may collapse requiring high pressures for reinflation.[23]

One theory related to accentuating atelectasis is the denitrogenation theory. Critically ill patients receiving high fractional oxygen concentrations (above 60 percent fraction of inspired oxygen, FIO_2) may not be able to maintain a Pao_2 above 50 to 60 mm Hg because of the denitrogenation process.[17] When high concentrations of oxygen are administered, there is a decrease in the amount of nitrogen inspired. Normally, inspired nitrogen remains in the alveoli and keeps the alveoli open. Nitrogen constitutes approximately 79 percent of breathable air. Alveoli that are underventilated (low ventilation-perfusion ratio $\dot{V}A/\dot{Q}$) are able to remain open because of the remaining volume of nitrogen gas in these units.[17] Giving high concentrations of oxygen results in lowering of alveolar nitrogen tensions. Thus, the loss of alveolar nitrogen *may* lead to the collapse of underventilated alveoli because the increased volume of oxygen being supplied can now be completely absorbed into blood and there will not be a sufficient supply of nitrogen to keep the alveoli inflated. Alveolar collapse from this process has been shown to be a significant clinical entity and is accentuated when the inspired oxygen is 60 percent or greater and the person has areas of low arterial ventilation-perfusion ($\dot{V}A/\dot{Q}$).[24,25] However, because of the use of large tidal volumes and PEEP, ventilator patients may be at a lesser risk for denitrogenation atelectasis.

Clinical Manifestations

The clinical features of ARDS usually include a history of a precipitating event that has led to a low blood volume state ("shock" state) 1 or 2 days prior to the onset of respiratory failure. The patient may complain of sudden marked respiratory distress.

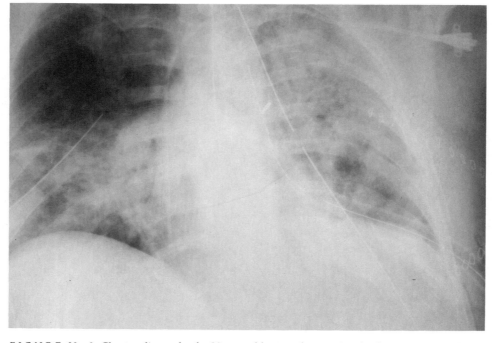

F I G U R E 22 – 2. Chest radiograph of a 28-year-old man who was involved in an auto accident. The patient presented with multiple bilateral rib fractures and bilateral pneumothoraces. Within 24 hours the patient developed severe ARDS (note diffuse "whiteout").

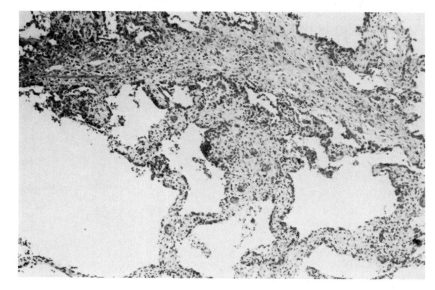

FIGURE 22–3. Photomicrograph of a lung specimen from a patient who died of ARDS, illustrating the fibrotic phase of the histopathology. The alveolar walls and intra-alveolar septa are thickened and contain increased amounts of collagen. The number of alveolar capillaries is markedly reduced, and the walls of the remaining capillaries are thickened. (Hematoxylineosin, ×70.) (From Meyrick B: Pathology of the adult respiratory distress syndrome. *Crit Care Clin North Am* 1986;2:411. Used with permission.)

Early signs and symptoms include a slight increase in pulse rate, dyspnea, and a low Pao_2. The initial presenting sign may be shallow, rapid respirations.

With progression of the disease, the patient demonstrates tachycardia, tachypnea, hypotension, marked restlessness, decreased mental status, and frothy secretions. On auscultation of lung fields, crackles and rhonchi are heard. The patient may be using accessory muscles to breathe and demonstrating intercostal and sternal retractions. A late sign is cyanosis.

Diagnosis

The hallmark of ARDS is **hypoxemia** that is refractory (does not respond) to delivery of increasing levels of Fio_2. Uncorrected hypoxemia is associated with hypotension, decreased urine output, respiratory acidosis, metabolic acidosis, and eventual cardiopulmonary arrest. Arterial blood gas determinations reveal **hypoxia,** acidosis, and **hypercapnia.** The chest radiograph shows a diffuse "whiteout" (Fig. 22–2) indicative of diffuse alveolar infiltrates.[26]

Pulmonary function tests show decreased FRC, decreased lung volumes, decreased lung compliance, and a $\dot{V}a/\dot{Q}$ mismatch with a large right-to-left shunt. Histologic changes found on open lung biopsy reveal atelectasis, hyaline membranes, cellular debris, and interstitial and alveolar edema (Fig. 22–3).

Treatment

The treatment of ARDS is primarily symptomatic and entails providing ventilator support, maintaining fluid and electrolyte balance, and providing adequate oxygenation with the use of a volume ventilator and PEEP. Treatment of the underlying disease process is essential. Because of increased permeability of the alveolar-capillary membrane, excessive fluid administration can produce or intensify pulmonary edema.

PEEP is used extensively in ARDS and other states of ARF resulting in hypoxemia. In the diseased state of ARDS, FRC decreases and alveoli collapse, which increases $\dot{V}a/\dot{Q}$ abnormalities and shunt, resulting in hypoxemia.[16] The FRC is the volume of gas left in the lungs at the end of a normal expiration. End-expiratory volume must remain above its critical volume (below which volume elastic forces will cause collapse) or many alveoli will collapse. The means by which PEEP relieves hypoxemia and reduces intrapulmonary shunting is not well established but is thought to be related to an increase in resting lung volume by increasing the transpulmonic pressure throughout expiration.[3,10,14] This in turn leads to increased FRC. The application of PEEP produces a positive distending pressure across the walls of airways and alveoli at end-expiration, thus maintaining their patency at an increased FRC.

Gattinoni et al (1986)[27] studied the effect of sequential increases of PEEP in ten patients with ARF while they were undergoing computed tomography. The application of PEEP showed increased cross-sectional surface area and decreased intraparenchymal densities. Increases in Pao_2 correlated well with decreased intraparenchymal densities (fluid). The recruitment and improved ventilation of previously nonventilated or underventilated alveoli increased the Pao_2. Another possible mechanism for the effectiveness of PEEP in reversing hypoxemia is that PEEP increases the air volume in the alveoli, thus decreasing the amount of fluid filling the alveoli. The remaining fluid then forms a layer on the surface of the alveolar wall, allowing some gas exchange to occur.[22]

The positive effects of PEEP include (1) increasing FRC, which leads to improvement in the Pao_2 by keeping alveoli open so that gas exchange is facilitated, (2) decreasing diffuse atelectasis, and (3) reducing shunting during the expiratory phase.[3,10,22,28]

The optimal ventilatory pattern and level of PEEP are widely debated and vary from patient to patient.[3] Most experts believe that PEEP should be regulated to preserve adequate cardiac output, maintain an FIO_2 at 0.6 or below, and maintain mixed venous oxygen tension ($P\bar{v}O_2$) above 30 mm Hg.[1–3,10,29,30] A large tidal volume (10–12 mL/kg) and a slow respiratory rate (10–12 breaths/min) *without* hyperinflation (sigh) are accepted ventilator settings for patients with ARF.

Complications associated with the use of PEEP include (1) decreased cardiac output, (2) subcutaneous emphysema, (3) decreased tissue oxygenation because of a low cardiac output, which leads to lactic acidosis, (4) increased intracranial pressure, (5) increased intraocular pressure, (6) decreased urine output associated with increased antidiuretic hormone production, and (7) pneumothorax.[12,14,30]

High-frequency jet ventilation has been used as a treatment for respiratory distress syndrome (RDS) in both the adult and the neonate. Hurst et al[31] evaluated high-frequency jet ventilation in 54 patients. All patients had improved CO_2 elimination, improved oxygenation, and lower mean airway pressures.

The use of corticosteroids remains controversial. Bone et al[11] found that patients given placebo had significantly better recovery and survival than those treated with methylprednisolone sodium succinate.

Bernard et al[32] compared 50 patients with ARDS taking methylprednisolone and 49 patients with ARDS taking placebo. The mortality was 60 percent in the methylprednisolone group, compared to 63 percent in the placebo group, not statistically significant.

The use of **surfactant** replacement in adult lungs is being currently researched.[33] Preliminary results in three patients using porcine surfactant showed a modest improvement in gas exchange. Further study is needed to show the long-term efficacy of surfactant replacement in adults.

KEY CONCEPTS

- **Adult respiratory distress syndrome (ARDS) causes profound hypoxemia and a greatly increased work of breathing, often requiring mechanical ventilation and high-level oxygen therapy to maintain PaO_2 above 60 mm Hg.**
- **ARDS occurs in association with other pathophysiologic process, such as trauma, sepsis, or shock. These disorders increase the risk of developing disseminated pulmonary inflammation leading to ARDS. ARDS is associated with a mortality rate of about 50 percent.**
- **ARDS is a consequence of widespread pulmonary *inflammation* leading to three major pathophysiologic processes:**
  1. **Noncardiogenic pulmonary edema associated with "leaky" pulmonary capillaries.**
  2. **Atelectasis associated with lack of surfactant. Surfactant normally decreases surface tension in small alveoli and prevents them from collapsing.**
  3. **Fibrosis (hyaline membranes) associated with inflammatory deposition of proteins.**
- **ARDS is associated with profound alterations in pulmonary function, including decreased vital capacity, decreased functional residual capacity, decreased compliance, and decreased tidal volume. Respiratory rate is increased and symptoms of tissue hypoxia may be profound.**
- **Noncardiogenic pulmonary edema is evident as "whiteout" on chest radiograph. Crackles and wheezing may be heard throughout the chest. Profound dyspnea and the use of accessory muscles are usual. Atelectasis and pulmonary edema result in right-to-left pulmonary shunting. Blood gas determinations show hypercarbia and hypoxemia, which do not improve much with oxygen therapy.**
- **Therapy is mostly supportive, to enhance tissue oxygenation until the inflammation resolves. Mechanical ventilation with PEEP and supplemental oxygen is the mainstay of therapy. PEEP is used to increase FRC and prevent alveolar collapse at end-expiration. PEEP may also force edema fluid out of the alveoli. High levels of oxygen (>60 percent) may contribute to ARDS because of toxicity to pneumocytes and absorption atelectasis. FIO_2 should be reduced as soon as possible.**

Infant Respiratory Distress Syndrome

Etiology

Infant respiratory distress syndrome (IRDS), also known as hyaline membrane disease, has features similar to those seen in ARDS. It is a syndrome of premature neonates characterized by hemorrhagic edema, patchy atelectasis, hyaline (glassy) membranes, and hypoxemia. The disorder occurs in 1 percent of all deliveries, or 1 in 6,000 births,[34] and occurs most commonly in neonates born before 25 weeks of gestation, although it may occur in full-term neonates. High-risk factors include birth prior to 25 weeks' gestation, birth at advanced gestational age, poorly controlled diabetes in the mother, deliveries after antepartum hemorrhage, and Rh incompatibility.

Pathogenesis

The primary cause of IRDS is lack of surfactant, leading to increased alveolar surface tension and decreased lung compliance. **Surfactant,** a phospholipid, is produced by the type II alveolar cells during the alveolar stage of fetal development (late fetal life). With IRDS, lung compliance is decreased to one fifth to one tenth of normal.[34–36]

The neonate with IRDS must generate intrathoracic pressures of (25–30 mm Hg) to maintain patent alveoli.[36] The premature neonate has a soft, compliant chest that is drawn inwardly with each inspiratory contraction of the diaphragm, thus making it difficult to maintain the high pressures necessary to maintain adequate oxygenation. The end result is increased work of breathing and decreased ventilation, which leads to progressive atelectasis, increased pulmonary vascular resistance, hypoxemia, and acidosis.

Surfactant also functions to maintain pulmonary fluid balance. Loss of surface tension forces maintained by surfactant causes further leakage of protein fluid into the alveoli. This proteinaceous fluid contains fibrin and cellular debris, which causes hyaline membrane formation.

A secondary cause of IRDS is immaturity of the capillary blood supply, which leads to $\dot{V}A/\dot{Q}$ mismatch, thus adding to the problems of hypoxemia and metabolic acidosis. In addition, a right-to-left shunt from an open foramen ovale or patent ductus arteriosus may increase the hypoxemia.

Histologically, there is a progressive damage to the basement membrane and respiratory epithelial cells. With increasing edema and loss of epithelial cells, patchy areas of atelectasis develop. Further cellular damage from the disease process, excess fluid administration, and high levels of F_{IO_2} lead to increased capillary permeability and leakage of high protein fluid into the alveoli.

Clinical Manifestations

The typical neonate presents with rapid, shallow respirations; intercostal, subcostal, or sternal retractions; diminished breath sounds; flaring of nares; hypotension; peripheral edema; low body temperature; oliguria; tachypnea (rate 60–120 breathes/min); and bradycardia.[34] Late findings include frothy sputum, central cyanosis, and an expiratory grunting sound. Nasal flaring is a physiologic response mechanism used to increase airway diameter in an attempt to increase air flow. An expiratory grunt is a physiologic response mechanism that attempts to create a physiologic PEEP by exhaling against a partially closed glottis. Paradoxical respirations ("seesaw" movement of the chest wall) may also be noted, indicating increased work of breathing.

During the first 48 hours of life, neonates with IRDS need progressively higher levels of F_{IO_2} to maintain adequate (60–80 mm Hg) oxygen levels.[35] As the work of breathing increases and oxygen levels decrease, metabolic acidosis occurs.

Diagnosis

Initial arterial blood gas determinations reveal hypoxemia and metabolic acidosis. As the disease progresses, hypercapnia and respiratory acidosis develop.[34]

The chest radiograph progresses from normal, shortly after birth, to a diffuse "whiteout" indicative of atelectasis and alveolar edema. Generalized hyperinflation of the lungs is also seen on the chest study.

Measurement of the lecithin/sphingomyelin (L/S) ratio and desaturated phosphatidylcholine (DSPC) concentration in amniotic fluid may be done to determine the ability of the fetus to secrete surfactant. If the L/S ratio is greater than or equal to 2:1, the incidence of RDS is less than 5 percent.[35,37] A DSPC equal to or greater than 500 mg/100 mL indicates a mature lung with an incidence of RDS of less than 1 percent.[37]

Treatment

The mainstay of therapy is mechanical ventilation with PEEP or continuous positive-airway pressure. The primary goal, as in the adult with ARDS, is to maintain adequate oxygen levels between 50 and 80 mm Hg.[34,35,37] The lowest F_{IO_2} settings should be used to maintain adequate arterial oxygen levels. High F_{IO_2} (100 mm Hg) delivered for extended periods of time may result in further alveolar damage and retrolental fibroplasia (failure of the peripheral retina to vascularize, leading to blindness).[34,35,37] Continuous monitoring of oxygen saturation by transcutaneous oxygen monitors has assisted the health care team in management of oxygen monitors has assisted the health care team in management of oxygen levels in the unstable neonate.

The use of exogenous surfactant in premature infants has been the focus of several research studies.[38–41] Gittin et al[38] assessed the use of bovine surfactant in 41 premature infants. Significant improvement in oxygenation status was found in the surfactant group as compared to the saline group.

Hallman et al[39] studied 64 newborn infants and determined that exogenous surfactant yielded positive results in infants with varying degrees of severity of RDS. They also found that the very small premature infants may require higher amounts of fluid volume than previously noted.

Raju et al[40] found similar results in a double-blind study of 30 premature infants. The researchers found significantly more patent ductus arteriosus in the control group and significantly less pneumothorax and pulmonary interstitial emphysema in the surfactant group.[40]

Davis et al[41] studied the effect of surfactant administration in 35 premature infants and determined that the shunt ratio was reduced by 56 percent. Other findings showed increased minute ventilation (38 percent), increased tidal volume (32 percent), increased dynamic compliance (29 percent); and increased inspiratory flow rates (54 percent).

Inositol dietary supplementation is also being tried in premature infants with IRDS.[42,43] Inositol is a sugar that is an important compound of phospholipids and functions to accelerate the production of surfactant. Treatment with inositol is associated with a more rapid recovery from IRDS at a lower F_{IO_2}.[42,43]

Extracorporeal membrane oxygenation (ECMO) is also used as a mode of oxygen delivery in some medical centers.[44] ECMO utilizes cardiopulmonary bypass to provide oxygen and remove carbon dioxide. Lotze et al[44] used ECMO in 13 infants with severe respiratory failure and noted improvement in lung compliance and oxygenation as compared to infants who received ventilator support.

High-frequency jet ventilation has proved to be effective in infants with severe RDS. Carlo et al[45] showed that infants ventilated with high-frequency jet ventilation required lower mean airway pressures and had better gas exchange than those ventilated conventionally.

General supportive therapy of adequate nutrition, fluid and electrolyte balance, and a neutral thermal environment should be maintained. Broad-spectrum antibiotics are prescribed for infections after cultures have been done.

Complications of RDS related to therapy include bronchopulmonary dysplasia, pneumothorax due to mechanical ventilation, oxygen toxicity, and retrolental fibroplasia due to high levels of oxygen therapy. In addition, the neonate is at high risk for the development of intracranial or intraventricular hemorrhage during the first few days of life.[34,35,37] The neonate is also at high risk for infections due to multiple invasive monitoring lines, catheters, and endotracheal intubation. Mortality statistics range from 30 to 50 percent.[46]

KEY CONCEPTS

- The symptomatology of infant respiratory distress syndrome (IRDS) is very similar to that of ARDS. IRDS occurs most commonly in premature infants born prior to adequate development of their surfactant-producing pneumocytes (25 weeks' gestation). Maturity of surfactant-producing cells can be estimated from the L/S ratio in amnionic fluid. An L/S ratio of less than 2:1 is associated with a higher risk of IRDS.

- Lack of surfactant causes atelectasis and increased work of breathing due to high alveolar surface tension. Leakage of inflammatory exudate into the alveoli results in formation of hyaline membranes.

- Symptoms of IRDS include nasal flaring, expiratory grunt, thoracic retractions, rapid shallow respirations, and bradycardia. Chest radiographs demonstrate a "whiteout." As in ARDS, blood gas values are poor, indicating severe hypoxemia and acidosis.

- Therapy for IRDS includes supportive measures such as mechanical ventilation with PEEP or CPAP and supplemental oxygen as well as specific measures to increase alveolar surfactant levels. Inositol supplementation may increase surfactant production by the immature lung. Surfactant administration may significantly enhance recovery from IRDS.

TABLE 22-3. Summary of Research Findings Related to ARDS and IRDS

Authors/Study	Findings
Adult Respiratory Distress Syndrome	
Gattinoni et al[27]	The researchers studied the effect of sequential increases in PEEP on ten patients with acute respiratory failure while undergoing CT scanning. The increases in PEEP led to decreased intraparenchymal densities, increased Pao_2, and increased cross-sectional surface and expansion.
Bone et al[11]	Seventeen medical centers studied 304 patients with sepsis and at risk for adult respiratory distress syndrome (ARDS). The study was a double-blind, randomized placebo-controlled clinical trial with methylprednisolone. ARDS developed in 32 percent of the methylprednisolone group and 25 percent of the placebo group. Mortality rates were 52 percent in the experimental group and 22 percent in the placebo group.
Bernard et al[32]	The researchers used a prospective, randomized, double-blind, placebo-controlled trial to study the effects of methylprednisolone on early ARDS. The methylprednisolone group ($n = 50$) had a 60 percent mortality rate. The placebo group had a 63 percent mortality rate.
Zarowitz et al[47]	The researchers studied 15 patients receiving 2 intravenous doses of theophylline about 10 hours apart. The data showed that there was a significant difference between absolute measurements of 0.15 L/kg between the first and second doses. This variability could result in underdosing or overdosing depending on the patients clearance of the drug.
Ghio et al[48]	The researchers evaluated 27 patients at least 1 year after onset of ARDS. Impairment was present in 18 to the 27 patients. Impairment was more severe in patients with a more severe case of ARDS.
Hurst et al[31]	The researchers evaluated high-frequency jet ventilation in 54 patients. All patients had improved CO_2 elimination, improved oxygenation, and lower mean airway pressures.
Richman et al[33]	Norcine surfactant replacement was used in three patients with ARDS. The patients showed a modest improvement in gas exchange. The Pao_2 increased 31 mm Hg, 37 mm Hg, and 26 mm Hg after 5 minutes in each patient.

TABLE 22–3. Summary of Research Findings Related to ARDS and IRDS Continued

Authors/Study	Findings
Infant Respiratory Distress Syndrome	
Gittin et al[38]	Bovine surfactant was used in premature infants with respiratory distress syndrome. Significant improvement was noted in oxygenation status when compared to the control group.
Hallman et al[42]	Inositol (a sugar) was tested as a dietary supplement in premature infants. Treatment resulted in a more rapid recovery with less inspiratory oxygen.
Hallman et al[39]	Human surfactant obtained from amniotic fluid was given intratracheally to 61 preterm infants; 51 control infants received air as a placebo. Fifty percent of the cases in the surfactant group required more than one dose. Mortality in the surfactant group of infants (gestational age 24–24 wks) dropped from 86 percent to 13 percent.
Davis et al[41]	Transpulmonary pressure was measured in infants before and after receiving calf-lung surfactant extract. The mean ratio of alveolar to arterial oxygen was reduced 56 percent after administration of surfactant. Minute ventilation increased 38 percent; tidal volume increased 32 percent; dynamic compliance increased 29 percent; and inspiratory flow rates increased 54 percent.
Lotze et al[44]	ECMO was used in 13 infants with severe respiratory failure (3 with ARDS and 9 with meconium aspiration, and 1 with sepsis). Significant positive correlations were noted between lung compliance and percent of bypass and between lung compliance and x-ray findings.
Carlo et al[45]	Forty-one infants with RDS were randomized to receive either high-frequency jet ventilation, at a rate of 250 per minute, or conventional ventilation for 48 hours. The infants receiving jet ventilation has lower mean airway pressures. Complications were similar in both groups.
Lewis et al[49]	A review of the literature with 181 references. Although the lung injury in adult RDS is more complex than in infant RDS, the authors contend that the lung dysfunction is exacerbated by alterations in endogenous surfactant in both cases. The authors describe the composition and metabolism of normal surfactant and the consequences of abnormal surfactant function. They present possible mechanisms of altered surfactant function. They describe various types of exogenous surfactant and their modes of administration. They are hopeful that treatment of ARDS victims with exogenous surfactant will dramatically decrease mortality rates.
Jobe[50]	A discussion of the uses of surfactants in the treatment of lung diseases, especially in infant RDS in preterm neonates. The author describes the timing of the use of surfactants and the acute effects of surfactants on the lungs. An excellent review of the uses, pharmicodynamics, and clinical implications of exogenous surfactants.
Rossaint et al[51]	Pulmonary hypertension and right-to-left shunting of venous blood are characteristics of ARDS. Inhalation of nitric oxide causes selectic vasodilation in regions of the lung being ventilated. The result is a decrease in mean pulmonary artery pressure and decreased intrapulmonary shunting. Arterial oxygenation is increased by improving the matching of ventilation to perfusion. The effects are limited to ventilated areas in the lung and no systemic vasodilation occurs.
Bone[52]	The author describes the basic pathophysiology of ARDS and describes the rationale for treatment protocols. Despite advances in ARDS treatment, mortality is still high. The author suggests that new treatments, which include inhalation of nitric oxide, hold great promise. The risks and benefits of nitric oxide inhalation are described.

Summary

Early diagnosis and treatment of acute respiratory failure is the ideal situation. The diseases presented in this chapter represent severe lung dysfunction, with significant mortality rates in adults. Table 22–3 presents an overview of current research regarding ARDS and IRDS.

REFERENCES

1. Kaplan JD: Acute respiratory failure, In Wooley M, Whelan A (eds): *Manual of Medical Therapeutics*, 26th ed. Boston, Little, Brown & Co, 1992, pp 179–195.
2. West JB: *Pulmonary Pathophysiology—The Essentials*, 4th ed. Baltimore, Williams & Wilkins, 1992.
3. Shoemaker WC: Pathophysiology and fluid management of post-operative and post-traumatic ARDS, in Shoemaker WC, Ayres S, Grenvek A, Holbrook PR, Thompson WL (eds): *Text-*

book of *Critical Care*, 2nd ed. Philadelphia, WB Saunders, 1989, pp 615–636.

4. Braun SR, Sufit RL, Giovannoni R, O'Connor M, Peters H: Intermittent negative pressure ventilation in the treatment of respiratory failure in progressive neuromuscular disease. *Neurology* 1987;37:1874–1875.

5. Stauffer J: Pulmonary diseases, in Schroeder SA, Tierney LM, McPhee SJ, Papadakios MA, Krupp MA (eds): *Current Medical Diagnosis and Treatment*. Norwalk, Conn, Appleton & Lange, 1993, pp 177–256.

6. Sugerman HJ, Olafsson KB, Pollock TW, Agnew RF, Rogers RM, Miller LD: Continuous positive end-expiratory pressure ventilation (PEEP) for the treatment of diffuse interstitial pulmonary edema. *J Trauma* 1972;12:263–274.

7. Pontoppidan H, Rie MA: Pathogenesis and therapy of acute lung injury, in Prakash O (ed): *Applied Physiology in Clinical Respiratory Care*. The Hague, Martinus Nijhoff, 1982.

8. Kumar A, Falke KJ, Geffin B, et al: Continuous positive pressure ventilation in acute respiratory failure. Effects of hemodynamic and lung function. *N Engl J Med* 1970;283(26):1430–1436.

9. Schumann L, Parsons GH: Tracheal suctioning and ventilator tubing changes in adult respiratory distress syndrome: Use of a positive end-expiratory valve. *Heart Lung* 1985;14(4):362–367.

10. Ayres SM, Schlichtig R, Sterling MJ: *Care of the Critically Ill*, 3rd ed. Chicago, Year Book Medical Publishers, 1988.

11. Bone RC, Fisher CJ, Clemmer TP, Slotman GJ, Metz CA: Early methylprednisolone treatment for septic shock and the adult respiratory distress syndrome. *Chest* 1987;92:1032–1036.

12. Alberts WM, Priest GR, Moser KM: The outlook for survivors of ARDS. *Chest* 1983;84(3)272–274.

13. Fanconi S, Kraemer R, Weber J: Long-term sequelae in children surviving adult respiratory distress syndrome. *J Pediatr* 1985;106(2):218–222.

14. Hopewell PC, Murray JF: The adult respiratory distress syndrome. *Am Rev Respir Med* 1976;27:343–356.

15. Thurlbeck WM, Miller RR: The respiratory system. In Rubin E, Farber JL (ed): *Pathology*. Philadelphia, JB Lippincott, 1993, pp 542–627.

16. Petty TL, Ashbaugh DG: The adult respiratory distress syndrome: Clinical features, factors influencing prognosis and principles of management. *Chest* 1971;60(3):233–239.

17. Shapiro BA, Harrison RA, Trout CA: *Clinical Application of Respiratory Care*. Chicago, Year Book Medical Publishers, 1977.

18. Slonim NB, Hamilton LH: *Respiratory physiology*, 5th ed. St. Louis, CV Mosby, 1987.

19. Cherniack RM, Cherniack L: *Respiration in Health and Disease*, 3rd ed. Philadelphia, WB Saunders, 1983.

20. Comroe JH: *Physiology of Respiration*, 2nd ed. Chicago, Year Book Medical Publishers, 1975.

21. Comroe JH, Forster RE, Dubois AB, Brisboe WA, Carlsen E: *The Lung*, 2nd ed. Chicago, Year Book Medical Publishers, 1977.

22. Sugerman HJ, Rogers RM, Miller LD: Positive end-expiratory pressure: Indications and physiologic considerations. *Chest* 1972;62:865–945.

23. Leftwich EI, Witorsch RJ, Witorsch P: Positive end-expiratory pressure in refractory hypoxemia. *Ann Intern Med* 1973; 79:187–192.

24. Ayres SM, Grave WJ: Inappropriate ventilation and hypoxemia as causes of cardiac arrhythmias. *Am J Med* 1969;46(4):495–505.

25. Dantzker DR, Wagner PD, West JB: Instability of lung units with low $\dot{V}_A/\dot{Q}$ ratios during O_2 breathing. *J Appl Physiol* 1975;38(5):886–895.

26. McLoud TC, Barasch PG, Ravin CE: PEEP: Radiographic features and associated complications. *Am J Roentgenol* 1977; 129:209–213.

27. Gattinoni L, Mascheroni D, Torresin A, et al: Morphological response to positive end expiratory pressure in acute respiratory failure; Computerized tomography study. *Intensive Care Med* 1986;12:137–142.

28. Angerpointer TA, Farnsworth AE, Williams BT: Effects of PEEP on cardiovascular dynamics after open-heart surgery: A new post-operative monitoring technique. *Ann Thorac Surg* 1977;23:555–559.

29. Rie MA, Pontoppidan H: Ventilatory complications: Prevention

and treatment, in Kinney JM, Bendixen HH, Powers SR Jr (eds): *Manual of Surgical Intensive Care*. Philadelphia, WB Saunders, 1977, pp 219–250.

30. Katz R: Respiratory distress syndrome and infection in infancy and childhood, in Shoemaker WC, Ayers S, Grenvek A, Holbrook PR, Thompson WL (eds): *Textbook of Critical Care*, 2nd ed. Philadelphia, WB Saunders, 1989, pp 636–641.

31. Hurst JM, Branson RD, DeHaven CB: The role of high-frequency ventilation in post-traumatic respiratory insufficiency. *J Trauma* 1987;27:236–241.

32. Bernard GR, Luce JM, Sprung CL, et al: High-dose corticosteroids in patients with the adult respiratory distress syndrome. *N Engl J Med* 1987;317:1565–1570.

33. Richman PS, Spragg RG, Robertson B, Merritt TA, Curstedt T: The adult respiratory distress syndrome: First trials with surfactant replacement. *Eur Respir J* 1989;2(suppl 3):109S–111S.

34. Snow J: Pulmonary disorders, in Hazinski MF (ed): *Nursing Care of the Critically Ill Child*, 2nd ed. St. Louis, CV Mosby, 1992, pp 253–333.

35. Stark AR: Respiratory disorders, in Cloherty JP, Stark AR (eds): *Manual of Neonatal Care*, 2nd ed. Boston, Little, Brown & Co, 1985, pp 167–173.

36. Klaus M: Respiratory function and pulmonary disease in the newborn, in Barnett H (ed): *Pediatrics*, 15th ed. New York, Appleton-Century-Crofts, 1972, pp 1255–1261.

37. Cloherty JP, Murphy WI: Management of the Newborn, II, in Graef JW, Cone TE (eds): *Manual of Pediatric Therapeutics*, 4th ed. Boston, Little, Brown & Co, 1988, pp 133–187.

38. Gittin JP, Soll RF, Parad RB, et al: Randomized controlled trial of exogenous surfactant for the treatment of hyaline membrane disease. *Pediatrics* 1987;79:31–37.

39. Hallman M, Pohjavuori M, Jorvenpaa AL, Bry L, Merritt TA, Pesonen E: Human surfactant in the treatment of respiratory distress syndrome. A spectrum clinical response. *Eur Respir J* 1989;3(suppl 2):77S–80S.

40. Raju TNK, Vidyasagar D, Bhat R, et al: Double-blind controlled trial with bovine surfactant in severe hyalaine membrane disease. *Lancet* 1987;1:651–656.

41. Davis JM, Veness-Meehan K, Notter RH, Bhutani VK, Kendig JW, Shapiro DI: Changes in pulmonary mechanics after the administration of surfactant in infants with respiratory distress syndrome. *N Engl J Med* 1988;319:476–479.

42. Hallman M, Arjemaa P, Hoppa K: Inositol supplementation in respiratory distress syndrome: Relationship between serum concentration, renal excretion and lung effluent phospholipids. *J Pediatr* 1987;110:604–610.

43. Hallman M, Jarvenpaa AL, Pehjavuori: Respiratory distress syndrome and inositol supplementation in preterm infants. *Arch Dis Child* 1986;61;1076–1083.

44. Lotze A, Short BL, Taylor GA: Lung compliance as a measure of lung function in newborns with respiratory failure requiring extracorporeal membrane oxygenation. *Crit Care Med* 1987;15:226–239.

45. Carlo WA, Chatburn RL, Martin RJ: Randomized trial of high-frequency jet ventilation versus conventional ventilation in respiratory distress syndrome. *J Pediatr* 1987;110:275–282.

46. Kersten LD: Restrictive pulmonary disease, in Kersten LD (ed): *Comprehensive Respiratory Nursing: A Decision Making Approach*. Philadelphia, WB Saunders, 1989, pp 121–158.

47. Zarowitz BJ, et al: Variability in theophylline volume of distribution and clearance in patients with acute respiratory failure requiring mechanical ventilation. *Chest* 1988;93:379–385.

48. Ghio AJ, et al: Impairment after adult respiratory distress syndrome: An evaluation based on American Thoracic Society recommendations. *Am Rev Respir Disease* 1989;139:1138–1162.

49. Lewis JR, Jobe AH: Surfactant and the adult respiratory distress syndrome. *Am Rev Respir Dis* 1993;147:218–233.

50. Jobe AH: Pulmonary surfactant therapy. *N Engl J Med* 1993; 328:861–868.

51. Rossaint R, et al: Inhaled nitric oxide for the adult respiratory distress syndrome. *N Engl J Med* 1993;328:399–405.

52. Bone RC: A new therapy for the adult respiratory distress syndrome. *N Engl J Med* 1993;328:431–432.

BIBLIOGRAPHY

American Thoracic Society, Medical Section of the American Lung Association: Withholding and withdrawing life-sustaining therapy. *Am Rev Respir Dis* 1991;144(3):726–731.

Bone RC: A critical evaluation of new agents for the treatment of sepsis. *JAMA* 1991;266(12):1686–1691.

Bone RC, Balk R, Slotman G, Maunder R, et al: Adult respiratory distress syndrome: Sequence and importance if development of multiple organ failure. *Chest* 1992;101(2):320–326.

Centers for Disease Control and Prevention. Update: Hontavirus infection—United States. *JAMA* 1993;270(4):429–432.

Collop NA, Sahn SA: Critical illness in pregnancy: An analysis of 20 patients admitted to a medical intensive care unit. *Ches* 1993;103(5):1548–1552.

Donnelly SC, Robertson C: Trauma, inflammatory cells and ARDS. *Arch Emerg Med* 1993;10(2):108–111.

Dunn MS: Surfactant replacement therapy: Prophylaxis or treatment. *Pediatrics* 1993;92(1):148–150.

Fields AI: Newer modes of mechanical ventilation for patients with adult respiratory distress syndrome. *Crit Care Med* 1993;21(9S):S367–369.

Fiser DH: Adult respiratory distress syndrome. *Pediatr Rev* 1993;14(5):163–166.

Gallup DG, Nolan TE: The gynecologist and multiple organ failure syndrome. *Gynecol Oncol* 1993;48(3):293–300.

Hudson LD: Fluid management strategy in acute lung injury. *Am Rev Respir Dis* 1992;145(5):988–989.

Jacobson W, Park GR, Saich T, Holcroft J: Surfactant and adult respiratory distress syndrome. *Br J Anaesth* 1993;70(5):522–526.

Pfenninger J: Adult respiratory distress syndrome in newborn infants. *Crit Care Med* 1993;21(9S):S362–S363.

Sassoon CSH: Positive pressure ventilation: Alternate modes. *Chest* 1991;100(5):1421–1429.

Seeger W, Gunther A, Walmrath HD, Grimminger F, Lasch HG: Alveolar surfactant and adult respiratory distress syndrome: Pathogenetic role and therapeutic prospects. *Clin Invest* 1993;71(3):177–190.

Slinger PD: Perioperative respiratory assessment and management. *Can J Anaesth* 1992;39(5–2):R115–R131.

Smith DW, Frankel LR, Derish MT, Moody RR, Black LE, Chipps BE, Mathers LH: High-frequency jet ventilation in children with the adult respiratory distress syndrome complicated by pulmonary barotrauma. *Pediatr Pulmonol* 1993;15(5):279–286.

Suchyta MR, Elliott CG, Jensen RL, Crapo RO: Predicting the presence of pulmonary function impairment in adult respiratory distress syndrome survivors. *Respiration* 1993;60(2):103–108.

Weinberger SE: Recent advances in pulmonary medicine. *N Engl J Med* 1993;328(20):1462–1470.

Wiedemann HP, Matthay MA, Matthay RA: Adult respiratory distress syndrome. *Clin Chest Med* 1990;11(3):575. Editorial.

Wood BP: The newborn chest. *Radiol Clin North Am* 1993;31(3):667–676.

Yang KL, Tobin MJ: A prospective study of indexes predicting the outcome of trials of weaning from mechanical ventilation. *N Engl J Med* 1991;324(21):1445–1450.

Zachariades N, Agouridakis P, Parker J: The adult respiratory distress syndrome: A review. *J Oral Maxillofac Surg* 1993;51(4):402–407.

CHAPTER 23
Other Respiratory Disorders

LORNA SCHUMANN and RICK MADISON

KEY TERMS

consolidation: The process of lung tissues becoming firm and solid as a result of pneumonia.

empyema: An accumulation of pus in the pleural space.

Ghon tubercle: A nodule or swelling containing *Mycobacterium tuberculosis*.

granulomas: Tissue that forms into a nodular mass as a result of inflammation, infection, or injury.

lysosomes: An organelle containing hydrolytic enzymes that function to digest intracellular materials.

opportunistic infection: An infection caused by organisms that are usually nonpathogenic, because of decreased function of the immune system.

pneumonia: An acute inflammation of lung tissue caused by an infectious agent or by aspiration of chemically irritating fluid.

T his chapter discusses respiratory infectious diseases, pulmonary vascular disorders, occupational disorders, and neoplasms that are not classified strictly as obstructive disorders (Chap. 20) or restrictive disorders (Chap. 21). The incidence of pulmonary disorders in these categories has been increasing over the past few years as a result of increased occupational hazards and environmental pollution.

Pneumonia

Etiology

The term **pneumonia** (from *pneumon*, the Greek word for lung) refers to an inflammatory reaction in the alveoli and interstitium of the lung, usually caused by an infectious agent. Pneumonia can occur from three different sources: (1) aspiration of oropharyngeal secretions composed of normal bacterial flora or gastric contents; (2) inhalation of contaminants (virus, *Mycoplasma*); or (3) contamination of the systemic circulation.

There are several ways to classify pneumonia. One of the most common methods is to separate bacterial pneumonia from viral pneumonia. The bacterial pneumonias may be grouped as either gram-positive or gram-negative, based on the staining characteristics of the organism. Staining involves applying a pigment or dye to the tissue to assist in demonstrating and classifying the organism. *Staphylococcus* and *Streptococcus* (including pneumococci) are the predominant gram-positive organisms. Gram-negative bacteria that may cause pneumonia include *Hemophilus*, *Klebsiella*, *Pseudomonas*, *Serratia*, *Escherichia coli*, and *Proteus*.

To assist the reader in differentiating among the various types of pneumonias, Table 23–1 presents the etiology; common clinical features, with age-related characteristics; diagnostic tests; and antibiotic therapies for 11 forms of the disease.

Pathogenesis

After microbial agents enter the lung, they multiply and trigger pulmonary inflammation. Alveolar air spaces fill with an exudative fluid, and inflammatory cells invade the alveolar septa. Bacterial pneumonia may be associated with significant ventilation-perfusion mismatching and poor blood gas values because inflammatory exudate collects in the alveolar spaces. Chapter 19 describes ventilation-perfusion mismatching in greater detail. Alveolar exudate tends to consolidate and becomes difficult to expectorate. Viral pneumonias do not produce exudative fluids. Figure 23–1 shows a cross-section of lung tissue in a patient with bronchopneumonia and histologic presentation of the same patient. Patients with chronic illnesses and those who are immobile or immunosuppressed are at highest risk for developing pneumonia. Disruption of the body's normal defense mechanisms leads to increased risk of pneumonia. Other patients at risk

are those who have undergone thoracic or abdominal surgery or anesthesia.

Clinical Manifestations

Clinically, pneumonia can be detected by auscultation of the lungs. Rales (crackles) and bronchial breath sounds can be heard over the affected lung tissue. In addition, the patient presents with fever, chills, cough, purulent sputum, and an abnormal chest radiograph.

Diagnosis

The chest radiograph demonstrates a lighter (whiter) shadow in the involved area, indicative of inflammatory alveolar processes.[1,2] In a patient with symptoms and clinical findings of pneumonia, a Gram stain of expectorated sputum should be obtained to distinguish bacterial from viral pneumonia and gram-negative from gram-positive organisms. If the patient had been previously healthy, the cause of the majority of these infections would either be viral, mycoplasma, or the gram-positive pneumococcal bacterium. However, if the patient had been hospitalized or has other illnesses such as emphysema, diabetes, or alcoholism, then gram-negative organisms should be suspected. Because 24 to 48 hours may be required to culture the etiologic agent, antibiotic therapy should be started empirically based on the results of the Gram stain and the patient's clinical history. Diagnosis is based on the chest radiograph, white blood cell count, and sputum culture, coupled with clinical features of fever with recurrent chills, cough, dyspnea, and rales.

Treatment

For pneumococcal pneumonia, penicillin is the drug of choice. If the patient is allergic to penicillin, erythromycin can be given in dosages of 250 to 500 mg four times per day, either intravenously (IV) or orally (PO).

If staphylococcal pneumonia is suspected as the etiologic agent, an alternative drug should be chosen because of the high incidence of penicillin-resistant strains. For staphylococcal pneumonia, either nafcillin, oxacillin, or methicillin may be used IV. Cephalosporins may also be chosen as a therapeutic alternative for staphylococcal pneumonia.

For gram-negative pneumonia, broad-spectrum antibiotic coverage is indicated until results of laboratory cultures are known. This may be accomplished either with a third-generation cephalosporin or an aminoglycoside. The incidence of side effects increases with the use of these drugs. Nephrotoxicity and ototoxicity are known complications of aminoglycoside therapy. Blood levels of the drugs must be monitored. These levels and the rate of infusion are usually measured from peak and trough blood samples. Peak refers to measurement of the drug at its highest level, and trough is a measurement done

TABLE 23–1. Differentiating Features of Pneumonias

Etiologic Organism	Common Clinical Features	Chest Radiograph	Antibiotic Treatment
Staphylococcus aureus	Follows upper respiratory infection; fever, chills, pleuritic chest pain, cough and yellow purulent sputum	Consolidation, may have cavitation	Nafcillin, oxacillin, or methicillin; alternative choice: cephalosporins
Streptococcus pneumoniae (*Pneumococcus*)	More common in alcoholics; fever, chills, pleuritic chest pain, cough, rusty colored sputum	Patchy infiltrates	Procaine penicillin G or aqueous penicillin G; alternative choice: erythromycin; prophylactic vaccine available
Haemophilus influenzae	Upper respiratory symptoms, fever, vomiting, irritability cough, purulent sputum, dyspnea. Affects children and older adults	Consolidation	Ampicillin alternative choices: chloramphenicol, second-generation cephalosporins, trimethoprim-sulfamethoxazole
Klebsiella pneumoniae	Seen frequently in middle-aged men and associated with alcoholism and diabetes mellitus	Consolidation	Aminoglycoside plus cephalosporin; alternative: chloramphenicol
Pseudomonas aeruginosa	Chronic obstructive pulmonary disease associated with COPD, cystic fibrosis, and mechanical ventilation; fever, chills, and copious greenish, foul-smelling sputum	Infiltrates, small pleural effusion	Aminoglycoside plus penicillin active against *Pseudomonas*
Escherichia coli	Complication of gastrointestinal surgery	Infiltrates, may have pleural effusion	Aminoglycoside; alternative: ampicillin, or third-generation cephalosporin
Virus	Fever, malaise, headache, nonproductive cough	Patchy infiltrates'	Amantadine
Legionella	Acute onset with fever, diarrhea, myalgia, and abdominal pain	Consolidation	Erythromycin; alternative: trimethoprim-sulfamethoxazole
Mycoplasma pneumoniae (atypical pneumonia)	Ages 5 to 25 years, most common in young adults; associated with otitis media and myringitis; sore throat, headache, myalgia, dry cough, fatigue and low-grade fever	Infiltrates	Erythromycin; alternative: tetracycline
Pneumocystis carinii	Immunosuppressed patients (infants, children, and adults); 60% of patients have acquired immunodeficiency syndrome (Schroeder)	Diffuse infiltrates, or chest x-ray may appear normal	Trimethoprim-sulfamethoxazole, pentamidine
Anaerobic Pneumonia (aspiration pneumonia)	Predisposition to aspiration, fever, weight loss, malaise; risk increases with decreased level of consciousness, artificial airway, and sedation	Infiltrates in dependent lung fields	Penicillin G; alternative choices: clindamycin, chloramphenicol, metronidazole, cefoxitin

Data from Stauffer JL: Pulmonary diseases, in Schroeder SA, Tierney LM, McPhee SJ, Papdakis MA, Krupp MA (eds): *Current Medical Diagnoses and Treatment.* Norwalk, Appleton-Lange, 1993, pp 177–256; *Nursing 84 Books: Controlling environmental disease.* Nurse's Clinical Library: Respiratory Disorders, Springhouse, Pa, Springhouse Corporation, 1984, pp 171–181; West JB: *Pulmonary Pathophysiology—The Essentials,* 3rd ed. Baltimore, Williams & Wilkins, 1987, pp 134–153; Kersten LD: Restrictive pulmonary disease, in *Comprehensive Respiratory Nursing: A Decision-Making Approach.* Philadelphia, WB Saunders, 1989, pp 121–158.

when the drug level is at its lowest point. The side effects of cephalosporins include phlebitis, hypersensitivity, and bleeding disorders. Once the organism has been cultured, specific antibiotic selection is based on sensitivity of the organism to different antibiotics.

Anaerobic bacteria may also cause pneumonia that may present clinically as a lung abscess, a necrotizing pneumonia, or empyema. These diseases are most often caused by aspiration of normal oral bacteria (such as *Bacteroides* and *Fusobacterium*) into the lung. Many clinicians use high doses of penicillin G as the drug of choice for such infections, but other antibiotics such as Flagyl (metronidazole), chloramphenicol, clindamycin, and cefoxitin are acceptable alternatives.

The most common cause of viral pneumonia is the influenza virus, and unfortunately, no antibiotics are currently available for its treatment. Amantadine,

an antiviral agent, may be effective in reducing symptoms; however, there have been no controlled studies testing the effectiveness of amantadine against influenza pneumonia.

Mycoplasma pneumonia is best treated with either erythromycin (first choice) or tetracycline. Mycoplasma is more commonly seen in the summer and fall in young adults.

Other causes of pneumonia occur less frequently in the general population. Legionnaire's disease, for example, is a severe systemic illness characterized by fever, diarrhea, abdominal pain, liver and kidney failure, and pulmonary infiltrates. The organism lives in water and is transmitted by means of potable water, condensers, and cooling towers.[3] The current treatment of choice is erythromycin.

Patients whose immune systems have been com-

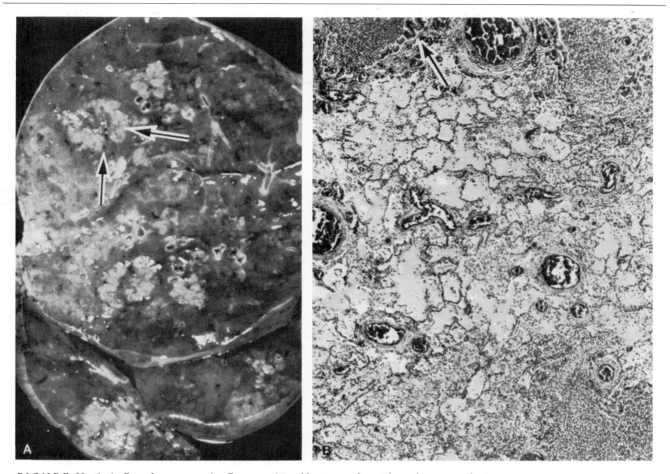

FIGURE 23–1. **A,** Bronchopneumonia. Gross section of lung reveals patches of gray purulent consolidation (*arrows*). **B,** Upper and lower parts of this histologic section are illustrative of the patchiness of inflammatory reaction. Note the edema fluid in less involved alveoli. *Arrow* points to bronchus with inflammation and ulceration. (From Cotran RS, Kumar V, Robbins SL: *Robbins Pathologic Basis of Disease*, 4th ed. Philadelphia, WB Saunders, 1989, p 781. Reproduced with permission.)

promised either by disease or by drug therapy may be susceptible to developing opportunistic pneumonias. These infections are caused by organisms that would ordinarily not cause disease in healthy people. For example, *Pneumocystis carinii* pneumonia, an opportunistic infection caused by a protozoon, is commonly found in cancer and patients with human immunodeficiency virus (HIV). Primary treatment is trimethoprim-sulfamethoxazole or pentamidine.

Aspergillus, an opportunistic fungus that is ubiquitous in nature, may cause progressive pneumonia. *Aspergillus* is liberated from walls of old buildings under reconstruction. Attention should be given to the renovation of old hospitals and the placement of susceptible patients in a reconstruction area. Treatment of *Aspergillus* pneumonia should be initiated with amphotericin B in slowly increasing dosages. 5-Fluorocytosine has also been used as an adjuvant to amphotericin B therapy and requires monitoring of renal function. Both of these pharmacologic agents are nephrotoxic. Please refer to a pharmacology textbook for special precautions in using these agents.

Actinomyces is an anaerobic gram-positive bacterium that may also cause opportunistic pneumonia. IV penicillin in dosages of 10 to 20 million units per day is used to treat this type of pneumonia.

Nocardia, a gram-positive bacterium that may be responsible for opportunistic infections, is sensitive to a number of antibiotics. Sulfonamides have been the standard therapy of choice, but ampicillin, erythromycin, and minocycline have also been used successfully.

Cryptococcosis is a systemic fungal infection. The infection is acquired by inhaling the encapsulated yeast *Cryptococcus* which is found in soil and dried pigeon dung. The fungus may cause pneumonia, which is treated with amphotericin B, 5-fluorocytosine, or ketoconazole. Spontaneous resolution of pulmonary complications has been reported.

KEY CONCEPTS

- Pneumonia is an inflammation of the lung that is usually associated with an infectious agent. The most common types of pneumonia are bacterial and viral. A productive cough is the primary differentiating feature between bacterial pneumonia and viral pneumonia, in which coughing is nonproductive.

- Bacterial pneumonia may be associated with significant ventilation-perfusion mismatching and poor blood gas values because inflammatory exudate collects in the alveolar spaces. Alveolar exudate tends to consolidate and becomes difficult to expectorate. Viral pneumonias do not produce exudative fluids.

- Manifestations of bacterial pneumonia include fever, chills, cough with purulent sputum, crackles, and areas of consolidation on chest radiograph. Dyspnea may be significant.

- The treatment of bacterial pneumonia centers on antibiotic therapy to eliminate the organism and supportive therapy to enhance ventilation and oxygenation. Most viral pneumonia (influenza) is treated symptomatically, as no effective antibiotic therapy is available.

- Fungal and protozoal pneumonias are uncommon and tend to occur in immunocompromised individuals.

Pulmonary Tuberculosis

Etiology

Although the incidence of tuberculosis is steadily declining in the United States, nearly 30,000 new cases occur each year in this country.[2] The majority of new cases occur in malnourished and aged populations. Over the past 20 years, there has been a shift in the care of such patients from specialized tuberculosis hospitals to outpatient therapy. Hospitalization of such patients may be necessary with isolation for a period of 2 to 4 weeks. Specialized tuberculosis hospitals were reopening owing to increasing resistance of the organism to treatment and increasing numbers of cases. Tuberculosis cases should be reported to local and state health departments.

Tuberculosis Pneumonia

Tuberculosis is caused by the bacterium *Mycobacterium tuberculosis*, an acid-fast aerobic bacillus. Any organ system can be affected by the disease, but the most common sites are the lungs and the lymph nodes. Tuberculosis is subdivided into two major classifications: primary and reactivating. Primary disease is the initial infection, and reactivation occurs with subsequent infections.

Entry into the body is by inhalation of small, 2 μm to 10 μm droplet nuclei of the bacterium. These droplets are produced by an infected person coughing, sneezing, and talking.

Pathogenesis

After entrance of the mycobacterium into the lung tissue, macrophages ingest and process the microorganisms. The organisms either are destroyed or persist and multiply. The infection spreads through the lymph system and circulatory system, becoming widespread prior to being walled off by **granulomatous** inflammation.[3] Dormant organisms persist for years. Reactivation may occur if the patient's immune system becomes impaired.

The pathologic manifestation of tuberculosis is the **Ghon tubercle** or complex, which has parenchymal and lymph components. The parenchymal component is composed of a well-circumscribed necrotic nodule that later becomes fibrotic and calcified. The lymph component is found in the lymph nodes. Figure 23–2 shows primary pulmonary tuberculosis.

Clinical Manifestations

Clinical features include a history of contact with an infected person, low-grade fever, cough, night sweats, fatigue, weight loss, and anorexia. As the disease progresses, the patient develops a productive cough with purulent sputum. Physical examination of the lung fields reveals apical crackles (rales), or

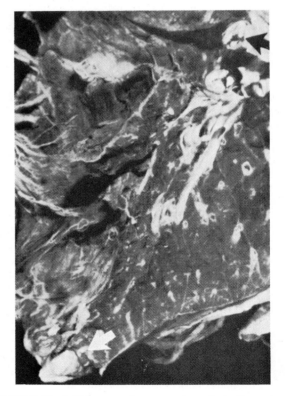

F I G U R E 23–2. Primary pulmonary tuberculosis. Parenchymal focus of white caseation is present in lower left corner (*arrow*) and caseated lymph nodes of drainage can be seen at upper right (*arrow*). (From Cotran RS, Kumar V, Robbins SL: *Robbins Pathologic Basis of Disease*, 4th ed. Philadelphia, WB Saunders, 1989, p. 787. Reproduced with permission.)

bronchial breath sounds over the region of lung **consolidation.** (Please refer to Chapter 10 for a discussion of the tuberculosis strain that occurs in HIV-infected patients.)

Diagnosis

Definitive diagnosis is made by results of sputum cultures. Serial morning cultures are usually done to identify the slow-growing acid-fast bacilli. Expectoration of sputum in the early morning is ideal because the sputum is more concentrated and more plentiful. Cultures require 6 to 8 weeks for determination. Gastric washings or bronchial washings may also be used for diagnostic culturing.

Chest radiographs usually show nodules with infiltrates in the apex and posterior segments of the upper lobes. The organism favors the apices because of the high oxygen content in the upper lung regions. Elderly patients may present with lower lobe infiltrates with or without pleural effusion. Figure 23–3 shows the radiographic appearance of a cavitary tuberculosis in a 23-year-old man.

Another primary diagnostic test is the tuberculin skin test (5 tuberculin units/0.1 mL of purified protein derivative [PPD] injected intradermally). This test does not distinguish between current disease and past infection. If the induration in a person with HIV infection is 5 mm or greater, the patient has close contact with individuals with tuberculosis, and if the patient has a chest radiograph consistent with tuberculosis, the likelihood of active disease is high.[3] An induration of 10 mm or greater is the reaction size for other high-risk individuals such as IV drug abusers, individuals who are debilitated or immunosuppressed, and individuals living in countries with a high incidence of the disease. An induration of 15 mm or greater is seen in all other persons.

False positive results may occur in persons with other mycobacterial infections or if they have received *Bacillus Calmette-Guérin*, a live attenuated strain of *Mycobacterium bovis* that provides active immunity against tuberculosis. False negative results may also occur in patients who are malnourished, elderly, or immunocompromised. Immunocompromised patients may not be able to mount a response (wheal) to injection of the organism. Pulmonary function tests are characteristic of restrictive diseases, with decreased lung volumes and decreased compliance.

Treatment

Primary therapy for active tuberculosis consists of isoniazid and rifampin for 9 months. If the organism is resistant to this therapy, ethambutol, streptomycin, or pyrazinamide are added to the drug regimen. Another method of treating resistant organisms is to treat for 6 months with isoniazid and rifampin and add an initial 2 months of pyrazinamide.[3]

Patients infected but without active disease should be considered for isoniazid prophylaxis for 12 months. Patients with positive results on tuberculin skin tests, such as household members, high-risk individuals, and individuals under the age of 35, should be given isoniazid. However, contacts with negative PPD skin tests should receive isoniazid for 3 months and then should be retested with the tuberculin skin test. If the test results are positive, isoniazid should be continued for another 9 months.[3]

KEY CONCEPTS

- **Tuberculosis is caused by inhalation or ingestion of the bacterium *Mycobacterium tuberculosis.* The organism spreads through the lymph and blood. Bacteria are ingested by macrophages and walled off by inflammatory proteins (granulomas). The organisms may not be killed, and can persist in a dormant state for years. These walled-off areas of inflammatory cells and bacteria become fibrotic and calcified, forming Ghon tubercles, the hallmark of tuberculosis.**

- **Symptoms are rather nonspecific: low-grade fever, cough, night sweats, fatigue, and weight loss. With progression of the disease the cough is productive of purulent sputum.**

- **The diagnosis is based on a positive PPD skin test for tuberculosis, positive sputum cultures, and characteristic nodules on chest radiographs.**

- **Isoniazid and rifampin are the agents of choice for treating tuberculosis. Drug therapy continues for 9 to 12 months for active disease and may be used for shorter periods in persons exposed to tuberculosis but having no active disease.**

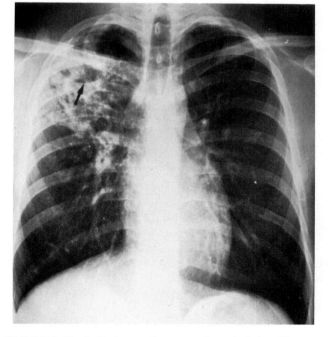

FIGURE 23–3. Cavitary pulmonary tuberculosis in a 23-year-old man. (From Kersten LD: *Comprehensive Respiratory Nursing.* Philadelphia, WB Saunders, 1989, p 146. Reproduced with permission.)

Neoplasms

Etiology

The incidence of lung cancer in the United States has been increasing for the past several years, with 150,000 new cases each year.[4,5] The four major types of lung cancer are large-cell carcinoma, small-cell carcinoma, squamous cell carcinoma, and adenocarcinoma. In 1990 cancer of the lung accounted for 35 percent of cancer deaths in men and 20 percent of cancer deaths in women.[3] Cigarette smoking is the major cause of lung cancer, with approximately 100,000 deaths reported per year. About 3,800 deaths per year are reported in nonsmokers who receive secondary smoke from the environment.[6] Individuals at highest risk for developing lung cancer are those who started smoking before the age of 25, have smoked one or more packs of cigarettes a day for 20 years, work in areas exposed to asbestos, and are over the age of 50.[6]

Pathogenesis

Large-cell carcinomas develop in the lung periphery and are similar to adenocarcinoma. The tumor cells are large and are arranged in nests or clusters. The tumor doubles in size about every 100 days and metastasizes to distant organs.[3]

Small-cell (oat cell) carcinoma tends to originate extrinsically in the central bronchus region, thus compressing and narrowing the bronchi. The narrowing may lead to signs and symptoms of obstruction of a central airway, leading to wheezing. This type of tumor grows rapidly and doubles in about 33 days.[3] Widespread metastasis is common with small-cell carcinomas, which are the most resistant to therapy.

Squamous cell carcinoma usually originates (in two thirds of cases) in the central bronchi near the hilus as an intraluminal growth.[3] Cytologic examination of sputum reveals the squamous cell carcinoma, leading to earlier detection of cancer than with other lung neoplasms. The tumor normally doubles its volume in 100 days and, as it advances, metastasizes to regional lymph nodes in the area.[3]

Adenocarcinomas usually appear in the periphery of the lung and are not as amenable to early detection as squamous cell carcinoma. Adenocarcinomas are characterized by acinar bronchoalveolar and papillary tumors. Doubling time is about 180 days, with metastasis occurring to distant organs, which may be due to aerosol transmission in the case of bronchoalveolar carcinoma.[3,6]

Clinical Manifestations

Clinical features vary with the type of tumor, location of the tumor, and whether the tumor has metastasized. Approximately 10 percent to 25 percent of cases are asymptomatic.[3] Signs and symptoms can be classified as intrathoracic or extrathoracic.

Extrathoracic manifestations are weight loss, anemia, and clubbing. Facial and upper extremity edema are noted in cases of tumor compression of the superior vena cava.

Intrathoracic manifestations are dyspnea, cough, chest pain, hemoptysis, and increased sputum with bronchoalveolar carcinoma. Hoarseness may be evident and is caused by pressure of the tumor on the recurrent laryngeal nerve. Phrenic nerve involvement (1 percent of lung cancer patients) leads to paralysis of the hemidiaphragm on the affected side with the potential for developing atelectasis and pneumonia. Abdominal breathing measures are taught to the patient who does not recover diaphragmatic function. Extension of the cancer cells to the pleural cavity may cause pleural effusion.

Diagnosis

Pulmonary function tests may show increased volumes in moderately advanced cases of bronchial carcinoma.[7] As the tumor blocks the airway, an obstructive pattern of pulmonary disease may lead to increased functional residual capacity (FRC) or decreased FRC due to the effect of the mass lesion.

The definitive diagnosis of cancer requires positive cytologic or histologic findings. Sputum samples derived from bronchoscopy are a simple way to diagnose lung cancer in patients whose lesions are centrally located. Pleural fluid samples show positive findings in 40 to 87 percent of patients with malignant pleural effusion.[3] Histologic examination of tissue after biopsy of the pleura, lung tissue, or mediastinal lymph nodes may also be helpful in diagnosing lung cancer. See Chapter 6 for further discussion of tumor classification.

Chest radiographs show abnormal findings in nearly all patients with lung cancer. Common findings are hilar (squamous cell) and/or peripheral (adenocarcinoma) masses, atelectasis, mediastinal widening, infiltrates, pleural effusions, and cavitation (squamous cell). Chest studies are helpful in evaluating tumor size and nodal involvement. Computed tomographic scans of the chest are used for staging and for follow-up study after treatment.

Treatment

Primary treatment options for pulmonary neoplasms are surgery, chemotherapy, radiation, and laser therapy for airway lesions. Immunotherapy is being used in research trials in major clinical settings. Patients are also strongly encouraged to stop smoking.

The treatment of choice for non-small-cell carcinoma is surgery. For nonoperable patients, radiation therapy is the secondary choice. Combination chemotherapy is the treatment of choice for small-cell carcinoma. (See Chapter 11 for a discussion of combination chemotherapy.) Combined chemotherapy and chest radiation therapy has proved effective as a cure for patients in whom disease was detected early. Radiation therapy is also used for palliation of symptoms.

KEY CONCEPTS

- Cigarette smoke is the major cause of lung cancer. Lung cancer is usually disseminated at the time of diagnosis and is associated with a high mortality.
- Lung cancers can develop in the bronchial tree (small cell, squamous cell) or in the parenchyma (large cell, adenocarcinoma).
- Lung cancer may be advanced before symptoms become troublesome. Manifestations include cough, hemoptysis, hoarseness, chest pain, and pleural effusion. The diagnosis is based on examination of cells from bronchial secretions or tissue biopsy. Pulmonary masses may be detected by plain radiography or CT of the chest.
- As with other cancers, treatment includes surgical removal of resectable tumors, followed by radiation therapy and/or chemotherapy.

Pulmonary Hypertension

Etiology

The normal pressure at the pulmonary artery (PA) is 25/10 mm Hg, with a mean of 15 mm Hg. Pulmonary hypertension is defined as a sustained increase in PA pressures above 30 mm Hg systolic or 18 mm Hg mean pressures. In some cases of pulmonary hypertension, systolic pressures may be as high as 60 to 110 mm Hg. Two broad types of pulmonary hypertension exist, primary and secondary. *Primary pulmonary hypertension* is rapidly progressive and occurs most commonly in young women in their 20s and 30s.[8,9] The cause is unknown, but the net effect is increased tone within the pulmonary arteries. The long-term prognosis is poor, and medical management is usually ineffective.

Pulmonary hypertension results from a variety of conditions that produce high pressures in the pulmonary blood vessels. Normally the pulmonary circulation is a high-flow, low-pressure system. Classification of pulmonary hypertension is either primary (idiopathic) or secondary owing to disease processes that produce the pulmonary hypertension.

Secondary pulmonary hypertension is the response to a primary disease process or pathophysiologic condition. Increased pulmonary blood flow, increased resistance to blood flow, and increased left atrial pressure are the three major mechanisms resulting in pulmonary hypertension. Of these, increased resistance to blood flow is the most common cause. Table 23–2 is a list of the major causes of secondary hypertension.

Pathogenesis

In fetal development, the walls of the pulmonary artery are thick, decreasing the internal vessel diameter.

TABLE 23-2. Mechanisms of Secondary Pulmonary Hypertension

Increased Pulmonary Vascular Resistance

Vasoconstrictive
    Alveolar hypoxia due to bronchitis or emphysema
    Acidosis
    High altitude
    Thromboembolic causes from obstruction or release of histamine, serotonin, or catecholamines
    Hypoxia due to neuromuscular disease, obesity, sleep apnea, kyphoscoliosis
Obstructive
    Embolism (blood clots, fat emboli, amniotic emboli, tumor cells, foreign body)
Obliterative (loss of capillary bed)
    Emphysema
    Arteritis
    Lung resection
    Pulmonary fibrosis

Increased Left Atrial Pressure

    Mitral stenosis
    Left ventricular failure
    Constrictive pericarditis

Increased Pulmonary Blood Flow/Viscosity

    Atrial septal defects
    Ventricular septal defects
    Polycythemia
    Patent ductus arteriosus
    Congenital heart disease

After the third day of life, the pulmonary arterial walls dilate and become very thin. Chronic exposure to the mechanisms listed in Table 23–2 (except primary pulmonary hypertension) results in morphologic changes within the arterial lumen. Initially, the walls of the small pulmonary vessels thicken because of an increase in the muscle mass of the media. This initial response is thought to occur as a result of local tissue hypoxia, acidosis, or both.

As the underlying pathologic process intensifies, the internal layer of the pulmonary arterial wall becomes fibrotic, with further muscle thickening. In addition, muscle development occurs in vessels that are normally nonmuscular. Pulmonary atherosclerosis is present in major pulmonary vessels, as well.

Sustained pulmonary hypertension (*mean* PA of 27 to 60 mm Hg) results in the formation of plexiform (network of blood vessels) lesions. These nodular lesions are composed of irregular, interconnecting blood channels which further impede an already compromised pulmonary vasculature. Tissue necrosis and hemorrhage often result.

The pathophysiologic mechanisms of pulmonary hypertension are as follows:

- Loss of at least two thirds of the pulmonary capillary bed[3]
- Increased pulmonary venous pressure
- Increased pulmonary blood flow
- Increased blood viscosity
- Primary pulmonary hypertension

Clinical Manifestations

The clinical manifestations of pulmonary hypertension vary according to the severity and duration of the underlying pathologic process. Because of the normal distensibility of pulmonary capillaries and the ability of the lung to recruit additional reserve capillary beds with increased pressure or flow, patients often remain asymptomatic until significant damage to pulmonary vasculature has occurred. Exercise intolerance (because of progressive loss of pulmonary capillary distention and recruitment capabilities) is often one of the earliest clinical symptoms. Patients may also experience syncope, increasing dyspnea, chest pain on exertion, fatigue, hemoptysis, and pulmonary edema. Eventually, cor pulmonale and right-sided heart failure will develop if persistent, severe pulmonary hypertension continues because of persistent backpressure to the right heart chambers. (Refer to the discussion of cor pulmonale and heart failure in Chapter 18.) Common signs of pulmonary hypertension are a systolic ejection click, narrowing or a splitting of S_2, and accentuation of the pulmonary component of the second heart sound (P_2).[3,10]

Diagnosis

Ideally, PA catheters would be used to obtain PA pressures in patients at risk while at rest and during exercise. Unfortunately, even if mild pulmonary hypertension is present, PA pressures are usually normal at rest. PA pressures measured in the exercising subject would be the optimal diagnostic tool. However, the feasibility of exercising a patient with invasive central line monitoring is problematic. The PA catheter could become wedged and necrosis could occur, or the catheter could slip back into the ventricle and irritate the myocardium, causing ventricular tachycardia. Stress testing without exercise may be done in the cardiac catheterization laboratory by using medications to test the stress response.

Chest radiographs, although usually normal, in cases of mild pulmonary hypertension, are one of the earliest diagnostic tests suggesting the presence of moderate to severe hypertension. Enlargement of the pulmonary arteries and right ventricle, as well as abnormal vessel contours, is indicative of hypertensive disease. Unfortunately, symptoms of the underlying disease process are usually identified before the clinical manifestations of pulmonary hypertension become apparent. The 12-lead electrocardiogram shows evidence of right ventricular hypertrophy. The two-dimensional echocardiogram (a noninvasive technique) can also provide evidence of pulmonary hypertension.

Treatment

The major treatment for pulmonary hypertension is early identification and control of the underlying disease process. In the case of left-to-right shunts, surgical closure of an atrial septal defect or patent ductus arteriosus may be indicated. Because the most common cause of pulmonary hypertension is related to increased pulmonary vascular resistance, treatment is often directed at reversing vasoconstriction by administering supplemental oxygen. Depending on the stage of hypertension, vasodilators and diuretics are commonly used in an attempt to control the symptoms. These medical regimens have produced inconsistent results.[9]

Advanced stages of primary pulmonary hypertension are irreversible. The only feasible intervention is lung or heart-lung transplantation.

KEY CONCEPTS

- Pulmonary hypertension usually results from conditions that increase the resistance of the pulmonary vasculature. Disorders that reduce the total cross-sectional area of the lung increase resistance and promote pulmonary hypertension. Destruction of capillaries (emphysema), blockage of vessels (emboli), and vasoconstriction (hypoxemia) are common examples.

- Pulmonary hypertension may occur when there is elevated left atrial pressure. Pulmonary artery pressure must increase in order to maintain the driving pressure necessary to propel blood through the pulmonary circulation. The excessive pulmonary blood flow that accompanies left-to-right shunting of blood through heart defects may also lead to pulmonary hypertension.

- Cor pulmonale (right ventricular hypertrophy) and right-sided heart failure may develop with sustained high pulmonary vascular resistance. Symptoms of pulmonary hypertension are few until the right side of the heart is affected.

- Treatment centers on efforts to ameliorate the underlying cause if possible (such as closure of heart defects, administration of oxygen to reduce hypoxic vasoconstriction). Vasodilators and diuretics may be used to reduce pulmonary artery pressure and reduce strain on the right side of the heart.

Occupational Lung Diseases

Specific occupational environments predispose workers to particular pulmonary pathologies. Occupational lung diseases result from the inhalation of toxic gases or foreign particles. According to the National Institute for Occupational Safety and Health, approximately 100,000 persons die annually from occupationally related pulmonary disease. In addition, an estimated 400,000 new cases develop yearly.[11]

Traditionally, occupational lung diseases included pathologies related to the effects of exposure to inhaled dusts. However, a holistic approach to these disease entities requires consideration of atmospheric pollutants as well as natural genetic resistance and compliance with health maintenance behaviors. The distinction between occupational and environmental respiratory diseases is becoming increasingly difficult. The integration of multiple environmental areas (home, work, and leisure) further compounds the complexity of occupational respiratory diseases.

Although atmospheric pollutants (toxic gases) are not discussed in detail here, their impact on occupational respiratory diseases must not be minimized. The sources, potential clinical manifestations, and potential disease pathologies associated with common atmospheric pollutants are presented in Table 23–3.

Etiology

Pneumoconiosis is defined as parenchymal lung disease caused by the inhalation of inorganic dust particles. Commonly, the greater the exposure to the dust, the worse are the pathologic consequences. Anthracosis (coal miner's lung or black lung), silicosis (silica inhalation), and asbestosis (asbestoses inhalation) are common examples of occupational lung diseases.[12] However, exposure to several other dusts may also induce respiratory changes. Included in this list are antimony ore, barium, iron, tin, fuller's earth (clay), kaolin (china clay), and talc. Inhalation of dusts from any of these inorganic compounds may result in impaired respiratory function.

Many workers are exposed to "pathogenic dust" through their job and the processing, packaging, or manufacturing of a specific product.[12] Predisposing factors such as preexisting lung disease, exposure to atmospheric pollutants, duration of dust exposure, amount of dust concentration, and particle size will affect the onset and severity of the respiratory impairment.

Pathogenesis

The respiratory tract is protected by two interrelated systems: the mucociliary escalator, and alveolar macrophages. The mucociliary system is composed of bronchial seromucous glands and goblet cells which secrete a mucoid, serous fluid and mucus. Covering the columnar epithelial tissue of the respiratory tract is a bilevel mucous film. The top layer consists of a sticky, tenacious gel that traps particles as they enter the airway. The bottom layer contains cilia and a more liquid mucous layer. Components of the bottom mucous film facilitate the active transport of dust particles up the mucociliary escalator and out of the respiratory tract.

The inhalation of inorganic particles has little effect on the mucociliary system. However, atmospheric pollutants (sulfur oxides, nitrogen oxides, and tobacco smoke) interfere with ciliary action. As a result, the escalator effect is impaired, and inorganic particles are unable to be removed.

Macrophages are debris-consuming cells located in the alveoli. Alveolar macrophages attempt to remove inorganic dust by one of the following methods: (1) engulfing dust and migrating to small airways to use the mucociliary escalator; (2) engulfing dust and exiting through the lymph and/or blood system; (3) engulfing dust and migrating through bronchial walls, depositing dust particles in extra-alveolar tissue; or (4) engulfing dust (specifically silica), with subsequent destruction of the macrophage.[7,12]

Macrophage impairment is the primary mechanism through which inorganic particles initiate lung diseases. In an attempt to maintain a sterile alveolar environment, macrophages secrete **lysosomes** to control foreign particle activity. These enzymes, released in response to the particulate stimuli, eventually damage the alveolar walls, which may cause deposition of fibrous materials. The resulting fibrosis is responsible for the restrictive lung movements causing ventilatory impairment.

Although the type of inorganic particle inhaled does individualize the pathophysiologic response, the general response is similar within the context of occupational lung diseases. Silica is one of the most toxic

TABLE 23–3. Common Atmospheric Pollutants Contributing to Lung Disease

Pollutants	Source	Clinical Manifestations	Potential Disease Pathologies
Carbon monoxide	Automobile exhaust (incomplete fossil fuel combustion)	Lethargy, mental status changes, cherry red mucous membranes, headache	Hypoxemia, respiratory failure
Sulfur oxides	Factories (corrosive, poisonous by-products of combustion of sulfur-containing fuels)	Inflamed mucous membranes, eyes, upper respiratory tract, bronchial mucosa; cough	Pulmonary edema, bronchitis
Photochemical oxidants (ozone)	By-product of exposure of hydrocarbons/nitrogen oxides (from fossil fuel combustion with high temperatures) to sunlight	Inflammation of eyes and upper respiratory tract; cough	Tracheitis, bronchitis, pulmonary edema
Cigarette smoke	Cigarettes (carbon monoxide, nicotine, "tars")	Impaired exercise tolerance, decreased mental activity, tachycardia, hypertension, sweating	Bronchial carcinoma, chronic bronchitis, emphysema, coronary heart disease
Particulate matter	Factories/power stations; small particles, visible smoke and soot	Cough; dyspnea; itchy, watery eyes; irritated mucous membranes	Bronchitis, tracheitis, asthma

particles to alveolar macrophages. Dense deposits of collagen material are formed around the silica particles, resulting in marked fibrotic tissue deposition and restrictive lung disease. Coal dust and asbestos initiate a similar response, although less severe. The pathologies and clinical features for each of the major occupational lung diseases are summarized in Table 23–4.

Clinical Manifestations

Pneumoconioses (anthracosis, asbestosis, silicosis) generally produce no symptoms in the early stages. No physical evidence is present until the pulmonary circulation is impaired or a pulmonary infection develops. Workers may remain symptom free for up to 10 to 20 years with chronic exposure.[3,7] Once again, symptom manifestation is dependent on the predisposing factors already presented.

As the pneumoconioses progress, patients present with a progressive, productive cough and dyspnea, especially with exercise. In addition, patients may complain of progressive weakness and fatigue. Clubbing of fingers may also be present. Late clinical features include chronic hypoxemia, cor pulmonale, and respiratory failure. Table 23–4 provides a summary of the major clinical features for each disease process.

Diagnosis

The reliability of pulmonary changes noted on chest radiographs varies with the severity of the disease. When the patient is symptom free, no changes may be noted. However, as the pneumoconioses progress, micronodular mottling and haziness become apparent. In addition, nodules, fibroses, and calcifications resulting from dust particle deposition are also noted. Pneumoconioses usually produce one of three radiographic findings: nodular, reticular, or linear. However, because of the insidious progression of occupational lung diseases, radiographs negative for lung disease do not exclude the presence of the disease process.

Pulmonary function tests may also be normal in the early stages of disease manifestations. However, as the condition worsens, decreases in forced expiratory volume and vital capacity occur. Changes in pulmonary function tests demonstrate predominantly restrictive impairment with a component of obstructive functional impairment, depending on the severity and type of dust inhalation.

Finally, hypoxemia is evident from arterial blood gas measurements in the late disease stages. Falling partial pressure of oxygen (Pao_2) levels are accompanied by decreased partial pressure of carbon dioxide ($Paco_2$) levels as the body initially compensates for the hypoxemia with an increased respiratory drive. However, as the disease progresses, both hypoxemia and hypercapnia are evident.

Treatment

Preventive measures are the key to limiting the onset and severity of occupational lung diseases. Adherence to federal standards for dust and particulate matter, as well as continuing education of workers and employers, will have a dramatic impact on the incidence of respiratory diseases. The use of respirators for miners and water sprays to decrease airborne particles in mines are two examples of common prevention techniques. Early evaluation of a work environment predisposed to occupational lung diseases is where "treatment" must begin.

Two primary goals in the treatment of active occupational lung diseases are to prevent further parenchymal damage and to relieve signs and symptoms, when possible. Ideally, if the problematic dust can be identified, the individual should be removed from the environment. However, if a job change is unrealistic, every possible measure must be implemented to prevent further inhalation of dust particles. Included in this treatment is the evaluation of current health maintenance behaviors.

TABLE 23–4. Major Occupational Lung Pneumoconioses

Pneumoconioses	Pathology	Clinical Features
Anthracosis (coal miner's lung)	*Early:* Collection of coal particles with small amount of dilation of airway	*Early:* Minimal to no symptoms. May be seen with dyspnea with cough, but often due to unrelated bronchitis or emphysema
	Late: Progressive, massive fibrosis, with condensed areas of black fibrous tissue noted	*Late:* Worsening dyspnea with excretion, productive cough, respiration failure
Silicosis	Dense collagen deposits in respiratory bronchioles, alveoli, and along lymphatics	*Early:* No symptoms noted
		Late: Productive cough, dyspnea, especially with exercise; increased risk for tuberculosis
Asbestosis	Fibrous deposits secondary to long, thin fibers allowing deep lung penetration	Progressive dyspnea on exertion, weakness, clubbing of fingers; pleural thickening with plaque development

Active signs and symptoms are treated with corticosteroids, bronchodilators, oxygen therapy, and respiratory treatments (intermittent positive pressure ventilation, postural drainage, and deep breathing). The effectiveness and utilization of these therapies depend on the patient's condition and the stage of disease. Rarely are disease pathologies reversed with medical treatment. The usual goal is to halt symptom progression.

KEY CONCEPTS

- Occupational lung diseases result from chronic inhalation of gases and inert particles. Commonly identified particles include coal, silica, and asbestos. Smoking and environmental pollutants may be contributing factors because they depress the ciliary function necessary to remove inhaled particles.

- The presence of inert particles in the alveoli initiates macrophage activity and inflammation. Inert particles cannot be digested by phagocytes, so they are walled off by deposition of fibrous proteins.

- Manifestations of pneumoconioses are related to the restrictive nature of the pulmonary dysfunction. Progressive dyspnea, decreased vital capacity and functional residual capacity, and increased respiratory rate are common. Blood gases show progressive hypoxemia; carbon dioxide levels may remain normal or low until late in the disease.

- Treatment includes prevention of further exposure and administration of corticosteroids, bronchodilators, and oxygen therapy.

Pulmonary Embolism

Etiology

Pulmonary emboli (PE) are undissolved materials that occlude blood vessels of the pulmonary vasculature. As a result, circulation distal to the obstruction is impaired. Approximately 500,000 patients are affected annually with an estimated 20 percent (100,000 patients) mortality rate. Of those who experience fatal PE, 80,000 die within 2 hours of the onset of initial symptoms.[1]

Pulmonary emboli are the sequelae of other pathologic changes in the body and not a primary disease process in themselves. The most common sources of PE are thrombi (blood clots). Ninety-five percent of thrombi form in the thighs and legs. Approximately 85 to 95 percent of PE arise from the iliofemoral veins.[12] Other sources of PE include fat, air, and amniotic fluid. The types of emboli and their causes are summarized in Table 23–5.

Virchow, a pathologist of the 1800s, discovered three physiologic factors that predispose patients to thrombus formation, increasing the risk of PE. The three factors, commonly referred to as Virchow's triad, are venous stasis/sluggish blood flow, hypercoagulability, and damage to the venous wall (intimal

TABLE 23–5. Embolism Types and Causes

Embolism Types	Etiology
Thrombotic	Blood clots develop in the venous system, predominantly in the thighs and legs
Fat	Globules of fat secondary to fractures of the pelvis or lower extremities
Amniotic fluid	Collections of fluid, hair, or other debris related to complicated labor, especially in older, multiparous women
Air	Venous access through IV catheters
Tumor	Fragments from malignant tissue
Foreign material	Foreign bodies (bullets, sutures, catheter tips, orally prepared medications injected IV)
Septic	Infected tissue or related substances
Parasitic	Parasites present in lung vasculature

injury). Several predisposing factors enhance the probability of thrombus development and the subsequent risk for PE. Using Virchow's triad, predisposing factors have been categorized under each of the three components. Table 23–6 provides a summary of the major predisposing factors using Virchow's framework.

Pathogenesis

Thrombi are dislodged from their point of origin by multiple mechanisms, including direct trauma, the effect of exercise and muscle action, and changes in blood flow. Once released into the venous system, thrombi are referred to as emboli and travel toward

TABLE 23–6. Factors Predisposing to Pulmonary Embolism in Virchow's Framework

Venous Stasis

Extended bed rest (delayed venous removal of activated clotting factors)
Immobility (activated clotting factors)
Vascular disorders (thrombophlebitis of the lower extremities and pelvic area)
Congestive heart failure (venous backflow/stasis)
Cardiac arrhythmias (atrial fibrillation)
Dehydration

Hypercoagulability

Oral contraceptives (estrogen therapy)
Pregnancy
Polycythemia (chronic high altitude; chronic pulmonary disease with decreased Pao_2 and increased $Paco_2$)
Malignant pathologies
Cigarette smoking

Damage to Vessel Wall (Intimal Injury)

Blunt trauma
Penetrating wounds
Bone fractures with soft tissue injury
Surgical procedures (hip, pelvic, abdominal, cardiovascular)
Obstetric manipulations during labor and delivery

the heart and lungs. Regardless of whether the emboli are actual blood clots or an alternative type of material (see Table 23–5), the undissolved material travels to the pulmonary vasculature. Most PE lodge in the right lower lobe of the lung owing to the normal increased blood flow to the lower lobes.[12]

The impact of PE on the cardiopulmonary circulation depends on the size and cross-sectional area of circulatory impairment. If the emboli occlude less than 25 percent of the pulmonary vessels in a healthy individual, no physiologic changes are seen. When the occlusive area approaches 25 to 30 percent, PA pressures may begin to rise, with potential right-sided heart failure.[1,12] In the patient without any underlying pulmonary pathology, 50 percent of the cross-sectional pulmonary circulation must be impaired before dangerously high PA pressures are generated. Because of the tremendous pulmonary capillary reserve, significant damage is necessary before pulmonary decompensation occurs.

PA pressures increase because of vasoconstriction from actual mechanical obstruction of blood vessels and the release of serotonin and neural sympathetic stimulation in a combined neurohormonal response. Right-sided heart failure occurs because of the high resistance generated by the pulmonary vasculature. Eventually, hypotension occurs as a result of diminished cardiac output.

Actual pulmonary infarction (death of lung parenchyma) occurs only in about 10 to 15 percent of the cases of PE.[1,12] Pulmonary necrosis is rare because there are three sources available for oxygen supply: the PA circulation, the bronchial arterial circulation, and the airways. Significant underlying pulmonary or cardiac impairment (chronic obstructive pulmonary disease, mitral stenosis) increase the risk for pulmonary infarctions to occur.[8]

Clinical Manifestations

Presenting symptoms depend on the size of the emboli as well as on any underlying cardiopulmonary pathologies. Initial symptoms may include restlessness, apprehension, and anxiety. In addition, tachycardia and tachypnea are often present. Sudden dyspnea and severe chest pain are usually associated with medium-sized or massive emboli. Hemoptysis may or may not occur. As the clinical picture worsens, patients experience heart failure, shock, and respiratory arrest.

Diagnosis

The ventilation/perfusion ($\dot{V}/\dot{Q}$) lung scan is the primary test performed to determine the presence of a PE. If capable, the patient is asked to breath xenon gas after being injected with labeled albumin. The lung scanning device determines if a mismatch exists between ventilation and perfusion. Adequate ventilation with impaired perfusion (blood flow) to the pulmonary vasculature (mismatch) is indicative of PE if the scan is performed within 8 hours of symptom onset.

Other screening tests such as arterial blood gases, electrocardiograms, chest radiographs, and cardiac enzyme determinations are valuable tools to rule out related pathologies. However, the only conclusive diagnostic test for PE is pulmonary arteriography. This invasive procedure involves the injection of radiopaque material into the pulmonary artery. If an intraluminal filling deficit can be identified, the test is considered diagnostic for PE.

Treatment

The primary treatment for PE is prevention. Patients who are at risk for developing one of the factors of Virchow's triad must be prophylactically treated. In the case of prolonged bed rest, active range-of-motion exercises as well as prophylactic low-dose subcutaneous heparin may be used. The treatment must be directed at eliminating or decreasing the specific predisposing factor(s) placing individuals at risk.

If prevention is unattainable, rapid, early detection of patients presenting with PE is vital. Unfortunately, owing to the variability of symptoms and size of emboli, PE are often undiagnosed. Therefore, identification of risk factors with the ability to integrate vague symptoms (anxiety, tachypnea) is the key to maximizing optimal patient outcomes.

Patients with suspected or confirmed PE are given supplemental oxygen with immediate activity limitations to decrease oxygen demand. The goals of treatment are to prevent lung parenchymal necrosis and return the pulmonary circulation to normal as rapidly as possible. Patients are given a bolus of heparin and started on a continuous heparin IV drip to maintain an activated partial thromboplastin time 1.5 to 2.5 times greater than the control. Although heparin does not dissolve the clot, formation of further clots is prevented. Heparin may also stimulate the intrinsic fibrolytic system, enhancing the degradation of PE. Thrombolytic therapy using streptokinase, tissue-type plasminogen activator, or Eminase may be used to dissolve the emboli. However, these compounds create an increased risk of bleeding, and unless the patient is extremely ill with a massive embolism, they are not used. Assuming a patient survives the acute phase, the key to treatment is the identification of the source and a proactive plan to prevent future occurrences.

Depending on the severity of the PE, ventilatory support may also be necessary. If patients are thought to be releasing multiple emboli despite adequate heparin therapy, an umbrella filter (Mobin-Uddin) or a "bird's nest" filter may be placed in the inferior vena cava to trap emboli as they migrate toward the pulmonary vasculature.[6] An embolectomy may be performed on an emergency basis, if the hemodynamic conseqeunces of the emboli are life-threatening.

KEY CONCEPTS

- Pulmonary emboli result in obstruction of blood flow through part of the pulmonary system. When emboli are large or multiple, a significant increase in pulmonary pressure may result, causing right ventricular failure.
- Emboli may be composed of fat, air, amniotic fluid, or thrombi (blood clot). Thrombi are the most common cause. Thrombi generally form in the leg under conditions of venous stasis, enhanced coagulation, or vascular trauma.
- Pulmonary embolism is suspected with sudden dyspnea and chest pain. Symptoms of right-sided heart failure may be present when emboli are large. A ventilation-perfusion scan may be done to confirm the diagnosis.
- Prophylactic anticoagulation in persons at risk for thrombus formation is important to prevent PE. Bed rest, oxygen, thrombolytic therapy, and anticoagulation are the mainstays of therapy for acute PE. Ventilator support and measures to improve the functioning of the right side of the heart may be necessary in severe cases.

Summary

This chapter has discussed a variety of respiratory diseases that do not strictly fit into the categories of respiratory obstructive diseases or restrictive diseases. Increasing environmental pollution and occupational hazards have led to increased numbers of patients with these diseases being seen by health care workers. A summary of research findings related to these respiratory diseases is presented in Table 23–7.

TABLE 23–7. Research Findings Related to Vascular, Neoplastic, Infectious, and Occupational Respiratory Diseases

Authors/Study	Findings
Lee et al[13]	Tuberculosis pleurisy was treated in 40 patients with either prednisolone or placebo. All patients were also being treated with isoniazed, rifampin, and ethambutol. Clinical signs and symptoms (fever, chest pain, dyspnea) subsided in 2.4 days in the treatment group as compared to 9.2 days in the placebo group. X-ray findings showed improvement in 54.5 days in the treatment group and 123.2 days in the placebo group.
Dutt et al[14]	A 4-month course of isoniazed and rifampin was used in 414 patients with positive tuberculin tests and abnormal x-rays but negative cultures. The rate of relapse was 1.2% in patients followed for a median of 44 months. This is comparable to the relapse rate in culture- and smear-positive patients who received therapy for 9 months.
Mehta et al[15]	Patterns of isoniazed use for preventive therapy in 32,722 contacts of infected persons during 1979–1985 were studied. Of infected contacts, 67% were given preventative therapy and only 37% were given therapy in 1985.
Stead et al[16]	The records of 52,000 residents of nursing homes in Arkansas were reviewed to determine the number of patients receiving isoniazed, duration of therapy, and evidence of hepatic toxicity. Data on 1,935 patients were analyzed. Therapy was discontinued in 84 patients for hepatic toxicity and 116 patients for drug intolerance. There were 135 deaths during therapy, but none related to isoniazed therapy.
Gorensek et al[17]	This study followed 50 heart or heart-lung transplant recipients for 34 months to determine risk factors associated with pneumonia development. The most significant factors were the need for reintubation and the use of large doses of steroids.
Kessler et al[18]	Forty-seven patients with PE were infused with 50 mg of tPA initially, followed by another 40 mg if lysis of the clot was not apparent. Nineteen patients showed improvement after 2 hr; the remaining 28 required 6 hr of infusion. Clinical improvement was noted in 44 patients, and 57% showed marked lysis of the clot.
Brownlee et al[19]	Hemodynamic data were collected while they were breathing room air and 95% FIO_2 15 and 30 min after nifedipine dosing. In children breathing room air after nifedipine, the mean PA pressure decreased 34% and the pulmonary vascular resistance decreased 49%. CO increased significantly.
Caporaso et al[20]	The risk of lung cancer was evaluated in smokers. Lung cancer patients ($n = 245$) were compared with controls ($n = 234$) having asthma, bronchitis, and emphysema. The ability of these patients to metabolize debrisoquine was studied. Patients who metabolized debrisoquine extensively had at a fourfold greater risk of lung cancer than poor metabolizers. The combined risk of high metabolization rate and occupational exposure to asbestos led to an 18-fold increase risk.
Pallares et al[21]	Data on 72 patients with penicillin-resistant pneumonia were collected: 24 in the treatment group (penicillin-resistant pneumococci) and 48 in the control group (penicillin-sensitive pneumococci). Mortality was 54% in the treatment group and 25% in the control group. Deaths occurred exclusively in patients with initial critical conditions.
Goodglick et al[22]	Mouse macrophages were exposed to crocadolite asbestos, which led to dose- and time-dependent increases in lipid peroxidation and cell death. Cell death was presented by the administration of superoxide dismutase plus catalase, deproxamine, vitamin E, and 3-aminobingamid.
Garcia et al[23]	Bronchoalveolar lavage was used to detect asbestos-induced alveolities in 93 patients exposed to asbestos, 12 smokers, and 10 nonsmokers. The 12 patients with clinical evidence of disease had increased neutrophils and eosinophils. These findings correlated well with pulmonary dysfunction and chest x-ray abnormalities. The release of the chemotoxin LTB_4 also correlated well with the severity of the disease.
Samet[24]	The author reviewed research literature related to exposure to radon and the development of lung cancer. Mixed results in the relationship of radon exposure to lung cancer risk were found.

Table continued on following page

T A B L E 23 – 7. Research Findings Related to Vascular, Neoplastic, Infectious, and Occupational Respiratory Diseases Continued

Authors/Study	Findings
Ernster[25]	Trends in smoking in the United States reveal that one fourth of the general population smokes. The decision to begin smoking occurs in the teenage years. An estimated 30% of all cancer deaths are associated with smoking.
Fielding et al[26]	In a review of the literature (13 studies) pertinent to the risk of lung cancer among nonsmokers married to smokers, nine studies showed a positive relationship.
Kawochi et al[27]	In New Zealand the estimated prevalence of exposure to passive smoking in the workplace is 34% for men and 23% for women. Estimates of lung cancer from passive smoking were 2.3% for both men and women at home and 2.2% for exposure at work. The estimated risks of ischemic heart disease from passive smoking were 2.3% for men and 1.9% for women.
Kurrer et al[28]	This cooperative international research study investigated the use of surgical resection for small-cell bronchial carcinoma in combination with one of two types of intensive chemotherapeutic regimens: a sequential alternating regimen or a standard nonalternating regimen. Differences between chemotherapeutic regimens were not significant.
Smit et al[29]	Etoposide was given to elderly patients with small-cell lung cancer. Seventy-one percent of 33 patients responded to therapy, and 6 went into remission. The incidence of bone marrow suppression was low, which has been a concern in elderly patients owing to toxicity.
Chan-Yeung et al[30]	A review of the literature related long-term exposure of workers (including farmers; grain elevator workers; dock workers; and feed, flour, and seed mill workers) to grain dust with a variety of respiratory syndromes. The report includes a discussion of the composition and physical and biochemical characteristics of grain dust. Such occupational exposure is linked to acute syndromes such as asthma, grain fever, acute respiratory disease, and skin and mucous membrane irritation syndrome as well as more chronic complications such as chronic bronchitis and emphysema. The authors also discuss relevant host factors such as atopy, smoking, α_1-antitrypsin deficiency, and nonspecific bronchial hyperresponsiveness in the pathogenesis of lung diseases.
Agostini et al[31]	A review of the literature on AIDS and its effects on the lungs. The authors describe how HIV-1 gains access to the lungs and infects host cells; the mechanisms by which the virus becomes latent and by which it is later reactivated; and the roles of the pulmonary and immune systems in normal body defenses. Impairment of these defenses after HIV infection leads to opportunistic infections. The authors suggest that the pulmonary immune response to HIV may play a role in the development of respiratory failure and propose models to explain the effect of HIV-1 on the lung.
Mulshine et al[32]	Reviews the literature on lung cancer initiation and promotion. The authors describe the early stages of cancer growth, including possible roles of oncogenes and tumor suppressor genes in initiation. Interventions with 13-cis-retinoic acid, anti-growth factors, and peptide hormone agonists may prevent or slow the spread of cancer in those at high risk for the disease, especially smokers and ex-smokers.
Richardson et al[33]	An overview of the latest information regarding lung cancer. Emphasis is placed on hormones produced by both cancerous and noncancerous lung cells that may somehow regulate growth in cancerous cells. The role of gene mutations and oncogenes is also described. An excellent though highly technical article.
Tang et al[34]	Treatment of lung cancer with the usual techniques of surgery, chemotherapy, and/or radiation has not led to improvements in mortality rates. The authors describe the advantages and mechanism of gene therapy in the treatment of lung cancers and identify specific genes that have been effective in animal systems. Gene therapy has tremendous potential for future use, but more refined delivery mechanisms must be developed and specific genes identified before this technology can be widely applied.

REFERENCES

1. Doyle J, Johantgen M, Vitello-Cicciu J: Vascular disease, in Kinney MB, Packa DR, Dunbar SB (eds): *AACN's Clinical Reference for Critical-Care Nursing*, 2nd ed. New York, McGraw-Hill, 1988, pp 727–755.
2. Hollander H: Infectious diseases: Mycotic, in Schroder SA, Tierney LM, McPhee SS, Papadakis MA, Krupp MA (eds): *Current Medical Diagnosis and Treatment*. Norwalk, Conn, Appleton & Lange, 1993, pp 1149–1157.
3. Stauffer JL: Pulmonary diseases, In Schroeder SA, Tierney LM, McPhee SJ, Papdakis MA, Krupp MA (eds): *Current Medical Diagnoses and Treatment*. Norwalk, Conn, Appleton & Lange, 1993, 177–256.
4. Minna JD: Neoplasms of the lung, in Wilson JD, Braunwald E, Isselbacher KJ (eds): *Harrison's Principles of Internal Medicine*. 2 vols. New York, McGraw-Hill, 1991.
5. Nursing 84 Books: Controlling Environmental Disease. *Nurse's Clinical Library: Respiratory Disorders*. Springhouse, Penn, Springhouse Corporation, 1984, pp 171–181.
6. Turley K: Thoracic wall, pleura, mediastinum, and lung, in Way LW (ed): *Current Surgical Diagnosis and Treatment*. Norwalk, Conn, Appleton & Lange, 1991, pp 307–348.
7. West JB: Occupation and other diseases, in West JB (ed): *Pulmo-nary Pathophysiology—The Essentials*, 3rd ed. Baltimore, Williams & Wilkins, 1987, pp 134–153.
8. West JB: Vascular diseases, in West JB (ed): *Pulmonary Pathophysiology—The Essentials*, 4th ed. Baltimore, Williams & Wilkins, 1992, 108–128.
9. Packer M: Vasodilator therapy for primary pulmonary hypertension: Limitations and hazards. *Ann Intern Med*. 1985; 103:258–270.
10. Mergner WJ, Trump BF: Hemodynamic disorders, in Rubin E, Farber J (eds): *Pathology*. Philadelphia, JB Lippincott, 1993, pp 252–273.
11. Smith W: Chronic lung disease, in *A Profile of Health and Disease in America: Respiratory and Infectious Diseases*. New York, Facts on File Publications, 1987, pp 88–98.
12. Kersten LD: Restrictive pulmonary disease, in *Comprehensive Respiratory Nursing: A Decision-Making Approach*. Philadelphia, WB Saunders, 1989, pp 121–158.
13. Lee CH, Wang WJ, Lan RS, et al: Corticosteroids in the treatment of tuberculous pleurisy: A double blind placebo-controlled, randomized study. *Chest* 1988;94:1256–1259.
14. Dutt AK, Moers D, Stead WW: Smear negative and culture positive pulmonary tuberculosis: Six-month short course chemotherapy with isonazid and rifampin. *Am Rev Respir Dis* 1990; 141:1232.

15. Mehta JB, Dutt AK, Harvill L, et al: Isoniazid preventive therapy for tuberculosis: Are we losing our enthusiasm? *Chest* 1988;94:138–141.

16. Stead WW, To T, Harrison RW, et al: Benefit-risk considerations in preventative treatment for tuberculosis in elderly persons. *Ann Intern Med* 1987;107:843–845.

17. Gorensek MJ, Steward RW, Keys TF, et al: A multivariate analysis of risk factors for pneumonia following cardiac transplantation. *Transplantation* 1988;46:860–865.

18. Kessler CN, Druy E, Goldhaber: Acute pulmonary embolism treated with thrombolytic agents: Current status of tPA and future implications for emergency medicine. *Ann Emerg Med* 1988;17:1216–1220.

19. Brownlee JR, Beekonen RW, Rosenthal A: Acute hemodynamic effects of nifedipine in infants with bronchopulmonary dysplasia and pulmonary hypertension. *Pediatr Res* 1988;24:186–190.

20. Caporaso N, Hayes RB, Dosemeci M, et al: Lung cancer risk, occupational exposure, the debrisoquine metabolic phenotype. *Cancer Res* 1989;49:3675–3679.

21. Pallares R, Gudiol F, Linares J, et al: Risk factors and response to antibiotic therapy in adults with bacteremic pneumonia caused by penicillin-resistant pneumococci. *N Engl J Med* 1987;317:18–22.

22. Goodglick LA, Pietras LA, Kane AB: Evaluation of the causal relationship between crocadolite asbestos-induced lipid peroxidation and toxicity to macrophages. *Am Rev Respir Dis* 1989;139:1265–1272.

23. Garcia JGN, Griffith DE, Cohen AB, et al: Alveolar macrophages from patients with asbestos exposure release increased levels of leukotriene B$_4$. *Am Rev Respir Dis* 1989;139:1494–1501.

24. Samet JM: Radon and lung cancer. *JNCI* 1986;81:745–747.

25. Ernster VL: Trends in smoking, cancer risks and cigarette promotion: Current priorities for reducing tobacco exposure. *Cancer* 1988;62:1702–1712.

26. Fielding JE, Phenow KJ: Health effects of involuntary smoking. *N Engl J Med* 1988;319:1452–1460.

27. Kawochi I, Pearce NE, Jackson RT: Deaths from lung cancer and ischemic heart disease due to passive smoking in New Zealand. *NZ J Med* 1989;102:337–340.

28. Kurrer K, Shields TW, Donck H, et al: The importance of surgical and multimodality treatment for small cell bronchial carcinoma. *J Thorac Cardiovasc Surg* 1989;97:168–176.

29. Smit EF, Carney DN, Harford D, et al: A Phase II study of oral etoposide in elderly patients with small cell lung cancer. *Thorax* 1989;44:631–635.

30. Chan-Yeung M, Enarson DA, Kennedy SM: The impact of grain dust on respiratory health. *Am Rev Respir Dis* 1992;145;476–487.

31. Agostini C, Trentin L, Zambello R, et al: HIV-1 and the lung: Infectivity, pathogenic mechanisms, and cellular immune responses taking place in the lower respiratory tract. *Am Rev Respir Dis* 1993;147:1038–1049.

32. Mulshine JL, Treston AM, Brown PH, et al: Initiators and promotors of lung cancer. *Chest* 1993;103:4S–11S.

33. Richardson GE, Johnson BE: The biology of cancer. *Semin Oncol* 1993;20:105–127.

34. Tang D, Carbone DP: Potential applications of gene therapy to lung cancer. *Semin Oncol* 1993;20:368–372.

BIBLIOGRAPHY

American Thoracic Society: Diagnostic standards and classification of tuberculosis. *Am Rev Respir Dis* 1990;142(3):725–735.

Athayde J, Shore ET: Invasive pulmonary aspergillosis presenting as massive hemoptysis in a nonimmunocompromised host. *Chest* 1993;103(3):960–961.

Barnes PF, Bloch AB, Davidson PT, Snider DE Jr: Tuberculosis in patients with human immunodeficiency virus infection. *N Engl J Med* 1991;324(23):1644–1650.

Bascom R: Occupational and environmental respiratory diseases: A medicolegal primer for physicians. *Occup Med* 1992;7(2):331–345.

Batra P, Brown K, Aberle DR, Young DA, Steckel R: Imaging techniques in the evaluation of pulmonary parenchymal neoplasms. *Chest* 1992;101(1):239–243.

Bradbury F: Comparison of azithromycin versus clarithromycin in the treatment of patients with lower respiratory tract infection. *J Antimicrob Chemother* 1993;31:153–162.

Carson JL, Kelley MA, Duff A, et al: The clinical course of pulmonary embolism. *N Engl J Med* 1992;326(19):1240–1245.

Dichter JR, Levine SJ, Shelhamer JH: Approach to the immunocompromised host with pulmonary symptoms. *Hematol Oncol Clin North Am* 1993;7(4):887–912.

Dichter JR: Drugs for tuberculosis. *Med Lett Drugs Ther* 1992;34(868):10–12.

Dutt AK, Moers D, Stead WW: Smear-negative, culture-positive pulmonary tuberculosis: Six-month chemotherapy with isoniazid and rifampin. *Am Rev Respir Dis* 1990;141(5):1232–1248.

Fang GD, Fine M, Orloff J, et al: New and emerging etiologies for community-acquired pneumonia with implications for therapy: A prospective multicenter study of 359 cases. *Medicine* 1990;69(5):307–316.

Ferson MJ: Infections in day care. *Curr Opin Pediatr* 1993;5(1):35–40.

Goldhaber SZ: Evolving concepts in thrombolytic therapy for pulmonary embolism. *Chest* 1992;101(4 suppl):183S–185S.

Goren A, Bibi H, Goldsmith JR: Prospective lung health monitoring in relation to a new power plant. *Public Health Rev* 1991–1992;19(1–4):103–108.

Hazuka MB, Bunn PA Jr: Controversies in the nonsurgical treatment of stage III non-small cell lung cancer. *Am Rev Respir Dis* 1992;145(4):967–977.

Hirsh J: Heparin. *N Engl J Med* 1991;324(22):1565–1574.

Hirsh J: Oral anticoagulant drugs. *N Engl J Med* 1991;324(26):1865–1875.

Little AG, Stitik FP: Clinical staging of patients with non-small cell lung cancer. *Chest* 1990;97(6):1431–1438.

Lopes AAB, Maeda NY, Aiello VD, Ebaid M, Bydlowski SP: Endothelial expression of von Willebrand factor in pulmonary hypertension. *Chest* 1993;104(5):1455–1460.

Maeda K, Nitta H, Nakai S: Exposure to nitrogen oxides and other air pollutants from automobiles. *Public Health Rev* 1991–1992;19(1–4):61–72.

McDonnell F, Zenick H, Hayes CG: U.S. Environmental Protection Agency's Ozone Epidemiology Research Program: A strategy for assessing the effects of ambient ozone exposure upon morbidity in exposed populations. *J Air Waste Management Assoc* 1993;43(7):950–954.

Mohs E, Rodriguez-Solares A, Rivas E, el-Hoshy Z: A comparative study of azithromycin and amoxycillin in paediatric patients with acute otitis media. *J Antimicrob Chemother* 1993;31:73–79.

Morales CF, Strollo PJ: Noncardiogenic pulmonary edema associated with accidental hypothermia. *Chest* 1993;103(3):971–973.

Nelson DM: Interventions related to respiratory care. *Nurs Clin North Am* 1992;27(2):301–323.

Pachon J, Prados MD, Capote F, Cuello JA, Garnacho J, Verano A: Severe community-acquired pneumonia: Etiology, prognosis, and treatment. *Am Rev Respir Dis* 1990;142(2):369–373.

Richards RJ, Oreffo VI: Respiratory tract epithelium and neoplasia. *Respir Med* 1993;87(3):175–181.

Ruben FL: Viral pneumonias. The increasing importance of a high index of suspicion. *Postgrad Med* 1993;93(7):57–60, 63–64.

Samet JM: Health benefits of smoking cessation. *Clin Chest Med* 1991;12(4):669–679.

Shamssain MH: Pulmonary function and symptoms in workers exposed to wood dust. *Thorax* 1992;47(2):84–87.

Shapiro ED et al: The protective efficacy of polyvalent pneumococcal polysaccharide vaccine. *N Engl J Med* 1991;325:1453.

Stark JM: Lung infections in children. *Curr Opin Pediatr* 1993;5(3):273–280.

Stein PD, Henry JW, Gottschalk A: Mismatched vascular defects: An easy alternative to mismatched segmented equivalent defects for the interpretation of ventilation/perfusion lung scans in pulmonary embolism. *Chest* 1993;104(5):1468–1471.

Strauss P, Orris P, Buckley L: A health survey of toll booth workers. *Am J Ind Med* 1992;22(3):379–384.

Tidwell BH, Cleary JD: *Pseudomonas aeruginosa*-acquired resistance to imipenem-cilastatin: Commentary on clinical implications of antibiotic resistance. *Pharmacotherapy* 1992;12(5):391–396.

Winterbauer RH: Atypical pneumonia syndromes. *Clin Chest Med* 1991;12:203. Editorial.

UNIT VII
Alterations in Fluid, Electrolyte, and Acid-Base Homeostasis

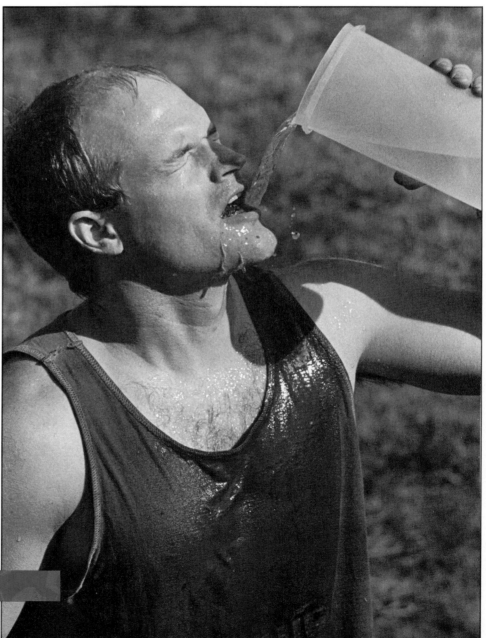

After intense exercise, a runner replaces fluid.

Photo by Kathleen Kelly

Humans are awash in fluids, and when they are not sufficiently awash, as is often the case with those who are extremely obese or with dehydrated elderly people, they have trouble living normally and are in danger of diseases that do not afflict those who maintain a normal amount and balance of fluids. This "sea within us" nourishes and cleanses the body, conducting essential minerals through the body and allowing for the exchange of nutrients and cellular excreta. The level of this sea is important for everyone and vitally important for some groups, such as the elderly, for whom dehydration causes common fluid or electrolyte imbalances.

The body's fluids are divided into intracellular, inside the cell, and extracellular, outside the cell membrane, compartments. The main extracellular electrolytes (dissolved minerals) include sodium, calcium, chlorides, and bicarbonate. The intracellular electrolytes are potassium, phosphate, and magnesium.

Sodium and potassium are the extracellular electrolytes that get most attention, but magnesium, calcium, and phosphorus also are important. One author calls them "the other electrolytes" and suggests that their presence in the ever-shifting volumes of water and electrolytes within the body is vital to the body's balance, or homeostasis. Too little or too much of any of these electrolytes can cause serious problems and be the sign of a multitude of disorders.

Magnesium, the most abundant intracellular electrolyte, is found in bones, in the extracellular fluid, and in other soft tissues. It influences neuromuscle activity, acts on skeletal muscle, and contributes to vasodilation in the cardiovascular system.

Magnesium's importance is suggested by the variety of consequences to the body when it is not present in adequate amounts, either through reduced intake or absorption or increased loss of the mineral. Malnutrition is one cause of lowered intake. Because it is absorbed in the lower gastrointestinal (GI) tract, disruptions in this system may decrease uptake. Fluid loss from the lower GI tract, through diarrhea, among other causes, can drain away essential magnesium.

Insufficient magnesium is most often found in the form of symptomatic hypomagnesemia among acute alcoholics, whose poor nutrition, impaired renal function, intestinal malabsorption, and diarrhea combine to deplete magnesium, producing an array of possible neuromuscular, neurologic, and cardiac symptoms.

Numbness, tingling in the extremities or around the mouth, muscle cramps in extremities, and abdominal muscle spasms may be signs of hypocalcemia, a serious deficiency of calcium seen more frequently in recent years among critically ill patients.

Calcium, researcher Judy Terry observes, "plays an active role in keeping us upright and moving" by strengthening our bones and teeth and by helping heart muscle tissue contract properly. She describes the system by which the calcium balance is maintained as being "very intricate." When extracellular fluid calcium declines, the parathyroid glands respond by producing a hormone that increases reabsorption of calcium from the renal tubules, increases absorption from the gastrointestinal tract, and prompts release of bone calcium phosphate. In contrast, if there is too much calcium in the body, the body acts to inhibit it.

FRONTIERS OF RESEARCH
The Cellular Environment
Michael J. Kirkhorn

The parathyroid also governs concentrations of phosphorus in the body. A severe shortage of phosphorus is common among alcoholics and has many of the same causes as alcohol-related magnesium deficit. Symptoms include weakness, irritability, apprehension, numbness, dysarthria, and ataxia. An excess of phosphorus often is caused by renal disease.

Conscious prevention will help patients avoid electrolyte imbalances, but when they do occur, treatment may require expert intravenous nursing care by health professionals who must know the signs, symptoms, causes, and treatments. Precise treatment is necessary because even offering a snack or a drink to a hospital patient with electrolyte imbalances could influence the balance and because imbalances can affect a number of body systems.

It is also necessary for health professionals to remind themselves of the influence of seasonal or regional variations. Extreme or persistent heat or dryness complicates the fluid balance picture and is especially crucial for the elderly and for other groups, such as children playing outside on hot days.

One researcher noticed a coincidence between a population living in extreme heat, which concentrates the urine, and a high incidence of urinary stones. The highly concentrated urine of dehydrated desert-dwellers in southern Israel contributes to the appearance of urinary stones, and renal diseases, sometimes fatal, may result.

As with many cases of preventive care, the solution seems obvious. Children should be taught to drink frequently, recharging the seas within them regardless of thirst, and protecting them from stones and renal disease.

CHAPTER 24
Fluid and Electrolyte Homeostasis and Imbalances

LINDA FELVER

KEY TERMS

body fluid: The water contained in the body plus the substances dissolved in it.

body water: All of the water contained in the body.

electrolyte: Substance that releases charged particles (ions) when dissolved.

extracellular fluid: Body fluid that is not inside the cells; includes vascular, interstitial, and transcellular fluids.

filtration: Movement of fluid across capillary walls, as a net result of opposing forces.

hypertonic fluid: Fluid that has a higher particle concentration (osmolality) than normal body fluid; causes a net flow of water out of the cell.

hypotonic fluid: Fluid that has a lower particle concentration (osmolality) than normal body fluid; causes a net flow of water across the cell membrane into the cell.

interstitial fluid: Fluid that lies between the cells; a component of extracellular fluid.

intracellular fluid: Fluid that is inside the cells.

ion: A charged particle, such as Na^+ or K^+ (cations) or Cl^- (anion).

isotonic fluid: Fluid that has the same particle concentration (osmolality) as normal body fluid.

osmosis: Movement of water across a semipermeable membrane to equalize the particle concentration of the fluid on both sides of the membrane.

transcellular fluid: Body fluid contained in special compartments such as the synovial or cerebrospinal compartments; a component of extracellular fluid.

vascular fluid: Fluid that is in blood vessels; a component of extracellular fluid.

---

*T*he fluid of the body flows in arteries, veins, and lymph vessels; it is secreted into specialized compartments as diverse as joints, cerebral ventricles, and the intestinal lumen; it both surrounds and permeates the cells. **Body fluid** serves as a lubricant and as a solvent for the chemical reactions that we call metabolism; it transports oxygen, nutrients, chemical messengers, and waste products to their destinations; it plays an important role in the regulation of body temperature. Because the fluid within the body is so widespread and serves so many functions, it is not surprising that abnormalities in the **volume** or **composition** of body fluid cause clinical problems.

Disorders of fluid or **electrolyte** homeostasis occur in persons who are experiencing many different pathophysiologic conditions. In severe cases, these disorders cause death. Although these disorders arise from many specific causes in different patient populations, these specific causes fall into general categories that arise from the principles of normal fluid and electrolyte homeostasis. This chapter first presents the principles of normal fluid homeostasis and then, building on that foundation continues with a discussion of fluid imbalances. Similarly, the principles of electrolyte homeostasis are explained before plasma electrolyte imbalances are presented.

Body Fluid Homeostasis

The term **body fluid,** as used in this chapter, pertains to water within the body and the particles dissolved in it. The body fluid is contained in two major compartments: extracellular and intracellular. Approximately 60 percent of body fluid is in the intracellular compartment (inside the cells). This **intracellular fluid** is relatively rich in potassium, magnesium, inorganic and organic phosphates, and proteins. It is relatively low in sodium and chloride. The other 40 percent of body fluid is extracellular fluid. The **extracellular fluid** lies between the cells (**interstitial** compartment), in the blood vessels (**vascular** compartment), in dense connective tissue and bone, and in several minor compartments that are collectively termed the transcellular fluids (for example, synovial, cerebrospinal, and gastrointestinal fluids). The extracellular fluid in the vascular and interstitial compartments is relatively rich in sodium, chloride, and bicarbonate and rela-

tively low in potassium, magnesium, and phosphates. The vascular portion of the extracellular fluid contains many proteins, while the interstitial and **transcellular** portions of the extracellular fluid contain very few proteins. Most **transcellular fluids** are secreted by epithelial cells; their composition varies according to their function. Total body water is the total of the water within all fluid compartments. The body fluid compartments are depicted in Figure 24–1.

The proportion of body weight that is water varies according to a person's age and proportion of body fat. A full-term newborn infant is about 75 percent water by weight. In a standard adult, **body water** is about 60 percent of body weight. The percentage is less (about 50 percent) in women because they have a greater proportion of body fat than men of the same weight. Obese adults, with a much larger proportion of body fat, have less of their body weight as water. Elderly adults typically have 50 percent of their body weight as water. The decrease in this percentage from that of middle age is due primarily to the relative increase in body fat that occurs with normal aging.

A liter (L) of water weighs 1 kg (2.2 lb). Thus, a lean, middle-aged, healthy adult male who weighs 70 kg (154 lb) has approximately 42 liters of body water. Of this amount, approximately 25 liters is intracellular water. The approximately 17 liters of extracellular water is distributed as 3 liters of plasma water, 8 liters of interstitial and lymph water, 5 liters trapped in dense connective tissue and bone, and 1 liter in transcellular water.

Fluid **homeostasis** is a dynamic process. In a healthy person, this process may be viewed as the net result of four subprocesses: *fluid intake, fluid absorption, fluid distribution, and fluid excretion.* In some persons who have pathophysiologic conditions, loss of fluid through abnormal routes also occurs. The interplay of these subprocesses is fluid homeostasis.[1]

Intake and Absorption

Fluid intake is entry of fluid into the body by any route. Healthy persons ingest fluids orally, both by drinking and by eating (water contained in food). They also synthesize a small amount of water through cellular metabolism of the foods they eat. Fluid intake by drinking is influenced by habit and social factors and by thirst. Additional routes of fluid intake that may occur in patients who have various pathophysio-

logic conditions include intravenous intake; tubes into the gastrointestinal tract, other body cavities, or subcutaneous tissue or bone marrow; rectal (such as tap water enema); and, occasionally, through the lungs (such as near-drowning). Fluid intake by these routes is often controlled by health care professionals.

Unless fluid intake occurs intravenously, the fluid must be absorbed before it reaches the vascular compartment. Fluid absorption from the gastrointestinal tract is dependent on osmotic forces generated by the absorption of **electrolytes** and other particles.

Distribution

Much of the fluid that reaches the vascular compartment is then distributed into other fluid compartments. *Fluid distribution between the vascular and interstitial compartments is the net result of* **filtration** *across permeable capillaries.* At the capillary level, two forces tend to move fluid from the capillaries into the interstitial compartment: *capillary hydrostatic pressure* (the push of the **vascular fluid** against the capillary walls) and *interstitial fluid osmotic pressure* (the pulling force of particles in the interstitial fluid). Concurrently, two forces tend to move fluid from the interstitial compartment into the capillaries: *capillary osmotic pressure* (the pulling force of particles in the vascular fluid) and *interstitial fluid hydrostatic pressure* (the push of the interstitial fluid against the outside of the capillary walls). The distribution of fluid between the vascular and interstitial compartments is analogous to two groups of people pushing on opposite sides of a swinging door—the strongest "push" will determine which direction the door will swing. Thus, at any one point along a capillary, the direction and amount of fluid flow between the vascular and interstitial com-

partments are determined by the net result of opposing forces. These forces are illustrated in Figure 24–1.

The distribution of fluid between the interstitial and intracellular compartments, on the other hand, occurs by **osmosis,** *rather than by filtration.* Cell membranes are permeable to water but not to electrolytes, many of which require specialized transport mechanisms to cross a cell membrane. For this reason, cell membranes are called semipermeable membranes. The movement of water by osmosis into or from cells is determined by the particle concentrations on the two sides of the semipermeable cell membrane. If the particle concentration (**osmolality**) of the interstitial fluid is higher than the particle concentration inside cells, water will move by osmosis from the cells into the interstitial fluid to equalize the osmolality in the two compartments. If, on the other hand, the osmolality of the interstitial fluid is lower than the osmolality of the intracellular fluid, then water will move from the interstitial compartment into the intracellular compartment. In this way, the osmolality of the interstitial and intracellular compartments controls the distribution of water between them.

The distribution of fluid between the intracellular and transcellular compartments is controlled by processes within the epithelial cells that secrete these fluids.

Excretion

The final component of fluid homeostasis in healthy persons is fluid excretion. The normal routes of fluid excretion are through urine, feces, the lungs, and the skin. Fluid is excreted through the skin as visible sweat (which may occur or not) and as insensible perspiration (which always occurs). Another obligatory route of excretion of water is through the lungs

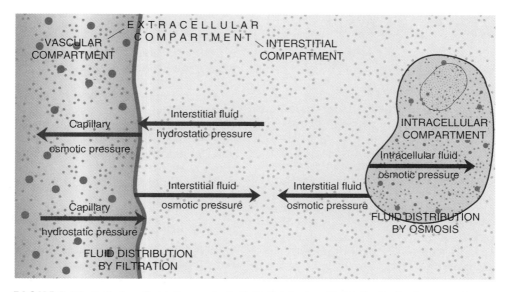

F I G U R E 24–1. Factors that influence body fluid distribution. Fluid distribution between the vascular and interstitial compartments is the net result of filtration across permeable capillaries. The distribution of fluid between the interstitial and intracellular compartments occurs by osmosis, rather than by filtration.

during exhalation. Fecal excretion of fluid increases dramatically in a person who has diarrhea. In a healthy person, the largest volume of fluid is excreted in the urine.

The amount of fluid excreted in the urine is controlled primarily by the hormones antidiuretic hormone (ADH), aldosterone, and atrial natriuretic factors, and to a lesser degree by minor hormones such as renal prostaglandins and by the renal sympathetic nerves. Antidiuretic hormone is synthesized by cells in the supraoptic and paraventricular nuclei of the hypothalamus. The axons of these cells extend down the median eminence of the pituitary stalk. The release of ADH thus occurs from the posterior pituitary gland. Factors that increase release of ADH into the blood include increased osmolality (concentratedness) of the extracellular fluid, decreased circulating fluid volume, pain, nausea, and physiologic and psychological stressors. The hormone circulates to the distal tubules and collecting ducts in the kidneys where, consistent with its name, ADH causes reabsorption of water. Reabsorption of water decreases the urine volume, thus decreasing fluid excretion. Factors that decrease ADH release (such as decreased osmolality of the extracellular fluid) allow a large urine volume.

Aldosterone is another hormone that influences urine volume. Aldosterone is synthesized and secreted by cells in the adrenal cortex. The major stimuli for its release are angiotensin II (from the renin-angiotensin system, which is activated by decreased circulating blood volume) and an increased concentration of potassium in the plasma. Aldosterone causes the renal tubules to reabsorb sodium and water (saline), so that it also decreases fluid excretion, although by a different mechanism than ADH. Decreased secretion of aldosterone promotes a larger urine volume.

Atrial natriuretic peptide (ANP) is secreted from cells in the atria of the heart when the atria are stretched. They cause **natriuresis** (sodium excretion in the urine), which is accompanied by water. Thus, ANP promotes fluid excretion. The urine volume that an individual produces is thus the end result of the action of several factors that respond to different stimuli and have different actions on the renal tubules.

Loss Through Abnormal Routes

Persons who have pathophysiologic conditions often experience loss of fluid through abnormal routes. Examples of these routes are emesis; tubes into the gastrointestinal tract or other body cavities; hemorrhage; drainage from fistulas, wounds or open areas of skin; and paracentesis. The fluid lost through abnormal routes may be a significant factor in disturbing normal fluid homeostasis.

If the body's physiologic mechanisms are functioning well, the processes of fluid homeostasis maintain normal body fluid status. If fluid intake is large, fluid excretion is increased by the mechanisms described previously that increase urine volume. If fluid intake is diminished, or if fluid is lost through abnormal routes, fluid excretion is decreased and thirst may cause an increase in fluid intake.

KEY CONCEPTS

- Habit and thirst are important regulators of fluid intake. Individuals who are unable to control their fluid intake (such as those receiving fluids intravenously, immobile patients, and unconscious patients) are at risk for fluid imbalance.
- Saline and electrolytes move by filtration across the capillary wall, and as a result, interstitial and serum levels of electrolytes are similar. Capillary hydrostatic pressure is the primary force promoting filtration. Plasma colloid osmotic pressure is the primary force opposing filtration from the capillary.
- Movement of electrolytes across cell membranes is highly regulated by membrane carriers and channels. Movement of water across cell membranes occurs through osmosis. Water moves from areas of low osmolality to areas of high osmolality.
- Fluid loss may be visible (urine, feces, emesis, sweat) or insensible (respiratory and skin). All routes must be taken into account to predict fluid balance accurately.
- The healthy kidney regulates fluid balance in response to blood pressure and several hormones. Urine output is normally a good indicator of body fluid balance. Aldosterone and ADH induce the kidney to conserve fluid; ANP (atrial natriuretic peptides) promotes fluid excretion.

Fluid Imbalances

If fluid homeostasis is disturbed by pathophysiologic processes or other factors (such as medications), fluid imbalances may result. Fluid imbalances fall into two major categories: imbalances of extracellular fluid *volume* (saline imbalances) and imbalances of body fluid *concentration* (water imbalances).

Extracellular Fluid Volume

In some circumstances, individuals have too much or too little extracellular fluid. These disorders are called extracellular fluid volume disorders because they involve a change in the *amount* (volume) of the extracellular fluid. These imbalances are also termed saline imbalances, because they are disorders of **isotonic** salt water. (Isotonic saline is salt water in the same concentration as the plasma concentration.) In an extracellular fluid volume imbalance, the *concentration* of the extracellular fluid may be normal; there is just too much or too little of it. Some persons have an extracellular fluid volume imbalance and an imbalance of body fluid concentration at the same time. In this case, both the volume and concentration (serum sodium) of the extracellular fluid are abnormal. In this section only the volume imbalances are discussed; the concentration imbalances are discussed separately because they may occur separately.

Volume Deficit

Extracellular fluid volume deficit is caused by removal of a sodium-containing fluid from the body. It is a decrease in saline (salt water) in the same concentration as the normal extracellular fluid, which is why the condition is sometimes termed *saline deficit*. In an uncomplicated extracellular fluid volume deficit, the serum sodium concentration is normal. The *composition* of the extracellular fluid is normal; the *amount* of the extracellular fluid is abnormally decreased. Specific causes of extracellular fluid volume deficit are listed in Table 24–1.

Clinical manifestations of extracellular fluid volume deficit include weight loss, postural blood pressure drop, flat neck veins (or veins collapsing with inspiration) when supine, increased small vein filling time, dizziness, and oliguria.[2] An extracellular fluid volume deficit that develops slowly may also be manifested by skin tenting when pinched up over the sternum, dryness of oral mucous membranes between cheek and gum, hard stools, soft sunken eyeballs, and longitudinal furrows in the tongue. Infants who develop extracellular volume deficit have a sunken fontanelle.

Rapid weight loss is a sensitive measure of extracellular fluid volume deficit. One liter of saline weighs 1 kg; therefore, a person who loses 1 kg in 24 hours has excreted 1 liter of fluid or lost it through an abnormal route. An extracellular fluid volume deficit may occur without a weight loss if fluid is sequestered somewhere in the body, as with ascites or intestinal obstruction.

A postural blood pressure drop denotes an inadequate circulating blood volume, which is the result of fluid depletion in the vascular compartment. If the systolic blood pressure decreases more than 15 mm Hg when a supine person stands or sits with legs dependent (hanging down) and the diastolic blood pressure decreases 10 or more mm Hg while the pulse rate increases, a postural blood pressure drop is present. A severe extracellular fluid volume deficit may lead to hypovolemic shock.

Volume Excess

An extracellular fluid volume excess is essentially the opposite of an extracellular fluid volume deficit. It is the condition in which the amount of extracellular fluid is abnormally increased. In an uncomplicated extracellular fluid volume excess, the *concentration* of the extracellular fluid is normal but an excessive *amount* of that fluid is present.

Extracellular fluid volume excess is caused by addition or retention of saline (salt water in the same concentration as the blood). For this reason, it is sometimes termed *saline excess*. As previously mentioned, the hormone aldosterone causes the kidneys to retain saline. Extracellular fluid volume excess, therefore, may be caused by conditions that involve excessive aldosterone secretion. For example, increased aldosterone secretion is a compensatory mechanism that commonly accompanies congestive heart failure and leads, in time, to extracellular fluid volume excess. Additional causes of extracellular fluid volume excess are presented in Table 24–2.

The signs and symptoms of extracellular fluid volume excess are rapid weight gain, edema, and manifestations of circulatory overload: bounding pulse, distended neck veins in a person in the upright position, rales, dyspnea, orthopnea, and even the frothy sputum of pulmonary edema. Infants who develop extracellular volume excess have a bulging fontanelle.

Body Fluid Concentration

In contrast to the extracellular fluid volume disorders just discussed, imbalances of body fluid concentration are disorders of the *concentration* rather than of the *amount* of the extracellular fluid. The serum sodium concentration reflects the **osmolality** (concentrated-

TABLE 24–1. Etiology of Extracellular Fluid Volume Deficit

Gastrointestinal Excretion or Loss of Sodium-containing Fluid

Emesis
Diarrhea
Gastric suction or intestinal decompression
Fistula drainage

Renal Excretion of Sodium-containing Fluid

Adrenal insufficiency
Salt-wasting renal disorders
Extensive diuretic use
Bed rest

Other Loss of a Sodium-containing Fluid

Hemorrhage
Massive diaphoresis
Third-space fluid accumulation
Paracentesis and similar procedures
Burns

TABLE 24–2. Etiology of Extracellular Fluid Volume Excess

Excessive Intravenous Infusion of Isotonic Solutions

Renal Retention of Sodium and Water

Primary hyperaldosteronism
Congestive heart failure
Cirrhosis
Chronic renal failure
Cushing's disease
Glucocorticoid therapy

ness) of the blood. Imbalances of body fluid concentration are recognized by abnormal serum sodium concentration. The normal serum sodium concentration is 135 to 145 mEq/L (may vary slightly with different laboratories). Many persons develop imbalances of both extracellular fluid volume and serum sodium concentration at the same time.

Hyponatremia

A serum sodium concentration below the lower limit of normal indicates **hyponatremia** (too little sodium in the blood). When hyponatremia is present, the extracellular fluid contains relatively too much water for the amount of sodium present; it is relatively too dilute.

Hyponatremia is caused by factors that produce a relative excess of water in proportion to salt in the extracellular fluid. Because the serum sodium concentration reflects the osmolality of the blood, the reduced serum sodium of hyponatremia indicates that the extracellular fluid has a reduced osmolality; it is relatively too dilute. Hyponatremia is also called **hypotonic** syndrome, hypo-osmolality, and water intoxication. All of these terms reflect the abnormal composition of the extracellular fluid that results when the normal proportion of salt to water in the extracellular fluid is disrupted.

A *gain of relatively more water than salt* will cause hyponatremia. As mentioned previously, the hormone ADH causes the kidneys to retain water (*not* salt and water) in the body. This hormone is part of the system that normally regulates the osmolality of the extracellular fluid. Circumstances that cause prolonged or excessive release of ADH, however, cause the kidneys to retain too much water, which effectively dilutes the blood; hyponatremia is the result. Antidiuretic hormone is elevated in the syndrome of inappropriate secretion of ADH (SIADH). It may also be produced ectopically. Small-cell (oat cell) carcinoma is a type of lung tumor that frequently synthesizes and releases ADH. This ectopic production of ADH from a tumor is not subject to the feedback inhibition of normal ADH release, so inappropriate amounts of ADH are released. With continually high levels of ADH being produced by the tumor, the kidneys retain excessive amounts of water—a gain of water relative to salt. Factors that cause a gain of water relative to salt are presented in Table 24–3.

Hyponatremia may also be caused by a *loss of relatively more salt than water*. If salt is removed from the body while water remains, then the extracellular fluid once again will become too dilute; hyponatremia results. Factors that cause hyponatremia by loss of salt relative to water are also presented in Table 24–3.

The clinical manifestations of hyponatremia are nonspecific manifestations of central nervous system dysfunction.[3] They vary from malaise, anorexia, nausea, vomiting, and headache to confusion, lethargy, seizures, and coma. Profound hyponatremia may be fatal. The signs and symptoms are caused by swelling

TABLE 24–3. Etiology of Hyponatremia

Gain of Relatively More Water Than Salt

Excessive antidiuretic hormone
Barbiturate overdose
Hypotonic irrigating solutions
Excessive intravenous infusion of D5W (5% dextrose in water)
Tap water enemas
Psychogenic polydipsia
Near-drowning in fresh water

Loss of Relatively More Salt Than Water

Diuretics
Salt-wasting renal disease
Replacement of water but not salt lost through emesis, diarrhea, gastric suction, diaphoresis, or burns

of neurons as a result of the decreased osmolality of the extracellular fluid. As the extracellular fluid becomes too dilute, the intracellular fluid is more concentrated. Therefore, water moves into cells by osmosis. The severity of the signs and symptoms depends on the rapidity of the development of hyponatremia as well as on the absolute value of the serum sodium concentration. A rapid decrease in osmolality produces more severe manifestations than a slow decline, other factors being equal.

Hypernatremia

Hypernatremia is indicated by a serum sodium concentration above the upper limit of normal (145 mEq/L). When hypernatremia is present, the extracellular fluid contains relatively too little water for the amount of sodium present; it is relatively too concentrated. Hypernatremia is also called water deficit, **hypertonic** syndrome, and hyperosmolality. These terms all reflect the relative deficit of water to salt in the extracellular fluid that occurs in hypernatremia.

Hypernatremia is caused by a *gain of relatively more salt than water* or by a *loss of relatively more water than salt*. Patients who receive concentrated tube feedings without enough water, especially elderly persons, are at high risk for hypernatremia because they gain relatively more solute than water, which causes an obligatory loss of more water than salt in the urine. Hypernatremia can be prevented in these patients by administering water between feedings. Other specific factors that cause hypernatremia are presented in Table 24–4 under the two major categories.

The signs and symptoms of hypernatremia are similar to those of hyponatremia in that they are nonspecific manifestations of central nervous system dysfunction.[4] In hypernatremia, the increased osmolality of the extracellular fluid causes neurons to shrivel because water moves from the cells into the interstitial fluid by osmosis. The dysfunction ranges from confusion and lethargy to seizures and coma. Thirst and oliguria (except for hypernatremia of renal origin) are common. Severe hypernatremia may cause death.

TABLE 24-4. Etiology of Hypernatremia

Gain of Relatively More Solute Than Water

Tube feeding
Intravenous infusion of hypertonic solution
Near-drowning in salt water
Overuse of salt tablets
Food intake with reduced fluid intake
    Difficulty swallowing fluids
    Prolonged nausea
    No access to water
    Inability to respond to thirst

Loss of Relatively More Water Than Salt

Diabetes insipidus
Osmotic diuresis
Prolonged diarrhea or diaphoresis without water replacement

Edema

Edema is an excess of fluid in the interstitial compartment. It may be a manifestation of extracellular fluid volume excess or it may arise from other mechanisms. The distribution of fluid between the vascular and interstitial compartments was explained previously in this chapter in the section under the heading Distribution. An increase in the forces that tend to move fluid from the capillaries into the interstital compartment or a decrease in forces that tend to move fluid from the interstitial compartment into the capillaries will cause edema by altering normal fluid distribution between the vascular and interstitial compartments. Thus, edema may arise from increased capillary hydrostatic pressure, increased interstitial fluid osmotic pressure, or decreased capillary osmotic pressure. *Increased capillary hydrostatic pressure* is caused by increased extracellular fluid volume, by the increased local capillary flow that accompanies inflammation, and by venous congestion. *Increased interstitial fluid osmotic pressure* occurs when inflammation increases capillary permeability and proteins leak into the interstitial fluid. Lymphatic drainage normally removes minute amounts of protein that enter the interstitial fluid. Blockage of lymphatic drainage (for example, by a tumor or parasites) also causes edema when the accumulation of protein increases interstitial fluid osmotic pressure. Edema resulting from increased interstitial fluid osmotic pressure is frequently localized. *Decreased capillary osmotic pressure* occurs when the plasma proteins are decreased, as in malnutrition, liver disease (decreased protein synthesis), or nephrotic syndrome (increased protein excretion). Edema from this cause may be extensive.

In summary, edema represents increased interstitial fluid volume, a condition that may be localized or more general. Edema may be a sign of extracellular fluid volume excess (which causes increased capillary hydrostatic pressure) or it may be caused by other factors that alter the distribution of fluid between the vascular and interstitial compartments.

KEY CONCEPTS

- **Saline deficit (extracellular volume deficit) occurs when sodium-containing fluids are lost from the body (e.g., hemorrhage). Saline deficit is characterized by *normal* serum sodium and manifestations of volume deficit (weight loss, hypotension, poor skin turgor, oliguria).**
- **Saline excess (extracellular volume excess) is commonly due to processes that disrupt normal kidney perfusion (such as low cardiac output). Saline excess is characterized by a *normal* serum sodium and manifestations of volume excess (weight gain, hypertension, edema, congestive heart failure).**
- **Water excess (hyponatremia) is associated with excessive ADH secretion or hypotonic fluid intake. Water excess is characterized by a *low* serum sodium. Clinical manifestations (confusion, headache, seizure, coma) occur because of cellular swelling.**
- **Water deficit (hypernatremia) is associated with inadequate water intake or excessive water loss. Water deficit is characterized by a *high* serum sodium. Clinical manifestations (confusion, lethargy, seizure, coma) occur because of cellular shriveling.**

Principles of Electrolyte Homeostasis

In a healthy individual, the *concentration* of an electrolyte in the plasma is the net result of four processes: *electrolyte intake, electrolyte absorption, electrolyte distribution, and electrolyte excretion.*[1] These processes work together in a dynamic fashion to maintain electrolyte concentrations within their normal limits. Thus, if electrolyte intake increases, electrolyte excretion also may increase, to normalize plasma levels. Similarly, if electrolyte intake decreases dramatically, electrolytes may be redistributed into the plasma to maintain the normal plasma concentration.

Intake and Absorption

Electrolyte intake normally occurs orally, through food and drink. It is important to remember that oral medications (for example, magnesium antacids) may be an important source of electrolyte intake. Intravenous fluids and hyperalimentation solutions are common sources of parenteral intake of electrolytes. Blood transfusions may provide significant amounts of electrolytes.[5] Less common, but important if it occurs, is intramuscular injection of the electrolyte magnesium. Some patients have electrolyte intake through tubes into body cavities. The most obvious examples are nasogastric and gastrointestinal feeding, but more unusual situations may cause significant electrolyte intake in specific individuals (such as irrigation of the renal pelvis with magnesium-rich solutions). Rarely, electrolyte intake may occur through such unusual routes as the lungs (for example, near-drowning in salt water, which is rich in magnesium) or the skin (for example, through application of ointments to large areas of broken or burned skin). Electrolyte intake is controlled by the individual and by health care providers.

If electrolyte intake occurs orally, the electrolyte must be absorbed before it is physiologically useful. The absorption of some electrolytes, such as potassium, depends on concentration gradients. The absorption of other electrolytes, such as calcium, depends on the availability of binding proteins, which is influenced by the activity of vitamin D.[6] The contents of the gastrointestinal tract may influence electrolyte absorption. Many agents will bind electrolytes and prevent them from being absorbed. For example, undigested fat in the intestines will bind calcium and magnesium from the dietary intake and prevent them from being absorbed. The pH of the intestinal fluid also influences the absorption of certain electrolytes. Medications often alter the absorption of electrolytes.

Distribution

Every fluid compartment contains electrolytes. However, the electrolyte concentration of these various compartments differs. The concentration of potassium, calcium, magnesium, and phosphate inside the cells is higher than in the fluid outside the cells. The bones serve as an important reservoir of calcium, phosphate, and magnesium. The cells and the bones are often called the electrolyte pools. The distribution of electrolytes between the extracellular fluid and the electrolyte pools is primarily influenced by hormones such as epinephrine and insulin. Certain medications will also influence electrolyte distribution. Significant movement of electrolytes between the cells and the extracellular fluid may occur within minutes.[7] In the absence of changes in electrolyte intake and excretion, a shift of electrolytes from the extracellular fluid into the electrolyte pools will decrease the plasma electrolyte concentration. Conversely, a shift of electrolyte from an electrolyte pool into the extracellular fluid will increase the plasma electrolyte concentration.

Excretion

Electrolyte excretion occurs through urine, feces, and sweat. The urinary excretion of some electrolytes is influenced by hormones (e.g., aldosterone increases potassium excretion), although factors such as the flow rate of renal tubular fluid are also influential. Many medications alter the rate of urinary excretion of electrolytes. Fecal excretion of electrolytes is influenced by the rate of fecal excretion. Diarrhea increases the rate of excretion of potassium and magnesium in particular. The composition of the feces also influences the amount of electrolyte excretion. Undigested fat in the intestines will bind both calcium and magnesium ions that are secreted into the gastrointestinal tract and cause them to be excreted in the feces.

Loss Through Abnormal Routes

When electrolytes exit the body through routes other than the normal urine, feces, and sweat, this may be termed abnormal electrolyte loss. This factor alters electrolyte homeostasis in patients who have diverse pathophysiologic conditions. Examples of abnormal electrolyte loss are vomiting, nasogastric suction, paracentesis, hemodialysis, wound drainage, and fistula drainage.[8] Abnormal loss of electrolytes may be uncontrollable or may result from therapeutic procedures.

Electrolyte homeostasis is a dynamic interplay between the processes of electrolyte intake, electrolyte absorption, electrolyte distribution, and electrolyte excretion. In some persons, electrolyte loss through abnormal routes becomes an important factor that requires adjustment of electrolyte intake and/or electrolyte excretion to prevent development of electrolyte imbalances. Patients who have acute or chronic illnesses have many factors that tend to cause electrolyte imbalances by disrupting or interfering with electrolyte intake, absorption, distribution, or excretion.

KEY CONCEPTS

- **The electrolyte composition of the body is maintained by a careful balance of electrolyte intake, absorption, distribution, and excretion. Electrolyte imbalances result from disruption of one or more of these regulatory mechanisms.**
- **Redistribution of electrolytes between cells and the extracellular fluid may contribute to serum electrolyte imbalance. Cells contain high concentrations of potassium, calcium, magnesium, and phosphate, whereas the extracellular fluid contains high concentrations of sodium, chloride, and bicarbonate ions.**

Electrolyte Imbalances

Electrolyte imbalances are widespread in many pathophysiologic conditions. An imbalance of an electrolyte may be a total body imbalance or it may be an imbalance in distribution of electrolytes within compartments, with the total body amount remaining normal. Based on the principles of electrolyte homeostasis explained in the previous section of this chapter, an excess of electrolytes in the extracellular fluid may be caused by increased electrolyte intake or absorption, shift of electrolytes from an electrolyte pool into the extracellular fluid, and decreased electrolyte excretion, either singly or in combination. Conversely, a deficit of electrolyte in the extracellular fluid may be caused by decreased electrolyte intake, shift of electrolytes from the extracellular fluid into an electrolyte pool, increased electrolyte excretion, abnormal loss of electrolytes, or some combination of these factors.[1]

Plasma Potassium

The normal concentration of potassium in serum is 3.5 to 5.0 mEq/L (may vary slightly with different laboratories), except in neonates, in whom it may be higher. Most of the potassium in the body is inside the cells; the standard serum potassium measurement gives only the concentration of the small portion of potassium that is in extracellular fluid. Because a number of factors cause potassium **ions** to move into or out of body cells, concentration of potassium in the plasma and total body potassium content are not necessarily correlated.[9] Whether or not they are accompanied by total body potassium imbalances, plasma potassium imbalances may cause clinically significant signs and symptoms.

Hypokalemia

Hypokalemia denotes a **decreased** potassium concentration in the **extracellular fluid.** A decrease in the *plasma* potassium concentration does not necessarily denote a decrease in *total body* potassium. Thus, hypokalemia may coexist with a total body potassium deficit, a total body potassium excess, or a normal total body potassium.

Hypokalemia is caused by factors that decrease potassium intake, shift potassium from the extracellular fluid into the cells, increase potassium excretion through the normal routes, and cause potassium loss from the body by some abnormal route. In many cases, a combination of factors leads to hypokalemia.[10] For example, some people follow a fad diet (decreased potassium intake) and abuse diuretics (increased potassium excretion) in an attempt to lose weight. The specific causes of hypokalemia are listed under their categories in Table 24–5.

The ratio of intracellular to extracellular potassium ion concentration is a major determinant of the *resting membrane potential* of muscle cells. For this reason, potassium imbalances cause altered function of muscles. In hypokalemia, both smooth and skeletal muscles are *hyperpolarized* (more electrical charge than usual across the cell membrane). Therefore, these muscles are less reactive to stimuli. The resulting clinical manifestations include abdominal distention, diminished bowel sounds, paralytic ileus, postural hypotension, skeletal muscle weakness, and flaccid paralysis. The skeletal muscle weakness of hypokalemia is bilateral weakness that typically begins in the lower extremities and ascends. It may involve the respiratory muscles, causing respiratory paralysis more commonly than does hyperkalemia.

Many types of cardiac arrhythmias arise from hypokalemia. Cardiac muscle cells usually become hyperpolarized with hypokalemia. However, with very low plasma potassium concentrations, *hypopolarization* of cardiac muscle occurs, most likely because of decreased potassium conductance. Hypokalemia also increases the rate of diastolic depolarization, which may give rise to ectopic beats, decreases conduction velocity in the atrioventricular node, prolongs cardiac ac-

TABLE 24–5. Etiology of Hypokalemia

Decreased Potassium Intake

Anorexia
NPO (nothing by mouth) orders and intravenous solutions without potassium
Fasting
Unbalanced diet

Shift of Potassium From Extracellular Fluid Into Cells

Alkalosis
Rapid correction of acidosis
Excess insulin (such as during hyperalimentation)
Excess beta-adrenergic stimulation
Hypokalemic familial periodic paralysis

Increased Potassium Excretion Through Normal Routes

Renal route
   Glucocorticoid therapy
   Potassium-wasting diuretics
   Parenteral carbenicillin or similar agents
   Hypomagnesemia
   Cushing's disease
   Hyperaldosteronism
   Excessive ingestion of black licorice
   Amphotericin B, cisplatin, or capreomycin
Fecal route
   Diarrhea
   Laxative abuse
Skin route
   Excessive diaphoresis

Loss of Potassium Through Abnormal Routes

Emesis
Gastric suction
Fistula drainage

tion potentials by decreasing the rate of repolarization, shortens the absolute refractory period, and prolongs the relative refractory period.[11]

Hypokalemia may also cause polyuria, by interfering with the action of ADH at the renal tubules. The plasma potassium concentration at which the various clinical manifestations of hypokalemia appear depends on individual responsiveness and the presence of other concurrent electrolyte and acid-base disorders.

Hyperkalemia

If the serum potassium concentration rises above 5.0 mEq/L (the upper limit of normal), hyperkalemia is present. Hyperkalemia denotes an elevation of potassium concentration in the *extracellular fluid.* As mentioned previously, most of the potassium in the body is within the cells and many factors cause potassium ions to move into or out of the cells. Thus, total body potassium may be increased, normal, or decreased in hyperkalemia, depending on its cause.

Hyperkalemia is caused by factors that increase potassium intake, shift potassium from the cells into the extracellular fluid, and decrease potassium excretion.[1] Large amounts of potassium released from cells after a crushing injury will elevate the potassium concentration of the extracellular fluid. Specific causes of hyperkalemia are summarized by category in Table 24–6.

As might be expected from the role of potassium ions in the establishment of the resting membrane potential of muscle cells, hyperkalemia causes muscle dysfunction. As hyperkalemia develops, the smooth muscle and skeletal muscle become *hypopolarized*. The main clinical manifestation at this stage is mild intestinal cramping and diarrhea, which occurs only in some persons. As hyperkalemia worsens, the skeletal muscle cells become so hypopolarized that their resting membrane potentials lie above their threshold potential; once they have discharged, they are unable to contract again. This situation results in the skeletal muscle weakness and flaccid paralysis that is typical in hyperkalemia.[12] This skeletal muscle weakness is an ascending weakness that appears first in the lower extremities. Both hypokalemia and hyperkalemia cause skeletal muscle weakness/paralysis, but the underlying alterations in the resting membrane potentials are different.

Cardiac muscle undergoes the same changes in resting membrane potential as skeletal muscle in hyperkalemia. In addition, hyperkalemia decreases the duration and rate of rise of cardiac action potentials and decreases conduction velocity in the heart. These pathophysiologic mechanisms underlie the cardiac arrhythmias of hyperkalemia.[11] In severe hyperkalemia, cardiac arrest occurs.

The plasma potassium concentration at which each of these clinical manifestations occurs varies, depending on the rapidity of rise of the potassium concentration, the causes of the hyperkalemia, and other concurrent electrolyte or acid-base imbalances. Patients who have chronic renal failure often undergo potassium adaptation and are relatively asymptomatic

T A B L E 24–6. Etiology of Hyperkalemia

Increased Potassium Intake

Excessive or too rapid intravenous potassium infusion
Insufficiently mixed intravenous potassium
Large transfusion of stored blood
Massive doses of potassium penicillin G

Shift of Potassium From Cells Into Extracellular Fluid

Acidosis caused by mineral acids
Insufficient insulin
Crushing injury
Cytotoxic drugs
Hyperkalemic periodic paralysis
β-adrenergic blockade

Decreased Potassium Excretion

Oliguria (such as in hypovolemia or renal failure)
Potassium-sparing diuretics
Adrenal insufficiency
Captopril use
Indomethacin use
Renin-deficient states

at high plasma potassium concentrations that would be disabling in other persons. Although the mechanisms of potassium adaptation are not completely understood, increased aldosterone levels in the presence of dysfunctional kidneys is believed to be an important part of the mechanism. This increased aldosterone increases potassium excretion in the colon and may alter potassium distribution between the extracellular fluid and the cells to normalize the resting membrane potentials.[13]

Plasma Calcium

The normal range of total serum calcium is 9 to 11 mg/dL or 4.5 to 5.5 mEq/L (may vary slightly with different laboratories). The calcium in the plasma is in three forms: some of the calcium ions are bound to plasma proteins (such as albumin); some of the calcium ions are bound to small organic ions (such as citrate); the remainder of the calcium ions are free (unbound). Only the free (ionized) calcium is physiologically active. Clinically significant calcium imbalances are caused by alterations in the plasma concentration of physiologically active calcium.

Hypocalcemia

Hypocalcemia occurs if the serum calcium concentration drops below the lower limit of normal or if the fraction of ionized calcium in the blood is decreased by an increase in calcium binding to plasma proteins or other organic ions.[14] In the latter case, the total serum calcium (the usual laboratory measurement) may be normal, but an *ionized* hypocalcemia is present and may cause signs and symptoms.

Hypocalcemia is caused by factors that decrease calcium intake or absorption, decrease the physiologic availability of calcium, and increase calcium excretion.[1] The hypocalcemia of pancreatitis arises from impaired fat digestion owing to lack of pancreatic lipase. Both dietary calcium and calcium secreted into the intestine from the extracellular fluid bind to undigested fat in the intestine and are excreted from the body. Thus, both decreased calcium absorption and increased calcium excretion play a part in hypocalcemia associated with pancreatitis. Table 24–7 is a list of the specific causes of hypocalcemia under these general etiologic factors.

The clinical manifestations of hypocalcemia are those of increased neuromuscular irritability: positive Trousseau's sign; positive Chvostek's sign; paresthesias; muscle twitching and cramping; hyperactive reflexes; carpopedal spasms; tetany; laryngospasm; seizures; and cardiac arrhythmias. The increased neuromuscular irritability of hypocalcemia is caused by a decrease in the threshold potential of excitable cells, so that action potentials are generated more easily. The cardiac effects of hypocalcemia are the result of prolongation of the plateau phase of the cardiac action potential, impairment of atrioventricular and

T A B L E 24 – 7. Etiology of Hypocalcemia

Decreased Calcium Intake or Absorption

Diet with insufficient calcium and vitamin D
Excessive dietary phytates or oxalates
Pancreatitis
Steatorrhea
Chronic diarrhea
Laxative abuse
Malabsorption syndromes

Decreased Physiologic Availability of Calcium

Hypoparathyroidism
Excessive phosphate intake
Tumor lysis syndrome
Hypomagnesemia
Alkalosis
Large transfusion of citrated blood
Rapid infusion of plasma expanders that bind calcium
Elevated plasma free fatty acids

Increased Calcium Excretion Through Normal Routes

Renal route
  Chronic renal insufficiency
Fecal route
  Steatorrhea
  Pancreatitis

intraventricular conduction, and impairment of myocardial contractility.[11]

A positive Trousseau's sign is occurrence of a carpal spasm after occluding arterial blood flow to the hand for approximately 3 minutes. A positive Chvostek's sign is spasm of muscles in the cheek and corner of the mouth produced by tapping the facial nerve in front of the ear. Positive Trousseau's and Chvostek's signs are general indicators of increased neuromuscular irritability from any cause, so they must be interpreted in the context of other clinical manifestations and specific risk factors. Chvostek's sign may be positive in neonates without electrolyte imbalances.

Hypercalcemia

Hypercalcemia occurs when the serum calcium concentration rises above the upper limit of normal (11 mg/dL or 5.5 mEq/L). It indicates an elevation of the calcium concentration of the extracellular fluid. Hypercalcemia is caused by factors that increase calcium intake or absorption, cause a shift of calcium from bone to the extracellular fluid, and decrease calcium excretion.[1] Many malignant tumors produce chemicals that are carried in the blood to cause release of calcium from the bones.[15] These bone-resorbing factors include osteoclast-activating factor, a parathyroid hormone–like substance, prostaglandins, and other substances not yet fully characterized. Humoral factors in malignancy may decrease the renal excretion of calcium, which also contributes to hypercalcemia.[16] Specific causes of hypercalcemia are listed by category in Table 24–8.

Clinical manifestations of hypercalcemia include anorexia, nausea, emesis, constipation, fatigue, polyuria, muscle weakness, diminished reflexes, headache, confusion, lethargy, personality change, and cardiac arrhythmias. The decreased neuromuscular irritability (diminished reflexes and muscle weakness) is caused by elevation of the threshold potential of excitable cells. The cardiac effects of hypercalcemia include shortened plateau phase of the action potential, increased rate of diastolic depolarization of sinus node cells, and delayed atrioventricular conduction.[11] Renal calculi may occur in hypercalcemia, owing to the high calcium concentration of the urine. Pathologic fractures may appear if hypercalcemia is caused by bone resorption.

Plasma Magnesium

The normal serum magnesium concentration is 1.5 to 2.5 mEq/L (may vary slightly with different laboratories). Similarly to calcium, magnesium is also present in the blood as bound (physiologically inactive) and ionized (physiologically active) forms. Plasma magnesium imbalances may occur concurrent with or in the absence of total body magnesium imbalances.

Hypomagnesemia

If the serum magnesium concentration decreases below the lower limit of normal (1.5 mEq/L), hypomagnesemia is present. Hypomagnesemia indicates a decreased magnesium concentration of the extracellular fluid and does not necessarily indicate a total body magnesium deficit (although the two may occur concurrently).

The major causes of hypomagnesemia are decreased magnesium intake or absorption, increased magnesium excretion, and loss of magnesium by an abnormal route.[1] Chronic alcoholism is a major risk

T A B L E 24 – 8. Etiology of Hypercalcemia

Increased Calcium Intake or Absorption

Milk-alkali syndrome
Vitamin D overdose

Shift of Calcium From Bone Into Extracellular Fluid

Hyperparathyroidism
Immobilization
Paget's disease
Bone tumors
Multiple myeloma
Leukemia
Non-osseous malignancies that produce bone-resorbing factors

Decreased Calcium Excretion

Thiazide diuretics
Familial hypocalciuric hypercalcemia

TABLE 24–9. Etiology of Hypomagnesemia

Decreased Magnesium Intake or Absorption

Chronic alcoholism
Malnutrition
Prolonged intravenous therapy without magnesium
Ileal resection
Chronic diarrhea
Malabsorption syndromes
Pancreatitis
Steatorrhea

Decreased Physiological Availability of Magnesium

Elevated plasma free fatty acids

Increased Magnesium Excretion Through Normal Routes

Renal route
    Diabetic ketoacidosis
    Chronic alcoholism
    Diuretic therapy
    Aminoglycoside (e.g., gentamicin) toxicity
    Amphotericin B, cisplatin, or capreomycin toxicity
    Hyperaldosteronism
Fecal route
    Pancreatitis
    Steatorrhea

Magnesium Loss Through Abnormal Routes

Emesis
Gastric suction
Fistula drainage

factor for hypomagnesemia because it is associated with decreased magnesium intake, altered physiologic availability of magnesium, increased urinary magnesium excretion, and magnesium loss through emesis.[17] Persons who present to health care providers with alcohol-related diseases frequently have hypomagnesemia. Hypomagnesemia often causes hypokalemia by increasing urinary excretion of potassium.[18] In such cases, correction of hypomagnesemia is necessary before the hypokalemia can be corrected. Specific causes of hypomagnesemia are listed in Table 24–9.

Magnesium ions in the extracellular fluid depress the release of acetylcholine at neuromuscular junctions. If there is too little magnesium present, excessive amounts of acetylcholine are released. Therefore, the clinical manifestations of hypomagnesemia are those of increased neuromuscular excitability. Such manifestations may include insomnia, hyperactive reflexes, muscle cramps and twitching, grimacing, positive Chvostek's sign, positive Trousseau's sign, nystagmus, dysphagia, ataxia, tetany, and seizures. Cardiac arrhythmias also occur. Hypomagnesemia causes decreased activity of Na^+-K^+ adenosine triphosphatase, so that intracellular potassium decreases in the myocardium. Increased spontaneous firing in the sinus node, shortening of the absolute refractory period, and lengthening of the relative refractory period contribute to the cardiac arrhythmias in hypomagnesemia.[11]

Hypermagnesemia

If the serum magnesium rises above the upper limit of normal (2.5 mEq/L), hypermagnesemia is present. Hypermagnesemia indicates an excess of magnesium in the extracellular fluid. The major causes of hypermagnesemia are increased magnesium intake and decreased magnesium excretion.[1] Shift of magnesium from the bones to the extracellular fluid is seen transiently in some stages of hyperparathyroidism. Hypermagnesemia from excessive intake of magnesium in cathartics and antacids may occur in elderly persons, who apparently absorb more magnesium from the gastrointestinal tract than do younger adults and in younger adults who take large doses of magnesium-containing antacids.[19,20] People who have oliguria are another high risk group for developing hypermagnesemia. Specific causes of hypermagnesemia are summarized in Table 24–10.

Too much magnesium in the extracellular fluid depresses neuromuscular function by decreasing the release of acetylcholine at neuromuscular junctions. Manifestations of hypermagnesemia thus include decreased reflexes, lethargy, hypotension, flushing, diaphoresis, drowsiness, flaccid paralysis, respiratory depression, bradycardia, cardiac arrhythmias, and even cardiac arrest. The mechanisms that cause the cardiac effects of hypermagnesemia include decreased cardiac conduction and depression of membrane excitability.[11]

Plasma Phosphate

The normal range of phosphate concentration in the plasma is 2.5 to 4.5 mg/dL (may vary slightly with different laboratories). Symptomatic phosphate imbalances are less common than other electrolyte imbalances, but, like other electrolyte imbalances, they may be fatal if untreated.

Hypophosphatemia

Hypophosphatemia is present when the phosphate concentration in the plasma decreases below the lower limit of normal (2.5 mg/dL). However, the clinical manifestations of hypophosphatemia are often not observed unless the plasma phosphate concentration is below 1.0 mg/dL. Persons whose plasma phosphate

TABLE 24–10. Etiology of Hypermagnesemia

Increased Magnesium Intake or Absorption

Ingestion or aspiration of sea water
Excessive ingestion of magnesium-containing medications (e.g., cathartics and antacids)
Excessive intravenous infusion of magnesium

Decreased Magnesium Excretion

Oliguric renal failure
Adrenal insufficiency

concentration is below 1.0 mg/dL) are said to have severe symptomatic hypophosphatemia.

Hypophosphatemia is caused by factors that decrease phosphate intake, shift phosphate from extracellular fluid into cells, increase phosphate excretion, and cause loss of phosphate through abnormal routes.[1] Frequently, many factors combine to produce severe symptomatic hypophosphatemia. Any factor that causes a rapid increase in cellular metabolism will cause phosphate to shift from the extracellular fluid into the cells. Patients who are severely malnourished (such as cancer patients with advanced disease) are at high risk for severe symptomatic hypophosphatemia for up to 10 days after total parenteral nutrition is started because of the increased cellular metabolism and previously depleted phosphate stores.[21] Specific factors that cause hypophosphatemia are summarized in Table 24–11.

Phosphate is an important component of adenosine triphosphate (ATP), the major source of energy for many cellular processes. The signs and symptoms of severe symptomatic hypophosphatemia are due, in part, to decreased ATP within the cells. Another contributing mechanism is tissue hypoxia caused by decreased 2,3-diphosphoglycerate within the red blood cells. These signs and symptoms include anorexia, malaise, paresthesias, hemolysis, diminished reflexes, muscle aching, muscle weakness, respiratory failure, confusion, stupor, seizures, coma, and impaired cardiac function.[22] The impaired cardiac function results from decreased cardiac contractility and stroke work concurrent with increased left ventricular end-diastolic pressure. Congestive cardiomyopathy may result.[11]

TABLE 24–11. Etiology of Hypophosphatemia

Decreased Phosphate Intake or Absorption

Chronic alcoholism
Chronic diarrhea
Malabsorption syndromes
Excessive or long-term use of antacids

Shift of Phosphate From Extracellular Fluid Into Cells

Refeeding after starvation
Total parenteral nutrition
Hyperventilation (respiratory alkalosis)
Insulin
Epinephrine
Intravenous glucose, fructose, bicarbonate, or lactate

Increased Phosphate Excretion Through the Normal Renal Route

Alcohol withdrawal
Diuretic phase after extensive burns
Diabetic ketoacidosis
Diuretic therapy
Hyperparathyroidism

Phosphate Loss Through Abnormal Routes

Emesis
Hemodialysis

TABLE 24–12. Etiology of Hyperphosphatemia

Increased Phosphate Intake or Absorption

Overzealous phosphate therapy
Excessive use of phosphate-containing enemas

Shift of Phosphate From Cells Into Extracellular Fluid

Tumor lysis syndrome
Crush injuries
Rhabdomyolysis

Decreased Phosphate Excretion

Oliguric renal failure
Adrenal insufficiency
Hypoparathyroidism

Hyperphosphatemia

Hyperphosphatemia is an increase of the serum phosphate concentration above the upper limit of normal (4.5 mg/dL). It may be caused by increased phosphate intake, shift of phosphate from the cells into the extracellular fluid, and decreased phosphate excretion.[1] Examples of specific causes in these categories are listed in Table 24–12.

The clinical manifestations of hyperphosphatemia depend on the effect of the elevated phosphate concentration on calcium ions. Typically, hyperphosphatemia causes hypocalcemia.[23] The signs and symptoms are thus the manifestations of increased neuromuscular excitability that were presented earlier in this section in the discussion of hypocalcemia. In some patients, however, especially those who have chronic renal failure, hyperphosphatemia causes deposition of calcium phosphate salts in the soft tissues of the body. These patients develop signs and symptoms such as aching and stiffness of joints and itching, depending on the areas where these salts precipitate.

KEY CONCEPTS

- **Abnormalities in serum electrolyte concentrations may profoundly affect cellular function. Excitable cells, such as nerve and muscle, are particularly sensitive to electrolyte imbalances.**

- **The manifestations of potassium imbalance are due to effects on resting membrane potential (RMP). Hyperkalemia causes depolarization of the RMP; hypokalemia causes hyperpolarization. Initiation of neuromuscular and cardiac action potentials is affected by both hyper- and hypokalemia, resulting in muscle weakness and cardiac dysrhythmias.**

- **The manifestations of calcium imbalance are due to effects on threshold potential of nerve and muscle cells. Hypocalcemia decreases the threshold, resulting in hyperexcitability (twitching, tetany); hypercalcemia increases the threshold, resulting in neuromuscular depression (hyporeflexia).**

- Manifestations of magnesium imbalances are quite similar to those of calcium imbalance. Hypermagnesemia depresses neuromuscular excitability (hyporeflexia), and hypomagnesemia increases excitability (twitching). Magnesium inhibits release of acetylcholine at the neuromuscular junction.

- Phosphate is important in the regulation of cellular enzymes and is a substrate for ATP synthesis. Phosphate deficiency is characterized by symptoms of generalized cellular energy deficiency. Hyperphosphatemia is associated with precipitation of calcium phosphate into soft tissues of the body.

Summary

In this chapter, the principles of fluid and electrolyte homeostasis and imbalances have been presented. Fluid and electrolyte homeostasis involves the continuous interplay of intake, absorption, distribution, and excretion of fluid and electrolytes. Loss of fluid and electrolytes through abnormal routes may also occur. When the normal mechanisms are impaired or overwhelmed, fluid and electrolyte imbalances occur. Fluid imbalances may involve the volume or the concentration of body fluid. Plasma electrolyte imbalances may be deficits or excesses and may or may not reflect total body electrolyte deficits or excesses. The pathophysiology of specific fluid and electrolyte imbalances can be derived from a working knowledge of normal fluid and electrolyte homeostasis.

REFERENCES

1. Felver L: Fluid and electrolyte balance and imbalances, in Patrick ML, Woods SL, Craven RF, Rokosky JS, Bruno PM (eds): *Medical-Surgical Nursing: Pathophysiological Concepts*, 2nd ed. Philadelphia, JB Lippincott, 1991, pp 228–271.
2. Reubi FC: Hemodynamic changes in isotonic dehydration. *Contrib Nephrol* 1980;21:55–61.
3. Pollock A, Arieff A: Abnormalities of cell volume regulation and their functional consequences. *Am J Physiol* 1980;239:F195–F205.
4. Simon R, Freedman D: Neurologic manifestations of osmolar disorders. *Geriatrics* 1980;35:71–83.
5. Simon G, Bove J: The potassium load from blood transfusions. *Postgrad Med* 1971;49:61–64.
6. Favus MJ: Factors that influence absorption and secretion of calcium in the small intestine and colon. *Am J Physiol* 1985;248:G147–G157.
7. Brown MJ: Hypokalemia from beta$_2$-receptor stimulation by circulating epinephrine. *Am J Cardiol* 1985;56:3D–9D.
8. Wiegand C, Davin T, Raij L, Kjellstrand M: Severe hypokalemia induced by hemodialysis. *Arch Intern Med* 1981;141:167–170.
9. Sterns RH, Cox M, Feig P, Singer I: Internal potassium balance and the control of the plasma potassium concentration. *Medicine* 1981;60:339–354.
10. Felver L, Pendarvis JH: Perioperative risk factors for hypokalemia. *Today's OR Nurse* 1988;10:26–32.
11. Felver L: Effect of electrolyte imbalances on the cardiovascular system, in Underhill S, Woods SL, Halpenny CJ, Sivarajan E (eds): *Cardiac Nursing*, 2nd ed. Philadelphia, JB Lippincott, 1989, pp 988–999.
12. Udezue EO, Harrold BP: Hyperkalemic paralysis due to spironolactone. *Postgrad Med J* 1980;56:254–255.
13. Sandle GI, Gaiger E, Tapster S, Goodship THJ: Enhanced rectal potassium secretion in chronic renal insufficiency: Evidence for large intestinal potassium adaptation in man. *Clin Sci* 1986;71:393–401.
14. Zaloga GP, Willey S, Tomasic P, Chernow B: Free fatty acids alter calcium binding: A cause for misinterpretation of serum calcium values and hypocalcemia in critical illness. *J Clin Endocrinol Metab* 1987;64;1010–1014.
15. Bringhurst FR, Bierer BE, Godeau F, Neyhard N, Varner V, Segre GV: Humoral hypercalcemia of malignancy. *J Clin Invest* 1986;77:456–464.
16. Ralston SH, Fogelman I, Gardner MD, Dryburgh FJ, Cowan RA, Boyle IT: Hypercalcemia of malignancy: Evidence for a nonparathyroid humoral agent with an effect on renal tubular handling of calcium. *Clin Sci* 1984;66:187–191.
17. Felver L: A protocol for nursing assessment of hypomagnesemia in chronic alcoholism. *Medicolegal Libr Drugs Alcohol* 1986;6:199–202.
18. Whang R, Flink E, Dyckner T, Wester P, Aikawa J, Ryan M: Magnesium depletion as a cause of refractory potassium depletion. *Arch Intern Med* 1985;145:1686–1689.
19. Ratzan R: Uncovering magnesium toxicity. *Geriatrics* 1980;35:75–86.
20. Lembcke B, Fuchs C: Magnesium load induced by ingestion of magnesium-containing antacids. *Contib Nephrol* 1984;38:185–194.
21. Knochel J: The pathophysiology and clinical characteristics of severe hypophosphatemia. *Arch Intern Med* 1977;137:203–220.
22. Insogna K, Bondley D, Caro J, Lockwood D: Osteomalacia and weakness from excessive antacid ingestion. *JAMA* 1980;244:2544–2546.
23. Glimp R, Angert J, Rodes A: Hypocalcemia associated with oral phosphate replacement therapy. *JAMA* 1980;243:731.

BIBLIOGRAPHY

Boelhower RU, Bruining HA, Ong GL: Correlations of serum potassium fluctuations with body temperature after major surgery. *Crit Care Med* 1987;15:310–312.

Cunningham SG: Fluid and electrolyte disturbances associated with cancer and its treatment. *Nurs Clin North Am* 1982;17:579–593.

Felver L: Severe symptomatic hypophosphatemia. *CEU Study Program*. Orange, Calif, National Critical Care Institute of Education, 1984;127:1–8.

Forster J, Querusio L, Burchard KW, Gann DS: Hypercalcemia in critically ill surgical patients. *Ann Surg* 1985;202:512–518.

Ladefoged K, Nicolaidou P, Jarnum S: Calcium, phosphorus, magnesium, zinc, and nitrogen balance in patients with severe short bowel syndrome. *Am J Clin Nutr* 1980;33:2137–2144.

Manning SH, Angaran DM, Arom KV, Lindsay WG, Northrup WF, Nicoloff DM: Intermittent intravenous potassium therapy in cardiopulmonary bypass patients. *Clin Pharmacol* 1982;1:234–238.

Rose BD: *Clinical Physiology of Acid-Base and Electrolyte Disorders*, 3rd ed. New York, McGraw-Hill, 1989.

Skorecki K, Brenner B: Body fluid homeostasis in man: A contemporary overview. *Am J Med* 1981;70:77–78.

Smith WO, Clark RM, Mohr J: Vertical and horizontal nystagmus in magnesium deficiency. *South Med J* 1980;73:269.

Szyfelbein SK, Lambertus JD, Jeevendra M: Persistent ionized hypocalcemia in patients during resuscitation and recovery phases of body burns. *Crit Care Med* 1981;9:454–458.

Thompson J, Hodges R: Preventing hypophosphatemia during total parenteral nutrition. *JPEN* 1984;8:137–139.

Vogelzang N, Nelimark R, Nath K: Tumor lysis syndrome after induction chemotherapy of small-cell bronchogenic carcinoma. *JAMA* 1983;249:513–514.

Weitzman RE, Kleeman CR: The clinical physiology of water metabolism. Part III: The water depletion (hyperosmolar) and water excess (hyposmolar) syndromes. *West J Med* 1980;132:16–38.

Whang R: *Potassium: Its Biological Significance*. Boca Raton, Fla, CRC Press, 1983.

Yu G, Lee D: Clinical disorders of phosphorus metabolism. *West J Med* 1987;147:569–576.

CHAPTER 25
Acid-Base Homeostasis and Imbalances

LINDA FELVER

Acid-Base Homeostasis
Buffers
Respiratory Contribution
Renal Contribution

Acid-Base Imbalances
Metabolic Acidosis

Respiratory Acidosis
Metabolic Alkalosis
Respiratory Alkalosis
Mixed Acid-Base Imbalances

Summary

KEY TERMS

acid: A substance that releases hydrogen ions in solution.

acidemia: The state in which body fluids are actually too acid.

acidosis: Presence of a condition that tends to make body fluids too acid.

alkalemia: The state in which body fluids are actually too alkaline.

alkalosis: Presence of a condition that tends to make body fluids too alkaline.

base: A substance that accepts hydrogen ions.

buffer: Chemicals that release hydrogen ions when a fluid is too alkaline and take up hydrogen ions when a fluid is too acidic.

compensation: A process that tends to restore the pH to normal by making other blood values abnormal.

correction: A process that tends to restore the pH to normal by fixing the original cause of an acid-base imbalance.

HCO_3^-: Bicarbonate ion; an indicator of the renal excretion of metabolic acids.

H_2CO_3: Carbonic acid; this acid is removed from the body in the form of carbon dioxide and water during exhalation.

metabolic acidosis: A condition that tends to cause a relative excess of any acid except carbonic acid.

metabolic alkalosis: A condition that tends to cause a relative deficit of any acid except carbonic acid.

Pa_{CO_2}: Partial pressure of carbon dioxide; an indicator of the effectiveness of respiratory excretion of carbonic acid.

pH: A measure of the degree of acidity of a solution; technically, the negative logarithm of the hydrogen ion concentration.

respiratory acidosis: A condition that tends to cause an excess of carbonic acid.

respiratory alkalosis: A condition that tends to cause a deficit of carbonic acid.

When the **pH** of body fluids becomes abnormal, cellular function is impaired. The pH of a fluid reflects its degree of acidity or alkalinity. Technically, pH is the negative logarithm of the hydrogen ion concentration. The normal hydrogen ion concentration of the blood is about 40 nanomoles per liter (40×10^{-9} moles/L), a very small number. The pH (negative logarithm) of this number is 7.40, which is easier to use in clinical settings.

An alteration of pH is a change in the hydrogen ion concentration. An **acid** releases hydrogen ions. The more hydrogen ions present, the more acidic is the solution. The normal pH range of the blood in children and adults is 7.35 to 7.45 (may vary slightly with different laboratories). The range is somewhat wider in young infants. If the blood and other body fluids become too acidic (reflected by a decreased pH), dysfunction occurs; if the pH of the blood falls below 6.9, death is likely to result. Similarly, if the body fluids become too alkaline, as reflected by an increased pH, dysfunction also occurs. If the pH of the blood rises above 7.8, death is again likely.

Cellular metabolism continually releases acids (carbonic and metabolic) that must be excreted from the body to prevent body fluids from becoming too acidic. This chapter presents a discussion of the normal mechanisms of acid-base homeostasis and the acid-base imbalances that arise when these homeostatic mechanisms become dysfunctional or overwhelmed.

Acid-Base Homeostasis

The acid-base status of the body is regulated by three major mechanisms: **buffers,** the respiratory system, and the renal system. Laboratory measurements, such as arterial blood gas values, are useful indicators of acid-base status of the extracellular fluids. The partial pressure of carbon dioxide in the arterial blood ($Paco_2$) is an indicator of the respiratory component of acid-base balance. The plasma bicarbonate ion concentration (HCO_3^-) is an indicator of the renal (metabolic) component of acid-base balance. The pH of the blood indicates the net result of normal acid-base regulation, any acid-base imbalance, and the body's compensatory responses. It is important to remember that the pH measured clinically is that of the blood and may not reflect the pH inside the cells or in the cerebrospinal fluid.

Buffers

Buffers are chemicals that help control the pH of the body fluids. Each buffer system consists of an acid, which releases hydrogen ions when the fluid is too alkaline, and a base, which takes up hydrogen ions when the fluid is too acidic. In this way, potential changes of pH are neutralized immediately by the action of buffers. All body fluids contain buffers. Chief among them are the bicarbonate buffers (in the extra-

cellular fluid), phosphate buffers (in intracellular fluid and urine), hemoglobin buffers (inside erythrocytes), and protein buffers (in intracellular fluid and the vascular compartment). These buffers are the first line of defense against pH disorders.

The bicarbonate buffer system is the most important buffer in the extracellular fluid. Bicarbonate ions (HCO_3^-) and carbonic acid (H_2CO_3), the two components of the bicarbonate buffer system, are in chemical equilibrium in the extracellular fluid. If too much acid (e.g., lactic acid) is present, the bicarbonate ions take up the hydrogen ions (H^+) released by the acid and become carbonic acid, which is then excreted through the respiratory system in the form of carbon dioxide and water. Thus, the excess acid is neutralized as bicarbonate ions are used in the buffering process.

$$HCO_3^- + H^+ \rightleftarrows H_2CO_3 \xrightarrow[\text{carbonic anhydrase}]{} CO_2 \uparrow + H_2O \uparrow$$

The pH of any fluid is determined by the relative amounts of **acids** and **bases** contained in it. In order for the pH of the blood to be within the normal range, the ratio of bicarbonate ion to carbonic acid must be 20:1. This means that there must be 20 bicarbonate ions for every carbonic acid molecule. This relationship is explained formally by the Henderson-Hasselbalch equation, which is the mathematical description of the pH of a buffered solution, here written specifically for the bicarbonate buffer system.

$$pH = pK_a + \log \frac{[HCO_3^-]}{[H_2CO_3]}$$

Square brackets, used throughout this chapter, are a standard notation for concentration. The pK_a is the dissociation constant for any particular acid; it equals 6.1 for carbonic acid.[1] If the normal 20:1 ratio of bicarbonate ions to carbonic acid is present, then the pH will be 7.4.

$$pH = 6.1 + \log 20$$
$$pH = 6.1 + 1.3$$
$$pH = 7.4$$

The 20:1 ratio of bicarbonate ions to carbonic acid necessary for a normal pH is an important concept in understanding the compensatory mechanisms for acid-base imbalances that will be discussed later in this chapter.

Respiratory Contribution

The *respiratory system* is the second defense against acid-base disorders. The lungs excrete carbon dioxide (CO_2) and water (H_2O) from the body. Together, CO_2 and H_2O make carbonic acid (H_2CO_3). Therefore, during the process of exhalation, the lungs are effectively excreting carbonic acid. In a healthy person, if too much carbonic acid begins to accumulate in the blood, the rate and depth of respiration increase and the excess carbonic acid is removed. If, on the other hand, too little carbonic acid is present in the blood, the rate and depth of respiration decrease to retain carbonic acid until it is once more present in normal amounts. Thus, the body's ability to **correct** a carbonic acid excess or deficit is dependent on the normal function of all components of the respiratory system.

The $Paco_2$ indicates how effectively the respiratory system is excreting carbonic acid. If the $Paco_2$ is elevated, carbonic acid has accumulated in the blood. If the $Paco_2$ is decreased below normal, the lungs have excreted more carbonic acid than usual.

The lungs can excrete only carbonic acid; they cannot excrete any other acids that may accumulate in the body. If another acid (such as lactic acid) accumulates in the blood, the rate and depth of respiration will increase. This hyperventilation does not excrete lactic acid (which would correct the problem), but it does remove carbonic acid from the blood. Removing carbonic acid from the blood when another acid is present in excess is an attempt to keep the pH from dropping too low. The respiratory response to an imbalance of any acid except carbonic acid is termed a **compensatory** response. A compensatory response does not *correct* a pH disorder but it does *compensate* for it by adjusting the pH back toward normal.

The compensatory response to a deficit of any acid except carbonic acid is hypoventilation.[2] By decreasing the rate and depth of respiration, the body retains carbonic acid. This carbonic acid accumulation helps to keep the pH of the blood from rising to a fatal level when another acid is deficient in the body. Respiratory compensation for an imbalance of metabolic acid requires at least several hours.

Renal Contribution

The third defense against acid-base disorders is the *kidneys*. The kidneys can excrete any acid from the body except carbonic acid (which is excreted by the lungs). Consequently, if a metabolic acid begins to accumulate in the blood, the kidneys increase their acid excretion mechanisms to correct the problem. If a metabolic acid is deficient in the blood, the kidneys slow down their acid excretion mechanisms to allow acid to accumulate to normal levels. The body's ability to correct an excess or deficit of a metabolic acid depends on normal function of the renal system. The renal response to a large acid load is less efficient in elderly adults.

The concentration of HCO_3^- in plasma is a reflection of the effectiveness of renal regulation of metabolic acids. If metabolic acids are accumulating in the blood, they will be buffered by HCO_3^- and the HCO_3^- concentration will then drop below normal. Thus, a decreased concentration of HCO_3^- in the plasma indicates a relative excess of metabolic acids. An increase of HCO_3^- concentration in the plasma indicates a relative deficit of metabolic acids (in the words, a relative excess of base).

Although the kidneys are unable to excrete carbonic acid, they can compensate for carbonic acid imbalances by adjusting the excretion of metabolic acids.

Thus, if carbonic acid accumulates in the blood, the kidneys can increase the excretion of metabolic acids. This compensatory action helps to keep the pH of the blood from becoming too abnormal. Similarly, if there is a prolonged deficit of carbonic acid in the blood, the kidneys will decrease the excretion of metabolic acids. As these metabolic acids accumulate in the blood, they will compensate for the lack of carbonic acid and return the pH of the blood toward normal. The body's compensatory response to an imbalance of one kind of acid thus returns the pH of the blood toward normal by creating an imbalance of another kind of acid. The renal compensatory response to an imbalance of carbonic acid requires several days to be fully effective.

KEY CONCEPTS

- The bicarbonate buffer system is the most important buffer in the extracellular fluid. Its chemistry is $H^+ + HCO_3^- \rightleftarrows H_2CO_3 \rightleftarrows H_2O + CO_2$. The normal ratio of base (bicarbonate) to acid (carbonic acid) is 20:1. Any deviation from this ratio will alter the pH of the blood, which is normally 7.40.

- The lungs control the concentration of carbon dioxide in the blood. This carbon dioxide (CO_2) combines with water (H_2O) to form carbonic acid (H_2CO_3). An increase in ventilation decreases the amount of carbon dioxide in blood and reduces the amount of carbonic acid. Hypoventilation allows carbon dioxide to accumulate and increases the amount of carbonic acid.

- The kidneys control the excretion of hydrogen ions (H^+) and bicarbonate ions (HCO_3^-). The concentration of HCO_3^- in serum is a reflection of the relative amount of metabolic acid in the blood. In conditions of acidosis, the kidneys excrete excess H^+ and retain HCO_3^-. With alkalosis, the kidneys retain H^+ and excrete HCO_3^-.

- The lungs compensate for acid-base disturbances resulting from altered levels of metabolic acids, and the kidneys compensate for altered levels of carbonic acid. With compensation, pH returns toward normal but $Paco_2$ and HCO_3^- levels are abnormal.

Acid-Base Imbalances

There are four primary acid-base disorders: **metabolic acidosis, respiratory acidosis, metabolic alkalosis,** and **respiratory alkalosis. Acidosis** is the presence of a condition that tends to decrease the pH of the blood below normal (to make the blood relatively more acid). If blood pH actually is decreased, then **acidemia** is also present. **Alkalosis** is the presence of any factor that tends to increase the pH of the blood above normal (to make the blood relatively more alkaline). The term **alkalemia** is used to denote an increased blood pH. The pathophysiology of the four primary acid-base disorders is based on an understanding of the principles of acid-base homeostasis.

Metabolic Acidosis

The term **metabolic acidosis** denotes a condition that tends to cause a relative excess of any acid except carbonic acid.[3] Metabolic acidosis may be caused by an increase of acid (not carbonic), by a decrease of base, or by a combination of the two. These mechanisms decrease the normal 20:1 ratio of HCO_3^- to H_2CO_3.

An increase of any acid except carbonic acid will decrease the normal ratio of bicarbonate to carbonic acid because the bicarbonate ions are used up in buffering the excess acid. For example, when there is insufficient caloric intake, as with prolonged fasting, the body begins to utilize its fat stores for energy. If there is no glucose intake, the fat is only incompletely metabolized, and ketoacids accumulate in the blood. This condition is termed starvation ketoacidosis.

Bicarbonate ions are a type of base. Any condition that causes excessive removal of bicarbonate ions from the body may cause metabolic acidosis. For example, the intestinal fluid is rich in bicarbonate ions, which are contained in the pancreatic secretions. Diarrhea causes removal of this base from the body and thus contributes to the development of metabolic acidosis.

Other causes of metabolic acidosis are listed in Table 25–1 under the two general mechanisms discussed: increase of acid (except carbonic acid) and decrease of base. Either mechanism tends to make the blood relatively too acid. The pathogenesis and etiology of these disorders that may cause metabolic acidosis are discussed in the pertinent chapters of this text.

The signs and symptoms of metabolic acidosis are headache, abdominal pain, and central nervous system depression (confusion, lethargy, stupor, coma). The central nervous system depression of metabolic acidosis results primarily from the decreased pH of the cerebrospinal fluid and interstitial fluid in the brain. When the interstitial fluid pH falls, intracellular pH decreases and protein structure and enzyme activity within cells are altered, causing dysfunction. Other factors specific to the cause of the acidosis may also cause central nervous system depression, such as hyperosmolality with diabetic ketoacidosis. Severe metabolic acidosis predisposes to ventricular arrhythmias (from myocardial intracellular acidity) and decreased cardiac contractility, which may be fatal.

TABLE 25–1. Common Causes of Metabolic Acidosis

Increase of Acid	Decrease of Base
Ketoacidosis (diabetes mellitus, starvation, alcoholism)	Diarrhea
Hyperthyroidism	Gastrointestinal fistula
Severe infection	Intestinal decompression
Burns	Renal tubular acidosis
Shock	
Tissue anoxia	
Oliguric renal failure	
Intake of acids or acid precursors	

Death from brain stem dysfunction occurs when the pH falls below 6.9.

The arterial blood gases in metabolic acidosis will show a bicarbonate concentration below normal. If the metabolic acidosis is uncompensated, the pH will also be below normal because the usual 20:1 ratio is decreased.

Uncompensated metabolic acidosis:

$$\frac{\text{Decreased } [HCO_3^-]}{\text{Unchanged } [H_2CO_3]} = \text{pH low}$$

The respiratory compensation for metabolic acidosis is hyperventilation. A decrease in pH of the blood stimulates the peripheral chemoreceptors, which then cause reflex stimulation of ventilatory neurons in the brain stem. The end response is increased rate and depth of respiration. As the rate and depth of respiration increase, more carbonic acid (carbon dioxide and water) is excreted. Although hyperventilation does not remove metabolic acid from the body, it does change the ratio of bicarbonate to carbonic acid in a favorable direction. Because the bicarbonate ion concentration is already decreased by the metabolic acidosis, the compensatory decrease of carbonic acid brings the ratio (and thus the pH) back toward normal.

The arterial blood gases of a person who has compensated metabolic acidosis will show decreased bicarbonate concentration (the primary imbalance), decreased $Paco_2$ (compensation), and a slightly decreased or even normal pH, depending on the degree of compensation. A flow chart for interpreting laboratory measures specific to acid-base imbalances is presented in Figure 25–1.

Compensated metabolic acidosis:

$$\frac{\text{Decreased (primary) } [HCO_3^-]}{\text{Decreased (compensatory) } [H_2CO_3]} =$$

pH slightly low (partially compensated)
or in normal range (fully compensated)

Respiratory Acidosis

Respiratory acidosis is the presence of a condition that tends to cause a carbonic acid excess.[4] Because carbonic acid is excreted by the lungs, in the form of carbon dioxide and water, during the process of expiration, this condition is aptly named.

Respiratory acidosis is caused by factors that impair the respiratory excretion of carbonic acid. Such factors include impaired gaseous exchange, inadequate neuromuscular function, and impairment of the respiratory control in the brain stem. Table 25–2 provides examples of these factors that may cause respiratory acidosis. These factors all decrease the normal 20:1 ratio of bicarbonate ion to carbonic acid (and thus decrease the pH of the blood) by increasing the carbonic acid portion of the ratio. Persons who have chronic obstructive pulmonary disease often develop chronic respiratory acidosis. If they develop pneumonia, their acidosis may become worse. Such a condi-

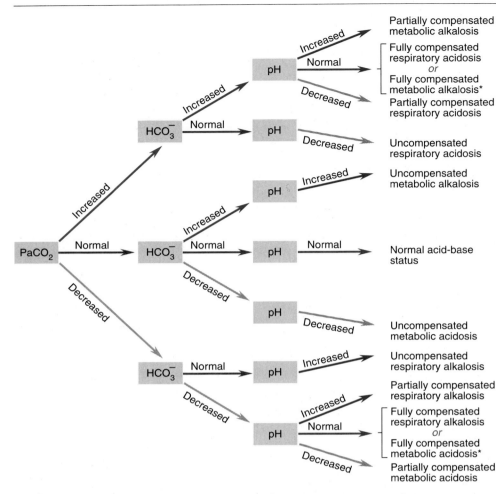

FIGURE 25–1. Flow chart for interpretation of laboratory measurements specific for acid-base imbalances. Use this flow sheet to determine the primary acid-base imbalance from a set of laboratory values. Begin on the left with the $Paco_2$ and follow the arrows. This flow sheet does not include mixed acid-base imbalances. *

*To differentiate between possible fully compensated imbalances with the pH in the normal range, look at the previous laboratory values for the patient. If no previous values are available, choose the acidosis if the pH is below 7.40 and the alkalosis if the pH is above 7.40.

tion may be termed acute-on-chronic respiratory acidosis.

The signs and symptoms of respiratory acidosis are headache, tachycardia, cardiac arrhythmias, and neurologic abnormalities such as blurred vision, tremors, vertigo, disorientation, lethargy, or somnolence. The headache occurs because of dilation of blood vessels in the brain. This cerebral vasodilation increases

TABLE 25–2. Common Causes of Respiratory Acidosis

Impaired Gaseous Exchange	Impaired Neuromuscular Function
Chronic obstructive pulmonary disease	Guillain-Barré syndrome
Pneumonia	Chest injury or surgery
Severe asthma	Hypokalemia
Pulmonary edema	Kyphoscoliosis
Adult respiratory distress syndrome	Respiratory muscle fatigue
Obstructive sleep apnea	**Impaired Respiratory Control (Brain Stem)**
	Respiratory depressant drugs (barbiturates, narcotics)
	Central sleep apnea

cerebrospinal fluid pressure; papilledema may result. Neurologic manifestations may be more prominent in respiratory acidosis than in metabolic acidosis because carbonic acid (in the form of carbon dioxide and water) crosses the blood-brain barrier relatively easily. The neurologic manifestations result from the decreased pH of the cerebrospinal fluid and interstitial fluid in the brain. This decreased interstitial fluid pH causes decreased intracellular pH, with resulting cellular dysfunction. Cardiac arrhythmias in respiratory acidosis are also a result of decreased intracellular (myocardial cell) pH. In severe respiratory acidosis, peripheral vasodilation may occur. Hypotension may result, especially if cardiac arrhythmias are also present.

The arterial blood gases in respiratory acidosis will show a $Paco_2$ above normal. If the respiratory acidosis is uncompensated, the pH will be below normal.

Uncompensated respiratory acidosis:

$$\frac{\text{Unchanged [HCO}_3^-]}{\text{Increased [H}_2\text{CO}_3]} = \text{pH low}$$

The compensatory mechanism for respiratory acidosis is increased renal excretion of metabolic acid. This mechanism requires several days to be effective.

Although the kidneys cannot excrete carbonic acid, their ability to excrete more metabolic acid changes the ratio of bicarbonate ion to carbonic acid in a favorable direction so that the pH moves toward normal. As the kidneys excrete more metabolic acid, the bicarbonate concentration will increase because fewer bicarbonate ions will be used for buffering. Because carbonic acid is already increased, the increase in bicarbonate concentration will tend to normalize the ratio of HCO_3^- to H_2CO_3. The arterial blood gases of a person who has compensated respiratory acidosis will show increased $Paco_2$ (the primary imbalance), increased bicarbonate concentration (compensation), and a slightly decreased or even normal pH, depending on the degree of compensation.

Compensated respiratory acidosis:

$$\frac{\text{Increased (compensatory) } [HCO_3^-]}{\text{Increased (primary) } [H_2CO_3]} =$$

pH slightly low (partially compensated) or in normal range (fully compensated)

Metabolic Alkalosis

Metabolic alkalosis is the presence of a factor that tends to cause a relative deficit of any acid except carbonic acid.[5] Metabolic alkalosis may be caused by an increase in base (bicarbonate), by a decrease of acid, or by a combination of the two. Bicarbonate may be ingested in antacids such as baking soda and over-the-counter bicarbonate products (e.g., Alka-Seltzer). With overuse of these agents, enough bicarbonate is absorbed from the gastrointestinal tract to increase the blood bicarbonate concentration, thus increasing the pH.

In addition to a gain of bicarbonate, metabolic alkalosis may also be caused by a decrease of acid. The stomach is a major reservoir of acid. Emesis and gastric suction remove acid from the body, creating a relative excess of base; this situation is, by definition, metabolic alkalosis. Increased renal excretion of acid with retention of bicarbonate occurs in extracellular fluid volume depletion. Hypokalemia causes hydrogen ions to shift into cells and also increases renal acid excretion.

The causes of metabolic alkalosis are summarized in Table 25–3. The pathogenesis and etiology of these disorders that may cause metabolic alkalosis are discussed in the pertinent chapters of this text.

TABLE 25–3. Common Causes of Metabolic Alkalosis

Increase of Base	Decrease of Acid
Intake of bicarbonate or bicarbonate precursors	Emesis
Massive transfusion with citrated blood	Gastric suction
	Extracellular fluid volume depletion
	Hyperaldosteronism
	Hypokalemia

The signs and symptoms in patients who have metabolic alkalosis may result from an extracellular fluid volume depletion that caused the alkalosis. Thus, postural hypotension may be present. Hypokalemia frequently coexists with metabolic alkalosis. As described previously, hypokalemia may cause metabolic alkalosis. In addition, metabolic alkalosis that arises from another cause frequently causes hypokalemia by shifting potassium ions into cells. Thus, the bilateral muscle weakness and polyuria of hypokalemia may be evident in patients who have metabolic alkalosis.

In patients who are symptomatic from the metabolic alkalosis itself, the initial manifestations are those of increased neuromuscular irritability. The increased interstitial pH causes increased irritability of nerve cell membranes. The fingers and toes may tingle; signs of tetany may progress to seizures. Persons who develop metabolic alkalosis may become quite belligerent. With severe metabolic alkalosis, initial excitation may change to central nervous system depression. Confusion, lethargy, and coma may ensue from dysfunction of brain cells. Death occurs when the pH is around 7.8. The plasma bicarbonate concentration is elevated in metabolic alkalosis.

Uncompensated metabolic alkalosis:

$$\frac{\text{Increased } [HCO_3^-]}{\text{Unchanged } [H_2CO_3]} = \text{pH high}$$

The compensatory mechanism for metabolic alkalosis is *hypoventilation*.[2] This shallow breathing retains carbonic acid within the body, thus increasing the lower portion of the bicarbonate ion to carbonic acid ratio. Because the upper portion of the ratio has been increased by the elevated bicarbonate concentration of metabolic alkalosis, the respiratory compensation tends to move the pH toward normal. Respiratory compensation for metabolic alkalosis is usually incomplete. The need for oxygen drives ventilation, even while the increased pH tends to depress it. Thus, the arterial blood gases of a person who has compensated metabolic alkalosis usually show increased bicarbonate concentration (the primary imbalance), increased $Paco_2$ (compensation), and a slightly increased pH.

Compensated metabolic alkalosis:

$$\frac{\text{Increased (primary) } [HCO_3^-]}{\text{Increased (compensatory) } [H_2CO_3]} =$$

pH slightly high (partially compensated)

Respiratory Alkalosis

Respiratory alkalosis is the presence of a condition that tends to cause a carbonic acid deficit. With a deficit of carbonic acid, the blood is relatively too alkaline.

Respiratory alkalosis is caused by *hyperventilation*. Carbonic acid is excreted during expiration; when the respirations are excessively rapid and deep (hyperventilation), too much carbonic acid is excreted. The resulting deficit of carbonic acid is respiratory alkalo-

TABLE 25–4. Common Causes of Respiratory Alkalosis (Hyperventilation)

Anxiety, psychological distress
Prolonged sobbing
Hypoxemia
Stimulation of the brain stem (salicylate overdose, meningitis, head injury)

sis. In gram-negative septicemia, the respiratory center in the brain stem is often stimulated abnormally, causing hyperventilation. Other causes of hyperventilation (and thus of respiratory alkalosis) are listed in Table 25–4.

The clinical manifestations of respiratory alkalosis are diaphoresis and increased neuromuscular irritability. Paresthesias (numbness and tingling) may occur in the fingers and around the mouth. Increased pH of the cerebrospinal fluid and cerebral interstitial fluid alters the function of brain cells. In addition, the increased pH has a direct effect of increasing membrane excitability of both central and peripheral neurons. Respiratory alkalosis also causes cerebral vasoconstriction, which reduces blood flow in the brain.

The increased excretion of carbonic acid in respiratory alkalosis causes the Pa_{CO_2} to be abnormally low. If the disorder is uncompensated, the pH will be abnormally high.

Uncompensated respiratory alkalosis:

$$\frac{\text{Unchanged [HCO}_3^-]}{\text{Decreased [H}_2\text{CO}_3]} = \text{pH high}$$

The compensatory mechanism for respiratory alkalosis is decreased renal excretion of metabolic acid. As metabolic acids accumulate in the blood, the bicarbonate ion concentration decreases because bicarbonate ions are used for buffering. Because the carbonic acid concentration is already decreased, renal compensation for respiratory alkalosis tends to return the ratio of bicarbonate ion to carbonic acid, and thus the pH, to normal. Renal compensatory mechanisms take several days to be fully effective. Many of the causes of respiratory alkalosis are short-lived and, for that reason, may not be compensated renally. The arterial blood gases of a person who has compensated respiratory alkalosis will show decreased Pa_{CO_2} (the primary imbalance), decreased bicarbonate concentration (compensation), and a slightly increased or perhaps normal pH, depending on the degree of compensation.

Compensated respiratory alkalosis:

$$\frac{\text{Decreased (compensatory) [HCO}_3^-]}{\text{Decreased (primary) [H}_2\text{CO}_3]} =$$

pH slightly high (partially compensated)
or in normal range (fully compensated)

Mixed Acid-Base Imbalances

In most patients, only one of the four primary imbalances discussed in this chapter will arise at a time. If the imbalance persists, a compensatory imbalance will arise as well. This situation has been discussed previously in this chapter. Occasionally, however, two primary imbalances will arise in the same person. This latter situation is termed a **mixed acid-base imbalance.**[6] For example, a patient who has bacterial pneumonia may develop respiratory acidosis. If this individual develops severe diarrhea at the same time, a concurrent metabolic acidosis may arise. In this mixed imbalance, the pH is likely to be very low, because the two types of primary acidosis will impair the effectiveness of the usual compensatory mechanisms. Specifically, the usual compensatory mechanism for metabolic acidosis is hyperventilation, which excretes more carbonic acid from the body. With bacterial pneumonia, however, the effectiveness of alveolar ventilation is already impaired and carbonic acid is being retained in the blood. Analogously, patients who have both types of primary alkalosis often have a very high pH, because their usual compensatory mechanisms are impeded by the concurrent acid-base disorders.

Mixed acid-base disorders may also occur with a nearly normal pH if a primary acidosis and a primary alkalosis are involved. An example of this type of mixed disorder is a head-injured patient whose treatment includes hyperventilation by mechanical ventilation to reduce intracranial pressure (respiratory alkalosis) but who at the same time has a metabolic acidosis from acute renal failure. In this situation, the Pa_{CO_2} will be decreased (respiratory alkalosis), the plasma bicarbonate concentration will be decreased (metabolic acidosis), and the pH will depend on the relative severity of the two imbalances.

KEY CONCEPTS

- A condition that tends to cause a relative excess of base is called alkalosis; a condition that tends to cause a relative excess of acid is called acidosis.
- Metabolic acidosis is characterized by a pH below 7.40 and abnormally low HCO_3^-. It is caused by processes that lead to metabolic acid accumulation (e.g., lactic acidosis) or loss of HCO_3^- (e.g., diarrhea). Compensatory hyperventilation will result in a decreased Pa_{CO_2} value on the arterial blood gas values.
- Metabolic alkalosis is characterized by a pH above 7.40 and an abnormally high level of HCO_3^-. It is caused by processes that lead to metabolic acid loss (e.g., vomiting) or gain of HCO_3^- (e.g., bicarbonate antacids). Compensatory hypoventilation will result in an increased Pa_{CO_2} on the arterial blood gas values.
- Respiratory acidosis is characterized by a pH below 7.40 and an abnormally high Pa_{CO_2}. It is caused by processes that lead to hypoventilation (e.g., decreased consciousness, lung diseases). Compensatory excretion of H^+ and production of HCO_3^- by the kidney results in increased HCO_3^- on the arterial blood gas values.
- Respiratory alkalosis is characterized by a pH above 7.40 and an abnormally low Pa_{CO_2}. It is caused by processes that lead to hyperventilation (e.g., hypox-

emia, anxiety). Compensatory retention of H^+ and excretion of HCO_3^- by the kidney results in decreased HCO_3^- on the arterial blood gas values.

- Mixed disorders are usually the result of simultaneous dysfunction of lungs and kidneys such that no compensation can occur. For example, cardiopulmonary arrest results in lactic acidosis, decreased kidney perfusion, and hypoventilation. The resultant mixed acidosis is identified by a low pH, increased $Paco_2$, and decreased HCO_3^- on the arterial blood gas values.

Summary

Acid-base homeostasis involves the interplay of the buffers, the respiratory system, and renal mechanisms. Metabolic acids are continually produced by cellular metabolism. These metabolic acids enter the blood, are buffered, and excreted by the kidneys. In healthy persons, the kidneys adjust the rate of excretion of metabolic acids to meet the demands of the acid load being produced. The concentration of bicarbonate ion in the blood indicates the effectiveness of renal excretion of metabolic acids. The carbon dioxide and water (carbonic acid) that are also produced by cellular metabolism are excreted by the lungs. In healthy persons, changes in respiratory rate and depth adjust the rate of excretion of carbonic acid. The $Paco_2$ indicates the effectiveness of respiratory excretion of carbonic acid.

If one of the acid-base regulatory mechanisms becomes dysfunctional or overwhelmed, another mechanism can produce a compensatory response that will help to normalize the pH of the extracellular fluid, even though it will not correct the acid-base imbalance. Thus, the kidneys adjust their excretion of metabolic acids when the respiratory excretion of carbonic acid is abnormally altered. Similarly, the respiratory system adjusts the rate of excretion of carbonic acid if the renal regulation of metabolic acids is impaired or overwhelmed. The pH of the blood at any one time is the net result of the operation of these regulatory and compensatory mechanisms.

Primary acid-base imbalances arise when the normal regulatory mechanisms for acid-base homeostasis become impaired or are overwhelmed by a large acid or alkaline load. Primary metabolic acidosis arises when the kidneys are unable to excrete enough metabolic acid or there is a loss of bicarbonate from the body. The compensatory response to metabolic acidosis is hyperventilation. Primary respiratory acidosis arises when the lungs are unable to excrete enough carbonic acid. The compensatory response to respiratory acidosis is increased renal excretion of metabolic acid.

Primary metabolic alkalosis arises when the kidneys excrete too much metabolic acid or there is a gain of bicarbonate. The compensatory response to metabolic alkalosis is hypoventilation. Primary respiratory alkalosis arises when the lungs excrete too much carbonic acid. The compensatory response to respiratory alkalosis decreased renal excretion of metabolic acid. The $Paco_2$ reflects the respiratory component of an acid-base imbalance, and the plasma bicarbonate concentration reflects the metabolic (renal) component of an acid-base imbalance.

A mixed acid-base imbalance occurs when two primary imbalances exist at the same time. The two primary imbalances may drive the pH to an extremely abnormal value or may nearly cancel each other's effect on the pH, although the $Paco_2$ and plasma bicarbonate concentration may still be very abnormal.

REFERENCES

1. *Merck Index*, 11th ed. Rahway, NJ, Merck Sharp & Dohme, 1989.
2. Javeheri S, Shore NS, Rose BD, Kazemi H: Compensatory hypoventilation in metabolic alkalosis. *Chest* 1982;81:296–301.
3. Kearns T, Wolfson A: Metabolic acidosis. *Emerg Med Clin North Am* 1989;7:823–835.
4. Molony DA, Schiess MC, Evanoff GV: Respiratory acid-base disorders, in Kokko JP, Tannen RL (eds): *Fluids and Electrolytes*, 2nd ed. Philadelphia, WB Saunders, 1990.
5. Toto RD: Metabolic acid-base disorders, in Kokko JP, Tannen RL (eds): *Fluids and Electrolytes*, 2nd ed. Philadelphia, WB Saunders, 1990.
6. Narins R, Emmett M: Simple and mixed acid-base disorders: A practical approach. *Medicine* 1980;59:161–187.

BIBLIOGRAPHY

Barcenas CG, Fuller TJ, Knochel JP: Metabolic alkalosis after massive blood transfusion. *JAMA* 1976;236:953–954.
Cohen J, Kassirer JP: Acid-base metabolism, in Maxwell M, Kleeman C (eds): *Clinical Disorders of Fluid and Electrolyte Metabolism*. New York, McGraw-Hill, 1980.
Done AK: The toxic emergency—acid-base disturbances: Aids to evaluation. *Emerg Med* 1981;13;159–171.
Dumier F: Primary metabolic alkalosis. *Am Fam Physician* 1981;23:193–197.
Felver L: Acid-base balance and imbalances, in Patrick ML, Woods SL, Craven RF, Rokosky JS, Bruno PM (eds): *Medical-Surgical Nursing: Pathophysiological Concepts*, 2nd ed. Philadelphia, JB Lippincott, 1991, pp 228–271.
Hobbs J: Metabolic acidosis. *Am Fam Physician* 1981;23:220–227.
Kokko JP, Tannen RL: *Fluids and Electrolytes*, 2nd ed. Philadelphia, WB Saunders, 1990.
Mandell H: Gases and 'lytes without anguish. *Postgrad Med* 1981;69:67–78.
Miller W: The ABCs of blood gases. *Emerg Med* 1984;16:37–58.
Mims B: Interpreting ABG's. *RN* 1991;54:42–46.
Missri J, Alexander S: Hyperventilation syndrome. *JAMA* 1978; 240:2093–2096.
Park R: Lactic acidosis. *West J Med* 1980;133:418–424.
Rose BD: *Clinical Physiology of Acid-Base and Electrolyte Disorders*, 3rd ed. New York, McGraw-Hill, 1989.
Shapiro B, Harrison R, Cane R, Kazlowski-Templin R: *Clinical Application of Blood Gases*. Chicago, Year Book Medical Publishers, 1989.
Winters RW, Dell RB: *Acid-Base Physiology in Medicine*, 3rd ed. Boston, Little, Brown & Co, 1982.
Wrenn KD, Minion GE: The syndrome of alcoholic ketoacidosis. *Am J Med* 1991;91:119–128.

UNIT VIII
Alterations in Intra- and Suprarenal Function

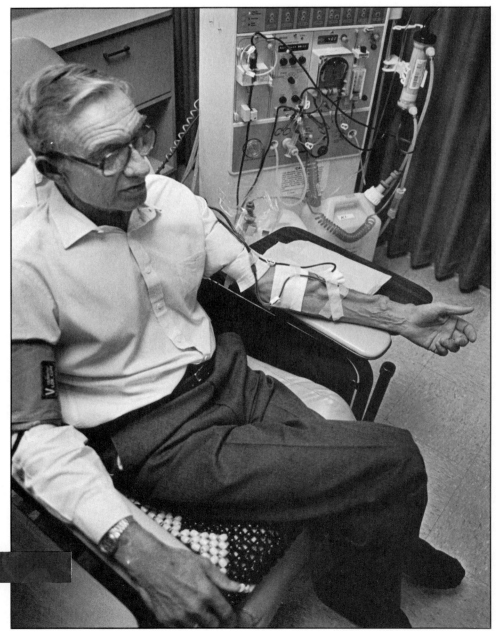

The process of hemodialysis removes toxic waste from the blood of a patient with renal failure. The complete dialysis cycle, performed three times a week, takes approximately three hours.

Photo by Kathleen Kelly

The kidneys are important regulators. The rate at which they dispose of extracellular fluid helps keep the arterial pressure at normal levels. When the arterial pressure rises, the kidneys respond by excreting extra water and salt to return the pressure to normal.

The kidneys help the body protect itself against a potentially lethal disease, hypertension, or high blood pressure, which may contribute to congestive heart disease, coronary heart disease, the rupture of major blood vessels in the brain, or hemorrhages in the kidneys, leading to kidney failure and uremia.

The two kidneys excrete urine through the activity of about 2 million nephrons, each of which is able to form urine. The nephron filters fluid from the blood and converts it to urine as it passes to the pelvis of the kidney. In this way kidneys clean unwanted substances—metabolic end products or excess ions of sodium, potassium, chloride, or hydrogen—from the blood plasma.

Because they regulate pressures within the body, the kidneys can be overpowered by imbalances, as they often are in a person with persistent, untreated hypertension. The body's organs are resilient, but continued resiliency often depends on a willingness to protect them from damage.

But the kidneys may also be damaged by congenital illnesses unrelated to the patient's weight, nutrition, exercise levels, or anxiety, all of which may contribute to hypertension. One of those illnesses is Bartter's syndrome, which is caused by a defect in sodium chloride reabsorption in the loop of Henle, a pathway through the kidney mass for fluids.

This syndrome suggests both the crucial functions and the vulnerability of the kidneys.

The kidneys filter 78 percent of the body's magnesium, and 95 percent of this amount is reabsorbed for use in the body. When sodium chloride reabsorption declines, urinary potassium loss increases. At the outset the effects of electrolyte imbalances may go undetected or may be confused with symptoms of a host of other diseases. The symptoms of hypokalemia (potassium deficit) may include fatigue, muscle tenderness, weakness or flabbiness, cardiac arrhythmias, or, in the gastrointestinal tract, anorexia, vomiting, dis-

FRONTIERS OF RESEARCH
Kidney Disease and Its Treatment
Michael J. Kirkhorn

tended abdomen, or paralytic ileus. The patient may also suffer from shortened or shallow breathing.

A patient with Bartter's syndrome may suffer from unsettling emotional symptoms as well as from physical debility. Therefore, care is complex. It will include medication, but it also may be desirable for the patient to have her family involved—the syndrome is more common among women—and perhaps to receive some psychological care.

Dialysis is a therapy used in patients with severely impaired kidney function. It is an expensive and, for the patient, an inconvenient therapy intended to restore red blood cell counts. In the future, a growth factor produced in the kidney, erythropoietin, isolated and cloned several years ago, might be used to return the red cell count to normal.

CHAPTER 26
Renal Function

CLEO RICHARD

KEY TERMS

autoregulation: Intrinsic ability of the kidney to maintain a constant glomerular pressure, by adjusting the tone of the afferent and efferent arterioles, as the mean arterial pressure fluctuates between 80 and 180 mm Hg.

blood urea nitrogen (BUN): Urea is an end product of protein metabolism, measured in the blood as BUN and excreted primarily by the kidney.

casts: Formed within the nephron during renal disease, composed of inflammatory substances surrounded by protein substance and excreted in the urine.

cortex: Outer portion of the kidney that is approximately 1 cm wide.

cortical nephron: Located in the renal cortex; 85 percent of the nephrons are this type.

creatinine: End product of muscle metabolism that is filtered freely through the glomeruli and excreted by the kidney only.

glomerular filtration: Movement of water and select substances through the glomeruli into Bowman's capsule that is dependent upon pressures in and anatomic features of the glomeruli and Bowman's capsule.

hilum: Concave portion of the kidney that faces the vertebral column through which nerves, blood vessels, and ureter enter and exit the kidney.

intravenous pyelography: Diagnostic test that determines the size, shape, and location of urinary tract structures and renal excretory function. Dye is injected intravenously and x-rays are taken.

juxtaglomerular apparatus: Responsible for storage and release of renin and composed of the macula densa cells in the distal convoluted tubule, afferent and efferent arterioles, and the juxtaglomerular cells located between these structures.

juxtamedullary nephron: Located mostly in the renal medulla, with a long loop of Henle, and has the ability to concentrate and/or dilute urine.

kidneys: Paired organs located in the retroperitoneal abdominal cavity on both sides of the vertebral column opposite the 12th thoracic vertebrae that form and excrete urine, produce hormones, and regulate many body processes.

medulla: Inner portion of the kidney that is approximately 5 cm wide.

nephron: Microscopic, structural-functional unit of the kidney that is composed of Bowman's capsule surrounding glomerular capillaries, proximal convoluted tubule, loop of Henle, distal convoluted tubule, and collecting duct.

nephrotoxic: Poisonous to the kidney.

renal biopsy: Diagnostic invasive procedure that obtains a piece of renal tissue for microscopic and immunofluorescence examination.

renin: Stored and released by the juxtaglomerular cells; converts angiotensinogen to angiotensen I.

retrograde pyelography: Diagnostic test that provides anatomical information about the urinary tract from the renal pelvis through the urinary meatus after dye is injected into the urinary tract and x-rays are taken.

ureters: Fibromuscular, mucosa-lined narrow tubes that connect the kidneys to the bladder.

urinary bladder: Muscular sac located in the anterior inferior pelvic cavity that holds urine until it is excreted through the urethra.

---

*T*his chapter is divided into three main sections: kidney structure, kidney function, and tests that assess kidney structure and function. The first two sections progress from macroscopic to microscopic and are foundational for Chapters 27 through 29. The anatomy and physiology sections provide rationale for therapeutic interventions. Embryology of the kidney is included so that the reader has a clearer understanding of the complexity of renal anatomy and physiology. In addition, embryology provides a basis for genetic and developmental renal disorders discussed in Chapter 27. Information about kidney changes throughout the life cycle provides a basis for individualizing care in order to protect or enhance renal function. Renal diagnostic tests and their potential complications are also described.

Kidney Structure

Macroscopic Anatomy

The urinary system consists of two kidneys, two ureters, one urinary bladder, and one urethra. The **kidneys** are located retroperitoneally in the posterior abdomen. *Retroperitoneal* means that the kidneys are behind and outside the peritoneal cavity. One kidney is on each side of the vertebral column between the level of the 12th thoracic and third lumbar vertebrae. Because the kidneys are in contact with the diaphragm, they move with ventilation. The right kidney is lower than the left kidney because the liver pushes it downward. The posterior upper portion of each kidney is protected by ribs. In addition, the kidneys are protected and surrounded by muscles, fascia, fat, and different abdominal organs and are not held rigidly in place. Therefore, they change position when the body changes from a supine to an erect position or vice versa (Fig. 26–1).

An adult kidney weighs approximately 140 grams and is 12 cm long, 6 cm wide, 2.5 cm thick, and shaped like a red kidney bean with the concave portion, termed the *hilum,* facing the vertebral column. A thin, cellophane-like *capsule* covers each kidney and contains blood vessels, lymphatic vessels, and nerve fibers, including pain receptors. Under the capsule the exterior surface of the kidney can be smooth but is usually slightly lumpy or lobulated. Interiorly the kidney is divided into two regions, the cortex and medulla (Fig. 26–2).

The **cortex,** the outer region, is approximately 1 cm wide and contains mostly nephrons, blood vessels, and interstitial tissue. (Nephrons and the other structures are discussed under Microscopic Anat-

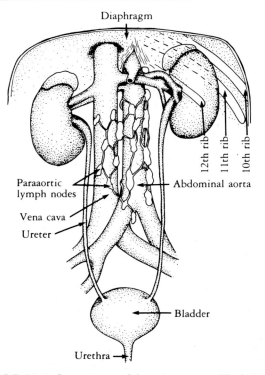

FIGURE 26–1. Components of the urinary tract. The kidneys are located in the dorsal abdominal cavity, in contact with the diaphragm and covered on the upper portions with ribs. An adrenal gland is immediately above each kidney. (From Richard CJ: *Comprehensive Nephrology Nursing.* Boston, Little, Brown & Co, 1986, p 10. Reproduced with permission.)

omy.) The **medulla** is the inner region. It is approximately 5 cm wide and contains some nephrons, blood vessels, interstitial tissue, and the collecting system. The nephrons and their blood vessels form triangular structures called pyramids. The pyramids are separated by cortical tissue known as the columns of Bertin.

The **collecting system** is composed of the papillae, minor calices, major calices, and renal pelvis. The collecting system is so named because it collects and transports urine but does not alter its composition. The papillae, also called the ducts of Bellini, are located at the base of the pyramids and are openings formed by the collecting ducts of the nephrons. The minor and major calices are tiny structures and the renal pelvis is only slightly larger, holding approximately 3 to 5 mL of urine. Urine is formed in the nephrons and flows through the following structures of the collecting system: papillae, minor calices, major calices, renal pelvis, ureter, bladder, urethra, and urinary meatus. Urine flows by gravity until it reaches the ureter, and then it moves by peristalsis through the lower urinary tract.

The **ureters** are fibromuscular, mucosa-lined, narrow tubes approximately 25 to 30 mm long that originate in the kidneys and terminate in the bladder. The **urinary bladder,** a muscular sac that holds approximately 300 to 500 mL of urine, is located in the pelvic region between the rectum and the pubic bone. The **urethra** is a mucosa-lined tube that connects the bladder to the urinary meatus. The urethra is shorter in

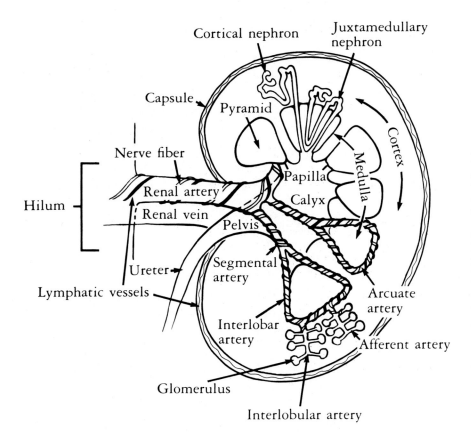

FIGURE 26–2. A longitudinal section through a kidney showing macroscopic and microscopic structures. The renal arterial vessels are shown. Nerve fibers and lymphatic vessels wrap around the arterial blood vessels and terminate in the cortex near the afferent arteriole. Another set of lymphatic vessels is depicted in the capsule. A cortical nephron and juxtamedullary nephron are shown. Note their relationship to each other and their positions in the cortex and pyramid. (From Richard CJ: *Comprehensive Nephrology Nursing.* Boston, Little, Brown & Co, 1986, p 12. Reproduced with permission.)

the female, approximately 3 to 5 cm long, than in the male, where it is approximately 20 cm long. Because the ureters, urinary bladder, and urethra are innervated with pain receptors, pain can be felt in any of these structures.[1]

Microscopic Anatomy

Nephron

The **nephron** is the structural and functional unit of the kidney. There are more than a million nephrons in each kidney. A nephron is composed of five parts: Bowman's capsule, proximal convoluted tubule, loop of Henle, distal convoluted tubule, and collecting duct. Actually, many distal tubules empty into one collecting duct. The beginning of each nephron, called **Bowman's capsule,** is shaped like a handleless cup. It surrounds a cluster of glomerular capillaries. These two structures together are often referred to as the **renal corpuscle.** The wall of Bowman's capsule is composed of two layers, the parietal and visceral epithelia. The parietal epithelium is the outer layer and the visceral epithelium is the inner layer. Both are composed of a single layer of cells and a basement membrane. The visceral epithelium is also the outer layer of the glomerular capillaries (Fig. 26–3).

Extending from each Bowman's capsule is the **proximal convoluted tubule.** It is called *proximal* because it is the segment nearest the tubule's origin from Bowman's capsule, and *convoluted* because it is

twisted. The proximal tubule narrows and becomes the descending limb of the **loop of Henle,** which later reverses directions and becomes the ascending limb of the loop of Henle. This widens and becomes the **distal convoluted tubule,** which terminates in a **collecting duct.** Many collecting ducts join and form the papillae.

The nephron wall is one cell thick and is reinforced by a basement membrane. Because it is composed of collagen and glycoproteins, which carry a negative charge, the basement membrane is negatively charged. Its function is to bind and support the tubular cells.[1]

There are two types of nephrons: 85 percent are cortical and 15 percent are juxtamedullary. Although both types have the same structures and participate in urine formation, the **juxtamedullary nephron** has a longer loop of Henle and greater ability to concentration and/or dilute urine. Because most of this nephron is located in the medulla, with only a small portion in the lower cortex, it was named juxtamedullary (*juxta* means close). The **cortical nephron** was so named because it is located only in the cortex. Although nephrons are packed closely together, they are separated by a variety of cells collectively referred to as the **interstitial tissue** or **interstitium** (see Fig. 26–2).

Blood Supply

The kidneys are very vascular and require a large blood supply for the high metabolic rate of the neph-

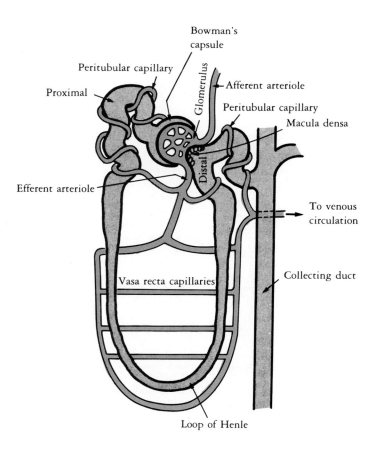

FIGURE 26–3. A nephron and its blood vessels. Bowman's capsule surrounds the glomerular capillaries. The proximal tubule, loop of Henle, distal tubule, and collecting duct compose the rest of the nephron. The peritubular capillaries surround the proximal and distal tubules and the vasa recta capillaries surround the loop of Henle. The small group of cells in the distal tubule are the macula densa. (From Richard CJ: *Comprehensive Nephrology Nursing.* Boston, Little, Brown & Co, 1986, p 14. Reproduced with permission.)

rons. Blood flows to the kidney from the abdominal aorta through the renal artery, which divides into several anterior and posterior segmental arteries. These divide into interlobar arteries, which travel adjacent to the pyramids toward the cortex. The arcuate arteries travel along the cortical medullary border parallel to the renal capsule. The interlobular arteries branch from the arcuate arteries, travel into the cortex, and divide into afferent arterioles. The afferent arteriole divides into glomerular capillaries, which unite to form the efferent arteriole. The efferent arteriole then divides into two branches, the peritubular and vasa recta capillaries. The peritubular capillaries wrap around the proximal and distal convoluted tubules and the vasa recta capillaries surround the loop of Henle and collecting ducts. Both capillary systems join together and drain into venules (Fig. 26–4).

Venous vessels accompany the arterial system and are named similarly. In the renal cortex the peritubular capillaries join to form the peritubular venules, and they and the vasa recta capillaries form the interlobular veins. The arcuate veins travel along the cortical medullary border parallel to the renal capsule. In the medulla the arcuate veins join, forming the interlobar vein, which travels adjacent to the pyramids toward the hilum. Multiple interlobar veins join and form segmental veins; the segmental veins form a renal vein that connects to the inferior vena cava.[2]

The glomerular capillaries are composed of four layers. Beginning with the capillary lumen, the layers

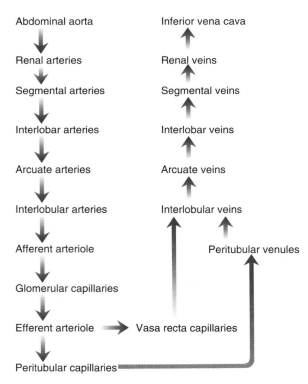

FIGURE 26–4. Blood flow through the kidney. The arterial blood enters the hilum and flows toward the renal cortex. Venous blood begins in the cortex and flows toward the hilum. *Arrows* indicate the direction of blood flow.

are the endothelium, which has fenestrations or pores; the mesangium, which has phagocytic cells; the basement membrane, which is composed of proteins and is negatively charged; and the visceral epithelium, which is composed of cells called podocytes with small pores between them. The visceral epithelium is the outer layer of the glomerular capillaries and the inner layer of Bowman's capsule (Figs. 26–5, 26–6).

Lymphatic and Nervous Systems

There are two lymphatic systems in the kidney. One system is composed of vessels that are located in the renal capsule and immediately under the capsule in the outer cortex. The other lymphatic system is composed of vessels that accompany and wrap around the arterial blood vessels. All the lymphatic vessels, as well as blood vessels and nerves, exit the kidney through the hilum, and lymph drains into the paraaortic lymph nodes. The lymphatics probably return excess protein and fluid to the circulation and transport renal hormones (see Fig. 26–2).

The kidneys are innervated by adrenergic and cholinergic fibers from the sympathetic division of the autonomic nervous system. The lesser splanchnic nerves come from the renal plexuses which are located next to the renal arteries. These nerve fibers travel with the renal arterial blood vessels and terminate in smooth muscle of the afferent and efferent arterioles. Stimulation of the sympathetic nervous system results in renal vasoconstriction and renin release. Because the renal capsule and all structures between the renal pelvis and urinary meatus are innervated with pain receptors or nocioreceptors, pain can be felt in any of these areas (see Fig. 26–2). Also see the section, Urinary Tract Pain, in Chapter 27 for further discussion.

Juxtaglomerular Apparatus

The **juxtaglomerular apparatus** (JGA) is composed of four structures: the macula densa in the distal convoluted tubule, afferent and efferent arterioles, and the juxtaglomerular cells, which are located between the afferent arteriole, efferent arteriole, and macula densa cells. The function of the JGA is explained later in this chapter.

Development of the Urinary System

The human body develops from three primary germ layers, the ectoderm, mesoderm, and endoderm. In general, the ectoderm gives rise to nervous tissue, mammary glands, and epidermis. The mesoderm gives rise to the musculoskeletal, circulatory, and genitourinary systems. The endoderm gives rise to the urinary bladder, urethra, and respiratory and gastrointestinal systems.

The human kidney develops in a series of stages from the following structures: pronephros, mesonephros, and metanephros. *Nephro* means kidney, *pro*

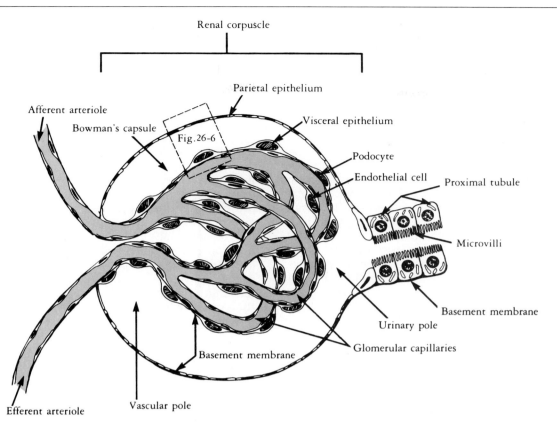

FIGURE 26–5. A renal corpuscle includes glomerular capillaries and Bowman's capsule. The basement membrane of the glomerular capillaries is continuous with the parietal epithelium of Bowman's capsule and the remainder of the nephron. (From Richard CJ: *Comprehensive Nephrology Nursing.* Boston, Little, Brown & Co, 1986, p 15. Reproduced with permission.)

means first or before, *meso* means in the middle, and *meta* means following something in a series. It is important to understand that one structure does not necessarily develop into another structure, but its

presence may induce or stimulate the formation of another structure. Usually two kidneys form at the same time bilaterally.[3,4]

During the early embryologic period, from con-

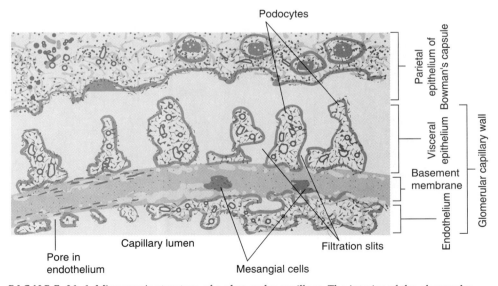

FIGURE 26–6. Microscopic structure of a glomerular capillary. The interior of the glomerular capillary, the lumen, is lined with endothelial cells bearing pores. Mesangial cells are found sporadically beneath the endothelium. The basement membrane is between the endothelium and visceral epithelium. There are filtration slits between the podocytes. Bowman's capsule surrounds the glomerular capillaries.

ception to 5 weeks, the **intermediate mesoderm** gives rise to the urogenital ridge, which gives rise to the nephrogenic ridge, which gives rise to the pronephros. The **pronephros** is nonfunctioning and regresses by the end of the fourth week but induces formation of the mesonephros. The **mesonephros** appears in the 5th week and may function until it degenerates by the end of the embryologic period (8th week). It induces formation of the metanephros.

The **metanephros** develops into the final kidney, mainly between the 5th and 14th to 15th weeks. The metanephros (metanephroi is plural) arises from two structures, the ureteral bud and the metanephric blastema. *Blastema* comes from a Greek word that means sprout. In embryologic terms, a blastema is a group of immature cells from which tissues or organs develop.[1]

The **ureteral bud** is located at the cloaca, which later becomes the urinary bladder. The ureteral bud undergoes multiple divisions and develops into the ureter. The anterior portion of the ureter dilates and gives rise to the renal pelvis, which grows and eventually differentiates into renal calices and collecting ducts.

The **metanephric blastema** is located near the developing collecting ducts and differentiates into the renal interstitium and glomerulus. The glomerular capillaries further differentiate into Bowman's capsule, the proximal convoluted tubule, the loop of Henle, and the distal convoluted tubule. The distal convoluted tubule and the collecting duct grow to meet each other and subsequently a nephron is formed that is continuous with the lower urinary system. The first nephrons originate in the medullary portion of the kidney. Subsequent nephrons originate in the cortical portion of the kidney.[1]

The intrarenal arterial blood vessels, starting with the renal artery and ending with the afferent arteriole, arise from the aorta. The intrarenal venous blood vessels likewise arise from the vena cava. After the afferent arterioles are linked carefully to the glomerular capillaries and the venous vessels are similarly linked, the intrarenal vascular system is complete.

Although the glomeruli and collecting system begin to mature first, by the 11th week there are sufficient numbers of functional nephrons to produce urine. The kidneys originate in the lower pelvic region. During this first growth period they rotate 90 degrees medially and start ascending to their adult position in the dorsal abdominal cavity (Fig. 26–7).

During the second and third growth periods, occurring between 14 and 32 weeks, the collecting system continues maturing. Collecting ducts elongate as they grow from the medulla toward the cortex and renal capsule. Simultaneously first-generation nephrons mature. Because they are attached to the medullary portion of the collecting duct, the nephrons can elongate their loops of Henle as the collecting ducts elongate. As new nephrons develop they are linked carefully to collecting ducts sequentially toward the cortex. Hence, each new nephron is closer to the renal capsule than the previous nephron. Juxtamedullary nephrons, therefore, originate during the early growth period and cortical nephrons during later growth periods (Fig. 26–8).

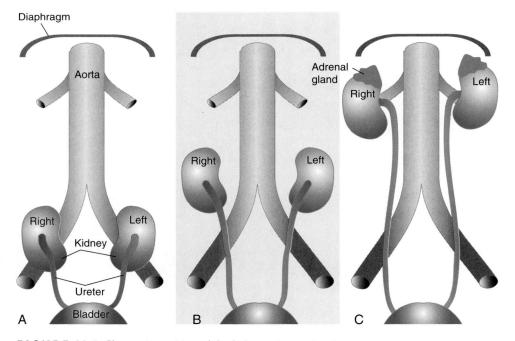

FIGURE 26–7. Change in position of the kidneys during development. **A**, Kidneys originate in the lower pelvic region. **B**, Kidneys ascending and gradually rotating medially. **C**, In the adult, the kidneys are adjacent to the diaphragm in the dorsal abdominal cavity. The kidneys have rotated 90 degrees medially during their ascent from the lower pelvic region. An adrenal gland is immediately above each kidney. The right kidney is slightly lower than the left kidney because the liver (not shown) pushes it downward.

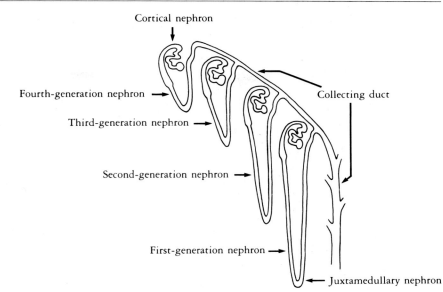

FIGURE 26–8. Development of nephrons. The short nephrons at the top of the figure are cortical nephrons and the long nephrons at the bottom are juxtamedullary nephrons. All the nephrons are attached to the same collecting duct. The first nephrons originate in the medulla. As the collecting duct grows toward the cortex, more nephrons are added. Juxtamedullary nephrons, therefore, develop first and cortical nephrons later. (From Richard CJ: *Comprehensive Nephrology Nursing.* Boston, Little, Brown & Co, 1986, p 18. Reproduced with permission.)

The fourth growth period begins between 32 and 36 weeks of gestation and lasts until the kidney is fully developed. Nephrons lengthen and become more tortuous, glomeruli enlarge, and the kidney surface changes from lumpy to smooth. The kidney reaches structural and functional maturity by the second year of life.[1]

The development of the urinary system is quite complex because there are three locations where two different structures must join successfully for the urinary system to be complete: the afferent arteriole must join to the glomerulus, the distal tubule must join to the collecting duct, and the ureter must join to the bladder. In fact, the first and second connections must occur over a million times, because there are more than a million nephrons! The third connection, however, occurs only twice, because there are only two ureters. It is helpful to understand the embryology of the urinary system because that provides insight into developmental abnormalities of the urinary system.

KEY CONCEPTS

- The kidneys are located in the retroperitoneal space, just under the diaphragm. The right kidney is lower than the left. The kidneys move with inspiration and expiration and changes in body position. The costovertebral angle is an external landmark useful for locating the kidneys.
- The kidney can be divided into two major anatomic sections, the cortex and medulla. The cortex is the outer portion and primarily contains nephrons. The medulla is the inner portion and contains some nephrons, juxtamedullary loops of Henle, and the collecting system.
- Nephrons are the functional units of urine formation. Most nephrons are located in the cortex (85 percent); the rest are juxtamedullary. Important parts of nephron structure include the glomerulus, proximal tubule, loop of Henle, distal tubule, and collecting duct.
- Blood is supplied to the kidneys by the renal artery, which divides into several branches. These branches divide again to form afferent arterioles. Each nephron has its own afferent arteriole, capillary tuft, and efferent arteriole. Efferent arterioles continue on to form peritubular capillaries, or vasa recta, which wrap around nephron structures and eventually drain into the renal veins.
- The kidneys are supplied with lymphatics to drain excess interstitial fluid and proteins, and with sympathetic neurons to regulate blood supply and renin release. Renin is released by juxtaglomerular cells located at the junction of the glomerulus and distal tubule.
- Development of the renal system progresses through an orderly sequence, resulting in functional nephrons by the 11th week of gestation. Juxtaglomerular nephrons develop first, followed by generations of cortical nephrons. The kidney reaches maturity by age 2 years.

Kidney Function

The kidneys are organs of regulation. They regulate many substances, such as water, electrolytes, nitrogenous wastes, acids, and bases, as well as bodily processes such as blood pressure. Regulation occurs through the production of urine and hormones.

Renal Blood Flow

Twenty to 25 percent of the cardiac output is delivered to the kidney. Approximately 90 percent of the renal blood volume circulates through the cortex at a rate of 4.5 mL/min, and 10 percent circulates through the medulla at a rate of 1 mL/min. Renal blood flow in both kidneys is approximately 1,200 mL/min. The hormonal systems that probably control renal blood flow are the renin-angiotensin system and the catecholamines of the sympathetic nervous system, which cause vasoconstriction, and the kinins and prostaglandins, which cause vasodilation.[5]

The organization of renal vessels is unique and purposeful because it is one of the few places where a capillary system is positioned between two arterioles. The glomerular capillaries are located between the afferent and efferent arterioles. The efferent arteriole branches into more capillaries—peritubular and vasa recta—and they join venules. This circulatory design provides a pressure system that accommodates the large renal blood volume and transport of many substances (see Fig. 26–4).

The pressure in the renal vasculature begins with 100 mm Hg in the renal artery, decreases to 50 mm Hg in the glomeruli, and decreases further to 5 mm Hg in the renal vein. The importance of this system is that the glomerular pressure, 50 mm Hg, is approximately double the pressure in other body capillaries, which is 25 mm Hg, whereas the pressure in the peritubular capillaries and vasa recta is less than the pressure in other body capillaries. The low pressure in the terminal renal capillaries supports the exchange of substances between the blood and tubular fluid. The high glomerular pressure is necessary for glomerular filtration. As pressure within the glomerular capillaries decreases, filtration also decreases and subsequently urine formation decreases.[6]

Autoregulation is the intrinsic ability of the kidney to maintain a constant glomerular pressure as the mean arterial pressure fluctuates between 80 and 180 mm Hg. Although the exact mechanisms of autoregulation are not fully understood, the following occurs. As the renal arterial pressure changes, the afferent and efferent arterioles change their diameters. For example, when the renal arterial pressure decreases, that will decrease blood flow to the glomerular capillaries, so that the afferent arteriole dilates and the efferent arteriole constricts. As the afferent arteriole dilates, more blood flows into the glomerular capillaries, and as the efferent arteriole constricts, there is more resistance to blood leaving the glomerular capillaries. These two physiologic actions maintain glomerular pressure.

Although both arterioles are innervated and neural mechanisms may participate in autoregulation, the process functions in a denervated kidney. When renal arterial pressure drops below 80 mm Hg, glomerular filtration decreases; filtration ceases at arterial pressures less than 40 to 60 mm Hg. Autoregulation is beneficial to stabilize renal circulation during exercise, postural changes, and emotional crises but not during severe blood loss such as hemorrhage.[7,8]

Urine Formation

There are two steps in urine formation, glomerular filtration and tubular processes.

Glomerular Filtration

Glomerular filtration, as the name implies, is a process that occurs in the glomerular capillaries and surrounding structures. As blood flows through the glomerular capillaries, water and many substances are filtered from the blood and pass through the capillary wall and into Bowman's capsule. Glomerular filtration is a passive process that is dependent on pressures in and the anatomic features of the glomerular capillaries and Bowman's capsule. The main driving force for filtration is hydrostatic pressure in the glomerular capillaries. The other three pressures are glomerular capillary colloidal osmotic pressure and Bowman's capsule hydrostatic and colloidal osmotic pressures (Fig. 26–9).

The *glomerular capillary hydrostatic pressure* exerts a force against the glomerular capillary walls. As blood

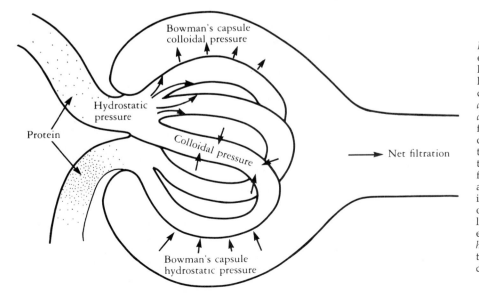

F I G U R E 26–9. Glomerular filtration entails the movement of water and select solutes through the glomerular capillaries and into Bowman's capsule. The direction of filtration is indicated by the *arrow* pointing toward net filtration. The *dots* represent proteins, which are not filtered usually. Their concentration increases in the efferent arteriole, as illustrated by the closeness of the dots, relative to a fluid loss with filtration. The four pressures that influence filtration are labeled in the figure and discussed in the text. *Arrows* indicate the direction of force for each pressure. Table 26–1 lists the approximate numerical value of each pressure. (From Richard CJ: *Comprehensive Nephrology Nursing.* Boston, Little, Brown & Co, 1986, p 23. Reproduced with permission.)

circulates through the capillaries the hydrostatic pressure pushes blood against the walls, and water and select substances are filtered out. The hydrostatic pressure exerts a force of approximately 50 to 60 mm Hg. This is the most significant of the four pressures that drives glomerular filtration. Glomerular filtration is dependent on capillary hydrostatic pressure, which is dependent on systemic blood pressure. So, for glomerular filtration to occur, systemic blood pressure must be maintained. If systemic blood pressure falls significantly, then glomerular filtration will decrease or even stop.

The *glomerular capillary colloidal osmotic pressure* exists because proteins are present in the blood. Plasma proteins are negatively charged and attract positive ions, which subsequently attract water. Because ions and water are attracted to the proteins and are not pushed against the capillary wall, the glomerular capillary colloidal osmotic pressure opposes filtration by holding water and ions in the capillaries. Because this pressure opposes glomerular hydrostatic pressure and glomerular filtration, its measurement is −30 mm Hg.

Bowman's capsule hydrostatic pressure exists because water and solutes are present in Bowman's capsule. Because this pressure exerts a force against the walls of Bowman's capsule and the glomerular capillaries, it opposes filtration and its measurement is −10 mm Hg. Normally plasma proteins do not filter into Bowman's capsule. If they do filter then they would create *Bowman's capsule colloidal osmotic pressure*. This pressure would enhance glomerular filtration because proteins attract cations and water. In a healthy kidney this pressure is negligible.

In summary, the total of all the pressures is approximately 10 to 20 mm Hg, and this represents the net filtration pressure. As blood leaves the afferent arterioles and enters the glomerular capillaries, the hydrostatic pressure is high and filtration begins. As blood passes through the capillaries, continued filtration lowers the hydrostatic pressure but at the same time leaves proteins in the capillaries, which raises the colloidal osmotic pressure. As blood reaches the efferent arterioles, filtration ceases because of the following pressure changes: decreased glomerular capillary hydrostatic pressure, increased capillary colloidal osmotic pressure, and increased Bowman's capsule hydrostatic pressure (Table 26–1).

Other factors that influence glomerular filtration are the structural integrity or permeability and the surface area of the glomerular capillaries and Bowman's capsule. In a healthy kidney, the filtrable surface area is approximately equal to the skin surface area. Although glomeruli are considerably more permeable than other capillaries in the body, they are semipermeable. Usually plasma proteins, erythrocytes, leukocytes, and platelets do not filter because they are either too large to pass through the pores and/or they are negatively charged and repelled by the basement membrane in the glomerular capillaries and Bowman's capsule. If these structures are diseased, the anatomy of the capillary walls is altered

TABLE 26–1. Pressures That Influence Glomerular Filtration

Pressure	Approximate Measurement (mm Hg)*
Glomerular	
Hydrostatic pressure	60
Colloidal osmotic pressure	−30
Bowman's capsule	
Hydrostatic pressure	−10
Colloidal osmotic pressure	0
Net filtration pressure†	20

*The −30 and −10 are shown as negative pressures because they oppose filtration.
†Net filtration pressure is the sum total of all the pressures.

and blood cells and proteins may filter and be found abnormally in urine. Usually proteins and circulating cells such as erythrocytes, platelets, and lymphocytes are not present in the urine. Proteinuria, or the occurrence of proteins in urine, is one sign of glomerular capillary disease.

The solution that is filtered through the glomerular capillaries into Bowman's capsule is termed the **glomerular filtrate** and is composed mostly of water, electrolytes, creatinine, sugars, nitrogenous wastes, and bicarbonate. The volume of glomerular filtrate and the rate at which it is filtered is called the **glomerular filtration rate** (GFR) and is approximately 125 mL/min. As glomerular filtrate leaves Bowman's capsule and enters the proximal tubule, the second step of urine formation begins—the tubular processes.

Tubular Processes

Throughout the length of the nephron, the tubular processes of reabsorption and secretion will selectively alter and reduce the glomerular filtrate and form urine. **Reabsorption** is the movement of substances from within the nephron to the surrounding capillaries (peritubular and/or vasa recta) and/or interstitial tissue. **Secretion** is the movement of substances from within the capillaries and/or interstitium into the nephron (Fig. 26–10). The following paragraphs briefly describe how tubular processes affect glomerular filtrate as it flows through the nephron (Fig. 26–11).

In the proximal tubule approximately 60 to 70 percent of the glomerular filtrate is reabsorbed. This filtrate includes water, most electrolytes, sugars, urea, and bicarbonate. Hydrogen ions and some drugs are secreted. In the descending loop of Henle a small volume of water is reabsorbed and urea is secreted. In the ascending loop of Henle chloride and sodium are reabsorbed.

In the distal tubule the transport of many substances is regulated by extrarenal hormones (Table 26–2). Aldosterone causes sodium reabsorption and potassium secretion. Generally, chloride follows the movement of sodium to maintain electroneutrality. Parathyroid hormone increases calcium reabsorption

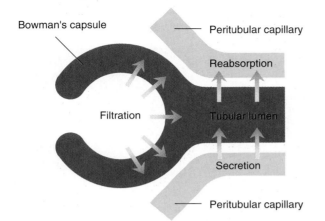

F I G U R E 26–10. Filtration, reabsorption, and secretion. *Arrows* indicate the direction of these processes. Filtration is the movement of substances from the glomerular capillaries into Bowman's capsule. Reabsorption is the movement of substances from the tubular lumen into the blood or interstitium. Secretion is the movement of substances from the blood or interstitium into the tubular lumen.

and decreases phosphate reabsorption. Calcitonin decreases phosphate and calcium reabsorption. Hydrogen ions and ammonia are secreted.

The collecting duct determines the final volume and composition of urine. Antidiuretic hormone (ADH), also called vasopressin, causes water reabsorption and consequently results in the formation of a concentrated urine. Without ADH, water is not reabsorbed and a dilute urine is excreted. Urea is reabsorbed or secreted, depending on its concentration in the interstitial tissues surrounding the collecting duct.

Creatinine, an end product of muscle metabolism, is a unique substance because it is freely filtered through the glomerular capillaries and is minimally affected by tubular processes. Therefore, the amount of creatinine filtered is found in the urine. Because creatinine is only excreted by the kidneys, it is very useful in diagnosing and evaluating renal disorders. Creatinine is discussed later in the chapter under Creatinine Tests.[1]

Acid-Base Regulation

With acid-base imbalances, the kidneys correct changes in pH that blood buffers and the lungs have

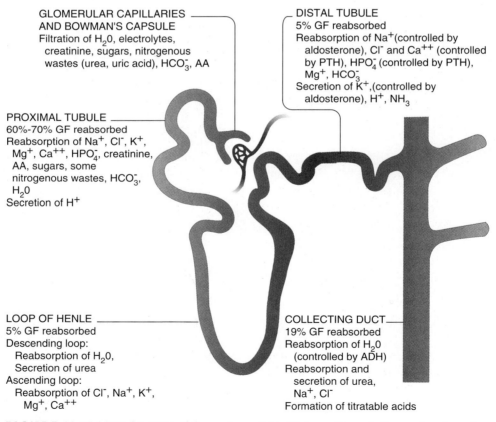

F I G U R E 26–11. Major functions of the nephron. Table 26–2 provides a further explanation of hormones that control the transport of substances throughout the nephron. AA, amino acids; ADH, antidiuretic hormone; Ca^{++}, calcium; Cl^-, chloride; GF, glomerular filtrate; H^+, hydrogen ions; HCO_3^-, bicarbonate; H_2O, water; HPO_4^-, phosphate; K^+, potassium; Mg^+, magnesium; Na^+, sodium; NH_3, ammonia; PTH, parathyroid hormone.

TABLE 26−2. Hormones and Their Effects on Renal Function

Hormone	Effects in Kidney
Aldosterone	Enhances sodium reabsorption in distal tubule (DT); enhances potassium secretion in DT
Parathyroid hormone	Enhances calcium reabsorption in DT; decreases phosphate reabsorption throughout nephron
Calcitonin	Decreases phosphate and calcium reabsorption
Vitamin D	Increases tubule reabsorption of phosphate and calcium in proximal tubule
Antidiuretic hormone/vasopressin	Increases water reabsorption in collecting duct
Atrial natriuretic peptide	Increases excretion of sodium
	Suppresses renin release from juxtaglomerular apparatus
Kinins and prostaglandins	Vasoactive substances
Angiotensin II and III	Influence renal hemodynamics—blood flow and distribution within the kidney; change tone of the renal vasculature

started to correct. The kidneys regulate the bicarbonate level and neutralize and excrete acids. The urinary pH can vary from acidic to alkaline (from pH 4 to 8), depending on the body's needs.

Sodium, chloride, bicarbonate, and phosphate are filtered into Bowman's capsule. In the cells of the proximal tubule, carbon dioxide (CO_2) combines with water (H_2O) and in the presence of carbonic anhydrase (CA) forms carbonic acid (H_2CO_3):

$$CO_2 + H_2O \xrightarrow{CA} H_2CO_3$$

The carbonic acid dissociates into hydrogen ions and bicarbonate (HCO_3):

$$H_2CO_3 \rightarrow H^+ + HCO_3^-$$

The hydrogen ions are secreted actively into the proximal tubule and sodium ions are reabsorbed actively to maintain electroneutrality. The hydrogen ions combine with the filtered bicarbonate and form carbonic acid. The carbonic acid dissociates into water and carbon dioxide. Carbonic anhydrase catalyzes this reaction. The water is reabsorbed or excreted in the urine and the carbon dioxide is reabsorbed.

All of the reactions that occur in the proximal tubule also take place in the distal tubule and collecting duct, only to a lesser degree. In addition, hydrogen ions are buffered by substances that form titratable acids, such as the filtered phosphate. Ammonia (NH_3) is formed in the cells of the distal nephron. Ammonia combines with hydrogen ions to form ammonium (NH_4), which is excreted in the urine. Figure 26–12 depicts the activity that occurs in the nephron with acid-base substances.

Water Regulation

The kidneys are the most important organs for regulating body water balance. Juxtamedullary nephrons participate more in diluting or concentrating urine because they have long loops of Henle that are located in the hyperosmotic medulla. Approximately 70 percent of the glomerular filtrate is reabsorbed in the proximal tubule, 5 percent in the descending loop of Henle, 5 percent in the distal nephron, and 19 percent in the collecting duct if ADH is present (Fig. 26–13).[1]

In the proximal tubule, 60 to 70 percent of the filtered solutes are reabsorbed, and water follows to maintain osmotic balance. The renal medulla is hyperosmotic because of the presence of sodium, chloride, and urea. In the descending loop of Henle, some water is reabsorbed because of the greater osmolality in the medulla than in the tubular fluid. A small amount of urea is secreted because there is more in the medulla than in the tubular fluid.

The thick ascending loop of Henle is impermeable to urea and water. The reabsorption of sodium, chloride, and potassium is driven by the sodium electrochemical gradient.[9] In the distal tubule solute reabsorption is controlled mostly by hormones. For example, aldosterone enhances sodium reabsorption and potassium secretion. A very small volume of water is reabsorbed because of the osmotic gradient between the tubular fluid and interstitial tissue.

The collecting duct is permeable to urea but not to water unless ADH is present. Urea moves bidirectionally, in and out of the collecting duct, until urea establishes a balance between the tubular fluid and the medulla. ADH changes the permeability of the collecting duct and allows water to be reabsorbed, because the medulla has a higher osmolality than the tubular fluid. Consequently a concentrated urine will be excreted. When ADH is not present, water cannot be reabsorbed and a dilute urine is excreted. The urine osmolality can vary from 300 to 1,200 mOsm/kg.

Renal Hormones

Renal hormones are hormones that are released by the kidney; they may or may not have an effect in the kidney. The hormones that are released from the kidney are erythropoietin, kinins, prostaglandins, and vitamin D. Their actions are summarized in Table 26–3.

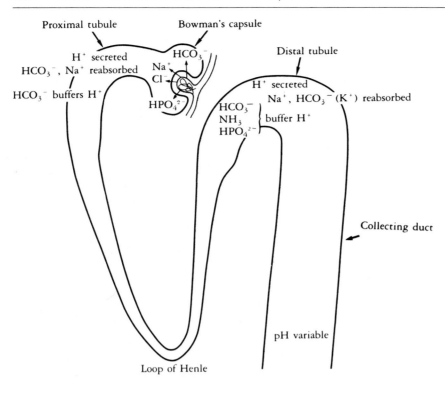

FIGURE 26–12. A summary of the transport mechanisms that buffer pH substances in the nephron. Bicarbonate (HCO_3^-), sodium (Na^+), chloride (Cl^-), and phosphate (HPO_4^{2-}) are filtered into Bowman's capsule. In the proximal tubule, hydrogen ion (H^+) is formed within the cell and secreted. Na^+ and HCO_3^- are reabsorbed. HCO_3^- buffers the secreted H^+ in the tubular lumen. In the distal tubule H^+ is formed within the cell and secreted. Na^+, HCO_3^-, and a small quantity of potassium (K^+) are reabsorbed. HCO_3^-, ammonium (NH_3), and HPO_4^{2-} buffer the secreted H^+ in the distal tubular lumen. The pH of urine is variable. (From Richard CJ: *Comprehensive Nephrology Nursing.* Boston, Little, Brown & Co, 1986, p 28. Reproduced with permission.)

Juxtaglomerular Apparatus

The **juxtaglomerular apparatus** is composed of the macula densa cells in the distal convoluted tubule, afferent and efferent arterioles, and the juxtaglomerular cells, which are located between the afferent arteriole, efferent arteriole, and the macula densa cells (Fig. 26–14). **Renin** is stored and released from the juxtaglomerular cells. Although the exact mechanisms that cause renin release are not clear, the following theories have been proposed. Renin is released when the baroreceptors in the afferent arteriole sense a decrease in pressure or volume, the sympathetic nervous system is stimulated, or the macula densa cells sense a change in sodium or chloride concentrations.[1]

Angiotensinogen is synthesized and secreted by the liver. Renin converts angiotensinogen to angiotensin I. As angiotensin I circulates through the lung, an enzyme there converts it to angiotensin II. Angiotensin II stimulates thirst, causes peripheral vasoconstriction, decreases renin secretion, and stimulates aldosterone release from the adrenal cortex. Aldosterone causes the plasma sodium level to rise by stimulating

TABLE 26–3. Renal Hormones

Hormone	Action
Erythropoietin	Stimulates formation of red blood cells in the bone marrow
Kinin	Vasodilation
Prostaglandins	Renal vasodilation; some cause constriction
Vitamin D	Increases calcium and phosphate absorption from the intestine, bone, and kidney

the reabsorption of sodium in the kidney, intestine, salivary glands, and sweat glands (Fig. 26–15). The above processes are frequently referred to as the renin-angiotensin-aldosterone mechanism and the overall goals are to maintain sodium, water, and blood pressure balances and renal perfusion.

Renal Changes Throughout Life

Fetus

The fetal kidney begins to excrete urine between the 11th and 12th week of development. Fetal urine is hypotonic to plasma because although ADH is present and the volume receptors and osmoreceptors are functional, the renal distal tubule is less sensitive to ADH than the adult nephron. Perhaps this is related to the immaturity of the distal tubule with inadequate binding sites for ADH and a low osmolality in the renal medulla. In addition, the placenta serves as a pseudo-kidney in regulating fetal fluid and electrolyte balance. Like other fetal organs, the kidney does not function independently until after birth.[4,10]

Infant

During the first week of postnatal life, the GFR is approximately 13 to 57 mL/1.73 m[2].[11] Renal blood flow is slow, the reabsorption of amino acids is limited, the ability to concentrate urine is minimal, and autoregulation is not fully achieved. Owing to an immature ability of the infant kidneys to regulate urine osmolality, infants are predisposed to volume deple-

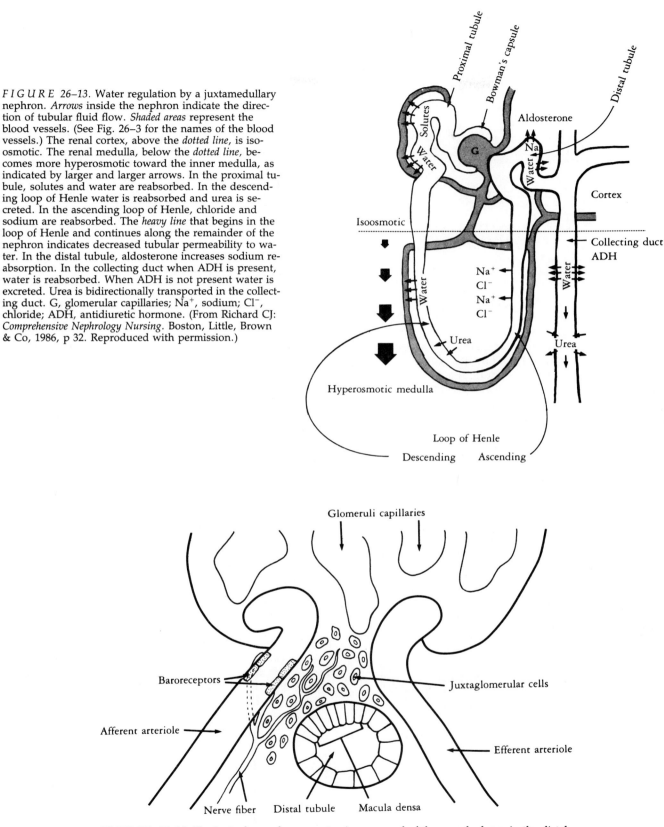

FIGURE 26–13. Water regulation by a juxtamedullary nephron. *Arrows* inside the nephron indicate the direction of tubular fluid flow. *Shaded areas* represent the blood vessels. (See Fig. 26–3 for the names of the blood vessels.) The renal cortex, above the *dotted line,* is iso-osmotic. The renal medulla, below the *dotted line,* becomes more hyperosmotic toward the inner medulla, as indicated by larger and larger arrows. In the proximal tubule, solutes and water are reabsorbed. In the descending loop of Henle water is reabsorbed and urea is secreted. In the ascending loop of Henle, chloride and sodium are reabsorbed. The *heavy line* that begins in the loop of Henle and continues along the remainder of the nephron indicates decreased tubular permeability to water. In the distal tubule, aldosterone increases sodium reabsorption. In the collecting duct when ADH is present, water is reabsorbed. When ADH is not present water is excreted. Urea is bidirectionally transported in the collecting duct. G, glomerular capillaries; Na⁺, sodium; Cl⁻, chloride; ADH, antidiuretic hormone. (From Richard CJ: *Comprehensive Nephrology Nursing.* Boston, Little, Brown & Co, 1986, p 32. Reproduced with permission.)

FIGURE 26–14. The juxtaglomerular apparatus is composed of the macula densa in the distal tubule, the afferent arteriole, and juxtaglomerular cells. Renin is stored and released from the juxtaglomerular cells. The function of the juxtaglomerular apparatus is explained in the text, and in Figure 26–15. (From Richard CJ: *Comprehensive Nephrology Nursing.* Boston, Little, Brown & Co, 1986, p 36. Reproduced with permission.)

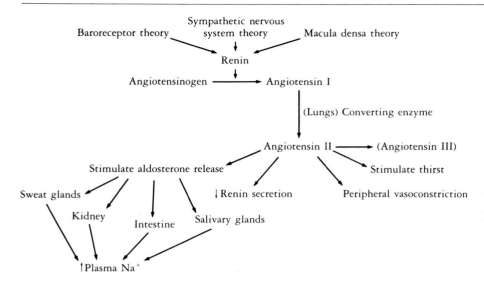

FIGURE 26–15. The renin-angiotensin-aldosterone system. Mechanisms that involve the baroreceptors, sympathetic nervous system, and macula densa lead to the release of renin. The theories that describe each of these mechanisms are presented in the text. The actions of renin, angiotensin II, and aldosterone are shown in the figure. NA$^+$, sodium. (From Richard CJ: *Comprehensive Nephrology Nursing.* Boston, Little, Brown & Co, 1986, p 36. Reproduced with permission.)

tion during fluid losses such as occur with diarrhea, fever, fluid restrictions, or decreased intake. These physiologic functions or abilities improve as the kidney matures. In addition, the glomerular and tubular basement membranes thicken, the glomeruli become increasingly permeable, and the loops of Henle lengthen. Systemic changes such as increased cardiac output and increased plasma proteins also influence the improvement in renal function. Between the first and second year of life, renal function essentially reaches maturity. Thereafter the kidney grows in proportion to overall body growth, reaching maximal size between 35 and 40 years of age.

Adult and Elderly

As part of the normal aging process, the kidney begins to diminish in size and function after the fourth decade and significantly by the middle of the sixth decade. By the sixth decade the kidney has shrunk 7 percent and by the eighth decade it has shrunk 20 percent. The shrinkage occurs mostly in the cortex and is primarily due to loss of glomeruli. After age 40 years, the number of glomeruli begins to decrease, and by age 80 it is estimated that at least 30 percent of the glomeruli have been lost. Adults less than 50 years old have zero to 7.2 percent sclerotic glomeruli, and people older than 50 have 0.5 to 36 percent sclerotic glomeruli. Reasons for the sclerotic glomeruli are not clear but a few suggestions are a high-protein diet and glomerular ischemia. Renal blood flow decreases after the fourth decade at an approximate rate of 10 percent per decade because of vascular changes, especially in the cortical blood vessels. The vasa recta are not as affected by the aging process.[1,12]

Because the GFR is related to the number of functioning glomeruli, and because the number of glomeruli decreases with age, a decrease in GFR is expected with age. After age 30 years the GFR declines approximately 7.5 to 8 mL/min per decade of life. Because creatinine clearance is a reflection of GFR, creatinine

clearance also decreases with age. By age 80 creatinine clearance is less than 100 mL/min (Fig. 26–16). There is a concomitant decrease in urinary creatinine excretion secondary to a decrease in muscle mass. Plasma creatinine levels, however, remain relatively constant throughout life.[12]

Other physiologic changes that occur in the adult are a decreased ability to conserve salt, a delayed response to an acid or base load, and a slight increase in ADH secretion, but a decreased responsiveness to ADH. Renin and aldosterone production falls by 30 to 50 percent. In addition, there is a significant loss in the kidney's ability to concentrate urine and conserve water, probably because the medulla is less concentrated and the collecting ducts are less responsive to ADH.[12] Table 26–4 summarizes the changes that occur in the kidney during the normal aging process.

Although renal function in the elderly appears to be physiologically inadequate, it is sufficient to meet its responsibilities to regulate and excrete certain substances. However, when the elderly experience stressful situations such as fever, surgery, or gastrointestinal diseases, the kidney does not have the capacity or speed to respond as though it were in a 25-year-old body. Therefore, elderly people are much more susceptible to fluid and electrolyte imbalances and renal damage. The elderly are also very susceptible to kidney damage while receiving drugs and medications, including contrast media. Consequently it is essential that renal function be evaluated before, during, and after they receive these agents or substances.

KEY CONCEPTS

- Renal function can be divided into two main processes, glomerular filtration and tubular processes. Kidneys also secrete important hormones and enzymes, including erythropoietin, active vitamin D, and renin.
- Glomerular filtration is a function of renal blood flow. The kidneys receive about 20 percent of the to-

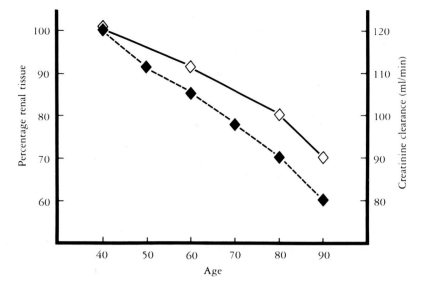

FIGURE 26–16. Renal changes through the life cycle. As the kidney decreases in size (*open diamonds*), there is a concomitant decrease in function, as evidenced by the decreasing creatinine clearance (*solid diamonds*). The decrease in kidney size and creatinine clearance is primarily related to a loss of glomerular capillaries. (From Richard CJ: *Comprehensive Nephrology Nursing.* Boston, Little, Brown & Co, 1986, p 38. Reproduced with permission.)

tal cardiac output (1,200 mL/min). Renal blood flow is determined by arterial blood pressure and renal arteriolar resistance. The kidneys are able to maintain renal blood flow despite large changes in arterial pressure by a process called autoregulation.

- Glomerular filtration in a particular nephron is determined by capillary hydrostatic pressure and Bowman's capsule oncotic pressure, which favor filtration, and by plasma oncotic pressure and Bowman's capsule hydrostatic pressure, which oppose filtration. Capillary permeability and surface area also determine filtration rate. Changes in any of these factors will affect the glomerular filtration rate (GFR). Filtration pressure is regulated by changes in afferent and efferent arteriolar diameter. Normal GFR is about 125 mL/min.

- The glomerular membranes are much more permeable than most other capillaries in the body. The composition of fluid leaving the capillary and enter-

ing Bowman's capsule is nearly identical to serum. Blood cells and large proteins do not pass through the membrane, but water, electrolytes, glucose, bicarbonate, and nitrogenous wastes pass freely.

- Filtrate formed by the glomerulus is modified by the epithelial cells that make up the nephron tubule. Substances are reabsorbed from and secreted into the filtrate as it passes through different tubule segments. In general, cations are actively reabsorbed while anions and water follow passively. The major tubular processes are summarized according to segment:

Proximal tubule: Reabsorption of two thirds of filtrate (water, sodium, chloride, potassium, bicarbonate, urea, calcium) and glucose. Secretion of hydrogen ions.

Loop of Henle: Descending: reabsorption of water. Ascending: reabsorption of sodium, chloride, and potassium.

Distal and collecting tubules: Reabsorption of sodium, chloride, calcium, and water; secretion of potassium and hydrogen ions. Sodium reabsorption and potassium excretion are regulated by aldosterone. Water reabsorption is regulated by ADH.

- Kidneys are important regulators of acid-base balance. Filtered bicarbonate ion is not directly reabsorbed but is first converted to carbonic acid by combining with secreted H^+. Carbonic acid then dissociates to CO_2 and H_2O, which are then reabsorbed into the tubule cell. A lack of secreted H^+ due to alkalosis will result in loss of bicarbonate ion in the urine, which helps restore acid-base balance. Excess H^+ ions due to acidosis combine with urine buffers (ammonia and phosphate) and are excreted.

- Renin release from juxtaglomerular cells occurs in response to sympathetic activation, decreased sodium in the distal tubule, and reduced renal blood

TABLE 26–4. Changes That Occur in the Kidney With the Aging Process

Decrease in kidney weight
Decrease in the number of glomerular capillaries
Increase in the number of sclerotic glomeruli
Decrease in renal blood flow
Interstitial tissue becomes more fibrotic
Decrease in the volume of the proximal tubule
Thickening of the glomerular and tubular basement membranes
Decrease in the glomerular filtration rate
Decrease in creatinine clearance
Decrease in production and activity of renin
Decreased ability to conserve sodium
Decreased ability to concentrate and conserve water
Decrease in the osmolality or concentration of the medullary tissue
Decrease in responsiveness to antidiuretic hormone by the collecting duct
Several vascular changes, especially in the renal cortex: blood vessels become less elastic and more twisted

flow. Renin is an enzyme that converts circulating angiotensinogen to angiotensin I. Angiotensin-converting enzyme then converts angiotensin I to II. Angiotensin II has vasoconstricting and sodium-reabsorbing actions. It also stimulates release of aldosterone.

- Renal function is impaired at both ends of the life span. Infants have reduced ability to make concentrated urine due to kidney immaturity. Aged individuals have reduced numbers of functioning nephrons, reduced renal blood flow and GFR, and decreased ability to conserve salt and water. Both age groups are at risk for fluid and electrolyte imbalances.

Tests of Renal Structure and Function

Urine

Although there are many reasons to analyze urine, this section will focus on urinalysis as it relates to structures, functions, and diseases of the urinary system. Additional information on urinalysis for specific conditions is presented in the following chapters. If the urine cannot be taken to the laboratory immediately after it is collected, it is refrigerated. Substances in the urine change at room temperature, which makes the results of the urinalysis inaccurate. For example, red blood cells hemolyze, bacteria grow and consume glucose, and the pH changes.

A routine or baseline urinalysis assesses urine color, clarity, odor, specific gravity and/or osmolality, pH, glucose, ketones, proteins and related substances, sediment (including cells, crystals, casts, and bacteria or other organisms), and possibly enzymes and electrolytes. The first urine voided in the morning is the most concentrated, due to the overnight fast, and therefore is the best specimen to use for a routine or baseline urinalysis, especially to assess pH, osmolality, and sediment.

A 24-hour urine collection measures the total quantity of a substance or substances excreted in a day. This is helpful for evaluating substances that are excreted in varying concentrations throughout the day, such as hormones, creatinine, protein, urea, and glucose.

A urine smear and culture and sensitivity tests assess the urine for microorganisms and accompanying cells, and the medications or drugs to which the organisms are most sensitive. For these tests, a few milliliters of urine are collected by the clean catch method and placed into a sterile container.

With a serial urine collection each voiding is saved in a separate container for a designated number of voidings, hours, days, or until some urinary characteristic is adequately assessed. The clean catch method is adequate and specimens can be assessed in a client's room, a utility room, a laboratory, or any combination of these.

Urinalysis

Urine is approximately 95 percent water and consists of excess water and excess substances that are the end products of body metabolism. Urine is a valuable body fluid to assess because it provides information about renal function as well as other bodily processes.

Freshly voided urine has a slight odor due to the breakdown of urea to ammonia. If urine stands for a period of time or has a large bacteria population, it will have a strong ammonia smell. The ingestion and excretion of certain foods, like asparagus, or of certain medications, like vitamins, will also cause urine to have a different odor.

The pale yellow to amber color of urine is due to the presence of urochrome pigments. Urine color can change because of the presence of cells and with an increased urine concentration. The presence of red blood cells, or hematuria, can cause urine color to range from yellow to bright red. White blood cells can make urine look whitish. Concentrated urine is usually dark yellow to orange. Certain foods and drugs can change urine color. For instance, if beets have been eaten, the urine may be burgundy in color, and if the individual has taken phenazopyradine (Pyridium), the urine may be orange.

Normally urine is clear and slightly acidic, although its pH range is 4.5 to 8.0. Urine allowed to stand undisturbed will become cloudy and alkaline because of the breakdown of urea to ammonia, which increases the pH. Cloudiness can result from the presence of cells, bacteria, crystals, casts, or fat substances.

The kidneys contribute significantly to regulating overall body fluid balance. They will excrete a concentrated urine when water needs to be conserved or will excrete a dilute urine when there is an excess of water. A measure of the kidney's ability to concentrate or dilute urine is **urine osmolality,** which ranges from 300 to 1,200 mOsm/kg H_2O. A very dilute urine is 300 mOsm/kg H_2O, whereas a very concentrated urine is 1,200 mOsm/kg H_2O. It is helpful to measure urine osmolality and blood osmolality simultaneously to assess if the kidneys are accurately regulating body fluid balance. Blood osmolality is approximately 290 mOsm/kg H_2O.

Urine specific gravity varies with the amount of solids in the urine such as cells, casts, and microorganisms, but urine osmolality is not affected by these substances, and that is why urine osmolality is a more accurate measure of the kidneys' ability to concentrate or dilute urine. The range for specific gravity is 1.005 to 1.030, with the higher number indicating a more concentrated urine. Usually urine osmolality and specific gravity vary somewhat throughout the day and from day to day. If they become fixed and remain the same over consecutive voidings and days, this could indicate renal disease.[13]

Urea, an end product of protein metabolism, is found in urine and varies with protein intake and fluid balance. A small amount of protein in the urine is insignificant, but excretion of more than 150 mg/24 hr should be investigated, as it could indicate glomerular capillary disease. Proteinuria can cause urine to be foamy.

The kidneys regulate electrolyte balance. They excrete a variable amount of electrolytes per day as well as throughout the day. Urinary electrolyte excretion is influenced by many factors and accurately assessed with a 24-hour urine collection and analysis of blood electrolytes.

Glycosuria, or glucose in the urine, is unusual except with hyperglycemia (elevated blood glucose), which can occur with diabetes mellitus or following an excessive ingestion of sugar. Rarely does glycosuria indicate renal disease.

A few epithelial cells—erythrocytes, leukocytes, and bacteria—are normally found in urine. An excess of any of these cells could indicate pathology anywhere along the urinary tract. The site of pathology can usually be identified with further assessment. For instance, erythrocytes that originate in the kidney are usually broken and found with red blood cell casts, whereas erythrocytes from the lower urinary tract are not as broken or found with red blood cell casts. Eosinophils are not usually found in urine and indicate a hypersensitivity reaction such as rejection of a transplanted kidney.

Crystals and stones are not usually found in the urine. Either one can originate any place along the urinary tract. If found in the urine, their composition should be identified and the urinary tract assessed for more crystals and stones. They may not be the result of urinary tract disease but can cause it by obstructing the flow of urine.

Casts are formed within the nephron and are unique to renal disease. There are many types of casts, each associated with certain renal pathologies. For example, white cell casts are composed of bits of leukocytes and are associated with renal inflammation such as pyelonephritis.

Creatinine Tests

Plasma Creatinine

Creatinine is an end product of muscle metabolism and is excreted only by the kidney. The plasma creatinine level averages approximately 0.7 to 1.3 mg/dL and is relatively constant throughout the day and from day to day. Creatinine levels are slightly higher in men than in women because of their larger muscle mass. A blood sample can be collected at any time to measure plasma creatinine.

Plasma creatinine is a reliable indicator of renal function because it is affected by only two factors: (1) the rate of creatinine produced from muscle, which is relatively constant in the absence of muscle breakdown, and (2) the rate of creatinine excreted by the kidney, which is determined by the GFR. Therefore, the GFR is reflected in the plasma creatinine level. For instance, when GFR decreases by half, the concentration of creatinine in the plasma will double. A rise in plasma creatinine indicates a decrease in renal function. For example, with a plasma creatinine level

above 9.0 mg/dL, there can be a 90 percent loss of renal function.[1,13]

Creatinine Clearance

Like the plasma creatinine level, the **creatinine clearance** is a very specific indicator of renal function, primarily the GFR. The test measures the amount of blood that is cleared of creatinine in 1 minute. Creatinine is filtered through the glomerular capillaries and passes through the rest of the nephron relatively unaffected. Therefore the rate at which creatinine is excreted in the urine is similar to the GFR. Normally the creatinine clearance rate is approximately 110 to 125 mL/min. A decrease in creatinine clearance indicates a decrease in renal function.[1]

To conduct the test, collect a 24-hour urine specimen and one blood specimen at the midpoint, the 12th hour, of the urine collection. The formula for creatinine clearance is:

$$\frac{\text{Volume of urine (mL/min)} \times \text{Urinary concentration of creatinine (mg/dL)}}{\text{Plasma concentration of creatinine (mg/dL)}}.$$

Blood Urea Nitrogen

Urea is an end product of protein metabolism. It is excreted primarily by the kidney and measured in the blood as **blood urea nitrogen** (BUN). The BUN averages approximately 10 to 20 mg/dL and rises with a decrease in renal function, a decrease in fluid volume, and an increase in catabolism and dietary protein intake. Because BUN is affected by multiple factors, it is correlated with changes in plasma creatinine to assess renal function. When renal function decreases, both plasma creatinine and BUN rise.

Kidney, Ureter, and Bladder Roentgenograms

A plain radiograph is taken of the abdomen to visualize the kidneys, ureters, and bladder (KUB) and serves as a screening test before most other procedures. A **KUB** study shows the position, shape, size, and number of macroscopic or gross renal, ureteral, and bladder structures and surrounding bones. In addition, foreign bodies, radiopaque objects, stones, and neoplasms can be seen on KUB.

Pyelography

Intravenous Pyelography

During **intravenous pyelography** (IVP), also called excretory urography, an iodine-containing radiopaque dye is injected into a vein, circulates through the kidney, and is excreted in the urine. A rapid series of radiographs is made as the dye is being excreted.

This test shows the size, shape, and location of urinary tract structures and can be used to evaluate renal excretory function. The dye is nephrotoxic, meaning poisonous to the kidney, and allergenic to some people. A hydrated state helps the dye pass through the kidney and prevents renal damage. Because fecal matter and gas in the intestinal tract will interfere with visualization of the kidneys and ureters on the radiographs, a laxative or enema may be indicated before IVP.

Retrograde Pyelography

Retrograde pyelography, also called retrograde urography, is an invasive procedure during which a catheter or cystoscope is passed into the bladder and smaller catheters are passed into the ureters. A radiopaque dye is injected into the urinary tract, and x-ray films are made. Additional films are obtained as the catheters are removed and should be obtained approximately 15 to 30 minutes after the initial set to make sure all the dye has been excreted. This test provides anatomic information about the urinary tract from the renal pelvis through the urinary meatus and is often done when an obstruction is suspected. If necessary, urine specimens may be obtained from each kidney before the dye is injected. Retrograde urography is often done in conjunction with cystoscopy.

Complications associated with retrograde pyelography are urinary tract infection from retrograde movement of organisms with catheter insertion and dye injection. Hematuria can be associated with urinary tract infection or can result from injury to the urinary tract mucosa from the catheter or cystoscope. Ureteral edema can result from manipulation of the catheters and obstruct urine flow. Signs and symptoms of ureteral edema include decreased urine output and possibly pain.

Although intravenous and retrograde pyelography (*pyelo* means pelvis) provide useful information about urinary tract structures and functions, these imaging studies can be hazardous to the urinary tract: the dye is nephrotoxic and allergenic, and there is the possibility of introducing microorganisms with instrumentation.

Radionuclide Studies

Renogram

A small amount of radioactive material, called an isotope, radionuclide, or radiopharmaceutical, is administered IV. It circulates through the kidney and is excreted in the urine. As the radionuclide circulates through the renal vessels and nephrons, a radiation detection probe counts the activity of the radioactive substance and simultaneously creates a graphic record or **renogram** of the activity. This test assesses renal function by measuring renal blood flow, glomerular filtration, and tubular secretion.

Renal Scan

A radionuclide is administered IV. It circulates through the kidney and is excreted in the urine. A scanning device such as a scintillator is passed over the client's back. It detects the radioactivity of the radionuclide and takes pictures of the kidney at timed intervals. The pictures or **renal scans** depict concentration of the radionuclide in the kidney and provide anatomic and some physiologic information. In the presence of tumors or nonfunctioning areas, the radioactive material will not be detected by the scan.

The renal scan is more useful for assessing renal structure and the renogram for assessing renal function. With either test, each kidney can be studied separately. Radionuclide studies are safe to use with young children and when a client is allergic to radiopaque dye. There is a low incidence of allergic reactions to radiopharmaceuticals. Additionally, because these substances are low-dose radiation, radionuclide studies can be repeated without deleterious effects.

Ultrasonography

Ultrasonography is a noninvasive, painless procedure that uses nonharmful, inaudible, high-frequency sound waves to image renal structures. Because the sound waves are at a frequency that is above the limit of human hearing, the waves are termed *ultrasound* (*ultra* means above). Ultrasound is used because its short wavelength produces a more detailed picture or image than other sound waves. A probe with a transducer inside is held against the back and emits ultrasound waves that travel through tissue to the kidney and reflect off the kidney, back to the probe. The reflective waves are echoes. The returning echoes are converted by the transducer into electrical signals that a computer plots as points of light on a screen. Eventually the points build into lines that form a picture or image.

Ultrasonography demonstrates gross renal anatomy, true kidney depth, structural abnormalities, and perirenal masses and can be used to distinguish between a fluid-filled cyst and a solid tumor. Ultrasonography may also be used for intrauterine detection of fetal genitourinary anomalies. Fetal kidneys may be detected as early as 12 weeks and the fetal bladder as early as 15 weeks.[14] Although ultrasonography is typically performed percutaneously, it can be done directly on the kidney, such as during an open renal biopsy.

Computed Tomography

Computed tomography (CT) combines roentgenograms with computer technology and is a noninvasive, painless procedure. Instead of using broad x-ray beams, CT uses thin x-ray beams, each about 10 degrees apart. The information obtained during scanning is transmitted to a computer, which constructs a tomograph and calculates its density. Because the

THE AGING PROCESS: CHANGES IN THE RENAL SYSTEM

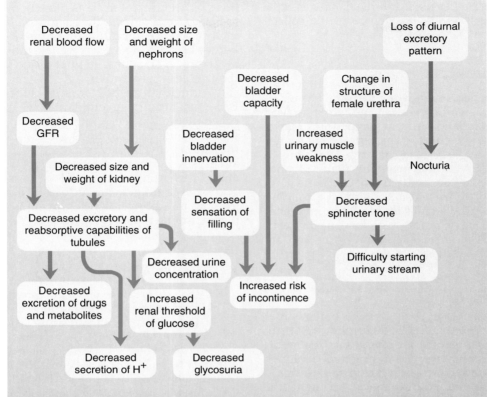

In the aging individual, there is a 30% to 50% decrease in the number, size, weight, and function of the nephrons with an accompanying reduction in the size and weight of the kidney. There is increasing interstitial fibrosis of the renal afferent arterioles. Loss of nephrons and diminished renal blood flow contribute to a decrease in the glomerular filtration rate (GFR).

There is also a decrease in the length and the excretory and reabsorptive capabilities of the tubules. The tubule changes affect the countercurrent mechanism, leading to significant changes in urine concentration, excretion, and absorption. Specifically, the changes include reduced urine concentration, decreased sodium retention, diminished drug and metabolite excretion, decreased hydrogen ion (H^+) secretion, and increased renal threshold for glucose. With aging, the kidney does not respond quickly to correct pH or sodium imbalances.

With aging, urinary muscles weaken, with decreased sphincter tone and bladder capacity. This increased muscular weakness can lead to a rise in the residual volume in the bladder and difficulty starting the urinary stream. The length of the urethra decreases. There is also less bladder innervation and a reduced sensation of filling. A loss of the diurnal excretory pattern induces nocturia.

Faith Young Peterson

kidneys are located deep within the abdominal cavity, they opacify better after an IV injection of a contrast agent. CT shows more detail than ultrasonography. CT can demonstrate perirenal and renal masses, renal vascular disorders, and filling defects of the collecting system.[1]

Magnetic Resonance Imaging

Magnetic resonance imaging (MRI) is a harmless, painless, noninvasive procedure. The job of an MRI scanner is threefold, and the term magnetic resonance imaging explains the three steps. First, the scanner applies a strong *magnetic* field that causes protons to align themselves with the magnetic field. Second, pulses of radio waves are emitted that cause the magnetic fields to rotate or *resonate*. Third, the rotating fields induce electrical signals that the computer analyzes and uses to create *images* or pictures on a screen. The renal images are available in all planes and are superior to the images achievable with CT.[7]

Renal Biopsy

The purpose of a kidney biopsy is to obtain renal tissue so that it may be studied to determine the nature and extent of renal disease for diagnosis, treatment, and prognosis. Tissue obtained during a renal biopsy is taken from the outer or cortical region of the kidney. The renal tissue is studied histologically by light and electron microscopy and immunofluorescence. Some indications for a kidney biospy are persistent proteinuria, hematuria originating from the kidney, unexplained acute renal failure, glomerular diseases, a renal mass, rejection of a transplanted kidney, and renal involvement in systemic disease.

Biopsy of the kidney may be accomplished by the open or closed method. Both are invasive procedures that require sterile technique. An **open renal biopsy** requires an operation with the subject under general anesthesia. An incision is made, the kidney is exposed, the biopsy needle is inserted into the kidney, a piece of tissue is extracted, and the area is closed and sutured. The advantages of an open biopsy are that the entire kidney is exposed and can be examined, and the biopsy site(s) can be selectively chosen, with or without the aid of an imaging technique such as ultrasonography. The disadvantages are all the complications associated with an operation.

A **closed renal biopsy,** also called a percutaneous renal biopsy (*percutaneous* means through the skin), is usually done in a radiology suite, although it can be done at the bedside. A local anesthetic is given and the client is placed in a prone position with a pillow under the abdomen. Clients who have undergone kidney transplantation are positioned to maximize access to the transplanted kidney, which is usually in the groin area. The client is instructed to hold his or her breath as the biopsy needle is inserted through the skin and into the kidney. Proof that the needle is in the kidney is movement of the needle as the client breathes, because the kidneys are in contact with the diaphragm and move with ventilation. Needle position in the kidney can also be confirmed with imaging techniques such as ultrasonography or fluoroscopy. Additionally, the client usually complains of intense pressure or dull pain as the needle enters the kidney because the renal capsule is innervated by pain receptors. A small fragment of tissue is obtained and the needle is withdrawn.

With either method of renal biopsy, hemorrhage is the most common complication. Hemorrhage may occur in the kidney, around the kidney, or in the urine. Other complications are infection, pain, clot formation in the kidney that could obstruct urine flow, aneurysm, intrarenal arteriovenous fistula, and laceration of adjacent organs or blood vessels.

Some contraindications to renal biopsy are hypertension, bleeding tendencies, documented renal neoplasm, solitary kidney, gross sepsis, and frequent coughing, sneezing, or both.

KEY CONCEPTS

- Urinalysis provides important information about kidney function. Normal urine is clear, pale yellow to amber in color, slightly acidic, and may contain a few cells. Urine osmolality and specific gravity normally vary over the course of the day, depending on fluid intake. Urine is abnormal if it is cloudy or malodorous or contains protein, red cells, crystals, stones, or casts. A fixed osmolality or specific gravity may indicate renal impairment.

- Serum creatinine and BUN are useful indicators of renal function. Serum creatinine is a more reliable indicator of renal function than BUN. In conditions of reduced GFR, serum creatinine and BUN increase. Creatinine clearance tests can be performed to evaluate GFR.

- Diagnostic studies used to evaluate kidney structure and function include plain radiography, pyelography, radionuclide studies, ultrasound, CT, and MRI. Renal biopsy may be performed to obtain tissue for histologic examination.

Summary

Although the kidneys are small, accounting for less than 1 percent of the total body weight, they are vital organs. Without the kidneys, life ceases within a few weeks.

The principal functions of the kidney are regulation and excretion. Blood pressure, fluid, electrolyte, and acid-base balances are regulated markedly by intrarenal processes. In addition, the kidney participates in hormone production, regulates extrarenal bodily processes, and excretes waste products and foreign substances.

Urine is formed within the nephrons and excreted as an end product of renal metabolism. Although the kidneys contain more than 1 million nephrons, all of which work together in unity, their function typically is explained as if there were only one large nephron. This precious structure performs numerous complex operations that adjust the composition of the blood to meet the body's needs. Intrarenal mechanisms such as autoregulation, and extrarenal mechanisms such as hormones and the nervous system, control renal function.

REFERENCES

1. Richard CJ: *Comprehensive Nephrology Nursing.* Boston, Little, Brown & Co, 1986.
2. Tortora GJ, Anagnostakos NP: *Principles of Anatomy and Physiology,* 6th ed. New York, HarperCollins, 1990.
3. Hildebrand M: *Analysis of Vertebrate Structure,* 3rd ed. New York, John Wiley & Sons, 1988.
4. Oppenheimer SB, Lefevre G Jr: *Introduction to Embryonic Development,* 3rd ed. Englewood Cliffs, NJ, Allyn & Bacon, 1989.
5. Leaf A, Cotran RS: *Renal Pathophysiology,* 3rd ed. New York, Oxford University Press, 1985.
6. Mountcastle VB: *Medical Physiology,* 14th ed. St. Louis, CV Mosby, 1980.
7. Gilbert BR, Leslie BR, Vaughan ED Jr: Normal renal physiology, in Walsh PC, Retik AB, Stamey TA, Vaughan ED Jr (eds): *Campbell's Urology,* 6th ed. Philadelphia, WB Saunders, 1992.
8. Valtin H: *Renal Function Mechanisms Preserving Fluid and Solute Balance in Health,* 2nd ed. Boston, Little, Brown & Co, 1983.
9. Moffett D, Moffett S, Schauf C: *Human Physiology: Foundations and Frontiers,* 2nd ed. St. Louis, Mosby–Year Book, 1993, p 546.
10. Moore KL: *Before We Are Born: Essentials of Embryology and Birth Defects,* 3rd ed. Philadelphia, WB Saunders, 1989.
11. Durate CG: *Renal Function Tests.* Boston, Little, Brown & Co, 1980.
12. Porush JG, Faubert PF: *Renal Disease in the Aged.* Boston, Little, Brown & Co, 1991.
13. Richard CJ: Assessment of renal structure and function, in Lancaster LE (ed): *Core Curriculum for Nephrology Nursing,* 2nd ed. Pitman, NJ, American Nephrology Nurses' Association, 1991.
14. Sanders R: Intrauterine detection of genitourinary anomalies by ultrasound. *Infect Control Urol Care* 1982;6(4):5–12.

BIBLIOGRAPHY

Berne RM, Levy MN: *Principles of Physiology,* 3rd ed. St. Louis, CV Mosby, 1993.
Brenner BM, Rector FC: *The Kidney,* 4th ed. Philadelphia, WB Saunders, 1991.
Corbett JV: *Laboratory Tests and Diagnostic Procedures with Nursing Diagnoses,* 3rd ed. Norwalk, Conn, Appleton & Lange, 1992.
Fischbach FT: *A Manual of Laboratory and Diagnostic Tests.* Philadelphia, JB Lippincott, 1992.
Guezzetta CE, Dossey BM: *Cardiovascular Nursing: Holistic Practice.* St. Louis, CV Mosby, 1992.
Kaptchuk TJ: *The Web That Has No Weaver: Understanding Chinese Medicine.* New York, Congdon & Weed, 1983.
Kee JL: *Laboratory and Diagnostic Tests with Nursing Implications,* 3rd ed. Norwalk, Conn, Appleton & Lange, 1991.
Llach F: *Papper's Clinical Nephrology,* 3rd ed. Boston, Little, Brown & Co, 1993.
Massary SG, Glassock RJ: *Textbook of Nephrology,* 2nd ed. Baltimore, Williams & Wilkins, 1989.
Monahan FD, Drake T, Neighbors M: *Nursing Care of Adults.* Philadelphia, WB Saunders, 1994.
Pernkopf E: *Atlas of Topological and Applied Human Anatomy,* 2nd ed. Philadelphia, WB Saunders, 1980.
Polin RA, Fox WW: *Fetal and Neonatal Physiology.* Philadelphia, WB Saunders, 1992.
Rolls BJ, Rolls ET: *Thirst.* New York, Cambridge University Press, 1982.
Scanlon VC, Sanders T: *Essentials of Anatomy and Physiology.* Philadelphia, FA Davis Co, 1991.
Schmidt-Nielsen K: *Animal Physiology: Adaptation and Environment,* 4th ed. New York, Cambridge University Press, 1990.
Stewart BH: *Operative Urology: The Kidneys, Adrenal Glands, and Retroperitoneum.* Baltimore, Williams & Wilkins, 1975.
Thibodeau GA, Patton KT: *The Human Body in Health and Disease.* St. Louis, CV Mosby, 1992.
Wallach J: *Interpretation of Diagnostic Tests,* 5th ed. Boston, Little, Brown & Co, 1992.
Whaley LF, Wong DL: *Nursing Care of Infants and Children,* 4th ed. St. Louis, Mosby–Year Book, 1991.
Yucha CB: Renal control of calcium. *ANNA J* 1993;20(4):440–446.
Yucha CB: Renal control of phosphorus and magnesium. *ANNA J* 1993;20(4):447–452.

CHAPTER 27
Intrarenal Disorders

PATTI STEC

KEY TERMS

azotemia: Increased levels of the waste product urea nitrogen in the blood, which indicates impaired renal clearance.

calculus: A mass of solid mineral or metabolic substance that has formed in the urinary tract.

cast: White or red blood cells that collect in the tubule and conform to the shape of the tubule; indicates damage to the nephron.

dermatome: An area of skin that is innervated by a specific spinal cord segment.

glomerulonephritis: Inflammation of the glomerular capillary walls causing decreased renal function.

hydroureter: Distention of a ureter with urine, usually resulting from an obstruction process.

intravenous pyelography: A diagnostic procedure in which an iodine-based contrast material is injected into the vascular system to image the kidneys and urinary tract.

lithotripsy: Shock waves delivered in a variety of ways to fragment renal calculi.

nephralgia: Renal pain.

nephrolithiasis: The presence of a stone or calculus anywhere in the urinary tract.

nephrotic syndrome: A common set of symptoms caused by damage to the glomeruli, in which proteins cross the capillary wall.

nociceptor: Pain receptor.

pyelonephritis: An infection of the kidney medulla or cortex.

reflux: Retrograde flow of urine from the bladder to the kidney.

urothelium: Epithelial lining of the urinary tract from the renal pelvis to the bladder.

---

*F*unctional kidneys are necessary for the removal of waste products from the blood and the maintenance of fluid, electrolyte, and acid-base balance despite wide variations in intake and nonurinary losses. Systemic disorders that alter the delivery of blood flow to the kidney may adversely affect the kidney's ability to perform its filtering and homeostatic functions. In addition, there are many disorders that occur primarily within the kidney that have the potential to result in renal insufficiency or failure. In general, these disorders can be categorized as (1) congenital, (2) infectious, (3) obstructive, and (4) glomerular. These disorders are characterized by insufficient filtering of wastes or excessive filtering of normally retained substances, and urinary tract pain. Careful assessment of the patient's history and pain symptoms aids in the localization and diagnosis of different intrarenal and postrenal disorders. A general description of urinary tract pain is presented as a preface to the discussion of specific disorders.

Urinary Tract Pain

Assessment of the location, onset, quality, quantity, and pattern of pain, as well as of interventions that relieve pain, helps to identify from which part of the urinary tract the pain is coming. Pain associated with the urinary tract may be perceived as coming from an area slightly below the ribs to the upper thighs and may be bilateral or unilateral. Typically bladder pain is felt in the suprapubic to upper thigh area, ureteral pain in the groin or genital area, and renal pain at the costovertebral angle in the back. Neither renal nor ureteral pain is altered by changing body position. Renal pain is also referred to as **nephralgia** (-*algia* is from the Greek *algos,* meaning pain).

Sympathetic nerves transmit information from renal and ureteral pain receptors or **nociceptors** (*noci* is from the Latin *nocere,* meaning to hurt or injure) to the spinal cord between T10 and L1. Because these sympathetic nerves enter the spinal cord at this level, the pain is felt throughout the corresponding T10–L1 dermatomes. A **dermatome** is an area of skin that is innervated by a specific spinal cord segment (Fig.

27–1). Visceral and cutaneous afferent fibers enter the spinal cord in close proximity and converge on some of the same neurons at the spinal, thalamic, and cortical levels. When visceral pain fibers are stimulated, concurrent stimulation of cutaneous fibers occurs and the visceral pain is felt as though it had originated in the skin.[1] Nerve fibers from the renal plexus communicate with the spermatic plexus, and because of this association, testicular pain may accompany renal pain.[2]

Extensive damage and even complete loss of a kidney can occur without nephralgia because most of the kidney is without pain receptors. The renal capsule, however, is innervated by nociceptors, and if it is distended, inflamed, or punctured, a dull to sharp pain is felt. Distention or inflammation of the renal capsule causes a dull, constant pain. Capsular stretching can result from intrarenal fluid accumulation such as occurs with inflammation with edema formation (pyelonephritis), inflamed or bleeding cysts, bleeding owing to blunt trauma, and neoplastic growth. In addition, whenever the renal capsule is penetrated (e.g., during biopsy or trauma), a dull pain or intense pressure is felt.

The lower portions of the collecting system, beginning with the renal pelvis and continuing throughout the rest of the urinary tract, are innervated by many pain receptors. Obstruction of the intrarenal collecting system causes pain if the obstruction leads to distention of the renal pelvis or capsule. Large calculi, however, can develop insidiously in the renal pelvis or calices and may be painless. Ischemia caused by occlusion of renal blood vessels (e.g., from an embolus, arteriosclerotic disease, or tumor), results in a constant dull or sharp pain.

Obstruction of the lower urinary system results in distention and intermittent sharp pain. The pain can be particularly intense if the obstruction develops rapidly. Movement of a stone down a ureter can cause renal colic and excruciating pain that can radiate from the flank into the genital area. **Renal colic** usually increases in intensity, plateaus and then decreases. *Colic* refers to spasm in a tubular or hollow organ accompanied by pain. Shock and circulatory collapse have been associated with renal colic.[1]

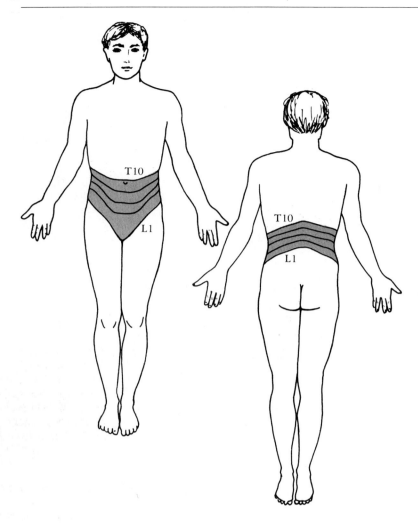

FIGURE 27-1. Dermatomes. Anterior and posterior views of the location of the T10 (thoracic) to L1 (lumbar) dermatomes. (From Richard CJ: *Comprehensive Nephrology Nursing.* Boston, Little, Brown & Co, 1986, p 44. Reproduced with permission.)

KEY CONCEPTS

- Renal pain is generally perceived at the costovertebral angle. Pain is transmitted to the spinal cord between T10 and L1 by sympathetic afferent neurons. Pain may be felt throughout the dermatomes corresponding to T10–L1. In men, testicular pain may accompany renal pain.

- Renal pain is usually due to distention and inflammation of the renal capsule and has a dull, constant character. Urinary tract pain involving the ureters is usually of an intermittent, sharp, and colicky character.

Congenital Disorders

Renal Agenesis

Renal agenesis, or failure of one or both kidneys to develop, can be found as a single entity or in combination with other congenital malformations.

Bilateral renal agenesis is found in approximately 1 in 3,000 to 4,000 live births. Males are affected more than females. Bilateral agenesis results from failure of the ureteral buds to develop or from an interruption in the progression of pronephros to metanephros formation in the fetus.[3,4] Bilateral renal agenesis is associated with **Potter's syndrome,** a collection of associated anomalies that includes (1) wide-spaced eyes with epicanthal folds, (2) low-set ears, (3) broad and flat nose, (4) hypoplastic lungs, and (5) limb anomalies.[4] This syndrome is incompatible with life outside the uterus, both because of the hypoplastic lungs and fluid volume excess and because death occurs within a few hours after birth. As many as 40 percent of infants born with bilateral renal agenesis are stillborn.

Unilateral renal agenesis is more common, affecting about 1 in 1,000 live births,[4] with males more often affected than females. The left kidney is usually the one that fails to develop.[3,4] The remaining kidney usually hypertrophies as a compensatory mechanism, occasionally to twice the normal volume. Unilateral agenesis is associated with several concurrent anomalies: (1) other genitourinary (GU) abnormalities (40 percent of cases), (2) skeletal abnormalities (30 percent), (3) cardiovascular and gastrointestinal (GI) abnormalities (15 percent), and (4) central nervous system (CNS) and respiratory system abnormalities (10 percent). If the single kidney is normal, life expectancy is normal; however, there may be an increased risk for hypertension and proteinuria.

Autosomal Recessive Polycystic Kidney Disease

Polycystic kidney disease, or kidneys with multiple fluid-filled cysts (Fig. 27–2), occurs in both adults and children. Although the pathogenesis is similar, adult autosomal dominant (ADPKD) and childhood autosomal recessive (ARPKD) forms of the disease are genetically different, with a different clinical course.

Etiology and Pathogenesis

Autosomal polycystic kidney disease is a recessive disease that begins in utero. The cysts affect primarily the collecting ducts, with virtually every collecting duct showing cystic change, accounting for the rapid decline in renal function. Cysts grow and develop due to increased epithelial cell proliferation, altered secretion, and abnormal extracellular matrix (the basement membrane is abnormally split).[5–7] Affected children also frequently have hepatic abnormalities such as hepatic fibrosis that may lead to cirrhosis, portal hypertension, or death from esophageal varices.

Clinical Manifestations

Infants with autosomal recessive polycystic kidney disease frequently die at birth or shortly thereafter of kidney failure or pulmonary hypoplasia. The kidneys may be large enough to account for 10 percent of the

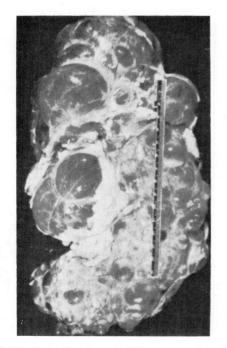

FIGURE 27–2. Adult polycystic kidney, more than 20 cm long. (From Cotran RS, Kumar V, Robbins SL (eds): *Robbins Pathologic Basis of Disease,* 4th ed. Philadelphia, WB Saunders, 1989, p 1020. Reproduced with permission.)

infant's body weight. About 25 percent of infants with autosomal recessive polycystic kidney disease survive into childhood. In childhood, presenting manifestations are abdominal masses, failure to thrive, urinary tract infections, hematuria, renal insufficiency, and hypertension.[4,6,7]

In extremely rare instances, children beyond infancy may demonstrate polycystic kidneys that arise from the autosomal dominant form of the disease.[2,3,5] In the usual course of ADPKD, affected individuals in childhood have only a very few small cysts. It is not until the fourth or fifth decade of life that the kidneys become greatly enlarged and produce symptoms such as microscopic hematuria, bilateral flank pain/masses, and hypertension.[2,5] End stage renal failure occurs in about half of those patients with ADPKD. The age at which renal failure ensues is extremely variable, but many patients are in the sixth or seventh decade of life.[3] Children who have ADPKD manifest multiple cysts, resulting in large kidneys and the same symptoms as older adults. The importance of determining the genetic cause of polycystic kidneys lies in the estimated progression of the disease. In the autosomal dominant form, only about 5 to 10 percent of all nephrons are affected by cystic formation, as contrasted by the autosomal recessive form, which involves virtually all nephrons.[3,5] The child who has ADPKD should experience a much slower disease progression, similar to the disease in adults. The child who has ARPKD experiences a much more rapid and lethal clinical course.

Diagnosis and Treatment

Diagnostic procedures include renal ultrasonography (US), intravenous pyelography (IVP), and occasionally open surgical biopsy of the right kidney and liver to distinguish between the recessive and dominant forms of the disease and multiple simple cysts or medullary sponge kidney.

Treatment is supportive for hypertension, cirrhosis, and renal failure. Renal dialysis and transplantation are both appropriate treatment modalities. In patients with hepatic fibrosis, cirrhosis, and portal hypertension, the prognosis is generally poor.

KEY CONCEPTS

- **Renal agenesis is relatively rare and, when present, is often associated with other congenital malformations. Bilateral renal agenesis is not compatible with life. Unilateral renal agenesis results in compensatory hypertrophy of the functional kidney. A single normal kidney is sufficient to perform renal function.**

- **Polycystic kidney disease is a genetically transmitted renal disorder. Autosomal recessive forms are evident at birth. Adult forms are autosomal dominant, with symptoms occurring later in life. The collecting ducts form cysts that progress to disrupt urine formation and flow. Renal failure is inevitable, necessitating dialysis or transplantation.**

Infectious Disorders

Normally, several mechanisms exist to protect the renal system from infection. Chemically, the acidic pH and the presence of urea in the urine produce a relatively hostile environment for bacterial growth. Mechanically, bacteria that may exist in small numbers are "washed out" from the system during micturition. **Reflux** of urine from the bladder to the kidney via the ureter is prevented by the contraction of the vesicoureteral junction that occurs when the bladder fills and pressure against the bladder wall constricts the junction into a closed position (see discussion under Vesicoureteral Reflux in Chap. 29). Bacteriostatic prostatic secretions in men also act as a protective mechanism.

The most common causative agents of renal system infection are gram-negative bacteria such as *E. coli, Pseudomonas,* and *Proteus* that are introduced into the kidney by a retrograde flow of urine from the bladder and ureter. Other causative organisms include gram-positive bacteria such as *Staphylococcus,* tuberculous bacilli, and fungi.

Acute Pyelonephritis

Pyelonephritis is an infection of the renal pelvis and interstitium.[8] Acute pyelonephritis frequently occurs after a lower urinary tract infection, but can occur independently. Other predisposing causes include vesicoureteral reflux (Fig. 27–3), pregnancy, neurogenic bladder, instrumentation (catheterization, cystoscopy), and female sexual trauma.[8,9]

Pathogenesis

Bacterial colonization commonly occurs in the renal papilla as a result of increased osmolarity of urine containing organisms. Increased osmolarity interferes with white blood cell (WBC) and complement function, allowing bacteria to multiply.[8,9] Abscesses or carbuncles (large localized multilocular abscesses) can form, particularly if the causative organism is *Staphylococcus* (Fig. 27–4). Perinephrenic abscesses associated with diabetes mellitus or renal calculi can develop if intrarenal abscesses rupture into the peritoneal cavity. Intra-abdominal abscesses usually require a complex treatment approach, frequently involving surgical drainage. In the absence of obstructive uropathy, usually only one kidney is involved, with the other remaining uninfected. However, if obstruction from any cause (gravid uterus, renal calculi, prostatic hypertrophy) is present, the potential exists for both kidneys to become infected.

Clinical Manifestations

Generalized symptoms of infection are usually present in acute pyelonephritis. Fever can be sudden, and the patient's temperature may rise to 38.9 to 40.6° C, accompanied by shaking chills. The patient may complain of generalized achiness, flank aching

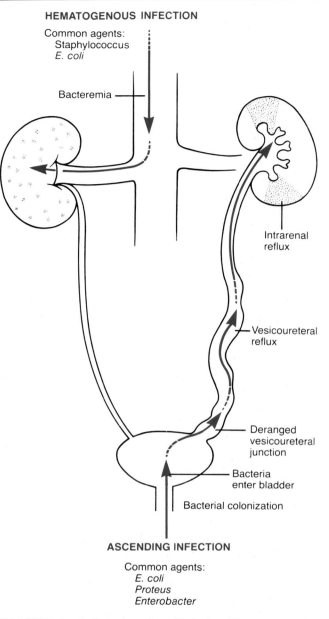

FIGURE 27–3. Pathways of renal infection. Hematogenous infection results from bacteremic spread. More common is ascending infection, which results from a combination of urinary bladder infection, vesicoureteral reflux, and intrarenal reflux. (From Cotran RS, Kumar V, Robbins SL: *Robbins Pathologic Basis of Disease,* 4th ed. Philadelphia, WB Saunders, 1989, p 1052. Reproduced with permission.)

or pain, or abdominal pain accompanied by nausea, vomiting, and fatigue. The hallmark symptom is tenderness or pain at the costovertebral angle on palpation. Lower urinary tract symptoms such as frequency and urgency of urination or hematuria may or may not be present.

Age-Related Considerations

Children may exhibit feeding difficulties, nausea and vomiting, irritability, or enuresis as well as fever. Uri-

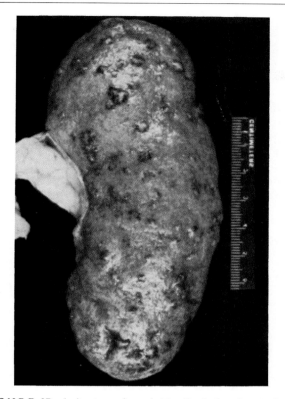

FIGURE 27–4. Acute pyelonephritis. Cortical surface is dotted with abscesses. (From Cotran RS, Kumar V, Robbins SL: *Robbins Pathologic Basis of Disease,* 4th ed. Philadelphia, WB Saunders, 1989, p 1054. Reproduced with permission.)

nary tract infections in children need close observation because significant dehydration can occur rapidly.

The elderly may have nonspecific or vague symptoms such as fever or malaise as the presenting complaint. Urinary tract infection should always be considered as a source of infection in the geriatric patient with fever.

Diagnosis and Treatment

The diagnosis of acute pyelonephritis is based on the patient's history, symptoms, physical examination results, and laboratory values. Urinalysis usually shows WBCs, occasional red blood cells (RBCs), and may show WBC casts. If the causative organism is fungal, commonly *Candida,* yeast will be found on urinalysis. Urine culture and sensitivity testing are usually done to identify the causative organism and to indicate which anti-infective agent may be suitable. A complete blood cell count may show an elevation in the total WBC count and an increase in the percentage of neutrophils, indicating a bacterial infection.

Urinary tract infections usually resolve with treatment in 10 to 14 days in the absence of obstruction or diabetes.[9] If antibiotic therapy (Table 27–1) is successful, bacteriuria should disappear in 24 hours, although symptoms may remain. Hydration adequate to maintain normal or near-normal glomerular filtration is essential for recovery of the kidney. An attempt

TABLE 27–1. Anti-infective Treatment for Pyelonephritis

Infection	Drug Formulation	
	Oral	*Parenteral*

Acute pyelonephritis	Sulfonamides
	Tetracycline
	Ampicillin
	Amoxicillin
	Cephlosporins
	Cotrimoxazole-
	  trimethoprim
		(Used if oral therapy
		  is not tolerated or
		  effective)
		Ampicillin
		Cephlosporins
		Aminoglycosides

Recurrent or chronic pyelonephritis	Cotrimoxazole- trimethoprim Nitrofurantoin	Aminoglycosides

should be made to eliminate any predisposing factors that are present. Prompt treatment of existing pyelonephritis and the prevention of future infections are important because renal scarring may occur during recovery, leading to intrarenal obstruction. Obstruction within the kidney predisposes the patient to recurrent or spreading infection.[10]

Chronic Pyelonephritis

Chronic pyelonephritis can be classified as active or inactive and occurs in about 1.5 to 3.0 percent of patients who have episodes of pyelonephritis.[8,11] Active chronic pyelonephritis involves patients with persistent or repeated complicated infections. Inactive chronic pyelonephritis is characterized by focal sterile scars of past infections that distort the renal structure (Fig. 27–5). Individuals at risk for chronic pyelonephritis have bacteriuria associated with obstructive uropathy, as in renal calculi or neurologic deficits, vesicoureteral reflux, or intrinsic renal disease.

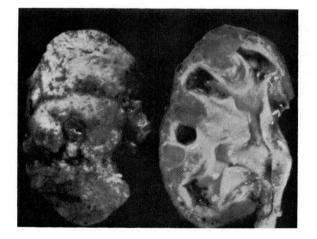

FIGURE 27–5. Chronic pyelonephritis. Surface (*left*) is irregularly scarred. Cut section (*right*) reveals characteristic dilation and blunting of calices. Ureter is dilated and thickened, consistent with chronic vesicoureteral reflux. (From Cotran RS, Kumar V, Robbins SL: *Robbins Pathologic Basis of Disease,* 4th ed. Philadelphia, WB Saunders, 1989, p 1056. Reproduced with permission.)

Pathogenesis

As a result of recurrent infections, chronic interstitial inflammation develops, with lymphocyte and plasma cell infiltration of the renal tissue. The interstitium has degrees of dilated or atrophic renal tubules with casts. Fibrosis of the interstitium, including renal tubules, decreases the number of functional nephrons. Tubercular pyelonephritis occurs as a secondary process, with the primary site of infection in the lung or other organ. Tubercular involvement causes a progressive caseous ulceration with extensive renal spread of inflammation, hydronephrosis, and eventually spread to the lower urinary tract. End-stage chronic pyelonephritis results in a shrunken and scarred kidney.[9] Chronic or recurrent pyelonephritis is the second leading cause of renal failure.

Clinical Manifestations, Diagnosis, and Treatment

The symptoms of chronic pyelonephritis may be minimal or similar to those of acute pyelonephritis. In general, frequency and urgency of voiding, dysuria (pain on urination), and flank pain that is vague and Less intense than in the acute disease may occur.

Diagnostic tests include urinalysis, IVP, and renal US. On urinalysis, bacteriuria may or may not be present, and WBC casts may be seen. On IVP the architecture of the kidney is distorted, with multiple wedge-shaped scars involving the cortex and papillae.[3] US shows a kidney smaller than normal, with "clubbing" of the affected calices.

Treatment is based on the underlying cause of the disease. Obstructive pathology must be resolved if present. Appropriate antibiotic treatment (see Table 27–1) is based on urine culture information. Chronic or recurrent disease may necessitate prolonged antibiotic therapy.

KEY CONCEPTS

- Pyelonephritis is an infection of the renal pelvis and interstitium that is most commonly due to an ascending urinary tract infection. Costovertebral angle tenderness is the hallmark symptom. It is accompanied by fever, chills, nausea, vomiting, and fatigue. Urinalysis usually shows evidence of an infective process. The presence of WBC casts is helpful in differentiating pyelonephritis from a lower urinary tract infection. Acute pyelonephritis usually responds to antibiotic therapy with little or no residual kidney damage.
- Chronic pyelonephritis is the second leading cause of chronic renal failure. Ascending urinary tract infections are usually associated with obstructive processes leading to chronic urine stasis. Chronic inflammation leads to fibrosis and scarring with associated loss of functional nephrons. The diagnosis is confirmed with ultrasonography and intrave-

nous pyelography. Urinalysis may or may not show evidence of an active infective process. Treatment includes correcting the underlying obstructive processes and providing antibiotics.

Obstructive Disorders

Obstructive disorders of the renal system or urinary tract interfere with the flow of urine. Obstruction can occur at any point in the system from the renal pelvis to the urethral meatus (Fig. 27–6). In general, an obstruction causes dilation of the tract proximal to the

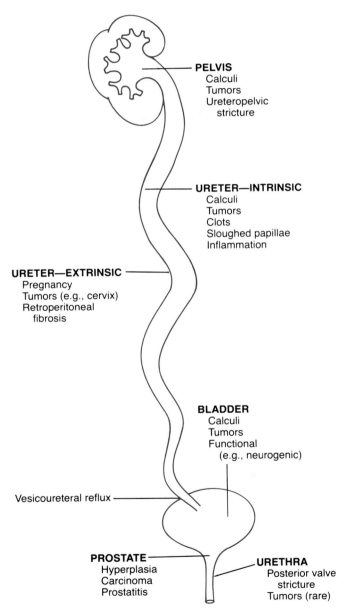

PELVIS
Calculi
Tumors
Ureteropelvic
   stricture

URETER—INTRINSIC
Calculi
Tumors
Clots
Sloughed papillae
Inflammation

URETER—EXTRINSIC
Pregnancy
Tumors (e.g., cervix)
Retroperitoneal
   fibrosis

BLADDER
Calculi
Tumors
Functional
   (e.g., neurogenic)

Vesicoureteral reflux

PROSTATE
Hyperplasia
Carcinoma
Prostatitis

URETHRA
Posterior valve
   stricture
Tumors (rare)

FIGURE 27–6. Obstructive lesions of the urinary tract. (From Cotran RS, Kumar V, Robbins SL: *Robbins Pathologic Basis of Disease,* 4th ed. Philadelphia, WB Saunders, 1989, p 1072. Reproduced with permission.)

TABLE 27–2. Causes of Renal System Obstruction

Type of Obstruction	Cause
Intraluminal obstruction	Calculi, clot
	Tumor: bladder/urethral/kidney
	Papillary necrosis
Extrinsic obstruction	Prostatic hypertrophy
	Retroperitoneal fibrosis
	Tumor: Pelvic, retroperitoneal
Acquired obstruction	Neurogenic bladder
	Ureteral stricture
	Urethral stricture

obstruction. Stasis of urine occurs and predisposes to infection and structural damage.

Disorders that are obstructive can be congenital or acquired. In children, urinary tract obstruction is usually due to anatomic abnormalities like ureteral valves, strictures of the urethral meatus, and stenosis at the ureterovesical or ureteral pelvic junction.[12,13] Obstruction in adults predominantly occurs as a result of acquired disorders and may be either intraluminal or secondary to extrinsic compression (e.g., by renal calculi or tumors) (Table 27–2).

Pathophysiology

Changes that occur within the urinary tract as a result of obstruction are dependent on (1) the degree of obstruction (i.e., partial or complete, unilateral or bilateral) and (2) the duration of the obstruction. Initially, hydrostatic pressure increases proximal to the collecting system of the kidney as a consequence of the continued glomerular filtration and obstruction to the flow of urine. Other structures proximal to the obstruction then begin to dilate. The lower or more distal (to the kidney) the obstruction, the less dilation is seen because of the increased surface area over which the pressure is diffused.

Complete obstruction of a ureter causes an accumulation of urine known as **hydroureter.** Pressure in the renal pelvis and tubules increase, causing dilation of both and a flattening of the renal papillae. The glomerular filtration rate (GFR) falls, and there is disruption of the junctional complexes between tubular cells. This disruption permits solutes to leak from the tubule to the capillary. Initially renal perfusion increases because of the effects of prostaglandins on vasodilation in the renal cortex.[10,12] After 4 to 6 hours, however, renal blood flow decreases to 10 to 15 percent of normal due to vasoconstriction. The kidney then becomes ischemic, and the nephrons that do continue to function have decreased filtration rates and are impaired in their ability to conserve sodium, secrete potassium, and acidify or concentrate urine. In 4 to 6 weeks, tubular atrophy and destruction of the medulla leaves connective tissue in place of the glomeruli. At this point, renal damage is irreversible.

Unilateral obstruction reduces the GFR to 50 percent of normal, and the serum creatinine level doubles.[12]

In partial obstruction, the renal pelvis may become very dilated but there may be little structural or functional disruption of the kidney. If partial obstruction is bilateral, as much as 2 to 3 liters of urine can accumulate in the system.[10] Functionally, partial obstruction can produce a slight to moderate decrease in blood flow and GFR, and inability to concentrate urine or secrete potassium and hydrogen ions. Normal or excessive volumes of urine may be seen despite a reduction in GFR. The risk of dehydration and metabolic acidosis increases because of sodium and bicarbonate wasting.

Postobstructive diuresis may occur after the obstruction has been corrected, particularly in lower tract and bilateral obstruction. This diuresis is temporary and results from excretion of the sodium, urea, and water that were retained during the obstructive period. The diuresis lasts until the composition and volume of the body's extracellular fluid *returns to normal,* so that symptoms of volume depletion (postural hypotension and tachycardia) do *not* appear. In some cases a true salt and water wasting occurs that depletes the extracellular volume. In these cases treatment is instituted to replace two thirds of the urine volume loss per day until the urine volume returns to normal. If salt and water losses are severe enough to result in signficant dehydration and decreased vascular volume, there is usually a defect in tubular reabsorptive function.[13]

Complications of urinary obstruction include infection, sepsis, progressive loss of renal function, and renal failure. The site, extent, and duration of obstruction determine the type of complication. Prolonged bilateral obstruction or severe partial obstruction leads to acute or chronic renal failure. If bilateral obstruction is relieved in 1 to 2 weeks,[12] a complete return to baseline renal function is possible. Infection can accompany obstruction at any point within the system but is more frequent with obstruction below the bladder.

Renal Calculi

Renal calculi consist of crystals combined with proteins that initially form in the calices or pelvis of the kidney.[15] These calculi then may migrate down the urinary tract, causing pain, obstruction, and infection. The presence of a stone or calculus anywhere in the urinary tract is termed **nephrolithiasis**.

Etiology and Pathogenesis

Renal calculi or nephrolithiasis occurs in 1 to 5 percent of the population in industrial countries.[14] The rate of recurrence once an individual has had calculus is 50 to 80 percent. Calculi are most common in white men[15] aged 20 to 50 years.[3] Women are less often affected than men. Calculi form due to supersaturation (increased concentration of the offending solute), an abnormal urine pH, or low urine volume. Hypercalciuria is the most frequent physiologic abnormality found in patients with nephrolithiasis. Calcium oxalate or calcium phosphate stones make up 75 to 90 percent of all renal calculi.[14–16] Uric acid, cystine, and struvite make up the remaining percentage of calculi.

Because the substances that compose renal calculi are normally present in urine and do not cause calculi in everyone, there appear to be mechanisms that normally inhibit crystallization and supersaturation. These inhibitors are thought to include pyrophosphate, citrate, magnesium, and certain macromolecules like glycoproteins.[14] Citrate appears to inhibit nephrolithiasis by forming a soluble complex with calcium and decreasing calcium activity.

When citrates and magnesium, substances in the urine that inhibit stone formation, are deficient, calcium-type calculi can form. The condition of hypocitraturia can be found in acidosis, chronic diarrhea, thiazide-induced hypocalcemia, and a diet high in animal protein. Hypomagnesiuria is usually found in conjunction with hypocitraturia and low urine volume. The cause of hypomagnesiuria is probably a diet deficient in magnesium. Hyperoxaluria is not common but can occur in a primary form (rare) or in the setting of pyridoxine deficiency, excessive ascorbic acid, and enhanced absorption of dietary oxalate (enteric hyperoxaluria).

Uric acid calculi are commonly found in primary gout, in conditions of low urinary pH (<5.5), and hyperuricosuria. Uric acid calculi may also be found in myeloproliferative states, glycogen storage diseases, and malignancy, which causes purine overproduction. Chronic diarrhea (ulcerative colitis, regional enteritis) may produce a net alkali deficit and decreased urine volume, precipitating uric acid calculi formation.

Cystinuria that causes cystine calculi results from an inborn error of metabolism of dicarboxylic acids. The urine may become supersaturated with cystine, particularly with a concurrently low urine pH. Struvite calculi form as a result of infection with urea-splitting organisms, usually *Proteus*.[16,17] Obstructed urinary drainage, instrumentation, surgery, and chronic antibiotic therapy predispose the patient to *Proteus* infection and struvite calculi.

Clinical Manifestations

While the calculi are in the renal pelvis there usually are no symptoms unless an infection or an obstruction of the kidney is present. As the calculi migrate from the renal pelvis into the ureter, pain known as **ureteral colic** occurs and is the hallmark symptom of this disorder. Ureteral colic usually has an abrupt onset. It is mild at first, then becomes more severe and sharp with time. The pain is unilateral and frequently starts in the flank area, radiating to the ipsilateral (same side) groin. It results from calculi obstructing the flow of urine in the ureter. Colicky type pain, or pain that is rhythmic and from contractions of the ureter, occurs as the ureter attempts to move the stone toward the bladder. Behind the stone the ureter becomes distended with urine and inflamed from the trauma of passage of the stone.

Diagnosis and Treatment

Evaluation of a patient for renal calculi includes a thorough history of the current pain episode, medical history (including prior episodes), dietary history, and medication history. Urinalysis is done to evaluate for hematuria, urine pH, and the presence of WBCs. Serum blood urea nitrogen (BUN) and creatinine levels are determined to assess renal function. A plain film (radiograph) of the abdomen is obtained to screen for the presence of calculi. Calcium and cystine calculi are radiopaque and may be seen on a plain film. Uric acid stones are radiolucent and usually are not seen. IVP may be needed to identify the site of obstruction.

The pain of ureteral colic is severe and is usually accompanied by nausea and vomiting. Acute treatment involves administration of narcotic analgesics and antiemetics and promoting a dilute urine with brisk diuresis. Dilution of the urine helps to decrease supersaturation of the involved mineral. Diuresis may facilitate the spontaneous movement of the calculi into the bladder. Generally, calculi less than 5 mm in diameter will pass spontaneously. Calculi of 5 to 10 mm in diameter may pass, while those larger than 10 mm will not pass spontaneously. When the stone is too large to pass spontaneously, is completely obstructing the ureter/kidney pelvis, or is accompanied by infection, it should be removed.[12] **Shock wave lithotripsy** is now widely used in the United States to fragment the calculus when it lies in the kidney, renal pelvis, or proximal ureter. The smaller fragments are moved down the ureter to the bladder by urine flow. Larger fragments may be extracted surgically. Lithotripsy can be performed extracorporeally or percutaneously. In extracorporeal shock wave lithotripsy the entire body, excluding the head and neck area, is submerged in water and the shock waves are administered from outside the body to precisely target and shatter the stones. In the percutaneous method a small incision is made in the patient's flank, a cystoscope or some other narrow tube is inserted, and the stone fragments are retrieved through the tube. Lithotripsy is replacing such open procedures as pyelolithotomy and ureterolithotomy.

After the acute episode has resolved, treatment is directed toward preventing the formation of new calculi. Treatment entails (1) diluting the urine to greater than 1 to 2 liters per day to reduce the concentration of calculi-forming substances, and (2) decreasing the amount of calculi-forming material in the urine by diet or medication.

KEY CONCEPTS

- Obstructive processes result in urine stasis, which predisposes to infection and structural damage. Common causes of obstruction include stones, tumors, prostatic hypertrophy, and strictures of the ureters or urethra.

- Complete obstruction results in hydronephrosis and ischemic kidney damage due to increased intraluminal pressure. The glomerular filtration rate falls because of increased pressure in Bowman's capsule. A period of diuresis generally follows relief of the obstruction.
- Stones tend to form in the urinary tract under conditions of high solute concentration, low urine volume, and abnormal urine pH. Certain substances in the urine (e.g., magnesium, citrate) are thought to inhibit stone formation. Deficiencies may predispose to stone formation.
- Most stones are made of calcium crystals. Other forms include uric acid, cystine, and struvite. Calcium and cystine stones are radiopaque and detectable on plain radiographs. Uric acid stones are usually undetectable on radiographs.
- Stationary stones in the renal pelvis are usually asymptomatic. When the stone migrates into the ureter, intense renal colic pain ensues. Pain is usually abrupt in onset and unilateral.
- Stones may pass spontaneously or may require dissolution by shock waves (lithotripsy) or surgical excision. Stones tend to recur, and attention toward prevention is indicated. High fluid intake to dilute the urine, dietary changes, and management of urine pH may be helpful.

Tumors

Renal tumors are divided into three groups: (1) benign, (2) primary neoplasms, and (3) secondary neoplasms (Table 27–3). All tumors distort the architecture of the kidney and renal system, hindering renal function. Malignant tumors also carry the threat of metastasis to distant sites.

TABLE 27–3. Renal Tumors

Benign

Adenoma
Oncocytoma
Mesoblastic Nephroma
Hamartoma
Leiomyoma
Hemangioma

Primary Neoplasms

Renal cell carcinoma
Nephroblastoma
Urothelial carcinoma
Sarcoma

Secondary Neoplasms

Primary sites are:
Adrenal carcinoma
Retroperitoneal sarcoma
Primary sites in the pancreas, colon, lung, stomach, or breast
Lymphoma, Hodgkin's Leukemia
Multiple Myeloma

Benign Renal Tumors

Benign renal tumors account for a small percentage of renal system tumors. The most common benign lesion is **renal adenoma.** Renal adenomas less than 3 cm in diameter are histologically similar to renal adenocarcinomas and therefore are treated as malignancies. **Renal oncocytomas** compose 5 to 7 percent of all renal tumors. Patients who have these tumors tend to be asymptomatic. **Mesoblastic nephroma** is a congenital tumor of infancy. Unlike Wilms' tumor (nephroblastoma), this tumor is diagnosed at birth or in the child's first few months. **Hamartoma-angiomyolipoma** type tumors are found in adults. The presenting complaint is flank pain, or lightheadedness/syncope due to a retroperitoneal hemorrhage. These tumors are found in multiple areas in both kidneys and are composed of vascular, adipose, and smooth muscle tissue.

Other benign renal tumors are **fibromas, lipomas, uromyomas,** and **hemangiomas.** Fibromas are fibrous masses of the renal medulla; they are usually found in females. Lipomas consist of adipose tissue within or around the kidney. Leiomyomas are retroperitoneal tumors that form from the renal capsule or vessels. Hemangiomas manifest with hematuria for which no other explanation can be found.

In general, the treatment for benign tumors is nephrectomy when symptoms of caliceal destruction are present. Asymptomatic tumors may be observed. Treatment for renal adenomas is radical nephrectomy because of the risk of progression to renal adenocarcinoma.

Renal Cell Carcinoma

Renal cell carcinoma accounts for approximately 85 to 90 percent of all primary renal neoplasms in adults, and for 6 percent of all malignancies. It results in 7,500 to 8,000 deaths per year.[18]

Etiology and Pathogenesis

Renal cell carcinoma appears in adults between 50 and 70 years of age. Males are affected two to three times as often as females. Associated risk factors include cigar and pipe smoking, disease in a family member, horseshoe kidney, autosomal dominant polycystic kidney disease (in adults), and acquired renal cystic disease from chronic (>3 years') hemodialysis.

Renal cell carcinoma arises from the epithelium of the proximal convoluted tubule. There are three cell types: clear cell, granular cell, and spindle cell sarcoid, which is rare. The clear cell variety consists of large cholesterol-filled cells with small nuclei and rare mitoses. Granular cell renal cell carcinoma has dark-staining cytoplasm with numerous mitochondria and more numerous mitoses. The spindle cell renal carcinoma has fusiform cells of variable cell size. The tumor itself is yellow in color with areas of hemorrhage, coagulation, necrosis, and cystic excoriation (Fig. 27–7).[3]

Clinical Manifestations

The classic triad of symptoms in renal cell carcinoma consists of hematuria, flank pain, and a palpable abdominal mass. This triad is found in only about 10 percent of cases and when the local tumor is advanced. The single symptom of hematuria, gross or microscopic, is found in about 60 percent of patients.

Systemic symptoms or **paraneoplastic syndromes** are present in about 50 percent of all patients with renal cell carcinoma.[18] Fatigability, weight loss, and cachexia are common. Fever, anemia, hypertension, hepatic dysfunction, erythrocytosis, hypercalcemia, and an increased erythrocyte sedimentation rate also occur. Hormone substances may be produced by renal cell carcinoma. Hypercalcemia, which is seen in 3 to 6 percent of patients, can be caused by an excess of parathyroid hormone and prostaglandins generated from the tumor. Hypertension may result from excess renin production in 20 to 40 percent of patients. Cushing's syndrome from increased glucocorticoids can also be found. Lower extremity edema may result from tumor invasion into the renal vein and inferior vena cava. Hepatosplenomegaly and ascites can de-velop from tumor extension into the hepatic vein or the inferior vena cava. Metastasis occurs in the lymph nodes, ipsilateral adrenal gland, lung, and long bones.

Diagnosis and Treatment

Urinalysis is the initial study done to evaluate hematuria, but IVP is the examination performed most often to detect a tumor. Renal US may be used to differentiate a cystic lesion from a tumor. Needle aspiration may be performed to obtain cyst fluid for cytology. Computed tomography (CT) and magnetic resonance imaging (MRI) are used in the diagnosis and staging of renal cell carcinoma.

Treatment includes radical nephrectomy, or the removal of the affected kidney, the ipsilateral adrenal gland, the fascia, and the local hilar lymph nodes. Survival rates for patients with no lymph node involvement and who undergo radical nephrectomy are 50 to 70 percent at 5 years. Patients with lymph node metastases have a 5-year survival rate of 15 to 35 percent. In patients with metastases to distant sites, such as the bone or lung, the 5-year survival rate is less than 5 percent. Metastatic disease is treated with radiation therapy, chemotherapy, and immunotherapy. Hormonal agents such as medroxyprogesterone, testosterone, and tamoxifen have been used.

Urothelial Tumors

Urothelial tumors are malignant tumors of the lining of the renal pelvis, calices, ureter, and bladder. They account for 8 to 10 percent of all renal cancers. The majority (90 percent) of these tumors are transitional cell carcinomas. The remaining 10 percent are squamous cell carcinomas and adenocarcinomas.

Etiology and Pathogenesis

Risk factors for transitional cell carcinoma include cigarette smoking, exposure to industrial chemicals such as aromatics and amines, and the chronic abuse of analgesics containing aspirin and phenacetin. Transitional cell carcinomas of the renal pelvis are found twice as often in males as in females. The peak age range of occurrence of renal pelvic transitional cell carcinoma is 50 to 60 years. Transitional cell carcinomas are multifocal and may occur simultaneously in more than one site. Patients who have a site of disease in the renal pelvis may also have tumors in the ureter and bladder or anywhere along the urothelium.[3,18] Transitional cell carcinoma grows slowly and is generally noninvasive; however, when metastasis occurs, it is usually to the lung and bone.

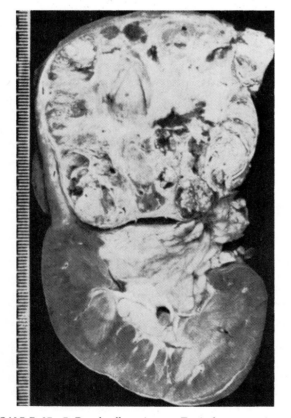

FIGURE 27–7. Renal cell carcinoma. Typical cross-section of spherical neoplasm in one pole of kidney. Note necrosis and hemorrhages in tumor. (From Cotran RS, Kumar V, Robbins SL: *Robbins Pathologic Basis of Disease*, 4th ed. Philadelphia, WB Saunders, 1989, p 1076. Reproduced with permission.)

Diagnosis and Treatment

Hematuria, either gross or microscopic, is the initial finding in more than 60 percent of patients. IVP shows a filling defect in the system. Renal US, cystoscopy, and retrograde pyelography are also used in the diagnosis. Urine cytology may isolate tumor cells but does not pinpoint the site of the tumor, for morphologically, urothelial transitional cell carcinomas are alike, regardless of where in the system they occur. CT and radionuclide scintigraphy are performed to evaluate the presence or extent of metastasis. Because these tumors tend to be multifocal, examination of the entire urinary tract, including the side opposite the initial tumor, is done prior to surgery.

The treatment for renal urothelial cancer is radical nephroureterectomy. This involves a radical nephrectomy and the removal of the entire ureter. Because the tumors are generally low-grade and noninvasive, the 5-year survival rate after surgery is 90 percent.[18] In patients with invasive or high-grade lesions, the 5-year survival rate is less than 15 percent. Chemotherapy is also used in metastatic transitional cell carcinomas.

Nephroblastoma

Nephroblastoma, or Wilms' tumor, is the most common malignancy of the kidney in children. Wilms' tumor can be found in adults but is rare in patients older than 10 years of age. Males and females are equally affected.

Clinical Manifestations
Nephroblastomas are initially identified by a parent or physician on routine physical examination. A tumor or mass of the flank or abdomen is palpable in about 80 percent of cases. Hypertension (60 percent), fever and pain (50 percent), and hematuria (10 to 20 percent) are found in patients with nephroblastoma.[4,19] Additionally, nausea and vomiting are concurrent findings in about 50 percent of patients.

Diagnosis and Treatment
The diagnosis of nephroblastoma is established with IVP, which usually shows caliceal distortion and occasionally calcification within the tumor mass. Renal US and CT are used to evaluate tumor extension and the possibility of bilateral tumors (found in 10 percent of patients).[19] Nephroblastoma may produce a tumor thrombus in the inferior vena cava, leading to decreased venous return and lower extremity edema. Metastasis occurs to the liver, lungs, and opposite kidney.[4,19]

Treatment entails complete removal of the primary tumor and kidney. Survival is estimated to be 85 percent if there is no distant metastasis. Radiation therapy and chemotherapy are useful postoperatively for single tumors[4] and preoperatively to shrink the size of bilateral tumors prior to resection.

KEY CONCEPTS

- The kidney can be host to a number of benign and malignant primary tumors. Symptoms depend on the location of the growth. Obstruction, hematuria, and flank pain may occur. Some tumors secrete hormones that alter fluid and electrolyte balance; examples are renin, parathyroid hormone, and glucocorticoids.
- Tumors are usually detected with IVP. Imaging studies and histology may be used to diagnose and stage the tumor. Treatment includes nephrectomy. Adjacent structures may also be removed if the tumor is malignant.

Glomerular Abnormalities

Glomerular abnormalities result from alterations in the structure and function of the glomerular capillary circulation. There are *primary glomerulopathies*, or disease states in which the kidney is the only or the predominant organ involved, and *secondary glomerulopathies*, which result from drug exposure or infection and glomerular injury in the setting of multisystem or vascular abnormalities. Alterations in glomerular capillary circulation may result in any of the following: (1) hematuria, (2) proteinuria, (3) decreased GFR, and (4) hypertension.

Glomerulonephritis

Glomerulonephritis, or inflammation of the glomeruli, may result from immunologic abnormalities, drug exposure, toxins, or vascular and systemic disease.

Acute Glomerulonephritis

Acute glomerulonephritis is defined as the acute or abrupt onset of hematuria and proteinuria in conjunction with **azotemia** (decreased GFR with increased serum BUN and creatinine levels) and renal salt and water retention.[20] The causes of acute glomerulonephritis are listed in Table 27–4.

TABLE 27–4. Causes of Acute Glomerulonephritis

Infectious	Primary Disease
Post-streptococcal glomerulonephritis	Berger's disease (IgA nephropathy)
Nonstreptococcal/postinfectious glomerulonephritis:	Mesangial proliferative
Bacterial:	Mesangiocapillary glomerulonephritis
Infective endocarditis	
Meningiococcemia	*Multisystem Disease*
Pneumococcal pneumonia	
Sepsis	Goodpasture's syndrome
Viral:	Henoch-Schönlein purpura
Hepatitis B	Systemic lupus erythematosus
Mononucleosis	Vasculitis
Mumps/measles	
Varicella	*Miscellaneous*
Parasitic:	
Malaria	Guillain-Barré syndrome
Toxoplasmosis	Serum sickness
	Irradiation for Wilms' tumor

Pathogenesis

In acute glomerulonephritis, the capillary walls are infiltrated by inflammatory cells. Once the antibody-antigen complex has been established in the glomerular capillary wall, complement is deposited and attracts neutrophils and monocytes. Lysosomal enzymes are then released and damage glomerular walls. This results in a reduction of the GFR by decreasing the capillary surface area available for filtering. Additionally, two other processes are thought to take place. Local vasoactive compounds like angiotensin and leukotrienes[20] contract mesangial cells and reduce perfusion to glomerular capillaries. Bowman's space may also be damaged as a result of fibrin deposition and crescent formation (accumulation of proliferating cells within Bowman's space in the form of a crescent). Water retention is due to two factors: a decrease in GFR, and distal tubule water and salt resorption. Water and salt resorption increase the vascular and extracellular fluid volume of the patient.

Hematuria results from erythrocytes crossing damaged glomerular or peritubular capillary walls into proximal tubule fluid (which is eventually urine). There appears to be a loss of capillary wall anionic charge of glomerular capillaries with a larger than normal pore radius. Either one of these alterations will permit the relatively large molecule of plasma protein to cross into the tubule, resulting in proteinuria.[20]

Clinical Manifestations

Urinary abnormalities may vary in severity. Gross hematuria, which manifests as smoky or coffee-colored urine, is the most common finding. Red cell casts may be present, representing erythrocytes that crossed from the glomerular capillary into the tubule and then assumed the shape of the tubule. White cell casts may also be present, particularly when inflammation is present in the glomerulus and interstitium.[20] Proteinuria, or the loss of more than 3 grams of protein per day, is generally present. If protein loss is extreme or continues for an extended period of time, the nephrotic syndrome may appear.

Systemically, disruptions related to fluid volume changes are the major manifestations. Edema is usually present, particularly in areas (periorbital) of low tissue pressure. However, edema may progress to dependent body areas, ascites, and pleural effusions. Edema occurs not only as a result of fluid volume excess but also as a result of protein loss causing a decrease in plasma oncotic pressure, which allows fluid to leave the vascular space for the extra- and intracellular spaces. Arterial diastolic hypertension results from increased extracellular fluid volume, increased cardiac output, and increased peripheral vascular resistance. Encephalopathy may accompany hypertension, particularly in children.[20]

Diagnosis and Treatment

Evaluation is based on the patient's history and on progression of the symptoms. Urinalysis looking for hematuria, proteinuria, and white or red cell casts is the initial diagnostic test. If the glomerulonephritis is thought to be post-streptococcal, exoenzymes such as antistreptolysin O (ASO) and antistreptokinase (ASK) are evaluated. Serum renal indicators such as BUN and creatinine levels are evaluated to estimate the extent of renal damage. Occasionally a renal biopsy may be done to evaluate the underlying lesion.

Treatment is based on the underlying causative mechanism. Commonly, azotemia is transient, with only a short period of oliguria (<400 mL of urine per 24 hours). A diuresis then occurs in days to weeks, and the GFR returns to normal or near normal. In general, infectious diseases tend to respond quickly to the appropriate anti-infective agent. However, there is always the possibility that the current episode will evolve into rapidly progressing or chronic glomerulonephritis.

Rapidly Progressing Glomerulonephritis

When renal failure develops in a short period of weeks to months, it is termed **rapidly progressing glomerulonephritis**. RPGN is also known by the term **extracapillary (crescentic) glomerulonephritis,** which is the actual lesion that causes the disease.

Etiology and Pathogenesis

Rapidly progressing glomerulonephritis is found primarily in adults. The causes fall into four general categories: (1) a complication of an acute or subacute infection, (2) a complication of a multisystem disease, (3) drug exposure, and (4) idiopathic.

The infections most commonly associated with rapidly progressing glomerulonephritis are post-streptococcal glomerulonephritis, infective endocarditis, visceral sepsis, and hepatitis B. The post-streptococcal state and infective endocarditis are by far the most common. Multisystem diseases that are associated with the disease are systemic lupus erythematosus, Henock-Schönlein purpura, systemic necrotizing vasculitis, and Goodpasture's syndrome. Drugs that may cause rapidly progressing glomerulonephritis are penicillamine, hydralazine, allopurinol in the setting of vasculitis, and rifampin.

Idiopathic rapidly progressive glomerulonephritis is found primarily in males, at a mean age of 58.[21] The pathologic lesion involves proliferation of epithelial cells and crescent formation, initiated by fibrin leaking into Bowman's space. The extent of the renal involvement varies but is between 50 to 100 percent of glomeruli.[21] In those patients with rapid (within weeks) progression of renal decline, more than 70 percent of the glomeruli are involved.[20]

Clinical Manifestations

Patients with rapidly progressing glomerulonephritis may experience viral-type symptoms in the prodromal period (arthralgias, myalgias, back and abdominal pain, fever, malaise). There may be only mild hypertension. Hematuria and proteinuria are present in conjunction with rapidly decreasing renal function. Nausea and vomiting as a result of azotemia also occur.

Diagnosis and Treatment

Urinalysis is done to screen for hematuria, proteinuria, and casts. Serum BUN and creatinine levels and a creatinine clearance time are determined to evaluate renal function. A streptococcal enzyme assay may also be performed to screen for that underlying mechanism. If infective endocarditis is suspected, a workup that includes blood cultures, echocardiography, and cardiac catheterization may be done. A renal biopsy may be needed to differentiate the mechanism of rapidly progressing glomerulonephritis.

At the time of presentation, up to 50 percent of patients are already significantly uremic and need immediate dialysis. The remaining patients need dialysis within weeks to months. If the disease is acute at the time of presentation, it is considered potentially reversible.

Methylprednisolone pulse therapy has been shown to be appropriate for patients with rapidly progressing glomerulonephritis. Large doses of the drug are given intravenously on a once daily or alternate-day basis three times, then followed by oral prednisone. Approximately 75 percent of patients have shown good improvement, reaching near-normal to normal renal function. A response to drug therapy is usually evident in 5 to 10 days. Nevertheless, in some patients the condition will eventually progress to renal failure. Plasmapheresis used in conjunction with prednisone and cyclophosphamide has shown improvement similar to methylprednisolone pulse therapy. Anticoagulants may be used to reduce fibrin deposition and crescent formation.

Chronic Glomerulonephritis

Chronic glomerulonephritis is defined as continuing or persistent hematuria and/or proteinuria resulting in slowly progressive deterioration of renal function.[20] The end result of chronic glomerulonephritis is hypertension, small (contracted) scarred kidneys, and renal failure.

Pathogenesis

The underlying structural lesions are classified into four groups: (1) proliferative (mesangial, or cells in the connective tissue that supports the glomerular capillaries; end-capillary and/or extracapillary; and focal/segmental), (2) sclerosing (focal and diffuse), (3) membranous, and (4) nonspecific. Tubular atrophy and dilation may also be seen.

Within the capillary filtration membrane there appear to be depositions of soluble antigen-antibody complexes or formation of anti-glomerular basement membrane antibodies. Biochemical mediators of inflammation (complement, leukocytes, and fibrin) then start to damage the glomerular wall. This series of events results in the changes in the renal system that were described under Acute Glomerulonephritis.

Clinical Manifestations

The clinical manifestations of chronic glomerulonephritis are similar to those of acute glomerulonephritis. Hematuria and proteinuria are present for the duration of the course of the disease. Systemically, edema, fluid volume excess, and hypertension develop more insidiously than in the acute form of the disease. The disease may run 10 to 20 years or more from onset to end-stage renal failure.

Diagnosis and Treatment

Evaluation includes urinalysis looking for hematuria, proteinuria, and casts. Serum BUN and creatinine levels, along with a creatinine clearance time, are determined to estimate the degree of renal damage. Renal biopsy may be needed to differentiate the underlying pathologic abnormality.

Treatment differs with the underlying mechanism. Antibiotics appropriate for the identified organism are used in infections. Avoiding nephrotoxic drug therapy or discontinuing identified toxins is advised. Steroids, cytotoxic drugs, nonsteroidal anti-inflammatory drugs and anticoagulants may be used, although clear evidence of efficacy is somewhat controversial.[20]

KEY CONCEPTS

- Glomerular disorders are inflammatory in nature. Damage is mediated by immune processes but is not directly due to infection. Often the glomerular basement membrane is damaged, leading to hematuria, proteinuria, decreased GFR, and hypertension.
- Glomerulonephritis may result from autoimmune processes, antigen-antibody deposition, and toxins. Inflammatory processes attract immune cells to the area, resulting in lysosomal degradation of the basement membrane. The GFR may fall, in part due to contraction of mesangial cells resulting in decreased surface area for filtration.
- Glomerulonephritis may be classified as acute, rapidly progressing, or chronic. Acute forms are usually due to post-streptococcal damage. The cause of the rapidly progressing form is often unknown, but it may be secondary to other disease processes. Chronic forms tend to be autoimmune.
- Treatment may include steroids, plasmapheresis, and supportive measures such as management of fluid balance and dialysis.

Nephrotic Syndrome

The **nephrotic syndrome** is a collection of symptoms caused by glomerular disease. It is characterized by an increase in the capillary wall permeability to serum proteins. The predominant abnormality in nephrotic syndrome is the loss of large amounts (>3 g/day) of

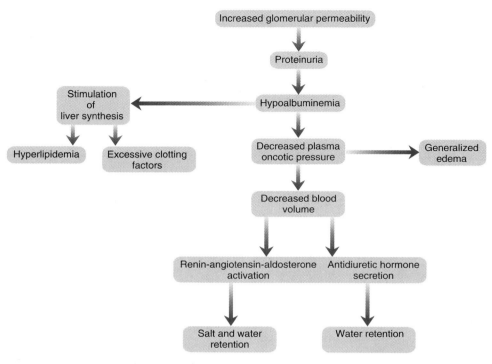

F I G U R E   27 – 8. Pathophysiology of nephrotic syndrome.

protein in the urine. Additionally, hypoalbuminemia, hyperlipidemia, edema, hypercoaguability, altered immunity, and lipiduria are present (Fig. 27–8).[20–22]

Pathogenesis

In a 24-hour day, plasma containing greater than 60,000 grams of protein perfuses the glomeruli. Normally, less than 150 mg of protein is lost in the urine. Barriers to protein molecule loss include the endothelial cells, basement membrane, and slit diaphragms. The protein molecule is too large to penetrate the normal openings in these barriers within the glomerular system. The electrical charge of the protein molecule also influences permeability. At normal physiologic pH, albumin (40 percent of urine proteins) is negatively charged, thus inhibiting permeability.[22]

Tubular reabsorption returns small proteins—peptides and immunoglobulin fragments—to the capillary circulation. When this reabsorptive mechanism fails or when the protein filter load exceeds reabsorptive capacity, proteins are lost in the urine. Immune mechanisms may cause a decrease in the net negative charge on the capillary wall, which allows albumin to be excreted in the presence of other proteins (selective proteinuria). In the setting of extensive capillary wall immune deposits or alterations of the basement membrane, all proteins are filtered at an increased rate (nonselective proteinuria).[20]

Clinical Manifestations

Hypoproteinemia results from **proteinuria**. The majority of the proteins lost are albumin, although other proteins, such as globulins, are also lost. Urinary protein loss may exceed 10 g/day and is greater than the rate at which the liver can synthesize new albumin (usually 12–14 g/day).

Edema results when there is an imbalance between hydrostatic and colloid oncotic pressures. Hydrostatic pressure on the arteriole side of the vascular tree is elevated and pushes fluid into the interstitial space. Colloid oncotic pressure on the venule side exerts an increased pressure that pulls fluid back into the vascular space. When serum protein levels are decreased, fluid remains in the interstitial space. Edema then forms in areas where hydrostatic pressure is high (dependent areas) and where interstitial pressure is low (periorbital areas). Although fluid movement favors the interstitial space, about half of patients with the nephrotic syndrome have normal or increased plasma volume. Renal retention of salt and water may account for some of this increased volume, but other factors may also contribute, among them (1) a relatively noncompliant interstitium, which resists excess fluid at a threshold, (2) the washout of interstitial oncotic pressure to less than vascular oncotic pressure as a result of increased lymph flow, which favors fluid remaining in the vascular space, and (3) the decreased capillary permeability to albumin in hypoalbuminemia.

Hyperlipidemia is inversely proportional to the serum albumin concentration. It appears that increased hepatic synthesis of cholesterol, triglycerides, and lipoproteins, which may be stimulated by decreased plasma albumin levels or decreased plasma oncotic pressure, accounts for hyperlipidemia. However, there may also be decreased catabolism of these substances. Lipiduria results from hyperlipidemia, but the level of lipiduria is more closely parallel to urine protein excretion.[21,22]

Hypercoagulability may be due to altered levels of clotting factors. A reduction in Factors IX, XI, and XII and elevated levels of Factors II, V VII, VIII, X, fibrinogen, and platelets may account for an increase in thromboembolic events in patients with the nephrotic syndrome. Renal vein thrombosis, once thought to be the cause of nephrotic syndrome, is actually secondary to hypercoagulability.

Decreased immune system competence has been described in nephrotic patients. Decreased IgG levels, which predispose patients to pneumococcal infections, occur as a result of urinary losses and increased catabolism.[22] There appears to be a depression of cell-mediated immunity that may be due to hypoalbuminemia, hyperlipidemia, or a zinc deficiency. In general, nephrotic patients are predisposed to and at risk for infection.

In **nephrosis,** T_3 and thyroid-binding globulins are decreased as a consequence of urinary loss. Trace metals (iron, copper, zinc) are deficient. There is a loss of cholecalciferol (vitamin D precursor), which leads to a vitamin D deficiency and secondary hyperparathyroidism, hypocalcemia, and renal osteodystrophy. Because many drugs are protein-bound, drug metabolism may be altered.

Diagnosis and Treatment

Evaluation is based on identifying the underlying pathologic mechanism, as described in previous sections. Continued assessment of symptoms and alterations is necessary in order to provide optimal treatment.

In children, **minimal change disease** (minimal pathologic change in the glomeruli) is the most common underlying disease. Steroids are used, and the child is usually free of proteinuria in about 4 weeks.

The management of *edema* is conservative. Treatment is not initiated unless the patient is symptomatic. Dietary sodium restriction, rest, and the judicious use of diuretics are the most common treatment options. Intravenous albumin may be used when aggressive diuresis is needed (severe ascites or pulmonary effusion). The additional albumin is lost in the urine within a short time, so this is only a temporary measure.

Dietary management varies from high-protein to normal protein diets, because some feel that an increased protein load only exaggerates protein loss. Diets low in sodium, with increased potassium, and low in saturated fats are commonly instituted. In patients on steroid therapy, adequate calorie and protein intake is essential.

Supplemental vitamin D and iron are used to replace losses. Prophylactic anticoagulation is generally not used. However, anticoagulation for pulmonary embolism is appropriate. The management of renal vein thrombosis is controversial.

The diseases that cause the nephrotic syndrome may progress to end-stage renal failure. Dialysis and renal transplantation are available as treatment options.

KEY CONCEPTS

- Nephrotic syndrome occurs because of increased glomerular permeability to proteins, resulting in a urinary protein loss of >3 g/day. Proteinuria leads to hypoalbuminemia and generalized edema as a result of decreased blood colloid osmotic pressure. Hyperlipidemia and hypercoagulability are thought to occur because of a generalized increase in liver activity stimulated by hypoalbuminemia.
- Management is conservative. Most cases resolve spontaneously. Protein supplementation and optimization of fluid balance are indicated.

Summary

Many disease entities can result in renal damage or failure. Any process that disrupts the normal architecture of the kidney will result in altered function, whether in the glomeruli, the vascular tree, or the collecting/draining system. Although the kidney has the capacity to respond to treatment and reverse the damage, ultimately any abnormality in the system has the potential to precipitate end-stage renal failure.

Glomerulonephritis and pyelonephritis are the first and second leading causes of chronic renal failure. Although glomerulonephritis is difficult to treat or prevent, pyelonephritis represents a potentially preventable cause of renal failure. Obstructive processes, including stones, tumors, and congenital malformations, may precipitate acute renal failure; however, they are often amenable to treatment if detected early.

REFERENCES

1. Franklin SS: *Practical Nephrology.* New York, John Wiley & Sons, 1981.
2. Richard CJ: *Comprehensive Nephrology Nursing.* Boston, Little, Brown & Co, 1986.
3. Schreiner GF, Kissane JM: *Anderson's Pathology,* 9th ed. St. Louis, CV Mosby, 1990, pp 804–870.
4. Gonzalez R: Urologic disorders in infants and children, in Behrman RE (ed): *Nelson's Textbook of Pediatrics,* 14th ed. Philadelphia, WB Saunders, 1992, pp 1359–1384.
5. Gabow P, Bennett WM: Renal manifestations: Complication management and long-term outcome of autosomal dominant polycystic kidney disease. *Semin Nephrol* 1991;11(6):643–652.
6. Gabow PA: Cystic disease of the kidney, in Wyngaarden JB, Smith LH (eds): *Cecil's Textbook of Medicine,* 18th ed. Philadelphia, WB Saunders, 1988, pp 644–647.
7. Grantham JJ: Polycystic kidney disease: I. Etiology and pathogenesis. *Hosp Pract* 1992;27(3):51–59.
8. Andriole VT: Urinary tract infections and pyelonephritis, in Wyngaarden JB, Smith LH (eds): *Cecil's Textbook of Medicine,* 18th ed. Philadelphia, WB Saunders, 1988, pp 628–632.
9. Stamm WE, Turck M: Urinary tract infection, pyelonephritis, and related conditions, in Wilson JD, Braunwald E, Isselbacher KJ, et al (eds): *Harrison's Principles of Internal Medicine,* 11th ed. New York, McGraw-Hill, 1988, pp 1189–1194.
10. Rector FC: Obstructive nephropathy, in Wyngaarden JB, Smith

LH (eds): *Cecil's Textbook of Medicine,* 18th ed. Philadelphia, WB Saunders, 1988, pp 614–617.

11. Kimmelstiel P, Kim OJ, Beres JA, Wellman K: Chronic pyelonephritis, in Schreiner GF, Kimmel JM (eds): *Anderson's Pathology.* St. Louis, CV Mosby, 1961, pp 1160–1171.

12. Turka LA: Urinary tract obstruction, in Rose BD (ed): *Pathophysiology of Renal Disease,* 2nd ed. New York, McGraw-Hill, 1987, pp 447–467.

13. Brenner BM, Milford EL, Seiffer JC: Urinary tract obstruction, in Wilson JD, Braunwald E, Isselbacher KJ, et al (eds): *Harrison's Principles of Internal Medicine,* 12th ed. New York, McGraw-Hill, 1991, pp 1206–1209.

14. Pak CYC: Renal calculi, in Wyngaarden JB, Smith LH (eds): *Cecil's Textbook of Medicine,* 18th ed. Philadelphia, WB Saunders, 1988, pp 638–641.

15. Premminger GM: Renal calculi: Pathogenesis, diagnosis and medical therapy. *Semin Nephrol* 1992;12(2):200–216.

16. Coe FL, Favus MJ: Nephrolithiasis, in Wilson JD, Braunwald E, Isselbacher KJ, et al (eds): *Harrison's Principles of Internal Medicine,* 12th ed. New York, McGraw-Hill, 1991, pp 1202–1206.

17. Coe FL, Parks LH: Pathophysiology of kidney stones and strategies for treatment. *Hosp Pract* 1988;23(3):185–189, 193–195, 199–200.

18. Garnick MB, Brenner BM: Tumors of the urinary tract, in Wilson JD, Braunwald E, Isselbacher KJ, et al (eds): *Harrison's Principles of Internal Medicine,* 12th ed. New York, McGraw-Hill, 1991, pp 1209–1212.

19. Williams RD: Tumors of the kidney, ureter and bladder, in Wyngaarden JB, Smith LH (eds): *Cecil's Textbook of Medicine,* 18th ed. Philadelphia, WB Saunders, 1988, pp 650–655.

20. Glassock RJ, Brenner BM: The major glomerulopathies, in Wilson JD, Braunwald E, Isselbacher KJ, et al (eds): *Harrison's Principles of Internal Medicine,* 12th ed. New York, McGraw-Hill, 1991, pp 1170–1180.

21. Couser WG: Glomerular disorders, in Wyngaarden JB, Smith LH (eds): *Cecil's Textbook of Medicine,* 18th ed. Philadelphia, WB Saunders, 1988, pp 582–602.

22. Wiseman KC: Nephrotic syndrome: Pathophysiology and treatment. *ANNA J* 1991;18(5):469–477.

BIBLIOGRAPHY

Johnson DL: Nephrotic syndrome: A nursing care plan for current pathophysiologic concepts. *Heart Lung* 1989;18(1):85–91.

Kaehny WD, Everson GT: External manifestations of autosomal dominant polycystic kidney disease. *Semin Nephrol* 1991; 11(6):661–670.

Lazarus JM: Uremia: A clinical guide. *Hosp Med* 1984;175–195.

Peterson RO: The urinary tract and male reproductive system, in Rubin E, Farber JL (eds): *Essential Pathology.* Philadelphia, JB Lippincott, 1990.

Ronald AR, Simonsch N: *Diseases of the Kidney,* 4th ed. Boston, Little, Brown & Co, 1988.

Rubin RH, Tolkoff-Rubin NE, Cotran RS: *The Kidney,* 3rd ed. Philadelphia, WB Saunders, 1986.

Walker PL: Shockwave lithotripsy. *AORN* 1984;40(4):560–563.

CHAPTER 28
Renal Failure

KAREN CARLSON

KEY TERMS

acute renal failure: An abrupt reduction of renal function accompanied by the progressive retention of waste compounds.

anuria: Absence of urine output.

azotemia: Presence of nitrogen-containing products in the bloodstream.

chronic renal failure: Gradual loss of renal function involving some or all of the nephrons.

dialysis: An artificial process that partially replaces renal function (i.e., eliminates wastes, fluid, and electrolytes).

diffusion: The process by which substances move from an area of greater concentration to one of lesser concentration.

diuresis: The excretion of large amounts of urine as a result of the actions of a diuretic.

glomerular filtration rate: Rate of filtration of blood through the glomerulus.

oliguria: Urine output less than 400 mL/day.

osmolality: Concentration of solute.

osmosis: A process by which water movement is encouraged across a semipermeable membrane in response to osmotic pressure.

polyuria: The excretion of large amounts of urine.

uremia: Clinical syndrome that accompanies the detrimental effects of renal dysfunction on the other organ systems.

*A*cute renal failure (ARF) is the most common renal problem that critically ill patients experience.[1] There is a 65 percent mortality associated with the development of ARF.[2] Chronic renal failure (CRF) complicates the clinical course of any other critical illness. Despite advances in the treatment of renal dysfunction, there has been little impact on mortality in the last 30 years.

Acute Renal Failure

Acute renal failure is defined as the abrupt reduction of renal function accompanied by the progressive retention of waste compounds (i.e., creatinine and urea). It is usually, although not always, reversible and accompanied by oliguria (urine output < 400 mL/day). Multiple causes of ARF exist and are classified into three groups: prerenal, intrarenal, and postrenal.[3] The etiology, pathogenesis, and clinical manifestations of each type of ARF differ. The differential diagnosis is important in determining treatment.

Prerenal Failure

Prerenal failure is characterized by physiologic conditions that lead to decreased renal perfusion (blood flow) without intrinsic damage to the renal tubules. The conditions that can lead to prerenal failure are listed in Table 28–1. Most forms of prerenal failure are easily reversed by removing the cause and enhancing renal perfusion.[4] The decrease in renal arterial perfusion leads to decreased afferent arteriole pressure, ultimately resulting in a decreased GFR. When the pressure in the afferent arteriole drops below 70 mm Hg, the protection of autoregulation is also lost, further decreasing the **glomerular filtration rate** (GFR), the rate of filtration of blood through the glomerulus.[5]

Renal tubular function, at this point, is still completely normal. The kidneys are unable to filter blood because of the decrease in GFR. Predictable changes

occur as a result of this decreased perfusion, regardless of the cause. If the decreased perfusion state persists, it can lead to irreversible damage to the tubules.

As a result of the decreased GFR, the filtrate moves more slowly through the renal tubules. Consequently, more sodium (Na^+) and water are reabsorbed, resulting in **oliguria.** Urine specific gravity increases while urine Na^+ concentration decreases (<20 milliequivalents per liter [mEq/L]). The blood urea nitrogen (BUN) to creatinine ratio is usually greater than 20 : 1. Urine osmolality (concentration of solute) is often greater than 500 milliosmoles per liter (mOsm/L).

The clinical presentation of the patient in prerenal failure differs with the cause. If the underlying problem is a decrease in circulating volume or an alteration in peripheral vascular resistance, the patient presents with tachycardia, hypotension, dry mucous membranes, flat neck veins, lethargy, and, as the disease progresses, coma. Patients in cardiac failure present with a decreased cardiac output, hypotension, tachycardia, and cool, clammy skin.

Intrarenal Failure

Primary damage to the renal tubule or blood vessels results in intrarenal failure. With a prolonged perfusion deficit, the kidneys gradually suffer damage that restoring perfusion does not improve.

Acute tubular necrosis (ATN) and acute glomerulonephritis are the most common pathologic conditions causing ARF. The extent of injury differs with the cause. The causes of intrarenal failure are varied and classified as nephrotoxic, ischemic, or inflammatory. Causes of intrarenal failure are listed in Table 28–2.

When the insult to the kidney is nephrotoxic, damage is done primarily to the epithelial layer. Because the epithelial layer has the ability to regenerate, rapid healing often occurs. When the insult is ischemic or inflammatory, the basement membrane is also damaged and regeneration is not possible.[5] These latter types of injury are more resistant to healing and often proceed to CRF.

TABLE 28–1. Causes of Prerenal Failure

Hypovolemia
  Burns
  Excessive use of diuretics
  GI losses (diarrhea, vomiting)
  Hemorrhage
  Third spacing (edema, ascites)
  Shock
Decreased cardiac output
  Dysrhythmias
  Cardiac tamponade
  Cardiogenic shock
  Congestive heart failure
  Myocardial infarction
  Pulmonary embolism
Altered peripheral vascular resistance
  Anaphylactic reaction
  Antihypertensive medications
  Neurogenic shock
  Septic shock

TABLE 28–2. Causes of Intrarenal Failure

Ischemic
  Prolonged decreased renal perfusion
  Septic shock
  Transfusion reaction
  Trauma or crush injury
Nephrotoxic
  Antibiotics
  Fungicides
  Pesticides
  Radiographic dyes
Inflammatory
  Acute glomerulonephritis
  Acute vasculopathy
  Acute interstitial nephritis

The underlying pathophysiologic abnormality in intrarenal failure is renal cellular damage leading to functional abnormalities. The glomerulus normally acts as a filter and does not allow large molecules to pass. When it is damaged, protein and cellular debris are allowed to enter the renal tubules. Intraluminal obstruction and back leak of the glomerular filtrate occur.

The diverse causes of intrarenal failure determine the clinical presentation of the patient. Renal failure can cause multiple organ dysfunctions and therefore manifests in a variety of ways. **Uremia** is the term used to describe the clinical syndrome that accompanies the detrimental effects of renal dysfunction on the other organ systems. The clinical presentation of the patient in uremia reflects the degree of nephron loss and, correspondingly, the loss of renal function.

As with prerenal failure, the patient often presents with oliguria. With intrinsic tubular damage, the kidney loses the ability to concentrate urine and reabsorb Na^+. As a result, urine specific gravity falls, urine osmolality is less than 350 mOsm/L, and urine Na^+ levels are high (>30 mEq/L). Both the BUN and creatinine concentrations will be elevated, resulting in an elevated BUN to creatinine ratio of 10:1.[1]

Initially, after the onset of oliguria, the clinical presentation is determined by the primary or underlying disease. As the renal failure progresses, the patient exhibits the clinical manifestations of uremia. The patient may be confused, lethargic, nauseated, vomiting, experiencing diarrhea or constipation, have deep, rapid respirations and pulmonary edema, have tachycardia, have hypo- or hypertension, and have dry skin. The patient also has an increased susceptibility to infection.[1]

Postrenal Failure

Postrenal failure occurs when there is any type of obstruction, partial or complete, of urine flow from the kidney to the urethral meatus. Partial obstruction increases renal interstitial pressure, which in turn increases Bowman's capsule pressure, opposing filtration. Diminished urine output is possible. Complete obstruction leads to urine backup into the kidney, eventually compressing the kidney. With complete obstruction, there is no urine output from the affected kidney.

Postrenal failure is caused by either mechanical or functional problems, as summarized in Table 28–3.

T A B L E 2 8 – 3. Causes of Postrenal Failure

Mechanical
Clots
Stones
Strictures
Tumors
Functional
Medications
Neurologic disorders

As the obstruction persists, BUN and creatinine concentrations are elevated. Specific gravity is variable, as is the urine Na^+ value.

The patient with bilateral obstruction presents as if in renal failure and has no urine output. Prompt removal of the obstruction usually brings relief of symptoms.

Clinical Phases

There are three clinical phases of ARF. The first phase is the oliguric phase, which usually begins within 48 hours of the insult to the kidney and is accompanied by an approximate rise in BUN of 20 mg/100 mL/day and a rise in creatinine of 1 mg/100 mL/day. The most common complications during this phase are fluid overload and acute hyperkalemia. The oliguric phase may range from a few days to several weeks but on the average lasts 12 days.[2] The longer the oliguric phase continues, the poorer is the patient's prognosis.

The diuretic phase follows the oliguric phase. During this phase, there is a gradual return of renal function. Although the BUN and creatinine concentrations continue to rise, there is an increase in urine output. The urine output is determined by the patient's state of hydration when entering this phase. Fluid overload leads to diuresis of up to 4 to 5 liters of urine a day.[2] There is marked Na^+ wasting. The average time of this phase is 2 weeks.[2] Patients must be observed carefully for complications from fluid and electrolyte deficits.

The recovery phase marks the stabilization of laboratory values. It can take 3 to 12 months for the recovery phase to be completed. Often, patients are left with some degree of renal insufficiency. Some patients do not recover and instead progress to CRF.

KEY CONCEPTS

- **Acute renal failure (ARF) is an abrupt reduction in renal function accompanied by accumulation of waste compounds in the blood. Oliguria is usually present. Acute renal failure is classified into three types, according to the site of disruption: prerenal, intrarenal, and postrenal. Distinguishing among the types of ARF is necessary to determine appropriate therapy.**

- **Prerenal failure is due to conditions that impair renal blood flow such as hypovolemia, hypotension, cardiac failure, or renal artery obstruction. Prerenal failure is characterized by manifestations of low GFR, including oliguria, high urine specific gravity and osmolality, and low urine sodium. Treatment is aimed at restoring renal perfusion and avoiding progression to acute tubular necrosis (ATN).**

- **Intrarenal failure is due to primary dysfunction of renal tubular cells, resulting in ATN. Intrarenal failure may occur with nephrotoxic, ischemic, or inflammatory insults. Intrarenal failure is characterized by manifestations of renal cell damage,** including proteinuria, low urine specific gravity and osmolality, and high urine sodium.

- Postrenal failure is due to obstruction within the urinary collecting system. Obstruction results in elevated Bowman's capsule pressures, impeding filtration. Specific gravity, urine sodium, and urine volume are variable, depending on the degree of obstruction. Untreated postrenal obstruction may lead to ATN.

- There are three characteristic phases of acute renal failure. The first phase, characterized by oliguria and progressive azotemia, lasts 1 to 2 weeks. Oliguria is followed by a diuretic phase that lasts about 2 weeks. During the diuretic phase, urine volume increases, but tubular function is impaired and azotemia continues. The recovery phase, lasting from 3 to 12 months, is characterized by gradual normalization of serum creatinine and BUN. Often a degree of renal insufficiency persists.

Chronic Renal Failure

Etiology and Pathogenesis

Chronic renal failure is the gradual loss of renal function involving some or all of the nephrons, depending on the basic disease process. The progress of the disease can sometimes be slowed but is ultimately irreversible, and culminates in end-stage renal disease. The mortality associated with end-stage renal disease is 100 percent if maintenance dialysis, transplantation, or both are not implemented.[6] The causes of CRF are summarized in Table 28–4. The differential diagnosis is important as treatment decisions are based on the underlying cause.

No matter what the cause is, nephron damage is always progressive. When damaged, nephrons are no longer able to participate in maintaining normal renal function. The intact nephrons compensate for the loss of the damaged nephrons by enlarging and increasing their clearance capacity. As a result of nephron hypertrophy, the kidneys are able to maintain relatively normal function with as many as 80 percent of nephrons nonfunctional.[6]

There are four stages of CRF, corresponding to the degree of nephron loss. The first stage is decreased renal reserve, representing nephron loss of approximately 50 percent. Usually the patient is asymptomatic and has a normal BUN and creatinine. The creatinine level may have doubled but is still within the normal range.[7]

The second stage of CRF is renal insufficiency. Approximately 75 percent of the nephrons have been lost at this point.[7] Evidence of decreased GFR and solute clearance is present. The concentrating ability is somewhat impaired. The patient exhibits signs of mild **azotemia** (the presence of nitrogen-containing products in the bloodstream) and may be developing anemia. The serum creatinine level in this phase is often four times the patient's baseline level.[7]

TABLE 28–4. Causes of Chronic Renal Failure

Developmental/congenital
  Renal agenesis
  Aplastic kidneys
  Renal hypoplasia
  Ectopic/displaced kidneys
  Fused kidneys
Cystic disorders
  Polycystic kidney disease
  Medullary cystic disease
Tubular disorders
  Renal tubular acidosis
  Diabetic nephropathy
  Hypertensive disease
Neoplasm
  Benign
  Malignant
  Wilms' tumor
Infections
  Pyelonephritis
  Renal tuberculosis
  Glomerulonephritis
Obstructions
  Nephrolithiasis
  Retroperitoneal fibrosis
Systemic disorders
  Diabetes mellitus
  Diabetes insipidus
  Hypertension
  Hyperparathyroidism
  Hepatorenal syndrome
  Gout
  Amyloidosis
  Scleroderma
  Goodpasture's syndrome
  Systemic lupus erythematosus

The third stage is end-stage renal disease, which corresponds to 90 percent nephron loss. All functions of the kidney are seriously impaired and the body is unable to maintain homeostasis. The BUN and creatinine concentrations are markedly elevated. The patient demonstrates anemia, hyperphosphatemia, hypocalcemia, metabolic acidosis, hyperuricemia, hyperkalemia, fluid overload, and is usually oliguric. All body systems are affected. Patients are evaluated for the number of systems affected and for the impact of the disease process on activities of daily living. Dialysis or transplantation needs to be considered. The main focus of care during this phase is maintaining remaining renal function and protecting the patient from complications that would cause loss of more nephrons.[7]

The final stage of CRF is the uremic syndrome. The symptoms in uremia are generally progressive and vary with the level of BUN and creatinine control achieved through the various therapies. Failure in other systems can be seen as a result of the kidney's failure.

Clinical Manifestations

The clinical presentation of the patient in CRF is determined by the rapidity with which the patient's renal function has deteriorated. The body is able to adapt if function is lost slowly, whereas if function is lost swiftly, the signs and symptoms will be more severe.

Patients demonstrate some combination of the following findings. They experience a decline in renal function and along with it, decreased ability to handle body salt and water. This may manifest as pulmonary or peripheral edema. Patients often become hypertensive. Anemia develops for several reasons. There is a deficiency of erythropoietin, so that fewer red blood cells (RBCs) are being produced by the bone marrow. The presence of waste products alters the internal environment, resulting in a decreased life span of the RBC as well as decreased platelet adhesiveness. These factors, in combination, make the patient more prone to coagulopathies. The effectiveness of circulating white blood cells (WBCs) is also altered, making the patient more prone to infections. The presence of waste products alters mucosal integrity, increasing the likelihood of vomiting, nausea, and itching. Because the kidneys play an important role in electrolyte balance, these patients manifest electrolyte disturbances. The most common imbalances are hyperkalemia, hyponatremia, hyperphosphatemia, and hypocalcemia. The impact of waste products on the cells of the brain results in changes in mentation and behavior.

KEY CONCEPTS

- Chronic renal failure occurs with a gradual loss of functional nephrons. Common causes are pyelonephritis, glomerulonephritis, and polycystic kidney disease. Four stages of chronic renal failure have been described according to the degree of nephron loss. The first stage, decreased renal reserve, corresponds to nephron loss of about 50 percent. Laboratory values are normal and the patient is usually asymptomatic. The second stage, or the stage of renal insufficiency, corresponds to nephron loss of about 75 percent. The patient has mild azotemia and may have polyuria and nocturia due to impaired urine concentration. End-stage renal disease occurs with about 90 percent nephron loss. BUN and creatinine concentrations are markedly elevated, and manifestations of fluid and electrolyte disorders are present. The uremic syndrome is the final stage.

- Manifestations of end-stage renal disease and uremia are due to decreased GFR (hypervolemia, hyperkalemia, water excess, hyperphosphatemia, azotemia), decreased secretion of H^+ (metabolic acidosis), decreased vitamin D production (hypocalcemia, osteodystrophy), and decreased erythropoietin (anemia). Azotemia is associated with itching, nausea, and altered mentation.

Patient Management

Ideally, a collaborative approach to the treatment of patients in renal failure begins by focusing on preven-

tion. Both physicians and nurses play a role in recognizing patients at risk for renal failure, developing and implementing plans to maintain perfusion, and taking steps to avoid further renal compromise.

There have been remarkable advances in prevention and treatment over the past 30 years. These advances have focused on prompt correction of hypotension and the early use of dialysis before the development of uremia. Aggressive management includes the appropriate use of medications, nutrition, electrolyte balance, and prevention or prompt treatment of infection. Infection is the leading cause of death in the renal failure patient. The objectives of management are listed in Table 28–5.

Once ARF has developed, the goal of treatment is to reestablish homeostasis as quickly as possible. Before homeostasis can be achieved, however, the insult must be removed.

Diagnostic Tests

A wide variety of diagnostic tests are available for use in determining the cause and location of renal dysfunction.[8] Tables 28–6 and 28–7 list the most frequently used blood and urine studies performed in a renal workup. The creatinine and BUN levels are closely monitored, as these levels and their relationship to each other (BUN : creatinine ratio) provide valuable information about the kidney's filtering ability. Urine Na^+ values vary as the kidneys attempt to retain or excrete water. Urine volume, specific gravity, and osmolarity are useful in identifying the kidney's ability to excrete and concentrate fluid. Test values associated with prerenal and intrarenal (acute tubular necrosis) dysfunction are compared in Table 28–8. These tests are valuable when attempting to establish the diagnosis.

Radiologic tests used in determining renal dysfunction are listed in Table 28–9, along with information about their individual purpose and a brief description of the test. The tests chosen by a physician may vary and are determined by the presentation of the patient.

Pharmacologic Management

There are two goals of pharmacologic intervention in the patient with renal failure: (1) to prevent or reverse

TABLE 28–5. Objectives of Patient Management

- Correction of fluid imbalance
- Prevention of hyperkalemia and other life-threatening electrolyte imbalances
- Treatment of acidosis
- Improvement of nutritional status
- Prevention of further nephrotoxicity by alterations in drug therapy
- Avoidance and treatment of infection
- Prevention of anemia

TABLE 28–6. Renal Function Tests—Blood

Test	Normal Value	Abnormal Trends Consistent With Renal Dysfunction	Significance for Renal Function
Creatinine	0.4–1.2 mg/dL	Increased	Most specific test of renal function
Blood urea nitrogen (BUN)	5–25 mg/dL	Increased	Provides information on renal function; less specific than creatinine
Potassium	3.5–5.0 mEq/L	Usually increased	Indicates renal tubular ability to excrete
BUN–creatinine ratio	20:1	Increased	Indicative of prerenal dysfunction
Osmolarity	280–300 mOsm/L	Increased or decreased	Indicates body water balance; imbalances may be water excess (decreased osmolarity) or water deficit (increased osmolarity)
Albumin	3.2–5.5 g/dL	Decreased	Degree of hypoalbuminuria depends on degree of glomerular capillary leakage, disease process, and nutritional status
Calcium	4.0–5.0 mg/dL (ionized) or 9.0–11.0 mg/dL (total)	Decreased	In renal failure, vitamin D is not converted to its active form, which is necessary for calcium absorption from the gut
Phosphorus	3.5–5.5 mEq/L	Increased	In renal disease, the kidney tubules are unable to excrete phosphate
Magnesium	1.4–2.2 mEq/L or 1.7–2.7 mg/dL	Increased	In renal failure, magnesium is not excreted by the renal tubules
Hematocrit	Female: 36–47/dL Male: 40–54/dL	Decreased	In renal failure, the kidneys do not secrete erythropoietin in normal amounts; erythropoietin stimulates the bone marrow to make red blood cells
pH	7.35–7.45	Decreased	Metabolic acidosis occurs in renal failure because of the renal tubule cells' inability to buffer H^+ ions

Adapted with permission from MacGeorge LL, Caniff R: Assessment of renal function, in Patrick ML, et al (eds): *Medical-Surgical Nursing: Pathophysiologic Concepts,* 2nd ed. Philadelphia, JB Lippincott, 1991, pp 1011–1013.

the renal insult before ARF occurs, and (2) once ARF is established, to support the patient to minimize morbidity and mortality. A number of pharmacologic agents have been proposed for use in preventing or treating ARF. Unfortunately, there is a lack of well-controlled studies to validate their success. As a result, many of the pharmacologic methods are considered to be controversial.[9]

Dosage Considerations

Because many medications are eliminated by the kidney, drug dosing must be altered in the patient with renal failure. Practitioners should be familiar with the excretory routes of the medications prescribed. Dosing decisions are based on the drug and the patient's degree of renal dysfunction. The phase of renal failure

TABLE 28–7. Renal Function Tests—Urine

Test	Normal Value	Abnormal Trends Consistent With Renal Dysfunction	Significance for Renal Function
Volume	1–2 L/24 hr	Decreased	Indicates kidney's loss of ability to excrete water
Specific gravity	1.005–1.025	Decreased or increased	Indicates kidney's loss of ability to concentrate urine
Osmolarity	100 mOsm 1,000 mOsm/L	Decreased or increased	Indicates body water status
Protein	Absent	Present	Indicates glomerular dysfunction
Blood	Absent	Present	Indicates trauma, infection, or dysfunction anywhere in the renal system
Bacteria	Absent	Present	Indicates infection
RBC, WBC, red cell casts	Absent	Present	Nonspecific indication of renal trauma, infection, or pathologic condition
Crystals	Absent	Present	Indicate potential for renal or urinary stones
Glucose and ketones	Absent	Present	Indicate metabolic status more than renal dysfunction
Creatinine clearance	60–120 mL/min	Decreased	Indicates filtration ability of kidney

Adapted with permission from MacGeorge LL, Caniff R: Assessment of renal function, in Patrick ML, et al (eds): *Medical-Surgical Nursing: Pathophysiologic Concepts,* 2nd ed. Philadelphia, JB Lippincott, 1991, pp 1011–1013.

TABLE 28–8. Differential Diagnosis of Renal Dysfunction

Test	Intrarenal (ATN)	Prerenal (Hypoperfusion)
Volume	<400 mL/L	<400 mL/L
Specific gravity	<1.010	>1.020
Osmolality	<350 mOsm/L	>500 mOsm/L
BUN	>25 mg/dL	>25 mg/dL
Creatinine	>1.2 mg/dL	Normal
BUN–creatinine ratio	10:1	>20:1
Sodium	>30 mEq/L	<20 mEq/L

and other treatments that a patient may be undergoing also assist in determining the appropriate dose of medication to be administered. It is important to remember that if a medication requires a loading dose, the loading dose must still be administered.

Drugs that are entirely dependent on renal function for elimination or that depend on both renal and hepatic elimination will require dosing modifications. Methods used in altering medication dosing are interval extension, dose reduction, or a combination of the two. Interval extension involves administration of the same dose with longer time periods between doses. This method results in wider fluctuations in blood

TABLE 28–9. Renal Diagnostic Tests

Radiologic Tests	Purpose	Procedure
Cystoscopy	Allows visualization of the urethra and bladder Structural abnormalities can be visualized and tissue biopsies obtained Urine flow from both ureters can be seen	Lighted cystoscope with a light is inserted through the urethra and into the bladder
Abdominal radiography (KUB)	Identifies gross renal abnormalities	Flat x-ray plate is placed over abdomen and x-ray film is taken
Excretory urography (intravenous pyelography—IVP)	Evaluates filling and emptying of urinary tract	Contrast dye is injected IV As the kidney filters and excretes the dye, x-ray films are taken at specific intervals
Retrograde pyelography	Allows visualization of the renal pelvis and ureters	Contrast dye is injected into each ureter through a cystoscope
Voiding cystourethrography	Film before voiding outlines the bladder wall Film during voiding outlines urethra and reflux of urine into ureters Film after voiding shows if bladder has emptied	Contrast medium is instilled into the bladder through a cystoscope and films are taken before, during, and after voiding
Renal arteriography	Allows visualization of the renal circulation	In the *translumbar* approach, a needle is inserted through the soft tissue in the lumbar region into the aorta; the dye is injected into the aorta In the *femoral* approach, the femoral artery is punctured, and a catheter is threaded up to the renal artery; contrast dye is injected into the aorta or renal artery Films are taken as the contrast dye passes through the renal circulation Contrast dye may also be injected IV; if so, the timing of x-rays depends on circulation time
Renography	Records the radioactive patterns that mark the outline of the kidney and allows visualization of intrarenal masses and the amount of renal blood flow Records the appearance and disappearance of radioactivity over both kidneys, which demonstrates the relative function of each kidney Used to detect vascular disease, obstructions, tumors, and malfunctioning kidneys Used frequently to detect rejection in renal transplant patients	Radioactive isotope with contrast dye is injected IV A nuclear medicine scanning machine or photography is used to follow the radioactive isotopes The tracer dose used negates the need for precautions against radioactivity
Computed tomography	CT scanners permit visualization of kidney and blood vessels Used to detect tumors, cysts, and change in size of kidney	Placement on machine table
Ultrasonography	Permits differentiation of solid masses and fluid collections Detects tumors, cysts, obstructions, abscesses	Machine passes sound waves into internal body structures Computer interprets tissue density based on sound waves and prints out in picture form

Adapted with permission from MacGeorge LL, Caniff R: Assessment of renal function, in Patrick ML, et al (eds): *Medical-Surgical Nursing: Pathophysiologic Concepts*, 2nd ed. Philadelphia, JB Lippincott, 1991, pp 1011–1013.

levels of the drug. Alternatively, the dose may be reduced while the same dosing interval is maintained. This method provides relatively constant blood levels. In addition to these changes in dose or interval, if a patient is being dialyzed, attention must be given to medication scheduling relative to the patient's dialysis schedule. Medications may be eliminated by dialysis or have their actions potentiated.

Commonly Used Medications

Diuretics and dopamine are commonly used in the treatment of the ARF patient in the critical care setting. Other medications used in the patient in renal failure may include antihypertensive agents, antimicrobial agents, and analgesics. Additionally, patients with CRF are often treated with vitamins, phosphate-binding agents, calcium supplements, human erythropoietin, and other antianemia agents.

Diuretics. Diuretics are substances that affect renal function and subsequently cause an increase in urinary output. The excretion of large amounts of urine is called **polyuria** (*poly* means many or much). Polyuria that results from the action of a diuretic is called **diuresis.** *Uresis* means to make water, also to urinate. Diuretics have different physiologic actions in the kidney and are classified by their actions, where the action occurs in the nephron, and if they are potassium-sparing or potassium-depleting. The more thoroughly nephron physiology is understood, the easier it is to understand the actions and side effects of diuretics.

Diuretics are commonly used in the prevention and treatment of renal failure. Diuretics are utilized to evaluate urine formation when the patient's fluid status is uncertain and in cases of fluid volume overload with edema and hypertension. Dosages may be increased in an attempt to determine the dose that will provoke a response. This is often done by doubling the dose (i.e., 20 mg, 40 mg, 80 mg, etc.) every 30 to 60 minutes until diuresis is achieved or a maximum dose is reached.

Table 28–10 lists some diuretics and Figure 28–1 illustrates the location in the nephron where diuretics exert their effect. The major action of each group of diuretics in the nephron will be discussed here. The reader is referred to the references for a complete discussion of the extrarenal effects of diuretics.

Mannitol and urea are filtered freely through the glomerular capillaries. Mannitol is unaffected by the tubular processes of reabsorption and secretion; hence, the amount of mannitol that is filtered is also excreted in the urine. The activity of urea in the nephron is discussed in Chapter 26. As mannitol and urea move into the proximal convoluted tubule, they increase the osmolality. For this reason they are called *osmotic agents.* Water stays in the proximal convoluted tubule and follows these osmotic agents instead of being reabsorbed with sodium. The tubular fluid is dilute, with a low concentration of sodium, and that diminishes the reabsorption of sodium. Mannitol causes vasodilation of the renal vessels and expands

TABLE 28–10. Diuretics

Agents	Site of Action in Nephron

Osmotic agents
  Mannitol (Osmitrol)
  Urea (Urevert)
	Proximal tubule

Carbonic anhydrase inhibitors
  Acetazolamide (Diamox)
  Dichlorpenamide (Daranide)
  Methzolamide (Neptazane)
	Proximal tubule

Inhibitors of chloride and sodium
  reabsorption
  Bumetanide (Bumex)
  Ethacrynic acid (Edecrin)
  Furosemide (Lasix)
	Ascending loop of Henle

Inhibitors of sodium reabsorption
  Chlorothiazide (Diuril)
  Hydrothiazide (Esidrix)
  Indapamide (Lozol)
  Metolazone (Diulo)
  Chlorthalidone (Hygroton)
  Bendroflumethazide (Naturetin)
	Distal tubule, proximal to site of potassium transport

Aldosterone inhibitors
  Spironolactone (Aldactone)
  Amiloride (Midamor)
  Triamterene (Dyrenium)
	Distal tubule, distal to site of potassium transport
	Collecting duct

Courtesy of Cleo Richard, R.N., Ph.C., Billings, Mont. See also Figure 28–1.

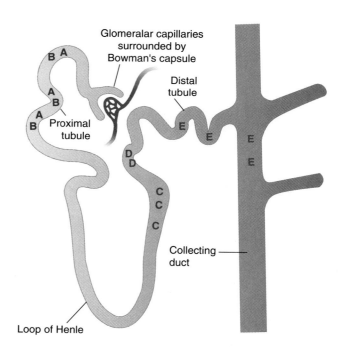

FIGURE 28–1. Sites of action of diuretics in the nephron. *A, B, C, D,* and *E* each represent a group of diuretics that act in the part of the nephron where the letter appears. (See Table 28–10 for names of specific diuretics.) *A,* osmotic agents that act in the proximal tubule. *B,* carbonic anhydrase inhibitors that act in the proximal tubule. *C,* diuretics that inhibit chloride and sodium reabsorption in the ascending loop of Henle. *D,* diuretics that inhibit sodium reabsorption proximal to the site of potassium transport in the distal tubule. *E,* aldosterone inhibitors that act distal to the site of potassium transport in the distal tubule and collecting duct. (Figure designed by Cleo Richard, R.N., Ph.C., Billings, Mont.)

vascular volume by enhancing movement of fluid from the interstitial space. The volume of tubular fluid also increases, in turn increasing the flow of the tubular fluid through the nephron. A fast tubular fluid flow rate enhances the diuresis because it decreases reabsorption of solutes and consequently water in distal parts of the nephron. The fast flow of the tubular fluid pulls or drags everything with it and does not allow time for solutes, such as potassium (K^+), and water to be reabsorbed.[10]

Mannitol is often used prophylactically in patients who are at risk of developing ARF in an effort to protect the kidney. The benefit from mannitol after ARF is established is unclear. It can contribute to fluid overload in the patient who has lost excretory renal function and so should be used cautiously.

Acetazolamide and like drugs are named *carbonic anhydrase inhibitors* because they block the action of this enzyme in the proximal tubule (see Acid-Base Regulation in Chap. 26). Subsequently hydrogen ions are not secreted into the proximal convoluted tubule and sodium is not reabsorbed. The concentration of sodium in the tubular fluid is high, and that attracts water. Therefore, the volume and flow rate of the tubular fluid increase.[11]

Ethacrynic acid, bumentanide, and furosemide are *loop diuretics*; they inhibit the reabsorption of chloride and subsequently sodium in the ascending loop of Henle. An elevated concentration of these electrolytes in the nephron increases the osmolality, attracting water. The tubular fluid volume and flow rate increase, leading to a decrease in potassium reabsorption in the distal tubule. Because potassium is excreted in the urine as a side effect of loop diuretics, they are termed *potassium depleting*.[12] Such agents are often used after ARF has been established in efforts to reduce fluid overload and the frequency of dialysis.

Thiazides and like substances (chlorothiazide through bendroflumethazide in Table 28–10) decrease sodium reabsorption in the distal tubule proximal to the site of potassium transport.[11] With an increased tubular concentration of sodium, water is not reabsorbed, leading to an increase in the volume and flow rate of the tubular fluid. Potassium reabsorption is decreased and kaliuresis results. These diuretics are also potassium depleting.

Spironolactone, amiloride, and triamterene inhibit the action of aldosterone in the distal tubule and collecting duct. Without aldosterone, sodium is not reabsorbed. Water subsequently stays with sodium, and once again, the volume and flow rate of the tubular fluid increase. *Aldosterone inhibitors* act distal to the site of potassium transport in the distal tubule. Therefore, potassium is reabsorbed and not excreted with the rapidly flowing tubular fluid. Consequently these diuretics are referred to as *potassium sparing*.[13]

Alcohol and caffeine suppress the release of antidiuretic hormone (ADH) from the pituitary gland. When ADH is not present in the collecting duct, copious, dilute urine is secreted.

The major *side effects* of diuretics are an exaggeration of their physiologic actions. For instance, all diuretics cause polyuria. With prolonged polyuria there is water loss, which can result in a fluid volume deficit. The signs and symptoms of fluid volume deficit are decreased weight, concentrated urine, hard stool, sunken eyeballs, dry mouth, poor skin turgor, dizziness, orthostatic hypotension, increased hematocrit, and increased plasma osmolality. If a fluid volume deficit becomes severe enough, blood flow to the kidney can be so reduced that renal failure results.[10]

The most reliable method to assess for body fluid changes is weight. Weigh the patient daily and, if possible, record fluid intake and output. Weigh the patient at the same time each day with the same amount of clothing and on the same scale. Before breakfast, after the bladder has been emptied, is usually a good time. Balance the scale before each weighing and use a metric scale if possible because it is easier to calculate fluid changes. Compare daily weight changes with fluid intake and output changes; the amounts should correlate. For example, if the weight from one day to the next day is a loss of 1 kg, the fluid change should be a loss of 1 liter (1 kg = 1 liter = 2.2 lbs). Teach patients how to weigh themselves and how to record fluid intake and output.

Once renal failure is established, diuretics may be used to assist in avoiding fluid overload and to potentiate the effects of antihypertensive medications. Most diuretics cause potassium depletion by interfering indirectly with reabsorption. Some diuretics directly affect the potassium-reabsorbing mechanisms. Other diuretics, especially those that act proximal to the distal tubule, cause an increase in the volume of fluid in the nephron. An expanded fluid volume increases the fluid flow rate; potassium and other substances are swept along so fast they do not have time to be reabsorbed. Signs and symptoms of hypokalemia are undue fatigue, weakness, loss of appetite, loss of muscle tone, muscle cramping in the legs, arrhythmias, constipation, and abdominal distention. It is, however, important to avoid the use of potassium-sparing diuretics, as the patient in renal failure has diminished ability to eliminate potassium.

Dopamine. Dopamine, often used in critical care areas, has dose-dependent effects on renal blood flow. At low doses (2–5 μg/kg/min), renal vasodilation occurs, while at higher doses (>10 μg/kg/min) vasoconstriction occurs.

Analgesics. Both narcotic and nonnarcotic analgesics may be used to treat pain in the patient with ARF. Acetaminophen is the drug of choice for the treatment of mild pain. It is metabolized in the liver and requires no dosage alteration.

Most narcotic analgesics do not require dosage adjustments and are usually not removed by dialysis. Meperidine is not recommended for use in the renal failure patient as its metabolites are eliminated by the kidneys and can accumulate in these patients.

Antihypertensive Agents. Hypertension is a major problem for many renal failure patients, often requiring the concomitant use of several antihypertensive agents for treatment. Most antihypertensive agents are not removed by dialysis. It is important to adjust the dosage schedule in the patient who is being dialyzed to avoid undue hypotensive episodes during dialysis. However, some antihypertensive agents are eliminated by the kidney. Therefore, dialysis patients receiving these medications require alterations in their dose or dosing schedule.

Antimicrobial Agents. Patients in renal failure are at high risk for infection and are commonly treated with antimicrobial agents. The antimicrobial agents must be carefully selected and monitored. Frequently, dose adjustment will be needed. Careful monitoring of both renal function and drug levels during antimicrobial therapy is imperative to avoid further renal damage.

Fluid Balance

Maintaining fluid balance in the patient in renal failure is challenging. A fine balance must be achieved in providing the fluid necessary for adequate renal perfusion while preventing fluid overload. It is often difficult to determine whether the patient is volume depleted or volume overloaded.

Correcting fluid balance is crucial in prerenal disease while the underlying problem is rectified. Fluid replacement must be matched with fluid loss, both in amount and composition, with insensible losses also considered. Volume loading with normal saline before a potential insult to the patient who is at risk for renal dysfunction is a widely accepted practice. Additionally, volume expansion is certainly beneficial in preventing a volume-depleted patient from developing ARF.

Managing fluid balance can become even more complex during the diuretic phase of renal failure, when the patient may require 1 to 4 liters of fluid a day to prevent hypovolemia while undergoing diuresis. Usually during this phase, the patient is allowed to diurese more fluid than is replaced, so that fluid will be pulled from the interstitial and intracellular spaces into the vascular space. For example, replacement of loss, with the exception of 500 to 1,000 mL, will provide the stimulus for this movement without leaving the patient in a hypovolemic state.

Throughout the care of the ARF patient, careful attention should be given to accurate determination of fluid intake and output as well as daily weights. Body weight should be allowed to drop by 0.2 to 0.3 kg/day as a result of catabolism. If the patient's weight is stable or increasing, volume expansion should be suspected. If weight loss exceeds these recommendations, volume depletion or hypercatabolism should be investigated.[9] Once the patient is normovolemic, daily fluid needs must be calculated carefully. It is uncommon for a patient to be able to tolerate more than 750 to 1,000 mL/day, which may place constraints on other therapies.

Electrolyte Balance

A number of electrolyte imbalances can occur in the patient in renal failure. The most common are hyperkalemia, hyponatremia, hypocalcemia, and hyperphosphatemia.

Of all of the potential electrolyte disorders, hyperkalemia is considered to be the most life-threatening secondary to K^+ effect on the heart. Hyperkalemia is also the most common reason for initiating dialysis in the ARF patient. Conservative management begins with a dietary restriction of 40 mEq/day. As the K^+ level rises, use of cation-exchange resins such as Kayexalate should be considered. Kayexalate is usually administered by mouth or enema with sorbitol. The sorbitol acts to draw fluid into the bowel, where the Kayexalate causes an exchange between Na^+ and K^+ ions. The K^+ is then eliminated from the body through feces.

When plasma K^+ levels exceed 6 mEq/L, other interventions are usually instituted as temporary measures to protect the heart from the negative effects of hyperkalemia. Hypertonic (50 percent) glucose infusions may be used with intravenous regular insulin. Insulin acts to drive K^+ into the cell on a temporary basis. Sodium bicarbonate infusions may also be used. This infusion also causes movement of K^+ into the cell, encouraging the exchange of H^+ ion inside the cell for the excess K^+ ion outside the cell. Calcium salts, such as calcium gluconate, may be administered to elevate the stimulation threshold, thereby protecting the patient from the negative myocardial effects and potential dysrhythmias. Dialysis is necessary when the patient's K^+ level cannot be controlled by other methods.

Hyponatremia is a manifestation of a water excess. Mild, asymptomatic hyponatremia often is not treated, or treated only with water restriction. Dialysis may be instituted if the patient is showing signs or symptoms of water intoxication. If central nervous system signs are present, careful infusions of hypertonic saline may be employed in conjunction with dialysis.

The ARF patient often demonstrates calcium (Ca^{++}) and phosphorus (PO_4^-) imbalances within 2 to 3 days of the onset of renal failure. Hypocalcemia is usually easily corrected by dialysis. If tetany or a positive Chvostek's sign develops, Ca^{++} supplementation may be instituted concurrently with the administration of PO_4^- binders such as aluminum hydroxide.

Acid-Base Management

The most common acid-base disorder in the patient in renal failure is metabolic acidosis. Additionally, patients often develop a mild respiratory alkalosis to compensate. The kidneys have lost their ability to reabsorb bicarbonate (HCO_3^-) and to excrete H^+. Treatment is usually not instituted until the serum HCO_3^- level drops below 15 mEq/L.[9] Even then, only half of the base deficit is replaced so as not to overcorrect the pH. Administration of excessive $NaHCO_3^-$ can cause tetany and lead to the development of pulmonary edema.

Nutritional Management

The challenge in managing the renal failure patient's nutrition is to provide a balance between sufficient calories and protein that will prevent catabolism, yet not create problems such as fluid and electrolyte imbalances or increased need for dialysis. Typically, the patient in renal failure is hypermetabolic, with caloric needs increased to twice normal. Additional stresses related to being critically ill can further elevate caloric requirements. As a result of uremia, these patients often experience nausea and vomiting, which decrease oral intake.

Because the patient in renal failure is unable to rid the body of wastes, fluid, and electrolytes, the diet is typically restricted in fluid, K^+, Na^+, and protein. The degree of these restrictions depends on the cause and severity of the disease. For example, the level of Na^+ restriction is determined by the cause of the renal failure. Some causes lead to Na^+ wasting and others to Na^+ retention. Phosphorus may need to be restricted and Ca^{++} supplemented if the Ca^{++} level is low in conjunction with normal PO_4^- levels. Additionally, vitamin supplementation is often necessary. Most commonly, supplementation of folic acid, pyridoxine, and the water-soluble vitamins is necessary. Dietary requirements change for patients, depending on their renal status and the severity of their underlying condition. Recommendations for diet in the patient with uncomplicated ARF who can take oral feedings are outlined in Table 28–11.

Patients who are critically ill or have more serious underlying conditions more often are hypermetabolic and catabolic, which relates to a poorer prognosis. Although the precise role of nutrition in ARF is controversial, it is felt that malnutrition increases morbidity and mortality in these patients.[14] Total parenteral nutrition in conjunction with daily dialysis has been shown to improve survival and promote healing of renal tubular cells. The usual approach to hypercatabolic states is to provide adequate proteins and carbohydrates to provide for resynthesis of damaged or lost tissue elements. Protein requirements may range initially from 0.5 to 1.0 g/kg/day and increase with dialysis to 1.0 to 1.5 g/kg/day.[15] Nonprotein calories, usually in the form of fat, are given for nonanabolic metabolic needs. Recommendations for the ARF patient who is hypermetabolic[16] are outlined in Table 28–12.

Careful monitoring of the patient's weight, fluid balance, and electrolyte balance is important. The nutritional interventions may need to be tailored daily as the patient's status changes. Dialysis treatments need to be taken into consideration when planning a patient's diet.

Dialysis

The general principles of dialysis are the same for both acute and chronic renal failure patients and are accomplished through either hemodialysis or perito-

TABLE 28–11. Dietary Recommendations for Patients With Acute, Uncomplicated ARF

Dietary Component	Amount
Protein	
Low-protein diet	0.55–0.60 g/kg/day ($\geq$0.35 g/kg/day of high-biologic-value protein)
RDA for dietary protein	0.80 g/kg/day (for noncatabolic patients with substantial residual renal function)
Hemodialysis diet	1.0–1.2 g/kg/day
Energy	$\geq$35 kcal/kg/day
Fat	30%–40%
Polyunsaturated/saturated fatty acid ratio	1 : 1
Carbohydrates	Rest of calories
Total fiber intake	20–25 g/day
Minerals	
Sodium	1,000–2,000 mg/day
Potassium	$\leq$50–70 mEq/day
Phosphorus	4–12 mg/kg/day
Calcium	800–1,000 mg/day
Magnesium	200–300 mg/day
Iron	10–18 mg/day
Zinc	15 mg/day
(Trace element supplements are generally not needed.)	

From Hirschberg RR, Kopple JD: Nutritional therapy in patients with renal failure, in Levine DZ (ed): *Care of the Renal Patient*, 2nd ed. Philadelphia, WB Saunders, 1991, p 178. Reproduced with permission.

neal dialysis. **Dialysis** is an artificial process that partially replaces renal function (i.e., eliminates wastes, fluid, and electrolytes). This removal is accomplished primarily through two processes—**diffusion,** a process by which substances move from an area of greater concentration to one of lesser concentration, and **osmosis,** a process by which water movement is encouraged across a semipermeable membrane in response to osmotic pressure. Through diffusion, substances are removed from and added to the blood. The hemodialysis membrane is similar to the glomerulus. It is selectively impermeable to large molecules such as plasma proteins, RBCs, and WBCs while being permeable to smaller particles such as urea and electrolytes.[17]

Dialysis is accepted treatment for the renal failure patient. The indications for dialysis fall into six general categories:

1. Volume overload
2. Uncontrollable hyperkalemia
3. Symptomatic uremia
4. Pericarditis (inflammation of the pericardial sac)
5. BUN > 100 mg/dL
6. Uncontrolled acidosis

These are general categories. Individual physicians make different decisions after evaluating specific patients. When the decision has been made to begin dialysis, the first step is to determine the method. There are advantages and disadvantages to each type of dialysis, which are beyond the scope of this chapter.

T A B L E 28 – 12. TPN Recommendations for Hypermetabolic Patients With ARF

TPN Constituent	Amount
Amino acids	Essential and nonessential free crystalline amino acids including branched-chain amino acids as 4.25%–5% solutions 0.55–0.60 g/kg/day (nondialyzed) 1–1.2 g/kg/day (hemodialysis) 1.2–1.3 g/kg/day (peritoneal dialysis)

Calories	35–50 kcal/kg/day or as calculated
	Energy sources:
	  Dextrose monohydrate: 3.4 kcal/g
	  Amino acids: 3.5 kcal/g
	  20% fat emulsion 2 kcal/mL

Fat	20% lipid emulsion: 250–500 mL/day, 500–1,000 kcal/day
Carbohydrates	70% dextrose monohydrate at a daily dose to complete the energy needs not provided by amino acids and fat
Minerals	
Sodium	40–50 mmol/L
Chloride	25–35 mmol/L
Potassium	about 35 mmol/day
Phosphorus	8 mmol/day
Calcium	5 mmol/day
Magnesium	4 mmol/day
Iron	2 mg/day
Vitamins	
Vitamin D	Varies
Vitamin K	7.5 mg/week (may be doubled during antibiotic therapy)
Vitamin E	10 IU/day
Niacin	20 mg/day
Thiamin HCl	2 mg/day
Riboflavin	2 mg/day
Pyridoxine HCl	10 mg/day
Pantothenic acid	10 mg/day
Ascorbic acid	60 mg/day
Biotin	200 mg/day
Folic acid	1 mg/day
Vitamin B_{12}	3 μg/day

Note: Patients must be monitored frequently for serum glucose and mineral levels and body water content, and the daily intake or use of insulin must be adjusted accordingly. When hyperkalemia, hyperphosphatemia, or plasma concentrations of other minerals are elevated at the onset of total parenteral nutrition, the intake of that mineral may be reduced or discontinued transiently.

From Hirschberg RR, Kopple JD: Nutritional therapy in patients with renal failure, in Levine DZ (ed): *Care of the Renal Patient*, 2nd ed. Philadelphia, WB Saunders, 1991, p 179. Reproduced with permission.

Peritoneal Dialysis

An alternative to hemodialysis is peritoneal dialysis. The *peritoneum* is a serous membrane that covers the abdominal organs and lines the abdominal wall. It is divided into two sections, parietal and visceral. The parietel peritoneum receives its blood supply from the arteries that feed the abdominal wall and drains into the systemic circulation. The visceral peritoneum receives its blood supply from the mesenteric and celiac arteries and drains into the portal vein. The peritoneum also has extensive lymphatic flow and drainage. Dialysis is performed using the peritoneal membrane as a semipermeable membrane.[18] Through diffusion, osmosis, and ultrafiltration, substances and water can be added to or removed from the blood supply.

Dialysis as a Therapy in Renal Failure

Most commonly, patients in ARF are hemodialyzed.[19] They are often unstable and may require some special adjustments to dialysis treatments.

There are four primary problems associated with dialyzing the unstable ARF patient: hypotension, bleeding, K^+ balance, and acidosis correction. Hypotension is the most common problem seen during dialysis.[20] If the patient is hemodynamically unstable, fluid removal with dialysis may be impossible. At times, fluid and vasopressor medications may be administered while the patient is dialyzing to support blood pressure to the extent that at least wastes can be removed from the body.

Alternatives to Dialysis

There are several alternatives to dialysis in the hemodynamically unstable patient. Continuous arteriovenous hemofiltration, also known as continuous arteriovenous ultrafiltration or slow continuous ultrafiltration, provides for uninterrupted blood flow from an artery to a vein through a filtering device that allows free water and noncellular plasma contents to drain off. The product is a protein-free ultrafiltrate of whole blood.[21] Patients appropriate for continuous arteriovenous hemofiltration are chosen after evaluating their clinical diagnosis, hemodynamic parameters, and metabolic status.

A second alternative to traditional dialysis is continuous arteriovenous hemodialysis. This is a slow form of hemodialysis that uses arteriovenous blood flow and a slow-flowing dialysate solution.[22]

Transplantation

Transplantation is a therapy for end-stage renal disease patients, not patients in ARF. The first successful renal transplant was performed in 1954.[23] Early projections estimated that by 1990 there would be more than 120,000 individuals with end-stage renal disease who would need dialysis or transplantation to live.[24]

KEY CONCEPTS

- Diuretics and dopamine are commonly used drugs for the evaluation and management of prerenal failure. Diuretics are used to evaluate the kidney's ability to make urine. Low-dose dopamine dilates renal arteries and may improve renal perfusion.
- Diuretics are used to increase urine excretion. They may be used diagnostically to test renal responsiveness or therapeutically to treat acute or chronic hypervolemia.
- Diuretics have different mechanisms of action, but they all promote diuresis (increased urine output). Diuresis may be accomplished by increasing renal blood flow, blocking reabsorptive transport processes, or creating an osmotic gradient that opposes reabsorption of water.

- Diuretics may result in fluid and electrolyte imbalances. Potassium wasting is a side effect of most diuretics. Excessive volume depletion or altered osmolality may also result. Serum potassium and sodium levels and body weight are important indices to be monitored during diuretic therapy. An acute change in weight of 1 kg corresponds to a volume change of 1 liter.

- Drugs to manage pain, hypertension, and infections are commonly used in renal failure patients. Dosing of medications must consider the route of excretion and timing of dialysis.

- The goals of fluid management are to maintain adequate renal perfusion while preventing fluid overload. Volume loading prior to a potential renal insult is commonly prescribed for patients with renal insufficiency. Prerenal oliguria is usually aggressively treated with fluids. However, once the patient enters the oliguric phase of ATN, fluids are usually restricted. Fluid administration during the diuretic phase is calculated to replace a percentage of urine output.

- Hyperkalemia is a potentially life-threatening complication of renal failure. Measures to reduce serum potassium include dietary restriction, cation-exchange resins (Kayexalate), glucose and insulin administration, and dialysis.

- Hypocalcemia and hyperphosphatemia often accompany renal failure due to decreased phosphate excretion by the kidney and decreased vitamin D production. Calcium supplementation and phosphate binders may be used.

- Metabolic acidosis is not usually treated unless the serum bicarbonate falls below 15 mEq/L. Patients usually compensate adequately by increasing ventilation.

- Dietary restrictions of fluids, potassium, sodium, phosphorus, and protein are commonly used in the management of renal failure. Total parenteral nutrition may be indicated for the acute renal failure patient to avoid protein catabolism.

- Peritoneal and hemodialysis may be used to substitute for renal function. Indications for dialysis include volume overload, hyperkalemia, symptomatic uremia, acidosis, and a BUN above 100 mg/dL. Complications of hemodialysis include bleeding, hypotension, and electrolyte and acid-base imbalances. Peritoneal dialysis may be complicated by peritonitis. Renal transplantation may be done as a definitive treatment for end-stage renal failure.

Summary

Renal failure is a prevalent problem across age groups. ARF has multiple causes and is classified into one of three categories, prerenal, intrarenal, and postrenal failure. Each category has unique pathophysiology, laboratory findings, and clinical presentation. Each of the three phases of ARF—oliguric, diuretic, and the recovery phase—requires different nursing interventions.

CRF is progressive, with the progression determined by the basic disease process. It is ultimately irreversible if the failed kidney is not replaced, and interventions focus on preserving renal function and maintaining as homeostatic an environment as possible. The clinical presentation of the patient in CRF is determined by the rapidity and severity of the failure.

There are many diagnostic tests available that provide the nurse with information about the patient's renal function. Key aspects of care include pharmacologic management; fluid, electrolyte, and acid-base balance; and nutritional management.

Patients in renal failure are often treated with renal replacement therapies. Hemodialysis, peritoneal dialysis, and continuous renal replacement therapies (CRRT) are all options. The therapy of choice is determined individually for each patient.

A clear understanding of the pathophysiology related to renal dysfunction is essential for nurses caring for patients with renal alterations. The impact that renal dysfunction has on all other body systems will present the nurse with many challenges.

REFERENCES

1. Stark JL: Acute renal failure, in Kinney M, Packa D, Dunbar S (eds): *AACN's Clinical Reference for Critical-Care Nursing,* 2nd ed. New York, McGraw-Hill, 1989, pp 873–885.
2. Butkus DE: Acute renal failure, in Hudak CM, Gallo BM, Benz JJ (eds): *Critical Care Nursing: A Holistic Approach,* 5th ed. Philadelphia, JB Lippincott, 1990, pp 450–467.
3. Baer CL, Lancaster LE: Acute renal failure. *Crit Care Nurs Q* 1992;14(4):1–21.
4. Baer CL: Acute renal failure, in Kinney M, Packa D, Dunbar S (eds): *AACN's Clinical Reference for Critical-Care Nursing,* 2nd ed. New York, McGraw-Hill, 1989, pp 885–901.
5. Stark JL: The renal system, in Alspach JAG (ed): *Core Curriculum for Critical Care Nursing,* 4th ed. Philadelphia, WB Saunders, 1991, pp 472–608.
6. Richard CJ, Lancaster LE: Causes of renal failure, in Lancaster LE (ed): *Core Curriculum for Nephrology Nursing.* Pitman, NJ, American Nephrology Nurses' Association, 1990, pp 55–78.
7. Stark JL, Kelleher R: Chronic renal failure. In Kinney M, Packa D, Dunbar S (eds): *AACN's Clinical Reference for Critical-Care Nursing,* 2nd ed. New York, McGraw-Hill, 1989, pp 886–909.
8. MacGeorge LL, Caniff R: Assessment of renal function, in Patrick ML, et al (eds): *Medical-Surgical Nursing: Pathophysiological Concepts,* 2nd ed. Philadelphia, JB Lippincott, 1991, pp 1011–1013.
9. Brezis M, Rosen S, Epstein FH: Acute renal failure, in Brenner BM, Rector FC (eds): *The Kidney,* 4th ed. Philadelphia, WB Saunders, 1991, pp 993–1061.
10. Richard CJ: *Comprehensive Nephrology Nursing.* Boston, Little, Brown & Co, 1986.
11. Gilman AG, Rall TW, Nies AS, Taylor P (eds): *Goodman and Gilman's The Pharmacological Basis of Therapeutics,* 8th ed. New York, Macmillan, 1990.
12. Shannon MT, Wilson BA: *Govoni and Hayes Drugs and Nursing Implications,* 7th ed. Norwalk, Conn, Appleton & Lange, 1992.
13. Kellick KA: Diuretics. *ACCN Clin Issues* 1992;3(2):472–482.
14. Hoffart N: Nutrition in renal failure, dialysis, and transplantation, in Lancaster LE (ed): *Core Curriculum for Nephrology Nursing.* Pitman, NJ, American Nephrology Nurses' Association, 1990, pp 145–166.
15. Mitch WE, Whitmore DW: Nutritional considerations in the treatment of acute renal failure, in Brenner BM, Lazarus JM (eds): *Acute Renal Failure.* New York, Churchill Livingstone, 1988, pp 743–767.

16. Hirschberg RR, Kopple JD: Nutritional therapy in patients with renal failure, in Levine DZ (ed): *Care of the Renal Patient*, 2nd ed. Philadelphia, WB Saunders, 1991, pp 169–180.
17. Keen M, Lancaster L, Binkley L: Concepts and principles of hemodialysis, in Lancaster LE (ed): *Core Curriculum for Nephrology Nursing*. Pitman, NJ, American Nephrology Nurses' Association, 1990.
18. Prowant B, Gallagher NM: Concepts and principles of peritoneal dialysis, in Lancaster LE (ed): *Core Curriculum for Nephrology Nursing*. Pitman, NJ, American Nephrology Nurses' Association, 1990, pp 277–322.
19. Ismail N, Hakim R: Hemodialysis, in Levine DZ (ed): *Care of the Renal Patient*, 2nd ed. Philadelphia, WB Saunders, 1991, pp 220–246.
20. Taylor T: Preventing complications from hemodialysis. *DCCN* 1990;9(4):210–215.
21. Price CA: Continuous arteriovenous ultrafiltration: A monitoring guide for ICU nurses. *Crit Care Nurs* 1989;9(1):12–19.
22. Lawyer LA, Velasco A: Continuous arteriovenous hemodialysis in the ICU. *Crit Care Nurs* 1989;9(1):29–41.
23. Cunningham N, Smith SL: Postoperative care of the renal transplant patient. *Crit Care Nurs* 1990;10(9):74–80.
24. Perryman JP, Stillerman PU: Kidney transplantation, in Smith A (ed): *Tissue and Organ Transplantation: Implications of Professional Nursing Practice*. St. Louis, Mosby–Year Book, 1990.

BIBLIOGRAPHY

American Society of Transplant Physicians: Statement of criteria for selection of ESRD patients for renal transplantation. Alexandria, VA, American Council on Transplantation, 1988.
Badalamenti J, DuBose T: Chronic renal failure, in Levine DZ (ed): *Care of the Renal Patient*. Philadelphia, WB Saunders, 1991.
Baer CL: Acute renal failure, in Hartshorn JC, Lamborn M, Noll M (eds): *Introduction to Critical Care*. Philadelphia, WB Saunders, 1992.
Bosworth C: SCUF/CAVH/CAVHD: Critical differences. *Crit Care Nurs Q* 1992;14(4):45–55.
Coloski D, Mastrianni J, Dube R, et al: Continuous arteriovenous hemofiltration patient: Nursing care plan. *DCCN* 1990;9(3):130–142.
Finn WF: Diagnosis and management of acute tubular necrosis. *Med Clin North Am* 1990;74(4):873–891.
Guyton A: *Textbook of Medical Physiology*. Philadelphia, WB Saunders, 1991.
Hakim RM, Lazarus JM: Hemodialysis in acute renal failure, in Brenner BM, Lazarus JM (eds): *Acute Renal Failure*. New York, Churchill Livingstone, 1988.
Lancaster LE: Manifestations of renal failure, in Lancaster LE (ed): *Core Curriculum for Nephrology Nursing*. Pitman, NJ, American Nephrology Nurses' Association, 1990.
Lievaart A, Voerman HJ: Nursing management of continuous arteriovenous hemodialysis. *Heart Lung* 1991;20(2):152–160.
Peeshman P: Acute hemodialysis issues in the critically ill. *AACN Clin Issues Crit Care Nurs* 1992;3(3):545–557.
Phillips K: Arterial hypertension, in Richard CJ: *Comprehensive Nephrology Nursing*. Boston, Little, Brown & Co, 1986.
Price C: Continuous renal replacement therapy: The treatment of choice for acute renal failure. *ANNA J* 1991;18(3):239–244.
Price CA: An update on continuous renal replacement therapy. *AACN Clin Issues Crit Care Nurs* 1992;3(3):597–604.
Robinson KJ, Robinson JA: Acute hemodialysis, in Boggs RL, Woolridge-King M: *AACN Procedure Manual for Critical Care*, 3rd ed. Philadelphia, WB Saunders, 1991.
Rubin R, Kaplan R, Bank N: Assessment of the patient with renal disease, in Levine DZ (ed): *Care of the Renal Patient*. Philadelphia, WB Saunders, 1991.
Schrier RW: *Renal and Electrolyte Disorders*, 4th ed. Boston, Little, Brown & Co, 1992.

CHAPTER 29
Disorders of the Bladder

PATTI STEC

KEY TERMS

bladder calculus: A solid mass formed from dead tissue and bacteria within the bladder.

cystitis: Inflammation of the urothelium (lining of the bladder) resulting from infection, irritants, foreign bodies, or trauma.

ectopic ureter: A single ureter that implants during fetal growth in any position other than normal, or an additional ureter.

neurogenic bladder: A bladder that does not fill or empty normally as a result of disruption of innervation to the bladder.

ureterocele: A congenital cystic dilation of the distal ureter.

vesicoureteral reflux: Retrograde movement of urine from the bladder to the kidney as a result of a disruption in the normal valvular mechanism at the ureter-bladder junction.

*T*he bladder serves as an expandable reservoir for the urine that is constantly produced by the kidney. A functional bladder assists in the one-way flow of urine from the kidney to the urethra. Disorders of bladder function can generally be classified as obstructive, infective, or congenital. These disorders are often overlapping because stasis of urine, which occurs with obstructive and congenital disorders, often leads to urinary tract infection. Disruption of the normal one-way flow of urine because of bladder dysfunction predisposes to infection and damage of the upper renal system. Pyelonephritis and acute postrenal renal failure are serious potential consequences of disorders of the lower urinary tract.

This chapter considers the normal structure and function of the bladder and selected bladder disorders in adults and children. Because of the interrelationship of the kidney and bladder, knowledge of bladder disorders and their treatment may prevent or decrease damage to the upper renal system.

Structure and Function of the Bladder

The function of the urinary bladder is to store urine until it is released during micturition. The bladder is primarily muscle, which allows bladder distention to hold urine and bladder contraction to allow urine to pass through the urethra.

There are two principal parts of the bladder, the body and the neck (Fig. 29–1). The **body** of the bladder, where urine collects, is made up of smooth muscle known as **detrusor muscle.** This muscle extends in all directions throughout the bladder. After the initiation of an action potential, the entire muscle contracts, allowing the bladder to empty in one contraction. **Ureters** enter the bladder obliquely through the detrusor muscle and then travel under the bladder mucosa for 1 to 2 cm, emptying into the bladder. The mucosal lining of the body of the bladder has folds known as **rugae.** Rugae allow the bladder muscle to distend to accommodate urine without friction.

The **neck** of the bladder also includes the posterior urethra. The wall of the bladder neck is composed of detrusor muscle with elastic tissue. The muscle of the bladder neck is also called the **internal sphincter.** When normal tone exists in the bladder neck, the bladder is prevented from emptying until the pressure in the body of the bladder rises above a threshold.

Innervation to the bladder is supplied by the pelvic nerves, which exit the spinal cord at S2 and S3 (see Fig. 29–1). Both sensory and motor nerve fibers are needed for bladder function. The sensory fibers detect stretch in the bladder wall. Signals from the posterior urethra are primarily responsible for initiating bladder emptying. The motor fibers are **parasympathetic** in nature.

Somatic nerve fibers, via the pudendal nerve, control the voluntary skeletal muscle of the **external bladder sphincter. Sympathetic innervation,** through the hypogastric nerves at L2, appear to stimulate blood vessels within the bladder. Sensations of fullness and pain may also be transmitted by the sympathetic fibers.

KEY CONCEPTS

- **The bladder is composed primarily of smooth muscle. The bladder body functions to store urine. The bladder neck leads to the urethra and contains the internal sphincter.**
- **Innervation of the bladder is supplied by pelvic nerves that exit the spinal cord at S2 and S3. Motor fibers to the bladder are supplied by the parasympathetic system. The somatic pudendal nerve innervates the external bladder sphincter. The sympathetic system innervates blood vessels via the hypogastric plexus (L2).**

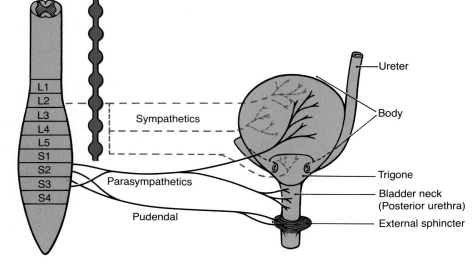

FIGURE 29–1. The urinary bladder and its innervation. (From Guyton AC: *Textbook of Medical Physiology,* 8th ed. Philadelphia, WB Saunders, 1991, p 352. Reproduced with permission.)

Neurogenic Bladder

The process of *micturition* is controlled by both the sympathetic and parasympathetic systems via the spinal cord. Any interruption of bladder innervation will cause a functional obstruction.

Pathogenesis

The degree and type of bladder impairment reflect the level of interruption in the central nervous system (CNS) or spinal cord. Upper motor neuron lesions occurring from the cortex to the sacral level of the spinal cord cause voluntary control of voiding to be lost. Lesions of the lower motor neurons disrupt the sacral reflex arc, causing loss of voluntary and involuntary control of micturition (Table 29–1).

In patients with reflex bladder, which results in involuntary voiding and incomplete emptying, urinary drainage may be accomplished with a catheter or condom catheter. Because the reflex arc remains intact, voiding may be stimulated by stroking the perineum, abdomen, or rectal area. Autonomous bladder may be managed by catheterization or urinary diversion. In the flaccid bladder (motor paralysis), the Credé maneuver or manual compression of the bladder may induce voiding. Bladder training to facilitate voiding on a scheduled basis can be used in people with sensory paralysis of the bladder.

Clinical Manifestations

In addition to the bladder function abnormalities listed in Table 29–1, urinary stasis predisposes to urinary tract infections and the development of renal calculi.[1] Urinary tract infections may be somewhat difficult to identify owing to interruption of the innervative pathways concerned with frequency, urgency, and dysuria. In general, a fever, decreased urinary output, or cloudy or foul-smelling urine indicate a probable urinary tract infection.

Treatment

Antibiotics appropriate for the identified organism are used in treating acute and chronic urinary tract infections. Increasing fluid intake to 2,000 to 4,000 mL/day will dilute the urine and flush bacteria out of the system. Renal calculi are treated by identifying the underlying cause (such as hypercalcemia from immobility or metabolic disorders) and increasing the fluid intake to dilute solutes. The use of intermittent catheterization in preference to indwelling catheters may decrease the incidence of calculous formation.

KEY CONCEPTS

- Upper motor neuron lesions generally result in loss of voluntary control of voiding. Lower motor neuron lesions that disrupt the sacral reflex arc result in disruption of both voluntary and involuntary micturition.
- Neurogenic bladder results in urine stasis and predisposes to infection and the development of renal stones.

Bladder Stones

Bladder stones are unusual but if present can cause symptoms of a urinary tract obstruction or infection.

TABLE 29–1. Neurogenic Bladder Classification

Lesion Type/Effect	Cause	Bladder Function
Upper Motor Neuron		
Uninhibited; loss of cortical inhibition	Multiple sclerosis Lack of voluntary control in infants	Decreased urine volume, incontinence, enuresis, frequency, urgency
Reflex	Lesions above T12 Complete transection of spinal cord Spinal cord tumors Multiple sclerosis	Incomplete emptying, involuntary voiding, urine retention, infection
Lower Motor Neuron		
Autonomous; loss of cortical inhibition Impaired spinal reflex arc	Lesions at the sacral level: trauma, tumors, herniated disk Transection of pelvic parasympathetic nerves	Bladder does not empty in response to stretch Incontinence due to overflow
Motor paralysis Flaccid bladder	S2–S4 lesions: trauma, tumors, polio	Lack of bladder contraction causing incontinence due to overflow; bladder never completely empties
Sensory paralysis	Lumbar posterior nerve root lesion Diabetes mellitus	Loss of sensation of bladder fullness, dribbling, overflow, incontinence

A stone in the bladder irritates the urothelium and may obstruct the bladder urethral orifice.[2]

Pathogenesis

Calculi are usually formed in the upper urinary tract or from a nucleus of dead tissue in the presence of bacteria. Stasis of urine in immobilized patients may also predispose to the formation of bladder calculi. Bladder stones are composed of uric acid, calcium oxalate, and ammonium acid urate.[3]

Bladder calculi are seen most frequently in Mediterranean and Far Eastern countries in which the diet is high in cereals. In industrialized nations, calculi in adults are usually calcium oxalate, calcium phosphate, or due to infection. Calculi in children are due to infections. Calculi occur more frequently in males than in females.

Clinical Manifestations

Bladder calculi cause general symptoms of urinary tract obstruction or infection. Irritation of the urothelial lining of the bladder causes hematuria, pyuria, and suprapubic pain. Bladder calculi can obstruct the bladder urethral orifice, causing a sudden interruption of the urinary stream. Exercise or movement will increase the suprapubic pain and obstruction that result from movement of the stone against the bladder wall.[2]

Treatment

Relief of urinary obstruction and treatment for infection are the primary goals of therapy. If the urethral obstruction can be eliminated or converted to a partial obstruction with a Foley catheter, then conservative treatment and determination of the underlying cause can proceed. The treatment of infections that precipitate or result from bladder stones is based on urine culture results and sensitivity. If relief of the obstruction cannot be accomplished with manipulation or catheterization, then surgical intervention to remove the stone may be necessary to avoid renal failure and sepsis.

KEY CONCEPTS

- Bladder stones are unusual, but when present may cause symptoms of obstruction or irritation of the bladder lining. Hematuria and suprapubic pain may occur. As with other obstructive processes, stasis of urine and infections may occur.

Cystitis

Cystitis, or inflammation of the bladder urothelium, may result from bacterial, fungal or parasitic infections, chemical irritants, foreign bodies (stones), or trauma.[3] Bacterial cystitis is generally secondary to an infection that began in the urethra. Most cystitis inflammations are uncomplicated and resolve spontaneously.

Symptoms of nonbacterial cystitis may be produced by the "acute urethral syndrome" or "irritable bladder." In these cases the urinalysis and culture results will be negative. Nonbacterial cystitis occurs most commonly in women aged 20 to 30 years. The cause of the urethral syndrome is not clear, but the syndrome is associated with dysfunction of the external sphincter, vaginitis, ureteritis, or inflammation of the glands adjacent to the vagina and urethra. Bacteria may or may not take hold after the initial symptoms develop.[4] Treatment is symptomatic. If bacteriuria develops, appropriate antibiotic therapy is initiated.

Pathogenesis

Normally, bacteria are cleared from the bladder by flushing and the dilutional effects of voiding. High urea and osmolarity in urine act to kill bacteria in a normal bladder environment. Cystitis is more common in women than in men because of the shorter urethra, the proximity of the urethra to the anal sphincter, and the presence of vaginal secretions, which contain bacteria that may migrate into the urethra. Individuals at increased risk for developing cystitis include sexually active or pregnant women and people with indwelling urinary catheters, diabetes mellitus, neurogenic bladder, poor hygiene, or any type of urinary tract obstruction. In men, prostatic secretions are antibacterial, which may account for the rarity of cystitis in men less than 50 years of age. However, prostatitis or ureteral obstruction due to prostatic hypertrophy can predipose the development of bacteriuria and cystitis in men.

The most common causative organisms are *E. coli, Klebsiella, Proteus, Pseudomonas,* and *Staphylococcus.* Less commonly, *Enterobacter* and *Serratia* are identified as causative agents. In catheterized patients or those with diabetes mellitus, *Candida* and other fungi are common causative agents.[4]

Clinical Manifestations

About 10 percent of individuals with bacteriuria are asymptomatic. The majority of patients with cystitis experience frequency, urgency, dysuria (painful urination), and pain in the suprapubic area or lower back, or both. Flank pain is usually more serious and can indicate an infection proximal to the bladder. Visually, hematuria or cloudy urine may be evident.

Treatment

Risk factors that predispose an individual to cystitis should be evaluated and treated. Urine is evaluated for bacteria, white blood cells (WBCs), red blood cells (RBCs), and nitrites. An elevated WBC count (>4-5 per high power field) or a positive nitrite test in a clean-catch urine sample, is usually indicative of a urinary tract infection. A wide-spectrum antibiotic is usually given when a positive urine sample is obtained. A urine culture is used to identify the specific bacterial or fungal cause of the infection and takes 24 to 48 hours to complete. Sensitivity testing to identify antibiotics that the organism is sensitive to is also done to indicate the best course of treatment. If the organism is not sensitive to the initial antibiotic prescribed, the prescription is changed. Relapsing infection may be present in about 25 percent of women with cystitis and requires prolonged antibiotic therapy.

Age-Related Considerations

Cystitis in the elderly, both men and women, is commonly asymptomatic, which may delay treatment and predispose these individuals to complications. Elderly individuals who are immobile are also at increased risk for developing urinary tract infections in general and cystitis in particular. In children, nighttime enuresis or daytime incontinence may be the presenting symptom associated with cystitis.

KEY CONCEPTS

- **Cystitis is an inflammation of the bladder lining that may be due to infection, chemical irritants, stones, or trauma. Most cases are infectious and result from bacterial invasion from the urethra.**
- **Factors predisposing to cystitis include female sex, catheterization, diabetes mellitus, and any disorder causing urine stasis. Manifestations include dysuria, cloudy urine, positive urine culture, and elevated urine levels of WBCs, RBCs, and nitrites.**
- **Cystitis in the elderly is commonly asymptomatic, which may delay treatment. Children may have daytime or nighttime incontinence as a presenting symptom.**

Tumors

Each year 40,000 new cases of bladder cancer are diagnosed. **Urothelial malignant tumors** account for 4 percent of cancers in men and 2 percent of cancers in women in the United States. About 90 percent or more of all bladder tumors originate from the transitional epithelium of the urinary tract.[5] **Transitional epithelium,** or **urothelium,** is the common lining found throughout the urinary tract. This may explain the propensity of tumors arising from this common lining to re-seed anywhere in the urinary tract.

Etiology and Pathogenesis

Approximately 20 to 30 percent of bladder tumors may be occupation related. Occupations involving chemicals and rubber are associated with bladder cancer. Sewage workers and laboratory technicians are also at increased risk for bladder cancer. There may be a lapse of 20 years or more between contact with carcinogens and the clinical appearance of a tumor.[6] Specific chemicals implicated are α- and β-naphthylamine, benzidene, and 4-aminodiphenyl. Cigarette smoke, phenacetin analgesics, and some antineoplastic drugs have been found to act as carcinogens. A malignant growth in the bladder and urinary tract may be associated with cell-mediated or humoral immune deficiency, because urothelial tumors occur primarily in patients over the age of 50 years and those receiving immunosuppressive therapy.

In children, the congenital anomaly of exstrophy of the bladder may predispose the development of bladder tumors, particularly adenocarcinomas. Repeated infections causing squamous metaplasia may also predispose to tumor development. Patients who have undergone urinary diversion for any reason also experience squamous metaplasia and are at risk for tumor development. Parasitic infections from schistosomiasis have been associated with squamous cell carcinoma as a result of urine-borne carcinogens formed during the infectious process and irritation by the parasitic ova.

Tumor Characteristics

Bladder tumors occur most often at the **trigone,** the ureteral orifices, and the posterior and lateral walls of the bladder. The tumor usually spreads by a direct route through the bladder wall to adjacent organs or through lymph nodes in the pelvis and abdomen. Once treated, tumors can recur at the original site, or an entirely new tumor may develop at another site. The most common sites of metastasis are the liver, lungs, bone, and adrenals; tumor cells are carried to these sites by the blood. Other sites of metastasis are the heart, brain, and kidney.

Four features are evaluated in bladder tumors: (1) the pattern of growth, (2) cell type, (3) tumor differentiation, and (4) depth of invasion. Tumor patterns include papillary, solid infiltrating, papillary and solid or noninvasive. Cell types include transitional, squamous, or glandular. Noninvasive tumor, or carcinoma in situ, may progress to a papillary or invasive tumor in a short period or may remain inactive for years.

In children, the most common bladder tumor is embryonal sarcoma, usually found at the base of the bladder. The distal ureters, prostate, and seminal vesicles may be involved by tumor in boys. In girls, masses at the introitus may be seen.

Clinical Manifestations

In the early stages of bladder tumor, about 75 percent of patients have either gross or microscopic hematuria as the presenting complaint. Dysuria, frequency, and urgency are also present in about 25 percent of patients.[6] Late presenting symptoms can include ureteral obstruction, pelvic pain, or metastatic symptoms (symptoms associated with metastatic sites in the liver, lungs, or bone). Diagnostic examinations such as urinary cytology, intravenous pyelography, mucosal biopsies, and direct visualization by cystoscopy are included in the evaluation. Abdominal computerized tomography (CT) may also be used for staging the tumor.

Treatment

Treatment protocols are based on the tumor's features. For noninvasive carcinoma in situ, endoscopic resection is usually used, with close follow-up every 3 to 6 months. If a recurrence of the original tumor is found, pharmacologic therapy with endoscopic resection is utilized. Invasive tumors are treated with radical or simple cystectomy and radiation therapy. The survival rate at 5 years is about 45 percent. Urinary diversions and the Koch pouch (Fig. 29–2) are utilized after cystectomy to provide for urinary drainage. In patients whose tumors have metastasized to distant sites, the life expectancy is about 2 years. Chemotherapy, which may include some combination of cisplatin, methotrexate, doxorubicin, cyclophosphamide, and vinblastine, is used to induce remission.

KEY CONCEPTS

- **Most bladder tumors originate from transitional epithelium lining the urinary tract. Occupational exposure to carcinogenic chemicals and repeated bladder infections are thought to be predisposing factors.**
- **Bladder tumors may cause manifestations of ureteral or urethral obstruction. Benign tumors may be surgically removed. Malignant tumors necessitate removal of the bladder and formation of an alternative route for urine elimination (ileal conduit, Koch pouch). In addition to surgery, radiation and chemotherapy may be used.**

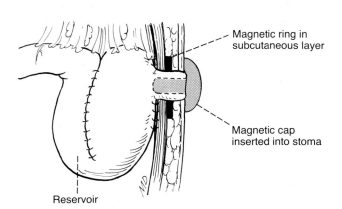

Magnetic ring in subcutaneous layer

Magnetic cap inserted into stoma

Reservoir

F I G U R E 29 – 2. Koch pouch. (From Black JM, Matassarin-Jacobs E: *Luckmann and Sorensen's Medical-Surgical Nursing: A Psychophysiologic Approach,* 4th ed. Philadelphia, WB Saunders, 1993, p 1645. Reproduced with permission.)

Congenital Disorders

Vesicoureteral Reflux

Reflux of urine from the bladder to the ureter and renal pelvis, known as **vesicoureteral reflux,** is usually due to incompetence of the valvular mechanism at the ureter-bladder junction. This condition is found in childhood, usually during evaluation for recurrent urinary tract infections.

Pathogenesis

Normally the ureters enter the bladder at an oblique angle and then continue 1 to 2 cm under the bladder mucosa before exiting inside the bladder cavity. As the bladder fills, pressure within the bladder increases against the muscle wall, closing the ureteral passageway. In vesicoureteral reflux, this process is not successful, and the urine flows backward into the ureters or the kidney. Reflux may lead to increased renal pelvis pressure and the migration of bacteria from the bladder to the kidneys. The end result can be ureteral dilation, dilation of the upper renal collecting system, and renal scarring. Reflux great enough to dilate ureters also prevents the bladder from emptying completely, causing bladder dilation and predisposing to infection. Reflux nephropathy (destruction of renal glomeruli) can result in end-stage renal disease (15–20 percent of all end-stage renal disease in children and young adults) and hypertension in children.[7]

There are two classifications of vesicoureteral reflux, primary and secondary. Congenital abnormalities at the ureterovesical junction are the cause of primary reflux. The mucosal ureteral tunnel is short, which decreases the efficiency of the valvular mechanism; the orifice is more lateral; and the trigone is not well developed. Primary reflux is also associated with other abnormalities of the urinary system, among them ureteral duplication, ureterocele with duplication, ureteral ectopia, and paraurethral diverticula (Fig. 29–3). Secondary reflux can occur from increased pressure within the vesical (neurogenic bladder, bladder outlet obstruction), inflammatory processes, and surgical procedures at or near the ureterovesical junction. The extent of reflux is graded from I to V (Table 29–2 and Fig. 29–4).

Clinical Manifestations

Most commonly reflux is discovered during evaluation for recurrent urinary tract infections in children.

T A B L E 29 – 2. Vesicoureteral Grading

Grade I	Reflux to the distal ureter
Grade II	Reflux into the upper collecting system
Grade III	Reflux into dilated ureter/calices
Grade IV	Reflux into a grossly dilated system
Grade V	Massive reflux with ureteral dilation and tortuous calices

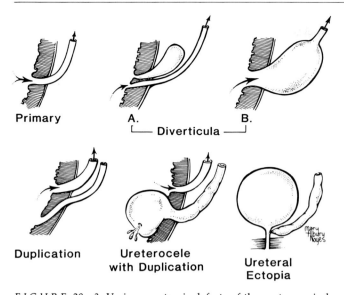

Primary

A.   B.
└── Diverticula ──┘

Duplication   Ureterocele
                   with Duplication   Ureteral
                                           Ectopia

FIGURE 29–3. Various anatomic defects of the ureterovesical junction associated with vesicoureteral reflux. (From Behrman RE: *Nelson Textbook of Pediatrics*, 14th ed. Philadelphia, WB Saunders, 1992, p 1364. Reproduced with permission.)

However, the child may present with voiding dysfunction, renal insufficiency, or hypertension. Diagnostic tests such as voiding cystourethrography, intravenous pyelography, radionuclide renal scintigraphy, and CT are performed to evaluate the status of the kidney and bladder system.

Treatment

Treatment depends on the grade of reflux. Grades I and II may resolve spontaneously. During the period of observation, low-dose antibiotics such as sulfamethoxazole-trimethoprim or nitrofurantoin are used to prevent infection. Urine cultures are performed every 3 months to ensure control of bacteriuria. If there is poor control of bacteriuria in a grade II reflux then surgical intervention may be needed. More than 50

percent of patients with grade III reflux will need surgical repair. Until surgery, management is much the same as for grades I and II. Grades IV and V are usually surgically repaired, particularly in infants and children less than 5 years old.

Obstruction of the Ureteropelvic Junction

Ureteropelvic junction obstruction is the most common childhood obstruction of the urinary tract. In the majority of cases, stenosis of the ureteropelvic junction is the cause of the obstruction.

Pathogenesis

Congenital stenosis of the ureteropelvic junction tends to cause increased pressure in the ureters. When the intraluminal pressure exceeds the renal pelvis pressure, dilation of the renal pelvis occurs, eventually leading to hydronephrosis. Obstruction may be unilateral or bilateral (about 20 percent of cases).

Clinical Manifestations and Diagnosis

The presenting symptoms include a palpable renal mass in a newborn infant, abdominal, flank, or back pain, or a urinary tract infection with fever or hematuria as a result of negligible trauma. Ureteropelvic junction obstruction may also be asymptomatic and found incidentally on renal ultrasonography (US) of the infant.

If unilateral hydronephrosis is found on neonatal US and the other kidney appears normal, no intervention is used. The infant is followed with renal US studies performed soon after birth and every 3 months for the first year of life to evaluate any changes in the system. If the opposite kidney and the serum creatinine level are normal, the child may be observed without invasive intervention. In older children, intravenous urography and renal US are used for diagnosis. Occasionally antegrade or retrograde pyelography is done during repair to locate the point of obstruction.

Treatment

Surgical repair involves removal of the stenosed area of the junction and anastomosis of the ureter and renal pelvis. Early surgical repair is indicated if function in the affected kidney decreases, in cases of bilateral obstruction, in cases of congenital single kidney with obstruction, or when renal function in general is decreased.

Ureteral Ectopy

An **ectopic ureter** is a single ureter implanted in a site other than normal, or a duplicate ureter (see Fig. 29–3). Alternate or duplicate sites of ureter implanta-

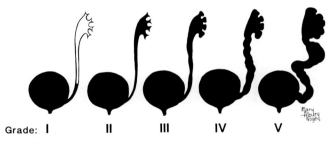

Grade: I   II   III   IV   V

FIGURE 29–4. Grading of a vesicoureteral reflux. Grade I: reflux into a nondilated distal ureter. Grade II: reflux into the upper collecting system without dilation. Grade III: reflux into dilated ureter and/or blunting of caliceal fornices. Grade IV: reflux into a grossly dilated ureter. Grade V: massive reflux, with ureteral dilation and tortuosity and effacement of the caliceal details. (From Behrman RE: *Nelson Textbook of Pediatrics*, 14th ed. Philadelphia, WB Saunders, 1992, p 1365. Reproduced with permission.)

tion predispose the patient to infection and the potential for reduced renal function.

Pathogenesis

Ureters may implant anywhere along the route of migration of the mesonephric duct during fetal development. In males, the ureter is usually single and can be found implanted in the bladder neck, the urethra, the seminal vesicle, or the vas deferens. In females, the ectopic ureter is commonly due to duplication of the collecting system. When associated with duplication, the ureter may implant in the bladder neck, urethra, vagina, or uterus.

Clinical Manifestations, Diagnosis, and Treatment

Significant obstruction of the urinary tract commonly occurs with ectopic ureters. Symptoms of infection are associated with males and females. Epididymitis may be a presenting problem in males, while females with implantation in the vagina or uterus may present with urinary incontinence or vaginal discharge.

The condition is diagnosed with intravenous urography, renal US, and endoscopy.

In the case of a single ectopic ureter, when the opposing kidney is normal, nephroureterectomy is the recommended course of treatment. If the involved kidney has adequate function, the ureter may be reimplanted in a more physiologically acceptable site.

Ureterocele

A **ureterocele** is a congenital cystic dilation of the distal ureter (see Fig. 29–3). The cystic structure pouches in the bladder and has an extremely small bladder orifice.

Etiology and Pathogenesis

Ureteroceles occur more commonly in females than in males. The embryonic development of the cystic structure is not well understood. Ureteroceles are classified as *simple* (not associated with duplicate collecting systems) or, more commonly, found in *duplicate systems with ectopic implantation.* Either type of ureterocele may be unilateral or bilateral. The small orifice of the ureter acts as an obstruction of the collecting system, causing ureteral and caliceal dilation. If the ureterocele is large, obstruction of the bladder outlet may be seen.

Clinical Manifestations, Diagnosis, and Treatment

Patients with ureteroceles often present with urinary tract infections. If the bladder outlet is obstructed, retention of urine may also be seen.

The procedure of choice for diagnosis is intravenous pyelography, which usually shows ureteral and caliceal dilation or a filling defect of the bladder.

Treatment varies according to the type of ureterocele and the degree of obstruction. Because most children with ureteroceles present with urinary tract infections, appropriate antibiotic therapy is utilized. Surgical manipulation of the defect varies and includes transurethral incision of the defect, excision of the defect with reimplantation of the ureter, or partial nephrectomy and ureterectomy. In an acutely septic patient, percutaneous nephrostomy to drain the upper collecting system may be needed.

KEY CONCEPTS

- Congenital abnormalities of the bladder include malimplantation of ureters, strictures, an extra ureter, and ureterocele. Most of these disorders cause problems by obstructing normal urine flow and predisposing to the retrograde flow of urine, urine stasis, and secondary infection.

Summary

Most disorders of the bladder are due to infectious processes or anatomic variations that disturb the normal flow of urine. Because of the close interrelationship between the bladder and the kidney, an abnormality or infectious process may affect the entire renal system, resulting in long-term disease and disability.

Urine stasis is a potential consequence of or a predisposing factor for nearly all lower urinary tract disorders. Measures to prevent or treat stasis of urine in lower urinary tract structures will minimize the likelihood of ascending ureteral and kidney disease.

REFERENCES

1. Walleck CA: Central nervous system: II. Spinal cord injury, in Cardona VD, Hurn PD, Bastnael Mason PJ, Scanlon AM, Veise-Berry SW (eds): *Trauma Nursing From Resuscitation Through Rehabilitation,* 2nd ed. Philadelphia, WB Saunders, 1994, pp 435–465.
2. Turka LA: Urinary tract obstruction, in Rose BD (ed): *Pathophysiology of Renal Disease,* 2nd ed. New York, McGraw-Hill, 1991, pp 447–468.
3. Schreiner GF, Kissane JM: The urinary system, in Kissane JM (ed): *Anderson's Pathology,* 9th ed. St. Louis, CV Mosby, 1990, pp 806–870.
4. Stamm WE, Turck M: Urinary tract infection pyelonephritis and related conditions, in Wilson JD, Braunwald E, Isselbacher KJ, et al (eds): *Harrison's Principles of Internal Medicine,* 11th ed. New York, McGraw-Hill, 1987, pp 1189–1194.
5. Garnick MB, Brenner BM: Tumors of the urinary tract, in Wilson JD, Braunwald E, Isselbacher KJ, et al (eds): *Harrison's Principles of Internal Medicine,* 12th ed. New York, McGraw-Hill, 1991, pp 1209–1212.
6. Coe FL, Brenner B: Approach to the patient with diseases of the kidneys and urinary tract, in Wilson JD, Braunwald E, Isselbacher KJ, et al (eds): *Harrison's Principles of Internal Medicine,* 12th ed. New York, McGraw-Hill, 1991, pp 1134–1144.
7. Behrman RG: *Nelson Textbook of Pediatrics,* 14th ed. Philadelphia, WB Saunders, 1992, pp 1359–1373.

BIBLIOGRAPHY

Brenner BM, Milford EL, Seiffer JC: Urinary tract obstruction, in Wilson JD, Braunwald E, Isselbacher KJ, et al (eds): *Harrison's Principles of Internal Medicine,* 12th ed. New York, McGraw-Hill, 1991, pp 1206–1209.

Garnick MB, Brenner BM: Tumors of the urinary tract, in Wilson JD, Braunwald E, Isselbacher KJ, et al (eds): *Harrison's Principles of Internal Medicine,* 12th ed. New York, McGraw-Hill, 1991, pp 1209–1212.

Peterson RO: The urinary tract and male reproductive system, in Rubin E, Farber JL (eds): *Essential Pathology.* Philadelphia, JB Lippincott, 1990, pp 488–509.

Rector JC: Obstructive nephropathy, in Wyngaarden JB, Smith LH (eds): *Cecil's Textbook of Medicine,* 18th ed. Philadelphia, WB Saunders, 1988, pp 614–617.

Williams R: Tumors of the kidney, ureter, and bladder, in Wyngaarden JB, Smith LH (eds): *Cecil's Textbook of Medicine,* 18th ed. Philadelphia, WB Saunders, 1988, pp 650–655.

UNIT IX
Alterations in Genitourinary Function

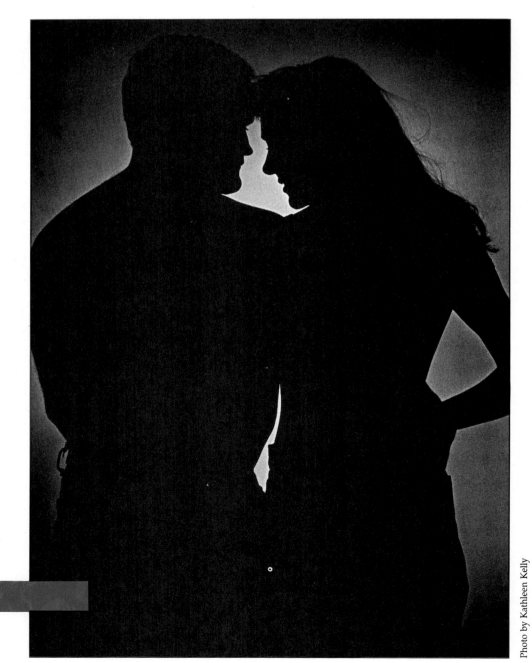

Touch and body language suggest intimacy and closeness.

Photo by Kathleen Kelly

Although the most common sexually transmitted diseases (STDs) have declined dramatically in other industrialized nations, they have been increasing among some urban populations in the United States. Social disintegration, persistent poverty, and prostitution, often exchanged for drugs, have increased the rates of gonorrhea, syphilis, and chancroid in American cities. And if that shameful fact were not enough—shameful because it is associated with long-unresolved social problems—drug-resistant bacterial infections and viruses that cause diseases not presently curable have complicated efforts to bring the United States into accord with conditions in the nations of Europe and with Japan, Australia, and New Zealand.

This is an area where the reduction or elimination of insidiously harmful diseases requires a linkage between scientific research, social policy, and strategies of public health care.

The implications of the return of STDs are ominous. In 1989, 4,714 cases of chancroid were reported in the United States. Chancroid causes genital ulcers and is associated with prostitution and having sex with prostitutes. This may not sound like an alarming number, but the bacterium that causes chancroid resists many antimicrobial drugs and the chancroid itself may facilitate the spread of human immunodeficiency virus (HIV). In those who have been exposed to HIV, the chancroid resists otherwise effective therapies. So HIV infection may help spread a bacterial STD, which in turn helps to spread HIV infection—a deadly cycle.

A fourth bacterial STD, chlamydiosis, has become more common than gonorrhea, syphilis, or chancroid. *Chlamydia* infects the urethra in men and the cervix in women. It is curable, but because of an ineffective public health response it is a major cause of infertility in women and increases their susceptibility to HIV infection. If the infection reaches the uterus and fallopian tubes it can cause serious symptoms, produce microscopic cervical ulcers, and scar the fallopian tubes, jeopardizing the woman's ability to have healthy children.

Unlike the other STDs, chlamydial infection is found frequently among the middle class of the United States. Apparently, programs intended to control chlamydiosis are not keeping pace with the spread of the disease. Where public health controls have been applied, infection has declined.

Viruses also cause STDs. The therapies applied to lesions caused by the human papillomavirus (HPV)—toxic chemicals, freezing, electrocautery, or laser treatment—cannot destroy a virus. Epidemiological studies based on tests that detect the proteins and DNA of STD-causing viruses now reveal widespread viral STD problems. The diseases include genital herpes and genital warts. A minority of HPV genital infections produce warts. Nevertheless, the number of consultations for genital warts increased from 169,000 in 1966 to more than 2 million in 1988.

Epidemiological studies based on tests that detect the proteins and DNA of STD-causing viruses now are disclos-

FRONTIERS OF RESEARCH
Sexually Transmitted Diseases

Michael J. Kirkhorn

ing, one report said, "the vast scope of the viral STD problem as well as the distribution and determinants of these infections."

Hepatitis B infection also is a viral STD. Researchers estimate there are 200 million carriers of hepatitis B virus in the world. The number of new cases diagnosed in the United States annually is estimated at 300,000.

The most prominent immunologic disease that can be transmitted by sexual contact is acquired immunodeficiency sydrome (AIDS), caused by HIV infection. AIDS has been associated with homosexual practices, but most of the cases now appearing in Africa and parts of the Caribbean have been transmitted heterosexually during vaginal intercourse. A growing proportion of cases of AIDS and HIV infection in Europe and Latin America have been transmitted heterosexually, and, a report said, "heterosexual HIV infections are now proliferating at explosive rates in parts of Thailand and India."

The risk of HIV infection is a greater hazard for those already infected with STDs. It appears that HIV infection prolongs infection for those who have genital and anorectal herpes ulcers, and it may account for failure of syphilis treatment and for altered manifestation of syphilis and gonorrhea. "We can therefore postulate that HIV and coexisting STDs may promote one another's spread," a recent *Scientific American* article reports.

CHAPTER 30
Structure and Function
of the Male Genitourinary System

DAVID MIKKELSEN

KEY TERMS

bulbourethral glands: Also called Cowper's glands, these two glands produce viscous fluid that is secreted into the urethra near the base of the penis.

epididymis: Tightly coiled tube in which sperm mature and develop the ability to swim; lies along the top of and behind the testes.

gonads: Derived from the urogenital ridge, the undifferentiated and primitive gonads become the testes in males and the ovaries in females.

Leydig cells: Clusters of interstitial cells within the testes that produce and secrete testosterone.

penis: Male organ of copulation and urinary excretion.

prostate: Gland located below the bladder; its secretion helps activate sperm and maintain their motility.

scrotum: Pouchlike sac containing the testes, epididymides, and spermatic cord.

semen: Male reproductive fluid that contains spermatozoa and is released at ejaculation.

seminal vesicle: Two glands that contribute rich nutrients to the seminal fluid.

Sertoli cells: Elongated cells that support and provide nutrition to the attached spermatid until they mature into spermatozoa.

spermatogenesis: Production of sperm cells.

spermatozoa: Mature sperm cells.

testis: The male gonad or reproductive gland that produces spermatozoa and houses the Leydig cells, which secrete testosterone.

testosterone: Male sex hormone produced by interstitial cells in the testes.

---

*T*his chapter will present the anatomy and embryology of the male genitourinary tract. The genitourinary tract refers to those organs involved in the processes of sexual reproduction and the elimination of nitrogenous wastes.

Because these organs derive from common embryologic structures, the anatomy and embryology of the male genitalia and urinary system will be initially presented. To facilitate understanding of both male and female anatomy, the differences in embryologic development will be briefly considered where they are pertinent.

The remainder of this chapter will deal with the physiology of male reproduction. The physiology of urinary elimination and of female reproduction are considered in other chapters.

Anatomy of the Genitourinary Tract

Upper Genitourinary Tract

The upper genitourinary tract consists of the kidneys and ureters. The kidneys are paired solid organs situated on each side of the midline in the retroperitoneal space. The position of the liver causes the right kidney to be lower than the left. The adult kidney weighs about 150 grams and measures about 12 cm by 7 cm, with a thickness of approximately 3 cm.

On longitudinal sections, the kidney is composed of an outer cortex, central medulla, and the collecting system, made up of the calices and renal pelvis (see Fig. 26–2). The cortex is homogeneous in appearance and contains the renal corpuscle, composed of the vascular glomerulus and Bowman's capsule. The renal corpuscle is contiguous with the proximal convoluted tubule of the nephron (see Fig. 26–3). The cortex also contains the distal convoluted tubule component of the nephron.

The medulla consists of numerous pyramids formed by the converging collecting ducts and the loops of Henle. The collecting tubules subsequently drain into the minor calices of the renal collecting system. The renal collecting system consists of the minor calices, which drain the numerous papillae of the renal pyramids, the major calices, which drain the minor calices, and the renal pelvis, which drains the bifurcating major calyces (Fig. 30–1).

Urine subsequently drains into the ureter, which propagates the urine down its tubular structure into the bladder by involuntary rhythmic smooth muscle contractions. The adult ureter is approximately 30 cm long. The ureteral lumen has several areas of relative narrowing, including the ureteropelvic junction, the pelvic brim, where the ureter passes over the iliac vessels, and the ureterovesical junction, where the ureter passes through the bladder wall. These positions are clinically relevant, as they provide the primary points of ureteral obstruction with passage of ureteral calculi (stones).

Histologically, the walls of the calices pelves, and ureters are composed of transitional cell epithelium under which lies loose connective and elastic tissue (lamina propria). External to the lamina propria is a mixture of spiral and longitudinal muscle fibers. The outermost or adventitial layer is composed of fibrous connective tissue.

The arterial blood supply of the kidney is usually provided by one renal artery that enters the medial concavity of the kidney (hilum) after branching from the aorta. The renal artery divides into an anterior and a posterior branch. The posterior branch usually supplies a middle segment of the posterior surface, whereas the anterior branch supplies the entire anterior surface as well as both upper and lower poles (Fig. 30–2).

The renal arteries further subdivide into interlobar arteries. The interlobar arteries ascend between the medullary pyramids and further subdivide into arcuate arteries (see Fig. 26–2). Smaller branches, the interlobular arteries, arise from the arcuate branches and give rise to afferent arterioles, which then pass into the glomeruli. From the glomeruli, efferent arterioles arise and subsequently form a peritubular capillary plexus that runs among the proximal and convoluted tubules of the kidney (see Fig. 26–3). Finally, the blood supply to the medulla arises from the vasa recta. These are straight branches that arise from the efferent arterioles of the juxtamedullary glomeruli and descend into the renal medulla, contributing side branches to a capillary plexus. This plexus is closely applied to the loop of Henle and collecting tubules.

The venous drainage of the kidney begins in the capillary plexus, which drains into the interlobular veins. Interlobular veins drain into arcuate veins, which parallel the course of arteries. The arcuate veins drain into the interlobar veins, which drain into the segmental vessels; the segmental vessels drain into the renal veins. The renal veins empty into the vena cava.

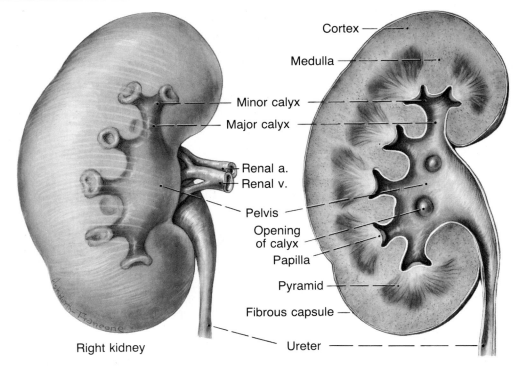

FIGURE 30–1. Entire and sagittal views showing relation of calices to kidney as a whole. (From Jacob SW, Francone CA: *Elements of Anatomy and Physiology*, 2nd ed. Philadelphia, WB Saunders, 1989, p 268. Reproduced with permission.)

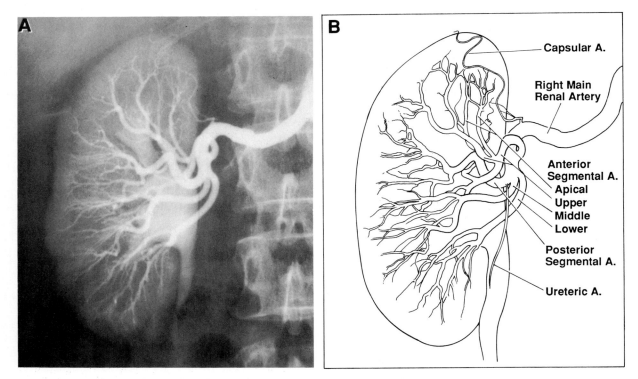

FIGURE 30–2. Segmental branches of the (right) renal artery demonstrated by renal angiogram. (From Walsh PC, Retik AB, Stamey TA, Vaughan ED (eds): *Campbell's Urology*, 6th ed. Philadelphia, WB Saunders, 1992, p 28. Reproduced with permission.)

The ureteral blood supply is derived from multiple sources. The renal pelvis and upper ureter are perfused by branches from the renal artery. The middle ureter is supplied by the internal spermatic artery, and the lowermost sections are usually served by branches from the common iliac, internal iliac, and vesical arteries (Fig. 30–3). The veins of the renal pelvis and ureter are usually paired with the arteries.

Lower Genitourinary Tract

Bladder

The bladder is a hollow muscular organ that serves as a reservoir for urine. The adult bladder normally has a capacity of 350 to 600 mL. When empty, the bladder lies behind the pubic symphysis and is mainly a pelvic organ. With overdistention or chronic urine retention, it may cause the abdomen to bulge and is easily palpable in the suprapubic region.

The ureters enter the bladder posteroinferiorly. The ureteral orifices are situated on a crescent-shaped ridge approximately 2.5 cm apart. The triangular area demarcated by this interureteric ridge and bladder neck is known as the trigone (Fig. 30–4). As will be discussed later in the chapter, it has a different embryologic origin from the rest of the bladder body or fundus, the trigone being composed of mesoderm and the fundus (body of the bladder) being composed of endoderm.

In males, the bladder lies adjacent to the seminal vesicles, vasa deferentia, ureters, and rectum posteriorly. The dome and part of the posterior bladder surfaces are covered by peritoneum and thus are in close proximity to the small bowel and the sigmoid colon. The neck of the bladder, which is the most inferior

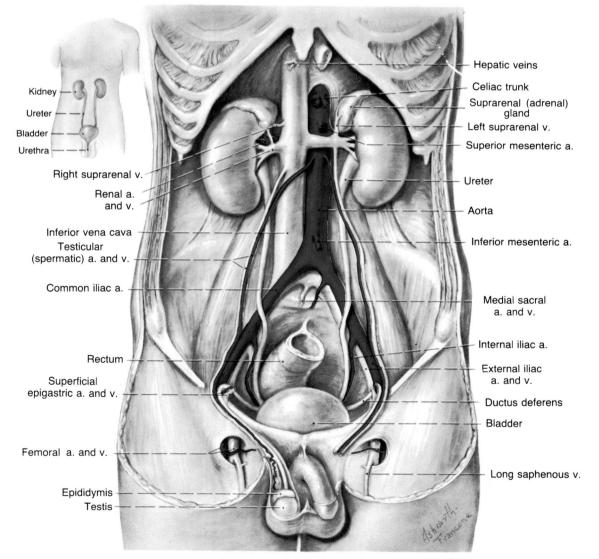

FIGURE 30–3. Posterior abdominal wall showing relationship of urinary system, genital system, and great vessels. (From Jacob SW, Francone CA: *Elements of Anatomy and Physiology*, 2nd ed. Philadelphia, WB Saunders, 1989, p 267. Reproduced with permission.)

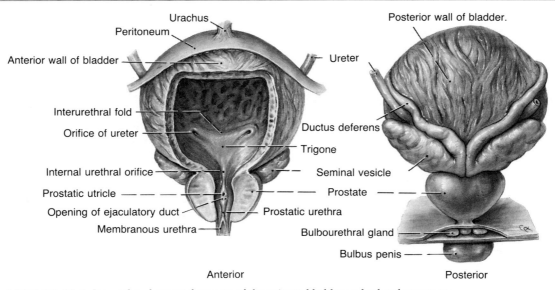

F I G U R E 30–4. Internal and external aspects of the urinary bladder and related structures. (From Jacob SW, Francone CA: *Elements of Anatomy and Physiology,* 2nd ed. Philadelphia, WB Saunders, 1989, p 272. Reproduced with permission.)

part, leads to the urethra. In males, the prostate lies between the bladder and the muscle layers of the pelvic floor that make up the urogenital diaphragm.

Histologically the inner lining or mucosa of the bladder is composed of transitional epithelium. Beneath this lies a layer of submucosa consisting of connective and elastic tissues. External to the submucosa lies a mixture of smooth muscle layers that compose the bladder muscle or detrusor. Although the bladder wall is often described as having three muscle layers—inner longitudinal, middle circular, and outer longitudinal coats—the detrusor fibers are probably arranged in a random pattern without a specific orientation except at the bladder neck, where they assume the previously described configuration.

The arterial blood supply of the bladder comes from the superior, middle, and inferior vesicle arteries, which originate from the anterior division of the hypogastric artery. Venous drainage is provided by a rich plexus of veins that surround the bladder and ultimately drain into the hypogastric vein.

The bladder and urethra receive a nerve supply from both the sympathetic and parasympathetic divisions of the autonomic nervous system. The sympathetic fibers, originating mainly from the lower thoracic and upper lumbar segments (T11–T12 and L1–L2), innervate the bladder and urethra as the hypogastric nerve. These sympathetic fibers are distributed more densely in the bladder base and proximal urethra than in the bladder dome. Studies have revealed differences in the sympathetic bladder muscle receptors, with β-adrenergic receptors concentrated in the fundus and α-adrenergic receptors present in the trigone and proximal urethra.

The parasympathetic nerve supply originates from the sacral segments (S2–S4), which proceed to form a plexus surrounding the bladder. In the male

a separate segment will reach the prostate, forming the prostatic plexus. From this plexus, nerves emerge to innervate the erectile tissue of the male penis and the clitoris of the female.

Branches of the bladder plexus penetrate the muscular coat of the bladder and become distributed throughout the detrusor. Parasympathetic muscle receptors are cholinergic in nature, and with parasympathetic stimulation a detrusor contraction occurs.

Urethra

The male urethra functions as a conduit for both the urinary and genital systems, extending from the bladder to the external opening (urethral meatus) at the tip of the penis. It is commonly divided into three segments—the prostatic, the membranous, and the penile or pendulous urethra (Fig. 30–5).

The prostatic urethra is the widest and most distensible part of the urethra. In the average male it is about 3 cm long. The most prominent landmark of this segment, the verumontanum, is a small elevation that is marked by a midline opening from the prostatic utricle, a remnant of the müllerian duct system. On either side of the utricular orifice lie the openings of both ejaculatory ducts, through which seminal fluid passes from the ejaculatory ducts to the prostatic urethra.

The membranous urethra is the urethral segment that passes through the muscular layers of the urogenital diaphragm (Fig. 30–6). On either side is one **bulbourethral** or **Cowper's gland.** Their ducts run distally for about 3 or 4 mm before they open into the urethra, depositing a mucoid secretion in the seminal fluid.

The penile urethra is the longest segment of the male urethra, being about 15 cm in length from

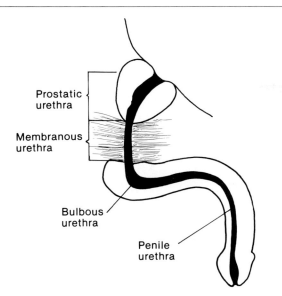

FIGURE 30–5. Urethral lumen, prostatic urethra, membranous urethra, bulbous urethra, and pendulous urethra, which opens into the external meatus after fusiform dilation of the navicular fossa. (From Walsh PC, Retik AB, Stamey TA, Vaughan ED (eds): *Campbell's Urology*, 6th ed. Philadelphia, WB Saunders, 1992, p 53. Reproduced with permission.)

the membranous urethra to the external meatus. The proximal portion of the penile urethra is called the bulbous urethra and is surrounded by the bulb of the urethra and bulbospongiosus muscle. Near the end of the penile urethra another area of widening, the fossa navicularis, is present.

Like the bladder, the proximal urethral mucosa is composed of transitional cell epithelium. Distal to the verumontanum it is composed of pseudostratified columnar and stratified epithelium.

Auxiliary Genital Glands in the Male

The auxiliary genital glands of the male consist of the prostate, the seminal vesicles, and the bulbourethral glands. These glands secrete products that contribute to the seminal fluid.

Prostate

The **prostate** lies below the bladder and has both a muscular and a glandular component. The normal prostate weighs about 20 grams and measures about 3.5 cm transversely and about 2.5 cm in its vertical and anteroposterior dimensions. The prostate is conical in shape. Its base is continuous with the bladder neck, and the inferior aspect of the prostate gland, or apex, lies adjacent to the urogenital diaphragm (Fig. 30–7). Behind the prostate lies the rectum and in front of the prostate a rich plexus of veins surrounded by fat lies between the prostate and the symphysis pubis.

The prostate consists of a thin fibrous capsule under which are circularly oriented smooth muscle fibers and collagenous tissue that surround the ure-

thra. Deep to this layer lies the prostatic stroma, composed of connective and elastic tissues, in which are embedded the prostatic epithelial glands. These glands drain into excretory ducts, which open chiefly on the floor of the urethra between the verumontanum and the vesical neck.

The main blood supply of the prostate is derived from the inferior vesical artery, a branch of the hypogastric artery. Besides the prostate, this artery also supplies the distal ureter, seminal vesicles, and part of the bladder. The venous drainage of the prostate is provided by a complex plexus, situated between the prostate and overlying tissues, that freely communicates with the inferior hypogastric veins.

Seminal Vesicles

The **seminal vesicles** are paired organs which lie cephalad to the prostate under the base of the bladder (See Fig. 30–7). Their coiled pouches secrete a fluid important to the survival of spermatozoa.

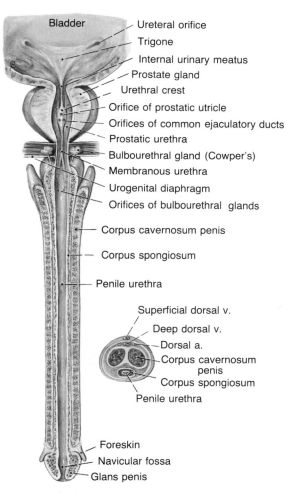

FIGURE 30–6. Section through the bladder, prostate gland, and penis. (From Jacob SW, Francone CA: *Elements of Anatomy and Physiology*, 2nd ed. Philadelphia, WB Saunders, 1989, p 283. Reproduced with permission.)

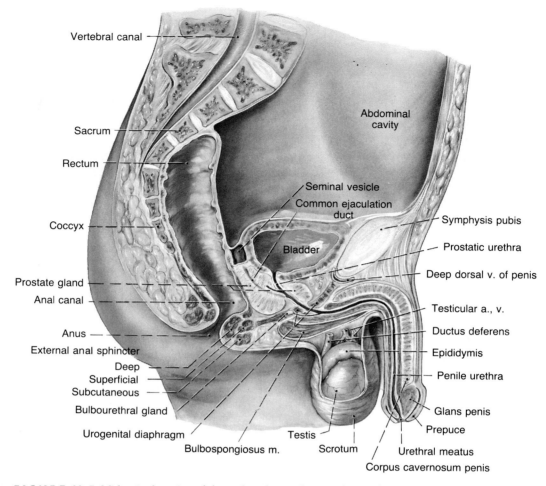

F I G U R E 30–7. Midsagittal section of the male pelvis and external genitalia. (From Jacob SW, Francone CA: *Elements of Anatomy and Physiology,* 2nd ed. Philadelphia, WB Saunders, 1989, p 281. Reproduced with permission.)

Bulbourethral Glands

The **bulbourethral** or Cowper's **glands** are located on each side of the membranous urethra within the urogenital diaphragm. They add a mucoid secretion to the semen.

External Genitalia of the Male

Scrotum

The **scrotum** (see Fig. 30–7) is a pouchlike sac that lies below the penis and pubic symphysis. Its two compartments are divided by a septum of connective tissue. Each compartment contains a male gonad or testis with its associated epididymis, as well as the lower portion of the spermatic cord and its coverings. The scrotum not only supports the testes but also, by relaxation and contraction of its muscular layer, helps to regulate their temperature.

The scrotal sac consists of several tissue layers. The scrotal skin overlies the dartos muscle layer, whose smooth muscle fibers are embedded in loose connective tissue. The dartos muscle functions to contract the scrotal pouch with cold and expand it with heat. Under the dartos layer several fascial layers exist (Fig. 30–8). These are continuous with the muscular layers of the abdominal wall and make up the coverings of the spermatic cord. The external spermatic fascia is continuous with the external oblique aponeurosis of the abdominal wall. A few slips of skeletal muscle derived from the internal oblique muscle layer make up the cremasteric muscle, which adds to the upper part of the cord. The internal spermatic fascia is a continuation of the transversalis fascia of the abdominal wall, with the transversus abdominis muscle not contributing to the cord layers. Finally, the peritoneum provides the tunica vaginalis layer, which is actually cut off from the abdominal cavity by the obliteration of the processus vaginalis.

The scrotum receives its blood supply from the external pudendal artery, a branch of the femoral artery. In addition, branches of the internal pudendal artery (which is itself a branch of the hypogastric ar-

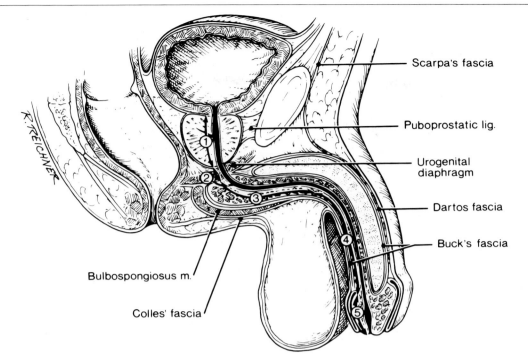

FIGURE 30–8. Diagram of the sagittal section of the penis and perineum illustrating the fascial layers. The divisions of the urethra are enumerated. (From Walsh PC, Retik AB, Stamey TA, Vaughan ED (eds): *Campbell's Urology*, 6th ed. Philadelphia, WB Saunders, 1992, p 2961. Reproduced with permission.)

tery) as well as the cremasteric and testicular arteries that traverse the spermatic cord also supply the scrotum.

Testes

The **testes** are the male reproductive organs responsible for sperm production. They average about 4 to 5 cm in length and 2 to 3 cm in thickness.

The testes lie within the scrotum and are suspended by the spermatic cord. They are covered by a thick fascial layer, called the tunica albuginea, which invaginates posteriorly to form the mediastinum testis. This fibrous mediastinum sends fibrous septa into each testis, separating it into many different lobules. Each lobule contains one to four seminiferous tubules which, if stretched to full length, would measure approximately 60 cm. It is in the epithelial lining of these tubules that the spermatozoa are formed (Fig. 30–9).

The seminiferous tubules have a basement membrane consisting of elastic and connective tissue that supports the seminiferous cells. The seminiferous cells are either **Sertoli cells** (supporting cells) or spermatogenic cells. Between the seminiferous tubules, and embedded in connective tissue, are the interstitial **Leydig cells** (Fig. 30–10). These cells are responsible for the production and secretion of testosterone. The tubules converge on the mediastinum testis. They are connected by the straight efferent ducts and drain into the head of the epididymis.

The testicular blood supply is derived from the internal spermatics, which arise directly from the aorta below the renal arteries. They course inferiorly through the spermatic cord and anastomose with the cremasteric arteries and the arteries of the vas; these vessels also contribute to the blood supply. The blood from the testis returns through a plexus of veins in the spermatic cord (the pampiniform plexus) that forms the spermatic veins. The left spermatic vein enters the renal vein, which subsequently enters the vena cava. The right renal vein enters the vena cava directly.

Epididymis and Ductus Deferens

The **epididymis** is a tightly coiled tube that lies along the top of and behind the testes. It is divided into the head, situated at the upper pole of the testes; the body, lying posterior to the testes; and the tail, which is attached to the inferior pole of the testes (see Fig. 30–9). The body and the tail of the epididymis are one continuous tube that serves as a conduit for maturing spermatozoa. In the epididymis sperm develop the ability to swim.

As the convoluted tube of the tail leaves its testicular attachments it increases in diameter, becoming a thick, muscular tube, the ductus (or vas) deferens. Leaving the spermatic cord, the vas follows an extraperitoneal course, passing caudally and laterally along the pelvic wall. As it passes medial to the distal end

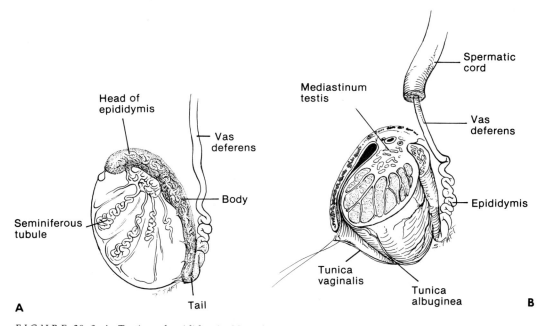

FIGURE 30–9. **A,** Testis and epididymis. Note the numerous compartments of the testis, filled with the seminiferous tubules gathering into the rete testis; they join to form a markedly convoluted tubule, which becomes the epididymis that leads to the vas deferens. **B,** Cross-section of the testis shows the several compartments and the mediastinum testis, as well as the coverings of the testis, with the tunica albuginea firmly adherent to its substance and the potential space surrounded by the tunica vaginalis. The epididymis attaches to the dorsomedial aspect of the testis, and the vas deferens joins the other structures of the spermatic cord. (From Walsh PC, Retik AB, Stamey TA, Vaughan ED (eds): *Campbell's Urology,* 6th ed. Philadelphia, WB Saunders, 1992, p 59. Reproduced with permission.)

of the ureter, it bends caudally to reach the midline and lies on the posterior wall of the bladder just medial to the seminal vesicles. It terminates in a dilated ampulla that courses underneath the base of the prostate. At this point the duct of the seminal vesicle joins with the duct of the ampulla, and the ejaculatory duct is formed. The ejaculatory ducts open in the prostatic urethra at the level of the verumontanum.

Penis

The **penis** is the male organ of copulation and urinary excretion. It is composed of three erectile bodies—two paired corpora cavernosa, which lie dorsally, and the corpus spongiosum, which contains the urethra (Fig. 30–11). Grossly, the penis is divided into three segments. The root of the penis consists of the proximal ends of the corpora cavernosa, which attach to the pelvic bones, and the proximal corpus spongiosum, which is attached to the undersurface of the urogenital diaphragm (Fig. 30–12). Together these attachments provide fixation and stability to the penis. The shaft of the penis consists of all three erectile bodies, the two cavernous bodies lying on the dorsum and the corpus, which occupies a depression on their ventral surface. Finally, the glans of the penis is the distal segment of the corpus spongiosum.

The three erectile bodies have the capability to become engorged with blood and enlarge considerably with erection. Microscopically these bodies have an internal spongelike network that consists of endothelium-lined spaces surrounded by smooth muscle.

Each corpus is enclosed in a fascia sheath, the tunica albuginea, and all are subsequently surrounded by a thick fibrous envelope know as Buck's

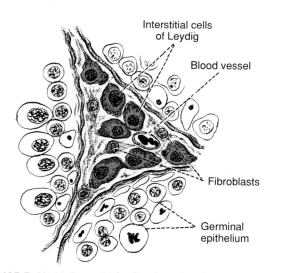

FIGURE 30–10. Interstitial cells of Leydig, the cells that secrete testosterone, located in the interstices between the seminiferous tubules. (From Guyton AC: *Textbook of Medical Physiology,* 8th ed. Philadelphia, WB Saunders, 1991, p 891. Reproduced with permission.)

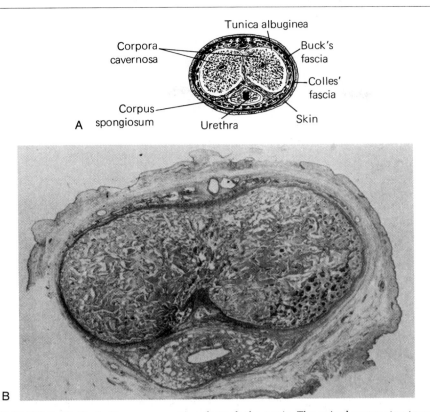

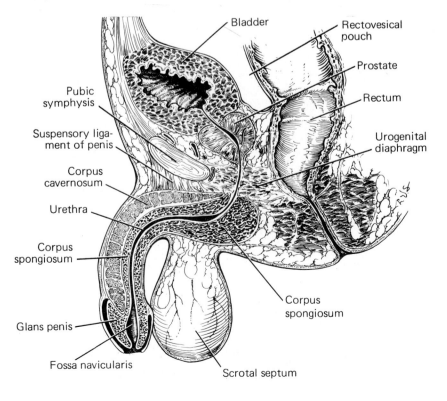

FIGURE 30-11. **A,** Transverse section through the penis. The paired upper structures are the corpora cavernosa. The single lower body surrounding the urethra is the corpus spongiosum. (From Tanagho EA, McAninch JW: *Smith's General Urology,* 13th ed. Norwalk, Conn, Appleton & Lange, 1992, p 9. Reproduced with permission.) **B,** Histologic cross-section of the adult male penis shows the main three spongy units—the two corpora cavernosa in the dorsum, and the corpus spongiosum with the urethra in its center. In the ventral portion, note the incomplete septum separating the two corpora cavernosa and the tunica albuginea as well as Buck's fascia surrounding the body of the penis. (From Walsh PC, Retik AB, Stamey TA, Vaughan ED (eds): *Campbell's Urology,* 6th ed. Philadelphia, WB Saunders, 1992, p 61. Reproduced with permission.)

FIGURE 30-12. Grossly, the penis is divided into three segments: the root, the shaft, and the glans. The root consists of the proximal ends of the corpora cavernosa, which attach to the pelvic bones, and the proximal corpus spongiosum, which is attached to the undersurface of the urogenital diaphragm. The shaft consists of the three erectile bodies (the paired corpora cavernosa and the corpus spongiosum). The glans is the distal segment of the corpus spongiosum. (From Tanagho EA, McAninch JW (eds): *Smith's General Urology,* 13th ed. Norwalk, Conn, Appleton & Lange, 1992, p 9. Reproduced with permission.)

fascia. The overlying skin of the penis is remarkable for its thinness and looseness of connection with the fascial sheath of the penis. The skin of the penis is folded upon itself to form the *prepuce* or *foreskin*. It is this penile skin that overlies the glans and is removed with circumcision.

The arterial blood supply is derived principally from the paired internal pudendal arteries, branches of the hypogastric arteries. Each internal pudendal artery branches several times in the penis. The deep or cavernous artery supplies the entire corpus cavernosum. The urethral artery supplies the corpus spongiosum, and the bulbar artery supplies the bulb of the corpus spongiosum. The dorsal artery continues along the dorsum of the penis, lying below Buck's fascia and between two dorsal veins. It provides additional supply to the glans (Fig. 30–13).

The venous drainage of the penis is through several channels. The cavernous veins drain the corpus cavernosum and the circumflex veins join the deep dorsal vein of the penis, also draining the corpora. The superficial dorsal vein drains the glans and part of the distal corpora. Finally, a bulbar branch drains the bulbar urethra and proximal corpus spongiosum. Together, these branches coalesce and pass through the urogenital diaphragm into the retropubic venous plexus of Santorini (Fig. 30–14).

The nerve supply of the penis is formed from both parasympathetic and sympathetic components. The parasympathetic fibers arise from S2–S4 and the sympathetic component derives from the hypogastric plexus. The parasympathetic fibers that form the pudendal nerve are responsible for erection. Although the final neurotransmitters have not been completely defined, parasympathetic stimulation results in relaxation of vascular resistance, which increases blood flow to the penis and creates an erection. Sensory fibers are also carried from the penis with the pudendal nerve and enter the sacral spinal cord.

The sympathetic neve fibers may contribute to erectile capacity but their role has not been proved conclusively. They do innervate the proximal involuntary sphincter of the bladder neck, where contraction prevents retrograde ejaculation of semen from the prostatic urethra into the bladder. They also innervate the muscles of the seminal vesicles and prostate, which, when stimulated, cause ejaculation of seminal fluid into the urethra.

KEY CONCEPTS

- Ureters transport urine from the renal pelvis to the bladder. Ureters have several points of narrowing that predispose to obstruction: the ureteropelvic junction, the pelvic brim, and the ureterovesical junction.

- The adult bladder has a normal capacity of 350 to 600 mL. With overdistention, the bladder may be palpable in the suprapubic region. The bladder is a muscular organ composed of several layers of muscle fibers. An important muscular landmark in the bladder is the trigone. Parasympathetic stimulation of the bladder results in bladder muscle contraction.

- The urethra extends from the bladder to the meatus at the end of the penis. In addition to transporting urine, the urethra has ducts that receive fluid from the prostate, seminal vesicles, and the bulbourethral glands.

- The scrotal sac supports the testes and regulates their temperature. Testes contain several cell types important in sperm production and the development of secondary sex characteristics. Sperm are produced in the testes from spermatogenic cells. Sertoli cells are supportive cells that nurture spermatogenesis. Leydig cells produce and secrete testosterone.

- The epididymis is a collecting conduit for sperm at the testes. The epididymis is continuous with the ductus (vas) deferens. The vas travels along the pelvic wall and joins with the seminal vesicle duct at the prostate to form the ejaculatory duct. The ejaculatory ducts open into the urethra.

- Skin overlying the penis is very loose, allowing for significant enlargement when the penis is engorged with blood during erection. Parasympathetic fibers forming the pudendal nerve are responsible for erection. Ejaculation is a function of the sympathetic nerve fibers.

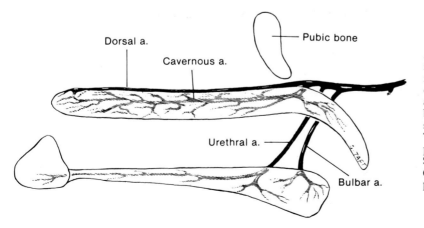

Dorsal a.

Cavernous a.

Pubic bone

Urethral a.

Bulbar a.

FIGURE 30–13. Arterial blood supply to the penis, where the two corpora cavernosa are separate from the corpus spongiosum. Note that the pudendal artery branches into the deep cavernous artery; also, it will give two other main branches, the bulbar artery and the urethral artery. The latter will supply the corpus spongiosum and the glans penis. The dorsal artery of the penis also sends blood supply to the glans penis. (From Walsh PC, Retik AB, Stamey TA, Vaughan ED (Eds): *Campbell's Urology*, 6th ed. Philadelphia, WB Saunders, 1992, p 61. Reproduced with permission.)

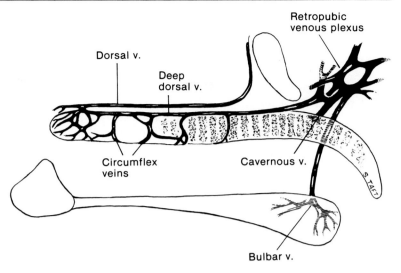

FIGURE 30–14. Venous drainage of the penis. Note that the cavernous spaces accumulate into one main vein, the cavernous vein, which is shown as a distinct body (in reality it is a very short segment) before it is joined by the deep dorsal vein, collecting all the circumflex veins. These two veins join the bulbar vein, and together they branch out into the dense retropubic venous plexus. (From Walsh PC, Retik AB, Stamey TA, Vaughan ED (eds): *Campbell's Urology,* 6th ed. Philadelphia, WB Saunders, 1992, p 62. Reproduced with permission.)

Embryology of the Genitourinary Tract

The development of the genital and urinary systems is intimately related. To facilitate understanding of the development, the two systems will be discussed in several subdivisions. The urinary system is divided into the nephric system and the vesicourethral unit. The genital system is divided into the gonads, the genital ducts, and the external genitalia.

Nephric System

The nephric system develops progressively through three distinct phases, the pronephros, mesonephros, and metanephros. The *pronephros* is the earliest state in humans, corresponding to the mature structure in primitive vertebrates. The pronephros consists of six to ten pairs of tubules connected by a pronephric duct. It grows caudally to join the cloaca, a blind end of the hindgut. The pronephros is a temporary structure and, except for its duct, disappears by the fourth week of intrauterine life (Fig. 30–15).

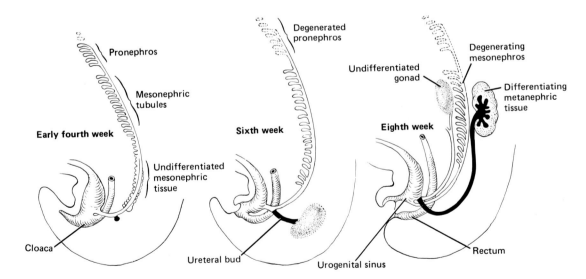

FIGURE 30–15. Schematic representation of the development of the nephric system. Only a few of the tubules of the pronephros are seen early in the fourth week, while the mesonephric tissue differentiates into mesonephric tubules that progressively join the mesonephric duct. The first sign of the ureteral bud from the mesonephric duct is seen. At 6 weeks, the pronephros has completely degenerated and the mesonephric tubules start to do so. The ureteral bud grows dorsocranially and has met the metanephrogenic cap. By the eighth week, there is cranial migration of the differentiating metanephros. The cranial end of the ureteric bud expands and starts to show multiple successive outgrowths. (From Tanagho EA, McAninch JW: *Smith's General Urology,* 13th ed. Norwalk, Conn, Appleton & Lange, 1992, p 18. Reproduced with permission.)

The *mesonephros* corresponds to the mature excretory organ of some amphibians. In humans, it begins developing at about the fourth week of gestation. The tubules of the mesonephros are more numerous and form a cuplike outgrowth into which capillaries push, forming a primitive glomerulus. The tubules communicate with the mesonephric duct, which is derived from the preceding pronephric duct. The mesonephros tubules reach a maximum number by about 8 weeks, then degenerate.

The final stage of development, the *metanephros*, begins in the fourth week when the ureteral bud grows out of the mesonephric duct. The bud elongates in a dorsocranial direction where it meets a mass of mesoderm, the nephrogenic cord, and begins to differentiate into the ureter and renal collecting system. The metanephros derived from the nephrogenic cord eventually differentiates into the mature mammalian kidney.

Vesicourethral Unit

The cloaca is formed from the blind end of the caudal hindgut and is separated from the outside by a thin membrane of tissue, the urogenital membrane. At about 4 weeks of gestation a septum grows downward, separating the cloaca into a posterior compartment that will become the rectum and an anterior compartment that will form the urogenital sinus.

The urogenital sinus receives the mesonephric duct, which is progressively absorbed into this structure. The mesonephric duct distal to the ureteral bud is absorbed into the sinus and its mesenchyme subsequently forms the bladder trigone. The ureter derived from the ureteral bud and the mesonephric duct that differentiated into the vas deferens become absorbed into the sinus as well. In a complex pattern of development, the opening of the ureteral bud, which will eventually become the ureteral orifice, migrates upward and laterally. The opening of the mesonephric duct, which will become the ejaculatory duct, migrates downward and medially (Fig. 30–16).

The urogenital sinus can be divided into two main segments. The ventral and pelvic portion, which receives the ureter, forms the bladder, part of the urethra in the male, and the whole urethra in the female. A phallic or urethral portion will receive the mesonephric ducts, and in the male will form a second part of the urethra. In the female, this portion receives the müllerian ducts, which fuse distally to form the uterus and upper vagina. The lower portion of the female urogenital sinus forms the lower vagina and vaginal vestibule (Fig. 30–17).

Gonads

The undifferentiated and primitive **gonads** are derived from the urogenital ridge, a dorsal region of thickening from which the primitive kidney also forms. The gonads are precursors to the testes in males and the ovaries in females. During the seventh

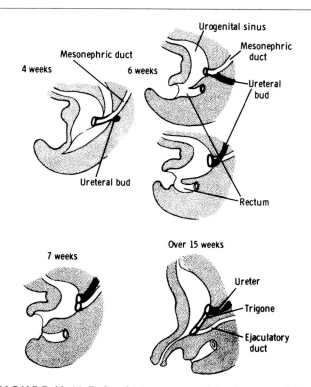

F I G U R E 30–16. Embryologic sequence of development of the urogenital sinus as it separates from the cloaca. Ureteral bud (First appearance at 4 weeks of gestation) is at the bend of the mesonephric duct; the common nephric duct becomes incorporated into the urogenital sinus when the latter separates from the rectum. When this separation is complete, the cloacal membrane will rupture to form two independent openings for the urogenital sinus and the rectum. (From Tanagho EA: Developmental anatomy and urogenital abnormalities, in Raz S (ed): *Female Urology.* Philadelphia, WB Saunders, 1983. Reproduced with permission.)

week, the gonad begins to assume characteristics of either testis or ovary.

If the gonad develops into a testis, the gland increases in size and the cells of the epithelium grow centrally into the organ's mesenchyme. These ingrowths become radically arranged, forming cords, and begin to converge on the posterior aspect of the testis. The cords eventually differentiate into the seminiferous tubules in which the spermatozoa are produced. The testes descend behind the abdominal cavity in the retroperitoneal space and into the scrotum, usually reaching this site by the eighth month.

If instead the gonad differentiates into an ovary, a cortex is formed from the germinal epithelium that ultimately gives rise to ovarian follicles containing ova. It descends only partially through the abdominal cavity and eventually lies adjacent to the fallopian tubes (Fig. 30–18).

Genital Duct System

As the embryo develops, two different but related kinds of ducts form beside the undifferentiated gonads. The mesonephric or **wolffian ducts,** as pre-

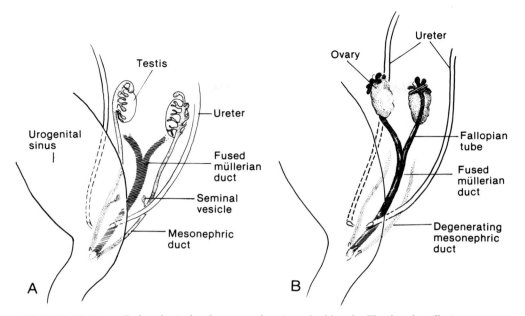

FIGURE 30-17. **A,** Embryologic development of an 8-week-old male. The fused müllerian ducts have already met the urogenital sinus at Müller's tubercle. On either side is the opening of the mesonephric ducts. The ureteral buds have started their ascent on the urogenital sinus; the gonads have started to differentiate and now connect to the mesonephric duct. **B,** Development of the fused müllerian ducts in an 8-week-old female embryo. Their cranial ends attach to the ovary, while the mesonephric ducts are degenerating. Again, the fused müllerian ducts already join the urogenital sinus at the level of Müller's tubercle. (From Walsh PC, Retik AB, Stamey TA, Vaughan ED (eds): *Campbell's Urology,* 6th ed. Philadelphia, WB Saunders, 1992, p 41. Reproduced with permission.)

viously explained, develop as nephric ducts but will go on to form male genital ducts. The **müllerian ducts** develop alongside the mesonephric ducts and are genital structures from the start.

Early in development, each of the two müllerian ducts arise lateral to the mesonephric ducts, either directly from the mesonephric ducts themselves or possibly from the adjacent epithelium of the primitive abdominal cavity. Both ducts grow caudally to enter the urogenital sinus.

If the gonad differentiates into a testis, the wolffian ducts subsequently develop into the male duct system, consisting of the epididymis, vas deferens, seminal vesicles, and ejaculatory ducts. The müllerian ducts, except for a few rudimentary fragments, rapidly degenerate.

If, on the other hand, the gonad develops into an ovary, the müllerian ducts proceed to form the uterus, fallopian tubes, and upper part of the vagina. The mesonephric or wolffian ducts fail to develop further and remain rudimentary.

External Genitalia

Development of the external genitalia begins at about 12 weeks. Prior to this point three small protuberances appear on the external aspect of the cloacal membrane. The genital tubercle is located anteriorly and the genital swellings are located on either side of the membrane. In the seventh week the urogenital mem-

brane ruptures, giving the urogenital sinus a separate opening on the undersurface of the genital tubercle.

In the male, the genital or labioscrotal swellings migrate and fuse centrally to form the scrotum. The fused genital tubercles elongate. The elongated fused tubercles form a cylindrical shape with a ventral groove communicating with the urogenital sinus. This groove subsequently becomes covered by folds of tissue to form the penile urethra.

The female external genitalia closely resemble those of the male until about the eighth intrauterine week. At this time the genital tubercle lags behind in growth and becomes the clitoris. The urogenital sinus shortens and widens somewhat, forming the vaginal vestibule, and the genital swellings form the labia majora. The urethral folds remain infused and form the labia minora.

KEY CONCEPTS

- During early embryonic development, genital structures of males and females are similar. Two important ductal systems are the mesonephric (wolffian) ducts and the müllerian ducts. The mesonephric ducts go on to form the kidneys and the genital duct in males. In the presence of a testis, the wolffian ducts develop into the epididymis, vas deferens, seminal vesicles, and ejaculatory ducts. In the presence of an ovary, the müllerian ducts de-

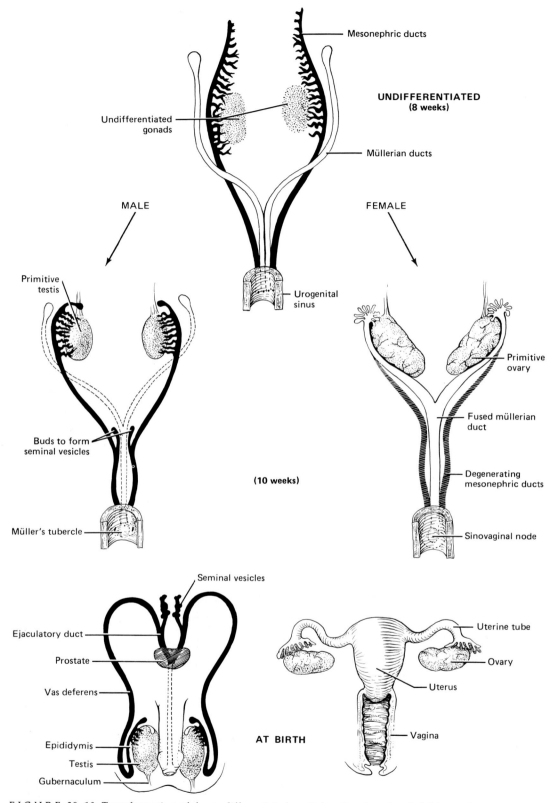

F I G U R E   30–18. Transformation of the undifferentiated genital system into the definitive male and female systems. (From Tanagho EA, McAninch JW: *Smith's General Urology,* 13th ed. Norwalk, Conn, Appleton & Lange, 1992, p 24. Reproduced with permission.)

velop into the uterus, fallopian tubes, and upper vagina, while the wolffian ducts fail to develop.

- **Development of the external genitals begins at about 12 weeks of gestation. In males the labioscrotal tissue fuses and elongates to form the scrotum and penis. In females, this tissue remains separated, forming the labia minora.**

Male Reproductive Function

Hypothalamic-Pituitary-Testicular Axis

To fully understand male reproductive function one must consider the endocrine function of the hypothalamic-pituitary-testicular axis. The components of this system function to maintain a constant level of the circulating hormones responsible for normal male sexual development and behavior as well as for the maturation of sperm necessary for fertility (Fig. 30–19).

The hypothalamus is the integrating center for this hormonal axis. At this organ, neural messages from the central nervous system and humoral (blood-borne) messages from the testis act to control the secretion of a small peptide hormone, gonadotropin-releasing hormone (GnRH). GnRH is transported to the pituitary gland, which lies caudal to the hypothalamus, by the pituitary stalk. A system of veins, the

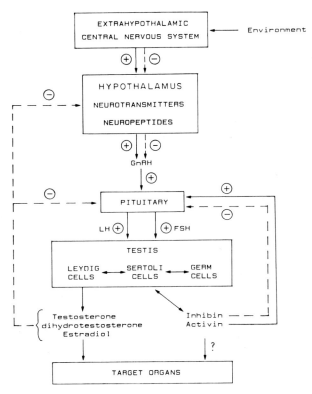

FIGURE 30–19. Diagram of the hypothalamic-pituitary-testicular axis. LH, luteinizing hormone; FSH, follicle-stimulating hormone. (From Walsh PC, Retik AB, Stamey TA, Vaughan ED (eds): *Campbell's Urology*, 6th ed. Philadelphia, WB Saunders, 1992, p 177. Reproduced with permission.)

pituitary portal system, traverses the pituitary stalk. This system of veins is responsible for transporting GnRH to the anterior portion of the pituitary gland.

In response to the secretion of GnRH, the pituitary synthesizes and releases two hormones, luteinizing hormone (LH) and follicle-stimulating hormone (FSH). These two hormones are named after their function in females. However, they are produced by both sexes and in males are secreted into the circulation and carried to the testes.

By binding to receptors on the surface of the testicular Leydig cells, LH is the mediator of testosterone synthesis. The binding of LH produces an increase in the conversion of adenosine triphosphate (ATP) to cyclic 3',5'-adenosine monophosphate (cAMP). This stimulates the production of other intracellular enzymes with the subsequent increased synthesis of testosterone. Testosterone is then released into the bloodstream and adjacent seminiferous tubules.

Besides testosterone, other steroid hormones are synthesized, among them dihydrotestosterone (DHT), 17-hydroxyprogesterone, and estradiol. DHT is responsible for the differentiation and maturation of the male external genitalia. In early puberty the production of androgen begins to increase, with normal adult plasma levels of testosterone and DHT being 300 to 1,200 mg/dL and 30 to 60 ng/dL, respectively.

The function of FSH in male reproduction is not completely understood. It appears, however, that the production of sperm in the seminiferous tubules (**spermatogenesis**) requires the presence of both high levels of androgen and FSH.[1,2]

A feedback inhibition exists to control the secretion of both LH and FSH. The production of LH is regulated by serum levels of testosterone and estradiol. The regulation of FSH is more hypothetical, with the proposed existence of a nonsteroid factor called inhibin produced by the seminiferous epithelium.[3,4] In addition to inhibin, sex steroids also modulate FSH secretion through feedback inhibition on the pituitary.[5,6]

Spermatogenesis

To understand spermatogenesis one must briefly consider the histology of the testis and its seminiferous tubules. As previously stated, the Leydig cells occur in clusters in the interstitial tissue between the seminiferous tubules. It is the Leydig cell that is responsible for the testicular production of testosterone.

The seminiferous tubules contain both germinal elements and supporting cells, which include the sustaining cells of the basement membrane and the Sertoli cells. The Sertoli cells rest on the basement membrane of the tubule and form a unique impermeable junction with each adjacent Sertoli cell. It is through this junction that the young germinal cells or primary spermatocytes migrate, passing from the basal compartment to the basement membrane and then to the central or adluminal compartment of the seminiferous tubule (Fig. 30–20). The junction is also responsible for

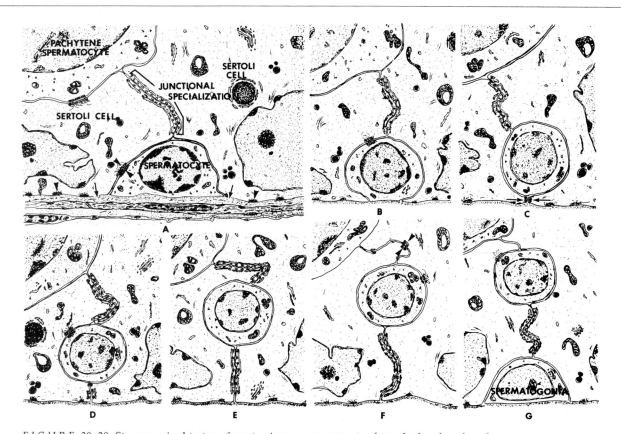

F I G U R E 30–20. Steps required to transfer rat primary spermatocytes from the basal to the ad-luminal compartment of the seminiferous tubule. **A** and **B,** Initially the Sertoli cells are attached to each other above the spermatocytes by tight junctions. **C** to **E,** Next, the Sertoli cells form new junctions below the spermatocytes, isolating the spermatocytes in an intermediate compartment, above and below which are tight junctions. **F** and **G,** The junctions above the spermatocytes then break down, and the spermatocytes enter the adluminal compartment. (From Russell L: Movement of spermatocytes from the basal to the adluminal compartment of the rat testis. *Am J Anat* 148:313, 1977. Copyright © 1977 John Wiley & Sons, Inc. Reprinted by permission of John Wiley & Sons, Inc.)

maintenance of the blood-testes barrier. This barrier ensures that the more mature spermatocytes and spermatids, located in the adluminal compartment, are behind the barrier and theoretically maintained in a constant intratubular environment.[7,8] This is important for the delicate development of the maturing sperm cell.

The process of sperm production is called **spermatogenesis** and involves several phases. The proliferative phase involves division of the young germinal cells near the basement membrane (spermatogonia), either to replace their numbers or to produce daughter cells that will form spermatocytes. Next, a meiotic phase occurs in which spermatocytes undergo a reduction division. This division reduces the number of chromosomes to the monoploid number of 23 from the diploid number of 46. Finally, a spermiogenic phase occurs when haploid spermatids undergo change to form mature spermatozoa (Fig. 30–21).

As sperm cells mature and move from the basement membrane to the adluminal compartment, the Sertoli cells play an important nutritional role in the spermatogenic process. As the spermatid matures, it elongates and develops a tail or *flagellum,* attaining a form similar to that of the mature spermtozoon. Mature spermatozoa are released into the tubular lumen and rapidly flow out to the **rete** testis and into the epididymis. Although each spermatogonium, one of the primitive male germ cells, requires about 70 days to develop into a mature sperm cell or spermatozoon, within each tubule there are spermatozoa in all stages of development. This allows new spermatozoa to be continuously produced.

Anatomy of Spermatozoa

The human spermatozoon is approximately 60 micrometers in length. The oval head contains a nucleus that is highly condensed and stabilized by cross-links between it molecules, making it very resistant to physical injury during its passage and storage in the epididymis. An outer membrane, the acrosome, contains enzymes required for the penetration of the female egg prior to fertilization.

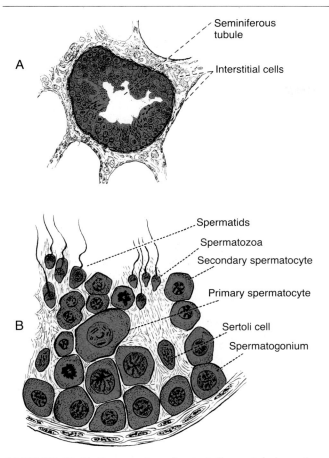

FIGURE 30–21. Cross-section of a seminiferous tubule, and the stages in the development of sperm from spermatogonia. (From Guyton AC: *Textbook of Medical Physiology,* 8th ed. Philadelphia, WB Saunders, 1991, p 886. Reproduced with permission.)

The tail accounts for 90 percent of the length of the spermatozoon and is divided into a middle piece, principal piece, and end piece. The spermatozoon derives its motile ability from the motor apparatus of the tail, called the *axoneme.* The axoneme, which runs the length of the tail, is composed of the central pair of tubules surrounded by a ring of nine pairs of tubules (the 9 + 2 pattern). This ring of tubules is surrounded by a supporting structure of nine noncontractile dense fibers. Within the middle piece, these outer dense fibers are surrounded by a circular sheath of mitochondria (Fig. 30–22).

The mitochondria contain the enzymes required for the production of ATP, the energy source for the cell. Within the axoneme, enzymes and structural proteins are contained. These enzymes are responsible for the conversion of chemical energy from ATP to the mechanical energy of sperm cell movement.[9]

Transport of Spermatozoa

Once mature spermatozoa are released from the Sertoli cells into the seminiferous tubules, they must pass through approximately 6 meters of duct in the male reproductive tract before leaving the urethral meatus

and being deposited in the vagina. From the seminiferous tubules, the spermatozoa are deposited into the *rete testis,* a collective chamber for all the seminiferous tubules. From the rete testis the sperm travels through the efferent ductules, 12 to 20 channels that pass into a single compact duct, the epididymis. The epididymis is a tightly convoluted duct that is divided into three regions: the caput (globus major), the corpus (body), and the cauda epididymis (tail, or globus minor). Unfolded and stretched, the epididymis would measure 12 to 15 feet in length.

After leaving the epididymis the sperm enter the ductus or vas deferens. Embryologically, this duct is derived from the mesonephric duct. It passes through the scrotum, traverses the inguinal canal into the pelvis, and then passes behind the bladder to enter the prostatic urethra at the ejaculatory ducts of the verumontanum. The terminal portion of the vas deferens is known as the *ampulla.* It is joined by the ducts of the seminal vesicle to enter the ejaculatory ducts.

As one passes proximal to distal from the efferent ducts to the vas deferens there is a gradual increase in the thickness of muscle. In the vas deferens, three interconnected smooth muscle layers form a thick muscular wall, making the ratio of wall thickness to lumen the greatest in any human structure.[10]

Aside from serving as a conduit and storage depot for spermatozoa, the epididymis probably sustains maturational processes. Several studies have demonstrated that sperm taken directly from the testes are incapable of fertilizing eggs. It appears that the development of motility and increased fertility are acquired during transit through the epididymis.[11,12]

Because epididymal sperm are probably immotile, other mechanisms must be involved in their transport. Initially, spermatozoa are carried into the efferent ducts by fluid from the rete testis. Within the efferent ducts, motile cilia within the lumen are reponsible for both reabsorption of testicular fluid and movement of spermatozoa into the epididymis. Within the epididymis, the spermatozoa are probably transported by rhythmic contraction of the smooth muscle cells.[13]

Ejaculation accelerates the passage of spermatozoa through the vas deferens and distal epididymis. In young men, approximately 200 million sperm can be found in the reservoir of the epididymis. About 50 percent are found in the cauda region. With ejaculation, sperm from the distal epididymis and vas deferens are deposited into the prostatic urethra, accounting for less than 10 percent of the normal ejaculate.[14]

Erection, Emission, and Ejaculation

In order to penetrate the vagina and deposit sperm, the penis must be erect. The physiology of erection is a complicated interaction of vascular, neurologic, and hormonal factors. Although erection has classically been thought of as a parasympathetic function, it is more complex. Erection may be mediated by either local stimulation, causing a reflexogenic erection through the sacral spinal cord, or psychic stimulation,

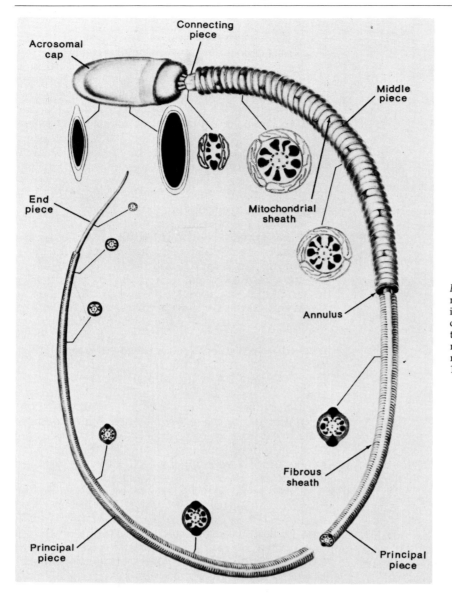

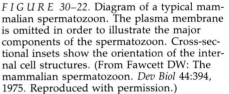

FIGURE 30–22. Diagram of a typical mammalian spermatozoon. The plasma membrane is omitted in order to illustrate the major components of the spermatozoon. Cross-sectional insets show the orientation of the internal cell structures. (From Fawcett DW: The mammalian spermatozoon. *Dev Biol* 44:394, 1975. Reproduced with permission.)

causing a psychogenic erection through cerebral centers. The presence of erections in spinal cord–injured patients attests to the presence of reflexic erections. In these patients an intact sacral spinal cord and its reflex arc of afferent and efferent nerves exist below the site of spinal cord injury.

The penis receives sensory innervation from the pudendal sensory nerves entering the sacral spinal cord. The pudendal nerve is a mixed nerve that provides motor innervation to the pelvic floor musculature and penile sensory fibers. The motor supply to the penis appears to be provided by sacral parasympathetic fibers. Although erection is possible in the spinal cord–injured patient, in the intact human it is a much more controlled process that is influenced to a great extent by the cerebral cortex. Impulses may traverse the spinal cord from the cerebral cortex in the lateral columns and exit the spinal cord through

sacral parasympathetic and possibly thoracolumbar sympathetic nerves as well.[15]

During erection, the vascular spaces that make up the spongy vacuous tissues of the corpus cavernosum and spongiosum fill with blood. The relaxation of smooth muscle tone in the corpus that allows filling and subsequent penile erection is modulated by an undetermined neurotransmitter. Although parasympathetic stimulation results in erection, the direct application of acetylcholine, the neurotransmitter of parasympathetic nerves, the corporal smooth muscle produces inconsistent erectile responses.[16,17] On the other hand, application of certain prostaglandins has been shown to induce smooth muscle relaxation, and in clinical applications intracorporeal injections are able to induce erection.

Ejaculation may be divided into two phases, emission and ejaculation. During emission secretions from the periurethral glands, seminal vesicles, and prostate are deposited with sperm from the vasa deferentia and the cauda epididymis into the prostatic urethra. The control of emission is primarily through sympathetic nerves, which stimulate contraction of smooth muscle in these organs.

With ejaculation, the bladder neck or internal sphincter closes. This closure is also mediated through the sympathetic nervous system. Next, the external sphincter relaxes and the perineal and bulbourethral muscles surrounding the bulb of the corpus spongiosum contract, expelling the ejaculate from the posterior urethra and through the urethral meatus.

The physiologic function of the secretory products of the accessory sex glands is uncertain. These secretions make up most of the seminal plasma, with the sperm and testicular fluid probably composing less than 10 percent of the final ejaculated semen volume. Although some investigators have demonstrated that sperm removed directly from the epididymis are capable of fertilization, these secretions most likely optimize conditions for sperm motility, survival, and transport in both the female and male reproductive tract.

Capacitation

Capacitation of the spermatozoa refers to the multiple changes that activate the sperm for the final processes of fertilization. Although sperm are anatomically complete and highly motile when ejaculated, the complex process of capacitation is necessary before the sperm are actually capable of fertilizing the egg. The capacitation process normally requires from 1 to 10 hours and occurs in sperm only after they have been introduced into the vagina of the female. Once the sperm are inside the female, the uterine and fallopian tube fluids wash away the various inhibitory factors that had suppressed sperm activity in the male genital ducts. During the time the spermatozoa were in the fluid of the male genital ducts, they were continually exposed to many floating vesicles from the seminiferous tubules containing large amounts of cholesterol. This cholesterol was continually donated to the cellular membrane covering the sperm acrosome, toughening this membrane and preventing release of its enzymes. After ejaculation, the sperm that are deposited in the vagina swim away from the cholesterol vesicles upward into the uterine fluid, and they gradually lose much of their excess cholesterol through the next few hours. As the cholesterol is lost, the membrane at the head of the sperm becomes much weaker.

The membrane of the sperm head also becomes much more permeable to calcium ions. The calcium that now enters the sperm in abundance is able to change the activity of the flagellum, giving it a powerful whiplash motion, in contrast to its previously weak undulating motion. In addition, the calcium ions probably also cause changes in the intracellular membrane covering the leading edge of the acrosome, making it possible for the acrosome to release its enzymes very rapidly and easily as the sperm penetrates the granulosa cell mass surrounding the ovum, and even more rapidly and easily as the sperm attempts to penetrate the zona pellucida of the ovum itself.[18]

The many changes of the capacitation process make it possible for the sperm to make its way into the interior of the ovum to cause fertilization.

Acrosome Reaction

The head of a sperm is essentially a highly compact package of genetic chromatin material covered by a specialized acrosome and acrosomal (head) cap. Stored in the acrosome of the sperm are large quantities of hydrolytic (water-splitting) enzymes that are released during capacitation. The specialized acrosomal enzymes first break down cervical mucus, allowing sperm to pass into the uterus and uterine tubes. If an ovum is present in the female reproductive tract when semen is introduced, continued release of acrosomal enzymes digests proteins in the structural elements of the outer covering of the egg. A high sperm count is essential for male fertility because the female ovum, once it is expelled from the ovarian follicle into the abdominal cavity and fallopian tube, carries with it multiple layers of granulosa cells. Before a sperm can fertilize the ovum, it must first pass through the granulosa cell layer, and then it must penetrate the thick covering of the ovum itself, the *zona pellucida*. It is believed that the acrosomal enzyme hyaluronidase plays an important role in opening pathways between the granulosa cells so that the sperm can reach the ovum.[19]

On reaching the zona pellucida of the ovum, the anterior membrane of the sperm binds specifically with a receptor protein in the zona pellucida. Then, rapidly, the entire anterior membrane of the acrosome dissolves, and all the acrosomal enzymes are immediately released. Within minutes, these open a penetrating pathway for passage of the sperm head through the zona pellucida.

The head at first enters the perivitelline space lying beneath the zona pellucida but outside the membrane of the underlying oocyte. Within 30 minutes, the membranes of the sperm head and the oocyte fuse; the sperm genetic material enters the oocyte to cause fertilization, and the embryo begins to develop.

KEY CONCEPTS

- **Normal male sexual development and spermatogenesis depend on the appropriate secretion of reproductive hormones. Gonadotropin-releasing hormone, secreted by the hypothalamus, induces the anterior pituitary gland to secrete luteinizing hormone (LH) and follicle-stimulating hormone (FSH). These hormones are secreted into the bloodstream and carried to the testes, where they bind to testicular cells.**

- **Leydig cells in the testes possess LH receptors and respond by increasing production of testosterone. Testosterone and related androgens are necessary**

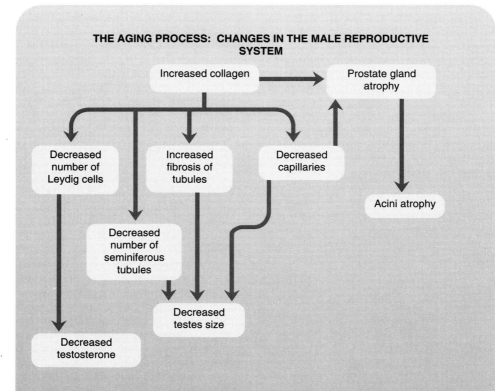

THE AGING PROCESS: CHANGES IN THE MALE REPRODUCTIVE SYSTEM

There is usually a decline in male fertility and reproductive organ function with aging. However, the functional decline of the male reproductive organs is variable. For example, there are some elderly men who maintain their fertility into their seventies and eighties.

Male reproductive organ variability is due to organ specific tissue changes. Active male germ cells continue to produce sperm (spermatogenesis), although the number of sperm produced declines proportionally over time. The testes become smaller as a result of increased connective tissue, fibrosis of the tubules, and decreased numbers of capillaries. The number of active seminiferous tubules declines with aging. The number of Leydig cells that produce testosterone decreases, leading to a decrease in testosterone with aging.

After age 50, the prostate gland undergoes atrophic changes with an increase in connective tissue, collagen, and smooth muscle fibers and a decreasing vascular supply. The acini may atrophy or become hyperplastic. Secretions within the gland may become calcified.

The arteries and veins in the penis become increasingly sclerotic. The penis itself becomes smaller, with an increase in fibroelastic tissue. There is decreased penile sensation. Sexually, the aging male has a longer refractory period after orgasm and decreased force of ejaculation.

Faith Young Peterson

for maturation of the male external genitalia. The function of FSH is less well understood, but it may be necessary for spermatogenesis.

- Spermatogenesis occurs when germinal cells within the seminiferous tubules undergo meiosis to form haploid (23 chromosomes) spermatids. Spermatids then develop into mature spermatozoa with the assistance of the Sertoli cells. Sperm require 70 days to mature, and they are continuously produced and released into the epididymis.

- Sperm are well formed to perform their function, having a highly stabilized nucleus that is resistant to physical trauma, a mobile tail (axoneme) for swimming, and specialized enzymes to enhance penetration of the female egg.

- Sperm traveling from their site of origin in the testes must traverse approximately 6 meters of tubules before arriving at the penile meatus. This tubular system includes seminiferous tubules in the testes, epididymis, vas deferens, and urethra. About 200 million sperm may be stored in the epididymal reservoir. Increased motility and fertility appear to be acquired by sperm as they pass through the epididymis. Sperm account for less than 10 percent of the ejaculate volume.

- The physiology of erection is a complex interplay of vascular, neurologic, and hormonal factors. The sacral parasympathetic nerves provide important innervation to the penis. Acetylcholine from parasympathetic nerves causes relaxation of the penile smooth muscle, resulting in engorgement. Prostaglandins are also able to induce erection when injected.

- Ejaculation is mediated by the sympathetic nervous system. Sympathetic actions include contraction of the internal sphincter to prevent retrograde ejaculation and relaxation of the external sphincter to allow emission.

- Once sperm are deposited in the female vagina, they undergo further changes (capacitation), which improves the chances of fertilization. Enzymes are released (acrosome reaction) that allow easier penetration of the ovum.

Summary

The genitourinary tract may be divided into upper and lower tracts, with the upper tract composed of the kidneys and ureters and the lower tract composed of the bladder and urethra. Auxiliary genital glands that lie adjacent to or surround the urethra include the prostate, seminal vesicles, and bulbourethral glands. The external genitalia of the male consist of the scrotum, testes, epididymides, and penis.

The embryologic development of the genital and urinary systems is closely related. The nephric system develops progressively through three distinct phases: the pronephros, mesonephros, and metanephros. The gonads are derived from the urogenital ridge, from which the primitive kidney also forms. Finally, the genital duct systems develop from two different but related ducts adjacent to the undifferentiated gonads, the müllerian ducts and the mesonephric or wolffian ducts.

Male reproductive function depends on an intact hypothalamic-pituitary-testicular endocrine axis. Spermatogenesis takes place within the seminiferous tubules. Spermatozoa mature in their transit through the male reproductive tract. Through erection, emission, and ejaculation, sperm are deposited in the female vagina. Through capacitation and the acrosome reaction, spermatozoa acquire the ability to fertilize ova residing within the female reproductive tract.

REFERENCES

1. Ewing LL, Davis JC, Zirkin BR: Regulation of testicular function: A spatial and temporal view. *Int Rev Physiol* 1980;22:41–115.
2. Dizerga GS, Sherins RJ: Endocrine control of adult testicular function, in Burger H, deKretzer D (eds): *The Testis*. New York, Raven Press, 1981, p 127.
3. van Thiel DH, Sherins RJ, Meyers GH, DeVita VT: Evidence for a specific seminiferous tubular factor affecting FSH secretion in man. *J Clin Invest* 1972;51(4):1009–1019.
4. Baker HW, Bremner WJ, Burger HG, et al: Testicular control of follicle-stimulating hormone secretion. *Recent Prog Horm Res* 1976;32:429–476.
5. Sherins RJ, Loriaux DL: Studies on the role of sex steroids in the feedback control of FSH concentration in men. *J Clin Endocrinol Metab* 1973;36(5):886–893.
6. Santen RJ: Is aromatization of testosterone to estradiol required for inhibition of luteinizing hormone secretion in men? *J Clin Invest* 1975;56(5):1555–1563.
7. Dym M, Fawcett DW: The blood-testis barrier in the rat and the physiological compartmentation of the seminiferous epithelium. *Biol Reprod* 1970;3(3):308–326.
8. Gilula ND, Fawcett DW, Alki A: The Sertoli cell occluding junctions and gap junctions in mature and developing mammalian testis. *Dev Biol* 1976;50:152–168.
9. Fawcett DW: The mammalian spermatozoon. *Dev Biol* 1975;44(2):394–436.
10. Baumgarten HG, Holstein AF, Rosengran E: Arrangement, ultrastructure and adrenergic innervation of the smooth musculature of the ductuli efferentes, ductus epididymis and ductus deferens of man. *Z Zellforsch Mikrosk Anat* 1971;120(1):37–39.
11. Orgebin-Crist MC, Danzo BJ, Davies J: Endocrine control of the development and maintenance of sperm fertilizing ability in the epididymis, in Hamilton KW, Greep RO (eds): *Handbook of Physiology*. Baltimore, Williams & Wilkins, 1975, section 7: *Endocrinology*, vol 5, *Male Reproductive System*, p 319.
12. Bedford JJ: Maturation, transport, and fate of spermatozoa in the epididymis, in Hamilton KW, Greep RO (eds): *Handbook of Physiology*. Baltimore, Williams & Wilkins, 1975, section 7: *Endocrinology*, vol 5, *Male Reproductive System*.
13. Johnson AL, Howards SS: Intratubular hydrostatic pressure in the testis and epididymis before and after long-term vasectomy in the guinea pig. *Biol Reprod* 1976;14(4):371–376.
14. Pabst RZ: Investigations of the construction and function of the human ductus deferens. *Z Anat Entwicklungsgesch* 1969;129(20):154–176.
15. Bors E, Comarr AE: Neurologic disturbance of sexual function with special reference to 529 patients with spinal cord injury. *Urol Surv* 1960;10:191–222.
16. Dorr LD, Brody MJ: Hemodynamic mechanism of erection in the canine penis. *Am J Physiol* 1967;213(6):1526–1531.
17. Penttila O: Acetylcholine, biogenic amines and enzymes involved in their metabolism in penile erectile tissue. *Ann Med Exp Biol Fenn* 1966;44(suppl 9):1–42.

18. Jeyendran RS, Van der Ven HH, Perez-Pelaez M, Crabo BG, Saneveld LJV: Development of an assay to assess the functional integrity of the human sperm membrane and its relationship to other semen characteristics. *J Reprod Fertil* 1984;70(1):219–228.

19. Lee MA, Trucco GS, Bechtol KB, et al: Capacitation and acrosome reactions in human spermatozoa monitored by chlortetracycline fluorescence assay. *Fertil Steril* 1987;48(4):649–658.

BIBLIOGRAPHY

Aumuller G, Seitz J: Protein secretion and secretory processes in male accessory sex glands. *Int Rev Cytol* 1990;121:127–231.

Benson CB, Doubilet PM, Richie JP: Sonography of the male genital tract. *Am J Roentgenol* 1989;153(4):705–713.

Ceccarelli FE: *Embryology of the Genitalia.* AUA Update Series, vol 1. Baltimore, American Urology Association, 1982.

Comhaire FH: Methods to evaluate reproductive health of the human male. *Reprod Toxicol* 1993;7(suppl 1):39–46.

Gibbs T: Genitourinary embryology and congenital malformation: Part 1. The kidneys and ureters. *Urol Nurs* 1990;10(3):16–24.

Gillenwater JY, Grayhack JT, Howards SS, Duckett JW: *Adult and Pediatric Urology.* St. Louis, Mosby–Year Book, 1991.

Heindel JJ, Treinen KA: Physiology of the male reproductive system: Endocrine, paracrine and autocrine regulation. *Toxicol Pathol* 1989;17(2):411–445.

Kapur DK, Ahuja GK: Immunocytochemistry of male reproductive organs. *Arch Androl* 1989;23(3):169–183.

Kelalis PP, King LR, Belman AB: *Clinical Pediatric Urology,* 3rd ed. Philadelphia, WB Saunders, 1992.

Macfarlane FJ: Genitourinary embryology and congenital malformations: Part 2. The lower urinary tract, gonads, and genital duct system. *Urol Nurs* 1991;11(1):8–14.

Tanagho EA: *Embryologic Development of the Urinary Tract.* AUA Update Series, vol 1. Baltimore, American Urology Association, 1982.

Tanagho EA, McAninch JW: *Smith's General Urology,* 13th ed. Norwalk, Conn, Appleton & Lange, 1992.

Wagner G: Aspects of genital physiology and pathology. *Semin Neurol* 1992;12(2):87–97.

Walsh PC, Retik AB, Stamey TA, Vaughan ED Jr: *Campbell's Urology,* 6th ed. Philadelphia, WB Saunders, 1992.

Wilson JD: Sexual differentiation of the gonads and of the reproductive tract. *Biol Neonate* 1989;55(6)322–330.

CHAPTER 31

Alterations in Structure and Function of the Male Genitourinary System

DAVID MIKKELSEN

KEY TERMS

benign prostatic hyperplasia: Noncancerous enlargement of the prostate gland.

cryptorchidism: Undescended testes.

fistula: An abnormal tubelike passage from a normal cavity or tube to a free surface or to another cavity.

hydrocele: Accumulation of fluid in the tunica vaginalis testis; one of the most common causes of scrotal swelling.

impotence: Failure to achieve and maintain an erection of the penis.

neoplasm: A new and abnormal formation of tissue growth. If malignant, the growth infiltrates tissue, metastasizes, and often recurs even after attempts at surgical removal.

phimosis: A condition in which the foreskin fits so tightly over the glans that it cannot retract.

stricture: A narrowing or constriction of the lumen of a tube, duct, or hollow organ such as the ureter or urethra.

torsion: Act of twisting or condition of being twisted. Applies to the state of the testes when abnormally rotated.

The male genitourinary system is susceptible to numerous congenital, acquired, and infectious conditions and, to a lesser extent, neoplasms. These disorders may interrupt the normal functions of urinary excretion and sexual function and fertility and directly affect the quality of life. This chapter will identify and explain the conditions most commonly seen in private practice.

Disorders of the Penis and Male Urethra

Congenital Anomalies

Micropenis

Micropenis is defined as a small, normally formed penis with a stretched length more than two standard deviations below the mean.[1] The normal range in newborns is 3.5 ± 0.7 cm, so micropenis may be defined as a stretched length less than 2.5 cm.[2]

Penile development and growth are both testosterone dependent. Because of this, micropenis may result from defects in testosterone production or a deficiency that results in poor growth of organs which are targets of this hormone. Patients with micropenis must therefore be evaluated for endocrine abnormalities. These may involve the hypothalamic-pituitary axis (Pader-Willi and Kallman's syndromes) or testicular disorders (Klinefelter's syndrome).[3]

Treatment depends on providing testosterone to stimulate penile growth, administered either intramuscularly (IM) or topically. This treatment requires caution, as growth may be altered by premature closure of the epiphyseal growth plates in the long bones. In rare cases, when micropenis fails to respond to testosterone, a female sex assignment is indicated.[3]

Urethral Valves

The vast majority of **urethral valves** are posterior in location, occurring in the distal prostatic urethra. They are the most common cause of urinary obstruction in male newborns and infants. These are mucosal folds that resemble thin membranes and cause obstruction when the child attempts to void.

Many theories have attempted to explain how valves develop. It has been suggested that several different processes may occur to form different posterior valves. Most commonly, posterior valves may result from an abnormal insertion and persistence of the distal wolffian ducts. Less frequently, a persistent urogenital membrane may result in valves and obstruction.[4]

Children with posterior valves may present with varying degrees of obstruction. In the most severe cases there may be intrauterine renal failure causing oligohydramnios (decreased amniotic fluid), pulmonary hypoplasia (incomplete lung development), and either stillbirth or extreme distress at the time of delivery. More frequently, inability to void is noted shortly after birth (normal voiding occurs within 48 hours after birth), or the infant has abdominal masses representing a thickened palpable bladder or hydronephrotic kidneys. Varying degrees of azotemia and renal failure occur with this scenario. Finally, urinary ascites (extravasated urine in the peritoneum) may occur, resulting from a urinary leak that is usually difficult to localize. In an infant with abdominal distention, the diagnosis of urethral valves is confirmed by a plain abdominal radiograph showing the bowel "floating" in the central abdomen.

Older infants with a urethral valve are less likely to present with a palpable kidney or ascites. Rather, there may be urinary infection, poor stream with straining to void, or occasionally hematuria. Urethral valves in these older male infants may not produce much obstruction, making the diagnosis more difficult.[5]

The management of posterior valves involves initial management of metabolic abnormalities with appropriate fluid management and electrolyte replacement. In patients with a urinary tract infection, drainage of urine with a urethral or occasionally a suprapubic catheter is necessary. Finally, ablation of the valves with an endoscopic resectoscope should be performed. In the infant, this step may be delayed until a cutaneous vesicostomy has been made to temporarily divert and drain the urine. This approach reduces the risk of traumatizing the infant's delicate urethra, which may create urethral stricture disease.

Rarely, urethral valves are located anteriorly in the penile urethra. Valves in this location are a very rare congenital anomaly and most likely represent urethral dilation or a diverticulum proximal to the valve.[6] Endoscopic resection will correct the problem.

Urethrorectal and Vesicourethral Fistulas

Urethrorectal and vesicourethral **fistulas** are rare and almost always associated with an imperforate anus. The fistula results from failure of the urorectal septum to develop completely, leading to a persistent communication between the rectum posteriorly and the urogenital tract anteriorly.

The child with a urethrorectal or vesicourethral fistula may pass fecal material and gas through the urethra. If the anus has formed normally with an external opening, urine may drain through the rectum. The diagnosis is made with cystoscopy and contrast-enhanced radiography to delineate a blind rectal pouch or communication. Surgery is needed to resect the fistula and open the imperforate anus.

Hypospadias

In **hypospadias** the urethral meatus is located on the ventral undersurface of the penis or on the perineum (Fig. 31–1). The condition may occur in varying degrees of severity. In the least severe cases, the meatus is located distally on the penis, either at the corona

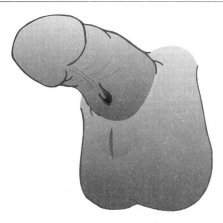

FIGURE 31–1. Hypospadias with chordee.

or on the undersurface of the glans. With increasing severity of the condition the meatus assumes a more proximal location and is more often associated with chordee, a curvature of the penile shaft.

Hypospadias is the result of incomplete fusion of the urethral folds, so that the meatus may be found anywhere along the phallus from the perineum to the glans. The majority of cases of hypospadias occur distally, with about 85 percent of all cases involving the glans or corona.[7] Because incomplete fusion of urethral folds may indicate insufficient masculinization, it is recommended that the more severe penoscrotal and perineal openings be evaluated for conditions of intersex.[8]

The treatment of hypospadias involves surgical repair. There are many procedures available, with several repairs indicated for each type of hypospadias. The goal of surgery is a good overall cosmetic appearance that will allow the patient to stand and direct his urinary stream and will also allow normal sexual function.

Epispadias

In **epispadias** the urethra opens on the dorsal aspect of the penis at a point proximal to the glans. Although much less common than hypospadias, it can be considerably more disabling.

The embryogenesis of epispadias is related to another congenital condition, extrophy of the bladder. In this condition, the abdominal wall fails to form below the level of the umbilicus. At birth, the back wall of the bladder is exposed to the external environment.[9] The development of epispadias is simply a mild degree of extrophy, with a deficiency of abdominal wall formation present inferiorly. Most commonly the defect extends proximally to involve the urinary sphincter, resulting in urinary incontinence. Less commonly the urethral meatus is located more distally along the dorsum of the penis and is accompanied by urinary continence because the sphincter is not affected.

Treatment of proximal epispadias with incontinence is difficult and involves staged surgical procedures to reconstruct a continent bladder neck and a functional urethra. The less common distal epispadias is usually managed with tubular reconstruction procedures similar to those used for the repair of hypospadias.

Acquired Diseases

Priapism

Priapism may be defined as a painful, persistent erection. The patient usually reports several hours of painful erection in which the corpora cavernosa are tense with congested blood. The corpus spongiosum and glans are characteristically soft and uninvolved.

The causes of priapism are multiple. Most cases are idiopathic, with the next most frequent etiology being sickle cell disease. Other causes include anticoagulant therapy, diabetes mellitus, leukemia, and the use of certain antidepressant medications.[10] Recently, intracavernosal injection of vasoactive substances for the treatment of impotence has been noted to cause priapism. Although multiple causes exist, the common abnormality is probably an obstruction of the venous drainage resulting in the buildup of viscous, poorly oxygenated blood in the corpora.[11] If the process is allowed to continue, fibrosis of the corpora cavernosa will eventually occur and may result in impotence.

The treatment of priapism may involve a combination of measures, depending on the cause and duration of the condition. Initial therapy for priapism secondary to sickle cell disease includes sedation and oxygen.[12] For the treatment of priapism secondary to other causes, initial measures may include aspiration of blood from the corpora as well as injection of α-adrenergic agents.[13] If the priapism remains refractory to these initial measures, a surgical shunting procedure may be necessary in which a shunt is created between the erect corpora cavernosa and the detumesced corpus spongiosum.

Phimosis and Paraphimosis

Phimosis occurs when the uncircumcised foreskin cannot be retracted over the glans of the penis (Fig. 31–2). This usually is the result of chronic inflammation and infection from poor hygiene. Calculi and squamous cell carcinoma may occur, though it is usually the presence of erythema, tenderness of the phimotic foreskin, or a discharge that prompts the patient to seek medical attention.[10] Management involves treating the infection with antibiotics, followed by circumcision.

Paraphimosis, on the other hand, occurs when the foreskin that has been retracted over the glans cannot be replaced in its normal position (see Fig. 31–2). This condition usually occurs secondary to a chronic inflammation under the foreskin. This creates a constricting ring of skin around the base of the retracted glans. The constriction causes venous conges-

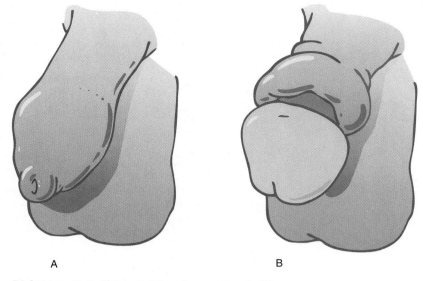

A   B

F I G U R E 31–2. Phimosis (**A**) and paraphimosis (**B**).

tion of the glans, with further swelling and edema making the condition worse. Treatment entails reducing the paraphimotic foreskin back over the glans. This can usually be accomplished by compressing the glans to reduce the edema. Occasionally a slit or formal circumcision is needed to manage the problem.

Peyronie's Disease

Peyronie's disease refers to the formation of palpable, fibrous plaques on the surface of the corpora cavernosa. These plaques subsequently cause curvature of the penis with painful, incomplete erections. There is no satisfactory treatment for this disease, though some cases may remit with time. Conservative therapies that have had limited success include the use of vitamin E or Potaba. In addition, several operative procedures have been developed. These procedures involve excising the plaque and repairing the corporal defect with a dermal graft.[14,15]

Urethral Strictures

Urethral strictures are fibrotic narrowings of the urethra and are usually composed of scar tissue. Most acquired strictures are due to a prior infection such as gonorrhea or trauma. Traumatic causes include both iatrogenic causes, such as large urethral catheters and instrumentation, as well as noniatrogenic causes, such as straddle injuries.

A decreased urinary stream is the most common complaint. Other common complaints include urethral discharges, bladder infection, and urine retention. The treatment of urethral strictures involves procedures to dilate, incise, or reconstruct the urethra, depending on the extent and duration of the stricture.

Impotence

The physiology of penile erection is a complex interaction of the vascular, hormonal, and neurologic systems. **Impotence,** or the inability to attain an erection, may be primary or secondary. Primary impotence refers to the inability to attain an erection throughout life and is often related to deep-seated psychiatric problems of some duration. Occasionally, vascular trauma sustained during early childhood or adolescence may account for primary impotence.[16]

Far more common than primary impotence is secondary impotence. The individual with secondary impotence is no longer able to achieve normal erections but did have normal erections in the past. The causes of secondary impotence are multiple and may be discovered by examining the patient's medical history. Common causes of secondary impotence are peripheral vascular disease, the use of certain medications, endocrine problems, trauma, iatrogenic causes, and psychological causes.

Arterial insufficiency of the penis may occur from obstruction of the arterial supply. Several processes may account for this obstructive arteriosclerosis. Stenosis of the arteries secondary to atheromatous plaques may be the most common etiology. Diabetes mellitus may not only result in occlusion of arterial vessels but may also cause a neuropathy of the pudendal nerve that might result in impotence.[17] Finally, some investigators have suggested that erectile dysfunction may result from excessive venous drainage from the penis.

The list of medications that may cause erectile dysfunction is long. Several antihypertensive agents, including propranolol, monoamine oxidase inhibitors, and thiazides, have been associated with varying degrees of impotence. Other medications linked to erectile dysfunction include the phenothiazines, antihistamines, and some antidepressants.[18]

Endocrinopathy accounts for a small percentage of impotence cases.[19] Pituitary dysfunction resulting in decreased or no secretion of luteinizing hormone (LH) may result in decreased secretion of testosterone. Primary failure of the testes may also occur, resulting in the decreased secretion of testosterone. Finally, an excessive secretion by the pituitary of the hormone prolactin may result in low testosterone levels.

Trauma to the penis resulting in penile fractures and damage to penile erectile tissue may occasionally lead to partial or complete impotence. More common injuries include pelvic fractures with subsequent damage to the penile vascular and nervous supply. Iatrogenic trauma secondary to several commonly performed operations, including aortoiliac vascular surgery, and radical pelvic cancer operations may also result in impotence.

Finally, it must be remembered that successful sexual function depends not only on intact vascular, hormonal, and neurologic systems but also on intact psychological and social responses. Several psychological factors may manifest as problems of low desire, erectile failure, or premature ejaculation. A discussion of the psychological contribution to impotence is beyond the scope of this chapter.

The treatment of erectile dysfunction requires an initial evaluation to differentiate organic causes from psychogenic causes. Further evaluation to distinguish among the various organic causes may then be needed. Once a psychogenic etiology has been ruled out, several therapeutic options exist. The surgical options include insertion of an inflatable or semirigid prosthetic device into the corpora cavernosa. In the past few years, several investigators have discovered that intracavernous injections of various vasoactive substances are able to cause an erection. Several of these substances, including papavarine, phentolamine, and prostaglandin E_1, are commonly used and afford a nonsurgical treatment option. Another nonsurgical alternative entails the use of a vacuum device to sustain an erection. Finally, in very specific cases of erectile dysfunction, surgical procedures may be done to revascularize the arterial supply of the penis or to ligate the penile venous drainage.

Infections Involving the Penis and Urethra

Gonococcal Urethritis

Gonococcal urethritis is associated with a gram-negative diplococcus, *Neisseria gonorrhoeae.* Most cases are acquired during sexual intercourse, with the incubation period lasting from 3 to 10 days. Gonorrhea classically produces a urethral discharge and a burning sensation during urination. The initial urethritis may resolve without treatment, but long-term complications may include urethral stricture, abscess, and fistula formation.

Management of this disease depends on the diagnosis, which is determined by culturing[9] urethral swab on special agar (chocolate blood agar). Recommended treatments include an IM injection of penicillin (4.8 million units), given along with 1 gram of probenicid orally. A poor response to penicillin suggests the possibility of a resistant form. These organisms may require other antibiotics (spectinomycin and cefotaxime).[20]

Nongonococcal Urethritis

Nongonococcal urethritis has several specific causes. The most responsible organism is probably *Chlamydia trachomatis. Chlamydia* is an intracellular organism that usually causes a urethral discharge and dysurea. A second organism, *Ureaplasma urealyticum,* has been implicated as a causative agent of nongonococcal urethritis. The treatment of nongonococcal urethritis involves oral antibiotics, either tetracycline or erythromycin, 500 mg four times daily for 7 days.[21]

Syphilis

Syphilis is caused by the organism *Treponema pallidum,* a spirochete that gains entrance to the body through the skin or mucous membranes. The initial site of involvement in males is usually the penis, where a characteristic painless, shallow ulcer (chancre) is formed. This primary chancre often becomes associated with enlarged inguinal lymph nodes.

The diagnosis of syphilis may be made by microscopic dark-field examination of serous drainage from the ulcer. In the absence of a dark-field microscope, the diagnosis may be made by either of two serologic tests, the rapid plasma reagin (RPR) test or the Venereal Disease Research Laboratories (VDRL) test. Treatment of early or primary syphilis involves an IM injection of benzathine penicillin G, 2.4 million units. For patients allergic to penicillin, tetracycline or erythromycin, 500 mg four times a day for 15 days, is the treatment of choice.[22]

Genital Herpes

Herpes simplex virus (HSV) is a double-stranded DNA virus that may cause persistent or latent infections. Two subtypes are recognized. The majority of patients with genital herpes have type II virus, whereas type I infections usually involve the oral cavity. Vesicles grouped together on an erythematous base are the typical lesion seen in genital herpes. To confirm the diagnosis, smears of the lesions to demonstrate intranuclear inclusions may be performed. In addition, viral cultures or tests to measure serum antibody to HSV may also be obtained. Acyclovir is one of the few drugs that have demonstrated efficacy in treating this disease. Given orally or IV, acyclovir acts to stop the formation of viral DNA chains by inhibiting viral DNA polymerase.

Genital Warts

Genital warts, or condylomata acuminata (singular: condyloma acuminatum), are caused by papillomavirus forms. The disease may be transmitted when viral particles from lesions come in contact with another person during sexual intercourse. A relationship between genital warts and cervical carcinoma in women have received considerable attention.[23] It is possible that this disease could cause significant, widespread problems.

Male patients may have warts anywhere on the external genitalia but commonly on the penile shaft or glans. Warts may also be found in the urethra as well as around or within the anus. Treatment involves the topical application of podophylline. The warts may also be removed with electrocautery or a carbon dioxide laser.

Neoplasms of the Penis

Although cancer of the penis is rare in the United States, accounting for fewer than 0.2 percent of cancer deaths, its prevalence fluctuates widely among various locations. Although the causes are poorly understood, phimosis of the foreskin accompanied by chronic inflammation has been thought to be the primary etiologic factor. The incidence of penile cancer among circumcised men is extremely low.[24]

The majority of penile cancer cases are squamous cell carcinoma (97 percent). They usually occur on the glans or the inner surface of the foreskin. Metastasis occurs by lymphatic dissemination, with initial involvement of the palpable inguinal lymph nodes. Death from penile carcinoma results from uncontrolled lymphatic spread and subsequent necrosis of the overlying skin, debilitation, and sepsis.

Penile carcinoma is staged as follows[25]:

Stage I: The lesion is limited to the glans or foreskin.
Stage II: The tumor involves the shaft of the penis.
Stage III: The inguinal nodes are involved but the lesion is operable.
Stage IV: Disseminated disease.

The lesion of penile cancer is usually ulcerative and fungating in appearance and may be associated with pain, bleeding, and urethral discharge. Inguinal adenopathy is present in more than 50 percent of patients at the time of diagnosis, although frequently the adenopathy represents an inflammatory response secondary to the lesion rather than metastasis.

Therapy for penile carcinoma depends on the stage of the lesion. Topical chemotherapy and radiation therapy may be considered for certain small superficial lesions. Larger distal penile lesions usually require partial penectomy, whereas proximal lesions may require total penectomy with creation of a perineal urethrostomy. Finally, removal of involved inguinal lymph nodes with an inguinal lymphadenectomy may be performed in cases of suspected Stage III disease.

The prognosis of penile carcinoma depends on the stage of disease. The 5-year survival rate for men with tumors localized to the penis is 65 to 90 percent. With inguinal node involvement, 5-year survival rates drop to about 30 to 50 percent, and if there are distant metastases, the 5-year survival rate is virtually zero.[24]

KEY CONCEPTS

- Congenital disorders of the penis may result from hormonal deficiencies or abnormalities of embryonic development. Micropenis, for example, is usually a result of testosterone deficiency. Urethral valves, fistulas, and malpositioning of the urinary meatus (hypospadias, epispadias) are related to abnormal development.

- Priapism is a persistent, painful erection, most commonly of unknown etiology. Priapism may occur in conditions that cause obstruction of venous drainage, including sickle cell anemia, anticoagulant therapy, diabetes mellitus, and certain antidepressant medications.

- Phimosis and paraphimosis are disorders of the foreskin. Phimosis is associated with chronic inflammation and poor hygiene, resulting in a foreskin that cannot be retracted. Paraphimosis refers to a foreskin that remains retracted and cannot be returned to its normal position.

- Uretheral strictures may be congenital or acquired. Most acquired strictures are secondary to gonorrheal infections or urethral trauma. Poor stream, bladder infections, and retained urine are common manifestations.

- Impotence is the inability to achieve a sustained erection. Causes of impotence are categorized as primary and secondary. Primary impotence is rare and usually related to adolescent vascular trauma or psychiatric problems. Secondary impotence may be due to a variety of factors, including vascular diseases, medications, endocrine disorders, trauma, and psychological distress.

- A number of infections are sexually transmitted and affect the penis and urethra. These include gonococcal urethritis, nongonococcal urethritis, syphilis, herpes, and genital warts. Gonococcal and nongonococcal urethritis and syphilis are effectively treated with antibiotics. Herpes and genital warts are associated with viruses and tend to be chronic, with intermittent recurrences.

- Penile neoplasms are rare, particularly in circumcised males. Phimosis and chronic inflammation may be important etiologic factors. Like other neoplasms, penile cancer has a better prognosis if treated prior to dissemination.

Disorders of the Scrotum and Testes

Congenital Disorders

Cryptorchidism

Cryptorchidism means "hidden testis" and refers to any testis that occupies an extrascrotal position. The cryptorchid testis may be incompletely descended and as such be located intra-abdominally, within the inguinal canal, or just external to the canal but above the scrotum. Occasionally the testis may emerge from the external ring of the inguinal canal and be misdirected into an abnormal extrascrotal position. In this situation the testis may be called ectopic. An ectopic testis may be located in any of several locations, but it is most commonly found in a superficical inguinal pouch (Fig. 31–3).[26]

The incidence of cryptorchidism is about 0.7 to 1.0 percent of male infants at 1 year of age. The etiology of the condition is uncertain but may be related to an intrinsic testicular defect or a subtle hormonal deficiency.[26]

The incompletely descended, cryptorchid testis undergoes deleterious changes. The tubules become fibrotic with a deficiency of spermatogenesis and subsequent infertility. More important is the increased incidence of testicular malignancy in cryptorchid testes.[27] Several studies have revealed an increased prevalence of testicular tumors in subjects with a history of cryptorchidism.

Because of the increased risk of malignancy and infertility, treatment at an early age to bring the testis into a normal scrotal position is recommended. This usually requires an operative procedure (*orchiopexy*), though in certain situations descent may be stimulated by the administration of human chorionic gonadotropin, which is given in a series of IM injections.[28]

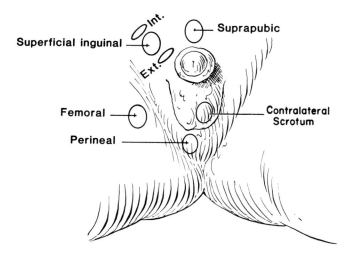

FIGURE 31–3. Schematic representation of sites of ectopic testes. Int., internal inguinal ring; Ext., external inguinal ring. (From Rajfer J: Technique of orchiopexy. *Urol Clin North Am* 9:422, 1982. Reproduced with permission.)

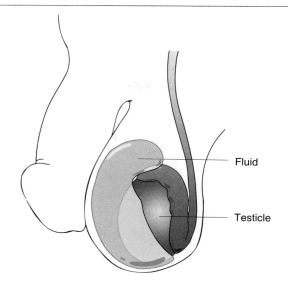

FIGURE 31–4. Hydrocele.

Acquired Disorders

Hydrocele

A **hydrocele** consists of a fluid collection surrounding the testicle or spermatic cord and contained within the tunica or processus vaginalis (Fig. 31–4). Scrotal swelling in infants or young boys may indicate a hydrocele. These congenital hydroceles exist because of a communication between the abdominal cavity and scrotum through the processus vaginalis. The scrotum is characteristically small and soft in the morning but larger and tense at night as it fills with fluid from the abdominal cavity.

Hydroceles may also develop secondary to scrotal injury, radiation therapy, infections of the epididymis, or testicular neoplasms. More commonly, however, the etiology is uncertain, with the hydrocele developing slowly over time and occurring in middle-aged or elderly men. These acquired hydroceles may vary in size and consistency from small and soft to large and tense. The fluid is usually clear and yellow.

Because hydroceles are a benign condition, treatment is required only if the fluid collection becomes uncomfortable for the patient. Occasionally a tense hydrocele might restrict circulation to the testicle. Treatment usually involves a surgical procedure to drain the fluid with either resection or plication of the hydrocele sac to prevent reaccumulation of the fluid. Aspiration of the hydrocele may be performed, although fluid often reaccumulates.

Spermatocele

Spermatoceles are painless, cystic masses containing sperm. Although they are usually small in size, they may be quite large and difficult to distinguish from a hydrocele. The etiology of spermatoceles is uncertain; they may arise from the tiny tubules that connect the epididymis to the testis (vasa efferentia) or from the epididymis itself. Like hydroceles, spermatoceles need not be treated unless they become large enough to trouble the patient. In that case an operative procedure to excise the spermatocele may be performed.

Testicular Torsion

Torsion of the testicle is described as a twisting of the spermatic cord with subsequent compromise of the testicular vascular supply and testicular ischemia, followed by infarction (Fig. 31–5). Although torsion may occur in the neonatal period, the majority of cases occur in prepubertal boys.

The diagnosis is suggested by the onset of severe pain in one testis, followed by swelling of the scrotum. Lower abdominal pain accompanied by nausea and vomiting may also occur. The condition may be differentiated from epididymitis (inflammation of the epididymis), which also presents with scrotal swelling, by the presence of vascular echoes detected using a Doppler ultrasound stethoscope. The torsed testis made ischemic by the event will not echo sound, whereas the inflammation of epididymitis and its hypervascularity increase the sound emission. Testicular nuclear scans are the most definitive test, with the torsed testes being avascular.

Treatment of torsion involves an operation to open the scrotum, untwist the torsed testis, and pex (secure) it to the scrotal wall. Because there is an increased chance of the contralateral testis also torsing, the contralateral testicle is pexed to the scrotal wall as well. If detorsion is accomplished within 12 hours of the event, the prognosis for testicular viability is usually good. If torsion has been present for more than 24 hours, viability of the testis is doubtful.

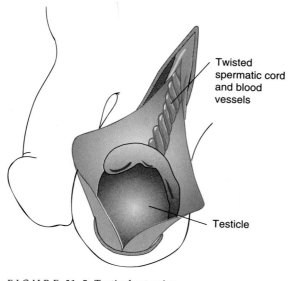

FIGURE 31–5. Testicular torsion.

Labels: Twisted spermatic cord and blood vessels; Testicle

Infectious Disorders

Epididymitis

Epididymitis, or inflammation of the testicle, has several causes. It may occur as a result of trauma or the reflux of sterile urine up the vas deferens. However, the majority of cases are probably secondary to a bacterial etiology, with both sexually transmitted organisms (*Neisseria gonorrheae* and *Chlamydia trachomatis*) and non-sexually transmitted organisms (*Pseudomonas* and *E. coli*) involved.

With epididymitis the scrotum may be enlarged, reddened, and tender. The pain may radiate along the spermatic cord into the inguinal area. Fever may also occur, as may urethral discharge, cystitis, and cloudy urine. Laboratory testing usually reveals an elevated white blood cell (WBC) count, and urine culture may reveal the infecting organism.

Treatment of the condition involves bed rest, scrotal support, and administration of antibiotics. In advanced cases, incision and drainage with the IV administration of antibiotics may be needed to effectively treat a resulting scrotal abscess.

Fournier's Gangrene

This severe though fortunately rare condition involves a gangrenous necrosis of the scrotum. Usually there is an underlying disease such as diabetes, alcoholism, or some other general debility that might predispose the patient to such an aggressive infection. Extravasation of infected urine from urethral trauma, a perforated urethral diverticulum, or a non-urinary tract source such as a perirectal abscess may act as the source of infection. Treatment, which must be instituted swiftly, includes incision and drainage of fluctuant areas and debridement of necrotic tissue.

Neoplasms of the Testis

Although testicular tumors are rare, occurring with a prevalence of 3.7 cases per 100,000 population, their peak incidence is in late adolescence to early adulthood. These neoplasms therefore represent the most common solid tumors of men between 20 and 34 years of age in the United States.[29]

Although the etiology of testicular tumors is uncertain, there is a strong association between cryptorchidism and the subsequent development of malignancy. Nevertheless, the majority of patients with testicular tumors have no history of cryptorchidism, which suggests that several other unrecognized factors may be contributing to the pathogenesis.

Histologically, testicular tumors may be considered in two groups. In the first group are nongerminal neoplasms, including those tumors which originate from either the Leydig cells or other stromal tissue cells of the testis. In the second group are germinal neoplasms, which are derived from the germinal cells of the testis. This group accounts for the vast majority

(95 percent) of testicular tumors. The germinal neoplasms may be further subdivided into five groups: seminomas, embryonal carcinomas, teratomas, choriocarcinomas, and yolk sac tumors.[29]

Although germinal tumors may consist entirely of one histologic subtype, many contain elements of more than one subtype. The treatment and prognosis vary according to the subtype of germinal tumor. For example, seminoma in its early stages is exquisitely sensitive to and easily cured with radiation therapy. On the other hand, nonseminomatous germ cell tumors in the early stage are usually successfully treated with surgery. The prognosis is also variable. Pure choriocarcinomas are usually first seen at an advanced stage with distant metastases. Treatment is usually less effective for this aggressive lesion. The majority of germ cell tumors, however, may be effectively treated even if lymph node metastases are present.

Except for choriocarcinomas, which disseminate by vascular means, testicular germ cell tumors usually metastasize through the lymphatic system. They usually disseminate in a stepwise manner, first involving the retroperitoneal lymph nodes lying adjacent to the great vessels. If untreated, the disease may progress to involve other lymph nodes and other organs such as the lungs.

There are multiple staging systems in existence to classify the extent of this disease. Most are a variation of the system proposed by Boden and Gibb in 1951.[30] One commonly used system is as follows:

Stage I: The tumor is confined to the testis.
Stage II: The tumor is spread to retroperitoneal nodes.
Stage III: The tumor is spread to nodes above the diaphragm
Stage IV: The tumor is spread to other organs.

Because the treatment of testicular tumors is complicated and somewhat controversial, a complete discussion here is not possible; however, several issues may be pointed out. After diagnosis of a testicular tumor, an operation to remove the testicle is performed. This procedure involves an inguinal incision with removal of the testis from the scrotum, followed by ligation and removal of the spermatic cord and testicle together. Histologic classification, further staging studies, and other factors then determine further treatment. This treatment may involve close observation with frequent radiologic studies to determine new progression, surgery to remove retroperitoneal lymph nodes (retroperitoneal lymphadenectomy), or chemotherapy. Some situations may call for a combination of these measures.

KEY CONCEPTS

- **Cryptorchidism refers to a testis located in a position other than the scrotum. Often the testis has failed to descend completely and is located in the inguinal canal. Undescended testes are associated with infertility and an increased risk of testicular malignancy.**
- **A hydrocele is a collection of fluid in the testicle or spermatic cord, commonly associated with a communication between the abdominal cavity and the scrotum (hernia). Hydroceles are a benign condition and are treated only if they become uncomfortable. A spermatocele is a cyst that contains sperm. Like hydroceles, they are benign and do not require treatment unless uncomfortable.**
- **Testicular torsion refers to a twisting of the spermatic cord with subsequent testicular ischemia and infarction. A sudden onset of severe testicular pain is common. If torsion is reduced within 12 hours, the testicle may be viable.**
- **Inflammation of the testicle, called epididymitis, is most commonly associated with infectious agents. Manifestations include a swollen, tender, reddened scrotum with associated bladder infection and cloudy urine. Antibiotics are indicated. Aggressive infections of the scrotum may result in Fournier's gangrene, manifested by gangrenous necrosis of the scrotum.**
- **Although rare in the population, testicular cancer is the most common solid tumor in men aged 20 to 34 years. The great majority of testicular neoplasms originate in the germ cells. Most germ cell tumors can be effectively treated even after lymph node metastasis. Treatment includes surgical removal of the testis and spermatic cord, with radiation and chemotherapy as indicated.**

Disorders of the Prostate

Prostatitis

Prostatitis, or inflammation of the prostate, has several causes and encompasses several syndromes. A common classification of prostatitis proposed by Drach et al in 1978 considers four types—acute bacterial prostatitis, chronic bacterial prostatitis, nonbacterial prostatitis, and prostatodynia.[31]

Acute bacterial prostatitis is characterized by the onset of fever, chills, low back pain, and the voiding symptoms of frequency, urgency, and dysurea. Rectal examination usually reveals a tender, swollen prostate, and subsequent urinalysis may reveal WBCs and bacteria.

The causative organism in bacterial prostatitis is usually *E. coli,* with species of *Proteus, Klebsiella, Enterobacter, Pseudomonas,* and *Serratia* occurring less commonly.[32] The possible routes of infection include ascending infection up the urethra, reflux of infected urine into the prostatic ducts, hematogenous infection, and invasion of rectal bacteria by direct extension or lymphogenous spread. Many cases of prostatitis occur from the periurethral infection associated with an indwelling urethral catheter.[33]

The diagnosis of bacterial prostatitis is usually suggested by the presenting symptoms and signs. Microscopic inspection of the urine and expressed prostatic secretions may reveal WBCs and bacteria. A urine culture with sensitivity testing for the offending organism is recommended to direct therapy with an appropriate antibiotic. In the event of high fever and an elevated WBC count, IV antibiotics are recommended.

Chronic bacterial prostatitis may manifest with variable symptoms. Although some men with chronic bacterial prostatitis may report a history of acute bacterial prostatitis, many have no prior history of this problem. Most men complain of voiding symptoms with pain localized to various areas, including the perineum, back, suprapubic area, and occasionally the testis. High-grade fever and chills are uncommon with this entity, as opposed to acute bacterial prostatitis.

In chronic bacterial prostatitis pathogenic organisms may persist in prostatic tissues, unaltered by the administration of several antibiotics. Because most antibiotics accumulate poorly in prostatic secretions, discontinuation of the antibiotic often results in reinfection and recurrence of symptoms. It is this occurrence of relapsing infections, often caused by the same organism, that is typical of chronic bacterial prostatitis. Several antibiotic agents, such as trimethoprim-sulfamethoxazole (Septra, Bactrim), when used for a prolonged period of time (4–6 weeks) have a better cure rate because of their ability to penetrate prostatic tissue.

Prostatitis may also occur secondary to a nonbacterial inflammation. In fact, nonbacterial prostatitis probably accounts for the majority of cases of prostatitis. The symptoms of this entity are variable but usually include irritative voiding symptoms of urgency, frequency, and nocturia, as well as occasional perineal and suprapubic pain. Although these symptoms are similar to those of bacterial prostatitis, patients have no prior history of positive urine cultures or urinary tract infections. Treatment may include a course of antibiotics, oral anti-inflammatory agents (e.g., ibuprofen), prostatic massage, and occasionally sitz baths. The symptoms are often intermittent in nature,

and patients should be reassured that the disease is not contagious and does not predispose to the development of cancer or other serious disease.

The final classification of prostatitis, prostatodynia, is typified by the patient who describes the symptoms of prostatitis but has no history of urinary tract infection and no evidence of inflammation in prostatic secretions. The etiology of this entity is uncertain and may involve spasm of the pelvic floor musculature. Treatment may involve use of α-adrenergic receptor blocking agents and occasionally diazapam (Valium).[33]

Benign Prostatic Hyperplasia

Benign prostatic hyperplasia (also referred to as benign prostatic hypertrophy) is a very common disorder. An estimated 80 percent of men older than 60 years of age experience some degree of BPH. It is important to recognize that BPH and prostate cancer are not related entities, and no study has demonstrated conclusively that BPH predisposes to the development of prostate cancer.[34]

Although the exact etiology of BPH is unknown, the occurrence of the disease with aging suggests a relationship to changes in the aging male endocrine system. The process involves hyperplasia of the glands surrounding the prostatic urethra (Fig. 31–6). As this tissue increases in size, it compresses the urethra and produces symptoms of bladder outlet obstruction.

Symptoms of obstruction may be minimal at first but may eventually progress to complete obstruction and urinary retention. A decrease in the force of the urinary stream, hesitancy or difficulty in initiating a urinary stream, and interruption of the stream may occur. Because the bladder may fail to empty completely, infection associated with residual urine may occur.

The diagnosis of BPH usually involves recognition of the characteristic symptoms. Rectal examination disclosing an enlarged prostate, urethral catheterization to document a post-void urinary residual, and intravenous pyelography to provide radiographic evi-

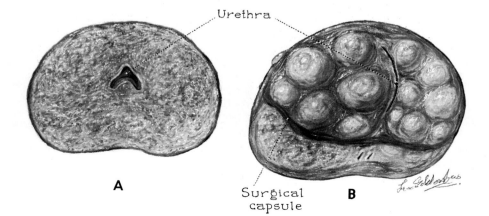

A   **B**

Urethra

Surgical capsule

FIGURE 31–6. Cross-sectional schematic illustration of (**A**) the normal prostate and (**B**) the prostate with established benign prostatic hypertrophy compressing the outer zones of the prostate, producing the surgical capsule. (From Walsh PC, Retik AB, Stamey TA, Vaughan ED (eds): *Campbell's Urology,* 6th ed. Philadelphia, WB Saunders, 1992, p 1011. Reproduced with permission.)

dence of hypertrophy and obstruction are some of the measures that may be employed to confirm the diagnosis.

Treatment involves a surgical procedure to remove the obstructing prostatic tissue. This may be performed transurethrally with an endoscopic resectoscope. The resectoscope utilizes a wire filament that cuts with the use of an electrical current. If the prostate is greatly enlarged, an open operation may be required. Endoscopic incision of the bladder neck, dilation of the prostatic urethra with balloon catheters, and several medications are newly developed treatment alternatives that may play a greater role in the future treatment of BPH.

Prostate Cancer

Prostate cancer is now recognized as the most prevalent form of cancer in men. About 100,000 cases are diagnosed annually in the United States, with approximately 35,000 deaths annually attributed to the disease. Cancer of the prostate rarely occurs in men younger than 50 years of age, and it increases in incidence with increasing age. The majority (95 percent) of prostate cancers are adenocarcinomas with abnormal proliferation of the prostatic glandular structures.[35]

The precise cause of prostate cancer is undetermined, although genetic, hormonal, dietary, and viral factors have all been suggested. Varying degrees of aggressiveness among the prostate cancers have been recognized, with different tumors expressing different malignant potential and ultimately carrying a different prognosis. Attempts to classify prostate cancer into different groups consider the structure and internal architecture of tumor cells and their pattern of proliferation. For example, the cells of the more aggressive or poorly differentiated prostate cancers have more indistinct cell borders, larger nuclei, and loss of the acinar (gland) formation.

Prostate cancer is staged as follows:

State A: The tumor is microscopic and intracapsular.

Stage B: The tumor is palpable on rectal examination but confined to the prostate.

Stage C: The tumor has extended beyond the capsule of the prostate.

Stage D: The tumor has metastasized to distant organs.

Prostate cancer may manifest with several clinical scenarios. The disease may be diagnosed after microscopic inspection of prostate tissue removed for treatment of presumed BPH. Prostate cancer may also be detected on rectal examination in patients with or without voiding symptoms. Occasionally patients present with urinary retention or even azotemia and renal failure secondary to obstructive nephropathy. Much interest has focused on the search for effective measures to detect prostate cancer in its early and most easily treatable stages. Two new techniques, a blood test for serum prostate-specific antigen and

transrectal ultrasonography, have generated considerable excitement within urology. Several initial investigations have shown efficacy in the early detection of prostate cancer.

Once the diagnosis of prostate cancer is made, the lesion must be staged. This usually involves a bone scan to rule out bone metastases, chest radiography to rule out lung metastases, and occasionally abdominal and pelvic computed tomography to rule out abdominal lymphadenopathy.

The treatment of prostate cancer depends on several factors, including the stage of the tumor as well as the age and health of the patient. A localized tumor without extension beyond the prostate is usually treated with radical surgery or radiation therapy. Advanced lesions may respond to hormonal manipulation. Orchiectomy, oral administration of estrogens, or IM injection of LH-RH agonists may reduce the patient's serum testosterone level. Many prostate cancers are androgen sensitive and may be temporarily controlled with androgen ablation. In more advanced cases which are no longer hormonally responsive, palliative measures such as spot radiation treatment of painful areas of bone metastasis and analgesics may be required.

KEY CONCEPTS

- Inflammation of the prostate, or prostatitis, is characterized by low back pain, urinary frequency, urgency, and dysuria. Fever and chills may also be present with acute bacterial prostatitis. E. coli is the most commonly associated organism. Prostatitis also may occur in the absence of infection.

- Benign prostatic hyperplasia is a common disorder, affecting about 80 percent of men over the age of 60 years. The prostate gland enlarges and progressively compresses the urethra, resulting in symptoms of obstruction. These include diminished force of the urinary stream, hesitancy, and poor bladder emptying. Transurethral resection of the obstructing prostatic tissue is the usual treatment.

- Cancer of the prostate is the most prevalent form of cancer in men, usually affecting those over age 50. Prostate cancer is usually detected as a lump or enlargement of the prostate gland. As with other cancers, early diagnosis is important for effective therapy. Surgical resection, radiation therapy, and hormone therapy (to reduce androgens) may be used.

Summary

Disorders of the penis and male urethra may be grouped into congenital and acquired anomalies, infections, and neoplasms. Common congenital anomalies include urethral valves and hypospadias. Common acquired disorders involve phimosis, urethral strictures, and impotence. Sexually transmitted diseases are some of the most common infections involving the penis and urethra; they include gonococcal urethritis, nongonococcal urethritis, syphilis, genital herpes, and genital warts. Neoplasms of the penis and urethra are relatively rare.

Congenital disorders of the scrotum and testes include cryptorchidism. This condition is one of the most common problems seen by pediatric urologists. Testicular torsion and Fournier's gangrene are two of the more immediate urologic emergencies. Finally, neoplasms of the testes, though rare, afflict younger men in the prime of life.

Disorders of the prostate account for a majority of the visits to a practicing urologist. Briefly, these can be divided into problems of prostatitis, benign prostatic hyperplasia, and prostatic cancer. Prostate cancer is the most frequently diagnosed cancer among men, with more than 100,000 cases diagnosed and 35,000 deaths yearly.

REFERENCES

1. Schonfeld WA, Beebe GW: Normal growth and variation in the male genitalia from birth to maturity. *J Urol* 1942;48:759–777.
2. Feldman KW, Smith DW: Fetal phallic growth and penile standards for newborn male infants. *J Pediatr* 1975;86(3):395–398.
3. Kogan SJ, Williams DI: The micropenis syndrome: Clinical observations and expectations for growth. *J Urol* 1977;118(2):311–313.
4. Stephens FD: *Congenital Malformations of the Rectum, Anus and Genitourinary Tracts.* Edinburgh, E & S Livingston, 1963.
5. King LR: Posterior urethra, in Kelalis PP, King LR (eds): *Clinical Pediatric Urology,* 2nd ed. Philadelphia, WB Saunders, 1985.
6. Williams DI, Retik AB: Congenital valves and diverticula of the anterior urethra. *Br J Urol* 1969;41(2):228–234.
7. Sweet RA, Schroot HG, Kurland R, Culp OS: Study of the incidence of hypospadias in Rochester, Minnesota 1940–1970, and a case controlled comparison of possible etiologic factors. *Mayo Clin Proc* 1974;49(1):52–58.
8. Aarskog D: Maternal progestins as a possible cause of hypospadias. *N Engl J Med* 1979;300(2):75–78.
9. Muecke EC: The role of the cloacal membrane in extrophy: The first successful experimental study. *J Urol* 1964;92:659–667.
10. McAninch JW: Disorders of the penis and male urethra, in Tanagho EM, McAninch JW (eds): *Smith's General Urology,* 13th ed. Norwalk, Conn, Appleton & Lange, 1992.
11. Fitzpatrick TJ: Spongiograms and cavernosograms: A study of their value in priapism. *J Urol* 1973;109(5):843–846.
12. Baron M, Leiter D: The management of priapism in sickle cell anemia. *J Urol* 1978;119(5):610–611.
13. Winter CC, McDowell G: Experience with 105 patients with priapism: Update review of all aspects. *J Urol* 1988;140(5):980–983.
14. Devine CJ Jr, Horton CE: Surgical treatment of Peyronie's disease with a dermal graft. *J Urol* 1974;111:44–49.
15. Wild RM, Devine CJ Jr, Horton CE: Dermal graft repair of Peyronies's disease: Survey of 50 patients. *J Urol* 1979;121(1):47–50.
16. Krane RJ: Sexual function and dysfunction, in Walsh PC, Gittes RF, Perlmutter AD, Stamey TA (eds): *Campbell's Urology,* 5th ed. Philadelphia, WB Saunders, 1986.
17. Faerman I, Glocer J, Fox D, Jadzins KG, Rapaport M: Impotence and diabetes: Histological studies of the autonomic nervous fibers of the corpora cavenosa in impotent diabetic males. *Diabetes* 1974;23(12):971–976.
18. Goldstein I: Drug-induced sexual dysfunction. *World J Urol* 1979;121:719.
19. Spark RF, White RA, Connolly PB: Impotence is not always psychogenic: Newer insights into hypothalamic-pituitary-gonadal dysfunction. *JAMA* 1980;243(8):750–755.
20. Harrison WO: Gonococcal urethritis. *Urol Clin North Am* 1984;11(1):45–53.
21. Bowie WR: Nongonococcal urethritis. *Urol Clin North Am* 1984;11(1):55–64.
22. Centers for Disease Control: Sexually transmitted disease treatment guidelines 1982. *MMWR* 1982;31:25.
23. Syrjanen KJ: Current views on the condylomatous lesions of the uterine cervix and their possible relationship to cervical squamous cell carcinoma. *Obstet Gynecol Surv* 1980;35(11):685–694.
24. Schellhammer PF, Grabstald H: Tumors of the penis, in Walsh PC, Gittes RF, Perlmutter AD, Stamey TA (eds): *Campbell's Urology,* 5th ed. Philadelphia, WB Saunders, 1986.
25. Jackson SM: The treatment of carcinoma of the penis. *Br J Surg* 1966;53(1):33–35.
26. Kogan SJ: Cryptorchidism, in Kelalis PP, King LR: *Clinical Pediatric Urology,* 2nd ed. Philadelphia, WB Saunders, 1985.
27. Martin DC: Malignancy in the cryptorchid testis. *Urol Clin North Am* 1982;9(3):371–376.
28. Bergada C: Clinical treatment of cryptorchidism, in Rierich JR, Giarola A (eds): *Cryptorchidism.* London, Academic Press, 1979, p 367.
29. Morse MJ, Whitmore WF: Neoplasms of the testis, in Walsh PC, Gittes RF, Perlmutter AD, Stamey TA (eds): *Campbell's Urology,* 5th ed. Philadelphia, WB Saunders, 1986.
30. Boden G, Gibb R: Radiotherapy in testicular neoplasms. *Lancet* 1951;2:1195–1197.
31. Drach GW, Fair WR, Meares EM, Stamey TA: Classification of benign diseases associated with prostatic pain: Prostatitis or prostatodynia? *J Urol* 1978;120(2):266.
32. Meares EM: Prostatitis syndromes; New perspectives about old woes. *J Urol* 1980;123(2):141–147.
33. Meares EM: Protatitis and related disorders, in Walsh PC, Gittes RF, Perlmutter AD, Stamey TA (eds): *Campbell's Urology,* 5th ed. Philadelphia, WB Saunders, 1986.
34. Walsh PC: Benign prostatic hyperplasia, in Walsh PC, Gittes RF, Perlmutter AD, Stamey TA (eds): *Campbell's Urology,* 5th ed. Philadelphia, WB Saunders, 1986.
35. Catalona WJ: Carcinoma of the prostate, in Walsh PC, Gittes RF, Perlmutter AD, Stamey TA (eds): *Campbell's Urology,* 5th ed. Philadelphia, WB Saunders, 1986.

BIBLIOGRAPHY

Bostwick DG, Cooner WH, Denis L, Jones GW, Scardino PT, Murphy GP: The association of benign prostatic hyperplasia and cancer of the prostate. *Cancer* 1992;70(suppl 1):291–301.

Brandell RA, Brock JW 3d: Common problems in pediatric urology. *Compr Ther* 1993;19(1):11–16.

Garnick MB: Prostate cancer: Screening, diagnosis, and management. *Ann Intern Med* 1993;118(10):804–818.

Gillenwater JY, Grayhack JT, Howards SS, Duckett JW: *Adult and Pediatric Urology.* St. Louis, Mosby–Year Book, 1991.

Gower PE: Urinary tract infections in men. *Br Med J* 1989;298:1595–1596.

Horoszewicz JS, Murphy GP: Prospective new developments in laboratory research and clinical trials in prostatic cancer. *Cancer* 1990;66(suppl 5):1083–1085.

Humphrey PA, Walther PJ: Adenocarcinoma of the prostate: I. Tissue sampling considerations. *Am J Clin Pathol* 1993;99(6):746–759.

Humphrey PA, Walther PJ: Adenocarcinoma of the prostate: Part II. Tissue prognosticators. *Am J Clin Pathol* 1993;100(3):256–269.

Kelalis PP, King LR, Belman AB (eds): *Clinical Pediatric Urology,* 3rd ed. Philadelphia, WB Saunders, 1992.

Krane RJ, Goldstein I, Saenz-de-Tejada I: Impotence. *N Engl J Med* 1989;321(24):1648–1659.

Lafferty PM, MacGregor FB, Scobie WG: Management of foreskin problems. *Arch Dis Child* 1991;66(6):696–697.

Lee PA, O'Dea LS: Primary and secondary testicular insufficiency. *Pediatr Clin North Am* 37(6):1359–1387.

Lindsey D, Stanisic TH: Diagnosis and management of testicular torsion: Pitfalls and perils. *Am J Emerg Med* 1988;6(1):42–46.

Mostofi FK, Davis CJ Jr, Sesterhenn IA: Pathology of carcinoma of the prostate. *Cancer* 1992;70(suppl 1):235–253.

O'Brien WM, Gibbons MD: Hypospadias. *Am Fam Physician* 1989;39(4):183–191.

Pienta KJ, Esper PS: Risk factors for prostate cancer. *Ann Intern Med* 1993;118(10):793–803.

Richie JP: Detection and treatment of testicular cancer. *CA* 1993;43(3):151–175.

Rotolo JE, Lynch JH: Penile cancer: Curable with early detection. *Hosp Pract Off Ed* 1991;26(6):131–138.

Tanagho EA, McAninch JW (eds): *Smith's General Urology*, 13th ed. Norwalk, Conn, Appleton & Lange, 1992.

Walsh PC, Retik AB, Stamey TA, Vaughan ED Jr (eds): *Campbell's Urology*, 6th ed. Philadelphia, WB Saunders, 1992.

CHAPTER 32
Structure and Function of the Female Reproductive System

JANE M. GEORGES

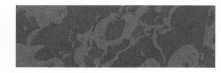

KEY TERMS

corpus luteum: Anatomic structure on the surface of the ovary that grows within the ruptured ovarian follicle following ovulation and that acts as a temporary endocrine organ that secretes estrogen and progesterone.

estrogen: One of a group of ovarian hormones that promote the development of female secondary sex characteristics. During the menstrual cycle, estrogen renders the female reproductive tract suitable for fertilization of the ovum, implantation of the zygote, and nutrition of the early embryo.

lactation: Formation and secretion of milk from the breasts for the nourishment of the infant.

menarche: The first menstrual period at the time of puberty, usually occurring around age 12 years in North America.

menopause: A process by which the supply of ovarian follicles and hormones declines, usually beginning between the ages of 45 and 52 years.

menstrual cycle: The rhythmic pattern of changes in hormonal secretions and in sexual organs occurring approximately every 28 days during a woman's reproductive years. The cycle culminates in the production of an ovum and the preparation of the uterus for implantation of a fertilized ovum.

morphogenesis: Arrangement of cells in a particular order during the development of complex organisms.

oogonia: The cells present in the female ovaries during prenatal development that ultimately develop into ova. The entire lifetime supply of ova is established prenatally; no new oogonia arise after birth.

placenta: A highly vascularized organ through which the fetus receives nutrients and via which wastes are removed. It also is an endocrine organ, producing several hormones, most notably human chorionic gonadotropin (HCG).

progesterone: Hormone that is produced by the corpus luteum and adrenal cortex during the luteal phase of the menstrual cycle and that promotes uterine changes essential for the implantation and growth of the fertilized ovum.

zygote: The developing ovum from the time it is fertilized until it is implanted in the uterus.

---

*T*he female reproductive system is complex, both in structure and in function. From birth to senescence, the organs of the female reproductive system function in concert with each other, with the brain, and with other endocrine organs. This integrated functioning constitutes some of the most intricate and elegant processes of the human body. This chapter presents an overview of these functions, beginning with a summary of the structures of the female reproductive tract.

The major processes related to the reproductive tract throughout life, including the menstrual cycle, pregnancy, lactation, and menopause, are then described, with an emphasis on recent research findings. Because the functioning of the female reproductive system has an enormous impact on the life of the individual woman, increasing importance is placed on the active involvement of women in understanding their own health care needs. Health care professionals are encouraged to include women as collaborators in decisions about their reproductive health.[1,2]

Reproductive Structures

Embryology

Until the sixth week of gestation, the gonads in both sexes are bipotential, meaning that the gonads present in the embryo may become either a testis or an ovary. In about the seventh week, the "indifferent" gonad begins to develop into either a male or female derivative. Recent research has demonstrated that a particular locus on the Y chromosome termed the testis-determining factor influences the indifferent gonad to organize into a testis. In a genetically female embryo, the gonad organizes into an ovary under the influence of one or more ovary-determining genes, which have not yet been identified.[3] The cortex of the gonad accumulates a nest of cells that differentiate into ovarian follicles, each containing a primary oocyte. The wolffian ducts, the primordial structures that are precursors to the male internal reproductive organs, begin to disappear, and the müllerian ducts, the struc-

tures that will develop into the female internal reproductive organs, become dominant.[3,4]

The external genitalia of both the male and female are identical until the eighth week of gestation. Like the gonads, the genitalia are bipotential until this time, having the potential to develop into organs of either sex. In the genetically male embryo, dihydrotestosterone (DHT), a metabolite of testosterone, binds to androgen receptors in the external genitalia and affects the differentiation of these structures into the male external genitalia. Without the influence of DHT, the bipotential external genitalia will spontaneously develop into female external genitalia.[3]

During the later period of fetal development, maternal hormones may have some influence on reproductive structures. Estrogens and progestins from the mother cause cervical enlargement, hypertrophy of the vaginal epithelium, and enlargement of the mammary gland of the female fetus. These alterations may be present at birth and usually subside during the first 1 to 2 months.[5]

Organization of the Female Reproductive Organs

The internal organs of the female reproductive system include the ovaries, oviducts (fallopian tubes), uterus, cervix, and vagina (Fig. 32–1). These organs are situated in the pelvic cavity and are supported and anchored in place by a series of ligaments (Fig. 32–2).

Ovaries

The two ovaries, which are the female gonads, are located close to the lateral walls of the pelvic cavity. When the ovary is in its normal position, its long axis is nearly vertical with respect to the horizontal axis of the body. The size of the ovary varies with age and with the stage of the menstrual cycle. It is somewhat larger before than after pregnancy, and will further reduce in size with the aging process.[6]

The ovary is covered with a single layer of epithelium. Underneath the epithelium is a layer of dense

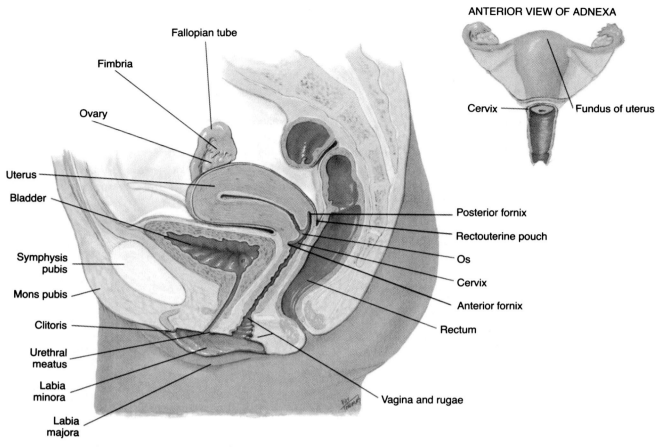

ANTERIOR VIEW OF ADNEXA

Cervix — Fundus of uterus

Fallopian tube

Fimbria

Ovary

Uterus

Bladder

Symphysis pubis

Mons pubis

Clitoris

Urethral meatus

Labia minora

Labia majora

Posterior fornix

Rectouterine pouch

Os

Cervix

Anterior fornix

Rectum

Vagina and rugae

F I G U R E 32–1. Cross-sectional view of the female reproductive system. (From Jarvis C: *Physical Examination and Health Assessment.* Philadelphia, WB Saunders, 1992, p 831. Reproduced with permission.)

fibrous connective tissue called the tunica albuginea. The tunica albuginea constitutes the outer portion of the cortex of the ovary. The remainder of the cortex consists of connective tissue called the stroma, which contains ova in various stages of maturation. The innermost part of the ovary, the medulla, consists of loose connective tissue that is richly supplied with blood and lymph vessels and nerve fibers.[7]

Before birth, hundreds of thousands of **oogonia** (cells that develop into ova) are present in the ovaries. Thus, the entire lifetime supply of ova is established during embryonic development; no new oogonia arise

after birth. Each oogonium is surrounded by a cluster of granulosa cells. The oogonium and its granulosa cells constitute a follicle. During prenatal development, the oogonia increase in size and become primary oocytes. By the time of full gestational development, the primary oocytes are in the prophase of the first meiotic division (Fig. 32–3). During childhood and into adult life, the oocytes enter a nonactive phase. With the onset of puberty, a few of the follicles develop every 28 days in response to follicle-stimulating hormone (FSH) secreted by the anterior pituitary gland. As the follicle grows in response to this stimula-

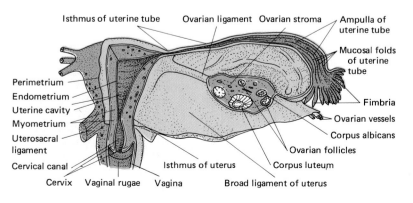

Isthmus of uterine tube   Ovarian ligament   Ovarian stroma   Ampulla of uterine tube

Mucosal folds of uterine tube

Perimetrium

Endometrium

Uterine cavity

Myometrium

Uterosacral ligament

Cervical canal

Fimbria

Ovarian vessels

Corpus albicans

Ovarian follicles

Corpus luteum

Cervix   Vaginal rugae   Vagina   Isthmus of uterus   Broad ligament of uterus

F I G U R E 32–2. View of female pelvis showing ovarian and uterine ligaments. (From *Physiology of the Human Body*, Sixth Edition, p 617, by Arthur C. Guyton, copyright © 1984 by Saunders College Publishing, reproduced by permission of the publisher.)

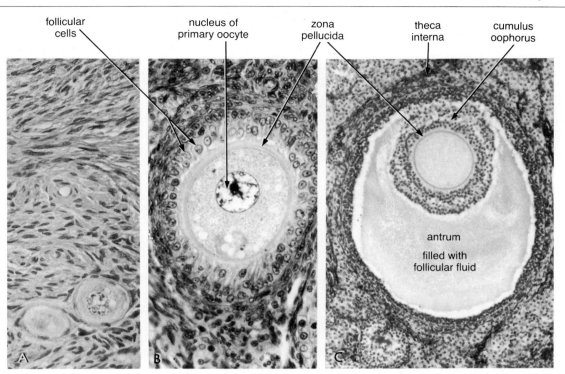

follicular cells nucleus of primary oocyte zona pellucida theca interna cumulus oophorus

antrum

filled with follicular fluid

FIGURE 32–3. Photomicrographs of sections from adult human ovaries. **A,** Ovarian cortex showing two primordial follicles containing primary oocytes that have completed the prophase of the first meiotic division. **B,** Growing follicle containing a primary oocyte. **C,** An almost mature follicle. (From Leeson TS, Leeson CR, Paparo AA: *Text/Atlas of Histology.* Philadelphia, WB Saunders, 1988. Reproduced with permission.)

tion, the primary oocyte completes its first meiotic division into a polar body and a secondary oocyte. The polar body later divides to form two polar bodies, which eventually disintegrate.[7] The secondary oocyte may continue to develop to an ovum and be ejected through the wall of the ovary in the process of ovulation, which is described in more detail under Menstrual Cycle.

Oviducts

The two oviducts, also called the fallopian or uterine tubes, are each about 10 cm long and are located in the upper margin of the broad ligament. Each oviduct runs laterally from the uterus to the uterine end of the ovary. The free end of the oviduct adjacent to the ovary is called the infundibulum. It is shaped like a funnel with long, fingerlike projections termed the fimbriae. The ampulla, the longest part of the oviduct, has an inner lining consisting of ciliated mucous membrane arranged in longitudinal folds. Beneath this ciliated lining is a double layer of smooth muscle, with a thick outer layer of peritoneal serosa. The oviduct plays an active role in propelling the ovum toward the uterus; the current created by the beating cilia and the peristaltic contractions of the muscular wall are powerful forces which move ova along the oviduct. Once inside the oviduct, the ovum is moved through the ampulla to the **isthmus** (the short, narrow portion near the uterus) and finally through the intramural passageway to the uterus. Fertilization of the ovum occurs in the upper third of the oviduct, and the **zygote** (fertilized ovum) begins developing as it moves through the oviduct. If no fertilization occurs, the ovum undergoes degeneration in the oviduct.[7]

Uterus

The uterus varies in size, shape, location, and structure during various phases of a woman's life and reproductive status. In the nonpregnant state, the uterus is about 8 cm long, 4 cm wide in its upper part, and 2 cm thick. The rounded part of the uterus, which lies above and in front of the openings of the oviducts, is called the fundus; the main portion of the uterus is the corpus, or body. The lower narrow portion of the uterus is the cervix, which extends downward to the opening within the vagina. The cervix contains a narrow canal that joins the uterine cavity at the internal os and opens into the vagina at the external os.

The wall of the body and fundus of the uterus consists of three layers—the endometrium, myometrium, and serosa (Fig. 32–4). The outermost layer of the uterus, the serosa, consists of a single layer of mesothelial cells supported by a thin layer of loose connective tissue. The middle layer, the myometrium, consists of three layers of smooth muscle, with muscle fibers arranged in a different direction in each layer.

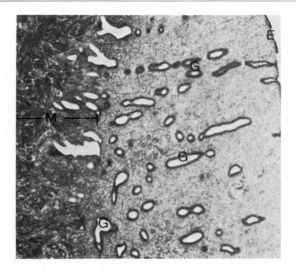

FIGURE 32–4. The uterine wall, consisting of an epithelial lining (E) from which uterine glands (G) extend through the full thickness of the mucosa. Beneath the endometrium, a small portion of myometrium (M) is shown. (From Leeson CR, Leeson TS, Paparo AA: *Atlas of Histology,* 2nd ed. Philadelphia, WB Saunders, 1985, p 261. Reproduced with permission.)

The innermost lining of the uterus, the endometrium, consists of two layers: a thin deep layer called the basilar layer, and a thick superficial layer referred to as the functional layer. During a woman's reproductive years, the endometrium displays a constant cyclic activity of alternating proliferation and sloughing of the functional layer in response to estrogen and progesterone secretion.[8] These changes will be discussed in more detail under Menstrual Cycle.

Vagina

The vagina is the sexual organ that enfolds the penis during sexual intercourse, serves as an exit for discarded endometrium, and comprises the lower end of the birth canal. It is located anterior to the rectum and posterior to the urethra and urinary bladder. The vagina surrounds the cervix at one end and opens to the vestibule at its other end. The vagina is a highly elastic muscle and is capable of considerable distention. Two longitudinal ridges run along the anterior and posterior walls, with numerous transverse folds called rugae. The vagina is lined by a mucous membrane of stratified squamous epithelium overlying a

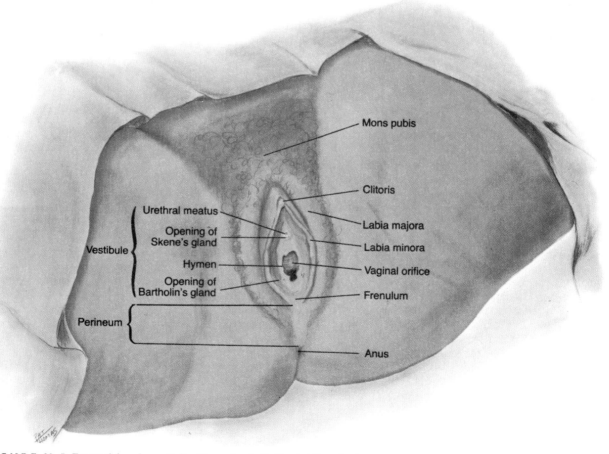

FIGURE 32–5. External female genitalia. (From Jarvis C: *Physical Examination and Health Assessment.* Philadelphia, WB Saunders, 1992, p 830. Reproduced with permission.)

layer of connective tissue. The vaginal wall is subject to thinning with aging; this and other age-related changes in the female sexual organs are described later under Menopause.

External Genitalia

The external female genital structures include the mons pubis, labia majora, labia minora, clitoris, and vestibule of the vagina (Fig. 32–5). The mons pubis is a rounded elevation in front of the pubis symphysis. It consists primarily of an accumulation of fat. After puberty, the skin over it is covered by coarse hair. The labia majora, which are homologous (that is, corresponding in structure) with the scrotum of the male, are folds of skin that run downward and backward from the mons pubis to the area behind the vaginal opening. Following puberty, the labia majora become pigmented and covered with hair. The labia minora are two small folds of skin located between the labia majora on either side of the vaginal opening. The vestibule of the vagina is the cleft between the labia minora and contains the openings of the vagina, the urethra, and the ducts of the greater vestibular glands (also called Bartholin's glands). These glands, along with the less vestibular or Skene's glands, secrete mucus that provides lubrication during sexual intercourse.[6,7]

The clitoris is a body of erectile tissue that projects from the anterior end of the vulva at the anterior junction of the labia minora. It is about 2 cm long and 0.5 cm in diameter and is covered by a fold of tissue the prepuce, formed by the merging of labial tissue. The glans of the clitoris is the rounded elevation on the free end of the body and is highly sensitive to stimulation. During sexual arousal, the erectile tissue of the clitoris becomes engorged with blood.[6,7]

KEY CONCEPTS

- Organs of the female reproductive tract include the ovaries, oviducts, uterus, cervix, and vagina. Ovaries contain a lifetime supply of ova at birth. After puberty a few of the ovarian follicles develop about every 28 days in response to secretion of follicle-stimulating hormone.
- The oviducts (fallopian tubes) actively propel the ovum toward the uterus by ciliary action and peristaltic contractions. The uterine lining undergoes a cyclic process of proliferation and then sloughing in response to estrogen and progesterone.
- External genitalia in the female include the mons pubis, labia majora, labia minora, clitoris, and vestibule of the vagina. The urinary meatus, vaginal opening, and vestibular gland ducts are located in the vaginal vestibule.

Menstrual Cycle

From menarche onward, the normal reproductive years of the female are characterized by rhythmic changes in hormonal secretion and corresponding changes in the sexual organs, which are called the target organs of the female hormones. This rhythmic pattern is called the menstrual cycle. Two significant results of the menstrual cycle are stimulation of the production of an ovum and preparation of the uterine endometrium for the implantation of a fertilized ovum at the appropriate phase of the cycle.

Although considerable variation exists among human females, an average menstrual cycle is 28 days long, with cycles as short as 20 days or as long as 45 days occurring in normal women. The first day of menstruation is considered the first day of the menstrual cycle. Ovulation occurs approximately 14 days before the next cycle begins; thus, in a 28-day cycle, ovulation occurs on about day 14 of the cycle.

The release of hormones and the accompanying response of the female sexual target organs are depicted in Figure 32–6. The principal female reproductive hormones are summarized in Table 32–1. As shown in Figure 32–6, the events of the menstrual cycle require precise synchronization between the activities of the pituitary, ovary, and uterus. Beginning on the first day of the menstrual cycle, or the first day of menstruation, these events can be summarized as follows. The thickened functional layer of the endometrium of the uterus is gradually sloughed off, resulting in a blood loss of about 35 mL. During this phase of the menstrual cycle, FSH is released by the pituitary gland, stimulating a group of follicles to develop in the ovary.

In the preovulatory phase, also called the proliferative phase, theca and granulosa cells in the developing follicles in the ovary secrete estrogen, which stimulates growth of the uterine endometrium once again. At about the midpoint of the cycle, an increase in estrogen secretion from the follicles occurs. This increase in estrogen is thought to render the anterior pituitary more responsive to luteinizing-releasing hormone (LRH) secreted by the hypothalamus. The anterior pituitary then produces a burst of luteinizing hormone (LH). FSH also increases about twofold at the same time, and these two hormones act synergistically to cause the extremely rapid swelling of the follicle that culminates in ovulation.[9] During the process of ovulation, the secondary oocyte is ejected through the wall of the ovary and into the peritoneal cavity. The free end of the oviduct is strategically located so that the ovum enters its fimbriated end almost immediately.[7]

After ovulation the postovulatory phase (also called the luteal phase) begins. During the luteal phase the site of the ruptured follicle becomes a corpus luteum (Latin, *yellow body*) that secretes estrogen and progesterone. These hormones stimulate continued thickening of the uterine endometrium. The cells of

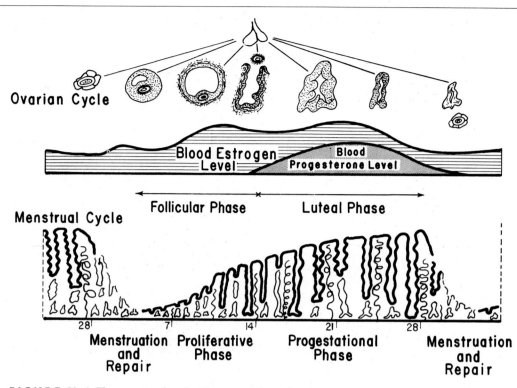

FIGURE 32–6. The menstrual cycle. The events that take place within the pituitary, ovary, and uterus are precisely synchronized. When fertilization does not occur, the cycle repeats itself about every 28 days. (From Leeson CR, Leeson TS, Paparo AA: *Atlas of Histology*, 2nd ed. Philadelphia, WB Saunders, 1985, p 253. Reproduced with permission.)

the corpus luteum become greatly enlarged and develop lipid, or fatty, areas that give the cells a distinctive yellow color. In the normal cycle, the corpus luteum grows to approximately 1.5 cm, reaching maximum development about 7 to 8 days following ovulation. If pregnancy does not occur, the corpus luteum begins to degenerate, and progesterone and estrogen levels in the blood fall markedly. Constric-

tion of the spiral arteries located in the uterine wall occurs, and the portion of the endometrium supplied by these arteries becomes ischemic. As the cells in the endometrium die, tissue is sloughed off and menstruation begins again. It is presently thought that prostaglandins liberated in the endometrium may play a role in stimulating the sloughing of endometrial tissue.[7]

If fertilization of the ovum does occur, the embryo

TABLE 32–1. Principal Female Reproductive Hormones

Hormone	Target Organs	Significant Actions
Estrogen	Multiple sites throughout the body, including reproductive structures, bone, fat, and muscle tissues	Development of reproductive organs during puberty Development of secondary sex characteristics, including breast maturation, widening of pelvis, and distribution of fat and muscle tissues in a distinctively female pattern Cyclical preparation of endometrium for implantation of ovum
Progesterone	Primarily uterus and breasts	Cyclical preparation and maintenance of endometrium for implantation of ovum Stimulation of development of breast lobules and alveoli
Follicle-stimulating hormone (FSH)	Ovary	Stimulates ovarian follicle development; with LH, stimulates secretion of estrogen and ovulation
Luteinizing hormone (LH)	Ovary	Stimulates final development of ovarian follicle; stimulates ovulation; stimulates development of corpus luteum

arrives in the uterus on about the fourth day of development. Small glands in the endometrium, stimulated by progesterone, produce a nutritive fluid for the developing embryo. On approximately the seventh day after fertilization, the embryo implants itself in the thick endometrium of the uterus, and development of the placenta occurs. The placenta secretes the hormone, human chorionic gonadotropin (HCG), which in turn signals the corpus luteum to continue to function. Subsequent events in pregnancy are described later in this chapter.

KEY CONCEPTS

- The monthly reproductive cycle averages about 28 days. Beginning on the first day of menses, the important events of the cycle are as follows:
  1. Sloughing of the endometrial layer occurs.
  2. Stimulation of ovarian follicles by pituitary FSH occurs.
  3. Estrogen is secreted from the developing follicles.
  4. Proliferation of the endometrium occurs in response to estrogen.
  5. At the midpoint of the cycle, a burst of LH and a doubling of FSH secretion from the pituitary stimulate ovulation.
  6. The ruptured follicle changes into a corpus luteum and secretes estrogen and progesterone.
  7. In the absence of pregnancy, secretion of estrogen and progesterone drops rapidly and the endometrial lining sloughs off again, completing the cycle.
- With fertilization and implantation of the ovum, the developing placenta secretes HCG, which in turn stimulates the corpus luteum to continue to secrete estrogen and progesterone, preventing endometrial sloughing.

Breast

The breast is an important accessory organ in sexual function and human reproduction. While its primary physiologic function is **lactation** (the production of milk) to nourish the human infant, the significance of the breast as a symbol of feminine sexuality in contemporary Western culture must also be recognized.

Structure of the Breast

The breasts are located anterior to the pectoralis major muscle and are separated from it by a layer of fat. The position of the breasts is maintained by fibrous bands called Cooper's ligaments, which are easily stretched, especially if the breasts are large. Lymph drainage from the breasts is mainly toward the axillary lymph nodes, with some drainage toward the substernal and diaphragmatic lymph nodes.[10,11]

Each breast consists of 15 to 20 lobes of glandular epithelial tissue and a duct system embedded in interstitial tissue and fat. The secretory cells that compose the glandular epithelium are arranged in grapelike clusters called alveoli (Fig. 32–7). Ducts or openings from each alveolus unite to form a single duct from each lobe. These main ducts then enlarge slightly into ampullae immediately before opening onto the surface of the nipple. The nipple, located at the center of the adult female breast, is composed of bundles of smooth muscle fibers with erectile properties. The areola that surrounds the nipple has a diameter of 1.5 to 2.5 cm. The openings from the lactiferous ducts are arranged radially under the areola; thus, there are 15 to 20 small openings on the surface of each nipple through which milk flows in the lactating female.[7]

Breast Development

The stages of development of the female breast are depicted in Figure 32–8. As shown in this figure, the breasts contain only rudimentary glands during childhood. At puberty, estrogen and progesterone, in the presence of growth hormone and prolactin, promote the development of the glandular tissue and ducts and the deposition of fat characteristic of the adult female breast. Throughout the reproductive years, some women note swelling of the breast around the latter part of each menstrual cycle prior to the onset of menstruation. The water retention and subsequent swelling of breast tissue during this phase of the menstrual cycle are thought to be due to high levels of circulating progesterone stimulating the secretory cells of the breast.[7,12]

Lactation

During pregnancy, high concentrations of estrogen and progesterone produced by the corpus luteum and the placenta stimulate the development of glands and ducts in the breast. During the first trimester of pregnancy, the ducts proliferate; in the second trimester, the ducts group together to form large lobules with new alveoli formation. In the third trimester, the existing alveoli dilate in preparation for lactation. Toward the end of pregnancy and until 1 to 3 days after childbirth, the mammary glands form colostrum, which contains protein and lactose but little fat. Following birth of the infant, the hormone prolactin secreted by the mother's anterior pituitary stimulates milk production, and milk is produced by the third day after delivery. The initiation and maintenance of lactation is a complex neuroendocrine process involving sensory nerves in the nipples and breast tissue, the spinal cord and hypothalamus, and the pituitary gland. The suckling movements of the infant on the breast stimulate the release of prolactin from the anterior pituitary gland and oxytocin from the posterior pituitary gland. These hormones in turn stimulate lactation and ejection of milk from the alveoli into the

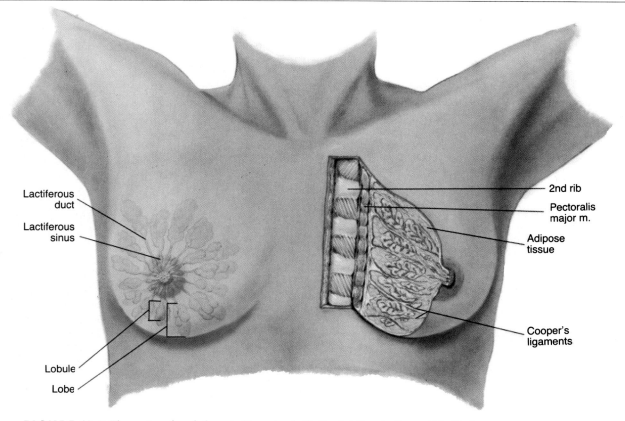

F I G U R E 32–7. The mature female breast. (From Jarvis C: *Physical Examination and Health Assessment.* Philadelphia, WB Saunders, 1992, p 443. Reproduced with permission.)

ducts, where it is accessible to the infant. Oxytocin then promotes the actual release of milk, called the "milk ejection reflex."[7]

KEY CONCEPTS

- At puberty, breast development occurs in response to estrogen and progesterone in cooperation with growth hormone and prolactin. During pregnancy, high estrogen and progesterone levels stimulate further development of the mammary glands and ducts.

- Milk production and release are stimulated by the pituitary hormones prolactin and oxytocin in response to suckling.

Pregnancy

During the 9 months of human gestation, the single-celled zygote gives rise to an infant with a complex set of physiologic systems. The fertilized ovum contains the entire genetic complement—or encoded genetic instructions—to develop into a fully functioning term infant, given adequate nutrition and time. Three basic developmental processes—growth, morphogenesis, and cellular differentiation—are involved in this transformation.[7] Growth denotes the proliferation

of new cells by mitosis, a necessary but not sufficient process for development. The arrangement of cells in a particular order is called *morphogenesis* and is essential to the elaboration of higher forms of life. In addition to growth and morphogenesis, cellular differentiation is needed for cells to specialize structurally and biochemically in a myriad of ways. This section describes the sequence of events in which growth, morphogenesis, and cellular differentiation function to transform a human zygote with encoded genetic information into a human infant. In addition, this section will describe the response of the mother's body to pregnancy. Information on genetic control of inheritance and genetic disorders is contained in Chapters 4 and 5, and the reader may wish to refer to these chapters for specific content in these areas.

Early Human Development

Fertilization of the ovum occurs in the oviduct. Within 24 hours after fertilization, the zygote begins a series of divisions, by the process of mitosis, which are referred to as cleavage (Fig. 32–9). From a two-cell entity the zygote soon divides multiple times, and its cytoplasm begins to be partitioned into specific cells that will serve as the building blocks of the embryo. As more cleavage takes place, the embryo is transported through the oviduct to the uterus. This process takes

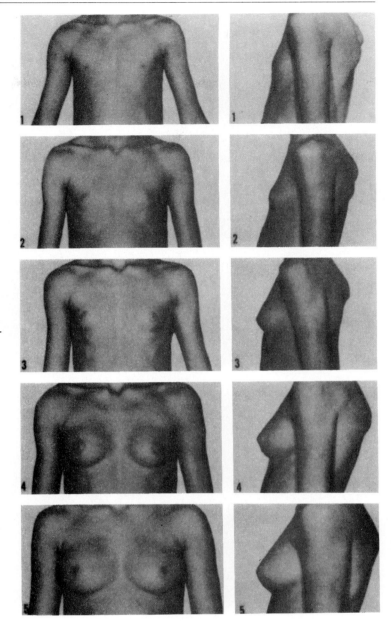

FIGURE 32–8. Development of the female breast. (From Tanner JM: *Growth at Adolescence*. Oxford, England, Blackwell Scientific Publishing, 1962. Reproduced with permission.)

about 6 days. The embryo receives nutrition during this time from secretions released by the epithelial cells lining the oviduct. After the embryo enters the uterus, the zona pellucida, the membrane surrounding the embryo, dissolves. At about day 6, the embryo arrives in the uterus and floats freely while receiving nutrition from secretions from the endometrial glands stimulated by progesterone.

At this point the cells of the embryo have arranged themselves into a hollow spherical structure called the blastocyst (Fig. 32–10). The outer cells of the blastocyst, called the trophoblast, will ultimately become the protective and nutritive membranes (chorion and placenta) that surround the developing embryo. The inner cell mass, a small cluster of cells that projects into the cavity of the blastocyst, will develop into the structures of the embryo itself. If at this point the inner cell mass divides into two separate groups of cells, identical twins with an identical genetic complement will result. (Fraternal twins develop when two ova are fertilized by two sperm cells and do not have an identical genetic complement.[5])

Implantation

On approximately day 7 after fertilization, the embryo attaches itself to the uterine lining and then implants itself into the endometrium. Enzymes secreted by the trophoblast erode a small portion of the uterine lining, and by day 10 of development the embryo has worked its way down into the endometrium completely. The

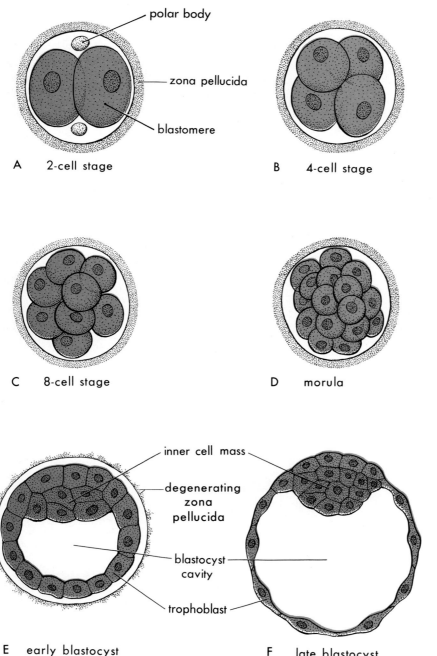

A   2-cell stage

B   4-cell stage

C   8-cell stage

D   morula

E   early blastocyst

F   late blastocyst

F I G U R E 32–9. Early human development. Drawings illustrate cleavage of the zygote and formation of the blastocyst. (From Moore KL: *The Developing Human: Clinically Oriented Embryology,* 5th ed. Philadelphia, WB Saunders, 1993, p 34. Reproduced with permission.)

opening in the uterine lining is closed, initially by a blood clot and then by the regeneration of the uterine epithelium; all subsequent development of the embryo takes place in the wall of the uterus.[7]

Fetal Membranes and Placenta

Fetal membranes serve to protect the developing embryo or fetus and to provide needed substrates for growth and development, particularly oxygen and nutrition. In addition, they serve the purpose of elimination of waste products of metabolism. All terrestrial vertebrates have four fetal membranes: the amnion, yolk sac, chorion, and allantois.[7] In the developing human, the yolk sac is usually thought to be a vestigial structure, although it serves as an important temporary center for the formation of blood cells between the second and sixth weeks. The allantois is also considered vestigial, although its blood supply does contribute to the formation of the umbilical vessels.

The amnion begins to develop at a very early stage and eventually expands to surround the entire embryo. The space between the amnion and the embryo is called the amniotic cavity and is filled with a clear amniotic fluid that keeps the embryo moist and pro-

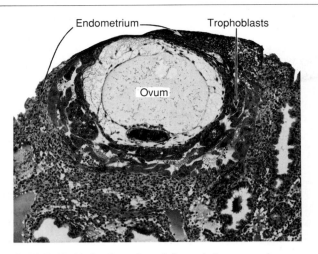

Endometrium — Trophoblasts

Ovum

FIGURE 32–10. Implantation of the early human embryo. (From Guyton, AC. *Textbook of Medical Physiology,* 8th ed. Philadelphia, WB Saunders, 1991, p 916. Courtesy of Arthur Hertig, M.D. Reproduced with permission.)

the infant through the pelvic structures during delivery. In addition to its role in providing early nutrition for the embryo, progesterone has the special effect of decreasing the contractility of the gravid uterus, thus preventing spontaneous abortion. In addition, progesterone may play a role in preparing the breasts for lactation, as described in an earlier section.

Of major importance in the role of the placenta as an endocrine gland is its production of HCG. From the time of implantation, the trophoblastic cells begin to secrete HCG, which sends a signal to the corpus luteum that a pregnancy has begun. The corpus luteum responds by increasing its size and its secretion of estrogen and progesterone, which then promote the continued development of the endometrium and the placenta. In the absence of HCG, the corpus luteum would disintegrate, as it does in a nonfertilized menstrual cycle, and the endometrium would deteriorate and be sloughed off along with the embryo. Thus, hCG is an essential element for continuation of the pregnant state.

vides a measure of protection against mechanical injury.

The placenta serves two basic functions. It is the organ of exchange between the developing fetus and the mother, by which nutrients are provided to the fetus and wastes removed, and it is also an endocrine organ and produces several hormones, most notably hCG. The placenta develops from both the chorion and the maternal uterine tissue. Following implantation, the chorion develops rapidly and forms highly vascularized villi as the embryonic circulation develops. The umbilical cord develops, connecting the embryo with the placenta. Two umbilical arteries arise in the umbilical cord and connect with a rapidly proliferating network of capillaries in the villi. The umbilical vein, also located in the umbilical cord, carries blood from the villi back to the fetus.

The placenta eventually consists of the portion of the chorion that develop villi, along with the uterine tissue between the villi that contains maternal capillaries and small pools of maternal blood. The placenta brings maternal blood adjacent to fetal blood, although the two circulatory systems are completely separate from each other. Thus, oxygen and nutrient substrates pass from the maternal blood through the placental tissue and diffuse into the blood of the fetus, where these substances can be used for growth and development of various body tissues. Waste products of fetal metabolism from fetal blood then pass through the placenta into the maternal blood supply and eventually are transported to the maternal kidneys for disposal.[7]

The placenta, like the corpus luteum, secretes both estrogen and progesterone during pregnancy. These hormones serve a variety of purposes in pregnancy. Estrogen promotes enlargement of the uterus and the growth of the ductal structure of the breast, as well as altering the elasticity of various pelvic ligaments and the symphysis pubis to allow passage of

Development of the Human Embryo and Fetus

The developing organism, from fertilization to the end of the eighth week, is referred to as an embryo; from the ninth week until birth, the developing baby is referred to as a fetus. Development of the fetus proceeds as an orderly sequence of complex events. With recent developments in fetal physiology, it is possible to predict which structures will begin their development or function on a particular day of development following conception. Table 32–2 describes some important developmental events from the time of fertilization to birth. Detailed information on the development of organ systems during fetal life is contained in the chapters in this book which focus on these organ systems; for example, Chapter 35 contains a description of the development of the gastrointestinal tract.

First Month

Rapid growth, morphogenesis, and cell differentiation occur early in the development of the human embryo. By 2½ weeks of development the notochord and neural plate, which eventually give rise to the central nervous system, are formed. In addition, the tissue that will form the heart has differentiated. By the end of the first month, an S-shaped heart beats about 60 times per minute, and the three primary vesicles of the brain have formed.

Second Month

Figure 32–11 shows an embryo in its seventh week. All the organs continue to develop during the second month, and the embryo becomes capable of movement. The major blood vessels assume their final posi-

TABLE 32–2. Summary of Developmental Events in Human Fetal Life

Time From Fertilization	Key Events
24 hr	Embryo has achieved two-cell stage
3rd day	Embryo reaches uterus
7th day	Implantation of embryo in uterine wall
2.5 wk	Differentiation of heart tissue; blood cell formation in yolk sac and chorion; formation of notochord and neural plate
3.5 wk	Formation of neural tube; heart tubes begin to beat; primordial eye and ear visible; respiratory system begins development; liver bud differentiates; blood vessels established
4 wk	Formation of three primary brain vesicles; limb buds appear
2nd mo	Embryo capable of movement; cerebral cortex differentiating; gonad identifiable as testis or ovary; bones begin ossification and muscles are differentiating; major blood vessels in final positions
3rd mo	Fetus performs breathing and sucking movements; sex is clearly identifiable
5th mo	Heartbeat is audible with stethoscope; fetus moves freely through the amniotic cavity
6th–9th mo	Rapid growth with final differentiation of tissues and organs
266 days	Birth

tions and the heart assumes its final shape. The brain begins to transmit impulses to regulate the function of its organ systems, and a few reflexes are now present. While sex cannot be distinguished externally, either an ovary or testis has begun to form internally. At the end of the second month, the rudiments of all organs are present and the embryo is now referred to as a fetus.[7]

Third Month

During the third month, the ears and eyes approach their final positions, and some of the bones become distinct. The fetus performs breathing movements, moving amniotic fluid in and out of the lungs, and can carry on sucking movements. By the end of the third month, the fetus is almost 56 mm in length and weights about 14 grams (Fig. 32–12).

Second Trimester

A trimester refers to a period of 3 months during pregnancy. During the second trimester, or months 4 through 6 of development, the fetus achieves independent mobility and can move freely through the amniotic cavity. The heartbeat of the fetus is now

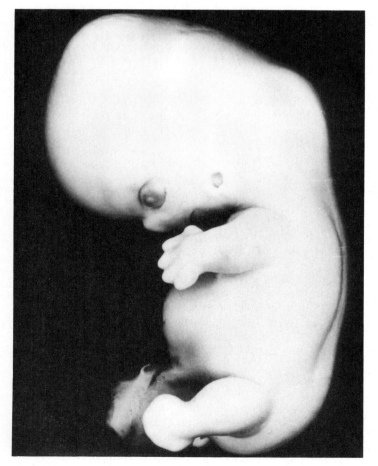

FIGURE 32–11. Human embryo in seventh week of development. (From Moore KL: *The Developing Human: Clinically Oriented Embryology,* 5th ed. Philadelphia, WB Saunders, 1993, p 85. Courtesy of Kazumasa Hoshino, M.D., former Professor of Anatomy and Director of the Congenital Anomaly Center, Faculty of Medicine, Kyoto University, Kyoto, Japan. Reproduced with permission.)

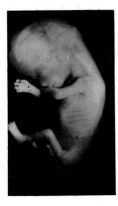

FIGURE 32–12. Photograph of human fetus at 10 weeks of development. (From Moore KL: *The Developing Human: Clinically Oriented Embryology*, 5th ed. Philadelphia, WB Saunders, 1993, p 98. Reproduced with permission.)

audible through a stethoscope and averages 150 beats per minute. By the fifth month of development, the fetus measures 250 mm (10 inches) in length, half its total length at birth.[7] Figure 32–13 shows a fetus in the second trimester at 17 weeks of development.

Third Trimester

By far the greatest growth of the fetus occurs during the third trimester. The weight of the fetus almost doubles during the last 2 months.[11] In addition, final differentiation of tissues and organs takes place. Survival of infants born prematurely during this time has increased markedly in the past few years due to an enhanced ability to sustain vital functions such as respiration and regulation of body temperature in neonatal intensive care settings.

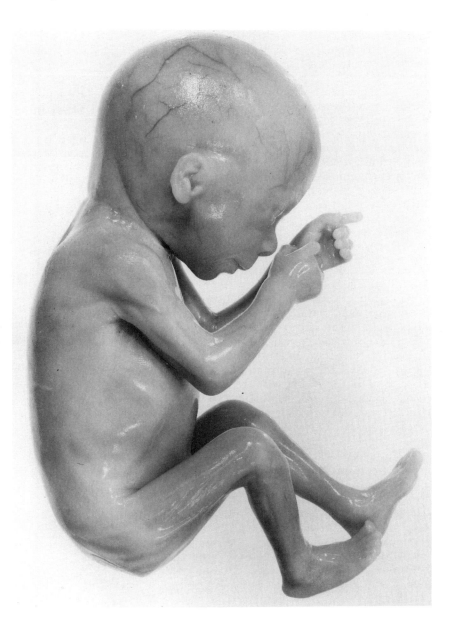

FIGURE 32–13. The human fetus at 17 weeks. (From Moore KL: *The Developing Human: Clinically Oriented Embryology*, 5th ed. Philadelphia, WB Saunders, 1993, p 100. Reproduced with permission.)

Parturition

Parturition refers to the process by which the infant is born. Toward the end of pregnancy, the uterus becomes progressively more excitable until it begins strong, rhythmic contractions that ultimately expel the infant.[11] At the present time, the exact cause of the increased uterine activity remains unknown. However, two sets of effects have been suggested as contributing to the increased excitability of uterine musculature at this time, progressive hormonal changes and progressive mechanical changes.[11,13]

Hormonal Changes

During the latter part of pregnancy, large amounts of estrogen, which have a definite tendency to increase uterine contractility, are secreted. Concurrent with this enhanced estrogen release, the secretion of progesterone, which inhibits uterine contractility, remains constant or may decrease slightly. Thus, it is hypothesized that the increased ratio of estrogen to progesterone secretion in the latter part of pregnancy may promote the increased contractility of the uterus.[11]

Oxytocin is a hormone secreted by the posterior pituitary that specifically causes uterine contraction and is thought to play a major role in promoting increased uterine contractility during parturition. The rate of oxytocin secretion is considerably increased at the time of labor (see the following discussion of mechanical changes), and the uterus exhibits an increased responsiveness to a given dose of oxytocin at this time.[11,13]

Mechanical Changes

Stretching smooth muscle organs increases their contractility; in addition, intermittent stretching of smooth muscle can elicit contraction. Thus, it is hypothesized that the stretch or irritation of the fetal head against the cervix begins a reflex action that causes the uterus to contract. As the cycle of stretching and contraction is repeated again and again, increased contractions result. In addition, stretching of the cervix causes release of oxytocin from the posterior pituitary. Oxytocin then stimulates additional uterine contractions, initiating another feedback cycle of stretching and contraction.[11,14]

Response of the Mother's Body to Pregnancy

The presence of a developing fetus in the uterus creates an extra physiologic load for the pregnant woman, with resulting effects on her basal metabolism and specific organ systems. Normal physiologic responses to pregnancy are described here; complications of pregnancy are discussed in Chapter 33.

Metabolism During Pregnancy

As a result of an increased secretion of many hormones, including thyroxine, adrenocortical hormones, and the sex hormones, the basal metabolic rate increases about 15 percent during the latter half of pregnancy.[11,15] This increase in metabolism results in alterations in many organ systems, including the circulatory, respiratory, and urinary systems.

Changes in the Female Reproductive Organs

The hormones secreted during pregnancy, either by the placenta or by the endocrine glands, directly promote alterations in body structures. In particular, the organs of the female reproductive tract increase markedly in size, with the uterus increasing from 30 to 1,100 grams and the breasts approximately doubling in size. Concurrently the vagina enlarges, with a widening of the vaginal introitus.

Changes in the Circulatory System

In the latter stages of pregnancy, about 625 mL of blood flows through the maternal circulation of the placenta each minute. This factor, along with a general increase in metabolism, causes an increase in maternal cardiac output of 30 to 40 percent above normal by the 27th week of pregnancy. However, for reasons not understood at the present time, the cardiac output decreases to a little above normal during the last 8 weeks of pregnancy, although the high uterine blood flow continues.[11]

As shown in Figure 32–14, an increase in maternal blood volume occurs, mainly during the latter half of pregnancy. This increase is mainly due to hormonal factors. Both aldosterone and estrogens, which are greatly increased in pregnancy, promote increased fluid retention by the kidneys. In addition, the bone marrow increases its activity to produce an excess of red blood cells to accompany the excess vascular volume. At the time of parturition, the mother has an additional 1 to 2 extra liters of blood in her circulatory system.[11]

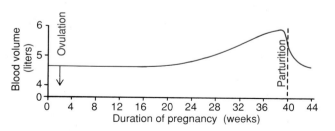

F I G U R E 32–14. Effect of pregnancy on blood volume. (From Guyton AC: *Textbook of Medical Physiology.* 8th ed. Philadelphia, WB Saunders, 1991, p 922. Reproduced with permission.)

Changes in the Respiratory System

The increased basal metabolic rate and size of the pregnant woman result is an increase in oxygen utilization to 20 percent above normal at the time of birth. Concurrently, a commensurate amount of carbon dioxide is formed. In addition, the growing uterus is pressing upward against the abdominal organs, which in turn press against the diaphragm, with a resulting decrease in diaphragmatic excursion. The net result of these changes is an increase in minute ventilation of approximately 50 percent and a decrease in arterial Pco_2 to slightly below normal.[11]

Changes in the Urinary System

Due to an increased load of excretory products, the rate of urine formation in pregnancy is usually slightly increased. In addition, other alterations in urinary function occur. Renal tubular reabsorption of sodium, chloride, and water is increased as a result of increased production of steroidal hormones by the placenta and adrenal cortex. Concurrently the glomerular filtration rate often increases as much as 50 percent, which serves to increase the rate of water and electrolyte loss in the urine. These two events tend to balance out each other, with the result that only a moderate excess of water and salt accumulation occurs under normal circumstances.[11] However, in the condition of toxemia of pregnancy, excess water and salt accumulation may occur, with life-threatening consequences.

Weight Gain and Nutrition During Pregnancy

The average weight gain during pregnancy is about 24 pounds, with most of this gain occurring during the last two trimesters. Approximately 7 pounds of this weight gain is the fetus, 4 pounds of the increased weight is amniotic fluid, placenta, and fetal membranes; 2 pounds represents an increase in uterine tissue; and another 2 pounds of the weight gain is an increase in breast tissue. Thus, an average of a 9-pound increase in the weight of the remainder of the woman's body occurs. Approximately 6 pounds of fluid may be excreted during the days following the birth, after the loss of the fluid-retaining hormones of the placenta.[11]

Appetite may be greatly increased during the latter part of pregnancy, in part due to fetal removal of food substrates from the mother's blood and in part due to hormonal factors. The developing fetus assumes priority in regard to many of the nutritional substrates of the mother's body fluids and will continue to grow even when maternal nutrition is inadequate. However, while fetal length may increase normally in the absence of adequate maternal nutrition, fetal weight will be considerably decreased, and abnormal bone formation and a decreased size of many bodily organs of the fetus may result.[11]

If the intake of nutritional elements during pregnancy is inadequate, a number of deficiencies can be present in the mother. In particular, deficiencies of calcium, phosphates, iron, and the vitamins may be present. As an example, approximately 375 mg of iron is needed by the fetus to form its blood, and an additional 600 mg is needed by the mother to form her own extra blood supply. As the normal store of nonhemoglobin iron in the mother at the beginning of pregnancy is often about 100mg and seldom above 700 mg, a pregnant woman will develop anemia without sufficient iron intake in her food.[11,16]

KEY CONCEPTS

- At about the seventh day after fertilization, the embryo attaches to the uterine lining. The placenta is the fetal lifeline, providing nutrients and oxygen and eliminating wastes. The placenta also secretes human chorionic gonadotropin, which is important in maintaining pregnancy.
- Normal gestation is about 9 months. Each 3-month period is called a trimester. By the end of the first trimester, fetal structures and organ systems are present. During the second and third trimesters, the fetus grows in size and weight.
- Near the end of the third trimester, an increase in estrogen production and mechanical stretching of the uterus and cervix are thought to induce parturition. Cervical stretching stimulates the release of oxytocin from the pituitary. Oxytocin stimulates uterine contractions.
- Pregnancy is associated with many physiologic changes. These include an increased basal metabolic rate (15 percent), increased cardiac output (30–40 percent) and blood volume (1–2 liters), increased oxygen consumption (20 percent) and minute ventilation (50 percent), increased glomerular filtration rate and tubular reabsorption of sodium and water, and increased body weight (24 pounds).

Menopause

Although **menopause** is defined specifically as the last menstrual period in a woman's reproductive life, the term is often used to denote the entire period of years before and after this event in which the function of the ovaries is in transition. The terms *climacteric* and *perimenopause* are used in the health care literature to describe this transitional period.[17] At about age 45 to 52 years, the supply of ovarian follicles declines, with the majority becoming atretic or degenerated. With the depletion of the ovarian follicles, secretion of estrogen and progesterone by the ovaries declines, and the menstrual cycle becomes irregular. When too little estrogen is secreted to cause endometrial growth, menstrual periods stop permanently.

The decline in ovarian hormone production that occurs in the perimenopause causes important physi-

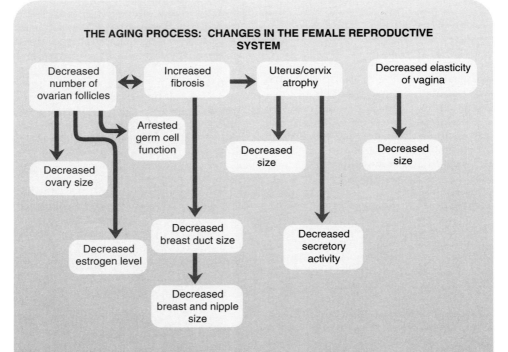

THE AGING PROCESS: CHANGES IN THE FEMALE REPRODUCTIVE SYSTEM

Female reproductive system function declines with organ specific tissue changes. Active female germ cells decline over time with variable function before they are arrested in menopause. The ovaries become smaller and increasingly fibrotic and have a smaller number of ovarian follicles.

The secretion of estrogen by the ovaries stops at menopause, resulting in a marked estrogen level decrease. The ovarian follicles become insensitive to gonadotropins (FSH and LH). However, the peripheral conversion of androgens to estrogen causes a small maintenance level of estrogen to persist at 10% to 30% of previous levels. The androgen producing ovarian cells (hilar and thecal) continue to remain active, leading to a slight increase in testosterone levels in post-menopausal women.

The follicles, uterus, and cervix undergo atrophy, with a decrease in size and secretory action. The vagina is reduced in size, with a loss of elasticity and atrophy of the vaginal epithelium. The vascular supply to the vaginal walls decreases with reduced glycogen and mucopolysaccharide. The pH of Bartholin gland secretions is increased or alkaline due to the loss of estrogen.

The breasts decrease in size. Breast ducts become smaller and are replaced by fat tissue. Some fibrosis and calcification may occur within the ducts. The nipples are smaller with less nipple pigmentation. The aging female's nipples may be normal or retracted.

Faith Young Peterson

ologic changes in a woman's body. The decline in plasma estrogen levels may result in a number of distressing symptoms, although many women experience no symptoms during this time. Hot flashes, described by women as an unpleasant sensation of sudden warmth sweeping upward over the abdomen, chest, neck, and face, are experienced by nearly 75 percent of postmenopausal women. Although the precise cause of hot flushes is still unknown, it is thought that decreased estrogen levels have an effect on the temperature-regulating center in the hypothalamus.[3] Hot flashes are often accompanied by other symptoms of autonomic nervous system instability, such as tachycardia, palpitations, and feelings of faintness. Other distressing symptoms, including pain and stiffness in the joints, sleep pattern disturbances, and changes in gastrointestinal function, have been noted by women in the perimenopausal period. These symptoms are presently the focus of many nursing research projects examining the health of aging women. While such psychological symptoms as increased nervousness have been reported in the medical literature as being related to hormonal imbalance in the menopause, it has been established that psychological symptoms are not directly related to estrogen deficiency.[18,19]

With the decline of estrogen associated with the perimenopause, many structural changes occur in various organs. The epidermis of the skin becomes thinner and less elastic throughout the entire body. The breasts may decrease in size; the labia may also lose their underlying fat and become thinner. The vaginal epithelium may become thin and atrophied, with the result that sexual intercourse may be painful. The decline in estrogen also leads to osteoporosis and decreased bone density, particularly in caucasian women, with resulting bone fractures. Exercise and supplemental calcium and vitamin D are recommended for postmenopausal women in order to prevent accelerated bone loss. At present, some authorities recommend estrogen therapy during perimenopause to prevent osteoporosis and relieve symptoms such as hot flashes and vaginal atrophy.[19,20] However, supplemental estrogen therapy has been associated with certain health risks. Women in perimenopause may wish to discuss the risks and potential benefits of estrogen therapy with their health care providers before making an informed decision about these medications.

KEY CONCEPTS

- Menopause begins at age 45 to 52 years and denotes the cessation of menstruation. Ovarian demise, with the loss of estrogen and progesterone production, results in irregular menses and then complete cessation of menstruation.

- Declines in estrogen production are associated with hot flashes, tachycardia, palpitations, faintness, joint pains, and sleep disturbances. Structural

changes with menopause include osteoporosis, thin skin, and atrophy of the vaginal structures and breast tissue.

Summary

This chapter has described the major processes related to the human female reproductive tract, including the menstrual cycle, pregnancy, lactation, and menopause. In approaching this material, the reader must view this information within the current context of social change in which women are taking an active role in meeting their health care needs. In addition, recent research in the area of reproductive endocrinology has yielded a rapidly expanding understanding of the reproductive structures and their function.

The female reproductive structures are a complex set of organs with multiple, integrated functions. A careful review of the section on the reproductive structures, including their embryologic development, will assist the reader in understanding the various alterations in these structures that occur throughout a woman's life. While the hormonal and structural changes occurring in the female reproductive organs may at first seem overwhelmingly complex to the student, some basic concepts will help in organizing this material. First, the **menstrual cycle** has two significant results: the production of an ovum and the preparation of the uterus for the implantation of the fertilized ovum. Second, the fertilized ovum contains the entire encoded genetic instructions to produce a unique human individual. Third, **pregnancy** consists of three basic developmental processes—growth, morphogenesis, and cellular differentiation—to bring about this transformation, which will also result in multiple changes in the body of the mother. The breast, with its function of **lactation,** is also a component of the reproductive system, and is subject to alterations throughout a woman's lifespan. Finally, **menopause** is not a discrete event but a *process* during which the supply of ovarian follicles declines. A review of these concepts will prepare the student for a better understanding of women's health concerns and provide a basis for approaching the next chapter, on alterations in reproductive function.

REFERENCES

1. Rodriguez-Trias H: Women's health, women's lives, women's rights. *Am J Public Health* 1992;82(5):663–664.
2. Senanayake P: Women's reproductive health—challenges for the 1990s. *Adv Contracept* 1991;7(2–3):129–136.
3. Steiner RA: Endocrine control of reproduction, in Patton HD, Fuchs AF, Hille B, Scher AM, Steiner R (eds): *Textbook of Physiology*, 21st ed. Philadelphia, WB Saunders, 1989.
4. Persaud TVN: Embryology of the female genital tract and gonads. In Copeland LJ (ed): *Textbook of Gynecology*. Philadelphia, WB Saunders, 1993.
5. Anbazhagan R, Bartek J, Monaghan P, Gusterson BA: Growth and development of the human infant breast. *Am J Anat* 1991;192(4):407–417.
6. Luckmann J, Sorenson KC (eds): *Medical-Surgical Nursing: A Psychophysical Approach,* 3rd ed. Philadelphia, WB Saunders, 1987.

7. Solomon EP: *Introduction to Human Anatomy and Physiology.* Philadelphia, WB Saunders, 1992.

8. Bartoli JM, Moulin G, Delannoy L, Chagnaud C, Kasbarian M: The normal uterus on magnetic resonance imaging and variations associated with the hormonal state. *Surg Radiol Anat* 1991;13(3):213–220.

9. Guyton AC: *Human Physiology and Mechanism of Disease,* 5th ed. Philadelphia, WB Saunders, 1992.

10. Forsyth IA: The mammary gland. *Baillieres Clin Endocrinol Metab* 1991;5(4):809–832.

11. Guyton AC: *Textbook of Medical Physiology,* 8th ed. Philadelphia, WB Saunders, 1991.

12. Ferguson JE, Schor AM, Howell A, Ferguson MW: Changes in the extracellular matrix of the normal human breast during the menstrual cycle. *Cell Tissue Res* 1991;268(1):167–177.

13. Blackburn ST, Loper DL (eds): *Maternal, Fetal, and Neonatal Physiology: A Clinical Perspective.* Philadelphia, WB Saunders, 1992.

14. Harbert GM: Assessment of uterine contractility and activity. *Clin Obstet Gynecol* 1992;35(3):546–558.

15. Katz VL: Physiologic changes during normal pregnancy. *Curr Opin Obstet Gynecol* 1991;3(6):750–775.

16. Beischer NA, Mackay EV, Purcal NK: *Care of the Pregnant Woman and Her Baby,* 2nd ed. Philadelphia, WB Saunders, 1990.

17. Utian WH: Menopause—a proposed new functional definition. *Maturities* 1991;14(1):1–2.

18. Bates GW, Boone WR: The female reproductive cycle: New variations on an old theme. *Curr Opin Obstet Gynecol* 1991; 3(6):838–843.

19. Barber HR: *Perimenopausal and Geriatric Gynecology.* New York, Macmillan, 1988.

20. Hacker NF, Moore JG (eds): *Essentials of Obstetrics and Gynecology,* 2nd ed. Philadelphia, WB Saunders, 1992.

BIBLIOGRAPHY

Beckmann CR: *Obstetrics and Gynecology for Medical Students.* Baltimore, Williams & Wilkins, 1992.

Berger H: *Vitamins and Minerals in Pregnancy and Lactation.* New York, Raven Press, 1988, Nestlé Nutrition Workshop Series, vol 16.

Butler RN: Improving older women's health. *Geriatrics* 1991; 46(11):15.

Callen PW (ed): *Ultrasonography in Obstetrics and Gynecology,* 2nd ed. Philadelphia, WB Saunders, 1988.

Fogel CI, Lauver D (ed): *Sexual Health Promotion.* Philadelphia, WB Saunders, 1990.

Gershenson DM, DeCherney AH, Curry SL (eds): *Operative Gynecology.* Philadelphia, WB Saunders, 1993.

Harlap S: The benefits and risks of hormone replacement therapy: An epidemiologic overview. *Am J Obstet Gynecol* 1992;166(6 pt 2):1986–1992.

Jacob S, Francone CA: *Elements of Anatomy and Physiology,* 2nd ed. Philadelphia, WB Saunders, 1989.

MacLaren A, Kenner CA: *Student Manual to Maternal, Neonatal, and Women's Health Nursing.* Springhouse, Penn, Springhouse Publishing Co, 1991.

Murtagh J, Krins T: Patient education: Your pregnancy. *Aust Fam Physician* 1991;20(12):1765.

Soares MJ, Faria TN, Roby KF, Deb S: Pregnancy and the prolactin family of hormones: Coordination of anterior pituitary, uterine, and placental expression. *Endocr Rev* 1991;12(4):402–423.

Sweet BR: *Mayes' Midwifery,* 11th ed. Philadelphia, WB Saunders, 1988.

Thompson ED (ed): *Introduction to Maternity and Pediatric Nursing.* Philadelphia, WB Saunders, 1990.

Weiner SM: *Clinical Manual of Maternity and Gynecologic Nursing.* St. Louis, Mosby–Year Book, 1989.

CHAPTER 33

Alterations in Structure and Function of the Female Reproductive System

JANE M. GEORGES

abruptio placenta: Premature separation of the placenta prior to delivery; the separation may be partial or complete, and may result in overt or concealed hemorrhage.

amenorrhea: Absence or suppression of menstrual bleeding, usually due to an altered pattern of hormonal functioning that interrupts the normal sequence of endometrial proliferation and sloughing.

cystocele: Protrusion of a portion of the urinary bladder into the anterior vagina at a weakened part of the vaginal musculature. Predisposing factors include obesity, aging, an inherent weakness, a history of heavy object lifting, or an injury during either childbirth or surgery.

dysfunctional uterine bleeding: Abnormal endometrial bleeding not associated with tumor, inflammation, pregnancy, trauma, or hormonal effects. It is most common around the time of menarche and menopause.

dysmenorrhea: Pain associated with menstruation, usually classified as either primary (unrelated to an identifiable disease) or secondary (related to the presence of an underlying disease).

endometriosis: Growth of endometrial tissue outside the lining of the uterine cavity; an abnormal condition with potentially destructive effects on the pelvic organs.

leiomyoma: Benign neoplasm of the smooth muscle of the uterus that is characteristically firm, well-circumscribed, and round. Uterine leiomyomas usually appear and exhibit growth activity during the reproductive years.

placenta previa: Conditions of pregnancy in which the placenta is implanted abnormally over the internal cervical os. It occurs in varying degrees of severity and may result in sudden massive hemorrhage following dilatation of the internal os.

pregnancy-induced hypertension: The rapid rise of arterial blood pressure associated with a loss of large amounts of protein in the urine occurring during pregnancy. Women at risk for pregnancy-induced hypertension (PIH) include teenagers and women in their late thirties and early forties. (PIH is also known as toxemia and pre-eclampsia-eclampsia.)

rectocele: Protrusion of the anterior rectal wall into posterior vagina at a weakened part of the vaginal musculature. It usually results from an injury during either childbirth or surgery, and it may also be the result of the aging process or an inherent weakness in the vaginal wall.

*T*he complex functioning of the female reproductive system described in Chapter 32 may be subject to alterations in structure and function throughout a woman's life that can have far-reaching effects on her health and well-being. This chapter is intended to be a survey of these alterations, and will describe the pathophysiologic basis of the most common disorders of the female reproductive system. In addition, current therapeutics for these alterations, including pharmacologic therapy, will be summarized. The information presented here is intended as an introduction to these complex areas, and the reader may wish to consult in-depth gynecology and obstetrics texts for more detailed information.

Perhaps no other function of the human body is so closely linked to psychological, social, and spiritual concerns as is reproductive function. Any alteration in reproductive status (or the perceived threat of such an alteration) may have profound effects on an individual. Clinicians caring for women experiencing alterations in the functioning of the reproductive system need to bear in mind the profundity of such alterations for the individual woman, and must also maintain an awareness of the context in which women seek help for such problems. A clinical approach in which information is freely shared between caregiver and client and in which mutual decision making is an integral part of the therapeutic environment is a necessary component of care for women seeking help for reproductive concerns. Previous clinical approaches in which women's concerns were labeled as unimportant or merely psychogenic often resulted in anger, frustration with health care providers, and withdrawal from the health care delivery system. Women consumers of health care are now seeking an active involvement in their care, and clinicians who care for women experiencing the alterations described in this chapter need to approach women's health concerns with sensitivity and openness.

Menstrual Disorders

Alterations in the normal functioning of the menstrual cycle include uterine bleeding disorders and dysmenorrhea, or painful menstruation. These disorders may be primary, meaning that no other recognizable physiologic disorder is present, or secondary, meaning that the abnormality is a sign of an underlying pathophysiologic process such as a neoplasm or blood coagulation disorder.

Uterine Bleeding Disorders

Amenorrhea

Amenorrhea is the absence or suppression of menstruation. Amenorrhea is normal before menarche (the first menstrual period at the time of puberty), after menopause, and during pregnancy and lactation.[1] At other times it is considered pathologic and may result from a wide range of pathophysiologic causes. In the majority of cases, amenorrhea is due to an abnormal pattern of hormonal functioning that interrupts the normal sequence of events in which the endometrial tissue lining the uterus proliferates and then sloughs off. The endometrial tissue must be stimulated and regulated by the proper quantity and sequence of the female sex hormones, estrogen and progesterone, and the gonadotropic hormones, follicle-stimulating hormone (FSH) and luteinizing hormone (LH). As described in Chapter 32, the menstrual cycle depends on essential changes in estrogen levels at key moments. The initial rise in LH and FSH in the menstrual cycle occurs in response to a decline in estrogen and progesterone; estrogen levels will then again rise in response to the actions of the gonadotropic hormones, and the endometrium proliferates again in response to estrogen secretion. Thus, events that prevent estrogen production, interfere with the normal fluctuations in estrogen levels, or block the actions of estrogen on the endometrium will result in abnormal or absent menstrual flow.[2] Such events may include physical or emotional stress, which can interfere with normal production of the gonadotropic hormones and alter the pattern of estrogen functioning. In addition, ovarian, adrenal, or pituitary tumors may interfere with the normal production of female sex hormones or LH and FSH. Neoplasms of the ovaries or adrenal and pituitary glands may result in an excess or deficit production of these hormones, with a consequent interruption in normal menstrual flow. Therapeutic strategies for amenorrhea are directed toward correcting the cause of the interruption in hormonal functioning, and may include the use of hormonal supplementation to reinstate a normal sequence of events in the menstrual cycle. If amenorrhea is the result of a neoplastic process, surgery may be indicated for tumor removal.

Abnormal Uterine Bleeding Patterns

Irregular or excessive bleeding from the uterus is one of the most common alterations in the female reproductive system. Uterine bleeding that varies from a woman's normal pattern either in quantity or in frequency may occur at any age and for a variety of reasons. The most common alterations in uterine bleeding patterns and their causes are described here. **Metrorrhagia,** or bleeding between menstrual periods, usually results from slight physiologic bleeding from the endometrium during ovulation but may also result from other causes, such as uterine malignancy, cervical erosions, endometrial polyps, or as a side effect of estrogen therapy.[1] **Hypomenorrhea,** or a deficient amount of menstraul flow, results from endocrine or systemic disorders that may interfere with the proper functioning of the hormones in the menstrual cycle, or may be due to partial obstruction of the menstrual flow by the hymen or a narrowing of the cervical os. **Oligomenorrhea,** or infrequent menstruation, usually reflects failure to ovulate due to an endocrine or systemic disorder with accompanying inappropriate hormonal function. Similarly, **polymenorrhea,** an increased frequency of menstruation, may be associated with an ovulation due to endocrine or systemic factors. **Menorrhagia,** an increase in the amount or duration of menstrual bleeding, usually results from lesions of the female reproductive organs such as uterine leiomyomas, endometrial polyps, and endometrial hyperplasia. It may also result from such inflammatory processes such as endometritis (an inflammatory condition of the uterine endometrium) or salpingitis (an inflammation or infection of the oviduct).[1,3]

The term **dysfunctional uterine bleeding** is used to describe abnormal endometrial bleeding not associated with tumor, inflammation, pregnancy, trauma, or hormonal effects. Dysfunctional uterine bleeding is most common around the time of menarche and menopause, and not as common in women between the ages of 20 and 35.[2,4] In adolescents, dysfunctional uterine bleeding is most often due to immaturity in the functioning of the pituitary and ovary, which have not yet properly orchestrated their activities.[5] Thus, an imbalance may be present in the ratio of estrogen to progesterone. Absent or diminished levels of progesterone will result in a thick and extremely vascular endometrium that lacks structural support. As a result of this fragile structure, spontaneous and superficial hemorrhage occurs randomly throughout the endometrium. In addition, the blood vessels in the endometrium fail to constrict to limit the extent and duration of the bleeding.[2] Uterine bleeding that is abnormal in both quantity and frequency can therefore occur in a noncyclic pattern.

In perimenopausal women, dysfunctional uterine bleeding may be the result of the progressive degeneration and failure of the ovary to produce estrogen. As ovarian follicles diminish in number, the production of estrogen by the ovary becomes unpredictable, and the secretion of LH and FSH may also assume an unpredictable pattern. As in the adolescent with dysfunctional uterine bleeding, diminished or absent production of progesterone may result in unopposed stimulation of the endometrium by estrogen, with subsequent unpredictable bleeding from a fragile endometrium.[2]

Dysmenorrhea

Dysmenorrhea is menstruation that is painful enough to limit normal activity or to cause a woman to seek health care. Dysmenorrhea is a widespread phenomenon that affects many women across the reproductive years, including high-school-age girls through perimenopausal women. Although symptoms of dysmenorrhea tend to decrease with age, the traditional notion that childbirth permanently decreases symptoms is unfounded. In addition, the contention that women with dysmenorrhea tend to be neurotic has been refuted in well-designed psychiatric research studies.[2] Recent research into the physiology of uterine contractions has enhanced our understanding of the causes of dysmenorrhea and led to better treatment.

Etiology and Treatment

Dysmenorrhea is usually classified as primary (not related to any identifiable pathology) or secondary (related to an underlying pathology). The cramps that occur with primary dysmenorrhea usually are located in the suprapubic region and are sharp in quality. The pain may radiate to the inner thighs and lower sacrum and may be accompanied by nausea, diarrhea, and headache.[2] Primary dsymenorrhea usually develops 1 or 2 years after menarche, when ovulatory cycles are established.[5] Under the influence of progesterone, increased amounts of prostaglandins, potent hormonelike unsaturated fatty acids, are released from the endometrium. Prostaglandins have significant effects on smooth muscle and vasomotor tone; when released from the endometrium, prostaglandins promote uterine contractions and ischemia of the endometrial capillaries, causing the cramping pain of dysmenorrhea.[3] Recent therapeutic strategies for management of primary dysmenorrhea have focused on the phenomenon of prostaglandin-induced enhanced uterine contractility. The use of prostaglandin synthetase inhibitors (PGSIs) such as ibuprofen and naproxen, which inhibit the formation of prostaglandins, has been very effective in many women experiencing dysmenorrhea.[2] Other approaches that use steroid hormones such as progestins or combined high-progestin/low-estrogen oral contraceptives have also been used. The rationale is that production of the high menstrual levels of prostaglandins needed to produce dysmenorrhea requires high levels of estrogen without progesterone in the proliferative phase of the menstrual cycle. Giving progestins, therefore, inhibits the production of prostaglandins and relieves the symptoms of dysmenorrhea.[2] However, the use of steroid hormones involves significant risks, which the individual client must weigh against the benefits of such therapy.

Secondary dysmenorrhea is characterized more often by dull pain that may increase with age. It is associated with pelvic disorders such as endometriosis, leiomyomas, or pelvic adhesions. Therapeutic strategies may involve diagnostic operative procedures such as laparoscopy, and medical and surgical therapy for the underlying condition.[3]

KEY CONCEPTS

- Amenorrhea, the absence of menstruation, is most commonly due to hormonal disturbances. Stress and neoplasms (ovarian, adrenal, or pituitary tumors) may interfere with the normal patterns of hormone secretion. Treatment is aimed at the underlying cause of the hormonal imbalance.

- Irregular or excessive uterine bleeding is a common problem. Metrorrhagia is bleeding between periods, hypomenorrhea is reduced menstrual flow, oligomenorrhea is infrequent menstruation, polymenorrhea is an increased frequency of menstruation, and menorrhagia is prolonged and heavy bleeding during menstruation. These disorders may be associated with hormonal imbalances or primary lesions of the reproductive tract.

- Dysfunctional uterine bleeding is common at menarche and menopause and is due to irregular secretion of reproductive hormones. Other causes of abnormal bleeding such as tumor, trauma, inflammation, and endocrine diseases are ruled out before the diagnosis of dysfunctional uterine bleeding is made.

- Dysmenorrhea is painful menstruation, generally described as sharp suprapubic cramping severe enough to limit activity. Dysmenorrhea may be treated with prostaglandin inhibitors. Dysmenorrhea secondary to pelvic disorders (endometriosis, adhesions) generally has a dull quality and may increase with age.

Alterations in Uterine Position and Pelvic Support

Alterations in uterine position and pelvic support may occur anytime during a woman's reproductive years. The major support for the uterus and upper vagina is provided by the thickenings of the endopelvic fascia known as the cardinal ligaments. Although tearing of the cardinal ligaments during labor and delivery is rare, they can be stretched abnormally during a difficult or prolonged delivery and subsequently fail to support the pelvic organs adequately.[4] In addition, congenital defects in the muscles of the pelvic floor may promote alterations in the position of the uterus and other pelvic structures. The two most common alterations in uterine position are **uterine prolapse** and **retrodisplacement** of the uterus. Other commonly occurring alterations resulting from a weakening of the vaginal and pelvic floor musculature are **cystocele** and **rectocele**.

Uterine Prolapse

The axis of the uterus normally forms an acute angle with the axis of the vagina. This anatomic feature itself tends to prevent a prolapse, or sinking, of the uterus from its normal position. Descent of the uterus occurs when supporting structures such as the uterosacral ligaments and the cardinal ligaments relax, altering the relationship of the uterus to the vaginal axis. This relaxation permits the cervix to sag downward into the vagina. If the support of the vaginal wall is also compromised, the pressure of the abdominal organs on the uterus will gradually force it downward through the vagina into the introitus.[4] Uterine prolapse may occur at any age. In female infants and in women who have never given birth, congenital defects in the basic integrity of the pelvic supporting structures are usually responsible. Trauma to the ligaments during childbirth is the cause of uterine prolapse in women who have given birth, particularly if multiple deliveries have occurred. Uterine prolapse is classified as first, second, or third degree according to the level to which the uterus has descended. In first-degree prolapse, the uterus is approximately halfway between the vaginal introitus and the level of the ischial spines. In second-degree prolapse, the end of the cervix has begun to protrude through the introitus. In a third-degree or complete prolapse, the entire body of the uterus is outside the vaginal introitus. Figure 33–1 shows a third-degree or complete uterine prolapse.

Clinical Manifestations

The symptoms of uterine prolapse will depend on the degree of severity of prolapse. The woman may become increasingly aware of a sensation of bearing down and discomfort in the vagina. If the prolapse has advanced to the second or third degree, she may note discomfort while walking or sitting and difficulty urinating. In addition, as the end of the cervix begins to protrude outside the body, it may be subject to trauma from friction and ulceration. Bleeding and ulceration of the cervix may be present.

Treatment

Surgical treatment of uterine prolapse is usually chosen. The faulty supporting structures are approached vaginally and a repair is made. In very old patients

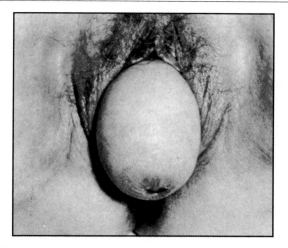

FIGURE 33–1. Complete uterine prolapse. (From Parsons L, Sommers SC: *Gynecology,* 2nd ed. Philadelphia, WB Saunders, 1978, p 1443. Reproduced with permission.)

who are a poor risk for surgery, a pessary, which is a small supportive device, is inserted to hold the uterus in place.[4]

Retrodisplacement of the Uterus

The term retrodisplacement refers to situations in which the body of the uterus is displaced from its usual location overlying the bladder to a position in the posterior pelvis.[4] As shown in Figure 33–2, the uterus may be in one of five positions: anteverted, midposition, anteflexed, retroflexed, or retroverted.

Retrodisplacement can be detected in 20 to 30 percent of all women.[4] It may be due to a congenital defect and therefore is present throughout a woman's entire life, or it may develop after childbirth when the supporting structures are injured.

Clinical Manifestations

In many women, no symptoms occur from uterine retrodisplacement. Symptoms of pelvic pain or pressure, dysmenorrhea, and dyspareunia (painful intercourse) may be present in other women. In addition, infertility has been associated with the presence of retrodisplacement.[4]

Treatment

If the woman has no symptoms, no treatment is indicated. The use of a pessary to support the uterus in a normal position may relieve symptoms. Surgical correction is sometimes indicated for severe symptoms.[4]

Cystocele

A cystocele is a protrusion of a portion of the urinary bladder into the anterior vagina at a weakened part

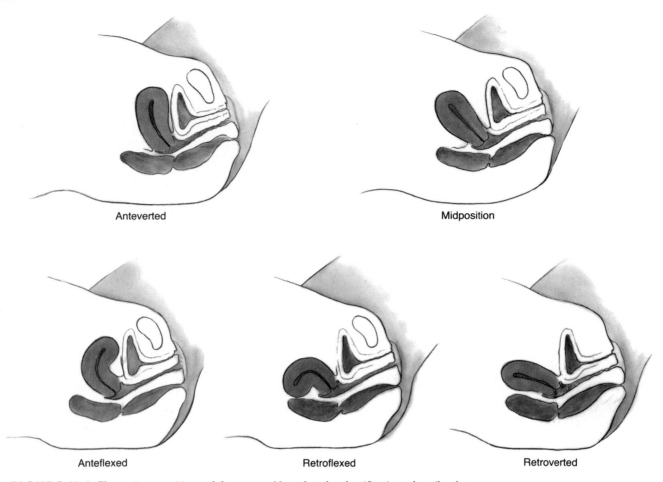

Anteverted

Midposition

Anteflexed

Retroflexed

Retroverted

FIGURE 33–2. The various positions of the uterus. Note that the classifications describe the position of the long axis of the uterus with respect to the long axis of the body. (From Jarvis C: *Physical Examination and Health Assessment.* Philadelphia, WB Saunders, 1992, p 852. Reproduced with permission.)

of the vaginal musculature (Fig. 33–3). The defect in the vaginal wall is usually caused by injury during childbirth or surgery but may also result from the aging process or as an inherent weakness. Other predisposing factors include obesity and a history of heavy-object lifting. The pressure created by this protrusion causes the anterior vaginal wall to bulge in a downward direction.[6]

Clinical Manifestations

A wide range of symptoms may be present, depending on the degree of severity of the cystocele. A mild degree of protrusion of the bladder may result in no symptoms. In moderate to severe cases, a sensation of pressure in the vagina is felt, along with dysuria and back pain. Fullness at the vaginal opening may be observed, as may a soft, reducible mucosal mass bulging into the anterior introitus of the vagina.[6]

Treatment

Surgical repair of the vagina is done to correct the cystocele and reestablish the support of the anterior vaginal wall. The bladder is restored to a normal position by reinforcing the weakened portion of the anterior vaginal wall.[6]

Rectocele

A **rectocele** (also called proctocele) is a protrusion of the anterior rectal wall into the posterior vagina at a weakened part of the vaginal musculature (see Fig. 33–3). As for a cystocele, the defect in the vaginal wall is usually caused by injury during childbirth or surgery but may also occur with aging or as an inherent weakness. Other predisposing factors for a rectocele include multiparity, obesity, and postmenopausal status. The rectocele forms a bulging mass

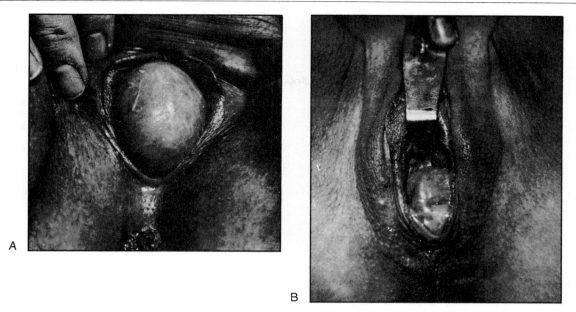

FIGURE 33–3. Cystocele (**A**) and rectocele (**B**). (From Huffman JW: *Gynecology and Obstetrics.* Philadelphia, WB Saunders, 1962. Reproduced with permission.)

beneath the posterior vaginal mucosa and pushes downward into the lower vaginal canal. Over time, the rectum may be torn from the fascial and muscular attachments of the pelvic wall. The levator ani muscles may also become stretched or torn.[6]

Clinical Manifestations

A wide range of symptoms may be present, depending on the degree of severity of the rectocele. The client may report a history of difficulty in bowel evacuation and may have experienced chronic constipation with laxative and enema dependency. A feeling of pressure may also be reported, along with painful sexual intercourse. Physical examination reveals a mass bulging into the posterior introitus of the vagina.[6]

Treatment

A surgical repair of the vagina is done to correct the rectocele and reestablish the support of the posterior vaginal wall. The rectum is restored to its normal location and the levator ani muscles are brought together in a proper position.[6]

KEY CONCEPTS

- Uterine prolapse occurs when supporting pelvic structures relax and the cervix sags downward into the vagina. Congenital defects, pregnancy, and childbirth are the usual contributing factors. Prolapse may be accompanied by a sensation of pelvic fullness and vaginal discomfort.

- Retrodisplacement of the uterus is common (20–30 percent of women) and may be associated with congenital defects, pregnancy, and childbirth. The body of the uterus is flexed or rotated into the posterior pelvis, leading to varied symptoms of pelvic pain or pressure, dysmenorrhea, and dyspareunia.

- A cystocele may result from weakness in the vaginal musculature that allows the urinary bladder to protrude into the anterior vagina. Contributing factors include childbirth, surgery, aging, obesity, and heavy lifting. Vaginal pressure, dysuria, and back pain may be present.

- A rectocele may result from weakness in the posterior vaginal musculature that allows the rectum to protrude into the vagina. Contributing factors are similar to those for cystocele. Symptoms include constipation, painful bowel evacuation, and painful intercourse.

Inflammation and Infection of the Female Reproductive Tract

Inflammatory and infectious processes of the female reproductive tract may have effects that range from discomfort to life-threatening situations. As the infectious agents responsible for inflammation and infection of the female genital tract may be sexually transmitted, there is some overlap in the discussion of these processes and sexually transmitted diseases. This chapter will describe the two principal inflammatory and infectious processes of the upper and lower female reproductive tract, pelvic inflammatory disease and vulvovaginitis. The reader may wish to refer to Chapter 34 for further information on sexually transmitted infections.

Pelvic Inflammatory Disease

Pelvic inflammatory disease (PID) is any acute, subacute, recurrent, or chronic infection of the oviducts and ovaries, with involvement of the adjacent reproductive organs. It includes inflammation of the cervix (cervicitis), uterus (endometritis), oviducts (salpingitis), and ovaries (oophoritis). The connective tissue underlying these structures between the broad ligaments may also be involved, a condition called **parametritis.**[1]

Approximately 1 million women are treated for PID each year in the United States.[2] In addition, significant reproductive health problems may occur as a result of PID. One fourth of all women who have had PID will go on to experience one or more long-term health problems. Infertility is present in 20 percent of women who have had PID, and the incidence of ectopic pregnancy is increased 6 to 10 times. Chronic pelvic pain, dyspareunia, pelvic adhesions, and chronic inflammation and abscesses of the oviducts and ovaries may all occur in women following PID.[2]

Etiology

Normally, cervical secretions provide protective and defensive functions for the reproductive organs. By providing a bacteriostatic barrier, cervical mucus prevents bacterial agents present in the cervix or vagina from ascending into the uterus. Therefore, conditions or surgical procedures that alter or destroy the cervical mucus may impair this bacteriostatic mechanism. PID may follow the insertion of an intrauterine device, pelvic surgery, abortion procedures, and infection during or after pregnancy. Bacteria may also enter the uterine cavity through the bloodstream or from drainage from other foci of infection, such as a pelvic abscess, ruptured appendix, or diverticulitis of the sigmoid colon.[1]

PID can result from infection with aerobic and anaerobic organisms. The aerobic organism *Neisseria gonorrhoeae* is the most common cause, as it readily penetrates the bacteriostatic barrier of cervical mucus. However, a variety of bacterial organisms may contribute to the development of PID, including the staphylococci, streptococci, diphtheroids, and coliforms such as *Pseudomonas* and *Escherichia coli*. These bacteria are commonly found in the cervical mucus, and PID can result from infection from one or several of these. In addition, PID may occur following the multiplication of bacteria in the endometrium, which are normally nonpathogenic. During parturition, the condition of the endometrium, which is atrophic and not stimulated by estrogen, favors the multiplication of bacteria.[1]

Clinical Manifestations

The associated signs and symptoms of PID vary with the affected part of the reproductive tract but generally include abdominal tenderness and tenderness or pain of the cervix or adnexa on palpation. In addition, the temperature may be elevated above 38° C and the white blood cell count elevated above 10,000/mm³. A pelvic abscess or inflammatory mass may be present on physical examination or ultrasound, and purulent vaginal discharge may be noted.[1,2]

Treatment

Early and aggressive use of antibiotic agents best suited for the causative organisms is essential in preventing the progression of PID. Various antibiotic regimens involving the use of multiple antimicrobial agents have been suggested by the Centers for Disease Control for use in PID.[2] Inpatient hospitalization may be indicated for patients with rapidly progressing PID and those requiring surgical drainage of pelvic abscesses. Rupture of a pelvic abscess is a potentially life-threatening condition, and a total abdominal hysterectomy (removal of the uterus) with bilateral salpingo-oophorectomy (removal of both oviducts and ovaries) may be indicated in this situation.

Vulvovaginitis

Vulvovaginitis is an inflammation of the vulva (vulvitis) and vagina (vaginitis). As the vulva and vagina are anatomically close to each other, inflammation of one location usually precipitates inflammation of the other. Vulvovaginitis may occur at any time during a girl or woman's life and affects most females at some point in life.[1]

Etiology

Infection from *Candida albicans* (also called *Monilia*) accounts for approximately half of all reported cases of vulvovaginitis (an infection from *Candida* is referred to as candidiasis).[2] *Candida albicans* is a fungus that requires glucose for growth; thus, its growth may be promoted during the secretory phase of the menstrual cycle when glycogen levels increase in the vaginal environment. In addition, other conditions in which the glycogen content of the vagina is enhanced may favor candidiasis, such as pregnancy and the use of oral contraceptives. Other predisposing factors for the development of vulvovaginitis from *Candida* infection include the use of estrogen supplementation and antibiotics. Women using estrogen supplementation in the perimenopausal period may be at greater risk for candidal infection of the vagina, as glycogen content of the vagina may increase with these therapies. The mechanism by which antibiotic use promotes candidiasis is presently unclear, but it is thought that the destruction of bacteria that normally exert the protective effect of consuming *Candida* results in an overgrowth of the *Candida* population with subsequent infection.[1,2]

Other infectious agents that may result in vulvovaginitis include *Trichomonas vaginalis, Hemophilus vaginalis,* and *Neisseria gonorrhoeae.* Viral agents that may cause vulvovaginitis include venereal warts (condylomata acuminata) or herpesvirus type II. These organisms can be transmitted during sexual intercourse and are discussed in more detail in Chapter 34.

In addition to infectious processes, vulvovaginitis may be promoted by conditions or agents that irritate the vulva and vagina. Chemical irritation or allergic reactions to detergents, feminine hygiene products, and toilet paper may be a causative factor. Trauma to the vulva or vagina or the atrophy of the vaginal wall that occurs postmenopausally may predispose to vulvovaginitis as well.[1]

Clinical Manifestations

Vulvovaginitis from candidiasis results in a thick, white discharge and red, edematous mucous membranes with white flecks adhering to the vaginal wall. Intense itching usually accompanies this discharge. Vulvovaginitis from other infectious agents may involve malodorous, purulent discharge. Irritation and subsequent inflammation of the vulva and vagina may be manifested by red, swollen labia, pain on urination and intercourse, and itching.

Treatment

Appropriate medical therapy for the causative organisms is usually instituted, including nystatin for vaginal candidiasis and local and systemic antibiotic therapy for vulvovaginitis caused by bacterial agents. Cool compresses and sitz baths provide relief of itching and burning of inflamed tissues. Avoiding factors that promote irritation of the vulva, such as drying soaps and tight clothing, is also of therapeutic benefit.[1]

KEY CONCEPTS

- Pelvic inflammatory disease (PID) refers to any infection of the oviducts, ovaries, and adjacent reproductive organs. It includes cervicitis, endometritis, salpingitis, and oophoritis. Manifestations and complications of PID include infertility, ectopic pregnancy, pelvic pain, dyspareunia, and abscesses.
- Intrauterine devices, abortion, and pelvic surgery predispose to PID. *Neisseria gonorrhoeae* is the most common organism. Treatment centers on aggressive antibiotic therapy.
- Inflammation of the vulva and vagina, or vulvovaginitis, is a common problem in women. Most cases are associated with fungal infection by *Candida albicans* and manifest with a white vaginal discharge and an irritated, itchy mucosa. Predisposing factors

include chemical irritation from feminine hygiene products, trauma, allergic reactions, and antibiotic therapy that inhibits the growth of normal flora.

Benign Growths and Aberrant Tissue of the Female Reproductive Tract

Benign growths and aberrant tissue in the female reproductive tract are not uncommon; for example, 20 percent of all women over age 35 develop uterine leiomyomas.[3] The presence of benign growths or aberrant tissue in the reproductive tract may cause no symptoms and go entirely unnoticed, or may cause symptoms ranging from debilitating to life-threatening. The diagnosis of these growths or tissue may cause anxiety in the individual woman experiencing them; in spite of their benign classification, their presence can have devastating effects on the underlying reproductive structures.[7] This section will focus on three of the most common forms of benign growths and aberrant tissue in the female reproductive organs: uterine leiomyomas, ovarian cysts, and endometriosis.

Uterine Leiomyomas

Uterine **leiomyomas,** which are also called myomas or fibroids, are the most common form of uterine growths that appear in women. Their actual incidence is difficult to establish, as many myomas are either too small or inaccessibly placed to be palpated. Uterine leiomyomas occur in approximately 20 percent of all women over age 35 and affect black women three times more often than caucasian women. Age appears to be a factor in their development, as myomas are not found before the onset of puberty and rarely exhibit growth activity after menopause.

Etiology

Uterine leiomyomas make their appearance and exhibit growth activity during the reproductive years. Therefore, while the actual cause of myomas is presently unknown, it is thought that estrogen and human growth hormone (hGH) may influence tumor formation by stimulating susceptible fibromuscular elements in the uterine wall. This theory is supported by the finding that tumor growth is enhanced by large doses of estrogen and the later stages of pregnancy, when hGH levels are high. In addition, uterine leiomyomas usually shrink or disappear after menopause, when estrogen levels decrease.[1]

Clinical Manifestations

Uterine leiomyomas can grow to large sizes (Fig. 33–4). Obviously, the presence of such a large mass within the uterus will cause symptoms of abdominal

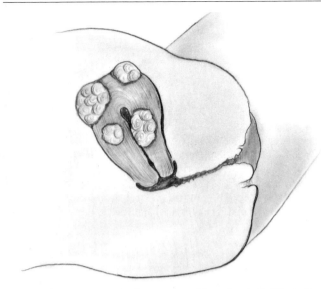

FIGURE 33–4. Uterine leiomyomas. (From Jarvis C: *Physical Examination and Health Assessment.* Philadelphia, WB Saunders, 1992, p 870. Reproduced with permission.)

pain and pressure, but smaller myomas can result in such symptoms as well. Other symptoms associated with leiomyomas may include abnormal vaginal bleeding and discharge, depending on the location of the mass. If the myoma is sufficiently large to cause pressure of the surrounding abdominal organs, backache, constipation, and urinary frequency or urgency may also be present.

Treatment

The treatment of uterine leiomyomas depends on such factors as the severity of symptoms, size and location of the leiomyoma, and the patient's age. Small myomas that cause no health problems generally are monitored carefully for growth patterns. Large or multiple masses that promote severe dysfunctional uterine bleeding or interfere with the function of the gastrointestinal tract are surgically removed, and hysterectomy may be indicated.[1]

Ovarian Cysts

Ovarian cysts are usually sacs on an ovary that contain fluid or semisolid material. Ovarian cysts can develop at any time between puberty and menopause, including during pregnancy.

Etiology

The cause of the formation of ovarian cysts is presently unknown. They can arise in several locations in the ovaries:

1. **Follicular cysts** result when a maturing ovarian follicle fails to rupture an ovum; instead, the follicle continues to enlarge and produce estrogen.

2. **Granulosa-lutein cysts** occur when the corpus luteum fails to degenerate normally; the cyst continues to grow and produce progesterone.
3. **Theca-lutein cysts** are commonly bilateral and filled with clear, straw-colored fluid. Often they are associated with hydatidiform mole, choriocarcinoma, or hormone therapy.[4]

Clinical Manifestations and Treatment

Normally, ovarian cysts produce no symptoms. They may be noted on periodic examination and may increase and decrease in size with the menstrual cycle. However, when an ovarian cyst ruptures, an ovarian vessel may tear, with massive intraperitoneal hemorrhage and severe abdominal pain. Immediate surgical intervention is indicated to control the hemorrhage and repair the site of rupture.[3]

Endometriosis

Endometriosis is the presence of endometrial tissue outside the lining of the uterine cavity. Since the only normal location for endometrial tissue is the endometrial lining of the uterus, the presence of this abnormal growth is associated with a variety of side effects ranging from mild symptoms to life-threatening consequences. These foci of abnormal endometrial tissue are called **endometriomas,** or endometrial implants, and usually occur within the pelvis. The most common sites of occurrence of endometriomas within the pelvis in order of frequency are the ovary, peritoneum of the cul-de-sac or pouch of Douglas, uterosacral ligaments, round ligament, oviduct, and the peritoneal surface of the uterus.[3] Less frequently, the endometrial implants occur in other body sites such as the bladder or large intestine. Although endometriosis is a benign disease, it possesses certain characteristics of malignant disease, such as the ability to grow, infiltrate, and spread. Symptoms of endometriosis may have an abrupt onset or may develop over many years.

The actual incidence of endometriosis is unknown, as it exists in many women without any significant symptoms. Endometrial implants have been identified in at least 20 percent of women undergoing gynecologic surgery.[3,8] Active endometriosis usually occurs between ages 30 and 40, particularly in women who have never given birth. Endometriosis is very rare in women younger than age 20 or after menopause. While some authorities report a higher incidence of endometriosis in caucasian women of higher socioeconomic levels,[3] these impressions may not be accurate, given the tendency of this group to delay childbearing and to have enhanced access to health care. The fertility rate for women diagnosed with endometriosis is about 66 percent, compared with 88 percent for the general population.[3]

Etiology

At the present time, three major theories exist regarding the etiology of endometriosis:

1. *Transportation.* Endometrial tissue flows backward through the oviducts during a normal menstrual period. Following this retrograde flow, endometrial fragments implant on the ovary, peritoneal surfaces, and other areas.
2. *Metaplasia.* Inflammation or a hormonal change triggers metaplasia (conversion of one kind of tissue into a form that is not normal for that tissue). Thus, coelomic epithelium at certain sites converts into endometrial epithelium.
3. *Induction.* In this theory, a combination of transportation and metaplasia takes place, and regurgitated endometrium chemically induces mesenchyma to form endometrial epithelium. (At present, this is thought to be the most likely cause.)[1,3,9]

Once the endometrial implants arise in their abnormal locations, they continue to be under hormonal influence, just as the endometrial lining of the uterus responds to hormonal influence. Thus, they periodically proliferate and bleed in response to hormonal stimulation. In some instances they may rupture, usually immediately before or after a menstrual period has occurred. Endometriomas are filled with brown blood debris; when they rupture, their contents spill out onto the sensitive pelvic peritoneum. This irritative discharge sets up a local chemical peritonitis, followed by the formation of fibrous tissue in the injured location. Dense tissue adhesions in the pelvis may result as the pelvic peritoneum undergoes repeated irritation by the cyclic activities of the endometrial implants.

Clinical Manifestations

The most prominent symptom of endometriosis is acquired dysmenorrhea, which produces pain in the lower abdomen and in the vagina, posterior pelvis, and back. The pain usually begins 5 to 7 days before menses reaches its peak and lasts for 2 to 3 days. It differs from the pain of primary dysmenorrhea, which is more cramplike and concentrated in the abdominal midline. Pain may be extremely severe, although the degree of pain does not necessarily indicate the extent of the disease. Dyspareunia and pain with defecation may also be present.[1] Significant changes in the pattern of menstrual flow may occur, with excessive bleeding that may progress to severe anemia and hemorrhagic shock.

Treatment

Treatment will vary according to the extent of the disease. Many women with endometrial implants never experience symptoms and require no treatment; others will experience a rapidly progressive set of severe symptoms requiring immediate intervention. Both medical and surgical treatment modalities may be utilized. Hormonal agents including progestational steroids and the antigonadotropic agents (Danocrine) may be used to produce a hormonal state similar to menopause. Because the endometriomas respond to cyclic hormonal functioning, it is thought that the use of hormones to interrupt this cyclical pattern may result in atrophy of the endometrial implants. Surgical intervention includes the removal of the endometriomas. If destruction of the pelvic organs is widespread and the disease is rapdily progressing, total abdominal hysterectomy with removal of the oviducts and ovaries is performed.[3,9]

KEY CONCEPTS

- Benign fibroid tumors, or leiomyomas, are the most common uterine tumor, affecting about 20 percent of women over age 35. Depending on their size, uterine leiomyomas may be characterized by abnormal vaginal bleeding, backache, constipation, and urinary frequency.
- Ovarian cysts are usually asymptomatic and may change in size with the menstrual cycle. Rupture of an ovarian cyst may result in severe abdominal pain and hemorrhage, necessitating immediate surgical intervention.
- Endometriosis occurs when endometrial tissue grows in areas other than the uterine lining. Endometriosis may involve the ovary, peritoneum, oviduct, outer uterus, bladder, and intestine. Although considered benign, endometriosis tends to infiltrate and spread to adjacent tissues. Endometriosis may be initiated by reflux of the uterine lining through the oviducts into the abdominal cavity during menses.
- Ectopic endometrial tissues periodically proliferate and bleed in response to fluctuations of reproductive hormones. Dysmenorrhea, with pelvic, back, and lower abdominal pain, usually begins 5 to 7 days prior to the peak of menses and last for 2 to 3 days. The pain is more diffuse than the pain of primary dysmenorrhea. Treatment may include induction of a menopause-like state with hormone administration or the surgical excision of affected structures.

Cancer of the Female Genital Structures

Malignant neoplasms occur in every part of the female reproductive system. This section describes the incidence and pathophysiologic aspects of the most common types of malignancies in the female genital structures. For further information about the process of neoplasm development, the reader may wish to refer to Chapter 6 of this text.

Cancer of the Cervix

Cancer of the uterine cervix is a neoplasm of the uterine cervix that can be detected in the early, curable stage by the Papanicolaou (Pap) test.[3] Invasive carcinoma of the cervix is responsible for 8,000 deaths annually in the United States alone.[1] Although the cause is unknown, several predisposing factors have been related to the development of cervical cancer: intercourse at a young age, multiple sexual partners, multiple pregnancies, and herpesvirus type II and other bacterial or viral venereal infections.[1] Improvements in genital hygiene and widespread screening with the Pap test have continued to decrease the mortality of cervical cancer. The American Cancer Society now recommends that, after two negative Pap tests 1 year apart, women over age 20 who are not at high risk should be tested at least every 3 years. Sexually active women under age 20 should also be tested at 3-year intervals. Women at risk are advised to have a Pap test every year.[3]

Etiology

Preinvasive cervical cancer produces no symptoms, although the Pap test can detect changes in cells of the cervical epithelium, which may be present for 10 years before invasive cancer develops.[1,3] Early invasive cancer causes abnormal vaginal bleeding, persistent vaginal discharge, and pain and bleeding after intercourse.[1] When symptoms appear, the cancer has usually progressed beyond its early stages. Squamous cell carcinoma accounts for 95 percent of all invasive cervical cancers diagnosed, and adenocarcinomas account for most of the rest. Invasive carcinoma of the cervix spreads by direct extension to the vaginal wall, laterally into the parametrium toward the pelvic wall, and anteroposteriorly into the bladder and rectum. Metastasis to the pelvic lymph nodes is more common than spread to distant lymph nodes.[3]

Treatment

The treatment utilized will depend on the clinical stage of the tumor at the time of diagnosis. Surgery, including cryocautery and laser surgery for mild dysplasia and hysterectomy for invasive carcinoma, may be indicated. Chemotherapy and radiation therapy are used in invasive disease. More than 55 percent of treated patients live 5 years. Radical surgery, including *pelvic exenteration,* or removal of all the pelvic organs, can now be performed safely with limited morbidity. The overall cure rate for cervical cancer is 29 percent.[3]

Other Cancers of the Female Genital Structures

Endometrial Cancer

Cancer of the endometrial lining of the uterus is less common than cervical cancer in young women, but both types of cancer occur with equal frequency in postmenopausal women.[3] Related factors include infertility, late menopause (after age 55), obesity, diabetes, and hypertension. Endometrial cancer occurs with higher frequency in urban, white, and Jewish women.[10] The most common initial symptom is bleeding between menstrual periods or postmenopausal bleeding. The diagnosis of endometrial cancer is based on histologic tissue examination. Treatment strategies for endometrial cancer include radiation therapy and total hysterectomy with removal of the ovaries and oviducts. The 5-year survival rate for patients diagnosed with early endometrial cancer is greater than 85 percent. The cure rate drops to 50 percent if the cancer has metastasized prior to diagnosis.[3]

Ovarian Cancer

Ovarian cancer has replaced cervical cancer as the leading cause of death from genital cancer.[11,12] The peak incidence is between 60 and 80 years of age.[3] As no symptoms occur until intra-abdominal metastasis has occurred, the mortality is high, with only a 34 percent survival rate.[3] When symptoms do occur, they are related to intra-abdominal metastasis and include increasing abdominal girth, weight loss, abdominal pain, dysuria or urinary frequency, and constipation. Treatment for ovarian cancer includes removal of the uterus, ovaries, and oviducts. Radiation therapy and chemotherapy may be used in conjunction with surgery.

Vaginal Cancer

Cancer of the vagina generally occurs in women in their early to mid-50s, although it has an increased incidence in young women whose mothers took diethylstilbestrol (DES) during pregnancy.[1] As the vagina is a thin-walled structure with rich lymphatic drainage, vaginal cancer may metastasize to the bladder, the rectum, vulva, pubic bone, and other surrounding structures. The primary signs and symptoms of vaginal cancer are vaginal spotting and discharge, pain, groin masses, and changes in urinary pattern.[3] Early-stage therapy is designed to treat the malignant area while preserving the normal parts of the vagina. Radiation therapy or surgery varies with the size, depth, and location of the tumor.[1] Preservation of a functional vagina is generally possible only in the early stages, although grafting from other body sites may be performed to avoid vaginal stenosis, particularly in younger women.[3]

Cancer of the Vulva

Cancer of the vulva accounts for approximately 5 percent of all gynecologic malignancies. It can occur at any age, including infancy, but has peak incidence in the mid-60s. Factors that seem to predispose to the disease include venereal disease, chronic pruritus of the vulva with swelling and dryness, obesity, hypertension, diabetes, and never having been pregnant.[1]

Leukoplakic changes (the presence of whitish, plaquelike or ulcerated lesions) in the vulva may precede the development of carcinoma. Once the carcinoma develops, vulvar masses may be present, with groin masses and abnormal urination and defecation later in the disease.[1] Treatment for vulvar cancer includes partial removal of the vulva to remove precancerous leukoplakic lesions, and total vulvar removal for advanced disease.[3]

KEY CONCEPTS

- Cervical cancer may be detected by evaluation of cervical cells (Papanicolaou test). Early-stage cervical cancer may be asymptomatic. When they appear, symptoms include abnormal vaginal bleeding and discharge. Cervical cancer may spread to the vaginal wall, pelvis, bladder, rectum, and pelvic lymph nodes. The overall cure rate is about 29 percent.
- Other cancers of the female reproductive tract include endometrial, ovarian, vaginal, and vulval cancers. There are no routine screening tests for these cancers. Ovarian cancer has a high mortality rate because it is usually diagnosed after it has metastasized.

Disorders of Pregnancy

Pregnancy results in a number of physiologic alterations in the mother that are usually well-tolerated, particularly if adequate prenatal care is available. However, pregnancy can result in a number of conditions that may be life-threatening to the mother and the developing fetus. The most common pregnancy-related disorders are described here; in addition, for information concerning diabetes in pregnancy, the reader may wish to consult Chapter 41, which covers the topic of diabetes in depth.

Pregnancy-Induced Hypertension

Pregnancy-induced hypertension (PIH) is known by other names such as toxemia and pre-eclampsia–eclampsia. Hypertension complicates 0.5 to 10 percent of pregnancies in the United States.[4] PIH is characterized by a rapid rise in arterial blood pressure associated with a loss of large amounts of protein in the urine. Women at risk for the development of PIH include teenagers and women in their late 30s and early 40s. In addition, the presence of multiple fetuses and the preexistence of hypertension, renal and cardiovascular disease, and diabetes may predispose to the development of PIH.[4]

Etiology

The exact causes of PIH are presently unknown, although poor nutrition, genetic, and immunologic factors have been suggested. PIH is characterized by salt and water retention by the kidneys, weight gain, and edema. In addition, arterial spasm occurs in many parts of the body, most significantly in the kidneys, brain, and liver. Both the renal flow and glomerular filtration rate are decreased, a condition exactly opposite to the normal changes in pregnancy. The renal effects are caused by a thickening in the glomerular tufts, which contain a fibrinoid deposit in the basement membranes.[13]

The severity of symptoms of PIH is closely related to the retention of salt and water and the degree of increase in arterial pressure. The increasing arterial pressure seems to promote a vicious cycle in which arterial spasm and other pathologic effects give rise to further increases in arterial pressure. These effects can be greatly delayed by drastic limitation in salt intake and bed rest during the latter months of pregnancy.[13]

In its severe form, PIH is characterized by extreme vascular spasticity throughout the body, clonic convulsions followed by coma, renal failure, liver malfunction, and extreme hypertension. Usually, this severe form occurs shortly before parturition. If PIH is left untreated, a high percentage of women experiencing it die. However, the immediate use of rapidly acting vasodilating drugs and cesarean section have reduced the mortality rate from PIH to less than 1 percent.[13]

Hyperemesis Gravidarum

Hyperemesis gravidarum is a Latin term for excess of vomiting in pregnant women. Although transient nausea and vomiting occur in about half of women in the first trimester of pregnancy, in a few women these symptoms continue throughout the entire course of pregnancy. In about 1 in 1,000 pregnancies, intractable vomiting, or hyperemesis gravidarum, occurs, sometimes with life-threatening consequences.[14] Severe dehydration and electrolyte imbalance, hepatic and renal damage, encephalopathy, and ultimately death may ensue if the vomiting cannot be controlled.

The causes of hyperemesis gravidarum are unknown, but it is thought that an abnormal response to the large production of chorionic gonadotropin by the placenta may be implicated.[13] Intravenous therapy to correct metabolic and nutritional abnormalities, antiemetic agents, and supportive care in a hospital environment may be needed to resolve the symptoms.[14]

Placenta Previa and Abruptio Placentae

Placenta previa is a condition in which the placenta is implanted abnormally over the internal cervical os. **Abruptio placentae** is the premature separation of the placenta before delivery of the fetus. Placenta previa occurs in approximately 1 to 200 deliveries and is more common in women with multiple pregnancies; at present, its cause is unknown. Placenta previa may occur in varying degrees of severity, and may range from partial to entire coverage of the internal cervical os. Abruptio placentae, or premature separation of the placenta, occurs after 20 weeks of gestation in about 1 percent of deliveries. The detachment may be partial or complete and may cause overt or concealed hemorrhage.[4] Abruptio placentae can be caused by trauma, a short umbilical cord, occlusion of the inferior vena cava, pregnancy-induced hypertension, or abnormal uterine structure. Therapeutic strategies for placenta previa and abruptio placentae include cesarean section for fetal distress or hemorrhage control. Medications designed to control preterm labor may also be utilized.[14]

Spontaneous Abortion

Spontaneous abortion is the expulsion of the products of conception from the uterus before the period of fetal viability. It is usually called a miscarriage by laypersons, and it is differentiated from elective abortion. Although the precise incidence is unknown, it is estimated that 10 to 15 percent of pregnancies end in spontaneous abortion. Abnormal development accounts for a large percentage of aborted pregnancies. Some 61 percent of abortions occurring in the first trimester demonstrate chromosomal abnormalities.[4] In addition, abnormal development may result from faulty implantation of the fertilized ovum or from an abnormality of the uterine environment. Maternal factors responsible for spontaneous abortion include both systemic and localized conditions. Infectious processes that may contribute to spontaneous abortion include cytomegalovirus, herpesvirus, and rubella infections. Abnormalities of the reproductive organs, endocrine malfunction, and physical and psychic trauma may all contribute to spontaneous abortion.[4,14]

Associated signs and symptoms of spontaneous abortion include vaginal bleeding and abdominal cramps. The cramps may intensify as the cervix dilates for expulsion of the uterine contents. If the entire contents are expelled, the bleeding and cramps subside. However, if any contents remain, an incomplete abortion has occurred, and medical intervention is needed to control bleeding and surgically remove the remaining uterine contents.[6]

KEY CONCEPTS

- Pregnancy-induced hypertension (PIH) is characterized by a rapid rise in blood pressure and proteinuria. Renal blood flow and glomerular filtration rate are reduced and the kidneys retain salt and water. When severe, PIH may be associated with convulsions and coma. Antihypertensive therapy may be indicated.

- Excessive vomiting during pregnancy is termed hyperemesis gravidarum. Dehydration, electrolyte imbalance, hepatic and renal damage and death may ensue. An excessive response to human chorionic gonadotropin may be responsible for hyperemesis.

- Placenta previa occurs when the placenta is implanted over the cervical os. Abruptio placentae is premature separation of the placenta. Both condi-

tions may interrupt fetal oxygen supply and cause maternal hemorrhage. Cesarean section is indicated.

- It is estimated that 10 to 15 percent of pregnancies end in spontaneous abortion. Fetal abnormalities, faulty implantation, infections, and trauma increase the risk of spontaneous abortion.

Disorders of the Breast

The breast is considered an accessory organ of the female reproductive tract and is affected by many of the same factors that promote alterations in the other reproductive organs. Women's breast health has become a critical concern in the United States, as the breast is the most common site of cancer in women between 25 and 75 years of age.[15] In addition, women are playing an increasingly important role in recognizing the symptoms of breast disease and are seeking earlier intervention with improved outcomes. It is essential that health care professionals continue to encourage this enhanced role and provide accurate information about breast health to their clients. This section includes information on the specific breast disorders involving reactive-inflammatory breast disorders, benign breast disorders, and carcinoma of the breast. Prior to reading this information, the reader may wish to review the section on the structure and function of the breast included in Chapter 32 of this text, and the specific information on neoplasm development included in Chapter 6.

Reactive-Inflammatory Breast Disorders

Breast disorders in which an inflammatory response occurs in reaction to irritation, injury, or infection include mammary duct ectasia, breast abscesses, fat necrosis, and reactions to injections or implantation of foreign materials in the breast.

Mammary Duct Ectasia

This syndrome is a chronic inflammatory process occurring in and around the terminal subareolar ducts of the breast (it is also referred to as periductal mastitis). It is more prevalent in older women, primarily postmenopausal women.[16] The Latin word *ectasia* means dilation, and in mammary duct ectasia the collecting ducts beneath the nipple and areola become dilated, thinned, and filled with secretions. Over time, the ducts become distended with cellular debris, and the debris begins to have an irritating effect on the duct walls. The inflammatory response is initiated, and a zone of granulation tissue is created around a small cavity filled with thick yellowish or brownish material. This area will be palpable as a mass in the central area of the breast, beneath or near the areola. By the time the duct ectasia has grown into a palpable mass, a reactive fibrosis in the tissue around the mass will also have occurred. This fibrous thickening of the surrounding breast tissue causes dimpling and distortion of the breast and nipple inversion (Fig. 33–5). However, a congenital inverted nipple is already present in some women with mammary duct ectasia, and it is thought that the presence of this nipple anomaly may in some way contribute to ductal wall irritation.[15]

In addition to a palpable mass and dimpling or distortion of the breast or areola, women with mammary duct ectasia may have persistent nipple discharge. These signs must be evaluated carefully, as they may also be indicative of a malignant breast mass. A biopsy is usually performed to rule out the presence of a malignancy. Following the confirmation of a diagnosis of mammary ductal ectasia, surgical excision of the dilated subareolar ducts is performed.[15]

Breast Abscesses

The majority of abscesses occurring in the breast are not associated with breast-feeding and are referred to as *nonlactational breast abscesses* (for a complete description of abscesses or mastitis related to lactation, the reader may wish to refer to an obstetric or maternity nursing text). Nonlactational breast abscesses are most often a recurring problem and usually affect persons with conditions that predispose to infections, such as diabetes, steroid therapy, or other skin le-

sions. Sign and symptoms of these abscesses include an area of tenderness, redness, and induration under the periareolar skin.[15]

Multiple factors may contribute to the formation of nonlactational breast abscesses. In some women, the presence of a congenital inverted nipple may predispose to abscess formation. Abscesses may also be part of the syndrome of mammary duct ectasia; in addition, women with the preexisting conditions listed above that predispose to infections may be at increased risk to develop an infectious process in the breast tissue. Unlike breast abscesses occurring during breast-feeding, in which *Staphylococcus aureus* is the most common causative organism, nonlactational breast abscesses usually yield multiple organisms when cultured. Unfortunately, nonlactational breast abscesses do not respond well to antibiotic therapy and often recur, and it is sometimes necessary to excise the major duct system beneath the areola in order to prevent further recurrence.[15]

Fat Necrosis

Necrosis refers to the death of a portion of tissue, and *fat necrosis* in the breast is the death of fat tissue following trauma or injury to the breast. The position of the breasts makes them vulnerable to trauma, particularly in larger women with pendulous breasts. This phe-

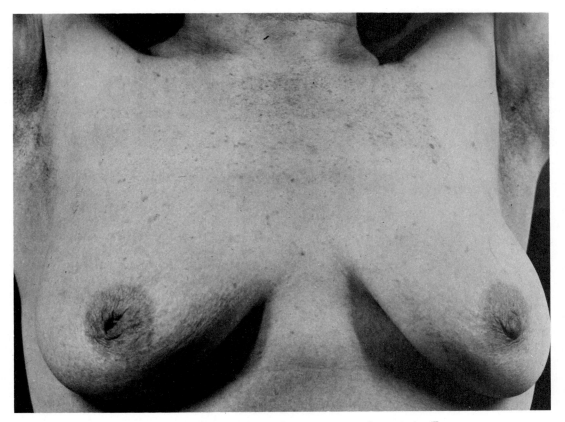

FIGURE 33–5. Nipple retraction of the right breast due to mammary duct ectasia. (From Haagensen CD: *Diseases of the Breast*, 3rd ed. Philadelphia, WB Saunders, 1986, p 359. Reproduced with permission.)

nomenon is important for health care professionals to assess, as fat necrosis may mimic or obscure carcinoma of the breast. Fat necrosis of the breast may have many of the same clinical signs as breast malignancy, including a painless mass in the breast that is firm, ill-defined, and poorly mobile. Skin thickening and retraction may also be present. In addition, a mammogram may not provide a clear diagnosis.[15] Unfortunately, many women with pendulous breasts frequently sustain injuries to the breast and may be unable to recall any specific trauma; thus, a diagnosis of fat necrosis may be difficult to make. If fat necrosis cannot be reliably distinguished from carcinoma based on clinical observation or mammography, an excisional biopsy must be performed.[15]

Reactions to Foreign Material

Surgery to enlarge the size of the female breast has become one of the most popular of all cosmetic surgical procedures in the past 25 years.[15] Since the early 20th century, a variety of materials have been used for breast augmentation. Silicone implants, which consist of silicone gel encased in polyurethane or other materials, have been the most widely used device for breast enlargement and have been implanted in more than 1 million women.[15] At present, controversy surrounds the use of silicone breast implants, as some side effects, including irritation at the implant area and other symptoms suggestive of an immune system response, have been reported.[17] Currently, the use of silicone implants for routine cosmetic breast augmentation is prohibited in the United States, and implants filled with a saline solution are now being used for this purpose. Health care professionals need to be aware of the reported side effects of silicone breast implants, as a substantial segment of the female population in the United States and Western Europe has undergone breast augmentation with these devices. In addition, persons with silicone implants who sustain blunt trauma to the chest are at risk for rupture of the implant, with subsequent leakage of the silicone gel into surrounding tissue. Following chest trauma, the communication of information regarding the presence of silicone breast implants to other health care professionals is an important consideration in planning care and preventing further tissue exposure to silicone.

Benign Breast Disorders

The term **benign breast disorders** encompasses a group of lesions affecting the breast. These disorders are usually divided into two categories: (1) fibrocystic breast disease and (2) specific benign neoplasms of the breast, such as fibroadenomas, adenomas, and papillomas. It is important for health care professionals to understand the clinical significance of these benign disorders. While these entities are ''benign'' in the sense of being differentiated from malignant breast neoplasms, clients experiencing them may be at risk for experiencing a psychological crisis, and may require teaching regarding their potential risk for breast malignancy.

Fibrocystic Breast Disease

Although the term **fibrocystic breast disease** is frequently used by health care professionals, it is important to understand that it is not a distinct disease entity.[15] Instead, it is a diagnosis classification that is applied to a condition in which there are palpable breast masses that fluctuate with the menstrual cycle and may be associated with pain or tenderness. A laboratory examination of this breast tissue shows macroscopic and microscopic cysts, along with a variety of alterations in tissue structure such as fibrosis or overgrowth of stromal fibrous tissue. However, these alterations in breast tissue are present to some degree in all female breasts, leading some authorities to question the use of the term *disease* for such a widespread condition.[15,18] Until a more precise system for classifying this type of benign breast disorder is widely adopted, however, fibrocystic breast disease will probably continue to be used to describe this phenomenon of tender breast masses that occur on a cyclic basis.

Etiology. Fibrocystic breast disease is thought to be due to hormonal imbalance in the reproductive years, specifically an excess of estrogen and a deficiency of progesterone during the luteal phase of the menstrual cycle. It is usually characterized by tenderness or pain in one or both breasts immediately before the onset of the menstrual period. On palpation, the cysts tend to be firm, regular in shape, and mobile. They are located most often in the upper outer quadrant of the breasts, and their size may fluctuate throughout the menstrual cycle.[15]

While it was previously thought that all women with fibrocystic breast disease were at increased risk for developing breast cancer, recent research has disproved this theory.[15,19] It is now known that only certain types of tissue changes may predispose a woman with fibrocystic breast disease to develop breast malignancy. The vast majority of women with fibrocystic disease do not have these alterations in breast tissue and therefore are not at a substantially increased risk of developing breast cancer.[15]

Treatment. Diagnostic studies, including needle aspiration of a cyst for histologic analysis, may be performed. Some clinicians have prescribed progestins to correct the progesterone deficiency thought to contribute to fibrocystic breast disease, although reports of the efficacy of this therapy have been mixed. Other supportive measures include the application of local heat and use of a support bra. Nutritional therapies have shown success in some women, particularly avoiding foods with methylxanthines such as tea, coffee, cola, and chocolate. It is thought that the methylxanthines tend to stimulate cyclic adenosine monophosphate and thus increase metabolic activity in the breast.[15]

Specific Benign Neoplasms

Specific benign neoplasms of the breast, such as fibroadenomas, adenomas, and papillomas, may occur at any time during a woman's life, from childhood through old age. These neoplasms behave in a clinically "benign" fashion, that is, they do not invade the surrounding tissue or metastasize to other sites. They generally appear as freely moveable, encapsulated masses that are sharply delineated from the surrounding breast tissue (Fig. 33–6).[15] However, it is important to have any breast mass evaluated, as biopsy and histologic examination may be needed to differentiate these benign neoplasms from breast carcinoma.

Carcinoma of the Breast

Carcinoma of the breast remains the most common form of cancer in women between 25 and 75 years of age, although lung cancer is increasing in prevalence in this group.[15] In the United States, it is the leading cause of death from all causes in women between the ages of 40 and 44 years. The incidence of breast carcinoma appears to be increasing in the United States, and the prevalence (the number of women with breast cancer in a given year) is approximately 100 per 100,000 women.[20] Although the disease is more common among white women, its incidence among blacks and Asians is rising.[15] Breast cancer does occur in males, but is 100 times less frequent.[20] While recent advances in early detection and treatment have afforded longer survival after diagnosis, invasive breast carcinoma remains an incurable disease that continues to take the lives of a large segment of the population.

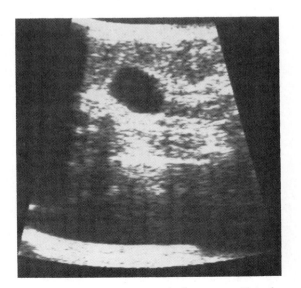

FIGURE 33–6. Ultrasound scan of a breast cyst. Note the smooth outline of this benign lesion. (From Donegan WL, Spratt JS: *Cancer of the Breast*, 3rd ed. Philadelphia, WB Saunders, 1988, p 149. Reproduced with permission.)

Etiology

Risk Factors. A substantial number of studies conducted in the past 20 years have begun to establish the risk factors and possible causes of breast cancer. Some factors that may place a woman at risk for developing breast cancer include hormonal influences, reproductive factors, dietary factors, family history, age, radiation exposure, and a previous history of cancer. It should be noted that helping a client to understand and interpret her personal breast cancer risk is a difficult task for a health care professional. The public media has given much attention to some of the risk factors for breast cancer but has not provided much context in which to interpret evaluations for individual risk factors.[15] **Risk factors** are characteristics related to the probability of a certain outcome—in this case, breast cancer. These risk factors may be either causally or correlatively associated with an outcome. For example, a factor may directly *cause* an outcome (as the smallpox virus causes smallpox), or may be *correlated* with an outcome (as not wearing a seat belt is correlated with an increased degree of injury in a motor vehicle accident). The distinction between causality and correlation is an important concept to impart to clients when discussing risk factors. A client may express concern, for example, that a certain risk factor will directly cause her to develop breast cancer. The ability of a health care professional to describe and discuss risk factors in a knowledgeable way will greatly enhance the client's ability to make decisions regarding such issues as hormonal replacement therapy following menopause.

Hormonal Factors. Hormones are now thought to play a major role in the etiology of breast cancer.[15] Length of exposure to the hormones secreted by the ovary (estrogen and progesterone) has been shown to affect the risk for breast cancer in the following way. If a woman has had an early (before age 12) onset of menses and a late (after age 55) menopause, her risk is increased. Put another way, women with 40 or more years of menstrual activity have twice the breast cancer risk when compared with women with fewer than 30 years of menstrual activity.[15] At the present time, controversy still exists regarding the effect of taking oral contraceptives or hormone replacements during menopause on breast cancer risk.[21] For many women, the known benefits of these medications continue to outweigh what presently appear to be relatively small effects on cancer risk.[15] Future research is needed to clarify the way in which hormonal exposure may foster breast cancer development, and the many interactive factors associated with taking hormonal medications.

Reproductive Factors. It has been observed in many research studies that giving birth at a young age (before age 18) is associated with a decreased risk of breast cancer, and that giving birth for the first time at or above age 35 increases the risk.[15] In addition, parity (the number of children a woman has given birth to) has been associated with risk, with low parity increasing risk and high parity having a protective effect.[15] However, it has been difficult for epidemiologists who study reproductive risk factors to determine the role these factors may play in a precise way. Other factors such as socioeconomic status are closely tied to the age at which a woman first gives birth and the number of children she has. The reader will gain a sense from this information of the complex nature of determining what factors truly can be said to be correlated with a given disease outcome.

Dietary Factors. The amount of fat in the diet has been suggested as a risk factor for breast cancer development.[15] Researchers who favor this theory point to the relatively low rates of dietary fat ingestion in countries with low rates of breast cancer. Although the media has given a great deal of attention to this issue, scientific data have been inconclusive thus far.[15] Countries in which low-fat diets are widespread are typically nonindustrialized countries in which other factors, such as age at first delivery or parity, differ from those in Westernized countries. No single dietary pattern or food has been shown to "cause" cancer, just as no specific food has been shown to prevent or cure it.

Family History. The role of heredity in contributing to breast cancer has long been recognized. Sophisticated genetic analysis has greatly improved the understanding of the role of heredity in contributing to breast cancer susceptibility. It is now known that certain families show a clear pattern of inheritance, but such families are comparatively rare.[15] It is more common to find families with one or two first-degree relatives (mother, sister) with a history of breast cancer. However, the role of genetic factors in increasing breast cancer risk remains unclear in these families. Because breast cancer tends to occur more often in older women, some authorities state that breast cancer may be occurring by chance, if the family members live long enough.[15] Still, research studies have indicated that women with a mother or sister with breast cancer do have an increased risk of developing it, and health care professionals need to consider carefully the family history of women when determining risk.[15]

Age. Breast cancer is an extremely rare disease among young women. The incidence of breast cancer begins to increase by age 25 to 30, and continues to increase with advancing age.[15]

Other Factors. Other factors, such as radiation exposure and a previous history of cancer, have been shown to be risk factors for the development of breast cancer.[15] Several potential factors have been suggested, such as exposure to low-frequency electric or magnetic fields, and a virus transmitted through lactation. More research is required to establish the role of these potential factors.

Clinical Manifestations

Breast cancer is most frequently discovered by the woman herself. She usually finds a single lump that is painless, hard, and poorly movable. Half of malignant tumors occur in the upper outer quadrant of the breast.[15] Other signs of advanced tumor development include dimpling of the skin (Fig. 33–7), nipple retraction, changes in breast contour, and bloody discharge from the nipple. Breast cancer is diagnosed by a number of techniques that utilize films (mammography, xerography) (Figs. 33–8, 33–9) and by thermography, a technique in which "hot spots" indicate increased metabolic activity. A person of any age with a suspect breast mass should undergo mammography and biopsy.

Most breast carcinomas arise in the epithelium of the glandular ducts of the breast. The lesion(s) have infiltrating edges, which begin to invade the normal breast tissue (Fig. 33–10). Following this invasion, malignant cells begin to scatter or **disseminate** into the lymph system of the axilla. The breast is in close

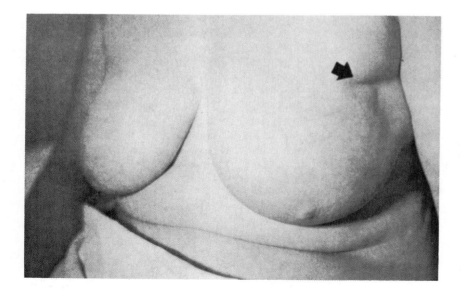

FIGURE 33–7. Skin dimpling caused by an underlying malignant tumor. (From Donegan WL, Spratt JS: *Cancer of the Breast,* 3rd ed. Philadelphia, WB Saunders, 1988, p 131. Reproduced with permission.)

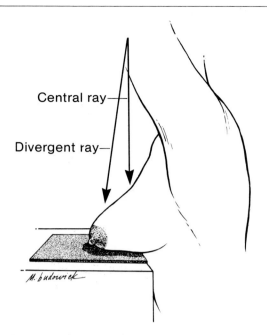

Central ray—

Divergent ray—

FIGURE 33–8. Placement of the breast for mammography, showing the direction of the x-rays. (From Egan RL: *Breast Imaging: Diagnosis and Morphology of Breast Diseases.* Philadelphia, WB Saunders, 1988, p 67. Reproduced with permission.)

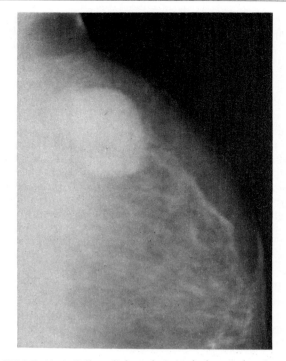

FIGURE 33–9. Full mediolateral view of a breast showing a lesion. (From Egan RL: *Breast Imaging: Diagnosis and Morphology of Breast Diseases.* Philadelphia, WB Saunders, 1988, p 64. Reproduced with permission.)

proximity to the large system of axillary lymph nodes, making easy dissemination of malignant cells possible. The major way by which breast carcinoma causes morbidity and death is through the dissemination of malignant cells to other body sites, most commonly to the lung, liver, and bone.[15] **Metastasis** (or spread of carcinoma) to these other body sites represents an extremely poor prognosis. The prognosis is vastly better for persons with no evidence of spread of malignant cells to the regional lymph nodes. The 5-year survival rate is 84 percent when no lymph node involvement is found at surgery but averages 56 percent when lymph node involvement is present.[15] The

more positive lymph nodes (nodes with malignant cells) that are found at operation, the less favorable is the patient's prognosis.

Treatment

Treatment for breast cancer includes surgery, chemotherapy, radiation therapy, and supportive measures. Surgical therapy is a controversial area, and various options are utilized. Removal of only the lesion is called a **lumpectomy;** removal of only the breast is a simple **mastectomy.** Other surgical interventions in-

FIGURE 33–10. Ultrasound scan of a carcinoma. Note the ragged appearance of this invasive, malignant lesion. (From Donegan WL, Spratt JS: *Cancer of the Breast*, 3rd ed. Philadelphia, WB Saunders, 1988, p 150. Courtesy of John R. Milbrath, M.D. Reproduced with permission.)

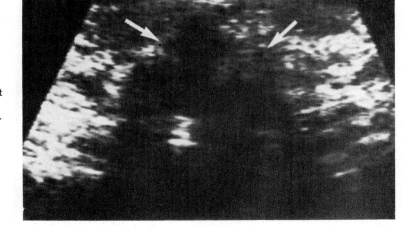

clude a **modified radical mastectomy,** in which the breast is removed and a portion of the axillary lymphatic system is dissected, and a **radical mastectomy,** in which the breast, lymphatic drainage, and underlying pectoral muscles are removed.[15]

Chemotherapy, in which a variety of hormonal and antineoplastic agents are administered, is also utilized. Malignant cells appear to have cytoplasmic hormone receptors that bind to hormone molecules, promoting cellular division and growth. Various hormonal agents are given to bind to these receptors and block this process. Antineoplastic agents such as fluorouracil (5-FU) are given to control the spread of malignant cells.[15]

Radiation therapy may be used as an adjunct to the above therapy and to control pain by shrinking large tumor masses. Other supportive measures in advanced disease include operations to reduce the bulk of tumors.[15]

Breast cancer is characterized by a wide variation in clinical course. Many patients who undergo treatment for breast carcinoma are able to achieve a satisfying quality of life. Educational and support programs for breast cancer patients and their families, both pre- and postoperatively, have been an important means of providing emotional support. Programs for continuing care following mastectomy have helped patients and families face the adaptive challenges of living with breast cancer. Follow-up care includes early detection of recurrent disease, with an emphasis on breast self-examination, yearly mammography, and regular contact with health care professionals for examination.

KEY CONCEPTS

- Chronic inflammation of the subareolar ducts may result in mammary duct ectasia. Fibrous thickening results in a palpable central mass, breast distortion and dimpling, and nipple inversion. Persistent nipple discharge may occur. These signs are similar to those of malignancy and are carefully evaluated by biopsy. Surgical excision may be done.
- Breast abscesses in nonlactating women are commonly associated with chronic infection, diabetes, and steroid therapy. These abscesses respond poorly to antibiotics and tend to recur.
- Fibrocystic breast disease is a condition in which palpable breast masses are present and fluctuate with the menstrual cycle. Breast cysts are firm, mobile, tender and most often located in the upper outer quadrant. There is no evidence that women with fibrocystic breasts are at higher risk for breast cancer. Progesterone, heat therapy, and avoidance of methylxanthines may be recommended.
- Breast cancer is the most common cancer in women between 25 and 75 years of age. Malignant tumors tend to be painless, hard, and fixed in place, in contrast to benign breast tumors, which are mobile and encapsulated. Risk factors for breast cancer include a high-fat diet, a first-degree relative with breast can-

cer, increasing age, radiation exposure, and a previous malignancy. In addition, reproductive factors such as the age at first pregnancy and the number of pregnancies may be associated with altered cancer risk.
- Breast cancer may spread to the regional lymphatics and disseminate to other sites. Localized breast cancer, without lymph node involvement, has an 84 percent 5-year survival rate. The survival rate falls to 56 percent when lymph nodes are cancerous. Depending on the extent of tumor spread, surgery may be done to remove the tumor only (*lumpectomy*), the affected breast and involved lymph nodes (*modified radical mastectomy*), or the breast, lymphatics, and underlying muscle (*radical mastectomy*). In addition, radiation therapy and chemotherapy may be initiated.

Summary

This chapter has described the most prevalent women's reproductive health problems at the present time. Any alteration in reproductive status may have profound implications for the individual; thus, the reader should carefully review this material to achieve the ability to distinguish the differences and similarities among these alterations.

Commonly occurring alterations in reproductive health for women may have serious consequences and require immediate intervention. Menstrual disorders may have multiple manifestations, and such disorders as amenorrhea and abnormal uterine bleeding disorders may occur at any time throughout a woman's life. Alterations in uterine position and pelvic support, including uterine prolapse, retrodisplacement of the uterus, cystocele, and rectocele, may result in severe symptoms and require surgical correction. Inflammation and infection of the female reproductive tract, including PID and vulvovaginitis, may have far-reaching effects for the individual woman experiencing them.

The reader will want to pay particular attention to the section on benign growths and aberrant tissue of the female reproductive tract, given the widespread nature and potentially serious consequences of these lesions. A thorough understanding of uterine leiomyomas, ovarian cysts, and endometriosis includes the ability to define these syndromes as described in this book, as well as an ability to explain them to clients. In addition, the reader is urged to review the material regarding the efficacy of the Papanicolaou smear in detecting cervical cancer at an early stage.

The section on disorders of pregnancy highlighted the most important aspects of this topic; the reader will probably wish to use this information as a basis for a more in-depth study of this area in a specialized course in maternal-child nursing. Finally, because of the widespread threat to women's health posed by disorders of the breast, particular attention should be paid to the final section. Specifically, the reader must be able to compare and contrast the differences between benign breast disorders and carcinoma of the breast, and discuss the meaning and importance of various risk factors for breast carcinoma in a knowledgeable way.

REFERENCES

1. Hacker NF, Moore JG: *Essentials of Obstetrics and Gynecology,* 2nd ed. Philadelphia, WB Saunders, 1992.
2. Glass RH: *Office Gynecology,* 4th ed. Baltimore, Williams & Wilkins, 1992.
3. Kim MH: Dysfunctional uterine bleeding, in Copeland LJ (ed): *Textbook of Gynecology,* Philadelphia, WB Saunders, 1993.
4. Wilson RJ, Carrington ER: *Obstetrics and Gynecology,* 9th ed. St. Louis, Mosby—Year Book, 1991.
5. Caufriez A: Menstrual disorders in adolescence: Pathophysiology and treatment. *Horm Res* 1991;36(3–4):156–159.
6. Nelson GL: Gynecologic surgery and cesarean birth, in Meeker MH, Rothrock JC (eds): *Alexander's Care of the Patient in Surgery,* 9th ed. St. Louis, CV Mosby, 1991.
7. Mitchell DG: Benign disease of the uterus and ovaries: Applications of magnetic resonance imaging. *Radiol Clin North Am* 1992;30(4):777–787.
8. Mahmood TA, Templeton A: Prevalence and genesis of endometriosis. *Hum Reprod* 1991;6(4):544–549.
9. Olive DL: Endometriosis: Advances in understanding and management. *Curr Opin Obstet Gynecol* 1992;4(3):380–387.
10. Makar AP, Trope CG: Endometrial and ovarian malignancies: Epidemiology, etiology, and prognostic factors. *Acta Obstet Gynecol Scand* 1992;71(5):331–336.
11. Daly MB: The epidemiology of ovarian cancer. *Hematol Oncol Clin North Am* 1992;6(4):729–738.
12. Petitti DB, Porterfield D: Worldwide variations in the lifetime probability of reproductive cancer in women: Implications of best-case, worst-case, and likely case assumptions about the effect of oral contraceptive use. *Contraception* 1992;45(2):93–104.
13. Guyton AC: *Textbook of Medical Physiology,* 8th ed. Philadelphia, WB Saunders, 1991.
14. Beischer NA, Mackay EV, Purcal NK: *Care of the Pregnant Woman and Her Baby,* 2nd ed. Philadelphia, WB Saunders, 1990.
15. Harris JR, Hellman S, Henderson IC, Kinne DW: *Breast Diseases,* 2nd ed. Philadelphia, JB Lippincott, 1991.
16. Haagensen CD: *Diseases of the Breast,* 3rd ed. Philadelphia, WB Saunders, 1986.
17. Mentor Corporation: Siltex Low-Bleed Gel-Filled Mammary Prosthesis (product insert). Goleta, Calif, Mentor Corporation, 1989.
18. Hughes LE: Classification of benign breast disorders: The ANDI classification based on physiological processes within the normal breast. *Br Med Bull* 1991;47(2):251–257.
19. Krieger N, Hiatt RA: Risk of breast cancer after benign breast diseases. *Am J Epidemiol* 1992;135(6):619–631.
20. Luckmann J, Sorenson KC: *Medical-Surgical Nursing,* 3rd ed. Philadelphia, WB Saunders, 1991.
21. Spicer DV, Pike MC: The prevention of breast cancer through reduced ovarian steroid exposure. *Acta Oncol* 1992;31(2):167–174.

BIBLIOGRAPHY

Blackledge GRP, Jordan JA, Shingleton HM: *Textbook of Gynecologic Oncology.* Philadelphia, WB Saunders, 1991.
Bland KI, Copeland III: *The Breast: Comprehensive Management of Benign and Malignant Disease.* Philadelphia, WB Saunders, 1991.
Breast disease: New approaches. *Br Med Bull* 1991;47(2):251–252.
Buchsbaum HJ, Schmidt JD: *Gynecologic and Obstetric Urology,* 3rd ed. Philadelphia, WB Saunders, 1993.
Burrow GN, Ferris TF: *Medical Complications During Pregnancy,* 3rd ed. Philadelphia, WB Saunders, 1988.
Donegan WL, Spratt JS: *Cancer of the Breast,* 3rd ed. Philadelphia, WB Saunders, 1988.
Egan RL: *Breast Imaging: Diagnosis and Morphology of Breast Diseases.* Philadelphia, WB Saunders, 1988.
Fu YS, Reagan JW: *Pathology of the Uterine Cervix, Vagina, and Vulva.* Philadelphia, WB Saunders, 1989.
Gerhenson DM, DeCherney AH, Curry SL: *Operative Gynecology.* Philadelphia, WB Saunders, 1993.
Keye WR Jr: *The Premenstrual Syndrome.* Philadelphia, WB Saunders, 1988.
Knuppel RA, Drukker JE: *High-Risk Pregnancy: A Team Approach.* Philadelphia, WB Saunders, 1993.
Murtagh J: Patient education: Endometriosis. *Aust Fam Physician* 1992;21(7):1023.
Prue LK: *Atlas of Mammographic Positioning.* Philadelphia, WB Saunders, 1994.
Saleh JW: *Laparoscopy.* Philadelphia, WB Saunders, 1988.
Zimny ME: Ovarian cancer: A nursing overview. *Oncology* 1991;5(8):147–53.

CHAPTER 34
Sexually Transmitted Diseases

JANE M. GEORGES

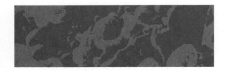

KEY TERMS

chancre: Painless, ulcerative lesion that arises at the original port of entry of the spirochete that causes syphilis.

chlamydia: Genus of a microorganism that lives as an intracellular parasite. *Chlamydia trachomatis* lives in the epithelium of the urethra and cervix and is responsible for the highly contagious systemic infection lymphogranuloma venereum.

condyloma acuminata: Benign epithelial tumors of the anogenital region with a wart-like appearance; predominately a sexually transmitted disease of the young, in which the causative organism has been identified as a type of human papilloma virus.

gay bowel syndrome: Transmission of and subsequent infection with enteric pathogens through sexual contact. These disorders are not limited to the homosexual community and may be transmitted among any individuals who engage in direct or indirect fecal-oral contact.

gonorrhea: Common sexually transmitted disease involving the inflammation of epithelial tissue by the organism *Neisseria gonorrhoeae.* Characteristic symptoms include urethritis, dysuria, purulent urethral discharge, and redness and swelling at the site of the infection.

herpesvirus infection: Important group of viral agents producing infections in humans. Two types of herpes simplex viruses, referred to as type 1 and type 2, may be sexually transmitted.

lymphogranuloma venereum: Highly contagious systemic infection caused by a number of strains of *Chlamydia.* It has progressive stages of development in which an initial lesion forms and systemic disease occurs following dissemination via the lymphatic system.

ophthalmia neonatorum: Purulent gonococcal conjunctivitis and keratitis of the newborn resulting from exposure of the infant's eyes to infected maternal secretions during the infant's passage through the vagina at birth.

sexually transmitted diseases: Large group of diseases that can be transmitted by sexual contact, regardless of whether the disease has manifestations in the genital organs (previously referred to as venereal diseases).

syphilis: Sexually transmitted disease that is caused by the spirochete, *Treponema pallidum,* and that is characterized by distinct stages of effects over a period of years.

---

*A*n epidemic of sexually transmitted diseases (STDs) currently exists in the United States. One million gonococcal infections are reported each year to the Public Health Service, and it is estimated that over 3 million chlamydial infections occur each year.[1] The true incidence of these infections is likely to be significantly higher, as many sexually transmitted infections go unreported. The cost of STDs, both in economic and in personal terms, is extremely high. It is estimated that the annual total costs associated with treating acute pelvic inflammatory disease associated with STDs in women amount to over $3 billion.[1] In addition, the personal costs to the individual experiencing an STD may include pain, disfigurement, and permanent sterility. Because of the epidemic status of these diseases and the enormous costs associated with them, it is imperative that health care providers become sufficiently knowledgeable to assess and educate clients about STDs in an accurate and compassionate manner.

The term **sexually transmitted diseases** refers to a large group of disease syndromes that can be transmitted sexually, regardless of whether the disease has manifestations in the genital structures.[2] In older texts, STDs are referred to as venereal diseases. Although STDs are more prevalent in the 19- to 25-year-old age group, they can occur at any age. These diseases are sometimes contracted by nonsexual transmission, as when a newborn infant contracts an STD from an infected mother during passage through the birth canal.[3]

A list of sexually transmitted organisms grouped according to type of pathogen is found in Table 34–1. As can be seen from this table, the list of pathogens that can be transmitted sexually is quite extensive, and the diseases which these pathogens can produce are equally extensive. Many pathogens produce multiple diseases, and many diseases may be caused by more than one pathogen. A useful approach to learning the complex pathophysiology of STDs is to group STDs according to the disease manifestations the client is most likely to exhibit when first seen by the care provider. These categories of STDs and the disease manifestations associated with them are listed in Table 34–2. This chapter will describe each of these categories and the pathophysiology associated with each relevant STD.

TABLE 34–1. Sexually Transmitted Organisms

Bacterial Agents	Viral Agents
Neisseria gonorrhoeae	Herpes simplex virus
Chlamydia trachomatis	Hepatitis virus
Mycoplasma hominis	AIDS-related virus
Ureaplasma urealyticum	Cytomegalovirus
Gardnerella vaginalis	Human papillomavirus
Hemophilus ducreyi	Molluscum contagiosum virus
Calymmatobacterium	
granulomatis	**Protozoan Agents**
Shigella	
Group B streptococcus	*Trichomonas vaginalis*
Treponema pallidum	*Giardia lamblia*
	Entamoeba histolytica
Fungal Agents	
Candida albicans	
Candida glubrata	

From Landers DV, Sweet RL: Sexually transmitted infections, in Glass RH (ed): *Office Gynecology,* 3rd ed. Baltimore, Williams & Wilkins, 1988. Reproduced with permission.

TABLE 34–2. Sexually Transmitted Diseases Categorized According to Disease Manifestations

Disease Manifestations	Disease
Urethritis, cervicitis, and salpingitis	Gonorrhea
	Nongonococcal urethritis
	Pelvic inflammatory disease
Ulcerative lesions with systemic involvement	Syphilis
	Lymphogranuloma venereum
	Herpes
Ulcerative lesions only	Chancroid
	Granuloma inguinale (donovanosis)
Nonulcerative lesions	Molluscum contagiosum
	Condylomata acuminata
Vulvovaginitis	Trichomoniasis
	Candidiasis
	Gardnerella vaginalis vaginitis
Systemic infections	Cytomegalovirus
	Hepatitis
	AIDS
Enteric infections	Giardiasis
	Campylobacter enteritis
	Shigellosis
	Amebic dysentery

Some diseases listed in Table 34–2 have been discussed elsewhere in this text but have been included here for completeness. In particular, the reader may wish to refer to Chapter 33 for more detailed information on pelvic inflammatory disease and vulvovaginitis. Also, certain systemic infections are potentially transmitted by sexual contact. Cytomegalovirus infection, hepatitis A and B, and acquired immunodeficiency syndrome (AIDS) have the potential for sexual transmission. These diseases are covered in detail in Units III and X along with more in-depth information concerning infectious processes and immune responses. Before studying this chapter, the reader may wish to review Chapters 1 and 8, emphasizing basic terminology such as incubation period and period of communicability. Health care providers caring for persons at risk for STDs need to be aware of the potential for acquisition of systemic diseases by sexual contact and include assessment of these diseases as part of their overall clinical evaluation.

Urethritis, Cervicitis, Salpingitis, and Pelvic Inflammatory Disease

Three types of STDs are manifested by *urethritis* (inflammation of the urethra), *cervicitis* (inflammation of the uterine cervix), and/or *salpingitis* (inflammation of the oviduct or fallopian tube). **Gonorrhea,** the most common sexually transmitted disease, is an inflammation of epithelial tissue by the organism *Neisseria gonorrhoea.* **Nongonococcal urethritis** refers to urethritis resulting from a pathogen other than the gonococcus, which is usually *Chlamydia trachomatis.* **Pelvic inflammatory disease** (PID), which was described in Chapter 33, is usually the result of an acute salpingitis caused by gonococccocal or nongonococcal infection that has extended into nearby pelvic tissues.[2,4]

Gonococcal Infection

Etiology

In gonorrhea, disease transmission occurs through contact with exudates from the mucous membranes of infected persons, usually by direct contact. The gonococcus then attaches to and penetrates columnar epithelium, producing a patchy inflammatory response in the submucosa with a polymorphonuclear exudate.[2] Although usually asymptomatic in women, gonorrhea may produce purulent vaginal discharge, dysuria, and abnormal vaginal bleeding. The most commonly affected areas in women are the cervix, urethra, Skene's and Bartholin's glands, and the anus. Gonococcal infections of the vagina are rare during the reproductive years but may occur in prepubescent girls and postmenopausal women. In men, symptoms of urethritis, including dysuria and a purulent urethral discharge, accompanied by redness and swelling at the site of infection, usually occur after a 3- to 6-day incubation period. In both sexes, infection and inflammation of the pharynx, conjunctivae, and anus may be present. Direct extension of the infection with gonococcus occurs by way of the lymphatic system. In the female, extension may spread unilaterally or bilaterally to the oviducts, with resulting salpingitis. In the male, direct extension of the infection most frequently occurs to the epididymis.[2,5,6]

Once the infection with gonococcus has spread to other areas, localized infection occurs, with the formation of cysts and abscesses. Purulent exudate containing the organism causes damage to tissue, and fibrous tissue replaces inflamed tissue. This hardened, fibrous tissue may result in scarring and narrowing of the urethra, epididymis, or oviducts. In women, the partial or complete closure of the oviducts results in sterility. Infection of the oviducts may also result in pelvic inflammatory disease as exudate is released into the peritoneal cavity.[1,7,8] As described in Chapter 33, pelvic inflammatory disease may be an acute or chronic condition causing widespread damage to the pelvic organs in the female.

Nongonococcal Infection

Etiology

Nongonococcal urethritis and cervicitis are most frequently caused by strains of *Chlamydia trachomatis* that act on columnar epithelium in a manner similar to gonococcus. The symptoms of infection with *chlamydia* are generally less severe than those of gonorrhea, and many infected persons, particularly women, may be entirely unaware of their infected status. As with gonorrhea, the infection may spread by extension to the oviducts, and pelvic inflammatory disease may eventually result. Transmission of *Chlamydia* during birth may result in ophthalmia neonatorum, or infection of the eyes in the newborn.[2]

Treatment

The classic treatment for gonorrhea has been penicillin; however, newer anti-infective agents are now being used in various combinations that may be more effective in treating the infection.[9] In pelvic inflammatory disease, a combination of antimicrobial agents is chosen after the agent or agents causing the infection have been identified.[2]

KEY CONCEPTS

- **Urethritis, cervicitis, salpingitis, and pelvic inflammatory disease are commonly due to gonorrhea or a chlamydial infection. Transmission is usually by direct contact with infected mucous membranes. The symptoms of chlamydial infection are usually less severe than those of gonorrhea.**

- **Gonorrhea may produce purulent discharge, dysuria, and abnormal vaginal bleeding. Cysts and abscesses may form in localized areas of infection, fol-**

lowed by scarring and fibrosis. Inflammation of the pharynx, conjunctivae, and anus may be present. Antibiotic therapy is indicated.

Diseases With Systemic Involvement

Several STDs cause a distinctive ulcerative lesion and disseminate throughout the body, affecting multiple organ systems. Most prominent of this type of STD are syphilis, herpesvirus infections, and lymphogranuloma venereum.

Syphilis

Syphilis is a systemic infection of the vascular system consisting of five distinct stages: incubation, primary and secondary stages, latency, and late syphilis.[2] Syphilis is communicable by persons with primary, secondary, or early latent syphilis.[1] The incidence of syphilis has been on the rise in the United States since 1958. An estimated 136,000 cases of primary and secondary syphilis occur annually. Although much of the increase in cases has occurred in the male homosexual population, an increasing rate has also been observed in heterosexual women.[3]

Etiology

Syphilis is caused by *Treponema pallidum,* an anaerobic spirochete. Syphilis is acquired when *Treponema pallidum* penetrates into intact mucous membrane or abraded skin during sexual contact (the process of the transmission of congenital syphilis is described below). Some of the *T. pallidum* pathogens remain at the original invasion site, while others migrate to regional lymph nodes within hours. During this incubation phase, *T. pallidum* is disseminated throughout the body and can invade and multiply in any organ system.[2]

During all stages of syphilis, the invasion of tissues by *T. pallidum* results in pathologic changes in the vascular system. The inflammatory response in the endothelial tissue causes the infiltration of lymphocytes and plasma cells, with subsequent endothelial swelling. The terminal arterioles and small arteries may become obliterated and no longer functional. Finally, the long-term inflammation of the vascular tissue results in the formation of hardened, fibrous thickening in the blood vessels and eventually tissue necrosis.[2]

Following the initial incubation period of 10 to 90 days, the primary phase begins with the formation of a **chancre,** a painless, ulcerative lesion that arises at the original spirochete portal of entry (Fig. 34–1). The chancre may go unnoticed in the female if it occurs on the cervix or in the vagina; in fact, most cases of syphilis in women go undiagnosed until recognized by positive testing of the blood in the latent phase. In males, the chancre may form on the genitalia; in

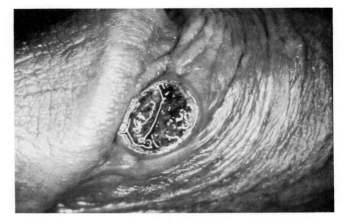

FIGURE 34–1. Typical syphilitic chancre, a painless, ulcerative lesion that arises at the original spirochete portal of entry. (From Gorbach SL, Bartlett JG, Blacklow NR (eds): *Infectious Diseases.* Philadelphia, WB Saunders, 1992, p 822. Reproduced with permission.)

both sexes, chancres may erupt on the anus, fingers, lips, tongue, nipples, tonsils, or eyelids.[4]

Untreated chancres will resolve spontaneously within 3 to 6 weeks and are followed by the secondary stage of syphilis, which is characterized by a low-grade fever, malaise, sore throat, headache, lymphadenopathy, and mucosal or cutaneous rash (Fig. 34–2). This secondary stage occurs as *T. pallidum* is spread throughout the bloodstream and lymphatic system. This secondary stage is also self-limiting and is followed by the latent phase, in which no symptoms are present. During the latent stage, the affected person will test positive for syphilis on serologic assays and may still experience infectious mucocutaneous lesions during the early latent stage. Thus, the early latent stage is considered contagious. The latent stage is of variable length and may last more than 40 years.[2] Approximately two thirds of patients remain asymptomatic and never have a recurrence of symptoms. If

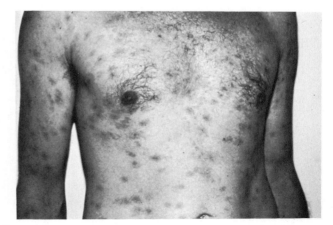

FIGURE 34–2. Typical generalized skin rash of secondary syphilis. (From Gorbach SL, Bartlett JG, Blacklow NR (eds): *Infectious Diseases.* Philadelphia, WB Saunders, 1992, p 823. Reproduced with permission.)

left untreated, approximately one third of affected people go on to develop late syphilis, the final, destructive phase of the disease.[4] The manifestations of late syphilis depend on the area of arterial lesions and the extent of circulatory insufficiency.[2] Body systems particularly at risk are the cardiovascular and central nervous systems. Damage to the cardiovascular system may include aortic necrosis and resulting aortic insufficiency; damage to the CNS may be progressively widespread, with degeneration of the cortical neurons and eventually paresis, blindness, and mental deterioration.[4,10]

Transmission of *T. pallidum* from the mother to the fetus may occur transplacentally at any point during pregnancy, but the fetus does not develop an inflammatory response to the pathogen until around the 15th week of gestation. Therefore, treatment of infected women before the 15th week may prevent damage to the fetus. Infection with syphilis before birth may result in physical deformities and developmental disabilities in the infant. If infants are born to untreated or inadequately treated mothers, they will have active infection and must be treated.[2,11]

Treatment

Penicillin is the first choice for the treatment of syphilis. If the affected person is allergic to penicillin, tetracycline or erythromycin is given. Treatment is administered to all individuals with positive evidence of syphilis on laboratory testing and to people who have had sexual contact with infected individuals.[1] Response to antibiotic treatment is monitored by repeating laboratory testing for evidence of syphilis at regular intervals up to 24 months following therapy.[4]

Lymphogranuloma Venereum

Lymphogranuloma venereum (LGV) is a highly contagious systemic infection caused by a number of closely related strains of *Chlamydia*. It occurs worldwide, although it has a slightly higher prevalence in the tropical and semitropical areas of South America, Africa, Asia, and the southeastern United States.[4] LGV develops more often in males than in females and has a higher incidence among sexually active young adults.

Etiology

Like syphilis, LGV has stages of development in which an initial lesion forms and systemic disease occurs following dissemination via the lymphatic system. Three stages occur in LGV: (1) a primary lesion, (2) regional inflammation of the lymphatic system (also called lymphadenitis), and (3) late complications resulting from progression of the lymphadenitis.[2]

Following the invasion of the mucosa by *Chlamydia* during sexual contact, a painless lesion appears on the genitalia after a 1- to 3-week incubation period. The lesion may range from a slight erosion to a small papule and often goes undetected. This lesion heals spontaneously in a few days. During this period, the pathogens are disseminated to regional lymph nodes, primarily the inguinal lymph nodes.

About 2 weeks after the appearance of the primary lesion, the inguinal lymph nodes begin to swell, and the systemic symptoms of fever and malaise develop. The nodal swelling is a manifestation of the inflammation of the lymphatic system in which lesions filled with polymorphonuclear leukocytes are forming in the lymph nodes. Spread of the inflammation throughout adjacent lymph nodes causes multiple nodes to become matted together and form a large abscess. These abscesses are said to be regional, as they develop in one or more areas along the lymphatic system. If LGV goes untreated, the abscesses rupture through the skin and other body cavities to create chronic fistulas. Thus, as the regional lymphadenitis progresses, complications such as perianal and rectovaginal fistulas develop, along with strictures of the rectum. Other complications include extreme swelling of the genitalia, as the normal lymph drainage of this area is now impeded (Fig. 34–3).[4]

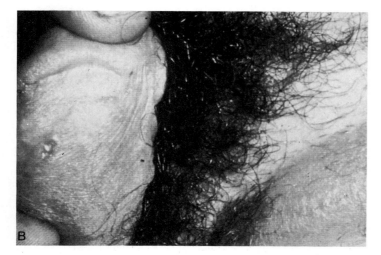

FIGURE 34–3. Lymphogranuloma venereum has a small, transient genital ulcer with swollen, extremely painful inguinal lymph nodes. (From Ronald AR, Alfa MJ, Chancroid, lymphogranuloma venereum, and granuloma inguinale, in Gorbach SL, Bartlett JG, Blacklow NR (eds): *Infectious Diseases.* Philadelphia, WB Saunders, 1992, p 848. Reproduced by permission of Willcox.)

Treatment

Anti-infective agents including tetracycline, doxycycline, and erythromycin are usually administered. Surgical treatment may include the aspiration of lymph nodes as needed; rectal strictures and fistulas may require surgical correction.[2]

Herpesvirus Infections

Herpesviruses are an important group of viral agents producing infections in humans. Two types of herpes simplex viruses (HSV), type 1 and type 2, may be sexually transmitted and are discussed in this section. **Herpes simplex virus type 1** is most often associated with herpetic infections above the waist, typically in the oral cavity and on the lips, but also in the eyes or on the epidermis. Although HSV type 1 has a potential for sexual transmission, it is present in saliva, stool, and urine and can be transmitted easily by nonsexual contact. The vesicles resulting from type 1 infections in the oral cavity are commonly referred to as cold sores or canker sores and often affect young children under age 5.[4] **Herpes simplex virus type 2** is implicated in 90 percent of genital, anal, and perianal herpes and is sometimes referred to as genital herpes for this reason. Type 2 HSV can also result in oral lesions following sexual contact. Although type 2 is primarily transmitted through sexual contact, pregnant mothers can transmit the infection to newborns during vaginal delivery.[2,12,13]

Etiology

HSV types 1 and 2 have certain characteristics in common. Both produce an initial infection that is self-limiting. The lesions produced by this infection heal, but HSV continues to be present in the body. Recurrence of the lesions, usually in the area of the initial infection, may take place as the virus is reactivated. Recurrence of either type may be triggered by an infectious disease, emotional stress, and immunosuppression.[2] The exact mechanism for the reactivation of the virus is presently unknown, but it is thought that ganglion neurons may contain latent forms of the virus, and may receive a trigger to stimulate the replication of the virus under certain conditions.[2,14]

Genital infection with HSV type 2 is manifested by fluid-filled vesicles that appear after a 3- to 7-day incubation period. In the female, the cervix is usually the primary infection site, although the labia, perianal skin, vulva, or vagina may also be involved (Fig. 34–4). In the male, the vesicles are located on the glans penis, foreskin, or penile shaft (Fig. 34–5). Extragenital lesions may appear on the mouth or anus. In both males and females, the vesicles, which are usually painless at first, may rupture and develop into extensive, shallow, painful ulcers.[15] The virus may enter the lymphatic system, creating localized lesions there; thus, the inguinal lymph nodes may be edematous and tender. Rarely, the virus spreads to visceral

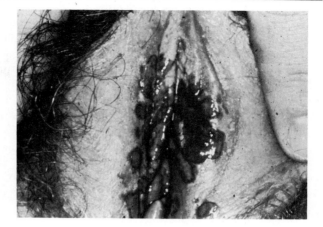

FIGURE 34–4. Primary genital herpes in the female. (From Oxman MN, Genital herpes, in Braude AI (ed): *Infectious Diseases and Medical Microbiology.* Philadelphia, WB Saunders, 1986, p 1043. Reproduced with permission.)

organs, producing areas of necrosis in the liver, adrenal glands, lungs, and CNS.[2,4] In newborns and people with weak immune defenses (particularly people with AIDS), HSV type 2 may result in severe damage to these organ systems, with a high mortality rate.[4]

HSV type 1 infections may appear as single or multiple fluid-filled, tender vesicles in the oral cavity or on the lips. Usually, the appearance of the lesions is preceded by 1 or 2 days of paresthesia before the "canker" or "cold sore" erupts. These lesions will usually crust and heal within 3 to 10 days.

Treatment

Normally, HSV type 1 lesions are self-limiting and respond to measures that promote good oral hygiene. HSV type 2 genital lesions are usually self-limiting but may be extremely painful. The use of anti-infective agents such as acyclovir has been shown to accelerate healing time and reduce the duration and severity of

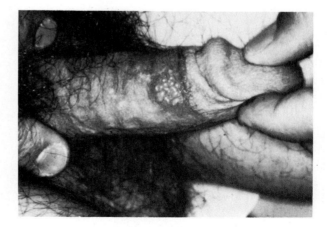

FIGURE 34–5. Recurrent genital herpes in the male. (From Oxman MN, Genital herpes, in Braude AI (ed): *Infectious Diseases and Medical Microbiology.* Philadelphia, WB Saunders, 1986. Courtesy of M.T. Jarratt, M.D. Reproduced with permission.)

symptoms in initial episodes of HSV type 2 infection. However, acyclovir has not been shown to influence the subsequent recurrence rate of genital herpes following the initial episode.[1,16]

If HSV type 2 lesions are active in a pregnant mother at term, a cesarean section may be recommended to avoid infection of the newborn.[17]

KEY CONCEPTS

- Syphilis is caused by an anaerobic spirochete that is transmitted sexually but disseminates throughout the body during incubation. Manifestations of early syphilis include chancre formation at the portal of entry that spontaneously resolves in 3 to 6 weeks if untreated. General malaise, fever, sore throat, and rash may then occur, followed by an asymptomatic latent phase. The latent phase may last more than 40 years. Late syphilis is characterized by central nervous system degeneration, blindness, and paresis.

- Lymphogranuloma venereum is a highly contagious systemic infection caused by strains of *Chlamydia*. An initial painless genital lesion appears after 1 to 3 weeks of incubation. The infection spreads to regional lymph nodes and is accompanied by fever and malaise. Infected lymph nodes become abscessed and may rupture through the skin and body cavities, causing fistula formation.

- Herpes simplex virus type 2 is implicated in 90 percent of genital herpes. Herpes lesions are fluid-filled vesicles that appear 3 to 7 days after infection. The virus may enter the lymphatics, causing inguinal lymph node tenderness. Although lesions may disappear, the virus remains in the body, predisposing to recurrences. Herpes may be transmitted from mother to newborn during birthing.

Diseases With Localized Lesions

Ulcerative Lesions

Two types of STDs result in the formation of ulcerative lesions but do not progress to systemic involvement. **Chancroid** (also called soft chancre) and **granuloma inguinale** both are manifested by ulcerative lesions, although their pathophysiologies differ.

Chancroid

Etiology. Chancroid is an ulcerative, infectious disease of the genital tract caused by the sexually transmitted anaerobic bacillus *Hemophilus ducreyi*. Chancroid was relatively rare in the United States until the past decade. Since 1981, small epidemic outbreaks of chancroid have been reported in the United States. Males usually outnumber females in a ratio of 10:1 in outbreaks in Western countries.[1]

Pathogenesis and Clinical Manifestations. H. ducreyi initially invades the genital skin or mucous membranes at sites traumatized by sexual contact; a preexisting abrasion may facilitate invasion. After a 4- to 7-day incubation period, a small papule with surrounding erythema develops at the site of entry. Within 2 to 3 days the lesion becomes pustular and ulcerates. Unlike the chancre in syphilis, the lesion in chancroid is painful and tender and is often multiple. Fresh lesions may occur from autoinoculation or the process of self-infection. The ulcerated lesions may enlarge and continue to erode (Fig. 34–6), producing destruction of surrounding tissues. In addition, inguinal lymph nodes may exhibit tenderness and pain, as the infection is disseminated to this region. If untreated, the enlarged lymph gland (called a *bubo*) may

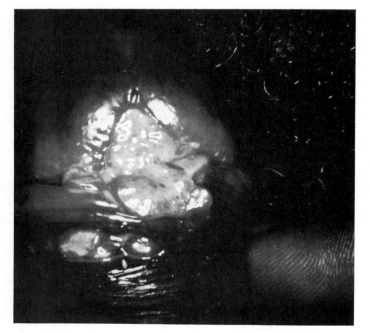

FIGURE 34–6. The eroded, purulent ulcer of chancroid. (From Ronald AR, Alfa MJ, Chancroid, lymphogranuloma venereum, and granuloma inguinale, in Gorbach SL, Bartlett JG, Blacklow NR (eds): *Infectious Diseases.* Philadelphia, WB Saunders, 1992, p 848. Reproduced by permission of A. R. Ronald.)

rupture, leaving a large inguinal ulcer. The infection is communicable until the lesions heal, which may be a period of weeks.[18,19]

Treatment. Anti-infective agents used for chancroid include erythromycin or ceftriaxone. Trimethoprim-sulfamethoxazole is also used.[1] As with all STDs, sexual partners should be treated simultaneously and reexposure avoided until therapy is completed. The aspiration of enlarged inguinal lymph nodes may also be indicated.[1]

Granuloma Inguinale

Etiology. *Calymmatobacterium granulomatis* is the causative agent in granuloma inguinale. This organism is a bacterium that is sometimes referred to as a Donovan body, and the disease as donovanosis. Granuloma inguinale is somewhat rare in the United States, with the highest incidence in homosexual males.[1,2]

Pathogenesis and Clinical Manifestations. The transmission of granuloma inguinale is not clearly understood. It is generally thought to be an STD, but the disease is also seen in adults who are not sexually active and in young children, possibly due to autoinoculation. The causative bacterium is found in the rectum of nondiseased persons, suggesting that the organism may be part of the normal gastrointestinal flora in some persons.[2] The communicability of the disease is relatively low, and it is generally believed that repeated exposure is necessary.[1]

The incubation period is variable, ranging from a few days to months. The initial sign of the disease may be a painless papule or nodule that subsequently ulcerates into an enlarging, granulomatous, red, velvety ulcer. The raised mass of granulation tissue may look more like a tumor than an ulcer; proliferation of the margins of the lesion may simulate the early epitheliomatous changes of cancer. Single or multiple lesions may coalesce, or lesions may spread to nearby tissue.[2] Secondary infection of the ulcers and expanding tissue necrosis in untreated lesions may lead to erosion of the genitals. In addition, the formation of scar tissue on genital structures during the healing process may produce urethral occlusion.[2] Lymph involvement is minimal, and inguinal swelling is usually due to the presence of subcutaneous granulomas.[1,20]

Treatment. Tetracycline therapy is the usual anti-infective agent and is given until all lesions are healed. Alternative therapies include streptomycin or gentamicin and chloramphenicol. Long-term follow-up should be provided in this disease, as it may recur.[1]

Nonulcerative Lesions

Molluscum contagiosum and **condylomata acuminata** (also called genital warts) are two prevalent types of STDs that produce nonulcerative lesions. Both are caused by viral agents that invade superficial layers of the epidermis during sexual contact.

Molluscum Contagiosum

Etiology. **Molluscum contagiosum** is a viral skin disease caused by a pox virus that is distinct from other pox viruses such as the smallpox virus. (The term "pox virus" refers to a viral agent that causes an eruption, or "pox," on the skin.) Its occurrence is worldwide, and 90 percent of all adults have antibodies.[2] Two forms of the disease exist. One affects children and is transmitted by skin-to-skin contact and indirect contact; the other affects young adults and is transmitted during sexual contact.[1]

Pathogenesis and Clinical Manifestations. Following invasion of the epidermis by the virus, pink to white lesions with an exudative core appear on the genitalia. The lesions are multiple and slow to develop, remaining stable for long periods of time. The disease is usually asymptomatic, tends to be self-limiting, and lasts 6 to 9 months.[1,2]

Treatment. The goal of treatment is primarily to prevent spread of the infection for cosmetic reasons. The lesions can be removed by minor surgery or frozen with liquid nitrogen. The sexual contacts of affected persons should be examined to prevent further spread.[1]

Condylomata Acuminata

Etiology. **Condylomata acuminata** (singular: condyloma acuminatum) are benign epithelial tumors of the anogenital region.[1] The wartlike appearance of these lesions has caused them to be referred to as genital or venereal warts. The causative agent for condyloma acuminata has been identified as a type of human papillomavirus (HPV). Condylomata acuminata are predominantly transmitted sexually in young adults, with the highest prevalence in the 16- to 25-year-old age group.[1] The risk of contracting the disease by sexual contact with an infected person is high; up to two thirds of the sexual contacts of affected persons will develop lesions. Nonsexual transmission has also been documented, and the lesions have been found in infants.[1] The period of communicability is unknown but is thought to last as long as the lesions persist.[2]

Pathogenesis and Clinical Manifestations. Following invasion of the epidermis by HPV, an incubation period of 1 to 20 months (usually about 4 months) precedes the appearance of the lesions. It is thought that the virus infects single epithelial cells and stimulates the cells to divide and proliferate into the wartlike lesions. The lesions are single or multiple, soft pink to brown, and usually elongated. They may occur in clusters and sometimes as large cauliflower-like masses (Fig. 34–7). The lesions are generally asymptomatic but may be friable and bleed considerably. In females, condylomata acuminata may be found in the vagina and cervix as well as in the anogenital area.[17] In males, they may occur in the anterior urethra and anogenital area.

Treatment. At present, therapies for condylomata acuminata include local excision, electrocautery, and

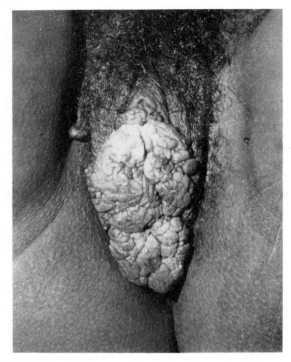

FIGURE 34–7. Clusters of condylomata acuminata form large, cauliflower-like masses on the vulva. (From Knuppel RA, Drukker JE: *High Risk Pregnancy: A Team Approach.* Philadelphia, WB Saunders, 1993, p 113. Reproduced with permission.)

cryosurgery. The advent of laser therapy and immunotherapy may bring enhanced treatment options for the disease. As malignant transformation to invasive carcinoma has been observed with some types of condylomata acuminata, it is generally agreed that affected persons should be treated and monitored carefully.[1]

KEY CONCEPTS

- Chancroid is caused by infection with an anaerobic bacillus. Initially the lesion is a small erythematous papule. After 2 to 3 days, the painful lesion ulcerates. Lesions resemble syphilis; however, the lesions of syphilis are painless.

- Granuloma inguinale is caused by an intestinal bacterium. The initial papule is painless and subsequently ulcerates into a growing granulomatous ulcer resembling a tumor.

- Molluscum contagiosum is associated with infection by a pox virus. Genital lesions are pink to white, with an exudative core. The disease is usually asymptomatic and self-limiting.

- Condylomata acuminata or genital warts are associated with infection by human papillomavirus. Warts are pink to brown, painless, and may occur in clusters. Human papillomavirus infection is an important risk factor for cervical cancer.

Enteric Infections

Until recently, information regarding the transmission of enteric infections of the gastrointestinal (GI) tract through sexual contact was limited. Recent research in this area has increased the knowledge base of health care providers, and the term gay bowel syndrome has been developed to describe the transmission and subsequent infection with enteric pathogens through sexual contact. It must be stressed that, despite the specific reference to homosexual males by the term gay, such disorders are *not* limited to the homosexual community. Enteric pathogens may be transmitted sexually among any individuals who engage in direct or indirect fecal-oral contact. Enteric organisms that may be transmitted through sexual contact include *Giardia, Campylobacter, Shigella,* and the agents causing amebic dysentery.[4]

The pathophysiology of enteric infections of the GI tract is described in Chapter 36, and the reader may wish to refer to this material. In general, persons who have acquired enteric infections by sexual contact will have variable manifestations. Some individuals may be asymptomatic, while others will have marked symptoms of enteritis or proctitis. All individuals who engage in oral-anal sexual practices should be monitored for the presence of enteric infections with laboratory studies and diagnostic examinations. Education for persons at risk for sexually transmitted enteric infections includes an emphasis on protective hygienic practices. Infected persons should avoid all sexual contact until all partners are examined and treated if necessary. Following completion of appropriate therapy for enteric infections, affected individuals should be retested for assessment of therapeutic effectiveness.[4]

Summary

Because of the epidemic nature of STDs, it is essential for readers preparing for careers in the health sciences to have a complete grasp of the material in this chapter. The STDs considered in the chapter are grouped according to the disease manifestations the client is most likely to exhibit. Gonorrhea, the most common sexually transmitted disease, nongonococcal urethritis, and pelvic inflammatory disease are manifested by urethritis, cervicitis, or salpingitis. A second group of STDs cause ulcerative lesions with systemic involvement. Syphilis, herpes, and lymphogranuloma venereum all cause a distinctive ulcerative lesion and go on to disseminate throughout the body, affecting multiple organ systems.

In reviewing the material on STDs related to ulcerative and nonulcerative lesions, the reader should compare and contrast the appearance of these lesions and consider the differing pathophysiologies of each type. Finally, consider how you will incorporate this material into your overall assessment process. Nurses and other health care providers caring for persons at risk for STDs need to be aware of the potential for acquisition of these diseases as well. Your overall goal in learning the material in this chapter is to be able to assess and educate clients with STDs in a comfortable and accurate manner.

REFERENCES

1. Landers DV, Sweet RL: Sexually transmitted infections, in Glass RH (ed): *Office Gynecology*, 3rd ed. Baltimore, Williams & Wilkins, 1988.
2. Csonka GW, Oates JK: *Sexually Transmitted Diseases: A Textbook of Genitourinary Medicine*. Philadelphia, WB Saunders, 1990.
3. Sweet RL, Gibbs RS: *Infectious Disease of the Female Genital Tract*, 2nd ed. Baltimore, Williams & Wilkins, 1990.
4. Gorbach SL, Bartlett JG, Blacklow NR (eds): *Infectious Diseases*. Philadelphia, WB Saunders, 1992.
5. Zenilman JM: Update on bacterial sexually transmitted disease. *Urol Clin North Am* 1992;19(1):25–34.
6. Horner PJ, Coker RJ, Turner A, Shafi MS, Murphy SM: Gonorrhoea: Signs, symptoms, and serogroups. *Int J STD AIDS* 1992;3(6):430–433.
7. Copeland LJ (ed): *Textbook of Gynecology*. Philadelphia, WB Saunders, 1993.
8. Wolner-Hanssen P: Pelvic inflammatory disease. *Curr Opin Obstet Gynecol* 1991;3(5):687–691.
9. Mogabgab WJ: Recent developments in the treatment of sexually transmitted diseases. *Am J Med* 1991;91(6A):140S–144S.
10. Hook EW 3rd, Marra CM: Acquired syphilis in adults. *N Engl J Med* 1992;326(16):1060–1069.
11. Sanchez PJ: Congenital syphilis. *Adv Pediatr Infect Dis* 1992; 7:161–180.
12. Maccato ML, Kaufman RH: Herpes genitalis. *Dermatol Clin* 1992;10(2):415–422.
13. Lycke E: The pathogenesis of the genital herpes simplex virus infection. *Scand J Infect Dis Suppl* 1991;80:7–14.
14. Thin RN: Does first episode genital herpes have an incubation period? *Int J STD AIDS* 1991;2(4):285–286.
15. Jarvis C: *Physical Examination and Health Assessment*. Philadelphia, WB Saunders, 1992.
16. Thin RN: Management of genital herpes simplex infection. *Int J STD AIDS* 1991;2(5):313–317.
17. Knuppel RA, Drukker JE: *High Risk Pregnancy: A Team Approach*, 2nd ed. Philadelphia, WB Saunders, 1993.
18. Levin SA: *The Clinician's Guide to Sexually Transmitted Diseases*. St. Louis, Mosby–Year Book, 1987.
19. Quinn TE: *Sexually Transmitted Diseases*. New York, Raven Press, 1992, *Advances in Host Defense Mechanisms*, vol 8.
20. Holmes K: *Sexually Transmitted Diseases*, 2nd ed. New York, McGraw-Hill, 1989.

BIBLIOGRAPHY

Buckley HB: Syphilis: A review and update of this "new" infection of the 90's. *Nurse Pract* 1992;17(8):25, 29–32.

Crane MJ: The diagnosis and management of maternal and congenital syphilis. *J Nurse Midwifery* 1992;37(1):4–16.

Fogel CI, Lauver D: *Sexual Health Promotion*. Philadelphia, WB Saunders, 1990.

Handsfield HH: Recent developments in STDs: Viral and other syndromes. *Hosp Pract* 1992;27(1):175–182.

Imperato PJ: Syphilis, AIDS, and crack cocaine. *J Community Health* 1992;17(2):69–71.

Keller ML, Jadack RA, Mims LF: Perceived stressors and coping responses in persons with recurrent genital herpes. *Res Nurs Health* 1991;14(6):421–430.

McMillan A, Scott G: *Sexually Transmitted Diseases*. New York, Churchill Livingstone, 1991.

Novotny PP: *What Women Should Know About Chronic Infections and Sexually Transmitted Diseases*. New York, Dell Books, 1991.

Parenti DM: Sexually transmitted diseases and travelers. *Med Clin North Am* 1992;76(6):1449–1461.

Paris-Hamelin A: Syphilis serology in 1991. *J Clin Neuro Ophthalmol* 1991;11(3):144–151.

Preventing sexually transmitted diseases. *Health News* 1992; 10(5):5–9.

Rothenberg RB: Those other STDs. *Am J Public Health* 1991; 81(10):1250–1251.

Soper DE: Surgical considerations in the diagnosis and treatment of pelvic inflammatory disease. *Surg Clin North Am* 1991; 71(5):947–962.

Tillman J: Syphilis: An old disease, a contemporary perinatal problem. *J Obstet Gynecol Neonat Nurs* 1992;21(3):209–213.

Wisdom A: *Color Atlas of Sexually Transmitted Diseases*. St. Louis, Mosby–Year Book, 1989.

UNIT X

Alterations in Gastrointestinal Function

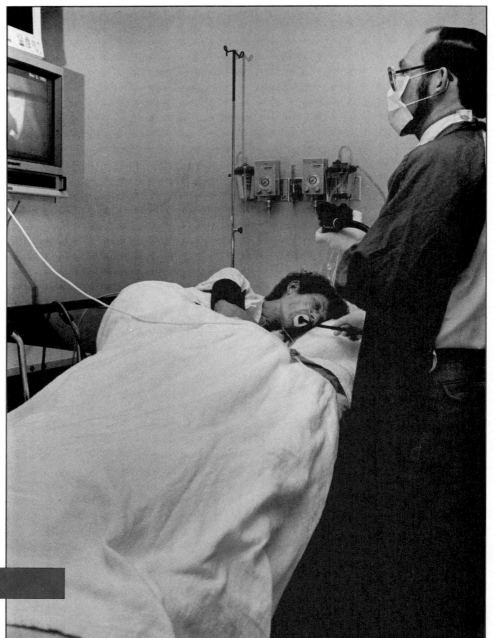

Visual examination of the upper gastrointestinal tract, using an endoscope.

Photo by Kathleen Kelly

When the gastrointestinal (GI) system is working properly, we are happy not to have to think about it. When it shows signs of stress or disease, we think about it only reluctantly. It seems so complicated—its coilings, its odd junctures, its paradoxical purposes—nourishing the body and disposing of wastes, sustaining life in two invaluable but seemingly contradictory ways.

The standard medical textbook listing of GI disorders is unappetizing: gastritis, peptic ulcer, pancreatitis, sprue, constipation, megacolon, diarrhea, vomiting, GI disruption, cancer.

Energetic research on a variety of GI diseases is leading medical scientists to better diagnosis and treatment of some of the more common and more drastic disorders.

Helicobacter pylori, an infectious GI bacterium, has drawn the attention of many medical researchers. Recent studies indicate that the eradication of *H. pylori* decreases basal acid secretion in duodenal ulcer patients and allows the ulcers to heal. The *Lancet,* the British medical journal, concluded a survey of recent experimentation intended to wipe out *H. pylori* in the intestinal tract of research subjects with the statement: "the great majority of duodenal ulcers will be determined by the coexistence of acid-induced gastric metaplasia in the duodenum and an *H. pylori*–associated antral gastritis."

Another study of the connection between high gastric cancer rates in 13 countries and the presence of *H. pylori* seems to some European researchers more than coincidence. The chain of causes seems to run this way: chronic gastritis, commonly caused by *H. pylori,* leads to atrophic gastritis, intestinal metaplasia, and finally gastric cancer. Here, the *Lancet* concludes, for "many cases of gastric cancer we can now safely conclude that *H. pylori* gastritis is a necessary though not sufficient cause."

Common, annoying, and sometimes dangerous as peptic ulcer may be, it is not, however, among the dread diseases of the GI system. Colon cancer is described as an epidemic in the United States, with an expected 149,000 new cases to be diagnosed in 1994. More than one third will result in the patient's death. Only lung cancer kills more Americans, and colon cancer attacks both sexes and all ethnic groups. Scientists are encouraged by their ability to cure colon cancer if the malignant polyps are detected early. They have also identified noncancerous lesions that are responsible for colon cancers and provide early warning because they often appear years before the cancer itself. Early screening, even of individuals without symptoms, will help detect the neoplastic polyps that precede cancer. The polyps may then be removed, reducing the possibility of colon cancer. Only 6 percent of colon cancers are inherited; for those, genetic studies promise an effective blood test.

The indispensable liver is another target of intense research. Part of the problem is alcohol or drug abuse. A British researcher reports that about 60 percent of patients suffering from severe, acute alcoholic hepatitis die during the first 6 weeks after hospitalization. Alcoholic hepatitis frequently is found in patients who eventually develop cirrhosis, a dangerous and often fatal liver disease.

Chronic hepatitis C is the most common cause of nonalcoholic liver disease, and, some researchers speculate, may be the most common form of liver disease in the United

FRONTIERS OF RESEARCH
Advances in Treatment of GI Disorders

Michael J. Kirkhorn

States. Of the 170,000 cases of acute hepatitis C that are diagnosed each year, more than 70 percent will develop into chronic hepatitis and may eventually develop into cirrhosis.

But researchers are encouraged by their improved ability to diagnose, treat, and manage a variety of liver diseases. Among these improvements are new developments in liver cell transplants, including the possibility of the grafting of transplanted tissue onto the diseased liver, allowing it to recover.

In the prosperous industrialized nations where advanced technology can be employed, new devices are aiding in the diagnosis of GI diseases. Computerized tomography can be used effectively to diagnose pancreatitis and with considerably less exactness indicate the cause of cases of acute pancreatitis, whether gallstones, fatty infiltration of the liver where alcohol is the culprit, or liver metastases in cases of pancreatic cancer.

There are also recent innovations in surgery that make it a little easier for patients to tolerate fairly common disorders. Each year more than 500,000 Americans undergo gallbladder surgery. A new technique, laparoscopic cholecystectomy, is intended to relieve the suffering of patients for whom gallbladder bile has crystallized in stones that block the cystic or common bile ducts through which it normally is released into the duodenum, where it helps digest fat. Rather than making a single large incision, surgeons remove the gallbladder and stones through four small abdominal incisions. Usually the patient is able to go home in a day or two.

CHAPTER 35
Gastrointestinal Function

JANE M. GEORGES

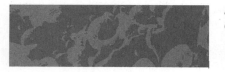

KEY TERMS

aspiration: Inadvertent entry of food substances, liquids, or gastric content into the respiratory system. This potentially life-threatening occurrence is normally prevented by the coordinated set of actions performed by the muscles in the pharynx during swallowing.

bolus: A round mass of food that has been softened and formed into an appropriate size for swallowing by the action of chewing.

brush border: Covering of the microvilli projecting from the intestinal villi. This fuzzy coating contains many digestive enzymes.

chyme: Viscous, semifluid contents of the stomach following the mixture of ingested nutrients with gastric secretions. Chyme then passes through the pylorus into the duodenum, where further digestion occurs.

intestinal villi: Fingerlike projections, numbering in the millions, that line the small intestine and that serve to increase the surface area of the intestine for digestion and absorption of nutrients.

intrinsic nervous system: Neural structures belonging entirely to the gastrointestinal (GI) system that control most GI functions and are responsible for many reflexes occurring locally in the GI tract. It is composed of two layers: the myenteric plexus, and the submucosal plexus.

peristalsis: The basic propulsive movement of the gastrointestinal (GI) tract. During normal functioning, this coordinated, rhythmic, serial contraction of smooth muscle propels the contents of the GI tract in a downward direction.

presbyesophagus: Presence of slow or disorganized esophageal motility in the older adult.

slow wave electrical activity: One of the basic types of electrical activity in the gut. Slow waves represent an ongoing basic oscillation in membrane potential occurring in the smooth muscle of the (gastrointestinal) GI tract between 3 and 12 times per minute.

spike potentials: Sudden increases in membrane potential in the smooth muscle of the gastrointestinal (GI) tract that appear on the peaks of slow waves in response to certain conditions, including stimulation by stretching or the effects of acetylcholine or parasympathetic excitation.

---

*T*he gastrointestinal (GI) tract is a major component of the GI system. The GI tract includes the mouth, pharynx, esophagus, stomach, and small and large intestines. These components can be thought of as a continuous tube about 5 meters in length running from the mouth to the anus. Other parts of the GI system that are located outside of the GI tract include the salivary glands, pancreas, and biliary system (liver, gallbladder, and bile ducts).[1,2]

The function of the GI system, illustrated in Figure 35–1, is to provide nutrients for the body. The process of ingesting nutrients, propelling them through the GI tract, and transforming them into a format capable of absorption into the body's internal milieu constitutes a remarkable interface of the human organism with the external environment. The general functions of the GI tract in providing nutrients for the body can be divided into (1) GI motility, including propulsive and mixing movements; (2) secretion of digestive juices; (3) digestion of nutrients; and (4) absorption of nutrients.[2,3] This chapter describes each of these functions in detail and provides an overview of the structure and organization of the GI tract and its growth and alteration across the life span.

Structure and Organization of the Gastrointestinal Tract

Embryology

As early as the fourth week of gestation, the GI system begins to form from the primitive gut structures of the foregut, midgut, and hindgut.[4,5] The foregut gives rise to the pharynx, esophagus, stomach, the duodenum proximal to the opening of the common bile duct, the hepatobiliary system, and the pancreas. The trachea and esophagus share a common develop-

mental origin, and an incomplete partitioning of these structures may lead to tracheoesophageal fistula, a developmental anomaly characterized by an abnormal connection between the trachea and esophagus. This anomaly may be accompanied by **esophageal atresia,** in which the esophagus is closed off in a blind pouch at some point. These disorders are two of the most

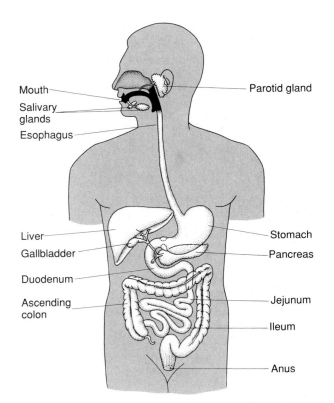

FIGURE 35–1. The gastrointestinal tract. (From Guyton AC: *Textbook of Medical Physiology,* 8th ed. Philadelphia, WB Saunders, 1991, p. 689. Reproduced with permission.)

701

serious surgical emergencies in newborns and require immediate diagnosis and correction. Esophageal atresia occurs in about 1 of every 4,000 live births, and about one third of the infants affected by this anomaly are born prematurely.[1]

The midgut gives rise to the small intestine (below the opening of the common bile duct), the cecum, the appendix, the ascending colon, and the proximal portion of the transverse colon.[2] If partitioning between the foregut and midgut fails to occur properly, **duodenal atresia,** a condition in which an obliteration of the lumen of the small intestine is present, may occur. This anomaly is the most frequent cause of intestinal obstruction in the newborn. If the midgut fails to develop or rotate properly with respect to the umbilical cord, **omphalocele,** a congenital herniation of viscera into the base of the umbilical cord, may be present.[2]

The hindgut gives rise to the distal part of the transverse colon, the descending and sigmoid colon, the rectum, and the superior portion of the anal canal.[2] Congenital malformations resulting from inappropriate development of the anorectal portion of the GI tract include **anal agenesis,** in which the rectal pouch ends blindly above the surface of the perineum. Other developmental anomalies of this portion of the GI tract include **anal stenosis,** in which the anal aperture is small, and **anal membrane atresia,** in which the anal membrane covers the aperture, creating an obstruction.[2]

Following its initial embryologic development, the GI tract continues to grow in length and caliber until somatic growth ends after puberty. The degree of the growth and development of the GI tract during childhood appears to depend on the same general factors as growth of the rest of the body. Such general factors as nutritional adequacy, insulin, growth hormone, thyroid hormone, cortisol, androgens, and estrogens may play a role in its development, as well as such specific factors as the direct effect of ingested nutrients, GI hormones, and secretions.[2,5]

Physiologic Anatomy

Each part of the GI tract is uniquely adapted for a specific function in the process of providing nutrients for the body, a process that continues from birth to senescence. Each major component of the GI tract is described as a basis for understanding the overall structure and innervation of the GI tract.

Oral Cavity and Pharynx

The mouth, or oral cavity, is the usual point of entry for nutrients and is the site of the initial breakdown of nutrient substances into a usable form. Food is pushed toward the side of the mouth by the tongue, facilitating chewing and grinding on the surfaces of the molar and premolar teeth. As the food is manipulated and broken down, it is moistened by **saliva,** secreted by three major pairs of salivary glands: the parotid, submandibular, and sublingual glands. Saliva serves three major functions which are important in the ingestion of nutrients: (1) By its moistening action, saliva allows the tongue to convert a mouthful of food into a bolus, or semisolid mass, that can be swallowed easily. (2) By its moistening action, saliva changes dry foods into a solute form and allows for taste perception by the papillae on the surface of the tongue, which are sensitive to chemical differences among food molecules. (3) The digestive enzyme contained in saliva, **salivary amylase** (also called ptyalin), initiates carbohydrate digestion by effecting the breakdown of **polysaccharides** (also called starch) into the simpler molecular structures of dextrin and maltose.[6–8]

The **pharynx,** or throat, is a muscular tube about 12 cm long that serves as the entryway for both the respiratory and the GI systems. The oropharynx is the portion of the pharynx posterior to the mouth and is separated from the nasopharynx, the portion of the pharynx posterior to the nose, by the soft palate. The laryngopharynx is the portion of the pharynx that opens into the larynx and the esophagus. During swallowing, the soft palate is pulled upward to close off the nasopharynx. The bolus of food being swallowed is propelled by reflex movements of muscles in the pharynx through the laryngopharynx and into the esophagus. Simultaneously the opening to the larynx is closed by the epiglottis. This coordinated set of actions prevents food substances and liquids from inadvertently entering the respiratory system, a potentially life-threatening occurrence referred to as **aspiration.**[3]

Esophagus

The esophagus is a muscular tube approximately 25 cm in length. Passage of food through the esophagus is greatly facilitated by mucus secreted by cells in the epithelial lining. Extremely rough or fibrous foods may potentially penetrate the mucous lining of the esophagus, causing damage. The stratified squamous epithelium lining the esophagus is constantly renewed by cells moving to the surface from below, thus providing a means of renewal for such damage.[3] The esophagus propels nutrients to the stomach by means of strong muscular contractions, a capability that may be affected by aging. Presbyoesophagus, or an abnormal esophageal motility pattern occurring with advanced age, is described in detail in a later section. When the body is in an upright position, gravity assists in the downward movement of food to the stomach. However, the muscular contractions of the esophagus are extremely strong and are sufficient to transport nutrients to the stomach even in the absence of gravity, as persons living (and eating) in the weightless conditions of space have demonstrated.[3,9]

At the lower end of the esophagus, about 2 to 5 cm above its juncture with the stomach, the circular muscle of the esophagus functions as a sphincter; this

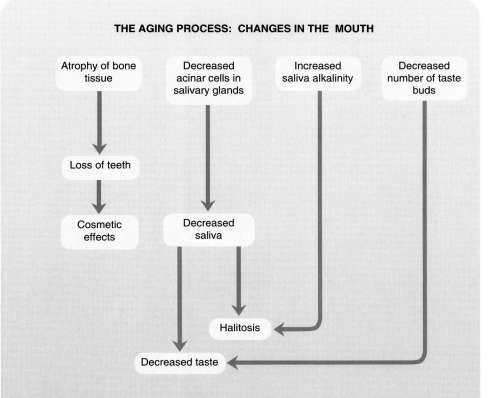

THE AGING PROCESS: CHANGES IN THE MOUTH

The elderly person experiences a decline in taste. This decline is due to both an increase in the sensation threshold for all four tastes and a decrease in the number of papilla. For example, children have more than 200 taste buds, whereas the elderly have less than 100. Of the four basic tastes, the elderly experience a particular decrease in salt and sugar tastes.

The elderly also experience a decrease in the number of acinar cells in the salivary glands, leading to a reduction in the amount and secretory rate of saliva. The saliva becomes more alkaline as well. The decrease in the amount of saliva and the increased alkalinity contribute to halitosis.

The loss of teeth in the elderly is due to atrophy of gum and bone tissue as well as actual tooth wear and tear. The enamel of the teeth may wear away, exposing dentin. As a result of secondary dentin deposition with aging, the size of the pulp chamber is decreased and the pulp is limited to the root cavity only. There is controversy as to whether the loss of gingival epithelial tissue is pathologic or a normal part of aging.

region is referred to as the **lower esophageal sphincter** (LES). Although anatomically this sphincter is no different from the remainder of the esophagus, it remains tonically constricted, in contrast to the mid- and upper portions of the esophagus, which are completely relaxed under normal conditions.[1,2] Thus, the LES serves to prevent the highly acidic gastric contents from moving in a retrograde motion back into the esophagus. Under certain conditions, the LES does not function properly, resulting in reflux of gastric contents into the esophagus. The resulting subjective sensation of irritation and spasms of the distal portion of the esophagus is often referred to as heartburn.[3]

Stomach

The stomach (Fig. 35–2) is essentially a food reservoir and is the site of the start of the digestive process. Under normal circumstances its capacity is 1,000 to 1,500 mL, although a capacity of as much as 6,000 mL is possible.[4] The portion of the stomach immediately below the LES is called the **cardia.** The **fundus** is the part of the stomach that continues lateral to and above the cardia; the body of the stomach extends from the cardia to the **antrum,** which stretches from the angulus to the pylorus. The antrum differs markedly from the rest of the stomach in function and is distinguished by the absence of **rugae,** the folds present in the mucous membrane of the other areas of the stomach. The **pylorus** is a muscular sphincter between the stomach and the duodenum that serves to control gastric emptying and limit the reflux of bile from the small intestine.[1,3,4]

The stomach is lined with simple columnar epithelium containing millions of gastric glands that extend down to the mucosa. A typical gastric gland is shown in Figure 35–3. As shown in this illustration, the gastric glands are lined by several types of specialized

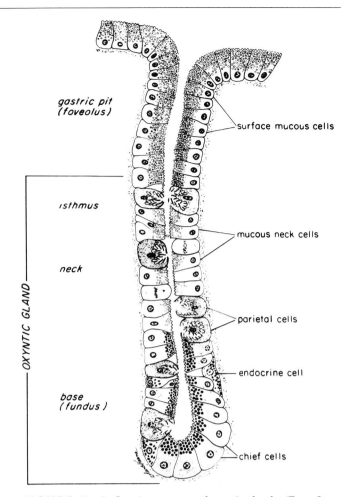

FIGURE 35–3. Gastric mucosa and gastric glands. (From Ito S: Functional gastric morphology, in Johnson LR, et al (eds): *Physiology of the Gastrointestinal Tract,* 2nd ed. New York, Raven Press, 1987, vol 1. Originally adapted from Ito S, Winchester RJ. The fine structure of the gastric mucosa in the bat. *The Journal of Cell Biology,* 1963, 16:541–578, by copyright permission of The Rockefeller University Press.)

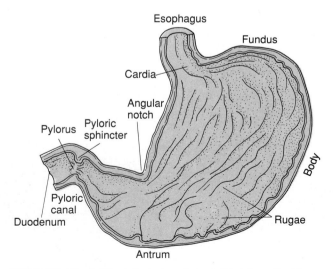

FIGURE 35–2. Physiological anatomy of the stomach. (From Guyton AC: *Textbook of Medical Physiology.* 8th ed. Philadelphia, WB Saunders, 1991, p. 701. Reproduced with permission.)

cells. The chief cells produce pepsinogen, the inactive form of the enzyme pepsin; the parietal cells produce hydrochloric acid and also a substance called intrinsic factor, which is needed for adequate intestinal absorption of vitamin B_{12}. Mucous cells produce an alkaline mucus that serves to shield the stomach wall and neutralize the acidity in the immediate area of the lining. A layer of mucus more than 1 mm thick continuously bathes the free surfaces of the gastric epithelial lining. In addition to these cells, gastrin cells are located in the antral epithelium and have surface microvilli that monitor the intragastric pH.[2,7,10] The role of these cells and the substances they secrete in the digestion of nutrients are described in detail in a later section of this chapter.

Small Intestine

The small intestine of the living adult is approximately 5 meters long, the longest portion of the GI tract. The

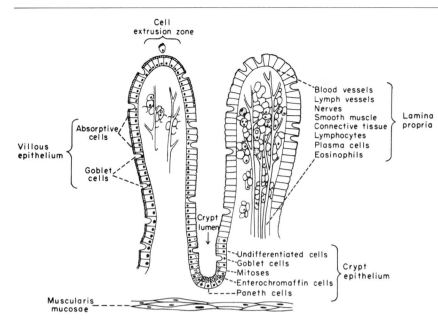

FIGURE 35–4. Villi of the small intestine. (From Sleisenger MH, Fordtran JS (eds): *Gastrointestinal Disease*, 5th ed. Philadelphia, WB Saunders, 1993, p 796. Reproduced with permission.)

duodenum composes the first 22 cm of its length, with the jejunum composing the next 2 meters and the ileum forming the remainder. The entire inner wall of the small intestine is marked by circular folds of a mucous membrane called the plicae circulares; these permanent ridges do not stretch out when the intestine is distended.[1,4]

On microscopic examination, the lining of the small intestine contains millions of fingerlike projections called **intestinal villi** (Fig. 35–4). Like the circular folds described above, these villi serve to increase the surface area of the intestine for digestion and absorption of nutrients. Each villus has its own microscopic projections called microvilli, which in turn are covered by a fuzzy coat (called the **brush border** because of its brushlike appearance when viewed with an electron microscope) containing many digestive enzymes. The combined effect of the circular folds, villi, and microvilli is to increase the surface area of the small intestine by about 600 times, creating a remarkably efficient milieu for nutrient digestion and absorption.[2,7,10] Figure 35–5 shows a microscopic section of the small intestine.

Between the villi are situated the intestinal glands, or crypts of Lieberkuhn. The intestinal glands secrete about 2 liters of fluid daily into the lumen of the intestine, but most of the fluid is quickly reabsorbed by the villi. Goblet cells throughout the intestinal mucosa secrete large amounts of mucus. In addition, specialized mucous glands called Brunner's glands, located in the first few centimeters of the duodenum, release a thick coating of mucus needed in that area to protect mucosa from the potentially damaging effects of acidic gastric juice that may enter through the pylorus.

Although the details of the process of digestion and absorption of nutrients occurring in the intestinal mucosa will be covered in greater detail in subsequent sections, a unique and salient feature of the villus

epithelial cells is described here. The villus epithelial cells have both digestive and absorptive functions, apparently dependent on their current stage of maturation. The rapidly dividing cells at the base of the intestinal glands are responsible for secretion, but as they migrate to the villus they mature into absorptive cells and are eventually pushed out of the villus tip. The turnover of cells in the small intestine occurs in 48 to 72 hours, one of the fastest cell turnover rates in the body. Therefore, conditions such as malnutrition or substances such as chemotherapeutic agents that interfere with cell replication or protein synthesis may adversely affect intestinal function.[4]

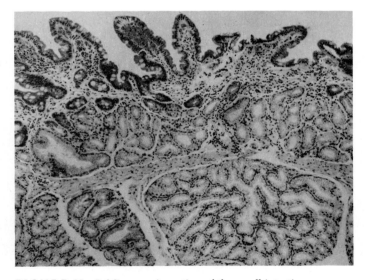

FIGURE 35–5. Microscopic section of the small intestine. (From Brandborg LL, Rubin GE, Quinton WE: A multipurpose instrument for suction biopsy of the esophagus, stomach, and small bowel. *Gastroenterology* 1959;37:1–16. Reproduced with permission.)

The **ileocecal valve,** a sphincter between the small and large intestines, is normally closed so that the contents of the large intestine cannot move in a retrograde fashion back into the small intestine. In response to a peristaltic contraction bringing intestinal contents toward it, the ileocecal valve opens.[1,3]

Large Intestine

The large intestine (Fig. 35–6) is termed "large" because of its 6.5-cm diameter, which is greater than the diameter of the small intestine. The large intestine is a 1.5-meter-long muscular tube that forms a frame around the small intestine. The vermiform appendix, which is attached to the cecum, is a worm-shaped blind tube containing specialized lymphatic structures. It is generally considered a vestigial structure that may have served a role as an incubator for bacteria that digested cellulose in the vegetarian past of the human species.[7] Inflammation of the appendix, or appendicitis, is a potentially life-threatening occurrence that can lead to peritonitis if not diagnosed and treated promptly.[3]

The portion of the large intestine from the cecum to the rectum is known as the colon. The ascending colon extends from the cecum straight up to the lower border of the liver; the transverse colon then extends across the abdomen, anterior to the small intestine. The descending colon then turns downward on the left side of the abdomen, finally becoming the S-shaped sigmoid colon, which empties into the rectum. The rectum has its outlet at the anus, the opening for the elimination of feces.

The mucosa of the large intestine has no villi and does not produce digestive enzymes. The epithelial surface of the colon consists of absorptive cells that predominantly absorb water and electrolytes.[11] Mucus-producing goblet cells line the glandular crypts present in the surface epithelium. Endocrine cells are also present, but the function of hormones in the large intestine is presently not well understood.

The turnover time of cells in the colonic mucosa is 3 to 8 days, comparatively longer than that of cells in the small intestine.[4]

KEY CONCEPTS

- Tracheoesophageal fistula, esophageal and duodenal atresia, and anal agenesis are congenital disorders that occur with abnormal development of the GI tract. These disorders usually present as obstructions.
- The major structures and corresponding functions of the GI tract can be summarized as follows:

  Mouth and salivary glands: Mastication, moistening, and beginning of starch digestion (by the enzyme salivary amylase) of foodstuffs.

  Pharynx: Transport of food to esophagus; protection of airway from aspiration of food particles.

  Esophagus: Movement of food to stomach by peristaltic waves. The lower esophageal sphincter prevents reflux of stomach contents.

  Stomach: Reservoir for food, mixing, and beginning digestion of proteins (by the enzyme pepsin). Secretion of hydrochloric acid, intrinsic factor, and gastrin. The pyloric sphincter prevents reflux of intestinal contents.

  Small intestine: Digestion and absorption of nearly all nutrients in the duodenum and jejunum. Absorption of bile salts in the terminal ileum. The brush border contains numerous digestive enzymes. Secretion of the enzymes secretin and cholecystokinin.

  Pancreas and gallbladder: The pancreas delivers digestive enzymes and bicarbonate to the duodenum. The gallbladder delivers bile salts to the duodenum.

  Large intestine: Reabsorption of water and storage of feces. Delivers feces to rectum for defecation.

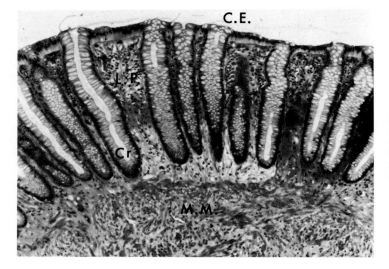

F I G U R E 35 – 6. Photomicrograph (×100) of the large intestine showing the columnar epithelium (CE), lamina propria (LP), crypt (Cr), and muscularis mucosae (MM). (From Sleisenger MH, Fordtran JS (eds): *Gastrointestinal Disease,* 5th ed. Philadelphia, WB Saunders, 1993, p 809. Reproduced with permission.)

Gastrointestinal Motility

The way in which nutrients and their eventual waste products are propelled through the GI tract is a complex and fascinating process involving an equisitely timed set of autoregulatory actions and responses. A summary of the characteristics of the intestinal wall, the innervation of the gut, and hormonal control of GI motility is presented as a basis for a description of the path taken by nutrients moving through the GI tract.

Characteristics of the Intestinal Wall

A typical cross-section of the intestinal wall is depicted in Figure 35–7. From the outer surface inward, there are five main layers: the serosa, a longitudinal muscle layer, a circular muscle layer, the submucosa, and the mucosa. A small layer, the muscularis mucosa, is located between the mucosa and submucosa. The muscular movements of the GI tract are performed mostly by the different layers of the smooth muscle, which extends from the distal esophagus through most of the large intestine. Skeletal muscle does play a key role in motility at both ends of the GI tract, however: motility from the mouth through the proximal esophagus at the upper end and through the external anal sphincter at the lower end is mediated by the action of skeletal muscle.[1,3,12,13]

The general characteristics of smooth muscle are covered in another part of this text. Specific characteristics of smooth muscle in the gut that render its function possible include the close proximity of these smooth muscle fibers to each other. In most areas of the GI tract, smooth muscle fibers are extremely close; about 12 percent of their membrane surfaces are actually fused with the membranes of other adjacent mus-

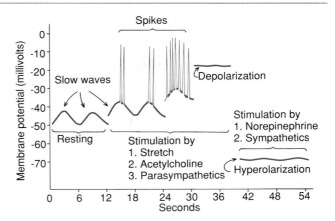

FIGURE 35–8. Membrane potentials in intestinal smooth muscle. (From Guyton AC: *Textbook of Medical Physiology*, 8th ed. Philadelphia, WB Saunders, 1991, p 689. Reproduced with permission.)

cle fibers to form a nexus, or junction. This close proximity of smooth muscle fibers in the GI tract allows intracellular current to travel very easily from one muscle fiber to another. Electrical signals originating in one smooth muscle fiber in the GI tract are generally propagated from fiber to fiber; the GI tract is said to be a *functional syncytium*, meaning that separate cells have the ability to function in concert with one another in a unified manner.[3]

Electrical Activity of Gastrointestinal Smooth Muscle

Electrical activity is almost constantly present in the smooth muscle layers of the GI tract. Two basic types of electrical wave activity have been identified in the gut, **slow waves** and **spikes,** the latter named for the spiking appearance of these sudden increases in membrane potential.[3] These two types of electrical wave patterns are shown in Figure 35–8. Slow waves represent an ongoing basic oscillation in membrane potential that occurs in the smooth muscle of the GI tract, especially in the muscle in the longitudinal layer. Normally, between 3 and 12 slow waves occur per minute. The slow waves can be any graded degree of intensity and are not an "all-or-nothing" type of action potential seen in other smooth muscle fibers in the body. In contrast to these nearly continuous slow waves, spikes occur under certain circumstances. When the muscle layer in the GI tract is stimulated by being stretched or by the effects of acetylcholine or parasympathetic excitation, the intracellular resting membrane potential of the muscle fibers becomes more positive. The entire potential level of the slow waves is raised, an effect called depolarization. As shown in Figure 35–8, when the depolarization rises above a certain level (around −40 millivolts), spikes, or sudden increases in the membrane potential, start to appear on the peaks of the slow waves. If the resting potential rises further, spikes appear more frequently. With very strong stimulation, the spikes generally disap-

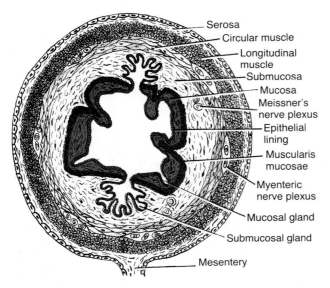

FIGURE 35–7. Typical cross-section of the intestinal wall. (From Guyton AC: *Textbook of Medical Physiology*, 8th ed. Philadelphia, WB Saunders, 1991, p 689. Reproduced with permission.)

pear, as the membrane now remains entirely depolarized. Figure 35–8 also illustrates the response of smooth muscle fibers to stimulation by norepinephrine or sympathetic excitation. In this situation, the resting membrane potential will be decreased, or *hyperpolarized,* so that electrical activity is almost abolished.[3,14,15]

Muscle Contraction of Gastrointestinal Smooth Muscle

In general, most contraction in the GI tract occurs in response to **spike potentials;** slow waves without superimposed spikes ordinarily do not give rise to contraction. Spike potentials occurring in the GI smooth muscle are analogous to action potentials in skeletal muscle and are responsible for the membrane changes that initiate contraction. As calcium enters the cell membrane to the interior of the smooth muscle, it initiates a reaction between actin and myosin,[3] a process described in detail in Chapters 16 and 49.

The electrical activity occurring in the smooth muscle of the gut gives rise to both tonic contractions and rhythmic contractions, both of which occur in most types of smooth muscle. Tonic contraction is continuous and is thought to be caused by a series of spike potentials. The intensity of tonic contraction may vary with the frequency of spike potentials. In turn, the intensity of tonic contraction in a specific segment of the gut will determine the amount of pressure in that segment. The degree of tonic contraction in the sphincters of the GI tract determines the amount of resistance to the movement of intestinal contents along the tract. Thus, the degree of contraction exerted by the pyloric, ileocecal, and anal sphincters serves to regulate the movement of nutrients through the GI tract.[3,12]

The degree of rhythmic contraction varies in different parts of the GI tract. These differing rhythmic frequencies are dependent on the rate of slow wave activity in a particular segment, and may occur at rates of 3 to 12 times per minute.[3,9] These slow wave–dependent contractions are responsible for the mixing and peristaltic propulsive movements present in the GI tract.

Neural and Hormonal Control

The movement of nutrients through the GI tract is controlled by the central nervous system (CNS) through its autonomic division and is modulated by numerous hormonal interactions.[16] In addition, the GI system has an intrinsic nervous system of its own that controls most GI functions. The **intrinsic nervous system** is composed of two layers: (1) the myenteric plexus, or Auerbach's plexus, which lies between the longitudinal and circular muscular layers, and (2) the submucosal plexus, or Meissner's plexus, which lies in the submucosa. The myenteric plexus is largely responsible for control of GI movements; the submucosal plexus serves to control secretion and also is

involved in many sensory functions, receiving information from the gut epithelium and stretch receptors in the intestinal wall. The entire intrinsic nervous system, including both the myenteric plexus and the submucosal plexus, is responsible for many reflexes that occur locally in the GI tract, such as reflexes causing the localized secretion of digestive juices by the submucosal glands or an increase in gut smooth muscle activity.[3,16–18]

In general, when the myenteric plexus is stimulated, activity in the GI tract increases. This stimulation results in four principal effects: (1) tonic contraction of the intestinal wall increases, (2) rhythmic contractions increase in intensity, (3) rhythmic contractions increase in rate, and (4) the velocity of conduction of excitatory waves along the intestinal wall increases. These excitatory **fibers** of the myenteric plexus are primarily **cholinergic,** meaning they secrete acetylcholine, in addition to one or more other excitatory transmitter substances. However, some myenteric plexus fibers have an inhibitory effect and may secrete purine-based transmitter substances, such as adenosine triphosphate (ATP).[3,16]

Autonomic Control

Input from the sympathetic and parasympathetic nervous systems can strongly affect the activity of the intrinsic nervous system. In general, sympathetic stimulation decreases its activity while parasympathetic stimulation increases its activity.

Parasympathetic Innervation

The parasympathetic supply to the GI tract is divided into cranial and sacral divisions. The cranial parasympathetic division is transmitted almost entirely in the **vagus nerves,** which provide extensive innervation to the esophagus, stomach, pancreas, and the first half of the large intestine (with little innervation of the small intestine). The sacral parasympathetic division originates in the second, third, and fourth sacral segments of the spinal cord and innervates the distal half of the large intestine. The sigmoidal, rectal, and anal regions of the large intestine are especially well supplied with parasympathetic fibers; these fibers play a key role in the defecation reflex.[3,16,19]

Sympathetic Innervation

The sympathetic fibers that innervate the GI tract have their origin in the spinal cord between T8 and L3. After exiting the cord, the preganglionic fibers enter the sympathetic chains and then pass through the chains to various ganglia located adjacent to the GI tract, such as the celiac ganglion and the mesenteric ganglia. From these locations, postganglionic fibers radiate out to all parts of the gut. The sympathetics supply essentially all parts of the GI tract, in contrast to the concentration of parasympathetic innervation at locations close to the entry and exit points of the gut.[3,16,20]

The sympathetic nerve endings in the GI tract secrete norepinephrine, which promotes the inhibitory effect of the sympathetic nervous system on the GI tract in the following ways. Norepinephrine acts directly on smooth muscle in the GI tract to inhibit activity; in addition, norepinephrine has an inhibitory effect on the neurons of the intrinsic nervous system of the GI tract. Strong stimulation of the sympathetic nervous system can effectively shut down motility in the gut and can block the movement of nutrients through the GI tract.[3,16]

Afferent Nerve Fibers

The GI tract is richly supplied with afferent nerve fibers arising from the gut that can transmit important information about the status of the GI tract. Afferent fibers that have their cell bodies in the submucosal plexus and terminate in the myenteric plexus transmit signals in response to irritation of the gut mucosa, excessive distention, or the presence of specific chemical substances. These signals can result in excitation or, in some circumstances, inhibition of intestinal motility or secretion. Other afferent fibers with cell bodies in the dorsal root ganglia of the spinal cord or cranial nerve ganglia can transmit signals to higher levels of the CNS, traveling along sympathetic or parasympathetic pathways. For example, the vagus nerves contain many afferent fibers that transmit signals to the medulla; this information is then used to initiate and modulate vagal signals that control many important functions of the GI tract.[3,16,18]

Hormonal Control

In the following section on secretory function of the GI tract, the role of hormones in controlling GI secretion is described in detail. It is important to note that many of these same hormones are involved in controlling motility in some portions of the GI tract. **Gastrin,** which is secreted by the mucosa of the stomach antrum in response to food entering the stomach, increases stomach motility. In addition, it promotes increased constriction of the LES, which serves to prevent reflux of stomach contents into the esophagus. Gastrin may also have a small effect in increasing motility of the small intestine and gallbladder.[3,21,22]

Cholecystokinin, which is secreted mainly by the mucosa of the jejunum in response to the entry of fatty substances, has an extremely strong effect in increasing the contractility of the gallbladder. This stimulation of gallbladder activity results in an outpouring into the small intestine of bile, which plays an important role in promoting fat digestion and absorption. Secretin, which is secreted by the mucosa of the duodenum in response to the entry of acidic gastric juice from the stomach, has a mild inhibitory effect on most of the GI tract.[3,22]

Gastric inhibitory peptide, which is secreted by the mucosa of the upper small intestine, primarily in response to the presence of fat but also carbohydrate, has a moderate effect in decreasing stomach motility. Thus, it serves to slow the emptying of stomach contents into the duodenum in circumstances in which the upper small intestine already contains an oversupply of nutrient substances.[3,22]

Types of Movement

There are basically two types of muscular activity involved in the digestive and absorptive functions of the GI tract, mixing movements and propulsive movements. In different portions of the GI tract, these movements may serve different functions to achieve proper digestion and absorption of nutrients. For example, mixing movements in the stomach and small intestine promote digestion by mixing the digestive juices with the food that enters from above. In the small intestine and proximal large intestine, mixing movements facilitate absorption by bringing newly arrived intestinal contents into contact with absorbing surfaces. In the case of propulsion, the rate at which nutrients are propelled through the GI tract may vary depending on the function of the different organs of the tract. For example, the passageway for nutrients from the mouth through the pharynx and esophagus is simply a conduit; essentially no digestive or absorptive function occurs here. Thus, the transit of nutrients through these regions is quite rapid. In contrast, transit from the stomach and through the small and large intestines is quite slow. This slow rate of passage allows for completion of the digestive and absorptive processes that occur in these portions of the GI tract.

While the characteristics of mixing and propulsive movements will differ in various parts of the GI tract and will be described separately in the next section, a description of the general characteristics of these movements is presented here.

Propulsive Movements

The basic propulsive movement of the GI tract is **peristalsis** (Fig. 35–9). Nutrients are propelled by the slow advancement of a circular constriction that squeezes the materials in front of the constricted area forward. Peristalsis is an inherent property of any smooth muscle tube that, like the intestine, is a functional syncytium. However, effective intestinal peristalsis requires the presence of an intact myenteric nerve plexus. The usual stimulus for peristalsis is distention of the intestinal walls. The entry and subsequent stretching of the intestinal wall by a bolus of food will have the effect of stimulating the gut wall 2 to 3 cm above this point, and a circular constriction will occur that then propels the food with a peristaltic movement. Although peristalsis can move in both directions in the gut (either toward the mouth or toward the anus), it normally moves toward the anus. The exact cause of this generally analward direction of peristalsis is still

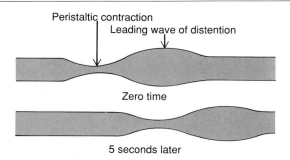

F I G U R E 35 – 9. Peristalsis. (From Guyton AC: *Textbook of Medical Physiology*, 8th ed. Philadelphia, WB Saunders, 1991, p 693. Reproduced with permission.)

being debated by physiologists; it is thought that the myenteric plexus may be organized in such a way that preferential transmission of signals downward occurs simultaneously with a relaxation of the portion of the intestine below the distended stimulus point. This posited ability of the GI tract to propel nutrients downward while relaxing an adjacent lower portion to receive these nutrients is sometimes referred to as the "law of the gut."[3,4,12]

Mixing Movements

Mixing movements that serve to keep the intestinal contents thoroughly mixed on a constant basis are caused by either peristaltic contractions or by local constrictive contractions of small segments of the gut wall. These movements may vary according to the specific function of each portion of the GI tract (see the discussion under Secretory Function).

Movement of Nutrients

The path taken by foods ingested into the GI tract as these nutrients travel down the tract, are digested and absorbed, and their waste products eventually excreted will be traced beginning with the mouth. Although this process is described here as a linear sequence, it is important to note that several steps may be occurring simultaneously. The individual steps involved in nutrient ingestion constitute a synergistic process, and an inability to perform one phase of the process will ultimately have a profound effect on the entire GI tract. In addition, different individuals may manifest a great deal of variability in such aspects of digestive function as tolerance of certain nutrients and defecation patterns. Such variations may represent age-related differences or conditioned responses to environmental cues.

Chewing

The entry of solid food into the mouth results in the action of chewing, an important first step in the process of nutrient digestion. The process of moving the food around in the mouth and mixing it with saliva

results in the stimulation of the taste buds and olfactory epithelia; this sensory input greatly increases the subjective enjoyment of eating. As the food is mixed with saliva, it becomes softened and formed into a mass of appropriate size (**bolus**) that can be swallowed. The action of the molars and premolars in crushing more rigid forms of foods serves to prepare rough substances for transport down the esophagus. Although the act of chewing is under voluntary control, it is also partly reflexive in nature. The entry of food into the mouth has been shown to stimulate chewing in animals in the absence of full cerebral function. The movements of the skeletal muscles responsible for chewing are coordinated by impulses traveling through cranial nerves V, VII, IX, X, XI, and XII.[1,3] The interruption of proper transmission of impulses through these nerve tracts will place an individual at risk for decreased voluntary control of chewing function.

Swallowing

Swallowing is the transport of material from the mouth to the stomach. The process of swallowing has been divided into three stages, which describe the regions the bolus of nutrients passes through on its way to the stomach: (1) the oral stage, (2) the pharyngeal stage, and (3) the esophageal stage.[1,3]

During the oral stage, the bolus is passed from the mouth through the isthmus of the fauces in the pharynx. The bolus, either solid or liquid, is rolled toward the back of the tongue, and the front of the tongue is then pushed up against the hard palate. Respiration is inhibited briefly in this phase as the pharyngeal muscles constrict to force the bolus of food into the pharynx. In the pharyngeal stage the bolus is passed through the pharynx into the esophagus, a process taking about one fifth of a second. The continued contraction of the pharyngeal muscles and the position of the tongue prevent reentry of the tongue into the oral cavity. The soft palate is pulled upward to close off the nasopharynx; simultaneously, food is prevented from entering the larynx by elevation of the larynx and the approximation of the vocal cords, both of which actions serve to close the glottis. As these openings are closed off, the pharyngeal constrictors contract and force the bolus of food into the esophagus. Respiration now is resumed, and pressure in the pharynx rises as a result of the muscular activities that have occurred.[1,3]

The muscular characteristics of the esophagus are of particular importance in effecting the third, or esophageal, stage of swallowing. The upper third of the esophagus consists of skeletal muscle, while the lower two thirds is composed of predominantly smooth muscle. In the normal resting stage, the upper part of the esophagus is closed by the tonic contraction of a band of skeletal muscle, which serves as the pharyngoesophageal sphincter. The pressure exerted by this sphincter in this region is normally about 20 to 40 cm H_2O above atmospheric pressure; this zone of high pressure acts to keep air from entering the esophagus during inspiration. Almost immediately following the initiation of a swallow, the sphincter relaxes and pressure in the region drops to atmospheric pressure, allowing the bolus to be forced into the esophagus by the pressure generated in the pharynx. Pressure in the pharyngoesophageal junction region then rises as the result of contraction of skeletal muscle in this area, thus preventing the reflux of food from the esophagus back to the pharynx. Pressure in this region then gradually subsides to a resting level as muscular relaxation occurs.[1,3]

If the bolus being swallowed is a liquid, it is propelled through the esophagus by the initial force of swallowing and travels by gravity to the stomach in about 1 second. If the bolus is a semisolid mass, it is propelled down the esophagus by means of a peristaltic wave. This esophageal peristalsis is a contraction of circular muscle that forces the bolus ahead of it toward the stomach, with a transit time of about 4 to 6 seconds.[1,3]

Although there is no well-differentiated muscular structure in the area where the esophagus joins the stomach, the region approximately 2 to 5 cm above the juncture with the stomach is referred to as the lower esophageal sphincter, and was described in a previous section. Almost immediately following the initiation of a swallow, pressure at the LES drops and remains low during the time a peristaltic wave is passing down through the lower esophagus. Once the bolus has passed through the lower esophageal region and pressure in the lower esophagus has fallen to a resting level, the pressure in the LES rises and remains elevated for about 10 seconds before falling to a resting level once more.[1,3]

Neural Control of Swallowing. Figure 35–10 illustrates the neural pathways involved in the swallowing mechanism. Swallowing receptors in the posterior mouth and throat transmit impulses in response to a stimulus to the mucous membranes in the mouth, such as the presence of a moderate amount of fluid. These impulses travel mainly through the trigeminal nerve into the reticular substance of the medulla oblongata, where the swallowing center is located. Once this center has been activated, the sequence of muscular reactions described above will occur automatically and usually cannot be voluntarily stopped. The swallowing center then sends impulses over a number of efferent nerves to the numerous skeletal and smooth muscles involved in the swallowing process, allowing the complete act of swallowing to occur in the appropriate sequence. The glossopharyngeal and hypoglossal nerves are primarily concerned with the oral and pharyngeal stages, while the vagus is important in activating the esophageal stage.[1,3,6]

Motor Functions of the Stomach

The motor functions of the stomach include the storage of ingested nutrients for variable lengths of time and the discharge of gastric contents into the small

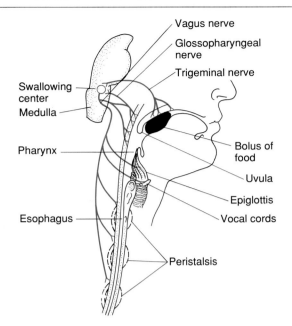

FIGURE 35–10. Neural pathways of the swallowing mechanism. (From Guyton AC: *Textbook of Medical Physiology,* 8th ed. Philadelphia, WB Saunders, 1991, p 699. Reproduced with permission.)

intestine at an appropriate rate for optimal digestion and absorption. The stomach also aids in the digestive process by its mixing movements, which convert large pieces of food into a finer, liquid consistency.

Gastric Filling and Storage. Upon entering the stomach from the esophagus, newly arrived food forms concentric circles in the body and fundus of the stomach, with the newest food lying closest to the esophagus and older food lying closer to the stomach wall. The smooth muscle in the fundus and body of the stomach can adapt to the volume of contents, so that relatively large contents can be introduced with little increase in intragastric pressure. The fundus and the body of the stomach maintain a certain pressure at all times. This tonic contraction continually presses on the food mass and aids in its delivery to the pyloric antrum.[1,3,6]

Peristaltic contractions occur in the stomach once every 20 seconds. These rippling peristaltic waves begin in the corpus and move at a velocity of about 1 to 2 cm per second. When they reach the more thickly walled pyloric antrum, they become much more vigorous and also increase in speed. These strong peristaltic contractions occurring in the pyloric antrum are largely responsible for mixing ingested nutrients with gastric secretions. As ingested food is churned and mixed to a greater degree of fluidity, the mixture takes on a milky white sludge appearance and is then called **chyme**.[1,3,4]

Emptying. As pressure in the antrum rises momentarily as the result of peristaltic contraction, a pressure differential exists between pressure in the antral pylorus and the duodenal bulb. The higher pressure in the antrum is sufficient to overcome the resistance of the pyloric sphincter, and the contents of the stomach are then propelled into the duodenum. Concurrently, the degree of constriction of the pyloric sphincter may increase or decrease, depending on several factors discussed below. As this process is dependent on the muscular activity of the antrum as well as pyloric muscle tone, gastric emptying is largely regulated by mechanisms that affect each of these regions.

Regulation of Gastric Emptying. Factors that may affect the rate at which the stomach empties include the degree of distention of the gastric wall and the release of the hormone gastrin in response to certain types of food in the stomach. Both of these factors increase the rate of gastric emptying by increasing the force of antral contractions while simultaneously inhibiting pyloric constriction. Distention of the gastric wall results in the stimulation of mechanoreceptors in the stomach with subsequent activation of reflexes over the vagus and the intrinsic nerve plexuses. These neural influences, along with contractile activity (which is a direct response to the stretch of gastric muscle), constitute a major mechanism in providing the stimulus for gastric emptying.[1,3,4]

Gastrin is a hormone released from the antral mucosa in response to stretching of the gastric wall as well as the presence of certain foods, particularly meat. The role of gastrin in promoting the secretion of highly acidic gastric juices will be discussed later. With respect to stomach emptying, gastrin plays a key role by enhancing peristalsis while at the same time relaxing the pylorus.[3,22]

In addition to these influences, many of the mechanisms that affect gastric emptying are initiated in the duodenum. Reflex nervous signals are transmitted from the duodenum back to the stomach in response to intraluminal stimuli; these signals probably play a key role in controlling both peristaltic activity and the degree of pyloric constriction. Stimulation of the duodenum in a variety of ways has the effect of slowing gastric emptying; both the chemical and physical properties of chyme entering the duodenum may affect the rate of gastric emptying. A variety of both duodenal cells and receptors, including osmoreceptors, mechanoreceptors, and chemoreceptors, respond to intraluminal stimuli to produce hormonal and reflex inhibition of gastric motor activity and enhancement of pyloric tone. The presence in the duodenum of chyme containing the breakdown products of proteins, and to a lesser extent fats, may impede gastric emptying. Also, the presence of a highly acidic or highly hypertonic or hypotonic chyme in the duodenum may inhibit the rate of gastric emptying. The degree of distention of the duodenum as well as the presence of any degree of irritation of the duodenum may serve to impede stomach emptying. Finally, the degree of distention in the duodenum may cause an inhibition of the rate of stomach emptying. These inhibitory mechanisms have a protective function and are effective in preventing the intestinal mucosa from overloading its digestive and absorptive abilities and from potential damage from chemical or mechanical sources.[1,3,4]

Although the regulation of gastric emptying is largely dependent on factors in the stomach and duodenum, gastric motility may be stimulated or inhibited reflexly from a variety of regions of the body. For example, stomach emptying in inhibited when the ileum is full and when the anus is mechanically distended. The stimulation of visceral and somatic pain receptors may result in inhibition of gastric motility. Various strong emotions, such as anger, fear, and anxiety, may produce changes in the motility of the stomach, but whether these states tend to predispose an individual to inhibition or excitation of gastric motility is not always predictable.[9,18]

Vomiting. Vomiting is the rapid emptying of the stomach of its contents into the esophagus through the pharyngoesophageal sphincter and into the mouth. The major force for vomiting is supplied by the skeletal muscle of the diaphragm and abdomen rather than by contraction of the muscle of the stomach wall. Vomiting is the result of an extremely complex set of neural events that are coordinated by a center located in the medulla. Afferent impulses from receptors in various regions of the body, including the sensory nerve endings of the pharynx, abdominal viscera, and the labyrinths, arrive at this center and the vomiting reflex is initiated. This reflex causes closure of the glottis and trachea, relaxation of the gastroesophageal sphincter, and contraction of the diaphragm and the abdominal muscles, which forcibly expels the contents of the stomach.[1,3]

Motility of the Small Intestine

What began as intact food entering the mouth has now been liquefied and partially digested in the stomach. It now enters the small intestine, where the major part of digestion and absorption occurs. As in other parts of the GI tract, the movements of the small intestine can be described as propulsive and mixing movements. Although this separation of types of movements is somewhat arbitrary in the small intestine, because all its movements may cause both propulsion and mixing simultaneously, these processes are usually described separately.

Propulsion. Chyme is propelled through the small intestine by peristaltic waves that move at a rate of 0.5 to 2 cm per second, with a faster rate at the proximal intestine and a slower rate in the terminal intestine. Approximately 3 to 5 hours is normally needed for the passage of chyme from the pyloric sphincter to the ileocecal valve, but this period may vary in some disease states. Peristaltic activity in the small intestine is greatly increased following the ingestion of a meal. The increase in contractile activity in the stomach caused by distention of the stomach wall is conducted principally through the myenteric plexus down along the wall of the small intestine. This so-called gastroenteric reflex serves to increase the activity of the small intestine, with an enhancement of both intestinal motility and secretion.[1,3,4]

The usual stimulus for peristalsis in the small intestine is distention of the intestinal walls; stretch receptors in the gut wall are sensitive to circumferential stretch and initiate a local myenteric reflex in response to this stimulation. The resulting contraction of longitudinal muscle, followed by contraction of the circular muscle, spreads downward in a peristaltic motion.

The peristaltic waves in the small intestine not only propel chyme downward toward the ileocecal valve but also spread out the chyme along the intestinal mucosa, thus facilitating the process of absorption of nutrients. As additional chyme enters the small intestine, this spreading process intensifies as peristalsis increases. When the chyme reaches the ileocecal valve, it is sometimes stationary for several hours until the individual eats another meal and a new gastroenteral reflex intensifies the peristaltic process and propels the remaining chyme through the ileocecal valve.

Certain disease states, particularly those that involve an intense irritation of the intestinal mucosa, may result in a peristaltic rush, a powerful peristaltic wave that travels long distances in the small intestine in a short period of time. The peristaltic rush clears the contents of the small intestine into the colon, thus relieving the small intestine of either irritating substances or excessive distention.[1,3,6]

Mixing. In addition to propulsive peristaltic movements, a set of movements characterized as **segmentation contractions** also occurs in the small intestine. The primary effect of these contractions is the progressive mixing of solid chyme particles with the secretions of the small intestine. As their name implies, segmentation contractions involve the contraction of the small intestine in regularly spaced segments that have the appearance of sausages (Fig. 35–11). As one set of segmentation contractions is completed a new set begins, with contractile points located at different locations along the small intestine. The segmentation contractions occur at a rate of 7 to 12 times per minute and effectively chop and mix the chyme, as well as assist in propelling the chyme toward the ileocecal valve (Figs. 35–12, 35–13).[1,3]

Control of Motility. There is a close association between the electrical and mechanical activities of the small intestine. Slow waves, as described previously

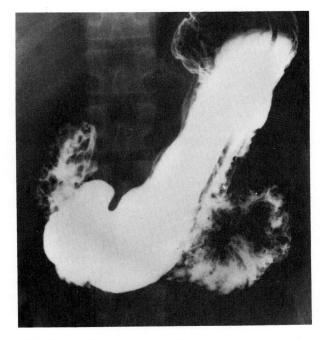

F I G U R E 35 – 12. Radiograph of the upper gastrointestinal tract. (From Sleisenger MH, Fordtran JS (eds): *Gastrointestinal Disease,* 5th ed. Philadelphia, WB Saunders, 1993, p 460. Courtesy of James W. Weaver, M.D. Reproduced with permission.)

in this chapter, occur at the membranes of the longitudinal smooth muscle, with frequencies of 11 to 12 per minute in the duodenum, decreasing to 7 to 9 per minute in the terminal ileum. The slow waves do not directly produce muscular contractions in the small intestine but serve to provide the conditions under which contractions can occur. Although the slow waves determine the velocity and direction of peristal-

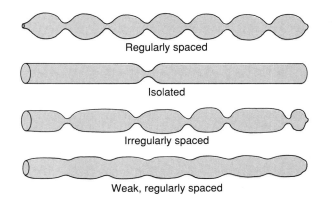

F I G U R E 35 – 11. Segmentation movements of the small intestine. (From Guyton AC: *Textbook of Medical Physiology,* 8th ed. Philadelphia, WB Saunders, 1991, p 704. Reproduced with permission.)

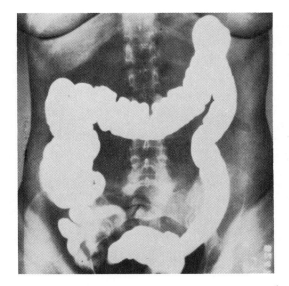

F I G U R E 35 – 13. Radiograph of the lower gastrointestinal tract. (From Berk JE (ed): *Bockus Gastroenterology,* 4th ed. Philadelphia, WB Saunders, 1985, vol 4, p 2388. Reproduced with permission.)

sis, other factors determine whether or not action potentials, and thus contraction, will occur. Local mechanical and chemical stimulation by chyme is probably largely responsible for the initiation and continuance of contraction in the small intestine. Thus, when the intestinal tract becomes overly distended or when the mucosa becomes irritated, myenteric reflexes enhance the electrical activity of the gut and spike potentials are superimposed on the slow waves. These spike potentials then spread through both the longitudinal muscle and the circular muscle and contraction results.[3]

Intestinal motility may also be influenced by stimulation from extrinsic sources. Stimulation of the vagus nerve generally causes increased intestinal motility, with sympathetic stimulation resulting in inhibition. Intestinal motility can be altered reflexly by stimulation of many sensory areas. For example, trauma to organs outside the GI tract, such as irritation of the peritoneum or urinary tract, may cause intestinal inhibition. A condition called paralytic ileus may occur following surgery to these areas, in which intestinal motility is inhibited as the result of reflex inhibition.[9,19]

Much current research is focused on the involvement of GI hormones in the regulation of GI tract motility. Cholecystokinin, a hormone that is released from the mucosa of the jejunum in response to fatty substances in the chyme, has been shown to block the increased gastric motility caused by gastrin. Another hormone, secretin, which is released mainly from the duodenal mucosa in response to gastric acid entering the duodenum, has the general effect of decreasing GI motility. A hormone called gastric inhibitory peptide, which is released from the upper small intestine in response to fat in the chyme but also carbohydrates, is known to inhibit gastric motility under some conditions.[13,22] These hormones will be described in more detail in the following section, Secretory Function.

Ileocecal Sphincter

The chyme that entered the small intestine has now been propelled down it and has arrived at the terminal ileum immediately proximal to the cecum, where the last 2 to 3 cm of the muscular coat is thicker than the rest of the ileum. This region, called the ileocecal sphincter, is normally closed; it is an area of high pressure, about 20 cm H_2O above atmospheric pressure. Distention of the lower ileum results in a lowering of pressure in the ileocecal sphincter. Thus, when intestinal contents are present in the terminal ileum and are ready to be propelled into the cecum, the sphincter reflexly relaxes and intestinal contents are pushed through the sphincter into the cecum by the propulsive movements of the distal small intestine. Subsequently, distention of the cecum following its filling with contents passing through the ileocecal valve results in an increased pressure in the sphincter, preventing reflux flow back into the ileum (Fig. 35–14).[1,3]

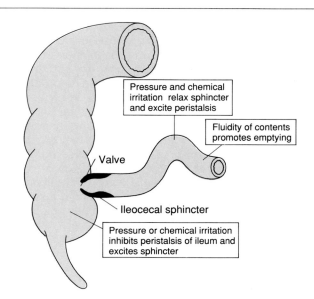

FIGURE 35–14. Emptying of the ileocecal valve. (From Guyton AC: *Textbook of Medical Physiology,* 8th ed. Philadelphia, WB Saunders, 1991, p 705. Reproduced with permission.)

Motility of the Colon

The movements of the colon are effective in promoting the two major functions of the colon: (1) the absorption of water and electrolytes from chyme, and (2) storage of the fecal mass until it can be expelled from the body by defecation.

Colonic Movements. For most of the time, the large intestine in humans is inactive. However, the presence of material in the proximal colon results in a type of mixing movement in the haustra (the outpouchings in the colon wall), termed **haustral churning,** that is similar to the segmenting movements in the small intestine. This is the major type of movement in the small intestine. Haustral churning exposes the contents of the large intestine to the mucosa, thus promoting the absorption of water. Normally, about 500 mL of chyme enters the proximal colon each day. Out of this total volume, 400 mL—mostly water and electrolytes—is reabsorbed before defecation takes place, with an average volume of 100 mL of feces remaining for eventual disposal from the body.[3,19]

At infrequent intervals of about three to four times a day, a strong peristaltic movement, termed a mass movement, occurs that propels the fecal material long distances. These strong contractions may reach a peak of 100 cm H_2O pressure in the segment undergoing the contraction. Fecal material may be transported all the way from the ascending colon to the descending colon by a mass movement. Feces then are stored in the distal colon until defecation takes place.[3,4]

Defecation. Under normal conditions, it takes about 18 hours for intestinal contents to reach the distal colon after leaving the small intestine. Fecal material is stored in the distal colon for varying lengths of time; defecation may take place 24 hours or longer after the ingestion of food. Ordinarily the rectum is empty, but fecal material is occasionally shifted into it after one of the mass movements, and the resulting distention of the rectum initiates the desire to defecate. The act of defecation is a combination of voluntary and involuntary movements. The contraction of the distal colon and the relaxation of the internal anal sphincter, which are regions composed of smooth muscle, are involuntary movements. The relaxation of the external anal sphincter, which consists of striated muscle, is a voluntary movement. Other voluntary movements that may assist in the act of defecation are contraction of the abdominal muscles and forcible expiration with closure of the glottis.[3,4]

Regulation of Colonic Motility. Movements in the proximal colon are largely initiated by distention in the colonic walls, which stimulates contractile activity by triggering short reflexes through the intrinsic nerve plexuses. Although the proximal colon receives extrinsic innervation via the vagus nerve, it functions in a relatively normal manner in the absence of extrinsic motor innervation and thus is a somewhat self-regulating structure. Extrinsic nerves may occasionally modify proximal colonic activity, however; for example, the entry of food into the stomach or duodenum may result in a mass contraction in the proximal colon. Sometimes termed the gastrocolic or duodenocolic reflexes, these strong mass movements are most evident after the first intake of nutrients in the morning and are often followed by a strong need to defecate.[3,19]

In contrast, the distal colon is somewhat more dependent on its extrinsic nerve supply, so that movements in this region, including the act of defecation, may be entirely abolished following some injury to these nerves. However, weak movements do return after a period of time, and defecation can still occur without voluntary control after the initial response to injury has passed.[9]

KEY CONCEPTS

- Movements of the GI tract are due to contraction of two layers of smooth muscle, the longitudinal and circular layers. Smooth muscle exhibits two types of electrical potentials: basic oscillations (slow waves), which do not result in contraction, and action potentials (spikes), which trigger calcium entry and result in contraction. Contraction of smooth muscle results in two types of intestinal motility: propulsive (peristalsis) and mixing (segmental).

- Gastrointestinal motility is regulated by the enteric nervous system, autonomic nervous system, and hormonal mediators. The enteric nervous system has two branches, myenteric and submucosal, that coordinate reflexive contraction and relaxation along the entire GI tract. Luminal distention is an important stimulus for reflexive motility. Sympathetic nervous system activity is generally inhibitory to GI motility (and secretion). Parasympathetic nervous system activity generally enhances motility. Regulatory hormones include gastrin (increased gastric motility), gastric inhibitory peptide (decreased gastric motil-

ity), cholecystokinin (gallbladder contraction), and secretin (decreased GI motility).

- Swallowing is a complex function coordinated by a swallowing center in the medulla. Swallowing is partially voluntary and partially involuntary. Cranial nerves IX, X, and XI mediate the various stages of swallowing.

- Regulation of gastric emptying involves gastric and duodenal factors. Gastric distention and the release of gastrin from gastric mucosa promote gastric emptying. Duodenal distention, acidity, hypertonicity, and high protein and fat concentration inhibit gastric emptying.

- Chyme spends 3 to 5 hours in the small intestine, where it is continually mixed by segmental contractions and slowly propulsed toward the ileocecal valve by peristalsis. Distention of the terminal ileum results in relaxation of the ileocecal sphincter, allowing contents to enter the large bowel.

- Segmental contractions (haustra) in the large intestine promote water absorption. About 18 hours is required for contents to traverse the large intestine and reach the distal colon. Three to four times a day a peristaltic mass movement occurs that sweeps fecal material along the colon. Mass movements may be initiated by entry of food into the stomach and duodenum (gastrocolic reflex).

- A desire to defecate is perceived when feces enters the rectum. Contraction of the distal colon and relaxation of the internal anal sphincter occur involuntarily as feces enters the rectum. The external anal sphincter is under voluntary control and inhibits defecation until voluntarily relaxed.

Secretory Function

Secretion of Gastrointestinal Juices

The many glands associated with the GI tract generally produce enzymes that participate in the digestive process to break down the major nutrient components of carbohydrates, fats, and proteins. The somewhat archaic term juices is still used to describe the fluids secreted in the GI tract, which contain a complex mixture of salts and protein enzymes. Thus, the glands located in the stomach are said to produce gastric juice, and the glands of the intestinal wall produce intestinal juice. Secretion of these digestive juices is stimulated by various factors, including mechanical and chemical stimulation by chyme, parasympathetic stimulation (in certain regions of the GI tract), and various hormones.

Gastrointestinal Hormones

Table 35–1 lists the major hormones of the GI tract, their sources, target organs, major actions, and factors that stimulate release. These hormones are released from the GI mucosa in response to distention or the

TABLE 35–1. Major Hormones of the GI Tract

Hormone	Source	Target Organ	Major Actions	Stimulated by
Gastrin	Stomach (mucosa)	Stomach (gastric glands)	Stimulates gastric glands to secrete specific substances	Distention of the stomach by food; other specific substances (e.g., partially digested proteins, caffeine)
Secretin	Duodenum (mucosa)	Pancreas	Stimulates release of the alkaline component of pancreatic juice	Acidic chyme acting on the duodenal mucosa
		Liver	Increases bile secretion rate	
Cholecystokinin	Duodenum (mucosa)	Pancreas	Stimulates release of digestive enzymes	Presence of fatty acids and partially digested proteins in the duodenum
		Gallbladder	Stimulates gallbladder contraction and emptying	
Gastric inhibitory peptide	Duodenum (mucosa)	Stomach	Reduces motor activity of the stomach; slows rate of gastric emptying	Presence of fat or carbohydrate in the duodenum

presence of certain nutrient substances. They are then absorbed into the blood and carried to glands in target tissues (i.e., tissues where they exert their effects), where they stimulate secretion. Chemically, the GI hormones are polypeptides or polypeptide derivatives.

Gastrin, secretin, cholecystokinin and gastric inhibitory peptide have been mentioned previously in this chapter as having additional roles in affecting the motility of the GI tract. Gastrin is secreted by the stomach mucosa and stimulates the gastric glands to secrete the specific substances produced by the different specialized cells of these glands. Secretin was one of the first of the many hormones of the body to be discovered. The most potent stimulus for secretin release is HCl, and the presence of acidic chyme acting on the mucosa of the duodenum promotes its release into the blood from the duodenal mucosa. It is carried to the pancreas, where it stimulates the secretion of a large volume of bicarbonate-rich juice, or the alkaline component of pancreatic juice. In the duodenum, sodium bicarbonate then neutralizes the HCl of the chyme, thus protecting the duodenal mucosa from potential damage and creating a slightly alkaline medium that is optimal for chemical digestion by pancreatic intestinal enzymes. Although the liver produces bile continuously, secretin is effective in increasing the rate of bile secretion. Hormonal regulation is the most important mechanism governing the activity of the pancreas, and cholecystokinin plays a key role in stimulating the release of large amounts of digestive enzymes from the pancreas. Cholecystokinin also stimulates the gallbladder to release the bile it stores. Gastric inhibitory peptide acts to slow stomach emptying by decreasing gastric motor activity.[3,22]

Histamine has also been shown to be a powerful stimulant of gastric acid secretion. The reader may recall that histamine is an amine with multiple roles in human physiologic processes, including its ability to constrict bronchial smooth muscle. Histamine is abundant in mast-like cells of the gastric mucosa and is released during an antigen-antibody reaction. Following its release, histamine diffuses readily into nearby parietal cells. Although less potent than gastrin, it causes the parietal cells to produce large amounts of gastric secretions. The exact mechanism by which histamine controls acid secretion is presently uncertain, although it is known that physical or emotional stress increases its release. The administration of certain medications that block its action (histamine-2 antagonists) is effective in reducing gastric acid secretions, and it is posited that histamine plays an important role in acid secretion.

Stimulation of the parasympathetic nerves to certain regions of the GI tract will also increase the rates of glandular secretion. Those glands in the upper portion of the GI tract that are innervated by the vagus and other cranial parasympathetic nerves, particularly the salivary, esophageal, and gastric glands, the pancreas, and some duodenal glands, are especially subject to parasympathetic stimulation. Glands in the distal portion of the large intestine are also affected by parasympathetic stimulation, as this region is innervated by the pelvic parasympathetic nerves. In the small intestine, the major stimulus for intestinal secretion is local and mechanical stimulation of the intestinal wall, which initiates the excitation of local myenteric reflexes and subsequent release of secretions.[1,3,17]

KEY CONCEPTS

- **Major secreting glands and secretions in the GI tract can be summarized as follows:**
  Salivary gland: Salivary amylase.
  Gastric glands: Chief cells secrete pepsinogen. Parietal cells secrete HCl and intrinsic factor. HCl activates pepsinogen to pepsin. Intrinsic factor enhances vitamin B_{12} absorption. Parietal cell secretion is stimulated by acetylcholine, histamine, and gastrin. G cells secrete gastrin into the bloodstream. Gastrin increases gastric motility and stimulates chief and parietal cell secretion.

Intestinal epithelium: Secretes brush border enzymes (peptidases, lipases, sucrase, lactase), secretin, which stimulates pancreatic secretion, and cholecystokinin, which stimulates gallbladder contraction.

Pancreas: Secretes bicarbonate-rich fluid containing amylase, trypsin, chymotrypsin, and lipase into the duodenum when stimulated by secretin.

Gallbladder: Secretes concentrated bile salts into the duodenum when stimulated by cholecystokinin.

Digestion and Absorption

Substances contained in foods that are important to the maintenance of the body include carbohydrates, proteins, fats (also called lipids), vitamins, inorganic salts, and water. Many of the nutrient constituents that make up intact food substances are structurally complex and cannot be easily absorbed from the GI tract in their original forms. During the process of digestion, digestive juices and the enzymes contained in these secretions convert these complex organic molecules to smaller molecules. These simpler compounds are then capable of absorption, or transfer across the wall of the small intestine into the blood and lymph, which in turn transport them to the cells of the body. This complex task of digestion and absorption of nutrients is the primary task of the GI tract. Inability to perform this function can compromise the health and existence of individuals experiencing interruptions in proper nutrient digestion and absorption. This section describes the mechanisms of digestion of the three major groups of nutrients, carbohydrates, lipids, and proteins, and then considers the absorption of these substances.

Digestion of Carbohydrates

In terms of calories, carbohydrates account for approximately one half of the American diet. The major digestible carbohydrate in food is the polysaccharide plant starch, a large molecule composed of straight and branched chains of glucose. A summary of carbohydrate digestion is presented in Table 35–2.

Digestion of starch begins in the mouth, as the enzyme salivary amylase breaks down polysaccharides to the much smaller disaccharide molecule maltose and dextrin. In the stomach, this action of salivary amylase continues until this enzyme is eventually inactivated by the acidic gastric juice. In the duodenum, the enzyme pancreatic amylase completes the task of splitting any remaining undigested polysaccharides and dextrins to small maltose units. Then maltase, an enzyme located in the brush border of the epithelial cells lining the duodenum, hydrolyzes each maltose molecule to two molecules of glucose. Other carbohydrates that are present in the diet in smaller quantities are the disaccharides sucrose, which is table sugar (glucose-fructose) and lactose, which is milk sugar (glucose-galactose). These two carbohydrates remain

TABLE 35–2. Summary of Carbohydrate, Protein, and Lipid Digestion

Location of Digestive Process	Source of Digestive Enzyme or Substance	Basic Digestive Process
Carbohydrates		
Mouth, stomach	Salivary glands (salivary amylase)	Polysaccharides $\xrightarrow{\text{salivary amylase}}$ maltose + dextrin
Small intestine lumen	Pancreas (pancreatic amylase)	Undigested polysaccharides/dextrins $\xrightarrow{\text{pancreatic amylase}}$ maltose
Brush borders	Intestine (maltase, sucrase, lactase)	Maltose $\xrightarrow{\text{maltase}}$ glucose + glucose
		Sucrose $\xrightarrow{\text{sucrase}}$ glucose + fructose
		Lactose $\xrightarrow{\text{lactase}}$ glucose + galactose
Lipids		
Small intestine	Liver	Lipid particle $\xrightarrow{\text{bile salts}}$ emulsified fat (triglycerides)
	Pancreas	Triglyceride $\xrightarrow{\text{lipase}}$ fatty acids + glycerol
Proteins		
Stomach	Stomach (gastric glands)	Protein $\xrightarrow{\text{pepsin}}$ polypeptides
Small intestine lumen	Pancreas	Polypeptides $\xrightarrow{\text{trypsin, chymotrypsin}}$ tripeptides + dipeptides $\xrightarrow{\text{carboxypeptidase}}$ free amino acids
Brush borders (and within cytoplasm of epithelial cells)	Small intestine	Tripeptides and dipeptides $\xrightarrow{\text{peptidases}}$ free amino acids

chemically unaltered until they reach the duodenum. There the enzyme sucrase in the brush border converts the sucrose to the monosaccharides glucose and fructose. Lactose is acted upon by lactase, which splits it into the monosaccharides glucose and galactose.[4,21]

Glucose is the major product of carbohydrate digestion, accounting for about 80 percent of the monosaccharides obtained from food, while fructose and galactose account for the other 20 percent. Humans do not secrete an enzyme capable of digesting cellulose, a plant polysaccharide found in the cell walls of plant cells and present in large amounts in fibrous vegetables. Although cellulose consists of glucose molecules, it contains molecular linkages different from those of starch. Thus, much of this complex carbohydrate passes through the digestive tract without being digested and is excreted in the feces.[1,4]

Digestion of Lipids

The **lipids** of the diet are mostly in the form of triglycerides but also include phospholipids, cholesterol, and vitamins A, D, E, and K. Lipid digestion occurs in the small intestine; neither the salivary nor the gastric enzymes appear to have any effect on triglycerides. The digestion of lipids begins in the duodenum, where they are emulsified by the action of bile. As the lipid particles enter the duodenum from the stomach, bile exerts a detergent action upon them in which the surface tension of the particles is decreased. This promotes the breakup of the particles into smaller particles as they are pushed around by the mixing movements of the small intestine. The emulsification process is an entirely mechanical action, as bile contains no enzymes and thus performs no chemical digestion.[4]

Eventually, the detergent action of bile salts reduces the particles of fat to tiny droplets, so that their surface area is greatly increased. This enhancement of surface area allows for maximum exposure to pancreatic lipase and enzyme, the latter (along with intestinal lipase, to a lesser extent) hydrolyzing the triglycerides to free fatty acids and glycerol. Some monoglycerides (glycerol with one fatty acid still attached) may still remain; in fact, some fat may escape digestion entirely or be reduced only to diglycerides (glycerol with two fatty acids attached).[4,23] A summary of triglyceride digestion is present in Table 35–2.

Cholesterol, a steroid type of lipid, is ingested in the form of cholesterol esters. These ester compounds cannot be directly absorbed. An esterase in the pancreatic juice degrades cholesterol esters to cholesterol and fatty acid, which can then undergo absorption.[4]

Digestion of Proteins

Proteins are composed of molecular subunits called amino acids that are linked together by peptide bonds. Protein that undergoes digestion in the small intestine includes both proteins from foods as well as from the desquamated cells and the many enzymes of the GI

tract. This protein of endogenous origin constitutes a sizable portion of the total protein utilized for digestion and absorption.[4,17]

Protein digestion involves breakage of the peptide bonds by hydrolysis and the release of free amino acids. Protein digestion begins in the stomach with the action of the enzyme pepsin, which is secreted by the gastric glands. By its action on peptide bonds, pepsin reduces most protein to intermediate-sized polypeptides. Pepsin is also capable of breaking down collagen, a protein component of intercellular connective tissue, thus rendering cellular proteins more accessible to enzymatic action in the GI tract. In the duodenum, trypsin and chymotrypsin contained in the pancreatic juice reduce the polypeptides to small peptides (tripeptides and dipeptides). Carboxypeptidase, which has its source in the pancreas, and peptidases in the brush borders of the intestinal epithelial cells split some of these peptides into free amino acids. Free amino acids, in addition to dipeptides and tripeptides, are absorbed into the intestinal epithelial cells. Within the cytoplasm of epithelial cells, the small peptides are then hydrolyzed by various peptidases into free amino acids prior to their passage into circulation. There are numerous proteolytic enzymes involved in protein digestion, as each enzyme acts on a slightly different type of peptide linkage.[4] Protein digestion is summarized in Table 35–2.

Absorption

Intestinal absorption is the movement of water and dissolved materials, such as the products of nutrient digestion, vitamins, and inorganic salts, from the inside of the small intestine through the semipermeable intestinal membrane and into the blood and lymph. A major feature of the intestinal absorptive surface is the villus, the small fingerlike projection lined with epithelial cells that was described earlier in this chapter. Within each villus is a network of capillaries that branches from a miniscule artery and empties into a miniscule vein. A central lymph vessel called a lacteal is also located in the villus. In the process of absorption, nutrient molecules must pass through the single layer of epithelial cells lining the villus and through the single layer of cells forming the wall of the capillary or lacteal. A number of transport systems specific to certain nutrient components function in the intestinal epithelium to promote this process of absorption.[4]

Energy for the operation of the intestinal transport systems is provided by certain chemical reactions occurring in the epithelial cells. These systems are capable of moving the products of nutrient digestion and inorganic salts from the intestinal lumen into the blood against electrochemical gradients (active transport). If the oxidative metabolism of the mucosal cells becomes inhibited, these active transport systems will be impeded. In addition to active transport, some molecules may move across the intestinal epithelium when a difference in concentration on the two sides of the epithelium exists. The rate of such molecular transfer based on diffusion gradients is dependent not only on the magnitude of the difference in concentration but also on the size of the molecules and the lipid solubility of the substances involved.[1,3,4]

Almost all substances capable of intestinal absorption disappear from the lumen of the small intestine by the time the intestinal contents reach the midjejunum. The ileum is not involved in absorption to any significant degree, as the proximal regions of the small intestine have usually done the work of absorption before intestinal contents reach the ileal region. Nevertheless, the distal small intestine has the capability of absorption, and may do so in situations in which absorption has not taken place in the proximal small intestine. Thus, about 50 percent of the small intestine can be surgically removed without compromising absorptive ability. However, it is important to note that vitamin B_{12} and the bile salts are absorbed specifically in the terminal ileum, and the surgical removal of this portion of the small intestine will result in impaired absorption of these substances.[3,4,9]

The intestinal contents arriving at the terminal ileum contain no digestible carbohydrate, very little fat, and only 15 to 17 percent nitrogen-containing substances. Most of the contents of the terminal ileum consist of bacteria, desquamated epithelial cells, digestive secretions, and the residues of foods which are undigested and therefore unabsorbed, such as the cellulose walls of fibrous plants and connective tissue from animal sources.[4]

Carbohydrates

Carbohydrates are absorbed in the form of monosaccharides. Polysaccharides and disaccharides lack the capacity for absorption; apparently the intestinal epithelium is impermeable to carbohydrates of such high molecular weight, and no transport systems exist for these types of carbohydrate molecules. The monosaccharides glucose and galactose are absorbed by an active, energy-requiring process in which a carrier molecule located on the luminal border of the epithelial cells transports glucose and galactose across the border. It is theorized that the same carrier molecule that ferries glucose and galactose also carries sodium, and that the carrier affinity for sugar is greatest when sodium is bound to the carrier. In contrast to the other monosaccharides, the monosaccharide fructose is absorbed passively by means of a diffusion gradient.[4]

Lipids

The absorption of lipid occurs by a highly complex, unique process. As fatty acids and monoglycerides are freed during digestion, they become dissolved in bile salt micelles, which are colloidal particles composed of many molecules. Within the micelles, the products of lipid digestion are now soluble, and can be absorbed far more efficiently. The bile salt micelles transport the lipid products to the epithelial brush borders, where the monoglycerides or fatty acids, which are highly soluble in the lipid cell membrane, diffuse into the epithelial cells, leaving the micelle behind. The micelle is now emptied of its cargo and can pick up more fatty acids and monoglycerides and transport them to the cell membrane.[4]

In the absence of bile, the amount of lipid absorbed in this manner is reduced by more than 25 percent. In this situation, the absorption of fat-soluble vitamins (vitamins A, D, E, and K), which are absorbed with fat, is compromised. The bile salts, which are required for micelle formation, are absorbed mostly in the terminal ileum and then recycled in the liver.[4,9]

The monoglycerides may be further degraded into glycerol and fatty acids by the enzyme lipase within the epithelial cell. Short-chain fatty acids (those with fewer than 12 carbon atoms) can be absorbed directly into the blood at this point. Longer-chain fatty acids and glycerol, however, are reassembled into triglycerides by the endoplasmic reticulum. These newly synthesized triglycerides are aggregated into droplets, which become progressively larger during passage through the cell. These lipid droplets are stabilized by enclosure with absorbed cholesterol and phospholipids and encased by a protein coat. The final product, called a chylomicron, passes out of the cell and into the lacteal of the villus. From the lacteal, chylomicrons pass through a series of lymph vessels that eventually drain into the general circulation.[4]

Proteins

Amino acids are transported across the epithelial membrane by means of an active transport carrier system, in much the same way as the monosaccharides are. It is currently thought that different carrier systems exist to carry the different chemical classes of amino acids (i.e., neutral, basic, dicarboxylic, imino acids). As is the case for transport of sugars, brush border membrane carriers are involved in the transfer of amino acids across the intestinal epithelial cell; these carriers require energy and are coupled to the transport of sodium. After being transported into the epithelial cells of the villi, amino acids diffuse through the base of the cell and into the blood. Both amino acids and the monosaccharides are transported directly to the liver by the hepatic portal vein.[4,7]

Water and Electrolytes

Water and inorganic ions, which are present inside the GI tract as the result of ingestion and secretion, are absorbed mainly from the small intestine and to a lesser extent from the colon. The process of absorption of water and ions is the same in both the small and large intestines: sodium is actively transported into the blood, and water follows passively in response to the osmotic gradient created by the removal of sodium from the intraluminal fluid. About 8,000 mL of water is absorbed every day by the small intestine and about 300 to 400 mL by the colon. Frequently,

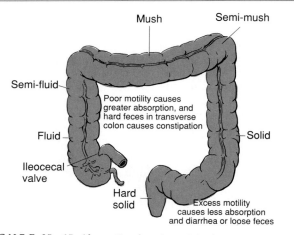

F I G U R E 35 – 15. Absorptive function of the large intestine. (From Guyton AC: *Textbook of Medical Physiology*, 8th ed. Philadelphia, WB Saunders, 1991, p 706. Reproduced with permission.)

diarrhea is the result of a failure of the small intestine to absorb water appropriately. If large quantities of water are allowed to enter the colon from the small intestine due to some malfunction of the small intestine's absorptive ability, the colonic absorptive mechanism may be overwhelmed, and diarrhea is the result (Fig. 35–15).[9,11]

KEY CONCEPTS

- Digestion, the process of converting large molecules to simpler forms, is accomplished by mechanical and enzymatic processes. Digestion is a necessary prelude to absorption because only simple molecules are able to cross the intestinal epithelia.

- Digestion of complex carbohydrates begins in the mouth, where salivary amylase begins to cleave large molecules into disaccharides. Pancreatic amylase continues this process in the small intestine. Disaccharides (maltose, sucrose, lactose) are cleaved into monosaccharides (glucose, fructose, galactose) by brush border enzymes on the intestinal epithelia (maltase, sucrase, lactase). Glucose and galactose are absorbed across the intestinal epithelia by a sodium-dependent cotransporter. Fructose is absorbed passively by facilitated diffusion. Monosaccharides then travel via the bloodstream to the liver.

- Lipid digestion begins in the small intestine where bile salts from the gallbladder mix and emulsify the fatty substances. Emulsification, mechanically separates the lipids into small drops that are more accessible to enzymatic digestion. Pancreatic lipase and brush border lipases digest the fats into free fatty acids and glycerol, which remain associated with the bile salts, forming micelles. Cholesterol is digested by pancreatic esterase. Fatty acids are transported to the intestinal epithelia by micelles. Free fatty acids diffuse out of the micelle and into the epithelial cell passively. Epithelial cells synthesize large protein-lipid complexes (chylomicrons) that enter the lymphatic system.

- Protein digestion begins in the stomach, where HCl from parietal cells activates pepsinogen to pepsin. Pepsin cleaves proteins into smaller polypeptides. Pepsin is neutralized in the duodenum, and pancreatic trypsin, chymotrypsin and carboxypeptidase take over protein digestion. Brush border peptidases split tri- and dipeptides into single amino acids. Amino acid transport into the intestinal epithelial cells is mediated by a sodium-dependent cotransport system similar to monosaccharide transport. Small peptides may also be endocytosed and cleaved into amino acids within the epithelial cells. Amino acids pass into the bloodstream and travel to the liver.

- Absorption of water occurs passively by osmosis. An osmotic gradient for water absorption is created as electrolytes are absorbed.

Gastrointestinal Function Across the Life Span

Maturation

During the first months of life, the newborn's GI tract undergoes many maturational changes. In the first 3 to 4 months of life, the sucking reflexes are present, and extrusion reflexes protect against the ingestion of solids that the immature GI tract is still unable to digest. The pressure in the LES remains low during this time, and the "spitting up" of gastric contents is common as the intragastric pressure often exceeds the pressure of the LES. Gastric motility is not well coordinated for the first 3 to 4 months, so that antral mixing is inadequate for the digestion of solid foods. At about 12 weeks of age, intestinal peristalsis similar to that in adults begins to develop, but it is one-third slower. This slower transit in infants may serve to improve nutrient digestion and absorption by increasing exposure of nutrient to the intestinal mucosa. The motor function of the large intestine appears to be fully developed at birth. During the first 2 years of life, the secretory and absorptive functions of the intestine mature and begin a pattern of functioning that continues into senescence.[4,9]

Age-Related Changes

Changes in GI function in older adults occur simultaneously with other age-related changes, such as a decrease in lean body mass and impaired homeostasis of multiple body systems. Within the GI tract, a variety of changes occur that may place the aging individual at risk for health problems related to GI functioning and nutrition. Loss of dentition and reduced taste and smell acuity may promote a decreased interest in food intake, as chewing may become difficult and the sensory enjoyment associated with food may be impaired. The older adult may develop a condition called **presbyesophagus,** in which esophageal motility

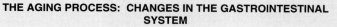

THE AGING PROCESS: CHANGES IN THE GASTROINTESTINAL SYSTEM

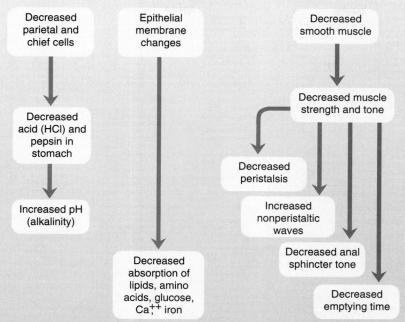

As a person ages, gastrointestinal muscle strength and movement decrease, leading to reduced peristalsis and decreased gastrointestinal motility throughout the system.

In the esophagus, the elderly person experiences greater numbers of muscle movements that do not propel the contents onward. These nonperistaltic waves are frequent in the lower esophagus. The phenomenon of presbyesophagus - in which the esophageal sphincter fails to relax and the lower esophagus becomes dilated - may not necessarily be normal in the elderly.

In the stomach, decreased numbers of parietal and chief cells result in diminished acid (HCl) and pepsin secretion. This leads to increased pH and a more alkaline secretion. The protective alkaline viscous mucus in the stomach is also decreased. The loss of smooth muscle in the stomach can delay emptying time, which increases and prolongs the exposure of gastric epithelial cells to the gastric contents.

The small intestinal smooth muscle, Peyer's patches, and lymphatic follicles are decreased. Normal intestinal absorption in the elderly is not well understood and may be influenced by a number of factors, including bowel motility, epithelial membranes, vascular perfusion, and gastrointestinal membrane transport. However, absorption of lipids, amino acids, glucose, calcium, and iron are known to be decreased. Normal changes in the large intestine have been difficult to determine. Owing to smooth muscle changes, anal sphincter tone decreases.

is slowed or disorganized. Presbyesophagus may be manifested as a difficulty in swallowing and may cause discomfort as the food passes through the esophagus. The incidence of hiatal hernia is also increased in the aging population, with 69 percent of persons over 70 years of age being affected. The transit time for intestinal contents to pass through the GI tract is decreased in older persons; this factor, coupled with a decreased perception of the sensory stimuli that produce the urge to defecate, may promote constipation in the aging population. Conversely, the confused or neurologically impaired older individual may experience fecal incontinence, as the sensation and tone of the rectum diminish with aging.[4,24,25]

KEY CONCEPTS

- Infants may experience GI dysfunction due to immaturity of the GI tract. Motility is not well coordinated until age 3 to 4 months, making digestion of solids difficult. Pressure in the lower esophageal sphincter is low, leading to "spitting up" with gastric distention. Maturation of the GI tract is complete by about age 2 years.
- Elderly individuals may experience GI dysfunction for a number of reasons. Poor dentition, loss of taste and smell acuity, and reduced esophageal motility may lead to poor intake of nutrients. Hiatal hernia and constipation are common in the elderly.

Summary

This chapter has described the structure of the human GI symptom and the process by which it provides nutrients for the body. A thorough understanding of the structure of the gastrointestinal tract, gastrointestinal motility, secretion of digestive juices, digestion of nutrients, and absorption of nutrients is needed as a basis for understanding other principles of health and disease.

Gastrointestinal motility is a complex process involving a set of carefully timed autoregulatory action responses. You may wish to trace the path and destiny of the apple you ate for lunch as an example of this process. As you track the movement of nutrients through the GI tract, consider the ways in which secretion of digestive juices occurs in response to the ingestion of your apple, which contains a great deal of carbohydrate (fructose), small amounts of protein, and minimal lipid. Consider also how digestion and absorption of these nutrients are occurring. What part of the apple will you use, for example, for energy to study this text? What part of the apple will your body "throw away," and how will this be accomplished? And finally, will your GI tract respond the same way to eating an apple when you are 85 years old? A careful review of the elegant and nearly automatic function of the human GI tract will prepare you to care for individuals experiencing interruptions in proper nutrient digestion and absorption.

REFERENCES

1. Guyton AC: *Human Physiology and Mechanisms of Disease*, 5th ed. Philadelphia, WB Saunders, 1992.
2. Solomon EP: *Introduction to Human Anatomy and Physiology*. Philadelphia, WB Saunders, 1992.
3. Guyton AC: *Textbook of Medical Physiology*, 8th ed. Philadelphia, WB Saunders, 1991.
4. Shils ME, Olson JA, Shike M (eds): *Modern Nutrition in Health and Disease*, 8th ed. Philadelphia, Lea & Febiger, 1993.
5. Facer P, Bishop AE, Moscoso G, et al: Vasoactive intestinal polypeptide gene expression in the developing human gastrointestinal tract. *Gastroenterology* 1992;102(1):47–55.
6. Patton HD, Fuchs AF, Hille B, Scher AM, Steiner R: *Textbook of Physiology*, 21st ed. Philadelphia, WB Saunders, 1989, pp 7–17.
7. Solomon EP, Phillips GA: *Understanding Human Anatomy and Physiology*. Philadelphia, WB Saunders, 1987.
8. Jacob S, Francone CA: *Elements of Anatomy and Physiology*, 2nd ed. Philadelphia, WB Saunders, 1989.
9. Sleisenger MH, Fordtran JS, Scharschmidt BF, Feldman M (eds): *Gastrointestinal Disease: Pathophysiology, Diagnosis, Management*, 5th ed. Philadelphia, WB Saunders, 1993.
10. Hollander D, Tarnawski A (eds): *Gastric Cytoprotection: A Clinician's Guide*. New York, Plenum Press, 1989.
11. Gebruers EM, Hall WJ: Role of the gastrointestinal tract in the regulation of hydration in man. *Dig Dis* 1992;10(2):112–120.
12. Johnson LR: *Gastrointestinal Physiology*, 4th ed. St. Louis, Mosby–Year Book, 1991.
13. Current concepts in research of gastrointestinal motility: International symposium, Aarhus, Denmark, July 18–20, 1991. *Dig Dis* 1991;9(6):321–443.
14. Huizinga JD: Action potentials in gastrointestinal smooth muscle. *Can J Physiol Pharmacol* 1991;69(8):1133–1142.
15. Sanders KM: Ionic mechanisms of electrical rhythmicity in gastrointestinal smooth muscles. *Annu Rev Physiol* 1992; 54:439–453.
16. McIntyre AS, Thompson DG: Review article: Adrenergic control of motor and secretory function in the gastrointestinal tract. *Aliment Pharmacol Ther* 1992;6(2):125–142.
17. Dockray GJ, Forster ER, Louis SM: Peptides and their receptors on afferent neurons to the upper gastrointestinal tract. *Adv Exp Med Biol* 1991;298:53–62.
18. Surrenti C, Maggi CA: Sensory nerves in the gastrointestinal tract: Changing concepts and perspectives. *Ital J Gastroenterol* 1991;23(2):94–99.
19. Karaus M, Wienbeck M: Colonic motility in humans—a growing understanding. *Baillieres Clin Gastroenterol* 1991; 5(2):453–478.
20. Holle GE, Hahn D, Forth W: Innervation of pylorus in control of motility and gastric emptying. *Am J Physiol* 1992;263(2 pt 1): G161–G168.
21. Marks V, Morgan L, Oben J, Elliott R: Gut hormones in glucose homeostasis. *Proc Nutr Soc* 1991;50(3):545–552.
22. Jenkins AP, Ghatei MA, Bloom SR, Thompson RP: Effects of bolus doses of fat on small intestinal structure and on release of gastrin, cholecystokinin, peptide tyrosine-tyronsine, and enteroglucagon. *Gut* 1992;33(2):218–223.
23. Titus E, Ahearn GA: Vertebrate gastrointestinal fermentation: Transport mechanisms for volatile fatty acids. *Am J Physiol* 1992;262(4 pt 2):R547–R553.
24. Marshall JC: The ecology and immunology of the gastrointestinal tract in health and critical illness. *J Hosp Infect* 1991;19(suppl C):7–17.
25. Shaffer E, Thomson AB (eds): *Modern Concepts in Gastroenterology*. New York, Plenum Press, 1992.

BIBLIOGRAPHY

Amidon GL, DeBrincat GA, Najib N: Effects of gravity on gastric emptying, intestinal transit, and drug absorption. *J Clin Pharmacol* 191;31(10):968–973.
Beck M, Evans NG (eds): *Gastroenterology Nursing: A Core Curriculum*. St. Louis, Mosby–Year Book, 1992.

Berk JE, Haubrich WS, Kalser MH, Roth JLA, Schaffner F (eds): *Bockus Gastroenterology*, 4th ed. Philadelphia, WB Saunders, 1985.

Berseth CL, Nordyke CK, Valdes MG, Furlow BL, Go VL: Responses of gastrointestinal peptides and motor activity to milk and water feedings in preterm and term infants. *Pediatr Res* 1992;31(6):587–590.

Black JM, Matassarin-Jacobs E: *Luckmann and Sorenson's Medical-Surgical Nursing Psychophysiological Approach*, 4th ed. Philadelphia, WB Saunders, 1993.

Drossman D (ed): *Manual of Gastroenterologic Procedures*, 3rd ed. New York, Raven Press, 1992.

Gitnick G: *Current Gastroenterology*. St. Louis, Mosby–Year Book, 1994, vol 14.

Grant M, Kennedy-Caldwell C: *Nutritional Support in Nursing*. Philadelphia, WB Saunders, 1987.

Heitkemper MM, Jarrett M: Pattern of gastrointestinal and somatic symptoms across the menstrual cycle. *Gastroenterology* 1991; 102(2):505–513.

Holt S: Upper gastrointestinal transit in humans. *J SC Med Assoc* 1991;87(10):493–498.

Kneisl CR, Ames SA: *Adult Health Nursing: A Biopsychosocial Approach*. Menlo Park, Calif, Addison-Wesley, 1986.

Miller LJ: A historical perspective of gastrointestinal endocrinology: The new age of molecular receptorology. *Gastroenterology* 1992;102(6):2168–2170.

Morriss FH: Neonatal gastrointestinal motility and enteral feeding. *Semin Perinatol* 1991;15(6):478–481.

Reuter SR, Redman HC, Cho KJ: *Gastrointestinal Angiography*, 3rd ed. Philadelphia, WB Saunders, 1986.

Thompson JC (ed): *Gastrointestinal Endocrinology: Receptors and Post-Receptor Mechanisms*. New York, Academic Press, 1990.

Turnberg LA: *Clinical Gastroenterology*. St. Louis, Mosby–Year Book, 1989.

CHAPTER 36
Gastrointestinal Disorders

JANE M. GEORGES

KEY TERMS

diverticulosis: The presence of diverticula, or outpouchings, in the wall of the colon.

dumping syndrome: The rapid emptying or "dumping" of stomach contents into the proximal small intestine due to loss of pyloric regulation of gastric emptying. This loss of function may occur following a gastrectomy.

dysphagia: Difficulty in swallowing as perceived by the individual. It may include the inability to initiate swallowing and/or the sensation of ingested substances sticking in the esophagus.

gastrectomy: The surgical removal of all or, more commonly, part of the stomach. This procedure may be used to remove a chronic peptic ulcer, to stop hemorrhage in a perforating ulcer, or to remove a malignancy.

gastritis: Inflammation of the stomach lining. It may occur following the ingestion of irritating substances or in the presence of viral, bacterial, or chemical toxins.

gastroenteritis: Inflammation of the stomach and intestines, which may occur on an acute or chronic basis.

inflammatory bowel disease: Term used to refer to either ulcerative colitis or Crohn's disease. These conditions may involve a life-altering chronic illness for persons experiencing them.

irritable bowel syndrome: The presence of alternating diarrhea and constipation accompanied by abdominal cramping in the absence of any identifiable pathology in the GI tract.

polyp: A general descriptive term used for any mass of tissue that protrudes into the GI tract. Polyps may be either benign or malignant, although the term polyp usually means a benign form.

steatorrhea: The presence of excess fat in the stool, characterized by frothy, foul-smelling fecal matter that floats. It is present in celiac disease, some malabsorption syndromes, and any condition in which fats are poorly absorbed by the small intestine.

Alterations in the function of the gastrointestinal (GI) tract may have far-reaching consequences in an individual's life. The ability to take in nutrients, convert them to usable forms for body functions, and dispose of their waste products goes beyond physiologic function and is intimately associated with social and psychological functioning. The person who is experiencing an alteration in GI function may be unable to participate fully in social activities, which in American society are largely centered on food consumption. Certain symptoms that may accompany GI disorders, such as chronic diarrhea and abdominal pain, may severely limit an individual's ability to maintain employment. Daily, approximately 200,000 people miss work because of GI-related problems.[1] In addition, GI diseases account for more hospital admissions in the United States than any other category of disease. Because many chronic GI conditions begin in midlife and continue into old age, their prevalence will increase as the U.S. population continues to age.[1]

This chapter describes the pathophysiology of the most common disorders of the GI tract and summarizes current treatments for these conditions. Because the knowledge of many GI disorders is expanding rapidly, some current research on selected GI conditions is described. Finally, because of the intimate relationship between GI function and the integrity and well-being of the person, a discussion of the psychological and emotional aspects of GI disorders across the life span is included.

Manifestations of Gastrointestinal Tract Disorders

As a basis for discussing individual types of GI disorders, a description of some common manifestations of these disorders and their pathophysiologic causes is presented. Common manifestations include dysphagia, esophageal and abdominal pain, intestinal gas, vomiting, and alterations in bowel patterns.

Dysphagia

Definitions and Categories

Dysphagia is difficulty in swallowing as perceived by the individual. It may include the inability to initiate swallowing or the sensation that the swallowed solids or liquids stick in the esophagus.[1] In certain disorders **odynophagia,** or pain with swallowing, may accompany dysphagia. The physiology of normal swallowing was described in Chapter 35; the reader may wish to refer to this information. The pathophysiologic basis for dysphagia usually falls into three major categories: (1) problems in delivery of the bolus of food or fluid into the esophagus as a result of neuromuscular incoordination, (2) problems in transport of the bolus down the body of the esophagus as a result of altered peristaltic activity of the esophagus, and (3) problems in bolus entry into the stomach as a result of lower esophageal sphincter (LES) dysfunction or obstructing lesions.[2]

In the first category of dysphagia, individuals have a decreased ability to accomplish the initial steps of swallowing in an orderly sequence. Pain, a neuromuscular disorder, or a lesion inside or outside of the esophagus may induce neuromuscular incoordination of the process of delivering food or fluids into the esophagus. Therefore, the normal sequence of pharyngeal contraction, closure of the epiglottis, upper esophageal sphincter relaxation, and initiation of peristalsis by contraction of the striated muscle in the upper esophagus is compromised or absent. Persons experiencing this type of dysphagia may cough and expel the ingested food or fluids through their mouth and nose or aspirate when they attempt to swallow. These symptoms are worse with liquids than with solids in this type of swallowing dysfunction.[1]

The second type of dysphagia may be the result of any disorder, structural or neuromuscular, in which the peristaltic activity of the body of the esophagus is altered. The presence of (1) esophageal **diverticula,** or outpouchings of one or more layers of the esophageal wall, (2) **achalasia,** a disorder of esophageal smooth muscle function, or (3) structural disorders such as neoplasms or strictures may interfere with proper peristaltic activity in the esophagus.[1] This alteration in peristalsis may be simply weak peristaltic activity, aperistalsis (the absence of all peristaltic activity), or disorganized and therefore ineffective peristalsis.[2] With this type of dysphagia the individual may have the sensation that food is "stuck" behind the sternum. Initially, dysphagia may be noted with solid foods; if the underlying pathology fosters a worsening of peristaltic ability, passage of liquids may also become impaired.

The third category of dysphagia, resulting from problems of bolus entry into the stomach, is secondary to any condition in which the LES functions improperly or is obstructed by a lesion. Tumors of the mediastinum, lower esophagus, and gastroesophageal junction may invade the myenteric plexus or produce an obstruction at the LES, thus interrupting normal LES function by neural invasion or direct obstruction.[1] In addition, motor disorders resulting from neuromuscular diseases or chronic inflammation of the lower esophagus from the reflux of acidic gastric contents may limit the ability of the LES to function properly.[1] This type of dysphagia may be manifested as tightness or pain in the substernal area during the swallowing process.[2]

Esophageal Pain

Two types of pain occur in the esophagus: (1) heartburn (also called pyrosis), and (2) chest pain located in the middle of the chest, which may mimic the pain of angina pectoris.[2] *Heartburn* is caused by the reflux of gastric contents into the esophagus and is a substernal burning sensation that may radiate to the neck or throat. Two possible mechanisms may be responsible

for the production of heartburn. First, the highly acidic gastric contents may be a noxious stimulant to sensory afferent nerve endings in the esophageal mucosa.[2] Second, heartburn may be produced by a spasm of the esophageal muscle brought on by acid stimulation.[2] It is probable that both of these mechanisms contribute to the development of heartburn.

Chest pain other than heartburn may be the result of esophageal distention or powerful esophageal contractions. These stimuli may arise from esophageal obstruction or a condition called **diffuse esophageal spasm,** in which high-amplitude, simultaneous contractions in the smooth muscle portion of the esophagus may occur, randomly interspersed with normal-appearing peristalsis.[1] This type of esophageal pain is similar to that of angina pectoris, particularly in its pattern of radiation into the neck, shoulder, arm, and jaw. Odynophagia may accompany diffuse esophageal spasm and may be indistinguishable from esophageal chest pain except that it is brought on specifically by swallowing.

Persons with herpetic or monilial esophagitis, infections of the esophagus that may be present in an immunocompromised state, may also experience a dull, aching chest pain. Swallowing may worsen the pain sensation and cause symptoms such as heartburn or chest pain.

Abdominal Pain

Pain in the abdominal region may be the first sign of a disorder of the GI tract and is often an important impetus to seeking medical care. While abdominal pain may result from GI tract disorders, it may also be the result of reproductive, genitourinary, musculoskeletal, and vascular disorders, as well as toxins or drug use. Abdominal pain is usually categorized into three types, although persons experiencing abdominal pain may manifest a combination of these types. (1) **Visceral pain** develops from stretching or distending an abdominal organ or from inflammation. The pain is diffuse and poorly localized and has a gnawing, burning, or cramping quality. (2) **Somatic pain** arises from the abdominal wall, the parietal peritoneum, the root of the mesentery, or the diaphragm. In contrast to visceral pain, it is sharper, more intense, and well localized. (3) **Referred pain** is felt at a location distant from the source of the pain but in the same dermatome or neurosegment. Referred pain is usually sharp and well localized, and may be felt in the skin or deeper tissues.[1,3]

Abdominal pain may be acute, with an instantaneous onset, signaling such events as a perforated ulcer or a ruptured internal organ. A more gradual development of abdominal pain may accompany such chronic states as diverticulitis or ulcerative colitis. Abdominal pain seldom occurs as a solitary manifestation of GI disorders but is usually accompanied by other manifestations such as vomiting or alteration in bowel patterns to a variable degree.[1]

mechanism of secretory diarrhea). In children and elderly people, fluid losses from diarrhea and vomiting can have serious consequences and may be life-threatening. Supportive treatment designed to eliminate the infective organism and provide fluid and electrolyte replacement may be required by these high-risk groups experiencing severe acute gastroenteritis.[1,2,6]

Peptic Ulcer Disease

The term *peptic ulcer disease* (PUD) refers to disorders of the upper GI tract caused by the action of acid and pepsin.[1] These disorders may include injury to the mucosa of the esophagus, stomach, or duodenum and may range from a slight mucosal injury to severe ulceration (Figs. 36–1 and 36–2, Color Plate III). Peptic disease seems to be the result of an increase in factors that tend to injure the mucosa over factors that tend to protect it. Factors such as the gastric mucosal barrier and the ability of the mucosa to perform epithelial renewal serve to protect it against injury. On the other hand, the presence of acid, which potentiates the actions of pepsin and other injurious substances, such as aspirin, will promote injury to the mucosa. Although it is known that some imbalance between these two sets of factors is implicated in the development of PUD, it is not known why one person may develop PUD and another may not.[1,2,6] In recent years, however, research suggests that the organism *Helicobacter pylori* may be key to the development of PUD.[10a] A brief review of the etiology and pathogenesis of PUD is presented as a basis for further discussion of the manifestations of and current therapy for PUD.

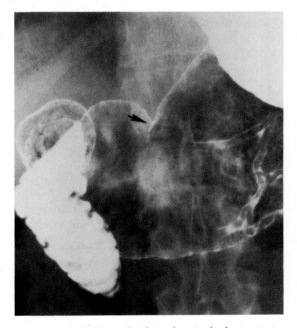

FIGURE 36–1. Radiograph of an ulcer in the lesser curvature of the stomach (*arrow*). (From Laufer I: *Double Contrast Gastrointestinal Radiology with Endoscopic Correlation.* Philadelphia, WB Saunders, 1979. Reproduced with permission.)

Etiology and Pathogenesis

Two different mechanisms for the development of PUD in the stomach and duodenum have been proposed. In the stomach, it is thought that a breakdown in the normally protective epithelial lining occurs. Under normal circumstances, flow of hydrochloric acid (HCl) from the lumen of the stomach into the epithelial cells is prevented by the presence of very tight, nonpermeable junctions between the epithelial cells and by the slightly alkaline layer of mucus that coats the surface of the gastric epithelium. In the formation of a gastric peptic ulcer, this diffusion barrier may be interrupted by the chronic presence of such injurious substances as aspirin, alcohol, and bile acids that may regurgitate back up from the duodenum. These substances apparently strip away the surface mucus and cause degeneration of the epithelial cell membranes, and massive diffusion of acid back into the gastric epithelial wall occurs.

The pathogenesis of duodenal peptic ulcers has a different proposed mechanism. It is thought that inappropriate, excess secretion of acid is primarily responsible for the development of PUD in the duodenum (Fig. 36–3, Color Plate III). Studies have documented that the activity of the vagus nerve is increased in persons with PUD of the duodenum, particularly during a fasting state and at night. The vagus nerve stimulates the pyloric antrum cells to release gastrin, which in turn travels via the bloodstream and acts on the gastric parietal cells to stimulate the release of HCl. The basal rate of firing of the vagus nerve is increased in people with PUD, thus resulting in an inappropriately high rate of HCl secretion.[6]

In addition to the erosiveness of HCl and other injurious substances, it is suspected that *H. pylori* plays a key role in both gastric and duodenal ulcer formation. Since identification in 1982, the organism has generated worldwide attention. It is reported that up to 90 percent of persons with duodenal ulcers and 70 percent of persons with gastric ulcers have *H. pylori* infection and active chronic gastritis.[10a] Eradication of the organism can result in resolution of gastritis with subsequent ulcer healing.

Currently, the relationship of stress to the development of PUD is in question. Substances called glucocorticoids, which are released in response to stress, may play some role in the promotion of excess acid production or the destruction of gastric mucosal defenses.[1]

Clinical Manifestations and Treatment

The manifestations of PUD include epigastric burning pain that is usually relieved by the intake of food or antacids. In some persons with gastric ulcers, pain may occur following a meal. Other manifestations that may occur in PUD include nausea, abdominal upset, and chest discomfort.[1]

Treatment strategies for PUD, which previously incorporated stress management techniques,[1] now include use of antibiotics and bismuth to eradicate

H. pylori. Research suggests that use of antibiotics and bismuth leads to marked reduction in the recurrence rate of PUD when compared with standard acid suppression methods.[10a] At the present time, no conclusive research has demonstrated that any specific diet has a therapeutic effect. Susceptible people are generally advised to avoid foods that seem to exacerbate symptoms. The use of histamine-2 antagonists, a group of medications that block the action of histamine, a potent stimulant of gastric acid secretion, may be useful in PUD in some cases.

Inflammatory Bowel Disease

The term **inflammatory bowel disease** is used in referring to the two separate disease entities of ulcerative colitis and Crohn's disease. The term is somewhat misleading, as many conditions may cause an inflammation of the bowel, such as gastroenteritis. Nevertheless, the health sciences literature uses inflammatory bowel disease (IBD) to denote these two conditions specifically, and the health practitioner may wish to make this distinction clear to clients experiencing these disorders of the GI tract.

IBD may be a life-altering chronic illness with serious consequences for people and their families who must cope with it. Both ulcerative colitis and Crohn's disease have their onset most commonly in childhood and young adulthood; the onset of these diseases during these life stages may have profound implications. This section describes the pathophysiology of ulcerative colitis and Crohn's disease separately; a later section in this chapter discusses the psychosocial aspects of IBD.

Ulcerative Colitis

Ulcerative colitis (Fig. 36–4, Color Plate III) is an inflammatory disease of the mucosa of the rectum and colon.[1] Most commonly it affects the most distal portions of the colon, but eventually it may extend to affect the entire colon. It is typically characterized by exacerbations and remissions; the disease is alternately active and inactive. The manifestations of ulcerative colitis are abdominal pain, diarrhea, and rectal bleeding.[2] Its causes are poorly understood. Recent research has focused on an immunologic basis for the disease; antibodies and lymphocytes from persons with ulcerative colitis have been shown to inflict damage on or are toxic to colon epithelial cells.[2] This immunologic basis for the disease is supported by the finding that ulcerative colitis is frequently accompanied by other conditions with an immunologic basis, such as systemic lupus erythematosus and erythema nodosum.

Etiology and Clinical Manifestations. Ulcerative colitis begins as an inflammation at the base of the crypts of Lieberkuhn. Damage to the crypt epithelium results, with eventual invasion of leukocytes and the formation of abscesses in the crypts. When multiple abscesses form in close proximity and begin to coalesce, large areas of ulcerations develop in the epithe-

lium. Concurrent with this destructive process, attempts at repair of damaged tissue occur, with the development of granulation tissue, which is fragile and highly vascularized. The manifestations of ulcerative colitis are the result of these processes. Bleeding occurs as a result of mucosal destruction and ulceration, along with damage to newly developed granulation tissue. Diarrhea is the result of the mucosal destruction in the colon, which leads to a decreased ability of the bowel to absorb water and sodium and an increased volume of fluid in the intestinal contents.[2,11,12]

The progression of ulcerative colitis may be highly variable. In some individuals it may have very mild manifestations; in others it may rapidly progress to a life-threatening disorder. Five to 10 percent of persons with ulcerative colitis have only one attack, with no further recurrence. However, 65 to 75 percent of persons with ulcerative colitis experience an intermittent series of exacerbations and remissions. For 10 to 15 percent of persons affected by ulcerative colitis, the disease is continuous and often has severe and life-threatening consequences.[2] An additional pathologic finding is an increased risk for the development of intestinal cancer in persons who have had ulcerative colitis for more than 7 to 10 years. Authorities recommend monitoring these individuals carefully.[1]

Crohn's Disease

Crohn's disease, also called regional enteritis and granulomatous colitis, is an inflammation of the GI tract that extends through all layers of the intestinal wall (Fig. 36–5, Color Plate III). It most commonly affects the proximal portion of the colon and, less often, the terminal ileum. It may affect multiple portions of the colon, leaving intervening normal areas in between the affected regions. The manifestations of Crohn's disease differ in some respects from those of ulcerative colitis, although some overlap may occur. In Crohn's disease, abdominal pain is often constant, and is usually in the right lower quadrant of the abdomen. A palpable abdominal mass may be present in the right lower quadrant. The stool may be bloody, although not to the extent that it often is in ulcerative colitis. The etiology of Crohn's disease is unknown at the present time, although a genetic influence may be involved. Up to 5 percent of people with Crohn's disease have one or more affected relatives.[6]

Etiology and Clinical Manifestations. Certain features of the pathogenesis of Crohn's disease differ from those of ulcerative colitis. Crohn's disease appears to be the result of a process in which the lymphoid and lymphatic structures of the GI tract become blocked. Subsequent engorgement and inflammation of surrounding tissues leads to the development of deep linear ulcers in the bowel wall. Eventually, all layers of the GI tract wall may become involved, and the portion of intestine that is affected may become thickened by fibrous scar tissue. Deep fissures may develop into fistulas, which may extend into adjacent bowel tissue of other tissue, such as the bladder wall or even the skin.[2]

COLOR PLATE III

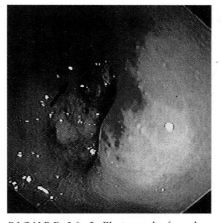

F I G U R E 3 6 – 2. Photograph of an ulcer.
(From Sleisenger MH, Fordtran JS: *Gastro-intestinal Disease,* 5th ed. Philadelphia, WB
Saunders, 1993, Color Plate V, #38.)

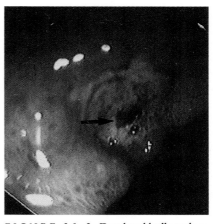

F I G U R E 3 6 – 3. Duodenal bulbar ulcer.
(From Sleisenger MH, Fordtran JS: *Gastro-intestinal Disease,* 5th ed. Philadelphia, WB
Saunders, 1993, Color Plate VI, #48.)

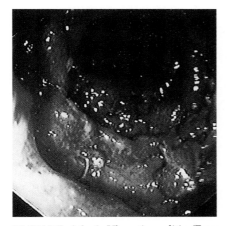

F I G U R E 3 6 – 4. Ulcerative colitis. (From
Sleisenger MH, Fordtran JS: *Gastrointestinal
Disease,* 5th ed. Philadelphia, WB Saunders,
1993, Color Plate XIII, #100.)

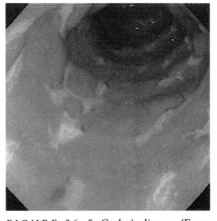

F I G U R E 3 6 – 5. Crohn's disease. (From
Sleisenger MH, Fordtran JS: *Gastrointestinal
Disease,* 5th ed. Philadelphia, WB Saunders,
1993, Color Plate XIV, #104.)

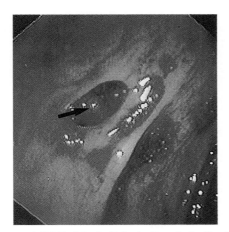

F I G U R E 3 6 – 6. Colonic diverticula. Small
outpouchings of colonic mucosa are noted
(*arrow*). (From Sleisenger MH, Fordtran JS:
Gastrointestinal Disease, 5th ed. Philadelphia,
WB Saunders, 1993, Color Plate X, #88.)

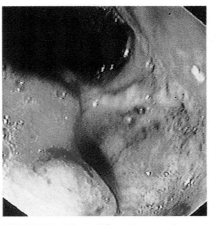

F I G U R E 3 6 – 7. Ulcerating gastric cancer.
(From Sleisenger MH, Fordtran JS: *Gastro-intestinal Disease,* 5th ed. Philadelphia, WB
Saunders, 1993, Color Plate IV, #33.)

COLOR PLATE IV

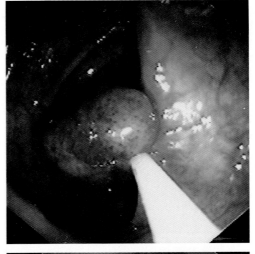

FIGURE 36–8. Photographs of colonic polyps. (Figure supplied by L.E. Copstead.)

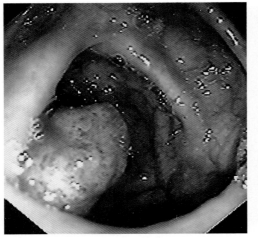

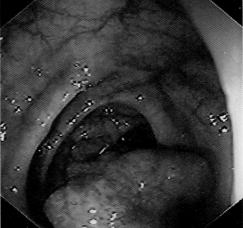

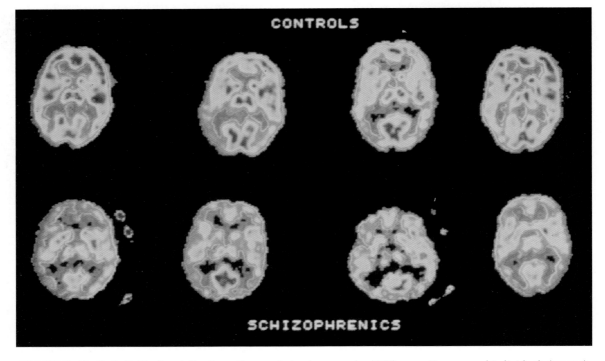

FIGURE 47–5. Individual variation in positron emission tomography (PET) scans. Four normal individuals (*top row*) and four schizophrenics (*bottom row*) show range of hypofrontality and diminished basal ganglia metabolism. (From Buchsbaum MS, Haier RJ: Functional and anatomical brain imaging: Impact on schizophrenia research. *Schizophrenia Bulletin* 1987:13(1):115-132. Reproduced by permission of Monte S. Buchsbaum, M.D., Mount Sinai School of Medicine, New York.)

The manifestations of Crohn's disease are the result of these pathologic changes, as the bowel becomes incapable of performing adequate absorption of intestinal contents. Complications such as perianal fissures, fistulas, and abscess are common in Crohn's disease and may be the symptoms that lead individuals to seek health care. The onset and course of Crohn's disease may vary a great deal; unlike ulcerative colitis, the symptoms present during a period of exacerbation may be subtle but persistent. At the present time, controversy exists concerning an increased incidence of cancer of the colon in persons with Crohn's disease.[2,13]

Treatment

Because the etiology of IBD is unknown, therapeutic strategies are focused on alleviating and reducing inflammation. Currently, various pharmacologic agents, such as sulfasalazine, are being used in both ulcerative colitis and Crohn's disease to reduce inflammation.[6] Future research may focus on the use of immunosuppressive agents for this purpose. A balanced, nutritious diet is recommended for persons with IBD. During a severe exacerbation of IBD, nutritional support by the intravenous route may be required.[4]

Enterocolitis

Two types of inflammatory conditions in which the intestinal tissue may undergo inflammation and necrosis are included here, as their incidence has increased in recent years. Pseudomembranous enterocolitis is an acute inflammation and necrosis of the small and large intestines, usually affecting the mucosa but sometimes extending to other layers. There is increasing evidence that antibiotics are a major factor predisposing to the development of this disorder.[2] Although the exact mechanism of its development is unknown, it is known that the necrosed mucosa is replaced by a pseudomembrane filled with staphylococci, leukocytes, mucus, fibrin, and inflammatory cells.[3,6] Resulting manifestations include diarrhea, abdominal pain, fever, and, rarely, rectal bleeding and colonic perforation. Persons at particular risk for the development of pseudomembranous colitis include debilitated or elderly persons who have received broad-spectrum antibiotics in the postoperative period.

Necrotizing enterocolitis is a disorder occurring most often in premature infants (less than 34 weeks' gestation) and infants with low birth weight (less than 5 pounds or 2.25 kg). This disorder is characterized by diffuse or patchy intestinal necrosis, accompanied by sepsis. Early manifestations include a distended abdomen, with gastric distention. The major complication of necrotizing enterocolitis is intestinal perforation, which may necessitate surgery. Various theories as to the etiology of necrotizing enterocolitis include perinatal oxygen deficit, with insufficient blood flow to the viscera, and the use of hypertonic feeding formulas in newborn infants.[6]

Appendicitis

The most common cause for emergency surgery to the abdomen, **appendicitis** is the inflammation of the vermiform appendix due to an obstruction. This inflammation may lead to necrosis of the appendix, with subsequent abscess formation and peritonitis. If left untreated, appendicitis will progress to a life-threatening situation. Appendicitis may occur at any age and affects both sexes equally, although its prevalence is higher in young males. The earliest manifestation of appendicitis is generalized or localized abdominal pain in the lower right abdomen, which is caused by distention of the serosa due to inflammatory edema. Edema compromises the vascular supply to the appendix and serves to increase the permeability of this segment of the intestine. Bacterial invasion of the wall of the appendix occurs, with resultant infection and inflammation. As the inflammatory process progresses, rupture of the appendix may occur and generalized peritonitis will develop.[2] Surgical removal of the appendix is the only effective treatment for appendicitis. Administration of antibiotics with replacement of fluid and electrolytes may be necessary.

Diverticular Disease

The term *diverticular disease* generally refers to **diverticulosis**, or the presence of diverticula, in the colon. **Diverticula** (the Latin plural form of diverticul*um*) are outpouchings in the wall of the colon (Fig. 36–6, Color Plate III) which probably result from high intraluminal pressure on areas of weakness in the bowel wall, particularly where blood vessels enter. Colonic diverticulosis is very common in Westernized countries and is thought to be associated with a diet low in fiber, which fails to provide enough bulk in the intestinal contents to provide a steady pressure against the walls of the intestine. The presence of diverticula increases with age; about 30 percent of the general population at age 60 and about 80 percent at age 80 will have diverticula in the colon.[1] Most persons experience no manifestations of diverticulosis, and of itself, diverticulosis is not considered a pathologic condition. However, when diverticula become inflamed, the condition is referred to as **diverticulitis** (see Table 36–1 for the terminology of diverticulosis).

TABLE 36–1. Terminology of Diverticulosis

Diverticulum: A single pouchlike herniation through the muscular layer of the colon.

Diverticula: More than one diverticulum (Latin plural form).

Divertic*ulosis*: The presence of one or more diverticula.

Divertic*ulitis*: Inflammation of one or more diverticula.

Diverticular disease: Complications related to the presence of diverticula.

The inflammation of the diverticula can lead to serious consequences, such as the development of abscesses in the bowel wall, peritonitis, and intestinal obstruction. Manifestations of diverticulitis include acute lower abdominal pain, fever, and tachycardia. During an acute episode of diverticulitis, the administration of broad-spectrum antibiotics and intravenous fluid and electrolyte support may be necessary. In the case of complications such as unresolved intestinal obstruction and fistula formation, surgery may be indicated.[1]

KEY CONCEPTS

- Alterations in intestinal wall integrity are generally a result of infection, inflammation, or weakness of the muscular layers. General symptoms include pain, bleeding, and diarrhea.

- Gastritis may be acute or chronic. Acute gastritis is generally precipitated by the ingestion of irritating substances, including alcohol and aspirin. Chronic gastritis may lead to atrophy of the gastric mucosa and the subsequent decreased production of HCl and intrinsic factor. Acute gastroenteritis is usually due to the ingestion of pathogenic organisms, which leads to a self-limited bout of diarrhea, vomiting, and abdominal pain.

- Peptic ulcer disease (PUD) may affect the esophagus, stomach and duodenum. Gastric ulcers are thought to be due to breakdown of the protective mucus layer that normally prevents diffusion of acids into gastric epithelia. Duodenal ulcers are due to excessive acid secretion that is mediated by increased vagal activity. The organism *H. pylori* has also been implicated in both gastric and duodenal ulcers. PUD is characterized by epigastric pain that is relieved by food or antacids. Perforation and bleeding are the major complications of PUD. Treatment for PUD is aimed at eradicating *H. pylori*.

- Ulcerative colitis and Crohn's disease are chronic inflammatory disorders of the bowel. Ulcerative colitis (inflammation and ulceration of the colon and rectal mucosa) manifests with bloody diarrhea and abdominal pain. An increased risk for colon cancer occurs in persons who have had ulcerative colitis for more than 7 to 10 years. Crohn's disease generally affects the proximal colon or terminal ileum. All layers of the intestinal wall are involved, which predisposes to fistula formation and malabsorption. Crohn's disease may result from blockage and subsequent inflammation of lymphatic vessels. Chronic abdominal pain and diarrhea are common. Treatment for ulcerative colitis and Crohn's disease is aimed at reducing inflammation.

- Acute inflammation of the intestinal wall may result in pseudomembranous enterocolitis or necrotizing enterocolitis. Abdominal pain, diarrhea, fever, and sepsis may result. The use of broad-spectrum antibiotics has been implicated in the etiology of pseudomembranous enterocolitis. Necrotizing enterocolitis, which occurs most often in infants, is thought to be due to bowel ischemia.

- Appendicitis is characterized by right lower quadrant pain, nausea and vomiting, and systemic signs of inflammation. Surgical removal of the appendix is necessary. Untreated appendicitis may result in rupture of the appendix, leading to peritonitis.

- Diverticula of the colon are very common in Western society because of a low intake of dietary fiber. Low-bulk stools result in the development of high intraluminal pressures and predispose to diverticula formation. Diverticulosis is generally asymptomatic. Inflammation of the diverticula, or diverticulitis, manifests with fever and lower abdominal pain.

Alterations in Motility of the Gastrointestinal Tract

Disorders of the GI tract that primarily alter its regular propulsive ability may have a negative effect on its ability to absorb nutrients. In these alterations in motility, the transit time of substances passing through the GI tract may be too fast to allow for adequate absorption. Conversely, a blockage or impedance of the GI tract may result in slowed or absent motility, which also prevents normal ingestion and processing of nutrient substances. As with alterations in the integrity of the GI tract wall, these alterations in GI motility may represent a chronic condition, with many implications for the person experiencing it, or may be a life-threatening, acute situation requiring immediate intervention.

Irritable Bowel Syndrome

The **irritable bowel syndrome** (IBS) is a complex entity that has been the focus of much recent research. A clear definition of this syndrome has not been agreed upon by all authorities; nevertheless, certain defining characteristics have been established. Typically, IBS is the presence of alternating diarrhea and constipation accompanied by abdominal cramping pain in the absence of any identifiable pathology in the GI tract.[6] Other terms that have been used for this syndrome include spastic colitis and irritable colon syndrome. It is important to differentiate irritable bowel syndrome, in which no pathology of the GI tract has been identified, from inflammatory bowel disease, in which pathology is identifiable. IBS is an extremely common disorder that is estimated to affect 17 to 20 percent of the U.S. population.[6]

Etiology and Pathogenesis

The etiology and pathogenesis of IBS are presently obscure. Most evidence seems to show that it is primarily a disorder of bowel motility. Research studies have demonstrated that the myoelectric activity of the colon of persons with IBS is altered. In particular, the slow wave activity of the colon, which usually occurs at a rate of three to six times per minute, is markedly increased in IBS.[1,6] Whether this altered pattern is the result of genetic factors or such environmental factors as level of stress or dietary patterns remains unknown.

Clinical Manifestations and Treatment

The manifestations of IBS may vary greatly, with some persons experiencing only diarrhea or constipation and others experiencing an alternating pattern of both. In addition to the abdominal cramping pain, other manifestations such as mucus in the stool and nausea may also be present.[14] The severity of manifestations may range from barely noticeable to incapacitating. Current therapy focuses on the use of antidiarrheal agents and antispasmodic medications as appropriate. Ingestion of a diet with increased amounts of fiber has proved useful in some cases and is thought to promote a more normal pattern of myoelectrical activity by providing a regular propulsive stimulus within the gut.[4,14]

Intestinal Obstruction

Intestinal obstruction is the partial or complete blockage of the intestinal lumen of the small or large bowel. In this situation, the contents of the intestine fail to propel forward through the lumen as a result of a mechanical or functional cause. Mechanical obstructions are caused by a blockage of the intestine by adhesion, hernia, tumor, inflammation and resulting stricture (as in Crohn's disease), impacted feces, volvulus, or intussusception. (Volvulus and intussusception are covered in more detail in the following section.) Functional obstruction refers to the loss of propulsive ability by the bowel and may occur following abdominal surgery or in association with hypokalemia, peritonitis, severe trauma, spinal fractures, ureteral distention, and the administration of some narcotic medications.[6,15]

Obstruction of the small bowel is most common (90 percent of cases). Intestinal obstruction is most common in persons who have previously undergone abdominal surgery or who have congenital abnormalities of the bowel.[15] The severity and types of symptoms initially accompanying an intestinal obstruction will vary with cause and location; if left untreated, however, an intestinal obstruction may result in death from shock and vascular collapse.

Etiology and Pathogenesis

With the obstruction of the bowel lumen, fluid and gas begin to accumulate proximal to the obstructed location. The distention caused by trapped fluids and gases causes the secretion of water and electrolytes into the obstructed lumen of the small bowel. Distention also results in the impedance of venous return, and the bowel wall becomes edematous. The absorptive ability of the bowel wall is compromised, and fluid and gas continue to accumulate as additional water and electrolytes are secreted into the lumen. As this self-perpetuating process continues, distention spreads to adjacent portions of the bowel, with resulting loss of absorptive ability. The pressure on the bowel wall exerted by the excess fluid and gas may result in leakage of fluid through the wall into the peritoneum, as well as necrosis of the bowel wall. Along with this process, abnormal bacterial growth may occur in the small intestine during an obstruction, leading to the production of additional gas and the transformation of small intestinal contents into feculent material.[15]

In addition to the process described above, other complications may be present with blockage of the intestinal lumen. Circulation to the bowel wall may be impaired during an obstruction; this occurrence is referred to as a strangulation obstruction. In a strangulation obstruction, the bowel wall becomes ischemic and the bowel responds to anoxia with increased peristalsis. Blood escapes from the engorged veins, and a significant loss of blood and plasma from the affected segment may result in the rapid development of shock. In addition, the strangulated segment may become gangrenous, with resulting peritonitis, or perforated, with the leakage of highly toxic bacterial material into the peritoneal cavity.[15]

Clinical Manifestations and Treatment

The manifestations of an intestinal obstruction depend on its site and duration. Obstructions in the upper jejunal area usually result in vomiting, dehydration, and electrolyte depletion. In obstructions of the distal small bowel or ileus, constipation may be an early manifestation, with the later massive accumulation of fluid in the lumen. Dehydration may progress to hypovolemic shock if the obstruction is left untreated. In obstructions of the colon, massive gas distention may be present. The fluid and electrolyte losses in a colonic obstruction may not be as severe as those of obstruction of the small bowel. Blockage of the colon by a tumor is the most common cause of colonic obstruction, and perforation of the bowel wall adjacent to the tumor may occur during an obstruction.

Therapeutic strategies for intestinal obstruction include surgical intervention to correct or remove the source of a mechanical obstruction. Supportive therapy, including decompression of the bowel using specialized tubes, and the administration of fluid and electrolyte replacement may be needed during an acute obstructive episode.

Volvulus

A **volvulus** is a twisting of the bowel on itself, which results in blood vessel compression. The two most common sites for the development of a volvulus are the cecum and the sigmoid colon. A volvulus may be the result of an anomaly of rotation, an ingested foreign body, or an adhesion; however, the cause is sometimes unknown.[6] With the sudden tight twisting of the bowel on its mesentery, blood flow to the bowel is impeded. Gangrene, necrosis, and perforation may develop, resulting in a life-threatening situation. If both ends of a bowel segment are twisted, a closed-loop obstruction results, with the manifestations described earlier for an intestinal obstruction. Treatment varies according to the severity and location of the volvulus and includes the therapeutic approaches described for intestinal obstruction.[3,6]

Intussusception

Intussusception is a telescoping or invagination of a portion of the bowel into an adjacent distal portion. It is most common in infants and occurs three times more often in males than in females.[6] Intussusception may be linked to viral infections, because its occurrence seems to coincide with the peak incidence of enteritis and respiratory tract infections. In most cases in infants, the actual cause is unknown, although in older children it may be associated with alterations in intestinal motility or a condition called Meckel's diverticulum, in which a congenital abnormality of a blind tube is present in the distal ileum. In adults, intussusception usually results from the presence of benign or malignant tumors.[6]

As a bowel segment undergoes intussusception, peristalsis acts to pull more bowel along with it. The resulting area of tightened, invaginated bowel becomes edematous; venous engorgement with hemorrhage may occur. Intestinal obstruction of the bowel may develop, with eventual gangrene, shock, and perforation of the bowel if treatment is delayed.[6,15]

Hirschsprung's Disease

Hirschsprung's disease is a congenital disorder of the large intestine in which the autonomic nerve ganglia in the smooth muscle are absent or markedly reduced. The **aganglionic** bowel segment contracts, but without the reciprocal relaxation needed to propel the intestinal contents forward. Stasis of stool and dilation of the proximal colon result in megacolon, or massive dilation of the colon. In 90 percent of people with Hirschsprung's disease, the aganglionic segment is in the rectosigmoid area, but occasionally the entire colon may be affected.[6] Hirschsprung's disease is believed to be familial, occurring in approximately 1 in 5,000 live births. It is more common in males than in females, with a ratio of 3.8 : 1. The disease often coexists with other anomalies, particularly Down's syndrome. Although Hirschsprung's disease is most commonly identified in infants and children, it may be present in adults as a long-standing undiagnosed condition.[6]

In infants, Hirschsprung's disease may have severe, life-threatening effects. Fecal stagnation may re-

sult in enterocolitis with bacterial overgrowth, profuse diarrhea, hypovolemic shock, and intestinal perforation.[6] Interventions such as colonic lavage may be performed to empty the bowel until the infant is stable enough to withstand surgical intervention.

KEY CONCEPTS

- **Irritable bowel syndrome is manifested with bouts of alternating diarrhea and constipation in the absence of identifiable GI pathology. The etiology is unclear; however the slow wave activity of the bowel is markedly increased. A high-fiber diet and antidiarrheal agents may be recommended.**

- **Intestinal obstructions may be mechanical or functional. Mechanical obstructions are due to adhesions, hernia, tumors, impacted feces, volvulus (twisting), or intussusception (telescoping). Mechanical obstructions are characterized by increased bowel sounds initially, accompanied by abdominal pain, nausea, and vomiting. Functional obstructions are due to conditions that inhibit peristalsis, such as narcotics, anesthesia, surgical manipulation, peritonitis, hypokalemia, and spinal cord injuries. Functional obstructions are characterized by absence of bowel sounds. Uncorrected obstructions may lead to intestinal wall edema, ischemia, and necrosis. Bowel gangrene, sepsis, and shock can result. Surgical intervention or decompression with an intestinal tube are often required.**

- **Hirschsprung's disease is a familial, congenital disorder of the large intestine in which the autonomic ganglia are reduced or absent. Stasis of stool and megacolon may occur in the abnormally innervated section of bowel.**

Malabsorption

Malabsorption refers to failure of the GI tract to absorb or digest normally one or more dietary constituents.[1] Malabsorption problems often manifest with diarrhea, as the passage of inappropriately processed intestinal contents may result in impairment of fluid absorption as well. Malabsorption may be associated with the presence of an opportunistic infection in the intestinal tract, as in acquired immunodeficiency syndrome. It may also be associated with radiation enteritis, an inflammation of the bowel wall that may occur following radiation therapy for cancer. In addition, malabsorption may be the result of lactase deficiency, which was discussed in Chapter 35. The types of malabsorption syndromes discussed here result from a mucosal disorder of the small bowel or from the surgical removal of portions of the stomach or small bowel.

Mucosal Disorders

A number of disorders of varying causes may affect the mucosa of the small intestine. Because the small intestine is the principal site of digestion and absorption of nutrients, a defect in the mucosa of the small intestine has the potential for causing the malabsorption of fat, protein, carbohydrate, vitamins, and minerals. Crohn's disease, which was described earlier, may result in damage to the mucosa of the distal ileum, which is the site of vitamin B_{12} and bile acid absorption. Thus, a deficiency in vitamin B_{12} and bile acid may be present in Crohn's disease. Other mucosal disorders of the small intestine that may result in malabsorption are celiac disease and tropic sprue.

Celiac Disease

Celiac disease (also called celiac sprue) is characterized by an intolerance of **gluten,** a protein in wheat and wheat products. Current research suggest that two mechanisms may be operant in the development of malabsorption in celiac disease: (1) the ingestion of gluten by a genetically susceptible individual may trigger an immunologic response, and (2) an intramucosal enzyme defect may result in inability to digest gluten. These defects in metabolism may promote tissue toxicity in the intestinal mucosa, with damage to the surface epithelium of the small bowel. The villi may atrophy, and a decrease in the activity and amount of enzymes in the surface epithelium may be present. The resulting malabsorption of ingested nutrients may promote malnutrition and severe debilitation.[16,17]

Celiac disease affects twice as many females as males and may have a familial inheritance pattern. The incidence in the general population is 1 in 3,000, and those affected are primarily of northwestern European ancestry. The onset of celiac disease may occur in infancy, when gluten-containing products are first introduced into the diet, and in the fourth and fifth decades.[16,17] Effective treatment may necessitate the elimination of all gluten from the diet, which results in significant improvements in the intestinal mucosa.

Tropical Sprue

In **tropical sprue,** the mucosa of the small intestine atrophies, with resulting malabsoprtion, malnutrition, and folic acid deficiency. At the present time, the cause of tropical sprue is unknown, and no single organism has been implicated in its development. It is thought that a bacterial cause may be operant in its development, as it often occurs in epidemics. Its incidence is high in persons living in or visiting tropical climates, and it appears to affect adults more often than children.

The atrophy of the small intestinal mucosa may have severe effects. Massive malabsorption may result from the failure of the mucosa to produce the enzymes needed for digestion. Manifestations include severe diarrhea with blood-tinged stools, abdominal distention, and **steatorrhea** (the presence of excess fat in the stool). Treatment includes antidiarrheal medication and prolonged antimicrobial therapy.[6]

Malabsorption Disorders Following Surgical Intervention

Surgical procedures in which a portion of the stomach or small bowel is removed may result in loss of the ability to absorb nutrients properly, either through a loss of appropriate motility patterns or through a loss of the surface area of the small bowel needed for adequate absorption. Two types of disorders of malabsorption may occur following surgical intervention on the stomach or small bowel: dumping syndrome and short bowel syndrome.

Dumping Syndrome

The **dumping syndrome** is a term used to describe the literal dumping of stomach contents into the proximal small intestine due to loss of pyloric regulation of gastric emptying. This loss of the normal function of gradual pyloric emptying may occur following the removal of part of the stomach (or **gastrectomy**), a procedure performed as part of treatment for peptic ulcer disease of cancer of the stomach. With the normal reservoir function of the stomach now impaired, a large volume of hyperosmolar food is dumped rapidly into the small intestine, with consequences that may be severe. The hyperosmolar contents of the small intestine draw water into the lumen and stimulate bowel motility. Manifestations of this process include diarrhea and abdominal pain. In addition, the rapid absorption of a large amount of glucose and a subsequent rise in blood glucose promote an excessive rise in plasma insulin. This elevated insulin level then causes a rapid fall in blood glucose levels 1 to 3 hours following a meal. This sudden rebound is referred to as "rebound hypoglycemia."[6,18]

Persons who have undergone a gastrectomy procedure may require specific instruction regarding eating small meals six to eight times a day, rather than three large meals. The restriction of carbohydrate intake may be needed to restrict glucose absorption. Medications to reduce bowel motility have been helpful in promoting a more normal pattern of bowel function in this population.[1]

Short Bowel Syndrome

Short bowel syndrome refers to the severe diarrhea and significant malabsorption that develop following the surgical removal of large portions of the small intestine. The severity of the manifestations will depend on the amount and location of the bowel resected. In particular, removal of the distal two thirds of the ileum and ileocecal valve may result in severe malabsorption. Because the ileocecal valve serves to increase the transit time of intestinal contents, its removal may promote a transit time that is too rapid for adequate absorption of nutrients to occur. In addition, removal of large portions of the small intestine will result in diminished ability to absorb water, electrolytes, protein, fat, carbohydrates, vitamins, and trace elements. The small intestine displays an amazing ability to adapt following a bowel resection, however. The remaining villi may enlarge and lengthen, increasing the absorptive surface area of the bowel. The presence of orally ingested nutrients is needed for this adaptive process to occur, and a gradual increase in oral intake following a bowel resection may promote an improvement in absorptive ability over time. The use of nutrients supplied intravenously has been an important supportive intervention for people in the initial stages of recovery from resection of the small bowel.[4]

KEY CONCEPTS

- Malabsorption occurs when the small bowel fails to absorb one or more dietary components. Diarrhea and abdominal discomfort are the usual manifestations. Malabsorption may occur because of mucosal dysfunction (Crohn's disease, celiac disease, tropical sprue), enzyme deficiencies, or surgical alterations that affect transit time and absorptive surface area.

- Celiac disease appears to be a familial intolerance of gluten-containing foods. Ingestion of gluten leads to inflammation and atrophy of the intestinal villi. A reduced surface area and decreased brush border enzymes impair nutrient absorption.

- Dumping syndrome occurs with loss of pyloric sphincter regulation, generally following gastric surgery for ulcers or cancer. Chyme is rapidly dumped into the duodenum, causing an osmotic shift of water into the lumen and diarrhea. Glucose absorption may be rapid, leading to overshoot of insulin secretion and rebound hypoglycemia.

- Short bowel syndrome follows surgical procedures that remove large sections of the small intestine. Rapid transit time and reduced surface area for absorption lead to diarrhea and malabsorption.

Neoplasms of the Gastrointestinal Tract

Neoplasms may develop in each region of the GI tract and vary in their severity and the ability to disrupt normal GI functioning. The most frequent neoplastic processes of the GI tract are summarized here; the reader may wish to refer to the chapter on neoplasms as a background for understanding these specific types of neoplasms occurring in the GI tract.

Esophageal Cancer

Esophageal cancer accounts for 1 to 2 percent of all cancers and affects men three times more often than women.[1] It usually develops in men over age 60. The 1-year survival rate is less than 20 percent.[1,19] Although the cause of esophageal cancer is presently unknown, several predisposing factors have been identified, including chronic irritation of the esopha-gus from heavy smoking and the use of alcohol. Chronic inflammation of the esophagus from gastric reflux and previous head and neck tumors are also considered associated factors in its development. Most esophageal tumors are squamous cell carcinomas; less than 10 percent are adenocarcinomas. Regardless of the cell type, the prognosis is extremely poor.[1,19] Tumors of the esophagus are usually infiltrating, and the disease may spread extensively to surrounding organs by way of the esophageal lymphatics at an early stage. Invasion of surrounding structures may lead to the formation of esophagobronchial or esophagopleural fistulas, with subsequent pneumonia or abscess. The tumor may partially constrict the lumen of the esophagus, and surgical and radiation therapy designed to maintain a patent esophagus may be instituted. If the individual survives the initial extension of the tumor, the liver and lungs are the usual sites of distant metastasis.[19]

Gastric Carcinoma

Gastric carcinoma is common throughout the world; however, certain population groups appear to be at higher risk than others for developing it.[1,19] In Japan, the prevalence of gastric cancer is about 10 times the prevalence in the United States. The incidence is higher in men over 30 than in other age and sex groups. The overall 5-year survival rate is approximately 10 percent, although the prognosis depends on the stage of the disease at the time of diagnosis.[1,19] Early gastric cancer is gastric cancer that has not penetrated the major muscle layer of the stomach wall and is associated with a more favorable survival rate than more advanced disease. Unfortunately, early gastric cancer typically has no manifestations and may not be identified at this stage. Advanced gastric cancer (Fig. 36–7, Color Plate III) is gastric cancer that has penetrated the muscle layer of the stomach. Most people in North America identified with gastric cancer already have the advanced form and have manifestations such as anorexia and GI bleeding. Although the cause of gastric cancer is unknown, dietary factors have been implicated, particularly an increased consumption of salt and dietary nitrates.[1] Other predisposing factors may include a reduced production of gastric acid and gastritis with gastric atrophy.[19]

Gastric carcinoma extends rapidly to regional lymph nodes and surrounding organs by way of the lymphatic system, the bloodstream, and direct extension through the wall of the stomach. Current treatment modalities include surgical resection of the tumor with appropriate surrounding margins of tissue.[19]

Small Intestinal Neoplasms

Neoplasms of the small intestine may be either benign or malignant. They are fairly unusual, accounting for less than 5 percent of GI tumors.[1] Tumors of the small intestine occur most often in persons over age 50. Depending on the extent and type of tumor, partial or complete obstruction of the small bowel may occur. If obstruction is chronic, stasis of intestinal contents may lead to bacterial overgrowth and malabsorption. If the tumor is located near the ampulla of Vater, the common bile duct may become obstructed, with resulting biliary stasis and jaundice. Bleeding and ulceration of small intestinal tumors are common manifestations. Treatment may include surgical intervention to remove the tumor and the affected portion of the small intestine.

Colonic Polyps and Cancer

Cancer of the colon and rectum is identified in over 100,000 men and women in the United States each year, with the incidence equally distributed between men and women.[19] It is second in cancer prevalence only to lung cancer in men, and third in prevalence in women, behind breast and lung cancer.[1] Although the relationship between the development of adenomatous polyps of the colon and colon cancer has been the subject of debate in the past, research has established that colonic polyps are a risk factor for the development of colon cancer.[1,20]

Colonic Polyps

The term **polyp** refers to any protrusion into the lumen of the GI tract. A *sessile polyp* is a raised protuberance with a broad base. A *pedunculated polyp* is attached to the bowel wall by a stalk that is narrower than the body of the polyp. Polyps may be either benign or malignant, although the term polyp usually means a benign form. Benign adenomatous polyps of the colon are believed to predispose to adenocarcinoma, or malignant carcinoma, of the colon. It is currently thought that some adenomatous polyps may already contain a focus of carcinoma, and that otherwise benign polyps may also eventually degenerate into cancerous lesions.[1,21] Many people with polyps have no manifestations, although polyps may cause occult or gross bleeding and abdominal pain. Treatment will vary according to the size and type of polyp and its location within the colon. Biopsy and subsequent removal of polyps may be performed during a sigmoidoscopy or colonoscopy procedure.[21] Figure 36–8 (Color Plate IV) shows various colonic polyps.

Colonic Cancer

Although no specific cause of colonic cancer has been identified, a number of risk factors have been identified. The risk of colon cancer increases with advancing age. After age 40, the annual incidence of colon cancer accelerates, doubling every decade until age 80.[1] Dietary factors also seem to increase the risk; a high-fat, low-fiber diet has been proposed as an associated factor. Certain bowel conditions may predispose an individual to colon cancer, including Crohn's disease, adenomatous polyps, and ulcerative colitis. A hereditary predisposition may also be present: the probability of colorectal cancer in a person who has a first-degree relative with the disease is over 15 percent, compared with a 5 percent risk in the general population.[1,20]

The manifestations of colonic cancer depend on the anatomic location and function of the bowel segment containing the tumor. On the right side of the colon, the site of water and electrolyte absorption, tumor growth tends to extend along the bowel, rather than surrounding the lumen (Fig. 36–9). While no signs of obstruction are present, black, tarry stools, which signify bleeding into the intestinal lumen, are a significant finding. On the left side of the colon, a tumor may cause manifestations of an obstruction in the early stages of its growth. Feelings of intermittent abdominal cramping and fullness may be present, and "ribbon" or pencil-shaped stools may occur. Typically, the individual may note that the passage of stool or flatus relieves the abdominal pain. As the tumor growth progresses, blood or mucus may be present in the stool. When the tumor is located in the rectum, early manifestations may include a change in bowel habits, often beginning with an urgent need to defecate upon awakening in the morning, or alternating constipation and diarrhea. Blood and mucus may also be present in the stool. Later in the progression of tumor growth, a sensation of rectal fullness and a dull ache may be felt in the rectum or sacral region.[19]

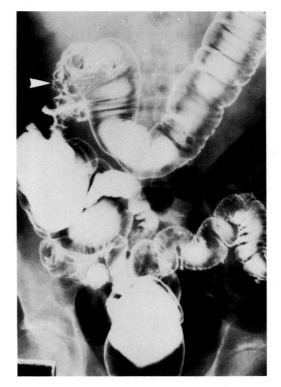

FIGURE 36–9. Barium enema demonstrating extensive mucosal destruction from a primary lymphoma of the right colon (*arrowhead*). (From Sleisenger MH, Fordtran JS (eds): *Gastrointestinal Disease*, 5th ed. Philadelphia, WB Saunders, 1993, p 1484. Reproduced with permission.)

The treatment and prognosis for colonic cancer depend on how extensively the tumor invades the colon and surrounding sites, as well as on the presence of distant metastasis. The 5-year survival rate is directly related to the extent of tissue invasion. A classification scheme based on the work of Dukes has been established which denotes the extent of tumor spread (Table 36–2).[1] The most effective treatment is surgery to remove the malignant tumor and adjacent tissues and lymph nodes that may contain cancer cells. The surgical formation of a colostomy, or an artificial opening of the colon on the abdominal wall, may be performed following the removal of the affected bowel segment. Chemotherapy and radiation therapy are used as supportive measures in addition to surgical intervention.

KEY CONCEPTS

- Warning signs for cancer of the GI tract include black, tarry, bloody, or pencil-shaped stools and a change in bowel habits. Risk factors for GI cancer include a low-fiber, high-fat diet, polyps, and chronic irritation or inflammation.
- The prognosis for GI cancer is related to the extent of spread in the body. Surgical removal of tumors followed by chemotherapy and/or radiation therapy is the usual treatment. Early detection is associated with better prognosis.

Psychosocial Aspects of Gastrointestinal Disorders

Gastrointestinal disorders may have profound effects on the psychosocial functioning of the affected individual and that person's family. Disorders of the GI tract that occur in the newborn, such as Hirschsprung's disease, may place great stress on the family attempting to cope with the demands of the infant's illness. The teenager affected by a chronic GI disorder, such as Crohn's disease, may be unable to participate in social eating activities and so may feel isolated from peers. Inflammatory bowel disease in the young adult who is beginning the most productive years of life may curtail his or her ability to function fully in the roles of spouse, parent, and wage earner. Finally, the onset of GI disorders, particularly a neoplastic process, in the middle-aged and older individual may not only limit that person's ability to perform activities of daily living but may also bring about an increased awareness of aging and mortality. The meaning of a disorder of the GI tract, or any health problem, to a particular person will be highly individualized, however. Nutrition and bowel elimination are behaviors that are dependent on cultural norms; changes in these basic areas of human activity brought about by a GI disorder may have a variety of meanings to different individuals.

In the past, much health care literature, including nursing texts, had a tendency to stereotype the individual experiencing chronic disorders of the GI tract as having abnormal psychological functioning. Abnormal psychological characteristics, it was thought, were somehow responsible for causing certain diseases of the GI tract, such as Crohn's disease and ulcerative colitis. It is now recognized that while certain chronic diseases of the GI tract may be aggravated by emotional factors, the pathogenic process is not the result of primarily psychological causes.[1,14] The stress of coping with a chronic, disabling illness may result in psychological trauma; in addition, any type of illness represents a threat to the integrity of the person. The person experiencing a chronic GI disorder may exhibit the psychological effects of such threats and will benefit from a sensitive approach to meeting his or her needs.

Summary

This chapter has described the major alterations in the GI tract that may occur across the human life span. Because of the strong links between cultural and psychological functioning and activities associated with the GI tract, an in-depth understanding of these alterations is essential for health care professionals.

Disorders of the GI tract may have many manifestations, including dysphagia, pain, vomiting, gas, and alterations in bowel elimination patterns. GI disorders may occur in any portion of the GI tract, from the mouth to the anus, and may be result of alterations in integrity of the GI tract wall (as in ulcerative colitis) or alterations in motility (as in the irritable bowel syndrome). Disorders of malabsorption, such as celiac disease, may seriously limit the individual's ability to utilize dietary nutrients and therefore are potentially life-threatening. Patients who have undergone surgery on the GI tract may also be at risk for malabsorption. Neoplasms of the GI tract are prevalent in the U.S. population, and the reader will want to review the associated risk factors for these very carefully.

T A B L E 36–2. Modified Dukes' Classification for Colorectal Cancer

Dukes' Category	Definition	5-year Survival (%) After Treatment
A	Cancer limited to mucosa or submucosa	90
B1	Cancer penetrates into but not through the muscularis propria	80
B2	Cancer penetrates through the muscularis	70
C1	Same as B1, plus lymph node metastases	50
C2	Same as B2, plus lymph node metastases	50
D	Distant metastases are present	<30

Finally, readers who are preparing for a career in health care should carefully consider the information provided on the psychosocial aspects of GI disorders and identify ways to provide optimal care for patients with these disorders.

REFERENCES

1. Eastwood GL, Avunduk C: *Manual of Gastroenterology.* Boston, Little, Brown & Co, 1988.
2. Greenberger NJ: *Gastrointestinal Disorders: A Pathophysiologic Approach,* 4th ed. St. Louis, Mosby–Year Book, 1989.
3. Ming S-C, Goldman H: *Pathology of the Gastrointestinal Tract.* Philadelphia, WB Saunders, 1992.
4. Shils ME, Olson JA, Shike M (eds): *Modern Nutrition in Health and Disease,* 8th ed. Philadelphia, Lea & Febiger, 1993.
5. McCallum RW, Champion M: *Physiology, Diagnosis, and Therapy of GI Motility Disorders.* Baltimore, Williams & Wilkins, 1989.
6. Sleisenger MH, Fordtran JS (eds): *Gastrointestinal Disease: Pathophysiology, Diagnosis, Management,* 5th ed. Philadelphia, WB Saunders, 1993.
7. Barrett KE: Mechanisms of inflammatory diarrhea. *Gastroenterology* 1992;103(2):710–711.
8. Gracey M: Recent advances in childhood diarrheal diseases. *Acta Paediatr Jpn* 1991;33(3):279–283.
9. Richter JE: Gastroesophageal reflux: Diagnosis and management. *Hosp Pract* 1992;27(1):59–66.
10. Jamieson GG, Duranceau A: *Gastroesophageal Reflux.* Philadelphia, WB Saunders, 1988.
10a. NIH Concensus Development Panel on *Helicobacter pylori* in Peptic Ulcer Disease: *Helicobacter pylori* in peptic ulcer disease. *JAMA* 1994;272(1):65–69.
11. Jayanthi V, Probert CS, Sher KS, Mayberry JF: Current concepts of the etiopathogenesis of inflammatory bowel disease. *Am J Gastroenterol* 1991;86(11):1566–1572.
12. Reddy SN, Bazzocchi G, Chan S, et al: Colonic motility and transit in health and ulcerative colitis. *Gastroenterology* 1991;101(5):1289–1297.
13. Mack DR: Epidemiology of IBD: Genetic versus environmental influence on the etiology of disease. *J Pediatr Gastroenterol* 1992;14(1):117.
14. Thompson WG: *Gut Reactions: Understanding Symptoms of the Digestive Tract.* New York, Plenum Press, 1990.
15. Welch JP: *Bowel Obstruction: Differential Diagnosis and Clinical Management.* Philadelphia, WB Saunders, 1990.
16. Kagnoff MF: Celiac disease: A gastrointestinal disease with environmental, genetic, and immunologic components. *Gastroenterol Clin North Am* 1992;21(2):405–425.
17. Trier JS: Celiac sprue. *N Engl J Med* 1991;325(24):1709–1719.
18. Hocking MP, Vogel SB: *Woodward's Postgastrectomy Syndrome,* 2nd ed. Philadelphia, WB Saunders, 1991.
19. Levin B (ed): *Gastrointestinal Cancer: Current Approaches to Diagnosis and Treatment.* Houston, University of Texas Press, 1988.
20. Levine R, Tenner S, Fromm H: Prevention and early detection of colorectal cancer. *Am Fam Physician* 1992;45(2):663–668.
21. Varma JR, Mills LR: Colon polyps. *J Fam Pract* 1992; 35(2):194–200.

BIBLIOGRAPHY

Ahlgren J, MacDonald J (eds): *Gastrointestinal Oncology.* Philadelphia, JB Lippincott, 1992.

Aitken TJ: Gastrointestinal manifestations in the child with cancer. *J Pediatr Oncol Nurs* 1992;9(3):99–109.

Beck M, Evans NG (eds): *Gastroenterology Nursing: A Core Curriculum.* St. Louis, Mosby–Year Book, 1992.

Berk JE, Haubrich WS, Kalser MH, Roth JLA, Schaffner F (eds): *Bockus Gastroenterology,* 4th ed. Philadelphia, WB Saunders, 1985.

Black JM, Matassarin-Jacobs E: *Luckmann and Sorenson's Medical-Surgical Nursing: A Psychophysiological Approach,* 4th ed. Philadelphia, WB Saunders, 1993.

Brady CE: AIDS-related diarrhea: What's a gastroenterologist to do? *Am J Gastroenterol* 1991;86(11):1685–1686.

Drossman D (ed): *Manual of Gastroenterologic Procedures,* 3rd ed. New York, Raven Press, 1992.

Farmer RG, Easley KA, Farmer JM: Quality of life assessment by patients with inflammatory bowel disease. *Cleve Clin J Med* 1992;59(1):35–42.

Feldman M, Maton PN, McCallum RW, McCarthy DM: Treating ulcers and reflux: What's new? *Patient Care* 1992;26(13):53.

Gitnick G: *Current Gastroenterology.* St. Louis, Mosby–Year Book, 1994, vol 14.

Grant M, Kennedy-Caldwell C: *Nutritional Support in Nursing.* Philadelphia, WB Saunders, 1987.

Heppner DG, et al: Treatment of gastrointestinal infections. *Curr Opin Gastroenterol* 1991;7(1):116–122.

Kauvar D, Brandt LJ: Treatment of common GI disorders in the elderly. *Physician Assist* 1992;16(2):105–108.

Kneisl CR, Ames SA: *Adult Health Nursing: A Biopsychosocial Approach.* Menlo Park, Calif. Addison-Wesley, 1986.

Sterling CE, Jolley SG, Besser AS, Matteson-Kane M: Nursing responsibility in the diagnosis, care, and treatment of the child with gastroesophageal reflux. *J Pediatr Nurs* 1991;6(5):331–336.

Whitehead WE: Behavioral medicine approaches to gastrointestinal disorders. *J Consult Clin Psychol* 1992;60(4):605–612.

Whitehead WE: Biofeedback treatment of gastrointestinal disorders. *Biofeedback Self Regul* 1992;17(1):59–76.

CHAPTER 37
Alterations in Function of the Gallbladder and Exocrine Pancreas

TIM BROWN

KEY TERMS

cholecystitis: Inflammation of the gallbladder wall; may be acute or chronic.

cholelithiasis: Formation of stones in the gallbladder.

gallbladder: A distensible sack of about 30 to 50 mL capacity which connects the common hepatic duct via the cystic duct to the common bile duct.

laparoscopy: Entering the abdominal cavity with a small incision to permit the insertion of a variety of optical scopes for diagnosis or therapy.

lithotripsy: Mechanical or chemical breaking up of gallstones, often while the stones are still in the gallbladder.

pancreatitis: Inflammation of the pancreas.

*S*tones have been discovered in the gallbladder of an Egyptian mummy, which suggests that gallbladder disease has been present in humans for thousands of years.[1] Over 500,000 cholecystectomies are performed annually in the United States and the incidence of new gallstones is 1 to 2 million cases per year. Most health care professionals will encounter diseases of the pancreaticobiliary system frequently. The incidence of acute pancreatitis varies according to geographic area but has been reported to be as high as 17 per 100,000 population in the Midwest. The incidence of chronic pancreatitis is about one-third to one-half that of the acute disease.

Structure and Function of the Pancreaticobiliary System

The pancreaticobiliary system is composed of the gallbladder and cystic duct, the intrahepatic, hepatic, and common bile ducts, and the ventral and dorsal pancreas. The extrahepatic biliary tree and the gallbladder form a controlled system for delivering bile to the intestinal tract.

The gallbladder is a distensible sack of about 30 to 50 mL capacity that connects the common hepatic duct via the cystic duct to the common bile duct. The common bile duct, which is about 3 inches long, runs behind the duodenum to terminate at the papilla of Vater, a complex mechanism that also forms the termi-

nating point of the main pancreatic duct. The pancreatic duct runs proximally in the pancreas, where it is joined by the dorsal pancreatic duct proceeding to the tail of the pancreas. The papilla of Vater forms the major aqueduct through which important digestive secretions enter the intestinal tract (Fig. 37–1).

Embryology of the Pancreaticobiliary System

In about the third or fourth week of gestation, the hepatic diverticulum forms from the primitive foregut.[2] It is composed of specialized liver cells that will eventually form the entire liver, biliary tree, and ventral pancreas. The dorsal pancreas forms from a separate outcropping of cells lying on the opposite side of the primitive foregut.

At 5 weeks, three buds can be seen in the hepatic diverticulum. The cranial bud contains specialized liver cells (hepatoblasts), which will form the liver. The liver sinusoids develop and feed into the developing bile canaliculi, which drain into intralobular ductules and then to interlobular ducts. The caudal bud develops into the gallbladder, which joins the common hepatic duct via the developing cystic duct to form the common bile duct. The gallbladder and the hepatic ducts are initially hollow, but fill in with development and become solid cords. With further differentiation they hollow out once again to become the tubes and reservoir for bile flow. During the sec-

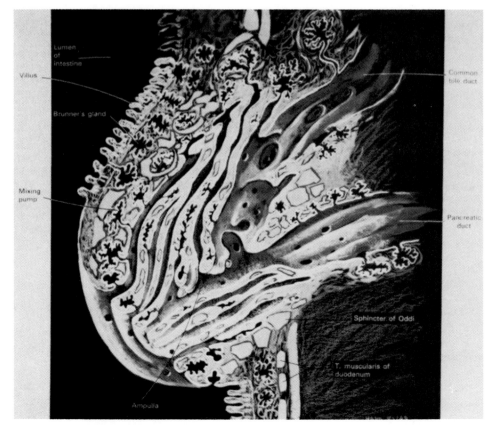

FIGURE 37–1. Detailed reconstruction of the papilla of Vater, showing junction of the common bile duct and the pancreatic duct in the ampulla and their investment by the smooth muscle of the sphincter of Oddi. (From Elias H: *Die Gallenwege.* Boehringer, Ingelheim, 1970. Reproduced with permission.)

ond trimester the fetus produces bile, which gives coloring to the fetal meconium. Finally, the basal bud transforms into the ventral pancreas (Fig. 37–2).

Physiology and Function of Bile Flow

Normal bile is composed primarily of water, electrolytes, and organic solutes. It has a low protein content, containing mainly bile salts, cholesterol, and phospholipids. Bile is formed in the canaliculi and then modified and stored in the gallbladder and bile ducts prior to secretion into the intestinal tract. The major functions of the bile are to aid in the digestion of lipids in the diet and to transport waste products (i.e., bilirubin), immunoglobulins (chiefly IgA), toxins, and cholesterol into the intestine for eventual disposal or reabsorption. After secretion into the bile canaliculi, bile then flows through the canals of Hering, ductules, interlobular ducts, septal ducts, right and left lobar ducts, and then into the common bile duct (Fig. 37–3). Bile salts consist mostly of primary bile salts (cholic and chenodeoxycholic acid) and secondary bile salts (deoxycholic, ursodeoxycholic, and lithocholic acids).

The gallbladder stores and concentrates hepatic bile in the fasting state. The muscular sphincter at the papilla of Vater is contracted at this time, promoting flow into the gallbladder. Only about half of the bile is stored during this time; the rest flows into the duodenum. At the same time that bile is flowing into the gallbladder absorption is also occurring so that within

4 hours up to 90 percent of water in bile can be removed, leaving a very concentrated mixture of sodium, bile salts, and other electrolytes.

With the first morning meal, a hormonally and possibly neurally regulated contraction of the gallbladder occurs, releasing the concentrated bile into the duodenum. Acids eventually may be absorbed again in the terminal ileum and travel by the portal circulation, where they are absorbed by the hepatocytes and secreted again into the bile. Bile acids may be reabsorbed two or three times. A small amount of the bile acid pool (less than 5 percent) enters the colon, where primary bile salts undergo bacterial transformation into secondary bile salts (Fig. 37–4).

After secretion into the bile, bile salts have dual properties, being hydrophilic (soluble in water) at one end and hydrophobic (insoluble in water) at the other. Therefore, these molecules tend to aggregate into micelles, which in turn can sequester lipids such as cholesterol and allow them to go into solution (Fig. 37–5). These micelles are not good stabilizers of cholesterol alone, but another molecule, lecithin, also secreted in large amounts in the bile is readily incorporated in the core of the micelle to greatly enhance the solubility of cholesterol. In this manner, bile is able to keep cholesterol partly solubilized. The capacity of the bile to keep cholesterol solubilized is often diagramatically represented by a triangle with the concentration of bile salts plotted against the concentration of cholesterol and lecithin. The line of cholesterol solubility suggests that precipitation of cholesterol from the bile

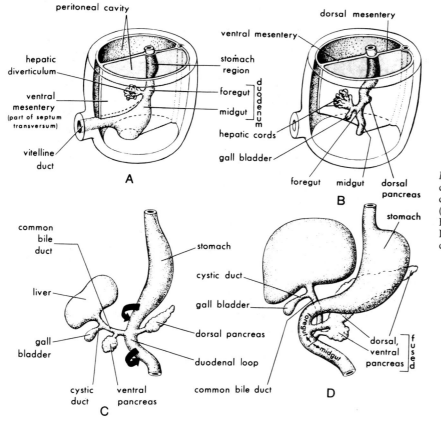

FIGURE 37–2. Stages in the embryologic development of the liver, gallbladder, pancreas, and duodenum at 4 weeks (**A**), 5 weeks (**B** and **C**), and 6 weeks (**D**). (From Moore KL, Persaud TVN: *The Developing Human,* 5th ed. Philadelphia, WB Saunders, 1993, p 241. Reproduced with permission.)

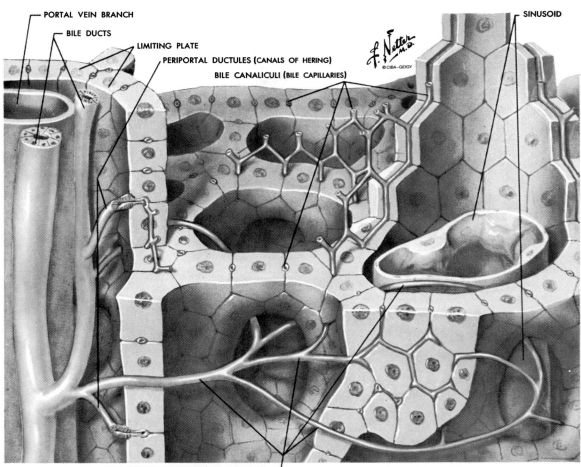

FIGURE 37–3. Three-dimensional schema of the intrahepatic biliary system. (© Copyright 1964 CIBA-GEIGY Corporation. Reprinted with permission from *The Ciba Collection of Medical Illustrations*, Volume 3, Digestive System, Part III, page 11. Illustrated by Frank Netter, M.D. All rights reserved.)

FIGURE 37–4. Enterohepatic bile salt recirculation is maintained by passive jejunal absorption of un-ionized bile salts, active ilial absorption of ionized bile salts, and colonic deconjugation and dehydroxylation of bile salts followed by passive absorption of lipid-soluble un-ionized secondary bile salt. The loss of unabsorbable bile salt is balanced by the de novo hepatic synthesis of bile salt from cholesterol. (From Cooper AD: Metabolic basis of cholesterol gallstone disease. *Gastroenterol Clin North Am* 1991;20(1):34. Reproduced with permission.)

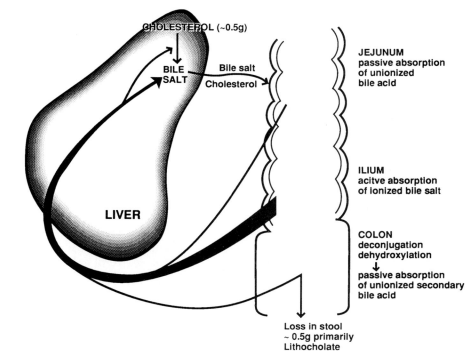

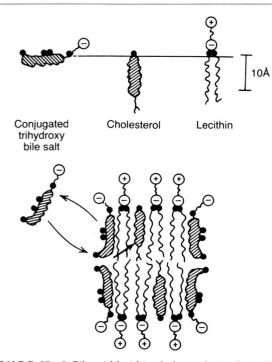

FIGURE 37–5. Bile acid-lecithin-cholesterol mixed micelle. Polar ends of bile acids and lecithin are oriented outward, whereas hydrophobic, nonpolar portions make up the interior. Cholesterol is solubilized within the hydrophobic, nonpolar center. (From Saunders KD, Cates JA, Roslyn JJ: Pathogenesis of gallstones. *Surg Clin North Am* 1990;70(6):1197–1216. Reproduced with permission.)

are composed of both active digestive enzymes (e.g., amylase, lipase) and precursor or proenzymes (e.g., trypsinogen). Their release during a meal is controlled by hormones secreted from the small intestinal mucosa: cholecystokinin (CCK) and secretin. When this regulation is deranged, enzymes may be released within the gland and produce an acute or eventually chronic pancreatitis.

KEY CONCEPTS

- Bile is produced by hepatocytes in the liver and stored in the gallbladder. Bile is composed of fluid, electrolytes, bile salts, cholesterol, and phospholipids. Bile salts are important for digestion and absorption of fats from the small bowel. Bile is an important route for excretion of waste products, particularly bilirubin. The gallbladder receives bile from the liver, concentrates bile by absorbing water, and then contracts to expel stored bile into the common bile duct, which terminates in the duodenum.

- The pancreas is both an endocrine organ, secreting insulin, glucagon, and somatostatin into the bloodstream, and an exocrine gland, secreting digestive juice into the duodenum. Some pancreatic enzymes are secreted in active form (amylase, lipase), while others are proenzymes that are activated in the duodenum (trypsinogen). Release of pancreatic enzymes is stimulated by cholecystokinin and secretin.

will occur in concentrations above the line of solubility (Fig. 37–6). Cholesterol can remain in suspension even above this line for a time because of the formation of cholesterol-lecithin vesicles, but because they are not as stable as micelles, cholesterol will eventually precipitate from the supersaturated solution, which may lead to nucleation of cholesterol crystals and then to the formation of gallstones.

Functional Anatomy of the Pancreas

The pancreas is really two organs in one: it functions as both an endocrine and an exocrine organ. On the one hand, hormones such as insulin, glucagon, and somatostatin are produced (characteristic of an endocrine organ); on the other hand, more than 1 liter of digestive juice is secreted via the sphincter of Oddi into the digestive tract (characteristic of an exocrine system).

Embryologically, the pancreas is composed of two fused organs: a dorsal and ventral pancreas (Fig. 37–7). The main pancreatic duct is a result of fusion between the ventral and dorsal ducts (Fig. 37–8).[3] Microscopically, the pancreas is somewhat lobular and arranged into exocrine glands. The pancreatic juices are secreted into the glandular acini, which eventually drain into the main pancreatic duct and then enter the intestinal tract. The juices themselves

Disorders of the Gallbladder

Pathophysiology of Cholesterol Gallstone Formation

In general, the formation of cholesterol gallstones (cholelithiasis) can be broken down into three phases: (1) saturation of bile with cholesterol, (2) nucleation of stones, and (3) stone growth.

The critical factor in the formation of cholesterol stones may not be the concentration of cholesterol in the bile but rather the relative concentrations of different biochemical elements containing cholesterol.[4] That is, the concentration of bile acids and phospholipids relative to cholesterol may determine whether the right conditions for stone formation exist. A complicating factor has recently been shown in the form of cholesterol-containing vesicles, which may help to solubilize cholesterol. The relation between cholesterol vesicle formation and the solubilization of cholesterol may modify stone formation and growth.[5]

If conditions are right for the formation of cholesterol gallstones, nucleation must then occur in which the cholesterol crystals aggregate together. This process is probably initiated by pronucleating agents—so far not definitely identified—that allow the tiny seed crystals to form. Continued growth then becomes a balance between cholesterol growth-promoting fac-

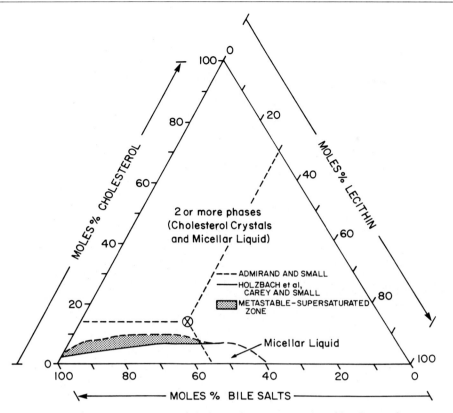

FIGURE 37-6. Determination of cholesterol saturation index (CSI). Tricoordinate phase diagram for representing by a single intersecting point ⊗ the relative concentrations of cholesterol, lecithin, and bile salt in bile. In this scheme, the relative concentration of each lipid is expressed as a percentage of the sum of the molar concentrations of all three. This manipulation permits representation of the relations between three constituents in two dimensions, the water content being invariant at, say, 90 percent (10 percent wet/vol solids).

In this figure, for example, at the point ⊗ the relative concentration of bile salt from its coordinate is 55 percent (indicating 55 percent of the sum of all three lipids), whereas that foclecithin is 30 percent, and that for cholesterol is 15 percent. The range of concentrations found consistent with a clear aqueous micellar solution is limited to a small region at the lower left. A solution having the composition represented by the point, on the other hand, would initially be visually turbid and contain precipitated forms of cholesterol crystals in addition to bile salt mixed micelles.

Lastly, a solution represented by a point falling in the *shaded area* below the *dashed line* would be unstable (i.e., metastable-supersaturated), meaning that by prediction it would be initially clear (micellar). Within a short time, however, vesicles and various precipitated forms of cholesterol crystals would form, and such a solution would then be visually turbid, similar to all solutions above the dashed line. (From Sleisenger MH, Fordtran JS (eds): *Gastrointestinal Disease: Pathophysiology/Diagnosis/Management*, 4th ed. Philadelphia, WB Saunders, 1989, p 1673. Reproduced with permission.)

tors and factors that tend to cause stone dissolution. One factor that may promote the continued growth of stones is stasis of bile within the gallbladder. Pregnancy and truncal vagotomy both produce stasis and are associated with an increase in gallstone formation.

Cholelithiasis and Cholecystitis

Etiology

Currently, about 20 million people in the United States have gallstones. The incidence of gallstones is related to age, sex, and a variety of medical factors. Gallstones are twice as frequent in women as in men. Native Americans are markedly susceptible to gallstones, caucasians less so. Obesity correlates with the development of gallstones, but so does rapid weight loss in an obese individual.

Population studies have shown that some individuals with gallstones have no symptoms or symptoms that are very mild and vague. Gracie and Ransohoff followed 123 asymptomatic patients for up to 24 years. Symptoms attributable to gallstones developed in 13 percent and complications of gallstones in 2 percent.[5] Other data have supported the conclusion that asymptomatic gallstones often remain so for many

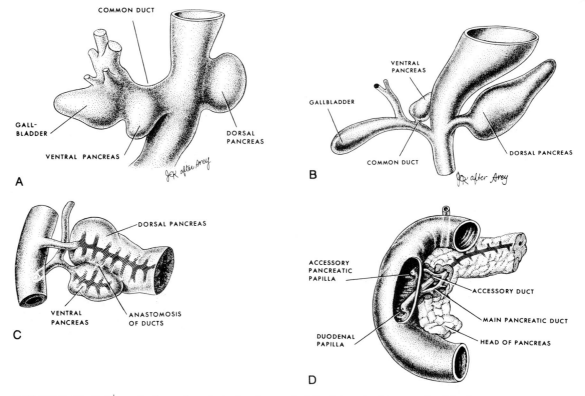

FIGURE 37–7. Stages in the embryologic development of the fetus. **A,** At approximately 4 weeks of gestation, dorsal and ventral buds are formed. **B,** At 6 weeks, the ventral pancreas extends toward the dorsal pancreas. **C,** By about 7 weeks, fusion of dorsal and ventral pancreas has occurred, and ductular anastomosis is beginning. **D,** At birth the pancreas is a single organ, and ductular anastomosis is complete. (From Sleisenger MH, Fordtran JS (eds): *Gastrointestinal Disease: Pathophysiology/Diagnosis/Management,* 4th ed. Philadelphia, WB Saunders, 1989, p 1772. Modified after Arey. Reproduced with permission.)

years, and when symptoms occur, they are usually "warning" symptoms, with complications occurring later. This implies that the aggressive treatment of cholesterol gallstones in an asymptomatic individual may not be warranted and that observation is appropriate, with intervention introduced selectively as symptoms develop. Whether there are certain high-risk subgroups that are predisposed to the development of complications is not clear. In the past, diabetes mellitus was thought to be associated with a more

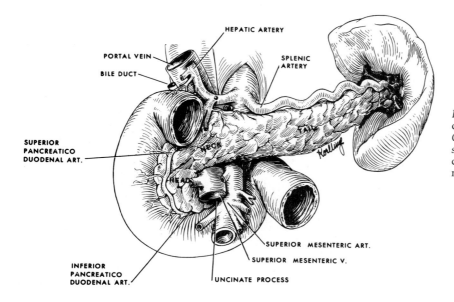

FIGURE 37–8. Anterior view of the pancreas. (From Sleisenger MH, Fordtran JS (eds): *Gastrointestinal Disease: Pathophysiology/Diagnosis/Management,* 4th ed. Philadelphia, WB Saunders, 1989, p 1766. Reproduced with permission.)

severe form of gallbladder disease. However, more recent studies have shown that this assumption is not correct[6] and that diabetes alone is not an indication for intervention in cholelithiasis.

Biliary Colic and Chronic Cholecystitis

Clinical Manifestations

Colic is the chief complaint of most patients with gallstone disease. "Chronic cholecystitis" may accompany these attacks of pain, consisting histologically of fibrosis and inflammatory changes in the gallbladder wall with varying amounts of thickening.[7] The pain is caused by intermittent obstruction of the cystic duct by a stone. Acute inflammatory change is not present in this setting.

Often pain is localized to the epigastrium or right upper quadrant and may radiate to the back. Symptoms may be precipitated by a meal, but often occur spontaneously and may occur at night. The pain will often increase steadily for 15 minutes and persist for an hour or more, then slowly decrease. Nausea, vomiting, and sweating are common. An attack that persists for more than several hours suggests acute cholecystitis. Attacks may recur on a frequent or infrequent schedule. Additional symptoms attributed to gallbladder disease include chronic dyspepsia (including fatty food intolerance, belching, flatus, bloating, and epigastric burning). These symptoms may occur frequently in patients without gallstones as well. However, removal of a diseased gallbladder may result in improvement of dyspeptic symptoms. The duration of relief may be short or long in a given individual.

Diagnosis and Treatment

Therapy for gallstone disease ranges from expectant management to emergency surgery, depending on the clinical circumstances. The emergence of a laparoscopic cholecystectomy has changed the standard management of gallstone disease in just the past 3 years. Nonoperative management, including chemodissolution, and a variety of interventional radiologic procedures have also been added to the therapeutic armamentarium.

Cholecystectomy was first performed in 1882.[8] Until the past few years, it was the standard of management for gallbladder disease. Indications for cholecystectomy include symptomatic cholelithiasis, including acute and chronic cholecystitis. Among asymptomatic patients, little rationale exists for prophylactic cholecystectomy except in a few special situations. Cholelithiasis in children is usually associated with symptoms, is often accompanied by additional diseases such as cystic fibrosis or sickle cell disease, and is an indication for gallbladder removal. Open cholecystectomy via laparotomy is an extremely safe operation with low morbidity and mortality. Hospital stay is usually 4 to 5 days, with an additional 2 to 3 weeks for convalescence.

Laparoscopic cholecystectomy was first performed in France in 1987[9] and since then has been popularized by the development of video laparoscopic instrumentation. The procedure is usually performed with four small incisions through which instruments are inserted. The gallbladder is freed using either electrosurgical or laser excision and then withdrawn through one of the small incisions. The advantages of the laparoscopic technique include (1) removal of the entire gallbladder, not just the stones; (2) less postoperative pain than after laparotomy; (3) small incision size, which allows rapid return to daily activities; (4) incisions cosmetically superior to the standard incision; and (5) discharge from the hospital on the day of or the day following surgery.[10]

Not all patients can be treated laparoscopically. Altered anatomy or scarring from previous surgery, anesthesia risk, or the presence of common bile duct stones may necessitate alternative therapies. Nonoperative methods to treat gallstones, such as chemodissolution with a variety of bile acids or organic solvents and shock wave lithotripsy, have been tried as alternatives to surgery.

Chemodissolution with a variety of pharmacologic agents began in 1971, when Danzinger demonstrated that the administration of a secondary bile salt, chenodeoxycholic acid (CDCA), to patients with gallstones resulted in dissolution of the stones.[11] CDCA suppresses an enzyme in the liver that regulates cholesterol synthesis and thereby reduces cholesterol in the bile, allowing the stones to dissolve slowly. Several major problems developed with the use of bile acid–dissolving agents. First, stones must be of the cholesterol type and must contain a minimum amount of calcium for dissolution to be effective. CDCA also causes diarrhea in about 50 percent of patients studied. A bile acid related to CDCA, ursodeoxycholic acid (UDCA), has been shown to be as effective as CDCA with almost no diarrhea, making it a preferred agent. Additional drawbacks to using bile acids in dissolving gallstones include limits on stone size (stones should be no larger than 2 cm in diameter), a low overall efficacy in dissolving stones in all patients with gallstones (15–20 percent, with higher success in carefully selected groups),[12] and a fairly high recurrence of stones after successful dissolution (up to 50 percent of cases). Because of these drawbacks, stone dissolution with bile acids is usually reserved for special situations in which surgery poses a high risk.

Dissolution of stones may also be achieved via extracorporeal shock wave lithotripsy (ESWL). The objective is to fragment stones into sizes small enough to be passed through the cystic duct, or small enough to allow bile acid dissolving agents to work. The devices in the United States all include three basic components: (1) an energy source to deliver a shock wave, (2) a focusing system to focus the shock wave on the gallstone, and (3) a targeting device to identify the gallstone to allow precise aiming of the shock wave. Shock waves may be generated by various devices. The most common use either a spark gap system or a piezoelectric crystal. With either type of generator, the object in lithotripsy is to focus pulses of energy on the gallbladder stones until they fragment. Thousands of pulses are delivered in a single session.[13]

The advantages of lithotripsy over surgery include the lack of a surgical scar and an abbreviated hospital stay. Often the procedure may be done without anesthesia. The disadvantages include restrictions on use in many patients, resulting in a low percentage of eligible patients. Stones are best fragmented if they are less than 2 cm in size and if there are fewer than three stones. The gallbladder also is left in place, allowing for possible recurrence of gallstones and necessitating the concurrent use of dissolving agents such as CDCA to prevent new stone formation. Exactly how long such therapy must be continued is not clear; lifetime therapy may be needed. Complications of ESWL include pancreatitis related to passage of stone fragments through the sphincter of Oddi, and damage to unrelated organs through which the energy wave must pass. Fortunately, these complications have not been common. Currently, lithotripsy for gallstones is still experimental in the United States, and its ultimate place in gallstone treatment is not entirely clear.

Additional techniques to obliterate gallstones are also being evaluated. These include contact dissolution of stones with the organic solvent methyl *tert*-butyl ether or another bile acid derivative, monooctanoin. A catheter is usually placed by a radiologist percutaneously into the gallbladder and then the agents are instilled. Various problems in using these agents have so far limited their use to special centers, and widespread application has not yet occurred.

In general, the problem with all nonsurgical techniques is that they leave the gallbladder in place and therefore allow for disease recurrence. In addition, all of these techniques are best applied to early gallstone disease in which the gallbladder is relatively free of inflammation and fibrosis. Most of them are not applicable to acute cholecystitis. The cost of these treatments is also of major concern. For the most part, in the near future the treatment of gallstone disease is likely to remain surgical, with standard or laparoscopic cholecystectomy being the major forms of intervention.

Acute Cholecystitis

Pathogenesis and Clinical Manifestations
Acute cholecystitis is defined as acute inflammation of the gallbladder wall, usually accompanied by abdominal pain, tenderness, and fever. The pathogenesis of cholecystitis is not well understood, and animal models of acute cholecystitis do not accurately depict cholecystitis in humans. Cholelithiasis is present in about 90 percent of patients with cholecystitis. Obstruction of the cystic duct is present in almost all cases, suggesting that stasis of bile in the gallbladder is important in the pathogenesis of the disease.

Ligation of the cystic duct in animal models does not necessarily result in cholecystitis. If the gallbladder is in the fasted state and distended with concentrated bile, ligation may lead to inflammatory change. This suggests that other factors must act to lead to inflammatory changes in the gallbladder. Candidates include cholesterol, prostaglandins, and lysolecithin and bile salts.[14] Bacterial infection may become a part of the pathologic process, although it is not thought to be active in its inception. Bacterial contamination of the bile will lead to suppurative cholangitis with empyema formation and possible rupture of the gallbladder.

The clinical manifestations of cholecystitis begin once the pathologic process of obstruction of the cystic duct and inflammatory change sets in. Initial symptoms include pain, usually in the upper abdomen. The location of the abdominal pain varies but is usually in the right upper quadrant. It may be intermittent at first but then becomes more constant as the inflammatory process worsens. Left upper quadrant pain may be present initially or occasionally may persist as the primary location of the pain. Radiation of the pain into the back is common. Fever and diaphoresis may occur. On abdominal examination, tenderness in the midepigastrium or right upper quadrant is common. The gallbladder may be palpable. Increasing pain in the right upper quadrant during inhalation leads to Murphy's sign—inspiratory arrest while the examiner palpates the right upper quadrant. Laboratory evaluation may reveal leukocytosis, mild jaundice, and occasionally elevated amylase levels.

Diagnosis
Evaluation for possible cholecystitis includes an appropriate history and physical examination, laboratory studies, and usually an imaging study designed to determine the status of the gallbladder and cystic duct. Abdominal ultrasonography (US) is usually performed early in the diagnostic evaluation. Typically the gallbladder will demonstrate evidence of cholelithiasis. Occasionally a thickened wall and either contraction or distention of the lumen may be noted. Very occasionally a cystic duct stone may be visualized as well. Criteria for gallstone identification in the gallbladder include an echogenic focus, which usually casts an acoustic shadow, and gravitational dependency. The mere presence of cholelithiasis and a thickened gallbladder wall is not definitive evidence acute cholecystitis, and so ancillary diagnostic tests are needed. One of the newer ancillary tests is biliary scintigraphy. A radioisotope of technetium coupled with iminodiacetic acid, is injected intravenously and its path through the gallbladder and bile ducts imaged. This study determines whether the cystic duct is patent. Acute cholecystitis is rare when the cystic duct is open. The liver and common hepatic and bile ducts will opacify first, followed by the gallbladder, usually within 45 minutes. Failure of the gallbladder to opacify suggests obstruction of the cystic duct and in an appropriate setting supports a presumptive diagnosis of acute cholecystitis. Unfortunately, false positive studies may occur, especially in a prolonged fasted state, such as in a patient on parenteral hyper-

alimentation. Oral cholecystography (OCG) is a time-honored means of evaluating the gallbladder. Iopanoic acid or a similar agent is given orally the night before the examination. The next day the gallbladder is imaged fluoroscopically and radiographs are taken. The time needed for this test and the numerous causes of nonvisualization of the gallbladder other than cholecystitis make the test less useful in the diagnosis of acute cholecystitis.

Treatment

Therapy for acute cholecystitis ranges from expectant management to emergency surgery, depending on the clinical course of an individual patient. In general, nonoperative methods are less effective in the acute setting because they leave an acutely inflamed gallbladder in place, take too long to accomplish the desired end point, or are not effective because of cystic duct obstruction and inflammation of the gallbladder. In general, whenever acute cholecystitis appears imminently likely to produce complications, surgical removal is indicated. Although surgery is usually performed through a laparotomy, the laparoscopic approach is occasionally successful in experienced hands. In the uncomplicated case, symptoms and signs of acute cholecystitis may resolve within a relatively short time. In this setting, therapy can be delayed for 6 to 8 weeks after recovery, which may or may not be beneficial. In general, early surgery has the advantages of eliminating progressive disease, requiring less total recovery time, and costing less. Surgery is no easier and may be more difficult if timing is delayed.[15]

KEY CONCEPTS

- Lecithin is an important part of bile that helps keep cholesterol from precipitating into crystals. Crystals of cholesterol may initiate gallstone formation. The relative concentrations of cholesterol, lecithin, and bile acids appear to determine the likelihood of cholesterol gallstone formation. Bile stasis contributes to growth of cholesterol stones.
- Gallstones occur more frequently in women than in men. Ethnicity, obesity, and rapid weight loss are predisposing factors. Gallstones may be asymptomatic or associated with symptomatic cholecystitis. Colicky pain due to intermittent obstruction of the cystic duct by a stone is the chief complaint. Symptoms of chronic cholecystitis include epigastric or right upper quadrant pain radiating to the back, nausea, vomiting, sweating, fat intolerance, bloating, and flatus.
- Acute cholecystitis is acute inflammation of the gallbladder associated with abdominal pain, leukocytosis, and fever. Cholelithiasis is present in about 90 percent of patients; obstruction of the cystic duct is present in nearly all cases.
- Treatment for cholecystitis includes surgical removal of the gallbladder (cholecystectomy), chemo-

dissolution, shock wave lithotripsy for stones, antibiotics if indicated, and management of pain. Cholecystectomy is the mainstay of therapy.

Disorders of the Pancreas

Acute Pancreatitis

Etiology and Pathogenesis

Acute pancreatitis is an inflammatory process involving the pancreas that may range from mild to severe. After an attack, the exocrine and endocrine functions of the pancreas may remain impaired for a variable period of time. The causes of pancreatitis are variable (Table 37–1), but in the United States the most common causes are biliary tract disease and ethanol-associated pancreatitis. Experimental models of pancreatitis do not perfectly mimic the human condition, making the disease more difficult to study. One hypothesis is that obstruction of the pancreatic duct by whatever mechanism results in release of digestive enzymes within the parenchyma, followed by enzyme activation and then autodigestion of the pancreas. There are certain problems with this model. Pancreatic tumors that block the pancreatic ducts often produce no sign of pancreatitis. In addition, ligation of the pancreatic duct often does not in itself produce pancreatitis.[16] Another popular model holds that reflux of duodenal contents into the pancreatic duct may induce pancreatitis. Animal models have demonstrated this potential. However, surgical sphincteroplasty performed in certain cases of recurrent pancreatitis allows free duodenopancreatic reflux, which does not result in recurrent pancreatitis. Other theories to explain the initiation of pancreatitis have included reflux of bile via a common channel into the pancreatic duct[17] and the possibility of hormonally

TABLE 37–1. Conditions Associated With Acute Pancreatitis

Cholelithiasis
Ethanol abuse } 90% of all cases
Idiopathic
Abdominal operations
Hyperlipemia
Injection into pancreatic duct
Trauma
Hypercalcemia
Pregnancy
Peptic ulcer
Outflow obstruction
Pancreas divisum
Organ transplantation
End-stage renal failure
Hereditary (familial pancreatitis)
Scorpion bite
Miscellaneous: hypoperfusion, viral infections, *Mycoplasma pneumoniae* infection, intraductal parasites

From Sleisenger MH, Fordtran JS (eds): *Gastrointestinal Disease: Pathophysiology/Diagnosis/Management*, 4th ed. Philadelphia, WB Saunders, 1989, p 1819. Reproduced with permission.

induced intracellular protease activation. Whatever the initiating mechanism, the final common path of injury appears to involve activation of the pancreatic proenzymes (such as trypsinogen) to active forms, followed by autodigestion of the gland, leading to the signs, symptoms, and complications of acute pancreatitis.

The role of alcohol in acute pancreatitis is not entirely clear. There is clearly an association of alcohol with pancreatitis, but the causal mechanism has not been determined. Up to 66 percent of first cases of pancreatitis are associated with alcoholism.[18] A major question regarding the alcoholic variety of pancreatitis is whether true acute pancreatitis occurs or whether the appearance of acute pancreatitis is really a first manifestation of chronic pancreatitis, which may be the true disease induced by ethanol.

Clinical Manifestations

The presentation of acute pancreatitis often begins with steady, boring pain in the epigastrium or left upper quadrant. It may radiate to the back and be accompanied by nausea and vomiting. Tenderness on palpation may be exquisite. Bowel sounds are reduced but not absent. Abdominal distention may be present. Fever is common but usually low grade initially. In more severe pancreatitis, this clinical picture is accompanied by signs of circulatory instability, respiratory insufficiency, and occasionally sepsis.

Diagnosis

The laboratory evaluation of acute pancreatitis begins with measurements of serum amylase, an enzyme released into the blood during the inflammatory process. The serum amylase level rises acutely during the first 12 hours and remains elevated for several days. Other enzymes such as lipase may also be elevated and can remain high for longer periods. Serum aminotransferases (AST, ALT) may also be elevated. Marked elevation of the alkaline phosphatase level should increase the suspicion of biliary disease. Serum bilirubin may rise, but marked elevations also suggest the possibility of biliary obstruction. Associated laboratory findings include leukocytosis, hyperlipidemia (which may be marked), and hypocalcemia.

The diagnosis of acute pancreatitis is based on the signs and symptoms, laboratory data, and imaging studies of the pancreas and surrounding organs. Plain radiographs of the abdomen may reveal an ileus pattern or the "sentinel loop"—a distended loop of small bowel in the area of the pancreas. US can provide a bedside technique to visualize the pancreas, gallbladder, common bile duct, and other abdominal structures. The disadvantage of US lies in the frequency of technically poor studies, often related to the presence of bowel gas. Computed tomography (CT) of the abdomen often shows the pancreas in remarkable detail, including edema, abscess or cyst formation, and the degree of peripancreatic involvement. The

differential diagnosis of acute pancreatitis includes perforated peptic ulcer, acute cholecystitis, mesenteric vascular disease, and a variety of other illnesses that may be associated with elevated amylase levels (Table 37–2).

Grading systems have been developed to allow prediction of the severity of acute pancreatitis. Several different schemes, such as the APACHE II scoring system, have been evaluated and have shown a degree of success in predicting the outcome of pancreatitis based on initial findings.[18,19] These grading systems use clinical assessment and simple biochemical measurements to determine severity (Table 37–3). Early monitoring in the intensive care unit is indicated for patients with a high number of risk factors. Once the diagnosis and severity rating of acute pancreatitis have been determined, attention may be directed to appropriate therapy.

Treatment

Conservative management is indicated for mild to moderate cases of acute pancreatitis. In general, with-

---

TABLE 37–2. Conditions Other Than Acute Pancreatitis Occasionally Associated With Hyperamylasemia

Group A	Chronic pancreatitis
	Pancreatic pseudocyst
	Carcinoma of pancreas
	Perforation of stomach, duodenum, jejunum
	Mesenteric infarction
	Opiate administration
	After ERCP
Group B	Common bile duct obstruction
	Acute cholecystitis
	Burn injury
Group C	Salivary adenitis
	Postoperative state
	Renal insufficiency
	Metabolic, including diabetic, acidosis
	Admission to intensive care unit
	Acute alcoholism
	Acute and chronic hepatocellular disease
	Anorexia nervosa, bulimia
	Ovarian neoplasm
	Salpingitis; ruptured ectopic pregnancy
	Incidental finding
	Upper gastrointestinal endoscopy
Group D	Macroamylasemia

Group A: Entry of pancreatic enzymes into blood stream directly from pancreas or via peritoneal surfaces. Indistinguishable from acute pancreatitis by measurements of serum pancreatic enzyme levels.

Group B: Generally minor total serum amylase elevation. Coexisting mild pancreatitis difficult to rule out without surgical exploration, US, or CT-scanning.

Group C: Minor total serum amylase elevation, mainly owing to elevation of salivary isoenzyme. Serum lipase and immunoreactive trypsin levels generally normal.

Group D: No symptoms of current pancreatic disease; low amylase-creatinine clearance ratio.

From Sleisenger MH, Fordtran JS (eds): *Gastrointestinal Disease: Pathophysiology/Diagnosis/Management*, 4th ed. Philadelphia, WB Saunders, 1989, p 1826. Reproduced with permission.

TABLE 37-3. Findings Correlated With Severe or Complicated Course and Increasing Mortality Risk in Pancreatitis

Acute, Ethanol-Associated Pancreatitis

At admission:
1. Age over 55 years
2. White blood cell count > 16,000 cells/mm³
3. Blood glucose > 200 mg/dL (no history of prior hyperglycemia)
4. Serum LDH > 350 IU/L (normal, up to 225 IU/L)
5. AST (SGOT) > 250 Sigma Frankel units/L (normal, up to 40 units/L)

During initial 48 hr:
6. Hematocrit drop > 10%
7. BUN rise > 5 mg/dL
8. Arterial Po₂ < 60 mm Hg
9. Base deficit > 4 mEq/L
10. Serum calcium < 8.0 mg/dL
11. Estimated fluid sequestration > 6 L

Acute Pancreatitis Not Related to Ethanol Intake

Any time during first 48 hr after hospitalization:
1. White blood cell count > 15,000 cells/mm³
2. Blood glucose > 180 mg/dL (no history of prior hyperglycemia)
3. BUN > 45 mg/dL (after adequate hydration)
4. Arterial Po₂ < 60 mm Hg
5. Serum calcium < 8.0 mg/dL
6. Serum albumin < 3.2 gm/dL
7. Serum LDH > 600 units/L (normal, up to 250 units/L)
8. AST (SGOT) or ALT (SGPT) > 200 units/L (normal, up to 40 units/L)

LDH, lactic dehydrogenase; IU, international units; AST, aspartate aminotransferase; BUN, blood urea nitrogen; ALT, alanine aminotransferase.
From Sleisenger MH, Fordtran JS (eds): *Gastrointestinal Disease: Pathophysiology/Diagnosis/Management*, 4th ed. Philadelphia, WB Saunders, 1989, p 1825. Reproduced with permission.

holding oral feedings, providing nasogastric suction for significant adynamic ileus, and providing careful volume replacement with IV fluids are indicated. Analgesics are administered parenterally. Morphine and codeine are usually avoided because of their effect on the sphincter of Oddi. This treatment is often sufficient when carried out for 3 to 7 days, after which the acute episode subsides and oral intake may gradually be resumed.

The more severe attack of acute pancreatitis may require monitoring in the intensive care unit. Monitoring of central venous pressure or pulmonary capillary wedge pressure may be required. Frequent determination of the urine output and laboratory values is necessary. Usually this type of severe attack is associated with more intense pancreatic necrosis. The extent of the necrosis may be visualized on contrast-enhanced CT. Bacterial contamination is the most important risk factor determining poor outcome in pancreatic necrosis.[20] The most common infecting agent is *Escherichia coli*. Treatment of severe pancreatitis with necrosis includes the standard measures for more moderate disease, plus consideration of more radical intervention. The most common interventions are

peritoneal lavage or laparotomy with debridement of devitalized tissue, or major pancreatic resection.[21,22] Postoperative drains are left in place to prevent the accumulation of loculated fluid. Additional supportive measures include calcium administration to reverse severe hypocalcemia, correction of magnesium deficiency, and control of hyperglycemia. Causes of death from severe pancreatitis include respiratory failure (usually associated with the adult respiratory distress syndrome), acute renal failure, and acute intraabdominal sepsis. Mechanical ventilation and hemodialysis may be required in prolonged cases.

Nutritional deficits develop rapidly with extensive catabolism and lack of caloric intake. The effect of total parenteral nutrition in the course of pancreatitis is not entirely clear. There appears to be no form of nutrition that can avoid pancreatic stimulation. Elemental diets are just as stimulating to the pancreas as other types of diet. Intravenous amino acids also stimulate gastric acid and pancreatic enzyme output. However, nutritional support is usually indicated when it is apparent that pancreatitis will not resolve within a few days, or if complications arise.

Localized complications of acute pancreatitis may result in prolonged morbidity for the patient. The most common localized complication is the pancreatic pseudocyst. This is a collection of fluid within or adjacent to the pancreas that often has a direct communication to the pancreatic duct. It is called a pseudocyst because, unlike a true cyst, there is no true epithelial lining. The failure of a patient to recover from an acute bout of pancreatitis may herald the development of a pseudocyst. The presentation often includes fever, tachycardia, and an abdominal mass and tenderness. CT is the modality of choice for demonstrating pseudocysts. Pseudocysts that are large or that persist for more than 6 weeks may fail to resolve spontaneously.[23] Complications of pseudocysts include infection leading to pancreatic abscess, spontaneous rupture, or hemorrhage. Treatment of pseudocysts includes either endoscopic or surgical drainage of the cyst either externally or internally, usually into the stomach or bowel.

Pancreatic abscess is a more severe localized complication of pancreatitis. An abscess may form from direct bacterial infection of pancreatic tissue during an acute episode of pancreatitis or by seeding of a formed pseudocyst in the pancreas. Detection of infected pancreatic tissue may be accomplished by CT-guided aspiration.[24] Treatment involves either percutaneous or surgical debridement of infected tissues. Broad-spectrum antibiotics are indicated in both settings.

Pancreatic ascites may occur and may represent a persistent leak in the main pancreatic duct. It is usually painless and often massive. The fluid may find its way into unusual places, and pleural effusions or mediastinal fluid may be found. Pancreatic ascites may be detected with CT and paracentesis, with analysis of the obtained fluid, including the amylase level. Treatment is often conservative with prolonged parenteral nutrition. Endoscopic visualization of the pancreatic duct is usually indicated. Occasionally improvement may occur following the endoscopic placement of a stent (a thin-walled tube) into the main pancreatic duct.

Other complications of acute pancreatitis include common bile duct obstruction, portal or splenic vein thrombosis, peptic ulcer disease, and chronic fistula formation.

Newer forms of treatment are emerging for acute pancreatitis associated with common bile duct gallstones. Pancreatitis associated with stones in the common bile duct may range from mild to severe. In more mild cases, traditional conservative therapy followed by endoscopic retrograde cholangiopancreatography (ERCP) is acceptable therapy. In more severe cases, ERCP and endoscopic extraction of stones is indicated emergently. Prospective studies have shown that ERCP is safe in the acute phase of the attack and that successful stone extraction may reduce the complication rate of pancreatitis.[25] After the common bile duct stones have been extracted, cholecystectomy performed either as open surgery or laparoscopically may be indicated.

Chronic Pancreatitis

Etiology and Pathogenesis

Chronic pancreatitis is defined as "the presence of chronic inflammatory lesions characterized by the destruction of exocrine parenchyma and fibrosis and, at least in the later states, the destruction of the endocrine parenchyma."[26] The most common form is chronic calcific pancreatitis. After a variable time most patients with chronic pancreatitis develop calcifications that become visible on radiologic films of the abdomen or CT. Chronic pancreatitis is most often associated with alcohol consumption, fat consumption, tobacco use, hypercalcemia, and in some tropical countries malnutrition. Additional causes include hyperparathyroidism (hypercalcemia), hereditary pancreatitis, posttraumatic chronic pancreatitis, and pancreas divisum. An additional major form of pancreatitis is associated with prolonged obstruction of the pancreatic duct, as with tumors, stenosis of the papilla of Vater, or scars secondary to acute pancreatitis.

The association of ethanol ingestion with chronic pancreatitis is profound. Autopsy studies have shown that the changes of chronic pancreatitis are present in 45 percent of alcoholics even without symptoms, and that this rate is 40 to 50 times higher than in nondrinkers.[23] Exactly how alcohol causes chronic pancreatitis is not known. One recent theory suggests that the initial factors include an increase in the protein concentration in pancreatic juice, coupled with reduction in a specific "pancreatic stone protein" that inhibits the formation of pancreatic protein plugs.[26] This biochemical situation allows the formation of protein plugs that can later calcify, in addition to causing obstruction to the flow of pancreatic juice. Another

facet of alcohol-associated pancreatitis is its tendency to progress after alcohol consumption is stopped.

All evidence suggests that repeated attacks of acute pancreatitis associated with gallstone disease rarely progress to chronic pancreatitis.

Clinical Manifestations

The presentation of chronic pancreatitis often includes bouts of acute pancreatitis superimposed on an irreversibly damaged organ. Alternatively, an insidious onset of pain in the epigastrium and radiating to the back may be the first symptom. About 10 to 15 percent of patients will not present with pain but rather with the sequelae of chronic pancreatitis, including diabetes mellitus, malabsorption, and weight loss. The mortality is 3 to 4 percent per year. Interestingly, the incidence of pancreatic carcinoma does not appear to be substantially increased in patients with chronic pancreatitis.[27]

The pain of chronic pancreatitis is often the major form of debility. Nerve fibers from the pancreas pass to the celiac plexus and then to spinal sympathetic ganglia. The events that actually trigger the pain are not well understood. There may be a relation to ductal pressures, or possibly ischemia in the pancreas. It is often accompanied by nausea and is steady and boring. The pain is usually located in the upper abdomen, particularly in the epigastrium, and radiates to the back in more than half of cases. In alcoholic pancreatitis, continued drinking affords temporary anesthesia but may foster recurrences of pain. Cessation of drinking may allow for a better long-term prognosis. After about 5 years of continual pain, many patients will note a decrease in the symptoms (the pain "burns out").[28]

Endocrine and exocrine pancreatic insufficiency lead to malabsorption, weight loss, and diabetes mellitus. Weight loss may be aggravated by poor intake as a result of pancreatic pain. Malabsorption of fat does not occur until pancreatic enzyme output drops 90 percent from normal. Along with the malabsorption of fat, the absorption of fat-soluble vitamins (A, D, K, and E) may be impaired, leading to coagulopathy and night vision problems. Diabetes mellitus arises from progressive loss of acinar cells. Diabetic ketoacidosis and nephropathy are unusual findings.

Diagnosis

The diagnosis of chronic pancreatitis is usually suggested by the clinical history, physical examination findings, and routine blood chemistries. Confirmation of the diagnosis is aided by plain radiographs showing calcifications in the area of the pancreas. ERCP shows the pancreatic duct to range from almost normal in early cases, to markedly dilated or beaded—the "chain-of-lakes" appearance. A common finding is truncation of the secondary branches of the pancreatic duct. The presence of strictures or focal dilation of the gland may allow specific therapeutic intervention to be undertaken. Barium studies and abdominal CT and US may also be of value in selected cases (Fig. 37–9).

Complications of chronic pancreatitis are similar to those of acute pancreatitis and include pseudocysts, pancreatic ascites, and obstruction of the common bile duct. Obstruction of the bile duct may lead to elevated values on liver function tests and the need to intervene either surgically or endoscopically. Alkaline phosphatase and bilirubin levels may become markedly elevated if obstruction is severe. Unusual complications include thrombosis of the portal and splenic veins. This may lead to GI hemorrhage from gastric varices. Peptic ulcer disease is also increased in patients with chronic pancreatitis. A definite causal relationship has not been established.

Treatment

The treatment for chronic pancreatitis is directed toward pain control, exocrine and endocrine insufficiency, and treating complications. By far the most challenging is the management of pain. For almost 40 years, analgesics and surgical intervention were the mainstay of pain control. With the advent of ERCP, newer, less drastic forms of therapy are now possible. Pancreatic sphincterotomy is indicated for the management of single or multiple stones. Endoscopic drains may be placed for pseudocysts of the pancreas if they are adjacent to the stomach or duodenum. Obstruction of the common bile duct can be treated with endoscopically placed biliary stents. Strictures of the main pancreatic duct can be managed with indwelling pancreatic stents. If endoscopic management fails or is not approriate in a given patient, surgery is still an option. Lateral fileting of the main pancreatic duct, or the Puestow procedure, is helpful when the main duct is diffusely dilated. This procedure allows drainage of the gland, theoretically reducing intraluminal pressure and reducing pain. Distal pancreatectomy may be helpful if there is a large mid-duct stricture that will not stay open after pancreatic stenting.[29]

Pancreatic enzyme therapy has recently been introduced for the management of chronic pain.[30] It has been determined that proteases (e.g., trypsin, chymo-

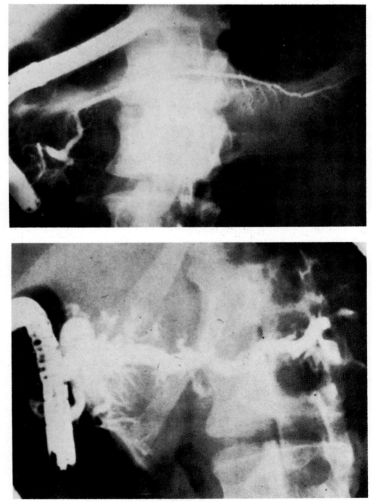

FIGURE 37–9. Top, normal retrograde pancreatogram obtained by endoscopic cannulation of the pancreatic duct. The main duct has opacified, along with the primary and some secondary branches. Bottom, Endoscopic retrograde pancreatogram in a patient with chronic pancreatitis. The duct is dilated throughout, with occasional points of narrowing. (From Sleisenger MH, Fordtran JS (eds): Gastrointestinal Disease: Pathophysiology/Diagnosis/Management, 4th ed. Philadelphia, WB Saunders, 1989, p 1853. Reproduced with permission.)

trypsin, and elastase) exert a controlling influence on pancreatic secretion. The exact mechanism has not been determined. The relief of pain following the oral administration of pancreatic enzymes is based on feedback regulation. Unfortunately, only 20 to 30 percent of patients with the typical alcohol-induced ("big duct") type of disease respond to such therapy. Responses are higher in patients with the small duct disease—perhaps 80 percent.[28] Treatment is simple: patients take a potent pancreatic enzyme supplement with each meal. The types of enzyme that work best are still under study. It is important that the enzymes be released in the duodenum where the approriate feedback mechanism can take place. This may require the use of antacids or H_2 receptor antagonists to reduce gastric acid, which may degrade enzymes in the stomach.

Treatment of exocrine insufficiency can usually be accomplished with low-fat diets and pancreatic enzyme supplementation. Likewise, endocrine insufficiency in the form of diabetes mellitus is managed with diet and either oral hypoglycemic agents or insulin.

KEY CONCEPTS

- Acute pancreatitis is commonly associated with biliary tract disease and excessive ethanol ingestion. Activation of pancreatic proenzymes to active forms within the pancreas leads to autodigestion and inflammation of the gland. The manifestations of acute pancreatitis may be mild or severe and include a steady, boring pain in the epigastrium or left upper quadrant, nausea, vomiting, a tender abdomen, reduced bowel sounds, and fever. In severe cases, circulatory shock may occur. Elevated serum amylase and lipase levels are indicative of pancreatitis.

- The treatment of acute pancreatitis is aimed at reducing pancreatic secretion. Since chyme entering the duodenum is the primary stimulus for pancreatic secretion, food is withheld and nasogastric suctioning may be instituted. Complications of acute pancreatitis include hyperglycemia, nutritional deficit, and pancreatic hemorrhage, infection, abscess formation, or necrosis. Antibiotics, fluid management, total parenteral nutrition, and insulin may be indicated to treat complications.

- Chronic pancreatitis is closely associated with alcohol use. Acute pancreatitis due to biliary obstruction rarely progresses to chronic pancreatitis. Chronic pancreatitis results in progressive destruction of endocrine and exocrine function. Manifestations of chronic pancreatitis are more insidious than acute. Epigastric pain, diabetes mellitus, malabsorption, and weight loss may be the presenting problems.

- The complications of chronic pancreatitis are similar to those of acute pancreatitis. Therapy is directed toward pain control, ameliorating endocrine and exocrine deficiency, and monitoring for and treating

complications. Surgery to correct obstruction of the pancreatic duct may be performed. Pancreatic enzyme therapy may be helpful in reducing pain by providing negative feedback, which reduces pancreatic secretion.

Summary

The pancreaticobiliary system is central to the digestion of food by providing necessary digestive enzymes and lipid-emulsifying agents that allow the intestine to absorb nutrients. This chapter has considered alterations in the function of the gallbladder and exocrine pancreas. A major disease of the pancreaticobiliary system is the formation of cholesterol gallstones, which can lead to acute and chronic cholecystitis and acute and chronic pancreatitis. New forms of surgical and nonsurgical interventions for the treatment of gallstone disease have become available in the past few years, with conventional open surgery remaining a useful option. These interventions, as well as interventions for acute and chronic pancreatitis, are the focus of much clinical research today.

REFERENCES

1. Duane WC: Pathogenesis of gallstones: Implications for management. *Hosp Pract* 1990;25(3):65.
2. Thaler MT: Biliary disease in infancy and childhood, in Sleisenger MH, Fordtran JS (eds): *Gastrointestinal Disease: Pathophysiology/Diagnosis/Management*, 4th ed. Philadelphia, WB Saunders, 1989.
3. Ermak TH, Grendell JH: Anatomy, histology, embryology and development anomalies, in Sleisenger MH, Fordtran JS (eds): *Gastrointestinal Disease: Pathophysiology/Diagnosis/Management*, 4th ed. Philadelphia, WB Saunders, 1989.
4. Saunders KD, Cates JA, Rosyln JJ: Pathogenesis of gallstones. *Surg Clin North Am* 1990;70(6):1197–1216.
5. Thistle JL, Cleary PA, Laclun JM, Tyor MP, Hersh T: The natural history of cholelithiasis: The National Cooperative Gallstone Study. *Ann Intern Med* 1984;101(2):171–175.
6. Ransohoff DF, Gracie WA, Wolfenson LB, Neuhayser D: Prophylactic cholecystectomy or expectant management for silent gallstones: A decision analysis to assess survival. *Ann Intern Med* 1983;99(2):199–204.
7. Way LA, Sleisenger MH: Cholelithiasis, chronic and acute cholecystitis, in Sleisenger MH, Fordtran JS (eds): *Gastrointestinal Disease: Pathophysiology/Diagnosis/Management*, 4th ed. Philadelphia, WB Saunders, 1989.
8. Wetter La, Way LW: Surgical therapy for gallstone disease. *Gastroenterol Clin North Am* 1991;20(1):157–169.
9. Dubois F, Icard P, Berthelot G, Levard H: Coelioscopic cholecystectomy: A preliminary report of 36 cases. *Ann Surg* 1990;211(1):60–62.
10. Soper NJ: Laparoscopic cholecystectomy: A promising new "branch" in the algorithm of gallstone management. *Surgery* 1991;109(3 pt 1):342–344.
11. Salen G, Tint GS, Shefer S: Treatment of cholesterol gallstones with litholytic bile acids. *Gastroenterol Clin North Am* 1991;20(1):171–182.
12. Maton PN, Iser JH, Reuben A, et al: Outcome of chenodeoxycholic acid (CDCA) treatment in 125 patients with radiolucent gallstones: Factors influencing efficacy, withdrawal, symptoms and side effects, and post-dissolution recurrence. *Medicine* 1982;61(2):86–97.
13. Garcia G, Young HS: Biliary extracorporeal shock-wave lithotripsy. *Gastroenterol Clin North Am* 1991;20(1):201–208.

14. Thomas CG Jr, Womack NA: Acute cholecystitis: Its pathogenesis and repair. *Arch Surg* 1952;64:590–600.

15. Jarvinen HJ Hasbacka J: Early cholecystectomy for acute cholecystitis: A prospective randomized study. *Ann Surg* 1980;191(4):501–505.

16. Nakamura K, Sarles M, Payan H: Three-dimensional reconstruction of the pancreatic ducts in chronic pancreatitis. *Gastroenterology* 1972;62(5):942–949.

17. Soergel KH: Acute pancreatitis, in Sleisenger MH, Fordtran JS (eds): *Gastrointestinal Disease: Pathophysiology/Diagnosis/Management*, 4th ed. Philadelphia, WB Saunders, 1989.

18. Jeffres C: Complications of acute pancreatitis. *Crit Care Nurse* 1989;9(4):38–50.

19. Steinberg WM: Predictors of severity of acute pancreatitis. *Gastroenterol Clin North Am* 1990;19(9):849–861.

20. Beger HG, Bittner R, Block S, Buchler M: Bacterial contamination of pancreatic necrosis: A prospective clinical study. *Gastroenterology* 1986;91(2):433–438.

21. Reynaert MS, Dugernier T, Kestens PJ: Current therapeutic strategies in severe acute pancreatitis. *Intensive Care Med* 1990;16(6):352–362.

22. D'Egidio A, Schein M: Surgical strategies in the treatment of pancreatic necrosis and infection. *Br J Surg* 1991;78(2):133–137.

23. Grendell JH, Cello JP: Chronic pancreatitis, in Sleisenger MH, Fordtran JS (eds): *Gastrointestinal Disease: Pathophysiology/Diagnosis/Management*, 4th ed. Philadelphia, WB Saunders, 1989.

24. Bradley EL III, Olson RA: Current management of pancreatic abscess. *Adv Surg* 1991:24:361–388.

25. Levelle-Jones M, Neoptolemos JP: Recent advances in the treatment of acute pancreatitis. *Surg Annu* 1990;22:235–261.

26. Sarles H, Bernard JP, Gullo L: Pathogenesis of chronic pancreatitis. *Gut* 1990;31(6):629–632.

27. Wynder EL, Mabuchi K, Maruchi N, Fortner JG: Epidemiology of cancer of the pancreas. *JNCI* 1973;50(3):645–667.

28. Pitchumoni CS, Toskes PP: Controversies, dilemmas, and dialogues: Is there an effective nonsurgical treatment for pain in chronic pancreatitis? *Am J Gastroenterol* 1991;86(1):26–29.

29. Cremer M, Deviere J, Delhaye M, Vandermeeren A, Baize M: Non-surgical management of severe chronic pancreatitis. *Scand J Gastroenterol* 1990;25(suppl 175):77–84.

BIBLIOGRAPHY

Babb RR: Managing gallbladder disease with prostaglandin inhibitors. *Postgrad Med* 1993;94(1):127–130.

Dickerman JL: Electrocardiographic changes in acute cholecystitis. *J Am Osteopath Assoc* 1989;89(5):630–635.

Duane WC: Pathogenesis of gallstones: Implications for management. *Hosp Pract Off Ed* 1990;25(3):65.

Everson GT: Gallbladder function in gallstone disease. *Gastroenterol Clin North Am* 1991;20(1):85–110.

Jacobs E, Ardichvili D, D'Avanzo E, Penneman R, Van Gansbeke D: Cyst of the gallbladder. *Dig Dis Sci* 1991;36(12):1796–1802.

Jacyna MR: Interactions between gall bladder bile and mucosa: Relevance to gall stone formation. *Gut* 1990;31(5):568–570.

Jebbink MC, Heijerman HG, Masclee AA, Lamers CB: Gallbladder disease in cystic fibrosis. *Neth J Med* 1992;41(3–4):123–126.

Jorgensen T, Teglbjerg JS, Wille-Jorgensen P, Bille T, Thorvaldsen P: Persisting pain after cholecystectomy: A prospective investigation. *Scand J Gastroenterol* 1991;26(1):124–128.

Lanzini A, Northfield TC: Assessment of the motor functions of the gallbladder. *J Hepatol* 1989;9(3):383–391.

Lee SP: Pathophysiology of gallstone formation. *Clin Ther* 1990;12(3):194–199.

Lichtenstein JE: The gallbladder: What if it's not stone disease? *Semin Roentgenol* 1991;26(3):209–215.

Middleton GW, Williams JH: Is gall bladder ejection fraction a reliable predictor of acalculous gall bladder disease? *Nucl Med Commun* 1992;13(12):894–896.

Miller FJ, Rose SC: Intervention for gallbladder disease. *Cardiovasc Intervent Radiol* 1990;13(4):264–271.

Mok HY, Ryan KG: Natural history of biliary stones. *Dig Dis* 1990;8(1):1–11.

Rosenthal RA, Andersen DK: Surgery in the elderly: Observations on the pathophysiology and treatment of cholelithiasis. *Exp Gerontol* 1993;28(4–5):459–472.

Taoka H: Experimental study on the pathogenesis of acute acalculous cholecystitis, with special reference to the roles of microcirculatory disturbances, free radicals and membrane-bound phospholipase A_2. *Gastroenterol Jpn* 1991;26(5):633–644.

Teplick SK: Diagnostic and therapeutic interventional gallbladder procedures. *Am J Roentgenol* 1989;152(5):913–916.

Williamson RC: A calculous disease of the gall bladder. *Gut* 1988;29(6):860–872.

CHAPTER 38
Liver Disease

ARNOLD COHEN

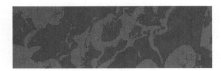

KEY TERMS

ascites: Abnormal accumulation of fluid in the peritoneal cavity. Causes include liver disease, heart failure, constrictive pericarditis, infection, malnutrition, pancreatitis, lymphatic obstruction or leakage, renal disease, hypothyroidism, collagen vascular diseases, and malignancy.

chronic hepatitis: Ongoing inflammation of the liver, usually of more than 6 months' duration, following viral hepatitis or due to autoimmune disease.

cirrhosis: A diffuse, irreversible scarring of the liver resulting in abnormal nodules of liver cells surrounded by fibrosis.

esophageal varices: Abnormally dilated blood vessels lying just below the mucous membrane of the esophagus that connect the hypertensive portal system with the systemic circulation. Esophageal varices may rupture, causing massive hemorrhage.

hepatocellular failure: Acute or chronic loss of essential liver function resulting in portal systemic encephalopathy and a variety of other problems, including coagulopathy, renal failure, bleeding, infection, hypoglycemia, respiratory failure, and death.

hepatitis: An inflammatory condition of the liver. Potential causes include viral, bacterial, fungal, and protozoal infections; drugs and toxins; autoimmune disorders; and metabolic disorders.

hepatoma: A primary liver cancer arising from cells normally found in the liver, not to be confused with cancer metastatic to the liver from a distant site.

portal hypertension: Abnormally high blood pressure in the blood vessels draining the intra-abdominal alimentary tract, pancreas, gallbladder, and spleen. It may be due to increased resistance to blood flow, as in cirrhosis, or, rarely, to abnormally increased blood flow, as in arteriovenous communications.

portal systemic encephalopathy: A neuropsychiatric syndrome caused by liver dysfunction and resulting in mental status changes ranging from mild cerebral dysfunction to deep coma (**hepatic coma**) and death.

The liver is one of the most frequently injured organs in the body. It is vulnerable to a wide variety of metabolic, circulatory, toxic, microbial, and neoplastic insults. In some instances the disease is primary to the liver, as seen in viral hepatitis and hepatocellular carcinoma. More often the hepatic involvement is secondary, a consequence of some of the more common diseases of man, such as cardiac decompensation, disseminated cancer, alcoholism, and infections. Liver disorders secondary to other conditions are discussed in the chapters on the primary organ system involved.

Structure and Function of the Liver

The liver is the largest parenchymal organ or the body, averaging 1,500 grams. It is located in the right upper quadrant of the abdomen, beneath the diaphragm, and is commonly divided into a right and left lobe, but may be further subdivided according to the pattern of its blood supply and biliary drainage. It is covered by a connective tissue capsule, Glisson's capsule, which in turn is covered by visceral peritoneum, reflections of which form the various suspensory hepatic ligaments. These demarcate the bare area of the liver directly in contact with the diaphragm (Fig. 38–1).

The liver has a dual blood supply. Arterial inflow from the aorta via the celiac trunk and hepatic artery provide 25 percent of the organ's blood supply. The remainder comes from the portal vein, which drains the capillary bed of the alimentary canal and pancreas (Fig. 38–2). This oxygen-depleted venous blood is rich in substances absorbed and secreted by the gut. These afferent blood vessels then arborize throughout the liver in association with the bile ducts, forming the portal triads. Eventually, blood from both the hepatic artery and the portal vein drains into the hepatic sinusoids, which surround sheets of liver cells, the hepatic plates (Fig. 38–3). This blood drains into the central

veins, which finally coalesce into the hepatic vein, emptying into the inferior vena cava. Any obstruction to the flow of blood may result in a rise in pressure proximal to the level of blockage. This is called **portal hypertension** and is a central pathophysiologic event in many liver diseases. The liver also has a rich and complex lymphatic drainage system.

The liver is the most metabolically active organ and may be viewed as a digestive organ, an endocrine organ, a hematologic organ, and an excretory organ (Table 38–1). All of these functions are elegantly interwoven with such redundancy that more than 80 percent of the liver may be destroyed before life is threatened.

General Manifestations of Liver Disease

Whether primary or secondary, all hepatic derangements tend to cause similar signs and symptoms that are directly attributable to loss of hepatocellular function or disruption of blood flow through the liver. Because of the liver's considerable reserve, however, manifestations appear only when the injury is significant and diffuse, or strategically located so as to obstruct biliary outflow.

Hepatocellular Failure

Hepatocellular failure results in a number of common manifestations of liver disease, including jaundice, muscle wasting, bleeding, hypoalbuminemia, glucose imbalance, osteomalacia, and feminization (Table 38–2). These manifestations are all attributed to loss of normal hepatic cell functions. The liver is primarily responsible for the production and excretion of bile. Loss of bilirubin conjugation and excretion leads to

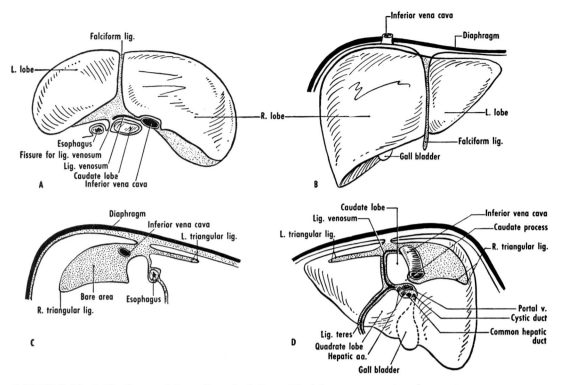

F I G U R E 38 – 1. The liver and its peritoneal relations. *Stippled areas* represent surfaces not covered with peritoneum. **A,** Superior view. **B,** Anterior view. **C,** The diaphragm, viewed from in front, showing the position of the bare area of the liver. **D,** Visceral surface of the liver, viewed from behind. (From Gardner E, Gray DJ, O'Rahilly R: *Anatomy: A Regional Study of Human Structure,* 3rd ed. Philadelphia, WB Saunders, 1969, p 414. Reproduced with permission.)

deposition of bilirubin in tissues, with resulting jaundice. Altered protein metabolism leads to decreased production of protein clotting factors, altered production of lipoproteins, muscle wasting, hyperlipidemia, and hypoalbuminemia. Decreased serum albumin in turn leads to generalized edema from decreased serum oncotic pressure. Abnormal uptake and release of glucose may result in bouts of either hyper- or hypoglycemia. Reduced production of bile salts by the liver impairs absorption of fat-soluble vitamins from the gastrointestinal (GI) tract. Lack of vitamin D may lead to osteomalacia; lack of vitamin K contributes to poor clotting factor production.

Hepatocellular failure is associated with impaired metabolism and detoxification of endogenous substances such as steroid hormones and the by-products of protein metabolism, as well as decreased clearance of exogenous drugs and toxins. Impaired metabolism of estrogen is associated with feminization (gynecomastia, impotence, testicular atrophy, female hair distribution, irregular menses), palmar erythema, and spider telangiectasis. Impaired conversion of ammonia to urea may lead to hepatic coma.

Portal Hypertension

Manifestations of liver disease not attributed to hepatocellular failure are mainly due to impaired blood flow through the liver as a result of increased resistance from fibrosis and degeneration of liver tissue. Sluggish blood flow through the liver results in increased pressure in the portal circulation (**portal hypertension**). With portal hypertension, venous drainage of much of the GI tract is congested. Anorexia, esophageal varices, hemorrhoids, and abnormal abdominal vascular patterns may result. Portal hypertension contributes to the accumulation of peritoneal fluid, or **ascites.** A serious consequence of portal hypertension is uncontrolled bleeding from esophageal varices, which are prone to rupture.

Portal Systemic Encephalopathy

Pathogenesis and Clinical Manifestations

Portal systemic encephalopathy is a complex neuropsychiatric syndrome characterized by symptoms ranging from mild confusion and lethargy with altered personality to stupor and coma. Some patients exhibit dementia, psychotic symptoms, spastic myelopathy, and cerebellar or extrapyramidal signs. The classic physical finding is asterixis or flap, a spastic jerking of the hands held in forced extension. Portal systemic encephalopathy is associated with fulminant hepatic failure or severe chronic liver disease, in which liver function is severely depressed and blood is shunted around the liver. Possible causes, including altered or false neurotransmitters, toxic short-chain fatty acids,

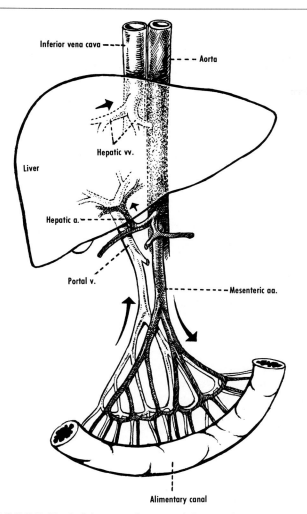

FIGURE 38–2. Schematic diagram of the portal circulation. Blood from the aorta supplies the alimentary canal. Venous blood from the intestine reaches the sinusoids of the liver by way of the portal vein. Venous blood from the liver reaches the inferior vena cava by way of the hepatic veins. (From Gardner E, Gray DJ, O'Rahilly R: *Anatomy: A Regional Study of Human Structure,* 3rd ed. Philadelphia, WB Saunders, 1969, p 417. Reproduced with permission.)

and altered ratios of plasma aromatic amino acids to branched-chain amino acids, remain under investigation. The arterial ammonia level correlates positively with the level of encephalopathy in most patients.

Portal systemic encephalopathy is usually precipitated by certain well-defined clinical developments, including hypokalemia, hyponatremia, alkalosis, hypoxia, hypercarbia, infection, use of sedatives, GI hemorrhage, protein meal gorging, renal failure, and constipation. In some patients, progressive liver failure leads to chronic encephalopathy without other exacerbating factors.

Treatment

Treatment of portal systemic encephalopathy consists of correcting any identifiable precipitating factors. More direct treatment must be employed to eliminate the toxic nitrogenous substances produced by the intestinal digestion of protein. The first step is temporary elimination of dietary proteins; simultaneously, the patient is purged to evacuate the colon. Magnesium citrate is classically used for the latter purpose. Standard precautions must be taken before any cathartic is administered. Bowel obstruction must be ruled out with plain radiographs of the abdomen, and any additional health problems must be identified. For patients in renal failure, cathartics containing magnesium, potassium, or large volumes of sodium may be harmful; cleansing enemas with close monitoring of sodium levels may be used in such cases. If the patient cannot swallow without aspiration, the cathartic may be administered by gavage.

Oral neomycin sulfate has been used for many years to suppress the intestinal flora and decrease endogenous ammonia production. Oral kanamycin may be used but has not achieved clinical popularity. The dosages range from 250 mg orally twice a day to 500 mg orally four times a day. Side effects and the interactions of these antimicrobial agents are discussed briefly in Chapter 8. In patients on chronic therapy, any diarrheal illness should be immediately evaluated for fecal leukocytes and stool *Clostridium difficile* toxin; endoscopy may be necessary. Should significant complications develop, neomycin should be stopped immediately. Because of these potential problems, neomycin is now considered second-tier treatment.

Presently, the primary agent for reducing ammonia levels is lactulose, a synthetic sugar that reaches the colon unchanged, where it is attacked by colonic bacteria and broken down primarily to lactic, acetic, and formic acids. This acidification and the increase in osmotic pressure cause an osmotic catharsis and stimulates increased excretion of ammonia in the stool. Some evidence suggests that lactulose-related change in pH also inhibits ammonia production by the gut flora. Colonic bacterial populations that produce less ammonia may also develop with chronic use. No serious adverse reactions have been reported with lactulose therapy, although flatulence and abdominal cramping may occur.[1,2] The dosage should be individually adjusted so that two soft, acidic stools are passed daily. It is neither necessary nor advisable to induce diarrhea. Most patients begin with 30 mL of lactulose by mouth or nasogastric tube every 4 hours until bowel movements occur. The dose is then adjusted down to the desired end point, usually 15 to 60 mL daily. Lactulose may also be administered as a retention enema by diluting 100 mL in a convenient volume of water. The procedure should be repeated every 4 to 6 hours, with standard precautions observed for giving enemas to patients with portal systemic encephalopathy.

During this time the patient should receive peripheral or central glucose infusions along with vitamins, especially thiamine. As the patient's ammonia levels drop, protein may be reintroduced into the diet. The initial amount of 20 g/day is increased by 10 or 20 g/day every few days to an ultimate 0.75 to 1.0 g

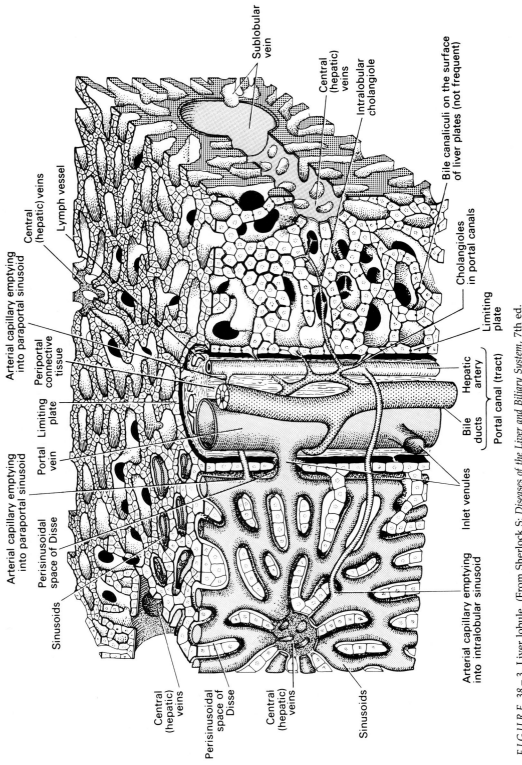
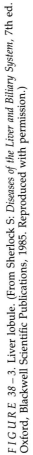

Arterial capillary emptying into paraportal sinusoid

Central (hepatic) veins

Lymph vessel

Sublobular vein

Central (hepatic) veins

Intralobular cholangiole

Bile canaliculi on the surface of liver plates (not frequent)

Periportal connective tissue

Limiting plate

Portal vein

Arterial capillary emptying into paraportal sinusoid

Perisinusoidal space of Disse

Sinusoids

Cholangioles in portal canals

Limiting plate

Hepatic artery

Bile ducts

Portal canal (tract)

Inlet venules

Central (hepatic) veins

Perisinusoidal space of Disse

Central (hepatic) veins

Sinusoids

Arterial capillary emptying into intralobular sinusoid

FIGURE 38–3. Liver lobule. (From Sherlock S: *Diseases of the Liver and Biliary System*, 7th ed. Oxford, Blackwell Scientific Publications, 1985. Reproduced with permission.)

TABLE 38-1. Summary of Normal Liver Function

The Liver as Digestive Organ

Bile salt secretion for fat digestion
Processing and storage of fats, carbohydrates, and proteins absorbed by the intestines
Processing and storage of vitamins and minerals

The Liver as Endocrine Organ

Metabolism of glucocorticoids, mineralocorticoids, and sex hormones
Regulation of carbohydrate, fat, and protein metabolism

The Liver as Hematologic Organ

Temporary storage of blood
Synthesis of bilirubin from blood breakdown products
Hematopoiesis in certain disease states
Synthesis of blood clotting factors

The Liver as Excretory Organ

Excretion of bile pigment
Excretion of cholesterol via bile
Urea synthesis
Detoxification of drugs and other foreign substances

---

of protein per kg of body weight daily. Observation for worsening encephalopathy is crucial at this time. Lactulose therapy should be continued during this period.

When protein is restricted, it is essential to provide at least 400 g of carbohydrate daily. Vegetable protein may be better tolerated than animal protein. High dietary fiber intake may help by decreasing constipation. If dietary measures fail, oral defined-formula feedings containing essential amino acids and enriched with branched-chain amino acids may be indicated.

Ascites

Pathogenesis and Clinical Manifestations

Ascites, or the pathologic accumulation of fluid within the peritoneal cavity, can occur in patients with advanced liver disease complicated by portal hypertension and hypoalbuminemia. Abdominal distention results from accumulation of sodium, water, and protein. A small amount of ascites may not require specific therapy. However, with increasing volumes, abdominal discomfort, respiratory embarrassment, abdominal or umbilical herniation, or infection may occur.

Other causes of ascites are malignancy, infection, pancreatitis, hypothyroidism, vasculitis, nephrosis, cardiac failure, constrictive pericarditis, Budd-Chiari syndrome, and portal vein thrombosis. Abdominal paracentesis should be performed in all patients with new ascites and in those with known ascites who have experienced a significant worsening of their condition. The fluid should be examined for fungal and bacteriologic organisms; total protein, albumin, amy-

lase, glucose, lipid, and lactate dehydrogenase (LDH) levels; and cell count and cytology.

Treatment

Dietary sodium should be restricted to 500 mg/day to 2.0 g/day in ascites patients. Bed rest and diuretics are useful. The aldosterone antagonist spironolactone works in the distal nephron as a weak diuretic that also inhibits potassium secretion, thus sparing the serum potassium. The usual starting dose is 50 to 100 mg/day. However, there may be a delay of 2 to 3 days before the full effect of the drug is seen, and the dosage should not be increased more frequently. As much as 1.0 g/day may be used. It is helpful to monitor both urinary sodium and potassium levels regularly. When the urinary sodium level exceeds the urinary potassium level, aldosterone is exerting its maximum effect. Serum potassium levels must be carefully controlled.

If spironolactone alone is unsuccessful, a loop diuretic such as furosemide or ethacrynic acid is added cautiously. The starting dose for furosemide is usually 40 mg on alternate days, slowly increased to as much as 120 mg/day. Occasional patients refractory to this regimen will respond to the addition of metholazone, a loop diuretic potentiator. In combination, metholazone and furosemide may result in unusually profound kaliuresis and natriuresis, so careful monitoring is essential. The goal is the loss of approximately 0.5 kg of body weight daily, although in patients with peripheral edema, a slightly more rapid weight loss is tolerable. More rapid losses may result in diuretic-induced renal impairment, intravascular volume depletion and severe electrolyte abnormalities, and portal systemic encephalopathy. Diuresis should be continued until the ascites is barely detectable (*not* until the patient is "dry"), and maintenance levels of diuretics should be prescribed.

In patients who do not respond to both diuretic therapy and sodium restrictions, the use of salt-poor albumin infusions may help initiate diuresis. However, the effect of this treatment is often short-lived and not without risk of overexpansion of the intravascular volume, with congestive heart failure, pulmonary edema, and precipitation of variceal hemorrhage all possible. Shunting procedures such as the LeVeen and Denver shunts have been used. These are one-way valves that connect the peritoneal space with the venous system, usually at the jugular vein.[3,4] These shunting procedures, while useful, carry significant risks, including the risk of intravascular volume expansion with pulmonary edema or ruptured varices, septicemia, and the initiation of disseminated intravascular coagulation. Central venous thrombosis, peritoneal fibrosis, bowel obstruction and, most commonly, shunt malfunction may occur. Recently there has been renewed interest in large-volume therapeutic paracentesis in otherwise refractory cases. This is a very rapid and effective treatment modality that can be safely instituted if the intravascular volume is

TABLE 38–2. The Pathophysiology Underlying Symptoms and Signs of Liver Disease

Symptoms/Signs	Pathophysiologic Mechanism
Weakness, fatigue, anorexia, weight loss, muscle wasting	Failure of multiple metabolic functions
Fever	Liver inflammation; decreased reticuloendothelial function with increased risk of infection
Bruising, increased bleeding	Thrombocytopenia due to splenic enlargement; decreased synthesis of clotting factors I, II, V, VII, VIII, IX, X
Palmar erythema, cutaneous spider telangiectases, gynecomastia, impotence, irregular menses; female body hair distribution, testicular atrophy	Altered metabolism of sex hormones; chronic debilitation
Hepatic encephalopathy	Abnormal protein metabolism
Fetor hepaticus	Decreased detoxification
Pruritus	Decreased bile salt excretion
Cyanosis	Arteriovenous shunts in lungs, liver
Jaundice	Biliary obstruction, decreased bilirubin synthesis, decreased bilirubin excretion
Hyperdynamic circulation Wide pulse pressure, tachycardia	Generalized vasodilation (? hormonally mediated)
Ascites, peripheral edema	Portal hypertension; sodium and water retention; low serum albumin due to decreased hepatic synthesis
Splenomegaly	Portal hypertension
Hepatomegaly	Cirrhosis (liver may be small, hepatitis, vascular congestion, bile duct obstruction, infection, benign infiltrative disease (e.g., fatty liver, amyloid, hemochromatosis), malignant infiltrative disease (e.g., metastatic cancer, lymphoma, large space-occupying lesions e.g., neoplasm, abscess)
Varices (esophageal, gastric rectal, ectopic) or abnormal abdominal vascular pattern (caput medusae, umbilical bruit)	Portal hypertension with collateral blood flow around hepatic block
Osteomalacia, hypocalcemia, night blindness, coagulopathy	Fat-soluble vitamin malabsorption and loss of fat-soluble vitamin reserves A, D, and K; loss of vitamin K metabolism (a cofactor for I, II, VII, VIII, IX, and X)
Anemia	Multifactorial: blood loss, chronic disease, B_{12} deficiency, splenic sequestration
Leukopenia	Hypersplenism due to portal hypertension
Hypoglycemia	Altered glycogenolysis, gluconeogenesis
Hyperglycemia	Portosystemic shunting with delayed hepatic uptake of absorbed glucose
Hypercholesterolemia	Obstructive jaundice with decreased cholesterol excretion

maintained by appropriate colloid infusions (25 percent albumin or hetastarch). Diuretic and dietary treatment should be continued, but in severe cases, large-volume paracentesis may be repeated as needed.

KEY CONCEPTS

• The liver is a vital, multifunctional organ located in the right upper quadrant beneath the diaphragm. Blood is supplied to the liver by the hepatic artery and the portal vein. The portal vein drains the capillaries of the alimentary canal and pancreas. Arterial and portal blood flows into the hepatic sinusoids, which have direct contact with hepatic cells.

• The functions of the liver are multiple and include the metabolism of fats, proteins, and glucose; the synthesis and secretion of bile salts; storage of vitamins and minerals; metabolism and detoxification of endogenous and exogenous substances; and urea synthesis.

• Manifestations of liver disease are attributable to hepatocellular failure and portal hypertension. Jaundice, decreased clotting factors, hypoalbuminemia, decreased vitamins D and K, and feminization are attributed to hepatocellular failure. Portal hypertension may result in gastrointestinal congestion with the development of esophageal or gastric varices, hemorrhoids, splenomegaly, and ascites.

• The symptoms of hepatic encephalopathy range from confusion and lethargy to coma. A spastic flapping tremor of the hands, called *asterixis,* is a classic finding. The severity of the encephalopathy correlates positively with serum ammonia levels. Encephalopathy may be precipitated by conditions that increase protein metabolism, such as gastrointestinal hemorrhage and increased protein consumption, and by conditions that further impair hepatocyte function. Treatment may include protein restriction, antibiotics to reduce ammonia production by intestinal organisms, and lactulose to enhance ammonia excretion in the stool.

- Ascites is a pathologic accumulation of fluid within the peritoneal cavity. It occurs commonly in liver disease because of the increased fluid transudation that occurs with portal hypertension and hypoalbuminemia. In severe ascites, treatment may be instituted to ameliorate pain and respiratory difficulty. Sodium restriction, diuretics, and intermittent paracentesis are commonly prescribed. Surgical shunting procedures that allow accumulated peritoneal fluid to flow back into the circulation through a one-way valve may be effective.

Hepatitis

Acute Viral Hepatitis

Etiology

Hepatitis is inflammation of the liver. Acute hepatitis may be caused by many viruses, among them cytomegalovirus, Epstein-Barr virus, rubella virus, herpes simplex virus, and the yellow fever, coxsackie, and Marburg viruses. However, the term **viral hepatitis** is usually applied to those illnesses caused by hepatitis virus A (HAV, or infectious, short-incubation hepatitis), hepatitis virus B (HBV, or serum, long-incubation hepatitis), and hepatitis virus C (HCV, or non-A, non-B virus). A fourth virus, known as the delta agent, is a defective RNA virus that requires the helper function of HBV. HDV coinfects with HBV and requires its presence for viral replication. Little is known about the fifth purported viral agent, hepatitis virus E. Even the immunoassay to detect its presence is experimental at this time (Table 38–3).[5]

Despite statistical variation in the symptoms, signs, and epidemiology of these diseases, it is often clinically impossible to differentiate them in a given patient without appropriate serologic tests.

Hepatitis A

Pathogenesis and Clinical Manifestations
Hepatitis virus A, an RNA enterovirus, is usually spread by the fecal/oral route, although parenteral transmission can occur. The infection has a 2- to 6-week incubation period. The illness may be asymptomatic or anicteric, with the patient exhibiting nonspecific flu or gastroenteritis symptoms. Icteric attacks range from mild to fulminant and fatal, although the latter are rare. Typical icteric hepatitis has a prodrome of 3 to 21 days, with malaise, anorexia, nausea, low-grade fever, and right upper quadrant pain. At the conclusion of the prodrome the urine grows dark and the patient jaundiced. After 1 to 4 weeks of jaundice

the patient recovers, although weakness and mildly abnormal results on liver function tests may persist for many months.

Treatment
Treatment is not expected to change the course of acute HAV infection. Supportive management includes avoidance of fatigue, a palatable and nutritious diet (often a high-carbohydrate, high-protein diet), and multivitamin supplements. Alcohol is prohibited. Steroids are not effective in this disease.

Isolation techniques are useless in limiting the community spread of hepatitis A as patients are infectious long before they display symptoms. Hepatitis A vaccine, perhaps the most effective approach to community prophylaxis, is still under development.[6] For now, immune serum globulin (γ-globulin, ISG) remains the prophylaxis of choice for exposed patients who are anti-HAV antibody negative. An intramuscular (IM) dose of 0.02 mL/kg of body weight should be given to close personal contacts of patients with acute HAV hepatitis. More casual contacts do not need prophylactic treatment. To be effective, ISG must be administered within the first half of the incubation period or within 1 to 2 weeks of exposure. Visitors to developing countries who may be exposed to poor sanitary conditions should receive 0.5 mg/kg of ISG, with a booster injection every 4 to 6 months. ISG given prophylactically usually provides passive immunity to both infection and illness. However, some patients may develop subclinical infections, and other patients develop a modified but clinically evident illness.

Hepatitis B

Pathogenesis and Clinical Manifestations
Acute hepatitis B is caused by a partially double-stranded DNA virus. It has an incubation period of 6 weeks to 6 months and is spread by parenteral contact with infected blood or blood products and by oral and sexual contact.

The prodrome of HBV hepatitis is often longer and more insidious than that of HAV hepatitis and may involve a variety of immune complex–related phenomena, including urticaria and other rashes, arthralgias and arthritis, angioedema, serum sickness, and glomerulonephritis. The jaundice phase may be identical to that of hepatitis A, only more severe, with a higher incidence of fulminant hepatitis and such other complications as aplastic anemia, pancreatitis, cardiomyopathy, neuropathy, and skeletal myopathy.

Treatment
The treatment of hepatitis B is similar to that for hepatitis A. Specific complications must be treated as they arise.

The administration of ISG containing high levels of hepatitis B surface antibody (HBsAb); hepatitis B immune globulin, HBIG, hyperimmune globulin affords effective postinoculation prophylaxis if given

TABLE 38–3. Immunologic Markers in Viral Hepatitis

Hepatitis A

Anti-HAV IgM	Acute infection with HAV, but may persist for months.
Anti-HAV IgG	Past infection with HAV.
	Implies immunity to the virus.

Hepatitis B

HBsAg	Surface protein coat of HBV.
(Hepatitis B surface antigen)	Implies active infection.
	Detectable 2–6 wk after infection.
	Remains present as long as infection is active.
HBsAb	Antibody to protein coat of HBV.
(Hepatitis B surface antibody)	Detectable shortly after or with clearance of HBsAg.
	Implies resolution of infection and immunity to HBV.
HBcAb IgM	Antibody to inner core protein of HBV.
(Hepatitis B core antibody IgM)	Detectable 3–5 wk after infection.
	Implies recent infection.
HBcAb IgG	As for HBcAb IgM, but implies past infection.
(Hepatitis B core antibody IgG)	
HBeAg	Soluble fraction of HBV.
(Hepatitis e antigen)	Detectable 2–6 wk after infection.
	Implies ongoing infection with high infectivity.
	May resolve independently of HBsAg.
HBeAb	Antibody to soluble fraction of HBV.
(Hepatitis B e antibody)	Detectable when HBeAg clears.
	Implies decreased infectivity.
HBV DNA	Assay for circulating viral particles. Detectable 6–10 wk after
(Hepatitis B virus DNA)	infection.
	Level of titer correlates with infectivity.
HBV DNA polymerase activity	Same significance as HBV DNA.

Hepatitis C

Anti-HCV	Antibody to HCV antigens.
	May not be detectable early in infection.
	Does *not* indicate immunity to the virus.
	Rapidly evolving area—many commercially available assays of
	different sensitivity and specificity.
	Many false positive and false negative results.
HCV RNA by PCR	Assay for level of viremia.
(Hepatitis C virus RNA by	Correlates positively with activity of infection.
polymerase chain reaction)	Clears with resolution of infection.
	Technically difficult; available through reference laboratories.

Hepatitis D (Delta)

HDAg	Assay for 35-nm RNA virus.
(Hepatitis delta antigen)	Detectable 2–10 wk after infection.
	Implies early infection.
Anti-HDV	Implies past or chronic infection.
	Does not indicate immunity to the virus.

within 7 days of exposure; it is thought that the sooner the globulin is given, the more effective it is.[7,8] The major indication for HBIG is postexposure prophylaxis after a single inoculation, oral ingestion, or mucous membrane contamination with material suspected or proven to be infectious. The usual dose is 0.05 to 0.07 mL/kg given IM, with the same dose repeated 25 to 30 days later. The immune status of the recipient may be determined prior to treatment to avoid unnecessary administration. For newborn infants of hepatitis B surface antigen (HBsAg)–positive mothers, HBIG is given in a dosage of 0.13 mL/kg IM immediately after birth and may be repeated every 3 to 4 months if the infant remains HBsAg negative.

Hepatitis B vaccine should be given concomitantly with HBIG to induce passive-active immunization.

Hepatitis B vaccine (Heptavax-B, Merck HBV) is a suspension of purified HBsAg particles. Minor soreness at the injection site and low-grade fever have been reported. There is no evidence of significant adverse effects or transmission of infectious disease, including acquired immune deficiency syndrome (AIDS), by the vaccine. However, in part to respond to fears of possible disease transmission, newer DNA recombinant vaccines of equal immunogenicity have been developed.

Adults are vaccinated IM with three doses of 1.0 mg (20 μg) of hepatitis B vaccine given at 0, 1, and 6 months after exposure. Immunocompromised patients should receive 2.0 mL doses. Simultaneous administration of HBIG and other vaccines neither increases nor decreases efficacy. After the full course, the antibody response rate is 96 percent. Field trials indicate 80 to 95 percent effectiveness in preventing disease.[9] The duration of protection is at least 5 years.

While hepatitis B vaccine is now a recommended part of childhood immunizations,[10,11] adults generally receive the vaccine only if they belong to one of the following high-risk groups: male homosexuals, Alaskan Eskimos, Southeast Asian immigrants and their descendants, users of illicit drugs, household contacts of HBV carriers, hemodialysis patients, residents of institutions, medical and dental personnel, patients needing frequent transfusions, and those planning to reside in high-risk areas (Far East and sub-Sahara Africa). If exposed to HBV, a susceptible person should receive one dose of HBIG and hepatitis B vaccine as soon as possible after exposure, and then complete the vaccination program. Universal vaccination is recommended by some experts, but the age at immunization and other specific guidelines are not yet available.

Hepatitis C

Pathogenesis and Clinical Manifestations
Not all cases of viral hepatitis are classifiable as A or B. The diagnosis of hepatitis C, or non-A, non-B hepatitis, is made when other causes of hepatocellular injury and all other known viral causes have been excluded and serologic tests for hepatitis C are positive. The tests for hepatitis C are rapidly evolving but usually consist of one sensitive test for screening followed by a more specific test for confirmation.

The mode of transmission of HCV closely resembles that of HBV. It is common after parenteral contact, occurs endemically, and appears to be spread by close contact, although in individual cases the mode of transmission is frequently obscure. It does not occur in epidemics, and frequently evolves into either a chronic illness or a carrier state. Its incubation period is about 8 weeks. Some data support the idea of two illnesses, one with a very short incubation period and another with a much longer incubation period.

HCV hepatitis is usually asymptomatic or mild, with transaminase levels rarely exceeding 1,000 IU/L. The course is erratic, with wide fluctuations on liver function tests. Patients may need to be retested periodically for up to 6 months to be sure of resolution. On biopsy, acute hepatitis, chronic persistent hepatitis, chronic active hepatitis, chronic lobular hepatitis (with histology resembling acute hepatitis), and occasionally cirrhosis are found. Most of these patients are not seriously ill, but fulminant hepatic failure has been reported, and progression to chronic liver disease is common.

Treatment
The treatment of acute HCV hepatitis is the same as for other acute viral strains, that is, supportive and expectant unless complications or subacute hepatic failure develop.

Prior to the development of immunologic tests for HCV, blood transfusions were a significant source of infection. Modern screening techniques, however, have dramatically reduced this risk. There is no good evidence that ISG given before or after transfusion decreases the incidence of the disease, although ISG is frequently recommended after accidental needlestick exposures to patients with known hepatitis C.

Delta Hepatitis

Pathogenesis and Clinical Manifestations
Delta hepatitis (HDV) coinfects with HBV and requires its presence for viral replication. Delta agent can infect a person simultaneously with HBV or can superimpose infection on a person already infected with HBV. Superinfection may coexist with chronic hepatitis B and may develop into a chronic carrier state.

The duration of HDV infection is determined by the duration of the HBV infection. However, chronic HDV infection appears to accelerate the progress of liver disease, causing additional damage to a liver that has already been compromised by chronic HBV infection.

Treatment and Control
The disease is primarily transmitted by parenteral routes and by intimate personal contact. In the United States and northern Europe, HDV infection is most prevalent in persons exposed to blood and blood products (e.g., drug addicts and hemophiliacs).

HDV can be introduced into a population through migration of people from endemic to nonendemic regions. Epidemics of severe hepatitis have occurred in remote South African villages as well as in urban America owing to population migration and percutaneous contact. No product is available for prophylaxis to prevent delta hepatitis superinfection in hepatitis B infection. Infection with HDV can be prevented by vaccinating susceptible persons with the hepatitis B vaccine.[12]

Case reporting to local health authorities for all types of viral hepatitis is mandatory.

Chronic Hepatitis

Etiology

Chronic hepatitis encompasses a group of diseases characterized by ongoing inflammation of the liver that lasts 6 months or longer. The condition may be idiopathic, autoimmune, or metabolic. It may also follow diseases such as viral hepatitis, or may be a result of hepatotoxic drugs or toxins.

Chronic Persistent Hepatitis

Chronic persistent hepatitis, also called triaditis or transaminitis, is a benign disease. The inflammation is confined to the portal triads without destruction of the normal liver structures, but the serum transaminase levels are elevated. The patient may be asymptomatic or may suffer mild nonspecific symptoms. Progressive liver disease does not develop, and no drug treatment is indicated. The illness has an excellent prognosis. However, more serious liver diseases may pass through a phase that is histologically indistinguishable from chronic persistent hepatitis.

Chronic Active Hepatitis

Pathogenesis and Clinical Manifestations

Chronic active hepatitis, on the other hand, is a progressive, destructive inflammatory disease that extends beyond the portal triad into the hepatic lobule (piecemeal necrosis). The disease may progress to macronodular or micronodular cirrhosis or may spontaneously arrest with any degree of fibrosis.

Symptoms may be typical of acute hepatitis or nonspecific, eventually culminating in jaundice or signs of significant liver disease (i.e., hepatosplenomegaly, easy bleeding, or ascites).

Four main subgroups of patients with chronic active hepatitis exist. Some patients, often younger women, exhibit a variety of immunologic markers including antinuclear antibodies, anti-smooth-muscle antibodies, liver/kidney microsomal antibodies, and hyperglobulinemia. In addition, they frequently suffer from a second autoimmune disease, such as Hashimoto's thyroiditis or Coombs-positive hemolytic anemia. The second subgroup includes patients who have histories of viral hepatitis or serologic evidence of unresolved HBV or HCV infection. In the third subgroup are patients with chronic hepatitis induced by therapeutic agents such as α-methyldopa or nitrofurantoin. In the fourth subgroup are patients with a metabolic liver disorder such as Wilson's disease. A small number of patients have neither a suggestive history nor any detectable markers that would place them in any of the four main groups.

Diagnosis

The diagnosis of chronic hepatitis is made with liver biopsy. Some patients may show elements of both chronic active and chronic persistent hepatitis on biopsy, and milder forms of the active disease may be difficult to distinguish from the persistent disease.

Treatment

Corticosteroids and immunosuppressive drugs have been used since the early 1960s in the treatment of autoimmune chronic active hepatitis. Their use is based on the assumption that immunologic mechanisms either cause or maintain ongoing hepatic inflammation. Corticosteroids have an anti-inflammatory effect, affecting capillary permeability and white blood cell function. None of these observations and assumptions, however, can fully explain the therapeutic action of corticosteroids in chronic active hepatitis.

Corticosteroids clearly lower mortality in chronic active hepatitis, most noticeably in symptomatic patients and those with very severe pathologic lesions demonstrated on liver biopsy. Patients with autoimmune chronic active hepatitis should be treated until a remission is induced (indicated by a significant improvement on liver function tests, and sometimes confirmed by liver biospy). After 6 months in remission, steroids may be tapered slowly, though full treatment must be reinstituted if relapse occurs, and relapse is common. In many patients the dosage cannot be tapered below a certain level without an exacerbation of the illness; these patients may require indefinite treatment at the lowest effective dose.[13] The sustained use of high-dose corticosteroids may be effective in patients whose condition does not respond to normal doses.

Prednisone is the customary corticosteroid prescribed for autoimmune hepatitis. Many dosage schedules have been proposed. Some clinicians begin with 40 mg/day of prednisone or its equivalent and reduce the dosage as improvement occurs; others prescribe a fixed daily dose of 20 mg, or 10 mg given with 50 mg of azathioprine. These daily schedules are considered to be equally effective, unlike alternate-day therapy, which is less so.

Azathioprine is an immunosuppressive drug that, when used alone, is not effective treatment for chronic active hepatitis. When used with corticosteroids, it allows a lower dose of steroid to be used (the steroid-sparing effect) with a resulting decrease in steroid side effects.

Chronic Viral Hepatitis

Pathogenesis and Clinical Manifestations

Chronic viral hepatitis may be caused by either HBV or HCV.

Chronic HBV hepatitis develops in approximately 5 percent of patients with acute HBV hepatitis. These patients show persistence of the viral marker HBsAg, and often demonstrate a marker of active viral replication, HBeAg (hepatitis B virus e antigen), which also indicates the patient is highly infective. Chronic hepatitis B may follow a very variable course, ranging from a mild elevation of liver-related enzymes with few symptoms to a rapidly progressive illness, leading to cirrhosis and hepatic failure. Even mild cases, however, can eventually lead to cirrhosis and an increased risk of liver cancer.

Chronic hepatitis C develops in 50 percent of acutely infected patients. The antibody to HCV merely indicates the patient was exposed to the virus and does not reflect the immune status. Chronic hepatitis C tends to follow a long and benign course, but it, too, may eventually lead to cirrhosis and hepatocellular carcinoma.

Treatment

Interferon (interferon-alpha-2b) has been approved in the United States for the treatment of chronic B and

C hepatitis.[14] Interferons are naturally occurring proteins and glycoproteins made in response to viral infections; they exert a variety of immunomodulating effects that favor viral clearance. The drug is given parenterally on a schedule determined by which virus is being treated. There are many potential adverse reactions, including severe flulike symptoms, fatigue, alopecia, bone marrow depression, mental status changes, hepatotoxicity, and worsening of endocrine disorders, especially thyroid disease. Treatment with interferon may exacerbate autoimmune hepatitis, so that a careful differential diagnosis is very important (and is sometimes difficult to achieve). It is essential to carefully follow patients receiving interferon with frequent examinations and appropriate laboratory studies.

Almost 50 percent of patients with chronic hepatitis B infection will respond to treatment and show long-term benefit.[15] Chronic hepatitis C patients exhibit a 40 percent response rate, but half of these relapse within 1 year of stopping treatment. Some experts believe that all patients will relapse in time. Protocols for retreatment and maintenance therapy are under evaluation. Antiviral drugs such as adenine arabinoside and ribavirin are also under investigation.

KEY CONCEPTS

- Acute viral hepatitis is generally classified as hepatitis A, B, C, or D (delta) infection. Modes of transmission and severity of symptoms differ among types.
  Hepatitis A is also known as infectious hepatitis because it is generally transmitted by ingestion of contaminated substances. Symptoms are flulike and tend to be less severe than those of hepatitis B. Early treatment with γ-globulin after exposure may be effective in preventing disease.
  Hepatitis B is also known as serum hepatitis because its usual route of transmission is through infected blood. The incubation period is longer and the severity of symptoms (particularly jaundice) greater than in hepatitis A. Immune serum globulin is effective post inoculation if given within 7 days of exposure. Hepatitis B vaccine is recommended as part of the childhood vaccination regimen and for high-risk individuals.
  Hepatitis C, also known as non-A, non-B hepatitis, closely resembles hepatitis B in its routes of transmission. Hepatitis C is usually asymptomatic or mild. Immune serum globulin does not appear to protect against hepatitis C.
  Hepatitis delta virus coinfects with hepatitis virus B and requires the presence of HBV to be active. Infection appears to accelerate and worsen hepatitis B symptoms. Prevention of hepatitis B also prevents hepatitis delta.
- Chronic hepatitis is characterized by persistent inflammation of the liver lasting 6 months or more. Chronic active hepatitis may progress to cirrhosis.

Autoimmune disease, viral hepatitis (B and C), and toxins may result in chronic hepatitis. Corticosteroids (prednisone) and immunosuppressants (azathioprine) are common therapeutics. Interferon-alpha may be used for chronic viral hepatitis.

Cirrhosis

Cirrhosis represents the irreversible end stage of many different hepatic injuries, including severe acute hepatitis, chronic hepatitis, the metal storage diseases, alcoholism, and toxic hepatitis.

Biliary Cirrhosis

Biliary cirrhosis is initiated by damage to the bile ducts. This may be due to chronic or recurrent large duct obstruction, as in gallstone disease, primary sclerosing cholangitis, or tumors, or damage to the microscopic ducts, as in primary biliary cirrhosis. The liver is scarred by diffuse and widespread fibrosis and regenerative nodule formation (nodules are islands of liver cell regeneration within the fibrosis). Consequences are portal hypertension with splenomegaly and esophageal varices, and liver failure with hepatic encephalopathy, jaundice, ascites, coagulopathy, and low serum albumin levels. The prognosis is improved with appropriate management of a treatable cause.

Alcoholic Liver Disease

Alcoholic liver disease manifests with fatty liver, hepatitis, and cirrhosis. One or more of these manifestations may be found in the alcoholic patient.

Alcoholic Fatty Liver

Alcoholic fatty liver (*steatosis*) is an accumulation of fat within the liver cells. It may be mild and asymptomatic or severe, involving liver enlargement, abdominal discomfort, abnormal liver function tests, and even portal hypertension. Steatosis is not exclusively alcohol related. Indeed, diabetes mellitus, obesity, and many other conditions may cause the same pathology.

Treatment involves stopping alcohol intake, providing appropriate nutrition, and controlling withdrawal symptoms.

Alcoholic Hepatitis

Alcoholic hepatitis is an active inflammation, especially of the centrilobular region of the liver. The liver cells also show pathologic changes. Clinically the illness ranges from mild to very severe, with the worse cases characterized by hepatomegaly, fever, peripheral leukocytosis, and mortality rates as high as 33 percent. This condition usually responds to the treatment suggested for fatty liver. In addition, corticosteroid therapy may be tried in critically ill patients, especially those in coma.

KEY CONCEPTS

- Cirrhosis is the irreversible end stage of many different hepatic injuries. The liver is fibrotic, scarred, and nodular. Symptoms of cirrhosis are due to hepatocellular failure and portal hypertension.
- Biliary cirrhosis is associated with chronic bile duct obstruction with resultant backup of bile in the liver. Gallstones, tumors, and primary intrahepatic bile duct inflammation are contributing factors.
- Alcoholic cirrhosis is associated with chronic alcohol ingestion, which may precipitate fatty liver, hepatitis, and finally cirrhosis. Alcohol metabolism in the liver results in the formation of acetaldehyde, which interferes with mitochondrial function and lipid metabolism.

Toxic Liver Disorders

Etiology

Various forms of pigment may accumulate in the liver. The two most important are hemosiderin and lipofuscin. The appearance of lipofuscin within cells is a marker of atrophy, and so is encountered in livers that have decreased in size and undergone what is called "brown atrophy." Hemosiderin is a hemoglobin-derived, golden yellow to brown granular or crystallin pigment containing iron. When there is a local or systemic excess of iron, as in gross hemorrhage or the myriad minute hemorrhages that accompany severe vascular congestion, ferritin forms hemosiderin granules, which are easily seen with the light microscope. The more extreme accumulations of iron in a disease called *hemochromatosis* are associated with liver and pancreatic damage resulting in liver fibrosis and diabetes mellitus.

Metal Storage Diseases

The metal storage diseases of the liver are specifically treatable disorders.

Hemochromatosis

Pathogenesis and Diagnosis
Hemochromatosis is an autosomal recessive inherited disorder associated with HLA-A3, B14, and B7. The mechanism of the disease is excessive and uncontrolled iron absorption by the GI system with subsequent deposition in liver parenchymal cells and other organs. In the liver, this results in fibrosis and macronodular cirrhosis. Ultimately the patient experiences multiple organ failure, skin melanosis, pseudogout, and an increased risk of hepatocellular carcinoma.

The diagnosis is suggested by an elevated serum ferritin level or an elevated serum iron and saturated total iron-binding capacity. The diagnosis is confirmed by liver biopsy.

Treatment
The mainstay of treatment for hemochromatosis is repeated phlebotomy. Patients who do not tolerate venesection may be treated with deferoxamine, a drug that chelates iron and facilitates its renal excretion. Subcutaneous or IM administration of deferoxamine is much less efficient than phlebotomy and requires adequate renal function. Intravenous use has been advocated, but too rapid administration carries the risk of hypotension and shock.[16]

Hepatolenticular Degeneration

Pathogenesis and Diagnosis
Hepatolenticular degeneration, or Wilson's disease, is a rare autosomal recessive disorder in which excessive amounts of copper accumulate in the liver or other organs. The condition may manifest with jaundice, intravascular hemolysis, chronic active hepatitis, macronodular cirrhosis, neuropsychiatric symptoms, renal tubular acidosis with a Fanconi-like syndrome, metabolic bone disease, and arthritis. The diagnosis is confirmed by slit-lamp examination of the cornea, and specifically by the appearance of brownish Kayser-Fleischer rings at the margin of the cornea. Low serum ceruloplasmin, low serum copper, and elevated urinary copper excretion are also typical. Liver biopsy material contains higher than normal amounts of copper.

Treatment
Since copper is plentiful in many foods as well as in certain local water supplies, dietary copper restriction is difficult. The use of oral potassium sulfide to bind dietary copper is only marginally effective.

D-penicillamine is the most effective copper-chelating drug. Patients receiving this medication early in the course of the disease will show significant improvement. Even patients with advanced Wilson's disease may expect some functional recovery.[17,18] The usual starting dose is 500 mg taken by mouth three times a day before meals; this dosage may be increased to as much as 4 g/day. Treatment success or failure is determined by 24-hour monitoring of urinary copper levels. Urinary copper excretion should rise above 2,000 μg/24 hr and gradually fall as total body copper falls. Lifelong treatment with an individually determined minimal effective dose is probably needed.

Unfortunately, D-penicillamine commonly causes serious side effects. Hypersensitivity reactions such as rashes and drug fever may be treated by temporarily withdrawing the drug and instituting systemic corticosteroid therapy.

Patients allergic to penicillin may experience cross-reactions to penicillamine. During penicillamine treatment, all patients require pyridoxine supplementation (50 mg/day). Mineral supplements, however, decrease the effectiveness of the drug. Short courses of iron may be required to combat iatrogenic iron deficiency. As penicillamine interferes with collagen formation, the dose must be reduced in surgical cases, at least until healing occurs.

Alternative but less effective treatments are BAL (dimercaprol, British antilewisite) or triethylenetetramine. Monitoring the hemogram, urinalysis, renal function tests, and physical examination results is important.

Acetaminophen Poisoning

Etiology

Many drugs and toxins cause liver damage. Unfortunately, treatment is often limited to withdrawing the offending agent and administering supportive care. Standard measures including gastric lavage, induced emesis, purging, and activated charcoal when appropriate are employed in cases of acute poisoning. Heavy metal intoxication may be treated with chelating drugs. Specific antidotes are few; however, acetaminophen overdose is an exception.

Pathogenesis and Clinical Manifestations

Acetaminophen is a widely used, nonprescription analgesic and antipyretic that is frequently implicated in suicide attempts and accidental poisonings. Oral acetaminophen is rapidly absorbed and metabolized. A toxic metabolite, N-acetyl-*p*-benzoquinone imine, is formed that is rapidly detoxified by reaction with glutathione. However, massive doses of acetaminophen may expose the liver to high levels of the toxic metabolite, resulting in hepatic necrosis. During the first 48 hours after ingestion, the patient experiences nausea, vomiting, and diarrhea. Within 5 days, progressive liver/kidney failure with jaundice, encephalopathy, hypoglycemia, coagulopathy, and even death occurs. Significant liver damage is rare if serum acetaminophen levels are less than 150 μg/mL and 37 μg/mL respectively 4 and 12 hours after ingestion. However, smaller doses of acetaminophen may be toxic if taken chronically, especially in association with alcoholism or malnutrition.[19-21]

Treatment

The proper use of acetylcysteine can prevent hepatic necrosis and its fatal consequences in many patients. Acetylcysteine, a mycolytic solution used in patients with bronchial diseases, is nontoxic but may cause rash and frequently induces vomiting because of its foul odor. The drug is given as one part 20 percent acetylcysteine mixed with three parts of cola or fruit juice, or it can be given by gavage. A loading dose of 140 mg/kg is given, followed by 70 mg/kg every 4 hours for 17 doses. Activated charcoal should not be used concurrently, as this interferes with acetylcysteine absorption.

KEY CONCEPTS

- The liver is subject to damage because of its role in storing and detoxifying potentially injurious substances. Metal storage diseases are genetic disorders in which excessive minerals are absorbed and subsequently deposited in the liver. Hemochromatosis is characterized by excessive iron absorption and manifests with elevated serum ferritin and iron levels. Phlebotomy is the usual treatment. Wilson's disease is due to excessive accumulations of copper in liver and other organs. Copper chelators are effective in preventing liver damage.

- Acetaminophen is converted to a toxic metabolic in the liver that is normally rapidly detoxified by liver enzymes. In acetaminophen overdose, the detoxification reaction may be overwhelmed, resulting in liver necrosis.

Liver Abscess

Pathogenesis, Clinical Manifestations, and Diagnosis

Pyrogenic **liver abscess** should be suspected in any patient with fever, anorexia, nausea, vomiting, and right upper abdominal or lower thoracic pain. Jaundice usually suggests biliary obstruction. Frequently there is tender hepatosplenomegaly and, sometimes, a palpable mass. Many patients experience leukocytosis, elevated erythrocyte sedimentation rate, and elevated alkaline phosphatase levels. Elevated hepatocellular enzyme levels indicate a poor prognosis.

Liver ultrasonography (US) and computed tomography (CT) have facilitated accurate and rapid diagnosis. US- or CT-guided thin needle aspiration of abscesses may provide necessary material for Gram stains and cultures. Blood cultures should also be obtained.

Causes of pyogenic liver abscess are as follows:

1. Infection ascending the bile duct secondary to cholecystitis, cholangitis, pancreatitis, and strictures of the biliary tree
2. Direct extension of infection from a neighboring structure
3. Secondary infection of necrotic liver neoplasms and cysts of benign or parasitic nature
4. Abdominal infections ascending the portal vein (e.g., appendicitis)

A microbiologic diagnosis is very valuable in determining therapy. If the patient's condition warrants immediate empirical therapy, then coverage for *Streptococcus, Staphylococcus, Pneumococcus, Escherichia, Proteus, Klebsiella, Pseudomonas*, and other gram-negative organisms is indicated. Anaerobes, including *Bacteroides* and *Clostridium* species, are found in more than 50 percent of abscesses and should be treated while awaiting culture results.[22] In some settings empirical antiamebic treatment may also be appropriate.

Treatment

A number of antibiotic combinations of one, two, or three drugs may meet treatment requirements. When possible, treatment should be guided by cultures and sensitivity results, modified according to the patient's allergies and other medical conditions, and continued for at least 2 months unless the abscess is surgically excised.

Large (>2.0 cm) solitary or multiple liver abscesses require drainage, traditionally a surgical procedure. However, recent developments allow CT- and US-guided percutaneous placement of drains, which may obviate surgery.

Trauma

Etiology and Clinical Manifestations

The liver is the most common organ to be injured by penetrating abdominal trauma of the abdomen (such as gunshot wounds, stab wounds, or rib fractures) and the second most commonly injured organ in blunt abdominal trauma. Damage or injury to the liver should be suspected whenever any upper abdominal or lower chest trauma is sustained. The liver is frequently injured by steering wheels in vehicular accidents. Common injuries to the liver include simple lacerations, multiple lacerations, avulsions, and crush injuries.

The liver is a highly vascular organ, receiving approximately 29 percent of the body's cardiac output. When hepatic trauma occurs, blood loss can be massive. The person may exhibit signs of hemorrhagic shock such as hypotension, tachycardia, tachypnea, pallor, diaphoresis, cool, clammy skin, and confusion. A decreased hematocrit may confirm suspected blood loss. Clinical manifestations include right upper quadrant pain with abdominal tenderness, distention, guarding, and rigidity. Abdominal pain exaggerated by deep breathing and referred to the shoulder may indicate diaphragmatic irritation.

Treatment

Treatment entails administration of fresh whole blood or packed red blood cells and fresh frozen plasma, as well as massive fluid infusion to maintain adequate intravascular volume and hematocrit. Postoperatively, the patient with hepatic trauma is admitted to a critical care unit and monitored for persistent bleeding. The complete blood cell count and coagulation parameters must be closely monitored for trends in changes.

Cancer

Etiology

Carcinoma of the liver usually develops as a metastatic process. Owing to the vascularity and lymphatic drainage of the liver, the organ is a common site for metastasis from primary cancers of the esophagus, stomach, colon, rectum, breasts, and lungs, or from a malignant melanoma—among many other possibilities.

Primary hepatic carcinoma (cancer originating within the liver) is rare in the United States, with an annual incidence of fewer than 4 cases per 100,000.[23] However, in other parts of the world, such as Africa, it is one of the most common malignancies. The geographic variation probably reflects the prevalence of chronic hepatitis B and C infection in other countries. HBV is thought to be the primary carcinogen in as many as 80 percent of patients with primary hepatic cancer worldwide.[24] Between 30 and 70 percent of patients with primary hepatic cancer also have cirrhosis, and the risk of hepatic cancer is 40 times greater in persons with cirrhosis.[25]

Primary hepatic cancer has also been associated with alcoholic cirrhosis, chronic hepatitis B and C, hemochromatosis, and exposure to carcinogens and hepatotoxins, including aflatoxin, thorium dioxide, and senecio alkaloids.

Clinical Manifestations and Diagnosis

The most common form of primary hepatic cancer is **hepatoma.** Signs and symptoms of hepatoma include hepatosplenomegaly, jaundice, ascites, fever, abdominal pain, weight loss, nonspecific GI complaints, and vomiting. The unusual manifestations of hepatoma include hypercalcemia, erythrocytosis, hypoglycemia, and hypertrophic osteoarthropathy (finger clubbing).

Space-occupying masses of the liver may first be suggested by abnormal liver-related enzymes, especially alkaline phosphatase. Definitive diagnosis requires imaging of the liver with US, CT, or magnetic resonance imaging. These studies also allow guided needle biopsy of the liver lesion. Radionuclide imaging, while providing less anatomic detail than the other studies, offers physiologic information not otherwise obtainable.

Treatment

The best treatment for hepatoma and some metastatic lesions is partial hepatic resection. Unfortunately, due to advanced diffuse liver disease or multifocal tumors, this is usually not possible. Other treatments include systemic chemotherapy and chemotherapy directed selectively to the liver via portal vein cannulation. Hepatic chemotherapay may employ a surgically implanted infusion pump, which enables controlled infusion for up to 14 days at a time. Other novel treatments include hepatic artery ligation, which is effective because most tumors derive their blood supply from the hepatic artery, whereas the normal hepatocytes derive 75 percent of their blood supply from the portal vein. Direct percutaneous injection of alcohol into hepatic tumors has also been used with some success. Transplantation is another but very controversial approach to treatment.

KEY CONCEPTS

- Liver abscesses are suspected in patients with fever, nausea, vomiting, and right upper quadrant pain. Ascending biliary infection, abdominal infections transported by the portal vein, and direct extension of infection from neighboring structures are usual sources of infection. Antibiotics and drainage are commonly prescribed.

- The liver commonly sustains injury during penetrating and blunt trauma to the abdomen. Because the liver is highly vascular, trauma may produce extreme blood loss and hemorrhagic shock. Liver trauma manifests with abdominal tenderness, distention, guarding, and rigidity.

- In the United States, cancer of the liver is usually metastatic and rarely primary. Tumors of the esophagus, stomach, colon, rectum, breast, and lung commonly seed in the liver. Primary liver cancer is more common in other parts of the world, with hepatitis B and C viruses suspected as important contributing factors.

Transplantation

The patient with end-stage liver disease that has not responded to conventional medical or surgical intervention is a potential candidate for **liver transplantation** (Table 38–4). In the adult, diseases treated by liver transplantation include end-stage cirrhosis from chronic active hepatitis or primary biliary cirrhosis; hepatic metabolic diseases such as protoporphyria and Wilson's disease; Budd-Chiari syndrome (hepatic vein obstruction impairing blood flow out of the liver); and sclerosing cholangitis. Liver transplantation is rarely performed for patients with malignant neoplasms, primarily because of tumor recurrence in immunosuppressed persons. Alcoholic cirrhosis and chronic hepatitis B are controversial indications for transplantation.

The potential transplant patient undergoes extensive physiologic and psychological assessment and evaluation by physicians and nurses to identify contraindications to the procedure. The patient with end-stage disease and multiorgan failure with life-threatening complications, such as sepsis, severe cardiovascular instability with advanced cardiac disease, hypertension, a known extrahepatic malignancy (especially if metastatic), and severe chronic lung disease, is not considered a candidate for transplantation. Additional identified risk factors include portal vein thrombosis, previous portal-systemic shunt operations, advanced catabolic state, active alcoholism, lack of knowledge and understanding of the procedure and required postoperative care measures, a poor psychosocial support system, and psychological instability. These are risk factors and do not necessarily preclude transplantation.

After the patient has been identified as a candidate and a donor organ has been procured, the actual surgical procedure can take 8 to 22 hours to complete. The procedure involves five anastomoses between recipient and donor organs, including the following vascular anastomosis sites: suprahepatic inferior vena cava, infrahepatic vena cava, portal vein, hepatic artery, and biliary tract. The biliary anastomosis site varies, depending on the patient's extrahepatic biliary tract.

The success of all transplants has greatly improved since the discovery of cyclosporin A, an immunosuppressant drug. This drug is widely accepted as the primary agent to prevent rejection of the donor organ. The blood level of cyclosporin must be carefully monitored because of the serious side effects associated with cyclosporin use. These include nephrotoxicity, hypertension, seizures, hepatotoxicity, and, most disturbingly, the development of lymphomas and lymphoproliferative syndromes in some patients.

The rejection response after liver transplantation most often occurs between the postoperative days 4 and 10. Clinical manifestations of acute rejection include tachycardia, fever, right upper quadrant or flank pain, diminished bile flow through the T-tube or a change in bile color, and increasing jaundice. Laboratory findings include elevated serum bilirubin, transaminase, and alkaline phosphatase levels and increased prothrombin time.

If the rejection is not controlled by immunosuppressive agents, including azathioprine, prednisone, cyclosporin A, antilymphocyte antibodies, and FK-506, a rapid deterioration in liver function occurs. Multisystem organ failure, including respiratory and renal involvement, develops, along with diffuse coagulopathies and portal-systemic encephalopathy. Chronic rejection, characterized by increasing cholestasis, may take months to become evident and does

---

TABLE 38–4. Clinical and Biochemical Indications for Liver Transplantation Candidacy

Acute Liver Failure

Bilirubin > 10–20 mg/dL and increasing
Prothrombin time > 10 sec above control and increasing
Progressive encephalopathy

Chronic Liver Disease

Cholestatic liver disease
    Bilirubin > 10–15 mg/dL
    Intractable pruritus
    Intractable bone disease
Hepatocellular liver disease
    Albumin < 2.5 g/dL
    Hepatic encephalopathy
    Prothrombin time > 5 sec above control
Factors common to both types of liver disease
    Hepatorenal syndrome
    Recurrent spontaneous bacterial peritonitis
    Intractable ascites
    Recurrent episodes of biliary sepsis
    Development of a hepatocellular carcinoma

From Van Thiel DH, Makowka L, Starzl TE: Liver transplantation: Where it's been and where it's going. *Gastroenterol Clin North Am* 1988;17(1):1–18. Reproduced with permission.

not respond to immunosuppressive therapy. The only alternative treatment is emergency retransplantation.

Infection is another potential threat. Immunosuppressant therapy, which must be used to prevent and treat organ rejection, significantly increases the patient's susceptibility to and risk for bacterial, fungal, and viral infections. In addition to the risks specific to immunosuppression and rejection, the transplant patient faces all of the usual potential complications attendant on long and complex operations. These include infection, vascular and biliary anastomotic disruption, renal failure, respiratory failure, cardiovascular decompensation, prolonged gut disfunction, and psychological maladjustment. A very worrisome long-term consequence of post-transplantation immunosuppression is the development of malignancies, especially Epstein-Barr virus–related lymphomas.

Summary

Disorders of the liver are diverse and complex. Because the liver is vital to most life processes, even mild disorders can cause life-threatening alterations. Health care professionals need a good understanding of hepatobiliary anatomy and physiology to appreciate the effects of these disorders on patients.

Many liver disorders are the consequence of lifestyle choices, such as alcoholism and drug abuse. Health care professionals are in a position to explain the risks of detrimental life-styles and their relationship to liver diseases in an effort to prevent the occurrence of these diseases.

Medical treatment entails the use of drugs from many different classes. Because the liver is central to the metabolism of many of these drugs, their use requires special attention. Before any drug is given to a patient with liver disease, it is essential to become completely familiar with it by consulting a good pharmacology text or drug information source.

REFERENCES

1. Schafer D, Jones EA: Hepatic encephalopathy, in Zakim D, Boyer TD (eds): *Hepatology*, 2nd ed. Philadelphia, WB Saunders, 1990, p 456.
2. Conn HO: Complications of portal hypertension. *Curr Hepatol* 1989;9:262–268.
3. LeVeen HH, Christondias CA, Ip M, Luft R, Falk G, Grosberg S: Peritoneo-venous shunting for ascites. *Ann Surg* 1974;180(4):580–591.
4. Lung RH, New Kirk JB: Peritoneo-venous shunting system for surgical management of ascites. *Contemp Surg* 1979;14:31.
5. Goldsmith R, Yarbough PO, Reyes GR, et al: Enzyme-linked immunosorbent assay for diagnosis of acute sporadic hepatitis E in Egyptian children. *Lancet* 1992;339:328–331.
6. Midthun K, Ellerbeck E, Gershman K, et al: Safety and immunogenicity of a live attenuated hepatitis A virus vaccine in seronegative volunteers. *J Infect Dis* 1991;163(4):735–739.
7. Alter HJ, Barker LF, Holland PV: Hepatitis B immune globulin: Evaluation of clinical trials and rationale for usage. *N Engl J Med* 1975;293(21):1093–1094.
8. Immunization Practice Advisory Committee: Postexposure prophylaxis of hepatitis B. *MMWR* 1984;33:285–290.
9. Szmunese W, Stevens CE, Harley EJ, et al: Hepatitis B vaccine: Demonstration of efficacy in a controlled clinical trial in a high risk population in the United States. *N Engl J Med* 1980;303(15):833–841.
10. Marwick C: Hepatitis B vaccine appears headed for pediatric immunization schedule. *JAMA* 1991;265(12):1502.
11. New recommendations for immunization against pertussis and Hepatitis B. *Med Let Drugs Ther* 1992;34(875):69–71.
12. Seeff L: Diagnosis, therapy, and prognosis of viral hepatitis, in Zakim D, Boyer TD (eds): *Hepatology*, 2nd ed. Philadelphia, WB Saunders, 1990, p 1005.
13. Maddrey WC: Chronic active hepatitis, in Zakim D, Boyer TD (eds): *Hepatology*, 2nd ed. Philadelphia, WB Saunders, 1990, p 1035.
14. First effective treatment for chronic hepatitis B now available in the United States. Letter to physicians. Kenilworth, NJ, Schering Corp, June 1992.
15. Product information: Intron A Interferon alpha-2b recombinant. Kenilworth, NJ, Schering Corp, 1992.
16. *Physicians Desk Reference*, 48th ed. Montvale, NJ, Medical Economics Data, 1994, p 818.
17. Sternlieb I, Scheringberg H: Wilson's disease, in Wright R, Alverta KGM, Karran S, et al (eds): *Liver and Biliary Disease*. London, Bailliere Tindall, 1985, p 949.
18. Sherlock S: *Disease of the Liver and Biliary System*, 7th ed. Oxford, Blackwell Scientific Publishers, 1985, p 378.
19. Licht H, Seeff LB, Zimmermann HJ: Apparent potentiation of acetaminophen hepatotoxicity by alcohol. *Ann Intern Med* 1980;92(4):511.
20. Seeff LB, Cuccherini BA, Zimmermann HJ, Adler E, Benjamin SB: Acetaminophen hepatotoxicity in alcoholics: A therapeutic misadventure. *Ann Intern Med* 1986;104(3):399–404.
21. Mitchell JR: Host susceptibility and acetaminophen liver injury. *Ann Intern Med* 1977;87(3):377–378. Editorial.
22. Spiro HM: *Clinical Gastroenterology*, 2nd ed. New York, Macmillan, 1977, p 1161.
23. *Cancer Facts and Figures*. Atlanta, American Cancer Society, 1991.
24. Dusheiko GM: Hepatocellular carcinoma associated with chronic viral hepatitis. *Br Med J* 1990;46(2):492–511.
25. Kew MC, Popper H: Relationship between hepatocellular carcinoma and cirrhosis. *Semin Liver Dis* 1984;4:136.

BIBLIOGRAPHY

Bayless T (ed): *Current Therapy in Gastroenterology and Liver Disease 1984–1985*. Philadelphia, BC Decker, 1984.

Fletcher LM, Kwoh-Gain I, Powell EE, Powell LW, Halliday J: Markers of chronic alcohol ingestion in patients with nonalcoholic steatohepatitis: An aid to diagnosis. *Hepatology* 1991;13:450–455.

Maddrey WC: Disorders that may stimulate chronic hepatitis. *DM* 1993;39(2):70–74.

Marsh WJ, Gordon RD, Stieber AC, et al: Critical care of the liver transplant patient, in Shoemaker CW, Ayres S, Grenvik A, Holbrook PR, Thompson WL (eds): *Textbook of Critical Care*. Philadelphia, WB Saunders, 1989, p 1328.

Millward-Sadler GH, Wright R, Arthur MJB (eds): *Wright's Liver and Biliary Disease: Pathophysiology, Diagnosis, and Management*, 3rd ed. Philadelphia, WB Saunders, 1992.

Poynard T, Aubert A, Bedossa P, et al: A simple biological index for detection of alcoholic liver disease in drinkers. *Gastroenterology* 1991;100:1397–1402.

Prytz H, Melin T: Identification of alcoholic liver disease or hidden alcohol abuse in patients with elevated liver enzymes. *J Intern Med* 1993;233(1):21–26.

Singer PA, Siegler M, Whitington PF, et al: Ethics of liver transplantation with living donors. *N Engl J Med* 1990;322(8):549–550.

Stibier H: Carbohydrate-deficient transferrin in serum: A new marker of potentially harmful alcohol consumption reviewed. *Clin Chem* 1991;37:2029–2037.

Takase S, Takada N, Enomoto N, Yasuhara M, Takada A: Different types of chronic active hepatitis in alcoholic patients: Does chronic hepatitis induced by alcohol exist? *Hepatology* 1991;13:876–881.

Todo S, Fung JJ, Starzl TE, et al: Liver, kidney, and thoracic organ transplantation under FK 506. *Ann Surg* 1990;212(3):295–305.

Van Thiel DH, Makowka L, Starzl TE: Liver transplantation: Where it's been and where it's going. *Gastroenterol Clin North Am* 1988;17(1):1–18.

Zakim D, Boyer TD: *Hepatology: A Textbook of Liver Disease*, 2nd ed. Philadelphia, WB Saunders, 1990.

UNIT XI

Alterations in Endocrine Function and Metabolism

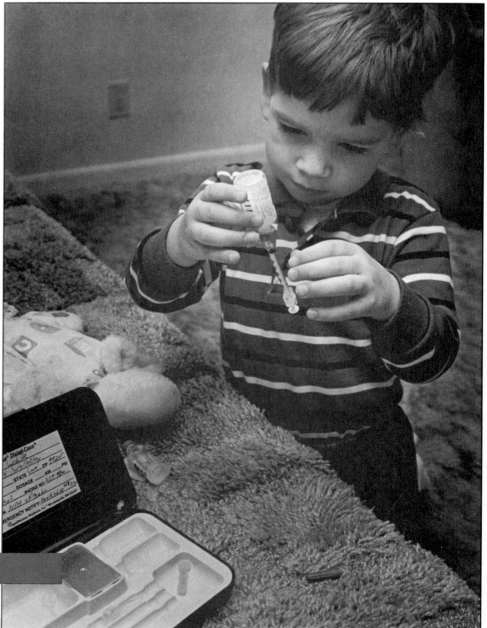

A diabetic child learns how to administer insulin.

Photo by Kathleen Kelly

There are different kinds of thirst. Medical professionals distinguish between the thirst of compulsive water drinkers, which may suggest a psychiatric disorder, the excessive thirst of patients with congestive heart failure or renal failure, the diminished thirst of the dehydrated older person, the thirst of a burn victim, and the symptomatic thirst found in a number of diseases.

Thirst is natural. The normal human body is 70 to 75 percent water. But there is a thirst, often an imperative thirst, sometimes made more urgent by a feeling that the throat is constricted and that water is needed to feed an "internal dryness." This is the thirst caused by diabetes.

For generations this thirst has been an alarming symptom of a disease that can contribute to or cause a number of disabling and sometimes fatal complications—blindness, kidney disease, arteriosclerosis, leg pains and ulcers, gangrene that requires limb amputation, and acidotic coma, which can lead to death within hours. The common form of this disease is diabetes mellitus, and it is one of the most pervasive disorders associated with the endocrine or hormonal system, which, along with the nervous system, regulates the functions of the body.

Diabetes mellitus is caused by decreased secretion of insulin by the beta cells of the exotically named islets of Langerhans in the pancreas. Insulin is vital. This small protein affects carbohydrate, fat, and protein metabolism. When it works as it should, it helps produce energy and plays a role in the storing of excess energy as glycogen, for example, in the liver and muscles.

Once secreted, insulin circulates in the blood. When it binds with receptors in the membranes of muscle, adipose, and other kinds of cells, their permeability to glucose, many amino acids, potassium, magnesium, and phosphate ions increases. Insulin's effect on the forming of new proteins and on the activity of intracellular metabolic enzymes is slower but no less decisive.

These are changes that can be sensed. When marathon runners eat high-carbohydrate meals before a race they can be assured that glucose absorbed into the blood not only nourishes straining muscles but increases the secretion of insulin, which energizes the body.

Diabetic patients, who lack insulin, may suffer from decreased glucose in body muscle cells, increasing blood glucose concentrations; abnormal release of fat from storage as the body shifts from carbohydrate to fat metabolism, depositing fat in arterial walls and causing arterial disease; and depleted protein.

The increase in fatty acids and an accompanying depletion of sodium in extracellular fluid, which is replaced by hydrogen ions, can cause the critical imbalance that produces one of the most ominous conditions of severely uncontrolled diabetes: acidotic coma.

Control is the issue, and recently sufferers have been able to take advantage of increasingly sophisticated methods of control and look forward to more innovations. Insulin was first isolated from the pancreas in 1922. That breakthrough meant that the diagnosis of diabetes was no longer a death warrant. But unless diabetes is controlled through careful and consistent monitoring, medication, and care, and through exercise and a healthful diet, preventing imbalances and obesity, diabetes still can restrict normal living and endanger life.

Late in 1993, the nation's 13 million diabetes sufferers, as well as many others who worry over possible inheritance of a susceptibility to the disease, learned from highly publicized research findings that diabetes could be further controlled in ways that reduce or prevent the disabling effects of the disease.

FRONTIERS OF RESEARCH
Diabetes Mellitus
Michael J. Kirkhorn

The results of a 10-year, $160 million investigation, supported by the National Institute of Diabetes and Digestive and Kidney Diseases, found that the diabetic patients enrolled in the research study who practiced "tight control"—that is, those who intended to keep blood sugars in the normal range all day by monitoring their blood glucose level four or more times and taking at least three injections of insulin each day, had 76 percent less diabetic eye disease, 60 percent less nerve damage, and 56 percent fewer kidney problems than those who practiced conventional therapy (i.e., one or two insulin injections and glucose monitoring two to three times a day). The goal of conventional therapy was to maintain clinical well being, and the goal of tight control was to achieve normalization of blood glucose.

It is estimated that health care for diabetes and its complications costs about $92 billion a year in the United States. In a nation deeply concerned about controlling health care dollars, research suggests that keeping patients on tight control may mitigate costly effects of the disease process.

Means also are being sought to restore the normal secretion of insulin by transplanting pancreatic tissue in animals. Several series of experiments employed a vascular shunt to provide the body with transplanted islets, which then would restore normal secretion of insulin. A selectively permeable tissue was used to isolate the transplanted tissue from the immune system of the recipient. The goal was to find ways to replace daily insulin therapy, which requires considerable discipline, with a biohybrid artificial pancreas.

The researchers found that pancreatic tissue transplanted through a device grafted onto the vascular system could maintain fasting glucose levels in animals at sufficient levels over a period of time.

Diabetes is not the only disease that concerns medical professionals and researchers concerned with the endocrine system. But it is one in which there is a growingly optimistic outlook for those who suffer diabetes, a prospect based on a range of countermeasures including preventive care, good nutrition, exercise, sound medical advice, increasingly knowledgeable monitoring and maintenance, and the possibility of a cure through research.

CHAPTER 39
Mechanisms of Endocrine Control and Metabolism

BARBARA BARTZ and DEBBY KAALAND

KEY TERMS

anabolism: The energy-requiring phase of metabolism through which molecules, cells, and tissues are created.

catabolism: The energy-releasing phase of metabolism through which molecules, cells, and tissues are broken down to simpler substances.

downregulation: A decrease in the number of cell receptors for a specific hormone resulting from the cell's prolonged exposure to high concentrations of the hormone. Downregulation results in a decrease in the target cell response to a hormone.

endocrine system: The cells and organs that produce and secrete hormones.

hormone: A blood-borne chemical messenger that affects target cells anatomically distant from the secreting cells.

hormone agonist: Chemicals that bind to hormone receptors and initiate intracellular activities identical to those caused by hormones. Some medications exert their therapeutic effects through this process.

hormone antagonist: Chemicals that compete with hormones for cell receptors. Antagonists bind to cell receptors and prevent the intracellular activities associated with hormone-receptor binding from occurring. Some medications produce their therapeutic effects through this process.

hormone receptors: Proteins on or within a target cell that bind to circulating hormones and allow the cellular response to a specific hormone. Hormone-receptor binding is the first step in the cellular response to a particular hormone.

metabolism: The synthesis and breakdown of molecules in a living organism. Metabolism involves both the use and the release of energy.

negative feedback: A decrease in the stimulus to secrete a hormone resulting from increased blood levels of the hormone. One of the body's most frequent means of regulating hormone concentration.

receptor specificity: The process that allows intracellular processes to be activated only by certain hormones. If a cell does not have the specific receptors for a hormone, it will not respond to the hormone.

upregulation: An increase in the number of cell receptors for a specific hormone resulting from chronically low concentrations of the hormone. Upregulation helps maintain the target cell response to a hormone, even when circulating hormone levels are low.

Communication between body cells and organs is maintained by the actions of and interactions between the nervous and endocrine systems. While the nervous system consists of anatomically connected elements, the **endocrine system** has a more loosely organized structure. It is composed of cells and organs that manufacture and secrete hormones; thus it is a functional rather than an anatomic system. The nervous and endocrine systems are closely coupled, affecting each other's functions and sharing some of the same chemical messengers, such as epinephrine and norepinephrine. They are also intimately related at the level of the hypothalamus. Anatomically part of the central nervous system, the hypothalamus produces and secretes hormones that determine the function of the pituitary gland, long considered the major coordinator for the endocrine system.

Although the nervous and endocrine systems are closely related, they are traditionally studied separately. This chapter covers general mechanisms of endocrine control and provides an overview of endocrine pathologies. Integration of the nervous and endocrine systems at the hypothalamus and pituitary gland is described. The latter part of the chapter discusses metabolic processes and related endocrine control.

Hormone Production, Secretion, and Action

Hormone Function and Classification

A **hormone** may be defined as a blood-borne chemical messenger that has an effect on target cells anatomically distant from the secreting cells. An **endocrine organ** or gland manufactures and secretes hormones. Major hormones, their primary gland of origin, and their major physiologic effects are listed in Table 39–1. Some of these hormone-secreting organs may have nonendocrine functions as well. For example, the atria of the heart secrete the sodium-controlling hormone atrial natriuretic hormone, although the primary activity of the heart is to function as a blood pump.[1] As noted in Table 39–1, more than one organ may secrete a particular hormone, and more than one hormone may be secreted by a particular organ.

Hormones must travel through the circulatory system to exert their actions. *Paracrines* are hormone-like substances secreted by one cell that affect cells adjacent to the secreting cell. Cells may also secrete hormone-like chemicals called *autocrines* that directly influence the cellular function of the secreting cell. Paracrines and autocrines are not usually included in discussions of hormone actions; however, it should be noted that chemicals that act as autocrines or paracrines in one instance may act as hormones in another.[2,3] For example, estrogen and testosterone act both locally and systemically. As endocrine research progresses, it is likely that substances now termed *candidate hormones* may prove to fit the classic hormone criteria.[3]

Function

Hormones control four broad categories of body functions: reproduction, growth and development, maintenance of homeostasis, and energy production during metabolic processes.[4] Endocrine control of reproduction is described in Chapters 30 and 32, regulation of growth in Chapter 40, and hormonal impact on general systemic homeostasis in Chapter 7. Hormonal control of energy production, storage, and use is described in the last part of this chapter.

An important point regarding hormonal control of various functions is that a particular hormone may have an effect on many body systems and functions. For example, among the effects of testosterone are growth and differentiation of the male genitourinary tract, growth of facial and body hair, promotion of muscle growth, and protein anabolism.[4]

A second important principle regarding endocrine effects is that one body function may require the coordinated action of many hormones. The plasma level of glucose is kept within a narrow range of normal by the complex interactions of insulin, glucagon, epi-

TABLE 39–1. Major Hormones and Their Functions

Major Function	Hormone	Primary Endocrine Gland
Anterior pituitary "tropic" hormones	Adrenocorticotropic hormone	Anterior pituitary
	Follicle-stimulating hormone	Anterior pituitary
	Luteinizing hormone	Anterior pituitary
	Thyroid-stimulating hormone	Anterior pituitary
Blood pressure control	Renin (angiotensin II)	Kidneys
Fluid and electrolyte balance	Aldosterone	Adrenal cortex
	Atrial natriuretic hormone	Atria of heart
	Calcitonin	Thyroid
	Parathyroid hormone	Parathyroid
	Vasopressin/antidiuretic hormone	Posterior pituitary
	Vitamin D	Kidneys
Gastrointestinal function	Cholecystokinin	Gastrointestinal tract
	Gastrin	Gastrointestinal tract
	Secretin	Gastrointestinal tract
Growth and metabolism	Cortisol	Adrenal cortex
	Epinephrine	Adrenal medulla
	Glucagon	Pancreas
	Growth hormone	Anterior pituitary
	Insulin	Pancreas
	Norepinephrine	Adrenal medulla
	Thyroid hormones	Thyroid
Hypothalamic releasing hormones	Corticotropin-releasing hormone	Hypothalamus
	Gonadotropin-releasing hormone	Hypothalamus
	Growth hormone–releasing hormone	Hypothalamus
	Prolactin release–inhibiting hormone	Hypothalamus
	Prolactin-releasing hormone	Hypothalamus
	Somatostatin	Hypothalamus
	Thyrotropin-releasing hormone	Hypothalamus
Immune response	Cortisol	Adrenal cortex
	Thymosin	Thymus
Red blood cell production	Erythropoietin	Kidneys
Reproduction and lactation	Chorionic gonadotropin	Placenta
	Estrogens	Ovaries and placenta
	Oxytocin	Anterior pituitary
	Progesterone	Ovaries and placenta
	Prolactin	Anterior pituitary
	Testosterone	Testes
Stress response	Cortisol	Adrenal cortex
	Epinephrine	Adrenal medulla
	Norepinephrine	Adrenal medulla

nephrine, norepinephrine, growth hormone, and cortisol. In addition, other hormones exert indirect effects on glucose levels by controlling appetite and nutrient absorption. The homeostatic implications are that there are backup systems and fine-tuning mechanisms such that even when portions of the system are dysfunctional, blood glucose levels continue to be maintained within normal or near-normal limits.[4]

Classification and Transport

Hormones may be classified as belonging to one of three groups, the amine, peptide, and steroid hormones. The **amines** are derived from the amino acid tyrosine and consist of the thyroid hormones and the catecholamines epinephrine, norepinephrine, and dopamine. The **peptides** are the largest group of hormones. Among the peptide hormones are atrial natriuretic hormone, growth hormone, luteinizing hormone, follicle-stimulating hormone, insulin, glucagon, vasopressin, and oxytocin. The various releas-

ing hormones and tropic hormones secreted by the hypothalamus and anterior pituitary are also peptide hormones. **Steroid hormones** are derived from the lipid cholesterol and include the androgens, estrogen, progesterone, cortisol, corticosterone, aldosterone, and vitamin D.[3–5]

A more functional way to categorize hormones is according to their solubility in water or lipids. The peptide hormones and the catecholamines are all water soluble. Functionally, this means that they can be transported easily by the circulation to target cells.[6]

The lipid-soluble steroid and thyroid hormones are not freely carried in blood; the majority of the hormone is bound to a transport protein that carries the hormone throughout the circulation. A small amount of the lipid-soluble hormone is carried in the *free (unbound)* state. It is the unbound hormone that is able to enter the cell and affect cell function. As free hormone is taken into the cell, bound hormone is released from the transport protein.[7]

Many lipid-soluble hormones have specific transport proteins. These proteins include thyroxine-binding, testosterone-binding, and cortisol-binding globulin. Hormones can also be carried by nonspecific proteins such as albumin.[7]

Hormone Synthesis, Secretion, and Metabolism

Hormone synthesis takes place within the cell organelles. Usually one organ produces the majority of the circulating hormone and is considered the endocrine organ for that hormone, although hormone synthesis and secretion may take place in many organs and types of cells. One organ may produce and release many types of hormones.

The stimulus for hormone synthesis and secretion may be closely coupled. The steroid hormones are not stored in large quantities, and once synthesized, they simply diffuse out through the cell membrane into the circulation. When there is a need for a steroid hormone, increased production of the hormone closely precedes hormone release into the circulation.[2,3]

Hormone synthesis may also precede secretion by several weeks, as is the case with the thyroid hormones. Triiodothyronine (T_3) and thyroxine (T_4) are synthesized and then bound to the protein thyroglobulin. Secretion occurs via cleaving of the thyroid hormone from the globulin in response to systemic needs.

Peptide hormones are not stored for long periods after synthesis. The initial forms of the peptide hormones are large molecules called *prohormones* or *preprohormones*. When needed, these large molecules are cleaved by specific enzymes, releasing the active form of the hormone.[2,3]

Factors Affecting Hormone Secretion

Secretion of hormone is dependent on the interplay of many factors. Many hormones are secreted in cyclic patterns. Cycles may occur over several minutes or hours; in 24-hour (circadian) periods; over longer periods such as the 28-day menstrual cycle; or over a lifetime, such as the hormones that control reproductive differentiation and maturity.[4] Immediate systemic needs or stressors can override cyclic patterns and modify hormone secretion. For example, the normal circadian rhythm of plasma cortisol is altered by insulin-induced hypoglycemia.[8]

Feedback Mechanisms

An almost universal process regulating hormone production and secretion is feedback control.[4] An excellent example of **negative feedback** is provided by the interaction between the hypothalamic-pituitary system and the organs whose hormone release is controlled by this system. Figure 39–1 illustrates this phenomenon for thyroid hormone. Thyroid-releasing hormone (TRH) is secreted by the hypothalamus in response to an inadequate supply of circulating thyroid hormones for cellular needs. TRH stimulates the

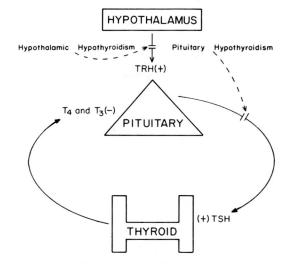

FIGURE 39–1. Negative feedback by the thyroid hormones inhibits anterior pituitary secretion of thyroid-stimulating hormone (TSH). (From Emerson CH: Central hypothyroidism and hyperthyroidism. *The Medical Clinics of North America* 1985:69(5): 1019–1034. Reproduced with permission.)

release of thyroid-stimulating hormone (TSH) from the anterior pituitary; TSH then stimulates the release of the thyroid hormones T_3 and T_4 from the thyroid gland. The resulting increase in plasma thyroid hormone concentration exerts an inhibitory effect, or negative feedback, on the release of TSH by the anterior pituitary. Negative feedback from an increased concentration of thyroid hormones also affects, but to a lesser extent, the hypothalamic release of TRH.[4] **Positive feedback**—a stimulus for more hormone release in response to an increased release of that hormone from the target cell—also occurs, but much less frequently than negative feedback.[3,9] The prevalence of feedback systems is one reason why evaluation of the level of one hormone alone is inadequate for diagnostic purposes where hormone excess or deficiency is suspected. For example, an elevated thyroid hormone concentration may be related to a disease process of the thyroid gland or to pathologically elevated levels of TSH or TRH. Assessment of the plasma concentrations of several hormones may be necessary to determine the cause of thyroid hormone pathology.

Hormone synthesis and release are also under the control of other types of feedback systems. Ionic changes in the extracellular fluid, increased or decreased amounts of the products of metabolism, osmolality, and extracellular fluid volume all act by feedback systems to regulate circulating hormone levels.[4] Table 39–2 summarizes factors that may affect hormone secretion.

Hormone Metabolism and Excretion

The plasma concentration of hormone depends not only on the rate of synthesis and release of the hormone, but also on how rapidly the hormone is metab-

TABLE 39–2. Factors Affecting Hormone Secretion

Cyclic rhythms
Stress (nervous system input)
Feedback mechanisms
    Hormonal feedback
    Extracellular ion concentration
    Metabolic by-products
    Osmolality
    Extracellular fluid volume

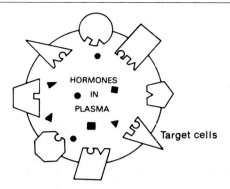

FIGURE 39–2. Receptor specificity: Hormones can bind only to those cells with appropriate receptors. (From Roth J, Lesniak MA, Megyesi CR, et al: Hormone receptors, human disease, and disorders in receptor design, in Sato GH, Ross R (eds): *Hormones and Cell Culture, Book A.* Cold Spring Harbor, NY, Cold Spring Harbor Laboratory, 1979, p 171. Reproduced with permission.)

olized and excreted. Like other compounds, hormones are frequently degraded and excreted by the liver and kidneys. Lipid-soluble hormones, which are bound to plasma proteins, are less readily metabolized by these organs and thus remain in the circulation for a more prolonged period than water-soluble hormones.[3] In addition to metabolism by the kidneys and liver, hormones can be degraded by the target cell after binding to target cell receptors.[6]

A final important point is that metabolism of a hormone may serve to increase hormonal activity. For example, the thyroid hormone T_4 is relatively inert; metabolism of T_4 converts it to T_3, the more biologically active form of thyroid hormone.[3]

Hormone Receptors

Tissue response to circulating hormone is only partially controlled by the amount of hormone present in the circulation. Although virtually all body tissues are exposed to the same concentration of circulating hormones, specific hormones elicit a response only from certain cells and tissues. The ability of a cell to respond to a particular hormone depends on the presence of specific receptors for that hormone on or within the cell. Cell **hormone receptors** are proteins that bind with the circulating hormone; hormone-receptor binding is the first step in eliciting a response from the cell.[10]

Receptor Specificity and Affinity

The concept of **receptor specificity** is an important one in understanding the endocrine system. As indicated in Figure 39–2, cells will respond only to those hormones for which they have receptors. Specificity explains why not all cells respond to all the hormones to which they are exposed.[10] Specificity cannot easily be separated from the concept of **affinity**. Affinity describes the degree of "tightness" of the hormone-receptor bond, or the inclination of the hormone to remain bound to the receptor. The potency of the hormone, or the amount of hormone required to elicit a cellular response, is dependent on the affinity of the receptor for a particular hormone. The higher the

affinity of the receptor for a hormone, the less hormone is needed to produce a response.[6]

There may be "cross-specificity" between hormones of similar structure. For example, growth hormone and the lactation-stimulating hormone prolactin both bind to the prolactin receptor. Under normal circumstances, the plasma concentration of growth hormone is not adequate to bind a significant number of prolactin receptors. However, in the condition called acromegaly, in which excessive concentrations of growth hormone lead to massive bone and tissue overgrowth, milk may be secreted from the mammary glands secondary to growth hormone stimulation of prolactin receptors.[11]

Downregulation and Upregulation

Another factor determining the degree of response to circulating hormone is the number of cell receptors available for hormone binding. When cells are exposed to high concentrations of hormone for a prolonged period of time, a common effect is a decrease in the quantity of receptors for that hormone. This is known as **downregulation**. An example of downregulation occurs with insulin receptors in obesity. An increase in the plasma insulin level commonly occurs in association with obesity; this does not result in an increase in those cellular activities regulated by insulin since the number of insulin receptors is decreased secondary to high plasma insulin concentration.[6,10] Downregulation probably serves a protective function: the cells are protected against excessive activity despite pathologies that cause excessive hormone levels.

Upregulation, or an increase in the number of receptors secondary to a chronically low hormone concentration, may also occur. This would make the cell more sensitive to the hormone, and hormone-dependent cellular activity could occur at normal or near-normal levels despite lower than normal hormone concentration.[6,10]

Permissiveness

Downregulation and upregulation are not the only means by which hormone receptors are controlled. One effect hormones may have on cells is to increase the number of receptors for other hormones, thus enhancing the effect of the second hormone. This phenomenon is known as **permissiveness.** For example, the effect of thyroid hormone on adipose cells is to increase the number of receptors for epinephrine. When the adipose tissue is subsequently exposed to epinephrine, a greater release of fatty acids (utilized in providing energy for cellular processes) takes place than would occur without the effect of thyroid hormone.[3] Permissiveness also allows cellular events to occur in sequence. One effect of estrogen, secreted early in the menstrual cycle, is to increase the numbers of uterine receptors for progesterone. The uterus is therefore sensitive to progesterone when it is present during the last part of the menstrual cycle, and normal proliferative changes take place.[3,9]

In addition to receptor specificity, affinity, and concentration, other factors also affect hormone-receptor binding. These include pH, ion concentration, and temperature.

Hormone Agonists and Antagonists

In order to produce a cellular effect, a hormone must bind to the receptor and initiate a series of events which lead to a change in cellular activity. A chemical may bind to a receptor without initiating this series of events; this chemical is described as a hormone **antagonist. Agonists** bind hormone receptors and cause the same series of intracellular events that would occur with hormone-receptor binding. The use of agonists and antagonists has important pharmacologic implications.[6] For example, medications that compete with epinephrine and norepinephrine for receptor sites are frequently used to block the cardiac stimulatory properties of these hormones and thus decrease cardiac work load. Conversely, medications that bind to the receptor sites for these adrenal hormones may be used to increase cardiac output and blood pressure in patients who have severe hypotension.

Mechanics of Hormone Action

Binding of hormone to receptor, or **receptor activation,** is only the first step in changing cellular activity. As the events after receptor activation vary according to whether the hormone is water soluble or lipid soluble, the postbinding activity of these different categories will be described separately.

Water-Soluble Hormones

Because water-soluble catecholamine and peptide hormones are unable to independently cross the lipid-containing cell membrane, receptors for these hormones are located in the outside portion of the cell membrane. A variety of activities may occur after hormone-receptor binding. Although the receptor for a specific hormone is the same no matter what the type of cell, postreceptor activity varies according to the cell type.[6]

Second Messengers

A problem for all hormone receptors located in cell membranes is how to relay the information that receptor activation has occurred to the intracellular components. The hormone is described as a "first messenger": the hormone carries the message from the secreting cell to the target cell. A "second messenger" in the cytoplasm must then be activated in order for the appropriate intracellular response to occur. A variety of second messengers have been identified.[3,10]

Cyclic AMP as a Second Messenger. The best researched second messenger is cyclic adenosine monophosphate (cAMP). As illustrated in Figure 39–3, hormone receptors, through the intermediation of an intramembrane protein known as a G-protein, activate the enzyme adenylate cyclase. Adenylate cyclase then allows the conversion of intracellular adenosine triphosphate (ATP) to cAMP. Cyclic AMP activates cAMP-dependent protein kinase, which then catalyzes the attachment of phosphate groups to intracellular proteins. Phosphorylation of intracellular proteins, which are most commonly enzymes, allows catalyzation of other intracellular functions such as secretion and contraction.[10]

For some intracellular proteins, phosphorylation will inhibit protein activity. Thus, the same initial hormone-receptor binding that results in activation of some intracellular proteins may lead to inactivation of other proteins. Frequently these intracellular activities are complementary. An example of a hormone utilizing cAMP as a second messenger is epinephrine. Epinephrine causes both the activation of intracellular enzymes that allow the conversion of glycogen to glucose and the inactivation of other enzymes that halt the intracellular synthesis of glycogen from glucose. The result of these combined effects is to free more glucose for energy needs.[3]

Other second messengers currently identified are listed in Table 39–3. In cellular location and activation, these second messengers differ from cAMP; however, all systems ultimately affect protein phosphorylation and lead to cellular responses. These second messengers do not act in isolation. Rather, they work competitively and synergistically, so that intracellular activity reflects the combination of many hormonal and second messenger effects.[6]

Amplification of Hormone Activity

The process of signal transduction explains why minute amounts of circulating hormone are able to have major cellular and tissue effects. Signal transduction occurs via a cascade effect. Progressively larger numbers of chemical reactions occur at each step so that activation of one molecule of adenylate cyclase (or

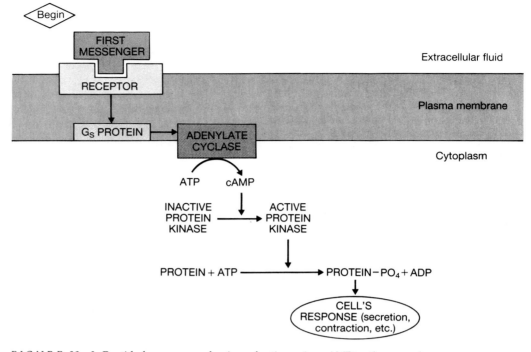

F I G U R E 39–3. Peptide hormone mechanism of action using cAMP as the second messenger. Hormone-receptor binding causes the creation of cAMP from ATP. Cyclic AMP catalyzes the phosphorylation of intracellular proteins, triggering intracellular activity. (From Vander AJ, Sherman JH, Luciano DJ: *Human Physiology: The Mechanisms of Body Function,* 5th ed. New York, McGraw-Hill, 1990, p 157. Reproduced with permission of McGraw-Hill, Inc.)

another enzyme) may lead to activation of many molecules of cAMP (or other second messenger), each molecule of cAMP activates many molecules of protein kinase, and so forth.[3,10]

Lipid-Soluble Hormones

The lipid-soluble thyroid and steroid hormones diffuse easily through the lipid-containing cell membrane. It is not known how the hormones then traverse the water-containing cytoplasm. Receptors for these hormones are located in the cytoplasm or, more frequently, the nucleus of the target cell. Binding of the hormone produces in the receptor an affinity for binding sites on deoxyribose nucleic acid (DNA) within the cell nucleus.[7,10]

As illustrated in Figure 39–4, gene expression is changed by binding of the hormone-receptor complex to DNA acceptor sites. The events that result from the interaction between nuclear DNA and the receptor include messenger ribose nucleic acid (mRNA) transcription, processing, and translation into specific proteins. Intracellular functioning and cellular growth and differentiation are altered by these proteins.[7,10]

Pharmacologic Hormone Concentrations

It is important to differentiate between physiologic and pharmacologic hormone concentrations. Pharmacologic levels of hormones can be defined as plasma hormone concentrations much greater than would normally be secreted by endocrine organs. Pharmacologic levels occur as a consequence of either pathologic processes or the administration of large doses of hormones. The kinds and amounts of cellular activity created by pharmacologic hormone concentrations may be radically different from those caused by physiologic levels of hormones.[3]

T A B L E 39–3. Second Messengers

Cyclic adenosine monophosphate (cAMP)
Cyclic guanosine monophosphate (cGMP)
Calcium
Inositol triphosphate
Diacylglycerol (DAG)

K E Y C O N C E P T S

- Hormones are chemical messengers that travel by the bloodstream to exert effects on target cells distant from the secreting glands. Hormones regulate four major body functions: reproduction, growth and development, homeostasis, and metabolism.

General Model of Steroid Hormone Action

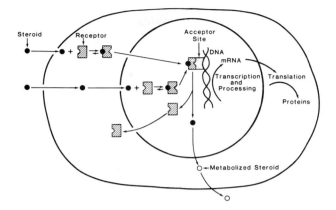

FIGURE 39–4. Steroid hormone action. Hormone-receptor binding leads to the creation of new intracellular proteins. (From Clark JH, Schrader WT, O'Malley BW: Mechanisms of steroid hormone action, in Wilson JD, Foster DW (eds): *Williams Textbook of Endocrinology*, 7th ed. Philadelphia, WB Saunders, 1985, p 34. Reproduced with permission.)

- Hormones may be classified according to chemical structure as amines (thyroid hormones, catecholamines), peptides, and steroids, and by solubility characteristics as water soluble (catecholamines, peptides) and lipid soluble (thyroid hormones, steroids).

- The hormone concentration depends on the rate of secretion and degradation. Lipid-soluble hormones are less readily metabolized because they are bound to protein carriers in plasma. Hormones are metabolized primarily by the liver, kidneys, and target tissues.

- Water-soluble hormones are transported in a free state in the bloodstream. They cannot effectively cross cell membranes and therefore exert their effects by binding with receptors on the target cell membrane. Only target cells displaying the corresponding receptor will respond to a hormone. Receptor activation leads to the production of second messengers within the cell (e.g., cAMP, Ca^{++}, inositol triphosphate) and alteration in activity of intracellular enzymes. Activation of surface receptors results in amplification of the first message because of the cascade effect.

- The number and affinity of hormone receptors on a cell's surface may be altered to adapt to changes in cell environment. High-affinity receptors are able to bind hormone at very low concentrations. Downregulation refers to a decrease in number of receptors at the cell surface in response to overstimulation by excessive hormone. Upregulation refers to an increase in number of receptors in response to lack of hormonal stimulation. Receptor number and responsiveness may be enhanced by the presence of other hormones (*permissiveness*). Chemicals other than the usual hormone may be able to bind to the hormone's receptors. Chemicals that bind receptors and block activity are antagonists; those that bind receptors and activate them are agonists.

- Lipid-soluble hormones are carried in the circulation by specific and nonspecific transport proteins. At the target cell, lipid-soluble hormones diffuse away from carrier proteins and pass directly through the lipid bilayer. Receptors in the cytoplasm or nucleus bind the hormone. Hormone-receptor complexes then bind to specific targets on nuclear DNA and alter gene expression.

- The secretion of most endocrine hormones is regulated by negative feedback mechanisms. Target gland hormones or chemical indicators of target gland function (such as glucose or calcium) feed back to inhibit secretion of the initial hormone.

Hypothalamic-Pituitary Control of the Endocrine System

The nervous system and endocrine system are most closely linked at the level of the hypothalamus and pituitary gland. Because endocrine function is affected in many ways by the hypothalamic-pituitary system, an understanding of the control exerted by this system is helpful in understanding endocrine effects in general.

The pituitary gland sits in the sella turcica, a pocket of bone at the base of the skull (Fig. 39–5). In adults, the gland is composed of distinct anterior and posterior lobes. The synthesis and secretion of the various pituitary hormones is controlled, directly or indirectly, by the hypothalamus.

Hormones of the Posterior Pituitary

The posterior pituitary gland consists of nerve axons whose neurons originate in the hypothalamus. In other words, the posterior pituitary can be considered an anatomic extension of the hypothalamus. Two major hormones, oxytocin and vasopressin (also known as antidiuretic hormone) are secreted from the posterior pituitary into the general circulation. These hormones are produced in the neurons of the hypothalamus and travel, packaged in vesicles, along the length of the nerve axons to the posterior pituitary. Release

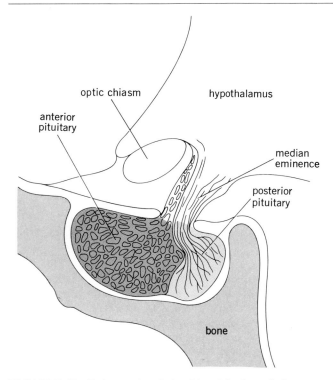

F I G U R E   39 – 5. Anatomic relationship of the hypothalamus and pituitary gland. (From Vander AJ, Sherman JH, Luciano DJ. *Human Physiology: The Mechanisms of Body Function,* 4th ed. New York, McGraw-Hill, 1985, p 244. Reproduced with permission of McGraw-Hill, Inc.)

of vasopressin or oxytocin occurs as a result of stimulation of the appropriate hypothalamic neurons.[12]

Hormones of the Hypothalamus and Anterior Pituitary

Although the hormones released by the posterior pituitary are actually manufactured in the hypothalamus, the effect of the hypothalamus on the anterior pituitary is less direct. Hypothalamic hormones are released into a capillary bed that is connected to a separate capillary bed in the anterior pituitary gland. The hormones secreted by the hypothalamus are called **releasing hormones** because they affect the release of other hormones from the anterior pituitary gland.[3,12]

Figure 39–6 illustrates the interactions between hypothalamic and anterior pituitary hormones and their target organs. As illustrated in the diagram, some anterior pituitary hormones act directly on target cells. Other anterior pituitary hormones, termed **tropic hormones,** stimulate the secretion of yet other hormones that finally act on target cells.

This multistep process provides a great deal of fine modulation of hormone actions on target organs. Further modulation of target cell activity comes from inhibition of anterior pituitary hormone release by some hypothalamic hormones. As illustrated in Figure 39–6, hypothalamic hormones may either inhibit or stimulate the release of hormones from the anterior pituitary gland. Secretion of anterior pituitary hormones is obviously dependent on whether inhibitory or stimulatory impulses predominate.

Hormone cross-sensitivity is also illustrated in Figure 39–6. Some hypothalamic hormones affect the secretion of more than one type of anterior pituitary hormone. For example, TRH stimulates the anterior pituitary release of both TSH and prolactin. Thus, in situations in which TRH is released, the potential for prolactin release is also present.

The hypothalamic and pituitary hormones exemplify the complexity of endocrine interactions. In addition to interactions between various hormones, other influences such as neuron activity, circadian rhythms, ion and metabolite concentrations, and temperature also affect endocrine function profoundly.[3]

Categories of Endocrine Disease

Endocrine pathologies can be divided into three general categories—diseases of hyposecretion, hypersecretion, and target cell hyporesponsiveness.

Hyposecretion

Primary hyposecretion occurs when an endocrine organ such as the thyroid gland releases an inadequate amount of hormone to meet physiologic needs. Secondary hyposecretion occurs when secretion of a tropic hormone such as TSH is inadequate to cause the thyroid gland to secrete adequate amounts of thyroid hormone. The diagnosis of hormone deficiency is complex, as knowledge of tropic and releasing hormone levels as well as the deficient hormone level is necessary. In a primary thyroid hormone deficiency, thyroid hormone would be low but TSH levels would be high, as the anterior pituitary would not be receiving negative feedback from thyroid hormone. However, in secondary thyroid hormone deficiency, thyroid hormone and TSH concentrations would both be abnormally low.

Hypersecretion

Hypersecretion disorders can also be either primary or secondary. When a gland is secreting an abnormally high amount of a hormone, the tropic hormone will be at unusually low plasma levels due to excessive negative feedback. If hypersecretion is secondary to elevated tropic hormone levels, the plasma concentration of both the hormone in question and its tropic hormone will be elevated. Excessive plasma hormone levels can also occur secondary to hormone secretion by an ectopic source, as sometimes occurs with malignancies.

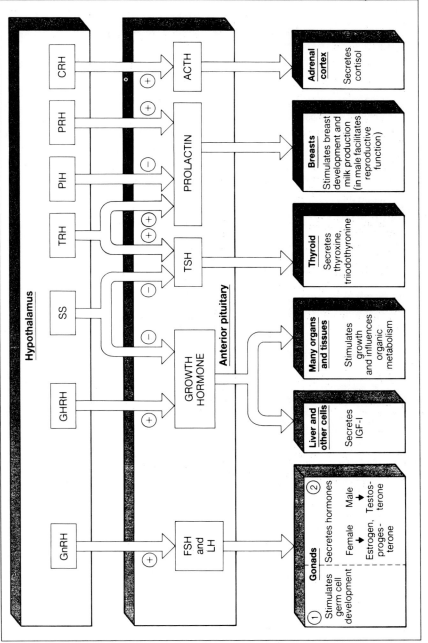

FIGURE 39-6. Relationship of the hypothalamic and pituitary hormones. GnRH, gonadotropin-releasing hormone; GHRH, growth hormone–releasing hormone; SS, somatostatin; TRH, thyroid-releasing hormone; PIH, prolactin-inhibiting hormone; PRH, prolactin-releasing hormone; CRH, corticotropin-releasing hormone; FSH, follicle-stimulating hormone; LH, leuteinizing hormone; TSH, thyroid-stimulating hormone; ACTH, adrenocorticotropic hormone; IGF-1, insulin-like growth factor 1. (From Vander AJ, Sherman JH, Luciano DJ: *Human Physiology: The Mechanisms of Body Function*, 5th ed. New York, McGraw-Hill, 1990, p 273. Reproduced with permission of McGraw-Hill, Inc.)

Hyporesponsiveness

Finally, hyporesponsiveness of the target organ will cause the same set of clinical symptoms as hyposecretion. The usual cause of hyporesponsiveness is lack of or a deficiency in receptors. If the target cell does not have appropriate receptors for a hormone, the clinical symptoms will be the same as if inadequate hormone levels were reaching the target cells. However, plasma concentrations of hormone would be expected to be normal or high, due to lack of negative feedback to hormone-secreting organs. For example, some diabetics have a lack of receptors for insulin. Despite high circulating insulin levels, these diabetics have high plasma glucose concentrations.[6]

The endocrine system allows communication and interactions to occur between anatomically distant cells. Virtually all body systems have some element of endocrine control. Hormones interact in complex ways during the most basic body process, that of obtaining energy for cellular reactions.

KEY CONCEPTS

- Oxytocin and vasopressin (antidiuretic hormone) are hormones of the posterior pituitary. They are synthesized in hypothalamic neurons that send axons to the posterior pituitary. Oxytocin is released during childbirth and suckling. Vasopressin is released in response to increased serum osmolality.

- Major hormones of the anterior pituitary are growth hormone, thyroid-stimulating hormone, prolactin, adrenocorticotropic hormone, and gonadotropins (luteinizing and follicle-stimulating hormones). The release of anterior pituitary hormones is regulated by releasing and inhibiting hormones secreted into pituitary portal blood by the hypothalamus. Many factor influence the release of releasing and inhibiting hormones, including circadian rhythms, hormone release from target cells, emotions, and pain.

- Endocrine disorders occur because of hyposecretion, hypersecretion, or lack of responsiveness by target cells. Hyporesponsiveness is clinically similar to hyposecretion and usually results from lack of functional receptors.

- Endocrine disorders may be due to abnormal tropic signals from the pituitary or to dysfunction of target glands (e.g., thyroid, adrenal cortex). Secondary disorders are due to abnormalities of pituitary hormone secretion. Primary disorders are due to abnormalities of the target gland. With secondary hypersecretion, pituitary hormone levels are high; with primary hypersecretion, pituitary hormone levels are low due to excessive negative feedback. With secondary hyposecretion, pituitary hormone levels are low; with primary hyposecretion, pituitary levels are high due to lack of negative feedback.

Metabolism

Each moment millions of chemical reactions occur within our body to create or expend energy to meet our physiologic needs. The total process, known as **metabolism,** utilizes energy to sustain the body's vital functions.[13] Metabolism involves the synthesis and breakdown of molecules with the resultant provision of energy. These interrelated and dynamic reactions occur to meet the obligatory function requirements of each body cell.[3]

Anabolism and Catabolism

Anabolism refers to the constructive phase of metabolism and involves the creation of organic molecules by cells. Larger molecules are built from smaller ones and in the process energy is used. Anabolism occurs during times of rest, healing, pregnancy, lactation, and growth. Hormonal secretions such as insulin and sex hormones may also trigger anabolism. Obesity, with the accumulation of adipose tissue, is anabolism taken to extreme.[14] Conversely, **catabolism** is the destructive phase of metabolism. Complex molecules are broken down into simpler substances with the concurrent release or production of energy. During times of disease, stress, fever, or starvation, or during the release of certain hormones such as thyroid hormone and cortisol, catabolism dominates the body's metabolic processes. Resultant tissue wasting leading to death occurs if excessive catabolism is left unresolved.[15] Anabolism and catabolism occur simultaneously and together create the dynamic balance of substance and energy known as metabolism.

The metabolic process requires nutrition in the form of carbohydrates, fats, and proteins. Each of these three nutrients is altered or broken down into simpler substances. The process may be accomplished by enzymes, or their coenzymes derived from vitamins and hormones, to produce glucose, fatty acids and amino acids. In this fashion the body's continual cellular energy requirements are met.[15]

The energy produced by metabolic processes is used to create the energy currency of the body known as **adenosine triphosphate.** ATP consists of adenine, ribose, and three phosphate radicals. Loss of one phosphate radical produces adenosine diphosphate (ADP), while loss of two phosphates produces adenosine monophosphate (AMP). Energy is produced with the destruction of the phosphate bonds. Located in the cytoplasm and nucleoplasm of all cells, ATP or other high-energy compounds provide the energy necessary for normal cellular function. Cells use ATP to release energy for the performance of mechanical work such as muscle contraction, transport of chemicals across cell membranes, and synthesis of chemical compounds. Continual cellular consumption of energy is enabled either by the release of high-energy phosphate bonds from ATP or by the re-creation of ATP through cellular oxidation of food.[15]

Cells use energy to perform essential body processes. **Energy** is measured in units of kilocalories (kcal); 1 kcal represents the amount of energy required to raise the temperature of 1 kilogram of water from 15° to 16° centigrade. During catabolism of fuel molecules, approximately 40 percent of the available energy is converted to ATP, with the remaining 60 percent being used for the production of heat.[3] The body, unable to use heat as an energy source, uses it for maintaining body temperature.

Metabolic Rate

Several factors determine the body's energy requirements or metabolic needs, including basal metabolic rate, activity level, and the energy necessary for digestion.[15]

Basal metabolic rate (BMR) refers to the rate of internal chemical activity of resting tissue. It is the measurement of the energy produced in the maintenance of the body at rest after a 12-hour fast.[15] It represents the energy used in maintaining basic body processes such as respiration, cellular metabolism, circulation, glandular activity, and the maintenance of body temperature.[15]

The body's BMR is determined by calculating oxygen use during a specific period of time. The normal range for BMR is generally between 0.8 and 1.43 kcal/min.[15] Several factors that affect an individual's basal metabolic rate are described in Table 39–4. Body stature and size affects BMR by the amount of heat lost from the body surface. Age is also an important determinant of BMR. The growing child's BMR is significantly higher than an adult's, primarily because of an increased rate of cellular reactions and the generation of new tissues.[15] Conversely, as one ages, the BMR gradually declines by about 2 percent per decade. Body composition, determined by the amount of fat tissue, also affects BMR. Muscle tissue requires more oxygen than adipose tissue, which explains why athletes have approximately a 5 percent higher BMR than nonathletes.[3] Women typically have a metabolic rate 5 to 10 percent less than men's, probably due to differences in body mass. Women also tend to have more adipose tissue than men, and fat is less metabolically active than muscle.[14] Pregnancy increases BMR by about 20 to 28 percent or 300 calories per day as a consequence of increased uterine and mammary gland size, fetal development, and additional cardiopulmonary work load.[15] Other factors affecting BMR include nutritional status, muscle tone, exercise, sleep, fever, environmental temperature, and stress.[3]

Almost any alteration in the body's normal homeostatic state will alter its energy requirements and BMR. Many diseases are known to dramatically increase the body's energy requirements; examples include chronic obstructive and restrictive pulmonary disease, hyperthermia, burns, cancer, diabetes, and Graves' disease (hyperthyroidism).

Nutrient Metabolism

Energy for the body is supplied by three classifications of nutrients: **carbohydrates, fats,** and **proteins.** These three groups of food sources supply the body with energy for ATP formation, but each acts in its own unique way. Metabolism in general is controlled by both the nervous system and the endocrine system. Four major hormones involved in substrate metabolism are insulin, glucagon, catecholamines, and cortisol. The effects of these four hormones on carbohydrate, fat, and protein metabolism are summarized in Tables 39–5 through 39–7. Both the nervous system and the endocrine system directly affect metabolism by the release of the catecholamines epinephrine and norepinephrine, which, during times of stress, inhibit insulin secretion. The liver and pancreatic hormones insulin and glucagon play a crucial role in the metabolic processes that govern the body's energy requirements. These hormones function antithetically, with insulin lowering blood glucose levels and glucagon ultimately increasing blood glucose levels.[3] Growth hormone affects metabolism by decreasing cellular uptake and use of glucose. High levels of growth hormone tend to decrease affinity for insulin at the receptor site such that even increased secretion of insulin by the pancreas has diminutive effects on blood glucose levels. Glucocorticoid hormones, primarily cortisol, stimulate gluconeogenesis by the liver. Blood glucose levels six to ten times normal may occur with significant cortisol secretion. Left uncorrected, diabetes mellitus may develop.[14]

Carbohydrates

Carbohydrates are the main energy source for the body and must be supplied in a fairly constant manner to meet energy requirements for normal body functioning. Approximately 45 percent of the typical American diet consists of carbohydrates, with almost half of that supplied in the form of simple sugars.[16] Dietary carbohydrates are starches or sugars and are composed of carbon, hydrogen, and oxygen molecules. Carbohydrates are classified into the three categories of **monosaccharides** (simple sugars), **oligosac-**

TABLE 39–4. Factors Affecting Basal Metabolic Rate

Increasing Metabolism	Decreasing Metabolism
Childhood growth	Aging process
Exercise	End-stage illnesses
Sympathetic stimulation	Starvation
Shivering	Sleep
Fever	Tropical climates
Thyroid hormone	
Muscle tissue	
Pregnancy	
Stress	
Male sex hormone	

charides (2 to 10 joined monosaccharide units), and **polysaccharides** (10 to 10,000 monosaccharide units). They range from very simple sugars consisting of three to seven carbons to incredibly complex polymers made up of repeating units of thousands of monosaccharides.[15]

Monosaccharides are the simplest form of carbohydrates. The most common in this category are the 6-carbon sugars of glucose, mannose, fructose, and galactose. Glucose, the most physiologically important of the group, is the form of sugar normally found in the bloodstream. Glucose is derived from the catabolism of more complex carbohydrates during the process of digestion. Fructose and galactose are also eventually converted to glucose by the liver. Once in the bloodstream, glucose is either oxidized to provide cellular energy or stored in the liver and muscles as glycogen. Blood sugar levels then reflect the difference between the amount of glucose released into the bloodstream by the liver and the amount of glucose taken up by the cell for energy.[14]

Intracellular Glucose Metabolism

Once in the cell, glucose undergoes additional breakdown, called **glycolysis,** which is the metabolic sequence that converts glucose to pyruvate and eventually yields the end products of carbon dioxide and water.[15] Catabolism of glucose may occur anaerobically along the Embden-Meyerhof pathway which, in a ten-step process, alters the chemical composition of glucose to pyruvic acid, resulting in a net gain of two ATP molecules for each molecule of glucose that enters the pathway. Pyruvic acid plays two important roles in the catabolic process of carbohydrates. It pro-

vides the body with acetyl coenzyme A, which is required for fatty acids to be converted to energy, and it is the initial step for the second stage of carbohydrate metabolism, the aerobically dependent Krebs cycle. The Krebs or citric acid cycle occurs in the mitochondria of the cell and provides approximately 90 percent of the body's energy. Though inherently complex, the Krebs cycle produces a total of 36 molecules of ATP for each molecule of glucose, ultimately yielding two carbon dioxide molecules and four hydrogen molecule pairs. Though other pathways do exist, the interrelated Embden-Meyerhof pathway and Krebs cycle produce nearly all the energy required for cellular functioning.[15] Figure 39–7 illustrates the metabolism of carbohydrates, fats, and proteins through the anaerobic Embden-Meyerhof and the aerobic Krebs pathways.

Just as glucose is constantly being catabolized for the production of energy, it is also continually being created. **Gluconeogenesis** refers to the process by which glucose is formed from noncarbohydrate sources, including amino acids supplied by muscle tissue and glycerol supplied from fat breakdown.[16] The glucose created through this mechanism may either be stored in the liver as glycogen or released into the bloodstream. During periods of fasting, gluconeogenesis provides the necessary glucose to meet the metabolic requirements of the brain and other glucose-dependent tissues.[14]

Hormonal Control of Glucose Metabolism

Many hormones affect glucose levels by either increasing or decreasing carbohydrate metabolism. The only hormone known to lower blood glucose levels is insu-

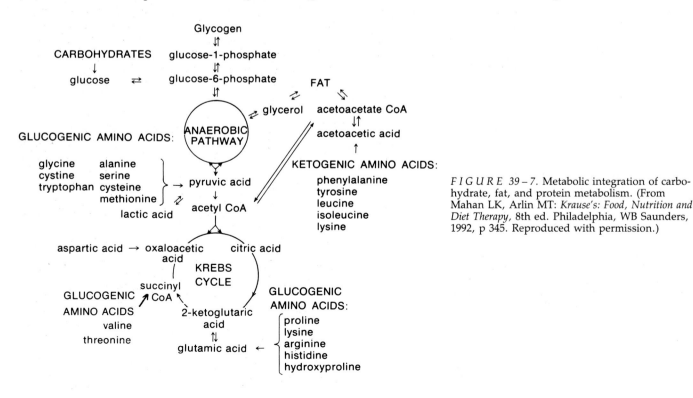

F I G U R E   3 9 – 7. Metabolic integration of carbohydrate, fat, and protein metabolism. (From Mahan LK, Arlin MT: *Krause's: Food, Nutrition and Diet Therapy,* 8th ed. Philadelphia, WB Saunders, 1992, p 345. Reproduced with permission.)

TABLE 39-5. Hormonal Actions on Carbohydrate Metabolism

Hormone	Actions
Insulin	Stimulates glucose uptake by the cells
	Stimulates glycolosis
	Inhibits gluconeogenesis
Glucagon	Stimulates glycogen breakdown
	Increases gluconeogenesis
Catecholamines	Maintain blood glucose level during stress
	Diminish glucose uptake by the cells
	Increase glycogen breakdown
Cortisol	Stimulates gluconeogenesis
	Diminishes glucose uptake by the cells

lin. Hormones that tend to raise blood glucose levels include glucagon, growth hormone, glucocorticoid hormones, epinephrine and norepinephrine, and thyroid hormone. Table 39–5 describes the major hormonal effects on glucose metabolism.

Insulin. Formed from its precursor proinsulin and synthesized by the beta cells in the pancreas, insulin is secreted in response to increased blood glucose levels. Minutes after ingestion of a meal, insulin levels in the blood rise significantly, peaking in 30 minutes and leveling off in about 3 hours. Between meals, when blood glucose levels tend to drop, insulin levels also remain low. At that time, glucose and amino acids stores are used for cellular energy requirements.[14]

Insulin directly affects glucose metabolism by promoting glucose uptake by the liver, which then favors the synthesis of glycogen. Glucose formation (**gluconeogenesis**) and the breakdown of glycogen to form glucose (**glycogenolysis**) are inhibited by insulin. The active transport of glucose across cellular membranes into the muscle and adipose tissues is facilitated by insulin. This has a direct lowering effect on blood glucose levels.[17] In diabetes mellitus there is either insulin hyposecretion or cellular hyporesponsiveness to insulin as a consequence of receptor downregulation. Obese and elderly persons are especially at risk for developing insulin receptor downregulation with resultant diabetes. Diabetes mellitus is discussed in Chapter 41.

Glucagon. The protein hormone glucagon is secreted by the alpha cells in the pancreas and also by some cells lining the gastrointestinal tract. Acting in a fashion exactly opposite that of insulin, glucagon increases blood glucose levels.[18] As blood glucose levels begin to drop, plasma glucagon levels begin to rise. The two primary effects of glucagon, then, are to promote the breakdown of liver glycogen with subsequent release of glucose into the bloodstream and to promote liver gluconeogenesis. These actions tend to bring serum glucose levels back to normal. Conversely, as glucose levels rise, glucagon secretion is diminished and serum glucose levels drop toward normal. This is a classic example of the negative feed-

back system discussed earlier in this chapter. The diametric actions of insulin and glucagon partially explain why increased glucagon secretion may also play a role in the elevated blood glucose levels as seen in diabetes mellitus.[3]

Catecholamines. In carbohydrate metabolism, the primary role of the catecholamines epinephrine and norepinephrine is to maintain blood glucose levels during times of stress. As the stress response occurs, catecholamines stimulate the conversion of glycogen to glucose in the muscles and liver. Although muscles, unlike the liver, cannot release glucose into the general circulation, mobilization of muscle glycogen frees up unused blood glucose for other tissues such as the brain and the peripheral nervous system. The second primary action of epinephrine during the stress response is to stimulate glucagon secretion and prevent insulin release from the pancreas, thereby preventing glucose movement into muscle cells. Epinephrine also promotes glycogenolysis by the liver and muscles and reduces uptake of glucose by muscle tissues. The role of catecholamines in glucose metabolism is very similar to that of glucagon and opposite that of insulin.[3]

Glucocorticoid Hormones. Cortisol, the primary glucocorticoid hormone secreted from the adrenal cortex, acts as an insulin antagonist to maintain serum glucose levels. During fasting, cortisol permissively enables other hormonal changes to occur, such as decreased insulin production and increased glucagon and epinephrine secretion. The end result is promotion of gluconeogenesis and lipolysis. If cortisol deficiency occurs simultaneously with fasting, hypoglycemic reactions significant enough to alter brain functioning can occur. A recent study indicated that cortisol deficiency may be a significant cause of morbidity and mortality in critically ill surgical patients, who frequently are poorly nourished.[19]

Growth Hormone. Although the role of growth hormone in carbohydrate metabolism is minor in comparison to its role in growth regulation and protein anabolism, it can have a significant impact under certain circumstances. Growth hormone's effects parallel those of cortisol; growth hormone increases gluconeogenesis in the liver and inhibits glucose uptake by muscle cells.[3] Elevated serum growth hormone levels tend to increase blood glucose levels. As a result, stimulation of the insulin-secreting beta cells in the pancreas occurs. If this process is not corrected, the beta cells will eventually be exhausted. It is for this reason that people with excessive growth hormone, as in acromegaly, eventually develop diabetes mellitus.[14]

Thyroid Hormone. The major physiologically active thyroid hormone is triiodothyrone (T_3). Thyroid hormone tends to raise blood glucose levels. In carbohydrate metabolism, the primary mode of action is to increase glucose absorption from the intestines and stimulate the release of epinephrine. Thyroid hormone also promotes the rate of insulin destruction. Ultimately, thyroid hormone exerts an influence to increase cellular oxygen consumption and the general metabolic rate of tissues.

Fats

Fats, the most concentrated form of energy, are derived from animal fats and vegetable oils. Fats supply 9 kilocalories of energy per gram, compared to 4 kilocalories from glucose and 4 kilocalories from protein. Fats are 98 percent **triglycerides.** Like carbohydrates, fats are made up of carbon, hydrogen, and oxygen. The bulk of each triglyceride molecule consists of fatty acids containing from four to 30 carbon atoms. Fats are frequently categorized as *saturated* or *unsaturated.* Figure 39–8 gives the chemical composition of some common saturated and unsaturated fatty acids. The degree of hydrogen **saturation** refers to the number of double bonds between the carbon atoms in the chain. If a fatty acid chain contains all the hydrogen molecules possible with no double bonds, it is called a *saturated fatty acid.* Those fatty acids with one double bond are typed as *monounsaturated* and those with several double bonds are *polyunsaturated fatty acids.*[15]

Fats in the form of triglycerides supply approximately two thirds of the cell's total energy requirements. Whereas the human body is able to economically store usable fats in adipose tissue, approximately 140,000 kilocalories, it can store only 24,000 kilocalories of protein and a mere 800 kilocalories of carbohydrates in the adult man.[18] Carbohydrates and amino acids not immediately used by the tissues are converted to fat and stored, along with ingested fat, as adipose tissue. Fat deposits are extremely important in the economical use of metabolites. If intake exceeds use, obesity results. During times of fasting, the body quickly reverts to the breakdown and use of fats as its energy source.[2] All tissues in the body, with the exception of brain cells, can metabolize and utilize fats as an energy source as effectively as glucose.[18]

Almost all fats are absorbed into the lymph system from the intestinal mucosa. They are then converted to a chylomicron consisting of 80 percent triglyceride, 9 percent cholesterol, 7 percent phospholipid, and 4 percent lipoprotein coat.[20] Chylomicrons empty into the venous blood at the thoracic duct and are carried to the liver for metabolism or assimilated into adipose tissue. Once in the liver, triglycerides are generally hydrolyzed into glycerol and fatty acids in a process known as **lipolysis.** Released, the fatty acids, bound to albumin, are quickly assimilated into the tissues. Oxidation in the tissues begins when acetylcoenzyme A binds to the end of a fatty acid. Progressing through a series of reactions known as beta oxidation, the fatty acid chain is shortened by two carbon atoms until all the carbon atoms have been transferred to coenzyme A. Acetylcoenzyme A then enters the Krebs cycle with each 2-carbon segment producing two molecules of carbon dioxide and 12 molecules of ATP. The average fatty acid contains approximately 18 carbon molecules, with 146 ATP molecules being produced during catabolism.[3] Unlike fatty acids, glycerol (the other component of triglycerides) can only be metabolized by a few tissues. Glycerol is generally carried to the liver, where it is either oxidized for energy or used to generate new triglycerides.

Within the liver, fatty acids are generally transformed to acetylcoenzyme A, which is further processed into one of three compounds collectively known as **ketone bodies.** Once released into the bloodstream, ketones play a critical role as an energy source for tissues able to oxidize them in the Krebs cycle. During a fasting state, tissues use ketones as a primary energy source, sparing glucose for brain metabolism. If the fasting state continues, many areas of the brain begin to use ketone bodies as an energy source. As the brain begins to use ketones, less protein is broken down to provide glucose. For this reason, the body is able to withstand periods of fasting with minimal protein breakdown and tissue disruption.[3]

The liver is the major organ responsible for lipid metabolism and regulation of serum lipid levels. The four primary functions of the hepatic system in regard to lipid metabolism are (1) synthesis of triglycerides from carbohydrates and proteins, (2) synthesis of phospholipids and cholesterol from triglycerides, (3) desaturation of fatty acids, and (4) utilization of triglycerides as an energy source.[15] Liver disease can significantly alter any of these processes, leading to serious metabolic disturbances. A fatty liver is characterized by fat deposits in the liver cells caused by either ingestion of hepatotoxic substances such as alcohol or halocarbons or by diets significantly low in proteins for a prolonged period of time. Infections treated with protein synthesis–inhibiting antibiotics such as tetracycline and malignancies may also lead to increased fat deposits within the liver by adversely affecting the hepatic cells or biliary tract. Increased mobilization of fatty acids from adipose tissue to the liver occurs in certain disease states such as diabetes mellitus or starvation, and in obesity where lipogenesis exceeds the ability of the liver to export the fat as lipoproteins.[21] Metabolic studies of critically ill patients indicate that fatty acid breakdown occurs at a much higher rate than patient caloric needs require. This excess lipolysis may cause fatty liver in these patients.[22]

Hormonal Control of Lipid Metabolism

Because carbohydrates and lipids may both be metabolized along the anaerobic Embden-Meyerhof pathway, hormones that affect carbohydrate metabolism also affect lipid metabolism. Table 39–6 describes those hormones that are considered to have the greatest effect on lipid metabolism. They include insulin, thyroid hormone, glucocorticoids, mineralocorticoids, growth hormone, epinephrine, and norepinephrine. Insulin prevents fat utilization by indirectly causing fatty

---

18-Carbon Fatty Acids

Stearic Acid	$CH_3(CH_2)_{16}COOH$ (saturated)
Oleic Acid	$CH_3(CH_2)_7CH=CH(CH_2)_7COOH$ (monounsaturated)
Linoleic Acid	$CH_3(CH_2)_4CH=CHCH_2CH=CH(CH_7)COOH$ (polyunsaturated)

F I G U R E 39 – 8. Chemical composition of some fatty acids.

TABLE 39–6. Hormonal Actions on Fat Metabolism

Hormone	Actions
Insulin	Increases fatty acid uptake by fat cells Promotes glucose uptake by fat cells
Glucagon	Promotes lipolysis in fat cells
Catecholamines	Increase fat mobilization Increase serum free fatty acid levels
Cortisol	Increases fat cell membrane permeability

acids to be taken up by adipose tissue and by decreasing the activity of hormone-sensitive lipase (HSL), which promotes the movement of fat out of adipose tissue. Glucocorticoids increase fat cell membrane permeability while mineralocorticoids increase the activity of HSL. Epinephrine and norepinephrine increase fat mobilization by stimulating the activity of HSL, thus increasing the serum free fatty acid level. Growth hormone increases fatty acid mobilization and use by tissues as an energy source.[15]

Proteins

Proteins are composed of nitrogen, carbon, hydrogen, oxygen, and occasionally sulfur. When hydrolyzed, they yield amino acids. Twenty-two amino acids have been identified in proteins, eight of which are essential—meaning that they must be supplied through the diet.[20] Muscle tissue, bones, teeth, skin, and hair are made up primarily of proteins. To function properly, most body processes require an adequate supply of proteins, many of which must be obtained through a balanced diet. Children, because of their rapid growth, require more protein per kilogram of body weight than adults. In addition, compared to adults, children also need a larger percentage of their dietary intake of proteins to contain essential amino acids.

Once ingested, proteins are broken down into amino acids or peptides and absorbed through the intestinal lumen. They are then carried to the liver through the portal vein. The liver regulates protein metabolism through the enzymatic breakdown of amino acids, the formation of nonessential amino acids from simple precursors, and the detoxification of ammonia, urea, uric acid, and other catabolic end products. Proteins are quickly synthesized and broken down by the liver, enabling a quick response to changing metabolic demands. Amino acids supplied in excess of metabolic requirements are degraded to by-products such as urea, uric acid, or creatinine, and the remaining carbon molecules are converted to carbohydrate and fat or oxidized for energy.[23] Of particular importance is the conversion of amino acids to fatty acids, which are carbohydrate-like in structure, created by the removal of the amino group during deamination. These keto acids may then enter the Krebs cycle, where they provide energy for liver metabolism, or they may be converted to fatty acids by the liver.

Protein metabolism can be measured in terms of **nitrogen balance.** If nitrogen intake approximates output, an equal nitrogen balance exists. If dietary intake of proteins exceeds output, a *positive nitrogen balance* occurs. Protein anabolism exceeds catabolism during periods of rapid growth, pregnancy, and during the formation of new tissue. Experimentally, positive nitrogen balance has been induced in malnourished patients through the administration of growth hormone.[24] A *negative nitrogen balance* occurs when protein breakdown exceeds daily protein intake and synthesis. If the daily caloric intake is insufficient, the body catabolizes dietary and tissue proteins for energy, as is the case after severe burns and during fever, illness, or stress.[3]

Hormonal Control of Protein Metabolism

Anabolic and catabolic protein metabolism is controlled by various hormones. Table 39–7 lists the major hormonal effects on protein metabolism. Hormones that also promote protein synthesis include growth hormone, especially during growth spurts; testosterone in specific reproductive organs during puberty; and indirectly thyroid hormone, by increasing the metabolic rate. Insulin also promotes the active transport of amino acids across cell membranes and accelerates protein synthesis within the cell. Insulin, in concert with growth hormone, is required for normal growth and development of children and adolescents. Glucagon, whose actions diametrically oppose those of insulin, promotes gluconeogenesis by stimulating the breakdown of proteins into amino acids and increasing their transport into hepatic cells. Glucagon also enables the conversion of amino acids into glucose precursors.

Aging and Metabolic Function

There is little doubt that the aging process has an effect on normal metabolism. It is sometimes difficult, however, to distinguish the effects of aging from the effects of chronic illness, drug therapy, or obesity.

There seems to be little difference in the ability of healthy people, young or old, to metabolize glucose, and little difference in insulin secretion by the beta cells in the pancreas. What does appear to occur with the aging process is a change in tissue sensitivity to insulin. Although many possible causes for this phenomenon have been proposed, such as reduced carbo-

TABLE 39–7. Hormonal Actions on Protein Metabolism

Hormone	Actions
Insulin	Actively transports amino acids into cells Accelerates cellular protein synthesis
Glucagon	Stimulates protein breakdown into amino acids Increases amino acid movement into hepatic cells
Cortisol	Increases protein catabolism

hydrate intake, decreased muscle mass, and lowered activity levels, the reason appears to lie in an alteration in the molecular makeup of insulin. The elderly have higher levels of circulating serum proinsulin than younger adults. It is also believed that the aging process alters the insulin receptor sites, rendering insulin less effective.[25]

Lipid metabolism may also be affected by the aging process as proportionate body fat increases. Although caloric intake generally decreases, a concurrent loss of lean body mass and a decline in energy expenditure begin with adulthood. A decline in resting metabolic rate also occurs with the aging process. This change is related to several factors such as reduced lean body mass, reduced lipogenic enzyme response to glucose, and decreased catecholamine secretion following a meal. Although cross-sectional studies demonstrate that cholesterol and triglyceride serum levels tend to rise with age, there is increasing evidence that this may be due more to obesity than to the aging process itself. As a risk factor, hyperlipidemia poses less threat for coronary artery disease and atherosclerosis with the aging process.[25]

A decrease in the quantity of skeletal muscle normally occurs with aging. Although this decrease in muscle is associated with factors such as physical inactivity and a decrease in the number of neurons to muscle cells, endocrine factors also influence the loss of muscle mass. Growth hormone secretion is decreased in elderly individuals, leading to decreased protein synthesis.[25]

KEY CONCEPTS

- Anabolism refers to energy-requiring processes that synthesize biomolecules; catabolism refers to energy-producing processes during which biomolecules are broken down into simpler forms. Metabolism refers to the dynamic state of simultaneously occurring anabolism and catabolism.
- The basal metabolic rate (BMR) is the rate of energy utilization when the body is at rest. Factors affecting the BMR include body size and composition, age, nutritional status, muscle mass, fever, stress, and pregnancy.
- Metabolism of carbohydrates, fats, and proteins provides energy to support the cell's energy-requiring processes and building blocks for synthesis of cellular biomolecules. The thyroid hormone primary hormonal regulators of nutrient metabolism are insulin, glucagon, catecholamines, cortisol, and growth hormone.
- Insulin is secreted from pancreatic beta cells in response to elevated serum glucose levels. Binding of insulin to receptors on target cells (muscle, adipose tissue) facilitates transport of glucose into cells and reduces blood glucose levels. Insulin inhibits lipolysis and gluconeogenesis.
- Glucagon is secreted from pancreatic alpha cells in response to low blood glucose levels. Glucagon promotes glycogenolysis and gluconeogenesis (from protein and glycerol) by the liver, thereby increasing blood glucose.

TABLE 39–8. Research in Endocrine Control and Metabolism

Research	Comments
Endocrine Control	
Streeten et al[8]	Baseline and stress-related activity of the hypothalamic-pituitary-adrenocortical system were studied in normal and abnormal subjects. In response to insulin-induced hypoglycemia, normal subjects exhibited an increase in plasma cortisol levels. Good correlation between the degree of hypoglycemia and the magnitude of the plasma cortisol response was obtained. Plasma cortisol response in abnormal subjects was significantly less.
Abi-Saad et al[19]	The presence of adrenal insufficiency (AI) was studied in critically ill surgical patients. Eight of 12 patients with high-risk criteria for AI were found to have AI. High-risk criteria were described as perioperative hypotension and the requirement for a vasopressor without a known etiology. Patients at high risk should be evaluated for AD and steroid replacement considered.
Metabolism	
Klein et al[22]	Lipolysis was measured in five critically ill patients. The potential energy released by fatty acid breakdown was almost double the rate of energy expenditure. The excess lipolysis would actually increase energy expenditure, as energy is required for reconversion of fatty acids to triglycerides in the liver. Stress-induced sympathetic nervous system activity was stated as the likely cause of the increase in lipolysis.
Ziegler et al[24]	The anabolic effects of growth hormone in malnourished surgical patients were studied. Administration of growth hormone resulted in significant weight gain, positive mineral and water balance, and positive nitrogen balance in patients receiving hypocaloric parenteral or enteral feedings.

THE AGING PROCESS: CHANGES IN THE ENDOCRINE SYSTEM

Decreased target organ sensitivity	Decreased levels of:	Decreased production and clearance of:	Increased levels of:
↓	Plasma somatomedin C	Thyroid hormones	Norepinephrine
Decreased receptor-ligand binding	T3	Cortisol	Parathyroid hormone
	Aldosterone	Aldosterone	Atrial natriuretic peptide
	Active renin	Inactive to active renin	Insulin
	Calcitonin	Norepinephrine clearance	Glucagon
	Arginine vasopressin		
	Glucose tolerance		
	Males: Nocturnal peak growth hormone		
	Females: Basal and nocturnal peak growth hormone		

Aging causes endocrine organ changes resulting in variable hormone activity, responsiveness, secretion rates, and target organ sensitivity. All endocrine glands in the elderly have an increased amount of connective tissue and changes in structure. For example, pituitary gland change is marked by increased pigment deposition, and adrenal gland change is identified by small cortex nodules.

Hormone secretion changes with age, but the change varies among the endocrine glands. For example with advancing age, adrenocorticotropic hormone (ACTH) secretion from the pituitary is unchanged while thyrotropic hormone (TSH) secretion increases and aldosterone secretion declines. And with aging, the rate of cortisol secretion (glucocorticoid) from the adrenal gland is decreased, but the basal level of cortisol is unchanged because of its prolonged degradation rate.

Blood osmolality receptors in the brain increase their sensitivity to antidiuretic hormone (ADH) secretion, but target organ (kidney) response to ADH declines with advancing age. In some instances, increased levels of hormones in the plasma are caused by decreased target organ responsiveness. For example, the levels of gonadotropins – follicle-stimulating hormone (FSH) and luteinizing hormone (LH) – continue to rise with age, but the ovaries and testes do not respond.

- Catecholamines increase glycogenolysis and gluconeogenesis by the liver, thereby increasing blood glucose levels. Catecholamines also stimulate lipolysis in adipose cells by enhancing the action of hormone-sensitive lipase. Glucagon secretion is enhanced and insulin secretion is inhibited by catecholamines.

- Cortisol enhances the actions of glucagon and catecholamines and promotes glycogenolysis, gluconeogenesis, and lipolysis, thus raising blood levels of glucose and fatty acids.

- Growth hormone increases blood glucose by inhibiting uptake by muscle cells and by stimulating gluconeogenesis in the liver. Growth hormone enhances cellular uptake of amino acids and stimulates protein synthesis.

- The main sources of cellular energy are glucose and fatty acids. Glucose is the primary energy source for the brain, although it can utilize ketones. Ketones are produced from fatty acids by the liver, particularly under conditions of decreased carbohydrate intake.

Summary

Metabolism is a dynamic and static process affecting every organ and physiologic process within the human system. The building phase of anabolic metabolism occurs concurrently with the energy-consuming and tearing-down phase of catabolic metabolism. All phases of metabolism either release or require energy in the form of ATP. The rate at which metabolism occurs within the resting human system is referred to as the basal metabolic rate, and the process releases both heat and energy. The metabolic fate of carbohydrates, proteins, and fats depends on cellular needs and systemic regulatory functions. The endocrine system greatly affects metabolism. Only one hormone, insulin, is known to lower serum glucose levels by decreasing liver glucose production and promoting the transfer of glucose into the cells. Although each works in a unique manner, growth hormone, cortisol, epinephrine, thyroid hormone, and glucagon all work in concert to maintain or raise blood glucose levels. Table 39–8 (page 794) summarizes recent research in endocrine control and metabolism.

The remaining chapters in this unit will discuss how abnormalities with the hormonal and metabolic systems can lead to physiologic abnormalities or illness. Alterations in growth and in thyroid and adrenal cortical hormones are examined, followed by a discussion of the pathophysiologic processes associated with diabetes mellitus.

REFERENCES

1. Cosgrove JA: Atrial natriuretic hormone: A new cardiac hormone. *Heart Lung* 1989;18(5):461–465.
2. Tepperman J, Tepperman HM: *Metabolic and Endocrine Physiology*, 5th ed. Chicago, Year Book Medical Publishers, 1987.
3. Vander AJ, Sherman JH, Luciano DJ: *Human Physiology: The Mechanisms of Body Function*, 5th ed. New York, McGraw-Hill, 1990.
4. Wilson JD, Foster DW: *Williams Textbook of Endocrinology*, 7th ed. Philadelphia, WB Saunders, 1985, pp 1–8.
5. Baxter JD: Principles of endocrinology, in Wyngaarden JB, Smith LH (eds): *Cecil Textbook of Medicine*, 18th ed. Philadelphia, WB Saunders, 1988, pp 1252–1268.
6. Roth J, Grunfeld C: Mechanism of action of peptide hormones and catecholamines, in Wilson JD, Foster DW: *Williams Textbook of Endocrinology*, 7th ed. Philadelphia, WB Saunders, 1985, pp 76–122.
7. Clark JH, Schrader WT, O'Malley BW: Mechanisms of steroid hormone action, in Wilson JD, Foster DW: *Williams Textbook of Endocrinology*, 7th ed. Philadelphia, WB Saunders, 1985, pp 33–75.
8. Streeten DHP, Anderson GH Jr, Dalakos TG, et al: Normal and abnormal function of the hypothalamic-pituitary-adrenocortical system in man. *Endocr Rev* 1984;5(3):371–394.
9. Rebar RW: The ovaries, in Wyngaarden JB, Smith LH (eds): *Cecil Textbook of Medicine*, 18th ed. Philadelphia, WB Saunders, 1988, pp 1424–1446.
10. Muldoon TG, Evans AC: Hormones and their receptors. *Arch Intern Med* 1988;148:961–967.
11. Fradkin JE, Eastman RC, Lesniak MA, Roth J: Specificity spillover at the hormone receptor: Exploring its role in human disease. *N Engl J Med* 1989;320(10):640–645.
12. Reichlin S: Neuroendocrinology, in Wilson JD, Foster DW: *Williams Textbook of Endocrinology*, 7th ed. Philadelphia, WB Saunders, 1985, pp 492–567.
13. Keesey RE: Physiological regulation of body weight and the issue of obesity. *Med Clin North Am* 1989;73:15–27.
14. Krause MV, Mahan LK: *Food, Nutrition, and Diet Therapy*, 7th ed. Philadelphia, WB Saunders, 1984.
15. Guyton AC: *Textbook of Medical Physiology*, 8th ed. Philadelphia, WB Saunders, 1991.
16. Hershman JM: *Endocrine Pathophysiology: A Patient-Oriented Approach*, 3rd ed. Philadelphia, Lea & Febiger, 1988.
17. Ignatavicius DD, Bayne MV: *Medical-Surgical Nursing: A Nursing Process Approach*. Philadelphia, WB Saunders, 1991.
18. Bray GA: Nutrient balance and obesity: An approach to control of food intake in humans. *Med Clin North Am* 1989;73(1):29–45.
19. Abi-Saad GS, Rivers EP, Horst HM, et al: Occult adrenal insufficiency in surgical intensive care patients. *Crit Care Med* 1991;19(4 suppl):S55. Abstract.
20. Mirtallo JM: Nutrient metabolism in health and disease, in DiPiro JT, Talbert RL, Hayes PE, Yee GC, Posey LM: *Pharmacotherapy: A Pathophysiologic Approach*. New York, Elsevier, 1989, pp 1151–1570.
21. McMurray WC: *Essentials of Human Metabolism: The Relationship of Biochemistry to Human Physiology*, 2nd ed. New York, Harper & Row, 1983.
22. Klein S, Peters EJ, Shangraw RE, Wolfe RR: Lipolytic response to metabolic stress in critically ill patients. *Crit Care Med* 1991;19(6):776–779.
23. Russe RM: Nutritional requirements, in Wyngaarden JB, Smith LH (eds): *Cecil Textbook of Medicine*, 18th ed. Philadelphia, WB Saunders, 1988, pp 1204–1208.
24. Ziegler TR, Young LS, Manson JM, Wilmore DW: Metabolic effects of recombinant human growth hormone in patients receiving parenteral nutrition. *Ann Surg* 1988;208(1):6–16.
25. MacLennan WJ, Peden NR: *Metabolic and Endocrine Problems in the Elderly*. London, Springer-Verlag, 1989.

BIBLIOGRAPHY

Bergstrom D: Hypermetabolism in multisystem organ failure: A nursing systems perspective. *Crit Care Nurs Q* 1992;15(3):63–70.
Carter LW: Influences of nutrition and stress on people at risk for neutropenia: Nursing implications. *Oncol Nurs Forum* 1993;20(8):1241–1250.
Dietz WH, Bandini LG, Morreli JA, Peers KS, Ching PLYH: Effect

of sedentary activities on resting metabolic rate. *Am J Clin Nutr* 1994;59:556–559.

Gianino S, St John RE: Nutritional assessment of the patient in the intensive care unit. *Crit Care Nurs Clin North Am* 1993;5(1):1–16.

Holmes S: Building blocks: How nutrients are assimilated. *Nurs Times* 1993;89(21):28–31.

Kelly KG: Advances in perioperative nutritional support. *Med Clin North Am* 1993;77(2):465–475.

Klesges RC, Shelton ML, Klesges LM: Effects of television on meta-bolic rate: Implications for childhood obesity. *Pediatrics* 1993;91(2):281–286.

Lehmann S: Nutritional support in the hypermetabolic patient. *Crit Care Nurs Clin North Am* 1993;5(1):97–103.

Rieg LS: Metabolic alterations and nutritional management. *AACN Clin Issues Crit Care Nurs* 1993;4(2):3888–3898.

Sikes P: Endocrine response to the stress of critical illness. *AACN Clin Issues Crit Care Nurs* 1992;3(2):379–391.

CHAPTER 40
Alterations in Endocrine Control of Growth and Metabolism

BRIDGET RECKER and LEE-ELLEN C. COPSTEAD

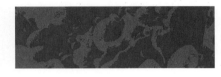

KEY TERMS

Addison's disease: Adrenal insufficiency, partial or total.

cretinism: Extreme hypothyroidism during infancy and childhood that causes mental and physical abnormalities.

Cushing's disease: Hyperfunctioning of the adrenal cortex with increased glucocorticoid (cortisol) secretion.

exophthalmos: Protrusion of the eyeballs.

glucocorticoids: A class of steroid hormones secreted by the adrenal cortex, necessary for use of sugars, fats, and proteins by the body and for the body's normal response to stress.

gluconeogenesis or glyconeogenesis: Formation of glucose or glycogen from protein and fats.

goiter: Enlargement of the thyroid gland.

Graves' disease: Hyperthyroid state characterized by exophthalmic goiter.

hormone: A chemical substance formed in an organ or other part of the body and carried in the blood to a distant organ or gland, where it acts to modify the structure or function of that organ or gland.

hyperthyroidism: Overactivity of the thyroid gland.

hypothalamus: A group of nuclei at the base of the brain concerned with regulation of body processes: temperature, thirst, hunger, satiety, and adaptive sexual behaviors.

hypothyroidism: Underactivity of the thyroid gland.

mineralocorticoids: A class of steroid hormones secreted by the adrenal cortex; regulate the mineral salts (electrolytes) and water balance in the body.

myxedema: Nonpitting edema caused by advanced hypothyroidism in adulthood.

panhypopituitarism: A condition of deficiency in all pituitary hormones.

pheochromocytoma: Tumor of the adrenal medulla that produces excess catecholamines.

---

*T*ogether with the nervous system, the endocrine system (the body's glands and their hormones) regulates body processes involving growth, maturation, metabolic functions, and reproduction. This regulation is carried out through the actions of the hormones produced and secreted by the endocrine glands. Endocrine glands release hormones directly into the bloodstream. **Hormones** are potent chemical messengers that exert a physiologic effect on specific target cells and tissues. In the healthy state, hormones are released by the glands when their action is needed and inhibited when their effect is attained. In disease, either hyperfunction (excessively high blood concentrations of a hormone, or conditions that mimic high hormone levels) or hypofunction (depressed levels, or conditions that mimic low hormone levels) exists.

This chapter discusses the anterior pituitary gland and alterations in growth hormone produced by the pituitary gland, the posterior pituitary gland and alterations in antidiuretic hormone produced by the posterior pituitary gland, the thyroid gland and alterations in thyroid hormone, the parathyroid glands and alterations in parathyroid hormone, and the adrenal glands and alterations in hormones secreted by the adrenal cortex and adrenal medulla. Table 40–1 lists the glands discussed in this chapter, the hormones produced by those glands, and the major actions of those hormones.

Basic Concepts of Endocrine Disorders

Hypothalamic-Pituitary Function

The **pituitary gland** is often called the master gland, in reference to its important role in stimulating other endocrine glands. It may be conceptualized as the orchestrator of endocrine function. The pituitary gland, or *hypophysis*, consists of a posterior lobe and an anterior lobe, sometimes referred to as the neurohypophysis and adenohypophysis, respectively. The anterior lobe of the pituitary is made up of three main types of cells: (1) the acidophils, or alpha cells, which secrete growth hormone (GH); (2) the basophils, or alpha and delta cells, which secrete thyroid-stimulating hormone (TSH), adrenocorticotropic hormone (ACTH), and gonadotropins (luteinizing hormone [LH], follicle-stimulating hormone [FSH]); and (3) chromophobes or gamma cells, which secrete prolactin (PRL).

The hormones produced by the anterior pituitary gland have direct actions on other endocrine glands in the body, with the exception of GH (Fig. 40–1).

Dysfunction, either hypo- or hypersecretion, may originate in the hypothalamic-pituitary unit, the hormone-producing gland, or the target organ (Fig. 40–2). The etiology of endocrine disorders may be

TABLE 40-1. Endocrine Glands, Hormones, and Major Actions

Gland	Hormone	Action
Pituitary Gland		
Anterior lobe	Growth hormone (GH), somatropin	Promotes growth of all tissues of the body capable of growing Increases rate of protein synthesis Decreases rate of carbohydrate utilization Increases mobilization of fats and use of fats for energy
	Thyrotropin-stimulating hormone (TSH)	Controls the rate of secretion of thyroxine by the thyroid gland
	Adrenocorticotropic hormone (ACTH)	Controls the secretion of some of the adrenocortical hormones
	Gonadotropins: Luteinizing hormone (LH) and follicle-stimulating hormone (FSH)	Control growth and reproductive activities of the gonads
	Prolactin (PRL)	Promotes mammary gland development, and initiation and maintenance of lactation
Posterior lobe	Antidiuretic hormone (ADH, vasopressin)	Important role in water conservation and maintenance of body fluid osmolality, blood volume, and blood pressure
	Oxytocin	Stimulates the flow of breast milk
Thyroid Gland	Thyroxine (T_4), triiodothyronine (T_3)	Regulate the body's metabolic rate
	Calcitonin	Can decrease blood calcium concentration
Parathyroid Gland	Parathyroid hormone (PTH)	Maintains normal calcium levels in the blood
Adrenal Glands		
Cortex	*Glucocorticoids:* Cortisol (major glucocorticoid)	Promotes gluconeogenesis by the liver, and storage of carbohydrate as glycogen
	Mineralocorticoids: Aldosterone (major mineralocorticoid)	Regulates electrolyte concentrations (Na^+, K^+) in the extracellular fluid
	Androgens: Dehydroepiandrosterone sulfate (DHS) Androstenedione (Δ_4) (major androgens)	Produce and maintain secondary sexual characteristics
Medulla	*Catecholamines:* Epinephrine	Actions are primarily inhibitory and metabolic: • increases excitability/contractility of the heart muscle • increases blood flow to muscle, brain • increases blood glucose levels • inhibits smooth muscle contraction
	Norepinephrine	Actions are excitatory: • vasoconstriction, increased blood pressure

congenital, infectious, necrotic, neoplastic, autoimmune, or idiopathic. The onset of the disorders can be slow and insidious or abrupt and life-threatening. The age at onset ranges from infancy to old age.

Classification of Endocrine Disorders

Endocrine disorders can be classified as **primary** (the result of glandular malfunction) or **secondary** (when an abnormal stimulus causes excess or inadequate hormone production). Measurement of pituitary and target gland hormones helps distinguish between primary and secondary endocrine failure. For example, inadequate ovarian estrogen secretion occurring with low LH and FSH levels indicates hypothalamic-pituitary disease, whereas a low estrogen level with elevated FSH and LH levels implies an ovarian disorder.

Endocrine disorders can also be classifed as **functional disorders caused by nonendocrine disease** such as chronic renal failure, liver disease, or heart failure. Dysfunction may arise if the end-organ fails to respond to the hormones. The presence of normal or elevated hormone levels without normal hormonal action indicates hormone resistance. This problem is also illustrated by diminished or absent response to the administration of exogenous hormones. The mechanisms of hormone resistance may be genetic or acquired and include defects at receptor sites, antibody reaction to hormone receptors, and defective postreceptor hormone action.

Abnormal hormone production frequently results from an inborn error of metabolism. Such defects include excessive production of hormone precursors due to a block in synthesis, and enzyme deficiencies that impair hormone synthesis. If such defects are not complete, increased stimuli may compensate by causing glandular hyperplasia, resulting in near-normal hormone levels.

In addition, hormones may be produced by nonendocrine tissue. Such ectopic hormone production is usually caused by a malignant tumor. Because pep-

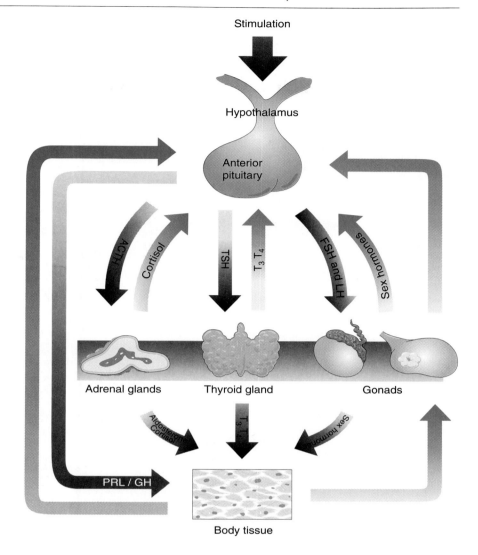

FIGURE 40–1. The hypothalamic-pituitary axis showing hormones, target glands and tissues, and negative feedback loops.

tides are more easily synthesized than steroids, most ectopic hormones are peptides. Although different tumors can produce hormones, some cell types are more commonly associated with specific tumors. For example, certain cells of endodermal origin, called amine precursor uptake and decarboxylation cells, are found in oat cell carcinomas of the lung and in tumors of the thymus and pancreas.[1]

Finally, some endocrine disorders may be induced by medical treatments such as therapy for a nonendocrine disorder or excessive therapy for an endocrine problem. These iatrogenic disorders can also be caused by chemotherapy, radiation therapy, or surgical removal of glands.

Clinical Manifestations and Treatment

Some endocrine disorders have such striking characteristics that recognition is obvious. Other symptoms of endocrine disease may be nonspecific and more difficult to detect. Observing and interviewing skills are important because, except for the thyroid and testicles, the endocrine glands cannot be directly exam-

ined. Laboratory diagnostic tests are especially important in assessing the endocrine system.

The treatment for endocrine disorders is varied and depends on the cause and classification of the problem. Methods such as surgical excision of tumor, radiation therapy, and hormonal replacement therapy may be employed.

KEY CONCEPTS

• Endocrine disorders occur because of hypersecretion, hyposecretion, or lack of responsiveness by target cells. *Hypersecretion* is usually due to secreting tumors or excessive stimulation of the gland by trophic signals. *Hyposecretion* may be due to congenital lack of glandular tissue, surgical removal of the gland, infarction, or lack of normal trophic signals. *Hyporesponsiveness* is clinically similar to hyposecretion and usually related to lack of functional receptors on the target cell.

• Endocrine disorders involving the hypothalamic-pituitary system are often classified as primary, secondary, and tertiary. *Primary endocrine disorders* re-

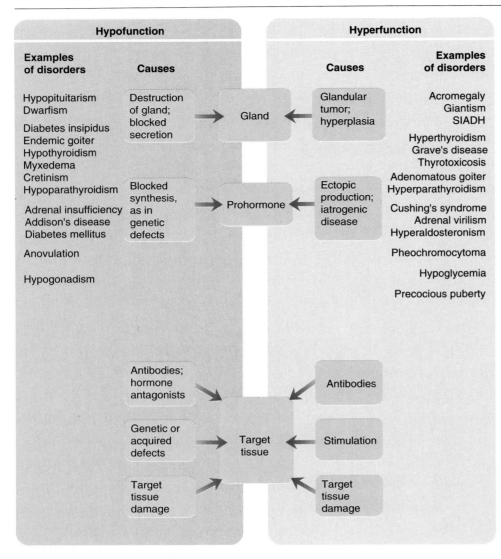

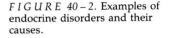

FIGURE 40-2. Examples of endocrine disorders and their causes.

sult from intrinsic defects within the target gland. *Secondary disorders* result from abnormal pituitary secretion of trophic signals. *Tertiary disorders* result from abnormal hypothalamic regulation of the pituitary gland. Manifestations of an endocrine disorder are due to abnormal target gland function and are therefore similar whether the etiology is primary, secondary, or tertiary.

Growth Hormone Disorders

Regulation and Actions of Growth Hormone

Pituitary GH secretion is controlled by hypothalamic release of growth hormone–releasing hormone (GHRH) and by the inhibitory control of somatostatin by somatotropin release–inhibiting hormone (SRIH). Defects or deficiencies in the secretion of GHRH or SRIH can result in decreased secretion of pituitary GH. Under normal physiologic conditions, the ante-

rior pituitary gland secretes small pulsatile amounts of GH each day. Approximately half the early production of GH in children occurs during the early night-time hours that follow the onset of deep sleep (stage 3 or 4).[2] Higher and more frequent pulses of GH release are noted during infancy and puberty. In adults, 24-hour studies reveal that half the GH released by the pituitary is in concentrations virtually undetectable with the current GH assay kits available.[3]

Growth hormone is a potent anabolic agent that causes the growth of all tissues of the body that are capable of responding to it. It promotes the increased size of cells and increased mitosis. It affects the body's metabolic processes by increasing the rate of protein synthesis, decreasing the rate of carbohydrate utilization, and increasing mobilization of fats and the use of fats for energy.[4] Generally, it is believed that GH indirectly regulates linear growth through its ability to stimulate production of growth factors (somatomedins), which in turn cause bone growth. Insulin-like growth factor 1 (IGF-1) is the main GH-dependent growth factor that stimulates linear growth in children. It is also involved in the negative feedback control of GH secretion.[2] Two thirds of pubertal growth is independent on GH secretion. In fact, testosterone-deficient boys grow well until puberty, and estrogen secretion in girls both stimulates GH secretion and inhibits skeletal growth.[2]

Growth Hormone Deficiency

Etiology and Pathogenesis

Alterations in GH secretion can be classified into four major categories: (1) decreased GH secretion, (2) defective GH action (structurally abnormal GH or defective GH receptor), (3) defective somatomedin generation, and (4) impaired response of cartilage to somatomedin (IGF-1). In the United States, GH deficiency occurs in 1 in 10,000 children.[5]

A birth history of prolonged labor or breech delivery is common.[5] GH deficiency may also be present in children who are born with midline craniocerebral defects, most likely due to congenital malformations or as sequelae of a chromosomal anomaly. There are data available that link pituitary stalk section defects (minor lesions or severing of the pituitary stalk) with GH deficiency.

The overall incidence of GH deficiency in adults is unknown, for usually only those who were diagnosed with GH deficiency as children are considered. Adults may become GH deficient after removal of brain tumors or after traumatic head injuries, but these adults are usually evaluated for deficiencies in pituitary hormones other than GH. GH is often excluded from evaluation because the action of GH in adults is less well understood than in children.

Classic GH Deficiency. Children with GH deficiency have a variety of presentations, depending on the cause of the deficiency, the age at onset, and the severity of the disorder. Idiopathic GH deficiency is more common than organic GH deficiency. The basis for this defect may be failure of the hypothalamus to stimulate pituitary GH secretion, or failure of the pituitary to produce GH.

Tumors. The most frequent tumors to influence hypothalamic pituitary function are midline brain tumors. These include gliomas of the optic nerve and craniopharyngiomas. Craniopharyngiomas are thought to arise from rests of squamous cells at the junction of the anterior and posterior pituitary gland. They are believed to be present at birth and are slow-growing. As the tumor increases in size, it compresses the pituitary gland.

Radiation. Radiation therapy for brain tumors or leukemia may cause damage to hypothalamic and pituitary function. The higher the dose of radiation, the greater is the risk of GH deficiency, because GH is the most radiation-sensitive hormone.

Trauma. Any insult to the skull or sella turcica may lead to impairment of pituitary function through damage to the gland itself or interruption of its flow of blood or hypothalamic stimulation.

Clinical Manifestations

GH-deficient infants usually have normal birth length and weight. They may experience hypoglycemia because GH, as well as cortisol, is necessary to maintain the euglycemic state. The hypoglycemia is generally related to prolonged fasting, which could be as short as 3 hours in an infant, and may be associated with the presence of ketone bodies in the blood and urine. During the newborn period, hypoglycemia may be associated with hyperbilirubinemias as well as with coexisting hypothyroidism. The tendency toward spontaneous hypoglycemia usually disappears between the second and fifth year of life. Recurrent episodes of hypoglycemia may lead to permanent cerebral damage and convulsive disorders. Additionally, closure of the anterior fontanelle is usually delayed.[2] Infants and children with GH deficiency usually are thin, and boys born with GH deficiency may have micropenis.

Infants in whom GH deficiency is not recognized or diagnosed during the newborn period usually achieve normal growth until 6 months of age. Children with GH deficiency may have a prominent forehead, poor development of the bridge of the nose, and truncal adiposity. Growth rates in affected children after 3 years of age are usually less than 4 cm/year. Older children with GH deficiency are overweight for height, and the skeletal age (bone age) in prepubertal children is always delayed. Delayed puberty is common, but puberty will occur if all other pituitary hormones are intact.[4] The skeletal age is usually proportional to the child's height age and delayed for the chronological age. Dental eruption is delayed, and the development and setting of the permanent teeth are irregular. The hair is thin, and the nail growth is poor. These children are usually healthy and have normal intelligence.

A craniopharyngioma can grow to a large size without producing typical signs of increased intracranial pressure (vomiting, headache, oculomotor abnormalities). In older children, growth failure may be the first symptom of a craniopharyngioma.[4]

Deficiencies in GH and other pituitary hormones need to be considered in any child with nystagmus or abnormalities of the optic disc and other midline or midfacial abnormalities such as cleft lip or palate.[6]

Little information exists regarding the manifestations of GH deficiency in adults. Adults with acquired pituitary deficiencies have rarely been studied for GH status. The data available come from mature individuals who were treated with GH in childhood for GH deficiency.

One study of adults who had been treated with GH in childhood reported their perceptions of their sense of well-being. In general, these adults indicated a poorer quality of life when compared to age- and sex-matched control subjects. They reported problems related to physical mobility, sleep, social isolation, pain, employment, sex life, interests, hobbies, and general health.[7] These findings must be interpreted with great caution, since these GH-deficient

T A B L E 40–2. Signs and Symptoms of Growth Hormone Imbalance

Growth Hormone Excess	Growth Hormone Deficiency
Children	*Children*
Increased linear growth and tall stature	Delayed growth Fine features Short stature, proportionate
Adults	*Adults*
Soft tissue hypertrophy Increased bone density Large hands, feet Coarse facial features Thick, leathery skin Weight gain Glucose intolerance	May be associated with hypo-secretion of other pituitary hormones

adults were shorter than average and had other pituitary hormone deficiencies that could explain their perceptions.[3]

Children's growth should be evaluated annually. If growth velocity is abnormal, an endocrinology evaluation and physiologic tests to stimulate GH release can be planned. There are many pharmacologic agents available that stimulate GH secretion in children, among them insulin, arginine, levodopa, and clonidine. Children's neurosecretory GH patterns can be studied by obtaining timed serum GH samples during a normal nighttime sleep cycle. Also, GHRH can be administered to stimulate GH secretion and clarify the presence of a hypothalamic defect of GH deficiency.

Diagnostic tests for adult-onset (acquired) GH deficiency are rarely done because it is unclear what the manifestations and implications are for adult health. Diagnostic tests are designed to stimulate the release of GH from the pituitary gland. The standard methods for diagnosing GH deficiency in children, as well the GH assay kits, must be adapted for assessing adults, because GH levels in adults are significantly lower than those found during normal growth and development.[8] Table 40–2 summarizes the signs and symptoms of GH imbalance.

Treatment

Hormonal replacement therapy for GH-deficient children has been available for about 30 years. In the early years, the supply of GH was limited and its use was under strict control. In the past decade, biosynthetic GH has become available. This advance has led to the earlier diagnosis and treatment of children with poor growth velocity and GH deficiency.

The most obvious effect of GH is stimulation of growth in children with bones that have not fused or closed. With treatment, children experience an increase in growth velocity as well as depletion of the fat stores noted in GH-deficient children. GH injections are given subcutaneously 3 to 7 days a week. Younger children appear to respond better than older

children, as do children with significantly delayed heights and bone ages.

Investigators are studying the effects of GH treatment on the growth of children with Turner's syndrome, chronic renal failure, and intrauterine growth retardation. Others are conducting trials of GH in healing and its effect on hospital length of stay in adult patients with burns, severe injuries, and postoperative wounds.

The success of GH replacement therapy can be measured by improved growth velocity and attainment of an adult height that is normal for the individual's genetic background. Parents and children need to discuss the benefits of treatment prior to its initiation. The family's concept of improved growth and ultimate adult height may not be realistic; therefore, this issue needs to be identified and clarified early in the course of treatment. Many children like being petite or small, as it may gain them special attention in school or at home. All children with GH deficiency should be evaluated by trained psychologists, because reports have indicated that GH-deficient children have a high incidence of academic underachievement, learning disabilities, or slightly lower IQ scores.[5]

Children with GH deficiency and their parents should be routinely seen by a nurse and a pediatric endocrinologist trained to work with children with hormonal deficiencies. This approach allows evaluation of the family's expectations and perceptions of the responses to treatment and will help in identifying new problems as they arise. Because the children appear much younger than their chronological age, friends, parents, teachers, and coaches need to be made aware that children with GH deficiency are older than they appear and should be treated and expected to perform as their age-matched peers.

The side effects of GH when given to GH-deficient children have been minor. There are reported cases of GH antibody formation, hypothyroidism, and measurable alterations in carbohydrate tolerance. Human pituitary GH, in use until 1985, was associated with Creutzfeldt-Jakob disease, caused by a slow-acting, fatal virus. Also, an association between GH and an increased incidence of leukemia has been reported by Japanese investigators.

It is important to identify very short and poorly growing children as early in life as possible, for a delay in the diagnosis and treatment of a child with GH deficiency can lead to the lack of attainment of a normal adult height and a loss of height potential.

Currently, the Food and Drug Administration (FDA) does not approve GH treatment for adults except in clinical research trials. In fact, GH replacement therapy in GH-deficient children is stopped once the stages of physical growth are completed.

Growth Hormone Excess

Etiology and Pathogenesis

Almost all cases of excess production of GH are caused by pituitary adenomas. This excess production of GH causes bones to grow large. The individual develops acromegalic features. **Acromegaly** (from the Greek *akron*, meaning extremity, and *mega*, meaning large) occurs with equal frequency in men and women during the fourth and fifth decades of life (Fig. 40–3). It is unknown whether GH-producing adenomas are primarily a pituitary disease or if they result from a hypothalamic dysfunction.

There are also cases of tall stature not linked to GH excess. Tall stature may be genetic. It may also be due to other conditions, including Marfan's syndrome, homocystinuria, Klinefelter's syndrome, and cerebral gigantism. Marfan's syndrome, characterized by arachnodactyly, is an inherited autosomal dominant disorder of connective tissue. In 65 to 75 percent of cases, one parent is also affected. Homocystinuria (a disorder of amino acid metabolism) is caused by a deficiency of cystathionine B-synthetase. This inborn error of metabolism is screened for during the early newborn period because it is inherited as an autosomal recessive trait. Klinefelter's syndrome occurs in 1 in 500 to 1 in 1,000 live male births. Klinefelter's syndrome is due to an abnormality in chromosome number in which two or more X chromosomes are present in male patients.

Clinical Manifestations

The signs and symptoms of GH excess (see Table 40–2) depend on the individual's age when excess secretion occurs. If it occurs when the epiphyses are open, linear growth can be tremendous. If it occurs during adolescence, acromegalic features develop, including enlargement of the lower jaw, hands, face,

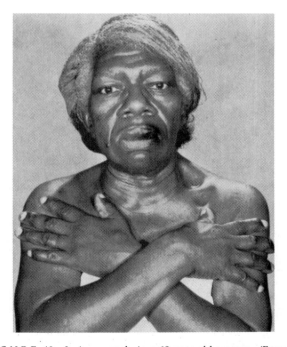

F I G U R E   40 – 3. Acromegaly in a 60-year-old woman. (From Cotran RS, Kumar V, Robbins SL (eds): *Robbins Pathologic Basis of Disease*, 4th ed. Philadelphia, WB Saunders, 1989, p 1210. Reproduced with permission.)

and feet. An adenoma, as it increases in size, may influence the secretion of other pituitary hormones, as well as cause impaired vision and visual field abnormalities.[9]

Children who are too tall for their age have heights above the 95th percentile of NCHS charts. Unusual height is usually of greater concern to females than males. Sometimes this bias may lead to the delayed diagnosis of tall stature problems. Birth length is usually normal, and body proportions are normal. Growth velocity is accelerated during early childhood, leading to very tall adult heights.

The clinical diagnosis of GH excess is made when an increase in the serum GH concentration is noted that is not suppressible by glucose given in a standard glucose tolerance test (1.75 g/kg of body weight, to a maximum of 100 g). The GH concentration should decrease to less than 2 ng/mL in normal individuals within 2 hours after oral glucose ingestion. IGF-1 levels would also be elevated.[10]

Twenty-five percent of individuals with GH excess will have some degree of glucose intolerance and hyperinsulinism.[11] When GH excess is known, the other pituitary hormones should be assessed for abnormalities. Neuroradiologic studies to determine the size and location of the pituitary adenoma are necessary.

Treatment

Treatment is focused on alleviating the adenoma that is producing the excess GH through transsphenoidal microsurgery. Radiation therapy has not been very successful except in reducing the size of the tumor, which reduces the complications of the surgical procedure. Pharmacologic management with a dopamine receptor agonist (bromocriptine, 10–20 mg/day given orally) has been used successfully in instances of documented GH excess. Unfortunately, total suppression of GH has not been achieved, but significant clinical improvement has occurred. Somatostatin, a short-acting GH inhibitor, and octreotide, an analogue of somatostatin (100–1,500 μg/day given subcutaneously in three to four divided doses), have been reported to cause a decrease in tumor size and clinical manifestations.[10]

KEY CONCEPTS

- **Growth hormone (GH) is an anabolic hormone that increases protein synthesis and fat utilization in most tissues of the body. GH is thought to act indirectly by stimulating the production of somatomedin growth factors such as IGF-1.**

- **Hyposecretion of GH results in decreased linear growth in children. In some cases decreased linear growth occurs despite normal GH levels, and abnormalities of somatomedin generation or responsiveness are suspected. Lack of GH in adults does not appear to cause significant alterations in growth.**

- GH deficiency may be idiopathic or related to tumors, irradiation, or trauma. The diagnosis is confirmed by measuring decreased GH levels in the blood and deficient GH release in response to hypoglycemia or other stimulants. Replacement therapy is indicated for children but not adults.

- Excessive GH production is usually due to pituitary adenoma. Excess GH during childhood results in increased linear growth and giantism. Excess GH after closure of bone epiphyses results in increased bulk and acromegaly. Other conditions characterized by tall stature (e.g., Marfan's syndrome, homocystinuria, and Klinefelter's syndrome) must be excluded.

- Features of acromegaly include a protruding jaw, increased bone density, increased growth of soft tissues (nose, ears), and large hands and feet. Symptoms of increased intracranial pressure from an expanding tumor (pituitary adenoma) may be present. An elevated GH level that is not suppressed by administration of glucose aids in the diagnosis. Excessive GH causes persistent hyperglycemia and increased insulin production in some individuals. Treatment entails surgical removal or pharmacologic palliation of the pituitary tumor.

Antidiuretic Hormone Disorders

Regulation and Actions of Antidiuretic Hormone

The posterior lobe consists of pituicytes (nervelike cells) that originate in the hypothalamus. Vasopressin (antidiuretic hormone, ADH) is derived from a precursor molecule that is synthesized primarily in the supraoptic and paraventricular nuclei of the hypothalamus. ADH is transported in neurosecretory granules through nerve fibers for storage in the posterior pituitary.

The most significant regulator of ADH release is the osmotic pressure of plasma, mediated by specialized neurons called osmoreceptors that are found in the hypothalamus. The osmoreceptors have a set point that influences the stimulation and suppression of ADH. Therefore, when body fluids become too concentrated, ADH is released, leading to increased reabsorption of water in the kidneys.

In the presence of ADH, the permeability of the collecting ducts and tubules to water increases greatly and allows most of the water to be reabsorbed as the tubular fluid passes through these ducts, thereby conserving water in the body.

The precise mechanism by which ADH acts on the ducts to increase their permeability is only partially understood. ADH causes special structural changes in the apical membranes of the tubular epithelial cells. This provides, temporarily, a pool of pores that allows free diffusion of water between the tubular and peritubular fluids (Fig. 40–4). Water is then absorbed from the collecting tubules and ducts by osmosis.

Antidiuretic Hormone Deficiency

Etiology and Pathogenesis

ADH acts directly on the renal collecting ducts and distal tubules. It increases membrane permeability for water and urea. Some pharmacologic agents, as well as injury to the posterior pituitary gland, can lead to abnormalities in ADH secretion (Table 40–3). The most common entity seen when there is damage to the posterior pituitary is **diabetes insipidus.** In adults with diabetes insipidus, 25 percent of cases are idiopathic, 17 percent are caused by the surgical treatment of brain tumors, 17 percent result from nonsurgical brain trauma, 13 percent are secondary to brain tumors, and 9 percent follow a hypophysectomy. ADH deficiency may be accompanied by other hypothalamic-pituitary hormone deficiencies. It also can occur as an autosomal recessive trait.[12]

The regulation of osmolality is based on control of water balance, which is dependent on the amount of water brought into the system (control of thirst) and renal conservation (influenced by ADH). ADH acts on vascular smooth muscle and in the kidney. Although ADH is a pressor agent, at physiologic levels it does not typically elevate blood pressure. ADH secretion is triggered by changes in osmolality; volume status has a weak effect on ADH secretion. (Changes in the renin-angiotensin-aldosterone system are sensitive to changes in volume and less responsive to changes in osmolality.) The most significant effect of ADH is its antidiuretic effect through its action in the kidney, where it is a major regulator of water management and maintenance of body fluid osmolality, blood volume, and blood pressure. In the absence of ADH, the permeability to water is diminished, resulting in the excretion of large volumes of hypotonic fluid. If the thirst center has been damaged, diabetes insipidus becomes a life-threatening illness, because increased water losses from the kidneys (due to the absence of ADH) are not counteracted by increased thirst and hydration.[13]

Diabetes insipidus results in hypernatremia. **Hypernatremia** is associated with serum sodium concen-

T A B L E 40 – 3. Agents Causing Alterations in Antidiuretic Hormone Secretion

Agents That Enhance Release	Agents That Suppress Release
Vincristine	Phenytoin
Cyclophosphamide	Alcohol
Prostaglandin E_2	α-Adrenergic agents
β-adrenergic agents	
Anesthetic agents	
Histamine	
Hypercapnia	
Morphine and narcotic analogues	
Nicotine	
Clofibrate	
Carbamazepine	
Barbiturates	
Hypoxia	

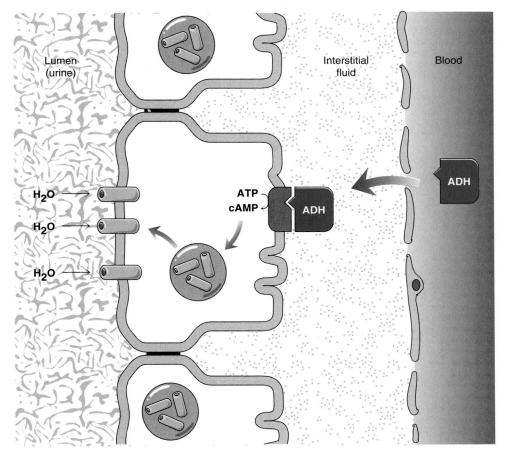

F I G U R E 40 – 4. The current hypothesis for the action of antidiuretic hormone on the water permeability of collecting duct epithelial cells.

trations in excess of 145 mEq/L. It usually indicates a body water deficit relative to sodium with hypernatremia; signs and symptoms are similar to those of dehydration and include thirst, disorientation, lethargy, and seizures. The neurologic symptoms are thought to be due to shrinkage and dehydration of cells.

Clinical Manifestations

The sudden development of **polyuria** (excessive urination) and **polydipsia** (excessive drinking) is the hallmark of diabetes insipidus. These symptoms persist at night (nocturia), interrupting normal sleep patterns. The individual's drive for excessive amounts of drinking water (or other fluids) often affects the amount of solid food (calories) he or she can ingest. This trend can lead to acute weight loss, dehydration, and skin turgor. It can have a direct impact on usual patterns of behavior and work habits.

Most sudden, critical presentations will be straightforward, with documented hypotonic polyuria, hypernatremia, and hypertonicity indicating a defect in secretion of ADH. Individuals presenting with the sudden onset of polyuria and polydipsia should undergo laboratory studies, including tests for urine and serum electrolyte, serum creatinine, and

blood urea nitrogen (BUN) levels. The results of these tests should exclude diabetes and kidney disease as the basis for the presenting complaints. A comparison of serum and urine osmolality is needed, as is a urine specific gravity measurement. Dilute urine in the presence of concentrated serum and hypernatremia along with (if possible) abnormally low ADH levels are diagnostic of diabetes insipidus.

A water deprivation test will confirm the diagnosis. When water intake is restricted, the individual will become dehydrated quickly, as the urine output is not diminished because of the inadequate or lack of ADH release by the pituitary. The osmolality of urine will remain fairly constant as serum osmolality increases rapidly. Once the serum osmolality exceeds 300 mOsm/kg (normal, 282–292 mOsm/kg), a single dose of DDAVP (desmopressin) should be administered intravenously (IV) or intranasally with continued monitoring of serum and urine osmolality. Following DDAVP administration, polyuria will diminish and thirst will be lessened. The urine osmolality should increase hourly by as much as 50 percent. The ADH levels, if measured, will remain low throughout the test.[14]

Magnetic resonance imaging or computed tomography (CT) of the hypothalamic-pituitary region should be performed to investigate possible causes of diabetes insipidus.

Treatment

Daily replacement of ADH is needed for the management of diabetes insipidus. DDAVP, a synthetic analogue of ADH, can be given by nasal insufflation tube. One dose lasts between 8 and 24 hours. Free access to fluids is necessary, and home testing of urine specific gravity may be useful for some individuals to allow them to adjust their dose of DDAVP independently. Careful education and follow-up of these individuals are needed.

Syndrome of Inappropriate Antidiuretic Hormone

Etiology and Pathogenesis

The ectopic production of ADH has been noted in association with many types of tumors. Nonmalignant lung tissue is capable of ADH synthesis, especially noted in pulmonary tuberculosis. Drug-induced ADH secretion occurs with the administration of chlorpropamide, carbamazepine, analgesics, and barbiturates. In adrenal insufficiency, the **syndrome of inappropriate ADH secretion (SIADH)** is induced by failure of cortisol-dependent ADH suppression.

SIADH results in **hyponatremia**, a condition in which the serum sodium concentration is decreased below the normal range (<136 mEq/L). In hyponatremia there is an excess of water relative to solute. Cells swell, and the effects of cellular swelling on neurons can be profound.

Clinical Manifestations

SIADH is characterized by hyponatremia. Urine osmolality is high and serum osmolality low (Fig. 40–5). Urine output decreases despite adequate or increased fluid intake, and the resultant water retention produces an acute gain in body weight.

The symptoms of SIADH include weight gain, weakness, muscle cramps, nausea and vomiting, postural blood pressure changes, poor skin turgor, fatigue, difficulty breathing, anorexia, and lethargy. In very severe cases, cerebral swelling can occur, causing confusion, hemiparesis (motor weakness on one side of the body), seizures, and coma. Laboratory findings include low serum sodium levels, hematocrit, and BUN levels as a result of expansion of the extracellular fluid volume.[15]

Treatment

Fluid restriction should be implemented for individuals with SIADH. Fluid restriction should result in loss of body weight and a steady rise in serum sodium levels and osmolality. If severe symptoms develop, IV administration of saline should be combined with furosemide therapy to minimize further expansion of intravascular volume. Hyponatremia should be corrected slowly.

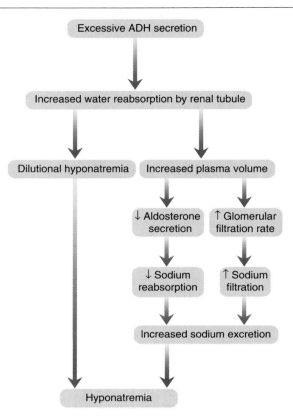

F I G U R E 40 – 5. The syndrome of inappropriate ADH secretion (SIADH) leads to hyponatremia by two mechanisms: (1) dilution of plasma and (2) increased excretion of sodium by the kidneys. Sodium excretion is increased because of the expanded plasma volume, which enhances sodium filtration and reduces sodium reabsorption.

KEY CONCEPTS

- **Antidiuretic hormone (ADH) secretion is primarily regulated by osmoreceptors in the hypothalamus that respond to changes in extracellular fluid concentration. An increase in osmolality stimulates secretion of ADH. Renal distal and collecting tubules respond to ADH by becoming more permeable to water. In the presence of ADH, water is reabsorbed from the urine filtrate, resulting in a concentrated urine.**

- **Diabetes insipidus is due to insufficient ADH secretion, which may be idiopathic or related to brain surgery, trauma, or tumor. Lack of ADH blocks water reabsorption in the kidney tubules, resulting in large volumes of dilute urine. Polyuria is accompanied by thirst, polydipsia, and increased serum sodium and osmolality. The resulting osmotic gradient causes cellular shrinkage and neurologic signs and symptoms. The diagnosis is confirmed from the formation of dilute urine despite water deprivation and a prompt decrease in urine output after administration of an ADH analogue (DDAVP). Diabetes insipidus is treated with hormone replacement therapy and fluid therapy.**

• The syndrome of inappropriate ADH secretion (SIADH) is associated with pulmonary tumors, tuberculosis, and certain drugs. Excess ADH stimulates the renal tubules to reabsorb water despite decreased blood osmolality and volume overload. Hyponatremia is associated with cellular swelling and neurologic dysfunction (e.g., confusion, coma). Fluid restriction and diuretics may be administered to treat volume overload and hyponatremia; however, detection and treatment of the underlying cause is paramount.

Thyroid Hormone Disorders

Regulation and Actions of Thyroid Hormone

The thyroid gland, a two-lobed gland, lies in the neck region on either side of and anterior to the trachea. It secretes the thyroid hormones **thyroxine** (T_4) and **triiodothyronine** (T_3). Thyroid hormones have marked effects on the metabolic rate of the body. When little or no thyroid hormone is secreted by the gland, a severe decrease in basal metabolic rate develops. Similarly, when excessive amounts of thyroid hormone are produced, a critical rise in the basal metabolic rate ensues. The amount of thyroid hormone released by the thyroid gland is controlled through thyroid-stimulating hormone (TSH) released by the anterior lobe of the pituitary gland as well by thyroid-releasing hormone (TRH) produced by the hypothalamus.

The secretion of thyroid hormone is regulated by the hypothalamic-pituitary-thyroid feedback system. The effect of this system is to maintain an almost constant concentration of free thyroid hormones in the circulating body fluids.

A well-vascularized gland, the thyroid is composed of follicular and perifollicular cells. Follicular cells contain a jellylike substance called thyroglobulin. Thyroglobulin is secreted by the columnar epithelial cells that line the follicle. Iodides are trapped from ingested foods, oxidized in the thyroid glandular cells, and combined with tyrosine, an amino acid, to form hormonally inactive iodotyrosines. The coupling of iodotyrosines forms hormonally active T_3 and T_4.[16]

The thyroid gland releases thyroid hormone in required amounts when the hypothalamic-pituitary-thyroid axis is intact. Any defect in the feedback mechanism of thyroid hormone can result in alterations in thyroid function. Thyroid hormone is an essential regulator of metabolic rate and growth.

Iodine is essential for the formation of T_4 and T_3, the two thyroid hormones that are necessary for maintenance of normal metabolic rates in all of the cells. About 50 mg of iodine is needed each year for the formation of adequate quantities of thyroid hormones.[17]

Lack of iodine prevents production of both T_4 and T_3 but does not stop the formation of thyroglobulin.[17]

As a result, insufficient hormone is available to inhibit production of TSH by the anterior pituitary. This imbalance allows the pituitary gland to secrete excessively large quantities of TSH. The TSH then causes the thyroid cells to secrete tremendous amounts of thyroglobulin (colloid) into the follicles, and the gland grows larger and larger, producing a **goiter** (Fig. 40–6).

Hypothyroidism

Etiology and Pathogenesis

Hypothyroidism may be congenital in origin or acquired later in life. Lymphocytic thyroiditis (Hashimoto's thyroiditis, or autoimmune thyroiditis) is the most common cause of acquired hypothyroidism. Other causes include irradiation of the thyroid gland, surgical removal of thyroid tissue, goitrogen ingestion, and iodine deficiency.[18] Some foods contain goitrogenic substances that have a propylthiouracil type of antithyroid activity, thus also leading to TSH-stimulated enlargement of the thyroid gland. Such goitrogenic substances occur in some varieties of turnips and cabbages.

Secondary hypothyroidism is caused by defects in TSH production, and tertiary hypothyroidism is caused by TRH deficiency. Individuals who have been exposed to severe trauma, neoplasms, infections, irradiation, and surgery can be left with secondary or tertiary hypothyroidism.

Acquired hypothyroidism can be iatrogenic (as a result of surgery or irradiation) in origin or, although rarely in the United States, can be due to dietary deficiencies of the iodine necessary to synthesize thyroid hormone. In these cases, abnormalities of the thyroid gland or thyroid gland function impair thyroid hormone synthesis and release.[18]

Lymphocytic thyroiditis (Hashimoto's disease, autoimmune thyroiditis) is characterized by an enlarged thyroid gland (see Fig. 40–6) caused by lymphocytic infiltration. Thyroid hormone production decreases, stimulating the release of TSH from the pituitary, indicating a hypoactive thyroid gland. Hypothyroidism and its clinical symptoms progress as the gland becomes fibrotic.

Clinical Manifestations

Individuals with hypothyroidism have decreased basal metabolic rates. The thyroid gland may become goitrous, the skin may be cool and dry, and constipation may be present. All metabolic processes are depressed. The subjective feelings of weakness, lethargy, cold intolerance, and decreased appetite may be experienced. A slowed heart rate, narrowing of the pulse pressure, and an unexpected weight gain may occur. Women with acquired hypothyroidism may experience menstrual irregularities. Table 40–4 summarizes the signs and symptoms of thyroid imbalance.

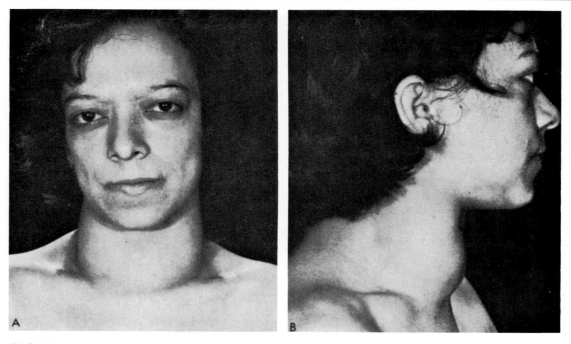

F I G U R E 40 – 6. An enlarged thyroid gland (goiter) can be present in both hypothyroid and hyperthyroid states. Note enlargement at the base of the neck. (From Wilson JD, Foster DW (eds): *Williams Textbook of Endocrinology*, 8th ed. Philadelphia, WB Saunders, 1992, p 425. Reproduced with permission.)

Myxedema refers to nonpitting edema that forms in severe thyroid deficiencies. The condition is noted more frequently in the elderly population. Individuals with myxedema usually present in an altered mental state, with alterations in thermoregulation and a history of a precipitating event such as sepsis, trauma, or the use of certain medications.[19] Figure 40–7 shows the typical features of patients with myxedema.

Myxedema coma is a rare, life-threatening clinical state associated with long-standing untreated hypothyroidism. The main cause of myxedema coma is the inability of an individual with hypothyroidism to adapt to functional or actual losses in blood volume or central nervous system (CNS) functional impairment.[19]

In individuals with typical presentations of hypothyroidism, the diagnosis can be confirmed by measuring thyroid hormone levels. Serum T_4 and free T_4 (unbound to thyroid-binding proteins) will be decreased (Table 40–5). When the TSH level is elevated in the presence of a low T_4, the diagnosis of hypothyroidism due to failure of the thyroid gland is made. A TRH test may differentiate primary hypothyroidism from other causes of hypothyroidism. In primary hypothyroidism, the TSH response to TRH is always increased. A test measuring thyroid uptake of radioactive iodine was used widely in the past, but it is less frequently used today because of cost, inconvenience, and radiation exposure.

Treatment

The goal of treatment is to return the individual with acquired hypothyroidism and thyroiditis to a euthy-

TABLE 40–4. Signs and Symptoms of Thyroid Imbalance

Hyperthyroidism	Hypothyroidism
Sleeplessness, nervousness	Lethargy
Muscle weakness, fatigue Susceptibility to infection	Weakness
Skin texture warm, silky, damp	Dry, pale, cool, coarse skin
Heat intolerance	Cold intolerance
Increased appetite with weight loss	Weight gain
Increased gastric motility	Constipation
Tachycardia, narrow pulse pressure, palpitations, angina	Bradycardia, wide pulse pressure
Dyspnea	Dyspnea, chest pain
Goiter	Thyroid shows diffuse enlargement or is not palpable
Hair silky, nail loose or detached from nail bed	Hair coarse
Hyperreflexia	Sluggish return of reflexes
	Mental impairment: slowed cognitive ability, poor memory, forgetfulness, depressed affect
	Deafness (in one third of population)
Eye symptoms: burning, tearing, diplopia, lid lag, prominent eyes (exophthalmia), stare, eyelid tremors when closed	Facial edema (especially periorbital)
Absence of forehead wrinkling on upward gaze	Thinned lateral aspect of eyebrows
Decreased or absent menses	Heavy, prolonged menses; infertility

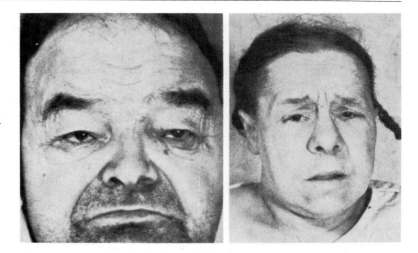

FIGURE 40–7. Typical facial puffiness and dull expression of patients with myxedema. (From Larsan PR, Ingbar SH: The thyroid gland, in Wilson JD, Foster DW (eds): *Williams Textbook of Endocrinology*, 8th ed. Philadelphia, WB Saunders, 1992, p 451. Reproduced with permission.)

roid state. When serum thyroid levels rise too quickly, individuals may become fretful and irritable and may have difficulty sleeping. Once treatment has begun, those individuals with a goiter usually experience a regression of the goiter.

Oral preparations of thyroid hormone (levothyroxine sodium) allow individuals diagnosed with hypothyroidism to maintain a euthyroid state. Before replacement therapy is started, a consideration of the cause of hypothyroidism is mandatory. If hypothyroidism is due to hypothalamic or pituitary disease, ACTH deficiency may coexist. If this is not investigated first, thyroid replacement therapy can precipitate adrenal failure, which was not a problem when the individual was hypothyroid.

Treatment of an individual with myxedema includes the rapid institution of therapeutic measures to stabilize the cardiovascular alterations, temperature balance, and other complications of the precipitating event. Also, if the myxedema is considered in the differential diagnosis, thyroid replacement therapy should be instituted. The rule is, "when in doubt, treat." No serious consequences have been reported when thyroid hormone replacement therapy was instituted in individuals presenting with possible myxedema who were in fact euthyroid.[19]

Hyperthyroidism

Etiology and Pathogenesis

Mechanisms that can produce thyrotoxicosis and hyperthyroidism include thyroid follicular cell hyperfunction with increased synthesis and secretion of T_4 and T_3, thyroid follicular cell destruction with release of preformed T_4 and T_3, and ingestion or administration of thyroid hormone or iodide preparations. The increased levels of serum thyroid hormones increase the metabolic rate (see Table 40–5).

Hyperfunction of thyroid follicular cells can be either autonomous or mediated through stimulation of thyrotropin receptors by substances such as thyrotropin (TSH) or thyrotropin receptor antibodies (TRAb). The basic abnormalities underlying autonomous hyperfunction are unknown. Autonomous hyperfunction can be caused by adenomas and thyroid carcinoma. Stimulation of thyrotropin receptors by TRAb leads to the diffuse toxic goiter of **Graves' disease.**[20]

The hyperthyroidism of Graves' disease seems to be mediated through the action of immunoglobulins of the IgG class. These immunoglobulins are thought to bind to their complementary antigenic regions on

TABLE 40–5. Thyroid Hormone Levels in Various States*

State	Serum $T_4(\mu g/dL)$, Range	Serum $T_3(ng/dL)$, Range	Serum TSH ($\mu U/mL$), Range
Euthyroid	4.5–11.5	60–180	0.5–4.5
Infants (<2 wk)	8.0–15.0	—	0.5–4.5
Children (prepubertal)	6.5–11.5	80–220	0.5–4.5
Hyperthyroid	>11.5	—	<0.15
Hypothyroid	<1.0–5.0	—	>10

* Because 90 percent of serum thyroid hormone is bound to thyroid-binding globulin (TBG), individuals with TBG deficiency may have low levels of T_4 and T_3 with TSH values in the expected range. In these cases, a serum free T_4 level (range, 0.8–1.8 ng/dL) may be a useful diagnostic measure. Laboratory normal ranges may vary.

the plasma membrane, leading to reactions resulting in thyroid growth and hyperthyroidism. This is more common in women than men, with increased occurrences during puberty, pregnancy, and menopause.

Inflammation of thyroid follicular cells can be associated with viral or autoimmune processes, and extensive destruction can release large amounts of T_3 and T_4. Examples are the toxic thyroiditis of Hashimoto's disease and subacute thyroiditis.

Acute or chronic ingestion of thyroid hormone preparations can produce excess levels of thyroid hormones. Ingestion or parenteral administration of iodides may also result in thyrotoxicosis.

Clinical Manifestations

Individuals with Graves' disease present with thyromegaly (**goiter,** enlarged thyroid), thyrotoxicosis, and often **exophthalmos** (Fig. 40–8). A diffuse toxic goiter or thyroid enlargement is the most common manifestations. Symptoms include changes in behavior, insomnia, restlessness, irritability, palpitations, heat intolerance, diaphoresis, nocturia, and an inability to concentrate that interferes with work performance (see Table 40–4). Spasm and retraction of the eyelids leads to widening of the palpebral fissure, resulting in exposed sclera. Lid lag develops, and severe, progressive exophthalmos may occur.[18]

Thyroid storm is a form of life-threatening thyrotoxicosis that occurs when an individual is not able to maintain adequate metabolic balances through compensatory mechanisms. The individual's clinical picture is the hallmark for distinguishing between severe hyperthyroidism and thyroid storm.

Thyroid storm presents with the clinical features of thyrotoxicosis in a more exaggerated state. Most individuals will have a goiter and, possibly, ophthalmopathy. Exceedingly elevated temperatures, significant tachycardia, cardiac arrhythmias, and congestive heart failure are frequent findings at presentation. Extreme restlessness, agitation, and psychosis may occur, with the situation possibly advancing to coma. The person may also experience vomiting, nausea, and severe diarrhea; jaundice may develop due to hepatic dysfunction.

Studies useful in the diagnosis of hyperthyroidism include measurements of hemoglobin and hematocrit, white blood cell count, liver profile, calcium, BUN, and thyroid function tests. Serum T_4 and resin T_3 uptake should be elevated. A 24-hour radioactive iodine uptake study can confirm the diagnosis of Graves' disease when the scan shows diffuse homogeneous uptake of tracer and can exclude the presence of thyroid neoplasms.

Treatment

Individuals should receive treatment to control hyperthyroidism through the use of antithyroid drugs, with or without iodide. Administration of β-adrenergic blockers may be tried to decrease the load on the cardiovascular system as suppression of the elevated thyroxine levels is begun with potassium iodide and thiosamides. Careful monitoring is needed to evaluate the response to treatment.

Individuals with Grave's disease may need long-term treatment with antithyroid drugs (propylthiouracil [PTU], methimazole, carbimazole). Appropriate dosages of these drugs can be expected to produce a gradual reduction in the basal metabolic rate and the disappearance of symptoms (decreased size of the gland). The exophthalmos that is present at diagnosis may not reverse. Monitoring of possible toxic reactions to these drugs is necessary. Frequently, rash and decreased WBCs develop, necessitating the consideration of other options for treatment. If these complications do not arise, the medical management of hyperthyroidism is usually successful. Radioactive iodine treatment to oblate the gland and therefore its ability to produce excess thyroid hormones is now the treatment of choice. Surgical removal of the thyroid gland increases the risk of secondary hypoparathyroidism. As with all the treatment options, suppression of thyroid hormone production will lead to hypothyroidism.

Because thyroid storm is a life-threatening form

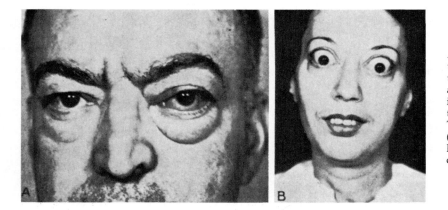

FIGURE 40–8. Patients with the usual ophthalmopathy found in Graves' disease. **A,** Patient with periorbital swelling, exophthalmos, and chemosis (edema). **B,** Woman with widening of the palpebral fissures owing to lid retraction and proptosis. (From Larsen PR, Ingbar SH: The thyroid gland, in Wilson JD, Foster DW (eds): *Williams Textbook of Endocrinology,* 8th ed. Philadelphia, WB Saunders, 1992, p 426. Reproduced with permission.)

of thyrotoxicosis, aggressive management to achieve metabolic balance is needed. All measures should be taken to block the production and binding of thyroid pathways. Antithyroid drugs such as propylthiouracil must be given orally or through a nasogastric tube because parenteral preparations are not available. Inorganic iodine may be given to further inhibit release of T_3 and T_4 only after an effective blockade of new hormone synthesis (with propylthiouracil) has been initiated. Beta blockers used for their antiadrenergic effects also inhibit the peripheral conversion of T_4 to T_3. Beta blockers are available in both oral and parenteral forms. Extremely careful monitoring of individuals receiving treatment for thyroid storm must be provided. Hyperpyretic therapy (cooling blankets, ice packs, acetaminophen) must be started to achieve peripheral cooling. Fluid replacement with dextrose and electrolytes must be provided and the cardiovascular status diligently monitored during stabilization of the individual. The addition of glucocorticoids to the pharmacologic regimen seems to improve survival. The mortality is between 20 percent and 50 percent; therefore, aggressive, multifocused preventive measures must be implemented early in individuals presented with thyroid storm.[21]

KEY CONCEPTS

- Thyroid hormone (T_3, T_4) is produced in follicular cells of the thyroid gland. The synthesis and secretion of thyroid hormone are stimulated by TSH from the pituitary. Thyroid hormone is an important stimulator of growth and cellular metabolism.

- Hypothyroidism may be primary (due to congenital agenesis, autoimmune destruction, irradiation, trauma, surgical removal of the gland, or iodine deficiency) or secondary to pituitary hyposecretion of TSH. The blood level of TSH is helpful in differentiating between primary (high TSH) and secondary (low TSH) causes of hypothyroidism. Low serum T_3 and T_4 levels confirm the diagnosis of hypothyroidism.

- Manifestations of hypothyroidism (myxedema) are due to a generalized decrease in metabolism. Untreated congenital hypothyroidism results in profound mental and physical retardation (cretinism). Manifestations of myxedema include nonpitting edema, slowed mentation, weight gain, dry skin, constipation, decreased heart rate, low blood pressure, lethargy, and loss of the outer third of the eyebrow. Severe hypothyroidism may lead to myxedema coma, characterized by bradycardia, hypothermia, hypotension, and decreased level of consciousness. Treatment centers on hormone replacement therapy.

- Hyperthyroidism may be primary (Graves' disease, autoimmune, tumor related, inflammatory) or secondary to pituitary hypersecretion of TSH. The blood level of TSH is helpful in differentiating primary (low TSH) from secondary (high TSH) causes of hyperthyroidism. High levels of T_3 and T_4 confirm the diagnosis of hyperthyroidism.

- The manifestations of hyperthyroidism result from a generalized increase in metabolism. Hyperactivity, irritability, insomnia, weight loss, increased appetite, heat intolerance, diarrhea, and palpitations are common. Most individuals have a detectably enlarged thyroid gland. Exophthalmos occurs with Graves' disease. Thyroid storm may be precipitated by stress or manipulation of the gland. It is characterized by tachycardia, hypertension, high temperature, and cardiac dysrhythmias. Treatment includes beta blockers to control cardiovascular symptoms, antithyroid drugs to reduce thyroid production, radioactive iodine to ablate the gland, and surgical removal of tumors.

Parathyroid Gland Disorders

Regulation and Actions of Parathyroid Hormone

The parathyroid glands are small glands located at the upper and lower poles of the thyroid. There are usually four parathyroid glands, although there are reports of fewer than four and more than four being found during surgery. The parathyroid glands help maintain homeostasis through the regulation of calcium concentrations in the blood (Fig. 40–9). Parathyroid hormone (PTH) is released and acts on bones, renal tubules, and intestinal mucosa. In the bone, PTH works with vitamin D to increase osteoclastic activity as it decreases osteoblastic activity. Resorption of calcium and excretion of phosphorus in the kidney occurs through the action of PTH by decreasing the reabsorption of renal tubular phosphate. PTH's effect on bone, kidney, and in the intestine is to raise the serum level of calcium. A decrease in serum calcium causes a release of PTH, which releases needed calcium from bone and decreases the kidneys' excretion of calcium. An elevated serum calcium level leads to suppression of PTH. A marked increase or decrease in serum PTH levels can have severe, often fatal consequences.[16] PTH is not part of the hypothalamic-pituitary feedback system.

Besides thyroid hormones (T_3 and T_4), the thyroid gland also produces a hormone called **calcitonin**. Produced by parafollicular cells (cells between the thyroid follicles), calcitonin influences the processing of calcium by bone cells. Calcitonin controls the calcium content of the blood by increasing bone formation by osteoblasts and inhibiting bone breakdown by osteoclasts. Calcitonin tends to decease blood calcium levels and promote conservation of hard bone matrix. PTH is an antagonist to calcitonin, since it has the opposite effects. Together, calcitonin and PTH help maintain calcium homeostasis.

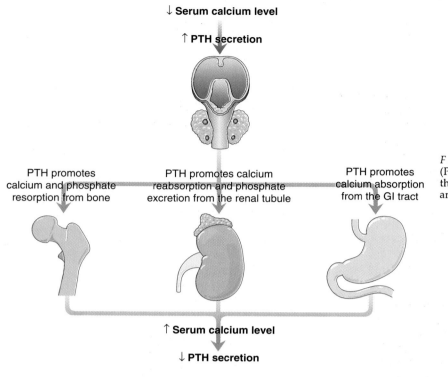

↓ **Serum calcium level**

↑ **PTH secretion**

PTH promotes calcium and phosphate resorption from bone

PTH promotes calcium reabsorption and phosphate excretion from the renal tubule

PTH promotes calcium absorption from the GI tract

F I G U R E 40 – 9. Parathyroid hormone (PTH) increases serum calcium level through its effects on bone, renal tubules, and intestine.

↑ **Serum calcium level**

↓ **PTH secretion**

Hyperparathyroidism

Etiology and Pathogenesis

The causes of primary hyperparathyroidism remain unclear. Despite an elevated serum calcium level, PTH continues to be secreted. Some forms of hyperparathyroidism can have a genetic origin. Hyperparathyroidism from a single parathyroid adenoma occurs in 80 percent of surgically proven cases. Hyperplasia of the parathyroid is found in the remainder of the cases.

In hyperparathyroidism, bone resorption and formation rates are increased. The abnormal regulation of PTH by calcium is not completely independent, for serum calcium levels do not rise uncontrollably. Its incidence is 1 in 1,000, with a 3:2 female-male predominance. Hyperparathyroidism occurs mostly during the fifth and sixth decades of life. Parathyroid carcinomas are rare, but when they are present, the levels of serum calcium are much greater (>14 mg/dL) than the usual elevations seen in hyperparathyroidism.[22]

A hyperparathyroid state during pregnancy leads to perinatal and neonatal complications. The newborn's PTH production will be suppressed by maternal hypercalcemia, and neonatal hypocalcemia and tetany can develop. This presentation in a newborn may be the first indication of the need for investigative studies in the mother if she was asymptomatic during pregnancy.[23] In chronic renal failure, secondary hyperparathyroidism may result from abnormal levels of phosphate and calcium.

Clinical Manifestations

The presentation of primary hyperparathyroidism is related to hypercalcemia and the hyperparathyroid state. Individuals are prone to kidney stones or to bone disease (demineralization). Hypercalcemia alone causes a wide variety of side effects, including a shortened Q-T interval on the ECG, anorexia, nausea, vomiting, constipation, and polyuria. Hyperparathyroidism may present as asymptomatic hypercalcemia.

Often mild cases of hyperparathyroidism are recognized on general serum chemistry laboratory reports that note mild elevations in serum calcium. The improved detection is why the incidence of hyperparathyroidism is apparently increasing. Serum calcium levels are elevated (>1 mg/dL above the laboratory normal range) and serum phosphorus levels are low to low normal. Urinary excretion of calcium and phosphate is elevated, as are serum PTH levels. Urinary cyclic adenosine monophosphate (cAMP) levels are increased, and 1,25-vitamin D levels may be elevated.[24]

Lithium and thiazides may increase serum calcium levels, negating the diagnosis of hyperparathyroidism.

Treatment

Surgical removal of the abnormal parathyroid gland is the treatment of choice. Individuals with asymptomatic hyperparathyroidism may defer or refuse surgery. In such cases, medical management may work for a time. Medical management includes hydration (to prevent kidney stone formation) and ambulation. Also, oral phosphate (K-Phos or Neutra Phos, equivalent to 2 grams of elemental phosphate per day) will lower serum calcium levels by 0.5 to 1.0 mg/dL.

Hypoparathyroidism

Etiology and Pathogenesis

Hypoparathyroidism most frequently occurs as a consequence of parathyroid or thyroid surgery as well as surgery in the area of these glands. The resulting hypoparathyroidism may be temporary or permanent. In some cases it may take years to develop.

Hypoparathyroidism can occur following the removal of a hyperfunctioning parathyroid gland. The hyperfunctioning gland suppresses the function of other glands, creating a temporary state of deficiency. Permanent hypoparathyroidism rarely follows initial surgery. Permanent hypoparathyroidism after thyroidectomy varies according to the type of thyroid lesion, the extent of surgical intervention, and the skill of the surgeon. Damage to the parathyroid glands can occur through manipulation of the gland or its blood supply during the surgical procedure.[25]

Idiopathic hypoparathyroidism can be a consequence of various rare disorders, including sporadic or familial defects that may become apparent over a wide time range, from early in the newborn period to later in adult life. The parathyroid glands may be targeted by other endocrine autoimmune disease processes such as Addison's disease.

Clinical Manifestations

The manifestations of acute hypocalcemia include circumoral numbness, paresthesias of the distal extremitities, muscle cramps, fatigue, hyperirritability, anxiety, depression, nonspecific electroencephalographic (EEG) changes, increases in intracranial pressure, and prolongation of corrected Q-T intervals on the ECG. Severe manifestations of hypocalcemia include carpopedal spasm, laryngospasm, and seizures. The clinical signs of hypocalcemia include neuromuscular irritability associated with tetany. Tetany is indicated by the Chvostek sign (ipsilateral contraction of the facial muscles that is elicited by tapping the facial nerve anterior to the ear) or Trousseau's sign (carpal spasm produced by pressure ischemia of the nerves in the upper arm during inflation of a blood pressure cuff for 3 to 5 minutes above the systolic blood pressure).[24,25]

Because hypocalcemia is a stimulus for PTH release, PTH levels should be increased in the presence of low serum calcium levels. Levels of antibodies to the parathyroid gland are high if an autoimmune mechanism is operant.

Treatment

Emergency treatment with IV calcium is needed if an individual presents in acute hypocalcemia crisis (tetany, laryngospasm, and convulsions). In adults, 10 to 20 mL of 10 percent calcium gluconate (equivalent to 93 mg of elemental calcium per 10 mL) may be infused slowly while serum calcium levels are monitored hourly until an acceptable serum calcium level is attained. Intravenous calcium preparations are very irritating, and care must be taken to prevent extravasation of the drug. Because bicarbonate and phosphate will form precipitates of calcium, their combined use should be avoided.[25]

Long-term treatment includes oral calcium supplements, vitamin D, or both. Serum calcium levels should be maintained in the low normal range in an attempt to avoid hypercalciuria.

KEY CONCEPTS

- Parathyroid hormone (PTH) is an important regulator of serum calcium levels. Low serum levels of ionized calcium are a potent stimulus for PTH release. PTH increases calcium absorption from the GI tract, the resorption of calcium and phosphate from bones, and the reabsorption of calcium from the urine filtrate. PTH also increases the excretion of phosphate by the kidney. Disorders of PTH secretion are manifested as alterations in serum Ca^{++} levels.

- Hyperparathyroidism may be idiopathic or may be due to a parathyroid adenoma. Its manifestations result from high serum calcium levels and bone demineralization. High serum calcium levels decrease neuromuscular excitability. Treatment entails removing the abnormal glands. Adequate hydration may help prevent the formation of kidney stones.

- Hypoparathyroidism may be idiopathic, autoimmune, or secondary to surgical removal of the parathyroid gland. The manifestations result from low serum calcium levels, which increase neuromuscular excitability. Paresthesias, cramps, spasms, tetany, and seizures may result. Elicitation of Chvostek's and Trousseau's signs indicates neuromuscular hyperexcitability. Treatment entails calcium (and vitamin D) supplementation rather than hormone replacement.

Adrenocortical Hormone Disorders

Regulation and Actions of Adrenocortical Hormones

The secretion of adrenal cortex hormones is regulated by pituitary adrenocorticotropic hormone (ACTH) through a system of negative feedback. The hormones produced by the adrenal cortex are called **steroids** and include (1) glucocorticoids (cortisol), (2) mineralocorticoids (aldosterone), and (3) sex steroids (androgens) (Fig. 40–10). Changes in the levels of any of these hormones cause a dysfunction in many body tissues and organs. The synthesis and secretion of these hormones, especially the glucocorticoids, are considered essential for life, regulating the body's response to normal and abnormal levels of physical, physiologic, and psychological stress. The activities of these three hormones can be remembered in terms of regulating the three S's—sugar, salt, and sex.

Glucocorticoids, principally cortisol, are named for their primary effect on glucose metabolism. They influence the way proteins and fats are utilized. **Glucocorticoids** are anti-insulin hormones whose overall effect is to raise blood sugar, making glucose immediately available. This is accomplished by decreasing glucose uptake by adipose and other tissue (decreased glycogenesis), and increasing glucose synthesis in the liver from amino acid and glycerol substrates in protein and fat stores (**gluconeogenesis,** glycogenolysis). Glucocorticoids also contribute to protein catabolism by releasing muscle stores, providing further amino acids for glucose production in the liver. Finally, glucocorticoids promote lipogenesis and increased blood cholesterol.[23]

Mineralocorticoids, principally aldosterone, function to maintain normal salt and water balance by promoting sodium retention and potassium excre-

tion in the distal renal tubules. Aldosterone, however, is not dependent on pituitary ACTH control. Its production is regulated primarily by the renin-angiotensin system associated with the juxtaglomerular cells of the kidney in response to a reduction in blood volume, and by a high serum potassium level (Fig. 40–11).

Androgenic hormone secretion by the adrenal cortex plays a relatively minor role in the development and maintenance of secondary sex characteristics except in children with adrenogenital syndromes, which produce virilization in the female and precocious sexual development in the male. Physiologically, adrenal androgens are the main source of androgens in the female. As with mineralocorticoids, there is no known feedback mechanism to suppress ACTH production associated with adrenal sex hormone plasma levels, but increased ACTH or adrenal hyperplasia may produce excessive amounts of these hormones.

Adrenocortical Insufficiency

Etiology and Pathogenesis

Hyposecretion of adrenocortical hormones can result from disease of the adrenal cortex (primary adrenocortical insufficiency, or **Addison's disease**) or from the deficient secretion of ACTH from the anterior pituitary (secondary adrenal insufficiency), or from a lack

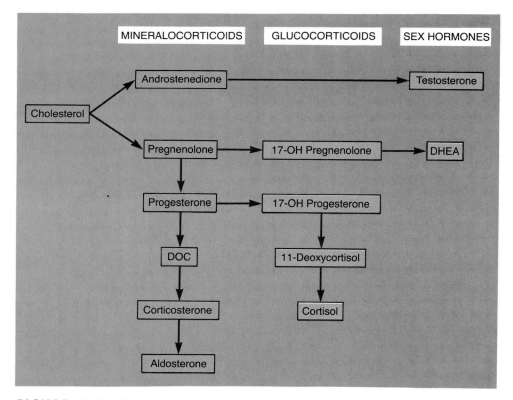

F I G U R E 40 – 10. Adrenal cortex hormone production. DOC, deoxycorticosterone; DHEA, dehydroepiandrosterone. (From Betz CL, Hunsberger M, Wright S (eds): *Family-Centered Nursing Care of Children,* 2nd ed. Philadelphia, WB Saunders, 1994, p 1957. Reproduced with permission.)

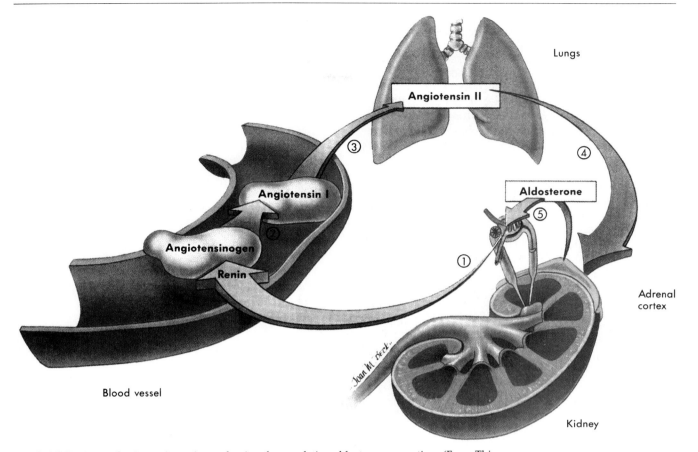

F I G U R E 40 – 11. Renin-angiotensin mechanism for regulating aldosterone secretion. (From Thibodeau GA, Patton K: *Anatomy and Physiology,* 2nd ed. St. Louis, CV Mosby, 1993, p 425. Reproduced with permission.)

of CRH corticotropin-releasing hormone (CRH) secretion from the hypothalamus due to hypothalamic malfunction or injury (tertiary disease). The levels of cortisol in plasma influence the secretion of CRH and ACTH through negative feedback. CRH stimulates ACTH secretion by the pituitary, which is released in a pulsatile diurnal rate. Stress induces increased hypothalamic-pituitary-adrenal axis activity. Aldosterone is necessary to maintain normal blood pressure levels and sodium, potassium, and water balance, but its release, although stimulated by ACTH, is mainly controlled by the renin-angiotensin regulatory system.

The syndrome of **congenital adrenal hyperplasia** is caused by specific enzymatic defects in the biosynthesis of cortisol by the adrenal gland and a resulting overproduction of ACTH, leading to hyperplasia of the adrenal glands.

The term *androgen* refers to any steroid hormone that has masculinizing effects, including testosterone. The adrenal glands secrete at least five different androgens, although the total masculinizing activity of all of them is normally so slight that they do not cause any significant masculine characteristics even in women, except for growth of pubic and axillary hair. But, when an adrenal tumor of the adrenal andro-

gen–producing cells occurs, the quantity of androgenic hormones becomes great enough to cause all the usual male secondary sexual characteristics.

If this occurs in a female, she develops such virile characteristics as growth of a beard, a much deeper voice, occasionally baldness (if she has inherited that genetic trait), masculine distribution of pubic hair, growth of the clitoris to resemble a penis, and deposition of proteins in the skin and muscles to yield typical masculine characteristics.[17]

In adult men, the virilizing characteristics of the adrenogenital syndrome are less obvious because male virilizing characteristics are normally associated with testosterone, which is secreted by the testes. Therefore, the diagnosis is difficult to make. In the prepubertal male, a virilizing adrenal tumor causes the rapid development of male sexual organs, secondary sex characteristics, and precocious sexual desires.

Primary adrenal insufficiency (Addison's disease) is caused by a destructive atrophy of the adrenal gland by idiopathic or autoimmune mechanisms, tuberculosis, trauma or hemorrhage in the areas of the adrenal glands (often associated with anticoagulant therapy), fungal disease (e.g., histoplasmosis), and neoplasia. Because of the high functional reserve, symptoms of adrenal insufficiency may or may not be recognized until nine tenths of the cortical tissue has been rendered nonfunctional.

The most common cause of adrenal insufficiency is sudden withdrawal of glucocorticoids or increased stress in individuals treated with exogenous steroids over prolonged periods of time. With prolonged supraphysiologic dosages, used for their anti-inflammatory and immunosuppressive effects in the treatment of profound illnesses, suppression of ACTH production with resultant hypoplasia of the adrenal cortex results.

A rare form of adrenal insufficiency is familial ACTH unresponsiveness. A defect in the ACTH receptor at the adrenal level has been identified as the cause of low cortisol levels in these children.[26]

In primary disease, cortisol, aldosterone, and androgen secretion may be decreased. In secondary disease only glucocorticoids are diminished, with aldosterone and androgens continuing to be produced by other mechanisms. There are two main causes of primary adrenal disease, autoimmune adrenal destruction and tuberculosis.

The primary glucocorticoid in humans is hydrocortisone. This hormone is essential for life. The syndrome of adrenal insufficiency is the manifestation of glucocorticoid prodution.

Primary adrenal insufficiency (Addison's disease) is caused by destruction of the adrenal gland itself. Addisonian crisis or acute adrenal insufficiency represents a true medical emergency caused by the effects of rapid withdrawal of glucocorticoids (and possibly mineralocorticoids) from the bloodstream. This may occur as the result of a slowly developing and unrecognized ACTH or adrenocorticosteroid deficiency in which secretion is adequate for the normal demands of life but inadequate for increased stress or trauma.[27]

In the newborn, classic congenital adrenal hyperplasia is a life-threatening condition. Infants are frequently diagnosed at birth because of the effects of the enzyme block on the genitals of the newborn. These enzymes are needed to synthesize cortisol and occasionally aldosterone. Failure to synthesize cortisol leads to increased production of ACTH and hyperplasia of the adrenal tissue. With the increase in ACTH stimulus, the pathway to androgen production is overstimulated. This leads to the virilization of a female fetus's genitalia but may not cause a recognizable change in a male fetus's genitalia (Fig. 40–12).[28]

Secondary adrenal insufficiency occurs following exogenous glucocorticoid administration and during Cushing's syndrome. For example, it may occur in a patient receiving long-term glucocorticoid therapy if the dosage is suddenly lowered drastically or if the patient is exposed to increased stress. It may also be the immediate result of bilateral adrenalectomy, or a medical or surgical hypophysectomy. It can also be caused by disorders in hypothalamic-pituitary function that result in diminished or deficient production of corticotropin (ACTH).

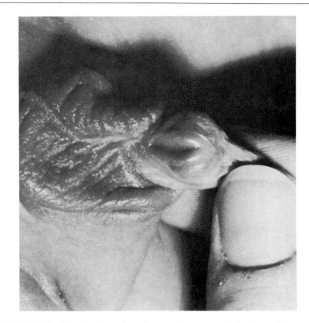

F I G U R E   40 – 12. Female infant with congenital adrenal hyperplasia demonstrating virilization of the genitalia. Note the enlarged clitoris and the fused labia, which resemble a scrotal sac. (From Hurwitz LS: Nursing implications of selected endocrine disorders. *Nurs Clin North Am* 1980;15(3):528. Reproduced with permission.)

Clinical Manifestations

The clinical manifestations of adrenal insufficiency may appear gradually or acutely. The signs and symptoms of adrenal insufficiency (Table 40–6) are the result of deficiencies in adrenocortical hormones, possibly accompanied by increased secretion of pituitary ACTH and melanocyte-stimulating hormone (MSH) in an attempt to stimulate cortisol production (Fig. 40–13). The acute presentation of adrenal crisis may be real or may represent a gradual deterioration in adrenocortical function the earlier signs of which were not recognized or were too vague.

Early signs of adrenal insufficiency include anorexia, weight loss, weakness, malaise, apathy, electrolyte imbalances, and hyperpigmentation of the skin caused by unsuppressed MSH production (Fig.

T A B L E   40 – 6. Signs and Symptoms of Adrenocortical Hormone Imbalance

Cushing's Syndrome	Adrenocortical Insufficiency
Truncal obesity	Weakness
Moon face	Hypotension
Buffalo hump	Hypoglycemia
Hirsutism	Hyperpigmentation (Addison's disease)
Muscle wasting	Hyperkalemia
Striae	Weight loss
Petechiae	
Glucose intolerance	
Hypertension	
Hypokalemia	

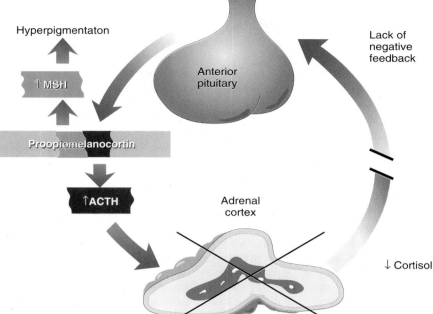

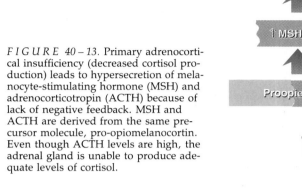

FIGURE 40–13. Primary adrenocortical insufficiency (decreased cortisol production) leads to hypersecretion of melanocyte-stimulating hormone (MSH) and adrenocorticotropin (ACTH) because of lack of negative feedback. MSH and ACTH are derived from the same precursor molecule, pro-opiomelanocortin. Even though ACTH levels are high, the adrenal gland is unable to produce adequate levels of cortisol.

40–14). Salt craving may be present due to sodium deficit. If the condition is unrecognized or left untreated, gastrointestinal symptoms can develop, including nausea, vomiting, diarrhea, and dehydration. The blood pressure and heart rate may be low for age.[29] Moodiness may progress to depression. Hypoglycemia with symptoms of shock suggests the diagnosis of acute adrenal hyposecretion, since blood glucose levels are elevated by the release of "stress

hormones" in persons with normally functioning adrenal glands.

In an emergency situation the triad of hypotension/shock, hyperkalemia, and hypoglycemia should trigger an evaluation for acute adrenal insufficiency. Diminished amounts of aldosterone from the adrenal cortex result in fluid and electrolyte imbalance because the distal tubules of the nephrons are unable to conserve sodium. As sodium loss increases through the

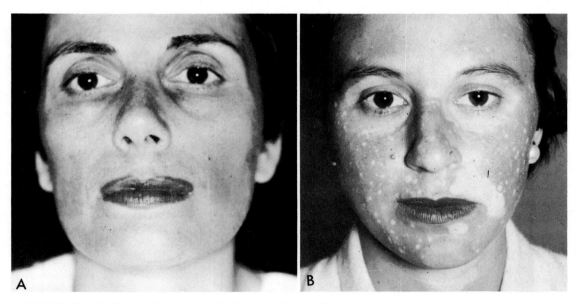

FIGURE 40–14. Altered pigmentation in adrenocortical insufficiency. **A,** Increased pigmentation across the bridge of the nose. **B,** Generalized hyperpigmentation with vitiligo. (From Bondy PK, Rosenberg LE: *Metabolic Control and Disease,* 8th ed. Philadelphia, WB Saunders, 1980, p 1462. Reproduced with permission.)

kidneys, the volume of extracellular fluid is depleted, and blood volume and blood pressure decrease. Serum sodium levels decrease (hyponatremia), and the potassium concentration increases (hyperkalemia) as a result of cation exchange in the distal tubules, which can no longer take place at a normal rate. Decreased amounts of cortisol from the adrenal cortex result in a decline in hepatic gluconeogenesis and an increase in tissue glucose uptake. Hypoglycemia results, leading the clinical symptoms.[26]

The diagnosis of adrenal insufficiency is made by comparing clinical and chemical abnormalities. In cases of acute insufficiency, hypotension and peripheral vasoconstriction occur. A serum sample for cortisol will demonstrate suppressed cortisol production of less than 20 μg/dL (normal during stress >20 μg/dL). Treatment should be started immediately with 100 mg of hydrocortisone given IV, along with measures to maintain blood pressure. Hydrocortisone, 100 mg IV, should be given every 6 hours until the crisis has resolved. The cause of the adrenal crisis should be explored when the individual is stable.

In cases of chronic adrenal insufficiency, an ACTH test should be given to the individual. Cosyntropin, a synthetic subunit of ACTH, 250 μg, is given IV, and serum samples of cortisol are measured 45 and 60 minutes after administration. Serum cortisol levels should increase to above 20 μg/dL following this stimulus. A slow ACTH infusion could also be given over 2 days and the excretion rate of some corticosteroids measured. ACTH levels could also be measured and compared with laboratory normal values; elevations would be consistent with primary adrenal insufficiency. Abdominal CT should be performed to determine the size of the adrenal glands. Large adrenals correlate with primary disease.

Aldosterone deficiency leads to the diagnosis of primary disease. This can be tested by the individual's ability to retain salt.

Treatment

The treatment of adrenal insufficiency entails replacing the absent or deficient hormones usually produced by the adrenal cortex, both glucocorticoids and, frequently, mineralocorticoids (aldosterone).

Aldosterone replacement, when needed, is in oral form (fludrocortisone acetate, Florinef) and must be taken daily. Fludrocortisone is basically equivalent to aldosterone and available only as an oral formulation. If the glucocorticoid replacement given does not have significant mineralocorticoid action (e.g., prednisone, dexamethasone) the dose of fludrocortisone needed will be higher. Aldosterone replacement tends to remain constant through adulthood. 9α-Fludrocortisone acetate (Florinef) will be effective only if salt is administered simultaneously. Therefore, sodium chloride supplement will be added if there is a sodium deficit.[28]

Cortisol is released when physiologic or psychological stress is experienced and frequently is referred to as the "flight-or-fight" hormone. Stress situations include acute illness (an increased temperature increases the body metabolic rate), injury (trauma, surgery, burns, etc.), and psychological episodes that affect an individual's ability to function normally (death of a significant relative). During these episodes of stress an individual may need double or triple the usual daily glucocorticoid dose. If illness or injury restricts the patient's ability to tolerate oral intake, hydrocortisone must be given IM or IV.[27]

Hypercortisolism

Etiology and Pathogenesis

Hyperfunction of a portion of the hypothalamic-pituitary-adrenal axis results in conditions characterized by **hypercortisolism.** Primary adrenocortical hyperfunction is caused by disease of the adrenal cortex. Secondary disease is caused by hyperfunction of the anterior pituitary ACTH-secreting cells, and tertiary disease is caused by hypothalamic dysfunction or injury. The term **Cushing's syndrome** is used to describe the clinical features of hypercortisolism, regardless of cause. **Cushing's disease** is the diagnosis reserved for pituitary-dependent conditions.

After age 8 years, hypercortisolism is frequently caused by the increased production of pituitary ACTH due to microadenomas or adenomas. Ectopic ACTH production by nonpituitary tumors can also stimulate the adrenal glands.[28] These types of tumor are very rare in children. The exogenous steroids used in the treatment of various diseases can also lead to Cushing's syndrome.

Clinical Manifestations

An individual with excess cortisol production will develop a round face with prominent, flushed cheeks, often referred to as "moon facies" (see Table 40–6). There is a noticeable weight gain with increasing total body fat, especially in the abdomen. A cervical pad ("buffalo hump"), capillary friability, and thinning of the skin with the formation of purple striae and ecchymoses over the abdomen, arms, and thighs develop. Muscle mass decreases and muscle weakness develops. Figure 40–15 shows the common clinical manifestations of Cushing's syndrome.

Hypertension may develop as a consequence of the salt-retaining activity of cortisol and of the increased blood volume. With chronic Cushing's syndrome, demineralization of the bones and resulting fractures may occur. Cerebral atrophy and neuropsychological defects have been found, for cortisol plays an important role in brain metabolism.

The cortisol excess may be accompanied by increased androgen production (excessive hair production, acne).

The diagnosis of adrenal cortical disease depends on reliable, accurate laboratory measurements. Urinary free cortisol levels may be elevated; the upper normal range is laboratory dependent. Following

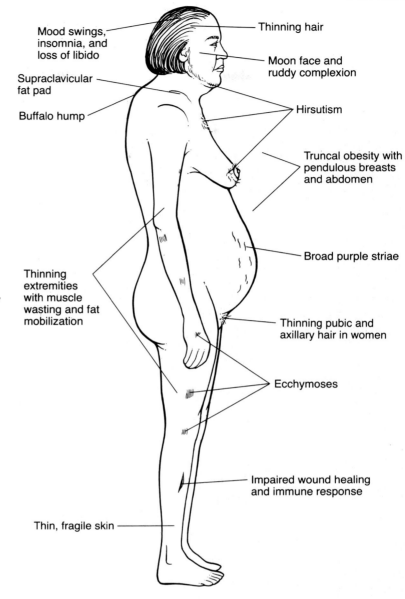

Mood swings, insomnia, and loss of libido

Supraclavicular fat pad

Buffalo hump

Thinning hair

Moon face and ruddy complexion

Hirsutism

Truncal obesity with pendulous breasts and abdomen

Broad purple striae

Thinning extremities with muscle wasting and fat mobilization

Thinning pubic and axillary hair in women

Ecchymoses

Impaired wound healing and immune response

Thin, fragile skin

F I G U R E 40 – 15. Common clinical manifestations of Cushing's syndrome. (From Monahan FD, Drake T, Neighbors M: *Nursing Care of Adults.* Philadelphia, WB Saunders, 1994, p 1290. Reproduced with permission.)

instruction for proper collection of specimens is paramount to obtaining reliable measurements. Measurement of the Porter-Silber chromogens or 17-hydroxycorticosteroids requires a 24-hour urine collection. The normal range is 4.5 mg/g of creatinine. Complete collections of urine are needed to exclude inappropriate diagnoses due to diurnal variations in cortisol production. Plasma cortisol levels should be monitored frequently during a 24-hour period because diurnal variations may show some normal values despite hypercortisolism.

Treatment

The choice of treatment for Cushing's disease is based on its cause. The transsphenoidal approach to the pituitary fossa has become the surgical treatment of choice. Figure 40–16 shows a woman before and after

treatment for Cushing's syndrome. Removal of the adrenal glands bilaterally is also an option. This would make the individual adrenal insufficient, and hormone replacement therapy for this condition would be instituted. Radiation therapy may be an option if surgery is contraindicated.

Hyperaldosteronism

Both primary hyperaldosteronism (excess production of aldosterone by the adrenal cortex) and excess levels of glucocorticoids (Cushing's disease or syndrome) tend to raise blood pressure. Aldosterone and glucocorticoids facilitate salt and water retention by the kidney; the hypertension that accompanies excessive levels of either hormone is probably due to this mechanism. Because aldosterone acts on the distal renal tubule to promote sodium exchange for the potassium

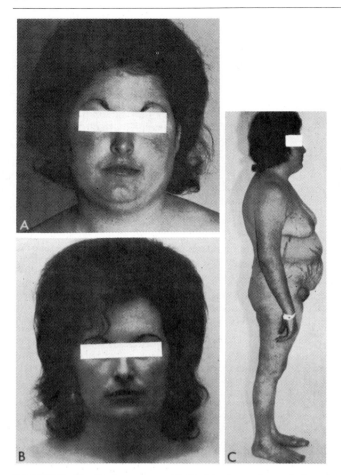

FIGURE 40–16. A woman with Cushing's syndrome before (**A, C**) and after (**B**) removal of an adrenal adenoma. (From Wyngaarden JB, Smith LH, Bennett JC (eds): *Cecil Textbook of Medicine,* 19th ed. Philadelphia, WB Saunders, 1992, p 1285. Reproduced with permission.)

lost in the urine, persons with hyperaldosteronism usually have decreased potassium levels (Fig. 40–17). The drug spironolactone is an aldosterone antagonist and therefore is useful in the medical management of persons with an aldosterone excess. Spironolactone increases sodium excretion and potassium retention.

KEY CONCEPTS

- The adrenal cortex produces three classes of steroid hormones: (1) glucocorticoids, (2) mineralocorticoids, and (3) sex steroids. Glucocorticoid synthesis is regulated by the pituitary secretion of ACTH. Mineralocorticoid synthesis is regulated by the renin-angiotensin system. The glucocorticoid cortisol provides the primary negative feedback mechanism to inhibit ACTH release.
- Adrenocortical insufficiency may be primary (Addison's disease), in which case it is characterized by high ACTH levels in the blood and hyperpigmentation of skin related to excessive pituitary secretion of melanocyte-stimulating hormone, or it may be secondary, in which case it is characterized by low

ACTH levels. Primary insufficiency may follow autoimmune destruction, surgical removal, or trauma to the gland. Exogenous administration of steroids suppresses ACTH, resulting in adrenocortical atrophy. The sudden withdrawal of exogenous steroids may result in adrenal insufficiency. A test dose of ACTH may be given to differentiate primary (no response) from secondary (increased cortisol level) insufficiency.
- Genetic defects in enzymes necessary for cortisol production may affect one or more of the steroid hormone synthesis pathways. Cortisol deficiency stimulates pituitary release of high levels of ACTH, which stimulate the adrenal gland to grow (congenital adrenal hyperplasia). Large amounts of androgens may be synthesized, leading to masculinization of females and precocious puberty in males.
- The manifestations of primary adrenocortical insufficiency include weight loss, salt wasting, volume depletion, low blood pressure, hypoglycemia, and hyperkalemia. Stress may lead to severe symptoms (Addisonian crisis), including circulatory shock, hyperglycemia, and hyperkalemia. Treatment includes hormone replacement therapy. Dosages are generally increased during periods of stress (e.g., surgery).
- Excess cortisol production due to pituitary hyperstimulation of the adrenal cortex is termed Cushing's disease. Hypercortisolism of any other cause is termed Cushing's syndrome. ACTH excess may be due to pituitary adenoma or exogenous production by nonpituitary tumors. Cushing's syndrome is commonly due to administration of exogenous steroids.
- The clinical manifestations of Cushing's disease and syndrome include moon facies, "buffalo hump," central obesity, thin extremities, weight gain, thin skin, striae, hypertension, and hyperglycemia. Plasma cortisol levels and the urinary excretion of cortisol metabolites are increased. Surgical removal of ACTH-producing tumors or removal of the adrenal gland is the usual treatment.
- Primary hyperaldosteronism is usually due to adrenal tumor. Secondary hyperaldosteronism is usually due to excessive circulating renin because of poor kidney perfusion. Congestive heart failure, chronic low cardiac output, and renal artery stenosis lead to aldosterone production. Aldosterone enhances sodium and water reabsorption and potassium excretion from the kidney, leading to hypervolemia, hypertension, and hypokalemia.

Adrenal Medullary Disorders

Etiology and Pathogenesis

The adrenal medulla secretes two important hormones, both of which are classified as nonsteroidal hormones called **catecholamines.** Epinephrine, or adrenaline, accounts for about 80 percent of the adre-

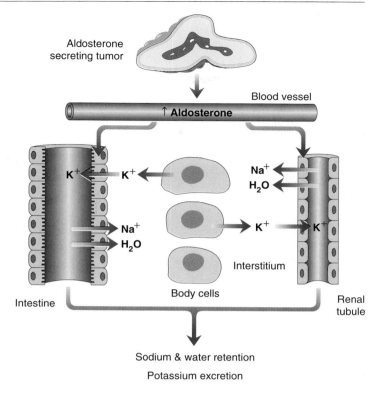

FIGURE 40–17. Hyperaldosteronism, regardless of the cause, results in sodium and water retention and potassium excretion.

nal medulla's secretion. The other 20 percent is nor-epinephrine. Norepinephrine is also the neurotransmitter produced by the postganglionic sympathetic fibers. Sympathetic effectors such as the heart, smooth muscle, and glands have receptors for norepinephrine. Both epinephrine and norepinephrine can bind to the receptors of sympathetic effectors to prolong and enhance the effects of sympathetic stimulation.

A tumor in the adrenal medulla can cause excess production of hormones. Stimulation of the sympathetic nerves to the adrenal medulla causes secretion of catecholamines (epinephrine and norepinephrine) into the blood. Pheochromocytomas occur in the adrenal medulla in 90 percent of cases. Rarely, they may occur in the paraganglia chromaffin cells of the sympathetic nervous system or in the organ of Zuckerkandl. The clinical manifestations change with variations in the amount of hormone released by the tumor. There are no known diseases or deficiencies caused by adrenal medullary insufficiency.[30]

Pheochromocytoma is an uncommon disease that results from the excessive production of catecholamines. A pheochromocytoma is a tumor of chromaffin tissue. It is usually found in the adrenal medulla, but it may also arise in other sites where there is chromaffin tissue, such as the sympathetic ganglia. Like adrenal medullary cells, the tumor cells of a pheochromocytoma produce and secrete the catecholamines epinephrine and norepinephrine. The massive release of these catecholamines results in hypertension. Thus, the hypertension in individuals with pheochromocytoma is influenced by the sympathetic

nervous system, the circulating catecholamine levels, and the cardiovascular response to these changes.

Clinical Manifestations

The most common symptom experienced by an individual with a pheochromocytoma is persistent hypertension. Headache and diaphoresis are very common consequences of the elevation in blood pressure. There may be episodic hypertensive episodes caused by stress, excitement, physical activity, certain drugs, and the smoking of tobacco products. Other, vaguer symptoms may include tachycardia, tremor, nervousness, emotionally labile, pallor, fatigue, generalized gastrointestinal complaints, and orthostatic hypotension. There may be signs of a hypermetabolic state such as fever, weight loss, polyuria, and polydypsia.[31] There are many other manifestations experienced by these individuals, but the presenting complaints frequently resemble those in other conditions such as renal disease, thyrotoxicosis, or psychological problems, if hypertension is intermittent. The final diagnosis may be delayed until symptoms worsens.

Uncontrolled hypertension can lead to decompensation of the vascular system, seizures, and congestive heart failure.

Treatment

In addition to α-adrenergic-blocking agents to control hypertension, an environment conducive to rest and essentially free of emotional stressors should be provided before unilateral or, if necessary, bilateral surgical removal of the adrenal gland is undertaken.

The only treatment for this condition is surgical removal of the tumor. Before surgery, antihypertensive drugs may be prescribed to manage blood pressure and relieve some of the symptoms related to this factor.

If both adrenal glands are removed, lifetime treatment for adrenocorticoid insufficiency is necessary. Because there is an increased risk of recurrence of the tumor in later years, annual follow-up by an endocrinologist should be planned. Pheochromocytomas are frequently inherited as an autosomal dominant trait. Family members should be informed, and preventive health care with specific attention to blood pressure monitoring should be suggested.

KEY CONCEPTS

- The adrenal medulla releases catecholamines into the bloodstream when stimulated by the sympathetic nervous system. Catecholamines increase heart rate, blood pressure, and glucose release from the liver.

- A pheochromocytoma is a catecholamine-secreting tumor that is usually located in the adrenal medulla. Excessive catecholamine release from the tumor causes intermittent or persistent hypertension, headache, tachycardia, tremor, and irritability. Most tumors are benign, and surgical removal relieves the disorder. Adrenergic blocking agents may be used to treat the hypertension until surgical treatment is accomplished.

Summary

Education is the key to maintaining an adequate state of health in individuals with an endocrine dysfunction. The individual with an alteration in endocrine function needs to understand the etiology, pathogenesis, clinical manifestations, treatment plan, prognosis, and consequences of proper as well as inadequate hormone replacement. The educational plan should be tailored to the individual's capacity to learn and understand. Often, it takes time for the person to understand all the facets of endocrine disorder; therefore, the educational process is ongoing throughout life.

Most of the hormones discussed in this chapter can be easily replaced. All nurses, physicians, and allied health care workers involved in the care of those with alterations in endocrine functioning recognize the importance of education in the treatment plan. Most endocrine hormones are replaced in patterns that mimic their natural release. Because lifelong treatment is usually necessary, people with alterations in endocrine function will at one time or another need concurrent treatment for other illnesses or diseases. The impact of other drugs on endocrine function must be recognized and adjustments made as appropriate.

REFERENCES

1. Endocrine disorders, in Nursing '84 Books. Springhouse, Penn, Springhouse Corp, 1984, p 21.
2. Bercu BB: Disorders of growth hormone neurosecretion, in Lifshitz F (ed): *Pediatric Endocrinology*, 2nd ed. New York, Marcel Dekker, 1990.
3. Vance ML: Growth hormone: non-growth-promoting uses in humans, in Mazzaferri EL (ed): *Advances in Endocrinology and Metabolism*. St. Louis, Mosby–Year Book, 1992, vol 3.
4. Kaplan SA: Growth and growth hormone, in Kaplan SA (ed): *Clinical Pediatric Endocrinology*. Philadelphia, WB Saunders, 1990.
5. Johanson AJ, Blizzard RM: Growth hormone treatment, in Lifshitz F (ed): *Pediatric Endocrinology*, 2nd ed. New York, Marcel Dekker, 1990.
6. Nishi Y, Masuda H, Nishimura S: Hereditary growth hormone deficiency, in Lifshitz F (ed): *Pediatric Endocrinology*. New York, Marcel Dekker, 1990, p 38.
7. Bjork S, Jonsson B, Westphal O, Levin J-E: Quality of life of adults with growth hormone deficiency: A controlled study. *Acta Paediatr Scand* 1989(suppl 356):55–59.
8. Hintz RL: Disorders of growth, in Harrison TR (ed): *Principles of Internal Medicine*, 12th ed. New York, McGraw-Hill, 1991.
9. Merimee TJ, Grant MB: Growth hormone and its disorders, in Becker KL (ed): *Principles and Practice of Endocrinology and Metabolism*. Philadelphia, JB Lippincott, 1990.
10. Thorner MD, Vance ML, Horjath E, Kovacs K: The anterior pituitary, in Wilson JD, Foster DW (eds): *Williams Textbook of Endocrinology*, 8th ed. Philadelphia, WB Saunders, 1992.
11. Frasier SD: Tall stature and excessive growth syndromes, in Lifshitz F (ed): *Pediatric Endocrinology*, 2nd ed. New York, Marcel Dekker, 1990.
12. Wells TG: The pharmacology and therapeutics of diuretics in the pediatric patient. *Pediatr Clin North Am* 1990;37(2):463–505.
13. Baylis PH, Thompson CJ: Diabetes insipidus and hyperosmolar syndromes, in Becker KL (ed): *Principles and Practice of Endocrinology and Metabolism*. Philadelphia, JB Lippincott, 1990.
14. Ginsberg L: Tolerance testing in children, in Lifshitz F (ed): *Pediatric Endocrinology*, 2nd ed. New York, Marcel Dekker, 1990.
15. Verbalis JG: Inappropriate antidiuresis and other hypo-osmolar states, in Becker KL (ed): *Principles and Practice of Endocrinology and Metabolism*. Philadelphia, JB Lippincott, 1990.
16. Recker BF: Anatomy and physiology of the endocrine system, in Jackson DB, Saunders RB (eds): *Child Health Nursing*. Philadelphia, JB Lippincott, 1993.
17. Guyton AC: *Textbook of Medical Physiology*, 8th ed. Philadelphia, WB Saunders, 1991.
18. Dallas JS, Foley JP: Hypothyroidism, in Lifshitz F (ed): *Pediatric Endocrinology*, 2nd ed. New York, Marcel Dekker, 1990.
19. Nicoloff JT, LoPresti JS: Myexedma coma: A form of decompensated hypothyroidism. *Endocrinol Metab Clin North Am* 1993;22(2):279–290.
20. Larsen PR, Ingbar SH: The thyroid gland, in Wilson JD, Foster DW (eds): *Williams Textbook of Endocrinology*, 8th ed. Philadelphia, WB Saunders, 1992.
21. Burch HB, Wartofsky L: Life-threatening thyrotoxicosis: Thyroid storm. *Endocrinol Metab Clin North Am* 1993;22(2):263–278.
22. Potts JR: Diseases of the parathyroid gland and other hyper- and hypocalcemic disorders, in Harrison TR (ed): *Principles of Internal Medicine*, 12th ed. New York, McGraw-Hill, 1991.
23. Recker BF: Pregnancy at risk: Metabolic and renal alterations, in Dickason EJ, Silverman BL, Schult MO (eds): *Maternal-Infant Nursing Care*, 2nd ed. St. Louis, Mosby–Year Book, 1994.
24. Aurbach GD, Mark SJ, Spiegel AM: Parathyroid hormone, calcitonin, and the calciferols, in Wilson JD, Foster DW (eds): *Williams Textbook of Endocrinology*, 8th ed. Philadelphia, WB Saunders, 1992.
25. Downs RW Jr, Levine MA: Hypoparathyroidism and other causes of hypocalcemia, in Becker KL (ed): *Principles and Practice of Endocrinology and Metabolism*. Philadelphia, JB Lippincott, 1990.
26. Clark KM: Nursing planning, intervention, and evaluation for altered endocrine function, in Jackson DB, Saunders RB (eds): *Child Health Nursing*. Philadelphia, JB Lippincott, 1993.

27. Werbel SS, Ober KP: Acute adrenal insufficiency. *Endocrinol Metab Clin North Am* 1993;22(2):303–328.
28. Migeon CJ, Lanes RL: Adrenal cortex: Hypo- and hyperfunction, in Lifshitz F (ed): *Pediatric Endocrinology*, 2nd ed. New York, Marcel Dekker, 1990.
29. New MI, del Balzo P, Crawford C, Speiser PW: The adrenal cortex, in Kaplan SA (ed): *Clinical Pediatric Endocrinology*. Philadelphia, WB Saunders, 1990.
30. Vorhees ML: Disorders of the adrenal medulla, in Lifshitz F (ed): *Pediatric Endocrinology*, 2nd ed. New York, Marcel Dekker, 1990.
31. Bravo EL, Gifford RW Jr: Pheochromocytoma. *Endocrinol Metab Clin North Am* 1993;22(2):329–342.

BIBLIOGRAPHY

Becker KL (ed): *Principles and Practice of Endocrinology and Metabolism.* Philadelphia, JB Lippincott, 1990.
Burrow GN, Oppenheimer JH, Volpe R: *Thyroid Function and Disease.* Philadelphia, WB Saunders, 1989.
Daughaday WH: Endocrine manifestations of systemic disease. *Endocrinol Metab Clin North Am* 1991;20(3):453–674.
Gagel RF: Multiple endocrine neoplasia type 1: Clinical features and screening. *Endocrinol Metab Clin North Am* 1994;23(1):1–18.
Harrison TR (ed): *Principles of Internal Medicine*, 12th ed. New York, McGraw-Hill, 1991.
Hershman JM (ed): *Endocrine Pathophysiology: A Patient Oriented Approach*, 3rd ed. Philadelphia, Lea & Febiger, 1988.

Jackson DB, Saunders RB (ed): *Child Health Nursing.* Philadelphia, JB Lippincott, 1993.
Kaplan SA (ed): *Clinical Pediatric Endocrinology*, 2nd ed. Philadelphia, WB Saunders, 1990.
Kappy MS, Blizzard RM, Migeon CJ: *The Diagnosis and Treatment of Endocrine Disorders in Childhood and Adolescence*, 4th ed. Springfield, Ill, Charles C Thomas, 1994.
Lifshitz F (ed): *Pediatric Endocrinology*, 2nd ed. New York, Marcel Dekker, 1990.
Mazzaferri EL: *Advances in Endocrinology and Metabolism*, 4th ed. St. Louis, Mosby–Year Book, 1993.
Moore WT, Eastman RC (ed): *Diagnostic Endocrinology.* Philadelphia, BC Decker, 1990.
Ober KP: Endocrine crisis. *Endocrinol Metab Clin North Am* 1993;22(2):181–446.
Parker LN: *Adrenal Androgens in Clinical Medicine.* New York, Academic Press, 1989.
Speroff L, Glass RH, Kase NG: *Clinical Gynecology, Endocrinology, and Infertility*, 4th ed. Philadelphia Williams & Wilkins, 1989.
Strauss JF III: Steroid hormones: Synthesis, metabolism, and action in health and disease. *Endocrinol Metab Clin North Am* 1991; 20(4):681–924.
Tindall GT, Barrow DL: *Disorders of the Pituitary.* St. Louis, CV Mosby, 1986.
Wilson JD, Foster DW (eds): *Williams Textbook of Endocrinology*, 8th ed. Philadelphia, WB Saunders, 1992.
Zaloga GP: Endocrine crises. *Crit Care Clin North Am* 1991;7(1): 1–252.

CHAPTER 41
Diabetes Mellitus

JACQUELINE SIEGEL

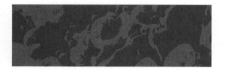

KEY TERMS

catecholamines: Hormones (epinephrine and norepinephrine) that stimulate glycogenolysis and gluconeogenesis.

corticosteroids: Hormones produced by the adrenal gland that stimulate gluconeogenesis and contribute to insulin resistance.

diabetes mellitus: An endocrine disorder characterized by glucose intolerance and affecting the metabolism of all the energy nutrients.

gestational diabetes: A disorder of glucose tolerance first diagnosed during pregnancy.

glucagon: Hormone produced by the alpha cells of the pancreas that stimulates glycogenolysis and gluconeogenesis in the liver.

gluconeogenesis: The production of glucose from amino acids and other substrates in the liver.

glycogenesis: The production of glycogen from glucose in hepatic and muscle tissue.

glycogenolysis: The production of glucose from the breakdown of glycogen in hepatic and muscle tissue.

glycolysis: The intracellular oxidation of glucose.

glycosylated hemoglobin: An index of glycemic control; the quantity of glucose attached to hemoglobin molecules, reflecting mean blood glucose values for a period of 120 days.

impaired glucose tolerance: A disorder of glucose tolerance that is not diagnostic of diabetes.

insulin: Hormone produced by the beta cells of the pancreas; has wide-ranging effects on energy metabolism and protein synthesis.

insulin resistance: The condition of requiring an increased amount of insulin for the same level of glucose utilization combined with lowered glucose utilization at all levels.

lipolysis: The production of free fatty acids from the breakdown of fat in adipose tissue.

pancreas: Gland located in the abdomen; has both endocrine and exocrine function. The endocrine pancreas produces insulin, glucagon, and somatostatin.

proinsulin: Precursor to insulin produced by the beta cells of the pancreas.

type I diabetes: Diabetes mellitus characterized by an absolute deficiency of insulin.

type II diabetes: Diabetes mellitus characterized by tissue insulin resistance and impaired insulin production by the pancreas.

*D*iabetes mellitus is an endocrine disease that is diagnosed by the presence of chronic hyperglycemia. Diabetes in fact alters the metabolism of all the energy nutrients and, with its complications, affects most organ systems. It is a highly prevalent disease: 6.8 million Americans have been diagnosed as having diabetes, a 1 million increase in 7 years, and it is estimated that at least 5 million additional Americans have undiagnosed diabetes. Current trends support the conclusion that the prevalence of diabetes is rising, particularly in the elderly.

Diabetes is a leading cause of death and disability in the United States. It increases the risk for heart disease, end-stage renal disease, blindness, amputation, and complications of pregnancy. Diabetes is ranked as the seventh leading cause of death and the 13th leading cause of premature death. Because diabetes disproportionately affects nonwhite and elderly patients, it is an important factor contributing to the excess mortality of black Americans.

Diabetes and its complications strain health care resources. The annual costs of diabetes have been estimated as at least $14 billion. The treatment of diabetic end-stage renal disease alone costs Medicare $330 million yearly.[1]

Regulation of Glucose Metabolism

Because diabetes affects the utilization of all the energy nutrients, it is helpful to review energy nutrient metabolism to understand the disease process of diabetes. The energy requirements of humans are predominantly met by glucose. Glucose is supplied to the bloodstream from the gastrointestinal tract, or produced from endogenous glycogen stores in the muscles and liver, or manufactured from such substrates as amino acids and lactate. Glucose is typically present in greater quantities in extracellular fluid than within the cells.

The plasma membranes of cells are variously permeable to glucose, and the diffusion of glucose in some cells is controlled by glucose transporters. Glucose transporters are specific to each tissue. The glucose transporters of neural tissue and erythrocytes do not require activation with the hormone **insulin.** Adipose and muscle cells possess insulin receptors on the cell membrane that bind to insulin and activate glucose transporters. Activated glucose transporters translocate to the cell membrane and facilitate the diffusion of glucose. Insulin plays an additional, as yet undefined role in glucose uptake.

Hormonal Regulation

Protein and fat metabolism are also affected by insulin. Insulin appears to increase the uptake and decrease the release of amino acids by skeletal muscle, thus inducing protein synthesis and preventing muscle breakdown. The amount of stored fats in the form of triglyceride is heightened by the action of insulin in preventing fat breakdown and inducing formation. Insulin also appears to play a role in growth by stimulating the secretion of somatomedin.

Normal glucose metabolism is usually described in reference to the fed and fasting or absorptive and postabsorptive states. The fed state occurs after ingestion of a meal and is characterized by utilization and storage of ingested energy nutrients. The fasting state is characterized by utilization of stored nutrients for the energy needs of the body.

In the fed state, glucose from ingested food provides the primary energy source (Fig. 41–1). The post-meal rise in blood glucose and the presence of certain

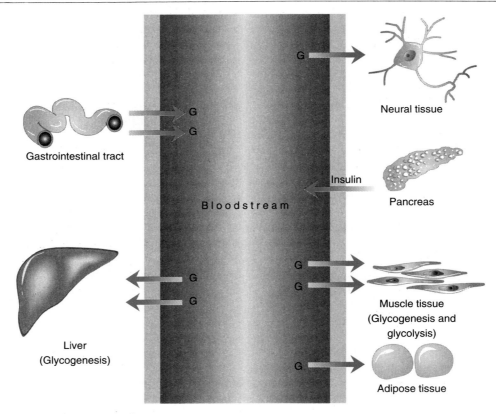

F I G U R E   41 – 1. Energy metabolism in the fed state. G, glucose.

gastrointestinal hormones stimulate the production of insulin. Initial stimulation produces a brief rise in insulin secretion, termed the *first phase*. The continued presence of increased glucose produces the *second phase* of insulin secretion, characterized by insulin synthesis.

Insulin is synthesized in the pancreas by the beta cells of the islets of Langerhans. The islets are groups of cells dispersed throughout the pancreas. Within the islets can be found beta cells that produce insulin in the form of **proinsulin,** alpha cells that produce **glucagon,** delta cells that produce somatostatin, and F-cells that produce pancreatic polypeptide.

Proinsulin is produced and packaged into granules. Enzymes within the granules cleave proinsulin into insulin and C peptide, with some remaining proinsulin. Granules release their contents into the bloodstream by exocytosis.

The presence of insulin stimulates diffusion of glucose into adipose and muscle tissue and inhibits production of glucose by the liver. After diffusion into the cell, glucose may be oxidized for the energy needs of the cell, a process termed **glycolysis.** Most ingested glucose is utilized in **glycogenesis** (the production of glycogen) in the muscle and the liver.

In the fasting state, glucose is produced by **glycogenolysis** (breakdown of stored glycogen) in the liver and muscles and **gluconeogenesis** (production of glucose from amino acids and other substrates) in the liver (Fig. 41–2). Insulin levels, no longer stimulated by an influx in ingested glucose, fall to a basal level. Glycogenolysis and gluconeogenesis are in fact stimu-

lated by the fall in insulin levels and a rise in glucagon levels. If insulin is the hormone that dominates the fed state, glucagon dominates the fasting. Glucagon-stimulated glycogenolysis and gluconeogenesis is responsible for up to 75 percent of glucose production in the fasting state.

The primary source of energy to the myocytes in the fasting state is free fatty acids produced by **lipolysis** (breakdown of fat from adipose tissue). Lipolysis is stimulated by the fall in plasma insulin. Neural tissue preferentially uses glucose.

Other hormones play a role in glucose metabolism in the fasting state. **Corticosteroids** stimulate gluconeogenesis and interfere with the action of insulin. **Growth hormone** increases peripheral insulin resistance and prevents insulin from suppressing hepatic glucose production. **Catecholamines** augment glucose production by prompting glycogenolysis and gluconeogenesis.

Exercise

Increasing activity requires increased fuel for muscle tissue. The onset of exercise precipitates a decrease in the production of insulin and an enhancement in the secretion of glucagon and catecholamines (Fig. 41–3).

In the first moments of exercise, under the influence of catecholamines, the muscle shifts from using primarily fatty acids for fuel to using stored glycogen. Lowered plasma insulin levels and increased produc-

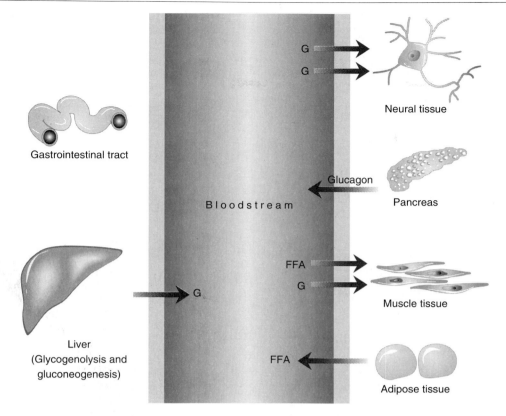

FIGURE 41–2. Energy metabolism in the fasting state. G, glucose; FFA, free fatty acids.

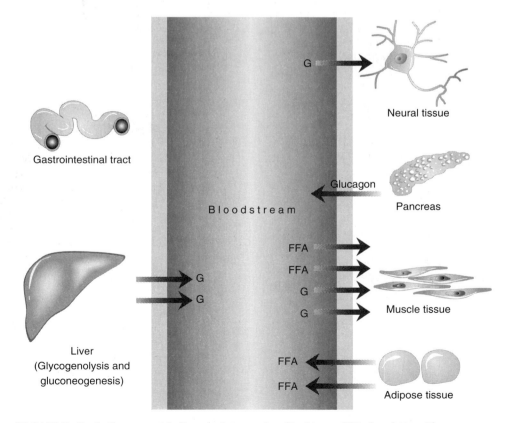

FIGURE 41–3. Energy metabolism during exercise. G, glucose; FFA, free fatty acids.

tion of glucagon are further stimuli to glycogenolysis and, more important, as exercise continues, to gluconeogenesis. After 10 to 40 minutes of exercise, blood glucose use by myocytes increases 7 to 20 times.

Catecholamines and the decrease in plasma insulin levels increase the production of free fatty acids. With increased duration of exercise, catecholamines cause a rise in hepatic glucose production. The interactions of hormones thus produce the mixture of glucose and free fatty acids used by muscle tissue during exercise.

Muscle tissue is affected by hormone levels and by exercise itself. The postreceptor activities of glucose transporters are enhanced by muscular contraction. The resulting increased insulin sensitivity can last as long as 16 hours.

Stress

During stress such as injury, illness, and pain, the stress hormones, including corticosteroids and catecholamines, interact to ensure continuous supplies of glucose. Corticosteroids increase the production of glucose from the liver and elevate the production of glucagon. Glucocorticoids also decrease the utilization of glucose by muscle tissue by diminishing the effect of insulin on glucose transporters and by generating a decline in the number of insulin receptors and their function.

Catecholamines increase serum glucagon levels, increase glucose production by the liver, and decrease the use of glucose by muscle and fat tissue. The production of fatty acids that is triggered by the action of catecholamines further inhibits glucose uptake in the periphery. The series of events produced by traumatic stress is referred to as *stress hyperglycemia.*

Psychological stress can produce comparable metabolic changes as physical stress. Deterioration in metabolic control has been noted in stressed diabetic subjects. An actual decrease in blood glucose levels has frequently been observed during acute stress.

KEY CONCEPTS

- **Plasma membrane permeability to glucose is determined by the type and density of glucose transport proteins in the membrane. In some tissues, particularly muscle and fat, the density of glucose transporters is regulated by insulin. Insulin binding to receptors on the cell surface results in translocation of glucose transporters to the cell surface. Glucose enters the cell passively by facilitated diffusion. Neurons and red cells have glucose transporters that do not require insulin.**

- **The metabolic effects of insulin include enhancing protein synthesis and inhibiting gluconeogenesis, enhancing fat deposition and inhibiting lipolysis, and stimulating cellular growth by enhancing somatomedin secretion.**

- **Insulin is synthesized in pancreatic beta cells as proinsulin. Proinsulin is stored in granules, where it is**

cleaved into insulin and C peptide. A postprandial rise in glucose stimulates the release of insulin into the bloodstream. During fasting, when blood glucose levels fall, insulin decreases and glucagon secretion increases, leading to lipolysis, glycogenolysis, and gluconeogenesis.

- **Exercise has complex effects on glucose metabolism. Insulin production decreases and glucagon and catecholamines increase, leading to elevated blood glucose levels. However, exercising muscle has increased insulin sensitivity, which facilitates glucose uptake for as long as 16 hours after exercise.**

- **A number of hormones released during stress increase blood glucose levels and oppose the effects of insulin. Catecholamines, glucocorticoids, and glucagon may precipitate "stress hyperglycemia."**

Etiology and Pathogenesis

Classification of Glucose Intolerance Disorders

Diabetes is probably not a single disease entity. As many as 30 different disorders may be called diabetes. Criteria for diagnosing the different conditions, all associated with glucose intolerance, were established by the National Diabetes Data Group of the National Institutes of Health in 1979.[2]

Accepted classifications include three clinical classes and two statistical risk classes (Table 41–1). The three clinical classes are diabetes mellitus (type I, type II, and other), impaired glucose tolerance (IGT), and gestational diabetes (GDM). Statistical risk classes are previous abnormality of glucose tolerance (PrevAGT) and potential abnormality of glucose tolerance (PotAGT.)

Diabetes Mellitus

Guidelines for the diagnosis of diabetes have been developed by the National Diabetes Data Group (Table 41–2).[3] The diagnostic criteria were designed to take normal aging changes into consideration. The

TABLE 41–1. Classifications of Glucose Metabolism Disorders

Actual Glucose Intolerance

Diabetes mellitus
　Type I (IDDM)
　Type II (NIDDM)
Diabetes associated with certain conditions or syndromes
Impaired glucose tolerance (IGT)
Gestational diabetes (GDM)

Statistical Risk of Glucose Intolerance

Previous abnormality of glucose tolerance (PrevAGT)
Potential abnormality of glucose tolerance (PotAGT)

go untreated for a time, resulting in persistent glycosuria with osmotic diuresis. Dehydration may
manifest as high osmolality and hemoconcentration
of red cells, proteins, and creatinine.

Clinical Manifestations and Complications

Acute Hyperglycemia

A primary concern of individuals with diabetes and
health care providers is avoiding the acute and chronic
complications of diabetes. Acute complications of diabetes include the signs and symptoms of hyperglycemia—polydipsia, polyphagia, and polyuria—and the
accompanying metabolic and fluid problems. Prolonged insulinopenia can result in ketoacidosis and
nonketotic hyperglycemic hyperosmolar coma with
the accompanying more severe electrolyte and fluid
derangements.

Acute complications of diabetes also include infections, most commonly of the skin, urinary tract, and
vagina. Infections that particularly affect elderly diabetic patients include malignant otitis externa, necrotizing faiscitis, and persistent candidal infections.
Tuberculosis infection and reactivation can be a particular problem in diabetic residents of extended-care
facilities.

Nausea, fatigue, and a generally decreased sense
of well-being frequently accompany hyperglycemia.
Blurred vision is a common short-term problem of
acute hyperglycemia. These symptoms can be quite
distressing and uncomfortable. Acute complications
are directly linked to hyperglycemia and recede as
euglycemia is approached.

Chronic Hyperglycemia

Chronic complications associated with diabetes are
extensive and are generally placed into two categories,
vascular and neuropathic. The vascular complications
are further subdivided into macrovascular and microvascular complications.

Vascular Complications

Macrovascular Complications. Macrovascular complications of diabetes include cardiovascular disease,
stroke, and peripheral vascular disease. The excess
mortality in diabetic individuals under the age of 70
is largely due to cardiovascular disease. Ischemic
cerebrovascular accidents (strokes) are more prevalent
in individuals with diabetes and have poorer outcomes. Diabetes is an independent risk factor for coronary artery disease. However, several important risk
factors for coronary artery disease—dyslipidemia,
free fatty acids, and triglycerides—are present in uncontrolled diabetes and decrease with improved blood
glucose control. Hypertension is more prevalent in
patients with diabetes and may, along with the charac-

teristic dyslipidemia of diabetes, be linked to the presence of the compensatory hyperinsulinemia of type
II diabetes.[12] The presence of very-low-density lipoproteins (VLDL) and insulin itself may induce the
proliferation of smooth muscle cells and lipids that
creates atherosclerotic disease. The use of exogenous
insulin may create immune complexes that damage
the arterial wall.

Control of the latter risk factors and of such other
risk factors as obesity and cigarette smoking may be
of greater benefit in reducing the incidence of macrovascular complications than improved glycemic
control.

Microvascular Complications. The microvascular
complications of diabetes, retinopathy and nephropathy, are thought to result from abnormal thickening
of the basement membrane in muscle capillaries. Capillary basement membrane thickening has been shown
to increase with the length of time after diagnosis and
with persistent hyperglycemia.[13]

Hyperglycemia has been shown to disrupt platelet
function and the growth of the basement membrane.
The presence of proteins altered by the presence of
high glucose levels (advanced glycosylation end products) is also believed to play a part in the pathogenesis
of microvascular complications. Thickening of capillary basement membranes has actually been shown
to decrease with improved glucose control.[14] Other
risk factors for microvascular disease include hypertension and smoking.

Basement membrane changes are implicated in
diabetic retinopathy, which affects 80 percent of all
individuals with diabetes 15 years after diagnosis.[3]
Retinopathy is the primary cause of new cases of
blindness in adults in the United States. The incidence
of diabetic retinopathy appears to correlate with the
duration of diabetes.

Nephropathy affects 30 to 40 percent of individuals with type I diabetes[15] and 5 to 10 percent of individuals with type II diabetes.[3] **Diabetic nephropathy** accounts for 25 percent of cases of end-stage renal
disease. Ethnic origin is a risk factor in the development of diabetic nephropathy, with black diabetic patients experiencing 2.6 times the rate of end-stage
renal disease as whites.[16] Nephropathy is also related
to changes in the basement membrane.

Neuropathic Complications

Some alteration in nerve function is present in all
individuals with diabetes. Neuropathic complications
produce symptoms in 25 percent of individuals with
diabetes. Partial or total disability because of pain or
dysfunction affects 12.5 percent of all individuals
with diabetes.

Diabetes in humans and experimentally induced
diabetes in animals are associated with decreased levels of myoinositol in peripheral nerves. There are several theoretical explanations for the myoinositol link
to neuropathy. Glucose appears to compete with myoinositol in transport into the cell. Degradation of glu-

cose to sorbitol and fructose (the polyol pathway) occurs in the nerves in the presence of hyperglycemia and insulinopenia. Increased activity of the polyol pathway also appears to be linked to reduced myoinositol in the peripheral nerves. Focal ischemic lesions of the nerves may also play a role in diabetic neuropathy.

Glycemic control has been shown to improve nerve function in animals and in humans and to decrease perceived pain. In addition to hyperglycemia, cigarette smoking, excessive alcohol use, male sex, and age are risk factors for the development of neuropathy.

Strong evidence linking prolonged hyperglycemia to neuropathy and the microvascular complications of diabetes was provided by the Diabetes Control and Complications Trial (DCCT), a 9-year multicenter prospective study designed to examine the effect of intensive insulin therapy on the development of retinopathy. Renal and neurologic indices were also examined. DCCT subjects were individuals with type I diabetes, with no or mild retinopathy at baseline. The experimental group was intensively treated with three or more insulin injections daily or with insulin delivered by a pump. The incidence of development of initial retinopathy was reduced by 76 percent and progression of existing retinopathy was reduced by 54 percent in the experimental group. Such indices of beginning nephropathy as microalbuminuria and albuminuria were reduced in the experimental group by 39 and 54 percent, respectively. Symptomatic neuropathy was reduced by 60 percent in the experimental group. Dilemmas presented by the DCCT include the presence of a significant increase in severe hypoglycemia in the experimental group, and some question as to the validity of extrapolating results to individuals with type II diabetes.[18]

Complications in Pregnancy

Pregnancy in women with type I diabetes has been complicated by an increased risk for perinatal infant mortality and congenital anomalies. Metabolic control during pregnancy reduces the risk of perinatal mortality to a rate approximating that of the general population.[19] An increased rate of congenital malformations continues to attend pregnancies in women with type I diabetes. Because the affected organs develop early in the first trimester, excellent glycemic control before conception is recommended.

Infants of women with gestational diabetes are at risk for macrosomia and perinatal hypoglycemia. A higher risk for congenital abnormalities may be present in the infants of women with gestational diabetes who need insulin treatment.[20]

KEY CONCEPTS

- The acute complications of hyperglycemia are hyperosmolar coma, ketoacidosis, and infections. Hyperglycemia may be associated with nausea, fatigue, and blurred vision.

- The chronic complications of hyperglycemia are primarily due to vascular and neuropathic dysfunction. People with diabetes are prone to vascular complications, including coronary artery disease, stroke, and peripheral vascular disease. These complications are related to dyslipidemia, hypertension, and immune-mediated damage. Retinopathy and nephropathy are thought to be due to hyperglycemia-induced thickening of retinal and glomerular basement membranes. Neuropathy presents as pain and loss of sensation. Excessive glucose is thought to interfere with myoinositol in neurons.

Treatment and Education

The usual treatment goals in diabetes are achieving metabolic control of blood glucose levels and preventing acute and chronic complications. The American Diabetes Association recommends as goals a fasting blood glucose level less than 140 mg/dL and a postprandial blood glucose level less than 200 mg/dL in type II diabetes.[3] For type I diabetes these goals are a fasting blood glucose level less than 120 mg/dL and a postprandial blood glucose level less than 180 mg/dL.[21] As a consequence of the findings of the DCCT, the American Diabetes Association has proposed a mean blood glucose value of 155 mg/dL as a reasonable goal.[22] The goals of treatment are accomplished by diet, exercise, medication, and such hygiene practices as daily foot care and smoking cessation. Each treatment involves life-style changes that are difficult to accomplish initially and challenging to maintain. Treatment must be individualized to the type of diabetes and the individual patient.

Nutrition

Nutrition has often been called the cornerstone of diabetes therapy. Ideas about the optimal dietary prescription have been far from constant throughout recorded history. From wheat, fruit, and beer in ancient Egypt, through blood pudding and rancid meats in 19th century France, to more recent investigations of fiber and fish oil, nutritional controversies are far from over.

In a position statement, the American Diabetes Association has listed seven recommendations for nutritional therapy for patients with diabetes (Table 41–5).[23] Accomplishing these recommendations raises questions concerning all the energy nutrients—carbohydrate, protein, and fat. A discussion of diabetes and nutrition must include a discussion of the proper combination, amount, and types of nutrients. Obesity and such eating disorders as bulimia are also important subjects.

Carbohydrates

Carbohydrates are categorized as monosaccharides (simple sugars) and polysaccharides (complex carbo-

TABLE 41–5. American Diabetes Association Recommendations for Nutritional Therapy

1. Restore normal blood glucose and optimal lipid levels.
2. Maintain normal growth rate in children and adolescents as well as the attaining and maintaining of reasonable body weight in adolescents and adults.
3. Provide adequate nutrition for the pregnant woman, the fetus and lactation.
4. Stay consistent in the timing of meals and snacks to prevent inordinate swings in blood glucose levels for people using exogenous insulin.
5. Determine a meal plan appropriate for the individual's lifestyle and based on a diet history.
6. Manage weight for obese people with non-insulin-dependent diabetes.
7. Improve the overall health of people with diabetes through optimal nutrition.

Data from American Diabetes Association: Nutritional recommendations and principles for individuals with diabetes mellitus: 1986. *Diabetes Care* 1987;10(1):126–32.

hydrates or starches). Carbohydrates contain four calories per gram. For many years, the American Diabetes Association recommended the restriction of carbohydrate, especially sucrose. The atherogenic potential of the resulting high-fat diet became a cause of concern. Epidemiologic studies have linked diets high in saturated fat to cardiovascular disease. A decrease in atherosclerotic lesions was found when carbohydrate and protein were substituted for fat.

Diets rich in carbohydrates have been postulated not only to protect against heart disease, but also to increase glycemic control. Since 1953, high-carbohydrate diets have been shown to decrease tissue insulin resistance in normal and diabetic subjects, resulting in lowered plasma glucose levels in patients with diabetes. Even high-sucrose diets have not been shown to cause deterioration in glycemic control in some studies.

Other studies have shown deterioration of glycemic control in diabetic patients on high-carbohydrate diets. High-carbohydrate diets have been associated with hypertriglyceridemia, decreases in high-density lipoprotein (HDL) cholesterol, and increases in low-density lipoprotein (LDL) cholesterol in some studies but not in others.[24,25]

The beneficial consequences of high-carbohydrate diets may be the result of substituting carbohydrate for saturated fat or the result of increasing dietary fiber content. Dietary fiber has been defined as plant carbohydrates found normally in foodstuffs that are not digestible by humans. Lowered blood glucose levels and improved lipid levels have been associated with diets rich in fiber, especially the soluble fiber found in legumes and oats.

Current recommendations include consumption of 55 to 60 percent of calories as carbohydrate, increasing the fiber content, and adding "modest" amounts of sucrose for diabetic patients in good glycemic control and at goal body weight. The use of artificial sweeteners is condoned at "established safe levels."

Protein

Protein is used in the repair and growth of tissues. Proteins are composed of amino acids and contain 4 calories per gram. The addition of protein to a meal will stimulate the secretion of insulin and blunt the postprandial rise in blood glucose levels in diabetic patients. Growth, development, and maintenance as well as glycemic control are considered to occur optimally at the recommended daily allowance of 0.8 g/kg of protein daily. Most Americans exceed this guideline.

Chronic high-protein intake is linked to heightened glomerular flow rates and renal hypertrophy. It is thought that continued renal hyperfunction can lead to nephropathy in diabetic patients. Restriction of dietary protein has been shown to improve renal function in patients with diabetes without adversely affecting metabolic control.[26]

Present recommendations call for not exceeding the RDA for protein except in cases of increased need, as in injury, gestation, and old age. A diet lower in protein may be prescribed for those at particular risk for renal disease.

Fat

Fats are composed of fatty acids and other substances. Fats contain 9 calories per gram. A high intake of dietary saturated fat has been associated with cardiovascular disease in animal and human epidemiologic studies. Dietary saturated fat and dietary cholesterol are strong stimuli to hypercholesterolemia. Elevated serum cholesterol levels have been identified as an important risk factor for cardiovascular disease. Hypertriglyceridemia is an independent risk factor for cardiovascular disease in diabetes.

Fat metabolism is dependent on the appropriate presence of insulin. Patients with diabetes often have multiple risk factors for cardiovascular disease, including dyslipidemia. Untreated diabetes is associated with hypertriglyceridemia, elevated VLDL levels, and lowered HDL levels. Although effective treatment of diabetes reduces the incidence of dyslipidemia, the risk of cardiovascular disease may not be affected.[27]

A lower incidence of cardiovascular lesions has been noted when serum cholesterol is lowered by drugs or by diet. The ideal diet for control of serum lipids continues to be a source of controversy. A high-carbohydrate, low-fat diet was discussed in the previous section. A diet high in monosaturated fat has been shown to lower serum triglycerides and VLDL cholesterol, raise HDL cholesterol, and promote euglycemia in patients with diabetes.[28] A similar diet was associated with decreased total cholesterol and LDL cholesterol in a nondiabetic population.[29]

Foods with plentiful omega 3 fatty acids (i.e., fatty fish) have been shown to reduce VLDL cholesterol and triglyceride levels and blood pressure in patients with diabetes,[30] and to reduce the incidence of second myocardial infarctions in cardiac patients.[31] Supplementation with omega 3 fatty acid capsules can result in deterioration of glycemic control and an increase in LDL cholesterol in individuals with diabetes.

Current recommendations on fat intake include limiting fat intake to less than 30 percent of total calories, with saturated fat composing less than 10 percent of total fat and polyunsaturated fat less than 10 percent of total fat. A reduction in cholesterol intake to less than 300 mg/day is suggested. The recommendations call for further research into omega 3 fatty acids and monosaturated fat.

Obesity and Eating Disorders

Obesity is the strongest risk factor for type II diabetes. Obesity is also a risk factor for cardiovascular disease in women. Weight loss is associated with suppression of glucose output from the liver and improvement of tissue glucose uptake. Fasting and postprandial glucose levels fall. Even a minor weight loss of 15 to 30 pounds can lead to marked improvement in glycemic control. Current recommendations for treatment of obesity include use of a nutritionally complete diet, a program of maintenance, and exercise.

Eating disorders such as bulimia and anorexia may be increased in women with type I diabetes. Inducing weight loss by reducing insulin has also been noted. Careful patient assessment is necessary to discover eating disorders for referral for treatment.

Exercise

Exercise is one of the oldest treatments for diabetes, having been prescribed in India in 500 B.C. Exercise can play a role in both type I and II diabetes in lowering blood glucose levels and promoting health maintenance. Exercise lowers such cardiovascular risk factors as high blood pressure and lipidemia, increases work capacity, reduces stress, prevents bone loss, and improves reaction time. Exercise may also be beneficial in weight reduction.

The effects of exercise on fuel utilization and insulin sensitivity are comparable to exercise-induced changes in normal metabolism. As glucose production increases and plasma insulin drops, the reduction in tissue insulin resistance can result in a net fall in blood glucose. Exercise has the potential to decrease insulin requirements in type I diabetes, decrease and possibly eliminate the need for pharmacologic agents in type II diabetes, and improve the health of all people with diabetes.

Although the benefits of exercise are numerous, there are associated risks. Individuals with type I diabetes are at risk for hypoglycemia and ketoacidosis. Exercise in individuals with type II diabetes can be associated with hypoglycemia, cardiac dysfuntion, orthopedic injury, and worsening of some complications.

When insulin or an oral hypoglycemic agent is used in the treatment of diabetes, the usual fuel metabolism of exercise is disturbed. Inappropriately high insulin levels result in decreased hepatic glucose production and increased tissue insulin sensitivity. The latter processes can lead to hypoglycemia. Replacement of expended glycogen and continued insulin sensitivity can result in hypoglycemia as long as 24 hours after activity.

When insulin levels are inappropriately low, hepatic glucose production is increased and tissue insulin sensitivity is decreased. The production of free fatty acids rises, probably due to the influence of exercise-stimulated production of catecholamines. Hyperglycemia and ketosis may be a result of exercise under insulinopenic conditions. Safeguards must be built into exercise programs to avoid hypoglycemia, ketoacidosis, injury, cardiac compromise, and exacerbation of diabetic complications.

The exercise prescription is as essential in diabetes treatment as the medication or nutrition prescription. To achieve metabolic and cardiovascular benefits, exercise must be performed for 20 to 45 minutes at least 3 days a week and must incorporate aerobic activity at 50 to 70 percent Vo_{2max}, which approximates 65 to 80 percent of maximum heart rate. Maximum heart rate is often estimated as 220 − age (years). Patients with autonomic neuropathy should be taught a method of judging exercise intensity by perceived exertion.

Before an exercise program is begun, a physical examination should rule out the presence of such limiting diabetic complications as retinopathy and neuropathic foot ulcers or malformations. Screening for cardiovascular problems should include an exercise-stress electrocardiogram in diabetic patients over the age of 35. To avoid orthopedic injury, the exercise session should be preceded by a warmup period involving mild activity or stretching. Exercise should be initiated at a low intensity and duration and gradually increased. Patients must be counseled to wear appropriate clothing and footwear and to carefully inspect the feet after the exercise session.

Individuals with type I diabetes are encouraged to eat additional carbohydrates or to reduce the dose of injected insulin when exercise is anticipated. A consistent exercise program can facilitate such adjustments. Additional food is not often necessary in type II diabetes; however, patients should be encouraged to have rapidly acting carbohydrate available should it become needed. Exercise should be avoided if the blood glucose level is less than 100 mg/dL or greater than 250 mg/dL when ketosis is present. Exercise when blood glucose values are over 250 mg/dL is safe when ketosis is not present.

Pharmacologic Agents

Oral Hypoglycemics

When diet and exercise have been ineffective in controlling hyperglycemia in type II diabetes, an oral hypoglycemic agent is usually the next treatment chosen. Sulfonylurea drugs have been used in the treatment of type II diabetes for over 35 years and are

TABLE 41–6. Oral Hypoglycemic Agents

Oral Hypoglycemic Agent	Onset*	Duration†	Comment†
Tolbutamide	1 hr	6–12 hr	Useful in renal disease
Chlorpropamide	1 hr	60 hr	Antidiuretic action
Acetohexamide	1 hr	12–18 hr	Uricosuric agent Contraindicated in renal disease
Tolazamide	4–6 hr	12–14 hr	Useful in renal disease
Glyburide	2–4 hr	24 hr	No disulfiram effect
Glipizide	1–1½ hr	Up to 24 hr	No disulfiram effect

*Data from Olin BR (ed): *Drug Facts and Comparisons.* St. Louis, Facts & Comparisons Inc., 1991.
†Data from Lebovitz HE: Oral hypoglycemic agents, *in* Ellenberg M, Rifkin H (eds): *Diabetes Mellitus: Theory and Practice,* 4th ed. New Hyde Park, NY, Medical Examination Publishing, 1990, pp 554–574.

currently the only oral hypoglycemic drugs sanctioned for use in the United States.

The sulfonylureas exert their hypoglycemic effect by inducing insulin release by the beta cells, augmenting the action of insulin in glucose disposal, diminishing insulin clearance by the liver, and reducing hepatic glucose production. Because sulfonylureas are ineffective in the management of type I diabetes, stimulation of the beta cells is a crucial factor in the action of these oral agents. Enhanced insulin secretion appears to be a short-term effect, possibly due to a reduction in insulin requirements as a result of the other hypoglycemic activities of sulfonylurea agents.

The so-called first-generation agents (those formulated earliest) are tolbutamide, chlorpropamide, acetohexamide, and tolazamide. Second-generation agents include glyburide and glipizide. Differences exist between the sulfonylureas in duration of action and in excretion (Table 41–6).[32,33] Second-generation agents are more potent than first-generation agents, possibly because of increased capacity to bind to the plasma membrane of the beta cell. Glyburide appears to characteristically increase basal secretion of insulin, and glipizide to heighten postprandial insulin production. However, neither second-generation agent has been shown to be effective after a first-generation agent has failed.

The side effects of sulfonylureas include hypoglycemia, nausea, dizziness, headache, allergic reactions, flushing with alcohol use (disulfiram effect), and other rarer blood disorders. Oral hypoglycemic agents that are metabolized by the liver to inactive compounds are considered safer for use in renal disease. Duration of action is another safety issue. Sulfonylureas are the major cause of severe hypoglycemia caused by a drug. The longer-acting sulfonylureas, chlorpropamide and glyburide, are responsible for the majority of cases of severe hypoglycemia and fatal hypoglycemic coma.

When prescribed along with an appropriate meal plan, sulfonylureas can be very effective in the treatment of type II diabetes. Primary failure of the drug is considered to have occurred when initiation of sulfonylurea therapy does not result in a significant decline in blood glucose levels. Primary failure can be due to misdiagnosis of type I diabetes or inadequate adherence to diet. Secondary failure, or hyperglycemia following an effective initial response to the drug, is often due to dietary nonadherence but may also be due to the progressive beta cell dysfunction of type II diabetes.

Other pharmaceutical agents are being studied to determine their efficacy in treating type II diabetes. Metformin, classified as a biguanide, has been used outside the United States for over 30 years. Metformin enhances glucose uptake by peripheral tissue without causing hypoglycemia. Metformin has been used alone and in combination with a sulfonylurea drug.

Acarbose, an α-glucosidase inhibitor, diminishes postprandial hyperglycemia by delaying carbohydrate absorption. It has been used alone and in combination with sulfonylurea drugs. Side effects include symptoms related to decreased gastrointestinal absorption (i.e., flatulence and diarrhea).

Insulin

Insulin therapy is required in 100 percent of patients with type I diabetes and 35 percent of patients with type II diabetes.[34] Patients with type I diabetes require replacement of the deficient hormone in as physiologic a manner as possible. The role of insulin in type II diabetes is more complex.

Because type II diabetes is a progressive disease, many if not most patients will likely need insulin at some time, either because of increasing insulin resistance or because of beta cell dysfunction. Glucose toxicity, a phenomenon in which insulin resistance and decreased production of insulin are worsened by hyperglycemia, may respond to insulin therapy. Insulin may be necessary in type II diabetes intermittently during times of physiologic stress that increase insulin requirements (e.g., intercurrent illness, surgery, weight gain). With the resolution of stress, the patient may be able to discontinue insulin use.

Porcine, bovine, and human preparations of insulin are available for use. Human insulin contains fewer noninsulin proteins than beef or pork insulin. Human insulin is recommended for pregnant women, patients with allergic or other adverse reactions to animal-source insulin, patients who use insulin intermittently, and all patients beginning insulin therapy.

T A B L E 41 – 7. Action of Insulin

Type of Insulin	Onset	Peak	Duration
Rapidly acting			
Regular	20 min	1½–2 hr	4–6 hr
Semilente*	½–1 hr	2–8 hr	5–8 hr
Intermediate acting			
NPH	1 hr	3–6 hr	11–16 hr
Lente	2 hr	4–8 hr	12–18 hr
Long acting			
Ultralente	4–6 hr	12–16 hr	>24 hr

*Kahn CR, Shechter Y: Insulin, oral hypoglycemic agents, and the pharmacology of the endocrine pancreas, in Gilman AG, Rall TW, Nies AS, Taylor P (eds): *The Pharmacological Basis of Therapeutics*, 8th ed. New York, Pergamon Press, 1990, pp 1463–1480.

Data from Skyler JS: Insulin pharmacology. *Med Clin North Am* 1988;72(6): 1337–1354.

Types of insulin are classified in three groups, based on their duration of action—short acting, intermediate acting, and long acting (Table 41–7). The most commonly used insulins in the short-acting category are regular and semilente; in the intermediate category, NPH and lente; and in the long-acting category, ultralente.[35]

Patterns of insulin use vary depending on diabetes type and degree of desired metabolic control (Fig. 41–6). For patients with type I diabetes, a minimum of two daily injections of a mixture of rapid- and intermediate-acting insulins has been used to control postprandial and fasting hyperglycemia. If hypoglycemia occurs during the night, the intermediate-acting insulin can be shifted to bedtime, producing a more intensive schedule. NPH and regular insulin may be mixed in the same syringe and given as one injection. Mixtures of regular and lente insulin are unstable. The latter insulins must be injected separately.

Intensive insulin schedules attempt to mimic normal insulin secretion closely and are considered important for optimal control. One such schedule calls for the use of regular insulin before meals and intermediate- or long-acting insulin at bedtime (or at breakfast and bedtime). In the latter schedule, the long- or intermediate-acting insulin stands in for basal insulin secretion. Insulin doses can be adjusted by the use of an algorithm based on capillary blood glucose monitoring or by an estimate of the carbohydrate content of the next meal.

Continuous subcutaneous insulin infusion (CSII) by means of an insulin pump has been used to approximate nondiabetic insulin secretion. CSII technology supplies a constant infusion of regular insulin and delivers a pre-meal bolus dose programmed by the user. Improvement in glycemic control has been noted with CSII. Complications associated with CSII therapy (infected infusion sites, ketoacidosis, and hypoglycemic coma) have resulted in a 27 to 50 percent rate of discontinuation of pump use.[36] A programmable implanted pump is in use on an experimental basis.

Other insulin delivery devices include jet injectors and insulin pens. Jet injectors, mechanisms that deliver a spray of insulin under the skin, increase the rate of insulin absorption. Further investigation has been proposed to determine risks and benefits of jet

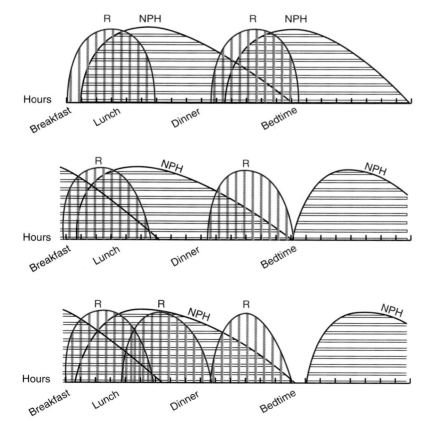

F I G U R E 41 – 6. Typical patterns of insulin use. *Top,* a mixture of R (rapid-acting) and NPH (intermediate-acting) insulin taken twice daily. *Middle,* a mixture of R and NPH insulin taken before breakfast, R taken before dinner, and NPH taken at bedtime. *Bottom,* NPH insulin taken twice daily, R taken before each meal. (Figure designed by Lisa Siegel.)

injector therapy. Insulin pens include the insulin, measuring devices, and needle in one pen-sized instrument. Delivery of insulin through the nasal route is under study.

Pancreas transplantation has been performed in patients with diabetes since 1966, with consistent improvement in patient outcomes. Pancreas transplantation restores normal metabolism but must be accompanied by lifelong treatment with immunosuppressive agents.

In the management of type II diabetes, insulin is prescribed when a management plan that includes an oral hypoglycemic agent no longer produces acceptable glycemic control. Two injections of rapid- and intermediate-acting insulins can be used. Premixed preparations of NPH and regular insulin facilitate the use of mixed doses, especially in the elderly. A mixture containing 70 percent NPH insulin and 30 percent regular insulin (70/30 insulin) is widely used in the United States, and 50/50 insulin (50 percent NPH and regular) has been introduced. A select group of patients may benefit from a bedtime dose of intermediate-acting insulin added to daytime sulfonylurea therapy. The use of an oral sulfonylurea in addition to insulin may improve metabolic control.[37]

The action of insulin is affected by many elements, including climate, alteration in blood flow, tobacco use, and injection site. Insulin is absorbed most rapidly from the abdomen, less rapidly from the arm, and slowest from the leg. Insulin is absorbed more rapidly from areas that are exercised or massaged after injection.

Hypoglycemia is the most frequent complication of insulin therapy, and the most hazardous. The incidence of hypoglycemia has been estimated at 4 to 6 percent of patients treated with sulfonylureas and 60 percent of insulin-treated patients. Severe hypoglycemia occurred in 8 percent of insulin-treated patients in a year in one study.[38] Hypoglycemia may cause or be a factor in 3 percent of deaths in patients with insulin-treated diabetes.[39]

Neural tissue depends on a constant supply of glucose for normal function. When insufficient food intake, unplanned activity, or an inappropriate insulin or sulfonylurea dose lowers blood glucose excessively, counterregulatory mechanisms are activated to ensure a continued supply of glucose to the brain. The production of glucagon, catecholamines, corticosteroids, and growth hormone is increased. The latter hormones increase glucose production by mechanisms outlined earlier in this chapter.

Symptoms of hypoglycemia produced by counterregulatory mechanisms include pallor, tremor, diaphoresis, palpitation, and anxiety. Neuroglycopenic symptoms noted in hypoglycemia are hunger, visual disturbance, weakness, paresthesias, confusion, agitation, coma, and death. In longstanding diabetes, neuropathy can alter counterregulatory mechanisms. Hypoglycemic unawareness, in which the diabetic patient does not experience counterregulatory symptoms, can be the result.

Alcohol interferes with counterregulatory processes by suppressing gluconeogenesis. Alcohol intake has resulted in fatal hypoglycemic coma even in the absence of other hypoglycemic drugs. The combination of alcohol and insulin or sulfonylurea drugs can be particularly dangerous.

Another typical complication of insulin therapy is lipodystrophy. Lipoatrophy has been linked to the use of animal-source insulins. Lipohypertrophy results from insulin-stimulated growth of adipose tissue at injection sites. Avoiding repeated injections at the same site is recommended to prevent lipodystrophy.

An acute complication of insulin use can be insulin edema, a localized or generalized accumulation of fluid. Weight gain can accompany initiation of insulin therapy, especially when glycemic control is improved. A third complicating factor in insulin therapy is insulin resistance. Insulin resistance is exacerbated by obesity and can necessitate the use of large insulin doses. An appropriate diet and exercise program is as important to insulin-treated patients as it is to other patients with diabetes.

Stress Management

Living with diabetes can be stressful. The tasks of blood glucose monitoring, medication administration, meal planning, and preventive care to avoid complications can be demanding. Fearing the onset of complications and the impact that complications may have, or living with complications, are parts of the psychological impact of diabetes. Stress management can play an important role in diabetes care by improving quality of life and reducing the possible impact of stress on glycemic control.

Assessment of Efficacy

Several measures are used by clinicians to determine the adequacy of glycemic control. One indirect but very useful indication of blood glucose levels is the level of glycosylated hemoglobin. Hemoglobin becomes glycosylated when glucose is nonenzymatically attached to one of its terminal amino acids. Four glycosylated hemoglobin products are formed: Hb A_{1a1}, Hb A_{1a2}, Hb A_{1b}, and Hb A_{1c}. The latter is produced in the largest quantity and is used in most assays.

As erythrocytes are freely permeable to glucose, the quantities of glycosylated hemoglobin formed are proportional to the quantity of glucose in the blood plasma. Glycosylated hemoglobin values will reflect mean blood glucose levels for the life of the average erythrocyte (100–120 days). Highly significant correlations have been found between mean Hb A_1 levels and mean blood glucose levels over a period of 8 months.[40] The presence of abnormal hemoglobins or hemolytic anemia can skew results. The normal value varies with laboratory technique but is usually around 6.5 percent.

Glycosylated hemoglobin values are used clinically to estimate long-term control and to set and evaluate therapeutic goals. Poor correlation with fasting blood glucose precludes glycosylated hemoglobin values from being used for short-term assessment and such changes in management as adjusting the dosage of hypoglycemic agents. Therefore, glycosylated hemoglobin values are not useful for day-to-day management of diabetes.

Venous blood can be drawn in a clinic or office and analyzed for glucose content. However, as Keen and Knight noted in 1962, "It is probable that many diabetics, who are thought to be well controlled will prove to have unexpected blood sugar fluctuation at times of day outside clinic hours."[41] Keen's proposal was to have patients collect blood samples from finger pricks on filter paper and mail them to his laboratory.

Keen was a man ahead of his time. The advent of capillary blood glucose monitoring in the late 1970s provided a solution to the problem of short-term evaluation of glycemic control. Individuals with diabetes and health professionals can use a drop of capillary blood applied to a glucose oxidase reagent strip to measure the blood glucose level. The treated strips are generally read in 1 or 2 minutes. Testing strips are read visually or by a meter. Some testing strips can be read both ways.

The Consensus Development Conference on Self-Monitoring of Blood Glucose, convened by the American Diabetes Association and other involved agencies, formulated several goals for the use of capillary blood glucose monitoring. The goals included use of capillary blood glucose monitoring to initiate and maintain a data base on client's glycemic status, provide guidelines for independent adjustment of therapy by clients alone or in communication with the health professional, assess the presence of such emergency situations as diabetic ketoacidosis and hypoglycemia and assist in treatment, and as a tool for education for individuals with diabetes and significant others.[42]

Capillary blood glucose monitoring has been shown to be an accurate reflection of venous blood glucose when performed by health professionals and by patients. However, unacceptable variation has been found in some studies.[43] Hematocrit and the presence of lipemia can affect results. Accuracy can be affected by such performance errors as under- or overloading the strip, incorrect placement of the sample, and improper sample removal. Training improves performance.

Patients with diabetes using capillary blood glucose monitoring have frequently reported enthusiasm and increased insight into the relationship between blood glucose and such factors as diet, exercise, and stress, or increased feelings of well-being. Capillary blood glucose monitoring has been associated with improved glycemic control.[44] Motivation may be an important factor especially during pregnancy, as evidenced in one study by deterioration in glycemic control post partum, although use of capillary blood glucose monitoring continued.[45] Capillary blood glucose monitoring is simply a biofeedback technique that can provide immediate information on the effects of a change in therapy.

There are hazards associated with the use of capillary blood glucose monitoring. Institutional use of capillary blood glucose monitoring involves potential handling of blood, with the concomitant risk or transmission of such blood-borne diseases as hepatitis B and HIV infection. The Centers for Disease Control has responded directly to the problem of performance of capillary blood glucose monitoring by providing guidelines in institutional use.[46] Patient use of capillary blood glucose monitoring has also been associated with such hazards as infection. Hand washing and using a fresh lancet for every test have been recommended to avoid finger infection.

Education

The individual with diabetes must meet physical and financial challenges and uncertainty about the future. The individual must also learn a variety of skills, some relatively easy to master, others more demanding. People with diabetes must learn to perform biological tests and interpret results correctly, measure and administer medication (often injectable medication), treat the side effects of medications, plan meals, design an exercise program, perform foot inspection and care, and accomplish other difficult tasks. Many of these tasks would require a license if performed on another person.

Few other chronic diseases make so many demands on patients. For this reason, diabetes education is considered an essential component of diabetes treatment. Participation in a diabetes education program has been shown to increase patient knowledge about diabetes, performance of self-care procedures, and psychological outlook. Benefit has been shown in such biochemical indices as blood glucose, glycosylated hemoglobin, and serum lipids. Systematic follow-up can improve continued adherence to self-care practices.[47,48]

The consequences of neglecting the education of diabetic patients can be grave. Hospitalization for complications of diabetes were shown to be primarily due to educational deficits in 27 percent of admissions and a contributing cause in an additional 20 percent in one study.[49] Several studies have confirmed the cost savings of diabetes education due to a decreased rate of hospitalization and outpatient medical visits.[50]

Many people with diabetes lack essential skills for performing diabetes self-care. Important knowledge deficits have been found in people with diabetes, including pregnant women. Deficits are greater in people not treated with insulin. It is the position of the American Diabetes Association that diabetes education is a critical constituent of diabetes care and should be an included benefit in third-party reimbursement.[51]

People with diabetes are a diverse group, with wide variations in age, ethnic background, years of disease duration, education, and intellectual abilities. For this reason, diabetes education must be tailored to the individual's needs. Newly diagnosed patients will need education in such survival skills as medication administration and the treatment of hypoglyce-

TABLE 41–8. Content Areas Stipulated by National Standards for Diabetes Patient Education

General facts
Psychological adjustment
Family involvement
Nutrition
Exercise
Medications
Relationship between nutrition, exercise, and medication
Monitoring
Hyperglycemia and hypoglycemia
Illness
Complications
Hygiene
Benefits and responsibilities of care
Use of the health care system
Community resources

Data from American Diabetes Association: National standards for diabetes patient education and American Diabetes Association review criteria. *Diabetes Care* 1990;13(suppl 1):60–65.

mia. More comprehensive education is best provided after the initial disturbance of the diagnosis has receded. Patients with low literacy skills will benefit from educational materials designed for their special needs. The education of elderly patients must take sensory deficits into consideration. The short attention spans of children implicate special guidelines for educating the young.

To ensure quality in diabetes education programs, national standards have been established by the American Diabetes Association. These standards define key content areas[52] and provide guidelines for assessment, setting objectives, follow-up, and other areas. Diabetes education programs able to demonstrate adherence to the national standards are officially recognized by the American Diabetes Association. The National Long-Range Plan to Combat Diabetes, formulated by a division of the U.S. Department of Health and Human Services, has set a goal of providing diabetes education to all patients with diabetes, preferably education that meets national standards (Table 41–8).[1]

KEY CONCEPTS

- **The mainstays of diabetic treatment are diet, exercise, and drug therapy. Education is an integral part of treatment to enable people with diabetes to follow the diabetic regimen and avoid complications. The efficacy of therapy can be assessed by following blood glucose levels and glycosylated hemoglobin levels. Blood glucose monitoring is useful for assessing short-term efficacy. Glycosylated hemoglobin is a better measure of long-term efficacy of therapy. A mean blood glucose level less than 155 mg/dL is desirable.**

- **The recommended diabetic diet includes 55 to 60 percent of calories from carbohydrate sources, less than 30 percent of calories from fat, and adequate intake of protein. High-protein intake may hasten the**

development of nephropathy. For type II diabetics, a diet geared toward weight loss may be beneficial. Even modest weight loss usually improves glycemic control.

- **Exercise has several benefits for the individual with diabetes. Insulin requirements may be reduced, weight loss facilitated, and the risk of cardiovascular complications decreased. Exercise may precipitate hypoglycemia, so insulin injections or dietary intake may need adjustment.**

- **Oral hypoglycemics may be successfully used in type II diabetes. The sulfonylureas exert their effects primarily by stimulating release of endogenous insulin. They also reduce insulin degradation and suppress release of glucose from the liver.**

- **Insulin replacement therapy is required in type I and about one third of cases of type II. Insulins are classified according to their onset, peak, and duration of action. A combination of insulins may be given to produce optimal control. Regular and NPH insulin are commonly used. Regular insulin is short acting. NPH is intermediate acting and may be given in combination with regular insulin.**

- **Hypoglycemia is the most common complication of pharmacologic therapy. Symptoms are mediated primarily by activation of the sympathetic nervous system stress response. Secretion of catecholamines, glucagon, corticosteroids, and growth hormone rises in an attempt to increase blood glucose. Pallor, tremor, diaphoresis, weakness, and decreased consciousness are the usual manifestations of hypoglycemia.**

Summary

Diabetes mellitus is the most common endocrine disorder, affecting at least 6.8 million Americans. Diabetes is characterized and diagnosed by chronic hyperglycemia, the result of a relative or absolute deficiency of insulin; however, the metabolism of all the energy nutrients is altered. There are four clinical classes of diabetes, the most common of which are type I and type II. Type I diabetes is the result of an autoimmune process leading to the destruction of the insulin-producing beta cells of the pancreas. Type II diabetes is characterized by insulin resistance (increased insulin requirement and decreased insulin responsiveness) and a reduction in insulin production, leading to a relative insulin deficiency.

Sequelae of insulin deficiency include the acute and chronic complications of diabetes. Acute complications include diabetic ketoacidosis in type I diabetes and nonketotic hyperglycemic hyperosmolar coma in type II diabetes. Chronic complications include cardiovascular disease, retinopathy, nephropathy, and neuropathy.

The goals of treatment are glycemic control and prevention of complications. Treatment is individualized and encompasses a low-fat, high-fiber diet, regular exercise, and appropriate use of such medications as oral hypoglycemic agents and insulin. The efficacy of treatment and the presence of complications of therapy are evaluated by capillary blood glucose monitoring. Patient education is an essential component in teaching skills associated with treatment.

REFERENCES

1. National Diabetes Advisory Board: *The National Long-Range Plan to Combat Diabetes*. NIH Publication No. 88–1587. U.S. Department of Health and Human Services. Bethesda, Md, Public Health Service, National Institutes of Health, 1987.
2. National Diabetes Data Group: Classification and diagnosis of diabetes mellitus and other categories of glucose intolerance. *Diabetes* 1979;28(12):1039–1044.
3. American Diabetes Association: *The Physician's Guide to Type II Diabetes (NIDDM): Diagnosis and Treatment*, 2nd ed. New York, American Diabetes Association, 1988.
4. Bruno G, Merletti F, Pisu E, Pastore G, Marengo C, Pagano G: Incidence of IDDM during 1984–1986 in population aged less than 30 yr. residents of Turin, Italy. *Diabetes Care* 1990;13(10):1051–1056.
5. Bougneres PF, Carel JC, Castano L, et al: Factors associated with early remission of Type I diabetes in children treated with cyclosporine. *N Engl J Med* 1988;318(11):663–670.
6. Eisenbarth GS: Type I diabetes mellitus: A chronic autoimmune disease. *N Engl J Med* 1986;314(21):1360–1368.
7. Solimena M, DeCamilli P: Spotlight on a neuronal enzyme. *Nature* 1993;366:15–17.
8. Bennett PH: Epidemiology of diabetes mellitus, in Ellenberg M, Rifkin H (eds): *Diabetes Mellitus: Theory and Practice*, 4th ed. New Hyde Park, NY, Medical Examination Publishing, 1990, pp 357–377.
9. Polonsky KS, Given BD, Hirsch LJ, et al: Abnormal patterns of insulin secretion in non-insulin dependent diabetes mellitus. *N Engl J Med* 1988;318(19):1231–1239.
10. Harris MI: Impaired glucose tolerance in the U.S. population. *Diabetes Care* 1989;12(7):464–474.
11. Abrams RS, Coustan DR: Gestational diabetes update. *Clin Diabetes* 1990;8(2):17–20.
12. DeFronzo RA, Ferrannini E: Insulin resistance. *Diabetes Care* 1991;14(3):173–194.
13. Jackson R, et al: Muscle capillary basement membrane changes in normal and diabetic children. *Diabetes* 1975;24(suppl 2). Abstract 32.
14. Peterson CM, Jones RL, Esterly JA, Wantz GE, Jackson RL: Changes in basement membrane thickening and pulse volume concomitant with improved glucose control and exercise in patients with insulin-dependent diabetes mellitus. *Diabetes Care* 1980;3(5):586–589.
15. Mogensen CE: Therapeutic interventions in nephropathy of IDDM. *Diabetes Care* 1988;11(suppl 1):10–15.
16. Cowie CC, Port FK, Wolfe RA, Savage PJ, Moll PP, Hawthorne VM: Disparities in incidence of diabetic end-stage renal disease according to race and type of diabetes. *N Engl J Med* 1989; 321(16):1074–1079.
17. National Institutes of Health: *Report of the National Commission on Diabetes to the Congress of the United States*. Vol 1: *The Long-Range Plan to Combat Diabetes*. DHEW Publication No. (NIH) 76–1018. U.S. Department of Health, Education and Welfare. Bethesda, Md, Public Health Service, National Institutes of Health, 1976.
18. The Diabetes Control and Complications Trial Research Group: The effect of intensive treatment of diabetes on the development and progression of long-term complications in insulin-dependent diabetes mellitus. *N Engl J Med* 1993;329(14): 977–986.
19. Coustan DR: Pregnancy in diabetic women. *N Engl J Med* 1988;319(25):1663–1665. Editorial.
20. Becerra JE, Pérez de Saliceti N, Smith JC: Diabetes mellitus during pregnancy and the risks for specific birth defects: A population-based case-control study. *Pediatrics* 1990;85(1):1–9.
21. American Diabetes Association: *The Physician's Guide to Type I Diabetes (IDDM): Diagnosis and Treatment*. New York, American Diabetes Association, 1988.
22. American Diabetes Association: Implications of the diabetes control and complications trial. *Diabetes Care* 1993;16(11): 1517–1520.
23. American Diabetes Association: Nutritional recommendations and principles for individuals with diabetes mellitus: 1986. *Diabetes Care* 1987;10(1):126–132.
24. Anderson JA: Effect of carbohydrate restriction and high carbohydrate diets on men with chemical diabetes. *Am J Clin Nutr* 1977;30:402–408.
25. Coulston AM, Hollenbeck CB, Swislocki AL, Reaven GM: Persistence of hypertriglyceridemic effect on low-fat high-carbohydrate diets in NIDDM patients. *Diabetes Care* 1989;12(2):94–101.
26. Zeller K, Whittaker E, Sullivan L, Raskin P, Jacobson HR: Effect of restricting dietary protein on the progression of renal failure in patients with insulin-dependent diabetes mellitus. *N Engl J Med* 1991;324(2):78–84.
27. American Heart Association: *Risk Factors and Coronary Disease: A Statement for Physicians*. Dallas, American Heart Association, 1980.
28. Garg A, Bonanome A, Grundy SM, Zhang ZJ, Unger RH: Comparison of a high-carbohydrate diet with a high-monosaturated-fat diet in patients with non-insulin-dependent diabetes mellitus. *N Engl J Med* 1988;319(13):829–834.
29. Ginsberg HN, Barr SL, Gilbert A, et al: Reduction of plasma cholesterol levels in normal men on an American Heart Association Step 1 diet or a Step 1 diet with added monounsaturated fat. *N Engl J Med* 1990;322(9):574–579.
30. Jensen T, Stender S, Goldstein K, Holmer G, Deckert T: Partial normalization by dietary cod-liver oil of increased microvascular albumin leakage in patients with insulin-dependent diabetes and albuminuria. *N Engl J Med* 1989;321(23):1572–1577.
31. Burr ML, Fehily AM, Gilbert JF, et al: Effects of change in fat, fish and fibre intakes on death and myocardial reinfarction: Diet and Reinfarction Trial. *Lancet* 1989;2:757–761.
32. Olin BR: *Drug Facts and Comparisons*. St. Louis, Facts & Comparisons Inc, 1991.
33. Lebovitz HE: Oral hypoglycemic agents, in Ellenberg M, Rifkin H (eds): *Diabetes Mellitus: Theory and Practice*, 4th ed. New Hyde Park, NY, Medical Examination Publishing, 1990, pp 554–574.
34. Galloway JA: Treatment of NIDDM with insulin agonists or substitutes. *Diabetes Care* 1990;13(12):1209–1239.
35. Kahn CR, Shechter Y: Insulin, oral hypoglycemia agents, and the pharmacology of the endocrine pancreas, in Gilman AG, Rall TW, Nies AS, Taylor P (eds): *The Pharmacological Basis of Therapeutics*, 8th ed. New York, Pergamon Press, 1990, pp 1463–1480.
36. Guinn TS, Bailey GJ, Mecklenburg RS: Factors related to discontinuation of continuous insulin-infusion therapy. *Diabetes Care* 1988;11(1):46–51.
37. Lebovitz HE, Pasmantier R: Combination insulin-sulfonylurea therapy. *Diabetes Care* 1990;13(6):667–675.
38. Casparie AF, Elving LD: Severe hypoglycemia in diabetic patients: Frequency, causes, prevention. *Diabetes Care* 1985; 8(2):141–145.
39. Campbell PJ, Gerich JE: Mechanisms of prevention, development, and reversal of hypoglycemia. *Adv Intern Med* 1988; 33:205–230.
40. Service FJ, O'Brien PC, Rizza RA: Measurements of glucose control. *Diabetes Care* 1987;10(2):225–237.
41. Keen H, Knight RK: Self sampling for blood sugar. *Lancet* 1962;1:1037–1040.
42. American Diabetes Association: Consensus statement on self-monitoring of blood glucose. *Diabetes Care* 1987;10(1):95–99.
43. Havlin CE, Parvin CA, Cryer PE: The accuracy of blood glucose monitoring devices. *Clin Diabetes* 1991;9(6):92–93.
44. Irsigler K, Bali-Taubald C: Self-monitored blood glucose: The essential biofeedback signal in the diabetic patient's effort to achieve normoglycemia. *Diabetes Care* 1980;3(1):163–170.
45. Skyler JS, Lasky IA, Skyler DL, Robertson EG, Mintz DH: Home blood glucose monitoring as an aid in diabetes management. *Diabetes Care* 1978;1(3):150–157.
46. Ludi MA: Blood-borne viruses and bgm: CDC responds. *Diabetes Educator* 1987;13(3):265. Letter.
47. Mazzuca SA, Moorman NH, Wheeler ML, et al: The diabetes education study: A controlled trial of the effects of diabetes patient education. *Diabetes Care* 1986;9(1):1–10.

48. Estey AL, Tan MH, Mann K: Follow-up intervention: Its effect on compliance behavior to a diabetes regimen. *Diabetes Educator* 1990;16(4):291–295.

49. Geller J, Butler K: Study of educational deficits as the cause of hospital admission for diabetes mellitus in a community hospital. *Diabetes Care* 1981;4(4):487–489.

50. American Diabetes Association Task Force on Financing Quality Health Care for Persons with Diabetes: *Diabetes Outpatient Education: The Evidence of Cost Savings.* New York, American Diabetes Association, 1986.

51. American Diabetes Association: Third-party reimbursement for outpatient diabetes education and counseling. *Diabetes Care* 1990;13(suppl 1):36.

52. American Diabetes Association: National standards for diabetes patient education and American Diabetes Association review criteria. *Diabetes Care* 1990;13(suppl 1):60–65.

BIBLIOGRAPHY

American Association of Diabetes Educators: *Diabetes Education: A Core Curriculum for Health Professionals.* Chicago, American Association of Diabetes Educators, 1993.

American Diabetes Association: *Medical Management of Pregnancy Complicated by Diabetes.* New York, American Diabetes Association, 1993.

American Diabetes Association: *Therapy for Diabetes Mellitus and Related Disorders.* New York, American Diabetes Association, 1991.

American Diabetes Association Clinical Practice Recommendations (1989–1990). *Diabetes Care* 1990;13(suppl 1):60–65. [Includes Position statements: Office Guide to Diagnosis and Classification of Diabetes Mellitus and Other Categories of Glucose Tolerance, Gestational Diabetes Mellitus, Screening for Diabetes, Standards of Medical Care for Patients with Diabetes Mellitus, Eye Care Guidelines for Patients with Diabetes Mellitus, Blood Glucose Control in Diabetes, Nutritional Recommendations and Principles for Individuals with Diabetes Mellitus, Use of Noncaloric Sweeteners, Insulin Administration, Continuous Subcutaneous Insulin Infusion, Bedside Blood Glucose Monitoring in Hospitals, Concurrent Care; Consensus statements: Diabetic Neuropathy, Role of Cardiovascular Risk Factors in Prevention and Treatment of Macrovascular Disease in Diabetes; Standards Review Criteria: National Standards for Diabetes Patient Education and American Diabetes Association Review Criteria.]

American Diabetes Association Council on Exercise: Diabetes mellitus and exercise. *Diabetes Care* 1990;13:(7):804–805.

Department of Health and Human Services: *The Prevention and Treatment of Five Complications of Diabetes.* Atlanta, Centers for Disease Control, 1991.

DeStefano F, et al: *Diabetes Surveillance.* U.S. Department of Health and Human Services, Atlanta, Public Health Service, Centers for Disease Control, Center for Chronic Disease Prevention and Health Promotion, Division of Diabetes Translation, 1990.

Ellenberg M, Rifkin H: *Diabetes Mellitus: Theory and Practice,* 4th ed. New Hyde Park, NY, Medical Examination Publishing, 1990.

Hirsch IB, Farkas-Hirsch R, Skyler JS: Intensive insulin. *Diabetes Care* 1990;13(12):1265–1283.

Horton ES: Exercise and diabetes mellitus. *Med Clin North Am* 1988;72(6):1301–1319.

Kreisberg RA: Aging, glucose metabolism and diabetes: Current concepts. *Geriatrics* 1987;42(4):67–72.

Rasmussen H, Zawalich KC, Ganesan S, Calle R, Zawalich WS: Physiology and pathophysiology in insulin secretion. *Diabetes Care* 1990;13(6):655–666.

Rossetti L, Giaccari A, DeFronzo RA: Glucose toxicity. *Diabetes Care* 1990;13(6):610–630.

Seltzer HS: Drug-induced hypoglycemia. *Endocrinol Metab Clin North Am* 1989;18(1):163–183.

Skyler JS: Insulin pharmacology. *Med Clin North Am* 1988;72(6):1337–1354.

UNIT XII
Alterations in Neural Function

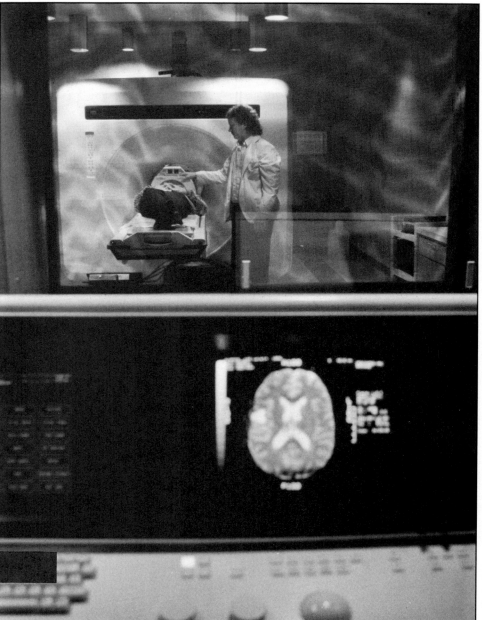

Magnetic resonance imaging (MRI) is used to evaluate neurological status. The MRI provides information about the chemical makeup of tissues, making diagnosis possible.

An editorial in *Science* announcing important advances in neuroscientific research noted that the brain is an organ of the body. The reminder is needed, the editorial writer said, because while most scientists are familiar with the organic nature of the brain, those who have not studied it sometimes prefer to believe that malfunctioning of the brain reveals other failures that have nothing to do with organic processes, even a demonic influence.

The popular view of at least some brain disease, *Science* said, was that it could be explained by "bad parenting, a poor environment, or evil spirits."

Because it is associated with an imponderable called "the mind," it is understandable that people who have not studied it might concoct a personal folklore about the brain but fail to appreciate what scientists learn better every week—that the brain is, as *Science* said, "such a difficult enterprise that it must be tackled by an enormous range of theories and techniques." They may resist the idea that in the brain the "distinction between a normal state and a pathological state is one between benign chemistry and malign chemistry."

But, says *Science*, with some confidence, "The aging Alzheimer's patient, the homeless schizophrenic, the aphasic child, the depressed adult—all those whose brains are not functioning properly—will benefit from advances in neuroscience."

The brain has an unpleasant function, one nevertheless indispensable to every human being and to the medical professionals who try to understand their symptoms: It produces pain. This "organ of the body" monitors the other organs and sounds the alarm when something has gone wrong.

Medical practitioners study pain not only to relieve it but because it is a useful diagnostic tool. The body senses danger in its external as well as internal environment with a network of pain receptors—free nerve endings—in the skin and in certain internal tissues. When they are stimulated, pain impulses move along two separate paths from the dorsal spinal roots into the spinal cord to various destinations in the brain. When the signals reach their destinations the outcome is clear: We hurt, we know how much and where and when the pain occurs. These signals monitored by the brain are so important that medical professionals are urged to take the patient's reports of pain very seriously.

But the brain's pain response is more than an alarm. The brain controls pain as well as signaling it.

Pain control resides in the analgesia system. It is capable of controlling the input of pain signals to the nervous system by blocking pain signals at their entry point to the spinal cord and by blocking other reflexes triggered by pain signals. The analgesia system and other areas of the brain have opiate receptors, which also dull pain. Researchers do not entirely understand the brain's opiate system, but it is clear that activation of the analgesia system either by nervous signals entering the periaqueductal gray area of the brain stem or by the administration of morphine-like drugs suppresses many pain signals.

Medical diagnosis depends on a sophisticated understanding of pain, and in the future it is expected that medical professionals who help the patient manage pain will play an important part in the control of pain in acute care.

Pain is pervasive in the United States. One estimate suggests that 97 million people have some form of chronic pain not associated with malignancy.

FRONTIERS OF RESEARCH
Pain and Its Control

Michael J. Kirkhorn

Cancer offers its own peculiar challenges because it often causes acute and lasting pain. As cancer advances in the body, pain becomes more acute. In the past, medical professionals were reluctant or at times unable to effectively control pain. A current study estimates, however, that "pain can be managed effectively by relatively simple means" for up to 90 percent of the 8 million Americans who have cancer or have had the disease.

Cancer patients are not the only ones who suffer pain that is difficult or impossible to endure without assistance. Women experience intense pain during childbirth, and burn patients nearly always experience severe pain. More than half of a sample of medical-surgical patients said they experienced "excruciating" pain.

The study of pain management is not far advanced. Studies show that recent nursing graduates were inadequately instructed about the assessment and control of pain. Pain management is hindered by a number of common misconceptions that prevent medical professionals from doing all they can to relieve pain. A 1990 study showed that more than half of nurses surveyed did not know that the patient's report of pain is the single most reliable indicator of pain, and many nurses failed to increase the dose of opioid analgesic when a weaker dose had failed to relieve pain and had caused no side effects.

Studies have shown that physicians and nurses have inaccurate knowledge about pharmacologic pain controllers and needless anxieties over the possibility that a patient given pain control drugs might become addicted to them. A recent survey of 2,459 nurses attending pain programs revealed that only about one in four knew that the incidence of addiction to opioid analgesics was less than 1 percent. About the same number thought that addiction would occur in more than 25 percent of all cases.

CHAPTER 42
Neural Development and Cortical Function

MARY SANGUINETTI-BAIRD

Elemental Function
of the Nervous System
Neuron Cell Types
Neurotransmission

Nervous System Organization
Primary Divisions

Embryologic Development
Formation of the Neural Tube
Cell Proliferation and the
   Development of the
   Nervous System
Spinal Cord Development

Development of the Rostral
   Neural Tube
Ventricular System

Meningeal Coverings
and Blood Supply

Cerebral Cortex
Cortical Organization
Regions of Localized Function
Association Cortex

Summary

KEY TERMS

afferent neuron: A primary sensory neuron whose distal axon originates at receptors in the peripheral nervous system. Sensory information is transmitted to the central nervous system by afferent neurons.

cytoarchitectonic: Refers to the layers of the cortex and the specific cell types found within the layers.

efferent neuron: A neuron that carries information away from the central nervous system to the muscle cells, glands, or postganglionic neurons.

ganglion: A cluster of neuronal cell bodies. Use of the term is generally restricted to neuronal clusters located outside the central nervous system.

neuroglia: A tissue derived from the neuroepithelium that supplies support to the nerve cells.

neuron: Within the central nervous system, the nerve cell is called a neuron. It includes the synapses (the receiving processes), the cell body, dendrites, and the axon (the transmitting process).

neurotransmitters: Highly specific chemical messengers that are released from the terminal end of an axon to bind to a specific membrane protein on a receptor. Neurotransmitters enhance, inhibit, or modify the activities of the receiving cell.

nuclei: A cluster of neuronal cell bodies in the central nervous system.

somatotopic: The sequential arrangement of neurons related to sensory or motor function for specific anatomic regions, e.g., foot-leg-trunk, hand-arm-face.

tract: A large bundle of myelinated nerve fibers in the central nervous system.

transsynaptic degeneration: Degeneration of a neuron or group of neurons whose function is dependent upon the stimulation of another neuron which has been injured and is degenerating. If the primary neuron degenerates, then the dependent neuron will also degenerate transsynaptically even though the dependent neuron was not exposed to the injury of the primary neuron.

wallerian degeneration: Complete disintegration of the distal portion of an axon that has been severed from the cell body. The axon, myelin sheath, and terminal arborization all disintegrate.

Study of the nervous system entails learning about the structure, function, and interrelationships of the brain, spinal cord, muscles, and nerves. Professionals practicing in this area of health care work with patients who are suffering from varying degrees of physiologic and psychosocial dysfunction. Someone with a neurologic disorder may have diminished ability to perform activities of daily living because of difficulties in cognitive processing, emotional expression and behavior, motor and autonomic function, communication, or the special senses of sight, smell, hearing, taste, and touch. The ultimate goal of the health care practitioner working with people who suffer from nervous system disorders is to provide quality patient care while facilitating the individual's return to a life that is as productive and independent as possible.

Elemental Function of the Nervous System

Neuron Cell Types

The human nervous system is extremely complex and highly organized. The fundamental unit of the nervous system is the nerve cell, or **neuron,** and the basis of function of the nervous system is interneuronal communication.

All cells, whether the simplest of one-celled animals or complex human nerve cells, communicate by responding to chemical and physical stimuli. This stimulus-response mechanism is the means by which information is transmitted from one cell to another and relayed throughout the organism. A neuron processes information via this response chain from cell to cell in a very rapid fashion. The total collection of neurons and supporting cells in an organism is called the **nervous system.**

Neurons are variable in shape and size but typically have four basic parts: the cell body (soma), dendrites, an axon, and an axon terminal. Dendrites are highly branched outgrowths of the cell body. The cell body and dendrites are the predominant sites of specialized junctions where impulses are received from other neurons. The axon, also called the **nerve fiber,** is a single process that extends from the cell body. The area where the axon joins the cell body is called the initial segment and is the site where most impulses are initiated. Once initiated, the impulse travels down the length of the axon to its terminal. Along its length the axon may branch into a multitude of collaterals. Each collateral has a terminal. The axon terminal is the site of stimulus transmission from one neuron to another (Fig. 42–1).

Cells of the nervous system are named according to the number of processes going to and from the cell body. Thus, a cell is said to be multipolar, bipolar, or unipolar. Neurons are also named according to their function. A neuron that is directly involved in the reception of specific stimuli such as touch or temperature is termed a **sensory neuron.** Those that end on either muscles or glands are called **motor neurons.** Neurons are termed **afferent** or **efferent** and are said to be of afferent or efferent divisions. At the peripheral end of an afferent neuron is a receptor that responds to chemical or physical stimuli, or both. When a receptor is stimulated, messages in the form of electrical impulses are transmitted from the receptor into the spinal cord and brain. Conversely, efferent neurons transmit electrical signals from the central nervous system (CNS) out to effector cells, which are muscles or glands. Strictly speaking, most nerve cells in the CNS are not afferent or efferent. Rather, they are interneurons that connect one neuron to another. Interneurons make up 99 percent of all nerve cells in the CNS.[1]

As in other cells, the neuron's cell body contains the nucleus and thus the genetic information neces-

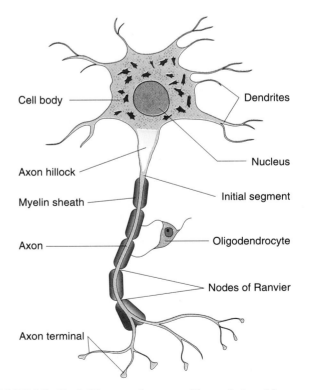

F I G U R E 42 – 1. Diagram of neuron. (Figure designed by Cindy Glover, Olympia, Wash.)

sary for protein synthesis. For the structure and function of the neuron and its processes to be maintained, proteins formed in the cell body must be transported down the axon to its terminal end. This method of transport is called **axonal transport** and occurs in both directions.[1]

Nonneural tissue that forms the interstitial tissue of the nervous system is called **neuroglia** and is derived from the neuroepithelium. Four of the most common cell types are oligodendroglial, astroglial, ependymal, and microglial cells. The functions of glial cells are varied. Some have structural functions, such as the oligodendroglia in the CNS and the Schwann cells in the peripheral system, which form myelin sheaths around axons that increase the speed of axonal transmission. Other glial cells are involved in metabolism, the destruction of foreign material in the CNS, and regulating the composition of extracellular fluids. About 40 percent of the brain and spinal cord is composed of neuroglia. Because these cells lack intracellular collagen and elastin, brain tissue has a jellylike texture. Unlike neurons, neuroglial cells divide mitotically. This is of clinical interest, as the neuroglial cells are the most common source of primary tumors in the CNS.[2]

Neurotransmission

Communication among the various neurons in the nervous system is vital to an organism's ability to function efficiently. Communication involves both intercellular and intracellular processes. Intracellular communication was described earlier in the discussion of axonal transport. The process of intercellular communication is more complex and starts when a nerve cell receives a stimulus that is strong enough to produce an action potential (a brief reversal in the cell membrane's electrical polarity). The stimulus may come from outside the organism, in which case it is received by a sensory receptor, or from an adjacent cell within the organism. The process is mediated by both chemical and electrical mechanisms.

The membrane of a cell has an electrical property and even at rest is a charged cell. This means that there is an electrical potential difference across its plasma membrane which keeps the inside of the cell negatively charged with respect to the outside of the cell. This is referred to as a resting membrane potential and is due to a steady-state ionic concentration.[3] The higher concentration of negative ions inside the cell is electrically attracted to the higher concentration of positive ions on the outside. While there are many ions involved in the maintenance of the membrane potential, sodium and potassium, because of their quantities, play the most significant role. Normally there is a high concentration of potassium inside the cell relative to outside the cell. Conversely, sodium has a high concentration outside the cell relative to the inside.

Several mechanisms are responsible for maintaining this balance between sodium and potassium ions. It is created by the interaction of the electrical charge and the diffusion properties of the individual ions. In a "resting" state the neuron interior is −60 to −70 mV with respect to the extracellular fluid. Although there is a pump transporting potassium into the cell, potassium moves relatively freely through the cell membrane. When the cell is at rest it is impermeable to sodium. In addition, there is a strong transport system called the sodium pump which continually picks sodium up from outside the cell and transports it inside the cell. As sodium is pumped in, potassium leaves the cell to maintain the resting state. When the cell surface receives a stimulus, it lowers the resting potential. If the stimulus is strong enough to make the membrane potential become less negative or closer to 0 than the resting potential (−60 to −70), the membrane becomes depolarized and its permeability is changed. The change in membrane permeability results in a sudden reversal in the flow of sodium and potassium. The movement of ions across the membrane is termed conductance and is inversely proportional to the resistance of the cell membrane (Fig. 42–2). In axons, conductance lasts about 1 msec and is called an action potential. Action potentials are generated in the soma at the point where the axon emerges and are propagated along the axon to its synaptic terminal. The speed of conduction of a transmission depends on the diameter of the axon and its associated myelin sheath. As the impulse passes, the membrane repolarizes and returns to the resting state.

At the axon terminal the propagating action potential causes an influx of calcium, which in turn stimulates the release of chemicals called **neurotransmit-**

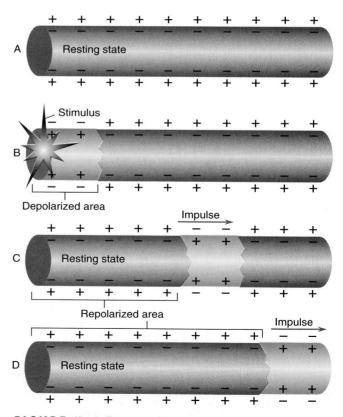

FIGURE 42–2. Diagram of an action potential. (Figure designed by Cindy Glover, Olympia, Wash.)

ters from the terminal end point. These chemical agents travel across the synaptic cleft and stimulate receptor sites on the postsynaptic membrane of an adjacent neuron. Although there are numerous neurotransmitters within the nervous system, neurotransmitters are highly specific to the type of axon from which they are released.

Almost all synapses responsible for signal transmission in the CNS are chemical synapses, which means they function by using neurotransmitters. A neurotransmitter is released from the synaptic terminal of one neuron, proceeds across the synaptic cleft, and acts on the receptor proteins in the membrane of the second neuron to excite, inhibit, or modify its activity. The response at the postsynaptic membrane depends on the type of ion channel that is opened or closed when the neurotransmitter binds to the receptor. The neurotransmitter is therefore a chemical messenger that stimulates a response that is built into the postsynaptic cell. Once neurotransmitters are released into the synaptic cleft, their potential to activate the postsynaptic receptors is limited by deactivation processes. Neurotransmitters are either actively transported back into the axon terminals for reuse or destroyed by enzyme activity.

Of the more than 40 neurotransmitters that have been identified the best known are acetylcholine, norepinephrine, dopamine, glycine, gamma-aminobutyric acid (GABA), glutamate, and serotonin. The following is a brief discussion of their actions.

Acetylcholine is a very common neurotransmitter that is secreted by neurons in many different areas of the brain, but largely by the large pyramidal cells of the motor cortex, some neurons in the basal ganglia, neurons that innervate skeletal muscles, preganglionic neurons of the autonomic nervous system, postganglionic neurons of the parasympathetic nervous system, and some postganglionic neurons of the sympathetic nervous system. Acetylcholine usually has an excitatory effect. In some instances, however, peripheral parasympathetic nerve endings have inhibitory effects. One such example is the inhibition of the heart muscle by the vagus nerve.

Norepinephrine is found in neurons whose cell bodies lie in the brain stem and the hypothalamus. The most prominent of these are norepinephrine-secreting neurons in the locus ceruleus in the pons. These neurons send fibers to widespread areas of the brain and help control brain activity and mood. In most instances, norepinephrine is an excitatory transmitter, but it, too, has inhibitory effects in some cases. It is secreted by most of the postganglionic neurons of the sympathetic nervous system and acts to excite some organs and inhibit others.

Dopamine is secreted by neurons whose cell bodies originate in the substantia nigra. These neurons terminate in the striatal region of the basal ganglia. Dopamine is an inhibitory neurotransmitter.

Glycine is thought to have inhibitory action. It is secreted primarily by cells with synapses in the spinal cord.

GABA has a widespread distribution, being secreted by synapses in the spinal cord, cerebellum, basal ganglia, and multiple sites in the cortex. It acts as an inhibitory transmitter.

Glutamate is believed to have excitatory influence. It is secreted by the presynaptic terminals in many of the sensory pathways and in numerous areas of the cortex.

Finally, *serotonin* is secreted by neurons that originate in the median raphe of the brain stem and project to many areas in the brain, notably the dorsal horn of the spinal cord and the hypothalamus. Serotonin acts to inhibit pain via the pathways in the spinal cord. It is also thought to be helpful in mood control and sleep.

The receptor sites on postsynaptic neurons are specific molecular binding sites for neurotransmitters. The transmitter–receptor interaction results in a response in the postsynaptic neuron. In the absence of neurotransmitter release, intercellular communication does not occur. When it does occur, transmission down a myelinated axon is very rapid, as the action potential does not need to travel the entire length of the axon. Instead it can "hop" along junctions in the myelin sheath called the *nodes of Ranvier* (see Fig. 42–1). This mechanism of hopping from node to node significantly increases the speed of impulse transmission. Many nervous system diseases (e.g., myasthenia gravis, multiple sclerosis) result from dysfunction in intercellular communication.

KEY CONCEPTS

- The fundamental unit of the nervous system is the neuron. Neurons have four basic parts: the cell body, dendrites, the axon, and the axon terminal. Nervous system function depends on specific communication between neurons through chemical synapses.

- Neuronal communication can be summarized as follows. Stimulation from other neurons occurs primarily at the dendrite and cell body. Action potentials are initiated at the axon hillock and conducted down the axon to the axon terminal where neurotransmitter is stored. Depolarization of the terminal opens voltage-gated calcium channels. Calcium influx mediates exocytosis of neurotransmitter into the interneuronal synapse. Neurotransmitter binds and activates specific receptors on the postsynaptic cell, changing its ion conductance. With sufficient depolarization of the postsynaptic cell, an action potential is generated.

- Common excitatory CNS neurotransmitters include acetylcholine, norepinephrine, and glutamate. Inhibitory neurotransmitters include dopamine, glycine, and gamma-aminobutyric acid. Serotonin has modulatory effects on pain, mood, and sleep.

- Conduction of action potentials is faster in large and myelinated axons.

- Neuroglial cells are supportive cells within the CNS. Oligodendroglial cells form insulating myelin sheaths, astroglial cells moderate extracellular fluid composition, microglial cells destroy foreign materials, and ependymal cells form cerebrospinal fluid.

Unlike neurons, glial cells are capable of proliferation.

Nervous System Organization

Primary Divisions

Discussions of the nervous system are often organized around convenient anatomic divisions. Understanding the function and purpose of the separate units facilitates an appreciation of the whole as a cooperative unit.

Humans have both a central and a peripheral nervous system. The CNS is composed of the brain and the spinal cord. The brain consists of the cerebrum, the diencephalon, the midbrain, the pons, the medulla, and the cerebellum. The midbrain, pons, and medulla collectively make up the brain stem. The fundamental units of the CNS are the neuron and its supporting glial cells. Within the human nervous system there are over 100 billion neurons and 10 times as many supportive or glial cells.[1-3]

The peripheral nervous system is composed of nerves that extend to (afferent) and from (efferent) the CNS. The fundamental unit of the peripheral nervous system is called a **nerve** instead of a neuron. Within this system there are 31 pairs of spinal nerves and 12 pairs of cranial nerves (Table 42–1). The afferent fibers convey information from receptors to the CNS. The cell bodies of peripheral nerves are located outside the brain and spinal cord in clusters called **ganglia.** From the cell body, one long process extends out to the receptor site. In the other direction a second process passes into the CNS. **Afferent fibers** enter the CNS from the dorsal (back) side of the spinal cord, forming the dorsal root and dorsal root ganglia. **Efferent fibers** exit from the front or ventral roots (Fig. 42–3). After leaving the spinal cord, the dorsal and ventral roots at the same level of the spinal cord combine to form a pair of spinal nerves. Within the efferent division of the peripheral nervous system there is further division between the somatic and the autonomic nervous system (ANS). Somatic nerves innervate skeletal muscles and autonomic nerves innervate smooth muscles, cardiac muscles, and glands.

The ANS is divided into sympathetic and parasympathetic branches. Sympathetic nerves originate in the spinal cord between segments T1 and L2 (Fig.

TABLE 42–1. Cranial Nerves

I	Olfactory
II	Optic
III	Oculomotor
IV	Trochlear
V	Trigeminal
VI	Abducens
VII	Facial
VIII	Auditory (vestibulocochlear)
IX	Glossopharyngeal
X	Vagus
XI	Spinal accessory
XII	Hypoglossal

42–4). Sympathetic fibers emerging from the cord first pass through the sympathetic chain ganglia, then travel on to various tissues and organs. Parasympathetic nerves are located in the sacral spinal segments and in cranial nerves III, V, VII, IX, and X (Fig. 42–5). Cranial nerve X, the vagus nerve, innervates the heart and gastrointestinal tract.

The CNS is divided into gray matter and white matter. The gray matter is composed primarily of cell bodies and dendrites. Dense areas of gray matter that are functionally related are often referred to as **nuclei.** White matter refers to axons coated with myelin sheaths. Myelin is mostly lipid and is white in appearance. Myelinated axons run longitudinally through the spinal cord in **tracts** or pathways. Tracts are organized according to specific functions. The name of a particular tract reflects its source and termination site. For example, the corticospinal tract originates in the cortex and terminates in the spinal cord. A cross-section of the spinal cord shows the separation of gray and white matter (see Fig. 42–3). Central gray matter contains interneurons, cell bodies and dendrites of efferent neurons, entering fibers of afferent neurons, and glial cells. Peripheral white matter is composed largely of myelinated afferent and efferent axons.

When a severe injury occurs in the peripheral nervous system, axons distal to the injury degenerate. They become irregular and beaded in shape, and after approximately 24 hours, neurofibrils within the axons disintegrate. Within a few days to a week, the axons break into irregular fragments: after 3 weeks they disappear completely. In the axonal segment proximal to the injury, disintegration occurs in the same fashion but to a lesser degree. If the nerve is myelinated, degeneration usually extends back to the next one or two nodes of Ranvier.

As axons and myelin sheaths degrade, Schwann cells of the injured nerve swell and divide. Over the next 2 to 3 weeks, continuous columns of short Schwann cells mark the course of the lost axons. If there is little separation between the ends of a divided nerve, the proliferating Schwann cells bridge the gap. If the divided ends are further apart, the proliferating Schwann cells form bulbous swellings at the end of the nerves. The ends of the surviving axons also form bulbous ending with the accumulation of mitochondria, lysosomes, and vesicles. Enzymes and mediators accumulate in these endings. After about 24 hours, fine fibrils begin to grow out of the ends of the axons, extending into the surrounding Schwann cells at random. Those fibrils that find a column of Schwann cells in the distal part of the nerve grow down the column at a rate of 2 to 5 mm/day. Initially these fibrils behave as unmyelinated axons. Eventually they will acquire a myelin sheath and their own Schwann cells. There is usually good functional return to the nerve secondary to this process. If continuity is not restored, the distal end gradually becomes replaced by collagenous tissue.

Within the CNS, axonal injury causes **wallerian degeneration,** much like the process in the peripheral nervous system. Damaged axons become irregular and beaded, break up, and disappear, but the process

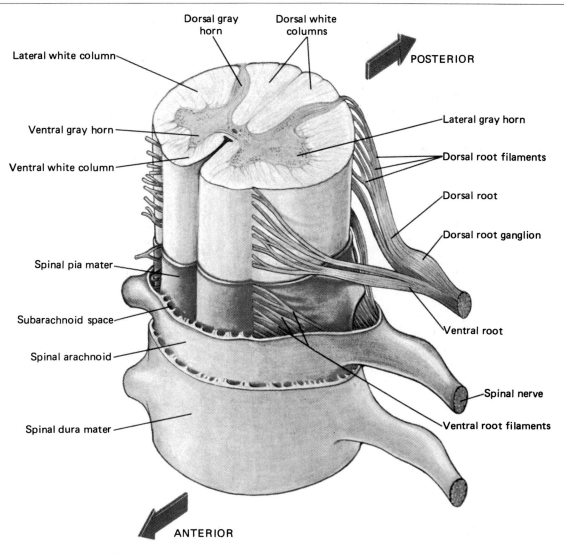

FIGURE 42–3. Diagram of spinal cord in cross-section demonstrating dorsal and ventral roots and showing the separation of gray and white matter. (From Guyton AC: *Basic Neuroscience: Anatomy and Physiology*. Philadelphia, WB Saunders, 1987, p 31. Reproduced with permission.)

is significantly slower. A large axon in the CNS system may not show evidence of degeneration for up to 30 hours after its separation from the cell body. Myelin sheaths of damaged axons become segmented and are gradually broken down into simpler lipids, eventually to neutral fats. It may be 3 months or more before all the myelin of the injured axon is converted to simpler lipids and 6 months before most of it is changed to neutral fats. Damaged axons in the CNS do not regenerate. A few small fibers may sprout from the proximal end of a damaged axon, but they are short and do not reestablish continuity with the distal end of the injured axon. If the neurons that have been lost were the principal source of stimulation to some other group of neurons, that other group of neurons is also likely to degenerate and disappear. This process is called **transsynaptic degeneration.**

Of interest to the health care provider, human function affected by disorders of the nervous system tends to cluster around specific divisions of the neuraxis.[4] The divisions of the neuraxis as described in

the American Association of Neuroscience Nurses' 1990 *Core Curriculum*[5] and the *AANN's Neuroscience Nursing*[4] will be used to describe neural structures in this unit. Axis I includes the cerebral hemispheres and diencephalon, Axis II includes the brain stem and cerebellum, Axis III includes the spinal cord, and Axis IV includes the peripheral nerves and junctions with innervated organs.

KEY CONCEPTS

- **The nervous system can be divided into two principal systems: (1) the central nervous sytem (CNS), consisting of the brain and spinal cord, and (2) the peripheral nervous system, consisting of 31 pairs of spinal nerves and 12 pairs of cranial nerves. Peripheral sensory afferents carry information to the CNS and motor efferents carry information from the CNS to muscles.**

- **The sympathetic nerves originate in spinal cord segments T1 to L2. The parasympathetic nerves emerge**

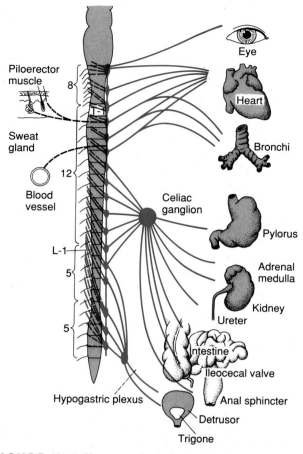

F I G U R E 42 – 4. The sympathetic nervous system. *Dashed lines* represent postganglionic fibers in the gray rami leading into the spinal nerves for distribution to blood vessels, sweat glands, and piloerector muscles. (From Guyton AC: *Textbook of Medical Physiology,* 8th ed. Philadelphia, WB Saunders, 1991, p 668. Reproduced with permission.)

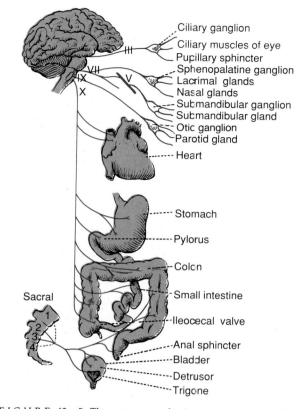

F I G U R E 42 – 5. The parasympathetic nervous system. (From Guyton AC: *Textbook of Medical Physiology,* 8th ed. Philadelphia, WB Saunders, 1991, p 669. Reproduced with permission.)

> from the sacral segments and also travel in cranial nerves III, V, VII, IX, and X.
>
> - Gray matter is composed of cell bodies and unmyelinated dendrites. Myelinated axons appear white.
> - Injured peripheral nerves can regenerate if the nerve tract remains intact. Injured CNS neurons do not regenerate.
> - The nervous system can be divided into functional units. Axis I includes the cerebral hemispheres and diencephalon; Axis II includes the brain stem and cerebellum; Axis III is the spinal cord, and Axis IV includes the peripheral nerves and terminal synapses.

Embryologic Development

Formation of the Neural Tube

The complexity and organization of the nervous system are quite evident in the examination of its embryology. The nervous system starts to take shape during the third week of embryonic development. At this time three primary tissues of the embryo are distin-guishable: the ectoderm, endoderm, and mesoderm. A thickened plate of ectoderm running longitudinally on the dorsal surface of the embryo, called the *neural plate,* gives rise to the central and peripheral nervous systems. The outer ectodermal layer is similar to the cells of the epidermis that cover the body surface.[6] Initially the neural plate is a single layer of cells. It proceeds through a stage of rapid proliferation, with the outer cells growing at a faster rate than those in the center, causing the plate to fold inward and form a neural groove in the midline with a neural fold on each side (Fig. 42–6). As proliferation of the cells continues, the folds curve toward one another. By the end of the third week the folds meet and start to fuse centrally along the dorsal midline. This fusion marks the beginning of the *neural tube.* Openings at either end of the neural tube are called neuropores (Fig. 42–7). As the tube continues to fuse in both rostral and caudal directions, the rostral neuropore closes on the 24th day and the caudal neuropore closes on the 26th day. The neural tube is the precursor of the future brain and spinal cord.

During formation of the neural tube, its lumen is connected with the amniotic cavity through both neuropores. Fusion of cells and formation of the neural tube starts in the cervical region of the future spinal cord, then progresses rapidly in a rostral direction toward the future brain. As the tube forms, it pinches off from the ectodermal surface. At the same time groups of cells from the crest of each neural fold are

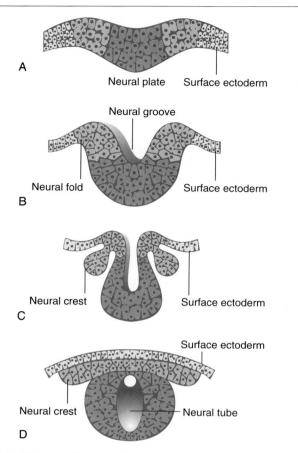

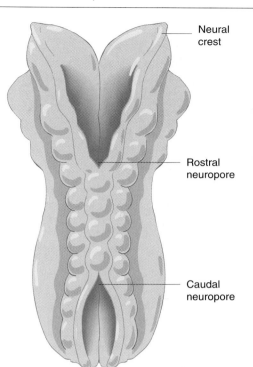

FIGURE 42–7. Diagram of neural tube with rostral and caudal neuropores. (Figure designed by Cindy Glover, Olympia, Wash.)

FIGURE 42–6. Diagram of transverse sections of embryonic development of the spinal cord. **A,** Neural plate. **B,** Development of neural fold and neural groove. **C,** Development of neural crest. **D,** Closure of neural tube. (Figure designed by Cindy Glover, Olympia, Wash.)

pinched off from the neural tube. Neural crest cells develop into a variety of cell types, among them the postganglionic neurons of the autonomic nervous system, Schwann cells and satellite cells of the peripheral nervous system, and sensory neurons of the ganglia of spinal and cranial nerves. Many of these cells even differentiate into non-nervous system tissues such as melanocytes of the skin and some bones and muscles. The neural tube eventually develops into the entire CNS. The cavity formed by the tube becomes the ventricular system of the brain.

Failure of the neural tube to close properly is a cause of congenital malformation of the nervous system. The initiation of closure of the neural tube is stimulated or "induced" by the cells above it. If this process fails to occur, the defects are known as defects of dorsal induction.[7] A fatal deformity known as craniorachischisis occurs when there is complete failure of the neural tube to close. In such instances the CNS looks like an open furrow along the dorsal surface of the fetus. The most common major CNS deformity results from failure of the rostral portion to close, a condition known as anencephaly. Anencephaly is incompatible with life.[7] Since 1970 occurrence rates have progressively declined in the United States. Re-

cently, British clinicians have discovered that rates can be further reduced with vitamin supplementation, specifically folic acid during pregnancy.[7] When the caudal portion of the neural tube fails to close, a defect known as myelomeningocele occurs. In this defect vertebrae do not form correctly and the caudal walls of the neural tube are continuous with the skin on the back. The spinal cord and meninges are displaced into a sac on the back. Although this defect is survivable, motor and sensory function below the level of the defect are lost.

Cell Proliferation and the Development of the Nervous System

Current thinking holds that when the neural tube closes, it initially consists of a single cell type, the neuroepithelial cell.[8] A pseudostratified epithelium is formed by neuroepithelial cells that extend from the innermost membrane of the neural tube to the external limiting membrane. After closure, the neuroepithelial cells give rise to another cell that no longer has the ability to reproduce, the primitive nerve cell or **neuroblast.** As neuroblasts are produced in increasing numbers, they surround the neuroepithelial cells, forming a layer of cells called the **mantle layer.** These cells start as apolar neuroblasts, then differentiate into bipolar neuroblasts with two cytoplasmic processes developing from opposite sides. One side develops into a primitive axon, and the other side develops several outgrowths that become primitive dendrites. At this stage of development the cell is a multipolar neuroblast. These processes extending from the cell form the outermost layer of the tube, which is also distinctive and is called the **marginal layer.** With further growth and development these cells will become adult nerves or neurons. As the neuroblasts mature, their axonal processes form synaptic connections with other neurons. The method in which they establish this contact with adjacent processes is selectively based on molecular mechanisms of cellular recognition.[6,8]

As cell proliferation continues in the now closed neural tube, areas of thickening become evident in both the anterior and posterior portions of the mantle layer. The anterior thickening will form the basal plates and ultimately the anterior gray horn or motor horn of the adult spinal cord. The posterior thickening is smaller and forms the alar plates and the future posterior gray or sensory horn of the adult spinal cord (Fig. 42–8).

Neuroblasts of the basal plate develop into the efferent peripheral neurons. Axons from these neuroblasts pass through the marginal layer and exit the spinal cord as ventral root fibers. Fibers of the ventral root go to autonomic ganglia, innervating visceral structures as well as providing direct innervation to skeletal muscle. Cells of the alar plate remain within the CNS. Within the CNS some of the neurons from the alar plate arch anteriorly, cross through the basal plate to the opposite side, enter the marginal layer,

and ascend or descend to variable distances. Some alar neurons remain on the same side but enter the marginal layer and ascend and descend to variable distances. Neurons that are confined to the CNS are called **central** or **intermediate cells.** Those that remain on the same side of the CNS are called **association cells,** and those whose axons cross to the opposite side are called **commissural cells.** The mantle layer increases in size to become the gray matter of the adult spinal cord. It is surrounded by the marginal layer, composed of ascending and descending axons of the central cells. With maturity, most of the processes in the marginal layer become myelinated and take on the glistening white appearance of the adult cord.

The expansion of the alar and basal plates medially leads to near approximation of the plates. The posterior median septum separates the posterior marginal layers and the anterior median fissure invaginates and separates them anteriorly. The anterior invagination greatly reduces the size of the central canal. At this stage the embryonic neural tube is transformed into the spinal cord.[1,6,8]

Spinal Cord Development

The **spinal cord** is a long cylindrical structure. It has an acute ventral curve, called the cervical flexure, where the spinal cord meets the hindbrain. Until the beginning of the third month of fetal development the spinal cord and the vertebral canal are of the same length. At this time the mesodermal tissue, responsible for the development of the cartilages and bones of the vertebral canal, grows faster than the spinal cord. As a consequence, at birth the caudal portion of the spinal cord, the conus medullaris, is at the level of the third lumbar vertebra. As the vertebral column grows, the sites where the spinal nerves exit do not change; instead, the root filaments of the nerves lengthen, notably in the cervical and thoracic regions. In the adult the conus medullaris lies between the first and second lumbar vertebrae. The tip of the conus is called the filum terminale. At the end of the spinal cord, the nerve rootlets extend down the canal, forming the cauda equina (Fig. 42–9).

Development of the Rostral Neural Tube

Most growth and differentiation occur in the rostral portion of the closed neural tube, as this will be the future brain. At the end of the fourth week of gestation three vesicles are evident at the rostral end of the neural tube—the prosencephalon, or forebrain; the mesencephalon, or midbrain; and the rhombencephalon, or hindbrain. During the fifth week, the first and third vesicles form two swellings each, resulting in five secondary brain vesicles. The prosencephalon forms the telencephalon and the diencephalon, the mesencephalon remains the same, and the rhombencephalon forms the metencephalon and the myelencephalon (Table 42–2).

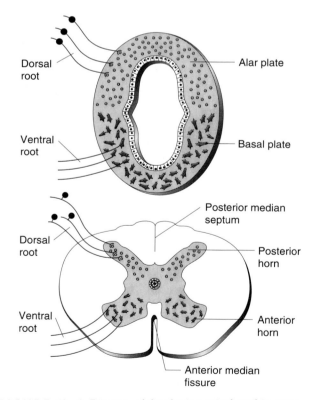

Dorsal root

Alar plate

Ventral root

Basal plate

Posterior median septum

Dorsal root

Posterior horn

Ventral root

Anterior horn

Anterior median fissure

FIGURE 42–8. Diagram of developing spinal cord in cross-section showing (*top*) alar and basal plates and (*bottom*) posterior horn/dorsal root and anterior horn/ventral root. (Figure designed by Cindy Glover, Olympia, Wash.)

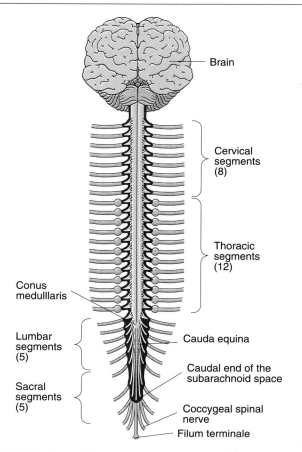

Brain

Cervical segments (8)

Thoracic segments (12)

Conus medulllaris

Lumbar segments (5)

Cauda equina

Caudal end of the subarachnoid space

Sacral segments (5)

Coccygeal spinal nerve

Filum terminale

FIGURE 42–9. Diagram of adult spinal cord. (Figure designed by Cindy Glover, Olympia, Wash.)

Most notable is Brodmann's map, which is based on histologic differences.[1] The specific function of the cerebrum will be discussed later in the chapter. The cerebral cortex, which is only a few millimeters thick, lies like a sheet over the entire surface of the cerebral hemispheres, each hemisphere almost a mirror image of the other. The cortex consists of neurons and their interconnections. Once of the amazing evolutionary features of the brain in mammals is the tremendous increase in size of the cerebral hemispheres. Throughout evolutionary time, as the hemispheres increased in size the outer surface became corrugated in appearance. This development provided a greater surface area of neurons and supportive cells without a comparable increase in brain size. One theory attributes the tremendous increase in size of the human cortex to the development of skills uniquely human such as abstract thought and complex language.[1] The cerebral cortex includes olfactory and limbic systems, both structures of ancient vertebrate lineage. The limbic system is involved in memory, emotions, and the influence of emotion on visceral functions via the autonomic nervous system.

At the base of each hemisphere are a number of dense nuclear bodies. The largest of these is the **corpus striatum,** which includes the caudate and the lentiform nuclei. The function of the corpus striatum is to modulate voluntary and automatic motor movements. It is part of the system that allows cognitive control over movement or motor planning. Lesions in this area can result in difficulties with initiating an activity as well as altering the course of activity as needed. Thus the corpus striatum are involved in cognitive as well as motor function. Another prominent mass at the base of the hemisphere is the **amygdala,** which is responsible for the semiautomatic visceral activities associated with eating (chewing, licking, salivating, gagging) and the visceral reactions to fear. Together the amygdala and the corpus striatum are called the basal ganglia.

The medullary center of the hemispheres is composed of millions of directional fiber tracts that not only travel to and from the cortex and the subcortical centers **(projection fibers),** but also connect the cortical areas of the same hemisphere **(association fibers)** and cross the midline to connect one hemisphere with

Regions of secondary brain swellings develop into distinctive structures, with the most dramatic growth and development occurring in the prosencephalon, or Neuro Axis I, which has divided into the telencephalon and the diencephalon. Together they will become the entire CNS above the midbrain. The telencephalon develops into the cerebral cortex, the corpus striatum, and the medullary center. The cerebral hemispheres are composed of paired lobes: frontal, parietal, temporal, and occipital. A number of scientists have mapped the hemispheres based on specific characteristics.

TABLE 42–2. Embryonic Sequence of Development From Primary Vesicles to Mature Brain Structures

Primary Vesicles	Secondary Vesicles	Mature Structures
Prosencephalon	Telencephalon	Cerebral cortex, corpus callosum, basal ganglia, rhinencephalon
	Diencephalon	Thalamus, hypothalamus
Mesencephalon	Mesencephalon	Midbrain
Rhombencephalon	Metencephalon	Pons, cerebellum
	Myelencephalon	Medulla oblongata

the other **(commissural fibers).** In general, afferent information comes from subcortical areas or from other cortical areas. Most information coming subcortically to the cortex comes from the thalamus.

Efferent fibers can also be connected to cortical or subcortical areas. Just below the cortical surface the millions of neuronal fibers leaving the cortex or arriving from the subcortical areas flow in fanlike fashion, forming the **corona radiata.** As they narrow and converge at the brain stem, this band of fibers becomes the **internal capsule.** Most subcortical efferent fibers exit the cortex by way of the internal capsule, the largest projection tract of all ingoing and outgoing cortical information. Cortical fibers traveling from the cortex to the brain stem and spinal cord pass through the internal capsule and continue through the **crus cerebri,** the equivalent of the internal capsule at the level of the midbrain. Fibers may continue downward to the spinal cord or synapse at junctions along the way. From the crus cerebri the tracts enter the medullary pyramids and the spinal cord (Fig. 42–10).

The cerebral hemispheres are separated longitudinally by the longitudinal fissure. Beneath the cortical surface they are connected by axonal commissures—the anterior and posterior commissures and the corpus callosum. The **corpus callosum** is the largest commissural band of fibers, containing more than 300 million axons.[1] Most of these axons connect mirror-image sites between the hemispheres. The commissural fibers passing to and from much of the temporal lobe travel through a portion of the corpus callosum called the anterior commissure. The corpus callosum allows stimuli that are initially presented to a sensory function in one hemisphere to be recognized when presented to the other hemisphere. For instance, a picture presented to the left visual field is readily recognized when presented to the right visual field.

Association fibers, those that connect cortical regions within the same hemisphere, can be short, connecting one convolution with another by way of the sulcus. They can also be long fibers, connecting different lobes to one another. The most prominent association tract is the cingulum. Lying on the medial aspect of the hemisphere, the cingulum connects regions of the frontal and parietal lobes with the parahippocam-

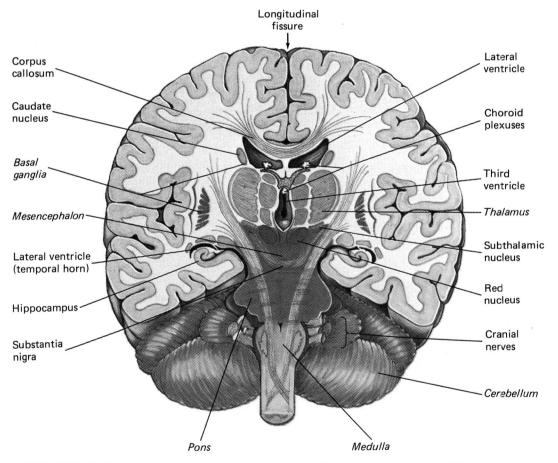

Longitudinal fissure

Corpus callosum

Caudate nucleus

Basal ganglia

Mesencephalon

Lateral ventricle (temporal horn)

Hippocampus

Substantia nigra

Lateral ventricle

Choroid plexuses

Third ventricle

Thalamus

Subthalamic nucleus

Red nucleus

Cranial nerves

Cerebellum

Pons

Medulla

FIGURE 42–10. A coronal view of the cerebrum looking from anteriorly backward. This section was made immediately anterior to the lower brain stem and through the middle of the thalamus. Efferent fibers are evident in their course from the cortex to the internal capsule, crus cerebri, and spinal cord. The bands of fibers can be seen in the subcortical white matter as they converge between the basal ganglia and the thalamus, through the mesencephalon, and into the medulla, where they cross. (From Guyton AC: *Basic Neuroscience: Anatomy and Physiology.* Philadelphia, WB Saunders, 1987, p 18. Reproduced with permission.)

pal and temporal cortical regions. The speed and effectiveness with which these fiber tracts pass impulses from one neuron to another ensures rapid integration of neuronal information throughout the brain.

The diencephalon develops from the caudal end of the prosencephalon. Early in embryogenesis, optic cups form on the lateral walls of the diencephalon. The central cavity of the prosencephalon narrows in the diencephalon, forming the third ventricle. Lying along the right and left sides of this ventricle is a small multinucleated structure called the **thalamus.** Much of thalamic function has to do with receiving sensory information and relaying it to appropriate areas of the cortex. The thalamus is involved in most exchanges between the cortex and subcortical connections and between sensory and motor or regulatory transactions, and it plays a significant role in the conscious experience of sensation. The thalamus functions as a cortical regulator, both in shifting and in focusing attention. It is also involved in complex mental processing and memory, and, through its connections with the limbic system, has a role in emotions.[9]

The hypothalamus is unique and critical for its supervisory role in the ANS. The ANS controls contractions of muscles that are not under voluntary control, such as the heart and smooth muscles in the blood vessels. It also has a controlling influence over secretions of the digestive system, sweat glands, and some endocrine organs. The regulatory mechanism of the ANS is different from that of the CNS in that the ANS influences large expanses of tissue and entire organs as opposed to single cells. In addition, the response to ANS stimulation is not necessarily instantaneous but can occur over time by hormonal influence. Within the hypothalamus are nuclei or clusters of cell bodies responsible for linking the ANS with the thalamus, cortex, olfactory cortex, and pituitary gland. This system influences visceral and somatic responses, such as the fight-or-flight response, fear, anger, and anxiety. The hypothalamus also regulates metabolic mechanisms, including the metabolism of fat, carbohydrate, and water. It regulates body temperature, controls appetite, influences genital functions, and influences sleep rhythms. Of note are two other areas of the diencephalon—the epithalamus, which is composed of small tracts and nuclei and the pineal gland, and the subthalamus, which includes sensory and motor circuits. The retina is a derivative of the diencephalon. The optic nerve and visual systems are related to this area of the brain.

The mesencephalon is part of Neuro Axis II. It is one of the original vesicles of the brain and does not divide. It develops into the midbrain and contains sensory and motor pathways and is the site of two cranial nerve nuclei (oculomotor and trochlear). The dorsal midbrain is called the tectum and is concerned with visual and auditory systems. It also includes two motor nuclei, the red nucleus and the substantia nigra. The cerebellum is attached to the midbrain by the superior cerebellar peduncles. The motor nuclei along with their cerebellar connections are involved in the smooth integration of muscle movements and in patterning of automatic posture. Lesions in this area can result in movement disorders, including tremor, rigidity, and uncontrolled movements of local muscle groups.

The rhombencephalon, also part of Neuro Axis II, divides into the metencephalon and the myelencephalon. The metencephalon is made up of the pons and the cerebellum. The dorsal portion of the pons includes sensory and motor tracts that are continuous with the midbrain above and the medulla below. The pons also contains the nuclei of four cranial nerves: the trigeminal, abducens, facial, and vestibulocochlear nerves. On the ventral portion of the pons are extensive connections between the cortex of the cerebral hemispheres and the contralateral cerebellar hemispheres. These connections contribute to the maximum efficiency of motor activities and form the structures known as the middle cerebellar peduncles.

The **cerebellum,** or "little brain," covers the posterior surface of the brain stem. The cerebellum, which is considered part of the motor system, actually has minimal direct effect on motor neurons. Rather, its role is to influence or modulate motor activities. The cerebellum receives and processes input from virtually every sensory system. It then sends messages by way of the deep cerebellar nuclei to various sites in the brain stem and thalamus that influence motor activity.

The cerebellar cortex is folded much as the cerebral cortex is folded, and in a way that significantly increases surface area. Its tightly folded shape gives it a banded appearance. The cortical ridges on the surface of the cerebellum are called folia. The white matter beneath is called the medullary center and is made up of fibers running to and from the cerebellar cortex.

The cerebellum is divided anatomically, first by the posterolateral fissure, which separates the flocculonodular lobe (the region immediately inferior to the middle cerebellar peduncles) from the main body, the corpus cerebelli. Another prominent landmark is the primary fissure, which subdivides the corpus cerebelli into the anterior and posterior lobes. From a longitudinal perspective, the midline body is called the vermis, and it is straddled on either side by the cerebellar hemispheres. The portion of the hemisphere that is adjacent to the vermis is called the paravermal zone.

The prominent tracts that attach the cerebellum to the brain stem are called the inferior, middle, and superior cerebellar peduncles. The inferior cerebellar peduncle is composed primarily of afferent fibers coming from the spinal cord and the brain stem. The middle peduncle contains afferents from the contralateral pontine nuclei. The superior cerebellar peduncle is different in that it is composed of major efferent pathways leaving the cerebellum.

Deep within the medullary center in each hemisphere are the cerebellar nuclei. The most lateral of these are the dentate nuclei, which receive most of their input from the lateral cerebellar hemispheres. Medial to the dentate lie the interposed nuclei, which consist of the emboliform and the globose nuclei. These nuclei receive input predominantly from the paravermal cortex. The most medial nuclear structures are the fastigial nuclei, which receive most of their input from the vermis. The functional role of the cerebellar nuclei is not entirely understood. Although it is known that they are the source of cerebellar output, it is increasingly clear that they also receive much of the sensory input that the cerebellar cortex receives, and it is likely that they are involved in feedback and modulation as well.

As a motor system, the cerebellum plays a role in maintaining equilibrium, muscle tone, postural control, and in the coordination of voluntary movements. As might be expected, it receives input from other areas of the nervous system also involved with these functions, namely, the spinal cord, cerebral cortex, and vestibular nucleus. Most of the vermal and paravermal regions receive spinal inputs. The major input into the lateral hemispheres comes from the cerebral cortex.

The lateral hemispheres form the biggest part of the cerebellum. Their major neural activity involves a feedback loop in which inputs from several areas of the cerebral cortex are received by the cerebellar hemispheres and dentate nuclei, then sent back to the motor and premotor cortex. This circuit is believed to influence the planning and programming of voluntary movements, especially learned, skilled movements—movements that become more rapid, precise, and automatic with practice.

The major inputs to the paravermal region, also called the intermediate cortex, are somatotypically arranged projections from the motor cortex and spinal cord. The primary output from this region is through the interposed nucleus to the red nucleus and also back to the motor cortex by way of the thalamus. The intermediate cerebellum therefore can influence spinal cord and motor neurons through the corticospinal tract and the rubrospinal tract, where it is involved in interpreting and responding to the position and velocity of the moving body.

The vermis receives inputs and contains representation of the trunk as conveyed by the spinocerebellar tracts. It sends outputs to the vestibular nuclei and the reticular formation by way of the fastigial nucleus and through direct projections to the vestibular nuclei. The vestibulospinal and reticulospinal tracts in turn influence spinal motor neurons. This area of the cerebellum, then, is most involved with regulation of posture and stereotyped movements that are programmed in the brain stem and spinal cord.

The flocculonodular lobe receives most of its transmissions by way of the inferior cerebellar peduncle from the vestibular nerve and nuclei. Because of this primary source of input, this lobe is often referred to as the vestibulocerebellum. Its role is to maintain equilibrium and mediate the slow eye movements needed for visual tracking.

The myelencephalon develops into the medulla, the lowest part of the hindbrain. This segment of the brain extends from the first spinal nerve of the spinal cord below to the beginning of the pontine flexure above. The last four cranial nerves—the glossopharyngeal, vagus, accessory, and hypoglossal nerves—have nuclei in the medulla. The medulla is the site of control centers for such basic life maintenance functions as respiration, blood pressure, and pulse. As the medulla develops, its walls shift laterally at its rostral portion owing to the expanding fourth ventricle. Diffusely organized within the medulla and extending upward to the diencephalon is the reticular formation. It is a network of nerve cell bodies and fibers that connects with all major neural tracts going to and coming from the brain. The reticular formation is responsible for mediating complex postural reflexes (turning motions of the trunk, turning and bending motions of the head, and postural motions of the limbs). It is involved in smooth muscle activity and helps to maintain muscle tone. Within the reticular formation is the reticular activating system (RAS), which controls waking and alerting mechanisms. Projections to the thalamus are particularly important, as activity in this pathway is essential for maintaining a normal state of consciousness. Neurons from the RAS terminate in the intralaminar nuclei of the thalamus and in turn project to widespread areas of the cortex. An intact RAS is a precondition to consciousness and the ability to attend to stimuli. In animals, stimulation of the mesencephalic and pontine portions of the reticular formation results in a high degree of wakefulness and increased muscle tone throughout the body. Lesions in this area result in disorders of consciousness such as coma or stupor.[9]

Ventricular System

Throughout vesicle development there is simultaneous expansion of the neural tube cavity. This cavity persists after the neuropores close and develops into the ventricular system of the adult brain. The ventricular system is lined with ependymal cells and is composed of a continuous, fluid-filled series of cavities that extends throughout all the major areas of the CNS. Large, dilated cavities that grow and change shape with development produce and bathe the brain and the spinal cord with cerebrospinal fluid (CSF), giving the brain buoyancy; help maintain the extracellular environment of neurons; and provide a route for neuroactive hormones in the CSF.[1,6] The large C-shaped lateral ventricles occupy the center of each hemisphere. They communicate with the third ventricle in the diencephalon by way of the intraventricular foramen, which in turn is linked to the fourth ventricle by way of the cerebral aqueduct, which lies between the pons and rostral medulla. The CSF leaves the fourth ventricle through the median or lateral aperture and moves slowly down and around the spinal cord and up over the cerebral hemispheres to the arachnoid villi, where it is absorbed into the venous system.

The rate of production of CSF is independent of blood pressure or intraventricular pressure. Thus, CSF will continue to be produced even when its path of circulation or absorption is blocked. If this occurs the amount of CSF increases, as do the size of the ventricles. This pathology is called **hydrocephalus.** Although hydrocephalus is most frequently caused by blockage of CSF pathways, it can also be caused by overproduction and malabsorption of CSF. Blockages can occur from tumors, congenital abnormalities of the fourth ventricle apertures, and adhesions outside the ventricular system. Congenital hydrocephalus can result in enlargement of the head, because the skull suture lines are not yet fixed. As the amount of CSF increases, the size of the head also increases to accommodate the increased fluid. Hydrocephalus can be diagnosed with computed tomography (CT) or magnetic resonance imaging (MRI) and can generally be treated with a ventriculoperitoneal shunt.

KEY CONCEPTS

- **The nervous system begins as a neural plate composed of ectoderm. As cells of the neural plate proliferate, a hollow tube with openings at either end is formed. The neural tube develops into the brain and spinal cord. Groups of neural crest cells pinch off the neural tube to become peripheral nerves, cranial nerves, and Schwann cells.**

- **As neural tube cells differentiate into primitive neurons, axonal and dendritic processes sprout and make specific connections with each other.**

- **The developing brain has five major divisions: the telencephalon (cerebral cortex, basal ganglia), diencephalon (thalamus, hypothalamus), mesencephalon (midbrain), metencephalon (pons, cerebellum), and myelencephalon (medulla, reticular activating system).**

  Telencephalon: Cerebral hemispheres are connected to each other by large commissural fiber tracts—the corpus callosum and the anterior and posterior commissures. Fiber tracts travel to and from the cerebral cortex and subcortical centers through the internal capsule. Still other axons, called association fibers, connect cortical areas within the same hemisphere. Basal ganglia are intimately involved in cognitive and motor function. Lesions of the basal ganglia result in difficulty initiating and adjusting movements.

  Diencephalon: The thalamus is a major relay station in the CNS. Sensory information is received, integrated, and relayed to appropriate areas of the cortex. Most transmissions from the cortex to subcortical centers pass through the thalamus. The hypothalamus is essential for controlling pituitary function and the autonomic nervous system. Cranial nerve II originates from the diencephalon.

  Mesencephalon: Midbrain structures include cranial nerves III and IV and attachments to the cerebellar peduncles.

  Metencephalon: The pons contains cranial nerves V, VI, VII, and VIII and attachments to the cerebellum. The cerebellum is involved in equilibrium, postural control, and coordination of voluntary movements. It receives projections for nearly all sensory input as well as cortical input.

  Myelencephalon: The medulla connects to the spinal cord below and the pons above. It contains centers for control of respiration, blood pressure, and heart rate. Cranial nerves IX, X, XI, and XII have nuclei in the medulla. The medulla also contains the reticular activating system, which controls waking and alerting. Lesions in this area result in impaired consciousness.

- **Expansion of the lumen of the neural tube results in formation of the ventricular system. CSF is produced in the ventricles and circulates through the ventricles and subarachnoid spaces of the brain and cord.**

Meningeal Coverings and Blood Supply

The CSF that bathes the brain and provides buoyancy also offers some protection from traumatic injury. Another mechanism of protection for the CNS is the hard skull and bony vertebral column, which house the soft brain and spinal cord, respectively. Yet another mechanism of protection is the meningeal covering of the brain and spinal cord.

The meninges are composed of three layers that act to suspend and maintain the shape and position of the nervous tissue during head and body movements. The brain is actually suspended within layers of meninges that are fixed to the skull. In this manner, the brain turns with the movement of the skull. The CSF circulates within the subarachnoid space, giving buoyancy to the brain and making an average 1,500-gram structure effectively weigh 50 grams. The brain is thus more resistant to distortion, which could occur from gravity alone were it not for the buoyancy effect.[1] The three meningeal layers are the dura mater, arachnoid and pia mater.

The dura mater, the outermost meningeal layer, is a thick, tough, collagenous membrane. It is composed of two layers, one contiguous with the periosteum of the skull, the other, adherent to the first, that covers the surface of the brain. The tough dura protects the soft tissue of the brain. Support and stability are also provided by dural septa that invaginate into the cranial cavity. The falx cerebri is a thin wall of dura that folds down between the cortex, separating the two hemispheres. The tentorium cerebelli is a septum that separates the cerebellum and brain stem from the rest of the cerebrum. The dural septa fix the brain in place by their tentlike structure and limit its movement within the skull. Venous sinuses which collect venous blood from cerebral veins are located between the two layers of the dura at the base of the septum.

Beneath and continuous with the dura is the arachnoid layer. The spaces between the dura and the skull and between the dura mater and the arachnoid are only potential spaces. Only during pathologic processes, notably epidural and subdural hemorrhages, do these spaces become evident. Unlike the dura mater, the arachnoid is a thin, delicate membrane. It is semitransparent and weblike in appearance, hence its name. From the arachnoid layer come strands of collagenous connective tissue called trabeculae that extend down to the pia mater, forming a subarachnoid space. In this space flows the CSF.

CSF is produced by the choroid plexus at a rate of approximately 500 to 700 mL/day. It is absorbed at about the same rate, so that only 150 to 175 mL is in circulation at any one time. CSF is absorbed by the arachnoid villi—small tufts of the arachnoid that invaginate into the dural sinus, especially along the superior sagittal sinus. These tufts bring CSF into close approximation with venous blood. CSF is able to flow into the venous system through one-way valves as a consequence of bulk flow or pressure gradient differences.

Although the CSF flows readily into the venous sinus, flow in the opposite direction cannot occur. That is, the fluid in the venous sinus cannot flow into the subarachnoid space. In fact, the CNS is protected from the rest of the body and actually functions within its own controlled environment. Part of that control stems from a system of barriers between the nervous system's extracellular space and the extracellular space in the rest of the body. One such barrier lies between the CSF in the subarachnoid space and the venous blood in the sagittal sinus. A system of tight junctions between cell bodies in the dura–arachnoid layer interface prevents the exchange of fluids or chemicals between these compartments.

Pia mater, the third meningeal layer, is also very thin, but unlike the other meningeal layers the pia closely follows the contours of the brain, over every sulcus and into every gyrus. Consequently the subarachnoid space between the arachnoid and the pia mater is not an evenly distributed space. The arachnoid meshes with the pia via the trabeculae in such a subtle manner that often it is difficult to differentiate one from the other. Consequently the two layers are often referred together as the **leptomeninges.** Many of the cerebral vessels traverse the subarachnoid space, lying on the pial surface before they enter the brain.

The meninges cover and provide protection to the spinal cord as well as the brain, with only a few variations. The spinal dura, for instance, has no periosteal layer, so it is a single rather than a double layer. It is continuous with the foramen magnum at the base of the skull and is separated from the spinal vertebral periosteum by an epidural space. Thus, in the spinal cord, the epidural space is a true space, unlike its counterpart in the cranium, which is only a potential space. Within this space lie fatty connective tissue and a vertebral venous plexus.

The spinal arachnoid, much like that covering the cerebrum, is closely adherent to the spinal dura. Between the arachnoid layer and the pial lining is another subarachnoid space filled with CSF. The spinal dura-arachnoid layer ends at approximately the second sacral vertebra. The spinal cord, on the other hand, ends between the first and second lumbar verte-brae (L1–L2). This results in a large subarachnoid cistern called the lumbar cistern, a favored place to obtain CSF samples. The spinal pia is much tougher and thicker than the cerebral pia. Projecting along the length of each side is the dentate ligament, which anchors the spinal cord to the arachnoid and through it to the dura. Another pial projection connects the end of the spinal cord (the cauda equina) at level L1–L2 to the caudal end of the spinal dural sheath, where it is tethered to the end of the vertebral column. This projection is called the filum terminale.

Brain metabolism is dependent on the oxidation of glucose. Twenty percent of the total body oxygen consumption is utilized for this purpose. At 750 mL/min the brain receives 15 percent of the total resting cardiac output. This is maintained at a relatively constant rate due to the body's autoregulatory mechanism. If the brain is without oxygen for 2 to 5 minutes, irreversible brain damage can ensue.

The entire cerebral blood supply arises from two pairs of arteries. The anterior circulation is supplied by the internal carotid arteries and the posterior circulation is supplied by the vertebral arteries. The left common carotid artery arises from the aortic arch and the right common carotid artery arises from the bifurcation of the brachiocephalic artery. The common carotid arteries bifurcate at the top of the thyroid cartilage to form the internal and external carotid arteries. The internal carotid arteries supply most of the hemispheres (excluding the occipital lobes, two thirds of the diencephalon, and the basal ganglia). Before entering the brain the internal carotids give off the tympanic and the ophthalmic arteries. Supplying the hemispheres are the terminal branches of the internal carotid, namely, the anterior and middle cerebral arteries and posterior communicating arteries. The anterior cerebral artery feeds the medial frontal and parietal lobes, adjacent cortex, and parts of the corpus callosum. The anterior communicating artery joins each anterior cerebral artery. The middle cerebral artery supplies the lateral surface of the four cerebral lobes. The posterior communicating artery connects the carotid circulation with the posterior cerebral artery. The meninges are richly supplied with arterial blood from the anterior, middle, and posterior meningeal arteries, which arise from the external carotid arteries.

The posterior circulation arises from the two vertebral arteries that originate from the subclavian arteries. The vertebral arteries enter the skull at the foramen magnum and join at the level of the pons to form the basilar artery. The basilar artery divides into two posterior cerebral arteries that join the posterior communicating arteries from the anterior circulation. The posterior cerebral arteries supply blood to the occipital lobes, the medial and inferior surface of the temporal lobes, and the midbrain and posterior diencephalon. The vertebral and basilar arteries supply the cerebellum, brain stem, and spinal cord. The ring of vessels that unites the anterior and posterior circulation at the base of the brain is known as the circle of Willis (Fig. 42–11).

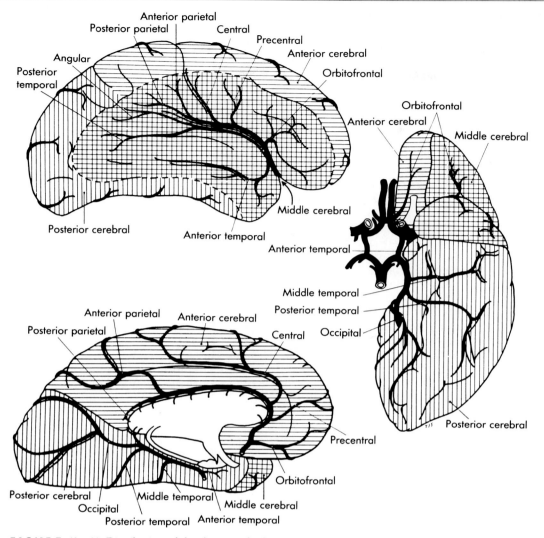

FIGURE 42–11. Distribution of the three cerebral arteries in lateral, medial, and inferior views of the cerebral hemisphere. The circle of Willis is evident in the inferior view. (Reproduced from Mettler, Fred A.: *Neuroanatomy*, 2nd ed. St. Louis, 1948, The C. V. Mosby Co.)

The venous system in the brain is unlike its counterpart in the systemic circulation, for it does not follow the arterial vessels. Instead, the cerebral veins drain into large vascular channels called sinuses that are formed by folds in the dura. From the sinuses, venous blood returns to the heart by way of the jugular veins.

KEY CONCEPTS

- Meninges affix the brain to the skull so that the brain is suspended and supported. Meninges have three layers. (1) The dura mater is the tough outer layer attached to the periostium of the skull. (2) The arachnoid is a delicate weblike membrane spanning the space between the dura and the pia mater. (3) The pia mater covers the contours of the brain surface. The spinal cord has the same arrangement of meningeal coverings.

- Blood is supplied to the brain by branches of the internal carotid and vertebral arteries. The internal carotids branch to form the anterior and middle cerebral arteries and the posterior communicating artery, which primarily supply the anterior aspects of the brain. The vertebral arteries join at the level of the pons to become the basilar artery, which branches to form two posterior cerebral arteries. Vertebral and basilar arteries supply the posterior cerebrum, cerebellum, and brain stem.

Cerebral Cortex

Cortical Organization

As embryonic neurons are developing, the means in which their processes synapse with those of other neurons is not haphazard. Rather, the development of interneuronal communication is systematic and extremely organized. This is exquisitely evident in the formation of six distinguishable horizontal layers of the cerebral cortex (Fig. 42–12). Each layer is notable for a predominance of a cell type or, as in the first layer, by the absence of cells. Laminar patterns are formed by the cell bodies of terminating afferents or the initiation of efferents as they respectively enter or exit within specific layers of the cortex or connect with adjacent or distinct cortical areas. This linkage underscores the interneuronal communication that is the principal role of the cerebral cortex and the fundamental element of human function. The ability to perform routine daily activities, to manage a job or balance a checkbook, is an outcome of the efficiency of this communication system. Health care professionals are often called on to evaluate and provide therapy for someone whose neural communication system is no longer fully intact and as a result is unable to perform with maximum independence. A basic understanding of cortical function and the mechanisms of interneuronal communication is useful to the professional attempting to facilitate an individual's return to a fully productive life-style. There is little question that all behavior is the result of underlying brain activity. The debate lies in the specificity of cortical location as it relates to a discrete behavior. Localization of brain function has been a much debated topic of research, as witnessed by the work of Head,[10] Kertesz,[11] and Luria.[12] Throughout the years, scientists of brain function have proposed at one extreme that all human function can be discretely attributed to areas or centers in the brain, and at the other extreme that human behavior is due to large cooperative areas of the cortex. While there is still insufficient evidence that would relate function to a **cytoarchitectonic** arrangement, from current research[13] it is known that some behaviors are related to distinct regions of the brain.

Luria[12] and Geschwind,[14] among others, can be credited with the establishment of current beliefs of nature of human function. From their work, as well as the more recent efforts of scientists like Damasio and Damasio,[15] it is understood that there are indeed areas of the brain responsible for particular behaviors. Disruptions of brain activity by lesions (localized cellular damage) in the same anatomic locations in most humans will disrupt behavior in a predictable fashion. This is true for such activities as movement of the index finger, the ability to perceive smells, the ability to comprehend speech, and the ability to reproduce a design. However, while precisely delimited activities can be attributed to the function of specific brain areas or even of certain cell groupings, processing and utilization of the activity require much larger areas of brain function. The ability to move the index finger and point to a specific area on a road map is not a function of a discrete area of the brain but requires numerous neural interactions with multiple areas of the brain. This is significant to health care professionals, who may find it useful to distinguish a deficit caused by a well-localized lesion from one that involves multiple or large areas of the brain as they plan appropriate therapeutic interventions. A patient with a well-circumscribed lesion in the left motor cortex that impairs the right upper extremity may be quite functional with occupational therapy and compensatory equipment such as utensils with built-up handles. However, if that same patient has a larger lesion in the left hemisphere resulting in a concurrent language impairment, it may be difficult to utilize the therapy and compensatory equipment because of poor comprehension of how and when to use the tools. In such a case, different rehabilitation strategies must be applied.

Regions of Localized Function

Scientists have named those functional areas of the cortex, that have direct connections to specific muscles or sensory receptors and are responsible for discrete movements or sensations (visual, auditory, or somatic) as *primary areas*. Surrounding the primary areas are *secondary areas* that elaborate or give greater definition to the functions of the primary cortex. For example, whereas the primary motor cortex is responsible for gross hand movements, it is the connections with supplemental, premotor cortex and basal ganglia that produce sufficient motor control to paint or handwrite. Besides the primary and secondary cortical areas there are large areas of cortex that are multimodal, involving interpretation of information from more than one primary and secondary area as well as subcortical areas. These large areas of cortex are called *association cortex*.

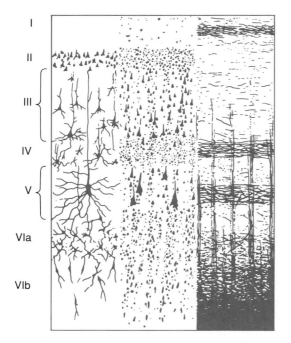

FIGURE 42–12. Structure of the cerebral cortex, illustrating distinguishing cell layers. (From Ranson and Clark [after Brodmann]: *Anatomy of the Nervous System*. Philadelphia, WB Saunders, 1959. Reproduced by permission.)

Acknowledging that the cerebral cortex has at once the properties of discrete function as well as those which are complex and interrelated, we will first examine areas of discrete localization. Cortex responsible for primary somatic sensation lies in the postcentral gyrus (Fig. 42–13), in Brodmann areas 3, 1, and 2. The **primary sensory cortex** is composed of long parallel strips on the postcentral gyrus, each structurally different from the other. All are **somatotopically** mapped such that distinct areas of the body are represented in a progression from tongue to contralateral leg along an inferior to superior line. Not only is each strip mapped separately, but in an anterior to posterior direction each strip responds to a different type of stimulus. Although other areas in the cortex are involved in sensation, this area is the most prominent, and is referred to as **S1**.[1] A second area that receives input from the thalamus and S1 lies in the inferior parietal lobe and into the lateral sulcus. This area is somatotopically mapped as well, but in reverse order, so that the area of facial representation in this area lies adjacent to the facial area in S1 on the parietal

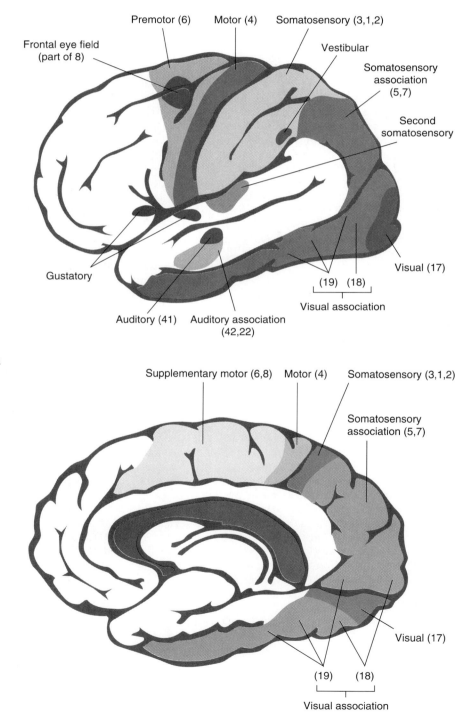

FIGURE 42–13. Diagram of the localization of function in the cerebral hemispheres. *Top,* lateral view; *bottom,* medial view. Various functional areas are shown in reference to areas of Brodmann. (Figure designed by Cindy Glover, Olympia, Wash.)

Premotor (6) Motor (4) Somatosensory (3,1,2)

Frontal eye field (part of 8)

Vestibular

Somatosensory association (5,7)

Second somatosensory

Gustatory

Visual (17)

(19) (18)

Visual association

Auditory (41) Auditory association (42,22)

Supplementary motor (6,8) Motor (4) Somatosensory (3,1,2)

Somatosensory association (5,7)

Visual (17)

(19) (18)

Visual association

lobe and the rest of the body lies in the lateral sulcus. Interestingly, this somatosensory area receives bilateral hemispheric innervation.

The distinct somatotopic mapping of the cortex is dependent on equally structured and organized delivery of sensory input from receptors in the periphery. As was discussed earlier in this chapter, information traveling to the cortex within the CNS does so by way of afferent projection fibers, and as part of a three-neuron circuit. The first nerve is a peripheral nerve fiber, which carries information from a sensory receptor to the CNS through the dorsal root ganglion. Upon entering the spinal cord, the axons of the sensory system become distinctly segregated into tracts. The tracts known as the **posterior columns** are made up of fibers responsible for carrying impulses of well-localized (epicritic) touch, posture, passive movement, and vibration, and are cirtical for temporal and spatial discrimination. With the sensory information provided by these fibers, it is possible to know the position of one's body, or separate parts of one's body, in space, without visual input. The primary neuron receptors of this tract are in the joint capsules, muscles, and skin (tactile and pressure), and they send impulses centrally to the cell bodies of the primary neurons that lie in the spinal ganglion. The central processes of primary fibers enter the cord and pass directly into the posterior white column on the same side without synapsing, then travel upward. As the fibers progress upward, they gradually move toward the midline, so that those corresponding to the lower extremities occupy the medial white column (fasciculus gracilis) and those representing the arm are more lateral (fasciculus cuneatus). The intermediate septum separates the two columns. Fibers for both the fasciculus gracilis and fasciculus cuneatus terminate and synapse with secondary fibers in the medulla oblongata at the nucleus gracilis and nucleus cuneatus, respectively.

From the nuclei in the medulla, axons of the secondary fibers cross to the opposite side as the arcuate fibers; travel up the brain stem, forming the medial lemniscus; and terminate in the ventral posterior lateral nucleus of the thalamus. In the thalamus, fibers synapse with tertiary neurons, which in turn pass upward in a great band of fibers known as the internal capsule, through the corona radiata and on to primary sensory cortex in the postcentral gyrus.

The **lateral spinothalamic tract** carries impulses for sensations of pain and temperature that originate from receptors throughout the body (excluding the face). Primary peripheral nerves are thin, myelinated or unmyelinated, with cell bodies in the spinal ganglion. Their central processes enter the spinal cord by way of Lissauer's fasciculus. They ascend at least one spinal segment before entering the posterior horn and synapsing with their secondary neuron. From the posterior horn cells, some secondary fibers ascend ipsilaterally in Lissauer's fasciculus all the way to the thalamus. Most fibers, however, cross the midline in the anterior white commissure and ascend as the lateral spinothalamic tract in the anterior portion of the lat-

eral white column. Fibers from the lower extremities and trunk are pushed laterally as they ascend in the spinal cord by the addition of fibers from the upper extremities and upper body, which enter medially. On their way to the thalamus, these fibers give off collaterals to the reticular formation of the brain stem and the periaqueductal gray matter in the midbrain, where it is believed that one of their functions is involved in pain inhibition. Secondary fibers of the spinothalamic tract terminate in several thalamic regions, including the ventral posterior lateral nucleus, the posterior region, and the intralaminar nuclei. Impulses for pain that ascend via the reticular formation terminate in the posterior region and the intralaminar nuclei. Tertiary neurons leave the thalamus and project to the postcentral gyrus by way of the internal capsule and corona radiata.

The **anterior spinothalamic tract** conducts impulses of light and poorly localized touch and is often considered part of the lateral spinothalamic tract and not a separate, distinct tract. Sensory receptors are in hairless areas of the skin, and the cell bodies lie in the spinal ganglion. The central processes of the primary neurons pass into the posterior horn and intermediate gray, where they synapse with secondary neurons that cross the midline in the anterior white commissure and enter the anterolateral white column. From here they ascend, forming the anterior spinothalamic tract. In the medulla the tract merges with the lateral spinothalamic tract. Because most of the sensory tracts cross the midline and terminate in the cortex opposite the side on which they entered the spinal cord, there is contralateral body representation in the cortex. Thus, lesions in the right hemisphere sensory cortex cause sensory loss in the left body.

The **primary visual cortex,** corresponding to Brodmann's area 17, lies in the calcarine sulcus of the occipital lobe. It receives **retinotopic** projections from the lateral geniculate nucleus in the thalamus regarding the contralateral visual field. The secondary visual cortex, in areas 18 and 19, is responsible for the detection of color, movement, and shape. The visual association cortex is found in the temporal and parietal lobes that juxtapose the occipital cortex. The primary visual cortex is critical, as destructive lesions in this area can result in loss of awareness of visual stimuli or functional blindness.

The **auditory cortex** is located on a portion of the superior surface of the temporal lobe. On the surface of this cortex there is a spectrum of audible frequencies that is discretely mapped. Although contralateral stimuli predominate, each hemisphere receives bilateral auditory innervation. Kinesthetic and vestibular functions are located on the inferior parietal lobe near the occipital and temporal boundaries.

Several of the senses, while not recognized as being mapped, are none the less located in specific areas of the cortex. **Gustatory sensation** is relayed from the thalamus to a discrete area on the inferior parietal lobe and anterior insula. **Vestibular function** is believed to be located on the parietal lobe adjacent to the representation of the head in the primary somatosensory cortex. And finally, **olfaction,** the sense of smell, is altogether different in that it is a function of the limbic system or old cortex.

The **primary motor cortex,** Broadmann's area 4, occupies the precentral gyrus. The motor cortex map closely mimics the somatotopic arrangement on the adjacent sensory cortex and similarly has contralateral body representation. Motor neurons in this area are primarily large pyramidal cells and make up the thickest area of cortex. Stimulation of cells in area 4 in a conscious patient results in discrete movements of a single muscle or a small group of muscles. Movements are always contralateral to the side stimulated except in the case of the palate, pharynx, masseters, and tongue, which have bilateral innervation. Area 6, the premotor cortex, is a secondary area involved in muscle movement but usually of larger muscle groups. This area is responsible for storage of information needed for controlling learned, skilled movements. At the lateral margin of the premotor cortex, anterior to the motor cortex, lies Broca's area (Fig. 42–14). Broca's area is responsible for the coordinated movements of the larynx and mouth necessary for speech production. It is often referred to as the speech center and in most people is in the left hemisphere. Finally, the supplementary motor area, located in the medial surface of the hemisphere, anterior to the representa-

tion of the foot in the primary motor cortex, is responsible for posture-related movements.

Although each of these areas is noted for its primary function, there is some crossover of function in adjacent areas. For instance, there is some motor representation found in the somatosensory cortex in the postcentral gyrus, and movement can be elicited by stimulation of the appropriate somatotopic neurons. The same is true for sensory representation in the primary motor cortex. As is the case throughout the cortex, destructive lesions result in the greatest damage when they involve the primary cortex. Lesions to area 4 result in initial flaccid paralysis of the contralateral body. This resolves fairly quickly into hemiparesis with mild spasticity, the distal muscles being much more involved than the proximal muscles. Lesions of the secondary motor cortex in conjunction with the primary cortex markedly increase the spastic element of dysfunction.

Motor impulses travel from the cortex to the spinal cord via efferent projection fibers. The **corticospinal tract** is the most important motor tract in the CNS and is responsible for voluntary motor control. In the upper extremities, this means control over the manipulation of objects, and in the lower extremities, control over locomotion. The corticospinal tract also functions

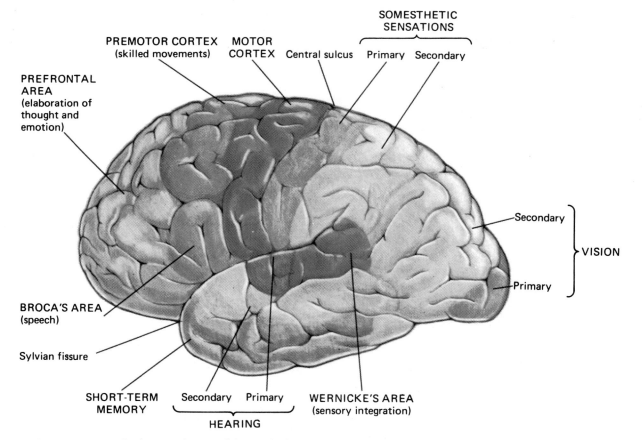

FIGURE 42–14. The functional areas of the cerebral cortex. Note Broca's and Wernicke's areas. (From Guyton AC: *Basic Neuroscience: Anatomy and Physiology.* Philadelphia, WB Saunders, 1987, p 13. Reproduced with permission.)

as a modifier or regulator of ascending sensory information.

Motor neurons arise in the cortex or subcortical nuclei and descend to lower motor neurons without synapsing. The corticospinal tract receives input from approximately 1 million neurons from each cerebral hemisphere. Those neurons that project to the anterior horn of the spinal cord are among the cells referred to as **upper motor neurons.** Many of the neuronal axons of this tract are unmyelinated, and their function is uncertain. Axons that are myelinated are small. Only 2 to 4 percent are large, rapidly conducting axons that arise from the giant pyramidal cells of Betz in the primary motor cortex. Their function is to inhibit antigravity tone of extensor muscles and allow motor action to occur.

Axons of the corticospinal tract leave the cortex and descend as part of the corona radiata, which narrows into the internal capsule just lateral to the diencephalon. In its descent, the corticospinal tract gives off collaterals to the diencephalon, traverses the base of the midbrain, and forms the major bulk of the crus cerebri. As the tract descends through the pons it is broken up into clusters by cells within the pons. The tract reassembles in the medulla, giving off collaterals and terminals, forming the pyramids. At the junction of the spinal cord and medulla a majority of the fibers in the pyramids cross or decussate to the contralateral side. After crossing, each tract forms a lateral corticospinal tract in the lateral funiculus of the spinal cord. Uncrossed fibers continue their descent in the anterior funiculus as the **anterior corticospinal tract.** The anterior corticospinal tract decussates at the cord segment in which it terminates, which is usually no further than the lower thoracic segments.

Approximately 50 percent of the corticospinal fibers terminate on neurons in the base of the posterior horn of the spinal cord and function to modify sensory input. The rest of the fibers terminate on the anterior horn motor neurons. The anterior horn motor neurons, their cranial nerve motor nuclei counterparts, and their axons terminate at the neuromuscular junctions of the muscles and form the final common pathway for the expression of voluntary motor movements.

Besides the corticospinal tract, there are tracts of upper motor neurons known as **extrapyramidal tracts,** which descend to the spinal cord from subcortical nuclei and are invovled in a cortical feedback loop with the corticospinal tract. They function by establishing a readiness state prior to individual motor acts initiated by the primary motor tract. One such tract is the **medial longitudinal fasciculus,** or MLF.

The MLF is composed of ascending and descending fibers that arise from several sources and have multiple termination points. Descending fibers arise from the medial vestibular nucleus in the rostral medulla and exert an inhibitory function on anterior horn motor neurons in the cervical cord. The descending fibers of the MLF also arise from the superior colliculus in the rostral midbrain, an area important for visual

reflexes, the accessory oculomotor nuclei of the rostral midbrain involved in visual tracking; the pontine reticular formation, which facilitates extensor muscle tone; and the vestibular nuclei of the medulla, which influence balance and equilibrium. Fibers of the MLF descend ipsilaterally in the anterior spinal cord with some fibers synapsing directly on the anterior horn motor neurons of the cervical cord. Axons of the anterior horn cells terminate primarily in the neuromuscular junction of neck muscles.

The ascending fibers of the MLF arise from the vestibular nuclei in the upper medulla and terminate in cranial nuclei responsible for eye movement: the oculomotor, trochlear, and abducens nuclei. Coordinated function of the MLF permits visual tracking of an object using eyes, head, neck, and trunk. It works in conjunction with the corticospinal tract for voluntary control over these otherwise reflexive activities.

The **vestibulospinal tract** is composed of input from the vestibular apparatus of the inner ear and the cerebellum. It is responsible for features of balance and coordination. Fibers in this tract descend ipsilaterally through the full length of the anterolateral spinal cord. Fibers terminate on anterior horn motor neurons. Motor neuron axons, in turn, terminate on neuromuscular junctions and muscle spindles. The vestibulospinal tract facilitates activity in extensor or antigravity muscles, facilitating basic posture and stance. The powerful influence of this tract is illustrated in cases of brain stem trauma in which the lesion occurs in the area just rostral to the vestibular nuclei. In such cases, cerebral inhibitory influence to the nuclei is lost, and the result is continuous extensor rigidity or decerebrate posturing.

Anterior horn cells are also influenced by two descending tracts from the brain stem, the **tectospinal** and **rubrospinal tracts.** The tectospinal tract arises from the superior colliculus of the midbrain, which is important for visual tracking and eye centering reflexes. Fibers in these tracts cross the midline and descend just anterior to the MLF. Terminal fibers end on interneurons that synapse on motor neurons in the spinal cord. The tectospinal tract blends the interaction of visual and auditory stimuli with postural reflex movements.

The rubrospinal tract arises from the red nucleus in the midbrain. Fibers cross the midline and descend in the spinal cord, where they are closely intermingled with the corticospinal tract. The rubrospinal tract descends as far as the thoracic level of the cord. The fibers of the rubrospinal tract terminate on interneurons in the anterior horn cells, which in turn terminate on both alpha and gamma motor neurons, which then end on neuromuscular junctions and muscle spindles. The rubrospinal tract is thought to be an alternate route from the cortex to the spinal cord. An important function is control of flexor muscle tone in the limbs. The actions of this tract is regulated by the cerebellum and the cerebral cortex based on sensory input.

The reticulospinal tracts originate from the brain stem reticular formation and act to modify motor and sensory functions of the spinal cord. Two tracts are recognized, the **pontine reticulospinal tract** and the **medullary reticulospinal tract.**

The pontine reticulospinal tract arises from cells in the pontine tegmentum. The tract descends through the brain stem and spinal cord as uncrossed fibers and gives off terminal fibers in route. These terminal fibers end in interneurons of the spinal cord. The interneurons project onto anterior horn alpha motor neurons, the axons of which terminate on neuromuscular junctions of extrafusal skeletal muscle fibers. They also project onto gamma motor neurons of the anterior horn cells, which innervate small intrafusal fibers of the muscle spindle.

The medullary reticulospinal tract originates in the medulla and descends through the brain stem and spinal cord as uncrossed fibers, giving off terminals to interneurons in the spinal cord. Interneurons of the cord receive influence from several corticosubcorticospinal tracts coming down from the brain stem. This influence is in turn projected to the alpha and gamma motor neurons of the anterior horn.

The reticular formation of the brain stem can inhibit or facilitate motor activity and muscle tone, influence the respiratory and circulatory systems, and affect the transmission of sensory impulses to higher centers. It appears that the medullary reticulospinal tract is involved in inhibition of motor activity, depression of cardiovascular responses, and stimulation of the inspiratory phase of respiration. The functions of the pontine reticulospinal tract are less clear but include facilitation of motor activity and cardiovascular responses.

Association Cortex

The discussion of cortical function thus far has focused on primary sensory and motor function. But what distinguishes humans from other mammals that also have such areas of specialized function? The difference is often referred to as "higher cortical function" and includes the ability to use language, create works of art and music, solve problems, and think in abstract terms. It is the ability to process information received from the primary cortical areas and direct behavior based on that information. Much of this activity is the function of association cortex. In fact, as the human brain has evolved over time, more of the cortex has become association cortex. Association cortex occupies large portions of the frontal and parietal lobes and responds to a multitude of sensory modalities. Responses may change relative to circumstances. These are considered multimodal association areas and related to high-level intellectual functions.

The most prominent of the association cortices are the parieto-occipitotemporal and the prefrontal association areas. The parieto-occipitotemporal cortex is a large area that lies between the somatic sensory cortex anteriorly, the visual posteriorly, and the auditory cortex laterally (see Fig. 42–13). This area is responsible for a high degree of interpretive function of the impulses it receives from the surrounding cortex. Although overlap of function is recognized even in the primary zones, overlap is a prominent feature of the association cortex. For example, the boundary between the occipital and parietal lobes is somewhat arbitrary, defined by a minor sulcus, the parieto-occipital sulcus. On either side of this boundary one does not find function that is distinctly visual or distinctly spatial. Rather, it is recognized as an overlap zone of visual and spatial function,[9] and the interpretation of impulses will be influenced by visual-spatial properties as well as by other sensory input. In fact, the area in the posterior parietal cortex and the superior occipital cortex is responsible for analysis of body position, where body parts are located in space, and the body's relationship to objects in the immediate environment. This ability requires the combined properties of visual, spatial, and proprioceptive input.

The area of cortex in the posterior part of the superior temporal lobe, behind the primary auditory cortex, is known as **Wernicke's area** and is responsible for language comprehension. This is perhaps the most significant region of the entire brain with respect to intellectual function, as almost all intellectual functions are language-based. Lesions selectively affecting this area and causing a pure Wernicke's aphasia are rare, but when they do occur they are devastating. The individual is able to understand very little of what is spoken to him, but his speech production remains intact. Many of these patients will prattle grammatically and syntactically correct nonsense. If the lesion is farther forward in the temporal lobe and more inferior, verbal memory can be impaired, with resulting problems of word recall. If severe enough, such a lesion can impair fluent speech and markedly restrict new learning.

Posterior to Wernicke's area, in the angular gyrus region of the occipital lobe, is an association area responsible for processing visual signals from written or printed words. Lesions in this area interrupt pathways that convey impulses from the visual cortex of both occipital lobes to the angular gyrus of the dominant hemisphere and result in the phenomenon of **alexia,** or the inability to understand written words.

The medial temporal lobe, including the hippocampus and the adjacent, anatomically related cortex of the entorhinal, perirhinal, and parahippocampal areas, has been identified as crucial for the function of memory and learning. It is involved in both immediate memory and in the establishment of long-term storage in the neocortex.[16]

The lateral portion of the anterior occipital lobe and posterior temporal lobe is an area responsible for naming objects. This area draws information about naming from the primary auditory cortex, and information about visual characteristics of the objects from the primary visual cortex. Naming is critical for language comprehension and intelligence.

The second most important area of association cortex is the prefrontal area. Neurons of the prefrontal cortex, while not responsible for motor movement, work in conjunction with the motor cortex to permit the performance of planned, complex motor sequences. The prefrontal cortex also receives input from the subcortical fibers that connect it with the parieto-occipitotemporal cortex, thus receiving processed sensory input. Output from the prefrontal cortex related to motor movement runs to the caudate and becomes part of the basal ganglia–thalamic feedback circuit which provides feedback impulses for the many sequential and parallel components in complex motor functions.

The prefrontal cortex is also critical for the behavioral display of emotions and intellectual functions. The lateral convexities of the prefrontal cortex receive input from the dorsomedial nucleus of the thalamus, which may relay some autonomic information and primitive affective components of consciousness, thus influencing the establishment and conditioning of emotional responses. The prefrontal cortex also receives input from the anterior temporal lobe via the uncinate fasciculus and the cingulum, as well as input from the parietal and occipitotemporal association cortex. Thus, the prefrontal cortex receives and consolidates information from throughout the brain. Although discrete areas of intellectual or emotional function are not localized, information about the role of the prefrontal lobe has been obtained by analyzing the effects of surgical injuries such as prefrontal lobotomy or leukotomy[17] and more recently from studies in patients with traumatic brain injury.[18] Lesions in the prefrontal cortex result in a reduced capacity for abstract thought, distractability, a lack of initiative, and poor reasoning and judgment. Patients have impaired mental concentration and capacity for sustained intellectual effort. Emotional behavior changes can result in a diminished ability to appreciate the feelings of others and a narrowed, focused attention on oneself. Patients may become careless with personal habits, may be unaffected by social norms, and may be unable to appreciate nonverbal cues. Reactions may be abrupt, transient, and superficial.[9]

In conclusion, localization of cortical function is defined by Stuss and Benson[13] as a "[series] of organized integrated fixed functional systems." Each system of the brain represents a broad functional skill such as language or movement. In addition to the functional skills, there exist more general systems such as sensory perception and motor function. Accordingly, the relationship of function to neuroanatomic location remains fairly constant or fixed in the population of normal adults. The system can be considered organized because it has component parts that operate separately but are intricately related to one another so that the whole operates in a smooth, consistent, successful fashion. A lesion in a particular area influences general function, but has specific characteristics related to the specific region of injury.

The notion of integration is important when one considers brain function. *Integration* means that all parts must be consistently connected in order for the whole to function properly. This contradicts the idea of isolated functional areas. Rather, areas in both hemispheres, the subcortical structures, and their connections must all be in place for successful function.

KEY CONCEPTS

- Many neurologic functions can be mapped to certain areas of the cerebral cortex. Areas with direct connection to sensory receptors or muscles are called primary areas. Secondary areas surround the primary areas and add complexity. Association areas are large areas of cortex involved in interpretation and integration.

- The best-characterized areas are the primary somatosensory cortex and the primary motor cortex. The body is somatotopically represented in both the sensory and motor cortex. Simulation of points in these areas results in discrete sensations or movements in the contralateral side of the body.

- Projections to the somatosensory cortex begin in receptors throughout the body. Receptors send axons to the spinal cord through the dorsal root. Sensations of touch and proprioception (posterior column) project up to the medulla on the ipsilateral side, then cross over and terminate in the thalamus. Sensations of pain (spinothalamic) usually cross the cord at the level of entry and travel up to the brain on the contralateral side. Sensory information is transmitted from the thalamus to the cortex by way of the internal capsule.

- The primary visual cortex is located in the occipital lobe. The primary auditory cortex is located in the temporal lobe.

- Projections from the motor cortex (corticospinal) travel by way of the internal capsule, cross over at the medulla, and travel down the contralateral spinal cord to synapse on alpha motor neurons in the anterior horn. Alpha motor neurons innervate skeletal muscle.

- Extrapyramidal tracts from subcortical nuclei innervate antigravity muscles and are primarily involved in balance, equilibrium, and coordination. Several pathways carry motor impulses to the cord from subcortical areas (e.g., the rubrospinal and reticulospinal tracts).

- An important area of association cortex is the language center (Wernicke's area), located at the junction of the parietal, occipital, and temporal lobes in the left hemisphere. Nearly all intellectual functions are language based, requiring an intact language center. Memory and learning are functions of the medial-temporal lobe and hippocampus. The prefrontal association cortex is involved in planning, reasoning, and judgment.

THE AGING PROCESS: CHANGES IN THE NERVOUS SYSTEM

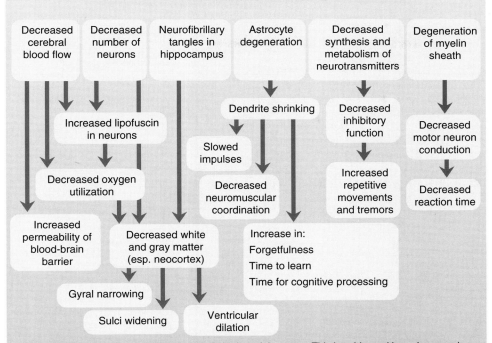

With aging, brain atrophy and a decrease in brain weight occur. This is evidenced by a decrease in white matter and gray matter up to 0.5% per year with gyral narrowing, sulci widening, and ventricular dilation. There is a gradual atrophy and loss of neurons in the brain and spinal cord over time. But neuron loss is not uniform within the brain. Most of the neuron loss is in the neocortex (20%), Purkinje cells of the cerebellum, substantia nigra, and locus coeruleus. Some parts of the brain, such as the vesticular nucleus, have no neuron loss. Blood supply to the brain is decreased owing to the decreased metabolic demands and brain atrophy. There is also increased permeability of the blood-brain barrier.

Intracellularly, there is an increase in lipofuscin, which hampers cellular oxygen use, crowds intracellular organelles, and decreases numbers of mitochondria. There are also neurofibrillary tangles in the hippocampus and neuritic plaques that are found only in the elderly.

Nerve fibers within the brain decrease and show signs of splitting or fragmentation. The cortex, subcortex, and cerebellar astrocytes degenerate. Nerve axons develop swellings near their ends called neuroaxonal dystrophy. The relevance of these swellings is unknown. Dendrites shrink, decreasing the number of messages received from other cells and synaptic linkages. This causes slowing of impulses and decreases neuromuscular coordination. These changes result in decreased short-term memory, reduced speed of learning, prolonged new information processing, increased reaction time, diminished abstract reasoning, and impaired perception.

Changes in the secretion and metabolism of neurotransmitters also impact the aging brain. There is a decrease in norepinephrine and dopamine secretion with an increase in monoamine oxidase (MAO). The reduction of dopamine leads to decreased inhibitory functions.

In the spinal cord, posterior root nerve fibers and sympathetic nerve fibers of the autonomic nervous system decline in number. Peripherally, there is degeneration of the motor nerve fibers and myelin sheath. Motor neuron axons remain intact. Decreasing motor neuron conduction velocity and prolonged muscle action potentials lead to decreased reaction times. Reflexes may be decreased or absent.

Faith Young Peterson

Summary

The human nervous system is a sophisticated communication network resulting in the efficient maintenance and monitoring of such homeostatic functions as cardiovascular function, temperature control, digestion, and hormonal balance. It is also involved in the control of sensory, motor, and higher cognitive functions that allow every one of us to carry out and appreciate our activities of daily living. Health care professionals play a key role in the care and education of patients and family members with nervous system dysfunctions. Knowledge of nervous system function and its role in daily living is essential in helping patients achieve maximum independent living and quality of life.

REFERENCES

1. Nolte J: *The Human Brain*. St. Louis, CV Mosby, 1988.
2. Hickey JV: *The Clinical Practice of Neurological and Neurosurgical Nursing*, 2nd ed. Philadelphia, JB Lippincott, 1986.
3. Vander A, Sherman A, Luciano DS: *Human Physiology: The Mechanism of Body Function*, 4th ed. New York, McGraw-Hill, 1985.
4. Mitchel PH, Hodges LC, Muwaswes M, Walleck CA: *AANN's Neuroscience Nursing*. Connecticut, Appleton & Lange, 1988.
5. American Association of Neuroscience Nurses: *Core Curriculum for Neuroscience Nurses*, 3rd ed. Chicago, American Association of Neuroscience Nurses, 1990.
6. Barr ML, Kiernam JA: *The Human Nervous System*. Philadelphia, JB Lippincott, 1988.
7. Menkes JH: *Textbook of Child Neurology*, 3rd ed. Philadelphia, Lea & Febiger, 1985.
8. Carpenter MB, Sutin J: *Human Neuroanatomy*. Baltimore, Williams & Wilkins, 1983.
9. Lezak MD: *Neuropsychological Assessment*, 2nd ed. New York, Oxford University Press, 1983.
10. Head H: *Aphasia and Kindred Disorders of Speech*. Oxford, Cambridge University Press, 1926.
11. Kertesz A: Issues in localization, in Kertesz A (ed): *Localization in Neuropsychology*. New York, Academic Press, 1983, pp 1–20.
12. Luria AR: *The Working Brain: An Introduction to Neuropsychology*. Haigh B, trans. New York, Basic Books, 1973.
13. Stuss DT, Benson DF: *The Frontal Lobes*. New York, Raven Press, 1986.
14. Geschwind N: Specializations of the human brain. *Sci Am* 1979;241:180–199.
15. Damasio H, Damasio AR: *Lesion Analysis in Neuropsychology*. New York, Oxford University Press, 1989.
16. Squire L, Zola-Morgan S: The medial temporal lobe memory system. *Science* 1991;253:1380–1386.
17. Guyton AC: *Basic Neuroscience: Anatomy and Physiology*, 2nd ed. Philadelphia, WB Saunders, 1991.
18. Rosenthal M, Griffith ER, Bond MR, Miller JD: *Rehabilitation of the Adult and Child With Traumatic Brain Injury*. Philadelphia, FA Davis, 1990.

BIBLIOGRAPHY

Adams RD, Victor M: *Principles of Neurology*, 3rd ed. New York, McGraw-Hill, 1985.

Bannister R: *Brain's Clinical Neurology*, 6th ed. Oxford, Oxford Medical Publications, 1986.

Blakesless TR: *The Right Brain*. Garden City, NJ, Doubleday, 1980.

Carpenter MB, Sutin J: The neuron, in *Human Neuroanatomy*, 8th ed. Baltimore, Williams & Wilkins, 1983, pp 85–133.

Daube JR, et al: *Medical Neuroscience*, 2nd ed. Boston, Little, Brown & Co, 1986.

DeArmond SJ, Fusco MM, Dewey MM: *A Photographic Atlas: Structure of the Human Brain*, 2nd ed. New York, Oxford University Press, 1976.

DeLisa JA: *Rehabilitation Medicine*. Philadelphia, JB Lippincott, 1988.

Dittman S: *Rehabilitation Nursing: Process and Application*. St. Louis, CV Mosby, 1989.

Haines DE: *Neuroanatomy: An Atlas of Structures, Sections and Systems*. Baltimore, Urban & Schwarzenberg, 1983.

Lemire RJ: *Normal and Abnormal Development of the Human Nervous System*. New York, Harper & Row, 1975.

Levin HS, Benton AL, Grossman RG: *Neurobehavioral Consequences of Closed Head Injury*. New York, Oxford University Press, 1982.

Lezak MD: *Neuropsychological Assessment*, 2nd ed. New York, Oxford University Press, 1983.

Volpe JJ: *Neurology of the Newborn*. Philadelphia, WB Saunders, 1987.

Wood RL: *Brain Injury Rehabilitation*. Rockville, Md, Aspen Publishers, 1987.

CHAPTER 43
Acute Disorders of Brain Function

MARY SANGUINETTI-BAIRD

KEY TERMS

arbovirus: Any of a large group of viruses transmitted by arthropods (mosquitoes, ticks), including the agents causing encephalitis, yellow fever, and dengue.

chromatolysis: The dissolution of chromophil (e.g., chromatin) material within a cell during cell destruction.

compliance: The ability of the brain to accommodate to changes in intracranial volume without a change in intracranial pressure.

elastance: In reference to brain tissue, the ability to be deformed yet resist deformity.

fibrinolysis: The normal breakdown of fibrin, usually by the enzymatic action of plasmin.

Glasgow Coma Scale: Scale developed by G. Teasdale and B. Jennett for the purpose of objectively assessing coma and impaired consciousness.

leptomeninges: Refers to the combined structures of the pia and arachnoid maters.

penumbra: An area in which something exists to a lesser or uncertain degree. In the case of stroke, a penumbra of viable tissue surrounds the necrotic core that can survive if optimal conditions exist and if it is not subject to further insults.

pyogenic: Producing or produced by fever.

sclerosed: In references to arteries, a thickened, hardened wall secondary to the formation and disposition of atheromatous plaques containing lipids and cholesterol, which narrow and roughen the surface of the vessel lumen.

The human nervous system is a group of interacting and interdependent elements that form a collective unit. Neuro Axis I structures (the cerebral hemispheres and the diencephalon) play an important role in this system, for they are responsible for receiving all sensory information from within the neuraxis and without, for maintaining homeostasis, and for directing human behavior based on this information. Patients experiencing dysfunction due to disease and trauma of Neuro Axis I structures can exhibit complex symptoms affecting the entire neuraxis, posing a challenge to health care professionals attempting to maximize these patients' function and quality of life. This chapter discusses some of the common disabilities of Neuro Axis I structures and their therapeutic management. Many Neuro Axis I disorders are associated with increased intracranial pressure, which is discussed first as a foundation for understanding neurologic assessment and specific Neuro Axis I disorders.

Increased Intracranial Pressure

Factors Affecting Intracranial Pressure

Intracranial pressure (ICP) is the pressure within the skull. Normal ICP is less than 15 mm Hg. Elevated ICP may occur in a variety of brain disorders, causing serious neurologic dysfunction.

The control of ICP has been the subject of abundant research and clinical focus. Attention to this particular complication of brain injury came about from its recognition as the most common cause of severe morbidity and mortality.[1] The intracranial compartment maintains a **pressure-volume equilibrium** among its components of blood, brain, and cerebrospinal fluid (CSF). As described by the modified Monroe-Kellie doctrine, under normal conditions, a volume increase in one component results in a reciprocal, compensatory decrease in volume in one or more of the other components, so that the total brain volume remains unchanged.[1] Maintaining normal pressure within the cranial vault is critical for the healthy functioning of brain tissue. The brain is both plastic (capable of being deformed) and elastic (capable of resisting deformity). As ICP rises above normal, the brain's **elastance** is compromised.

Each of the cranial components has a varying capability to compensate for an increase in compartment volume. The brain's elastic properties provide some protection to neural tissue. Cerebral blood vessels have the capability to reduce volume by vasoconstriction. The CSF compartment is capable of the most significant compensation, as it can shunt CSF down into the subarachnoid space around the spinal cord or into the venous system by way of the arachnoid villi. Unfortunately, there is only minimal and finite capability for compensation by any one of the intracranial components, and when that capability is exhausted, pressure within the cranium rises.

The impact of expanding volume on ICP varies among individuals, depending on the amount of increase that occurs, the effectiveness of compensatory mechanisms, and cerebral elastance. The relationship of volume and pressure is illustrated in Figure 43–1. Intracranial pressures of 0 to 15 mm Hg are thought to be normal in humans, and in the healthy individual, the transient increases in ICP that occur with straining, coughing, and the Trendelenburg position are well tolerated without symptoms. In the case of intracranial injury, volume increases are most often due to increases in blood volume or edema. ICP initially stays the same as compensation take place. When pressures are maintained by this method, elastance is said to be low and compliance is high. **Compliance** refers to the brain's ability to accommodate to changes

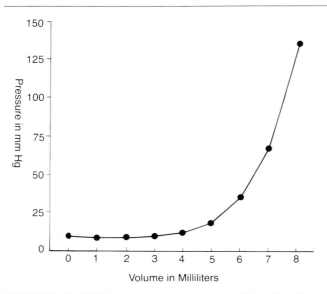

FIGURE 43–1. Volume-pressure index curve. (From Marshall SB, Marshall LF, Vos HR, Chestnut RM: *Neuroscience Critical Care: Pathophysiology and Patient Management.* Philadelphia, WB Saunders, 1990, p 149. Reproduced with permission.)

in intracranial volume without a change in ICP. Even though ICP remains unchanged, the intracranial system becomes less able to tolerate additional increases in volume without a corresponding change in pressure. This means that compliance is reduced, and correspondingly the brain's elastance increases. As elastance increases the brain tissue is less able to resist deformity. If the contents of the cranium expand faster than can be handled adequately by the mechanisms of compensation, these mechanisms become exhausted, and pressure within the cranium increases. As reflected in Figure 43–1, with the increasing loss of compliance, pressure within the cranium rises exponentially and is life-threatening. Increased ICP causes compression of blood vessels and brain tissue, which results in cellular ischemia and brain damage. If ICP continues to rise, brain tissue will move along the path of least resistance and herniate, typically by pushing the medial portion of the temporal lobe through the incisura tentorii, causing compression and ischemia of the brain stem and death. Assessment of intracranial compliance is therefore critical in the care of brain-injured patients.

Absolute values of ICP do not necessarily signify a life-threatening condition, as any one patient may be able to tolerate a given rise in intracranial volume, depending on his or her state of compliance. Compliance has long been recognized for its clinical significance and was first quantified as a **pressure-volume index** by Miller and Pickard in 1974.[2] They calculated the pressure-volume index by measuring brain compliance response to the brisk injection of 1 mL of fluid into the intraventricular space. Because this maneuver measures only a single moment in time and is potentially dangerous for the patient, current measures of compliance rely on the indirect method of monitoring ICP waveforms.

Pressure Waveforms

Pressure-volume index studies have demonstrated that increased ICP is a dynamic process. Although not a direct measure of compliance, ICP waveforms are a reflection and critical indicator of a patient's status. ICP patterns were first described in 1960 by Lundberg,[3] who identified these patterns as waves and correlated them with changes in cerebral blood volume, respiratory patterns, and changes in arterial blood pressure. Waveforms are typed as A, B, and C (Fig. 43–2). Currently ICP monitoring is used to evaluate pressure-volume relationships, compliance, pulse pressure, plateau waves, and cerebral perfusion pressure.

The **A** or **plateau wave** is believed to reflect severe pathologic increases in ICP due to changes in cerebral blood volume. A waves are steep, steplike increases in ICP to a plateau that lasts 15 to 20 minutes. ICP elevations during A waves can reach 40 to 50 mm Hg. After the plateau period the ICP slowly decreases but usually remains elevated above baseline. A waves reflect a potentially life-threatening situation, and if the pathologic process is not stopped, a cycle of increased ICP followed by vasodilation to maintain constant blood flow through swollen tissues continues, which in turn further increases ICP. A waves are associated with ischemia and brain damage and are frequently accompanied by neurologic symptoms, including changes in level of consciousness, alteration in respiratory patterns, headache, nausea, vomiting, pupillary changes, and motor paresis.

B waves are also pathologic but reflect less severe elevations in ICP and generally last for a much shorter time. B waves are sharp, rhythmic oscillations lasting 30 seconds to 2 minutes. ICP elevations of 20 to 50 mm Hg are common during B waves. B waves are associated with respirations and frequently occur just before A waves.

C waves reflect changes in arterial pressures and are thought to be less significant than A or B waves in terms of pathology.

Autoregulation of Cerebral Blood Flow

The brain in a nonpathologic state uses about 750 mL of oxygen per minute, or 15 percent of the resting cardiac output. Unlike other tissue in the body, cerebral tissue has very little capacity for anaerobic metabolism. The stores of oxygen and glycogen in the brain are very slight, enough for about 2 minutes. Therefore, brain metabolism depends on the continued delivery of oxygen and glucose by the blood. A sudden disruption in the supply of oxygen to the blood results in loss of consciousness within 5 minutes. Although the brain has minimal capacity for energy storage, it has a powerful mechanism known as **autoregulation,** which attempts to ensure the delivery of continual and adequate substrates necessary for metabolism.

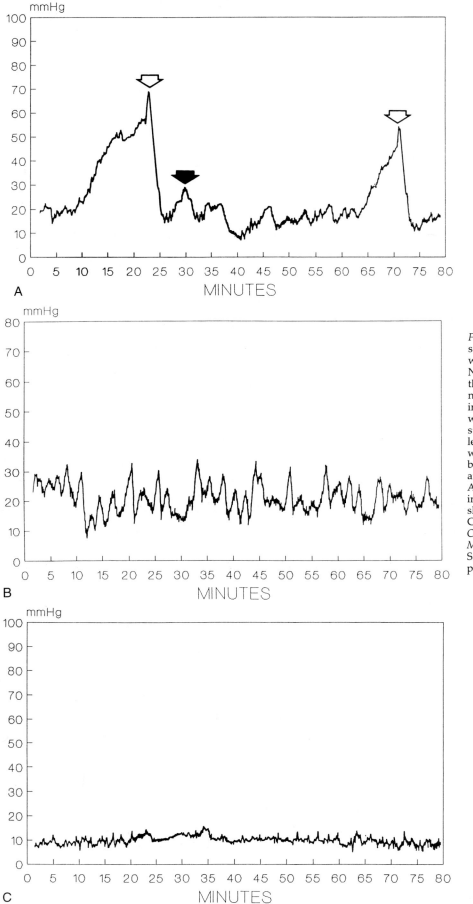

FIGURE 43–2. Intracranial pressure waves. **A,** Two classic A waves are shown (*open arrows*). Note that when the ICP falls after the A wave (*closed arrow*), it does not return to the baseline preceding the first wave. **B,** Multiple B waves are shown. The ICP rise is steep and rapid but to heights less than those observed with A waves and much briefer. **C,** Lundberg C waves. The ICP changes are much less impressive than in A or B waves and reflect changes in arterial pressure. (From Marshall SB, Marshall LF, Vos HR, Chestnut RM: *Neuroscience Critical Care: Pathophysiology and Patient Management.* Philadelphia, WB Saunders, 1990, pp 156–157. Reproduced with permission.)

Effects of Blood Pressure

Pressure autoregulation responds to changes in systemic blood pressure by dilation or constriction of cerebral blood vessels to ensure delivery of adequate substrates. Normally, blood flow to the brain remains constant despite wide fluctuation in mean arterial blood pressure (50–160 mm Hg). At either end of this range autoregulation is lost and cerebral blood flow is passively dependent on systemic blood pressure. If systemic blood pressure drops below 50 mm Hg, the normal response of cerebral blood vessels to vasodilate will not provide adequate cerebral blood flow, and ischemia occurs. If systemic blood pressure rises above 160 mm Hg, vasoconstrictive mechanisms cannot be controlled, and critical intracranial hypertension ensues. Loss of autoregulation can occur throughout the brain or may be limited to local areas of injury. The degrees of disruption reflects the severity of the injury.[4]

Effects of Arterial CO₂ and O₂

Autoregulation is influenced by the partial pressures of carbon dioxide ($Paco_2$) and oxygen (Pao_2) in the arterial blood. The response to a change in $Paco_2$ is very brisk: as $Paco_2$ falls, cerebral vessels constrict, and as $Paco_2$ levels rise, the cerebral vessels dilate. A rise in $Paco_2$ from 40 mm Hg to 80 mm Hg will increase cerebral blood flow by almost 100 percent.[1] The response to changes in Pao_2 is much less dramatic.

The changes in cerebral vessel diameter induced by changes in $Paco_2$ and Pao_2 are referred to as **chemical autoregulation.** Chemical autoregulation remains robust except in severely brain-injured patients and can be used to help manipulate cerebral blood flow and ICP when pressure autoregulation is lost. The clinical implications of chemical autoregulation have resulted in the use of mild hyperventilation as a standard protocol in the management of patients with increased ICP. Hyperventilation cannot be utilized without caution, however. Because a reduction in $Paco_2$ results in vasoconstriction and lowers cerebral blood flow, there is a potential for tissue ischemia if cerebral blood flow is reduced in an area that is already compromised by decreased flow.

Effects of Metabolism

A significant factor contributing to increased ICP and cerebral ischemia after traumatic brain injury is an increase in cerebral blood flow. Cerebral blood flow itself appears to be influenced by several mechanisms. Since the 1890 hypothesis of Roy and Sherrington,[5] it has been accepted that there is a coupling relationship between cerebral blood flow and metabolism according to which cerebral blood flow rapidly responds to the needs of cerebral metabolism. The exact coupling mechanism, however, remains unknown. Silver[6] in 1978 reported that local blood flow can be increased as soon as 1 second after neuronal excitation. This increase is limited to 250 μm from the site of the increased neural activity. Thus, flow can be adjusted rapidly at the microvascular level to accommodate metabolic demands. Obrist et al[7] found similar results using radioactive xenon injected into the carotid arteries of animals. They recorded as many as 256 different areas in the cortex that could respond independently and simultaneously, depending on the local metabolic demand. In pathologic conditions, namely cerebral hemorrhage and traumatic brain injury, this relationship between cerebral blood flow and metabolism becomes uncoupled;[8,9] in areas of damaged brain, cerebral metabolism or tissue demand for substrates can no longer influence the supply of blood. The potential risk under such circumstances is that cerebral blood flow will be insufficient to meet cerebral metabolic oxygen demand and ischemia will develop. On the other hand, if cerebral blood flow is increased in excess of metabolic demand, brain swelling and dangerous increases in ICP may occur, also resulting in ischemia.

Brain Swelling

In brain injury, brain swelling appears to be a common cause of increased brain bulk and therefore is an important factor contributing to increased ICP. Brain swelling can result from either an increase in blood flow or by an increase in water content in the tissues **(edema).** Brain swelling is identified on computed tomography (CT) as a decrease in ventricular size and compression or absence of the mesencephalic cisterns and cortical sulci.[1] Cerebral edema results from a breakdown in the blood-brain barrier. It becomes injurious only if it interferes with tissue perfusion or results in increased ICP. Edema is usually secondary to increased capillary pressure or damage to the capillary wall from a sudden increase in vascular pressure beyond autoregulatory limits. This results in extravasation of electrolytes, proteins, and blood, which in turn pulls water out of the vascular compartment and into the intercellular space. This condition is known as **vasogenic edema.** A second type of edema, **cytotoxic** or **cell injury edema,** occurs when ischemic tissue swells because of membrane pump failure. The extra fluid collection in this case is intracellular.

Cerebral edema, when severe, can start a feedback cycle that promotes further edema of increasing severity and contributes to increased ICP. As edema fluid collects, it compresses local vessels and cell tissues, preventing adequate blood and oxygen from reaching the cells. This results in ischemia, which in turn triggers vasodilation and increased capillary pressure, further fluid leakage into the injured tissue, and increased edema. Vasogenic edema tends to be a delayed process in terms of the secondary effects of brain injury, progressively worsening during the first several days after injury.

Clearance of brain edema occurs primarily by bulk flow into the CSF.[10,11] One advantage to using an intraventricular ICP monitor is the ability to facilitate the reduction of edema by lowering pressure in the ventricular space.

Current research on the scavengers of oxygen free radicals offers some possibilities for the treatment of brain swelling. The formation of free radicals of oxygen has been implicated as a causative factor in cerebral edema. Using animal models of traumatic brain injury researchers have found that the production of oxygen free radicals after injury correlates with damage to endothelial cells, disruption of the blood-brain barrier, structural changes in neurons and glial tissue, and the subsequent development of cerebral edema.[11,12] Research in animals has also successfully demonstrated that the introduction of free-radical scavengers prevents the development of both vasodilation and vasogenic edema.[13]

KEY CONCEPTS

- Pressure within the cranium is a product of the volume of brain tissue, blood, and cerebrospinal fluid (CSF). Increases in any one component are offset by reductions in the others to maintain intracranial pressure (ICP). Blood volume is reduced by vasoconstriction. CSF volume is reduced by shunting to the spinal cord.

- Normal ICP ranges from 0 to 15 mm Hg. Transient increases are well tolerated, but chronically increased ICP results in compression of vessels and brain tissue, leading to cellular ischemia and brain damage. High ICP may precipitate herniation of brain tissue through bony compartments leading to brain stem ischemia and death.

- Monitoring of ICP waveforms allows assessment of ICP changes. A waves are steep increases in ICP to a plateau that lasts 15 to 20 minutes, followed by a slow decline in pressure. A waves are associated with neurologic signs and indicate significant pathology.

- Autoregulation of cerebral blood flow achieves appropriate flow to meet metabolic needs despite changes in blood pressure and metabolism. The mechanisms are largely unknown. Autoregulation is effective over a range of mean arterial pressure from 50 to 160 mm Hg. Hypoxia and high $PaCO_2$ result in vascular dilation. Hyperventilation to reduce $PaCO_2$ results in cerebral vasoconstriction.

- Brain swelling is a common cause of increased ICP. Edema may result from changes in vascular competency that lead to transudation of fluid into intercellular spaces, or from cellular swelling to deficient cell membrane integrity. Cellular swelling secondary is usually due to dysfunctional membrane pumps because of cellular ischemia.

Neurologic Evaluation

When a patient with a neurologic emergency arrives in the emergency room, the airway and **ventilation** are the first areas of assessment and intervention.

Hypoxia should be suspected in any patient who presents with unconsciousness, anxiety, or apprehension, or who is combative or uncooperative. Even if the individual appears to be breathing normally, studies indicate that patients are often hypoxic, with PaO_2 values of 65 mm Hg or less.[17] All patients who are in coma should be intubated and hyperventilated. Arterial blood gas values are optimal at a PaO_2 of 80 mm Hg or greater and a $PaCO_2$ of 27 to 30 mm Hg. **Hemodynamic stabilization** with fluid resuscitation and maintenance of blood pressure is critical for adequate supply of substrates and prevention of ischemia.

Glasgow Coma Scale

Once the vital signs have stabilized, critical assessment of the patient's neurologic status is necessary. This is done using the **Glasgow Coma Scale** (Table 43–1). The Glasgow Coma Scale is a standardized tool developed for the purpose of assessing the level of consciousness in acutely brain-injured patients. It can also be used to evaluate patients with an altered level of consciousness as a result of other neurological insults such as hemorrhage or craniotomy. Numerical scores are given to arousal-directed responses of eye opening, verbal utterances, and motor reactions. The best response is scored, bilateral responses are recorded for motor reactions, and consistent application of a painful stimulus is required for accuracy.[18] When used correctly, the Glasgow Coma Scale avoids ambiguous terms and has a high degree of inter-rater reliability.

TABLE 43–1. Glasgow Coma Scale

The Glasgow Coma Scale is a practical means of monitoring changes in level of consciousness based upon eye opening and verbal and motor responses. The responsiveness of the patient can be expressed by summation of the figures. The lowest score is 3, the highest is 15.

Eyes Open	Spontaneously (eyes open, does not imply awareness)	4
	To speech (any speech, not necessarily a command)	3
	To pain (should not use supraorbital pressure for pain stimulus)	2
	Never	1
Best Verbal Response	Oriented (to time, person, place)	5
	Confused speech (disoriented)	4
	Inappropriate (swearing, yelling)	3
	Incomprehensible sounds (moaning, groaning)	2
	None	1
Best Motor Response	Obeys commands	6
	Localizes pain (deliberate or purposeful movement)	5
	Withdrawal (moves away from stimulus)	4
	Abnormal flexion (decortication)	3
	Extension (decerebration)	2
	None (flaccidity)	1
	Total Score	_____

From Marshall SB, Marshall LF, Vos HR, Chestnut RM: *Neuroscience Critical Care: Pathophysiology and Patient Management.* Philadelphia, WB Saunders, 1990, p 98. Reproduced with permission.

Eye Opening

The **eye opening response** is simple and assesses whether or not the eyes open spontaneously. If not, do they open in response to verbal stimuli? This implies any verbal stimuli, not necessarily a command to the patient to open the eyes. Finally, do they open in response to painful stimuli? If not, the eye response is scored as absent. In patients with acute mass lesions, eye opening is usually depressed in conjunction with impaired response to pain and motor function. Spontaneous eye opening in the acute phase is an encouraging sign, as it implies that the arousal mechanism in the brain stem is intact.

Verbal Response

The **verbal response** on the Glasgow Coma Scale makes a distinction between arousal and orientation. A full score in this category indicates that the patient is alert and fully oriented: the patient knows his or her name, current location, and the time of day. In the next level down the patient is awake and can pay attention to a certain degree, but is confused as to who he or she is and does not know the time or the location. If attention is poor and the verbal responses consist of yelling and swearing (inappropriate response), the score is lower. Incomprehensible verbalizations are unintelligible sounds or mumbling. The final level in this category includes no sounds at all.

Motor Response

Motor response has been identified as the most powerful predictor of outcome.[1] Motor response indicates the best or highest level of response the patient is able to perform. Each extremity is evaluated and recorded independently. At the highest level, the patient can obey a command such as "show me two fingers" or "put your foot in my hand." At the next level down the patient is unable to obey commands, but when a painful stimulus is applied the patient can reach in a purposeful manner toward the stimulus; the patient is able to "localize pain." As status deteriorates, the patient cannot localize but will make an attempt to withdraw his or her limb from the painful stimulus. This is not a purposeful response to the stimulus. Further deterioration results in abnormal motor movements. The highest level of abnormal movement is called decorticate or abnormal flexor response. A bilateral response includes a posture of the arms and wrists in flexion and the legs and feet extended and internally rotated. The level below decorticate posturing is called decerebrate or abnormal extension; a bilateral response includes arms extended with external rotation of the wrists. The legs and feet are extended and internally rotated. The final level in motor response is no response to painful stimuli, that is, flaccidity in all four limbs. It is important to emphasize that all limbs must be tested separately, as motor responses may be preserved on one side only and levels of involvement may vary from side to side (Fig. 43–3).

Level of consciousness is a continuum reflected by the ranges in Glasgow Coma Scale scores from mild (scores 9–14), to moderate (scores 6–8), to severe (3–5), and is only a single measure of the patient's status. Vital signs and Glasgow Coma Scale scores are not enough to determine the status of the patient with an acute insult to the brain. Integrity of brain stem function is also vital and is assessed from pupillary findings and eye movements.

Pupillary Assessment

Pupillary assessment provides important information about the function of the brain stem and cranial nerves II and III. The normal pupillary response to light results from an intact afferent cranial nerve II stimulating the intact efferent cranial III. The response of the pupil to light, both in terms of its shape and reactivity, is a function of cranial nerve III. Cranial nerve III has both parasympathetic and sympathetic innervation. The sympathetic branch contracts the pupilodilator muscle and causes the pupil to enlarge. The parasympathetic branch, on the other hand, contracts the pupiloconstrictor muscle and causes pupil constriction. Normally, both branches work in concert. The second cranial nerve's afferent response to light transmits the light impulse from the retina to the superior colliculus of the midbrain. The oculomotor nucleus of cranial nerve III in the midbrain then transmits impulses to the pupillary muscles.

The pupillary response to light is recorded by noting pupil size in millimeters, shape, and reactivity. Careful monitoring of the pupillary response to light during the acute phase is critical, as a failing response may be the first indication of impending brain herniation. Mild dilation of a pupil with sluggish or absent light response is ominous. This phenomenon results from stretching of the oculomotor nerve by the uncus during herniation and impairment of the parasympathetic efferent signal for pupillary constriction and dominance of the sympathetic response of dilation. An **oval pupil** may be the first indicator of dangerously poor compliance and transtentorial herniation.[19] According to Marshall et al[19] the oval pupil represents a transitional pupil that will return to normal responsivity if ICP is controlled. If ICP is not controlled and uncal or central herniation progresses, the result is full mydriasis, ptosis, and paresis of the medial rectus and other ocular muscles innervated by the oculomotor nerve. At this stage, the same response in the contralateral pupil and ocular muscles will occur.

Other pupillary responses indicate damage to the optic nerve. The **afferent pupillary defect** is a paradoxical response detected with the swinging light test. As the examiner swings a light from the normal eye to the abnormal eye, the abnormal pupil responds by dilating instead of constricting. This occurs because the light signals transmitted to the Edinger-Westphal nucleus in the midbrain through the injured optic nerve are insufficient to maintain constriction brought on by stimulation of the normal eye. Bilaterally small

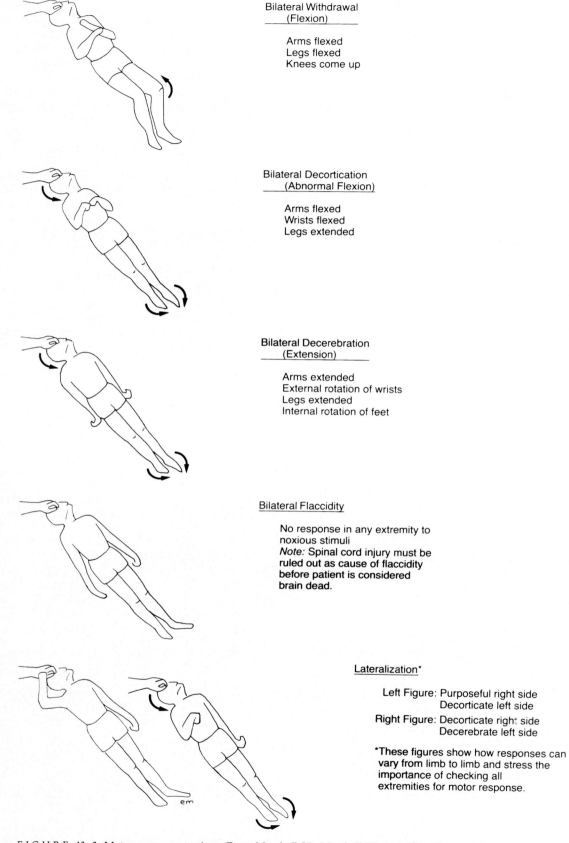

Bilateral Withdrawal
__(Flexion)__

Arms flexed
Legs flexed
Knees come up

Bilateral Decortication
__(Abnormal Flexion)__

Arms flexed
Wrists flexed
Legs extended

Bilateral Decerebration
__(Extension)__

Arms extended
External rotation of wrists
Legs extended
Internal rotation of feet

Bilateral Flaccidity

No response in any extremity to
noxious stimuli
Note: Spinal cord injury must be
**ruled out as cause of flaccidity
before patient is considered
brain dead.**

Lateralization*

Left Figure: Purposeful right side
Decorticate left side
Right Figure: Decorticate right side
Decerebrate left side

*These figures show how responses can
vary from limb to limb and stress the
importance of checking all
extremities for motor response.

FIGURE 43–3. Motor response testing. (From Marshall SB, Marshall LF, Vos HR, Chestnut RM: *Neuroscience Critical Care: Pathophysiology and Patient Management.* Philadelphia, WB Saunders, 1990, p 102. Reproduced with permission.)

pupils suggests a destructive lesion in the pons or the presence of certain drugs. **Horner's syndrome** results from disruption of the sympathetic pathway between the hypothalamus and the upper thoracic cord and the apex of the lung to the eye. It includes a small pupil and ipsilateral ptosis and, depending on the site of the disruption, may include loss of sweating on the ipsilateral face. **Bilaterally fixed and dilated pupils** suggest inadequate cerebral perfusion. This could be related to hypotension or increased ICP. If perfusion is not interrupted too long, a normal pupillary response returns with adequate flow.

Eye Movements and Position

Eye movements are important indicators of brain stem function. The interactions between cranial nerves III, IV, and VI are responsible for normal eye movements. Abnormalities of eye movement are useful in localizing the site of brain dysfunction.

Examination begins with assessment of the eyelids, which in the comatose patient are closed as a result of tonic contraction of the orbicularis oculi muscles. If the lids are manually opened, then released they will gradually close.

Abnormal eye movements seen in the brain-injured patient include nystagmus, dysconjugate eye movements, and ocular palsies. **Nystagmus** is a persistent rhythmical or jerky movement in one or both eyes and is not useful in localization. **Dysconjugate movements** almost always represent a structural lesion in the brain stem. **Ocular palsies** also are not localizing but often are a consequence of increased ICP and nerve compression by herniation.

A gross test of brain stem function in the unconscious patient is the **oculocephalic** or "doll's eye" **response** (Fig. 43–4). This test is performed only in patients in whom a lateral spine radiograph has been obtained to rule out spinal injury. The test is performed by holding open the patient's eyelids and suddenly rotating the head from one side to the other. If the brain stem is intact, the eyes will deviate to the side opposite the direction in which the head was turned. If the eyes do not move in conjugate fashion or are asymmetric, the response is abnormal and brain stem function is impaired. If the eyes do not move at all, the response is said to be absent.

The **oculovestibular response** is a similar test of brain stem function that requires the instillation of 20 mL of ice water against the intact tympanic membrane

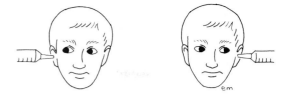

FIGURE 43–5. Oculovestibular response. (From Marshall SB, Marshall LF, Vos HR, Chestnut RM: *Neuroscience Critical Care: Pathophysiology and Patient Management.* Philadelphia, WB Saunders, 1990, p 108. Reproduced with permission.)

of an unconscious patient (Fig. 43–5). If the brain stem is intact, the normal response will be a tonic deviation of both eyes toward the side that is irrigated. It is abnormal if there is dysconjugate or asymmetric eye movement. If there is no eye movement, the response is absent. Testing of the oculovestibular response is one of the essential examinations performed in patients who are suspected of being brain dead.[1] Patients with depression of brain function due to metabolic abnormalities usually retain an intact oculovestibular response. A note of caution must accompany the interpretation of this response, as it is recognized that certain drugs, such as barbiturates and high doses of Dilantin, can severely depress the response.

Eye position in the alert and oriented patient should be directed straight ahead without involuntary movement. In the unconscious patient with bilateral diffuse hemispheric injuries without direct destruction or compression of the brain stem, the eyes should be directed forward without involuntary movements except for occasional slow, roving eye movements. The oculocephalic and oculovestibular responses are intact. In patients with midbrain lesions the eyes are immobile and directed straight ahead. Conjugate deviation of the eyes results from either an ipsilateral hemispheric lesion or a lesion in the contralateral pons.

Loss of Consciousness

Loss of consciousness from a brain injury is a result of damage to the **brain stem reticular formation**, its inputs from the sensory systems, and its projections to the thalamus, hypothalamus, limbic system, and neocortex. Such damage usually results from diffuse lesions involving large areas of both hemispheres, a localized hemispheric lesion large enough to cause mass effect and encroachment on diencephalic struc-

FIGURE 43–4. Oculocephalic response. (From Marshall SB, Marshall LF, Vos HR, Chestnut RM: *Neuroscience Critical Care: Pathophysiology and Patient Management.* Philadelphia, WB Saunders, 1990, p 108. Reproduced with permission.)

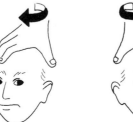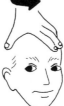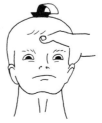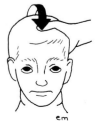

tures, or a direct injury to the reticular activating system in the brain stem.[20,21] Lesions that result in mass effect and acute dynamic changes in ICP are poorly tolerated and, depending on cerebral compliance, place the patient at risk for cerebral ischemia and potential herniation. Lesions localized to one compartment can produce areas with different levels of compliance. Under such circumstances, the areas of lower compliance will push and distort areas with greater compliance and produce hernias. If hernias block the incisura or the foramen magnum, intolerable pressures result within the cranium, and brain tissue is pushed through these openings, resulting in ischemia to the brain stem and death.

Herniation

Cingulate Herniation

Cingulate herniation will occur when a lesion in one hemisphere is large enough to cause a lateral shift across the midline of the intracranial cavity, forcing the cingulate gyrus under the falx cerebri. This results in distortion and compression of the internal cerebral vein. Cingulate herniation can be asymptomatic. The greatest danger results from compression of blood vessels, particularly the ipsilateral anterior cerebral artery, which can cause cerebral ischemia and edema and contribute to the ICP problem (Fig. 43–6).

Central Herniation

Central (transtentorial) herniation results from expanding lesions in the frontal, parietal, and occipital lobes that force a downward displacement of the hemispheres and basal nuclei and compression of the diencephalon and adjoining midbrain through the incisura. This can also occur with extracranial lesions at the vertex or frontal-occipital poles. Central herniation should be thought of as an end result that compresses and eventually buckles the diencephalon and the adjoining midbrain structures through the tentorial notch. The initial signs are changes in level of con-

sciousness, then changes in eye movements with a loss of upward gaze, and bilateral decorticate and decerebrate posturing.

Transtentorial herniation can occur rapidly or more slowly, depending on the type of lesion. The speed with which the process is recognized plays a critical role in patient survival. A slowly dilating pupil or one that is oval is an ominous sign of impending herniation, and emergency interventions are necessary if the process is to be stopped. The goal in treating increased intracranial hypertension is to prevent compression of the third cranial nerve and midbrain, as once compression occurs, mortality is significantly increased.[1] Hernias in the supratentorial compartments are dangerous and not tolerated because they initiate vascular and obstructive processes, which then contribute to the existing problem of ischemia and hypertension.

Uncal Herniation

Uncal herniation typically occurs with expanding lesions in the temporal lobe. As the lobe shifts, the basal edge of the uncus and the hippocampal gyrus bulge over the edge of the incisura. In the process the third cranial nerve and the posterior cerebral artery are crushed by the overhanging swollen uncus. Thus the pupil on the same side of the lesion becomes fixed and dilated. Flattening of the midbrain interferes with the ascending reticular activating system and depresses the level of consciousness. The ipsilateral cerebral peduncle is also compressed, resulting in contralateral motor dysfunction. Compression of the contralateral cerebral peduncle is also common, leading to the confusing symptom of ipsilateral motor dysfunction.

Tonsillar Herniation

Tonsillar herniation is less common than the other herniation syndromes and involves the shift of the cerebellar tonsils through the foramen magnum and compression of the medulla and upper cervical cord (Fig. 43–7). This typically occurs in patients with cerebellar hemorrhage. Because of the proximity of the

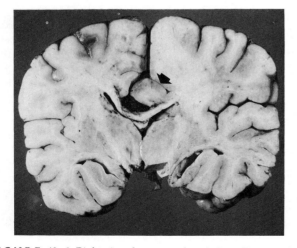

F I G U R E 43–6. Right cingulate gyrus herniation. (From Becker DP, Gudeman SK: *Textbook of Head Injury.* Philadelphia, WB Saunders, 1989, p 529. Reproduced with permission.)

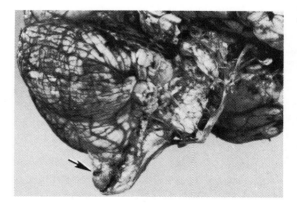

F I G U R E 43–7. Tonsillar herniation. (From Becker DP, Gudeman SK: *Textbook of Head Injury.* Philadelphia, WB Saunders, 1989, p 529. Reproduced with permission.)

cerebellum to the brain stem, tonsillar herniation evolves very rapidly and can result in death in a matter of minutes. Signs usually include precipitous changes in blood pressure and heart rate, small pupils, distrubances in conjugate gaze, ataxic breathing, and quadriparesis.

KEY CONCEPTS

- The Glasgow Coma Scale is used to assess level of consciousness by scoring alertness (eye opening response), orientation (verbal response), and motor control (movements). The highest score is given to demonstration of spontaneous eye opening, full orientation, and obeying motor commands.
- Pupillary responses indicate the function of the brain stem and cranial nerves II and III. Changes in size, shape, and reactivity of the pupil may be an early indicator of impending brain herniation.
- Eye movements controlled by cranial nerves III, IV, and VI may be impaired with increased ICP. Nystagmus, dysconjugate gaze, and ocular palsies may be evident. A positive "doll's eyes" response when the subject's head is turned or an abnormal response to activation of the oculovestibular reflex by instilling cold water into the ear are very poor prognostic signs.
- Pressure changes in the cranium can result in shifting of brain tissue through rigid structures in the cranial vault. This is generally termed herniation and carries a poor prognosis. Cingulate, transtentorial, uncal, and tonsillar herniations may occur. With herniation, changes in level of consciousness generally occur first, followed by eye and pupillary dysfunction, then decorticate and decerebrate posturing.

Head Injury

Etiology

Attempts at determining the exact occurrence rate of head injury are complicated by the historical absence of systematic data collection. Definitions vary across institutions regarding the type and severity of the injury. Added to this is the difficulty in gathering data on the number of head-injured people who do not seek medical treatment. Just as collecting figures on the true incidence of this public health problem is fraught with problems, so too is establishing public concern and financial support for the health care needs of the victims. Yet head injury is one of the most critical problems facing the health care system today. A number of localized studies[22–24] have extrapolated the annual incidence of head injury as over 7 million in the United States each year, with 500,000 of these individuals requiring hospitalization. Head injury is involved in over two thirds of all auto accidents and is the cause of death in about 70 percent of the fatal cases. Trauma is the third leading cause of death, primarily for those under the age of 38. Of those requiring hospital care, about 20 percent are either moderately or severely impaired. In 1980 the estimated economic cost of caring for the head injured was about $4 billion per year.[25] This figure has continued to rise, as has the incidence rate.

Most head injuries are acquired in motor vehicle accidents, frequently associated with alcohol. Other common causes are falls and sports accidents. The prevalence is highest in those under the age of 38, notably between the years of 16 and 25, with males involved three times as frequently as females. Most often the victim is single, either unemployed or at the lower end of the economic scale, and not highly educated.[26] Interestingly, the second most frequently involved age group is the population over the age of 75, who tend to acquire head injuries during falls. Developing and providing care that is appropriate for such diverse patient types poses a challenge for the health care worker. Efforts must focus on identifying the special care needs of each patient group within the acute setting, the appropriateness and timing of rehabilitation, and targeting preventive education relative to the risks involved for each group.

Classification

A classification of head injury provides the opportunity to compare outcomes among group types and levels of severity, as well as the opportunity to provide data on which to base prognosis and intervention, both in the acute and rehabilitation stages. Although the absence of a systematic approach has made epidemiologic studies difficult, current efforts strive for standardization and consistency.

Efforts to clearly define the pathology and stages of head injury have been largely facilitated by the development and widespread use of the Glasgow Coma Scale (see Table 43–1). This standardized tool has greatly increased prognostic skill and assisted medical practitioners in the appropriateness and timeliness of their interventions. The Traumatic Coma Data Bank (TCDB) collects data on head injury based on Glasgow Coma Scale classification. The TCDB identifies all patients with a score of 8 or less after nonsurgical resuscitation and those whose condition deteriorates to that level within the first 48 hours after admission as having a *severe head injury*. *Moderate head injury* is defined as Glasgow Coma Scale scores of 9 to 12, and *mild head injury* as scores above 12. These scores naturally apply only to those who reach the hospital alive. U.S. and Australian studies note that in urban areas almost two thirds of head injury deaths occur before the victims reach the hospital. In rural areas this figure may be as high as 90 percent.[1] The TCDB has recently adopted a classification system that describes the patient's intracranial pathology in terms of CT findings (Table 43–2). Although it doesn't solve all the problems encountered in head injury classification, this system can provide greater consistency in description across institutions, thereby enhancing the validity of the data collection.

TABLE 43–2. TCDB Diagnostic Categories of Abnormalities Visualized on CT Scanning

Diffuse injury I	No visible intracranial pathology seen on CT
Diffuse injury II	Cisterns are present with shift 0–5 mm and/or lesion densities present
	No high or mixed density lesion > 25 cc
	May include bone fragments and foreign bodies
Diffuse injury III (with swelling)	Cisterns compressed or absent
	Shift 0–5 mm
	No high or mixed density lesion > 25 cc
Diffuse injury IV (with shift)	Shift > 5 mm
	No high or mixed density lesion > 25 cc
Evacuated mass lesion	Any lesion surgically evacuated
Nonevacuated mass lesion	High or mixed density lesion > 25 cc, not surgically evacuated

From Marshall SB, Marshall LF, Vos HR, Chestnut RM: *Neuroscience Critical Care: Pathophysiology and Patient Management.* Philadelphia, WB Saunders, 1990, p 172. Reproduced with permission.

Pathogenesis

The pathogenesis of traumatic head injury is complex. The first step in examining this process is to distinguish between direct or primary injury and indirect or secondary injury. Damage to neural tissue and structures that occurs from the direct impact of trauma is referred to as **primary injury.** Any further insult to the already compromised cerebral tissue as a result of the body's response to the injury (e.g., hypoxia, ischemia, hypercapnia, hypotension) is referred to as **secondary injury.**

Secondary injury has been identified as a significant cause of morbidity and mortality in the head-injured patient.[1,27,28] The importance of secondary injury cannot be overemphasized because unlike the primary injury, which can only be targeted through preventive education, secondary injury often occurs while the patient is in the care of health professionals. Thus, it is addressed through attempts of early diagnosis of mass lesions and rapid medical and surgical interventions as a means of minimizing the ultimate impairment of the patient.

When considering the pathogenesis of primary and secondary head injury it is important to recognize that any type of injury to the brain is influenced by its preexisting condition. Factors such as individual variations in size and shape of the skull, the thickness of the scalp, and ability of the dura to pull free from the skull can affect the potential for skull fracture, epidural hematoma, or infection. The location and size of an intracranial lesion, the configuration of the tentorium cerebelli, and the size of the tentorial notch will determine the risk of life-threatening herniation. Any preexisting cerebral injury such as stroke, head injury, or dementia will have a cumulative effect on the outcome of the acute injury.

Primary Injury

Primary injury is the result of the initial impact on neural tissue. It is commonly described as focal, polar, or diffuse. Although such injuries rarely occur in pure form, for simplification they are discussed separately.

Focal injuries are those that are localized to the site of impact of the skull. The extent of the damage is quite variable. Injuries may include contusion and laceration. They may be superficial or extend deep into the brain matter. Local injury to the brain can result in specific neurologic symptoms, depending on the site. An injury over the motor cortex may result in contralateral weakness of the face and arm, whereas an injury to the frontal lobe can lead to apraxia, abulia, impulsive behavior, and poor judgment. On the other hand, localized hemorrhages (epidural, subdural, or intracerebral) or significant edema may act as space-occupying lesions and result in pathologic intracerebral hypertension, brain shift, and herniation. In such cases symptoms may include a decrease in the level of consciousness, ipsilateral oculomotor or abducens nerve palsies, and contralateral weakness.[1,27]

Polar head injuries occur as a consequence of the brain shifting within the skull and meninges during the course of an acceleration-deceleration movement. This is commonly the case in motor vehicle accidents in which the head, traveling at the same high speed as the motor vehicle, is abruptly stopped by an obstacle such as the windshield. As a result, the frontal and temporal poles are crushed against the anterior and middle cranial fossae, damaging the tips and inferior surface of the temporal and frontal lobes. Damage may be contusional or hemorrhagic and, combined with edema, may result in significant intracerebral mass lesions. Most forces to the head have a lateral rotational component; thus, one side of the brain typically is more severely injured than the other. Edema and the resulting mass effect may not be symptomatically evident for 2 to 3 days and often are the reason for delayed deterioration in brain-injured patients.[1,27] Patients with polar injuries may or may not need significant acute care, depending on the severity of the injury. Polar injuries can, however, play a significant role in the extent of subsequent cognitive impairment, affecting rehabilitation and long-term recovery.

Diffuse head injury is also a function of movement of the brain within the cranial cavity. As noted for polar injuries, in addition to the acceleration-deceleration force, the brain is often subject to a rotational effect during injury. The combined force causes stretching and shearing of the axonal white matter known as **diffuse axonal injury.** The injury is typically widespread and has a devastating impact on function. Patients with diffuse axonal injury frequently are comatose from the time of injury, with symptomatic abnormal posturing of the extremities. Coma is a consequence of axonal damage in the reticular activating center in the brain stem and can be prolonged. Recovery is frequently limited to a severely disabled or vegetative state.[29]

At the cellular level, primary injury results in swelling of the cell body, dissolution of the Nissl bodies, and movement of the nucleus to the periphery of the cell. This is called **chromatolysis** (dissolution of chromatin). Nissl body degeneration begins at the center and progresses peripherally. Histochemical changes within the degenerating neurons result in a reduction in glucose metabolism, a breakdown in Golgi bodies, and a tremendous increase in cell volume as water rushes into the cell. If the cells are to survive the initial injury, an optimum environment for metabolism and protein synthesis is critical. Further insult by secondary injury obstructs the fragile process and dramatically affects morbidity and mortality.

Secondary Injury

Secondary injury is an insult to the nervous tissue that occurs as a consequence of the original injury and has a compounded effect on the already damaged cellular structure. Recent research examining the effects of trauma from the cellular perspective has led to a greater understanding of the process that leads to cellular disruption and frequently destruction. Perhaps the most interesting discovery is that the product of traumatic injury is due to a metabolic chain of events triggered by the initial event. From a health care perspective this discovery is very exciting, as the implication is that the outcome may not be inevitable. There may be opportunities to intervene at different points in the chain of events to block the cascade and limit the extent of injury.

It seems clear from research that the initial response to a catastrophic event such as a traumatic injury or a stroke is a massive release of the excitatory neurotransmitter, glutamate.[30,31] Normally this agent is stored within the cell. Its release and re-uptake are carefully balanced, and high-energy phosphates are needed to pump it across cell membranes. After trauma, glutamate spills uncontrollably from the cells, quickly overpowering the uptake receptors. **Glutamate overstimulation** prompts the next step in the cascade, which is a rush of ions, notably calcium, via NMDA receptor-mediated channels into the cell and an outpouring of potassium from the cell. This ion shift results in **electrolyte imbalance** and **cellular edema.** Normally the cell has sufficient high-energy sources available to maintain ionic balance. However, the tremendous influx of calcium into the cell apparently overburdens the normal mechanisms. In response to the increased energy demand for pumping ions across the cell membrane, the glycolytic energy pathway is triggered. Indeed, immediately after injury there is a period of hyperglycolysis. However, dependence on this anaerobic pathway leads to a buildup of lactic acid inside the cell, a lowering of cellular pH, and acidosis. The buildup of lactic acid in the neuronal cells appears to be the key element in destruction. As long as the calcium influx into the cell is uncontrolled, it further depletes any available adenosine triphosphate (ATP) necessary for pumping it out of the cell and restoring ionic balance. Further

demand on the glycolytic energy pathway results in the buildup of lactic acidosis. In this setting, cells die.

Another key element in this metabolic cascade is the **breakdown of the cell membrane.** In trauma and stroke, this occurs within seconds. A breakdown product of the cell lipoprotein membrane is arachidonic acid. The metabolism of arachidonic acid results in the production of oxygen free radicals. Oxygen free radicals are a form of oxygen with unpaired electrons, making them highly reactive. Free radical atoms or molecules actively combine with other molecules and in so doing can alter cellular structure or function. In the normal, healthy brain, the production and destruction of oxygen free radicals is adequately controlled by enzyme mechanisms. In the setting of traumatic injury, the change in cellular metabolism and the buildup of lactic acidosis increases the production of oxygen free radicals. In large numbers these radical atoms easily overwhelm the enzyme system and are very destructive to nervous tissue. Oxygen free radicals are attracted to the proteins and lipids in the cell membranes, and will attack and break apart the membranes. If there is inadequate means of deactivating the oxygen free radicals, this process of breaking apart the cell membrane and the subsequent lipid peroxidation becomes self-propagating. Nearby membranes, not damaged by the original injury, when exposed to circulating free radicals are damaged, and more oxygen free radicals are produced.[32] Free radical production has been implicated in the mediation of the cerebral arteriolar abnormalities seen in brain injury, which can result in increased ICP, brain ischemia, and death.[12,33]

This destructive metabolic cascade that occurs as a consequence of brain injury and stroke seems to offer many points for intervention. If mechanisms can be found to interrupt the cascade of events, perhaps the ultimate consequence of the brain injury may be reduced. One example is the encouraging investigational trials using synthetic steroids called **lazaroids.** Lazaroids are oxygen free radical scavengers that bind the molecules and thus protect the cell membrane from the destructive by-products of cell injury.[32] Current research is also focused on the use of calcium antagonists and mechanisms to block glutamate neurotoxicity. Because the uncontrolled influx of calcium into the cells is an early step in the cascade, interruption of this process may significantly reduce the extent of cellular destruction.[30]

The process of cellular injury described above has examined cerebral disruption at a basic cellular level. Derangements are also evident in the mechanisms that control cerebral blood flow, cerebral metabolism, and the maintenance of intracerebral pressure, as discussed in the previous section on intracranial pressure. In addition, changes in cerebral blood flow can be influenced by autonomic responses.

Sympathetic Response

Head injury results in complex cerebral blood flow derangements that can result in either ischemia or hyperemia.[4,14] Complicating factors such as hypoxia and hypotension occurring at the time of the injury play a role in the complexity of these derangements, as does the type of structural damage incurred. Studies using xenon CT and looking at blood flow patterns during the first 24 hours after head injury indicate that flow patterns change as a function of time and are related to the severity of injury and the type of lesion.[15] In patients without surgical mass lesions, low blood flow is common in the first few hours after injury and is then followed by a hyperemic phase. The pattern of low blood flow followed by high blood flow is most consistently seen in patients with low Glasgow Coma Scale scores. Surgical mass lesions tend to be associated with high-flow states.

The phases of changing blood flow patterns are also influenced by what has been termed a **catecholamine surge** or "storm"[15,16] occurring at the time of or immediately after injury. Although the role of this catecholamine surge remains unclear, theories based on animal research and humans with spinal cord injury implicate this phenomenon as a critical factor in injury due to brain swelling. Extreme catecholamine levels are recognized as a stress response and are related to the severity of injury. In animals, the systemic response to traumatic brain injury is immediate hypertension, bradycardia, and apnea. With increased severity of injury, tachycardia is a much more predominant finding. Interestingly, the rise in systemic blood pressure is followed shortly by a fall in blood pressure to relative hypotension. The initial surge in systemic arterial blood pressure correlates with the catecholamine surge and is thus directly related to the severity of the injury. In animal models, norepinephrine has been noted to increase as much as 100-fold above normal baseline values and epinephrine has increased 400- to 500-fold within seconds of the injury.[16] If the stress is eliminated, the catecholamine levels drop logarithmically. However, stresses such as convulsions, hypoxia, or apnea appear to cause further catecholamine surges and act to maintain elevated catecholamine levels.[16]

Myocardial depression has been associated with this massive release of catecholamines. Rosner et al[16] noted three phases in the cardiovascular response to brain injury which are related to severity and time. In mild injury, there is an initial period of bradycardia, a mild decline in blood pressure, and little or no change in catecholamine level. In more severe injuries, there is a massive rise in systemic pressure, tachyrhythmia-bradyrhythmias, and very high circulating catecholamine levels. The cause is thought to be massive sympathoadrenal discharge via the spinal sympathetic nervous system involving adrenal tissue and peripheral vasoconstrictive sympathetic nerve terminals. The third phase is cardiovascular collapse, associated with varying arrhythmias, progressive hypotension, and moderately elevated catecholamine levels. The concurrent release of opiates from the adrenal glands in addition to the catecholamine release may be related to subsequent cardiovascular collapse.

Catecholamine peaks were also associated with hyperglycemia. Although the importance of hyperglycemia in the pathophysiology of head injury is unclear, there is some speculation that it may influence cellular and tissue lactic acidosis. Because the initial sympathetic surge occurs at the scene of injury, little can be done to limit its impact on the brain. Recognition of its potential implications for cardiovascular and neurologic function, however, makes assessment, monitoring, and timely interventions critical to the care of the patient.

Treatment

From this review of the pathophysiology of head injury, it is clear that the management of the patient with a traumatic head injury is a complex task. The ability to maintain an optimal environment for cellular repair is tenuous and dependent on the interrelationship of multiple factors.

Probably the greatest impact on patient outcome has come about through improved prehospital care, primarily in airway and blood pressure management and spinal stabilization. The care that the individual receives within the first hour after injury dramatically affects outcome.[34-36] Because secondary injuries, especially intracranial hypertension, have a devastating impact on patient outcome, much effort in acute management is focused on preventing secondary injuries.

For those who recover from brain injury, the final outcome depends on the premorbid status of the brain, the degree of damage suffered during the primary insult, and how quickly the health team can intervene to lessen the cumulative effect of the primary and secondary injuries. The basic brain and life support that an individual victim receives in 1 hour can reduce the cost of later hospital and rehabilitation care by hundreds of days, thousands of man-hours, and tens of thousands of dollars.[36]

Important factors in outcome are rehabilitation resources, the timing of their application, and the appropriateness of the intervention. Because most of the victims of head injury are young, the cost of their care continues for many years, as does their lack of productivity. The long-term effect on the financial, emotional, physical, vocational, and psychosocial stamina of the family can be devastating. Although medicine has made tremendous strides in saving and prolonging the lives of these victims, the community has not matched these efforts in resources.

An interesting outcome of a study in Virginia[26] was the identification of risk factors for head injury other than sex, age, and socioeconomic status. It was found that 24 percent of the brain-injured population had a history of treatment for alcoholism, 20 percent had heart disease, 11 percent had a psychiatric history, 4 percent had a history of seizures, and 4 percent had a history of drug abuse. Identifying these individuals as the ones most at risk for head injury should provide an impetus for preventive education supported on all community and governmental levels.

For the health care worker involved in the care of the head-injured patient, the goal is the same as in all long-term neurologic disabilities: to help the patient achieve the highest degree of quality and independent function as possible. In addition, health care workers might adopt a more active role in advocating legislative support for efforts at education and prevention, much like those that have focused on seat belt and helmet use.

KEY CONCEPTS

- Most head injuries are incurred in motor vehicle accidents, falls, and sports accidents. Young males ages 16 to 25 are the most common victims. The seriousness of head injury can be classified according to Glasgow Coma Scale scores as severe (<8), moderate (9–12), or mild (>12).

- Injury due directly to the initial impact is called primary injury. Primary injuries are classified as focal, polar, or diffuse. *Focal injuries* are localized to the site of skull impact. *Polar injuries* are due to acceleration-deceleration movement of the brain within the skull, resulting in double injury. *Diffuse injury* is due to movement of the brain within the skull, resulting in widespread axonal injury.

- Secondary injury is a consequence of the body's response to the primary injury. Massive release of glutamate may be the initiating event in secondary injury. Glutamate stimulation increases the influx of calcium ions into neurons, precipitating electrolyte shifts and cellular edema. Loss of membrane integrity is associated with the formation of highly destructive oxygen free radicals. Accumulation of lactic acid within the cell further disrupts function.

- Massive sympathetic discharge after a brain injury is associated with immediate hypertension, bradycardia, and apnea. Dysrhythmias and cardiovascular collapse may follow.

- The treatment of head injury is directed primarily toward reducing brain damage from secondary injury. Administration of steroids as free radical scavengers and prevention of ICP are important components of this treatment.

Cerebrovascular Disease

Etiology

There are over 500,000 new cerebrovascular accidents (CVAs) each year in the United States, and it is the third leading cause of death. In the past three decades significant advances have been made in the area of prevention of cerebral infarction and care for its associated diseases. Unfortunately, mortality in the acute phase of stroke has not changed appreciably.[37] There is no sex prevalence for cerebrovascular disease, although it occurs more frequently with advancing age and it more frequently affects blacks than caucasians. Of interest to the health care provider, although there are over 500,000 new cases each year, 150,000 of these victims survive and require long-term care. There are over 2 million survivors of CVAs in the United States today.[38,39] Although prevention of the disease remains a concern, current research is primarily focused on reducing the morbidity and mortality in the acute phase of stroke.

Cerebrovascular disease includes several pathologic processes involving the cerebral vasculature and the brain tissue it supplies. The neurologic manifestation of cerebrovascular disease is a syndrome called **cerebrovascular accident** or **stroke,** which is characterized by a sudden onset of neurologic dysfunction due to insufficient cerebral blood supply. The etiology of cerebrovascular accident is generally threefold: embolic, thrombotic, and hemorrhagic. In this context hemorrhage refers to intracerebral hemorrhage. Subarachnoid hemorrhage, that caused by arteriovenous malformations and aneurysm, will be discussed later in the chapter.

The most common cause of CVA is a **thrombus** formation. Patients most at risk for experiencing a thrombotic event are those who have hypertension, hyperlipidemia, atherosclerosis, diabetes mellitus, or have a history of transient ischemic attacks (TIAs). In each of these disease states there is a progressively injurious change to the lining of the blood vessels. Also at risk, but not as significant, are individuals with hypovolemia, polycythemia, sickle cell anemia, obesity, or smoking habits.

The second etiological source of CVA is an **embolic event,** the primary causes of which are cardiac arrhythmias, atrial fibrillation, heart valve replacement, and oral contraceptive use by women over 35 years of age.

Intracerebral hemorrhage is the third source of CVAs. Hemorrhagic strokes are the cause of 15 to 25 percent of all CVAs and usually occur under conditions of extreme hypertension.[1,3]

Pathogenesis

Thrombotic Disease

The pathogenesis of CVA depends on the etiological nature of the event. Specific symptoms are related to the area of brain involved. In thrombotic disease, the process starts with endothelial injury in the cerebral arteries. Cerebral arteries are similar in construction to systemic arteries, having an intima, media, and adventitia layer, but the layers are thinner and less elastic. Sclerosed arteries, whether due to diabetes, hypertension, or atherosclerosis, provide a roughened surface that slows blood flow and provides an opportunity for platelet adherence and aggregation. In atherosclerosis, areas of thickening develop along the inner wall of the arteries and further narrow the lumen in which blood flows. An insidious process of lipid and calcium salt deposition in the intima results in hypertrophy, then atrophy of the media layer. This pathologic process continues, limiting the blood flow to the brain and eventually resulting in coagulation and thrombus formation.

As the progressive occlusion lowers the cerebral perfusion pressure, a compensatory hyperemia or "luxury" perfusion in collateral vessels results in congestion, edema, and additional brain ischemia, as well as a risk of hemorrhage. Insufficient blood flow to brain tissue results in oxygen deprivation and rapid cerebral deterioration. Neurologic deficits become evident after just 1 minute of insufficient oxygen. If the ischemia continues for 2 to 5 minutes, irreversible cellular damage can occur. With further progression large areas of gray and white matter become necrotic or infarcted. Initially, normal fibrinolysis may prevent full occlusion of the affected arteries and allow adequate blood flow to reach the tissues. If arterial pressure or fibrinolysis resolves an occlusion and the deficits completely disappear, this event is called a **transient ischemic attack** (TIA). The neurologic symptoms of a TIA typically last only minutes but may last as long as 24 hours. Symptoms resolve completely without evidence of neurologic dysfunction. TIAs are important warning signs of thrombotic disease and the potential for a cerebral catastrophe. Between 25 percent and 50 percent of thrombotic strokes are preceded by TIAs,[38] usually within 5 to 10 years.

Like TIAs, **reversible ischemic neurologic deficits** (RINDs) are ischemic events in which symptoms completely resolve, but typically over a period exceeding 24 hours. They are also significant warning signs that immediate medical intervention is necessary to ward off potential disaster. Patients who present with TIAs or RINDs should undergo evaluation aimed at discovering the origin of their symptoms. Many of these patients are started on daily aspirin therapy, although the efficacy of this approach is still being investigated.[40] Recent research demonstrates that the effectiveness of aspirin on platelet aggregation varies among individuals.[41,42] Carotid endarterectomy may prevent stroke in a subset of patients experiencing TIAs. The North American Symptomatic Carotid Endarterectomy Trial data indicated benefit of carotid surgery in patients with carotid artery stenosis of greater than 70 percent of the vessel diameter.[43]

Embolic Disease

A narrowed atherosclerotic vessel is a vulnerable area for emboli to lodge, the second etiological process in stroke. Emboli can be air or fat; however, they are most often a result of heart disease. The most common source is **atrial fibrillation** in an enlarged left atrium. Mural thrombi tend to form at this spot and then shed emboli into the systemic circulation. Unlike a thrombotic event, an embolic stroke evolves very quickly, in seconds to minutes. Most emboli enter the carotid system and typically enter the left middle cerebral artery because it is a straighter vessel.[5] Entry via the vertebral system often affects the posterior cerebral artery.

Hemorrhagic Disease

Intracerebral hemorrhage occurs in the context of severe and often long-standing **hypertension.** It carries a 50 percent mortality, with death occurring within minutes to hours. Most hemorrhagic strokes occur in the basal ganglia or thalamus. If the hemorrhage is large, the mass effect results in increased ICP which, if uncontrolled, progresses to herniation and death. The prognosis for hemorrhagic stroke depends on the patient's age, the location and size of the hemorrhage, and how rapidly the hemorrhage produces brain distortion and shift.

In stroke, as in head injury, ischemia and cell injury stimulate the same metabolic cascade of cellular destruction and vascular disruption. Intracranial hypertension is usually a problem only in hemorrhagic stroke, where the patient is managed in the intensive care unit. Clinical trials of free radical scavengers are now being extended to stroke patients, as are investigational trials of calcium antagonists.

Timeliness of intervention in stroke and head injury is critical. Cerebral blood flow studies using positron emission tomography have revealed the existence of a **penumbra** of ischemic tissue surrounding the infarcted area after a stroke. For a limited time this area can survive in a state of functional deficit, from which it is able to recover if blood flow is promptly restored.[44,45] In animal models, this therapeutic window occurs at 4 to 8 hours.[44] Thus, therapy designed to reduce the impact of secondary injury must be initiated within this time frame.

Clinical Manifestations

Specific symptoms of neurologic dysfunction are related to the cerebral vasculature involved. To understand the deficits, recall the areas of function and the vascular distribution discussed in Chapter 42 (see Fig. 42–11). Occlusion of the **internal carotid artery** may cause widespread damage, as this artery supplies an entire cerebral hemisphere. Thus, symptoms can include contralateral motor and sensory loss, profound hemispheric functional deficit (e.g., deficits in language processing, perception, vision, and cognition), and repeated attacks of blindness or visual blurring in the ipsilateral eye, called amaurosis fugax.

Occlusion of the **anterior cerebral artery,** with its primary distribution in the medial, frontal, and parietal lobes, can result in confusion, personality changes, and incontinence, as well as contralateral motor and sensory loss in the leg and difficulty with eye tracking.

Occlusion of the **middle cerebral artery** is most common. Involvement of its main stem results in a massive infarct in most of the involved hemisphere. There may be initial vomiting, then the rapid onset of coma, which may last for weeks. Cerebral edema is usually quite extensive. Neurologic deficits include contralateral motor and sensory loss, with the arm more involved than the leg; contralateral motor loss in lower face; contralateral visual field loss; aphasia with involvement of the dominant hemisphere; affect and spatial-perceptual deficits in the nondominant hemisphere; and vasomotor paresis.

The **posterior cerebral artery** supplies the occipital and inferior temporal lobes as well as the thalamus and some deeper structures. Occlusion of this artery results in some contralateral sensory loss, homonymous hemianopsia, and problems with color blindness and depth-of-field perception. Perseverative behavior and memory impairment are also common. If the thalamus is involved, there may be sensory loss of all modalities, spontaneous pain, and intentional tremors. If the cerebral peduncle is involved, there may be oculomotor nerve palsy with contralateral hemiplegia. Brain stem involvement can result in conjugate gaze deficits, nystagmus, and pupillary abnormalities, with possible ataxia and postural tremors.[46]

CVA is diagnosed from the history and clinical findings. The history includes familial and preexisting risk factors. Physical examination looks at both cardiac and neurologic condition. In addition, diagnostic procedures may be ordered, including blood studies, CT, magnetic resonance imaging (MRI), Doppler studies, and electrocardiography.

Treatment

In all cases of stroke management, a thorough neurologic evaluation and serial assessments are essential. The examiner looks for any indication of deterioration in status that might reflect progression of the stroke or cerebral edema. Medical management of the acute stroke focuses on establishing the type and cause of the stroke and implementing measures to restore cerebral circulation and control or reverse pathologic processes. Patients who experience severe stroke, notably a hemorrhagic event, and those whose require surgical intervention will need critical care management in the intensive care unit. Ventilation, hemodynamic monitoring, and blood pressure management are essential. Patients who have experienced a hemorrhagic stroke secondary to hypertensive disease often have extremely high blood pressures. Bringing their blood pressure into normotensive ranges could result in ischemia. In these circumstances it is best to keep the patient mildly hypertensive with the goal of normalizing the blood pressure once the patient is medically stable. Patients who have experienced cerebral hemorrhage are at risk for increased intracranial hypertension and should be managed and assessed much as the patient with a traumatic head injury.

Most patients who experience an occlusive stroke are managed in the medical unit unless there is a loss of consciousness and ventilation is compromised. It is critical to prevent further cerebral hypoxia or ischemia. Thus, volume depletion, hemoconcentration, hypotension, and arterial obstruction must be avoided. As with the hemorrhagic patient, careful blood pressure management is critical. The judicious use of antihypertensives and management of fluid volume are important part's of patient care. Fluid intake, both oral and intravenous, must be carefully monitored to avoid overhydration. Excessive fluid volume can compromise cardiac and respiratory function. It can also result in cerebral edema in the ischemic area of the brain and raise ICP. Patients who are taking fluids by mouth should have their ability to swallow evaluated *before* they take any food or liquids orally. Injury to cranial nerves V, VII, IX, X, or XII can place a patient at risk for aspiration and further compromise the individual's health and potential for recovery.

Anticoagulation therapy is frequently used in ischemic stroke, especially if the event is progressive. A stroke is termed *progressive* if an initial focal deficit worsened or fluctuated before hospital admission, or deteriorated on serial examinations after admission. The therapeutic effectiveness of anticoagulation therapy under these conditions is still being explored.[47] Throughout the course of therapy, it is essential to monitor clotting parameters and recognize the potential for hemorrhage into the ischemic area.

The treatment of **embolic stroke** centers on managing the underlying cardiac abnormality. Interventions depend on the cause and may include careful cardiac and blood pressure monitoring, control of cardiac arrhythmias, anticoagulation therapy, anti-platelet aggregation medication, or the placement of a Greenfield filter to prevent emboli from reaching the cerebral circulation. The most common cause of embolic stroke is atrial fibrillation. Nonvalvular atrial fibrillation is responsible for approximately 75,000 strokes each year in the United States. Thrombotic material is formed in the stagnant left atrium and is embolized to the systemic and cerebral circulation.[48] Unlike the mixed reports on anticoagulation therapy in progressive ischemic stroke, in the case of nonvalvular atrial fibrillation, a beneficial effect from both warfarin and aspirin in preventing ischemic stroke and systemic embolism has been demonstrated.[49]

Thrombus lysis using tissue-type plasminogen activator remains controversial but has proved successful in patients with coronary artery disease and in animal models of cerebral disease.[48,50] Hemodilution is also a subject of research and experimentation. Success with this therapy depends on the timing of the intervention and the size of infarct and accompanying edema.[1] Drugs that enhance the integrity of or dilate the blood vessels are also among current investigational clinical trials, as is cerebral angioplasty. Some patients who have easily accessible atherosclerotic plaques may be candidates for surgical intervention.

Medical management of the stroke patient does not stop once the patient has been stabilized and is ready for rehabilitation. One must take into consideration that the survivor of a stroke is at risk for a subsequent stroke, as the initial precipitating factors are still present. Patients who have experienced thrombotic strokes are also at significant risk for other catastrophic vascular events, such as myocardial infarctions or systemic embolism.[39] In the presence of co-morbidities such as cardiac disease or diabetes mellitus, the risk of a second stroke can double.[39] One study found that the most common primary cause of death between 2 and 4 weeks after the initial stroke event was pulmonary embolism, followed by recurrent cerebrovascular disease, cardiac events, and bronchopneumonia.[51] Thus, in addition to the medical interventions already discussed, secondary prevention must be an ongoing health care focus for individuals who survive the initial stroke. Secondary prevention includes patient education on antiplatelet or anticoagulation medications, blood pressure control, diet or medication management of hyperlipidemia, smoking cessation, and exercise.

Stroke Sequelae

Motor Deficits

Recovery from stroke is a product of time, the degree of impairment, and appropriate rehabilitative interventions. Three of the most common neurologic deficits experienced after a stroke are motor, language, and cognitive impairments.

Motor impairment from a stroke is initially characterized by **flaccidity,** a decrease in or absence of muscle tone. Foot drop, outward rotation of the leg, and dependent edema are common features in the lower extremity. In the upper extremity, the arm may sublux from the shoulder if not supported, and it, too, will be subject to dependent edema due to poor vascular tone. Muscles in the affected limbs tend to atrophy from lack of tone and use. Many of the complications can be limited with therapeutic interventions, including frequent range of motion exercises, elevation of edematous limbs, the use of elastic stockings, and maintenance of body alignment.

Starting at about 6 weeks after the stroke, recovery of motor function is evident by the onset of **spasticity.** Spasticity is the resistance of muscle groups to passive stretch with an increase in tone. Increased flexor tone is usually seen in the upper extremities and increased extensor tone in the lower extremities. Passive or active range of motion exercises and positioning are critical to maintenance of function, as uncontrolled spasticity can result in **contractures** of the limbs, including adduction of the shoulder, pronation of the forearm, and finger flexion. In the lower extremity the patient may have problems with hip and knee extension. If spasticity is not evident within 3 months, function is not likely to return to the affected limb.

Language Deficits

Aphasia is an integrative disorder that occurs secondary to brain damage and involves all language modalities. Characteristics of aphasia include a reduced vocabulary, reduced verbal attention span, and reduced ability to use learned linguistic rules. Aphasia is associated with lesions in the primary language centers (Broca's area and Wernicke's area) as well as in adjacent cortical areas (see Fig. 42–14). Aphasia is categorized according to the location of the lesion and the linguistic deficit. The following is a brief description of those categories.

Broca's aphasia, also known as verbal motor or expressive aphasia, results from a lesion in the third frontal convolution of the left hemisphere. Patients speak with poorly articulated and sparse vocabulary and in the simplest grammatical constructions. Written language patterns are the same as oral patterns but are usually more impaired.[52,53]

Wernicke's aphasia, also known as sensory, acoustic, or receptive aphasia, is characterized by impaired auditory comprehension and speech that is fluent but empty of content. This form of aphasia is caused by lesions in the posterior portion of the first temporal gyrus of the left hemisphere. Speech is frequently circumlocutious or tangential and contains paraphasic errors and jargon. Word finding and naming difficulties are a prominent feature of this disorder. Patients with Wernicke's aphasia are unable to monitor their own language production and cannot comprehend or monitor the language production of others.[52,53]

Anomic aphasia results from lesions in the parietotemporal area in proximity to the angular gyrus. This is a fluent aphasia with intact grammatical structure. Patients have greater word-finding difficulties than those with Wernicke's aphasia but do not make paraphasic errors and have intact comprehension. Their speech, however, is typically devoid of substantive words.[52,53]

Conduction or **central aphasia** is associated with increased paraphasic errors and a reduced ability to repeat words. It is associated with a lesion in the arcuate fasciculus in the left hemisphere. Patients are well aware that they are making language errors. However, the more they struggle to find the correct words, the more likely they are to repeat paraphasic errors.[52,53]

Cognitive Deficits

Cognitive disorders after a stroke are in fact often **cognitive-linguistic disorders** and are experienced by patients with space-occupying lesions, cerebral degenerative disorders, and head traumas as well. Patients experience impairments of language skills due to diffuse cortical or subcortical injuries that affect the ability to be alert, to concentrate or attend to stimuli, to remember, and to reason. Hagen[54] describes the cognitive-linguistic disorders as appearing "similar to the aphasia disorders. Symptoms reflect an underlying impairment, release, suppression and/or disorganization of the cognitive process which support language processing."

Cognitive impairment is relative to the area of the brain involved and the severity of the injury. There is also an assumed **hierarchy of cognitive function.** This hierarchy identifies arousal or alertness as the most basic function, as it is a prerequisite to all other cognitive abilities. Therefore, injuries that disturb an individual's ability to maintain an alert status are the most severe. The next most basic skill is the ability to *attend* or concentrate on a stimulus. Increasing cognitive skill is necessary for the function of memory and the ability to learn and associate, to discriminate, to separate, and to categorize various stimuli. The highest levels of cognitive function include analysis, synthesis, and reasoning abilities. A deficit at any level of cognitive function can impair efficiency in language.[54]

Regardless of the cause of the stroke, once the patient has stabilized and the medical management is no longer acute, rehabilitation services are essential to facilitate the patient's return to productive function. As each patient's level of dysfunction is individual, so too must be the plan for recovery. A complete assessment and therapy program should be planned by all health professionals involved, as well as by the patient and family. In addition to what health care professionals do in the hospital and rehabilitation centers, we must also be advocates for the patient when they return to the community. In the past few years there has been a significant increase in community resources for the disabled. However, access to these resources or the appropriateness of the resources do not always match the needs of the patient. Seventy percent of stroke victims survive the first 30 days, and 90 percent of those continue to survive with varying degrees of deficits. At any one time there are over 2.5 million survivors of stroke in the United States.[38] Clearly, cerebrovascular disease has a tremendous impact not just on our communities but on our entire health care system.

KEY CONCEPTS

- Cerebrovascular disease may lead to cerebrovascular accident (CVA), or stroke, which is the sudden onset of neurologic dysfunction due to focal brain ischemia. The most common cause of CVA is thrombosis, followed by embolization and intracranial hemorrhage.

- Thrombi form at atherosclerotic plaques, causing sudden occlusion of an already narrowed vessel. If the clot is quickly lysed, the deficits may completely disappear, a phenomenon associated with a transient ischemic attack (TIA). Emboli are usually a consequence of clots from within the heart chambers due to disease or dysrhythmia. Hemorrhage is usually associated with hypertension.

- Stroke symptoms depend on the area of brain affected, which in turn depends on the vessel occluded: internal carotid, anterior cerebral, middle cerebral, or posterior cerebral artery. Common manifestations include contralateral motor and sensory loss, aphasia, and partial visual field loss.

- Treatment is mostly symptomatic and supportive. Assessment of gag and swallow reflexes before oral intake may prevent aspiration. Blood pressure management, anticoagulation, hemodilution, and thrombolysis may be instituted.

- Stroke is associated with long-term deficits in motor, language, and cognitive abilities. Initially, affected muscles are flaccid, with spasticity occurring after about 6 weeks. Prevention of contractures is a major concern. Aphasia may be described as expressive or receptive. Most individuals with aphasia have impaired integrative ability involving all language modalities. Concentration, memory, and reasoning may be impaired.

Cerebral Aneurysm and Subarachnoid Hemorrhage

Aneurysms

Etiology

Subarachnoid hemorrhage (SAH) is an arterial bleed into the subarachnoid space from a ruptured arteriovenous malformation (AVM), hypertensive hemorrhage, head injury, or, most commonly, a ruptured **intracranial aneurysm.** Aneurysm rupture occurs in about 15,000 Americans each year, or 6 per 1,000,000 (Fig 43–8).[38] The prevalence is higher in women than in men, and rupture most often occurs between the ages of 30 and 60 years. Ninety-five percent of ruptured aneurysms occur on the circle of Willis, and of those, 94 percent involve the anterior circulation. In 10 to 20 percent of these cases, the aneurysms are multiple.[55]

Warning leaks before an aneurysm rupture often produce severe headaches, which is typically described by the patient as "the worst headache I have ever had," and if recognized can significantly influence the morbidity in these patients. Patients may also complain of photophobia and stiff neck. A stiff and painful neck results from meningismus caused by the irritating properties of blood in the CSF. After rupture, the onset of symptoms is very rapid. Sudden injection of blood into the subarachnoid space raises

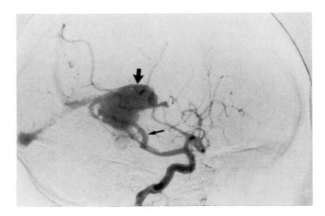

FIGURE 43–8. Vein of Galen aneurysm (*large arrow*) supplied by branches of the posterior cerebral artery (*small arrow*). (From Drayer B, Hayman LA, Taber KH, Lownie SP: Nontraumatic intracranial hemorrhage. *Neuroimaging Clin North Am* 1992;2:205. Reproduced with permission.)

ICP and distorts intracranial structures. **Secondary cerebral vasospasm,** a pathologic narrowing of the major vessels around the area of rupture, typically occurs from day 4 to day 14. This process significantly reduces cerebral blood flow and results in increased cerebral ischemia and possibly infarction. It is the leading cause of morbidity and mortality in this disease process.[56] The next most serious consequence of the initial rupture is rebleeding. The risk for rebleeding in an unclipped aneurysm is highest in the first 14 days. The surgical strategy is to clip the aneurysm before the hemorrhage renews itself.

Diagnostic procedures for detecting aneurysm include CT to confirm an SAH. In the absence of bleeding, MRI is most helpful. The presence of **xanthochromic cells** in a lumbar puncture is also indicative of an SAH, and in those who experienced an SAH, an angiogram demonstrates the location of the aneurysm in about 80 percent of cases.

Pathogenesis

An aneurysm is a lesion of the blood vessel that results in dilation of the vascular lumen. The dilation is caused by weakness, which allows the components of the vessel wall to yield. Although the exact pathogenesis is not fully understood, saccular aneurysms are believed to result from congenital defects. The defect is a localized absence of the media layer in the vascular wall. This structural weakness permits gradual ballooning at the site as a consequence of arterial pressure effects over years. A common location for saccular aneurysms is the arterial bifurcations, where turbulent blood flow might have a greater impact on a weakened vessel wall.

Saccular aneurysms generally are round. They may have a broad-based attachment to the vessel wall or be attached to the mother vessel by a narrow stalk. Rarely, these aneurysms might have a narrow and cylindric configuration. The aneurysmal sac is composed of thickened intima and adventitia, the media layer having abruptly ended at the sac edge. It is common to find that atherosclerosis has developed prematurely in the wall and that thrombosis partially obliterates the vessel lumen.[55] Rupture of the aneurysm generally occurs from the dome of the sac or at the edge of the atheromatous plaque.

Treatment

The primary treatment for an aneurysm is surgical stabilization, either by clipping or covering, and aggressive treatment of vasospasm. Current practice is to operate as soon as possible, as overall management mortality is less. This is contingent on receiving the patient immediately after the initial hemorrhage. If the patient does not go to the hospital until several days after the initial hemorrhage, the surgical risk is much greater because of ischemia induced by vasospasm.[1] Although a variety of techniques are used, in general vasospasm is managed by hypertensive-

hypervolemic or normotensive-hypervolemic therapy, a balance between the administration of hypertensive agents, volume expanders, maintenance of optimal cerebral perfusion, and blood pressure.[56] The patient with an aneurysm is most often cared for in the intensive care unit. In addition to hemodynamic monitoring, careful and frequent neurologic assessments are essential to monitor stability and recognize the first signs of deterioration so that rapid intervention can occur.

Arteriovenous Malformations

Pathogenesis and Clinical Manifestations

Arteriovenous malformations (AVMs) are the second most common cause of spontaneous subarachnoid hemorrhage (Fig. 43–9).[57] Sixty-four percent of AVMs are diagnosed in patients before the age of 40 years. By contrast, only 26 percent of symptomatic saccular aneurysms occur in the same age range.[57] Ninety per-

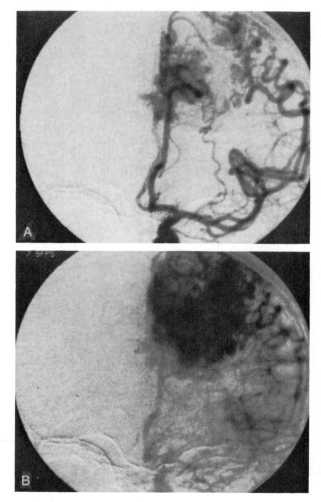

FIGURE 43–9. Digital subtraction angiogram of a brain arteriovenous malformation supplied by the anterior and middle cerebral arteries. (From Drayer B, Hayman LA, Taber KH, Jacobs JM: Nontraumatic intracranial hemorrhage. *Neuroimaging Clin North Am* 1992;2:98. Reproduced with permission.)

cent of AVMs are found in the cerebral hemispheres. Typically, AVMS are in the shape of a cone with its base in the cortex and the apex pointing toward the lateral ventricle. These are congenital vascular lesions that begin to evolve between the fourth and eighth week of embryonic development. The vessel wall defect is similar to that found in saccular aneurysms. Gaps can be found in the endothelium. The subendothelial basement membrane, on the other hand, is thick, reticulated, or multilaminated. Degenerative changes are often evident in the muscle walls.[57]

In the normal vascular system, the capillaries control cerebrovascular resistance by preventing arterial blood from directly entering the veins. In this condition the capillary system is missing. Consequently, arterial blood is shunted directly into the venous system. As the venous system becomes a high-pressure system, the vessels involved in the lesion progressively enlarge, as do the arteries and veins that feed and drain the lesion. Eventually the AVM becomes a lesion of congested, enlarged vessels of varying sizes. Because of their abnormal structure and the high pressure, AVMs are vulnerable to hemorrhage. The brain surrounding the lesion has been found to develop important pathologic changes associated with the AVM. Changes commonly seen include recent or old hemorrhage, extensive gliosis, dysplastic brain tissue, foci of chronic inflammation, and parenchymal calcification.[57]

AVMs may symptomatically manifest as progressive neurologic dysfunction as a result of ischemia in normal tissue caused by abnormal shunting of blood into the lesion. The AVM may also present secondary to a hemorrhage. In contrast to the high mortality from aneurysm rupture, mortality after an AVM is only 10 to 15 percent. The clinical presentation is often a function of age. Adults frequently present with seizures and hemorrhage. Children experience hemorrhage more often than seizures, and neonates may present with high output cardiac failure. The incidence of clinically recognizable hemorrhage from an AVM is 2 to 4 percent per year. The risk of rebleeding within the first year after an initial hemorrhage increases to 6 percent.[57]

Treatment

AVMs that cannot be surgically removed may sometimes be selectively irradiated. Other nonsurgical interventions include the introduction of catheters to selectively occlude the lesion with glue, or **embolization**. Surgical treatment is fairly straightforward for small lesions on the cortical surface. Large and deep AVMs pose greater intraoperative hazards. One of the greatest risks with a large AVM is reperfusion breakthrough hemorrhage when large volumes of blood are returned to vessels that are not used to the volume or pressure. Hemodynamic control is essential in such instances. Recovery from intracranial hemorrhage is similar to recovery from stroke. Once stabilized, the patient must be assessed and an appropriate interdisciplinary rehabilitation program developed.

KEY CONCEPTS

- Subarachnoid hemorrhage is arterial bleeding into the subarachnoid space. Bleeding may be precipitated by hypertension, head injury, an intracranial aneurysm, or an arteriovenous malformation.

- Blood in the subarachnoid space is associated with headache, stiff neck, and secondary cerebral vasospasm. Vasospasm, which leads to cerebral ischemia, is the primary cause of morbidity and mortality.

- Aneurysms are caused by congenital weakness in the arterial walls that leads to dilation and increased intraluminal pressure. Treatment is surgical stabilization. The aggressive treatment of secondary vasospasm includes hypervolemia and elevated blood pressure.

- Arteriovenous malformations are congenital malformations in which arterial blood is shunted directly into the venous system, causing high venous pressure. The AVM enlarges and may compress adjacent structures or rupture. Surgical treatment or glue embolization to occlude the AVM may be done to prevent bleeding.

Central Nervous System Infections

Infections of the central nervous system (CNS) pose an interesting challenge to the health care provider. Only the most common, namely, meningitis, encephalitis, and abscesses, will be discussed here. Depending on the disease entity and its degree of severity, health care can run the continuum from monitoring the safety of a mildly confused patient to preventing life-threatening intracranial hypertension. Severe infection is often accompanied by a **change in level of consciousness.** This initial depression is a response to cellular invasion of the organism and the presence of toxins.[1] Increasing inflammation can result in occlusion of arteries and veins, especially along cortical surfaces. This can result in edema, infarction, and intracranial hypertension and often determines the ultimate outcome. A frequent consequence of bacterial infections is obstructive hydrocephalus as the bacteria, white blood cells, and cellular debris block CSF reabsorption in the arachnoid villi.

All invading organisms of the CNS must have a portal of entry. These include the bloodstream, by direct extension from a primary site, the CSF, by extension along peripheral and cranial nerves, the mouth, and the nasopharynx, and through maternal-fetal connections. Factors contributing to infections include such conditions as immunocompromise, debilitation, poor nutrition, radiation therapy, steroid therapy, and contact with vectors.

Meningitis

Meningitis is the most common sequela to bacterial invasion of the CNS. Most frequently meningitis is bacterial in origin, but it can also be viral or fungal. AIDS patients who have an increased susceptibility to infection, also have an increased prevalence of meningitis of viral, fungal, and parasitic origin. Interestingly, in animal studies the subarachnoid space is resistant to infection in normal animals. The risk of infection appears to increase with changes in CSF pressure due to bacteremia.[9]

Etiology

The bacteria most frequently involved in causing meningitis are *Streptococcus pneumoniae* and *Neisseria meningitidis*. *Hemophilus influenza* type B is most often the causative agent in children. The bacteria that cause meningitis most frequently reach the CNS by way of the bloodstream or by extension from cranial structures such as the paranasal sinuses or ears. Some of the organisms responsible for causing meningitis may be normal inhabitants of the nasopharynx. Pathogens can also gain access to the CNS through breaks in the barrier system, as occur with penetrating head wounds or skull fractures or following neurosurgery in which the dura is penetrated.

Pathogenesis and Clinical Manifestations

Bacterial meningitis is a **pyogenic infection** that invades the **leptomeninges** and the subarachnoid space. Because of its involvement in the subarachnoid space, the infection travels readily around the brain and spinal cord. The accumulation of exudate frequently results in **obstructive hydrocephalus** and exudative invasion into the sheaths of the blood vessels and spinal and cranial nerves. If the perivascular space is involved, an accompanying encephalitis ensues.[1,58] Vascular changes are not uncommon and can result in venous and arterial thrombosis. Necrotizing vasculitis is evident in some cases. Small cortical or subcortical infarcts or hemorrhages may result from these vascular changes.[59]

The diagnosis of meningitis is usually made by lumbar puncture. Gram stain of the CSF will reveal the causative organism in 75 percent of patients. In addition to the causative organism, classic CSF findings include white blood cell counts between 100 and 15,000 cells/mm^3 with a predominance of polymorphonuclear leukocytes. CSF glucose is reduced and often extremely low, and patients with bacterial or fungal meningitis have increased protein levels.

Infection is usually experienced as an acute onset with fever, stiff neck, and headache. Deterioration in level of consciousness is progressive and often rapid. Patients who deteriorate rapidly often demonstrate dramatic tachypnea. About one third of patients experience seizures. Cranial nerve involvement is also common and is most often seen as ocular palsies, facial weakness and/or deafness, and vertigo.

Obstructive hydrocephalus is a risk and, in combination with edema, can result in pathologic intracranial hypertension and herniation. If the disease process cannot be stabilized and regressed, the effects of increased ICP, venous and arterial thrombosis, and the accumulation of exudate result in a reduction in cerebral blood flow and utilization of oxygen. Cerebral autoregulation can be lost, with a resulting fall in cerebral perfusion pressure. The mortality from CNS infections correlates with the loss of cerebral perfusion pressure.[58]

Treatment

Recovery from bacterial meningitis depends largely on how quickly effective treatment is started. Treatment includes general supportive care, intravenous antibacterial drug therapy targeting the specific pathogen for at least 10 days, and management of any complications. Even with the use of antibiotics, meningitis still carries a high morbidity and mortality, each about 20 percent. Complications from meningitis can include visual impairments, optic neuritis, deafness, headache, seizures, personality changes, motor weakness, hydrocephalus, endocarditis, and pneumonia.[1]

An important role for the health care worker is not only to manage the care of patients with meningitis but also to play an active role in prevention. Indirect involvement includes public education promoting prompt and appropriate treatment of sinusitis, mastoiditis, ear infections, and pneumonias. A more direct role is the observation of policies for strict aseptic techniques for all procedures involving a break in the CNS barrier system, involvement of the infectious control department in your institution, and the incorporation of isolation as needed.

Encephalitis
Etiology and Pathogenesis

Encephalitis, an inflammation of the brain, can be caused by the same infectious agents as meningitis, although viruses are most often the pathogen. Viruses are obligate intracellular parasites. The process of cellular infection by viruses is complex and includes the following stages: (1) absorption of the virus to the cell membrane, (2) penetration of the cell and viral uncoating, (3) translation of immediate early proteins, (4) replication of viral neucleic acid, (5) transcription and translation of late, structural proteins, (6) virus assembly, and (7) release of mature virions.[45] The pathogenesis of encephalitis has not been established unequivocally for all viral pathogens. Interestingly, nearly all encephalitic infection-causing viruses enter the body and initiate replication at a nonneural site. In the nonimmune host, viral replication results in viremia, and the viral infection is spread hematogenously to the CNS and other organs. Most viruses causing encephalitis cause neurologic impairment by direct infection of neural cells. In some instances immunologic responses to the infection contribute to the neurologic dysfunction.[60]

Western Equine Encephalitis

The two most common types of viral encephalitis in the United States are the western equine encephalitis and herpes simplex encephalitis.[1] **Western equine encephalitis** is one of the most common **arboviral** infections. The principal epidemic vector is a mosquito, *Culex tarsalis*. In the western United States, *C. tarsalis* breeds in sunlit grassy marshes, ground pools and streams, then readily infects humans. Birds are the preferred host, and humans are not usually infected unless the population of *C. tarsalis* far outnumbers the bird host population. In the eastern United States, western equine encephalitis is carried by the mosquito vector, *Culex melanura*. Here its distribution is restricted to swamps and therefore rarely results in human infections. Western equine encephalitis is primarily a disease of the summer months, typically May to September. It most often infects the very young and those over the age of 50 years.

In fatal cases of this disease, the brain may appear normal or may have demonstrable vascular congestion. Lesions are not limited to a specific region of the brain, although the basal ganglia are often the most severely involved. It affects both gray and white matter. Inflammatory reactions include proliferation of neutrophils and mononuclear cells, which form perivascular cuffs around small arteries and veins. Neutrophils frequently invade the vessel walls and extend into the perivascular tissues, forming microabscesses. These lesions are not restricted to the perivascular region but can be found in diffuse or focal areas scattered throughout the brain. Vascular involvement is variable. Hemorrhages of varying degree may or may not occur. White matter usually shows patchy demyelination. In general, the meninges are not involved.

The incubation period for western equine encephalitis is 5 to 15 days. Onset of symptoms is typically rapid, and symptoms include general malaise, mild headache, and often nausea and vomiting. The patient develops a moderately elevated temperature and the headache usually becomes severe. Lethargy and irritability are often present after a few days. In an uncomplicated infection symptoms will persist for about 10 days, then gradually subside. In severe cases, lethargy progresses to stupor alternating with extreme restlessness. In fatal cases the progression of disease is rapid, culminating in coma and death. The CSF of infected individuals typically demonstrates a mononuclear pleocytosis with a cell count of up to 200 cells/mm^3. The diagnosis of western equine encephalitis is made by serologic evaluation.[60]

Herpes Simplex Encephalitis

Herpes simplex encephalitis is the most important cause of sporadic and often fatal (70 percent) encephalitis in the United States.[59] It results from spread of the herpes simplex virus type I (HSV-1) from neural tissue to the CNS. This can occur as a primary or secondary infection or as a reactivation of latent virus. The trigeminal ganglia have been shown to harbor latent HSV-1. It may be that the virus, once reactivated, travels down the trigeminal fibers that innervate the middle and anterior fossae.[60] If so, it might explain the unique distribution of the disease to the mesotemporal and orbital frontal cortex.

There is no seasonal incidence of this disease. In adults with herpes simplex encephalitis there are no accompanying cutaneous or visceral lesions associated with this fulminating and febrile disease. In premature infants who contract the disease during delivery from genital lesions on their mother, there is an acute encephalitis as well as disseminated visceral lesions.[59] Most often this is an acute hemorrhagic necrotizing encephalitis. There is typically massive tissue necrosis with petechial and confluent hemorrhages. The initial lesions become masses of lipid-laden macrophages that evolve into collapsed gliotic scars.

Herpes simplex encephalitis produces a variable impact on the patient. The patient may initially complain of flulike symptoms. Subsequent lethargy, confusion, and delirium are common and may evolve into coma. Some patients may experience a much more rapid course with an acute necrotizing encephalitis and widespread destruction of white matter and extensive brain edema. Herpes simplex encephalitis is typically associated with a profound memory impairment and changes in personality, reflective of the unique anatomic distribution of this disease.[61]

The diagnosis is usually made from the history, clinical findings, and lumbar puncture in which there is usually an elevated WBC count, a small increase in protein, and a normal glucose. Electroencephalography and MRI may be performed; and, in the case of herpesvirus, a brain biopsy offers the only measure of definitive diagnosis.

Treatment

In general, the management of encephalitis is supportive and symptomatic. As with all severe illnesses, respiratory and cardiovascular support is imperative. Patients with encephalitis must be carefully hydrated as they frequently develop signs and symptoms of excessive antidiuretic hormone. Those with moderate to severe disease will need careful and ongoing neurologic assessment. Seizures are common complications in encephalitis secondary to hypoxia, tissue destruction and toxic encephalopathy, inflammatory vasculitis and hyponatremia.[61] All patients with moderate to severe illness should be monitored for intracranial hypertension. Although there is no definitive drug treatment, steroids are often given to control edema, anticonvulsants to prevent seizures, analgesics for headache, and antipyretics for hyperthermia. The exception to this general protocol is the patient with herpes encephalitis. Patients in whom herpes simplex encephalitis has been diagnosed should be treated with **antiviral acyclovir,** as it can dramatically improve their outcome.[46,58]

Although CNS inflammatory processes were relatively uncommon in the past, with the exception of meningitis, the increased number of patients with human immunodeficiency virus infection has increased the incidence of CNS infection in intensive care patients. The care and recuperation of these patients can be lengthy. Once the patient has stabilized, the health care team needs to focus on rehabilitation.

Brain Abscess

Etiology

A brain abscess is a localized suppuration within the brain parenchyma. Pyogenic pathogens reach the brain by a number of routes, including (1) penetrating wounds, (2) by direct extension or retrograde thrombophlebitis of an infected neighboring structure (e.g., mastoiditis, sinusitis), or (3) by blood-borne dissemination from a distant infected site (e.g., lungs). Most brain abscesses are bacterial and frequently arise from anaerobic organisms. Historically, most brain abscesses originated from infections in the sinus or middle ear, and staphylococci and pneumococci were the most frequently isolated pathogens. Today, brain abscesses are more frequently the result of pulmonary empyema, cardiac valvular disease, and immunosuppression.[59] Streptococci, both aerobic and anaerobic, are the most common pathogens when infection is from a distant source. Staphylococci are the most common pathogens involved in direct, traumatic lesions. Gram-negative aerobic and anaerobic pathogens are also commonly found in the primary focus of infection. In the immunocompromised patient, *Toxoplasma gondii* is a frequent cause of chronic inflammatory abscesses.

Pathogenesis

A brain abscess may pursue a very quiet course or one that is more progressive, with rapid deterioration in level of consciousness and associated focal neurologic deficits and seizures. Extensive edema is common with abscess and can result in hemispheric shifts and the potential for herniation.

Most patients become symptomatic 1 to 4 weeks after the initial infection. The process of abscess formation follows several stages. Initially the abscess is a focal septic encephalitis, or **cerebritis,** in which the central portion contains an abundance of polymorphonuclear leukocytes and tissue debris. The peripheral portion of the abscess is made up of inflammatory granulation tissue. Around the abscess is perifocal edema with proliferation of surviving astrocytes. In the chronic phase the core of the abscess is liquefied and the peripheral portion forms a collagenous capsule that in turn is surrounded by fibrous gliosis.

An abscess formation may be an isolated lesion or multiple ring-enhanced lesions, as seen on CT (Fig. 43–10). CT is critical before a lumbar puncture can be performed in these patients because of significant lesion- and edema-induced cerebral hypertension. Lumbar puncture typically reveals mildly elevated

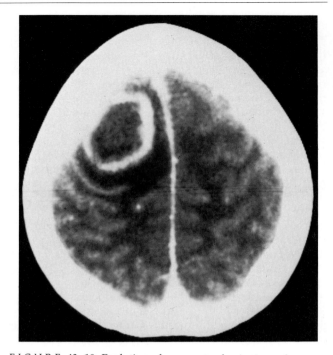

F I G U R E 43–10. Evolution of process to classic ring enhancement with contrast infusion typical of brain abscess. (From Marshall SB, Marshall LF, Vos HR, Chestnut RM: *Neuroscience Critical Care: Pathophysiology and Patient Management.* Philadelphia, WB Saunders, 1990, p 269. Reproduced with permission.)

protein levels, normal glucose levels, a mild leukocytosis, and, infrequently, the pathogenic organism. More often the causative agent can be isolated from the serum.

Treatment

The treatment of a brain abscess depends on its location and accessibility, and will most often involve drainage or **excision.** A critical feature in management is the administration of intravenous antibiotics, which is required for at least 1 month. Treatment failure is most often due to an inadequate course of antibiotics.[46] Recently, the management of patients with brain abscess has become increasingly challenging because of the increase in unusual bacterial, fungal, and parasitic infections, particularly in immunosuppressed patients. Postinfection care must address residual neurologic deficits of cognitive, motor, or sensory function.

KEY CONCEPTS

- **Meningitis is usually a consequence of bacterial infection in the CNS. Infection is usually introduced via the bloodstream or by invasion from infected sinuses or ears. Fever, stiff neck, and headache are common. Seizures may occur. The diagnosis is based on elevated CSF white cell count and the presence of bacteria in the CSF. Obstructive hydrocephalis is a serious complication of meningitis that leads to increased ICP. Antibiotics are used for treatment.**

- **Encephalitis is inflammation of the brain that is most commonly due to viral infection. Two common causes of viral encephalitis are western equine encephalitis and herpes simplex virus. Western equine encephalitis is transmitted by mosquitoes. Symptoms include malaise, headache, fever, and lethargy. Herpes simplex encephalitis is associated with flulike symptoms, memory impairment, and personality changes. Treatment is symptomatic and includes steroids, anticonvulsants, analgesics, and antipyretics. Antiviral agents (acyclovir) are helpful in the treatment of herpes simplex encephalitis.**

- **Brain abscesses are usually due to bacteria, often anaerobic types. Patients may be asymptomatic for weeks, then show manifestations of a space-occupying lesion. Drainage or excision and antibiotics are indicated.**

Summary

Current medical technology is responsible for a significant decline in mortality from such pathologic disorders as head trauma, stroke, or CNS infections. Unfortunately, many of those who are saved have long-term deficiencies in sensory, motor, or cognitive function. A common thread to all of the Neuro Axis I disorders mentioned in this chapter is the long-term impact of the disability on the patient, the family, and the community. Today's health care practitioners face the challenge of knowing not just the management of the acute illness but of assessing residual disability and facilitating the patient's return to maximum function and quality of life. Finally, the health care worker is responsible for being an advocate for the patient in the local community as well as the legislature, striving for the acquisition of resources necessary for providing adequate care.

REFERENCES

1. Marshall SB, Marshall LF, Vos HR, Chesnut RM: *Neuroscience Critical Care*. Philadelphia, WB Saunders, 1990.
2. Miller JD, Pickard JD: Intracranial volume/pressure studies in patients with head injury. *Injury* 1974;5:265–268.
3. Lundberg N: Continuous recording and control of ventricular fluid pressure in neurosurgical practice. *Acta Psychiatr Neurol Scand Suppl* 1960;149:1–193.
4. Bruce DA, Langfitt TW, Miller JD, et al: Regional cerebral blood flow, intracranial pressure, and brain metabolism in comatose patients. *J Neurosurg* 1973;32(2):131–144.
5. Roy CW, Sherrington CS: On the regulation of the blood supply of the brain. *J Physiol* 1890;11:85–108.
6. Silver IA: Cellular microenvironment in relation to local blood flow, in Elliott K, O'Connor M (eds): *Cerebral Vascular Smooth Muscle and Its Control. Ciba Found Symp* 1978;56:49–61.
7. Obrist WD, Langfitt TW, Jaggi JL, Cruz J, Gennarelli TA: Cerebral blood flow and metabolism in comatose patients with acute head injury: relationship to intracranial hypertension. *J Neurosurg* 1984;61(2):241–253.
8. Raichle ME, Grubb RL Jr, Gado MH, Eichling JO, Ter-Pogossian MM: Correlation between regional cerebral blood flow and oxidative metabolism. *Arch Neurol* 1976;33(8):523–526.
9. Lou HC, Edvinsson L, MacKenzie ET: The concept of coupling blood flow to brain function: Revision required? *Ann Neurol* 1987;22(3):289–297.
10. Reulen HJ, Tsuyumu M, Tack A, Fenske AR, Prioleau G: Clearance of edema fluid into cerebrospinal fluid: A mechanism for resolution of vasogenic brain edema. *J Neurosurg* 1978;48(5):754–763.
11. Reulen HJ, Graham R, Spatz M, Klatco I: Role of pressure gradients and bulk flow in dynamics of vasogenic brain edema. *J Neurosurg* 1977;46(1):24–35.
12. Kontos HA, Enoch PW: Superoxide production in experimental brain injury. *J Neurosurg* 1986;64:803–807.
13. Zimmerman RS, et al: Reduction of intracranial hypertension with free radical scavengers, in Hoff JT, Bet AL (eds): *Intracranial Pressure VII*. Berlin, Springer-Verlag, 1989, pp 804–808.
14. Miller JD: Head injury and brain ischemia: Implications for therapy. *Br J Anaesth* 1986;57:120–129.
15. Marion DW, Darby J, Yona SH: Acute regional cerebral blood flow changes caused by severe head injuries. *J Neurosurg* 1991;74(3):407–414.
16. Rosner MJ, Newsome HH, Becker DP: Mechanical brain injury: The sympathoadrenal response. *J Neurosurg* 1984;61(1):76–86.
17. Frost EA: The physiology of respirations in neurosurgical patients. *J Neurosurg* 1979;50:699–714.
18. Teasdale G, Jennet B: Assessment of coma and impaired consciousness. *Lancet* 1974;2(872):81–84.
19. Marshall LF, Barba D, Toole BM, Bowers SA: The oval pupil: Clinical significance and relationship to intracranial hypertension. *J Neurosurg* 1983;58:566–568.
20. Plum F, Posner JB: *The Diagnosis of Stupor and Coma*, 3rd ed. Philadelphia, FA Davis, 1982.
21. Mitchel PH, Hodges LC, Muwaswes M, Walleck CA: *AANN's Neuroscience Nursing*. Norwalk, Appleton & Lange, 1988.
22. Kraus JF, Black MA, Hessol N, et al: The incidence of acute brain injury and serious impairment in a defined population. *Am J Epidemiol* 1984;119(2):186–201.
23. Jennet B: Scale and scope of the problem, in Rosenthal M, Griffith ER, Bond MR, Miller JD (eds): *Rehabilitation of the Head Injured Adult*. Philadelphia, FA Davis, 1983, p 3.
24. Pollack IW, Kohn H: Rehabilitation of cognitive function in brain-damaged persons. *J Med Soc NJ* 1984;81(4):311–315.
25. Anderson DW, McLaurin RL: Report on national head and spinal cord injury conducted for NINCDS. *J Neurosurg* 1980;Suppl:S1–S43.
26. Rimel RW, Jane JA, Bond MR: Characteristics of the head injured patient, in Rosenthal M, Griffith ER, Bond MR, Miller JD (eds): *Rehabilitation of the Adult and Child With Traumatic Brain Injury*. Philadelphia, FA Davis, 1990, pp 8–16.
27. Becker DP, Gudeman SK: *Textbook of Head Injury*. Philadelphia, WB Saunders, 1989.
28. Rose J, Valtonen S, Jennett B: Avoidable factors contributing to death after head injury. *Br Med J* 1977;2:615–618.
29. Gennarelli JA, Thibault LE, Adams JH, et al: Diffuse axonal injury and traumatic coma in the primate. *Ann Neurol* 1982;12:564–574.
30. Choi D: Methods for antagonizing glutamate neurotoxicity: *Cerebrovasc Brain Metab Rev* 1990;2(2):105–147.
31. Hovda DA, Becker DP, Katayama Y: Secondary injury and acidosis. *J Neurotrauma* 1992;9(suppl 1):47–60.
32. Hall ED, Younkers PA, Andrus PK, et al: Biochemistry and pharmacology of lipid antioxidants in acute brain and spinal cord injury. *J Neurotrauma* 1992;9(suppl 2):425–441.
33. Wei EP, Kontos HA, Dietrich WD, et al: Inhibition by free radical scavengers and by cyclooxygenase inhibitors of pial arteriolar abnormalities from concussive brain injuries in cats. *Circ Res* 1982;48:95–103.
34. Jeffreys RV, Jones JJ: Avoidable factors contributing to death of head injury patients in general hospitals in Mersey region. *Lancet* 1981;2:459–461.
35. Klauber MR, Marshall LF, Toole BM: Cause of decline in head-injury mortality rate in San Diego County. *J Neurosurg* 1985;62:528–531.
36. Pentland B, Berrol S: Early evaluation and management, in Rosenthal M, Griffith ER, Bond MR, Miller JD (eds): *Rehabilitation of the Adult and Child with Traumatic Brain Injury*. Philadelphia, FA Davis, 1990, pp 21–51.
37. Fieschi C: Antithrombotic and protective therapy of stroke. *Stroke* 1990;21(8):6–7.

38. American Association of Neuroscience Nurses: *Core Curriculum for Neuroscience Nurses,* 3rd ed. Chicago, American Association of Neuroscience Nurses, 1991.

39. Goldberg F: Secondary stroke prevention. *Phys Med Rehabil Clin North Am* 1991;2(3):517–527.

40. Lowenthal A: European stroke prevention study. *Acta Neurol Belg* 1988;88:14–18.

41. Grotemeyer KH, Schutt P: Aspirin-nonresponder under additional treatment with metoprolol. Presented at the 18th International Joint Congress on Stroke and Cerebral Circulation, Miami Beach, FL, Feb. 11–13, 1993. Abstract 60.

42. Helgason CM, Kondos GT, Hoff JA, et al: Platelet aggregation studies, aspirin, coumadin, and atrial fibrillation. Presented at the 18th International Joint Congress on Stroke and Cerebral Circulation, Miami Beach, FL, Feb.11–13, 1993. Abstract 61.

43. Alexandrov AV, Bladin CF, Maggisano R: NASCET index or NASCET stenosis. Presented at the 18th International Joint Congress on Stroke and Cerebral Circulation, Miami Beach, FL, Feb. 11–13, 1993. Abstract 51.

44. Weinstein PR, Anderson GG, Telles DA: Neurological deficit and cerebral infarction after temporary middle cerebral artery occlusion in unanesthetized cats. *Stroke* 1986;7:173–178.

45. Jaggi JL, Obrist WD, Gennarelli TA, Langfitt TW: Relationship of early cerebral blood flow and metabolism to outcome in acute head injury. *J Neurosurg* 1990;72(2):176–182.

46. Hickey JV: *The Clinical Practice of Neurological and Neurosurgical Nursing,* 2nd ed. Philadelphia, JB Lippincott, 1986.

47. Slivka A, Levy D: Natural history of progressive ischemic stroke in a population treated with heparin. *Stroke* 1990;21:1657–1662.

48. Zivin FM, Fisher M, DeGirolami U, Hemenway CC, Stashak JA: Tissue plasminogen activator reduced neurological damage after cerebral embolism. *Science* 1985;230:1289–1292.

49. Anderson DC: Progress report of the stroke prevention in arterial fibrillation study. *Stroke* 1990;11:12–17.

50. Bednar MM, McAuliffe T, Raymond S, Gross CE: Tissue plasminogen activator reduces brain injury in a rabbit model of thromboembolic stroke. *Stroke* 1990;21(12):1705–1709.

51. Viitanen M, Winblad B, Asplund K: Autopsy-verified causes of death after stroke. *Acta Med Scand* 1987;222(5):401–408.

52. Goodglass H, Kaplan E: *The Assessment of Aphasia and Related Disorders.* Philadelphia, Lea & Febiger, 1972.

53. Goodglass H, Kaplan E: *The Assessment of Aphasia and Related Disorders,* 2nd ed. Philadelphia, Lea & Febiger, 1983.

54. Hagen C: Diagnosis and treatment of language disorders secondary to closed head injury. Presented at the Rehabilitation of the Brain-Injured Young Adult conference, Leesburg, VA., 1983.

55. Okazaki, H: *Fundamentals of Neuropathology.* Tokyo, Igaku-Shoin, 1983, pp 62–72, 107–109.

56. Mitchell SK, Yates RR: Cerebral vasospasm: Theoretical causes, medical management and nursing implications. *J Neurosci Nurs* 1986;18(6):315–324.

57. Vinuela F: Update on intravascular functional evaluation and therapy of intracranial arteriovenous malformations. *Neuroimaging Clin North Am* 1992;2(2):297–289.

58. Weil ML. Infections of the nervous system, in Menkes JH (ed): *Textbook of Child Neurology.* Philadelphia, Lea & Febiger, 1985, pp 316–431.

59. Bale JF Jr: Encephalitis and other virus-induced neurologic disorders, in Joynt RJ (ed): *Clinical Neurology,* Philadelphia, JB Lippincott, 1993, pp 1–86.

60. Stuss DT, Benson DF: *The Frontal Lobes.* New York, Raven Press, 1986.

BIBLIOGRAPHY

Damasio AR, Damasio H: Brain and language. *Sci Am* 1992;267(3):89–95.

Fischbach GD: Mind and brain. *Sci Am* 1992;267(3):48–57.

Goodman CS, Jessell TM: Development. *Curr Opin Neurobio* 1992;2(1):1–141.

Heilman KM, Valenstein E: *Clinical Neuropsychology.* New York, Oxford University Press, 1985.

Kandel ER: Brain and behavior, in Kandel ER, Schwartz JH (eds): *Principles of Neural Science,* 2nd ed. North Holland, Elsevier, 1985, p 3.

Kandel ER: Synapse formation, trophic interactions between neurons and the development of behavior, in Kandel ER, Schwartz JH (eds): *Principles of Neural Science,* 2nd ed. North Holland, Elsevier, 1985, p 743.

Kandel ER, Hawkins RD: The biological basis of learning and individuality. *Sci Am* 1992;267(3):78–86.

Kolb B, Whishaw IQ: *Fundamentals of Human Neuropsychology.* San Francisco, WH Freeman, 1980.

Meier M, Benton A, Diller L: *Neuropsychological Rehabilitation.* New York, Guilford Press, 1987.

Noback CR, Demarst RJ: *The Human Nervous System: Basic Principles of Neurobiology,* 2nd ed. New York, McGraw-Hill, 1975.

Restak RM: *The Mind.* Toronto, Bantam Books, 1988.

Shatz CJ: The developing brain. *Sci Am* 1992;267(3):61–67.

Wilson BA: *Rehabilitation of Memory.* New York, Guilford Press, 1987.

CHAPTER 44
Chronic Disorders of Neurologic Function

DEBRA WINSTON-HEATH and LEE-ELLEN C. COPSTEAD

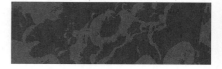

KEY TERMS

brain stem: Portion of the brain made up of the midbrain, pons, and medulla oblongata.

cerebellum: Portion of the brain, attached to the brain stem, that plays an essential role in maintaining muscle tone and coordinating normal movements.

cerebral dysrhythmia: An abnormality in an otherwise normal rhythmic pattern, as seen on electroencephalography.

cerebrospinal fluid: Fluid found in the cavities and canals of the brain and spinal cord.

cerebrum: Portion of the brain that controls consciousness, memory, sensations, emotions, and voluntary movements. The largest part of the brain, it consists of two hemispheres.

diencephalon: "Between" brain; parts of the brain between cerebral hemispheres and the midbrain.

electroencephalogram: Graphic tracing of brain's action potentials; used to evaluate nervous tissue function.

epileptogenic focus: Cellular focus with the capacity to induce epilepsy.

hypothalamus: Portion of diencephalon; vital neuroendocrine and autonomic control center.

limbic system: A group of structures surrounding the corpus callosum that produces various emotional feelings.

meninges: Membranes surrounding the brain and spinal cord.

paroxysm: A sudden outburst or change from the norm, as in a sudden burst of electrical activity, seen on electroencephalography, as occurs with seizure activity.

reticular formation: Fibers within the brain stem that arouse the cerebrum.

thalamus: Portion of diencephalon; mass of gray matter involved in relay of sensory information, emotion, arousal, and complex reflexes.

ventricles: Fluid-filled spaces within the brain.

Chapters 42 and 43 described the interdependence of the structure and function of the central nervous system. Such interdependence is especially evident in the communication that exists within all the neuraxes. This neural communication results in the processing of sensory information, maintenance of homeostasis, and purposeful human behavior.

Patients experiencing neurologic dysfunction from chronic disease states present a challenge to health care professionals, who must strive to maximize the patients' function and quality of life. A similar challenge is faced by professionals working with individuals with disorders of brain function. This chapter focuses on common disabilities of the neuraxes due to chronic disease states.

Epilepsy

Epilepsy is a disorder characterized by recurrent paroxysmal episodes of abnormal or excessive cortical electrical discharges. Epilepsy may be manifested in disturbances of skeletal motor function, sensation, autonomic visceral function, behavior, or consciousness. The disorder is said to be paroxysmal because the symptoms are not constant and the length of time between epileptic episodes is extremely variable. Because epilepsy is a component of more than 50 diseases, it is often referred to as a *syndrome* instead of an isolated disease.[1]

It is difficult to estimate the prevalence of epilepsy because it is not a reportable disease. It is believed that epilepsy affects 0.5 to 2.0 percent of the U.S. population, and that 80 percent of all epileptic episodes occur before the age of 20.[2] As epilepsy is a chronic condition, these statistics are even more impressive. In fact, epilepsy is the second most common neurologic disorder, surpassed only by stroke. With appropriate anticonvulsant management, 50 to 80 percent

of people with epilepsy can have their disease controlled.

Etiology

There are numerous causes of the syndrome of epilepsy. The etiological variables are briefly discussed here, and the reader is referred to the reference list for more detailed information.

Under the right circumstances, anyone can experience an epileptic event or seizure.[1] For some individuals, however, there appears to be a genetic tendency toward **cerebral dysrhythmia.** In such cases the threshold for seizure activity is lower than normal. Interestingly, not all individuals with cerebral dysrhythmia as demonstrated by **electroencephalography** (EEG) experience seizures.

Epilepsy can be acquired as a consequence of cerebral injury or other pathologic processes. Some acquired pathologic conditions that can result in epilepsy are due to structural lesions; examples are head injury, infections, space-occupying lesions, and cerebrovascular disorders. When epilepsy develops as a consequence of a structural injury, the temporal onset is not predictable. In some cases epilepsy may not develop for months or years after the initiation of the structural change (e.g., trauma, tumor growth) as the evolution of structural alterations in the involved cellular tissue may be very gradual. Metabolic and nutritional disorders that cause epilepsy include electrolyte and water imbalance, hypoxia, acidosis, pyridoxine deficiency, and toxins (e.g., heavy metals, street drugs, theophylline overdose). Finally, in some individuals no explanation for the disorder can be found. These individuals are classified as having an idiopathic epileptic disorder.

An epileptic event is often triggered by specific stimuli, usually unique for each individual. Physical inducements include specific sensory stimuli such as flashing lights, loud noises, and rhythmic music. Fever, physical exhaustion, inadequate nutrition, menses, hyperventilation, injury, and drugs can also

---

The section on epilepsy was contributed by Mary Sanguinetti-Baird.

prompt a seizure. Psychosocial factors include family and environmental stress, shock, and emotional stress.

Pathogenesis

Epilepsy is due to an alteration in membrane potential that makes certain neurons abnormally hyperactive and hypersensitive to changes in their environment. These physiologically abnormal neurons form an **epileptogenic focus,** that is, an area from which the seizure emanates. The epileptogenic focus functions autonomously, emitting excessively large numbers of **paroxysmal discharges.** The focus can be enhanced or suppressed, depending on the neurotransmitter at the postsynaptic membrane. Nerve cells in the epileptogenic focus can recruit neurons in adjacent areas as well as synaptically related neurons in distant areas, greatly enhancing the number of neurons involved in the seizure activity. Recruitment can also incorporate neurons in the opposite hemisphere by way of connecting pathways.[3] Clinical symptoms become evident when a sufficient number of neurons has been excited. Seizures are classified according to these clinical symptoms and the EEG features. It is important to realize that abnormal electrical discharges may occur in the absence of clinical manifestation. As with other pathologies of Neuro Axis I, the nature of the clinical manifestation depends on the area of the brain involved, both the area of origin and the area to which the seizure spreads.

Classification

Seizures are known as **partial** when they involve part of the brain. Partial seizures are further divided into simple and complex. In **simple partial seizures,** the individual does not lose consciousness. Seizures may be characterized by motor symptoms limited to one part of the body. On the other hand, a *jacksonian march* results in a systematic topographic spread of motor involvement along the motor strip of the cortex. Simple partial seizures may also be sensory in nature, resulting in somatic experiences such as tingling or numbness, or may involve the special senses, producing auditory, olfactory, or visual manifestations. Autonomic and psychic forms are also common in simple partial seizures.

Complex partial seizures begin as simple partial seizures that progress to impairment of consciousness. At the onset of consciousness impairment, the individual often displays automatisms such as lip smacking or repetitive or semipurposeful movements. There may be a display of aggressive behavior as well, especially if bystanders attempt to restrain the individual. Partial seizures that initially involve a focal area and then spread to involve the entire brain are said to secondarily generalize. All seizures preceded by an *aura* are referred to as partial seizures that secondarily generalize.

Episodes in which the entire brain is involved from the onset of the seizure are referred to as **generalized seizures.** Spread to the thalamus and reticular activating system results in loss of consciousness. This category includes absence, atypical absence, myoclonic, atonic (drop attack), clonic, tonic, and tonic-clonic (grand mal) seizures. Metabolic or toxin-induced seizures tend to be generalized; however, if the underlying cause is removed, these seizures usually do not recur.

Absence or **petit mal seizures** usually occur only in children. They are very brief (2–10 seconds) and characterized by staring spells that last only seconds. During the spell the individual is unaware of the surrounding environment and usually motionless; however, it is not uncommon for the person to continue walking or performing a routine motor task. **Atypical absence seizures** have accompanying myoclonic jerks and automatisms with the staring spell. The EEG patterns are unique to each syndrome. **Myoclonic seizures** are extremely brief and are characterized by a single jerk of one or more muscle groups. **Atonic seizures** or **drop attacks** are sometimes associated with myoclonic episodes. **Clonic seizures** involve jerking of muscle groups, while **tonic seizures** result in stiffening of muscle groups.

Some people may have a subjective sense of an impending seizure. This *prodromal period* may be characterized by any one of several phenomena, such as a type of movement, palpitations, or epigastric sensations, which may precede the actual seizure by several hours. In about half of cases there is some type of movement or odd sensory experience that occurs seconds before consciousness is lost and is remembered by the individual after recovery from the seizure. This experience is known as an *aura.* Although the individual may interpret the aura as an indication that a seizure is about to occur, in fact it is the beginning of the seizure episode. Auras can be significant, as they may be a clue to the location of the epileptogenic focus.

In a **grand mal seizure,** the person experiences a loss of consciousness and falls to the ground. The initial motor signs include opening of the mouth and eyes, extension of the legs, and adduction of the arms. Then the jaws snap shut, often resulting in tongue biting, and the individual emits a high-pitched cry as the whole musculature is seized in a spasm and air is forced out of the lungs through closed vocal cords. Breathing is impossible, as respiratory muscles are caught in the tonic spasm. Within seconds, the skin and mucous membranes become cyanotic. The bowel and bladder may empty at this time. This is the *tonic phase* and lasts about 10 to 15 seconds.

The transition to the *clonic phase* initially manifests with trembling that rapidly progresses to violent, rhythmic, muscular contractions. During this phase the eyes roll, the face grimaces, and the pulse accelerates. If the tongue has been lacerated, bloody, frothy saliva may seep through closed lips as salivation increases and bathes the lacerated tongue. The individual sweats profusely. The entire clonic phase lasts 1 to 2 minutes, with a gradual decline in amplitude and frequency of clonic jerks. The individual remains apneic until the end of the clonic phase, which is marked by a deep inspiration.

The *terminal phase* (postictal phase) is marked by absence of movement. The individual is limp and in deep coma. This lasts for about 5 minutes at which time the person will start to open the eyes but is clearly disoriented and confused. If allowed, the individual will readily fall into a deep sleep for several hours, only to awaken with a headache and sore muscles and tongue but no recollection of the incidence except for the aura if it was present. During the seizure the person is at risk for injury from both the initial fall after losing consciousness and from the violent muscle contractions of the clonic phase.

A potentially life-threatening situation known as **status epilepticus** occurs in some seizure disorders. Status epilepticus is a continuing series of seizures without an intercritical period of recovery between seizure episodes. It can occur with all type of seizures but is most common in generalized convulsions. Studies in animals have revealed that the increased metabolic activity that occurs during status epilepticus results in ischemic brain damage if the state continues untreated for 30 to 40 minutes.[4] Thus, not only is it imperative to ensure an adequate airway and ventilation, but the seizures themselves must be stopped.

Diagnosis and Treatment

The diagnosis of epilepsy is typically based on the history, physical and neurologic examination results, and EEG studies. EEGs may be normal between seizures, so activation techniques (sleep deprivation, hyperventilation) may be used to elicit the pathology. Laboratory studies are frequently used to investigate metabolic abnormalities as well as therapeutic serum levels in those already using anticonvulsants. Initial studies ruling out structural causes may include computed tomography (CT) or magnetic resonance imaging (MRI).

Management of an individual experiencing a seizure is concentrated on maintaining an airway and protecting the individual from injury. Recording the course of the seizure episode is useful for identifying the location of the epileptogenic focus, and for noting any change in the pattern and general management of the condition. The information recorded should include the time of onset, the duration of the seizure, precipitating factors, the presence of an aura, the sequence of seizure activity, autonomic signs, the level of consciousness, and the postictal state.

Long-term management depends on the cause. If possible, as in epilepsy due to metabolic abnormalities, infection, or tumors, the precipitating source is removed. If the epilepsy is due to irreversible factors, anticonvulsant medications specific to the type of seizure are the best management. The objective of therapy is to achieve seizure control with minimal side effects. This is a form of control, not a cure. Manage-

ment also includes patient education in the avoidance of activating factors (e.g., stress, loud noises, alcohol). For some individuals with intractable epilepsy, surgical excision of the seizure focus may be an option.

Life-style adjustments are often necessary when someone is given the diagnosis of epilepsy. As with all chronic conditions, patients may be frightened and resistant to therapeutic recommendations. Compliance with healthy life-style patterns and medication routines can be greatly facilitated by appropriate education and the availability of resources and support groups. Counseling may be useful for the person who is having difficulty with self-image or coping with illness. Health care workers involved with educating patients and their families are faced with the challenge of helping individuals maintain dignity, social involvement, and maximum independence even as they provide education on the pharmacologic management, side effects from medicines, and, perhaps most important, the safety implications relative to working environments, driving, and sports activities. Another very important activity for the health care worker is educating the public regarding the disorder in an attempt to dissolve prejudices and foster resources for support.

KEY CONCEPTS

- Epilepsy is characterized by recurrent episodes of abnormal electrical impulses in the brain (seizures). Some individuals appear to have a lower than normal threshold for seizure activity. Seizure activity may occur in anyone, given the right conditions. Head injury, meningitis, brain tumors, and metabolic disorders (electrolyte imbalance, fever, acidosis) may predispose to seizure.

- Initiation of seizure activity may occur in a particular brain area, the epileptogenic focus. Nearby and distant neurons may then be recruited into the seizure. When sufficient neurons are involved, the seizure becomes clinically evident as involuntary movement or unusual sensations.

- Seizures are classified as partial and generalized. Partial seizures involve a part of the brain, generalized seizures involve the entire brain at the onset. Partial seizures are further classified as simple, in which consciousness is retained, and complex, in which consciousness is impaired. Seizures may begin as partial and then generalize to affect the entire brain. Generalized seizures include absence, myoclonic, atonic, and tonic-clonic types. Consciousness is always impaired. The quality of an aura may be an important clue to the location of the epileptogenic focus.

- Status epilepticus is a serious condition in which seizures occur continuously, resulting in intense brain metabolism. Ischemic brain damage may result. Management of a seizure in progress is aimed at maintaining the individual's airway and protecting the person from trauma. Close attention is given to the quality and progression of seizure activity. Anticonvulsant medications are used to suppress seizure activity.

Dementia

Epidemiology

Dementia is a progressive degenerative disease state associated with deterioration of memory and additional cognitive functions. Adams and Victor[5] suggest that this definition is too narrow, as personality and behavior changes accompany the cognitive deterioration, and that many causes exist for this disorder. Because the onset of dementia is insidious, the affected individual may initially appear disinterested or lacking in initiative, with the gradual development of forgetfulness. Additional cognitive functions, language, and physical abilities are impaired as the disease progresses. Frequently, in the late stages of dementia, the individual is bedridden. Death is commonly due to infection.

Accurate data on the prevalence of dementia are not available; however, it is estimated that 4 to 5 percent of the U.S. population over 65 years of age have severe dementia, and an additional 10 percent have mild to moderate dementia.[6] If one considers the affected population by various age cohorts, the prevalence rates become even more interesting. For example, in the 65- to 70-year-old age group, the prevalence of severe dementia is only 1 percent; however, in those 85 years old or older, the prevalence rate increases to above 15 percent. These numbers are particularly impressive when one considers that the cohort of people aged 85 years or older is one of the fastest growing segments of our society.[7] If the current rate of increase remains unchanged, it is estimated that by the year 2040, 45 percent of the population will be at risk of developing dementia at some point in their lives.

Etiology

Multiple types of dementia exist, and a full discussion of each is beyond the scope of this chapter. Some examples of dementing diseases are dementia of the Alzheimer's type, multi-infarct dementia, and dementia associated with alcoholism, intracranial tumors, normal-pressure hydrocephalus, or Huntington's disease. Because the dementia of Alzheimer's disease is the most frequently occurring type of dementia in adults,[5] the following discussion of pathophysiology will focus on this disease. The subsequent discussion of the management of people with dementia will be more general, for the care issues are similar regardless of the type of dementia.

Pathogenesis

Structural lesions of the cerebral hemispheres and diencephalon are associated with dementia. Although the neuronal damage may be diffuse, the temporal and frontal lobes are frequently involved in dementing diseases.[5] At autopsy, the brain of the patient with Alzheimer's disease reveals two major neuropathologic lesions, neurofibrillary tangles and amyloid deposits in the form of senile plaques and cerebrovascular accumulations. The appearance of tangles seems to represent dying neurons in several degenerative neurologic diseases. The amyloid plaques, however, occur only in Alzheimer's disease, Down's syndrome, and normal aging. The number of senile plaques seems to correlate well with the degree of dementia in the Alzheimer patient.[8] Gross examination of the brain of the Alzheimer patient after death also finds that it is atrophic, often weighing less than 1,000 grams, compared with a normal brain weight of approximately 1,380 grams. The temporoparietal and anterior frontal regions of the brain are chiefly affected, exhibiting enlarged sulci and atrophic gyri.[9]

The pathophysiology of the various dementias remains under investigation; however, much interest exists in the neurotransmitter systems in relation to Alzheimer's disease.[10] Several studies have found abnormalities in the cholinergic system, including reduced activity of choline acetyltransferase (the enzyme necessary for acetylcholine synthesis) and decreased acetylcholine synthesis. Fortunately, as the neurobiology of Alzheimer's disease becomes better understood, progress in the search for therapeutics is under way.[11] One new experimental agent is tacrine (Cognex), which has been designed to increase brain acetylcholine levels. Additional investigators have found correlations with early-onset disease and more severe dysfunction of the cholinergic system.[7] The degeneration of cells in the nucleus basalis, a band of gray matter in the ventral portion of the medulla oblongata, has been linked to the diminished levels of acetylcholine in the cerebral cortex, a finding that provides further evidence for the significant role of the cholinergic system in Alzheimer's disease. Genetic factors have been found to play a role in some cases of dementia of the Alzheimer's type.[12] A major key to decoding the etiology of Alzheimer's disease has been provided by the discovery of beta protein, which is the major component of the amyloid fibrils of the plaques and cerebral vessels as well as the neurofibrillary tangles. Similar lesions in elderly patients with Down's syndrome are also composed of beta protein. Genes for beta protein and familial Alzheimer's disease have been localized to chromosome 21.[9] Further study of the genes responsible for Down's syndrome on chromosme 21 may provide information on the series of events causing dementia of the Alzheimer's type.[12]

Besides this abnormal protein theory, two other major theories about the etiology of Alzheimer's dementia have been posited. The *slow virus theory* suggests that certain viruses with an incubation period of 2 to 30 years enter the brain through a disruption in the blood-brain barrier. Some investigators theorize that head trauma disrupts the blood-brain barrier, producing a portal of entry for the virus. This possibility has some support, since a history of head trauma has been associated with the subsequent development of Alzheimer's dementia in certain individuals. Nevertheless, transmission of a slow virus is difficult to prove.

The *aluminum toxicity theory* is based on the findings of aluminum deposits in the brains of patients with Alzheimer's disease. Although aluminum intoxication produces similar pathology, its role in the etiology of Alzheimer's disease remains unclear.

Treatment

The initial management of a patient thought to have dementia of any type begins with thorough evaluation by a skilled clinician to rule out treatable conditions that might explain the presenting symptoms. At some point in the evaluation, input from responsible family members is necessary to validate existing data and supply additional information regarding the presenting problem. Of note, a potentially reversible psychiatric condition is found in almost 1 in 20 patients evaluated for dementia in a neurology center. Other treatable causes of dementia include brain tumor, chronic drug intoxication, cryptococcosis, neurosyphilis, normal-pressure hydrocephalus, pellagra, subdural hematoma, and certain endocrine and metabolic disorders.[5,13] A complete review of the patient's current medications should be included in this evaluation, as many medications, including antihistamines, barbiturates, benzodiazepines, cimetidine, digoxin, diuretics, ibuprofen, and levodopa, have been reported to affect memory.[7]

When all treatable causes of dementia have been ruled out, the treatment focuses on patient wellness and symptom management. People in the early stages of a dementing disease should be provided with information regarding surrogate decision makers and advance directives regarding their preferences for health care decisions. Such information is invaluable as the disease progresses, as it is difficult for healthy individuals to determine the quality of life of a demented person without knowledge of that peron's wishes. Efforts directed at wellness include optimal management of existing medical conditions (e.g., chronic pulmonary disease, diabetes), nutritional management, and protecting the patient from injury. Recent efforts in treating depression in demented persons has resulted in increased function for these persons.[14] Optimal management of existing chronic conditions can have a tremendous effect on the demented brain, as the diseased brain has a decreased ability to adapt to metabolic changes (e.g., changes in arterial blood gas values or temperature). This decreased adaptive ability of the brain may be readily observed in the decline in cognitive function or behavioral changes in the demented person with a fever.

Because the majority of demented persons in the United States live at home with caregivers until the later stages of disease, there is much that the health care professional can do to assist the caregiver with patients' daily management. Efforts to assist the caregiver have been outlined by Hall[15] and include (1) education for patients and family regarding the disease and its progression, (2) the development of routines and strategies to enhance optimal behavior, (3) simplification of daily care activities, (4) resource location and network development, and (5) social support and patient advocacy. Such educational efforts might include teaching the caregivers about stressors that may aggravate dysfunctional behavior in demented patients. Among these stressors are changes in routine, excessive demands, fatigue, overwhelming stimuli, and physical stressors (e.g., illness).[15] The functional losses due to a dementing illness may be all-encompassing, eventually affecting all aspects of human function as the dementia progresses. Initial functional deficits may begin with simple forgetfulness and progress to cognitive functions (e.g., problem solving and decision making), behavioral changes, communication, swallowing and nutrition, self-care, elimination, sleep, and safety.

KEY CONCEPTS

- **Dementia refers to progressive degeneration of cognitive function due to organic causes. In many instances the cause is unknown. There is no definitive treatment for dementia, and it is important to first rule out treatable causes of mental impairment.**

- **The dementia of Alzheimer's disease is characterized by degeneration of neurons in temporal and frontal lobes, brain atrophy, and amyloid plaques. The synthesis of brain acetylcholine is deficient. The etiology of Alzheimer's disease is unknown. Several theories have been proposed, including a viral origin and aluminum toxicity.**

- **The behavioral problems of people with Alzheimer's disease may be exacerbated by changes in routine and excess stimulation. Alzheimer's disease progresses from forgetfulness to total inability to care for self. Depression may be significant.**

Parkinson's Disease

Epidemiology

Parkinson's disease is a disorder of mobility that affects nearly 1 percent of the U.S. population older than 50 years. The disease occurs in adults from the ages of 40 to 70 years, with onset most frequently occurring in the sixth decade of life. The disease exists in all countries and all ethnic and socioeconomic groups.[5]

Etiology

Parkinson's disease may be idiopathic or acquired. Idiopathic cases of Parkinson's disease are those in which no demonstrable cause is identified. Common causes of acquired parkinsonism include infection and intoxication.[16] Infectious cases of Parkinson's disease date back to the early 1900s and were associated with an epidemic of encephalitis lethargica. Interestingly, no cases were reported before the period 1914–1918, and no additional cases have been reported since 1930; thus, postencephalitic parkinsonism has essentially disappeared. Rare cases of parkinsonism have since been reported in association with coxsackievirus group B and Japanese B encephalitis.

Typically, parkinsonism due to drug toxicities evolves rapidly, unlike the slow, insidious onset of the idiopathic disease. Side effects of drugs of the phenothiazine class (e.g., chlorpromazine, prochlorperazine, and thioridazine) and butrophenone class (e.g., haloperidol) may manifest in a parkinsonian syndrome at toxic levels. Stopping the medication generally results in improvement in the symptoms of masked facies, tremor, slowness of movement, shuffling gait, and generalized rigidity. However, use of the anticholinergic antiparkinsonian drugs may aid in more rapid recovery. Recently, a neurotoxin derived from meriperidine analogues (known as MPTP) has been associated with an irreversible form of parkinsonism.[5]

Pathogenesis

Parkinson's disease affects the basal ganglia of the extrapyramidal system, specifically the substantia nigra, caudate, and putamen nuclei. Dopamine levels in the brains of patients who die of Parkinson's disease are less than 10 percent of the levels found in normal brains. Additional studies have found lower than normal levels of the enzymes needed for the metabolism of dopa to dopamine in the same basal ganglia nuclei. Interestingly, microscopic changes found in the brains of parkinsonian patients with dementia include amyloid plaques and neurofibrillary tangles similar to those found in the brains of individuals with Alzheimer's disease. The prevalence of dementia in parkinsonian patients has been estimated to be between 30 percent and 50 percent.[46]

Clinical Manifestations and Treatment

Because of the insidious onset, earlier evidence of Parkinson's disease may be discovered in a thorough history taken by an expert clinician. Frequently, the very early signs of the disorder (loss of flexibility, aching, and fatigue) are overlooked by the patient or are attributed to the aging process. Often the characteristic tremor (4–10 cycles per second) of the disease, though absent in approximately 30 percent of the patients,[16] is the initial symptom that prompts the patient to seek medical assistance. Additional early signs of the disease include bradykinesia, rigidity, and hypokinesia (loss of facial expression and infrequent eye blinking) (Fig. 44–1). Again, these symptoms may be overlooked by the patient, but they are usually apparent to observant family members.

As the disease progresses additional functional changes are noted. The patient's handwriting may become small (micrographia) and cramped, with evidence of tremor. Speech may become low in volume, monotonous, and dysarthric. There may be a "mumbling" quality to the speech. The effects of bradykinesia are evident in the patients' swallowing function, ability to initiate activity, and mobility. Swallowing becomes delayed, so much so that the individual cannot keep up with the normal flow of saliva and will frequently drool. Impaired swallowing function results in substantially lengthened meal times as the disease progresses, in addition to an increased risk of aspiration. The effect of the disease on the ability to initiate activity is evident when the individual rises from a chair or begins to walk from a standing-still position. Many people with Parkinson's disease, however, are able to act quickly in times of emergency, such as a fire. This phenomenon is known as paradoxical kinesia.

Additional difficulties in mobility are evident from the lack of spontaneous position changes while the individual is sitting in one position, from the decreased or absent arm swing while the individual is walking, and from the shuffling gait. Impairment of postural reflexes presents particular safety problems for the individual with Parkinson's disease in maintaining balance, as evidenced by propulsive or retropulsive gaits. Involvement of the autonomic nervous system may result in orthostatic hypotension, which adds yet another risk to the individual's health. Because of these various impairments, falls are a frequent problem. Patients with these functional problems often benefit from consultation with a speech pathologist for speech and swallowing difficulties, with a physical therapist for mobility and balance problems, and with an occupational therapist to enhance their self-care abilities.

Because there is no known cure for Parkinson's disease, treatment focuses on the delicate balance of medications to minimize side effects while yielding optimal function.[17] Classes of drugs utilized in the treatment of Parkinson's disease include dopamine precursors, dopamine agonists, anticholinergics, antihistamines, monoamine oxidase inhibitors,[18] and antidepressants. The side effects of postural hypotension and hallucinations may occur with the dopamine precursors and the antihistamines. These side effects directly affect the safe function of the individual with Parkinson's disease. Research involving transplantation of autologous adrenal medulla tissue into the caudate nucleus as treatment for Parkinson's disease has not been as promising as once hoped, and the transplantation of fetal tissue remains controversial.[19] The rationale for transplanting adrenal medulla tissue is to reestablish a physiologic source of dopamine to the brain. The extent to which this graft reintegrates into the neural circuitry varies, as does the long-term survival and function of the transplanted nerve cells.[20] Other neurosurgical techniques to be considered in the treatment of Parkinson's disease include subthalamotomy and pallidotomy. These techniques represent an attempt to ameliorate symptoms of Parkinson's disease by interrupting one or more neuronal path-

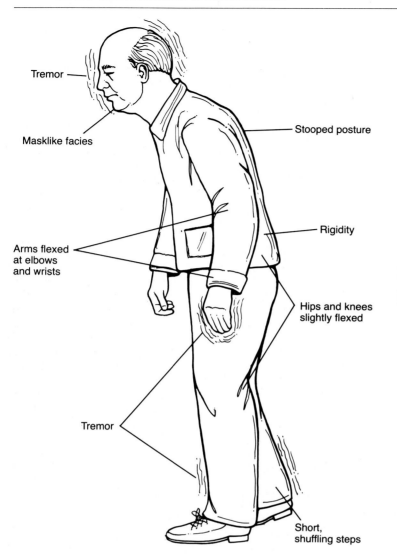

Tremor

Masklike facies

Stooped posture

Rigidity

Arms flexed
at elbows
and wrists

Hips and knees
slightly flexed

Tremor

Short,
shuffling steps

FIGURE 44–1. Clinical manifestations of Parkinson's disease. (From Monahan FD, Drake T, Neighbors M: *Nursing Care of Adults.* Philadelphia, WB Saunders, 1994, p 1513. Reproduced with permission.)

ways through electrocoagulation or freezing the ventrolateral nucleus of the thalamus. Sympathalamotomy and pallidotomy have been shown to relieve contralateral tremor and rigidity in the limbs. These areas demonstrate a great potential for expanded knowledge of the pathology underlying neurodegenerative diseases and also, perhaps, the definitive therapies.

KEY CONCEPTS

- Parkinson's disease may be idiopathic or a consequence of certain drugs. Dopamine deficiency in the basal ganglia (substantia nigra, caudate, and putamen) is associated with symptoms of motor impairment. Difficulty initiating and controlling movements results in akinesia, tremor, and rigidity. Tremor occurs at rest and in the hands may be described as pill-rolling movements. Attempts to passively move the extremities are met with cogwheel rigidity. There is a general lack of movement, loss of facial expression, drooling, propulsive gait, and absent arm swing.

- Treatment is aimed at restoring brain dopamine levels or activity by administration of dopamine precursors, dopamine agonists, monoamine oxidase inhibitors, and anticholinergics.

Multiple Sclerosis

Epidemiology

Multiple sclerosis (MS) is a demyelinating disease of the CNS that causes significant disability in young adults. MS is the third most common cause of disability in people between the ages of 15 and 60 years,[21] and probably accounts for more disability, health care costs, and lost wage earnings than any other neurologic disease in this age group. The age at onset ranges from 10 to 50 years, and the disease tends to have a predilection for persons of northern European descent.[21] Studies by Kurtzke and associates[5,22] have confirmed an increased risk of acquiring MS with increasing geographic latitude. The prevalence rate of

MS in the United States is 57.8 per 100,000. Above the 37th parallel, the prevalence is reported at 68.8 per 100,000, and below it is reported at 35.5 per 100,000.[21]

Etiology

Despite much research and increased knowledge over decades, the etiology of MS remains unknown. However, there is evidence to suggest that exposure to some environmental agent in genetically susceptible individuals with immune system abnormalities[23] may result in the development of MS. A variety of studies have documented abnormalities in the immune system of individuals with MS. Some of these abnormalities include a selective increase in certain immunoglobulins (primarily IgG, less frequently IgM or IgA),[24] abnormalities in immunocompetent cells (T-helper/inducer lymphocytes, T-suppressor/cytotoxic lymphocytes, macrophages, and B-cells),[21,25] and a significant association with certain human leukocyte antigen (HLA) complexes. The HLA complex is concerned with the genetic control of the immune system.[21,25] Considerable research has focused on viruses and the immune response. However, many unanswered questions remain concerning the special role of the immune system in lesion formation.[22,26]

Pathogenesis

Although much has been learned about MS since the development of the experimental model of the disease in the early 1930s, the pathogenesis of the disease remains poorly understood. Demyelination may occur throughout the CNS. The structures most frequently involved are the optic nerves, oculomotor nerves, and the corticospinal, cerebellar, and posterior column systems.[21] Because myelin facilitates nerve conduction, lesions in the stated structures may result in visual loss, diplopia, disorders of eye movement, motor weakness, spasticity, gait disturbance, coordination problems, and sensory deficits.

Clinical Manifestations and Treatment

Because there is no conclusive test for MS, the diagnosis is based on clinical characteristics and laboratory evidence. Clinical characteristics include objective abnormalities of CNS function in two parts of the CNS and a temporal sequence of at least two attacks that were remitting and relapsing or followed a slow stepwise progression over at least 6 months. The classic criteria for the diagnosis of MS by Schumacher and co-workers[27] have been adapted to include the laboratory data of oligoclonal bands and an elevated IgG index in the cerebrospinal fluid.[27] Oligoclonal bands are present in 77 to 93.5 percent of people with MS, and IgG is elevated in approximately 90 percent of people with MS.[28] Technological advances have increased the value of data from evoked potential recording (visual, brain stem, and somatosensory) and from neuroradiographic studies, specifically MRI, in the diagnostic workup for MS.[29,30]

MS presents in a wide spectrum of severity in different individuals. It is estimated that 30 percent of individuals with MS have a benign form, in which they experience one or two symptomatic attacks and enjoy functionally complete recovery of the symptoms. Roughly 10 percent of the MS population have a progressive form of the disease, in which they experience a malignant course from disease onset to severe disability within years.[21] Because demyelination may occur throughout the CNS, the presenting symptoms will correspond to the affected neuroanatomic structures. Losses in visual acuity and color perception may result from involvement of the optic nerves. Abnormalities of eye movements may result from oculomotor nerve involvement, and patients with abnormal eye movements may complain of seeing double images. Involvement of the motor system may manifest with spasticity and weakness. Patients may describe stiffness, spasm, or pain. Weakness may initially be noticed as difficulty in completing physical tasks of long duration, with eventual complaints of clumsiness. Coordination difficulties due to cerebellar involvement may be particularly disabling for individuals with MS. Stability of the trunk and gait may be affected, in addition to upper extremity function.[21] Speaking and swallowing function may also be impaired with cerebellar involvement. Impairment of bladder function has been estimated to occur in 50 to 80 percent of people with MS at some point during the course of the disease. Symptoms of bladder dysfunction may include urgency, frequency, incontinence, and retention.[31] Sensory symptoms may result from involvement of the sensory pathways. Patients may complain of "pins and needles"; sensory loss, although less common, may also be reported. Additional sensory symptoms may include impairment of two-point discrimination, graphesthesia, position sense, and vibratory function. Neurobehavioral symptoms commonly reported in MS patients include depression, emotional lability, memory impairment, sexual dysfunction, and fatigue.[21]

Recent interest has focused on the cognitive deficits in persons with MS. Memory problems, especially the retrieval function, are common.[32] Neuroimaging techniques suggest that disruption in the cortical-subcortical connections may be the cause of these deficits.[33]

Management of symptoms frequently enlists participation from multiple disciplines in the care of individuals with MS. These disciplines usually include medicine, nursing, speech pathology, occupational therapy, physical therapy, neuropsychology, social services, and vocational services. Treatment with an array of medicines such as antispasmodics, anticholinergics, antidepressants, and antimicrobials may be effective in symptom management. A variety of agents and regimens have been tried to manage acute exacerbations of this disease; however, effective treatment remains limited. Short-term treatment with corticosteroids (steroids) or adrenocorticotropic hormone

(ACTH) may benefit those experiencing an acute exacerbation of the disease.[31] Long-term use of steroids or ACTH is not recommended in the management of MS, as the risks outweigh the benefits. Additionally, there is some evidence to suggest that the effects of steroids decrease with repeated use. The role of immunotherapies in the treatment of MS is under investigation.[21,34–36]

KEY CONCEPTS

- Multiple sclerosis (MS) is a demyelinating disease of the CNS that primarily affects young adults. The risk of contracting MS is greater for persons living above the 37th parallel. The etiology of MS is unknown, but immunologic abnormalities and environmental factors are suspected.

- Demyelination can occur throughout the CNS but most frequently affects the optic and occulomotor nerves and spinal nerve tracts. In most cases symptoms are slowly progressive, marked by exacerbations and remissions. Symptoms include double vision, weakness, poor coordination, and sensory deficits. Bowel and bladder control may be lost. Memory impairment is common.

- Treatment is symptomatic. Short-term steroid therapy may be helpful during acute exacerbations.

Amyotrophic Lateral Sclerosis

Epidemiology

Amyotrophic lateral sclerosis (ALS) is a progressive degenerative disease affecting the motor system. The annual incidence is approximately 1.5 to 2.0 cases per 100,000, and the male-female ratio is about 1.7 : 1. The disease occurs worldwide. Typically, the onset of ALS occurs between ages 40 and 70 years; patients younger than 30 and older than 60 years make up only 10 percent of the cases.[37]

Etiology

The cause of ALS remains unknown, and no single hypothesis about etiology has been widely accepted. Proposed etiologies have included virions, immunologic factors, and environmental toxins.[38] Neuropathologic findings include degeneration of the motor neurons in the cortex, lower brain stem, and spinal cord.

Clinical Manifestations and Treatment

The classic sporadic form accounts for 90 to 95 percent of cases of ALS in the United States. Approximately 40 percent of these cases begin with weakness and wasting of the upper extremities; fewer than 20 percent begin with symptoms in the lower extremities.[39] Symptoms may be asymmetric in presentation. Dysarthria and dysphagia may result with involvement of the motor nuclei in the lower brain stem. Respiratory

function becomes compromised as the neural control of respiration is affected. The mean duration of survival for patients with ALS is 3 years, although longer survival rates have been reported.[40]

Because no cure exists, treatment is symptomatic and supportive. Patients with ALS frequently benefit from a multidisciplinary approach to care. In addition to medicine and nursing, speech pathology, nutritional services, physical therapy, occupational therapy, respiratory therapy, social services, and psychology may assist patients and their families in achieving optimal daily function. A discussion of advance directives regarding health care decisions is appropriate with ALS patients, preferably before they become dyspneic and their ability to communicate is severely impaired.

KEY CONCEPT

- The cause of amyotrophic lateral sclerosis remains unknown. Weakness and wasting of the upper extremities usually occur, followed by impaired speech, swallowing, and respiration. There is no effective treatment. The mean survival time is about 3 years from the time of diagnosis.

Guillain-Barré Syndrome

Epidemiology

Guillain-Barré syndrome, also known as acute infectious polyradiculoneuritis, is an inflammatory disease affecting the peripheral nervous system. The annual incidence of Guillain-Barré syndrome in the United States was reported to be 1.7 cases per 100,000 population in the United States National Surveillance Study. Slightly higher rates were noted among males than females, among whites than blacks, and in those more than 45 years old.[41] This disease affects all age groups and both sexes. It occurs worldwide and does not follow any seasonal pattern.[5]

Etiology

The cause of Guillain-Barré syndrome is unknown; however, much interest exists regarding immunologic events and their role in this disorder. Patients report a viral infection (lasting days or a few weeks) preceding the onset of symptoms in approximately 50 percent of the cases. Patient history, lack of association with a specific virus, and mononuclear cell infiltration with segmental demyelination suggest an immunologic reaction directed at the peripheral nerve.[5]

Clinical Manifestations and Treatment

As with other neurologic illnesses, an important part of the diagnostic workup is a careful history to rule out exposure to toxins or other metabolic conditions. Examination of the CSF and electrodiagnostic studies of nerve conduction provide additional valuable information. Typically, the CSF protein level rises and peaks 4 to 6 weeks after the initial onset of symptoms, and nerve conduction velocities are slowed.[5] The major symptom, weakness, develops over a period of a few days to a couple of weeks. Owing to the rapid development, most cases reach their peak severity in 10 to 14 days. Muscle atrophy is not evident. In the majority of cases, the weakness is ascending in nature, beginning with the lower extremities. Proximal and distal muscles are affected, with eventual involvement of the muscles of the trunk, thorax, neck, and those innervated by the cranial nerves. Sensory abnormalities, such as paresthesias and muscle discomfort, occur in some cases.[5] It is estimated that approximately half of people with Guillain-Barré syndrome experience the autonomic symptoms of altered blood pressure and cardiac arrhythmias.[41]

Spontaneous recovery is experienced by the majority of patients, although approximately 7 to 22 percent of patients are left with some residual disability. The reported mortality in adults ranges from 2 to 7 percent.[5,42] Similar data are not available for children; however, evidence suggests that the residual impairment is less severe.[42]

Treatment is primarily supportive, with the focus on excellent nursing and respiratory care. Symptoms due to weak muscles of respiration and swallowing present a great challenge to all concerned. A controlled multicenter study of 245 cases of Guillain-Barré syndrome examined the use of plasmapheresis in the acute management of this disease.[43] Results indicate that treatment within 2 weeks of onset decreased the length of time that the patients needed ventilatory support. Although plasmapheresis remains the best studied of the immunodulatory therapies for Guillain-Barré syndrome,[44] the use of intravenous immune globulin is under investigation.[45,46] Rehabilitation therapy programs are often helpful in assisting patients on the road back to a functional recovery.

KEY CONCEPT

> • Guillain-Barré syndrome is characterized by ascending muscle weakness that begins in the lower extremities and moves upward. The etiology is unknown; however, postviral immunologic mechanisms are suspected. Treatment is supportive and spontaneous recovery usually occurs.

Spinal Cord Injury

Spinal cord injury continues to be a major consequence of trauma. Although efforts have been increased to prevent spinal cord injury, the number of victims per year has remained the same for the last decade.[47]

Cervical spine injuries are devastating to the patient. Marked changes in life-style are required for the survivors of such injuries. Medical advances in the

treatment of spinal cord injury and its associated complications have been successful in increasing survival from the initial injury. Continuing research is focused on minimizing the mortality and morbidity of spinal cord injury.

Epidemiology

Spinal cord injury occurs most frequently in young people, with 80 percent of patients under age 40 and 50 percent between ages 15 and 25. The "typical" victim with spinal cord injury is a young man injured in a motor vehicle collision. Motor vehicle collisions account for 55 percent of all cases of spinal cord injury, followed by falls (21 percent) and sports injuries (18 percent).[47,48] Penetrating wounds are responsible for about 15 percent of all spinal cord injuries, but children experience a higher percentage of these injuries. The spinal cord of an infant can, while passing through the birth canal, be injured. Breech deliveries cause hyperextension of the head, and injury of the spinal cord and brain can result. The overstretched cord develops an hourglass narrowing at the cervical-thoracic juncture. In adults, especially middle-aged to elderly individuals, the spinal cord can be compressed by herniated intervertebral disks (slipped disks) or by spurs of bone that protrude between vertebral bodies degenerated by osteoarthritis. Injuries to the spinal cord are classified by level, degree (complete or incomplete), and mechanism of injury (Table 44–1).

Etiology

Spinal cord injury results from compression, contusion, or transection of the spinal cord. The major mechanisms of injury are hyperflexion, hyperextension, and compression (Fig. 44–2). Flexion injury with tearing of the posterior ligaments and dislocation is the most unstable injury and is often associated with severe neurologic deficits. Hyperextension injury is

TABLE 44–1. American Spinal Injury Association Impairment Scale

Classification	Description
A = Complete	No motor or sensory function is preserved in the sacral segments S4–S5.
B = Incomplete	Sensory but not motor function is preserved below the neurological level and extends through the sacral segments S4–S5.
C = Incomplete	Motor function is preserved below the neurological level, and the majority of key muscles below the neurological level have a muscle grade less than 3.
D = Incomplete	Motor function is preserved below the neurological level, and the majority of key muscles below the neurological level have a muscle grade greater than or equal to 3.
E = Normal	Motor and sensory function is normal.

From *Standards for Neurological and Functional Classification of Spinal Cord Injury*, American Spinal Injury Association, Chicago, Illinois, 1992. Reproduced with permission.

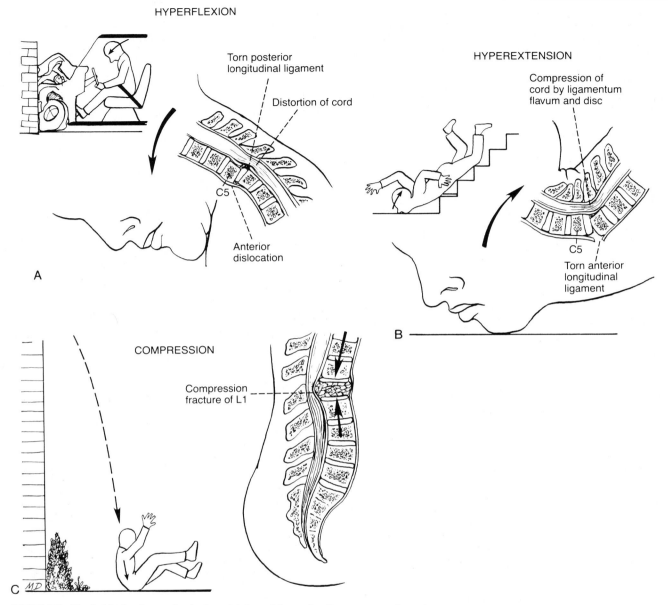

F I G U R E 44 – 2. Mechanisms of spinal cord injury. Many situations may produce these consequences. This figure shows examples only. (From Black JM, Matassarin-Jacobs E (eds): *Luckmann and Sorensen's Medical-Surgical Nursing: A Psychophysiologic Approach.* 4th ed. Philadelphia, WB Saunders, 1993, p 795. Reproduced with permission.)

the most common. After injury, hemorrhage and necrosis of the spinal cord often ensue. Compression of the cord and disruption of the cord blood vessels may follow.

Pathogenesis

Actual damage to the spinal cord is caused by a variety of factors, including morphologic damage to the spinal cord, hemorrhage, vascular damage, ischemia, structural changes in the gray and white matter, and other biochemical responses to the trauma.[49,50] The systemic hemodynamic changes that occur after spi-

nal cord injury are a major factor in the resulting damage to the spinal cord. Blood flow to the cord is profoundly decreased because of the loss of autoregulation immediately after the injury, which causes an overriding ischemic injury to the cord. The ischemia causes changes in tissue oxygen tension that ultimately affect all of the metabolic functions of the cells. As blood flow continues to be compromised, free radicals are released from the ischemic areas, increasing the area of the original injury. The optimal time for intervention to limit or reverse these destructive processes is within 4 hours of the injury, preferably within 60 to 90 minutes.[51]

The necrotic process consumes approximately 40 percent of the cross-sectional cord at the level of injury within 4 hours of trauma, and 70 percent of the cord may be destroyed within 24 hours.[52] After the necrotic process is complete, all of the cross-sectional level of the cord will be included in the necrosis, which will also extend several millimeters above and below the level of injury.

Clinical Manifestations and Treatment

Spinal Shock

Spinal shock is a physiologic disruption of the function of the spinal cord that accompanies spinal cord injury. It is a temporary suspension of function and reflexes below the level of injury. Symptoms include flaccid paralysis of all skeletal muscles, loss of all spinal reflexes; loss of pain sensation, proprioception, and other sensations; bowel and bladder dysfunction with paralytic ileus; and loss of thermoregulation. Spinal shock usually occurs at the time of the injury, but it may emerge up to 1 week after the injury. Spinal shock usually lasts 7 to 10 days after the injury, although it may be prolonged by infection or other complications.[51] A return of reflexes indicates the end of spinal shock. As spinal shock dissipates, flaccidity gives way to spasticity in the affected muscle groups.

Neurogenic Shock

In patients with a cervical or upper thoracic cord injury, another type of shock has been identified, neurogenic shock. **Neurogenic shock** is a form of distributive shock caused by the loss of brain stem and higher center control of the sympathetic nervous system. The loss of sympathetic outflow results in hypotension caused by peripheral vasodilation, bradycardia (secondary to the overriding parasympathetic influence), loss of cardiac accelerator reflex, and loss of the ability to sweat below the level of injury. The patient may be hypothermic because of the loss of impulses from the temperature regulatory center in the hypothalamus and the sympathetic nervous system.[52]

Patients who suffer cervical spinal cord injury with neurogenic shock need critical care for at least 3 days or until hemodynamic stability is reached. In addition to supporting hemodynamic stability, emphasis on supporting the patient's respiratory function is a component of the initial care. Ongoing assessment is critical. Systematic, methodical motor-sensory checks are important in determining improvement or deterioration in neurologic function. Monitoring of cardiovascular and respiratory status is critical. Skin and mobility assessments are necessary during this phase to identify potential complications early.

As the patient progresses, and once neurogenic and spinal shock have resolved, the rehabilitative process begins. Rehabilitation emphasizes independence and self-care. Levels of injury and expected functional ability are summarized in Table 44–2.

Autonomic Dysreflexia

Autonomic dysreflexia (hyperreflexia) is a serious condition occurring in spinal cord injuries at or above T6. It is characterized by a sudden episode of hypertension, headache, bradycardia, upper body flushing and lower body vasoconstriction, piloerection, and sweating. The usual stimulus initiating autonomic dys-

TABLE 44–2. Levels of Injury and Expected Functional Ability

Level	Normal Activity	Functional Expectation
C4	Head control Mouth control Shoulders/scapular movement Diaphragm movement	Use of a mouthstick for turning pages, typing, or writing
C5	Shoulder flexion Elbow flexion Increased scapular function	Feeds self with special adaptive devices Able to move wheelchair for short distances, does better with electric wheelchair Assists a little in self-care
C6	Good elbow flexion Wrist extension Shoulder rotation and abduction	Independent in feeding and some grooming with adaptive devices Weak hand grasp Can roll over in bed Can drive a car with hand controls Can assist in transfer
C7	Elbow extension Strong wrist extension Good shoulder movement	Transfers independently to chair Independent in most activities of daily living Excellent bed mobility
T1	Normal hand strength Normal upper extremity strength	Bed and wheelchair independent Performs self-catheterization Wheelchair independent

From Walleck C: Neurotrauma: spinal cord injury, in Barker E (ed): *Neuroscience Nursing*. St. Louis: Mosby–Year Book, 1994, p 355. Reproduced with permission.

reflexia is activation of visceral or cutaneous pain receptors below the level of injury. A full bladder is the most common initiating event.

Stimulation of afferent pain receptors causes activation of sympathetic efferents in the cord and reflex vasoconstriction. Sustained activation of sympathetic neurons below the level of cord injury increases blood pressure significantly. High blood pressure produces the symptom of headache and also initiates the baroreceptor response. Baroreceptors mediate inhibition of heart rate and vasodilation of vessels above the level of injury. Vasodilation is responsible for upper body flushing. Descending signals from the brain cannot pass the cord injury, so inhibition of sympathetic neurons below the level of injury does not occur. Continued vasoconstriction of the lower body is sufficient to sustain high blood pressure despite bradycardia and upper body vasodilation. Blood pressure may be dangerously high and may precipitate intracranial hemorrhage.

Treatment is aimed at removing the source of irritation. If the hypertension does not resolve, adrenergic receptor–blocking agents may be used. Removal of leg wraps and upright positioning will induce pooling of blood in the extremities and may assist blood pressure reduction.

Understandably, there is a terrific adjustment process with spinal cord injuries. During the rehabilitative phase, the patient begins to deal with the realities of a disability. The grieving process is a natural and expected part of rehabilitation. Anyone who cares for a patient with spinal cord injury must recognize the range of possible behaviors, which include withdrawal, extreme anger, and verbal abuse to physical demonstrations of frustration. These behaviors are a result of the injury and represent attempts of the injured person to deal with life alterations. Often support groups, patient-advocacy groups, and peer groups can serve as support for the patient and family. As the patient begins to adapt to a new life-style, the team approach to care becomes increasingly significant. Physical therapists, occupational therapists, nutritionists, psychologist, nurse, and physician work together to ensure optimal recovery. Reintegration into the community can be difficult. The ability to return to work can be complicated by the amount of time it takes to perform simple activities of daily living. In discharge planning, all aspects of life must be considered, including future hopes and desires. The needs and concerns of the patient's significant others must also be addressed throughout the hospitalization and during the discharge planning. Independence and self-care must be reinforced. Ongoing participation in care and counseling may be appropriate to provide the family and significant others the help they need to be able to support each other.

KEY CONCEPTS

- Spinal cord injury is usually traumatic, a result of motor vehicle accidents, falls, penetrating wounds or sports injuries. The cord may be compressed, transected or contused. Further injury may result from hemorrhage, swelling and ischemia post injury.
- Spinal shock occurs immediately following injury and is characterized by temporary loss of reflexes below the level of injury. Muscles are flaccid and skeletal and autonomic reflexes are lost. The end of spinal shock is noted when reflexes return and flaccidity is replaced by spasticity.
- Neurogenic shock may occur post spinal cord injury due to peripheral vasodilation. Hypotension and circulatory collapse may occur. High spinal cord injuries may also affect respiratory muscles leading to ventilatory failure.
- Autonomic dysreflexia is an acute reflexive response to sympathetic activation below the level of injury. Visceral stimulation (full bladder or bowel) or activation of pain receptors below the injury are common initiating stimuli. Manifestations include hypertension, bradycardia, flushing above the level of injury and clammy skin below the level of injury. Prompt removal of the offending stimulus is indicated.

Summary

A traumatic event such as a spinal cord injury or a chronic neurologic disease such as dementia can transform an individual from a relatively healthy state to one of almost complete dependence. At best, chronic neurologic states may require some life-style adjustment, but often they also require lifetime rehabilitation. Follow-up neurodiagnostic studies may be needed to augment the history and physical assessment findings.

The process of life care planning includes taking stock of current health status, future health care concerns, approriate resources, and associated costs to address lifelong disability/illness management. Many of the chronic neurologic diseases discussed in this chapter require life care patient planning.

In general, rehabilitation strives to increase self-care and promote a meaningful life-style that incorporates the neurologic disability. The primary goal is to help maintain the highest possible level of wellness while living with a disability.

REFERENCES

1. Hickey JV: *The Clinical Practice of Neurological and Neurosurgical Nursing*, 2nd ed. Philadelphia, JB Lippincott, 1986.
2. American Association of Neuroscience Nurses: *Core Curriculum for Neuroscience Nurses*. Chicago, American Association of Neuroscience Nurses, 1991.
3. Marshall LF, Barba D, Toole BM, Bowers SA: The oval pupil: Clinical significance and relationship to intracranial hypertension. *J. Neurosurg* 1983;58:566–568.
4. Marshall SB, Marshall LF, Vos HR, Chesnut RM: *Neuroscience Critical Care*. Philadelphia, WB Saunders, 1990.
5. Adams RR, Victor M: *Principles of Neurology*, 3rd ed. New York, McGraw-Hill, 1985.

6. Terry RD, Katzman R: Senile dementia of the Alzheimer type. *Ann Neurol* 1983;14:497–506.
7. McDermott JR, Fraser H, Dickinson AG: Reduced choline acetyltransferase activity in scrapie mouse brain. *Lancet* 1978;2:318–319.
8. Tanzi RE: Molecular genetics of Alzheimer's disease and the amyloid beta peptide precursor gene. *Ann Med* 1989;21(2):91–94.
9. Glener GG: The pathobiology of Alzheimer's disease. *Annu Rev Med* 1989;40:45–51.
10. Palmer AM, DeKosky ST: Monoamine neurons in aging and Alzheimer's disease. *J Neural Transm* 1993;91(2–3):135–159.
11. Davis RE, Emmerling MR, Jaen JC, Moos WH, Spiegel K: Therapeutic intervention in dementia. *Crit Rev Neurobiol* 1993;7(1):41–83.
12. Schellenberg GD, Bird TD: The genetics of Alzheimer's disease. *Biomed Pharmacother* 1989;43(7):463–468.
13. Arnold SE, Kumar A: Reversible dementias. *Med Clin North Am* 1993;77(1):215–230.
14. Kramer SI, Reifler BV: Depression, dementia, and reversible dementia. *Clin Geriatr Med* 1992;8(2):289–297.
15. Hall GR: Care of the patient with Alzheimer's disease living at home. *Nurs Clin North Am* 1988;23(1):31–46.
16. NcDowell FH, Cedarbaum JM: The extrapyramidal system and disorders of movement, in Joynt RJ (ed): *Clinical Neurology.* Philadelphia, JB Lippincott, 1993.
17. Koller WC: Initiating treatment of Parkinson's disease. *Neurology* 1992;42(1 suppl 1):33–38, 57–60.
18. Goetz CG, De Long MR, Penn RD, Bakay RA: Neurosurgical horizons in Parkinson's disease. *Neurology* 1993;43(1):1–7.
19. Koller WC, Giron LT Jr: Selegiline HC1: Selective MAO-type B inhibitor. *Neurology* 1990;40(10 suppl 3):58–60.
20. Yurek DM, Sladek JR: Dopamine cell replacement: Parkinson's disease. *Annu Rev Neurosci* 1990;13:415–440.
21. Weinfeld FD, Baum HM: The National Multiple Sclerosis Survey: Background and economic impact. *Ann NY Acad Sci* 1984;436:469–471.
22. Kurtzke JF, Hyllested K: Multiple sclerosis in the Faroe Islands: Clinical and epidemiological features. *Neurology* 1979;5:6.
23. Herndon RM, Rudick RA: Multiple sclerosis and related conditions, in Joynt RJ (ed): *Clinical Neurology.* Philadelphia, JB Lippincott, 1990, pp 1–61.
24. McDonald WI: The mystery of the origin of multiple sclerosis. *J Neurol Neurosurg Psychiatry* 1986;4(2):113–123.
25. Tourtellotte WW, Potvin AR, Fleming JO, et al: Multiple sclerosis: Measurement and validation of central nervous system IgG synthesis rate. *Neurology* 1980;30:240–244.
26. Antel JP, Amason BG, Medof ME: Suppressor cell function in multiple sclerosis: Correlation with clinical disease activity. *Annu Neurol* 1979;5:338–342.
27. Shumacher GA, Beebe G, Kibler RF, et al: Problems of experimental trials of therapy in multiple sclerosis: Report by the Panel on the Evaluation of Experimental Trials of Therapy in Multiple Sclerosis. *Ann NY Acad Sci* 1965;122:552–568.
28. Posner CM, Paty DW, Scheinberg L, et al: New diagnostic criteria for multiple sclerosis: Guidelines for research protocols. *Ann Neurol* 1983;13(3):227–231.
29. Rieumont MJ, DeLuca SA: Neuroimaging evaluation in multiple sclerosis. *Am Fam Physician* 1993;48(2):273–276.
30. Bodis-Wollner I: Sensory evoked potentials: PERG, VEP, and SEP. *Curr Opin Neurol Neurosurg* 1992;5(5):716–726.
31. Catanzaro M, Winston-Heath D: Alterations in elimination: Bladder, in Snyder M (ed): *A Guide to Neurological and Neurosurgical Nursing.* Albany, Demar, 1991, pp 183–200.
32. Pozzilli C, Gasperini C, Anzini A, Grasso MG, Ristori G, Fieschi C: Anatomical and functional correlates of cognitive deficit in multiple sclerosis. *J Neurol Sci* 1993;115(suppl):S55–S58.
33. Mahler ME: Behavioral manifestations associated with multiple sclerosis. *Psychiatr Clin North Am* 1992;15(2):427–438.
34. Noseworthy JH: Clinical trials in multiple sclerosis. *Curr Opin Neurol Neurosurg* 1993;6(2):209–215.
35. Achiron A, Pras E, Gilad R, et al: Open controlled therapeutic trial of intravenous immune globulin in relapsing-remitting multiple sclerosis. *Arch Neurol* 1992;49(12):1233–1236.
36. Panitch HS: Interferons in multiple sclerosis: A review of the evidence. *Drugs* 1992;44(6):946–962.
37. Kurtzke JF: The current neurologic burden of illness and injury in the United States. *Neurology* 1982;32:1207–1214.
38. Rowland LP, Layzer RB: Muscular dystrophies, atrophies, and related diseases, in Joynt RJ (ed): *Clinical Neurology.* Philadelphia, JB Lippincott, 1990, pp 1–109.
39. Pascuzzi RM: Amyotrophic lateral sclerosis. *Indiana Med* 1988;81(7):607–612.
40. Jurtzke JF, Kurland LT: Epidemiology of neurologic disease, in Joynt RJ (ed): *Clinical Neurology.* Philadelphia, JB Lippincott, 1990, pp 1–142.
41. Mitchell PH, Dowling GA: Common neurologic health problems: The phenomena of neuroscience medicine, in Mitchell PH, Hodges LC, Muwaswes M, Walleck CA (eds): *AANN's Neuroscience Nursing.* Norwalk, Conn, Appleton & Lange, 1988.
42. Koski CL, Khurana R, Mayer RF: Guillain-Barré syndrome. *Am Fam Physician* 1986;34(3):198–210.
43. The Guillain-Barré Syndrome Study Group: Plasmapheresis and acute Guillain-Barré syndrome. *Neurology* 1985;35:1096–1107.
44. Hund EF, Borel CO, Cornblath DR, Hanley DF, McKhann GM: Intensive management and treatment of severe Guillain-Barré syndrome. *Crit Care Med* 1993;21(3):433–446.
45. van der Meche FG, Schmitz PI: A randomized trial comparing intravenous immune globulin and plasma exchange in Guillain-Barré syndrome. Dutch Guillain-Barré Study Group. *N Engl J Med* 1992;326(17):1123–1129.
46. Urtaun M, Lopez de Munain A, Carrera N, Marti-Masso JF, Lopez de Docastillo G, Mozo C: High-dose intravenous immune globulin in the management of severe Guillain-Barré syndrome. *Ann Pharmacother* 1992;26(1):32–33.
47. Young JS, Northrup NE: *Statistical Information Pertaining to Some of the Most Commonly Asked Questions About Spinal Cord Injury.* Phoenix, National Spinal Cord Injury Data Center, 1981.
48. Krause JF: Epidemiological aspects of acute spinal cord injury: A review of incidence, prevalence, causes and outcomes, in Becker DP, Powlishock J (eds): *Central Nervous System Trauma Status Report 1985.* Bethesda, NINCDS/NIH, 1985.
49. Albin MS, White RJ: Epidemiology, physiopathology, and experimental therapeutics of acute spinal cord injury. *Crit Care Clin* 1987;3:441–452.
50. Carol MO, Ducker TB: Spinal cord injury and spinal shock syndrome, in Siegel JH (ed): *Trauma Emergency Surgery and Critical Care.* New York, Churchill-Livingstone, 1987.
51. Geisler FH: Acute management of cervical spinal cord injury. *Trauma Q* 1988;4(3):1–22.
52. Chilton J, Dagi TF: Acute cervical spinal cord injury. *Am J Emerg Med* 1985;3(4):340–351.

BIBLIOGRAPHY

Ahlskog JE: Cerebral transplantation for Parkinson's disease: Current progress and future prospects. *Mayo Clin Proc* 1993;68(6):578–591.
Anderson DK, Hall ED: Pathophysiology of spinal cord trauma. *Ann Emerg Med* 1993;22(6):987–992.
Appel SH: Excitotoxic neuronal cell death in amyotrophic lateral sclerosis. *Trends Neurosci* 1992;16(1):3–5.
Appel SH, Smith RG, Engelhardt JI, Stefani E: Evidence for autoimmunity in amyotrophic lateral sclerosis. *J Neurol Sci* 1993;118(2):169–174.
Brooks DJ: PET studies on the early and differential diagnosis of Parkinson's disease. *Neurology* 1993;43(12 suppl 6):S6–S16.
Calnet DB: Treatment of Parkinson's disease. *N Engl J Med* 1993;329(14):1021–1027.
Coons DH: The therapeutic milieu: Concepts and criteria, in Coons DH (ed): *Specialized Dementia Care Units.* Baltimore, Johns Hopkins University Press, 1991.
Coyle JT, Price DL, DeLong MR: Alzheimer's disease: A disorder of cortical cholinergic innervation. *Science* 1983;219:1184–1189.
Cummings JL, Benson DF: *Dementia: A Clinical Approach.* Stoneham, Mass, Butterworth, 1992.
Ditunno JF Jr, Formal CS: Chronic spinal cord injury. *N Engl J Med* 1994;330(8):550–556.
Dixon AY: Environments of care for the patient with Alzheimer's disease. *J Adv Med Surg Nurs* 1989;1(2):48.

Eisen A, Calne D: Amyotrophic lateral sclerosis, Parkinson's disease and Alzheimer's disease: Phylogenetic disorders of the human neocortex sharing many characteristics. *Can J Neurol Sci* 1992;19(suppl 1): 117–123.

Eisen A, Krieger C: Pathogenic mechanisms in sporadic amyotrophic lateral sclerosis. *Can J Neurol Sci* 1993;20(4):286–296.

Farrell K: Classifying epileptic syndromes: Problems and a neurobiologic solution. *Neurology* 1993;43(11 suppl 5):S8–S11.

Fenstermaker RA: Acute neurologic management of the patient with spinal cord injury. *Urol Clin North Am* 1993;20(3):413–421.

Folstein MF, Ross C: Cognitive impairment in the elderly, in Kelly WN (ed): *Textbook of Internal Medicine.* Philadelphia, JB Lippincott, 1992.

French J: The long-term therapeutic management of epilepsy. *Ann Intern Med* 1994;120(5):411–422.

ffrench-Constant C: Pathogenesis of multiple sclerosis. *Lancet* 1994;343(8892):271–275.

Glendinning DS, Enoka RM: Motor unit behavior in Parkinson's disease. *Phys Ther* 1994;74(1):61–70.

Gutierrez PA, Young RR, Vulpe M: Spinal cord injury: An overview. *Urol Clin North Am* 1993;20(3):373–382.

Gwyther LP: *Care of Alzheimer Patients: A Manual for Nursing Home Staff.* Chicago, Alzheimer's Disease Association and the American Health Care Association, 1985.

Homberg V: Motor training in the therapy of Parkinson's disease. *Neurology* 1993;43(12 suppl 6):S45–S46.

Jenner P, Schapira AH, Marsden CD: New insights into the cause of Parkinson's disease. *Neurology* 1992;42(12):2241–2250.

Jorm AF: *A Guide to the understanding of Alzheimer's Disease and Related Disorders.* New York, New York University, 1987.

Katzman R: Differential diagnosis of dementing illness, in Hutton JT (ed): *Neurologic Clinics: Dementia.* Philadelphia, WB Saunders, 1986.

Koller WC: When does Parkinson's disease begin? *Neurology* 1992;42(4 suppl 4):27–31.

LeWitt PA: Levodopa therapeutics: New treatment strategies. *Neurology* 1993;43(12 suppl 6):S31–S37.

Lombardo MC: Degenerative and other disorders of the nervous system, in Price P, Wilson L (eds): *Pathophysiology: Clinical Concepts of Disease Processes,* 4th ed. St. Louis, Mosby–Year Book, 1992.

Mathew LJ, Sloane PD: Care on dementia untis in five states, in Sloane PD, Mathew LJ (eds): *Dementia Units in Long-Term Care.* Baltimore, Johns Hopkins University Press, 1992.

Merrill JE, Graves MC, Mulder DG: Autoimmune disease and the nervous system: Biochemical, molecular, and clinical update. *West J Med* 1992;156(6):639–646.

Oksenberg JR, Begovich AB, Erlich HA, Steinman L: Genetic factors in multiple sclerosis. *JAMA* 1993;270(19):2362–2369.

Rabins PV: Psychological aspects of dementia. *J Clin Psychiatry* 1988;49(suppl 5):29–31.

Ropper AH: The Guillain-Barré syndrome. *N Engl J Med* 1992;326(17):1130–1136.

Saint-Cyr JA, Taylor AE, Lang AE: Neuropsychological and psychiatric side effects in the treatment of Parkinson's disease. *Neurology* 1993;43(12 suppl 6):S47–S52.

Shorvon SD: Medical assessment and treatment of chronic epilepsy. *Br Med J* 16 1991;302:363–366.

So EL: Update on epilepsy. *Med Clin North Am* 1993;77(1):203–214.

Stenger KM: Surveillance of spinal cord motor and sensory function. *Nurs Clin North Am* 1993;28(4):783–792.

Stern MB: Parkinson's disease: Early diagnosis and management. *J Fam Pract* 1993;36(4):439–446.

Swash M, Schwartz MS: What do we really know about amyotrophic lateral sclerosis? *J Neurol Sci* 1992;113(1):4–16.

Willison HJ, Kennedy PG: Gangliosides and bacterial toxins in Guillain-Barré syndrome. *J Neuroimmunol* 1993;46(1–2):105–112.

Wyler AR: Modern management of epilepsy: Recommended medical and surgical options. *Postgrad Med* 1993;94(3):97–98, 103–108.

CHAPTER 45
Alterations in Special Sensory Function

DEBRA WINSTON-HEATH and LEE-ELLEN C. COPSTEAD

KEY TERMS

adaptation: Changes in receptor potential in response to continuous stimulation.

chemoreceptor: Receptor that responds to certain chemicals.

cochlea: Spiral tube in the inner ear; contains hearing receptors.

equilibrium: Sense of balance.

gustatory: Pertaining to sense of taste.

mechanoreceptor: Receptor activated by mechanical stimuli.

nociceptor: Pain receptor.

olfactory: Pertaining to sense of smell.

photoreceptor: Receptor found only in the eye; responds to light.

refraction: Bending of light rays.

retina: Innermost coat of the eyeball; contains visual receptors.

rhodopsin: Photopigment found in the rods.

There are countless sense organs in the human body. The sense organs fall into two main categories: general sense organs and special sense organs. Of these, by far the most numerous are the general sense organs or **receptors.** Receptors function to produce the general or somatic senses (such as touch, temperature, and pain) and to initiate various reflexes necessary for maintaining homeostasis. Special sense organs, by comparison, function to produce the specialties of hearing, balance, vision, smell, and taste. This special sensory function allows us to experience our environment in a variety of dimensions.

Alterations in special sensory function may be acute or progressive and may result from factors such as genetics, disease, infection, trauma, and normal aging. Changes in special sensory function require prompt assessment, evaluation, and treatment from appropriate health care professionals. Equally important is an assessment of how the sensory impairment affects the individual's daily function. This chapter discusses special sensory function with regard to physiology, sensory impairments, and common interventions.

Hearing

Normal hearing results from a complex system of communicating neurons found in the cerebral auditory cortex, brain stem, pons, and thalamus. The sound stimulus (sound waves) received by the outer ear is transmitted by vibration to the tympanic membrane. Further amplification of the sound stimulus by the ossicles (incus, malleus, and stapes) occurs in the middle ear, where the sound is then transmitted to the oval window (Fig. 45–1). The action of the stapes on the oval window results in movement of the perilymph in the scala vestibuli. Perilymph is fluid contained within the space separating the membranous

from the osseous labyrinth of the ear. The scala vestibuli, scala media, and scala tympani are three parallel coiled tubes that form the **cochlea.** Movement of the perilymph through the scali vestibuli and the scala tympani eventually is dissipated by movement of the round window. The sound stimulus from the scali vestibuli is also transmitted to the vestibular membrane, resulting in displacement of the endolymph (the fluid contained in the membranous labyrinth) of the scala media and the basilar membrane (Fig. 45–2).

Neuronal Pathways

Dendrites of neurons whose cell bodies lie in the spiral ganglion and whose axons make up the cochlear nerve terminate around the bases of the hair cells of the organ of Corti, and the tectorial membrane adheres to their upper surfaces. The movement of the hair cells against the adherent tectorial membrane stimulates these dendrites and initiates impulse conduction by the cochlear nerve to the brain stem (Fig. 45–3). Before reaching the auditory area of the temporal lobe, impulses are relayed through nuclei in the medulla, pons, midbrain, and thalamus.[1,2]

Etiology and Pathogenesis

Hearing impairment commonly affects the ability to measure the volume and frequency of sound. Individuals with a decreased sensitivity to sound have a **conductive hearing impairment.** Disorders affecting the external and middle ear may result in this impairment. Among the disorders that commonly affect the external ear are excessive accumulation of cerumen and infections. Fluid effusion in the middle ear cleft, infection (otitis media), tumors, disease, and otosclerosis are examples of middle ear disorders that may affect the sound threshold.[2] These middle ear disorders may

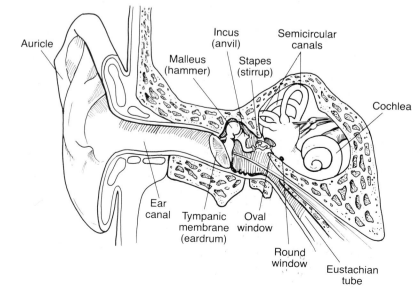

Auricle

Incus (anvil)

Semicircular canals

Malleus (hammer)

Stapes (stirrup)

Cochlea

Ear canal

Tympanic membrane (eardrum)

Oval window

Round window

Eustachian tube

FIGURE 45–1. Anatomic structure of the ear. (From Monahan FD, Drake T, Neighbors M: *Nursing Care of Adults*. Philadelphia, WB Saunders, 1994, p 1628. Reproduced with permission.)

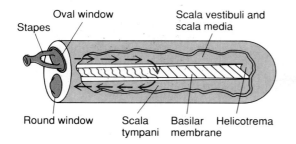

FIGURE 45–2. Movement of fluid in the cochlea following forward thrust of the stapes. (From Guyton AC: *Textbook of Medical Physiology*, 8th ed. Philadelphia, WB Saunders, 1991, p 572. Reproduced with permission.)

affect the ability of the joints of the ossicles to function smoothly.

Individuals with difficulty in detecting frequencies may perceive the sounds they hear as distorted. Difficulty in detecting sound frequencies commonly occurs with **sensorineural hearing impairments,** in which the hearing mechanism is disturbed in the inner ear or brain. Acquired sensorineural hearing impairment due to chronic, repeated exposure to loud sounds is common in the U.S. population. Fortunately, this damage to the sensorineural hearing mechanism may be preventable with limited exposure to excessively loud sound and the use of ear protectors; however, the need for continued education for all ages remains paramount. Ototoxic medications, frequently aspirin, the aminoglycoside antibiotics, and some of the diuretics, including furosemide, ethacrynic acid, and acetazolamide, contribute to sensorineural hearing impairment.[2] The hearing impairment caused by aspirin usually resolves when the medication is discontinued. Monitoring drug levels in patients receiving aminoglycoside antibiotics and testing patients before, during, and after drug therapy are suggested to decrease the risk of ototoxicity.[3]

Clinical Manifestations and Diagnosis

The symptoms of hearing impairment may be manifested in certain behaviors such as inattention, speaking out of turn in conversations, withdrawal from social situations, increased volume of voice when speaking, increased volume of radio or television required for participation, confusion, postural changes, loss of reaction to loud sounds, and emotional outbursts.[4,5] Children with hearing impairment may demonstrate inattentiveness and difficulty with articulation and the development of speech.[6] Most public school systems screen hearing function before kindergarten or the first grade; however, if screening is not done or if a hearing impairment is suspected, the child should be tested before starting school. Undiagnosed or untreated hearing impairment in school-aged children may lead to problems with social and academic development.

Hearing impairment is found across the age spectrum. Severe sensorineural hearing loss has been estimated to exist in 1 in 380 to 1 in 750 live births, and deafness has been estimated to occur in 1 in 1,000 births. The incidence of hearing loss in former patients of neonatal intensive care units has been reported to be 1 in 25 to 50 infants.[7] Impaired hearing function continues into adulthood and has been estimated to occur in over 25 percent of those more than 65 years of age.[2] When one considers the rapidly growing elderly population in America, the prevalence of hearing impairment is overwhelming.

Assessment of the person with suspected hearing impairment begins with a patient history that includes a description of the presenting problem, a physical examination, and diagnostic testing. Appropriate history questions include an assessment of repeated exposure to loud noises and a review of medication history with particular attention to aspirin, aminoglycoside antibiotics, and selected diuretics. In the case of children with suspected hearing impairment, questions regarding family and birth history and infection are important to ask.

The physical examination should include inspection of the outer ear to detect excessive collection of ear wax, which commonly contributes to hearing impairment. Basic assessment of hearing function can be readily performed at the bedside. Techniques include assessment of the individual's ability to hear a watch ticking, his or her reaction to loud noises (e.g., hand clapping in various parts of the room), the ability to understand what is said when not spoken to directly (observe for lip reading when the individual is spoken to directly), and the ability to distinguish high-frequency sounds that are similar (e.g., *feel, catch, thumb, heap, wise, wedge, fish, shows, bed, juice*).[5] Health care professionals familiar with the Rhine and Weber tests may add these tests to the bedside examination. Communication of assessment data to appropriate persons so that the need for further, more sophisticated assessment can be determined is essential to identify and treat the hearing impairment and to maximize daily function.

Treatment

Awareness of special sensory dysfunctions, knowledge of basic assessment techniques, and the prescrip-

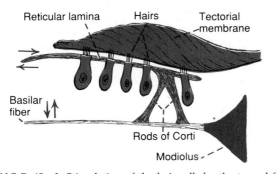

FIGURE 45–3. Stimulation of the hair cells by the to-and-fro movement of the hairs in the tectorial membrane. (From Guyton AC: *Textbook of Medical Physiology*, 8th ed. Philadelphia, WB Saunders, 1991, p 574. Reproduced with permission.)

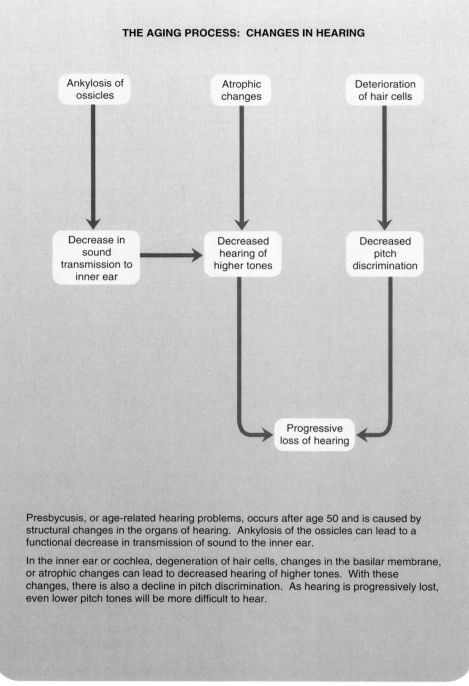

THE AGING PROCESS: CHANGES IN HEARING

Presbycusis, or age-related hearing problems, occurs after age 50 and is caused by structural changes in the organs of hearing. Ankylosis of the ossicles can lead to a functional decrease in transmission of sound to the inner ear.

In the inner ear or cochlea, degeneration of hair cells, changes in the basilar membrane, or atrophic changes can lead to decreased hearing of higher tones. With these changes, there is also a decline in pitch discrimination. As hearing is progressively lost, even lower pitch tones will be more difficult to hear.

Faith Young Peterson

tion of practical interventions for affected individuals are essential skills for health care professionals.

Zeeger[4] suggests teaching hearing-impaired elderly people the following three strategies to enhance hearing function: compensate with other senses, alter the stimulus and behavior, and modify the environment whenever possible. Compensating with other senses might include using safety alarms adapted with a colored flashing light, or a vibrator placed under a pillow to coincide with a wakeup alarm. In order to alter the stimulus and behavior, hearing-impaired individuals may request that other people use simple gestures, facial expressions, and eye level positioning. Such alterations will enhance communication. It is often more helpful for persons who are speaking with hearing-impaired individuals to lower their voice pitch because speaking louder may distort the message received. Additional examples of changing the stimulus and behavior include requesting that others decrease the rate of their speech delivery, use short sentences with pauses, and allow adequate time for the affected individual to process and respond to the information. Suggestions that focus on modifying the environment might include amplifying the ring of the telephone and lowering the pitch of timers, doorbells, and so forth. Decreasing background noise and the use of acoustic material to absorb excess noise are additional ways to enhance hearing ability.[4]

KEY CONCEPTS

- Perception of sound requires that sound waves be transmitted through the outer ear canal, across the tympanic membrane, and through the bones of the middle ear to the oval window. Movement of the oval window initiates movement of perilymph, followed by motions of the round window. Finally, the round window initiates movement of the endolymph that bathes the neurosensory organs of hearing, the hair cells. Bending of hair cells induces action potentials in the cochlear nerve, which projects to the brain stem. Neural projections to the auditory area in the temporal lobe result in sound perception.

- Hearing loss may occur from interruptions in any part of the sound transmission pathway. Disorders of the outer and middle ear are generally termed conductive because sound waves are not conducted reliably to the sensory organs of hearing. Accumulation of wax in the outer ear, ossification of bones, and middle ear infection and edema may result in conductive hearing loss. Conductive hearing loss is amenable to treatment.

- Sensorineural hearing loss is due to dysfunction of the hair cells or neural pathways to the brain. Chronic exposure to loud noise, ototoxic drugs, head trauma, and aging changes may lead to sensorineural hearing loss. Sensorineural hearing loss is not amenable to treatment.

- Meniere's disease is a chronic inner ear disease of unknown etiology characterized by vertigo and progressive unilateral nerve deafness.

Balance

The ear has dual sensory functions. In addition to its role in hearing, it also functions as the sense organ of balance or **equilibrium.** The stimulation, or "trigger," responsible for hearing and balance involves activation of the specialized hair cells called **mechanoreceptors.** Sound waves and movement are the physical forces that act on hair cells to generate receptor potentials and then nerve impulses, which are eventually perceived in the brain as sound or balance.

The sense organs involved in the sense of balance are found in the vestibule and semicircular canals of the inner ear. Nerve damage can occur in **Meniere's disease,** a chronic inner ear disease of unknown etiology. Meniere's disease is characterized by tinnitus, progressive nerve deafness, and vertigo (sensation of spinning).

Vision

Healthy vision requires three basic processes: the formation of an image on the retina, the stimulation of rods and cones, and the conduction of nerve impulses to the brain. Malfunction of any of these processes can disrupt normal vision.

The visual system is composed of *nonneural structures,* located in the eye, and *neural structures,* located in the retina, thalamus, hypothalamus, and cerebral cortex.

Nonneural Structures

The outermost membrane of the eye, the cornea, is transparent and functions to focus the light stimulus inside the eye. The white sclera to which the cornea is attached is a tough supporting tissue that encloses the eye completely, except where it connects with the optic nerve. Affixed to the sclera are the extraocular muscles, which control eye movements. The colored iris controls the size of the pupil, the central opening through which the light stimulus is transmitted to the posterior portion of the eye. Directly behind the iris is the lens, which focuses the light stimulus on the retina. The lens is supported by the ciliary body. Behind the ciliary body and lens is the vitreous humor, a clear, gelatinous substance that fills the space in front of the retina, thus supplying support and shape to the eye. Between the sclera and the retina lies the vascular choroid, which nourishes the retina and lessens the dispersion of light inside the eye.[1]

Neural Structures

The **retina,** a neural structure, is composed of multiple layers of cell types that are essential to the function of the visual system. Among the specialized cells of the retina are two types of **photoreceptors,** rods and cones. The cones are responsible for daylight vision, color vision, and visual acuity. The rods are important

RETINAL CELL TYPE

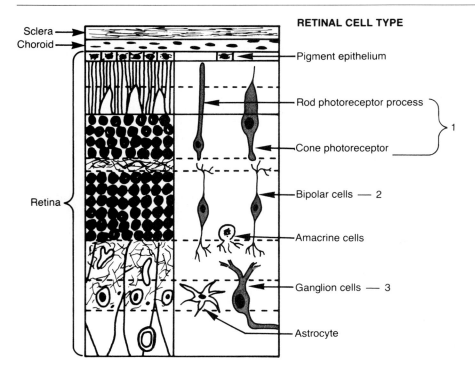

FIGURE 45 – 4. A schematic representation of the basic three-neuron organization of the retina. The three neuron types are (1) photoreceptors (rods or cones) and (2) bipolar cells that interconnect the photoreceptors with (3) the ganglion cells, whose axon processes transmit the signal to the brain. (From Cotran RS, Kumar V, Robbins S (eds): *Robbins Pathologic Basis of Disease*, 4th ed. Philadelphia, WB Saunders, 1989, p 1459. Reproduced with permission.)

for nighttime and peripheral vision.[8] Rods outnumber cones by nearly 20 to 1.

Action potentials from the rods and cones are communicated throughout the cellular components of the retina. The ganglion cells of the retina communicate the impulse through the optic nerve to connections in the thalamus, with the final connection in the occipital (visual) cortex via the geniculocalcarine tract (Fig. 45–4).[8]

Visual Impairment

Etiology and Pathogenesis

Visual impairment may occur or become evident any time during the life span. Common causes of visual impairment have been discussed by Adams and Victor[9] according to age groups. Frequently in late childhood or early adolescence, nearsightedness (**myopia**) exists, whereas farsightedness (**presbyopia**) is common in the middle-age years. In both of these conditions the eye is unable to focus images correctly, resulting in poor visual acuity.

Focusing a clear image on the retina is essential for good vision. In the normal eye, light rays enter the eye and are focused into a clear, upside-down image on the retina (Fig. 45–5). The brain can easily right the upside-down image in conscious perception but cannot correct an image that is not sharply focused. If the eye is elongated, the image focuses in front of the retina rather than on it. The retina receives only a fuzzy image. This condition, called myopia or nearsightedness, can be corrected with concave contact lenses or glasses (see Fig. 45–5). If the eye is

shorter than normal, the image focuses behind the retina, also producing a fuzzy image. This condition, called hyperopia or farsightedness, can be corrected with convex lenses (see Fig. 45–5).

Various other conditions can prevent the formation of a clear image on the retina. For example, aging-related inability to focus the lens properly (**presbyopia**) can be corrected by the use of reading glasses when near vision is needed. An irregularity in the curvature of the cornea or lens, a condition called **astigmatism** (Fig. 45–6), can also be corrected with glasses or contact lenses that are formed with the opposite curvature.

To make visual perceptions meaningful, the visual images in the two eyes normally fuse with each other on corresponding points of the two retinas. **Strabismus,** also called squint or cross-eyedness, means lack of fusion of the eyes. Strabismus is often caused by an abnormal "set" of the fusion mechanism of the visual system. In the early efforts of the child to fixate the two eyes on the same object, one of the eyes fixates satisfactorily but the other fails to fixate, or they both fixate satisfactorily but never simultaneously. Soon the patterns of conjugate movements of the eyes become abnormally set so that the eyes never fuse.

Broadly speaking, conditions that alter vision may be divided into those that affect the nonneural structures and those that affect the neural structures of the visual system. A brief discussion of some of the common conditions that affect the nonneural structures of the visual system will be presented first, followed by a discussion of common conditions that affect the neural structures.

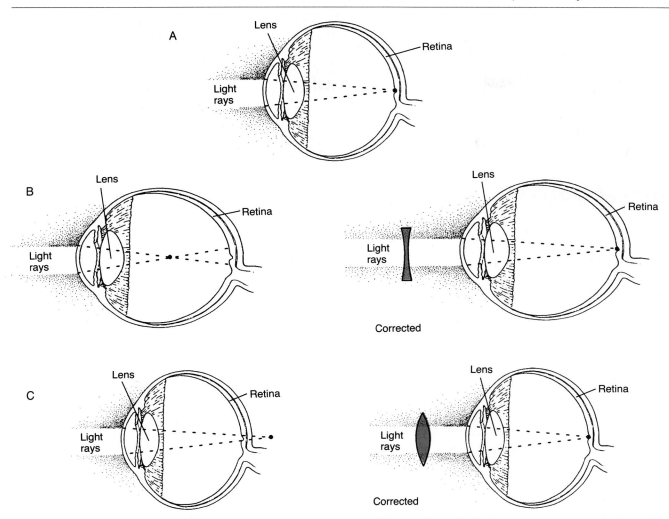

FIGURE 45–5. **A,** Light rays are focused directly on the retina, resulting in a clear visual image (emmetropia). **B,** In myopia, light rays are focused in front of the retina. A concave lens moves the focus back onto the retina and results in a clear image. **C,** In hyperopia, light rays are focused behind the retina. A convex lens moves the focus forward so that the light rays fall directly on the retina. (From Monahan FD, Drake T, Neighbors M: *Nursing Care of Adults*. Philadelphia, WB Saunders, 1994, p 1599. Reproduced with permission.)

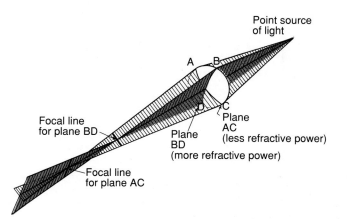

FIGURE 45–6. Astigmatism. In this condition, light rays focus at one focal distance in one focal plane and at another focal distance in the plane at right angles. (From Guyton AC: *Textbook of Medical Physiology*, 8th ed. Philadelphia, WB Saunders, 1991, p 540. Reproduced with permission.)

Lesions Affecting Nonneural Structures

Infection and trauma are frequent causes of **corneal scarring,** thus affecting the cornea's function of focusing light. Infections of the eye also have the potential to impair vision, sometimes permanently. Most eye infections begin in the conjunctiva, producing an inflammation response known as "pink-eye" or **conjunctivitis.** A variety of different pathogens can cause conjunctivitis. For example, the bacterium *Chlamydia trachomatis* that commonly infects the reproductive tract can cause a chronic infection called chlamydial conjunctivitis, or **trachoma.** Because *Chlamydia* and other pathogens often inhabit the birth canal, antibiotics are routinely applied to the eyes of newborns to prevent conjunctivitis. Highly contagious acute bacterial conjunctivitis, characterized by drainage of mucous pus, is most commonly caused by bacteria such as *Staphylococcus* and *Hemophilus.* Conjunctivitis may produce lesions on the inside of the eyelid that can damage the cornea and thus impair vision. Occasionally infections of the conjunctiva spread to the tissues of the eye itself and cause permanent injury and even total blindness. Besides infection, conjunctivitis may be caused by allergies. The red, itchy, watery eyes commonly associated with allergic reactions to pollen and other substances results from an allergic inflammatory response of the conjunctiva.

An interruption of the normal flow of the aqueous fluid from the anterior chamber of the eye may result in damage to the optic disc and thus visual loss. This condition affecting the anterior chamber, **glaucoma,** is a common cause of visual loss in older adults.[9] Glaucoma is excessive intraocular pressure caused by abnormal accumulation of aqueous humor. As fluid pressure against the retina increases above normal, blood flow through the retina slows. Reduced blood flow causes degeneration of the retina and thus loss of vision. Although *acute narrow-angle glaucoma* can occur, most cases of glaucoma develop slowly over a period of years. This chronic form, *open-angle glaucoma,* may not produce any symptoms, especially in its early stages. For this reason, routine eye examinations typically include a screening test for glaucoma. As chronic glaucoma progresses, damage first appears at the edges of the retina, causing a gradual loss of peripheral vision. Blurred vision and headaches may also occur. As the damage becomes more extensive, "halos" are seen around bright lights. If untreated, glaucoma eventually produces total, permanent blindness.

The lens is another structure that is commonly affected by disease and aging, both of which may result in visual impairment. **Cataract formation** may result in opacity of the lens and scattering of the light stimulus, both of which contribute to the degree of visual impairment in affected individuals. Cataract formation is frequently associated with aging, but may also occur in younger persons with diabetes mellitus.[10] **Rupture of a ciliary or retinal vessel** into the vitreous humor of the eye due to trauma also commonly causes visual impairment.[9]

Lesions Involving Neural Components

A variety of lesions involving the neural components of the visual system may result in visual impairment. Damage to the retina impairs vision because even a well-focused image cannot be perceived if some or all of the light receptors do not function properly. For example, in a condition called **retinal detachment** (Fig. 45–7), part of the retina falls away from the supporting tissue. This condition may result from aging, eye tumors, or from sudden blows to the head, as in a sports injury. Common warning signs include the sudden appearance of floating spots that may decrease over a period of weeks and odd flashes of light that appear when the eye moves. If the condition is left untreated, the retina may detach completely, causing total blindness in the affected eye.

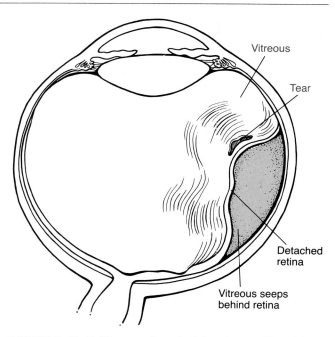

F I G U R E 45 – 7. Diagram of a retinal detachment. (From Monahan FD, Drake T, Neighbors M: *Nursing Care of Adults.* Philadelphia, WB Saunders, 1994, p 1613. Reproduced with permission.)

Vascular disease affecting the blood supply to the retina may result in conditions ranging from infarction to hemorrhage. Such conditions may be associated with diabetes mellitus, hypertension, or leukemia. In **diabetic retinopathy,** the diabetes causes small hemorrhages in retinal blood vessels that disrupt the oxygen supply to the photoreceptors. The eye responds by building new but abnormal vessels that block vision and may cause detachment of the retina. Diabetic retinopathy is one of the leading causes of blindness in the United States. A specific result of a vascular condition, **amaurosis fugax,** is episodic in nature and may be due to internal carotid artery disease or migraine headaches. **Retinal degeneration,** an important cause of visual loss in the elderly, may be idiopathic or may be associated with a number of disorders, including Paget's disease, sickle cell anemia, acromegaly, syphilis, or tuberculosis.[9]

Tumors, vascular and demyelinating lesions occurring along the visual pathway may result in a wide range of visual impairments. In general, damage to or degeneration of the optic nerve, the brain, or any part of the visual pathway between them can impair vision. For example, the pressure associated with glaucoma can also damage the optic nerve. Diabetes, a cause of retinal damage, can also cause degeneration of the optic nerve.

Damage to the visual pathway does not always result in total loss of sight. Depending on where the damage occurs, only a part of the visual field may be affected. For example, a certain form of neuritis often associated with multiple sclerosis can cause loss of only the center of the visual field, a condition called **scotoma.**

Cerebrovascular accident (stroke) can cause visual impairment when the resulting tissue damage occurs in one of the regions of the brain that process visual information. For example, damage to an area that processes information about colors may result in a rare condition called **acquired cortical color blindness.** This condition is characterized by difficulty in distinguishing any color—not just one or two colors, as in the more common forms of color blindness.

Aging

Concerns specific to the aging eye have been discussed by several authors.[4,5,9] In summary, these concerns include increased sensitivity to glare, decreased light sensitivity, decreased dark-light adaptation, and decreased color vision and depth perception. Common causes of visual impairment in the elderly include **cataracts, retinal detachments or hemorrhages,** and **macular degeneration.** Macular degeneration or loss of central vision, the area of clearest vision, affects 30 percent of those older than 65, and the percentage increases gradually with succeeding decades.[11] The person with loss of central vision is unable to read fine print, sew, or do fine work, and may have difficulty distinguishing faces. The peripheral vision is not affected.

Changes in the aged lens, cornea, and vitreous humor impair the ability of the eye to focus the light stimulus on the retina, resulting in a scattering of light and the development of glare. The smaller pupil and changes in the lens limit the amount of light allowed to enter the eye. On the globe itself, the cornea may show an infiltration of degenerative lipid material around the limbus (**arcus senilus**).

Typically, the elderly require a greater intensity of light for detailed work; however, intense light may also contribute to increased glare. Aging changes in the eye resulting in a myotic pupil and loss of rod cell receptors contribute to the increased time needed for light to dark adaptation. Difficulty seeing at night, called **nyctalopia,** or "night blindness," can also be caused by a deficiency of vitamin A. Vitamin A is needed to make retinal, a component of **rhodopsin.** A deficiency of rhodopsin impairs the function of the rod cells that are needed for dim light vision.

Loss of lens flexibility alters visual acuity, and the yellowing of the lens results in the changes in color vision that are experienced by many elderly. Generally, the aged eye discriminates warm primary colors (yellow, red, orange) more easily than cool, muted shades. In addition to changes in color vision, the degenerative changes in the rod cell receptors adversely affect depth perception.[4]

Clinical Manifestations and Diagnosis

Inspection of the eye can often reveal additional cues suggestive of visual impairment, such as excessive or inadequate tearing and lesions or crusts around the eyelid. The presence of these cues merits further investigation. Attention to the placement of the eye in the eye socket as the individual looks ahead may provide useful information regarding visual fields. Loss of subcutaneous fat surrounding the eye or ptosis of the eyelid may limit the horizontal and vertical gaze of vision.[4]

Basic visual function can be readily tested at the bedside. The examiner may begin with an assessment of cranial nerves II, III, IV, and VI, which test pupils for equality and reactivity to light and accommodation, visual fields, and extraocular movements. Visual acuity may be tested with the use of a Snellen eye chart or, if that is not available, with newsprint held at 14 inches. Colored pictures of familiar objects may be used as tools for testing visual function in children, the illiterate, or those with a marked impairment in visual acuity.[11] An assessment of color discrimination may be included. Environmental factors to be considered in this examination include adequate lighting, patient comfort, and decreasing glare.

Treatment

Once the visual impairment of an individual has been thoroughly investigated, specific interventions may be prescribed. It is important to note whether the client's problem is primarily one of visual acuity or visual field deficit, as the interventions for each impairment differ.

Interventions may be thought of in three general categories: assistive devices, environment, and behavior. Prosthetics and assistive devices offer aid to many individuals with visual impairment. Proper care and cleaning of contact lenses and eyeglasses directly influences the effectiveness of the prosthesis. Tinted lenses are generally available and may be effective in reducing glare for some individuals. Pocket magnifiers are frequently useful for persons with an acuity impairment. Large print is now available on many household items (e.g., watches, playing cards, telephones, books), and various textures are used in further modifications for the visually impaired. Additionally, some health care items such as blood glucose monitoring devices are available with alterations for those with visual impairment.[4,11] Further information regarding resources for the visually impaired may be obtained by contacting the local Council for the Blind. Assistive devices have limited use among persons with visual field deficits; however, the use of bright primary colors and cues to encourage these individuals to look to the affected field has had some success.

An unchanging, structured environment where items are kept in fixed locations familiar to the visually impaired person promotes safety and independence. Attempts to structure temporary environments, such as by introducing personal items into a hospital room, might yield positive results if consistently considered by the staff. Attention to adequate lighting, glare reduction, and the appropriate use of contrasting colors enhances safety and independent function for those with visual impairment. Behavioral techniques for the health care professional and visually impaired persons can promote client comfort, safety, and indepen-

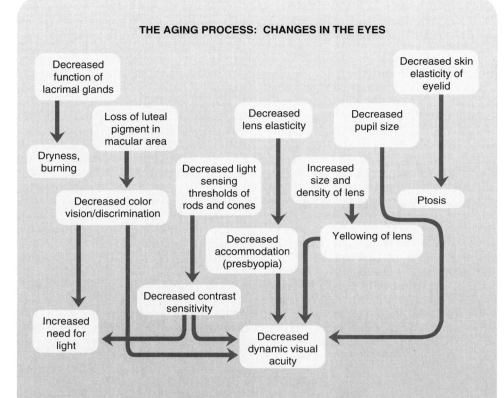

THE AGING PROCESS: CHANGES IN THE EYES

Aging affects all parts of the eye. Minor changes include decreased skin elasticity, changes in lacrimal gland function, and shrinking of the vitreous body. The changes in the lens and retina of the eye are more significant. These changes cause a decrease in color vision and discrimination, reduced contrast sensitivity, and diminished accommodation. As a result, the elderly need brighter light to see and do not differentiate color well. The elderly also have less dynamic visual acuity.

The retina is affected by a loss of the luteal pigment in the macular areas as well as reduced light sensing thresholds of the rods and cones. This leads directly to a slowing of dark adaptation and a decrease in the ability to discern brightness and colors, particularly shorter light wavelengths such as blues and greens.

A primary change in the aging eye is the development of presbyopia. This is due to a decrease in the elasticity of the lens and a decrease in the effectiveness of the ciliary muscle, leading to an inability to focus on near objects.

Faith Young Peterson

dence. Such techniques for the professional include announcing oneself upon all interactions and explaining sensory occurrences (e.g., the breeze of an open window). Approaching clients and placing items within their field of vision are considerations when working with clients with visual field deficits. Encouraging independence and social interaction often benefits affected individuals, as they may experience anger, frustration, or changes in self-concept as a result of their visual deficit. Visually impaired persons may be taught to wait several minutes for changes in dark-light adaptation and to avoid abrupt changes in lighting. Discourage individuals from looking directly into bright lights to decrease glare. Persons with visual field deficits can be taught to turn their head to scan the environment, and those with diplopia may benefit from the use of an altering eye patch. Assessment of the individual's ability to summon help in the health care and home environments is advised.

KEY CONCEPTS

- Visual acuity depends on the formation of discrete patterns of light on the retina. Errors of refraction, such as myopia and hyperopia, cause light from an image to focus in front of or behind the retina. Irregular curvature of the cornea results in astigmatism. These disorders are correctable with lenses to refract light to the appropriate retinal location.

- Strabismus occurs when both eyes do not focus together to form a single image. If not corrected, the image from one eye may be ignored by the brain to avoid double-imaging.

- Cataracts are due to opacification of the lens that blocks and scatters light. Cataracts may be congenital, traumatic, or associated with aging.

- Glaucoma is increased intraocular pressure due to excessive accumulation of aqueous humor. Drainage of intraocular fluid may be blocked chronically (open-angle glaucoma) or acutely by pupil dilation (narrow-angle glaucoma). Glaucoma is usually painless. Pressure on the retina leads to progressive loss of vision if not treated.

- Retinal detachment is a serious disorder associated with head trauma, tumor, and aging. Floaters and loss of a portion of the visual field are the usual symptoms.

- Systemic vascular disorders (hypertension, diabetes) may affect the blood supply to the retina, resulting in characteristic signs.

- The aging eye normally has a loss of lens accomodation that impairs near vision (presbyopia). Macular degeneration is also common, resulting in loss of central (clear) vision, while peripheral vision is unimpaired.

Smell and Taste

The senses of smell and taste allow separation of noxious or even lethal agents from those that are desir-

able. The sense of smell has a protective function in signaling danger: animals use smell to recognize the proximity of other animals, and humans use smell to sense harmful odors in the environment. The sense of taste allows a person to select food in accordance with desire and perhaps also in accordance with tissue needs. Both senses are strongly tied to primitive emotional and behavioral functions of the nervous system. Although these chemical senses are interrelated, they will be described separately.

Smell

The **olfactory system** is composed of a group of neurons and their connections located at the supratentorial level of the neuraxis (Fig. 45–8). The sense of smell begins with chemical stimulation of the olfactory receptor cells in the superior nasal mucosa. Axons of the receptor cells pass through the cribriform plate of the skull, traveling in groups of fibers that synapse with the neurons in the olfactory bulb. The olfactory bulb is a small elongated structure that lies below the frontal lobe at the anterior end of the olfactory sulcus. Olfactory bulb fibers form the olfactory tract, which divides into lateral and medial striae with connections in the medial temporal lobe and the medial basal frontal lobe, respectively.[1]

Disorders of Smell

Etiology and Pathogenesis

Olfactory disorders range from loss or reduction in the sense of smell to distortions and olfactory hallucinations. Commonly the sense of smell is diminished due to smoking and conditions in which there is congestion and swelling of the nasal mucosa, such as

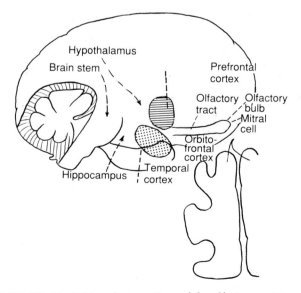

FIGURE 45–8. Neural connections of the olfactory system. (From Guyton AC: *Textbook of Medical Physiology,* 8th ed. Philadelphia, WB Saunders, 1991, p 584. Reproduced with permission.)

allergies and sinusitis. Head trauma often results in the loss of smell due to the actual shearing of the neuronal fibers as they traverse the cribriform plate. Tumors and large cerebral aneurysms of the anterior cerebral and anterior communicating arteries are lesions capable of diminishing the olfactory sense. Epilepsy and psychiatric disorders may be associated with olfactory hallucinations.[9]

Clinical Manifestations and Diagnosis

Individuals with smell dysfunction frequently complain of a diminished ability to taste. They may experience a decreased appetite and use excessive amounts of salt, sugar, or other seasonings on their foods. These individuals may stop reacting to strong odors and not notice their own bodily stench. Smell dysfunction increases the risk of accidents, as these individuals may not detect signs of imminent danger such as gas or smoke. Additionally, spoiled food may be ingested, and there are health risks from the excessive use of salt. Assessment of the sense of smell is done by asking the individual to smell different odors while keeping the eyes closed. Allow adequate time between test items presented, and test each nostril separately. Familiar, nonirritating items (coffee, peppermint, vanilla, etc.) should be used. Irritating substances such as ammonia should be avoided, as they stimulate the trigeminal nerve.[9]

Treatment

Interventions for those with smell dysfunction can be thought of in terms of augmenting the stimulus, teaching the individual to rely on other senses, and changing the environment. Individuals with a decreased ability to smell are encouraged to smell the aroma of food before eating and to consider the use of pleasant-smelling colognes and lotions.[4] Because their sense of smell is unreliable in identifying spoiled foods, people with smell dysfunction are encouraged to adhere to a strict schedule for discarding leftovers and to follow expiration dates on food products. As there can be significant nutritional problems associated with smell dysfunction, it is important to educate and monitor the individual's diet. Smoke alarms should be liberally installed in all rooms where smell-impaired persons are apt to fall asleep, and instructions never to light matches in areas that might contain gas are reinforced to these individuals.[12]

Taste

Taste is the last of the special senses to be covered in this chapter. Like the stimuli for smell, the stimuli for taste are chemical. Food particles dissolved in fluid stimulate the sensory receptors (taste buds) located on the surface of the tongue and in lesser density on the palate, pharynx, and larynx.[9] Stimulation from the sensory receptors is conducted through the cranial nerves of taste (VII, IX, X) to connections in the brain stem and thalamus with eventual termination in the gustatory cortex in the parietal lobe.[8] The gustatory sensory receptors have a heightened sensitivity for one of the primary taste sensations (sweet, salty, sour, or bitter); however, they are able to respond to a variety of stimuli. The sensory receptors decrease in number with age.[9]

Disorders of Taste

Etiology and Pathogenesis

A decreased gustatory sense can result from heavy smoking and from extreme dryness of the tongue and mucous membranes. A variety of medications are known to alter the sense of taste, including amitriptyline, griseofulvin, and antithyroid, antirheumatic, and anticancer medications. In addition, influenza-like illnesses and lesions on the thalamus and parietal lobe may impair taste sensation.[9]

Clinical Manifestations and Diagnosis

Assessment of the gustatory sense should include the primary taste sensations in appropriate areas of the tongue, with the surface of the tongue wiped clean between substances.[9] Questions regarding the individual's food preferences, use of salt and sugar, weight loss, and appetite add valuable information to the assessment data.

Treatment

Interventions for those with an impaired sense of smell should include education and monitoring of their dietary intake because of the influence of taste on nutrition. The creative use of flavor extracts, vinegars, lemon juice, and herbs can augment taste. Foods of a variety of textures and attractively served may enhance appetite. Individuals with taste impairment are encouraged to avoid blended foods and to practice frequent oral hygiene. Like the person with smell dysfunction, the person with taste impairment should adhere to expiration dates on foods, discard leftovers on a scheduled basis, and inspect canned goods for bulges.[4]

KEY CONCEPT

- Changes in smell and taste most commonly result from smoking and inflammation due to colds, sinusitis, or allergies. A change in smell or taste sensation in the absence of obvious etiology may indicate brain tumor and should prompt a thorough neurologic evaluation.

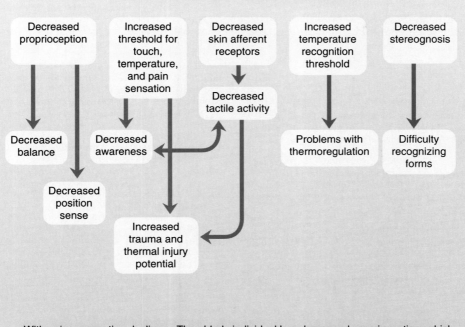

THE AGING PROCESS: SENSORY CHANGES

With aging, sensation declines. The elderly individual has decreased proprioception, which is one's perception of body position. This loss can result in decreased or absent position sense and loss of balance. Aging also results in a reduction of vibration sense. There is an increased threshold for touch, temperature, and pain sensation, leading to reduced sensory and environmental awareness.

Aging decreases the body's ability to respond well to temperature changes, resulting in increasing difficulty with thermoregulation. The temperature recognition threshold is increased, which can lead to late or absent fever when ill. There is decreased stereognosis, with subsequent difficulty recognizing forms.

Faith Young Peterson

Summary

Alterations in the special senses can affect individuals throughout the age span and those suffering from other conditions. In many cases, these sensory alterations may be permanent, yet the quality of the life of sensory-impaired individuals may be enhanced by health care professionals. Methods of enhancing these lives begin with timely assessment, intervention, and continued evaluation.

REFERENCES

1. Daube JR, Reagan TJ, Sandok BA, Westmoreland BF: *Medical Neurosciences*, 2nd ed. Boston, Little, Brown & Co, 1986.
2. Ruben RJ, Kruger B: Hearing loss in the elderly, in Katzman R, Terry RD (eds): *The Neurology of Aging*. Philadelphia, FA Davis, 1983, pp 123–147.
3. Koegel L: Ototoxicity: A contemporary review of aminoglycosides, loop diuretics, acetylsalicylic acid, quinine, erythromycin, and cisplatinum. *Am J Otol* 1985;8:190–199.
4. Zeeger LJ: The effects of sensory changes in older persons. *J Neurosci Nurs* 1986;18:325–332.
5. Kopac CA: Sensory loss in the aged: The role of the nurse and the family, *Nurs Clin North Am* 1983;18:373–384.
6. Lamb C: When hearing impairment occurs. *Patient Care* 1983;17:147–167.
7. Mandell JR: Identification and treatment of very young children with hearing loss. *Infants Young Children* 1988;1:20–30.
8. Barr ML, Kiernan JA: *The Human Nervous System: An Anatomical Viewpoint*, 5th ed. Philadelphia, JB Lippincott, 1988.
9. Adams RD, Victor M: *Principles of Neurology*, 3rd ed. New York, McGraw-Hill, 1985.
10. Wright BE, Henkind P: Aging changes and the eye, in Katzman R, Terry RD (eds): *The Neurology of Aging*. Philadelphia, FA Davis, 1983, pp 149–165.
11. Wolanin MO, Phillips LRF: *Confusion: Prevention and Care*. St Louis, CV Mosby, 1981.
12. Davidson TM: The loss of smell. *Emerg Med* 1988;20:104–108, 111–116.
13. Blainey CG: Alterations in the peripheral senses, in Mitchell PH, Hodges LC, Muwaswes M, Walleck CA (eds): *AANN's Neuroscience Nursing*. Norwalk, Conn, Appleton & Lange, 1988, pp 385–395.

BIBLIOGRAPHY

Alexander LJ: Age-related macular degeneration: The current understanding of the status of clinicopathology, diagnosis and management. *J Am Optom Assoc* 1993;64(12):822–837.
Ashmore JF: The electrophysiology of hair cells. *Annu Rev Physiol* 1991;53:465–476.
Bartoshuk L: Clinical evaluation of the sense of taste. *Ear Nose Throat J* 1989;68(4):331–337.
Bell GR: Biomechanical considerations of high myopia: Part I. Physiological characteristics. *J Am Optom Assoc* 1993;64(5):332–338.
Bell GR: Biomechanical considerations of high myopia: Part II. Biomechanical forces affecting high myopia. *J Am Optom Assoc* 1993;64(5):339–345.
Bell GR: Biomechanical considerations in high myopia: Part III. Therapy for high myopia. *J Am Optom Assoc* 1993;64(5):346–351.
Brown NA: The morphology of cataract and visual performance. *Eye* 1993;7(pt 1):63–67.

Caprioli J: Correlation of visual function with optic nerve and nerve fiber layer structure in glaucoma. *Surv Ophthalmol* 1989;33(suppl):319–330.
Dakkis P: The active cochlea. *J Neurosci* 1992;12(12):4575–4585.
Dulon D, Schacht J: Motility of cochlear outer hair cells. *Am J Otol* 1992;13(2):108–112.
Eybalin M: Neurotransmitters and neuromodulators of the mammalian cochlea. *Physiol Rev* 1993;73(2):309–373.
Flock A: Do sensory cells in the ear have a motile function? *Proc Brain Res* 1988;74:297–304.
Hadol JB Jr: Does the eye grow into focus? *Nature* 1990;345:477–478.
Hudspeth AJ: How the ear's works work. *Nature* 1989;341:397–404.
Jackson WB: Differentiating conjunctivitis of diverse origins. *Surv Ophthalmol* 1993;38(suppl):91–104.
Janda AM: Sudden nontraumatic visual loss: The challenge in primary care. *Postgrad Med* 1992;91(5):111.
Kimmelman CP: Clinical review of olfaction. *Am J Otolaryngol* 1993;14(4):227–239.
Lichtenstein MJ: Hearing and visual impairments. *Clin Geriatr Med* 1992;8(1):173–182.
Litwak AB: Evaluation of the retinal nerve fiber layer in glaucoma. *J Am Optom Assoc* 1990;61(5):390–397.
Marion RW: The genetic anatomy of hearing: A clinician's view. *Ann NY Acad Sci* 1991;630:32–37.
Mott AE, Leopold DA: Disorders in taste and smell. *Med Clin North Am* 1991;75(6):1321–1353.
Murray T: Strabismus: Challenges and trends. *Eye* 1993;7(pt 3):332–340.
Newman NJ: Neuro-ophthalmology: The afferent visual system. *Curr Opin Neurol* 1993;6(5):738–746.
Reed RR: Mechanisms of sensitivity and specificity in olfaction. *Cold Spring Harbor Symp Quant Biol* 1992;57:501–504.
Richer SP: Is there a prevention and treatment strategy for macular degeneration? *J Am Optom Assoc* 1993;64(12):838–850.
Roberts SP: Visual disorders of higher cortical function. *J Am Optom Assoc* 1992;63(10):723–732.
Ronnett GV, Snyder SH: Molecular messengers of olfaction. *Trends Neurosci* 1992;15(12):509–513.
Saunders JC, Cohen YE, Szymko YM: The structural and functional consequences of acoustic injury in the cochlea and peripheral auditory system: A five year update. *J Acoust Soc Am* 1991;90(1):136–146.
Schiffman SS, Gatlin CA: Clinical physiology of taste and smell. *Annu Rev Nutr* 1993;13:405–436.
Scott AE: Clinical characteristics of taste and smell disorders. *Ear Nose Throat J* 1989;68(4):297.
Scott AE: Medical management of taste and smell disorders. *Ear Nose Throat J* 1989;68(5):386.
Smith DV: Assessment of patients with taste and smell disorders. *Acta Otolaryngol Suppl Stockh* 1988;458:129–133.
Souder E, Yoder L: Olfaction: The neglected sense. *J Neurosci Nurs* 1992;24(5):273–280.
Teas DC: Auditory physiology: Present trends. *Annu Rev Psychol* 1989;40:405–429.
Thibos LN, Bradley A: New methods for discriminating neural and optical losses of vision. *Optom Vis Sci* 1993;70(4):279–287.
Vader LA: Vision and vision loss. *Nurs Clin North Am* 1992;27(3):705–714.
Van Buskirk EM, Cioffi GA: Glaucomatous optic neuropathy. *Am J Ophthalmol* 1992;113(4):447–452.
Weiffenbach JM, Bartoshuk LM: Taste and smell. *Clin Geriatr Med* 1992;8(3):543–555.
Weiss AH: Chronic conjunctivitis in infants and children. *Pediatr Ann* 1993;22(6):366.
Whitmore WG: Congenital and developmental myopia. *Eye* 1992;6 (pt 4):361–365.
Woods S: Macular degeneration. *Nurs Clin North Am* 1992;27(3):761–775.

CHAPTER 46
Pain

LORIE RIETMAN WILD and LESLIE A. CLARK EVANS

KEY TERMS

acute pain: Pain that results from tissue injury and resolves when the injury heals, usually in less than 3 months.

afferent: In reference to direction of neuron travel, from the peripheral nervous system toward the brain.

agonist: Opioid, either exogenous or endogenous, that produce analgesia and other central nervous system effects by binding to specific receptors in the encephalon and spinal cord.

antagonist: A chemical that reverses the effects of an agonist by binding with specific receptors. A drug may be agonistic at one receptor type and antagonistic at another. These drugs are called mixed agonist-antagonists. Naloxone is the best-known antagonist.

ascending neural pathway: The method of transmission of nerve "messages" (e.g., nociception) from the spine to the thalamus. The most prevalent pain pathways are the spinoreticulothalamic and spinothalamic pathways.

chronic pain: Exists when pain lasts longer than several months beyond the expected healing time.

efferent: In reference to direction of neuron travel, from the brain to the lower levels of the nervous system, in the opposite direction from the afferent nerve fibers.

endogenous opioids: Opioid-like chemicals created within the body that decrease pain. Endorphin is an endogenous opioid.

endorphins: A potent endogenous opioid peptide derived from cells in the hypothalamus, also found in the periaqueductal gray matter of the brain. β-endorphin has been found to have analgesic properties.

ischemic pain: Pain resulting from a sudden and profound loss of blood to the tissue in a particular part of the body.

neuropathic pain: Pain resulting from dysfunctional abnormalities of the nervous system. Nerve injury due to surgery, tumor growth, metastasis, radiation or chemotherapy, or trauma often causes neuropathic pain.

nociception: Activation of nociceptors by potentially tissue-damaging stimuli.

nociceptor: Receptor stimulated by tissue injury.

opioid: Any of a group of drugs with an affinity for opioid receptors in the central nervous system. Morphine is the standard opioid with which others are compared for characteristics and potency.

pain: An unpleasant sensory and emotional experience associated with actual or potential tissue damage, or described in terms of such damage.

pain behavior: Result of nociception and suffering, observable in actions such as splinting, moaning, limping, taking pain medications, or ceasing to work.

referred pain: Pain that emanates from the source of injury to another location in the body.

stress-induced analgesia: Inhibition of pain by an environmental stimulus, such as the stress of athletic competition or the stress of battle.

substantia gelatinosa: Another name for lamina II, one of the six subdivisions of the spinal cord where neurons synapse. The cells in this lamina are thought to be excitatory in response to primary afferent input.

wide dynamic range neurons: Neurons in lamina V that respond to a wide range of input—chemical, thermal, and mechanical.

---

*P*ain is a complex phenomenon. Pain is a personal experience; no two people will be alike in their response to either pain or its treatment. Because of the uniqueness of each person's pain, defining pain can be difficult. Merskey defined pain as "an unpleasant sensory and emotional experience associated with actual or potential tissue damage or described in terms of such damages."[1] McCaffery offers an expanded definition: "Pain is whatever the experiencing person says it is, existing whenever the experiencing person says it does."[2] Clearly, pain is most meaningful to the individual who is experiencing it.

Defining a Complex Phenomenon

Model for Pain

As a complex phenomenon, the experience of pain cannot be explained by pathophysiologic models. A comprehensive model of pain includes psychological and environmental factors as well as physiologic factors (Fig. 46–1).[3] When a mechanical, thermal, or chemical injury occurs, a sequence of neurologic events takes place that transmits the message of tissue injury to the central nervous system (CNS). The receptors stimulated by tissue injury are known as **nociceptors,** and activation of these receptors by potentially tissue-damaging stimuli is known as **nociception.**

Pain, the perception of nociceptive events, usually results from nociception, although the correlation is not absolute. Pain can occur without nociceptive input, as in the clinical conditions of postherpetic neu-ralgia or postparaplegic pain. In these cases the nervous system reacts as if nociception occurs when in fact it does not.

An affective component of pain is **suffering.** Suffering is associated with the emotional response to pain and usually involves a perceived loss of objects or function. Stress, anxiety, and depression may also play a role in suffering. Frequently we use the language of pain to express suffering.

Pain behavior usually results from each of the preceding aspects. Pain behaviors may include actions such as splinting, moaning, limping, taking pain medications, or ceasing to work. Because the intensity of nociception, pain, and suffering cannot be adequately measured, in the clinical setting we are often limited to a subjective assessment of pain and quantifying pain behaviors.

Types of Pain

Pain is often categorized as being either acute or chronic. Pain associated with cancer usually involves components of each type. **Acute pain** results from tissue injury and resolves when the injury heals, usually in less than 3 months. Acute pain is typically accompanied by clinical signs and symptoms of pain that result from stimulation of the sympathetic nervous system.

Chronic pain exists when pain lasts more than several months beyond the expected healing time. When chronic pain is not due to a malignancy, its cause is often difficult to ascertain. Chronic pain is

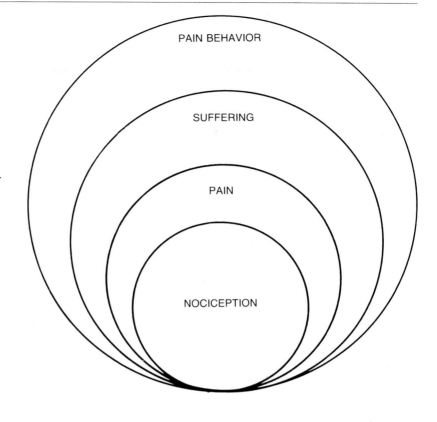

FIGURE 46 – 1. A model of pain including psychosocial, environmental, and physiologic factors. (Reprinted with permission from Loeser JD: Concepts of pain, in Stanton-Hicks M, Boas R (eds): *Chronic Low Back Pain.* New York, Raven Press, 1982, p 146.)

not always manifested by signs and symptoms of sympathetic activity such as elevated blood pressure and respiratory and heart rates (see Table 46–4). As the body becomes accustomed to pain, the nervous system desensitizes itself to the noxious input; therefore symptoms are more often psychological in nature. Lack of sleep because of pain causes fatigue and irritability. Loss of a job or loss of body image because of pain causes personal and family difficulties. Treatment failures may create a sense of hopelessness or distrust of caregivers. In chronic pain situations, it becomes increasingly important to listen to the client, to assess function and mood, and to consider the myriad life-style changes that contribute to the total chronic pain picture.

Cancer pain is usually a subcategory of chronic pain, although it may be acute. Malignant pain differs from nonmalignant chronic pain in that it often has an identifiable etiology. Pain associated with cancer may result from infiltration of organs or compression of structures by an expanding tumor, or it may occur as a result of radiation therapy or chemotherapy, which often damages tissue. In the cancer pain patient, clinical signs and symptoms are often a mixture of sympathetic nervous system activation and behavioral changes.[4]

KEY CONCEPT

- **Pain is a subjective personal experience, best defined as whatever the experiencing person says it is.**

Physiologic Mechanisms

The physiologic mechanisms involved in the pain response are numerous and complex. The body orchestrates a multilevel response to tissue injury. To explain these intricate mechanisms, this discussion will follow the pathway of pain transmission from the periphery to the CNS, including the spinal cord and brain, as well as the efferent modulation and control of pain. Much of the research that scientists report deals with the mechanisms of acute pain. Therefore, this discussion will focus on the physiologic mechanisms associated with acute pain; however, differences in the mechanisms of acute and chronic pain will be addressed when they are known.

Peripheral Mechanisms

Nociceptors are found in skin, muscle, connective tissue, the circulatory system, and abdominal, pelvic, and thoracic viscera.[4,5] Tissue injury lowers the threshold of nociceptors such that even a mild stimulus activates the receptors.[6] Stimulation can be the result of direct damage to nerve endings or chemicals released at the site of injury, although the precise mechanism of nociceptor stimulation is unknown.[5] Numerous substances released at the site of injury participate in the transmission of nociceptive impulses.[7-9] Damaged cells release electrolytes such as potassium and hydrogen; lactic acid accumulates as

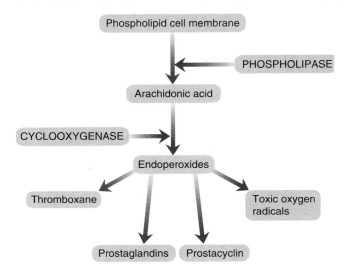

FIGURE 46-2. Tissue injury results in the release of prostaglandins from the breakdown of phospholipid cell membranes.

damaged cells cease to function. Norepinephrine sensitizes nociceptors in the setting of tissue injury or inflammation.[10] Substance P is then released from nerve terminals, causing vasodilation and the release of histamine and serotonin. With continued nociception, levels of histamine and serotonin in the extracellular fluid rise, causing an expanding area of pain known as hyperalgesia.

Several of the agents listed above have a key role in the inflammatory process, explaining the relationship between inflammation and pain. Of particular interest in this process are the prostaglandins. Recall that cells have a phospholipid component to their membranes. When cells are damaged, the enzyme phospholipase breaks down the phospholipid, converting it to arachidonic acid (Fig. 46-2).[9] Arachidonic acid undergoes further breakdown by the enzyme cyclooxygenase, creating endoperoxides, some of which are the prostaglandins. Sensitization by prostaglandins lowers the threshold of nociceptive fibers so that stimuli that would not be "painful" under normal circumstances are now pain producing.[10] The role of prostaglandins in pain transmission is important, especially when one is considering analgesic therapies. For example, the nonsteroidal anti-inflammatory drugs (NSAIDs) prevent prostaglandin production by inhibiting the action of cyclooxygenase, and thus are potent analgesics,[9,10] acting in the peripheral nervous system.

Afferent Transmission

Stimulated nociceptors transmit impulses to the CNS by means of specialized sensory fibers. The primary sensory fibers involved in the transmission of nociceptive impulses are the A-delta and C fibers.[4,5,7,8] The characteristics and function of these fibers are summarized in Table 46-1. In general, the large, myelinated A-delta fibers transmit the nociceptive impulses very quickly as an initial response to tissue injury. The nature of the pain carried by the fast-traveling A-delta fibers is pain that is sharp, stinging, and highly localized.[11] In contrast, unmyelinated C fibers transmit pain more slowly. Pain transmitted by C fibers is poorly localized and has a dull or aching quality that lingers long after the initial sharp pain abates.[11] The majority of pain sensations travel via C fibers.

It was only discovered in the past 30 years that infants have an abundance of C fibers at birth and even in utero. Prior to that time, it was thought that the nervous system was essentially incomplete until about age 2 years, which prompted the appalling myth that nociception could not occur in infants, and thus they could not feel pain. Indeed, children have undergone surgery without analgesia based on this myth, and some have died from the pain. Hopefully, clinicians working with neonates and children in pain now have the education and compassion to treat this vulnerable population in a humane and appropriate fashion. While it is true that A-delta fibers are still being manufactured in the first few months of life, it has been proved that C fibers are abundant in the newborn.

Most sensory afferent fibers enter the spinal cord by way of the posterior nerve roots. Although once thought to carry only efferent fibers, a small number of sensory afferent fibers enter the spinal cord by the anterior nerve roots.[6,8] The cell bodies of these unipolar sensory neurons are located in the posterior or dorsal, root ganglion.

Spinal Cord Modulation

The majority of primary sensory afferent neurons (A-delta and C fibers) enter the spinal cord via the posterior nerve roots and terminate in the posterior

TABLE 46-1. Afferent Sensory Pain Fibers

	A-delta Fibers	C Fibers
Structure	Myelinated	Unmyelinated
Amount	10%	90%
Source	Mechanical stimuli	Polymodal stimuli (mechanical, thermal, chemical)
Speed	Fast traveling, 5–10 m/sec	Slower traveling, 0.6–2 m/sec
Sensory quality of pain mediated	Sharp, stinging, cutting, pinching	Dull, burning, aching

horn of the spinal cord.[5] However, as the afferent neurons enter the posterior horn, collateral branches also spread in a segmental fashion by way of the **tract of Lissauer.** The collateral fibers spread in both rostral and caudal directions, involving two to three spinal segments in each direction. Although the majority of the afferent sensory neurons enter the spinal cord by way of the posterior nerve roots, there is evidence as well for the presence of C fibers in anterior root fibers.[5]

Sensory afferent neurons synapse with interneurons, anterior motor neurons, and sympathetic preganglionic neurons in specified, anatomically distinct regions of the spinal cord (Fig. 46–3).[5,12] A-delta and C fibers carry excitatory impulses from cutaneous receptors in small, localized areas of the skin to lamina I. Many of the neurons originating in lamina I cross the spinal cord to ascend to the brain via the spinothalamic tract.

Laminae II and III represent a key anatomic region involved in pain mechanisms known as the **substantia gelatinosa.** Laminae II and III are characterized by the presence of multiple synaptic connections among primary sensory afferent neurons, interneurons, and spinothalamic ascending fibers.[5]

Lamina IV receives input from the substantia gelatinosa interneurons as well as primary sensory afferents. Neurons projecting from lamina IV extend to other laminae and to ipsilateral ascending fibers.[5]

Another key synaptic area involved in nociception is lamina V. Numerous A-delta and C fibers deliver somatic input from mechanical, thermal, and chemical receptors in the periphery to lamina V. Sensory afferent neurons from visceral receptors also terminate in lamina V. The convergence of both somatic and visceral fibers in lamina V may help to explain the phenomenon of referred pain.[5] Neurons originating in lamina V project primarily to the contralateral anterior spinothalamic tracts.[5]

The remaining, deeper laminae VI through VIII receive sensory input from muscles, joints, and visceral afferent fibers. In contrast to the narrow receptive fields carrying sensory information from cutaneous structures that terminate in laminae I through

V, the receptive fields for laminae VI through VII are extensive.[5] These neurons with their large receptive fields are known as **wide dynamic range neurons** and are concentrated in laminae V through VIII.[13]

As with the transmission of nociception in the periphery, numerous agents are involved in the continued transmission of sensory input at the level of the spinal cord.[13] The key nociceptive transmitter is **substance P** and is active in both the dorsal root ganglion and the substantia gelatinosa. Another neurotransmitter for nociception is **calcitonin gene–related peptide** (CGRP). Even though CGRP does not provoke pain on its own, it strongly facilitates the effect of substance P and causes neurogenic inflammation. Glutamate is another excitatory peptide active in the spinal cord.

Ascending Spinal Pathways

The ascending spinal pathways carry nociceptive information from the level of the spinal cord to various areas within the brain. Nociceptive impulses become pain impulses after they have reached the brain and have been interpreted as pain by the cerebral cortex. There are two major ascending pathways connecting the spinal cord with higher centers in the brain: the **spinothalamic tract** (STT) and the **spinoreticulothalamic tract** (SRT). Sometimes the STT and the SRT are referred to as the neospinothalamic tract and the paleospinothalamic tract, respectively, based on their phylogenetic age (that is, time of genetic development).[4] The descriptive nature of the terms STT and SRT helps explain both the origin and termination areas of the neurons involved.

The STT is a discriminative path that informs the body about the pain and where it is. The cell bodies of the neurons composing the STT are located primarily in lamina I through V. Axons of these neurons then ascend through the lateral and anterior portions of the spinal cord and project directly to the thalamus, where they synapse (Fig. 46–4). From the thalamus, axons project to sensory regions of the cerebrocortex

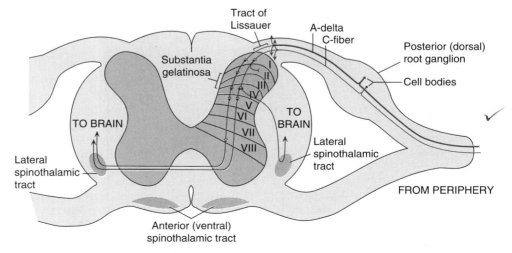

FIGURE 46 – 3. Posterior horn of the spinal cord with primary afferent input.

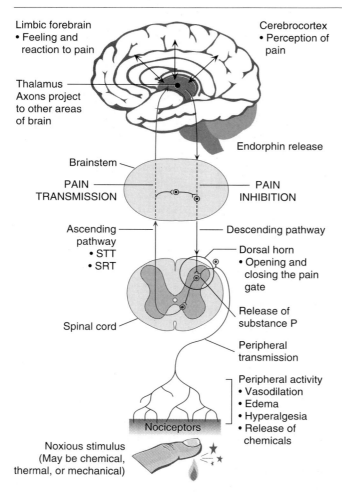

Limbic forebrain
• Feeling and reaction to pain

Cerebrocortex
• Perception of pain

Thalamus
Axons project to other areas of brain

Endorphin release

Brainstem

PAIN TRANSMISSION — PAIN INHIBITION

Ascending pathway
• STT
• SRT

Descending pathway

Dorsal horn
• Opening and closing the pain gate

Release of substance P

Spinal cord

Peripheral transmission

Peripheral activity
• Vasodilation
• Edema
• Hyperalgesia
• Release of chemicals

Nociceptors

Noxious stimulus (May be chemical, thermal, or mechanical)

FIGURE 46–4. Ascending and descending nociceptive pathways.

located in the parietal lobe.[4,5] The cortical areas of the brain are involved in the perception of pain and painful stimuli.

The SRT is a nondiscriminative pathway that connects the spinal cord and the brain. The SRT is responsible for the body's aversive reaction to pain. The cell bodies of the neurons composing the SRT lie primarily within laminae I and V. The SRT travels with the STT in the anterolateral spinal cord to the level of the medulla, then sends diffuse projections to the reticular formation, the mesencephalon, and, finally, the thalamus.[4,5] From the thalamus, further projections to the cerebral cortex, limbic system, and basal ganglia occur.[14]

Two additional pathways that ascend through the posterior spinal cord are the spinocervical tract (SCT) and the dorsal column pathway. The neurons of the spinocervical tract originate in lamina IV and project to the lateral cervical nucleus and ultimately to the thalamus.[4,5,11] The SCT carries information mostly from mechanoreceptors associated with hair follicles.[5] The dorsal column pathway has neurons that originate in laminae II and IV and project to the dorsal column nuclei and then the thalamus.[4,5,11] The dorsal column pathway has generated a great deal of scien-

tific and clinical research interest, resulting in the development of dorsal column stimulators as a pain management technique for both chronic and cancer pain.[4]

Descending Pathways

Descending pathways from the brain to the lower regions of the spinal cord are also involved in the pain response. The purpose of the descending tracts is to control or modify the afferent sensory input.[11] The corticospinal tract conveys information from the cortex to the brainstem and on to the spinal cord, where it terminates in laminae I through VIII.[15] The reticulospinal tract predominantly projects to laminae I and V, but also to laminae II and VI.[15]

The periaqueductal gray (PAG) region of the brain is active in the descending control of pain. Information from the cortex, limbic system, and thalamus stimulates the PAG of the midbrain. Pathways extend from the PAG to the raphe magnus in the medulla, and finally to the posterior horn of the spinal cord via the dorsal longitudinal fasciculus (DLF).[4,5,11] The DLF terminates in laminae I, II, and IV, where the descending control attenuates the afferent input entering the spinal cord in these areas. Also, at the level of the mesencephalon, the pathway contains serotonin, an inhibitory neurotransmitter active in the pain response.[11]

Norepinephrine is also an active substance in the descending control of pain. Serotonin and norepinephrine are the primary neurotransmitters active at the level of the pons, where neurons project to the posterior horn, also via the DLF.[5] At the level of the spinal cord, stimulation of the sympathetic ganglia leads to the release of norepinephrine at the periphery. The role of the sympathetic nervous system in both pain transmission and modulation is an area of growing research interest.

Endogenous Opioid System

Specific receptors for opioids within the brain, especially within the region of the PAG and the amygdala, were identified in the early 1970s.[16] Also discovered around this time were naturally occurring morphine-like substances, or **endorphins,** within the brain and spinal cord. The word *endorphin* is a combination of two words, *endogenous* (coming from within the body) and *morphine* (from the Latin word *morpheus,* meaning "sleep inducing"). The term endorphins actually refers to two groups of naturally occurring peptides: enkephalins, which are pentapeptides, and three types of larger polypeptides, α-, β-, and γ-endorphin. Of these, most is known about β-endorphin.[16] The endorphins play a key role in the neuromodulation of pain transmission (Fig. 46–5). The endorphins may affect neurotransmission of afferent nociceptive impulses as well as modulating descending responses to those impulses.[5,17]

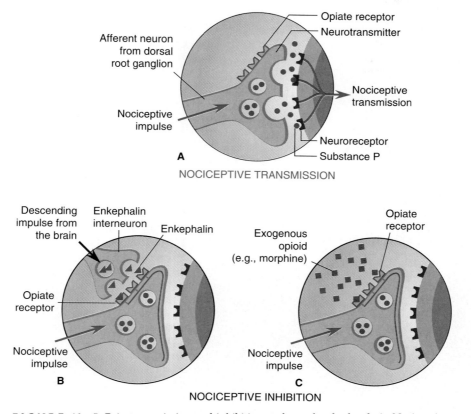

FIGURE 46 – 5. Pain transmission and inhibition at the molecular level. **A,** Nociceptive transmission to higher levels of the central nervous system. **B,** Nociception inhibited through binding of endogenous opioids (e.g., enkephalin). The release of substance P is prevented. **C,** Nociception inhibited through binding of exogenous opioid (e.g., morphine). The release of substance P is prevented.

During times of extreme stress, pain, or emotion, the body may create its own analgesia. This is known as **stress-induced analgesia.** Environmental stimuli become a physiologic trigger of the individual's intrinsic pain-inhibiting processes. It is not known how this occurs, but stress-induced analgesia has been shown to be sensitive to naloxone, suggesting the involvement of endogenous opioid peptides.[18] As β-endorphin is highly concentrated in the pituitary gland, it is probable that the release of pituitary opioids and adrenocorticotropin, which occurs in times of stress, is accompanied by the release of endorphin.[19] Similarly, the adrenal glands produce endogenous opioids as a sympathetic response to stress.[20]

Unfortunately, in chronic pain states, an individual's capacity to produce endogenous opioids may become diminished.[21] Research in the area of pain and depression points to a possible correlation between endogenous opioids, depression, and resultant pain, although the results are conflicting. In some studies CSF endorphin levels are low,[22,23] while in others they are normal.[24,25]

Opioid Receptors

The opioid receptors appear to be of greater clinical relevance than the endogenous opioids. At least four types of opioid receptors have been identified: mu, kappa, sigma, and delta.[6,14] The distribution of the specific opioid receptors varies throughout the body. For example, mu and sigma receptors are found in high concentration in the brain but occur at much lower concentrations in the spinal cord. There is growing evidence that mu receptors may also be present in the periphery. Mu receptors appear to have a greater affinity for opioids than other receptor types. Kappa receptors are concentrated primarily in the spinal cord, while delta receptors are primarily supraspinal.[14] The clinical significance of the opioid receptors is twofold: first, researchers have identified characteristics unique to the different receptors (Table 46–2), and second, both endogenous and exogenous opioids have varying affinities for the specific receptor sites (Table 46–3).[7]

Theories to Explain Pain

Gate Control Theory

A useful theoretical schema for understanding the intricacies of pain and the factors that facilitate and inhibit its perception is the **gate control theory.** The gate control theory was proposed by Melzack and Wall in 1965.[26] At the core of the theory is the capacity

TABLE 46–2. Opioid Receptor Activity

Opioid Receptor	Activity
mu	Analgesia
	Sedation
	Respiratory depression
	Pupil constriction
	Nausea and vomiting
	Constipation
	Urine retention
	Pruritus
kappa	Analgesia
	Sedation
	Respiratory depression
	Pupil constriction
	Diuresis
sigma	No analgesia
	Vasomotor stimulation
	Tachypnea
	Pupil dilation
	Psychotomimetic effects (hallucinations, paranoia, delirium)
delta	No analgesia
	Respiratory depression
	Nausea and vomiting
	Pruritus

of the organism to alter the intensity of painful stimuli at a perceptual level by means of a "gating system" at the level of the spinal cord.[11,27] The gate control theory proposes that cells within the substantia gelatinosa modulate incoming stimuli before they reach what Melzack and Wall termed transmission or T-cells. The T-cells facilitate the central transmission of nociceptive impulses. The number of nociceptive impulses that arrive at the T-cells depends on the activity of large fibers (A-beta), small fibers (A-delta and C fibers, discussed previously), and descending influences from the brain. Large fibers stimulate the cells in the substantia gelatinosa and inhibit central transmission by the T-cells. Perceived pain intensity is a result of the balance of myelinated and unmyelinated nerve fiber input. In other words, for pain transmission to take place, a number of small fibers carrying nociceptive impulses enter the posterior horn of the spinal cord. When left unopposed, small fiber impulses progress directly through an "open gate" to the T-cells and beyond. In contrast, when large fibers are also activated, they can "take over" or "close the gate" in the substantia gelatinosa and inhibit the transmission of pain impulses by the T-cells. Some of the descending control systems that originate in the PAG, as described above, can also "close the gate" by exerting an inhibitory influence on the T-cells.

Because the gate control theory proposes that large-fiber stimulation helps modulate the pain response, activities, therapies, or procedures that stimulate large-fiber activity should be beneficial.[28] Cutaneous stimulation is believed to stimulate large fibers. Also, the presence of competing sensory information in the brain may provide a modulatory response, owing to the inhibitory effects of descending control on the T-cells in the posterior horn of the spinal cord.[11,27,28]

Other Theories

Basic scientists in the area of pain discovered an intriguing concept involving repeated noxious stimuli.

TABLE 46–3. Receptor Affinity of Commonly Used Opioids

Drug	Receptor Affinity	Agonist		Antagonist	
		Pure	*Partial*	*Pure*	*Partial*
Morphine, meperidine, hydromorphone, methadone, fentanyl	mu	×			
	kappa (*morphine only*)		×		
	delta		×		
Buprenorphine	mu		×		
	kappa	×			
Butorphanol	mu				×
	kappa	×			
	sigma	×			
Nalbuphine	mu				×
	kappa	×			
	sigma		×		
Pentazocine	mu				×
	kappa	×			
	sigma	×			
Naloxone	mu			×	
	kappa			×	
	sigma				
	delta				
Naltrexone	mu			×	
	kappa			×	

In rat models, repeated stimuli were found to cause a nociceptive response that was much more profound than expected.[29] The phenomenon is referred to as **windup.** The spinal cord seems to become barraged with nociceptive input even though the repeated stimulus is no stronger than the first stimulus. Windup is induced only by C fiber input, but A fibers can enhance the effect. The pain is characterized by **allodynia** (pain caused by a stimulus that should not cause pain, such as a light touch). Although humans have not shown the exact response in research,[30] the theory of windup may explain why people complain of intense pain when the noxious input is not intense but is constant.

It has been found that the excitatory amino acid glutamate, a neurotransmitter, carries the nociceptive message from primary afferent fibers to secondary neurons. A nonopioid receptor, the *N*-methyl-D-aspartate (NMDA) receptor, appears to have a major role in the increase of receptive fields of nociception (hyperalgesia). Drugs that inhibit glutamate production may impede the windup response, thereby controlling pain before it crescendos to an unbearable state. If glutamate cannot be assuaged, there is evidence that ketamine (an NMDA receptor antagonist), administered before the first incision is made in the operating room and again before the end of the operation, may decrease postoperative pain by preventing windup.[30]

Neural plasticity is another recent theory of great use to scientists and clinicians alike. Plasticity refers to the hyperexcitability of dorsal horn neurons that follows severe pain and inflammation. In the first phase of plasticity, an injury occurs in the peripheral nervous system and input from surrounding neurons that are *not* damaged relays a nociceptive impulse to the CNS. This also results in *hyperalgesia,* or pain surrounding the area of injury.

The second phase occurs when nociceptive reflexes are inhibited by these neurons. This is said to modulate or change the pain. An example of pain modulation in this phase is the prevention of a local withdrawal response.

In phase three, commencing within 10 minutes and lasting up to 3 months after an injury, sensitization to noxious stimuli is increased and locomotion is decreased. This is termed the period of recuperation. The action of plasticity and windup suggest that drugs with an affinity for certain receptors (not opiate receptors) which could block the release of glutamate could be effective in pain control.[29]

Clearly, pain theories are an attempt to make understandable the diverse and complex physiologic occurrences that make up the pain experience. No one theory is complete or beyond scrutiny. Psychosocial, environmental, and developmental factors are particularly difficult to encompass in a theory that deals in such concrete neurophysiologic concepts. Ongoing research in this area continues to advance knowledge of pain types and their peripheral and central transmission.

KEY CONCEPTS

- Pain sensation is transmitted from nociceptors to the cerebral cortex by neurons. Nociceptor activation is enhanced by prostaglandins and other chemicals that directly stimulate or lower the threshold for stimulation. Nociceptor activity is transmitted to the spinal cord by two types of neurons: large, myelinated A-delta fibers, which transmit sharp, localized sensations, and small, unmyelinated C fibers, which transmit dull, aching, poorly localized sensations.

- Most afferent fibers enter the cord through the posterior horn and synapse on interneurons, motor neurons, and sympathetic neurons. Neurons originating in the cord may then cross the cord and project centrally on the contralateral side (spinothalamic tract) or project centrally on the ipsilateral side. Neurotransmitters such as substance P and calcitonin gene–related peptide are active in pain transmission at the cord level.

- There are two divisions of afferent fibers that ascend from the contralateral side of the cord: the spinothalamic (neospinothalamic) division, which projects directly to the thalamus and then the sensory cortex, and the spinoreticulothalamic (paleospinothalamic) division, which projects diffusely to the reticular formation, mesencephalon, and then the thalamus.

- Afferent fiber activity can be modulated at several levels. Descending pathways project from the periaqueductal gray area to neurons in the spinal cord. Ascending pain impulses may also be modulated in the brain stem. Endogenous opioids (enkephalins, endorphins) also moderate pain perception. Specific receptors for opioids are located within the spinal cord and brain.

- The gate control theory proposes that afferent pain impulses are "gated" or modulated at the level of the spinal cord before they are conducted centrally by transmission neurons (T-cells). Activity in other neuronal pathways, such as cutaneous touch fibers, can inhibit pain transmission by "closing the gate."

- No one pain theory is capable of explaining the intricacies of the pain phenomenon. Future neurophysiologic research may refute existing theories. Moreover, psychosocial and cultural pain research will most assuredly demonstrate the inadequacy of theories based entirely on laboratory and clinical data.

Manifestations of Different Types of Pain

In addition to a general overview of pain mechanisms and theory, the next section provides an overview of three specific types of pain: referred pain, neuropathic pain, and ischemic pain. Although the basic mechanisms of pain transmission are similar to those dis-

cussed previously, the characteristics of these types
of pain are unique.

Referred Pain

Referred pain is pain that emanates from the source
of injury to another location in the body. It is often
felt at some distance from the point of arisal. A familiar
example is the pain of myocardial infarction that is
felt in the jaw or left arm. The mechanism of this type
of pain is not clearly understood, although it has been
studied for over a century. Other examples of referred
pain include shoulder pain following pelvic laparoscopic procedures or with liver metastasis in cancer,
and cutaneous pain experienced with visceral irritation or tension (Fig. 46–6). There is evidence supporting the presence of dual innervation of somatic (e.g.,
skin, muscle) and visceral (e.g., hollow organs, membranes) structures by common afferent fibers. Also, a
growing body of evidence suggests convergence of
visceral nociceptor activity with primary somatic afferents within the posterior horn of the spinal cord and
the spinothalamic tract.[4,31] For example, the diaphragm is innervated largely by the fourth cervical
nerve (C4), as is the shoulder. In the case of diaphragmatic irritation, shoulder pain often coexists because
the spinal cord and the brain interpret the nociceptive
input as originating from C4 and cannot distinguish
the specific origin of the impulse.

Knowledge of where pain tends to be referred can
be helpful in diagnosis and treatment. For example,
trigger points are tender points in a band of muscle
fibers that are painful when palpated, most commonly
seen in the neck or back. These points may refer pain
to the head, which to the untrained observer would
be identified as a headache.[32]

Neuropathic Pain

Neuropathic pain results from dysfunctional abnormalities of the nervous system. Nerve injury due to
surgery, tumor growth, metastasis, radiation therapy
or chemotherapy, or trauma often causes neuropathic
pain. It is characterized by constant aching sensations
that may be interrupted by bursts of burning or shocklike pain in the affected area.[4] A mild stimulus such
as stroking the affected area causes pain, a condition
termed **allodynia.** After the initial injury, neuropathic
pain is not often felt immediately. Days, weeks, or
even months later, after the tissue-damaging source
of pain has resolved, the onset of neuropathic pain
initiates a new and complex pain state.

The pathophysiology of neuropathic pain is now
thought to result from altered central processing of
nociceptive input. In one proposed model of neuropathic pain for pain states where mechanically stimulated allodynia is a chief complaint, ongoing afferent
fibers from the periphery appear to maintain an abnormal processing of the pain message in the CNS.[33] In
earlier models, neuropathic pain was thought to arise
primarily from the efferent activity of sympathetic

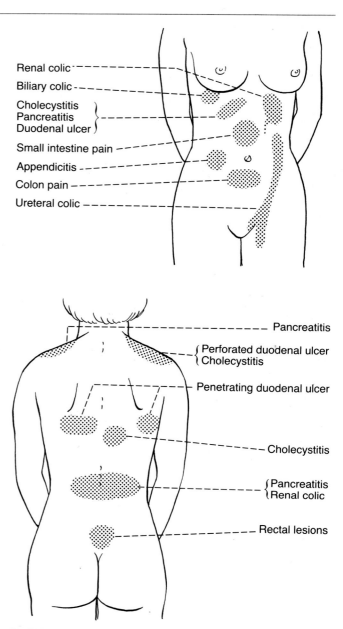

F I G U R E 46 – 6. Areas of referred pain. (From Black JM, Matassarin-Jacobs E: *Luckmann and Sorensen's Medical-Surgical Nursing: A Psychophysiologic Approach,* 4th ed. Philadelphia, WB Saunders, 1993, p 322. Reproduced with permission.)

nerves. Convincing studies support the concept of
altered central processing of afferent fibers,[34,35] although this model is not meant to explain all neuropathic pain, and more research is necessary to identify
the etiology of the numerous neuropathic pain states.

Examples of neuropathic pain include **postherpetic neuralgia,** epidural spinal cord compression,
cauda equina compression, plexus injuries, and neuropathies. Phantom limb pain may fall into this category as well. The pathophysiology of phantom pain
is still in the hypothesis phase, but several theories
involve dysfunction of either the peripheral or central
nervous system.[36] The facts that nociceptive input is
no longer a factor after healing of an amputation and

that pain may persist as a burning, shooting intermittent pain lead to the belief that this is indeed a neuropathic process.

Sympathetically maintained pain is a unique type of neuropathic pain that may occur in the absence of nerve injury.[4,31] The pathophysiologic mechanisms of an individual's pain that fit into this category are numerous and diverse. Recently, the term sympathetically maintained pain has been contrasted with sympathetically independent pain, chronic pain that can be identified as *not* having sympathetic nervous system involvement.[37] Thus, sympathetically maintained pain is an operantly based diagnosis for a particular group of patients.

In the scenario of sympathetically maintained pain, the sympathetic nervous system becomes hyperactive. The diagnosis may be made on the basis of improved analgesia with sympathetic blockade or aggravation of pain with sympathetic nerve stimulation. Not all sufferers exhibit the same symptoms, but most prevalent are *allodynia* (painful sensation to normal touch), *hyperalgesia* (painful area surrounding the injured area), *atrophy* of the affected extremity (in which it usually occurs), *coldness* in the affected area, and *dystrophic changes,* most often evidenced by hair loss and a shiny quality to the skin.

A model for the basic mechanisms of sympathetically maintained pain has been proposed and involves both the peripheral and central nervous systems.[31] The salient elements of the model suggest that nerve or soft tissue injuries result in α-adrenergic activity or peripheral nociceptors, with the localized release of norepinephrine activating the nociceptors. This process sensitizes the cells in the posterior horn of the spinal cord such that they can respond to a larger range of nociceptive input. In response to the increased pain, sympathetic discharge also increases, aggravating the initial problem. There is no doubt some nociceptive input in sympathetically maintained pain as well, because people frequently complain of a "deep, aching" component to the pain.[38]

Neuropathic pain is difficult to treat. It is frequently unresponsive to opioid or other pharmacologic therapy. Subsequently, both laboratory and clinical researchers continue to seek answers to questions regarding the mechanism of and treatment for this complex pain phenomenon.

Ischemic Pain

Pain resulting from a sudden and profound loss of blood to the tissue in a particular part of the body may be described as **ischemic pain.** As ischemia worsens, the inflamed tissue impinges on nerves, rendering them unable to function. **Paresthesia** (burning, prickling) usually develops as a result. An interesting characteristic of ischemic pain is that it may have similar symptoms as referred pain, neuropathic pain, or acute somatic pain.

The symptoms of ischemic pain depend on the origin of the ischemia. If cardiac in origin, the pain is visceral, radiating to the arm or jaw. This pain is perceived as being deep, aching, diffuse, and pressing. It most often has a sudden onset.

Ischemia resulting from acute deep venous occlusion is also aching and has a deep quality and gradual onset. Acute arterial occlusion may be felt as either burning or aching, but has a sudden onset.[39]

Arteriosclerosis obliterans occurs over a period of time as plaque develops in the intima of the arteries, most often of the lower extremities. In early stages, the pain is intermittent and has a cramping quality. In severe cases, ischemic neuropathy may ensue, as evidenced by a burning, shooting pain in the leg or foot.

The treatment of ischemic pain is multifaceted. Pharmacologic therapy may be sufficient to restore blood flow, thus decreasing pain. NSAIDs, possibly combined with a weak opioid, may be effective if pain control is the specific goal. If ulcers develop, if the pain of ischemia increases, or if gangrene becomes a threat, vascular surgery is indicated, followed by either local anesthetics or intraspinal opioids in the postoperative phase.

Life-style changes can have a dramatic effect on early ischemic diseases. Cessation of smoking, weight loss, and exercise regimens are often recommended because of their positive cost and risk-benefit ratio. Accurate diagnosis and astute observation of pain symptoms are critical for early and effective treatment of all three types of pain, neuropathic, referred, or ischemic.

Physiologic Responses to Pain

The purpose of pain is to serve as a warning system to the body. The autonomic nervous system is responsible for much of the physiologic response to pain. The autonomic nervous system response includes both the sympathetic and parasympathetic divisions. As discussed previously, norepinephrine is an active neurotransmitter in the pain response. Norepinephrine and epinephrine play important roles in the stimulation of the sympathetic nervous system as a physiologic response to pain. Activation of the autonomic nervous system (sympathetic division) results in a predictable cluster of physical signs and symptoms, including elevated heart rate, blood pressure, and respiratory rate, as well as dilated pupils, perspiration, and pallor (Table 46–4).[6,8,11,40–42] Sympathetic stimulation results in blood shifts from superficial vessels to striated muscle, the heart, the lungs, and the nervous system; bronchodilation; increased cardiac contractility; and increased circulating blood glucose. In addition, although gastrointestinal motility and secretion decrease, sphincter tone increases.[11] Nausea, vomiting, and even ileus may develop. Hypomotility of the bladder and ureters can also result from sympathetic activation, leading to urine retention.[7]

Supraspinal involvement in the pain response also leads to a hormonal response to pain. Pain stimulates the release of numerous hormones in addition to

T A B L E 46 – 4. Physiologic Responses to Pain*

Criteria	Response
Signs and symptoms	↑ Heart rate
	↑ Blood pressure
	↑ Respiratory rate
	Dilated pupils
	Pallor and perspiration
	Nausea and vomiting
	Urine retention
Physiologic response	Blood shifts from superficial vessels to striated muscle, heart, lungs, and brain
	Bronchioles dilate to ↑ oxygenation
	↑ Gastric secretions
	↓ Gastrointestinal motility
	↑ Circulating blood sugar
	Hypomotility of the bladder and ureters

*Result from sympathetic activation.

Adapted with permission from Wild L: Pain management. *Crit Care Clin North Am* 1990;2(4):538.

endogenous catecholamines. The hormones secreted include antidiuretic hormone (ADH), aldosterone, and cortisol.[6,8,11]

Even though the predominant physiologic responses to pain are the result of sympathetic stimulation, the body cannot sustain this level of activation for prolonged periods of time. Eventually physiologic adaptation occurs and the observed sympathetic response to pain abates.[11,28] Thus, heart rate, blood pressure, and respiratory rate return to normal or baseline. However, pain can be present even in the absence of overt physiologic signs and symptoms of sympathetic activation. One example is chronic pain. Another clinical example is the post-acute injury or postoperative period, during which the sympathetic stimulation caused by uncontrolled pain masks other underlying problems such as hypovolemia.[41]

KEY CONCEPTS

- Pain usually results from stimulation of nociceptors located throughout the body. Acute pain results from tissue injury and generally resolves when the injury resolves. The clinical manifestations of acute pain result from activation of the sympathetic nervous system (elevated heart rate, blood pressure, and respiratory rate, dilated pupils, perspiration, and pallor).

- Chronic pain lasts several months beyond the expected healing time and often is not associated with sympathetic manifestations of pain, owing to physiologic adaptation. Instead, changes in personality or life-style may occur. Individuals may experience acute and chronic pain simultaneously.

- Referred pain is a painful sensation perceived at some distance from an injury but generally within the same dermatome. Referred pain is thought to occur because of convergence of visceral nociceptor activity with primary somatic afferents in the posterior horn of the cord.

- Neuropathic pain results from injury to peripheral or central nerves as a consequence of surgery, tumor, trauma, or drugs. Neuropathic pain is generally constant, achy, or shocklike. The sympathetic nervous system may mediate neuropathic pain by releasing an excitatory neurotransmitter, norepinephrine, onto nociceptors.

- Ischemic pain occurs when there is a sudden and profound loss of blood to the tissue in a particular part of the body. It may be manifested in a variety of ways: as referred pain, neuropathic pain, or acute somatic pain.

Treatment Modalities

Many pain management treatments are available. By understanding the basic mechanisms of pain transmission, one can readily identify potential sites where various types of treatment modalities could interrupt pain transmission and perception. In other words, available treatments alter pain transmission at specific points in the pain pathway. Pain management interventions can be directed at four points: (1) interrupting peripheral transmission of nociception, (2) modulating pain transmission at the spinal cord level, (3) "closing the pain gate," or (4) altering the perception and integration of nociceptive impulses in the brain.

Interrupting Peripheral Transmission of Pain

Modalities that interrupt the peripheral transmission of nociceptive impulses are the first step in controlling pain. The basic action of splinting an injured limb or area of the body alters the peripheral transmission of pain by minimizing or reducing tissue injury. Applying heat or cold to an injured area also helps to reduce peripheral nociception by increasing blood flow to the area or by reducing swelling in the area, respectively.[28]

Pharmacologic treatments such as NSAIDs or local anesthetic agents also exert their analgesic effects by interrupting, at an early stage, the peripheral transmission. The use of NSAIDs and local anesthetic agents as a primary intervention for pain management has grown rapidly. The inhibition of prostaglandin production by NSAIDs reduces the number of neurotransmitters for pain available to conduct nociception in the peripheral tissues. Without adequate numbers of nociceptive neurotransmitters, pain transmission cannot continue.[42] The role of prostaglandins in the pain response was described earlier. The NSAIDs include but are not limited to drugs such as indomethacin, ibuprofen, naproxen, sulindac, piroxicam, and ketorolac. However, blocking the production and action of prostaglandin also has other effects on the body. For example, prostaglandins are also responsible for maintenance of the gastric mucosa, and blocking their actions can result in gastrointestinal bleeding.[9] Prostaglandin inhibition can also lead to decreased platelet aggregation and renal insufficiency. Knowledge of the risks and prescribing guidelines is essential for safe patient care, especially for prolonged periods of time.

Local anesthetic agents can be applied either to nerve endings at the site of injury or to the nerve plexus supplying the area. By providing localized or regional blockade, peripheral pain transmission is interrupted.[7,42,43] Local anesthetic agents diminish or block conduction of the nociceptive impulses by blocking sodium influx during phase 0 of the action potential. The degree of blockade achieved with local agents depends on the amount of drug applied and hence the extent of sodium channel blockade. Local infiltration of wounds with local anesthetic agents such as bupivacaine or lidocaine is now common practice for many health care professionals.

Modulating Pain Transmission at the Spinal Cord

Numerous procedures and agents are used to modulate pain transmission at the level of the spinal cord. The effective techniques and drugs are those whose primary action is to close the pain gate. Nonpharmacologic techniques that close the gate include all types of cutaneous stimulation. Recall that cutaneous stimulation activates and recruits large fibers and inhibits the central progression of a nociceptive transmission at the T-cells. Examples of cutaneous stimulation include transcutaneous electrical nerve stimulation (TENS), massage, acupuncture, application of heat or cold, and therapeutic touch.[11,28,42]

Pharmacologic measures that act at the level of the spinal cord include epidural and intrathecal analgesia. Intraspinal analgesia (i.e., epidural or intrathecal approaches) can be achieved using opioids, local anesthetics, and, more recently, α-adrenergic blocking agents.[42,44-46] Intraspinal opioids work by binding with opioid receptors in the posterior horn of the spinal cord, thereby decreasing the release of neurotransmitters such as substance P. Without an adequate number of pain neurotransmitters present in the substantia gelatinosa, central transmission cannot progress. The mechanism of action for intraspinal local anesthesia agents is like that described earlier except that these agents block nerve conduction at the posterior nerve root. Epidural administration of an α-adrenergic blocking agent such as clonidine is a promising analgesic tool. The mechanism of action for epidural clonidine is in blocking some of the sympathetically mediated pain transmission.

Finally, dorsal column stimulators, sometimes used in chronic pain management, also work at the level of the spinal cord to close the pain gate. This particular technique, still relatively new, modulates descending input from the brain to the spinal cord.

Altering the Perception and Integration of Pain

The traditional modality for managing pain is the administration of systemic opioids. This pharmacologic intervention has stood the test of time. Opioids work at specific receptor sites that are located throughout the body but are highly concentrated in the brain. The opioid analgesic agents such as morphine and other derivatives alter the perception of pain at the level of the brain.

Other, nonpharmacologic techniques of pain management include such activities and procedures as distraction, imagery, biofeedback, and hypnosis. With distraction, the number of generalized stimuli reaching the brain increases. Because the brain has a limited capacity to sort and attend to multiple and varied stimuli, it is less able to integrate the pain experience when other competition is present.[11,42] Imagery also alters the perception of painful stimuli in the higher centers of the brain. A second benefit of imagery is that it often produces relaxation as well as analgesia. Biofeedback is a conditioned response that can be learned as a pain control. Biofeedback helps control pain by increasing blood flow (usually as a consequence of relaxation), as directed, to target body areas. The increased blood flow decreases the concentration of neurotransmitters in the area.[11] Biofeedback may also increase the amount of endorphins produced and released.

KEY CONCEPTS

- Treatment is aimed at moderating pain transmission at specific points along the pain pathways. Potential sites of pain moderation are at the peripheral nociceptor, spinal cord, and brain.
- Nociceptor activation can be altered by prostaglandin inhibitors (NSAIDs), heat and cold, and local anesthetics that block sodium influx through fast channels.
- Spinal cord transmission can be altered by cutaneous stimulation (gate control theory) and intraspinal analgesics (opioids, local anesthetics, α-adrenergic blockers).
- The perception of pain can be altered within the brain with systemic opioids and by nonpharmacologic means such as hypnosis, distraction, and biofeedback.

Summary

Pain is a complex human experience that is also a normal and expected phenomenon, particularly in response to injury. Although pain is a challenging experience for both the affected individual and those who are charged with treating it, it is also a gift. Without pain, our bodies would be without an alarm system that alerts us to problems within. Pain as a specialty in the biological sciences, medicine, and nursing is still relatively new. As we learn more about the intricacies of pain mechanisms and human responses to pain, the options for relieving pain and suffering will grow.

REFERENCES

1. Merskey H: IASP Subcommittee on Taxonomy: Pain terms. A list with definitions and notes on usage. *Pain* 1979;6:249.
2. McCaffery M: *Nursing Practice Theories Related to Cognition, Bodily Pain, and Man-Environment Interactions.* Master's thesis, University of California, Los Angeles, 1968.
3. Loeser JD: Concepts of pain, in Stanton-Hicks M, Boas R (eds): *Chronic Low Back Pain.* New York, Raven Press, 1982, pp 145–148.
4. Payne R: Pathophysiology of cancer pain, in Foley KM, Bonica JJ, Ventafridda V, Callaway MV (eds): *Proceedings of the 2nd International Congress on Cancer Pain. Adv Pain Res* 1990;16:13–26.
5. Casey K: Neural mechanisms of pain: An overview. *Acta Anaesth Scand* 1982;74(suppl):13–20.
6. Benedetti C: Acute pain: A review of its effects and therapy with systemic opioids, in Benedetti C, Chapman CR, Giron G (eds): Opioid analgesia: Recent advances in systemic administration. *Adv Pain Res* 1990;14:367–424.
7. Benedetti C, Bonica JJ, Bellucci G: Pathophysiology and therapy of postoperative pain: A review, in Benedetti C, Chapman CR, Moricca G (eds): *Recent Advances in the Management of Pain. Adv Pain Res* 1984;7:373–407.
8. Puntillo K: The phenomenon of pain and critical care nursing. *Heart Lung* 1988;17:262–273.
9. Paice JA: Unraveling the mystery of pain. *Oncol Nurs Forum* 1991;18:843–849.
10. Basbaum AI: Peripheral mechanisms of sensitization and hyperalgesia, in Stanley TH, Ashburn MA, Fine PG (eds). *Anesthesiology and Pain Management.* Dordrecht, Kluwer Academic Publishers, 1991, pp 31–37.
11. Abu-Saad H, Tesler M: Pain, in Carrieri VK, Linsey AM, West CM (eds): *Pathophysiological Phenomena in Nursing: Human Responses to Illness.* Philadelphia, WB Saunders, 1986, pp 235–269.
12. Sundsten JW: The peripheral nerves, spinal cord, and brainstem, in Patton HD, Sundsten JW, Crill WE, Swanson PD (eds): *Introduction to Basic Neurology.* Philadelphia, WB Saunders, 1976, pp 4–48.
13. Basbaum AI: The central nervous system substrate for the transmission of "pain" messages, in Stanley TH, Ashburn MA, Fine PG (eds): *Anesthesiology and Pain Management.* Dordrecht, Kluwer Academic Publishers, 1991, pp 67–72.
14. Bullingham R: Physiological mechanisms in pain, in Smith G, Covino B (eds): *Acute Pain.* London, Butterworths, 1985, pp 1–21.
15. Wallace KG: The pathophysiology of pain. *Crit Care Nurse Q* 1992;15(2):1–13.
16. Huhman M: Endogenous opiates and pain. *Adv Nurs Sci* 1982;62:71.
17. Terenius L, Tamsen A: Endorphins and the modulation of acute pain. *Acta Anaesth Scand* 1982;74(suppl):21–24.
18. Willer JC, Dehen H, Cambier J: Stress-induced analgesia in humans: Endogenous opioids and naloxone-reversible depression of pain reflexes. *Science* 1981;212:689–691.
19. Axelrod J, Reisine TD: Stress hormones: Their interactions and regulations. *Science* 1984;224:452–459.
20. Lewis JW, Tordoff MJ, Sherman JE, Liebeskind JC: Adrenal medullary enkephalin-like peptides may mediate opioid stress analgesia. *Science* 1982;217:557–559.
21. Terenius LY: Biochemical assessment of chronic pain, in Kosterlitz KW, Terenius LY (eds): *Pain and Society.* Basel, Verlag Chemie, 1980, pp 355–364.
22. Baldi E, Salmon S, Anselmi B, et al: Intermittent hypoendorphinaemia in migraine attack. *Cephalgia* 1982;2(2):77–81.
23. Hargreaves KM, Flores CM, Dionne RA, Mueller GP: The role of pituitary β-endorphin in mediating corticotropin-releasing factor–induced antinociception. *Am J Physiol* 1990;258:E235–E242.
24. Bach FW: Beta-endorphin-related peptides in human cerebrospinal fluid, in AR Genazzani, Negri M (eds): *Opioid Peptides in Biological Fluids.* Parthenon, Carnforth, 1989, 17–25.
25. Bach FW, Langemark M, Secher NH, Olesen J: Plasma and cerebrospinal fluid β-endorphin in chronic tension-type headache. *Pain* 1992;51(2):163–168.
26. Melzack R, Wall PD: Pain mechanisms: A new theory. *Science* 1965;150:971–974.
27. Wolf ZR: Pain theories: An overview. *Top Clin Nurs* 1980;2:9–18.
28. McCaffery M, Beebe A: *Pain: Clinical Manual for Nursing Practice.* St. Louis, CV Mosby, 1989.
29. Willis W: *Hyperalgesia and Allodynia.* New York, Raven Press, 1992, pp 259–266.
30. Ho G, Evans S, Yaksh TL, Clark LA, Shapiro HM: The effects of intraoperative ketamine on postoperative opioid requirements: A randomized double-blind study. 1993. Unpublished manuscript.
31. Cousins MJ: Pain and the sympathetic nervous system: A clinical perspective, in Stanley TH, Ashburn MA, Fine PG (eds): *Anesthesiology and Pain Management.* Dordrecht, Kluwer Academic Publishers, 1991, pp 61–66.
32. Mense S: Referral of muscle pain. New aspects. *APS J* 1994;3:1–9.
33. Gracely RH, Lynch SA, Bennett GJ: Painful neuropathy: Altered central processing maintained dynamically by peripheral input. *Pain* 1992;51(2):175–194.
34. Woolf CJ: Recent advances in the pathophysiology of acute pain. *Br J Anaesth* 1989;63:139–146.
35. Dubner R: Neuronal plasticity and pain following peripheral tissue inflammation or nerve injury, in Bond MR, Charlton JE, Woolf CJ (eds): *Pain Research and Clinical Management.* Vol 4: *Proceedings of the VIth World Congress on Pain.* Amsterdam, Elsevier, 1991, pp 263–276.
36. Wesolowski MS, Lerma ML: Phantom limb pain. *Reg Anesth* 1993;18:121–127.
37. Campbell JN, Meyer RA, Rafa SN: Is nociceptor activation by alpha-1 adrenoreceptors the culprit in sympathetically maintained pain? *APS J* 1992;1:3–11.
38. Roberts WJ, Kramis RC: Adrenergic mediation of SMP: Via nociceptive or non-nociceptive afferents or both? *APS J* 1992;1:12–15.
39. Bonica JJ: Pain due to vascular disease, in Bonica JJ (ed): *The Management of Pain.* Philadelphia, Lea & Febiger, 1990, pp 502–537.
40. Puntillo KA: The physiology of pain and its consequences in critically ill patients, In Puntillo KA: *Pain in the Critically Ill: Assessment and Management.* Gaithersburg, Md, Aspen, 1991, pp 9–29.
41. Wild L: Transition from pain to comfort: Understanding the hemodynamic risks. *Crit Care Nurs Q* (in press).
42. Wild L: Pain management. *Crit Care Clin North Am* 1990;2:537–547.
43. Armitage EN: Local anesthetic techniques for prevention of postoperative pain. *Br J Anaesth* 1986;58:790.
44. Cousins MJ, Mather LE: Intrathecal and epidural administration of opiates. *Anesthesiology* 1984;61:276–310.
45. Behar M, Olshwang D, Magora F, Davison JT: Epidural morphine in the treatment of pain. *Lancet* 1979;1:527–529.
46. Wang JK, Nauss LA, Thomas JE: Pain relief by intrathecally applied morphine in man. *Anesthesiology* 1979;50:149–151.

BIBLIOGRAPHY

Acute Pain Management Guideline Panel: *Acute Pain Management: Operative or Medical Procedures and Trauma. Clinical Practice Guideline.* AHCPR Pub. No. 92-0032. Rockville, Md, Agency for Health Care Policy and Research, Public Health Service, US Department of Health and Human Services, 1992.

Acute Pain Management Guideline Panel: *Acute Pain Management in Infants, Children, and Adolescents: Operative and Medical Procedures. Quick Reference Guide for Clinicians.* AHCPR Pub. No. 92-0020. Rockville, Md, Agency for Health Care Policy and

Research, Public Health Service, US Department of Health and Human Services, 1992.

Casey KL: Nociceptors and their sensitization: Overview, in Willis W (ed): *Hyperalgesia and Allodynia.* New York, Raven Press, 1992, pp 13–17.

Ferrante FM, VadeBoncouer TR: *Postoperative Pain.* New York, Churchill Livingstone, 1993.

Fields HL: *Pain.* New York, McGraw-Hill, 1987.

Harkins S: Pain in the elderly, in Dubner R, Gebhart G, Bond M (eds): *Proceedings of the Fifth World Congress on Pain.* Amsterdam, Elsevier, 1988, pp 355–357.

Henriksson KG: Have new aspects on referral of muscle pain and on hyperalgesia any bearing on the pathogenesis of chronic widespread muscle pain and tenderness? *APS J* 1994;3:13–16.

International Association for the Study of Pain: Task Force on Acute Pain: Ready LB, Edwards WT (eds): *Management of Acute Pain: A Practical Guide.* Seattle, IASP Publications, 1992.

Kanner R: *Diagnosis and Management of Pain in Patients with Cancer.* Basel, Karger, 1988.

Levine JK, Taiwo YO, Heller PH: Hyperalgesic pain: Inflammatory and neuropathic, in Willis W (ed): *Hyperalgesia and Allodynia.* New York, Raven Press, pp 117–125.

Management of Cancer Pain Guideline Panel: *Management of Cancer Pain. Clinical Practice Guideline, Number 9.* AHCPR Pub. No. 94–0592. Rockville, Md, Agency for Health Care Policy and Research, Public Health Service, US Department of Health and Human Services, 1994.

Patt R: *Cancer Pain.* Philadelphia, JB Lippincott, 1993.

Price DD: *Psychological and Neural Mechanisms of Pain.* New York, Raven Press, 1988.

Sabbe MB, Yaksh TL: Pharmacology of spinal opioids. *J Pain Symptom Management* 1990;5:191–203.

Wallace KG: The pathophysiology of pain. *Crit Care Nurs Q* 1992;15:1–13.

UNIT XIII
Alterations in Neuropsychological Function

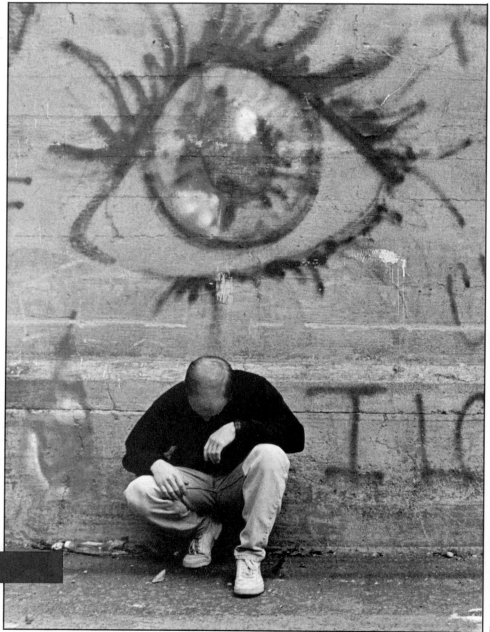

Disordered thinking, posturing, and altered mood may characterize persons affected by neuropsychological dysfunction.

We prefer to believe that happiness is an attainable ideal in the lives of most people, but happiness's antithesis, depression, is pervasive. Depression is not just unhappiness. It is a disease that inhibits the impulse to live with satisfaction and pleasure. Medical professionals encounter it in many different settings, no matter what their specialties or practices may be. Research over the past few decades has produced greater understanding of the biological basis of depression and raised the prospect that it might be treated genetically.

Researchers have identified categories of people who are most likely to be depressed. The number and variety of these categories suggest that depression is a common problem. As many as 8 million Americans may suffer serious depression at any one time.

Recent epidemiological studies have demonstrated that young women are more than twice as likely to suffer depression than young men. Depression among the elderly is common, especially if they suffer other illnesses, as many depressed people do. But it may be overlooked unless caregiving professionals who have frequent contact with older people notice cases and obtain diagnosis and treatment so that therapy or drugs can be used to treat the condition.

People suffering chronic illnesses may also suffer chronic depression. Depression has been found increasingly among persons suffering from multiple sclerosis, in which it is studied both as a possible symptom or a precipitating factor in the disease. Depression also is commonly found among persons suffering from dementia of the Alzheimer's type, which is characterized by memory loss and intellectual disabilities.

Differences in depressive behavior have also been noted by researchers in the emotional outlook of persons who have suffered single ischemic strokes to their right and left hemispheres. Those with right hemisphere damage were found to have less anxiety than those with left hemisphere stroke. Researchers speculated that misunderstanding of the lower anxiety of patients suffering damage to the right hemisphere may have accounted for clinical descriptions of their seeming indifference and failure to recover as expected.

Research also indicates a relationship between depression and immunity. One study argues that indexes of immunocompetence are lower among depressed people.

Inquiries of various kinds suggest that the use of biological markers in the assessment of depression will be important in the future. Researchers expect that molecular genetics will contribute to an increased understanding of the biochemical nature of depression and how it is inherited. Neurologists have shown interest in research that reveals that depression produces observable changes in some brain systems.

Like depression, schizophrenia can be a severely disabling disease characterized by serious brain dysfunction, perhaps in many areas of the brain. Over the past generation, researchers have followed a hypothesis that suggests that schizophrenic patients suffer from functional changes in the central dopaminergic systems of their brains. As research continues, this hypothesis is being refined with new diagnostic devices, and other theories are emerging.

Although researchers agree that schizophrenia is caused

FRONTIERS OF RESEARCH
Biological Basis of Psychiatric Illnesses

Michael J. Kirkhorn

by brain dysfunction—a relief for many researchers if only because it allows them to dismiss the notion that mental illness is a myth or that harmful parenting or some other warping experience might cause schizophrenia—there is still no clear agreement exactly how and where the brain harbors the disease.

Dopaminergic mechanisms help mediate the symptoms of schizophrenia, but exactly what they do is unclear. The research, one study says, supports "both increased and decreased dopamine function in schizophrenia." New diagnostic devices, such as functional brain imaging, have confirmed abnormal frontal cortex functioning in schizophrenia, but subcortical pathology also seems to be involved, and this is not clearly understood.

Other disorders that resemble schizophrenia harm the health and prospects of many Americans. One recent article reported that research that studied the evidence from a number of medical perspectives found that schizotypal personality disorder is closely related to chronic schizophrenia, and may be one disorder in a "continuum of schizophrenia-related disorders."

The study of patients suffering from schizotypal personality disorder, often overlooked but "probably more prevalent than more severe forms of schizophrenia," indicated to researchers that personal and social impairment may be associated with altered cortical, particularly frontal cortical, function. But psychotic symptoms seem to be related to "increases in dopaminergic activity." The researchers speculate that these two dimensions of schizotypal disorder "may represent partially distinct but potentially interactive pathophysiologic processes that may converge and interact to result in chronic schizophrenia."

CHAPTER 47
Neurobiology of Psychotic Illness

ANNE ROE MEALEY, MARTHA J. SNIDER, and JO ANNALEE IRVING

KEY TERMS

affect: An immediate expression of an emotion.

anhedonia: Loss of interest in and withdrawal from all regular and pleasurable activities, often associated with depression.

blunted affect: A severe reduction in the intensity of externalized feelings.

clang associations: Association of words similar in sound but not in meaning; words have no logical connection, may include rhyming and punning.

delusion: A fixed, false belief that is held despite considerable contradictory evidence.

flat affect: Absence of emotional expression.

hallucination: A perception for which there are no real sensory data.

illusion: The misperception of a real sensory stimulus.

libido: Sexual drive; feeling of sexual desire.

loosening of association: Flow of thought in which ideas shift from one subject to another in a completely unrelated way. When severe, speech may be incoherent.

mood: Sustained expression of an emotion that affects one's outlook.

mood swings: Oscillations between periods of euphoria and depression or anxiety.

neologism: New word created by the person, often from combining syllables of other words; or a word given special or private significance.

perseveration: Persisting response to a prior stimulus after a new stimulus has been presented.

poverty of speech: Speech that gives little information owing to vagueness, empty repetitions, or obscure phrases.

reality testing: The ability to evaluate and appreciate the differences between internal experiences and external events.

Psychosis is the term used to describe the most serious and debilitating of mental disorders. The hallmarks of psychosis are delusions and hallucinations, inappropriate emotional responses, thought disorders, and inappropriate social activity. Recent research points to both structural and biochemical abnormalities in the brain as possible causes of these symptoms.

The major discoveries about the brain's effects on pathologic behavior were accidental. Although for centuries scientists have inferred brain-behavior relationships, the impetus for the inclusion of hypotheses about the pathophysiology of mood disorders and schizophrenia emerged from discoveries in the 1950s of psychoactive drugs that affected the exacerbation and remission of psychiatric signs and symptoms. Working from observations about what certain drugs did chemically, researchers observed a logical progression. The serendipitous nature of breakthroughs in psychopharmacologic research and treatment led to hypotheses about the etiologies of certain mental disorders or suggested final common pathways in the brain.

This chapter focuses on the three most prevalent psychoses: schizophrenia, delusional disorder, and the major affective (mood) disorders.

Schizophrenia

Schizophrenia is a syndrome or collection of diseases with similar presentations. Schizophrenia has been described for thousands of years. It occurs in all cultures and affects about 1 percent of the world's population.

The word *schizophrenia* is derived from Greek and means "split mind," but this is a misnomer, because the disorder does not result in a split mind or a multiple personality disorder. Eugene Bleuler coined the term to describe the symptoms of a break with reality and disordered thinking.

The symptoms of schizophrenia may be classified as either positive or negative depending on their response to treatment. If a symptom is responsive to antipsychotic drug therapy, it is classified as a positive symptom. Negative symptoms are less responsive to treatment. Disorganized thinking, delusions, and hallucinations are positive symptoms. Negative symptoms include social withdrawal and flat affect.

Etiology and Pathogenesis

Researchers have long speculated about the effects of prolonged stress and the development of schizophrenia. Because much of the harm from stress relates to the person's interpretation of the meaning of the stress, individual sensitivity to increased stress may act in concert with an inherited predisposition to produce the disease. Although physical and sexual abuse during vulnerable periods of development may certainly be a precipitating factor, even these noxious events in the absence of other conditions do not in every case act as pathogenic agents. Schizophrenia often develops without any psychopathology in the family system. It is also likely that some mental disorders would never reach full expression without the impetus of destructive exogenous events.

There is little question that certain factors may improve the ability of an individual to cope with schizophrenia. These factors are found in most psychosocial theories about behavior and personal vulnerabilities. A sense of safety and security and a self-appraisal leading to the conclusion that one is adequate, worthwhile, loving and loved, and belongs somewhere or to some group with common values all appear to have importance. Additionally, favorable perceptions of life and environment appear to enhance character armor. A sense of order, predictability, and meaning supports personal identity and continuing growth.

There is some evidence that the rates of schizophrenia are higher in the lower socioeconomic classes and in the more Westernized societies.[1] These findings are supported by two commonly accepted hypotheses. First, it is assumed that stressors besetting persons in the lower classes are greater in number, intensity, and complexity, and that the availability of personal strategies to deal with stress may be diminished. A second hypothesis is related to the notion of downdrift. That is, persons with schizophrenia fail to move up the class ladder because of particular behavioral deficits or, possibly, persons in the middle and upper classes who develop schizophrenia tend to drift downward in class because of the characteristic difficulties inherent in the disorder. Industrialized societies have higher rates of schizophrenia, and cultures becoming more technologically complex note a rise in the incidence and prevalence of the disorder.

Approximately 2 million Americans bear the diagnosis of schizophrenia, with about 200,000 new cases diagnosed every year.[1] The constancy of the total number may be due to higher mortality rates in people with the illness. Suicide may contribute to the higher mortality rate. Additionally, people with schizophrenia seem to be more vulnerable than others to a host of naturally occurring illnesses that end in death. Until recently, the reproductive rates of people with schizophrenia were lower than those of the general population.

Most persons with schizophrenia are between 15 and 54 years old. The age at onset is between 25 and 35 years for women and between 15 and 25 years for men.[1] Birth dates of schizophrenics show a modest peak during the late winter and early spring months above that found in the general population.[1]

Genetic Factors

Although the etiology of schizophrenia remains unknown, current scientific opinion, in the main, favors a biological explanation for the behaviors associated with this illness. There are also indications that psychosocial factors may act as precipitants in otherwise vulnerable persons. Vulnerability may be related to genetic predisposition, as noted in the first-degree relatives of persons with schizophrenia, and much research has been devoted to this aspect.

Ever since the very early studies of monozygotic and dizygotic twins in the early 1900s, a genetic predisposition to the development of schizophrenia has been widely accepted. Identical twins of schizophrenic parents reared apart from their parents had an incidence of 50 percent, whereas the incidence in dizygotic twins reared apart from their parents was only 14 percent.[2] Although these figures are impressive, they do not explain the fact that 86 percent of the predisposed offspring did not develop the syndrome. Further, in no case was there evidence of how genetic factors could explain the pathophysiology and phenomenology of schizophrenia. In particular, no genetic etiologic factors have been identified to account for the earlier age at onset of schizophrenia in men or for differences between paranoid and nonparanoid subtypes. No consistent evidence of linkage between a specific gene locus and a putative schizophrenia susceptibility locus has been documented. However, knowledge of the human genome is rapidly advancing, and genetic linkage studies of schizophrenia are only in their beginning stages. Any valid etiologic hypothesis of schizophrenia will have to explain the consistent finding of substantial genetic influences as risk factors for schizophrenia.

Gestational Factors

Given evidence such as the seasonality-of-birth phenomenon in schizophrenia, researchers from the University of Southern California (USC) and the University of Helsinki investigated the possible influence of viral infections during gestation on the subsequent development of adult schizophrenia.[3] Helsinki suffered a severe epidemic of Asian flu in October 1957. If the connection between fetal exposure to influenza and the subsequent development of adult schizophrenia exists, it was hypothesized, those fetuses exposed to the virus should correspond to records of hospitalization for schizophrenia. Indeed, "the results were striking; individuals whose *sixth* month of gestation overlapped a month with an unusually high level of influenza had a significantly elevated risk of succumbing to schizophrenia in adulthood."[3] British researchers O'Callaghan and colleagues reported that mothers "exposed to the 1957 flu epidemic in the fifth month of gestation had almost twice the risk of adult schizophrenia in comparison to controls."[4]

Kovelman and Scheibel (1984)[5] reported pathophysiologic changes in the hippocampus of brains of long-term schizophrenics (Fig. 47–1). The pyramidal cells were not lined up like a "picket fence," as in nonschizophrenic clients, but were rotated 70 to 90 degrees. Because these cells migrate in the second trimester of gestation and become adhered by neuronal cell adhesion molecules (N-CAMs), research focused on possible developmental faults in the disarray of the pyramidal cells and the adhesive qualities of the N-CAMs. Results also demonstrated that pregnant women in Scandinavia and England exposed to the 1957 flu epidemic "during the second trimester produced 300 percent as many children who were diagnosed with schizophrenia as did women who experienced the flu during the first or third trimesters."[5] These findings are significant for two reasons: (1) neuronal migration reaches its peak during the second trimester, and (2) the influenza virus is one of a very few that produce capsular neuraminidase, an enzyme that can change the adhesive properties of N-CAMs.[5]

The cells in the hippocampus, parahippocampus gyrus, and the amygdala process information and emotional expression. Therefore, it is possible that the symptomatology of schizophrenia is due to failed neuronal connections that distort the interpretation of messages into the brain and produce an inability to filter out extraneous stimuli.

In an effort to explain why a gestational factor, such as exposure to influenza, would wait to manifest many years later in young adulthood, a longitudinal study by USC and Danish researchers[6] followed 207 Danish children born to severely schizophrenic mothers for 29 years. The team examined reports of elementary school behavior in an attempt to identify behavioral indications of dysfunction during childhood. The study revealed that children who later developed the negative schizophrenic symptoms of withdrawal, isolation, and passivity as young adults had also been described by their elementary school teachers in these same terms. Children who later demonstrated the positive schizophrenic symptoms of hallucinations, delusions, and inappropriate behavior had been identified by elementary school teachers as having behavior problems; they were high-strung and aggressive. Evidently, problematic childhood behaviors could be interpreted as precursor symptoms of schizophrenia. Rather than the constellation of symptoms having a sudden onset in young adulthood, it may be that schizophrenia actually occurs much earlier.

Despite considerable compelling evidence that prenatal exposure to influenza constitutes a risk factor for schizophrenia, further research is needed. Susser and colleagues in 1994[7] were unable to successfully replicate this finding. Their careful comparison of Dutch birth cohorts that were and were not exposed during the second trimester of gestation to the 1957 A2 influenza epidemic did not reveal a higher risk of schizophrenia among the exposed birth cohort. This important finding may suggest a co-factor that varies across populations. Such a factor (for example, over-the-counter medication used by pregnant mothers who had contracted influenza) could have been more common in England, Scandinavia, and Wales than in Holland in 1957.

Neurologic Factors

Neurologic signs in schizophrenics suggest brain damage at earlier ages. These signs include abnormal facial movements; unusually high or low rates of

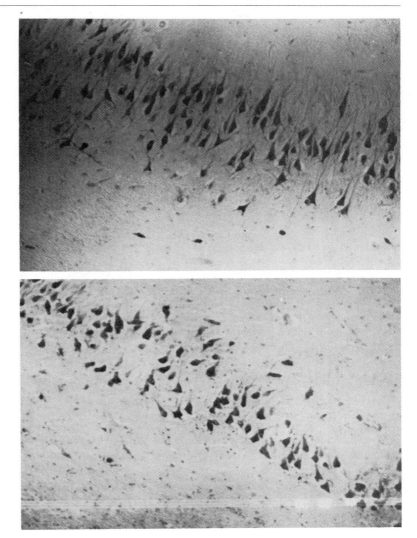

FIGURE 47–1. Photographic comparison of control (*top*) and chronic schizophrenic (*bottom*) hippocampal tissue at CA 2/3 interface. Original magnification of the Nissl-stained tissue is 100 ×. (Reprinted by permission of Elsevier Science Inc. from A neurohistological correlate of schizophrenia, by JA Kovelman and AB Scheibel, *Biological Psychiatry*, 19:1601–1621. Copyright 1984 by the Society of Biological Psychiatry.)

blinking; staring and avoidance of eye contact; absent blink reflex in response to a tap on the forehead; episodes of deviation of the eyes to the right, accompanied by speech arrest; bursts of jerky eye movements; poor visual pursuit of a smoothly moving object; inability to move the eyes without moving the head; poor pupillary light reactions; and continuous elevation of the brows, causing characteristic horizontal creasing of the forehead. Some monozygotic twins discordant for schizophrenia reflect possible brain injury in a difficult delivery for the schizophrenic twin.

Magnetic resonance images show larger lateral and third ventricles in chronic schizophrenics than in nonschizophrenic subjects, as well as reduced gray matter in the temporal lobes[5] (Fig. 47–2). Other brain imaging findings include a reduction in blood flow to the frontal lobes and a relative decrease in metabolic activity in the same areas. Prefrontal cortical deficits have emerged most consistently in patients when studies were carried out under conditions that might stress or impose a physiologic load on the prefrontal cortex. These studies included situations that might involve psychological stress, contingency planning, or divergent thinking as well as cognitive tasks that

required these capacities and are specifically linked to prefrontal cortex[5] (Fig. 47–3). The fact that prefrontal cortical dysfunction in schizophrenia may be condition dependent is consistent with the clinical picture of a psychopathology that waxes and wanes under various circumstances.

Dopamine Hypothesis

The discovery of chlorpromazine (Thorazine) in 1950 by Paul Carpentier, a French chemist, made it possible to treat the positive symptoms of schizophrenia. Thorazine is thought to achieve its antipsychotic effects by blocking dopamine D_2 receptors. By doing this it eliminates the positive symptoms of schizophrenia; delusions and hallucinations decrease or disappear.

Another way to look at the dopamine hypothesis is to look at the category of drugs known to *produce* the positive symptoms of schizophrenia. These are dopamine agonists such as amphetamines and cocaine.

Because dopamine antagonists reduce the positive symptoms of schizophrenia and dopamine ago-

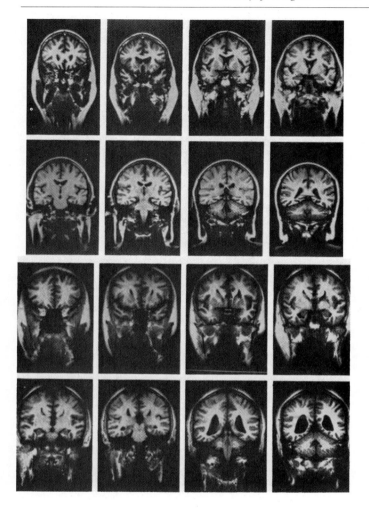

FIGURE 47–2. A set of MRI scans in the coronal plane showing (*top two rows*) normal structure in a normal volunteer and (*bottom two rows*) an abnormal scan from a patient with schizophrenia and nearly complete agenesis of the corpus callosum. In the abnormal scan, temporal lobes are also distorted, and the posterior ventricular horns are markedly enlarged. (From Andreasen NC: Brain imaging: Applications in psychiatry. *Science* 1988;239:1381–1388. Copyright 1988 by the AAAS. Reproduced with permission.)

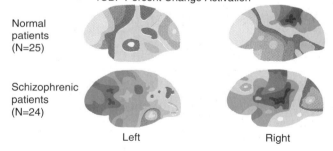

National Institute of Mental Health Clinical Neuropsychiatry rCBF Percent Change Activation

Normal patients (N=25)

Schizophrenic patients (N=24)

Left   Right

FIGURE 47–3. Regional cerebral blood flow (rCBF) study. Regional cerebral blood flow (rCBF) maps showing lateral views of cerebral cortex with frontal pole at left, occipital pole at right. Lateral view of left and right hemisphere percent change in rCBF during the Wisconsin Card-Sorting (WCS)/number matching tasks. Data are for 25 normal subjects (*top*) and 24 patients with schizophrenia treated with neuroleptics (*bottom*). Note that the normal subjects show striking rCBF increases during WCS/number matching tasks. (Redrawn with permission from Berman KF, Zec RF, Weinberger DR: Physiologic dysfunction of dorsolateral prefrontal cortex in schizophrenia II. *Arch Gen Psychiatry* 1986; 43:126–135.)

nists produce them, abnormalities in dopaminergic pathways may contribute to the pathogenesis of schizophrenia. The neurons that secrete dopamine are located in the ventral tegmentum of the mesencephalon, medial and superior to the substantia nigra. They give rise to the so-called mesolimbic dopaminergic system, which projects nerve fibers mainly into the medial and anterior portions of the limbic system, and especially into the nucleus accumbens, the amygdala, the anterior caudate nucleus, and the anterior cingulate gyrus of the cortex, all of which are powerful behavior control centers (Fig. 47–4). When patients with Parkinson's disease are treated with L-dopa, which releases dopamine in the brain, they sometimes develop schizophrenia-like symptoms, also indicating that excess dopaminergic activity can cause dissociation of a person's drives and thought patterns. Almost certainly there are other factors in schizophrenia besides excess secretion of dopamine; nevertheless, the symptoms of schizophrenia are similar to the behavioral effects of excessive dopamine.

Positron emission tomography (PET) has enabled researchers to further examine the dopamine hypothesis. PET studies suggest low rates of glucose metabolism in the frontal lobes and in the dopamine areas

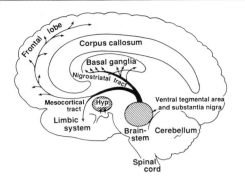

FIGURE 47–4. Schematic drawing showing probable dopamine projections in the human brain. Two main projections arise in the ventral tegmental area. The nigrostriatal tract projects to the basal ganglia, while the mesocortical tract projects to the temporal and frontal lobes. Reciprocal connections are not shown. Hyp, hypothalamus. (From Andreasen NC: Brain imaging: Applications in psychiatry. *Science* 1988;239:1381–1388. Copyright 1988 by the AAAS. Reproduced with permission.)

of the brain[5] (Fig. 47–5). In addition, different areas of the brain have different dopamine receptors. Researchers believe this fact may explain why dopamine D_2 receptors respond better to standard neuroleptic drugs, whereas D_1 receptors may respond better to other medications such as clozapine (Clozaril) or risperidone (Risperdal).

Clinical Manifestations

Although no single sign or symptom characterizes all persons with schizophrenia at all times, a generally accepted behavioral hallmark is disorganization from a previous level of functioning. There is some degree of impairment in work, relationships, and self-care.

A frequent observation made of the person with schizophrenia is a disturbance in language and communication. The nature of this disturbance resides in the failure to conform to the semantic and syntactic rules governing the person's native tongue; these discrepancies cannot be attributed to low intelligence, educational level, or culture and do reflect underlying problems in thinking. Some characteristic speech manifestations of disorders of thought form include tangentiality, the use of words with private or approximate rather than generally accepted meanings, non sequiturs, and **neologisms.**[8] Neologisms are new words created by the person, often by combining syllables of other words. Sometimes neologisms are ordinary words given special or private significance by the affected individual. **Loose associations,** or an apparent unrelatedness between and among ideas, may be present as well. Table 47–1 summarizes some of the neuropsychological abnormalities in schizophrenia.

Dysfunctions in thought content are reflected by **delusions,** or fixed, false beliefs that persist despite considerable evidence to the contrary. These beliefs, ideas, and attributions of meaning to stimuli are,

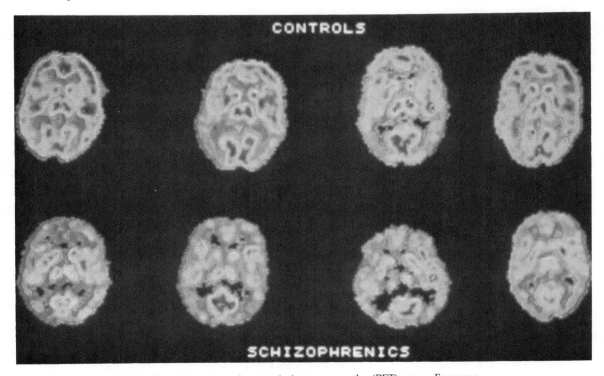

FIGURE 47–5. Individual variation in positron emission tomography (PET) scans. Four normal individuals (*top row*) and four schizophrenics (*bottom row*) show range of hypofrontality and diminished basal ganglia metabolism. See Color Plate IV. (From Buchsbaum MS, Haier RJ: Functional and anatomical brain imaging: Impact on schizophrenia research. *Schizophrenia Bulletin* 1987;13(1):115–132. Reproduced by permission of Monte S. Buchsbaum, M.D., Mount Sinai School of Medicine, New York.)

TABLE 47–1. Selected Neuropsychological Abnormalities in Schizophrenia

High distractibility
Slow information processing
Decreased mental flexibility
Poor tactile problem solving
Decreased memory for stories and designs
Loosening of association
Perseveration
Poor language processing

Data from Grebb JA, Cancro R: Schizophrenia: Clinical features, in Kaplan HI, Sadock BJ (eds): *Comprehensive Textbook of Psychiatry V*, 5th ed. Baltimore, Williams & Wilkins, 1989, vol I, p 767.

therefore, opposed to reality and do not merely reflect the person's cultural background.

The types of delusions vary among persons with schizophrenia. Common types are grandiose, persecutory, and somatic. There may be beliefs that one is being poisoned, spied on, bombarded with radioactivity, harassed, or plotted against, or that one is the victim of an unknown but powerful group. Fearful convictions that one's thoughts, feelings, or actions are being controlled by others may prevail. A sense of having one's thoughts broadcast may also be present. On the other hand, the person may believe that he or she controls the thoughts, feelings, and actions of others. Delusions having the themes of control and passivity are often included in what are referred to as first-rank symptoms. It is interesting to note that delusional content, while arising from the personal history and experience of the person, is usually congruent with current events. Other functional thought process deficits may include blocking, poverty of ideas, and the like.

A breakdown in perceptual selectivity is a common feature; there is grave difficulty encountered by the person with schizophrenia in sorting out sensory information. Perceptions for which there are not objectively discernible stimuli, or **hallucinations,** reflect this breakdown. Hallucinations are usually auditory but may affect any sensorial sphere. The person, in clear consciousness, may hear his or her own thoughts, or hear known or unknown voices, arguing, commenting, comforting, threatening, or evaluating. Disorganized thinking, delusions, and hallucinations are classified as *positive symptoms.*

The *negative symptoms* of schizophrenia include social withdrawal, flat affect, poverty of speech, and ritualistic posturing or immobility and are thought to be related to dopamine D_1 receptors.[9] They are called negative symptoms because they do not readily respond to treatment.

Affect, or emotional tone, may be blunted, shallow, flat, inappropriate, or silly. Flat affect is characterized by an unchanging facial expression, poor eye contact, limited gestures, or absence of vocal inflection. **Anhedonia,** the absence of joy or pleasure that may also be observed in depression, can take the form

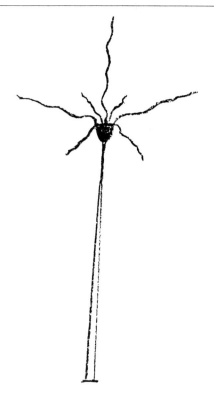

FIGURE 47–6. An actively psychotic person was asked to draw a tree. Black was chosen from a selection of colors. The slender tapered tree trunk may represent the instability of the ego. The branching structure is reminiscent of religious symbolism and poverty of hope. (Figure supplied by Chris Rost, RNC, MN, Spokane, Washington.)

of a decrease in or lack of interest in sexual activity, close relationships, and recreational interests.

Disturbances in the sense of self may often manifest as a compromised ability to differentiate one's physical self from the environment (Fig. 47–6). This can take the form of a cosmic feeling of being one with the universe, or being limitless. This is related to the perceptual and cognitive failure to appreciate boundaries of the self (Fig. 47–7). One's sexual identity may become difficult to ascertain or validate as a consequence.

The external world can be a source of confusion, anxiety, and emptiness for the person with schizophrenia. **Autism** is the development of a process of detachment from the world. In autism, the real world is essentially traded in for a highly personal, private, and illogically constructed one. It is possible that what the observer refers to as inappropriate affect is only a manifestation by autistic persons of an emotional response to an unshared, inner world.

Motor behavior is affected in the person with schizophrenia. Posturing, mannerisms, bizarre rituals, clumsiness, grimacing, and aimless activity may be elements of deficits in psychomotor behavior (Fig. 47–8). It is often the case that some of these behaviors can be related to the effects of antipsychotic medications.

A common sleep disturbance in people with acute schizophrenia is inability to fall asleep. Anxiety and

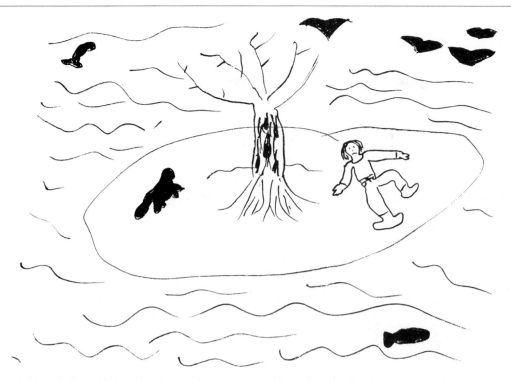

FIGURE 47-7. This schizophrenic drawing (created by a thought disordered person) demonstrates absence of boundaries between sky and sea. The isolation and powerlessness are underscored by the island and body position of the person. Negation of vital life is represented by the decaying tree. The fish and birds and squirrel maintain a menacing quality. Although a full color range of markers was available, the person utilized only black. (Figure supplied by Chris Rost, RNC, MN, Spokane, Washington.)

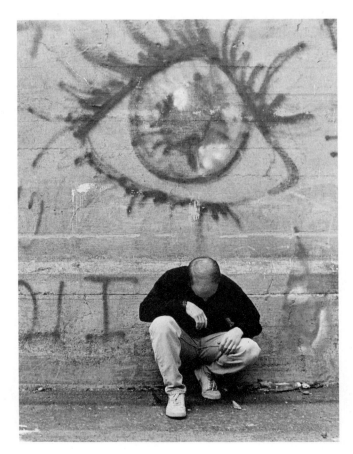

FIGURE 47-8. Model exhibiting catatonic posturing. (Photographer: Kathleen Kelly, Spokane, Washington.)

increased motor activity, heightened by delusions and hallucinations, keep agitated people awake for hours. Once asleep, they may spend close to normal amount of time in bed, but their sleep is usually disturbed by frequent awakenings. As a result, schizophrenic persons' arising time might gradually shift from morning to afternoon.

All of these signs and symptoms do not consistently characterize every person who has schizophrenia. The same individual may produce markedly different behavior day by day or hour by hour. It follows, then, that the person with schizophrenia is not psychotic every second of the day, nor is he or she simply a set of signs and symptoms.

Treatment

Positive symptoms are more responsive to antipsychotic drug intervention and are manifested in the more acute stages of schizophrenia. Negative symptoms are less responsive to treatment. A recent study suggested that the biological deficits or abnormalities responsible for producing these two categories of symptoms may differ. It was concluded that persons with high genetic risk, delivery complications, and autonomic nervous system nonresponsiveness were at increased risk for negative symptom behavior.[10] An interesting notion that complicates the negative-positive symptom issue relates to men who have schizophrenia. Using sex as the critical variable, a recent study concluded that schizophrenic men have less schizophrenia in their families, have poorer premorbid functioning, have an earlier onset of illness, show more evidence of social withdrawal and emotional inexpressiveness, and have poorer ultimate outcomes. It was also noted that there is more left hemisphere abnormality in schizophrenic men.[11]

A functional excess of dopamine at certain sites, excess postsynaptic dopamine receptors, and hypersensitivity of dopamine receptors, either as single entities or in combination, have been postulated as significant neuropathologic states in persons with schizophrenia. Drugs that are effective in treating positive schizophrenic symptoms, such as chlorpromazine (Thorazine), haloperidol (Haldol), and thiothixene (Navane), all decrease the secretion of dopamine by the dopaminergic nerve endings and thus decrease the effect of dopamine on the subsequent neurons. The new agents risperidone (Risperdal) and clozapine (Clozaril) appear to help alleviate some of the negative symptoms through serotonergic effects and D_1 blockade.

KEY CONCEPTS

> • Schizophrenia is characterized by altered perceptions of reality and disordered thinking. Genetic predisposition and environmental factors are thought to interact to produce biological changes in the brain, in particular the hippocampus, temporal lobes, and dopaminergic pathways that project to

the limbic system. Exposure to influenza virus during the fifth to sixth months of gestation appears to predispose to schizophrenia.

> • The age at onset is 15 to 25 years for men and 25 to 35 years for women. There is a higher incidence in industrialized societies. Stress and childhood experiences may affect the expression of schizophrenia. Lack of safety, security, order, and predictability and low self-worth are probable contributing factors.

> • Neurologic abnormalities found in schizophrenics and preschizophrenic children include abnormal blinking and blink reflex, abnormal pupil reflex and facial movements, enlarged lateral and third ventricles, reduced temporal gray matter, decreased blood flow, and decreased glucose metabolism in frontal lobes.

> • The *positive symptoms* of schizophrenia are thought to be due to excessive dopamine D_2 receptor activation in the brain. Disorganized thinking (inability to connect thoughts logically), disorganized speech (rambling, tangentiality), delusions (fixed system of false beliefs), and hallucinations (sensory perceptions when no apparent stimulus exists) are typical positive symptoms. Delusions are often persecutory, grandiose, or controlling. Hallucinations are most often auditory, but may also be visual, olfactory, or tactile. Positive symptoms respond to drugs that decrease dopamine activity in the brain (e.g., chlorpromazine, haloperidol).

> • The *negative symptoms* of schizophrenia are less amenable to treatment. Negative symptoms are thought to be mediated by dopamine D_1 receptors in the brain. Drugs that block D_1 receptors (clozapine) may alleviate some of the negative symptoms, which include social withdrawal, flat affect, poverty of speech, ritualistic posturing, and autism.

Delusional Disorder

Delusional disorder does not present a clinical picture that is patently schizophrenic. This disorder is characterized by a behavioral constellation dominated by a system of fixed, false beliefs that are tenacious and typically refractory to contrary evidence. Unlike the delusions observed in schizophrenia, there is a systematic framework to the themes and to the process. Other features usually associated with formal thought disorder are absent, as is pervasive involvement of the full range of life activities.

Etiology and Pathogenesis

The presence of a delusional system suggests some relationship with schizophrenia or a schizophrenic spectrum disorder.[12] However, it appears that the delusional disorder is not related to the more pervasive illness of schizophrenia. Although it is logical to assume that some biological substrates exist that presage the full expression of this slowly developing disorder, the evidence is not definitive. A more fruitful area of exploration is found in the character traits of the person who develops this disorder. The learning of suspiciousness because of interpersonal hurts and other stressful situations may be a more common finding. There may originally be some justification for some of the delusions developed, the so-called grain of truth. However, the elaboration of slights, misfortunes, failures, and disappointments into an unassailable system of fixed beliefs cannot be validated by an observer. The readiness of the individual to add neutral experiences or coincidental events into a web of proof is beyond that which one would view as adaptive and mentally intact. Constant failure and reminders of personal inadequacies may lead to delusional disorder as a massive effort to defend one's self-esteem from injury.

Clinical Manifestations

The hallmark of a delusional disorder is the fixed belief system of delusional proportions that may or may not have a bizarre character. Generally, the beliefs of the person could possibly happen, but not probably. Most functions, other than the disturbance in thought process as manifested by the delusional system, are intact. **Reality testing,** the ability to evaluate and appreciate differences between internal experiences and external events, is affected by definition, since the falsity of the person's beliefs fails to yield to compelling evidence that would logically refute those beliefs. Predominant themes characterizing the delusional system may include beliefs that a well-known person is secretly in love with the individual. Grandiose systems might include beliefs that the individual has great power, knowledge, or a special relationship with God. Jealousy themes related to a sexual partner's unfaithfulness can predominate. Litigiousness, or the propensity of the individual to take legal action for alleged wrongs or slights, is possible. It is noteworthy that the individual who believes that he has been wronged or slighted could resort to violence in retaliation, and this potential propensity is always of concern to clinicians.

The incidence of this disorder is believed to be three to four cases per 100,000 and the prevalence is less than a tenth of a percent. It is reasonable to conclude that it is a rare disorder, though the predilection of persons with the disorder to avoid psychiatric treatment may contribute to an underestimate.

The age at onset has a range from 25 on, with an average of 40 years. Women may be slightly more likely to be diagnosed than men; they tend to be married, employed, and members of lower socioeconomic strata.[9]

KEY CONCEPTS

- Delusional disorder is a psychotic illness dominated by a tenacious system of false beliefs. It is a slowly developing disorder that may begin with a "grain of truth," then escalate to delusional proportions by assigning false meaning to life experiences. Delusional beliefs often have themes of jealousy, secret loves, grandiosity, persecution, and legal retaliation for perceived wrongs (litigiousness).
- The biochemical and structural basis of delusional disorder is unknown. Some commonality with schizophrenia is suspected.

Major Affective Disorders

The third category of psychosis is the major affective disorders. Whereas schizophrenia and delusional disorder involve disordered thoughts, affective disorders involved disordered emotions or affects.

The *Diagnostic and Statistical Manual of Mental Disorders*, fourth edition (DSM-IV), describes two major types of major affective disorders. The first is **bipolar disorder,** which is characterized by alternating periods of mania and depression. These periods of mania can occur from a few days to many months, and the following depression usually lasts three times as long as the mania.

The second type is **unipolar depression,** which is depression without periods of mania, often called **endogenous depression** because it arises from characteristics *within* the person. Another type of depression is termed **reactive depression,** usually a *reaction to sad events* in the person's life.

These mental disorders are among the most common, particularly major depression. It is believed that the lifetime risk for women is approximately 20 percent, and for men, 10 percent. The risk for bipolar disorder is much less, 1 percent, and is almost equally distributed between men and women. Generally, clinicians see more persons with bipolar disorder in treatment settings than persons with major depression, few of whom (25 percent) are treated. Depressed people, on the other hand, generally use more health services and are less productive than might be expected of people in general.

The proportion of depressions noted in women is about twice that observed in men. The reasons for the different distribution are not clear. Major depressions have a median age at onset in the usually productive years between 20 and 50, with 40 as the average age. Bipolar disorders occur earlier, with an average age at onset of 30 years. Race and ethnicity do not appear to be highly significant variables in relation to the mood disorders. Social class is not related to major depression, but a trend does appear between bipolar disorder and the upper classes. Bipolar disorder may be more common in divorced and separated people, whereas major depressions are thought to be more common in persons without close intimate relationships or who are divorced, separated, or widowed. Table 47–2 summarizes risk factors for major affective disorders.

Many psychosocial theories have been generated to explain the development of mood disorders. Most

TABLE 47–2. Risk Factors for Major Depressive and Bipolar Disorders

Risk Factor	Major Depression	Bipolar Disorder
Lifetime prevalence	Female 5–9% Male 2–4%	.6–.9%
Male/Female ratio	1:2	1:1.2
Age at onset	Mid to late 30s	Late teens to early 20s
Social class	No relationship	Slight increase in upper classes
Race	No relationship	No relationship
Family History		
% Major depression in relatives	17%	15%
% Bipolar depression in relatives	2–3%	8%

From Hirschfeld RMA, Goodwin PR: Mood disorders, in Talbott JA, Hales RE, Yudofsky SC (eds): *The American Psychiatric Press Textbook of Psychiatry.* Washington DC, American Psychiatric Press, Inc., 1988, p 410. Reproduced with permission.

include the concepts of loss and low self-esteem as central features. The behavioral dynamics posited by Freud associated vulnerability to depression with the revocation of the original infantile response to each subsequent loss of life. He placed the original psychic conflict in the oral phase of development, pointing to the orality inherent in both depression and mania. The loss of loved ones, or the loss of persons on whom one is dependent, is responded to with feelings of guilt and inadequacy because of unconscious hostility toward the lost person. Depression occurs in adulthood whenever a psychologically vulnerable person is faced with a real, anticipated, or perceived loss. Mania is considered to be a massive defense, through denial and activity, of the underlying sense of depression.

Learned helplessness is a concept derived from the cognitive theorists. Here, individuals in stressful situations, when unable to alter a painful stimulus, tend to withdraw and make no further efforts to alter the stimulus or to avoid it even when opportunities to mitigate the situation are clearly available. Depression results from repeated experiences in which the person cannot control the outcomes of negative events, and that person develops the conviction that action is futile.[9]

The ubiquitous human response of sadness and some of the previously described symptoms in abbreviated form tend to reinforce the notion that depression is almost always a normal reaction to loss and that grief and depression are synonymous. The consideration of the full range of signs and symptoms reflected by the true mood disorder refutes this notion. Although the causes of mood disorders have yet to be delineated for every case, it would seem logical to infer that biochemical vulnerability precedes the

psychosocial events which are readily identified as those stressors which are experienced as loss.

Depression

Etiology and Pathogenesis

Monoamine Hypothesis. Depression is related to insufficient levels of monoaminergic neurons. The major monoamines identified are **norepinephrine** and **serotonin.** It is unclear if there is an alteration in the production of neurotransmitters, functioning of the receptor site, or involvement of the secondary messenger systems postsynaptically. Possibly all three mechanisms are involved.

Because direct measures of serotonin in the central nervous system (CNS) are not reliable or stable, recent focus has been on 5-hydroxyindoleacetic acid (5-HIAA), a reliable, measurable component of the product of serotonin breakdown. The primary methodological difficulty has been the need to use spinal taps to measure CNS 5-HIAA levels. Decreased CNS levels of 5-HIAA in depressed persons imply either that less serotonin is released in the brain or that there is excessive postreceptor uptake of serotonin. Significantly lower levels of CSF 5-HIAA have been identified in attempted suicides, and 20 percent of clients with levels of 5-HIAA below the median killed themselves; no clients with levels above the mean committed suicide (Fig. 47–9).

Role of Sleep Abnormalities in Depression. Persons with endogenous depression show reduced slow-wave delta sleep (stages 3 and 4) and increased stage 1 sleep. Rapid eye movement (REM) sleep latency is shortened, with an increased number of REM periods early in the night (Fig. 47–10). Family studies of endogenous depression have linked these abnormalities of REM sleep to depression.[13] Though no symptoms of depression surfaced in first-degree relatives of de-

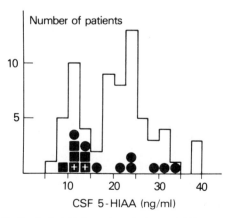

FIGURE 47–9. Suicidal acts in relation to 5-HIAA in CSF. Suicidal attempts with sedative drugs (*circles*); attempts with other means (*squares*). Patients died from suicide (*crosses*). (From Asberg M, Traskamn L, Thoren P: 5-HIAA in the cerebrospinal fluid—A biochemical suicide predictor? *Arch Gen Psychiatry* 1976;33:1193–1197. Copyright 1976, American Medical Association. Reproduced with permission.)

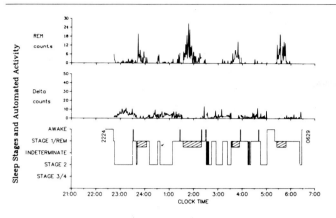

Sleep, REM, and Delta Patterns

FIGURE 47-10. Sleep histogram depicting an increase in the number of arousals during the night, a decrease in Stages 3 and 4 sleep, and a redistribution of rapid eye movement (REM) sleep into the first half of the night. (From Reynolds CF III, Kupfer DJ: Sleep disorders, in Talbott JA, Hales RE, Yudofsky SC (eds): *The American Psychiatric Press Textbook of Psychiatry.* Washington DC, American Psychiatric Press, Inc., 1988, p 741. Reproduced with permission.)

pressed persons, studies showed the short REM sleep latency in family members. Those with the lowest rates had the greatest potential for developing the disorder.

PET studies have also focused on sleep abnormalities in depressed persons who respond to sleep deprivation and in nonresponders. Some individuals experience a lifting of the depression after a night with little or no sleep; however, relapse occurs after sleeping. Responders showed a significantly elevated rate in the cingulate gyrus (the same area identified with anxiety and hostility in normal dreaming). PET studies also showed that the overall metabolic rate was much higher in depressed patients.

Circadian Rhythms and Depression. Because sleep disturbance is one of the hallmark symptoms of depression, research has also focused on the role of circadian rhythms. One condition related to circadian rhythms is the disorder called **seasonal affective disorder** (SAD). Persons suffering from SAD report lethargy and the "blahs" when seasonal changes result in less daylight and nights are longer. The theory underlying the condition is that light serves as a *Zeitgeber*—a synchronizer of the biological clock—to the day-night cycle. Because circadian rhythms of sleep and wakefulness are regulated by the suprachiasmatic nucleus of the hypothalamus, it is hypothesized that clients with SAD require a stronger *Zeitgeber* to synchronize their biological clock.

Symptoms of SAD are somewhat different from those of endogenous depression. During the winter, clients report decreased activity, decreased pleasure, craving for chocolate, weight gain, and a feeling of body discomfort at room temperatures of 70°F, although they are comfortable at this temperature in summer. Some theorize the phenomenon is related to hibernation in animals. The treatment of SAD by

increased bright light for several hours daily has improved the mood of clients.

Other Factors Contributing to Depression. Animal models have focused on the effects of specific stressors such as separation from the mother, and the resultant exhibition of vegetative signs of depression. These signs reflect those of depression, such as sleep disturbance and decreases in appetite, weight, libido, and motor activity. Considerable research related to neuroendocrine and neurotransmitter abnormalities is now moving toward a theory of hypothalamic-pituitary-adrenal axis dysfunction.

Genetic factors, stressful life events, coping strategies, social support, and cognitive processing styles have been implicated for their effects on dysregulation of the hypothalamic-pituitary-adrenal axis. However, controversy exists as to whether these factors are causes, results, or concomitants of depression.

Clearly, there are many more hypotheses than facts related to the development of depression. However, the multiple effects of heritability, biological rhythms, monoamine metabolism, and other factors suggest that many entities work together to produce this diagnosis.

Clinical Manifestations

Depression was described in the ancient literature. An association with endogenous or exogenous factors, or both, has been proposed. The hallmarks of major depression include depressed mood or anhedonia over a specific period of time. These features are relatively constant as experienced by the individual or observed by others. That is, the mood and outlook peculiar to this disorder are present almost all the time. It is important to note that the quality of depression is different from the normal affect of sadness. Moreover, depression is different from the normal mood state experienced by an individual as bereavement. Occasionally, the person's expressions of sadness, bleakness, and hopelessness are perceived by others as a general aura of painful irritability or dissatisfaction. The posture is stooped, the facial expression sad and forlorn. Early in the illness, crying may occur, though this is not particularly seen in the more severe stages of the illness. Anhedonia may be defined as an inability to experience joy, pleasure, or satisfaction from occupational, recreational, or relational activities that were previously sources of positive feelings. Anhedonia develops early in depression.

Low levels of energy usually accompany the sadness and joylessness. Activities that once were almost automatic come to be insurmountable and ominous tasks. The least amount of energy necessary to engage in activities is expended, and it becomes more and more difficult to initiate tasks as the illness increases in severity. Eventually the depressed person may not even respond to external events.

There may also be, in some individuals, agitation and restlessness. Moaning, rocking, pacing, and hand-wringing may predominate rather than the motoric slowing down previously described.

The ability to concentrate, attend, and think is affected in depressed persons. Thoughts slow down, are difficult to maintain, and are dominated by depressive themes that become recurrent and constant. A consequence of the slowing down and narrowing of thought content is a marked reduction in decision-making ability. As the illness progresses, making the most minor choices or stating simple preferences becomes disproportionately difficult.

Low self-esteem is a psychological hallmark of depression. The appraisal of self-worth is replete with references to feelings of guilt, helplessness, and hopelessness. Guilt, in particular, may assume delusional proportions. That is, the expressed degree of guilt is markedly disproportionate to the reported misdeed, and evidence to the contrary is ignored or discounted and may result in greater tenacity and escalation in depressive thought processes and content.

The perceptions of one's life, future, and prospects correlate highly with the negative self-appraisal. That is, life is perceived as futile, empty, and without value. The future is equally gloomy and bleak, and the subject's prospects for a change in status are projected to be virtually nil. The impairment in judgment is variable but related to the severity of the depression. Should the disorder be of psychotic proportions, then it is certain that the impairment will be marked and will, by definition, affect reality testing. Hallucinations, when present, are usually congruent with the depressed mood.

Vegetative Symptoms. Sleep disturbances are common complaints in almost all persons with major depression. Insomnia is a frequently described event and may range from difficulty falling asleep to the more common terminal insomnia. Terminal insomnia is characterized by waking in the early hours of the morning and inability to fall asleep again. The individual does not feel refreshed on awakening. A milder form of this problem may be waking up 1 or 2 hours before the usual time. The more severe the illness, the shorter is the period of time between sleep onset and waking. Hypersomnia may be the reported sleep disturbance, though this isn't as common as terminal insomnia.[13]

Appetite disturbances typically occur in major depression. Food comes to be tasteless and uninteresting. There may be diminished saliva and diminished gastric activity. The latter may be associated with complaints of feelings of heaviness in the abdomen. Occasionally there may be increased appetite, though this is relatively uncommon in a typical major depression. Weight loss is a consequence of decreased intake, though weight loss may occur when there has been no or only a minor change in intake.

Libido, or sexual drive, is typically disturbed. Interest in sex diminishes rather soon after the onset of depression and may continue even when other symptoms are reported to be abating. Women may also complain of irregular or decreased menstruation.

The vegetative phenomena, when present, are hallmarks of melancholic depression. In addition to depressed mood or anhedonia, these characteristic changes in sleep, appetite, libido, and psychomotor activity are specifically associated with a typical major depression. The preferential response of this disorder to antidepressant drugs led researchers to the formulation of hypotheses about the pathophysiologic substrates of what had been a so-called functional illness.

Dysthymia. **Dysthymia** is a chronic mood disorder characterized by consistently depressed mood for at least 2 years, accompanied by less severe degrees of several of the previously described signs and symptoms. Two subcategories, primary and secondary dysthymia, have significant differences. *Primary dysthymia* is not associated with any other disorder. It is neither a prelude to major depression nor a state existing between episodes of a cyclic form of mood disorder. *Secondary dysthymia,* conversely, is associated with some other nonmood disorder, which may be a classic mental disorder such as anorexia nervosa or a physical illness germane to a psychiatric treatment plan.

Treatment

A principal reason for believing that depression is related to diminished activity of the norepinephrine and serotonin systems is that drugs that block the secretion of norepinephrine and serotonin, such as the drug reserpine, frequently cause depression. Conversely, about 70 percent of depressive patients can be treated very effectively with one of two types of drug that increase especially the excitatory effects of norepinephrine at the nerve endings, and perhaps of serotonin as well: (1) monoamine oxidase inhibitors, which block destruction of norepinephrine and serotonin once they are formed, and (2) tricyclic antidepressants, which block reuptake of norepinephrine and serotonin by the nerve endings, so that these transmitters remain active for longer periods of time after secretion. A third type of drug, selective serotonin reuptake inhibitors, includes such newer agents as Prozac, Paxil, and Zoloft. Chemically unrelated to the tricyclics, these drugs are selective for serotonin, having little affect on other neurotransmitters such as norepinephrine.

Mental depression can also be treated effectively by electroconvulsive therapy, commonly called shock therapy. In this therapy, an electric shock is used to cause a generalized seizure similar to that of an epileptic attack. This has also been shown to enhance norepinephrine transmission efficiency.

Bipolar Disorder

Etiology and Pathogenesis

Hypotheses about the familial transmission of bipolar disorder have strong support. Where some hypotheses suggest that mania and depression are polar opposites, the complexity of the neurochemistry of the brain considerably weakens the notion that too much of a single substance results in mania and too little results in depression. It may be concluded that there is a bit more known about the why of mania than of depression, and a bit more known about what happens in depression. It is entirely likely that mood disorders are related to both brain and environmental factors, either inborn, acquired, or both, that in some combinations yield a mood disorder in vulnerable individuals (Fig. 47–11).

Genetic Factors. There is considerable evidence that bipolar disorder is familial. More first-degree relatives (parents, children) of persons with bipolar forms of mood disorder have bipolar forms of mood disorder and unipolar disorders than the general population. Moreover, in experimental subjects in whom control of environmental variables was possible, heritability of mood disorder has been demonstrated.[14]

A relationship between a gene on chromosome 11 and bipolar disorder in a group of Old Order Amish subjects has been reported.[15] It has been suggested that a dominant gene with incomplete penetrance (i.e., not all persons having a susceptible genotype will develop the illness) was present in this pedigree, but other factors were necessary for the behavioral expression of the gene.

Other studies have suggested a relationship between the genes for color blindness and glucose-6-phosphate deficiency on the X chromosome and bipolar illness in a cohort of Sephardic Jews.[16] The chromosomal findings in these two pedigrees have not been replicated in other populations. This suggests that more than one gene is responsible for the inheritance of bipolar disorder.

Use of the new molecular genetic technology to detect a gene for mood disorders is in its infancy. But, now that the techniques are available, it seems reasonable for researchers to use a combination of strategies for applying molecular genetic techniques to this illness, including studies of unrelated patients and controls, families or larger pedigrees, and affected sibling pairs. If major genes for mood disorders exist, they may be found in the foreseeable future.

While less dominant a finding, there does appear to be a relationship between a family history of mood disorders and major depression in an individual. This does not suggest that the familial transmission is entirely due to genetics. It is also possible that environment plays a role, although the exact nature of the relationship has yet to be described.

Biological Vulnerability Traits. A number of studies have attempted to identify biological factors that are inherited in mood disorders. Ideally, an inherited biological factor would be a variant (such as an altered protein) that could be assigned a specific locus on an identifiable chromosome. Because stable biochemical differences may suggest genetic variation, virtually any stable biological finding that is clearly associated with a tendency toward mood disorder may be studied as a possible genetic trait, even if the association is limited to a subgroup of patients. The converse is also valid: genetic strategies may be used to demonstrate the validity of a particular biological component of the mood disorders even without an established mechanism of genetic transmission. One possible genetic vulnerability trait for mood disorders is the lithium erythrocyte-plasma ratio—an index of lithium transport. Data from one study[14] suggest that there is a difference between the transport of lithium in affected persons and controls. If the study's conclusions can be replicated with larger numbers of lithium studies of ill individuals, the finding would have important diagnostic and preventive implications.

Neurotransmitter Involvement. An early hypothesis regarding the etiology of mood disorders is often referred to as the **catecholamine hypothesis.** This model suggested that abnormally low catecholaminergic neurotransmission led to depression and abnormally high catecholaminergic neurotransmission led to mania. An underlying assumption was that depression and mania were biochemically opposite states.[17]

A second hypothesis related to the indoleamine, serotonin, reflects the relationship between it and norepinephrine. The **permissive hypothesis** posits that poor dampening by serotonin of other neurotransmitter systems (e.g., norepinephrine and dopamine) allows wide variations in mood. The serotoninergic functional deficit is a necessary precondition that also seems to require a simultaneous increase or decrease in norepinephrine before signs and symptoms of depression or mania emerge.

The **cholinergic-noradrenergic imbalance hypothesis** suggests that a relative increase in the ratio of acetylcholine activity to norepinephrine activity produces depression and that mania is the result of a relative increase in the ratio of norepinephrine activity over acetylcholine activity.

Sleep Disturbances. Disorders of initiating and maintaining sleep (DIMS) associated with affective

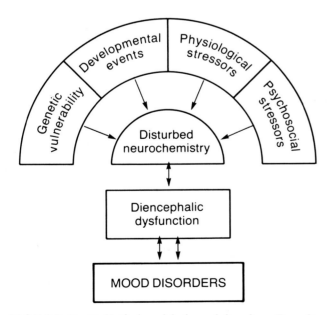

FIGURE 47–11. Unified model of mood disorders. (From Stuart GW, Sundeen SJ: Disturbances of mood, in Stuart GW, Sundeen SJ (eds): *Principles and Practice of Psychiatric Nursing*, 4th ed. St. Louis, Mosby–Year Book, 1991, p 429. Reproduced with permission.)

disorders compose two types of severe insomnias that are characteristic of the disorders: in depression, the ability to fall asleep, but sleep maintenance disturbance, "early morning" premature arousals, and shortened REM sleep latency; in mania, sleep-onset insomnia and short sleep. Bipolar depression may also be associated with excessive sleep.

Clinical Manifestations

There are two bipolar disorders. The more severe is the occurrence of one or more manic episodes that cycle with a major depressive episode. The second is that characterized by manic episodes only. This disorder has the chief characteristic, in the manic phase, of a sustained period of elevated mood. Less frequently, irritable mood is present. The individual is characteristically cheerful, full of enthusiasm and optimism, but the buoyant mood is disproportionate to events and surroundings. Self-esteem is markedly inflated such that the individual's self-appraisal brooks no criticism or contradiction. This opinion of self can assume delusional proportions with regard to one's importance, power, and prospects.

Energy levels are reported by the individual to be very high. Hyperactivity and constant shifting of the focus and uses of energy are remarkable. There may be a dangerously low sensitivity to fatigue, injury, and pain. The individual is at the mercy of every stimulus; even as the individual verbalizes myriad plans and interests and starts many activities, nothing is completed.

Speech is pressured, loud, rapid, and constant. Early on, there is an adroit and humorous play on words. Jokes, rhymes, and puns may be produced in abundance. **Clang associations,** or the continuity of thought associated with word sounds, may occur. Eventually, speech may become incoherent.

Perceptions and thoughts are generally congruent with mood. Auditory and visual hallucinations may occur. **Illusions,** or the misperception of real stimuli, tend to be more characteristic; misidentification of stimuli based on the euphoric mood is also more common than hallucinations. Thinking is dominated by mood in both content and process. Thoughts may be generated in a constant fashion, with relationships between thoughts based on understandable connections. As thoughts accelerate, the connections become difficult to identify.

Given the hyperresponsiveness to stimuli, it is predictable that the person is easily distractible and attends to anything that draws the most momentary focus. The inability to concentrate is a consequence of that distractibility. While there is seemingly endless mental and physical activity, the themes in thought content are recurrent. These themes are mood-congruent and may pertain to self-importance, wealth, special talents or abilities, and the like. Sometimes these thoughts may reach delusional proportions.

In obvious contrast to people with major depression, sleep, appetite, and libido are affected differently. Appetite is increased, though food intake is not necessarily increased because of the person's constant activity. There is weight loss to some degree, possibly due to the ratio of activity to caloric intake.

Sleep is disturbed or, in the extreme, almost absent. Although brief naps may be taken from time to time, very little sleep is possible in the severe stages of this disorder. Libido is increased and, when combined with poor judgment, may lead to promiscuous behavior.

Hypomanic episodes are similar to manic episodes but are not nearly as severe. While there may be minor impairment in functioning, there is notable absence of characteristics associated with psychosis, such as delusions and hallucinations.

The consequences of these dysfunctional behaviors for judgment, decision making, and reality testing are numerous. There is poor impulse control and inability to realistically appraise one's abilities. Potentially damaging choices can be made with regard to sexual partners, projects, money, and commitments.

Treatment

Drugs that diminish the formation or action of norepinephrine and serotonin, such as lithium compounds, can be effective in treating the manic condition of bipolar illness. Therefore, it is presumed that the norepinephrine system, and perhaps the serotonin system as well, normally functions to provide motor drive to the limbic system to increase a person's sense of well-being and to create happiness, contentment, good appetite, appropriate sex drive, and psychomotor balance. In support of this concept is the fact that the pleasure and reward centers of the hypothalamus and surrounding areas receive large numbers of nerve endings from the norepinephrine system.

When encountering a patient with psychotic symptoms, everything reasonable must be done to rule out common physical causes. Many medical problems have psychiatric as well as physical symptoms. Thus, patients with mood or psychotic disorders require careful physical screening to be certain of the basis of the disorder. Appropriate treatment depends upon correct diagnosis. For example, an elderly person who presents symptoms of mental depression may actually have influenza. Once the influenza is treated, the depression lifts. A correct diagnosis of influenza prevents inappropriate antidepressant treatment. At the time of the initial recognition of symptoms, a thorough evaluation to rule out other medical disorders is indicated. Primary medical conditions and drug reactions that can cause mood disorders, anxiety, or paranoia are presented in Table 47–3.

KEY CONCEPTS

- Affective disorders are due to disordered emotions or affect. Included in this category of psychoses are bipolar disorder (periods of mania and depression) and unipolar depression. The average age at onset is 30 years for bipolar disorder and 40 for unipolar

TABLE 47–3. Selected Physical Illnesses and Drug Reactions Associated With Psychiatric Conditions Continued

Cause	Psychiatric Symptoms Associated With Specific Disorders			
	Depression	*Mania*	*Paranoia*	*Anxiety*
Infectious processes	Influenza Viral hepatitis Infectious mononucleosis General paresis (tertiary syphilis) Tuberculosis	Influenza St. Louis encephalitis Q fever General paresis (tertiary syphilis)		
Endocrine disorders	Myxedema Cushing's disease Addison's disease	Hyperthyroidism	Addison's disease Cushing's disease Hypothyroidism Hyperthyroidism Hypoparathyroidism Hyperparathyroidism	Hyperadrenalism (Cushing's disease) Hyperthyroidism Hypothyroidism
Neoplastic disorders	Occult abdominal malignancies (e.g., carcinoma of head of pancreas)			Secreting tumors (carcinoid, insulinoma, pheochromocytoma)
Collagen disorders	Systemic lupus erythematosus	Systemic lupus erythematosus Rheumatic chorea Systemic lupus erythematosus		Systemic lupus erythematosus
Neurological disorders	Multiple sclerosis Cerebral tumors Sleep apnea Dementia Parkinson's disease Nondominant temporal lobe lesions	Multiple sclerosis Diencephalic and third ventricular tumors	Brain tumors Temporal lobe epilepsy Alzheimer's disease Pick's disease Huntington's disease Parkinson's disease Multiple sclerosis Cerebral atherosclerosis Hypertensive encephalopathy Multi-infarct dementia	Encephalopathies (infectious, metabolic, toxic) Essential tremor Intracranial mass lesions Postconcussive syndrome Complex partial seizures Vertigo
Nutritional states	Pellagra Pernicious anemia		Vitamin B_{12} deficiency	Caffeine Monosodium glutamate Vitamin-deficiency diseases Anemias
Reactions to drugs	Steroidal contraceptives Reserpine Alpha-methyldopa Physostigmine Alcohol Sedative hypnotics Amphetamine withdrawal	Steroids Levodopa Amphetamines Methylphenidate Cocaine Monoamine oxidase inhibitors Tricyclic antidepressants Thyroid hormones	Amphetamine Cocaine Hallucinogens (LSD, PCP) Marijuana Mescaline Withdrawal syndromes (alcohol, sedative-hypnotics, barbiturates, benzodiazepines)	Akathisia (secondary to antipsychotic drugs) Anticholinergic toxicity Digitalis toxicity Hallucinogens Hypotensive agents Stimulants (cocaine, amphetamines, related drugs) Withdrawal syndromes (alcohol, sedative-hypnotics) Bronchodilators (theophylline, sympathomimetics)
Metabolic disorders			Hypoglycemia Liver failure Uremia	Hyperthermia Hyponatremia Hyperkalemia Hypocalcemia Hypoglycemia Menopause Porphyria (acute intermittent)

Table continued on following page

TABLE 47–3. Selected Physical Illnesses and Drug Reactions Associated With Psychiatric Conditions *Continued*

	Psychiatric Symptoms Associated With Specific Disorders			
Cause	*Depression*	*Mania*	*Paranoia*	*Anxiety*
Cardiovascular disorders				Angina pectoris Arrhythmias Congestive heart failure Hypertension Hypovolemia Myocardial infarction Syncope (of multiple causes) Valvular disease Vascular collapse (shock)
Respiratory disorders				Asthma Chronic obstructive pulmonary disease Pneumonia Pneumothorax Pulmonary edema Pulmonary embolism

Data from: Whybrow P, Akiskhal H, McKinney W: *Mood Disorders: Toward a New Psychobiology.* New York, Plenum Press, 1984; Hyman SE, Jenike MA: *Manual of Clinical Problems in Psychiatry.* Boston, Little, Brown and Co, 1990; Rosenbaum JF: The drug treatment of anxiety. *N Engl J Med* 1982;306(7):401–404.

depression. Depression affects women twice as often as men.

- A biochemical basis for bipolar disorder is supported by observations that brain monoamines (norepinephrine, serotonin) are below normal or the ratio of norepinephrine to serotonin is altered. Depression is thought to occur when serotonin and norepinephrine activity in the brain is low. Mania may be due to a relative excess of norepinephrine in the context of low serotonin or acetylcholine activity. Plasma membrane transport of small molecules such as lithium also is different. Bipolar disorder has a familial pattern of expression, suggesting a genetic etiology.
- Psychosocial factors that may affect the development and expression of mood disorders include loss (real, anticipated, or perceived) and low self-esteem. Sleep disorders accompany both extremes of mood. Depression is associated with altered REM sleep and decreased slow-wave sleep. Mania is associated with short sleep and reduced fatigue.
- Depression is manifested by low energy, inability to experience joy, difficulty initiating tasks, reduced decision-making ability, difficulty sleeping, poor appetite, weight loss, and decreased libido. Thoughts may be occupied by guilt, futility, emptiness, hopelessness, helplessness, and suicide. The treatment of unipolar depression is aimed at increasing norepinephrine and serotonin activity in the brain: monoamine oxidase inhibitors reduce the rate of neurotransmitter destruction; tricyclic antidepressants inhibit reuptake; newer agents (Prozac) selectively prevent serotonin reuptake.

- Mania is manifested by high energy, inflated self-esteem, hyperactivity, inability to focus or concentrate, low sensitivity to fatigue, injury or pain, rapid or incoherent speech, illusions, delusions, increased appetite and libido, decreased time sleeping, poor judgment, and poor impulse control. Mania is treated by lithium, a compound that inhibits the action of norepinephrine and serotonin in the brain.

Considerations for the Elderly

Schizophrenia and delusional disorder may continue into old age or may manifest for the first time only during senescence.

Symptoms such as delusions of control, thought insertions, and third-person auditory hallucinations are quite common in elderly delusional patients and in DSM-IV would be classified as late-onset schizophrenia or delusional disorder.[18]

More important factors are previous deviant personality and deafness. Up to 70 percent of late-onset schizophrenic persons have been characterized as "eccentric people, with related low marriage and fertility rates."[9] Deafness has been registered in 30 percent of aged schizophrenic persons, as opposed to 11 percent of aged depressives.[10] Deafness is due to long-standing ear diseases rather than to age-linked degeneration.

Psychiatric admissions of the elderly are characterized by significantly more major depression and less dysthymia than are seen in younger adults. The

The incidence of bipolar disorder in the geriatric age group should approach that of lifetime risk. It is extremely rare for the onset of bipolar disorder to occur after age 60, and all bipolar disorder patients who survive to old age continue to be vulnerable to that illness.

The causes of mood disorders in the elderly are more likely to be associated with concomitant illnesses or their treatments. In part, this is because the elderly are more likely to have a medical disorder and also because the aged brain is more sensitive to physiologic disturbances.

Some physiologic correlates of aging that are not considered pathologic may nevertheless increase vulnerability to depression. In particular, brain levels of metabolites of serotonin (5-hydroxyindoleacetic acid) norepinephrine (3-methoxy-4-hydroxyphenyglycol), and dopamine (homovanillic acid), as well as γ-aminobutyric acid, decrease with age in humans as in other animals.[19] Monoamine oxidase levels increase with age, which may account in part for the reduced levels of catecholamines (which are necessary for maintenance of normal mood).

Treatment

The altered physiology that affects pharmacokinetics in this age group influences the choice and course of pharmacologic therapies. Glomerular filtration rate, hepatic blood flow, and hepatic hydroxylation and demethylation are all decreased. When considering pharmacotherapy for an aged person, it is wise to assume an increase in drug half-life. Additionally, the CNS is more sensitive to a given drug blood level. Therefore, lower doses should be given initially to older persons. Because of wide variations in drug metabolism from person to person, however, some older patients may tolerate and need high doses to achieve therapeutic effects.

Antidepressant blood levels are not specifically established for elderly persons. They may serve as a useful guideline for dosage adjustment, because the toxic dose is certainly not elevated in this age group. Therefore, blood levels are obtained to document the safety of increasing the dosage to higher ranges. Nothing replaces careful clinical observation for potential signs of toxicity: confusion, ataxia, impaired memory, or cardiovascular symptoms. Because any antidepressant medication may affect cardiac function, during pretreatment evaluation, and periodically thereafter, it is wise to obtain an electrocardiogram (ECG) and sitting and standing blood pressures to seek orthostatic changes. People with bipolar disorder continue to need prophylactic as well as acute treatment with lithium or other anticycling agents. Neurotoxic signs often are apparent in the elderly at drug blood levels that are usually considered normal. Therapeutic effects may be achieved at lithium levels usually considered subtherapeutic (0.3–0.6 mEq/L) in younger persons.

Summary

Clinical manifestations, hypotheses regarding etiologies, and the pathogenesis of schizophrenia, major depression, and bipolar disorder have been presented. Each of the disorders has the potential to seriously disable an affected individual in the critical areas of work, relationships, self-care, and survival. It is important to remember that these disorders do not exhaust the category of psychoses. This chapter has presented an overview of those psychiatric disorders about which most has been identified in terms of neurophysiologic concomitants.

REFERENCES

1. Tien AY, Eaton WW: Psychopathologic precursors and sociodemographic risk factors for the schizophrenic syndrome. *Arch Gen Psychiatry* 1992;49:37–46.
2. Suddath RL, Christison GW, Torrey EF, Casanova MF, Weinberger DR: Anatomical abnormalities in the brains of monozygotic twins discordant for schizophrenia. *N Engl J Med* 1990; 322(12):789–794.
3. Mednick SA, Machon RA, Huttanen MO, Bonett D: Adult schizophrenia following prenatal exposure to an influenza epidemic. *Arch Gen Psychiatry* 1988;45:189–192.
4. O'Callaghan E, Sham P, Takei N, et al: Schizophrenia after prenatal exposure to 1957 A2 influenza epidemic. *Lancet* 1991;337:1248–1250.
5. Kovelman JA, Scheibel AB: A neurohistological correlate of schizophrenia. *Biol Psychiatry* 1984;19:1601–1621.
6. Weinberger D: Implications of normal brain development for the pathogenesis of schizophrenia. *Arch Gen Psychiatry* 1987; 44:660–669.
7. Susser E, Lin SP, Brown AS, Lumey LH, Erlenmeyer-Kimling L: No relation between risk of schizophrenia and prenatal exposure to influenza in Holland. *Am J Psychiatry* 1994;151:922–924.
8. Jampala VC, Taylor MA, Abrams R: The diagnostic implications of formal thought disorder in mania and schizophrenia: A reassessment. *Am J Psychiatry* 1989;146(4):459–471.
9. Talbott JA, Hales RE, Yudofsky SC (eds): *The American Psychiatric Press Textbook of Psychiatry.* Washington, DC, American Psychiatric Press, 1988, p 367.
10. Cannon TD, Mednick SA, Parnas J: Antecedents of predominantly negative- and predominantly positive-symptom schizophrenia: A reassessment. *Arch Gen Psychiatry* 1990;47(7): 622–632.
11. Goldstein JM, Tsuang MT, Faraone SV: Gender and schizophrenia: Implications for understanding the heterogeneity of the illness. *Psychiatry Res* 1989;28:243–253.
12. Kendler KS: Familial aggregation of schizophrenia and schizophrenia spectrum disorders. *Arch Gen Psychiatry* 1988; 45:377–383.
13. Giles DE, Biggs MM, Rush AJ, Roffwarg HP: Risk factors in families of unipolar depression: I. Psychiatric illness and reduced REM latency. *J Affect Disord* 1988;14(1):51–59.
14. Blehar MC, Weissman MM, Gershon ES, Hirschfeld RM: Family and genetic studies of affective disorders. *Arch Gen Psychiatry* 1988;45:289–292.
15. Egeland JA, Gerhard DS, Pauls DL, et al: Bipolar affective disorders linked to DNA markers on chromosome 11. *Nature* 1987;325:783–787.
16. El-Badramany MH, Farag TI, al-Awadi SA, et al: Familial manic-depressive illness with deleted short arm of chromosome 21: Coincidental or causal? *Br J Psychiatry* 1989;155:856–857.
17. Winokur G, Clayton P (eds): *The Medical Basis of Psychiatry*, 2nd ed. Philadelphia, WB Saunders, 1994.
18. American Psychiatric Association: *Diagnostic and Statistical Manual of Mental Disorders*, 4th ed. Washington, DC, American Psychiatric Association, 1994, p 281.

19. Golden RN, Potter WZ: Neurochemical and neuroendocrine dysregulation in affective disorders. *Psychiatr Clin North Am* 1986;9(2):313–326.

BIBLIOGRAPHY

Dawson G: *Human Behavior and the Developing Brain.* New York: Guilford Press, 1994.

Flaherty JA, Davis JM, Janicak PG: *Psychiatry: Diagnosis and Therapy,* 2nd ed. Norwalk, Conn, Appleton & Lange, 1993.

Gold PW, Goodwin FK, Chrousos GP: Clinical and biochemical manifestations of depression: Related to the neurobiology of stress. *N Engl J Med* 1988;319(6):348–353.

Haber J, McMahon AL, Price-Hoskins P, Sideleau BF: *Comprehensive Psychiatric Nursing,* 4th ed. St. Louis, Mosby–Year Book, 1992.

Hersen M, Turner SM (ed): *Adult Psychopathology and Diagnosis,* 2nd ed. New York, John Wiley & Sons, 1991.

Irving S: *Basic Psychiatric Nursing,* 3rd ed. Philadelphia, WB Saunders, 1983.

Kaplan HI, Sadock BJ (eds): *Comprehensive Textbook of Psychiatry V,* 5th ed. Baltimore, Williams & Wilkins, 1989.

Kaplan HI, Sadock BJ (eds): *Synopsis of Psychiatry: Behavioral Sciences, Clinical Psychiatry,* 6th ed. Baltimore, Williams & Wilkins, 1991.

Leach AM: Negative symptoms. *Curr Opin Psychiatry* 1991; 4(1):18–22.

Nicholi AM (ed): *The New Harvard Guide to Psychiatry.* Cambridge, Harvard University Press, 1988.

Reid WH: *The Treatment of Psychiatric Disorders.* New York, Brunner/ Mazel, 1989.

Sims ACP: *Symptoms in the Mind: An Introduction to Descriptive Psychopathology.* Philadelphia, WB Saunders, 1988.

Taylor CM: *Essentials of Psychiatric Nursing,* 14th ed. St. Louis, CV Mosby, 1994.

Winokurt G, Clayton P (eds): *The Medical Basis of Psychiatry,* 2nd ed. Philadelphia, WB Saunders, 1994.

CHAPTER 48
Neurobiology of Nonpsychotic Illness

JO ANNALEE IRVING, ANNE ROE MEALEY, and MARTHA J. SNIDER

KEY TERMS

agoraphobia: Irrational fear of open spaces. In panic disorder, agoraphobia is a fear of any place or situation in which assistance would be unavailable in case of an unexpected panic attack. Agoraphobia is also known as *phobic avoidance.*

anorexia: Loss of appetite.

anorexia nervosa: Intense fear of becoming obese.

anticipatory anxiety: Anxious anticipation of another panic attack.

bulimia: Excessive and insatiable appetite.

bulimia nervosa: Recurrent episodes of binge eating followed by self-induced vomiting or diarrhea, excessive exercise, strict dieting or fasting, and an exaggerated concern about body shape and weight.

compulsions: Repetitive ritualistic behaviors that have a driven quality.

dysphoria: The constant experience of unpleasant feelings.

histrionic: Theatrical, dramatic.

impulsivity: Spontaneous acting out of impulses accompanied by failure to plan ahead, predict consequences, or consider other possibilities.

narcissistic: Self-absorbed.

obsessions: Powerful, persistent, intrusive thoughts, impulses, or images that dominate the mental life of the individual to the extent that there is serious interference with the normal progression of life.

schizoid: Indifferent to social interaction and possessing a limited range of emotional experience and expression.

Mental disorders are often mistakenly identified only with psychotic behavior. That is, there is a common misconception that the person who has a mental disorder is out of touch with reality, sees or hears things that aren't there, or believes that he is some famous person. A related misconception is that people with mental disorders are only encountered in psychiatric facilities. Although these misconceptions are understandable, the truth of the matter is that many persons with nonpsychotic mental disorders are able to get along without hospitalization. Many are unrecognized by or unknown to mental health clinicians.

Mental disorders that are only rarely associated with psychotic behavior tend to dominate the nomenclature. Those selected for presentation in this chapter include representative subsets of three large categories of illness—the anxiety disorders, the personality disorders, and the eating disorders.

Anxiety disorders are characterized by irrational fears and have great potential to cause disability in persons so affected. Panic disorder, agoraphobia, and obsessive-compulsive disorder will be discussed.

The personality disorders, unlike the anxiety disorders in several ways, represent immature, inflexible, and persistently maladaptive ways of dealing with both intrapersonal and interpersonal demands of life. These disorders are recognized by adolescence; in some cases they may be perceived as extensions of certain childhood disorders. This is a broad category that is highly controversial for its inclusion or exclusion of certain behavioral phenomena. The two disorders discussed from this category are borderline personality disorder and antisocial personality disorder.

Finally, the eating disorders of anorexia nervosa and bulimia nervosa will be presented.

In this chapter, disorders are characterized by hypotheses about etiology and pathogenesis. Clinical manifestations are also presented.

Anxiety Disorders

Three major diagnoses are recognized under the diagnosis of **anxiety disorders:** panic disorder, generalized anxiety disorder, and obsessive-compulsive disorder.

Panic Disorder and Generalized Anxiety Disorder

Panic disorder is a psychiatric diagnosis. People with panic disorder experience episodes of acute anxiety, fear, and panic, often accompanied by a belief that they may be having a heart attack, or are unable to breathe, or that death is imminent.

Panic disorder is a common illness that affects 1.6 to 2.9 percent of women and 0.4 to 1.7 percent of men. The disorder usually begins in the third decade of life, with a mean age at onset of 26.6 years. Most affected people experience the first panic attack before the age of 30, although there are some cases with onset well past that age. Women appear to have the disorder twice as often as men.[1]

Persons with panic disorder often develop **anticipatory anxiety** related to fear of another panic attack. Because no single precipitating event can be correlated with the actual panic attack, clients live in dread that anything or everything could cause a repeat of their symptoms. As a means of controlling this anticipatory anxiety, clients often develop **agoraphobia**—a fear of open spaces. It is a fear of being in a place where help may not be attainable if a panic attack develops. These clients severely restrict their activities, sometimes even remaining in their homes for years.

Etiology and Pathogenesis of Panic Disorder

Some evidence of heritability of panic disorder has been established. Thirty percent of first-degree relatives of a person diagnosed as having panic disorder show symptoms of the disorder.[2] Monozygotic twins have a higher concordance rate than dizygotic twins. Researchers have suggested the possibility of a single, dominant gene.

Physiologically, panic attacks in susceptible clients can be precipitated by intravenous infusion of 0.5 molar sodium lactate or by breathing air with elevated carbon dioxide levels. Magnetic resonance spectroscopy has revealed that lactate crosses into the brain from the blood. Blood flow evaluated by positron emission tomography (PET) has also shown a rise in activity at the anterior ends of the temporal lobes during an attack. Studies in laboratory animals also have suggested that the temporal lobes are activated in anxiety reactions. These temporal poles provide important input to the amygdala, which is thought to be involved in severe emotional reactions. Other studies have focused on serotonin function in anxiety disorders but so far have been inconclusive.

The pathogenesis of the acute attack may differ from the pathogenesis of the anticipatory anxiety and phobic avoidance components. Panic attacks may be generated by massive neural discharge in the locus ceruleus. The evidence for this is based primarily on the ability of certain chemical agents to produce acute attacks in persons with the disorder but not in persons without the disorder. When given sodium lactate in a laboratory setting, diagnosed subjects complain first of palpitations, then dyspnea, dizziness, light-headedness, paresthesias, and diaphoresis. Additionally, they report a feeling of overwhelming fear and dread that something terrible is going to happen. This does not happen to control subjects.[3]

Anticipatory anxiety is proposed to react to the stimulation of the limbic lobe by activation of irritable areas in the brain stem. This component of the disorder could also be related to changes in cerebral blood flow that result from acute hyperventilation.

Phobic avoidance is believed to be a learned phenomenon. That is, higher brain centers are involved in the elaboration of anticipatory anxiety, which might occur when these centers interpret attacks as directly resulting from or associated with neutral events that occurred at the same time as the distressing physical symptoms.[3] There is some evidence that persons who develop panic disorder have an inordinate number of stressful life events historically than do other people before the onset of the first panic attack.[4] It is also possible that, through conditioning, people vulnerable to the development of panic disorder from a neurologic standpoint overlearn fear as a response to changes in the body.[5]

Clinical Manifestations of Panic Disorder

During the first panic attack, the person experiences the feelings already noted. Concurrent physical symptoms include dyspnea, palpitations, a sense of smothering, chest discomfort and tightness, dizziness, derealization, light-headedness and faintness, sweating, tremors, and hot and cold flashes. There may be fears that one is having a heart attack, or is dying, or is losing control.[1] The attack may last from 5 to 30 minutes.[3] The individual then returns to preattack behavioral functioning. Panic disorder is usually diagnosed when these attacks occur with some frequency. Either four attacks have occurred within a month's time, or the attacks have been followed by a period of anticipatory anxiety.[6] Other critical variables in the diagnosis include the presence of a relatively neutral context within which the first attack occurs.

Three distinct elements to panic disorder have been identified. The first of these, the attack itself, has already been described. The second feature is anticipatory anxiety. This is characterized by the individual worrying about having another of these frightening attacks. The anxiety becomes, in many cases, a chronic affective state. In a subset of persons with panic disorder, a third characteristic occurs. This is phobic avoidance and is referred to as agoraphobia. Persons become so anxious about having another phobic attack that they begin to avoid situations where, should they have an attack, they could not escape or would not have anyone who could help them. This avoidance may range from staying away from a few selected situations to the much more severe form of avoiding leaving the home. The avoidance may persist for years. Not all persons with panic disorder have agoraphobia, though the points of differentiation are not well understood.

Generalized Anxiety Disorder

Panic disorder is not the same as generalized anxiety disorder. This illness is characterized by the continual presence of a moderate degree of anxiety without discrete periods of acute attacks. **Generalized anxiety disorder** symptoms include chronic anxiety and tension accompanied by physical coordinates of headaches, abdominal problems, or sleep problems. Agoraphobia is rarely seen in generalized anxiety

disorder, and there is far less evidence regarding familial transmission.[7]

Treatment

Anxiety disorders have been successfully treated with benzodiazepines, particularly clomipramine. Based on the effectiveness of benzodiazepines, one etiologic hypothesis is that the disorder may reflect decreased numbers of benzodiazepine receptors or a neuromodulator that is opposite in its effect to benzodiazepine.

Mitral valve prolapse is a common finding in people with panic disorder, with or without agoraphobia. Dyspnea and palpitations lead to fear and associated sympathetic response, which may aggravate symptoms by a feedback loop. The diagnosis is corroborated by echocardiography. Explanation of the cause of symptoms and of the usually benign consequences generally relieves most of the symptoms. Antidepressants may be helpful but may also cause cardiac arrhythmias in some persons, compounding the problems. In the emergency situation, alprazolam or propranolol reduces symptoms of mitral valve prolapse.

Obsessive-Compulsive Disorder

This is a chronic anxiety disorder characterized by obsessions and compulsions that impair functioning and create distress in the individual. **Obsessions** are powerful, persistent, intrusive thoughts, impulses, or images that dominate the mental life of the individual to the extent that they seriously interfere with the normal progression of life. The individual perceives these thoughts to be generated from his or her own mind, but appraises them as senseless and not congruent with his or her usual mental life.

Compulsions are repetitive ritualistic behaviors that have a driven quality. These behaviors may be related to the obsessions within a context of control; that is, they occur to ward off or neutralize the obsessive thoughts. The individual realizes that the compulsive behaviors are unreasonable, senseless, or extreme.

Etiology and Pathogenesis

Some evidence has suggested that a genetic origin is the basis of obsessive compulsive disorder. Family studies show that the disorder often occurs in later life in families in which Tourette's syndrome has afflicted some member during childhood. Tourette's syndrome consists of uncontrollable muscular and vocal tics. This correlation in families is thought to be related to a single dominant gene; however, it is unclear why some members develop obsessive-compulsive disorder and others show symptoms of Tourette's syndrome. Other researchers have identified that some form of brain trauma preceded the development of the obsessive-compulsive disorder.

PET has shown increased glucose metabolism in the frontal lobes, caudate nucleus, and cingulate gyrus. These structures are closely connected and are involved in severe emotional reactions. As a last resort in treatment, some clients have been treated by cingulectomies.

Several hypotheses have sought to explain the pathogenesis of this disorder. Biological abnormalities are now believed to be far more significant than they once were. The most recent explanation of the illness is that the pathways that link the frontal lobes to the basal ganglia are dysfunctional. This proposition rests on the observed relationships with other illnesses that have a known etiology related to areas of the brain that control certain cognitive and motor tasks.[8] Specific pathology has been identified indicating that there is dysregulation of the basal ganglia/limbic circuits that modulate neuronal activity in posterior portions of the orbitofrontal cortex and the associated medial thalamic nuclei.[9] The dysfunctional status of the neurotransmitter serotonin has also been identified as a possible source of this disorder.

Contrary to earlier beliefs, most persons with this disorder do not have premorbid traits that once were associated with so-called anal traits. These included, but were not limited to, orderliness, obstinateness, stinginess, and the like. These traits are certainly not pathologic unless taken to extremes that result in dysfunctional performance in work and relationships. Obsessions and compulsions could, in a sense, be avoidance behaviors that fail. These symptoms develop almost an independent ability to generate anxiety, or at least psychic discomfort.

Clinical Manifestations

Obsessions are thoughts that repeatedly intrude into a person's mind. Individuals who have obsessive thoughts recognize that the thoughts are not sensible but are unable to prevent them from coming into their awareness.

Compulsions, on the other hand, are behaviors that the person feels compelled to perform. These compulsive behaviors are usually related to counting, checking (such as locks or the stove), cleaning (even to the point of damaging the skin by washing hundreds of times daily), or by avoidance behaviors (of sources of possible danger). If the individual is prevented from performing the rituals, a high degree of anxiety ensues. The rituals can become so consuming of the person's life that employment or usual activities of daily living are interfered with.

The incidence of this disorder is somewhat difficult to ascertain because it is generally accepted that people are quite secretive about having compulsions. Lifetime prevalence rates are believed to be between 2 and 3 percent, though this is probably an underestimate. A recent study reported that the median age at onset was 23 years, with the age range of highest risk between 15 and 39 years. There does not appear to be a difference between males and females in prevalence,

although childhood onset may be more common in males. The disorder is more frequent in the upper classes and in people with higher levels of intelligence.[1] There is some evidence of a familial component, either in the illness itself or in character traits of lesser degree.

There is a relationship between this disorder and Tourette's syndrome and major depression. These relationships have yet to be definitively identified, although certain pharmacologic agents are cross-effective.[1]

Treatment

Drug treatment has been the most effective therapy. Clomipramine, fluoxatine, and fluroxamine are the drugs of choice. Although these medications are categorized as antidepressants, their action is primarily to block uptake of 5-hydroxytryptophan, and they are known as serotonergic agonists.

KEY CONCEPTS

- Anxiety disorders are characterized by irrational and debilitating fears. The three major categories of anxiety disorders are panic disorder, generalized anxiety disorder, and obsessive-compulsive disorder. These disorders show some evidence of heritability, and biochemical correlates are suspected. Defects in serotonin pathways have been proposed as etiologic factors.

- Panic disorder is characterized by acute episodes of severe anxiety accompanied by dyspnea, chest pain, and a sense of impending doom. Palpitations, hyperventilation, dizziness, paresthesias, and diaphoresis may occur during an attack, which may last 5 to 30 minutes. Mitral valve prolapse is a common finding in persons experiencing panic. Once symptoms are attributed to a specific cause, panic attacks may cease. People with panic disorder may develop anticipatory anxiety and phobic avoidance. Efforts to avoid future episodes may result in agoraphobia.

- Generalized anxiety disorder is characterized by a continuous but moderate degree of anxiety without discrete periods of acute attacks. Agoraphobia rarely develops, but chronic headaches, muscle tension, abdominal discomfort, and sleep disturbances are usual.

- Obsessive-compulsive disorder is characterized by obsessive thoughts and compulsive behaviors. Obsessions (persistent, intrusive, compelling thoughts) commonly have themes of committing violent acts, being a victim of violence, or fear of contamination. In contrast to schizophrenia, the person realizes that the obsessive thoughts are from his or her own mind but is helpless to control them. Compulsions (repetitive, ritualistic behaviors) include such actions as excessive washing and grooming, repeated checking to ensure safety, and elaborate measures

- to avoid contact with dirt or bodily wastes. If the individual is prevented from performing compulsive rituals, a high state of anxiety ensues.
- Benzodiazepines and antidepressants may be used to treat anxiety disorders.

Personality Disorders

Personality disorders are disturbances in ways of handling life. The behaviors that constitute this category are composed of inflexible and maladaptive propensities of individuals to deal with the usual stresses and events that require everyone to act or respond. The patterns of response are recognizable by adolescence and are believed to be more discomforting to those around the individual than to the individual himself. There are three diagnostic clusters of personality disorders. In the first cluster are the schizotypal, schizoid, and paranoid disorders. Histrionic, narcissistic, antisocial, and borderline disorders are in the second cluster, and the compulsive, dependent, avoidant, and passive-aggressive disorders are in the third cluster. Two diagnostic entities, borderline personality disorder and antisocial personality disorder, have been selected for presentation. They illustrate many of the common theoretical problems in definition, as well as problems in differentiation in personality disorders.

Borderline Personality Disorder

Borderline personality disorder has a long history of identity problems from a conceptual point of view. In the early literature, the border referred to was schizo-phrenia. More recently, some overlap with depression has been suggested. It is probably accurate to say that the borderline personality disorder enjoys its own identity, although some relationship to other disorders is likely (Fig. 48–1).

Etiology and Pathogenesis

Recent research has focused on dysregulation of the serotonergic system, which correlates with impulsiveness, aggression, and suicidal ideation. Cerebrospinal fluid shows an inverse relation between serotonergic level and those behaviors. However, so many of the personality disorders are similar to other psychiatric conditions that it has been difficult to differentiate distinct neurobiological abnormalities.

The behaviors associated with this disorder may overlap with other personality disorders. A recent study of discriminating features of the person with borderline personality disorder concluded that some characteristics were typically specific: quasi-psychotic thought, self-mutilation, manipulative suicide attempts, abandonment/engulfment/annihilation concerns, demandingness/entitlement, and some specific difficulties in psychotherapy.[10]

It is conceded that the themes and issues in the dysfunctional relationships that characterize borderline personality disorder may have some basis in the early mother–child relationships. It has been suggested that an increased sensitivity to loss may occur because of early separations, which interact in some way with a more basic dysregulation in brain areas associated with the regulations of affect; many of these same areas are also related to mood disorders.

It is possible that there is some deficit in mood regulation that could disrupt early bonding or exag-

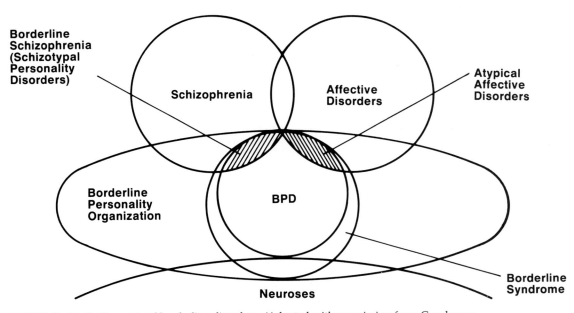

FIGURE 48–1. Concepts of borderline disorders. (Adapted with permission from Gunderson J: *Borderline Personality Disorder.* American Psychiatric Press, Washington, DC, 1984, p 12.)

gerate the child's response to normal frustrations. This would or could presage a hostile and conflictual relationship with the major caretaker. A low threshold for excitability in the limbic system could also relate to mood lability and impulsivity.

Many theorists believe that the early family environment contributes significantly to the development of borderline personality disorder. It is possible that the individual has a constitutional inability to regulate affect and that the impulsivity associated with the dysregulation predisposes to disorganization under stress; this tendency emerges in childhood. It is also proposed that the individual may have a tendency to alternately devalue and idealize the same individual. Such splitting between devaluing and idealizing arises from early experiences that failed to allow the child to learn to perceive the parent as both good and bad, giving and withholding, simultaneously. When the child confronts the reality of the coexistence of good and bad, anxiety is raised, and through the use of primitive defenses against anxiety, this difficulty continues into adulthood and affects all future relationships. These propositions rest on clinical inference but have been validated to relatively consistent degrees.

A strong association has also been suggested between borderline personality disorder and a reported history of childhood abuse. The strength of the association suggests that it is an important factor but not alone sufficient to account for all the psychopathology. It is possible the trauma is most pathogenic for children with vulnerable temperaments or for those most lacking protective factors such as positive relationships with caretakers or siblings.[11]

Clinical Manifestations

Borderline personality disorder is characterized by interpersonal relationships that are intense, unstable, and dependent. The person with this disorder tends to express desires for sole or exclusive possession of another through clinging behavior. A noteworthy manifestation is the tendency of the person to alternately devalue and idealize the same individual. This is expressed by directly or indirectly undermining and discrediting the personal assets of the other. Devaluation is motivated on the surface by anger in response to threats of abandonment, the setting of limits by someone who has some power over the person, or confrontation.

Covert means are used to control the behavior of others or to induce another to meet the individual's needs. These manipulative behaviors may be characterized by complaints of serious physical illness, provocative acts that result in the person being able to play the victim, misleading another in a deliberate fashion, and self-destructive behaviors.

Self-destructive behaviors occur frequently and may be motivated by the wish to elicit rescue behaviors from the other person. These behaviors can include wrist slashing, hitting walls or other hard surfaces with one's head, taking pills, and the like. This is a highly dangerous characteristic, since the obvious consequence can be death.

The person with borderline personality disorder is terrified of being abandoned and may panic when left alone. Fears of abandonment may be defined as an ever-present dread that the person on whom one is dependent may leave. There is typically great expenditure of energy in making sure that one is never alone.

A common feature in this disorder is dysphoria, or the constant experience of unpleasant feelings. The display of feelings is intense, and the feelings are often anger, sadness, or frustration. There are complaints of loneliness, emptiness, and boredom. The person may not be able to relate to a sustained period of life when feelings of satisfaction and contentment prevailed.

A feature of the borderline personality that is almost ubiquitous is the tendency of the affected person to transiently lose the sense of reality, referred to as derealization, when in situations of ambiguity or little structure. This tendency is short-lived and mitigated by the imposition of structure.

Impulsiveness in a variety of areas is commonplace. This propensity is reflected in episodic substance abuse, promiscuity, fighting, and the like. The response to stressful situations may be flight.

Unstable role performance, disturbances in identity, absence of goals in life, and general underfunctioning round out the picture of the person with borderline personality disorder.

Prevalence data for borderline personality indicate a rate of 1 to 2 percent of the population. Women are twice as likely as men to have this disorder. The families of borderline patients have a tendency to major depression, alcoholism, and other substance abuse. As with all personality disorders, the behavioral pattern can be identified in adolescence.

Antisocial Personality Disorder

This disorder generally comes to mind when one thinks of a "character" disorder. The antisocial disorder is a more modern concept of the category once referred to as the sociopathic personality. Even earlier, the appellation constitutional psychopathic disorder was used. Historical descriptions once referred to moral insanity. All these terms refer to the same group of behaviors.

Etiology and Pathogenesis

Both psychosocial and constitutional factors have been identified as the putative causes. The failure to develop and internalize a set of values consistent with the larger culture indicate difficulties with the parental relationships from an early age. Emotional deprivation because of loss, physical or psychological absence of adults in the environment, and inconsistency in the system of rewards and punishments may have some bearing on the development of this disorder.

Faulty parental models are also mentioned as having etiologic significance from an environmental point of view.

Relatively consistent findings in studies of persons with antisocial personality disorder and their parents show electroencephalographic abnormalities. It is possible that this is predisposing rather than causative, however. A childhood history of attention deficit disorder and hyperactivity has also been associated with later development of antisocial personality disorder. Although the specific causes are unknown, it is generally agreed that the final common pathway is related to failure to acquire the conditioned responses that are necessary for the learning of avoidance behaviors, conventional morality, and socialized positive responses to others.

Clinical Manifestations

Common behavioral and trait lists almost always include an apparent lack of anxiety and guilt as hallmarks of the antisocial personality disorder. More elaborate descriptions of the affect in this disorder also remark that callousness, insensitivity, and cold-bloodedness are observed. Additionally a lack of compassion, incivility, and careless indifference to what happens to others are noted.[14] Deficits in personal loyalties and in value organization are notable.

The person with antisocial personality disorder is able to project a charming facade to impress and exploit others. The person tends to blame others for his or her own behavior.

Impulsivity is a major source of difficulty for others. The spontaneous acting out of impulses is accompanied by failure to plan ahead, predict consequences, or consider other ways of achieving the same positive outcomes in other ways.

The individual is unable to learn from his or her mistakes and is likely to repeat the same misdeeds and heedless activities several times. Irresponsibility is a feature observed in the adult antisocial person, and includes failure to meet marital, parental, occupational, and financial obligations. Children and spouses may be abused.[12]

A long history of difficulty with the legal system and participation in illegal pursuits is diagnostic in this disorder. Contempt for social norms, authority figures, rules, and role expectations dominate the person's behavior.

Antisocial personality disorder is the only clinical entity in which diagnostic psychiatry uses historically based criteria. The onset of this disorder must be documented by a detailed history of antisocial acts and behaviors before age 15, along with failure to present adequate occupational history after 18 years.[3]

The reported prevalence of the antisocial personality disorder is 3 percent in men and less than 1 percent in women. The disorder seems to be more common in highly mobile residents of poor urban areas. Prisons are also primary sources of residence for persons with antisocial personality disorder. There

is evidence, authorities believe, that antisocial personality disorder is related to having a sociopathic and alcoholic father, whether or not the child is reared with that parent. It is not always the case that the person with antisocial personality disorder has experienced cultural conflict, deviant companions, social-class inner city homes, or brain damage, at least as primary factors. It is likely that the genetic link with deviant parents who are depriving, nonaffectionate, and abusive is more critical.[13]

KEY CONCEPTS

- Personality disorders are characterized by behaviors deemed "inappropriate" or deviant within the cultural context. Behavioral patterns are recognizable by adolescence and include paranoid, schizophrenia-like; narcissistic, self-absorbed, antisocial; and compulsive, passive-aggressive, dependent.
- Borderline personality disorder is characterized by unstable and dependent interpersonal relationships. Exclusive possession of another person is desired. To this end the individual may exhibit clinging, manipulation (complaints of illness, threatened suicide), self-destruction, and lying. Fear of abandonment may be ever-present. Impulsiveness, substance abuse, loneliness, and lack of life goals are common. Psychosocial and biochemical factors are thought to be contributory: Poor early mother–child relationships, child abuse, separation, or abandonment are significant contributing factors. Biological deficits in mood regulation could contribute to poor child–parent bonding.
- Antisocial personality disorder is characterized by failure to internalize moral and ethical values consistent with societal norms. Lack of anxiety and guilt, cold-bloodedness, and careless indifference or contempt for others are hallmarks of the disorder. Antisocial personality disorder is diagnosed based on repeated antisocial behavior before age 15 along with failure to establish an occupational history after age 18. Psychosocial and biological factors are thought to be contributory and include lack of adequate parental role models, child abuse, inconsistent parenting, emotional deprivation, and having an alcoholic parent. A genetic component has been proposed.

Eating Disorders

Anorexia nervosa and bulimia nervosa are apparently related eating disorders. They are typically illnesses of young adult women. Anorexia nervosa has the earlier onset.

Anorexia Nervosa

Anorexia nervosa is generally characterized by dietary restrictions that are imposed by the individual, significant weight loss, peculiar and ritualistic ways of handling and relating to food, and an intense, irrational fear of gaining weight and becoming obese. The body image is grossly disturbed such that the individual perceives herself to be overweight even when she is emaciated.

Etiology and Pathogenesis

The specific etiology of this disorder is unknown. The obvious mechanisms that have generated hypotheses include phobic avoidance, neurotransmitter dysregulation, and hunger-satiety psychological and physiologic interactions. An early theoretical formulation held that fear of oral impregnation led to phobic avoidance. The relation of perceptual and cognitive deficits to the proper assessment of body image was, for a time, a more measurable hypothesis than the psychodynamic model. The relationship of a hypothalamic dysfunction to amenorrhea continues to be of interest, as is the possibility of dysregulation of norepinephrine, serotonin, and dopamine.

Family studies in anorexia nervosa suggests a genetic predisposition and an association with mood disorders (although not with eating disorders) in first-degree relatives in twin studies. This finding in particular is consistent with a final common pathway in which the manifestations differ but the neuropathology is the same.

Clinical Manifestations

Most of the behavior that is directed toward weight loss occurs in secret. Weight loss of at least 15 percent of body weight is required for diagnosis.[6] Anorexia nervosa is also characterized by hiding food or carrying food on the person, collecting recipes, and fixing elaborate meals for friends and family. Low-calorie foods may constitute the diet of the individual, whereas the meals cooked for others are not particularly low in fats or carbohydrates. At the table, the person will dawdle over each bite, cut food into very small portions, and take very small bites. When confronted, the individual typically denies the unusual nature of this behavior.

The suppression of appetite and eating is not always successful, so that binging and then purging through self-induced vomiting and laxative use can coexist with this disorder. Most adolescents who develop this disorder have delayed psychosexual growth. Amenorrhea is a characteristic that relates to delayed development. After severe weight loss has occurred, the person presents with hypothermia, dependent edema, bradycardia, hypotension, and languor. Anorexia nervosa causes death in about 5 to 18 percent of confirmed cases.[14]

Significant laboratory findings in this disorder include failure to suppress cortisol by dexamethasone, elevated basal growth hormone levels, hypokalemia, and electrocardiographic changes. Arrhythmias may occur and are usually the cause of death in this disorder. The laboratory findings are state dependent and apparently return to more normal values when the starvation phase of the illness is reversed. The vast majority of people with anorexia nervosa are female. The incidence of the disorder has increased markedly over the past three decades. The average age at onset of anorexia nervosa is 13 to 15 years.

Bulimia Nervosa

Bulimia nervosa is characterized by episodes of uncontrollable, compulsive, and rapid ingestion of huge amounts of calories in a short period of time. Abdominal pain, nausea and vomiting, or exhaustion terminate the eating binge. Following the eating event, the individual feels guilt and disgust, usually over her or his inability to control the behavior.

Etiology and Pathogenesis

Although the specific etiology of this disorder has yet to be delineated, there is some evidence that strict dieting that precipitates binging may affect the hunger-satiety mechanisms such that the perception of these states is disturbed.[15] There does seem to be a relationship between mood disorder and bulimia, although this is not causal. The majority of bulimics have depressive symptoms. Alcohol or other drug abuse is not uncommon.

Clinical Manifestations

Laxatives and self-induced vomiting are used to get rid of the caloric intake. The person with bulimia nervosa is usually of normal or a little over normal weight and has a reasonably accurate body image, at least in comparison to the person with anorexia nervosa. During binges, the kind of food ingested is sweet, soft, and high in calories. Bulimics are conscious of how they look to other people, are sexually active, and are concerned about their body image. The prevalence of bulimia nervosa varies between 4 and 9 percent; approximately 10 to 15 percent of bulimics are male. The average age at onset of bulimia is 18 years.

KEY CONCEPTS

- Anorexia nervosa is an eating disorder characterized by excessive dietary restriction, significant weight loss (>15 percent), irrational fears of gaining weight, and disturbed body image. The disorder appears to have a genetic predisposition and affects females almost exclusively. The average age at onset is 13 to 15 years. Afflicted individuals tend to be secretive about their food restrictions. Self-induced vomiting and laxative abuse may also occur. Manifestations of anorexia nervosa include amenorrhea, hypothermia, edema, hypotension, and fluid and electrolyte imbalance. Potassium imbalance may lead to the serious consequence of cardiac dysrhythmias.

- Bulimia nervosa is characterized by episodes of binging, or the uncontrollable ingestion of large quantities of food. Binging may precipitate efforts to rid the body of ingested calories through self-induced vomiting or laxative use. Strict dieting, depressive mood disorders, and poor self-concept may be contributing factors. Perception of body image is accurate. Age at onset is about 18 years. Most bulimics are female.

Summary

Hypotheses regarding etiology and pathogenesis, clinical manifestations, and implications for treatment of representative subsets of two large categories of illness have been presented. An understanding of the psychophysiology of these illnesses is particularly useful for the health care professional.

It is important to recognize that these conditions represent mixtures of biological, psychological, social, and situational factors. The success of pharmacologic treatments has reinforced the concept of chemical dysregulation. However, researchers have yet to unlock the mysteries surrounding the neurobiology of nonpsychotic illness. Although many people with nonpsychotic mental disorders are able to get along without hospitalization, these disorders are serious, significant, and often unrecognized or unknown to mental health clinicians.

REFERENCES

1. Wesner R: Panic disorder and agoraphobia. *Primary Care* 1987;14(4):649–656.
2. Hollander E, Liebowitz MR, Gorman JM: Anxiety disorders, in Talbott JA, Hales RE, Yudofsky SC (eds): *The American Psychiatric Press Textbook of Psychiatry*. Washington, DC, American Psychiatric Press, 1988.
3. Gorman JM: A neuroanatomical hypothesis for panic disorder. *Am J Psychiatry* 1989;146(2):148–160.
4. Farvelli C, Pallanti S: Recent life events and panic disorder. *Am J Psychiatry* 1989;146(5):622–626.
5. Brown DR, Eaton WW, Sussman L: Racial differences in prevalence of phobic disorders. *J Nerv Ment Dis* 1990;189(7):434–440.
6. American Psychiatric Association: *Diagnostic and Statistical Manual of Mental Disorders*, 4th ed. Washington, DC, American Psychiatric Association, 1994.
7. Appenheimer T, Noyes R: Generalized anxiety disorder. *Primary Care* 1987;14(4):635–648.
8. Rapoport JL: *The Boy Who Couldn't Stop Washing: The Experience and Treatment of Obsessive-Compulsive Disorder*. New York, Dutton, 1989.
9. Modell JG, Mountz JM, Curtis GC, Greden JF: Neurophysiologic dysfunction in basal ganglia/limbic striatal and thalamocortical circuits as a pathogenetic mechanism of obsessive-compulsive disorder. *J Neuropsychiatry* 1989;1(1):27–36.
10. Zanarini MC, Gunderson JG, Frankenburg FR: Cognitive features of borderline personality disorder. *Am J Psychiatry* 1990;147(1):57–63.
11. Herman JL, Perry JC, van der Kolk BA: Childhood trauma in borderline personality disorder. *Am J Psychiatry* 1989;146(4):490–495.
12. Millon T: A theoretical derivation of pathological personality, in Millon T, Klerman GL (eds): *Contemporary Directions in Psychopathology*. New York, Guilford Press, 1986.
13. Gunderson JG: Personality disorders, in Nicholi AM (ed): *The New Harvard Guide to Psychiatry*. Cambridge, Harvard University Press, 1988, pp 337–357.
14. Carson RC, Butcher JN, Coleman JS: Psychological factors and physical illness, in *Abnormal Psychology and Modern Life*, 8th ed. Glenview, Ill, Scott Foresman, 1988, p 121.
15. Pope HG, Hudson JI: Eating disorders, in Kaplan HI, Sadock BJ (eds): *Comprehensive Textbook of Psychiatry V*, 5th ed. Baltimore, Williams & Wilkins, 1989.

BIBLIOGRAPHY

Berger PA, Brodie HKH: *American Handbook of Psychiatry*. Vol 8, *Biological Psychiatry*. New York, Basic Books, 1986.
Gardner DL, Cowdry RW: Suicidal and parasuicidal behavior in borderline personality disorder. *Psychiatr Clin North Am* 1985;8(2):389–402.
Kaplan HI, Sadock BJ (eds): *Comprehensive Textbook of Psychiatry V*, 5th ed. Baltimore, Williams & Wilkins, 1989, vols 1 and 2.
Kernberg OF: *Severe Personality Disorders: Psychotherapeutic Strategies*. New Haven, Yale University Press, 1984.
Maxmen JS: *Essential Psychopathology*. New York, WW Norton, 1986.
Melges FT, Swartz MS: Oscillations of attachment in borderline personality disorder. *Am J Psychiatry* 1989;146(9):1115–1120.
Nicholi AM (ed): *The New Harvard Guide to Psychiatry*. Cambridge, Harvard University Press, 1988.
Reich J: Personality disorders. *Primary Care* 1987;14(4):725–736.
Swartz MS, Blazer DG, George LK, Winfield I, Zakris J, Dye E: Identification of borderline personality disorder with the NIMH diagnostic interview schedule. *Am J Psychiatry* 1989;146(2):200–204.
Talbott JA, Hales RE, Yudofsky SC (eds): *The American Psychiatric Press Textbook of Psychiatry*. Washington, DC, American Psychiatric Press, 1988.
Weissman MM, Klerman GL, Markowitz JS, Ouellette R: Suicidal ideation and suicide attempts in panic disorder and attacks. *N Engl J Med* 1989;321(18):1209–1214.
Winokur G, Clayton P (eds): *The Medical Basis of Psychiatry*, 2nd ed. Philadelphia, WB Saunders, 1994.

UNIT XIV

Alterations in Musculoskeletal Support and Movement

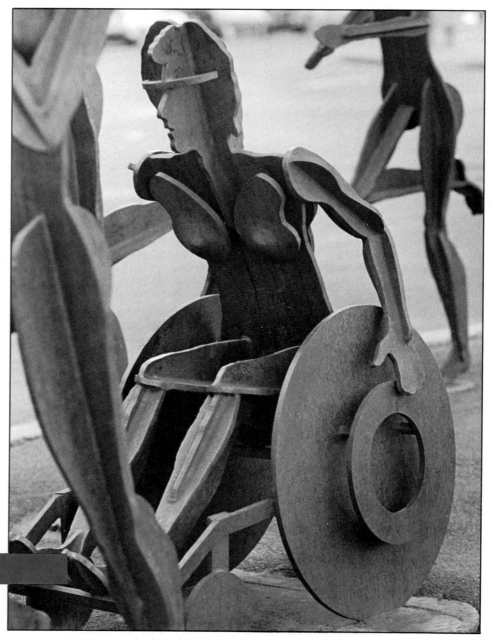

The runners sculpture pays tribute to the strength and agility of people. Wheelchair athletes compete in a race despite altered musculoskeletal function.

Photo by Kathleen Kelly

When health professionals find themselves caring for one or another of the 2 million Americans who each year suffer fractures of the long bones—the humerus, radius, ulna, metacarpals, femur, tibia, fibula, or metatarsals—they are preoccupied with the patient's comfort or medication, with the alignment of the reset bones, with the possibility of infection, and with the patient's outlook. They are participating in the process of healing, which requires attention to the injury but also a watchful concern for the patient's morale, nutrition, and general health.

Hurrying from one chore or one patient to the next, they have little time to be concerned about common misperceptions of the bone, of the reputation of bones. They are not alone. Perhaps because our boniness is always with us, conspicuously, whether we are walking or sitting, stretching, or rapping our "funny bone," we tend to take the skeleton for granted, for the wrong reasons.

We may notice one person's cheekbones, or say that another has a "rawboned" look. But we are not much aware of the bones' processes, of their life, as we are bound to be, for example, when the gastrointestinal or the genitourinary systems remind us of their processes. Most of the time, bones live quietly in the body.

For some fairly obvious reasons we regard our connected armature of bones as a durable but lifeless framework for the body. After dinner, at least for the carnivorous human, what is left? The bones of the fish. When a tourist visits Dinosaur National Monument, there, carefully revealed by decades of scientific effort, are the prehistoric fossilized skeletal remains, evidence of life long ago destroyed, evidence of lifelessness.

Their durability reminds us that bones are strong. One writer observes that bones are constructed like reinforced concrete, a combination of fibers and crystals, with a compressed strength greater than that of reinforced concrete and a tensile strength nearly as great.

But there is much more to the bone than its boniness.

The skeleton is the sturdy framework of each human life. As long as humans have walked the planet they have been supported by this armature, and as they watch their children grow they take special pleasure in the straight, strong growth of the bones.

The skeleton supports life, and protects the organs, and as a person grows older and perhaps suffers a degenerative bone disease such as osteoporosis, the loss of that protection may expose the organs to other kinds of degeneration or disease. An elderly person who breaks a hip and requires surgery must be carefully observed so that her weakness will not invite infection.

But the skeleton itself exists in delicate balance. When women began to worry about calcium deficiency, they took doses of calcium, only to learn that calcium made it more difficult for them to absorb iron. When we set out with deliberate intention to strengthen ourselves, we sometimes learn that we have upset our balance even when we are dealing with a framework as seemingly impervious as the skeleton.

Some scientists interested in helping people resist brittle bone disease might be drawn to the other end of the spectrum, where bones are formed. Research interest in degeneration and disease can provoke a deeper interest. Age-adjusted osteoporosis has been increasing in Western nations, and this fact—the brittleness of aging bones—has led to research on how diet, exercise, and modern life-styles affect bone growth and condition. Researchers assume that

FRONTIERS OF RESEARCH
Advances in Treatment of Musculoskeletal Disorders

Michael J. Kirkhorn

high peak bone mass may be a defense against the eventual development of osteoporosis. Scientists assume that calcium intake during childhood is a major determinant of bone development, but they are far less certain about the relationships between calcium sources, total daily calcium intake, hormonal levels, physical activity, and bone mass.

Here again, new technology has allowed researchers to understand important factors. Dual-energy x-ray absorptiometry and its low-radiation exposure has helped in the development of studies that are needed to determine peak bone mass.

The skeleton moves through the contraction of the muscles that adorn the armature, give it power, and mobility. Stripped of its musculature, and therefore of its mobility and power, the skeleton becomes, as it does on Halloween, a reminder of the final immobility, death.

Gene therapy offers promising directions for some muscle diseases, as it does for many other diseases as genetic research continues to progress.

Duchennne type muscular dystrophy (DMD) is a degenerative disorder that first attacks skeletal muscle and proceeds to loss of ambulation, respiratory and cardiac dysfunction, and early death. It also affects the brain. It is the most common form of muscular dystrophy in children. DMD is the first muscular dystrophy for which the defective gene was cloned and characterized and the corresponding protein identified. Therefore it is a model for muscle gene therapy research.

Encouraging results have been reported as functional dystrophin minigenes have been constructed in the laboratory that would compensate for the loss of dystrophin, a cytoskeletal protein, in DMD patients due to dystrophin gene mutations. Animal studies indicate that "recombinant dystrophin can substitute functionally for native dystrophin, a requisite for attempts at human in vivo correction," researchers reported.

CHAPTER 49
Structure and Function of the Musculoskeletal System

GARY SMITH

KEY TERMS

articular cartilage: A connective tissue of firm consistency and little or no vascularity. Tolerates extreme compression stress. Lines the ends of bones that comprise many of the synovial joints.

collagen: The major protein of the white fibers of connective tissue. Collagen's important mechanical properties are its resistance to tension stress and its strength.

epiphyseal plate: A segment of a long bone developed from a center of ossification and distinct from the shaft. An area of growth in a bone.

ground substance: Composed of protein polysaccharides or glycosaminoglycans, this material serves as the "cement" between layers of collagen fibers.

immobilization: A mechanical action of limiting or preventing movement at a joint. Prolonged immobilization may cause a shortening of connective tissue, a breakdown of cartilage, a weakening of ligaments, and a decrease in the muscles' ability to contract.

joint capsule: Dense layers of connective tissue surrounding synovial joints. The capsule is solidly attached to the periosteum of the adjacent bony components. The joint capsule provides strength to the joint and, through its neural receptors, detects motion, compression, tension, vibration, and pain.

skeletal muscle: Comprising 40 percent of total body weight, skeletal muscle enables bones to move at the joint and provides strength and protection to the skeleton by distributing and absorbing shock.

skeletal system: Rigid system of bony structures designed to protect internal organs, provide bony attachments for muscles and ligaments, and presents rigid levers to allow for functional movement of the body and its separate parts.

synovial fluid: Similar to blood plasma but contains hyaluronic acid and a glycoprotein. Synovial fluid reduces friction between the capsule and joint surfaces, lubricates the surface of the cartilage, resists shear forces, and provides nourishment for the cartilage.

trabecular system: The alignment of cancellous bone cells in response to mechanical stress placed upon the bone. The configuration of bone cells increases the strength of the bone.

Movement is one of the most characteristic and visible aspects of human life. Ease of movement adds to each individual's sense of self-worth and well-being, for the ability to move is closely interrelated with independence. A working knowledge of the system responsible for bodily movement is imperative to the health care provider. Basic characteristics of the firm support of bone and joint structures that make motion possible, and the properties of skeletal muscles that actually move the body's framework, are examined in this chapter.

Structure and Function of Bone

The purpose of the skeletal system is to protect internal organs, provide bony attachments for muscles and ligaments, and present rigid levers to allow functional movement of the body and its separate parts. Bone is an extremely hard structure but is metabolically active from birth to death. Bone is highly vascular and is well suited for self-repair.

Composition

Structurally, bone is able to adapt and alter shape and density in response to the mechanical demands placed on it.[1] A specialized connective tissue, bone has a high content of inorganic material (mineral salts) that combines with an organic matrix. This combination provides for a hard, rigid structure that is both flexible and resilient.

The mineral portions of bone, mainly calcium and phosphate, account for 65 percent to 75 percent of the dry weight of bone and give bone its solid structure. Bone is also a reservoir for essential minerals, especially calcium. Bone mineral is embedded in fibers of protein collagen, the fibrous aspect of the extracellular matrix. Collagen fibers are quite tough but pliable and resistant to stretching. Collagen composes approximately 95 percent of the extracellular matrix and accounts for 25 to 30 percent of the dry weight of bone.[1] Collagen is the chief fibrous component of the musculoskeletal system.

A ground substance surrounds the collagen fibers in the structure of bone. The **ground substance** consists of protein polysaccharides, or glycosaminoglycans (GAGs), mainly in a molecule called proteoglycans (PGs). The GAGs serve as the cement between layers of collagen fibers.

Water comprises approximately 25 percent of the weight of live bone. The majority of the water is found in the organic matrix surrounding the collagen fibers and the ground substance. Another 15 percent of the water is located in the canals that carry nutrition to the bone tissue.[1]

Microscopic Composition

Microscopically, the basic unit of bone is the **osteon** or the **haversian system** (Fig. 49–1). The haversian canal lies at the center of each osteon and contains blood vessels and nerve fibers. A concentric series of lamellae of mineralized matrix surrounds the central canal. Bordering the lamellae are small cavities (lacunae) that contain a bone cell, the **osteocyte.** Many small channels, the canaliculi, connect adjacent lamellae with each other and eventually with the main haversian canal. This canal system allows nutrients from blood vessels in the haversian canal to reach the osteocytes. Collagen fibers connect one lamella to another within the osteon and increase the mechanical strength of bone.[2]

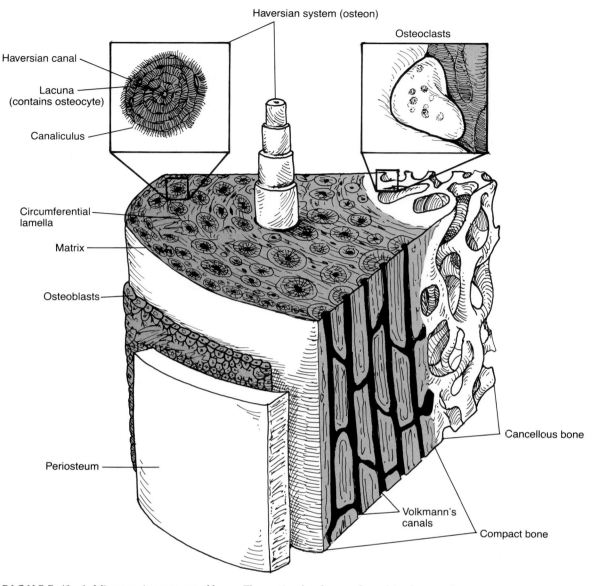

Haversian system (osteon)

Osteoclasts

Haversian canal

Lacuna
(contains osteocyte)

Canaliculus

Circumferential
lamella

Matrix

Osteoblasts

Periosteum

Cancellous bone

Volkmann's
canals

Compact bone

F I G U R E 49 – 1. Microscopic anatomy of bone. The section has been enlarged to show perios-teum, osteoblasts, haversian system, lacunae, and osteoclasts. (From Monahan FD, Drake T, Neighbors M (eds): *Nursing Care of Adults.* Philadelphia, WB Saunders, 1994, p 1343. Reproduced with permission.)

Macroscopic Composition

At the macroscopic level, bones are composed of two types of tissue: **compact,** or **cortical,** bone and **cancellous,** or **trabecular,** bone (Fig. 49–2). Compact bone is quite resistant to compression and is dense in structure. Compact bone is laid down in concentric layers. Cancellous bone is formed in thin plates called **trabeculae.** Trabeculae are laid down in response to stress and actually remodel their shape to accommodate loads placed on the bone.[3] All bones are covered by a tough fibrous membrane called the **periosteum.** The periosteum is highly vascularized and provides nutrition for the bone via Volkmann's canals (see Fig. 49–1). An inner layer of the periosteum is composed of **osteoblasts,** which are responsible for bone growth

and repair. The periosteum covers the entire bone except for the ends of bones, which are covered by hyaline cartilage.

In the longer bones, a central cavity (**medullary cavity**) is present (see Fig. 49–2). This cavity is covered by a thin membrane called the **endosteum**. The central cavity is filled with fatty marrow. The endosteum contains osteoblasts[4] and osteoclasts,[5] which play a role in resorption of bone.

Growth and Ossification

Bones grow in length by a process involving endochondral ossification and grow in width by intramem-

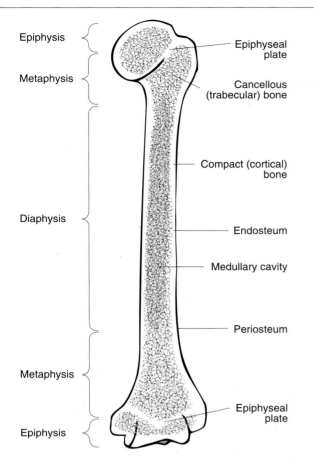

F I G U R E 49 – 2. Structure and composition of a typical long bone.

branous ossification. Interstitial growth is impossible in bone.[6] Bone can grow in length only by a process of growth within cartilage, followed by endochondral ossification. Two sites of cartilage growth are available in a long bone: articular cartilage and epiphyseal plate cartilage.[6] In the longer bone, the epiphysis provides the only growth plate for the entire bone.

Continuous Growth

The **epiphyseal plate** (see Fig. 49–2) allows for lengthening of the metaphysis and diaphysis of a long bone. The plate is the site of continuous growth. Growth and thickening of cartilage cells of the plate move the epiphysis away from the metaphysis. Calcification and replacement of cartilage occur on the metaphyseal surface (endochondral ossification).

The function of the epiphyseal plate in the growth process may be illustrated by examining the zones (Fig. 49–3) of the plate and their contribution to the growth process.[6] The **zone of resting cartilage** maintains adherence of the plate to the epiphysis. Immature chondrocytes and vessels penetrate the first zone from the epiphysis, providing nourishment to the plate. The **zone of young proliferating cartilage** is the section of the epiphyseal plate demonstrating the

most active cartilage cell growth. The **zone of maturing cartilage** contains the enlarged and mature cartilage cells as they migrate toward the metaphysis. The final zone of the epiphyseal plate, the **zone of calcifying cartilage,** is a very thin line of chondrocytes. The chondrocytes in this zone are no longer living, owing to calcification of the matrix. The zone of calcifying cartilage is the weakest segment of the epiphyseal plate.

Bone is also deposited quite actively on the metaphyseal side of the plate. With the addition of new bone, the metaphysis becomes longer.

Osteoblasts located in the inner layer of the periosteum are responsible for the growth in width of bones. This process is called **intermembranous ossification.** Resorption of bone, through a process of osteoclastic resorption, causes the medullary cavity to enlarge, thus causing additional widening of the bone.

Response to Injury, Stress, and Aging

The ability of bone to remodel after injury is important. Although remodeling of bone continues throughout life, death of the osteon or removal of calcium from bone requires that new bone be deposited to retain strength and function.

Physical stresses lead to realignment of bone trabecular systems and to the deposition of additional bone at the site of increased stress. The response of bone to stress is summarized in **Wolff's law,** which states that bone is laid down where it is needed and resorbed where it is not needed.[7] If bone is immobilized or not subjected to mechanical stresses, periosteal and subperiosteal bone is resorbed[8] and strength decreases.[9] This diminution in strength is an important clinical consideration because it means that recently immobilized patients have a lowered tolerance for mechanical stress.

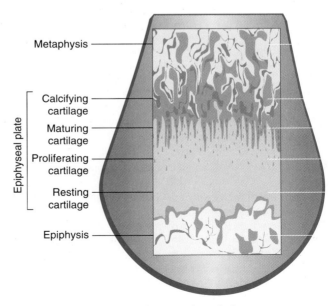

F I G U R E 49 – 3. Zones of the epiphyseal plate.

Internal fixations of a fracture may also cause decreased bone strength. With metal implants, mechanical stress is dispersed from the bone and carried by the implant. Bone resorption occurs under the plate, and "stress relief" osteoporosis may occur. Care must be taken once implants are removed and the bone must be protected until strength returns.

With aging, a progressive loss of bone density can be identified.[10] A decrease in the amount of cancellous bone and cortical bone has been noted. With age, bone deposition does not keep pace with resorption. As bone tissue decreases, a subsequent decrease in bone strength occurs.

KEY CONCEPTS

- Bone is a hard, metabolically active tissue that is capable of altering its shape and density in response to mechanical demands. The primary components of bone are calcium, phosphorus, collagen, and fluid.
- The osteon is the basic unit of bone. A central haversian canal contains blood vessels and nerve fibers. Concentric circles of mineralized matrix are formed by bone cells, or osteocytes, within the osteon.
- Bone tissue may be dense and compact (cortical) or more light and trabecular. Trabecular bone forms and remodels in response to mechanical stress. Highly vascularized periosteum covers the bones, and the center region of bone is filled with marrow.
- In long bones, the epiphyseal plate is the site of linear growth. This plate is characterized by zones, including (1) the zone of resting cartilage, (2) the zone of proliferating cartilage, (3) the zone of maturing cartilage, and (4) the zone of calcifying cartilage. The zone of calcifying cartilage is the weakest segment of the plate. Increases in bone width are mediated by osteocytes in the periosteum.
- Bone is a *dynamic tissue,* undergoing constant remodeling. Remodeling is the result of two simultaneous processes, bone deposition and bone resorption. Bone cells responsible for deposition are called osteoblasts; osteoclasts mediate bone resorption. In general, bone is deposited in areas of mechanical stress and resorbed from areas of disuse. Absence of bone stress due to immobility or altered weight-bearing leads to demineralization.

Structure and Function of Joints

Coordinated movement is only possible because of the way bones are connected to one another in joints and the way muscles are attached to those bones. The joints permit complex, highly coordinated, and purposeful movements. A **joint,** also called an **articulation,** is a point of contact between bones. Functional articulations between bones in the extremities such as the shoulder, elbow, hip, and knee contribute to controlled and graceful movement.

The type and configuration of a joint depend on the functional demands placed on that joint. As is the case with all aspects of the musculoskeletal system, structure determines function. When considering the human joint or articulation, it is also important to remember that once the articulation has developed, the configuration of the joint surface will determine the movement of the joint. Any aberrant joint movement has the potential to disrupt function and cause a breakdown in joint integrity.

Articulations can provide more than a single function, such as flexion and extension. Flexion, extension, adduction, abduction, and rotation may all be functional movements of a joint. The more complex the movement, the more complex is the joint structure.

Broadly speaking, the articulations or arthroses in the human body may be divided into two categories, based on the makeup of the joint and the method in which the joints unite the body components. The two categories are **synarthroses,** or fibrous and cartilaginous joints, and **diarthroses,** or synovial joints.

Synarthroses

Interosseous connective tissue connects the bony components in synarthrodial joints. The two types of synarthrodial joints are the fibrous and cartilaginous joints.

Fibrous Structure

In the fibrous joint, the bones are united by fibrous tissue. Three types of fibrous joints are found in the human body: suture joints, gomphosis joints, and syndesmosis joints. A *suture joint* unites the bones with a thin but dense layer of fibrous tissue. The interlocking bony ends overlap and increase stability. Suture joints are found only in the skull (Fig. 49–4).

The joint that is found between a tooth and the mandible or maxilla is the only *gomphosis joint* in the human body. The best description of a gomphosis joint is that of a peg implanted into a hole. Fibrous tissue stabilizes the two bony structures and permits little movement.

A *syndesmosis joint* is a joint in which the two bony components are joined by ligament or interosseous membrane. These joints normally allow slight movement and are quite functional in the kinematics of the joint. The interosseous membrane, joining the fibula and the tibia, is an example of a syndesmosis joint (Fig. 49–5).

Cartilaginous Structure

Bony segments connected by fibrocartilage or hyaline growth cartilage are classified as cartilaginous joints. Symphysis joints and synchondrosis joints are the two types of cartilaginous joints in the body.

A *symphysis joint* connects the bony segments by a fibrocartilaginous plate or disk. The symphysis pubis

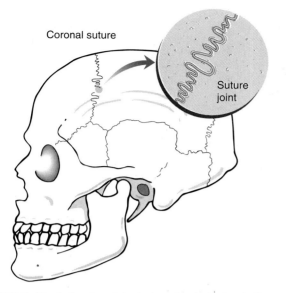

FIGURE 49–4. A suture joint is found only in the skull.

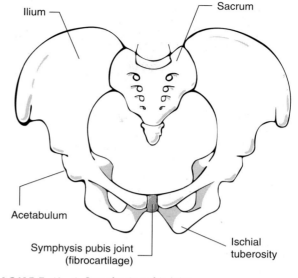

FIGURE 49–6. Symphysis pubis joint.

joint (Fig. 49–6) joins the two pubic bones of the pelvis. This joint is a weight-bearing structure and is important in the transmission of stress and providing stability.

In a synchondrosis joint, cartilage connects the bony components. This joint allows bone growth while providing stability. This type of joint can be found at growth sites of the body. The first sternocostal joint is an example of a synchrondrosis joint (Fig. 49–7).

Diarthroses

Joints designed to allow mobility are classified as **diarthroses,** or **synovial joints.** These joints are covered with a **joint capsule,** or synovial sheath. Movement in these joints is provided by the contraction of the muscle-tendon unit, and control is provided by the joint capsule and ligaments. The stability of the synovial joint is enhanced by additional soft tissue structures—the menisci, disks, and labra. Synovial fluid secreted into the mobile joints provides the lubrication necessary to reduce friction between the articulating surfaces. In the diarthrodial, or synovial, joint the bony ends are free to move because no cartilaginous tissue connects the adjacent bony surfaces. The synovial joint connects the adjacent bony surfaces through a joint capsule that surrounds the joint.

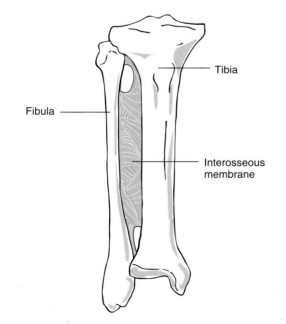

FIGURE 49–5. The interosseous membrane joining the fibula and the tibia is an example of a syndesmosis joint.

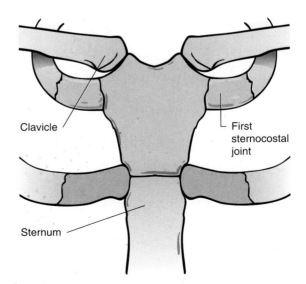

FIGURE 49–7. First sternocostal joint.

Synovial Structure

The consistent features of the synovial joint include (1) the fibrous joint capsule, (2) a joint cavity, (3) a synovial membrane that lines the inner surface of the capsule, (4) the lubricating synovial fluid, and (5) hyaline cartilage, which covers the joint surface (Fig. 49–8).

Many synovial joints also have accessory structures within the joint capsule. Menisci, disks, fat pads, and ligaments are a few of the structures situated in the capsule that are important to the proper function of the joint.

Joint Capsule. The **joint capsule** is composed of two layers of connective tissue. The outer layer or stratum fibrosum is quite dense and encapsulates the entire joint. This dense tissue is solidly attached to the periosteum of the adjacent bony components. Although the stratum fibrosum is poorly vascularized, it is innervated by joint receptors. The joint receptors are able to detect motion, compression, tension, vibration, and pain.[11]

The inner layer or stratum synovium is highly vascularized but is poorly innervated.[12] The stratum synovium is not pain sensitive. Specialized cells called synoviocytes synthesize the hyaluronic acid component of synovial fluid.[12] The inner layer of the joint capsule is the entry point for nutrients and the exit for waste material.

Synovial Fluid. **Synovial fluid** is similar to blood plasma but contains hyaluronic acid and a glycoprotein (lubricin).[13] The hyaluronic acid provides for viscosity and reduces the friction between the capsule and the joint surfaces. Lubricin provides for the lubrication between the surfaces of the cartilage. Synovial fluid resists shear loads,[12] keeps the surfaces lubricated to reduce friction, and provides nourishment for the cartilage.

Range of Movement

Synovial joints can be divided into three main categories according to the visible movement allowed at the joint: uniaxial, biaxial, and triaxial.

A *uniaxial joint* allows motion around a single axis of movement. Two types of uniaxial diarthrodial joint can be identified in the human body, hinge joints and pivot joints. A hinge joint permits flexion and extension; an example is the interphalangeal joint of the finger (Fig. 49–9A). A pivot or trochoid joint allows rotation as its single axis movement. The superior radioulnar joint of the elbow is an example of a pivot joint (Fig. 49–9B).

A *biaxial joint* has two axes of movement and permits movement in two planes. Two kinds of biaxial joint are found in the body, condyloid joints and saddle joints. The metacarpophalangeal joint of the hand is an example of a condyloid joint; it permits flexion and extension at one axis and adduction and abduction around another axis (Fig. 49–10A,B). A saddle joint is a joint in which the surfaces are convex in one plane and concave in the other. The surfaces of a saddle joint fit together as a saddle fits a horse. The carpometacarpal joint of the thumb is a saddle joint; it permits both flexion-extension and adduction-abduction movements (Fig. 49–10C).

Triaxial joints permit movement around three axes so that motion can occur in three planes. A plane joint permits gliding movement between two bones and is exemplified by the carpal joints of the hand. The carpal joints may glide or rotate relative to the adjacent surfaces. A ball-and-socket joint is formed by a ball-like surface fitting into a concave socket. Ball-and-socket joints permit flexion-extension, adductionabduction, and rotational movements. The hip joint is an example of a ball-and-socket joint (Fig. 49–11).

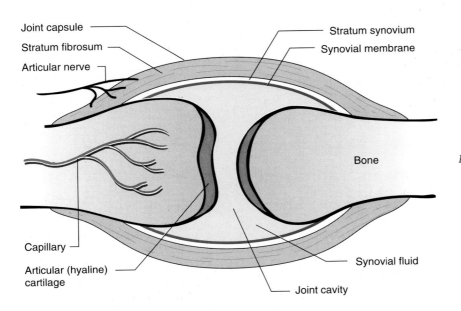

FIGURE 49–8. Typical synovial joint.

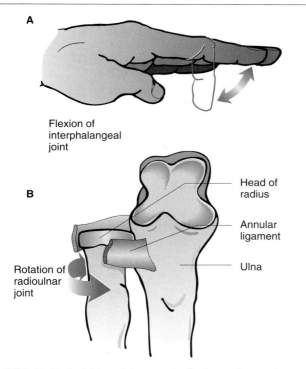

FIGURE 49 – 9. A hinge joint permits flexion and extension and is represented by the interphalangeal joint of the finger (**A**). A pivot joint allows rotation and is represented by the superior radioulnar joint of the elbow (**B**). Both the hinge joint and the pivot joint are considered uniaxial joints because they allow motion around a single axis.

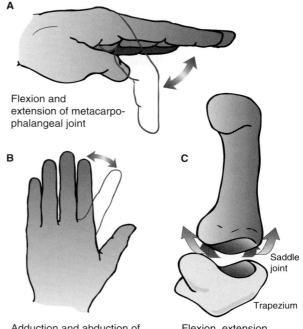

FIGURE 49 – 10. A condyloid joint permits flexion and extension at one axis and adduction and abduction around another axis; it is represented by the metacarpophalangeal joint of the hand (**A** and **B**). Because of its convex and concave surfaces, a saddle joint allows for flexion and extension and adduction and abduction; it is represented by the carpometacarpal joint of the thumb (**C**). Both the condyloid joint and the saddle joint are considered biaxial joints because they have two axes of movement and permit movement in two planes.

KEY CONCEPTS

- Joint configuration dictates the possible motions of a joint. The kinds of joint movement possible include flexion, extension, adduction, abduction, and rotation. Joints that allow these types of movements are called diarthroses (synovial joints). The ends of the bones in synovial joints are held together by a joint capsule composed of two layers of connective tissue. The capsule contains synovial fluid, which reduces friction and provides nutrients.

- Synovial joints are classified according to the visible movements they allow:

  Uniaxial: Movement in one plane only (e.g., distal hinge joints of fingers).

  Biaxial: Movement in two planes (e.g., thumb saddle joint).

  Triaxial: Movement in three planes (e.g., ball-and-socket hip joint).

- Some bones are held together by joints that allow little or no movement. These joints are called synarthroses (nonsynovial joints). Examples include sutures between the skull bones, tooth-jawbone joints, and the symphysis pubis joint.

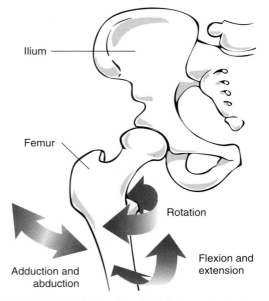

FIGURE 49 – 11. A ball-and-socket joint permits flexion and extension, adduction and abduction, and rotation; it is represented by the hip joint. A ball-and-socket joint is considered a triaxial joint because it permits movement around three axes; motion can occur in three planes.

Structure and Function of Articular Cartilage

Any discussion of the musculoskeletal system demands a description of articular cartilage. **Articular cartilage** is a specialized tissue designed to withstand the stress imposed by movement of the bony structures of the skeleton. Articular or hyaline cartilage covers the ends of each bone. It functions to distribute joint loads over a wide area to decrease the stress of prolonged compression due to contracting joint surfaces[14] and to allow movement of the joint surfaces with minimal friction and wear.[15] Articular cartilage is devoid of blood vessels, lymph channels, and nerves. If a mechanical defect is present, however, this avascular structure can cause major disruption of joint movement.

Composition

Chondrocytes or **cartilage cells** account for less than 10 percent of the tissue volume of articular cartilage.[16] Although sparsely distributed, chrondrocytes manufacture the organic component of the matrix. This organic matrix is composed of a network of collagen fibrils encased in a solution of PGs. The collagen content of cartilage tissues is between 10 and 30 percent, with the PG content composing between 3 to 10 percent.[17] The remaining 60 to 80 percent is composed of water, inorganic salts, and other proteins, glycoproteins, and lipids.[18]

Functional Properties

Collagen fibers in articular cartilage are highly structured to provide stability (Fig. 49–12). The most important mechanical properties of collagen fibers are strength and tensile stiffness. By themselves, collagen fibrils tolerate tension but not compression.

In order to increase tolerance to compression, cartilage PG associates with hyaluronate to form PG aggregates.[19] This PG aggregation promotes immobilization of the PGs within the collagen meshwork, adding structural rigidity and increased compression tolerance to the extracellular matrix.[16]

The importance of PGs and the interaction with collagen does not end with an increase in tolerance to compression. PGs have also been shown to be closely associated with collagen as a bonding agent to stabilize the cross-links between collagen fibers.[20] PGs are thought to maintain the ordered structure and mechanical properties of collagen fibers to assist in increasing strength.[20]

Articular cartilage also requires a sophisticated lubrication process to ensure a decrease in friction between joint surfaces. Without correct lubrication, the articular cartilage will begin to break down as a result of the mechanical action of the joint. The fluid component of articular cartilage is extremely important to articular cartilage. The joint fluid also assists in provid-

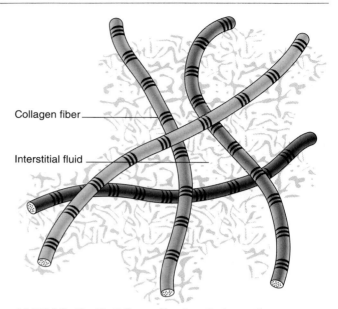

Collagen fiber

Interstitial fluid

F I G U R E 49 – 12. Collagen fiber in articular cartilage.

ing nutrition to the cartilage. Because this tissue is avascular, the fluid component of articular cartilage provides a mechanism for the influx of nutrients and the elimination of waste products.[21] Water, the most abundant component, contains mobile cations such as sodium and calcium, which are important in the mechanical behavior of cartilage. The majority of water in articular cartilage is found in the intermolecular space. Water is quite mobile and increases and decreases in response to pressure gradients. This movement of fluid supports the mechanical behavior of cartilage and provides joint lubrication.[22]

Response to Injury, Stress, and Aging

Articular cartilage may begin to wear through three primary mechanisms: interfacial wear due to the interaction of weight-bearing surfaces, fatigue wear due to deformation secondary to weight-bearing,[1] and intolerable stress on the joint matrix if loads are superimposed faster than internal fluid redistribution can occur.[23] Interfacial wear occurs when the joint surfaces come into direct contact as a result of the lack of lubricating film. The nonlubricated surfaces are quite abrasive to each other, and the joint surface may wear down. Fatigue wear occurs due to an accumulation of microscopic injuries from repeated stress. The third type of wear to articular cartilage occurs if loads on the joint matrix become intolerable.

Unlike bone, articular cartilage has a limited capacity for repair and regeneration. With trauma to the cartilage, a loosening of the collagen network allows for tissue swelling,[24] a decrease in cartilage strength, and an increase in permeability.[18] With abnormal joint function, stress to the joint surface increases, predisposing the cartilage to failure and the development of osteoarthritis.

THE AGING PROCESS: CHANGES IN THE SKELETAL SYSTEM

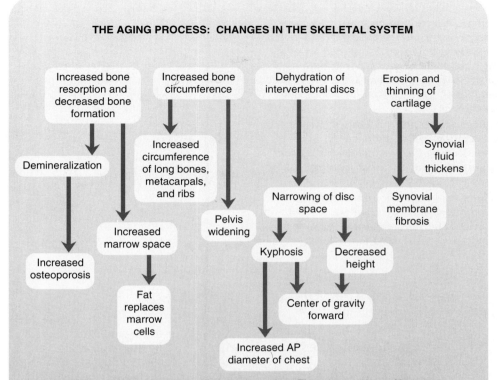

With aging, bone absorption exceeds bone formation. There is a net loss of bone mass and bone protein matrix. The interior of the long and the flat bones is absorbed faster than that of other bones. Trabecular bone destruction is greater than cortical bone loss. Aging females have a greater amount of bone loss than aging males. The bone marrow space is decreased, with fat replacing marrow cells.

While interior bone is lost, the circumference of the bones increases. This occurs because osteoblasts on the exterior bone beneath the periosteum continue bone formation. The long bones, metacarpals, and ribs become bigger around while the pelvis becomes wider and the skull thicker.

There is dehydration of the intervertebral discs with narrowing of the disc space, leading to a decrease in height of between 3 cm and 5 cm. There is an increase in the thoracic curve, resulting in kyphosis and anterior scapular displacement. This leads to an increase in the anteroposterior diameter of the chest. A decrease in the lordotic curve results in lumbar flattening and a decrease in lumbar flexibility. There is greater flexion of the knees and hips. There is also a change in the relationship between the pelvis and the femoral head and neck.

Fissuring, erosion, and thinning of cartilage occur. With the loss of cartilage, the subchondral bone must withstand greater pressures, resulting in increased density and the formation of joint margin osteophytes. The synovial membrane undergoes fibrosis and the synovial fluid thickens.

Faith Young Peterson

KEY CONCEPTS

- The ends of bones are covered with articular cartilage, which helps distribute mechanical loads placed on the joint and minimize friction and wear. An important component of articular cartilage is collagen, which provides strength and tensile stiffness. A second component, proteoglycan, increases compression tolerance.
- Articular cartilage is avascular and relies on synovial fluid for nutrition and waste removal. Synovial fluid lubricates the articular surfaces, reducing friction and minimizing wear. Articular cartilage has limited capacity for repair and regeneration.
- Interfacial joint wear occurs because of insufficient lubrication. Fatigue wear occurs because of repetitive stress injuries. The sudden imposition of excessive stress may also cause trauma to the joint matrix.

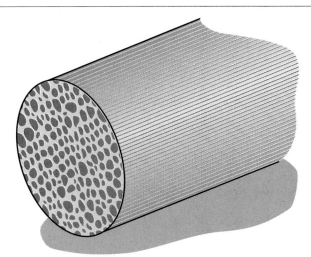

FIGURE 49–13. Parallel bundles of collagen fiber in tendons.

Structure and Function of Tendons and Ligaments

Approximately 200 bones in the human skeleton are connected by joints. These joints must not only allow for movement but also for dynamic stability. Ligaments, tendons, and joint capsules provide essential stability. Tendons, ligaments, and joint capsules, although not contractile structures causing movement, are nevertheless very significant. Without joint stability, no movement of the limbs would be possible.

Ligaments and joint capsules connect bone to bone, provide mechanical stability to the joints, and guide joint motion. Tendons, through attachment to a contractile structure (muscle) and a rigid object (bone), assist in the generation of movement. Because injuries to ligaments and tendons are common, an understanding of their function and properties is especially important.

Composition

Tendons and ligaments are dense connective tissue in which the collagen fibers are positioned in parallel alignment (Fig. 49–13). Figure 49–14 shows a schematic representation of a tendon. Tendon and ligament tissue is composed of few cells (**fibroblasts**) and large amounts of extracellular matrix. Approximately 20 percent of the total tissue is fibroblastic and 80 percent of the structure consists of the extracellular matrix. Of the matrix, 70 percent is water and 30 percent is solid material. The solids consist of collagen (75 percent), ground substance, and small amounts of elastin. Collagen content is greater in tendons than ligaments.[25]

Collagen molecules are formed into a triple-helix formation (Fig. 49–15), with hydrogen-bonded water bridges or cross-links providing stability of the molecule. The cross-links give strength to the tissue and increase tolerance for mechanical stress.

Another substance found in tendons and ligaments is the protein **elastin.** This protein provides for some elasticity or extensibility in function. With the exception of the ligamentum flavum, the majority of tendons and ligaments contain very little elastin, and minimal stretch is allowed. Unlike these stiffer tendons and ligaments, the ligamentum flavum connects the laminae of adjacent vertebrae and provides stretch and stability to the spine. The ligamentum flavum has a 2:1 ratio of elastin to collagen fibers.[26]

The ground substance in ligaments and tendons consists of a large amount of PGs along with glycoproteins and plasma proteins. The PG aggregate binds the extracellular water in the matrix and acts as a glue to stabilize the collagen fibers and enhance the strength of the ligaments and tendons.[1]

Functional Properties

Tendons and ligaments are quite interesting relative to function. Tendons are extremely strong but are able to angulate around bony prominences. This ability enables the pull of the muscle to change direction and, thus, improve mechanical leverage. Ligaments

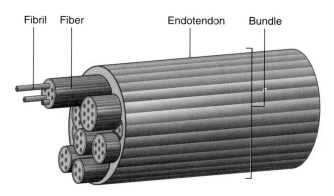

FIGURE 49–14. Schematic representation of a tendon.

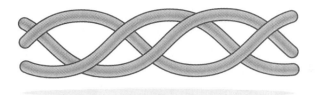

FIGURE 49–15. Triple helix formation of collagen molecules.

are supple and flexible but at the same time rigid. Ligaments stabilize the joint through their inextensibility but allow mechanically correct movement of the joint due to their suppleness.

The strength of tendons and ligament is determined by the number and quality of the cross-links within the collagen molecules. As a child matures into a young adult, the number and quality of cross-links increase, causing a subsequent increase in the strength of the tendon and ligament.[27]

Response to Injury, Stress, and Aging

As aging progresses, the collagen plateaus and then begins to diminish. With the aging process, the tensile strength and stiffness of ligaments and tendons decreases.[27] Tolerance to stress is also compromised during pregnancy and the postpartum period. During pregnancy, a laxity of the tendons and ligaments is noted[28] with a subsequent increased potential for injury.

Similar to bone, ligaments and tendons respond to mechanical demands placed on them. Increased stress causes these structures to become stronger and tolerate higher mechanical loads. With a decrease in stress, ligaments and tendons become weaker and less stiff.[29] Immobilization has also been demonstrated to decrease the tensile strength of ligaments.[30]

KEY CONCEPTS

- **Ligaments and joint capsules connect bones to bones and provide stability to joints. Tendons attach bones to muscles to allow movement. Tendons and ligaments are composed of dense connective tissue formed by fibroblasts. Collagen and elastin are the primary protein components. Most tendons and ligaments have little elastin, making them strong but not very compliant. An exception is the ligaments that connect adjacent vertebrae, which have more elastin than collagen.**

- **Ligament and tendon strength is determined by the quantity and quality of collagen cross-links. Maximal strength is achieved in young adulthood; pregnancy and aging reduce collagen strength. Ligaments and tendons respond to increased functional demand by increasing strength. Disuse results in weakened structures.**

Structure and Function of Skeletal Muscle

Approximately 40 percent of the total body weight is composed of skeletal muscle.[11] Muscle not only enables the bones to move at the joint but also provides strength and protection to the skeleton by distributing loads and absorbing shock.

Composition

The structural unit of skeletal muscle is the muscle fiber (Fig. 49–16). A skeletal muscle is composed of thousands of muscle fibers. Each fiber is a single muscle cell enclosed in a membrane called the sarcolemma. Muscle fibers are grouped together in bundles called fasciculi. Individual muscles are composed of many fasciculi. The sarcolemma of the individual muscle fiber is surrounded by connective tissue called the endomysium. Connective tissue surrounding the fasciculi is called the perimysium. The connective tissue surrounding the entire muscle is called the epimysium. The epimysium runs continuously with the endomysium and the perimysium (Fig. 49–17A). Tendons are attached to bones by Sharpey's fibers, which are continuous with the perimysium.

The arrangement of fasciculi varies among muscles and can present a specific visual effect of the muscle (Fig. 49–17B). Fasciculi, which lie parallel to each other, are often found in muscles that function to generate larger range of motion of joints. Muscles designated as strap or spiral have fibers situated in parallel arrangements. Fibers situated in an oblique pattern relative to the long axis of the muscle are called unipennate, bipennate, or multipennate muscles. Pennate (Latin for feather) muscles usually contain a large number of muscle fibers and are able to transmit a large amount of force to the muscle tendon. Examples of pennate muscles include the gastrocnemius muscle (a bipennate muscle), the deltoid (a multipennate muscle), and the flexor pollicis longus (a unipennate muscle).

The cytoplasm of the muscle fiber is called the

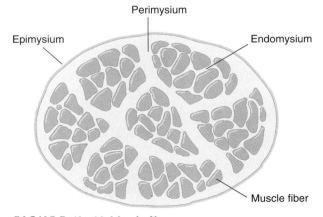
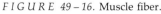

FIGURE 49–16. Muscle fiber.

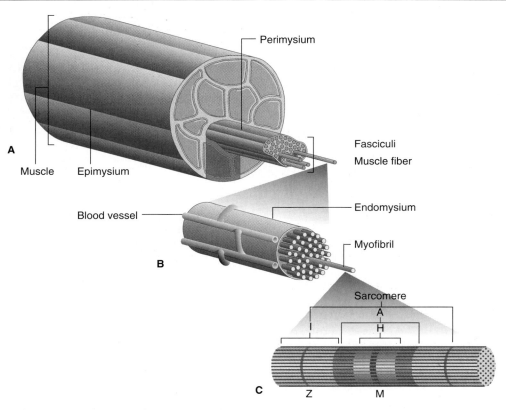

FIGURE 49–17. Muscle fiber. **A,** The epimysium runs continuously with the endomysium and the perimysium. **B,** The arrangement of fasciculi varies among muscles. **C,** The banding pattern apparent on microscopic inspection of a muscle cell results from the organized structure of the proteins (myofibrils) of the contractile apparatus.

sarcoplasm. Structures composing the sarcoplasm include ribosomes, glycogen, and the mitochondria, which are required for cell metabolism. Muscle contraction is accomplished by protein filaments of the contractile apparatus.

Contractile Apparatus

Microscopic inspection of a skeletal muscle cell reveals a typical pattern of banding called striation. This striated appearance is due to an organized structure of the proteins (myofibrils) of the contractile apparatus (Fig. 49–17C). The contractile proteins actin and myosin are called filaments because they are long and narrow. Myosin filaments are larger and are referred to as thick filaments. Thin filaments are actually composed of three different types of proteins bundled together. **Actin** is the primary constituent of thin filament, with smaller amounts of the proteins tropomyosin and troponin bound to it.

The thick and thin filaments are specifically arranged in contractile units called sarcomeres (Fig. 49–18). Sarcomeres are defined by dark bands called Z lines that lie perpendicular to actin and myosin filaments. A sarcomere extends from one Z line to the next. Thin actin filaments are attached to Z lines and extend from them. The I bands (isotropic) are light in color and correspond to the position of thin actin

filaments extending in both directions from the Z line. Thick myosin filaments lie parallel to and in between the thin filaments. Each myosin filament is actually surrounded by six thin filaments. The dark A band corresponds to an area where the actin and myosin filaments overlap. An M line marks the center of the

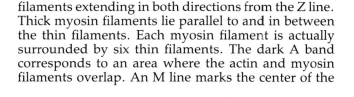

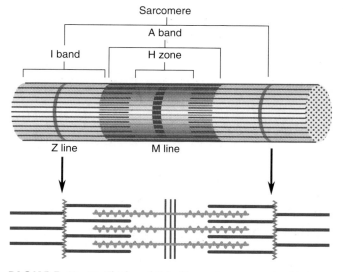

FIGURE 49–18. Thick and thin filaments are organized into contractile units called sarcomeres.

A band and the midpoint of the myosin filaments. One other zone, the H zone, corresponds to a region occupied solely by myosin filaments with no actin filament overlap. An efficient, synchronized contraction is enhanced by this precise arrangement of contractile elements. (See Chapter 16 for a detailed description of contractile filament structure.)

KEY CONCEPTS

- Muscles are composed of bundles of muscle fibers called fasciculi. A single muscle fiber is one elongated muscle cell, packed with contractile proteins and cytoplasmic organelles. Connective tissue encases each fasciculus (endomysium) and the muscle as a whole (perimysium). Tendons that attach muscle to bone are continuous with the perimysium.

- The arrangement of fibers within a muscle may be parallel or oblique. A parallel arrangement occurs in muscles having greater range of motion. Oblique patterns occur in muscles with large force potential.

- Skeletal muscle is striated because of an orderly arrangement of contractile proteins within muscle cells. Myosin is the primary component of the thick filament. Thin filaments are composed mainly of actin, with smaller amounts of the regulatory proteins troponin and tropomyosin.

Mechanics of Muscle Contraction

To accomplish the powerful shortening, or contraction, of a muscle fiber, several processes are necessary. Contraction allows muscle tissue to pull on bones and thus body movement is possible. The molecular basis of muscle contraction is described by the sliding filament or crossbridge theory.

Sliding Filament Theory

The **sliding filament** or **crossbridge theory** of muscle contraction is suggested by the anatomic configuration of the sarcomere. Muscle shortening is accomplished by increasing the amount of overlap of actin and myosin filaments. The Z lines at the ends of the sarcomere move closer together as interdigitating actin and myosin filaments slide past one another. Myosin head groups grip binding sites on the actin filaments and pull the thin filaments toward the sarcomere's center. Each time a myosin head binds an actin bead, it forms a so-called **crossbridge.**[31] Flexible myosin heads move in a ratchet-like manner to tug on the actin filaments. Myosin heads bend back and forth, binding and pulling on the actin filaments in steplike fashion. Actin filaments are prevented from slipping back to their original position because some myosin-actin bonds are forming while others are releasing. The making and subsequent breaking of each actin-myosin crossbridge requires one molecule of ATP. Consequently, tremendous quantities of ATP are hydrolyzed with each muscle contraction.

Role of Calcium

Muscle contraction depends on an adequate amount of calcium ion in the cytoplasm. In the absence of free intracellular calcium, no muscle contraction will take place even though myosin head groups have high affinity for actin-binding sites. This phenomenon can be explained in the following way. Myosin heads are prevented from binding to actin by tropomyosin proteins, which lie on top of actin-binding sites. The position of tropomyosin protein is controlled by troponin. When calcium is absent, troponin induces tropomyosin to cover the actin-binding sites. When calcium is present, troponin allows tropomyosin to move over and uncover the binding sites (Fig. 49–19). Crossbridge formation immediately ensues because myosin heads have a high affinity for these sites in the relaxed state.

Electromechanical Coupling

The nerve impulse that a muscle fiber receives to begin contraction is transmitted through the alpha motor neuron (Fig. 49–20). The cell body of the neuron is located in the anterior horn of the spinal cord. The axon extends from the cell body to the muscle and divides into many small branches. Each branch ends in a structure called a *motor end-plate.* The end-plate is positioned near the sarcolemma of a single muscle fiber. All muscle fibers innervated by a single motor neuron are part of one motor unit (see Fig. 49–20).

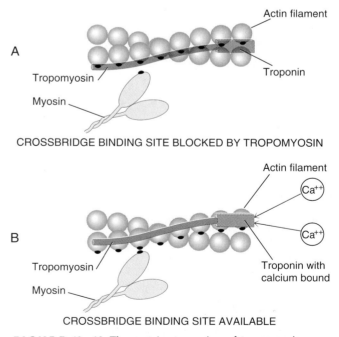

FIGURE 49–19. The proteins troponin and tropomyosin regulate the ability of actin and myosin to form crossbridges. **A,** In the absence of calcium, tropomyosin covers the binding sites on actin and inhibits crossbridge formation. **B,** In the presence of calcium, troponin induces the tropomyosin to "uncover" the actin-binding sites and allows crossbridge formation.

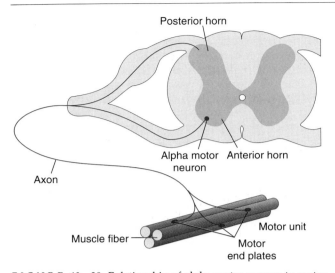

F I G U R E 49 – 20. Relationship of alpha motor neuron to motor unit of muscle. The nerve impulse that a muscle fiber receives to begin contraction is transmitted through the alpha motor neuron. All muscle fibers innervated by a single motor neuron are part of one motor unit.

After the nerve impulse is transmitted from the cell body, it passes along the axon to the motor endplate. Acetylcholine is released into the neuromuscular synapse and diffuses across to bind with receptors on the skeletal muscle cell. More than enough acetylcholine is released with a single action potential to ensure depolarization of the muscle cell. Acetylcholine binding opens channels in the membrane that allow Na^+ to flow into the cell. Depolarization of the motor endplate area to threshold then opens voltage-gated channels, leading to an action potential. Enzymes (acetylcholinesterase) located within the synapse quickly degrade acetylcholine to stop receptor activation. The sarcolemma is depolarized and an action potential spreads along the surface of the sarcolemma and into the interior of the fiber through the transverse tubules (T tubules). The sarcoplasmic reticulum, a calcium-storing structure, fills the space between myofibrils and forms sacs. The sacs, the terminal cisternae, are positioned closely with the T tubules. When the action potential passes down the T tubules, free calcium from the terminal cisternae is released into the myofibrils. The release of the calcium ions stimulates the actin-myosin crossbridge, causing muscle tension. After depolarization, or when the sarcolemma becomes electrically stable, calcium ions rebind in the sarcoplasmic reticulum and the muscle fiber relaxes.[1]

The motor unit is the functional unit of skeletal muscle and consists of the alpha motor neuron and all of the muscle fibers it innervates. When stimulated, all of the muscle fibers innervated by a motor unit will respond as one. This response is called the all-or-none response, meaning that the motor unit will contract to its maximum or it will not contract. The size of the contraction of the muscle depends on the number of motor units recruited. The greater the demand placed on the muscle or the more stimulus provided, the greater the number of motor units firing. The fibers of each motor unit are not in contact with each other but are dispersed throughout the muscle and intermixed with other fibers. If a single motor unit is stimulated, a large section of the muscle visibly contracts. If additional motor units of the nerve are stimulated, the muscle is able to contract with greater force. *Recruitment* is the term used for calling in more motor units in response to an increase in stimulation of the motor nerves.

Types of Muscle Contraction

Electromyography (EMG) is used to evaluate muscle contraction. With EMG, aspects of the contractile process, such as time relationships between the beginning of electrical activity and the actual contraction of the muscle, may be studied. The mechanical response of a muscle to electrical stimulation causes movement in the joint, control of joint motion, or joint stabilization.

Twitch Contraction

The fundamental unit of recordable muscle activity on the electromyography is the muscle twitch. A **twitch** is the mechanical response to a single stimulus of a motor unit. Following stimulation, there is a latency period before tension in the muscle fibers begins to increase. This latency period represents the time required for elastic structures to tighten to prepare for the development of tension. The time from initial tension development to peak tension is called the *contraction time*. The *relaxation time* is the period between peak tension and zero tension.

An action potential in a muscle lasts only a fraction of a second. It is possible for a series of action potentials to be initiated prior to the completion of the first twitch. The mechanical response to repetitive stimuli is known as *summation*. The term *refractory* refers to the period in which a second stimulus occurs during the latency period of the first muscle twitch, and no additional response of the muscle occurs.

The frequency of motor unit stimulation is quite variable. The greater the frequency of stimulation, the greater is the tension produced in the muscle. A muscle is able to achieve higher levels of work when it shortens immediately after being stretched.[32] The elastic components of the muscle do not account entirely for this phenomenon. Some energy must be stored in the contractile component of the muscle. If the stimulus is so great as to exceed the ability of the muscle to increase tension, the muscle is said to be in tetanus. In this situation, the speed of stimulation is faster than the contraction-relaxation time of the muscle. Little relaxation occurs prior to the next contraction.

The variable grade of contraction demonstrated by muscles is quite important. The repetitive twitching of all recruited motor units develops a summation of contractions of the muscle, which is responsible for the smooth movements of the skeletal muscle.

Concentric, Eccentric, and Isometric Contractions

Contraction of a muscle exerts a force that causes a torque or turning effect on the joint involved. When the muscle force generates sufficient tension to overcome the resistance of the limb of the body segment, the muscle will shorten, and joint movement occurs. This shortening contraction is called a **concentric contraction.** Lifting a cup of water to one's mouth is an example of a concentric contraction. If the load is greater than the amount of tension the muscle is able to generate, the muscle will lengthen even though the muscle is contracting. A lengthening contraction is termed an **eccentric contraction.** Walking down stairs is an example of an eccentric contraction of the quadriceps muscle. A third type of contraction is an **isometric contraction.** No movement occurs, and the muscle maintains its specific length. Holding a weight in the hand with the elbow flexed is an example of an isometric contraction.

The combined actions of concentric, eccentric, and isometric contractions provide the body the ability to control movement and function in the environment. Activities such as walking, eating, or lifting all require the interaction of various types of contractions to provide for smooth and coordinated activity. In a rehabilitative situation, it is interesting to note that isometric contractions generate greater tension than concentric contractions. Eccentric contraction may generate higher levels of tension than isometric contractions.[33] When using strengthening programs in rehabilitation settings, a working knowledge of the requirements of strengthening and the tolerance of the traumatized tissue is imperative to ensure safe reconditioning.

Mechanical Principles

The amount of tension that a muscle is able to generate is dictated by a number of mechanical concepts or principles of relationship. These principles include the length-tension relationship, load-velocity relationship, force-time relationship, and the effects of muscle temperature and muscle fatigue. A brief review follows.

Length-Tension Relationship

Maximum tension is produced when the muscle is at its usual resting length since this position allows the actin and myosin filaments to overlap and provide the maximum number of crossbridges between the filaments.[34] At a short resting length, little tension or muscle shortening is possible.

Load-Velocity Relationship

The velocity of shortening of a muscle is inversely related to the load applied.[35] The lower the weight, the higher is the velocity. The greater the weight, the slower is the contraction of the muscle. An isometric contraction occurs when the load equals the amount of force that the muscle exerts. If the load exceeds the force generated by the muscle, an eccentric contraction occurs. The greater the load, the faster the eccentric lengthening occurs.

Force-Time Relationship

The longer the time of contraction, the greater is the force the muscle is able to generate, until the muscle reaches its point of maximum tension. An increase in duration of force allows higher levels of tension to be produced by the contractile structures.

Effects of Temperature Change

Conduction velocity across the sarcolemma increases with a rise in muscle temperature.[36] Temperature elevation increases the enzymatic activity of muscle metabolism and the elasticity of collagen in elastic components. Both of these changes increase the amount of force that a muscle is able to produce.

Effects of Fatigue

Muscle is able to contract and relax only when adenosine triphosphate (ATP) is available. Prolonged activity of muscles can be sustained only when the muscle has an adequate supply of nutrients and oxygen to synthesize ATP. If activity is of high enough intensity to deplete ATP faster than it can be replaced, muscle tension will gradually weaken and, at some point, drop to zero. When muscle returns to its original state, creatine phosphate, a major storage form of energy in muscle, must be resynthesized and glycogen stores replaced. This revitalization process requires energy, so the muscle will continue to consume oxygen at high rates even after termination of activity. Heavy, rapid breathing continues after a period of strenuous exercise to provide adequate oxygen for ATP synthesis.

Response to Movement and Exercise

Immediate or early motion may prevent muscle atrophy after surgery or injury. With early motion, muscle fibers position themselves in a more parallel alignment as opposed to fibers in the immobilized individual. With movement, capillarization occurs more rapidly and tensile strength improves more quickly.[37] With immobilization, the cross-sectional area of muscles decreases and the oxidative enzyme activity is reduced.[38] Early motion prevents atrophy, and the afferent impulses from the muscle spindles increase, improving the stimulation of certain muscle fibers.[39]

Physical training and conditioning increase the cross-sectional area of muscle fibers. With the increase in area comes a concomitant increase in muscle bulk and strength.[38] Stretching programs provide other benefits. Stretching not only is effective in preventing injury and improving performance,[40] it also increases muscle flexibility, maintains and improves joint motion, and enhances the elasticity and length of the musculoskeletal unit.[41]

KEY CONCEPTS

- The fundamental unit of muscle contraction is the sarcomere. A sarcomere extends from one Z line to the next and consists of interdigitating thick and thin filaments. Muscle contraction occurs when myosin head regions bind to sites on the actin filament, forming crossbridges. After binding, myosin tugs on the actin filament, causing thick and thin filaments to overlap more. Myosin then releases and proceeds to bind at another point farther along the actin filament. Each crossbridge cycle requires one molecule of ATP.

- For contraction to occur, there must be sufficient calcium ions in the cytoplasm. In the absence of calcium, tropomyosin covers binding sites on the actin filament and prevents crossbridge formation. Another regulatory protein, troponin, controls the position of tropomyosin. When calcium is bound to troponin, tropomyosin is moved to expose binding sites on actin, and crossbridge formation ensues. Calcium ions are stored in the sarcoplasmic reticulum and released into the cytoplasm when the muscle cell depolarizes during an action potential.

- A group of skeletal muscle cells innervated by a single motor neuron is called a motor unit. All the cells in the unit contract together when the motor neuron depolarizes. An action potential in the alpha motor neuron releases acetylcholine at the motor end-plate. Acetylcholine binds to receptors on the muscle cell membrane and triggers an action potential in the cell. To generate more force in the muscle, a greater number of motor units can be activated, a process termed *recruitment*.

- Activation of a motor unit by a single action potential results in a brief twitch contraction. A train of action potentials in the motor neuron results in a sustained contraction. This occurs because calcium is released into the cytoplasm faster than it is being removed. Sustained contraction in response to repetitive stimulation is termed *summation*.

- Muscle contraction does not always result in muscle shortening. Isometric contraction refers to contraction with no change in muscle length. Eccentric contraction occurs when the muscle lengthens while contracting (due to high load). Muscle shortening with contraction is termed concentric. Isometric contraction generates greater tension than concentric; eccentric contraction may generate the highest tension.

- The behavior of contracting muscle is described by several physiologic relationships:

  Length-Tension Relationship: Up to a point, a greater resting length of the muscle generates a greater force of contraction. Optimal actin-myosin overlap occurs at about the usual resting muscle length.

  Load-Velocity Relationship: The velocity of muscle shortening is inversely related to the applied load.

  Force-Time Relationship: A longer contraction is associated with a greater force of contraction.

- Creatine phosphate is a storage form of energy that is quickly converted to ATP when cellular ATP levels fall. Fatigue results when energy and nutrient supply are insufficient. A higher rate of muscle oxygen consumption occurs during and for a period of time after muscle activity.

- Lack of muscle use (disuse) leads to a reduction in muscle mass and a slowing of oxidative enzyme activity. Early activity after injury is associated with quicker recovery of tensile strength, less atrophy, and better circulation.

Summary

The musculoskeletal system provides humans the ability to function within a gravity restricted environment. The flexibility to place body and limbs in desired positions in space ensures daily survival: the ability to eat, work, exercise, and play. Alterations in the function of the musculoskeletal system that decrease the efficiency of movement often magnify the stress placed on noninvolved structures and increase the potential for degeneration, joint laxity, and pain.

Health care providers need a solid understanding of the anatomy, physiology, and biomechanics of movement. Such knowledge will make diagnosis of aberrant movement and function easier and will help in planning the necessary care for and education of patients. Too often, in attempts to provide relief for patients with musculoskeletal dysfunction, the tissue involved or the mechanism of activity causing the injury is not properly identified. Short-lived relief may be provided for the pain through the use of analgesics. Return to activity, however, exacerbates the pain and restriction of movement present prior to medical care.

Familiarity with the musculoskeletal system also allows health care providers to identify the basic tissues involved in the injury or disease. Such awareness empowers the clinician to provide relief of pain as well as address quality of life issues. Determination of the type of activity that creates the problem and identification of the segments of the musculoskeletal system affected provide the basis to achieve positive long-lasting improvement. Weakness, instabilities, or decreased motion of the structures involved in the

THE AGING PROCESS: CHANGES IN THE MUSCULAR SYSTEM

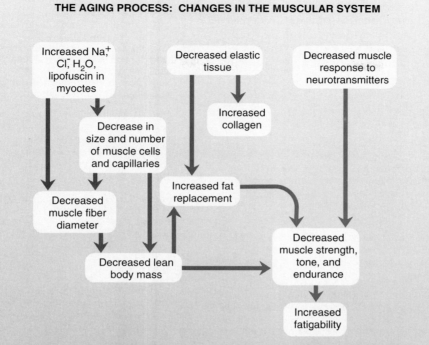

With aging, there is a decrease in the size and number of muscle cells. The remaining muscle cells experience atrophy, decreased muscle fiber diameter, and reduced elastic tissue. These changes result in reduced muscle mass. Within muscle cells, there is an increase in extracellular sodium, chloride, water, and lipofuscin pigment, with diminished intracellular potassium. The loss of muscle protein may not be obvious because of increased collagen and fat replacement.

Fewer capillaries are available to supply the muscles, causing decreased removal of metabolites. There is decreased hormonal stimulation of muscle by testosterone, somatotropin, and thyrotropin, as well as reduced muscle uptake of glucose during exercise.

Muscle response to nervous system stimulation is decreased with decreased muscle norepinephrine. There is also less responsiveness of the muscle to neurotransmitters including acetylcholine at the myoneural junction, as well as decreased cholinesterase activity.

The muscle, neural, and hormonal changes in aging that affect the muscular system lead to a functional decrease in muscle strength of between 30% to 50%, reduced muscle endurance, diminished muscle tone, and increased fatigability. Muscular decline rises with increasing age and usually occurs earlier in males; however, the extent of muscular system decline varies. An elderly individual with good nutritional balance and protein intake combined with adequate active exercise maintains muscle function and strength.

Faith Young Peterson

dysfunction must be identified. The analysis of physical limitations can lead to patient education and referral to sources able to reduce the impact of physical limitations. In addition, the use of tested exercise, modification of living and working environments, education of family members, and medical management will help the patient achieve optimal motor function and prevent reinjury.

REFERENCES

1. Nordin M, Frankel V: *Basic Biomechanics of the Musculoskeletal System,* 2nd ed. Philadelphia, Lea & Febiger, 1989.
2. Dempster WT, Coleman RF: Tensile strength of bone along and across the grain. *J Appl Physiol* 1961;16:355–360.
3. Carter DR, Orr TE, Fyhie DP: Relationship between loading history and femoral cancellous bone architecture. *J Biomech* 1989;22(3):231–244.
4. Vaughn J: *The Physiology of Bone,* 3rd ed. New York, Oxford University Press, 1981.
5. Hanaoka H: The origin of the osteoclast. *Clin Orthop* 1979;145:252–263.
6. Salter RB: *Textbook of Disorders and Injuries of the Musculoskeletal System,* 2nd ed. Baltimore, Williams & Wilkins, 1984.
7. Wolff J: *Des Gesetz der Transformation der Knochen.* Berlin, Hirschwold, 1892.
8. Jenkins DP, Cochran TH: Osteoporosis: The dramatic effect of disuse of an extremity. *Clin Ortho* 1969;64:128–134.
9. Kazarian LL, Von Gierke HE: Bone loss as a result of immobilization and chelation: Preliminary results in *Macaca mulatta. Clin Orthop* 1969;65:67.
10. Siffert RS, Levy RN: Trabecular patterns and the internal architecture of bone. *Mt Sinai J Med* 1981;48(3):221–229.
11. Guyton A: *Human Physiology and Mechanisms of Disease,* 5th ed. Philadelphia, WB Saunders, 1992.
12. Hettinga DL: Normal joint structures and their reaction to injury. *J Orthop Sports Phys Ther* 1979;1:1.
13. Simkin PA: Joints: Structure and function, in Schumacher HR Jr (ed): *Primer on the Rheumatic Diseases,* 9th ed. Atlanta, Arthritis Foundation, 1988, pp 18–23.
14. Askew MJ, Mow VC: The biomechanical function of collagen ultrastructure of articular cartilage. *J Biomech Eng* 1978;100:105. Editorial.
15. Armstrong CG, Mow VC: Friction, lubrication, and wear of synovial joints, in Owen R, Goodfellow J, Bullough P (eds): *Scientific Foundation of Orthopaedics and Traumatology.* London, William Heinemann, 1980, pp 223–232.
16. Muir H: Proteoglycans as organizers of the intercellular matrix. *Biochem Soc Trans* 1983;11(6):613–622.
17. Muir H: The chemistry of ground substance of joint cartilage, in Sokoloff L (ed): *Joints and Synovial Fluid.* New York, Academic Press, 1980, vol II, pp 27–94.
18. Armstrong CG, Mow VC: Variations in the intrinsic mechanical properties of human articular cartilage with age, degeneration, and water content. *J Bone Joint Surg [Am]* 1982;64A(1):88–94.
19. Rosenberg L, Hellmann W, Kleinschmidt AK: Electron microscopic studies of proteoglycan aggregates from bovine articular cartilage. *J Biol Chem* 1975;250(5):1877–1883.
20. Poole AR, Pidoux I, Reiner A, Rosenberg L: An immunoelectron microscope study of the organization of proteoglycan monomer, link protein, and collagen in the matrix of articular cartilage. *J Cell Biol* 1982;93(3):921–937.
21. Mankin HAJ, Thrasher AZ: Water content binding in normal and osteoarthritic human cartilage. *J Bone Joint Surg [Am]* 1975;57A(1):76–80.
22. Mow VC, Holmes MH, Lai WM: Fluid transport and mechanical properties of articular cartilage: A review. *J Biomech* 1984;17(5):377–394.
23. Mow VC, Kuei SC, Lai WM, Armstrong CG: Biphasic creep and stress relaxation of articular cartilage in compression: Theory and experiments. *J Biomech Eng* 1980;102(1):73–84.
24. McDevitt CA, Muir H: Biochemical changes in the cartilage of the knee in experimental and natural osteoarthritis in the dog. *J Bone Joint Surg [Br]* 1976;58B:94.
25. Amiel D, Frank C, Harwood F, Fronek J, Akeson W: Tendons and ligaments: A morphological and biochemical comparison. *J Orthop Res* 1984;1(3):257–265.
26. Nachemson AL, Evans JH: Some mechanical properties of the third human lumbar interlaminal ligament (ligamentum flavum). *J Biomech* 1968;1:211.
27. Vogel HG: Influences of maturation and age on mechanical and biochemical parameters of connective tissue of various organs in the rat. *Connect Tissue Res* 1978;6(3):161–166.
28. Rundgren A: Physical properties of connective tissue as influenced by single and repeated pregnancies in the rat. *Acta Physiol Scand* 1974;17(suppl 4):6–138.
29. Noyes FR: Functional properties of knee ligaments and alterations induced by immobilization. *Clin Orthop* 1977;123:210–243.
30. Amiel D, Woo SL, Harwood FL, Akeson WH: The effect of immobilization on collagen turnover in connective tissue: A biochemical-biomechanical correlation. *Acta Orthop Scand* 1982;53:325–332.
31. Huxley HE: The mechanics of muscle contraction. *Science* 1969(886):1358–1365.
32. Ciullo JV, Zarins B: Biomechanics of the musculotendinous unit: Relation to athletic performance and injury. *Clin Sports Med* 1983;2(1):71–86.
33. Norkin C, Levange P: *Joint Structure and Function: A Comprehensive Analysis.* Philadelphia, FA Davis, 1983.
34. Crawford GN, James NT: The design of muscles, in Owen R, Goodfellow J, Bullough P (eds): *Scientific Foundation of Orthopaedics and Traumatology.* London, William Heinemann, 1980, pp 67–74.
35. Brobeck JR: *Best and Taylor's Physiological Basis of Medical Practice,* 10th ed. Baltimore, Williams & Wilkins, 1979, pp 59–113.
36. Phillips CA, Petrofsky JS: *Mechanics of Skeletal and Cardiac Muscle.* Springfield, Ill, Charles C Thomas, 1983.
37. Jarvinen M: *Healing of a Crush Injury in a Rat Striated Muscle: With Special Reference to Treatment by Early Mobilization or Immobilization.* Thesis. Finland, University of Turku, 1976.
38. Haggmark T, Jansson E, Eriksson E: Fiber type area and metabolic potential of the thigh muscle in man after knee surgery and immobilization. *Int J Sports Med* 1981;2(1):12–17.
39. Haggmark T, Eriksson E: Cylinder or mobile cast brace after knee ligament surgery: A clinical analysis and morphologic and enzymatic study of changes in quadriceps muscle. *Am J Sports Med* 1979;7(1):48–56.
40. Jacobs M: Neurophysical implications of slow, active stretching. *Am Corr Ther J* 1976;30(5):151–156.
41. Huxley AF: Muscle contraction. *J Physiol* 1974;243(1):1–43.

BIBLIOGRAPHY

Armstrong CG, Mow VC: Friction, lubrication, and wear of synovial joints, in Owen R, Goodfellow J, Bullough P (eds): *Scientific Foundation of Orthopaedics and Traumatology.* London, William Heinemann, 1980, pp 223–232.

Armstrong CG, Mow VC: Variations in the intrinsic mechanical properties of human articular cartilage with age, degeneration, and water content. *J Bone Joint Surg [Am]* 1982;64A(1):88–94.

Crawford GN, James NT: The design of muscles, in Owen R, Goodfellow J, Bullough P (eds): *Scientific Foundation of Orthopaedics and Traumatology.* London, William Heinemann, 1980, pp 67–74.

Guyton A: *Human Physiology and Mechanisms of Disease,* 5th ed. Philadelphia, WB Saunders, 1992.

Hettinga DL: Normal joint structures and their reaction to injury. *J Orthop Sports Phys Ther* 1979;1:1.

Mow VC, Holmes MH, Lai WM: Fluid transport and mechanical properties of articular cartilage: A review. *J Biomech* 1984;17(5):377–394.

Muir H: The chemistry of ground substance of joint cartilage, in Sokoloff L (ed): *Joints and Synovial Fluid.* New York, Academic Press, 1980, vol II, 27–94.

Nordin M, Frankel V: *Basic Biomechanics of the Musculoskeletal System,* 2nd ed. Philadelphia, Lea & Febiger, 1989.

Norkin C, Levange P: *Joint Structure and Function: A Comprehensive Analysis.* Philadelphia, FA Davis, 1983.

Noyes FR: Functional properties of knee ligaments and alterations induced by immobilization. *Clin Orthop* 1977;123:210–243.

Salter RB: *Textbook of Disorders and Injuries of the Musculoskeletal System,* 2nd ed. Baltimore, Williams & Wilkins, 1984.

Schumacher HR: *Primer on the Rheumatic Diseases,* 9th ed. Atlanta, Arthritis Foundation, 1988.

Vaughn J: *The Physiology of Bone,* 3rd ed. New York, Oxford University Press, 1981.

CHAPTER 50
Alterations in Musculoskeletal Function: Trauma, Infection, and Disease

GARY SMITH

KEY TERMS

cancellous bone: Bone with a spongy or lattice-like appearance, found in the interior of bones. Cancellous bone does not tolerate compression stress.

contractile tissue: Tissues involved in the contraction of muscle, including not only the muscle belly but also the tendon and bony insertion.

cortical bone: The dense cortex or outer shell of the bone, designed to tolerate compression and shearing forces.

fibrositis-fibromyalgia syndrome: A syndrome of musculoskeletal pain within a broad spectrum of nonarticular rheumatism. Complaints of generalized pain, joint and muscle pain, swelling, weakness, stiffness, fatigability, and tender points are common but few or no objective findings are present.

fracture: A structural break in the continuity of a bone, an epiphyseal plate, or cartilage.

inert tissue: Soft tissue that possesses no ability to contract or relax, includes the joint capsule, ligament, bursa, fascia, dura mater, and nerve root.

muscular dystrophy: A group of genetically determined myopathies characterized by progressive degeneration of muscle fibers.

osteoporosis: A reduction in bone mass resulting from bone resorption proceeding at a rate faster than new bone formation.

scoliosis: A lateral deviation of the spine resulting in an S- or C-shaped spinal column. The disorder, most common in adolescent girls, can be a consequence of congenital, connective tissue, or neuromuscular disorders.

soft tissue injury: Any trauma to soft tissue with disruption of circulatory and lymphatic systems.

A smoothly functioning musculoskeletal system facilitates a complete range of human actions, including walking, talking, running, breathing, and the myriad physical activities that are under the willed control of the individual. Any abnormality in the musculoskeletal system decreases the efficiency of movement and increases mechanical stress. The ballistic requirements of many sports and occupations, such as skiing and driving an automobile, have increased the potential for trauma. Diseases also disrupt the integrity of the musculoskeletal system. Infectious processes, genetic abnormalities, and nutritional deficiencies may all affect movement.

Clinicians who work with patients experiencing dysfunctions of the musculoskeletal system must have a solid background in the evaluation and treatment of such disorders. Without this preparation, interventions will not be sufficient to promote maximum functional return. This chapter discusses lesions particular to the musculoskeletal system as they affect the skeletal frame, soft tissue, and muscles.

Bone Disorders

The skeletal system is subject to alterations in function due to mechanical stress and infection. The purpose of the skeletal system is to protect internal organs, provide rigid kinematic links and muscle attachment sites, and facilitate muscle action and body movement.[1] Bone, one of the body's hardest structures, is also one of the most dynamic and metabolically active tissues in the body. Bone, a highly vascular tissue with a capacity for repair, adapts to the mechanical demands placed on it and is able to alter its properties and configuration in response to those mechanical stresses.[1,2]

Fracture

A **fracture,** whether of a bone, an epiphyseal plate, or a cartilaginous joint surface, is simply a structural break in continuity.[2] Trauma generating enough energy to fracture a bone will also produce force sufficient to traumatize soft tissue. With that concept in mind, the remainder of this section will address the injury to the bony component of the musculoskeletal system.

Two types of bone are present in the human body: cortical bone and cancellous bone. **Cortical bone** forms the cortex or outer shell of the bone. Cortical bone is designed to tolerate compression and shearing forces. Tension forces may exceed the tolerance of the cortical bone. Salter states that the majority of fractures represent tension failures in which the bone is actually pulled apart.[2] With bending, twisting, or straight tension, the stress may exceed tolerance, and a fracture will occur on the convex side of the bend. **Cancellous bone** is bone with a spongy or latticelike appearance, found in the interior of bones. Unlike cortical bone, cancellous bone does not tolerate compression stress.

Types of Fracture

The type of fracture that occurs reflects the type of tension stress placed on the bone (Fig. 50–1). A **transverse fracture** occurs in a straight line perpendicular to the bone. **Spiral fractures** are the result of rotational forces and cause the bone to separate in the form of an S. **Longitudinal fractures** split the bone along its length. **Oblique fractures** result from a rotational force but, unlike the spiral fracture, the break is along an oblique course and does not rotate around the

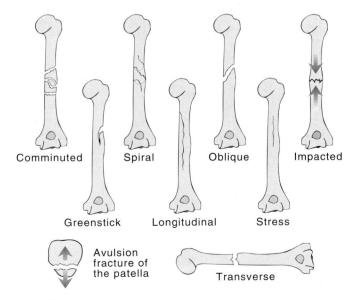

FIGURE 50–1. Types of fracture.

entire bone. **Comminuted fractures** consist of three or more fragments at the fracture site. Comminuted fractures often present considerable problems in care because of the large amount of associated soft tissue damage and the multiple fragments of bone. An **impacted fracture** is caused by excessive forces that compress or force the bony ends into one another. A **greenstick fracture** is an incomplete break in the bone. The cortex and a portion of the cancellous bone are traumatized, but the fracture does not extend completely across the shaft. The term *greenstick* refers to the appearance of a green branch of a tree when it is bent beyond tolerance, but not broken in two. A **stress fracture** is a failure of the cortex of the bone, often the result of repetitive activity. Without proper treatment, a stress fracture can expand to a complete fracture. An **avulsion fracture** is a separation of the bone fragments. This type of fracture may occur with a sudden contraction of a muscle that causes a portion of bone to separate or *avulse* from the main segment.[3]

Of special concern are fractures at or near a joint line in children. This location of a fracture may suggest an epiphyseal growth plate fracture (Fig. 50–2). With epiphyseal injuries, the potential for retardation of growth of the long bones is present. Cancellous bone does not tolerate compression stress, and therefore **crush** or **compression fractures** (Fig. 50–3) are consistent with cancellous bone trauma. In children, a compression injury of the cancellous bone of the metaphysis of the long bone is identified as a *buckle fracture*. In the adult, compression fractures are often found in a vertebral body of the spine.

Extent of Fracture

Fractures can be classified relative to the extent and depth of the fracture. A **complete fracture** is one in

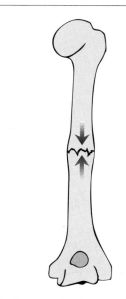

FIGURE 50–3. Compression fracture.

which the bone has broken completely across (Fig. 50–4). In an **incomplete fracture** a segment of the bone has fractured, but not the entire bone. Fractures can also be classified as **open** (compound) or **closed** (simple) (Fig. 50–5). An open fracture occurs when the sharp edges of the broken ends of the bone penetrate through the skin or a projectile penetrates the skin and fractures the bone. A closed fracture is a fracture in which the skin is not broken.[4]

Healing Process

Healing in a Cortical Bone. At the time of fracture in a cortical bone, the blood vessels in the haversian

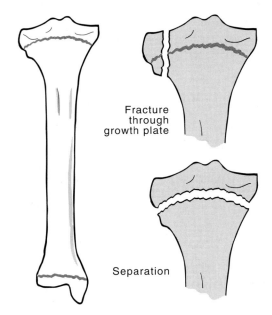

Fracture through growth plate

Separation

FIGURE 50–2. Epiphyseal injury.

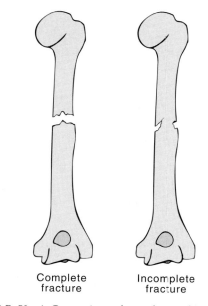

Complete fracture

Incomplete fracture

FIGURE 50–4. Comparison of complete and incomplete fractures.

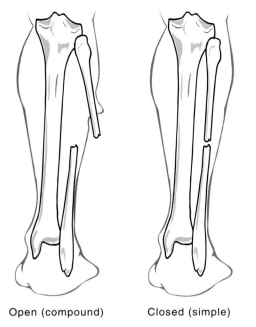

Open (compound)   Closed (simple)

FIGURE 50–5. Comparison of open and closed fractures.

systems are torn. After a period of bleeding, clotting will occur at the fracture site and for a short distance on either side of the fracture. Because of the lack of circulation, a small section of bone will die (Fig. 50–6). The avascular bone will eventually be replaced by living bone through resorption and bone deposition. The majority of bleeding occurs from the arteries in the periosteal sleeve.

The hematoma that forms becomes the medium for the early stages of healing. Osteogenic cells, which develop from the periosteum, form the external and internal callus. If the periosteal sleeve of the bone is severely torn, the healing cells must proliferate from the mesenchymal cells of the surrounding soft tissue. During the early stages of repair, the amount of osteogenic tissue is extensive. Within the first few weeks, the thick mass of osteogenic tissue has formed a fracture callus.

During the initial stages of **callus formation,** there are no bone cells within the matrix. The callus is quite soft but becomes progressively more firm. With the consolidation of the fracture callus, new bone formation begins. Initially the new bone forms at the edges of the periosteum, where the blood supply is more substantial. Where the blood supply is sufficient, the osteogenic cells differentiate into osteoblasts and primary woven bone. Near the fracture site, where the blood supply is less adequate, the osteogenic cells initially differentiate into chondroblasts (cartilage).

As the external and internal callus hardens from the cartilage stage through the process of ossification, the fracture site becomes firm and stable. No movement is detected by the medical evaluator or the client. At this point the fracture is said to be clinically united. Although stable, cartilage and primary woven bone may be found at the site of healing.

With time, the primary callus is replaced by mature bone, and any excess callus is reabsorbed. When all of the immature bone cells have been replaced by mature lamellar bone, the fracture is said to be consolidated (radiographic union).

Healing in a Cancellous Bone. Cancellous fracture healing occurs mainly through the development of an internal callus. The rich blood supply present in cancellous bone prevents necrosis of the bone at the fracture site. If the fracture is undisplaced, the healing process is much more rapid in comparison to healing of cortical bone. The osteogenic cells in the trabeculae form the primary woven bone in the internal fracture hematoma (Fig. 50–7). The internal callus fills the open space of the cancellous bone and crosses the fracture site. Woven bone develops and is eventually replaced by lamellar bone. As noted earlier, cancellous bone is susceptible to compression forces, and the majority of injuries incurred are compression-type fractures. With a compression fracture, the fragments of bone are impacted together, giving a more suitable environment for healing of the cancellous bone.

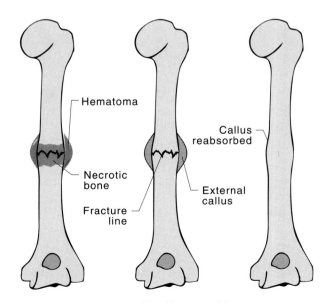

Hematoma

Callus reabsorbed

Necrotic bone

External callus

Fracture line

FIGURE 50–6. Stages of healing cortical bone.

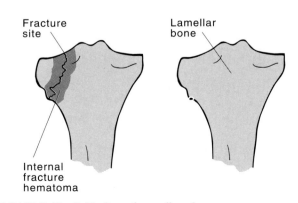

Fracture site

Lamellar bone

Internal fracture hematoma

FIGURE 50–7. Healing of cancellous bone.

The medical treatment of a fracture consists of stabilization of the fracture site until healing is sufficient to allow stress to be placed on the structure. Rehabilitation of a patient with a fracture really begins at the time of release from treatment of the fracture. Time is the treatment of a fracture, but the bone is not the only structure injured at the time of the initial trauma. Soft tissue is subjected to insult with stress of sufficient magnitude to cause a fracture. Soft tissue is also stressed with the immobilization requirements of a healing fracture. Rehabilitation of a fracture site is, in reality, the rehabilitation of the soft tissue surrounding the site.

Dislocations and Subluxations

Two additional mechanical alterations in the musculoskeletal system to be addressed are dislocations and subluxations. A **dislocation** is a complete separation or disunion of the joint articulating surfaces. A **subluxation** is a partial dislocation in which an incomplete separation between the articulating surfaces occurs. A dislocation or subluxation can occur when forces cause one aspect of the joint complex to move beyond its normal anatomic limit.[3] A considerable amount of tissue damage occurs in dislocation and subluxation. Treatment must include consideration of soft tissue trauma and healing. With any dislocation, especially the first-time dislocation, evaluation for a fracture is necessary. The highest incidence of dislocation involves the fingers, followed by the shoulder.

According to Arnheim,[3] signs and symptoms consistent with a dislocation are:

- Loss of limb function. The individual is unable to move the body part.
- Deformity is almost always present. In heavily muscled individuals, it may be necessary to palpate the joint to determine a difference in body contour relative to the opposite side.

- Swelling and point tenderness are immediately present.

Alterations in Bone Mass and Structure

Scoliosis

Scoliosis is a lateral deviation of the spine resulting in an S- or C-shaped spinal column. Scoliosis most commonly occurs in adolescent girls. Scoliosis can be a consequence of numerous congenital, connective tissue, and neuromuscular disorders. The majority of cases have no known cause and are classified as idiopathic.

Mild scoliosis is termed **postural scoliosis** and does not involve permanent structural changes of the vertebra. Conditioning exercises to strengthen muscles and correct posture are used to treat postural scoliosis. **Structural scoliosis** is more serious, involving deformity of the vertebrae and asymmetric changes in the hip, shoulder, and rib cage positions. Structural scoliosis generally requires intensive therapy or surgical intervention to halt progression and correct deformities.

Scoliosis is detected by typical asymmetric changes (Fig. 50–8), including (1) uneven shoulders or hips, (2) shoulder or scapular prominence, (3) rib or chest hump when bending over, and (4) C- or S-shaped spine. The diagnosis is confirmed by radiographic examination of the spine. The degree of curvature is determined from radiographs and is classified as right or left, depending on the direction of convexity. Definitive corrective therapy is indicated for curvatures of 40 degrees or greater. Less significant degrees of curvature may be treated conservatively with exercise and frequent reevaluation to assess progression to more significant deformity.

In addition to body image disturbances, scoliosis predisposes to a number of physiologic problems. Respiratory difficulties from restricted expansion of the

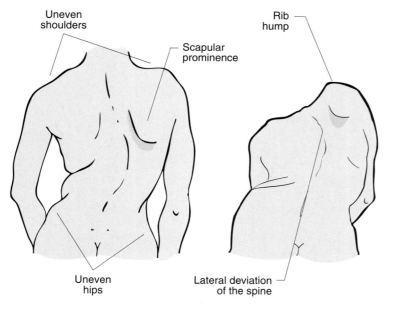

F I G U R E 50 – 8. Scoliosis.

lungs may occur. Severe forms may be associated with significant pain. Gastrointestinal dysfunction can result from compression of abdominal organs. If uncorrected, scoliosis may progressively worsen with age owing to increased upper body weight and gravitational forces that exacerbate vertebral deformity.

The treatment of structural scoliosis is aimed at correcting spinal malalignment. Nonsurgical measures include braces and neuromuscular stimulators. Bracing applies constant pressure to the spinal convexity, straightening out the curve. Braces must be worn for prolonged periods each day to be effective, and compliance is a major difficulty. Surgical intervention includes spinal realignment, fusion, and bracing with internal appliances. A number of different surgical bracing methods are in use, including Harrington rods, segmental bracing, and three-dimensional stabilization. Most surgical procedures require prolonged body immobilization postoperatively.

Osteoporosis

Osteoporosis is an extremely common disorder characterized by a reduction in the bone mass that may prejudice its structural integrity and predispose to fractures.[5] In osteoporosis the loss of bone results from an imbalance between bone resorption and bone formation. The cause of osteoporosis is unclear, but estrogen deficiency in women and androgen deficiency in men are immediately present as possible factors.

Clinically, the individual suffering from osteoporosis complains of bone pain, especially back pain. Fractures are common and include vertebral crush fractures, distal radius fractures, and femoral neck fractures. Prior to a fracture, however, radiologic evaluation and tests to determine the levels of serum calcium, phosphorus, and alkaline phosphatase assist in detecting the loss of bone. Attempts to decrease the loss of calcium and bone should be initiated promptly, before the disease progresses.

Disuse osteoporosis may occur with prolonged bed rest, which leads to an increase in osteoclastic activity and resorption of bone. Osteoporosis may also occur when collagen formation is impaired in such conditions as scurvy, protein deficiency, or Cushing's syndrome.

Rickets and Osteomalacia

Rickets and **osteomalacia** are characterized by deficits in the mineralization of newly formed bone matrix with resulting soft osteopenic bone. Vitamin D deficiency prevents the maintenance of normal levels of calcium and phosphorus. In rickets, the cartilage that occurs in the growing epiphyses fails to calcify. Cartilage is not replaced by bone and continues to enlarge. Bone is poorly calcified and quite weak. Kyphosis, genu valgus ("knock knee"), and bowing of the bones are common deformities.

Osteomalacia is the adult counterpart of rickets. With vitamin D deficiency, calcification fails to occur, and the bone consists mainly of osteoid, causing the bone to be soft. All bones are affected, but the weight-bearing structures may collapse and cause compression-type fractures.[5,6]

Infectious Processes

Paget's Disease

Paget's disease of bone (osteitis deformans) is characterized by a progressive enlargement and deformity of many bones. An unexplained deposition and resorption of bone is noted in this disease. The etiology is thought to be a slow virus, but precise information is not available. Paget's disease is more common in men over the age of 40 years.

In the initial stages of Paget's disease the bones soften and tend to bend. As the disease progresses, irregular subperiosteal bone formation occurs, causing the bone to become thick and hard. Thickening of the cranial bones may cause compression of the cranial nerves, resulting in blindness, deafness, headaches, and facial paralysis.[7] During the active stages of the disease, treatment focuses on preventing deformity, fracture, and managing pain.

Pyogenic Osteomyelitis

Pyogenic osteomyelitis is an infection of both bone marrow and the bone itself. The infectious agents may be introduced by blood from infection elsewhere in the body (*hematogenous osteomyelitis*) or by direct traumatic introduction, including surgically (*exogenous osteomyelitis*). *Staphylococcus aureus* is the most common organism isolated in cases of hematogenous osteomyelitis.

In children, acute hematogenous osteomyelitis manifests with a high fever and pain at the site of bone involvement. Muscle spasms, redness, and swelling are common, and the child may refuse to move the limb. In adults, hematogenous osteomyelitis is more difficult to detect. The symptoms are vague and may include fever, malaise, anorexia, and weight loss. Pain at rest is common. The diagnosis may be confirmed by radiographic signs of bone destruction.

The signs and symptoms of exogenous osteomyelitis involve the soft tissue, since entry was through the skin. Inflammation of soft tissue, abscesses, low-grade fever, local pain, swelling, and lymphadenopathy are present. Due to the infection, large areas of the periosteum may cause necrosis of fragments of the bone, known as *sequestrum*. If the infection becomes walled off, a localized abscess, called *Brodie's abscess*, may form. This abscess has the potential to develop a site of chronic infection.[2]

During the acute phase, prompt administration of antibiotics is essential. Analgesics for pain management is required. Splinting, bed rest, and traction may be used to protect the weakened bony structure. If an abscess develops, drainage may be necessary.

Tuberculosis

Tuberculosis of bone, although not a significant problem in the United States, is found in many developing countries. **Tuberculosis osteomyelitis** usually occurs by the hematogenous route. This type of infection tends to develop insidiously and extends into the joint space to cause widespread destruction. The long bones of the extremities and the spine (Pott's disease) are common sites of tuberculosis osteomyelitis.[5]

Tumors

The majority of tumors in the bone are metastatic but a number of primary tumors of bone can be identified.[2,8]

Osteochondroma

Osteochondroma or exostosis is a benign lesion and is considered to be a developmental aberration, as opposed to a neoplasm. The lesions develop from epiphyseal cartilage, are composed of orderly bone, and are capped by a layer of cartilage. Exostoses are usually asymptomatic and found by chance. Pressure on surrounding soft tissue may cause pain.

Chondroma

Chondroma or enchondroma is a benign neoplasm located within the interior of the bone. It is believed to arise from remnants of epiphyseal cartilage. Chondromas arise most often in the small bones of the hands and feet but can develop in other areas. The growth may erode the cortex of bone and expand the contour.

Osteoid Osteoma

Osteoid osteoma is a painful but benign neoplasm. This small lesion is often found within the cortex of the tibia and femur, but any bone may be involved. Radiographs show the lesion enclosed in a sclerotic shell. These lesions are normally cured by excision.

Giant Cell Tumor

The **giant cell tumor** is normally benign but has a tendency to recur after removal. In some cases, giant cell tumors undergo transformation to sarcomas. Giant cell tumors commonly occur between the ages of 20 and 40 years. There is no sex preponderance. The area of development includes the distal femur, proximal tibia, distal radius, and proximal humerus. Pain is the presenting complaint of the client.

Osteosarcoma

Osteosarcoma is an extremely malignant neoplasm that develops in the metaphyseal region of the long bones. The majority of victims are children, adolescents, and young adults. The most active epiphyseal growth areas—the distal femur, proximal tibia, fibula, and humerus—are the common sites of involvement.

The osteosarcoma grows rapidly and is quite destructive, destroying the cortex of the metaphyseal region and predisposing it to pathologic fracture. Metastasis to the lungs is noted early in the disease development. Pain is consistent and progressively more intense. Joint function may be compromised as a result of the proximity of the metaphysis. Amputation may be necessary, but conservative surgery, radiation therapy, and chemotherapy have provided positive results, with a 60 percent 5-year survival rate.

Chondrosarcoma

A **chondrosarcoma** is a malignant cartilaginous skeletal tumor that arises in adults over the age of 30. These tumors develop slowly, so that pain is not a prominent clinical symptom. Even with the slow rate of development, the tumor will eventually metastasize, typically to the lung. Chondrosarcomas tend to develop in the pelvic and shoulder girdles and the proximal long bones.

Ewing's Sarcoma

Ewing's sarcoma is a relatively uncommon but rapidly growing malignant neoplasm. This tumor most often develops in the long bones of children between the ages of 10 and 15 years. Ewing's tumor begins in the medullary cavity and soon perforates the cortex of the shaft, separating the periosteum from the shaft. This tumor metastasizes quite early in its development to the lungs and other bones. Because of the rapid rate of growth, pain is a dominant symptom that increases in severity. Tenderness and fever are also features of Ewing's sarcoma.

KEY CONCEPTS

- Bones are subject to different types of fracture, depending on the type of tension stress imposed. Fractures can be classified according to the orientation of the break as transverse, longitudinal, oblique, or spiral. A *comminuted fracture* consists of three or more fragments. A *greenstick fracture* is an incomplete break. Fractures are classified as *open* or *compound* when the skin is penetrated and as *closed* or *simple* when the skin is not broken.

- Healing of fractured cancellous bone occurs more quickly than healing of cortical bone. Trauma causes hematoma formation, followed by *callus formation.* The callus is initially soft and cartilaginous, then progressively ossifies to become firm and stable. The fracture is clinically stable when no movement at the break is detectable. Radiographically apparent union occurs when the callus has been completely replaced by mature bone. Healing of fractured bone is dependent on stabilization and time.

- Complete separation of joint articulating surfaces is termed dislocation. Subluxation refers to partial separation. Soft tissue damage is the primary problem.
- Scoliosis is a lateral deformity of the spinal column that is detected from asymmetry of the shoulders, hips, and chest wall. Severe scoliosis can compromise lung expansion and lead to a restrictive respiratory disorder.
- Bone density is a product of the rate of bone resorption and bone deposition. A reduction in bone mass predisposes to fractures. Hormone deficiencies (estrogen, androgen), poor calcium intake, and lack of use are common causes of osteoporosis. Vitamin D deficiency is associated with rickets and osteomalacia, disorders characterized by soft, weak bones.
- Bone infections may be from blood-borne organisms or direct traumatic infection. Viruses (Paget's disease) and bacteria (*S. aureus* and tuberculosis) are typical causative organisms. Antibiotic therapy is useful in bacterial infections; however, abscess formation and chronic infection may occur.
- Most bone tumors are secondary to metastasis from other sites. Osteochondroma, chondroma, osteoid osteoma, and giant cell tumors are benign, primary bone tumors. Malignant bone tumors include osteosarcoma, chondrosarcoma, and Ewing's sarcoma.

Soft Tissue Injuries

In addition to injuries of the bony skeleton, soft tissue may also be traumatized. At times it is difficult to differentiate among the types of soft tissue. Cyriax, in an attempt to determine the exact site of a lesion, described two types of soft tissue, contractile and inert.[9] **Contractile tissue** is composed of the structures involved in the contraction of muscle and includes not only the muscle belly but also the tendon and bony insertion. Although not involved in a pure contraction, as is the muscle belly, the tendon and its insertion into the bone are mechanically linked to the tension generated by the muscle. According to Cyriax, pain may be elicited by active contraction and by passive stretching in the opposite direction.[9] Pain with resisted contraction may also be caused by a fracture site near a muscular insertion or a lymphatic gland, bursa, or abscess situated under a muscle.

Inert Soft Tissue Injuries

Inert or **noncontractile tissue** possesses no ability to contract or relax. Inert soft tissues include joint capsules, ligaments, bursae, fasciae, dura mater, and nerve roots. Passive stretching provokes pain from inert tissue. Evaluation of inert tissue lesions requires identification of all structures involved: the capsule of a joint, a section of a ligament or a nerve, or the mechanical displacement of the meniscus. It is interesting that the literature is now beginning to identify injuries to the musculoskeletal system as neuro-orthopedic disorders.[10]

Ligament Injuries

A ligament is a dense connective tissue with parallel-fibered collagenous tissues designed to connect bone to bone. Ligaments augment the mechanical stability of the joint, guide motion, and prevent excessive motion.[1] Injuries to the ligament occur when loading exceeds the physiologic range of motion. Microfailure precedes total failure of the ligament. With total failure of a ligament, damage to surrounding soft tissue will occur. O'Donoghue[11] has categorized ligament injuries into three types:

- **Mild** (first degree): A few fibers of the ligament are damaged, but there is no loss of strength of the ligament. Little treatment is necessary. Treatment is only for relief of symptoms.
- **Moderate** (second degree): A definite tear in some component of the ligament with loss of strength of the ligament exists. There is no wide separation of the fibers. Treatment is primarily to protect the ligament.
- **Severe** (third degree): The ligament is completely torn and no longer functions. There is potentially a wide separation of fragments of the ligament. Treatment is to restore ligament continuity.

Joint Capsule Injuries

Another inert structure that is intimately involved in stabilization of a synovial joint is the **joint capsule** (Fig. 50–9). The joint capsule is composed of two layers. The inner layer (stratum synovium) of the joint capsule is highly vascularized but has minimal innervation.[12] The stratum synovium is important because it synthesizes the hyaluronic acid component of the synovial fluid, produces matrix collagen, and is essential for nutrition of the joint.[13] The outer layer of the capsule is attached to the periosteum of the bones through Sharpey's fibers. The capsule is reinforced by ligaments and musculotendinous structures. The outer layer of the capsule is poorly vascularized but richly innervated by joint receptors. Joint receptors are able to detect the rate and direction of motion, compression and tension, vibration, and pain.[14]

An injury to the joint capsule results in an increase in vascularity and the development of fibrous tissue—a thick capsule. Any effusion into the joint cavity may lead to stretching of the capsule and its associated ligaments. The joint capsule, like the ligaments, provides stability to the joint. The capsule, however, has an interesting mechanical adaptation, a capsular

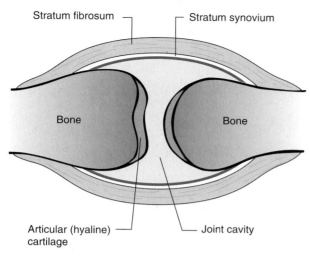

FIGURE 50–9. Joint capsule.

redundancy. This redundancy is extremely important in joint function and joint motion. An example of the importance of the redundancy has been identified by Hettinga[15]: "The inferior medial portion of the shoulder joint capsule is a loose, redundant sac that becomes tense only when the shoulder is fully abducted or flexed. The posterior capsule of the knee is loose in flexion but so tight in extension that it becomes an important stabilizer."

Capsular redundancy provides for a stable joint at the end ranges of movement. Any injury or edema into the joint that causes a scarring in the lax section of the capsule prevents achievement of full range of motion. Prolonged immobilization of a joint causes loss of the mobility and extensibility of the capsule, with subsequent loss of motion. An example of such a restriction is the loss of function in the shoulder following even a minor injury. With an injury to any component of the shoulder complex, inflammation or thickening of the capsule may ensue. The result may be the development of an **adhesive capsulitis,** a very painful and functionally restrictive disorder of the glenohumeral joint. Any injury to the joint may cause edema into the joint cavity and distention of the capsule. Capsular tightness leads to a loss of movement and an increase in pain. Excessive joint motion may cause a tearing of the capsule, similar to a ligamentous tear, and render the joint unstable.

Internal Joint Derangement

Internal joint derangement caused by injury to inert soft tissue structures is also seen clinically. Meniscal tears at the knee, labrum tears at the glenohumeral joint, and disk tears in the temporomandibular joint all cause restrictions of the joint and may lead to soft tissue dysfunction in the form of weakness, loss of motion, or pain.[13,15,16]

Injuries to Fasciae and Bursae

Fasciae and **bursae** may also be causes of pain and restriction of movement of the musculoskeletal system.

Fasciae. When the connective tissues of the body are arranged in sheaths that envelop muscles, the tissue is designated as *fascia*. Fascia may assist in dynamic stabilization (lateral raphe of the thoracolumbar region[17]) or in the dynamics of function (plantar fascia of the foot[13]). Individual muscles are surrounded by a thin fascia called the *perimysium*. This is especially important in situations in which muscles are adjacent to one another. The fascia provides a fluid between the tissues and acts as a lubricant to allow free movement.[18] Trauma to the fascia, as with any soft tissue, may cause edema and scarring. Restrictions in movement of the fascia cause a restriction in joint function.

Bursae. In many locations between muscles or between muscle or tendon and bone, connective tissue forms a pocket lined with synovium and containing fluid. These pockets are identified as bursae. Bursae are located in areas of high friction and are designed to dissipate some of the stress. With faulty mechanics of the joint, repetitive movement, or direct trauma, the bursal sac may become inflamed (bursitis) and extremely painful. Bursitis, because of its strategic position at stress points of muscle function, causes major disruption of movement. An inflamed bursa may restrict any movement of the joint and lead to restriction in capsular function or muscle dysfunction. Bursitis is commonly seen in the following regions: olecranon, prepatellar regions, psoas, retro-Achilles, retrocalcaneal, subacromial, subcoracoid, trochanteric, and pes anserinus.[19]

Injuries to Nerve, Nerve Root, or Dura Mater

Trauma to any soft tissue may lead to adhesive restriction in the movement of the nerve, nerve root, or dura mater.[10] Tethering of a nerve causes pain that radiates along the structures innervated by that nerve. Loss of function, weakness, and diminished reflexes may result from trauma to these essential soft tissue components of the musculoskeletal system.

Contractile Soft Tissue Injuries

Injury to Tendons

Injury to tendons occurs along a continuum from minor strain, in which a few fibers of the tendon are torn, to a complete tear or rupture. The sheath in which a tendon slides may also be traumatized. Inflammation of the tendon within the sheath is called **tendinitis.** Tendons are injured when the stresses placed on them are greater than the fibers can tolerate. Muscle tendons subjected to high tensile stress or compression are more prone to injury. Frequently injured tendons (Fig. 50–10) include the following:

- Extensor pollicis brevis and abductor pollicis longus (de Quervain's syndrome)
- Rotator cuff of the shoulder
- Biceps brachii tendon
- Tendons of the patellar complex
- Quadriceps tendon
- Hamstring tendon
- Achilles tendon
- Posterior tibialis muscle (shin splints)

Muscle and Tendon Strains

Muscle trauma compromises the contractile unit. As in the case of the injury to a tendon, tears in a muscle may range from a minor tear to complete rupture. The majority of injuries to muscle are produced by an abnormal muscle contraction.[3] Muscle and tendon strains are often categorized by the severity of injury[16]:

- Grade I: Minute tear of the connective tissue and muscle fiber.
- Grade II: A large portion of the contractile unit is torn, but a segment is still intact.
- Grade III: Total rupture of the contractile structure.

Blunt Trauma

A contusion or crush injury of soft tissue also compromises the contractile structure. Any blunt trauma that causes bleeding into the muscle belly may lead to inability to contract the muscle. Hemorrhage within a muscle belly has the potential to coagulate and calcify. This abnormal calcification within a muscle is a painful condition called **myositis ossificans.** Calcification prevents a normal and strong contraction of the muscle involved.

Compartment Syndrome

A **compartment syndrome** is trauma to the soft tissue caused by the unyielding structure of inert tissue. With an injury, edema will cause an increase in pressure within the fascia surrounding the muscle. Because volume is expanding in a confined area, the pressure reduces capillary flow. The muscle becomes ischemic, with a resultant excruciating pain. Besides pain, the skin looks pale, the pulse may be absent, and sensation is diminished. A compartment syndrome is a medical emergency. Nerves can survive only 2 to 4 hours of ischemia and muscles approximately 6 to 8 hours. Muscles, however, do not have the ability to regenerate, and if the muscle become necrotic, it will be replaced by fibrous tissue.[8] Compartment syn-

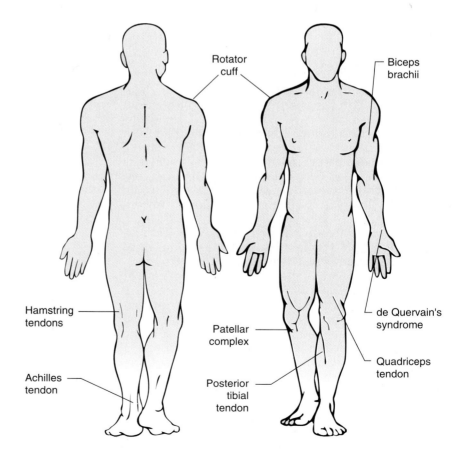

FIGURE 50–10. Frequently injured tendons.

dromes are noted in the forearm, fingers, hands, calf muscle, and the muscles of the anterior aspect of the lower leg.

Evaluation of Contractile Injuries

Cyriax has provided a functional guide to the evaluation of contractile injuries.[9] The patterns of function deal with pain and strength rather than excessive motion noted during evaluation of the ligamentous injury.

- **Strong and pain free:** Indicates there is no lesion of the contractile structure being tested, regardless of how tender the muscle is on palpation. The muscle functions painlessly and is not the source of the patient's pain.
- **Strong and painful:** Indicates a local lesion of the muscle or tendon. Previously listed as a grade I or II muscle strain. No limitation of passive movement is noted unless secondary joint restriction from disuse is present. The stiffness in the joint would then take precedence in treatment.
- **Weak and painful:** Indicates a severe lesion around the joint, such as a fracture. Weakness is usually due to reflex inhibition of the muscles around the joint.
- **Weak and pain free:** Indicates a rupture of a muscle or involvement of the nerve supplying the muscle.

If all movements are painful, pain may be due to fatigue, emotional hypersensitivity, or emotional problems.

Soft Tissue Healing After Trauma

Trauma to soft tissue results in disruption of the circulatory and lymphatic systems. Hemorrhage, fluid loss, and cell death result. With an injury, blood vessels at the site of trauma constrict and thus diminish blood loss from the affected area.[20] Norepinephrine mediates this initial constriction response, which may last a few minutes. Serotonin, contained in mast cells of connective tissue, and platelets released into the interstitial fluid with bleeding may prolong vasoconstriction.[21]

Platelets adhere to collagen fibers and release serotonin and the chemical adenosine diphosphate (ADP). ADP causes platelets to adhere to the traumatized endothelial wall and form a platelet plug that temporarily decreases bleeding.[20] Trauma to the endothelial surface triggers an enzyme that initiates clotting by converting prothrombin to thrombin, which converts fibrinogen to fibrin. During this period, the endothelial surfaces of small vessels are compressed and occlude the lumen, ensuring that the vessels remain closed after vasoconstriction has ceased.[22] In the early stages of inflammation, the endothelial margins of the venules may be covered with neutrophilic leukocytes, a process called neutrophilic margination. At this point, histamine is released from mast cells,

basophils, and platelets, causing vasodilation and increased permeability of venules.[21] With the increase in permeability, serous fluid containing cells and plasma proteins accumulates as edema in tissue spaces (Fig. 50–11). This edema fluid contains fibrinogen, which, through an interaction with thrombin, forms fibrin. Fibrin seals damaged lymphatics and confines the inflammatory reaction to the area in close proximity to the injury.[22]

The inflammatory response prepares injured tissue to progress to the healing process of repair and reorganization. Figure 50–12 provides a summary of the phases of wound repair. The acute response lasts approximately 2 weeks and the subacute phase another 2 weeks. At the time when the wound is clear of foreign substances, an infiltrate of macrophages and fibroblast is noted. A matrix of collagen, hyaluronic acid, and fibronectin develops. Lymphatics form in the matrix and prevent additional edema and assist in preventing infection. This granulation tissue develops in the wound space. Macrophages play an important role in wound repair. The chemical and cellular substances that promote formation of granulation material have not been identified.[23,24]

Next in the process of wound repair is reepithelialization of the wound surface. One mechanism of healing suggests that the epidermal cell migrates over previously implanted epidermal cells until the defect is closed.[25] The formation of basement membrane is next in sequence. This membrane is first laid down at the wound periphery and then progresses to the center of the wound. A strong bond forms between epidermal cells and the newly formed basement membrane to complete the reepithelialization stage (granulation tissue formation).[26]

Wound tensile strength develops through the deposition of collagen.[27] Collagen production begins approximately 5 days after myofibroblast migration into the wound space. Hyaluronic acid, found in the extracellular matrix, assists the glycosaminoglycans to

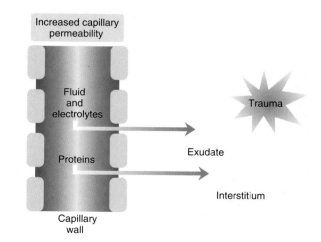

F I G U R E   50 – 11. Edema formation. With trauma, increased capillary permeability and dilation cause leaking into tissue space. Initially clear, the exudate in the tissue space becomes more viscous with an increase in plasma protein.

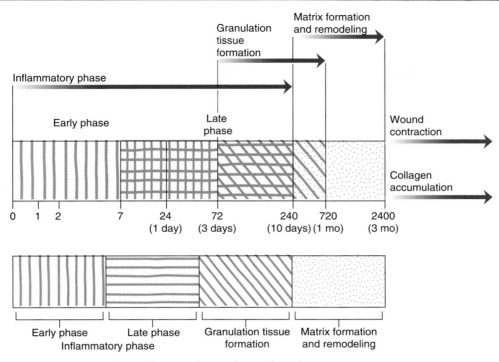

FIGURE 50-12. The overlapping phases of wound repair.

stimulate the process of fibroplasia.[28] Myofibroblasts secrete an extracellular matrix that induces cell migration and proliferation, and synthesizes proteoglycans that stimulate collagen formation and increase tissue resilience and tensile strength. By the end of the first month, tensile strength begins to increase, but a number of months are required to achieve the maximum level. Collagen reaches its maximum strength at approximately 3 months after injury. This maximum tensile strength, however, is only 70 percent to 80 percent of pre-injury levels.[5]

Revascularization (matrix formation and remodeling) must take place to ensure survival of the new tissue. Vascularization occurs through the development of new circulatory networks in the wound and the reattachment or recoupling of existing vessels.[21] Extracellular matrix, endothelial cell development, lactic acid, and heparin are a few of the factors that stimulate revascularization.

Wound closure or contraction is the final segment of healing in soft tissue injuries. Contraction begins rapidly after an injury and is complete in approximately 2 weeks.[21] Myofibrils assist in the process of wound closure. An interaction between the extracellular matrix and the granulation tissue results in the development of a contractile unit called a fibronexus.[29] Cytoplasmic actin binds to the fibronexus and draws the tissue together.[30] The contraction ensures a stable wound. As tension increases across the wound, reorientation of collagen fibers occurs and collagen phagocytosis increases.[31] Normal organization and concentration of collagen may require over 40 weeks to complete.[32] In the case of rupture or severance of soft tissue structures, surgical intervention may be neces-

sary to ensure that the traumatized tissue is in close enough proximity to allow healing.

KEY CONCEPTS

- Soft tissue injury refers to injuries of noncontractile elements (joint capsule, ligament, bursa, fascia, dura mater, and nerve root) and contractile elements (muscle and tendons). Passive stretching causes pain in noncontractile tissue injury, whereas active contraction is painful in contractile injury.
- Noncontractile tissue injuries generally cause altered range of motion around a joint due to pain, edema, adhesion, or fibrosis. Contractile tissue injuries are characterized by decreased muscle strength.
- Compartment syndrome is a dangerous complication of soft tissue injury due to swelling of injured tissue within a restrictive fascia. Unless pressure is quickly reduced, compressed tissue may become ischemic and necrotic. Manifestations include severe pain, pulselessness, and diminished sensation.
- Soft tissue injury results in local inflammation and initiates the process of wound healing. Strength within the injury is improved by the deposition of collagen. Normalization of collagen may require over 40 weeks to complete.

Diseases of Skeletal Muscle

Skeletal muscle is the most abundant tissue in the human body, accounting for approximately 45 percent of the total body weight.[5] Skeletal muscle performs dynamic work (locomotion) and static work (posture). As with other tissue of the musculoskeletal system, muscle atrophies in response to disuse and immobilization and hypertrophies when subjected to increased stress.

Muscular Dystrophy

Muscular dystrophy comprises a group of genetically determined myopathies in which there is progressive degeneration of muscle fibers.

Duchenne's Muscular Dystrophy

Duchenne's muscular dystrophy is inherited as an X-linked trait and therefore afflicts only males. The disease begins at birth with initial involvement of the pelvic girdle and progression to the shoulder. The calf muscles of an individual with Duchenne's muscular dystrophy are noticeably enlarged due to an infiltration of fat cells and a degeneration of muscle fibers. The individual suffering from this dystrophy dies by the age of 30 years.[6]

Fascioscapulohumeral Muscular Dystrophy

Fascioscapulohumeral muscular dystrophy is an inherited autosomal dominant trait that affects the muscles of the shoulder girdle and the face. The onset of disease is in adolescence, with a slow progression. Life expectancy is normal.[5]

Myasthenia Gravis

Myasthenia gravis is an autoimmune disease characterized by profound muscle weakness and fatigability. The disease starts at about 20 years of age, with women more often affected than men. Characteristically, weakness affects the ocular and cranial muscles. The limb muscles can also be involved. During times of emotional stress, the respiratory muscles may be included.

In myasthenia gravis, antibodies are produced that affect the acetylcholine receptors of the muscle end-plate of the neuromuscular junction. The antibodies impair the transmission of acetylcholine across the junction. The result is the muscle weakness and fatigability so prevalent in this disease.[5]

Anticholinesterase agents (e.g., neostigmine) may by used to inhibit breakdown of acetylcholine in the neuromuscular synapse. Increased synaptic acetylcholine enhances the activation of postsynaptic receptors and improves skeletal muscle contraction force. Because myasthenia gravis is an autoimmune disorder, steroids, plasmapheresis, and cytotoxic agents may be used to suppress the immune system. In severe cases, respiratory muscle fatigue may necessitate mechanical ventilation.

Fibrositis-Fibromyalgia Syndrome

Fibrositis-fibromyalgia, which occurs predominantly in women with onset in the teenage years, refers to a syndrome of musculoskeletal pain within a broad spectrum of nonarticular rheumatism.[33] The etiology remains elusive. No laboratory abnormalities have been found, nonspecific muscle biopsies are present, and patients are normal on psychological testing.

Patients with fibrositis complain of musculoskeletal pain, stiffness, and fatigability. Generalized pain is a common complaint. Joint pain and swelling are perceived by the patient, but the swelling cannot be documented. Complaints of muscle pain and weakness are expressed without objective demonstrations. In addition to stiffness and fatigue, sleep disturbances are a common complaint. The examination of a patient with fibrositis is characterized by an excessive number of reported symptoms with minimal objective findings. Tender points in fibrositis occur in precise locations. Eight paired tender points have been identified[34]:

- Insertion of the nuchal muscles into the occiput
- Midportion of the upper trapezius
- Pectoralis muscle (lateral to second costochondral junction)
- Two centimeters below the lateral epicondyle
- The upper gluteal area
- Two centimeters posterior to the greater trochanter
- Medial knee (anserine bursa)
- Gastrocnemius–Achilles tendon junction

Attempts at rehabilitation must be delicately balanced between increasing activity and preventing fatigue. Too aggressive a program results in an increase in symptoms. Gentle pool therapy seems to provide relief of symptoms without exacerbation of complaints.

KEY CONCEPTS

- Muscular distrophy comprises a group of genetic disorders characterized by degeneration of skeletal muscle. Duchenne's muscular dystrophy is inherited as an X-linked disorder and affects only males. Fascioscapulohumeral muscular dystrophy is an autosomal dominant disorder in which degenerating muscle fibers are replaced by connective tissue such that muscles may gain in bulk even though muscle strength is lost.

- Myasthenia gravis is an autoimmune disorder characterized by progressive weakness as the muscles are used. Antibodies against acetylcholine receptors in the motor end-plate interrupt neuromuscular transmission.

- Fibrositis-fibromyalgia syndrome is a poorly characterized disorder associated with generalized pain, stiffness, and fatigability.

Summary

A solid working knowledge of the anatomy, physiology, and biomechanics of movement is extremely important when dealing with any type of alteration in the musculoskeletal system. With a grasp of the mechanics involved in function, the clinician is able to approach each aberration with an awareness of the time requirements for healing, stress tolerances, and expected management outcomes.

The injuries and diseases discussed in this chapter are but a small representation of the many dysfunctions that may afflict the musculoskeletal system. The ability to determine the specific type of tissue involved (contractile or inert) allows the clinician to be cognizant of activities that would aggravate trauma, types of injury that require supportive devices, and injuries that respond to medical intervention.

An awareness of tissue response to healing enhances the clinician's evaluative skills and provides a signal as to when the intervention has achieved the expected results within an appropriate time frame. It is the responsibility of the practitioner to become knowledgeable about the variety of dysfunctions that occur. This knowledge base must continue to expand as technological advancements provide increasingly complex levels of information and new diagnostic tools become available.

REFERENCES

1. Nordin M, Frankel V: *Basic Biomechanics of the Musculoskeletal System*, 2nd ed. Philadelphia, Lea & Febiger, 1989.
2. Salter RB: *Textbook of Disorders and Injuries of the Musculoskeletal System*, 2nd ed. Baltimore, Williams & Wilkins, 1983.
3. Arnheim DD: *Modern Principles of Athletic Training*, 6th ed. St. Louis, CV Mosby, 1985, pp 251–252.
4. Gradisar IA: Fracture stabilization and healing, in Gould J (ed): *Orthopaedic and Sports Physical Therapy*. St. Louis, CV Mosby, 1990, pp 119–135.
5. Kumar V, Cotran RS, Robbins SL (eds): *Basic Pathology*, 5th ed. Philadelphia, WB Saunders, 1992.
6. Walter JB: *An Introduction to the Principles of Disease*, 3rd ed. Philadelphia, WB Saunders, 1992.
7. Guyton A: *Human Physiology and Mechanisms of Disease*, 5th ed. Philadelphia, WB Saunders, 1992.
8. Apley GA, Solomon L: *Apley's System of Orthopaedics and Fractures*. London, Butterworth, 1986.
9. Cyriax J: *Textbook of Orthopedic Medicine: Diagnosis of Soft Tissue Lesions*, 8th ed. London, Bailliere Tindall, 1982.
10. Butler D: *Mobilization of the Nervous System*. London, Churchill Livingstone, 1993.
11. O'Donaghue DH: *Treatment of Injuries to Athletes*, 3rd ed. Philadelphia, WB Saunders, 1976.
12. Hettinga DL: Normal joint structures and their reaction to injury. *J Orthop Sports Phys Ther* 1979;1:1.
13. Norkin C, Levangie P: *Joint Structure and Function: A Comprehensive Analysis*, 2nd ed. Philadelphia, FA Davis, 1992, pp 52–91.
14. Guyton AC: *Basic Human Physiology: Normal Function and Mechanism of Disease*. Philadelphia, WB Saunders, 1977.
15. Hettinga DL: Inflammatory response of synovial joint structures, in Gould J (ed): *Orthopedic and Sports Physical Therapy*, 2nd ed. St. Louis, CV Mosby, 1990, pp 87–117.
16. Richardson JK, Iglarsh ZA: *Clinical Orthopedic Physical Therapy*. Philadelphia, WB Saunders, 1993.
17. Poterfield J, DeRosa C: *Mechanical Low Back Pain: Perspectives in Functional Anatomy*. Philadelphia, WB Saunders, 1991.
18. Jenkins D: *Hollinshead's Functional Anatomy of the Limbs and Back*, 6th ed. Philadelphia, WB Saunders, 1991.
19. Magee D: *Orthopedic Physical Assessment*, 2nd ed. Philadelphia, WB Saunders, 1992.
20. Vander AJ, Sherman JH, Luciano DS: *Human Physiology: The Mechanics of Body Function*, 3rd ed. New York, McGraw-Hill, 1980, pp 319–324.
21. Kloth LC, Miller KH: The inflammatory response to wounding, in Kloth L, McCullock J, Feeder J (eds): *Wound Healing: Alternatives in Management*. Philadelphia, FA Davis, 1990, pp 3–12.
22. Peacock E: *Wound Repair*, 3rd ed. Philadelphia, WB Saunders, 1983.
23. Werb A, Gordon S: Secretion of a specific collagenase by stimulated macrophages. *J Exp Med* 1975;142:346–360.
24. Werb A, Gordon S: Elastase secretion by stimulated macrophages. *J Exp Med* 1975;142:361–377.
25. Krawczyk WS: A pattern of epidermal cell migration during wound healing. *J Cell Biol* 1971;49(2):247–263.
26. Winstanley EW: Changes in epithelial thickness during healing of excised full thickness skin wounds. *J Pathol* 1974;114(3):155–162.
27. Madden JW, Peacock EE: Studies on the biology of collagen during wound healing: Rate of collagen synthesis and deposition in cutaneous wounds of the rat. *Surgery* 1968;64:288–294.
28. Rollins BJ, Culp LA: Glycosaminoglycans in the substrate adhesion sites of normal and virus-transformed murine cells. *Biochemistry* 1979;18(1):141–148.
29. Singer II, Paradisco PR: A transmembrane association of fibronectin-containing fibers and bundles of 5mm filaments in hamster and human fibroblasts. *Cell* 1979;16:675–685.
30. Singer II, Kawka DW, Kazazis DM, Clark RA: In vivo co-distribution of fibronection and actin fibers in granulation tissue: Immunofluorescence and electron microscope studies of the fibronexus at the myofibroblast surface. *J Cell Biol* 1984;98:2091–2106.
31. McGaw WT: The effect of tension on collagen remodeling by fibroblasts: A stereological ultrastructural study. *Connect Tissue Res* 1986;14(3):229–235.
32. van der Meulen JCH: Present state of knowledge on the processes of healing collagen structures. *Int J Sports Med* 1982;3(suppl 1):4–8.
33. Yunus MB, Masi AT: Juvenile primary fibromyalgia syndrome: A clinical study of 303 patients and matched normal controls. *Arthritis Rheum* 1985;28(2):138–145.
34. Wolfe F, Cathey MA: The epidemiology of tender points: Prospective study of 1,520 patients. *J Rheumatol* 1985;12(6):1164–1168.

BIBLIOGRAPHY

Butler D: *Mobilization of the Nervous System*. London, Churchill Livingstone, 1993.
Cyriax J: *Textbook of Orthopedic Medicine: Diagnosis of Soft Tissue Lesions*, 8th ed. London, Bailliere Tindall, 1982.
Guyton A: *Human Physiology and Mechanisms of Disease*, 5th ed. Philadelphia, WB Saunders, 1992.
Guyton AC: *Basic Human Physiology: Normal Function and Mechanisms of Disease*. Philadelphia, WB Saunders, 1977.
Hettinga DL: Inflammatory response of synovial joint structures, in Gould J (ed): *Orthopedic and Sports Physical Therapy*, 2nd ed. St. Louis, CV Mosby, 1990, pp 87–117.
Jenkins D: *Hollinshead's Functional Anatomy of the Limbs and Back*, 6th ed. Philadelphia, WB Saunders, 1991.
Kloth LC, Miller KH: The inflammatory response to wounding, in Kloth L, McCullock J, Feeder J (eds): *Wound Healing: Alternatives in Management*. Philadelphia, FA Davis, 1990, pp 3–12.
Kumar V, Cotran RS, Robbins SL (eds): *Basic Pathology*, 5th ed. Philadelphia, WB Saunders, 1992.
Magee D: *Orthopedic Physical Assessment*, 2nd ed. Philadelphia, WB Saunders, 1992.

Nordin M, Frankel V: *Basic Biomechanics of the Musculoskeletal System,* 2nd ed. Philadelphia, Lea & Febiger, 1989.

Norkin C, Levangie P: *Joint Structure and Function: A Comprehensive Analysis,* 2nd ed. Philadelphia, FA Davis, 1992, pp 52–91.

Poterfield J, DeRosa C: *Mechanical Low Back Pain: Perspectives in Functional Anatomy.* Philadelphia, WB Saunders, 1991.

Richardson JK, Iglarsh ZA: *Clinical Orthopedic Physical Therapy.* Philadelphia, WB Saunders, 1993.

Salter RB: *Textbook of Disorder and Injuries of the Musculoskeletal System,* 2nd ed. Baltimore, Williams & Wilkins, 1983.

Walter JB: *An Introduction to the Principles of Disease,* 3rd ed. Philadelphia, WB Saunders, 1992.

CHAPTER 51

Alterations in Musculoskeletal Function: Rheumatic Disorders

GARY SMITH

KEY TERMS

ankylosing spondylitis: An arthritis of the sacroiliac joints that may often involve the entire spine. Marked limitation of motion develops, and a flexed spinal posture with flexed hips and knees may predominate.

gout: A condition caused by lack of the enzyme uricase and the inability to oxidize uric acid into a soluble compound; characterized by recurrent attacks of articular and periarticular inflammation, the accumulation of tophi (crystalline deposits) in bony and connective tissue, renal impairment, and uric acid calculi.

Lyme disease: A complex illness caused by a tick-borne spirochete, characterized by the development of a red papule that may form an annular lesion; this lesion becomes red and warm but not painful. Headache, neck stiffness, fever, chills, myalgias, arthralgias, malaise, and fatigue accompany the skin involvement, and arthritis of the large joints may develop.

osteoarthritis: A common degenerative joint disease characterized by progressive loss of articular cartilage and by changes in joint structures and subchondral bone.

Raynaud's phenomenon: Blanching or cyanosis of fingers or hands on exposure to cold or emotional stress. The phenomenon is attributed to vasospasm and structural disease of blood vessels. Puffiness and swelling of the hands and fingers are noted clinically.

Reiter's syndrome: A seronegative arthritis that appears 2 to 6 weeks after the onset of an infection and characterized clinically by diffuse swelling of fingers and toes, swelling in the Achilles tendon or plantar fascia, and low back pain.

rheumatoid arthritis: A systemic inflammatory disease of unknown etiology. Enzymes are released into the joint fluid, causing inflammation, proliferation of synovium, and tissue damage. The hands, wrists, knees, and feet are most commonly involved.

systemic lupus erythematosus: A chronic inflammatory disease resulting from an immunoregulatory disturbance. Arthralgias and synovitis are common features. Skin lesions are often present as a butterfly rash.

---

*A*rthritis is the most common disabling musculoskeletal condition in the United States. The National Arthritis Foundation estimates that over 37 million people have arthritis, and 125,000 are newly diagnosed with arthritis each year. More than 100 defined rheumatologic diseases have been identified. This chapter discusses the more common rheumatologic diseases.

Local Disorders of Joint Function

Osteoarthritis

Osteoarthritis (degenerative joint disease) is the most common rheumatic disease. Characterized by a progressive loss of articular cartilage and by changes in joint structure and subchondral bone, osteoarthritis becomes more prevalent with increasing age. Individuals over 65 years of age constitute a high-risk group. Occupation, life-style, and genetic factors may be predisposing factors.[1-4] Obesity may be a contributing factor owing to the additional mechanical stress placed on weight-bearing structures.[5]

Repetitive stress has not been consistently related to the development of osteoarthritis. Some research has suggested an increase in osteoarthritis in the dominant hand[6] and shoulders[7] of bus drivers, yet other studies of pneumatic hammer drillers[8] and marathon runners[9] have not demonstrated any increase in arthritic changes.

Etiology and Pathogenesis

Biomechanical, biochemical, inflammatory, and immunologic factors may all be involved in the development of osteoarthritis (Fig. 51–1). A primary injury occurs that releases proteolytic and collagenolytic enzymes from the chondrocytes.[10] A breakdown of the matrix of proteoglycan and collagen occurs. Subsequent to the damage, the water content of cartilage increases.[11] Collagen fatigue and fracture occur with the stress of weight bearing. Microfractures of the

subcortical bone lead to a decrease in the ability of the structure to absorb shock.[12] Breakdown of joint integrity overloads the capacity of repair, with resultant degenerative changes. Inflammatory responses may also cause an increase in the degenerative responses, which accelerates the destruction of the osteoarthritic cartilage.[13]

Structural breakdown of the cartilage involves fissuring, pitting, and erosion. Erosion can become so extensive that the articular surface denudes the full thickness of the cartilage. Osteophyte spur formation, sclerosis of subchondral bone, and cyst formation are also examples of structural changes present in osteoarthritis. Synovitis is common in advanced cases. This inflammation of the affected joint is a reaction to tissue breakdown.

Clinical Manifestations

Enlarged joints, crepitus with movement, and pain with function are typical clinical manifestations. These signs and symptoms are usually local. Any joint of

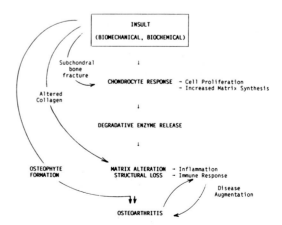

F I G U R E 51 – 1. Representation of pathogenesis of osteoarthritis. (From the *Primer on the Rheumatic Diseases*, ninth edition, copyright 1988, p 173. Used by permission of the National Arthritis Foundation.)

the body may be affected. Mechanical dysfunction, anatomic anomalies, or trauma may cause the breakdown of the joint surface. It is imperative to establish a differential diagnosis and to rule out a systemic or medical problem. If systemic, a connective tissue disease must be considered. Radiologic abnormalities are normally consistent with the clinical symptoms.

The most common deformation in the hands occurs in the distal interphalangeal (DIP) joints (Fig. 51–2). The enlargement is caused by spurs (Heberden's nodes) formed on the dorsolateral and medial aspects of the joint. Similar enlargements in the proximal interphalangeal joints are called Bouchard's nodes. The knee is also a common location for osteoarthritis. Local tenderness, crepitus, and muscle atrophy are common findings. Loss of cartilage in the medial or lateral compartments of the knee may lead to the structural changes of genu valgus or varus (Fig. 51–3).

Pain is relieved by rest during the initial stages. Because cartilage does not contain nociceptors (pain receptors), pain originates from intra- and periarticular structures. An acute inflammatory response is often the result of a specific traumatic incident and may cause synovitis in the joint capsule. As the breakdown

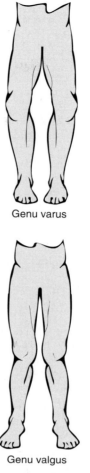

Genu varus

Genu valgus

FIGURE 51–3. Genu varus and genu valgus.

in structure progresses, even very slight activity elicits discomfort, and pain at night is quite common. Pain and crepitus in the joint with movement are frequently noted. Synovitis causes an enlargement of the joint and is accompanied by local tenderness.

Treatment

Initial treatment is designed to decrease stress on the joint and protect it from additional trauma. Analgesics and anti-inflammatory drug therapy decrease swelling and pain. Range of motion activity and gentle strengthening exercises prevent loss of function. Assistive devices, such as a cane or crutches, afford mechanical relief of weight-bearing stress. Surgical intervention may be necessary if the joint surface loses enough integrity to prevent joint function.

Infectious Arthritis

Any infectious agent may cause arthritic changes in the joint. Bacterial arthritis is the most destructive form of infectious arthritis. Most cases of bacterial arthritis result from hematogenous infection in the joint. Because of the vascularity of the synovium, or-

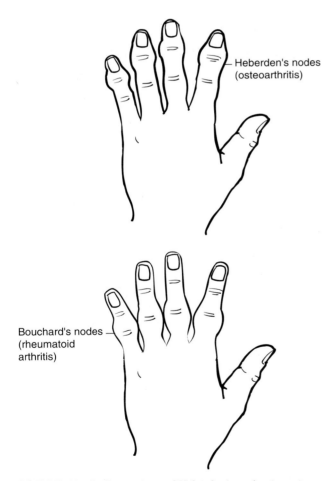

Heberden's nodes (osteoarthritis)

Bouchard's nodes (rheumatoid arthritis)

FIGURE 51–2. Comparison of Heberden's nodes (seen in patients with osteoarthritis) with Bouchard's nodes (seen in patients with rheumatoid arthritis).

ganisms in the blood may be trapped in the synovial space, providing an environment conducive to multiplication. Advancing infection causes a breakdown of synovium and cartilage.[14]

Etiology and Pathogenesis

The basic cause of bone and cartilage destruction is the interaction of antigenic bacterial cell wall components, the toxic effects of bacteria, the destruction caused by the purulent inflammatory exudate, and the local immune-mediated synovial or cartilage response. Untreated, the bacterial infection can rapidly destroy the cartilage and cause a fibrous or bony ankylosis of the joint.[15]

Clinical Manifestations

A warm and swollen joint is symptomatic of any type of infectious arthritis. Usually only a single joint is involved, but at times two joint structures may be infected. A low-grade fever is present in most patients. The diagnosis is established by recovering bacteria from the synovial fluid. Blood cultures are also used to provide a medical diagnosis.

Staphylococcus aureus is the most common nongonococcal bacterium involved in bacterial arthritis. Many of these infections occur in the elderly.[16,17] More septic joint infections due to anaerobic bacteria have also been noted.

Anaerobic bacterial arthritis is often seen in patients following total joint replacements or fractures and in patients with rheumatoid arthritis.[18] Approximately 2 percent of the 150,000 total hip and knee replacements in the United States are complicated by an infection.[19] Generally, a prosthetic joint infection requires removal of the prosthesis. If revisions fail, excision arthroplasty and complete joint debridement may be necessary.[20]

KEY CONCEPTS

- Osteoarthritis is a local degenerative joint disorder associated with aging and wear and tear from repetitive stress. It is characterized by loss of articular cartilage, wear of underlying bone, and the formation of bone spurs. The process is noninflammatory. Weight-bearing joints are often affected. Signs and symptoms are localized (not systemic) and include joint pain and crepitus with movement.

- Joint infection may be due to a variety of infectious agents, but bacteria are most problematic. The route of infection is usually by way of the bloodstream. Signs and symptoms are due to localized infection and the systemic manifestations of inflammation.

Systemic Disorders of Joint Function

Immune-Mediated Disorders

Rheumatoid Arthritis

Rheumatoid arthritis (RA) is a systemic inflammatory disease. In the United States approximately 0.3 percent to 1.5 percent of the population are affected. Women are two to three times more likely to develop RA, with a peak incidence between the fourth and sixth decades.[21]

Etiology and Pathogenesis

Most recent research has focused on a viral cause for RA. In fact, current theory suggests that several viruses may trigger the disease.[22] In RA, the normal immune protective process is diminished. Immune complexes activate a change in the chemical makeup of tissue and increase vascular permeability. Hydrolytic enzymes are released into the joint fluid, causing inflammation, proliferation of synovium, and tissue damage.

Rheumatoid factors or antibodies may augment the inflammatory response and increase fixation, alter the size of immune complexes, and render the joints and synovial tissue more susceptible to destruction by phagocytic cells.[23]

Early in the disease process, a breakdown of the microvascular structures occurs with edema of subsynovial tissue and cell proliferation of the synovial lining. As the disease progresses, phagocytosis is noted in synoviocytes and large mononuclear cells.[24] In advanced RA the synovium becomes edematous and projects into the joint cavity. Vascular changes include venous distention and capillary obstruction.[25]

Two immunologic processes seem to explain the inflammation and tissue destruction. In the synovial fluid, the process is initiated by the interaction of antigens and antibodies.[23] This interaction of antigens and antibodies in the tissue causes reduced levels of synovial fluid, increased vascular permeability, and an increase in cellular blood elements. Polymorphonuclear leukocytes ingest the immune complexes and cause a release of hydrolytic enzymes, oxygen radicals, and acid metabolites, which are responsible for inflammation and tissue damage.

Immunoglobulin molecules and rheumatoid factors are also found in the superficial layers of articular cartilage. Pannus is the most destructive component of rheumatoid arthritis. *Pannus* is granulation tissue composed of proliferating fibroblasts, small blood vessels, and inflammatory cells. Collagen and proteoglycans are dissolved in the region adjacent to the pannus.[22] Synovial pannus attacks the articular cartilage as a result of the chemical attraction of the immune complex deposits on the phagocytic cells in the proliferating synovium.[26]

Destruction of the articular cartilage, ligaments, tendons, and bone characterizes chronic RA. Digestants in the synovial fluid and granulation seem to be causative factors in the breakdown.[27] The pathologic changes are quite variable and may arrest at any stage. In chronic disease, adherence of adjacent articular surfaces may cause an adaptive shortening of the fibrous tissue and prevent movement of the joints. Capsular adhesions may also prevent joint mobility. Rupture of tendons may also occur. With the breakdown of joint integrity and dysfunctional mechanical pull, characteristic deformities occur.

Clinical Manifestations

Rheumatoid arthritis has a number of clinical features. Malaise, fatigue, and diffuse musculoskeletal pain are common manifestations during periods of acute flare-ups of the disease. Interestingly, symmetric patterns involving the joints of the hands, wrists, elbows, and shoulders are noted. The DIP joints are usually spared. This symmetry and the noninvolvement of the DIP joint assist in making the diagnosis of RA.

The hands, wrists, knees, and feet are most commonly involved. In the spine, the upper cervical area is most often affected. However, any diarthrodial joint is potentially at risk. The synovium of the joint is the site of joint deterioration. The development of pannus followed by inflammatory destruction of the soft tissue leads to laxity of the ligaments and tendons and results in biomechanical dysfunction. This mechanical stress causes the typical deformities of RA.

Swelling in the hands is a typical sign of proximal interphalangeal (PIP) joint involvement, as is swelling of the metacarpophalangeal joints. Pain is elicited on palpation of the joints. Laxity in the soft tissue allows for an ulnar deviation of the fingers (Fig. 51–4). In advanced situations a swan-neck deformity develops in the fingers. This deformity consists of a hyperextension of the PIP joints and flexion of the DIP joints. A boutonniere deformity, consisting of flexion of the PIP joints and extension of the DIP joints, is also a fairly common dysfunctional position (Fig. 51–5). Loss of strength and the ability to achieve a good pinch is frequently noted in the hand affected by RA. A rup-

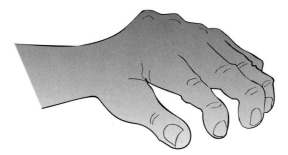

F I G U R E 5 1 – 5. Boutonniere deformity.

ture of tendons and loss of the ability to extend one's fingers are common findings in later stages of the disease.

The wrist is commonly involved. The synovium around the wrist becomes boggy and affects the tendon sheaths. Limitation of movement, especially dorsiflexion of the wrist, is often noted. Proliferation of the synovium on the volar or palmar aspect of the wrist may cause compression of the medium nerve and the development of carpal tunnel syndrome. Flexion contractures and swelling of the elbow are other common manifestations. Loss of joint space and an increase in joint laxity allow the possibility of dislocation of the elbow. In later stages of the disease, shoulder involvement is common. Typical signs of shoulder involvement are limitations of movement and pain on palpation in the area of the coracoid process. Dislocation, subluxation, or rupture of the joint capsule may occur as the disease progresses.

Involvement of the upper cervical vertebrae is yet another common finding. The destruction of the structures of the atlantoaxial vertebrae creates the potential for subluxation of this joint and endangerment of the spinal cord. The laxity in the cervical region may also allow compression of the vertebral artery, leading to vertebrobasilar insufficiency. Limitation of motion, especially rotation, pain on palpation, and headache in the occipital region are common.

Abnormalities in gait and limitations of movement are signs noted when RA affects the hip. Groin pain due to capsular involvement may be present. If synovitis of the hip becomes extensive, severe pain may be noted on evaluation. RA involvement in the knee is often extensive. Effusion, quadriceps atrophy, and synovitis of the semimembranous bursa (Baker's cysts) may be observed. Destruction of the articular surface, bone, and soft tissue may result from joint instability. The most common clinical sign of involvement of the foot is a retrocalcaneal bursitis. Other common signs of foot involvement include a cocking-up of the toes due to a subluxation of the metatarsal heads (claw toes), and lateral deviation of the first through fourth toes.

These clinical manifestations may develop rapidly or progress over many years. Normally, the symptoms develop over weeks and months. Initially the patient may feel fatigued or chronically tired and may

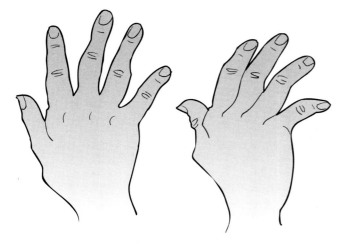

F I G U R E 5 1 – 4. Typical deformity of the hand seen in patients with rheumatoid arthritis. Note ulnar deviation.

complain of systemic aching in the musculoskeletal system. Specific joint pain, tenderness, swelling, redness, and nodules are quite common. Joint pain is normally symmetric and often involves the hands, wrists, elbows, and shoulders.

Prolonged inactivity such as sitting causes complaints of stiffness and swelling. As the disease progresses, walking, climbing stairs, opening jars or door, and precise movement of the digits become quite difficult. Weight loss, depression, and a low-grade fever often are noted in these patients.

It is imperative that a definitive differential diagnosis be developed. RA may be confused with a number of disease entities such as Lyme disease, systemic lupus erythematosus, or gout. RA may also cause subcutaneous nodules and present with cardiac, pulmonary, and ophthalmologic manifestations.

Systemic Lupus Erythematosus

Systemic lupus erythematosus (SLE) is a chronic inflammatory disease. Its development seems to result from an immunoregulatory disturbance related to an interaction of genetic, hormonal, and environmental factors.[28]

Etiology and Pathogenesis

Genetic involvement has been demonstrated in familial occurrences of SLE.[29] The incidence is also higher in specific ethnic groups.[30] Environmental situations such as sunlight, thermal burns, and other types of physical stress may initiate the development of SLE. Autoantibodies have been found not only in blood relatives but also in individuals sharing the same residence.[31] Medications such as hydralazine, procainamide, some anticonvulsants, and some foods such as alfalfa sprouts may be linked to the development of SLE.[32,33] SLE is more common in women, suggesting hormonal involvement.[34,35]

Clinical Manifestations

SLE typically affects multiple organ systems. Not all systems are affected simultaneously. The characteristic clinical course is one of exacerbation and remission. A remission may last for many years.

In the joints, tendons, and bones, arthralgias and synovitis are common features of SLE. Most patients complain of joint pain at some time during the course of the disease. Swelling, tenderness, pain on movement, and morning stiffness are noted. The involvement of the capsule, ligaments, and tendons can be extensive, causing deformities in the hands and feet. Deformities range from contractures of the fingers, hyperextension of the interphalangeal joint of the thumb, to subluxation of the metacarpophalangeal joint of the thumb. With steroidal therapy, tendon rupture is not uncommon.

Skin lesions may be quite extensive in SLE. Acute cutaneous lupus erythematosus often manifests with a classic butterfly rash (Fig. 53–15B shows the butterfly rash). The skin lesion may exacerbate during systemic flare-up. Swelling and redness are noted, and sunlight or artificial ultraviolet light may initiate a response. Skin involvement may occur on the shoulders, upper arms, upper back, chest, and neck. Scales or plaques develop on the scalp, ears, face, and neck. A latticelike venular skin change (livedo reticularis) is a very common skin manifestation.

A number of systemic manifestations may also be present. Cardiac complications include pericarditis, myocarditis, and congestive heart failure. Lung and pleural involvement includes pleuritis or pleural effusion. Renal involvement is common. Necrosis may develop on the fingertips, elbows, toes, and surfaces of the arms. Central nervous system involvement has also been recognized.[36] Lymphadenopathy occurs in 50 percent of all patients with SLE during the course of the illness.[20,28]

Scleroderma

Systemic sclerosis is a generalized disorder of connective tissue. Degenerative and inflammatory changes leading to fibrosis are characteristic. The skin, blood vessels, synovium, skeletal muscles, and internal organs may be affected.[37] Systemic sclerosis has a worldwide distribution. It affects women three to four times more frequently than men. Onset is most common between 30 and 60 years of age.

In systemic **scleroderma,** the skin becomes thick and fibrous. Plaques may occur at a specific site, or the disease may be widespread and affect many areas of the skin.

Clinical Manifestations

Clinical manifestations include Raynaud's phenomenon and swelling or puffiness of the fingers. Polyarthritis involving the small joints of the hands is common. A few months after the initial complaints, thickening of the skin may be noted.

Raynaud's phenomenon is present in approximately 75 percent of patients with diffuse scleroderma.[38] Exposure to cold and emotional stress may induce characteristic vasospasm, causing blanching or cyanosis of the fingers.

Evaluation of the skin discloses bilateral swelling of the fingers, hands, and, periodically, feet. After a few weeks or months, the edema is replaced by thick skin. Normal skin folds are lost and a shiny appearance is noted. Hyper- and hypopigmentation are also possible. Thickening of the skin can spread to the arms, face, and trunk.[39]

Joints and tendons become involved. Polyarthralgias or arthritides affect both small and large joints. Tenosynovial involvement may be seen in the presence of carpal tunnel syndrome and on the palpation of thickened tendons in the forearm. Flexion contractures may be quite severe.[40]

Patients with scleroderma may present with disuse atrophy of the muscle due to limitation of motion secondary to involvement of the skin and joints; atrophy and overall weakness are common. Gastrointestinal involvement is present in a majority of patients. The musculature of the esophagus is involved and leads to difficulties in swallowing. Involvement of the esophageal sphincter musculature may result in reflux of gastric contents and the development of peptic esophagitis. Malabsorption problems may also result from intestinal dysfunction.[20]

Pulmonary involvement may cause a reduced vital capacity and pulmonary arterial hypertension. The manifestations of myocardial involvement include congestive heart failure and a variety of atrial and ventricular arrhythmias.[20] Renal involvement is the major cause of death. Malignant arterial hypertension may rapidly progress to renal insufficiency without immediate treatment.[41]

Ankylosing Spondylitis

Ankylosing spondylitis (AS) is an arthritis of the sacroiliac joints that often involves the entire spine and, to some extent, the peripheral joints.[42] Age at onset is less than 40 years. Historically considered a disease found predominantly in men, recent studies suggest a more uniform distribution between men and women.[43,44] The disease in women tends to manifest in the peripheral joints, whereas in men there is equal spinal involvement.[45,46]

Clinical Manifestations

Clinical features include the insidious onset of discomfort, and morning stiffness that persists for more than 3 months. Some improvement with exercise is noted. Evaluation of the spine suggests an increase in muscle tone and a loss of normal lordosis. Marked limitation of mobility is noted in both anterior and lateral planes. With limitation of movement and a position of spinal flexion, the hips and knees must compensate, creating lower extremity deformities. Because of the restricted postural position and the decreased chest expansion, tidal volume may be diminished.[42] A typical postural position for AS is shown in Figure 51–6.

The primary objectives of treatment are to relieve pain, decrease inflammation, and strengthen and maintain posture and function.

Polymyositis and Dermatomyositis

Polymyositis and **dermatomyositis** are idiopathic inflammatory myopathies.[47] Proximal limb and neck weakness and associated muscle pain are clinical signs of these illnesses. Most patients initially complain of hip and leg weakness and difficulty with climbing stairs and rising out of a chair. Later in the progression of the disease, weakness in the arms prevents functional overhead activity. Anterior neck weakness makes lifting the head from the pillow very difficult.

Clinical Manifestations

During the physical examination, manual muscle testing reveals weakness in the proximal limb muscles.

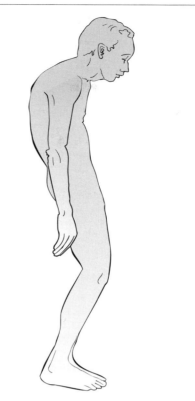

FIGURE 51 – 6. Typical posture of patient with ankylosing spondylitis.

Contractures are not usually present but may develop. Facial and ocular muscle weakness seldom occurs, distinguishing myositis from myasthenia gravis.

In dermatomyositis, cutaneous manifestations may develop with the muscle involvement. Common findings are flat-topped papules overlying the dorsal surface of the interphalangeal joints of the hands (Gottron's papules). These areas will atrophy and develop hypopigmentation. A more common finding is the development of an erythematous smooth or scaly patch over the dorsal interphalangeal or metacarpophalangeal joints of the elbow, knees, or medial malleoli area.[20]

Cardiac involvement is often noted. Dysrhythmias, congestive heart failure, conduction defects, ventricular hypertrophy, or pericarditis are typical. Weakness of the respiratory muscles and lung pathology can cause pulmonary disease.

Postinfectious Systemic Disorders

Reiter's Syndrome

Historically, Reiter's syndrome consisted of three types of clinical problems: arthritis, urethritis, and conjunctivitis. Currently, Reiter's syndrome is defined as a seronegative arthritis that follows urethritis, cervicitis, or dysentery. Possible associated problems include inflammatory lesions, oral ulcers, and keratoderma.[48] The male-female ratio is approximately 5 : 1.[49]

Clinical Manifestations

Clinically, an arthritis typically appears 2 to 6 weeks after the onset of the infectious episode. This acute arthritis onset predominantly affects the knees and ankles. Three features of musculoskeletal manifestations are typical: diffuse swelling of entire fingers or toes (sausage digits); swelling at the Achilles tendon insertion, or plantar fascia; and low back pain, especially in the sacroiliac region.

Involvement of the genitourinary system is not uncommon in Reiter's syndrome. Prostatitis and clinical cystitis are noted in a segment of the population.[50] The most common eye involvement is noninfectious conjunctivitis. Iritis, uveitis, episcleritis, and corneal ulceration could cause permanent impairment of vision.[51]

Cutaneous lesions related to Reiter's syndrome include the development of small, shallow, painless ulcers on the glans penis and urethral meatus. A hyperkeratotic skin lesion (keratoderma blennorrhagicum) may form on the soles of the feet and palms of the hands. Hyperkeratosis (extreme thickening beneath the nails) can occur.[20]

Acute Rheumatic Fever

Acute rheumatic fever is an inflammatory disease induced by an antecedent Group A streptococcal pharyngeal infection.[52] The incidence of acute rheumatic fever has greatly decreased in the United States. Attempts to alleviate poverty and crowded conditions and the early recognition and treatment of the infection have led to a decline in its severity.[53]

Clinical Manifestations

The clinical aspects of acute rheumatic fever depend on the age of the affected individual. Children and teenagers present with polyarthritis and carditis. Polyarthritis is usually the only manifestation in the adult. Fever between 101° and 104°F is present in most patients.[20]

Arthritis is the most common symptom noted in patients with acute rheumatic fever.[54] Pain may be quite severe and usually reaches its maximum in 12 to 24 hours. Synovial effusion, inflammation, and erythema may be noted.[55] The knees and ankles are affected most often. The shoulders, hips, elbows, wrists, and small joints of the hands and feet may also be compromised.[54] Numerous joints (mean of seven joints) may be involved. Joint symptoms usually respond rapidly to treatment.

Approximately 75 percent to 90 percent of children and teenagers and 15 percent of adults with acute rheumatic fever develop carditis.[54] The signs of carditis include murmurs, cardiomegaly, congestive heart failure, and pericarditis. Mitral valve regurgitation is the most common murmur, followed by aortic regur-

gitation. Evidence of rheumatic heart disease may not be apparent for many years after the acute incident.[56]

A rash is noted in approximately 10 percent to 20 percent of the children affected by acute rheumatic fever. The rash begins as small, pink, blanching macules over the trunk and proximal regions of the extremities. Painless nodules may cover the extensor surfaces. Chorea—abrupt, purposeless movements that interfere with voluntary activity—occurs in less than 5 percent of children affected by this disease entity.[20]

Postparasitic Disorders

Lyme Disease

Lyme disease is a complex illness caused by a tickborne spirochete.[57] This disease has been recognized in 32 states, 18 countries, and four continents.[58]

Clinical Manifestations

The tick bite produces a red macule or papule that may expand to form an annular lesion. The lesion may expand and become quite red. The lesion is warm to the touch but not painful, and is often accompanied by severe headache, neck stiffness, fever, chills, myalgias, arthralgias, malaise, and fatigue.[59] Systemic involvement may consist of lymphadenopathy, splenomegaly, hepatitis, nonproductive cough, testicular swelling, and conjunctivitis.

Musculoskeletal symptoms occur early in the illness and follow a pattern of migratory pain in joints, tendons, bursae, muscle, or bone. Minimal swelling is noted. About 60 percent of the patients develop frank arthritis with involvement of the large joints, especially the knee.[60] Erosion of cartilage and chronic involvement of the joints occur in approximately 10 percent of patients.[20]

Neurologic abnormalities suggest meningeal irritation. After a period of time, neurologic abnormalities may increase to include meningitis, cranial neuritis, motor and sensory radiculoneuritis, and chorea.[61]

Cardiac involvement may be noted, including atrioventricular blocks, left ventricular dysfunction, or cardiomegaly. Cardiac involvement lasts only a few weeks but can be fatal.[62]

KEY CONCEPTS

- **A number of immune-mediated systemic connective tissue diseases result in joint dysfunction, including rheumatoid arthritis, lupus, and scleroderma. Most are classified as autoimmune disorders of unclear etiology. The signs and symptoms of systemic joint disorders are generalized but involve multiple joints and usually other connective tissue structures.**

- **Differentiation among types of systemic joint disorders is based on patterns of joint dysfunction, immunologic factors (e.g., rheumatoid factor), and related lesions (e.g., the butterfly rash of lupus).**

- Joint destruction in systemic joint disorders is inflammatory in nature and involves the synovial membrane, cartilage, joint capsule, and surrounding ligaments and tendons.
- Rheumatic fever and Lyme disease are inflammatory joint disorders associated with a known organism. Rheumatic joint disease is a sequela of Group A streptococcal infection. Lyme disease is associated with a spirochete carried by ticks.

Joint Dysfunction Secondary to Other Diseases

Psoriatic Arthritis

Studies have confirmed an increase in the prevalence of inflammatory arthritis in association with psoriasis.[63] The disease apparently involves a complex relationship among genetic, environmental, and immune factors.

Clinical Manifestations

The pattern of joint involvement seen clinically varies. The majority of patients have peripheral joint involvement in the form of asymmetric arthritis. A smaller percentage have a polyarthritis that is difficult to distinguish from RA.[20]

Commonly, psoriatic arthritis is characterized by a combination of soft tisue and peripheral joint disease. Inflammation occurs not only in the joints, but also in the periosteum, along the tendons, and at tendon insertions into bone. Edema in the digits is common.[64]

Evidence of skin or nail changes, typical of psoriasis, is noted in psoriatic arthritis. These skin changes include macular or papular lesions with characteristic scales. Nail involvement includes pitting and transverse or longitudinal ridging. Subungual hyperkeratosis and oil droplet discoloration suggest psoriasis.[65] Eye inflammation is also present.[66]

Patients with psoriatic arthritis must not place excessive pressure on inflamed joints through stressful activity. Range of motion exercises preserve joint mobility and need to be performed.

Enteropathic Arthritis

Enteropathic arthritis refers to the articular manifestations of two inflammatory bowel diseases, **ulcerative colitis** and **Crohn's disease.**[67]

Clinical Manifestations

The articular manifestations include peripheral arthritis, spondylitis, and involvement of the muscle and the bone. Peripheral arthritis is most commonly noted in the knees and ankles. Synovial inflammation may be mild to quite severe. The development of granuloma in patients with Crohn's disease may cause destruction of the articular surfaces of the joint.[20] Spondylitis can cause extensive spinal involvement, similar to the features seen in patients with ankylosing spondylitis.

Other features associated with enteropathic arthritis include hypertrophic osteoarthropathy, granulomatous bone, and muscle involvement.[68–70] A number of cutaneous, mucosal, serosal, and ocular manifestations such as leg ulceration, thrombophlebitis, mouth ulcers, and ocular inflammation are noted with this disease.[71,72]

Neuropathic Osteoarthropathy

Commonly called Charcot joint, **neuropathic osteoarthropathy** is a neurologic disease that leads to bone abnormalities and joint involvement. The mechanics of disease development are probably a combination of neurovascular and neurotraumatic processes.[73] Neurovascular changes desensitize the joint. With repetitive trauma, injury to the joint causes a breakdown in structure. Motor neuron involvement can affect both upper and lower motor neurons. Diabetes, tabes dorsalis, and syringomyelia are the three most prevalent disease processes that lead to neuropathic osteoarthropathy.

Clinical Manifestations

Clinically, the patient presents with a swollen, deformed, and unstable joint. Radiologic findings demonstrate advanced joint destruction and pathologic fractures.[74] Management requires protection of the involved joint through immobilization and a decrease in weight bearing. Surgical intervention has had poor results because of non-union, dislocation, or infection.

Hemophilic Arthropathy

Bleeding into joints, as noted in hemophilia, causes extension of the joint capsule and a limitation of movement. Chronic synovitis causes changes in the synovial lining and eventually leads to destruction of the joint.[75]

Clinical Manifestations

Three stages of hemophilic arthropathy are described. The acute stage manifests with bleeding in the joint and occurs as the child begins to walk. Bleeding into the confined area of the capsule causes the joint to be positioned in flexion and increases stress to the articular structures. The second stage is the result of repetitive hemorrhages into the joint. Chronic synovitis and proliferation of connective in the joint capsule are seen in the second stage. The third stage is characterized by destruction of joint integrity.[75–77]

The larger joints are affected more frequently than the smaller joints. Seldom are the structures of the wrist involved. The elbow, hip, and knee are subject to major destruction. Medical care to enhance clotting is imperative. A critical component of care in hemophilia is education and the prevention of deformity.[20]

Gout

Gout in humans arises from lack of the enzyme uricase and the subsequent inability to oxidize uric acid to a soluble compound. Inability to oxidize uric acid increases the possibility of the deposition of crystalline forms of urate.[78] The acute attack is often triggered by a traumatic event, a surgical procedure, an acute illness, or the use of alcohol or drugs.

Clinical Manifestations

The prevalence of gout in the United States is approximately 275 per 100,000 population. The risk of developing gout increases with age and with an increase in serum urate concentrations. Clinically, acute gouty arthritis is the form most frequently observed. Gouty arthritis is noted mainly in middle-aged men and postmenopausal women.[20]

Manifestations of gout include recurrent attacks of articular and periarticular inflammation (acute gouty arthritis), accumulation of tophi (crystalline deposits) in bony and connective tissue, renal impairment, and uric acid calculi.[79] The evolution of gout can be identified in four phases: asymptomatic hyperuricemia, acute gouty arthritis, intercritical gout, and chronic tophaceous gout.[80]

Asymptomatic Hyperuricemia. In asymptomatic hyperuricemia there are no clinical signs, but the serum urate level is elevated. In the male, hyperuricemia can begin at puberty. In women, hyperuricemia usually does not appear before menopause.

Acute Gouty Arthritis. Gouty arthritis is the most common early clinical sign. The affected joints are warm, red, and tender to palpation and weight bearing. The metatarsophalangeal joint of the great toe is most often involved. The ankle, tarsal, and knee joints are often affected. The first episode of acute gouty arthritis is often an intense pain that wakens the patient from a sound sleep. A diffuse periarticular erythema will often accompany the attack.

The initial attacks subside within 3 to 10 days and the patient is symptom free until the next episode. The attacks tend to become more frequent and to involve more joints. Mild arthralgias between attacks may be caused by the gout.

Intercritical Gout. Intercritical gout is the name for the disease in the intervals between acute attacks. Even during asymptomatic periods, urate crystals can be aspirated from the involved joints.

Chronic Tophaceous Gout. Tophaceous gout is an advanced stage of gout. Tophi begin to appear approximately 10 years after the initial onset of gout. Tophi occur commonly in the synovium, subchondral bone, olecranon bursa, and the infrapatellar and Achilles tendons. Tophi have been noted in the walls of the

aorta, the valves of the heart, nasal cartilage, cornea, sclerae, and in the central nervous sytem.[81]

As a result of the deposition of crystals and chronic inflammation, deforming arthritis can develop. Development of tophi in the tendon sheaths of the hand and the wrist can cause a trigger finger or carpal tunnel syndrome.

Patients with gout may have involvement of the kidneys and develop renal malfunction. These individuals have a higher frequency of arterial hypertension, diabetes mellitus, and cardiac and cerebral atherosclerosis. Hypertriglyceridemia occurs more frequently in the patient diagnosed with gout.[82]

Adult-Onset Still's Disease

Adult-onset Still's disease is a form of seronegative polyarthritis with a number of symptoms similar to Still's disease in children (see discussion under Pediatric Joint Disorders).[83] Adult-onset Still's disease may follow the diagnosis of RA.

Clinical Manifestations

A high-spiking fever and a rash on the trunk and extremities are clinical features.[84] Polyarthritis usually affects the PIP and MCP joints of the hands. Arthritic changes are also noted in the wrist, knees, hips, and shoulders. Fusion of the carpometacarpal and intercarpal joints is characteristic.[85] Visceral involvement includes hepatic insufficiency, chronic respiratory failure, cardiac tamponade, congestive heart failure, and anemia.[84,86–88]

KEY CONCEPT

> • Neurovascular, hematologic, and metabolic disorders may lead to associated disorders of joint function. Diabetes, for example, results in neurovascular changes that desensitize the joint and predispose to traumatic joint dysfunction. Hemophilia predisposes to intra-articular bleeding. Altered uric acid metabolism leads to deposition of uric acid crystals in joints, causing inflammation and gouty arthritis.

Pediatric Joint Disorders

Pediatric rheumatic diseases include approximately 110 illnesses associated with arthritis and musculoskeletal syndromes.[89] Recent changes in pediatric rheumatology have recognized that soft tissue pain and restrictions constitute a major proportion of the cases.

Nonarticular Rheumatism

Growing pain or **nonarticular rheumatism** is a common soft tissue syndrome in children. Nocturnal pain, usually occurring in the calves, shins, and thighs, is the most common symptom. This problem seems to be benign, but medical consultation and education concerning the problem is essential.[90]

Hypermobility of Joints

Hypermobility of joints is a common cause of complaints of pain in the joints. Mobility may be excessive in any joint but is most apparent in passive apposition of the thumb to the forearm, hyperextension of the fingers parallel to the forearm, and excessive extension (greater than 10 degrees) of the knees and elbows. Education, restriction of activities causing irritation, and reassurance that improvement is forthcoming are some useful treatment approaches.[91]

Juvenile Rheumatoid Arthritis

Juvenile rheumatoid arthritis (JRA) begins with synovial inflammation of unknown etiology and affects approximately 60,000 to 200,000 children in the United States.[92] Two subtypes of juvenile rheumatoid arthritis are included in this discussion, Still's disease and polyarticular onset JRA.

Still's Disease

Clinical Manifestations

Systemic-onset JRA or **Still's disease** is noted in approximately 20 percent of children with JRA. Clinical indications include spiking fevers, a centripetal rash, lymphadenopathy, hepatosplenomegaly, and pericardial or pleural effusions. Fatigue, muscle atrophy, and weight loss can be severe. Musculoskeletal findings in the early stages of the disease include recurrent arthralgias, myalgia, and transient arthritis, which are consistent with fever spikes. Polyarthritis develops within weeks to months after the onset of the disease. Severe chronic arthritis may continue after the systemic symptoms subside.[89]

Polyarticular Onset

Clinical Manifestations

A **polyarticular onset** of JRA is seen in approximately 40 percent of patients. Malaise, growth retardation or weight loss, low-grade fever, organomegaly, adenopathy, and anemia are manifestations of this disease.[20] Both systemic and polyarticular JRA can cause general growth retardation. Inflammation in the area of the epiphyseal plates can result in changes in the growth of the long bones.[93]

Treatment

It is imperative to achieve early diagnosis and apply appropriate treatment to minimize deformity and disability. Education and counseling are also important.[94] Relief of symptoms and the maintenance of joint position and muscle function are immediate goals of treatment.

Pharmacologic intervention is an important component of the treatment regimen. Drug therapy is instituted to decrease pain and arrest progression of the disease. The following categories of drugs are used: (1) nonsteroidal anti-inflammatory drugs (NSAIDs), (2) corticosteroids, and (3) disease-modifying drugs.[95] Physical and occupational therapy assessment and treatment plans are important, and daily activity needs to be an integral part of the child's life-style. Contractures may be prevented by support and physical activity.[96]

KEY CONCEPT

> - Juvenile rheumatoid arthritis has two subtypes: Still's disease, which has more systemic manifestations, including rash, high fever, lymphadenopathy, splenomegaly, and fatigue, as well as polyarthritis; and polyarticular arthritis, in which symptoms are primarily localized to the joints.

Summary

This chapter has provided an overview of the major rheumatic disorders. Broadly speaking, interventions must assist in controlling the disease activity, manage pain, minimize deformity, and maintain or restore function. Depending on the stage of the disease, the correct intervention must be implemented using a knowledge of joint physiology biomechanics and the pathologic changes caused by the disease.

The challenge to the health professional is to ensure that an inflammatory response is not exacerbated while the body structures are being stimulated to increase strength, enhance nutrition, and improve tolerance to stress. Long periods of immobilization, bed rest, and sedentary habits are counterproductive in the patient with arthritis.[97] Lack of activity poses particular problems in people with arthritis. Deleterious effects on muscle strength, reflexes, connective tissue extensibility, and cardiovascular fitness are identifiable in the immobilized arthritic patient.[98] It is imperative that the health professional look beyond disease-specific interventions and prescribe a well-developed exercise program for people with arthritis. The achievement or retention of as much function possible is the ultimate goal for an individual with arthritis. Every level of intervention must be directed toward the achievement of specific performance goals co-developed by the clinician and the patient.

REFERENCES

1. Solomon L, Beighton P, Lawrence JS: Rheumatic disorders of South African Negro: Part II. Osteo-arthrosis. *S Afr Med J* 1975;49(42):1737–1740.
2. Mukhopadhorya B, Barooak B: Osteoarthritis of the hip in Indians: An anatomical clinical study. *Indian J Orthop* 1967; 1:55–62.
3. Hoaglund FT, Shiba R, Newberg AH, Leung KY: Diseases of the hip: A comparative study of Japanese oriental and American white patients. *J Bone Joint Surg* 1985;67(9):1376–1388.

4. Solomon L, McLaren P, Irwig L, et al: Distinct types of hip disorders in Mseleni joint disease. *S Afr Med J* 1986;69(1):15–17.

5. Hartz A, et al: The association of obesity with joint pain and osteoarthritis in the HANES data. *J Chronic Dis* 1986;39:311–319.

6. Acheson R, Chan Y, Clemmett A: New Haven survey of joint diseases: Distribution and symptoms of osteoarthritis in the hands with reference to handedness. *Ann Rheum Dis* 1970;29:265–286.

7. Lawerence J: Generalized osteoarthrosis in a population sample. *Am J Epidemiol* 1969;90:381–389.

8. Burke M, Fear E, Wright V: Bone and joint changes in pneumatic drillers. *Ann Rheum Dis* 1977;36:276–279.

9. Puranen J, Ala-Ketola L, Peltokallio P, et al: Running and primary osteoarthrosis of the hip. *Br Med J* 1975;2:424–425.

10. Pelletier J, Martel-Pelletier J, Howell D, et al: Collagenous and collagenolytic activity in human osteoarthritis cartilage. *Arthritis Rheum* 1983;26:63–68.

11. Maroudas A, Venn M: Chemical composition and swelling of normal osteoarthritic femoral head cartilage. *Ann Rheum Dis* 1977;13:399–406.

12. Radin E, Martin R, Burr D, et al: Effects of mechanical loading on the tissues of the rabbit knee. *J Orthop Res* 1984;2:221–234.

13. Moskowitiz R, Kresina T: Immunofluorescent analysis of experimental evidence for selective deposition of immunoglobulin and complement in cartilaginous tissue. *J Rheumatol* 1977;13:391–396.

14. Smith R, Merchant T, Schurman D: In vitro cartilage degradation by *Escherichia coli* and *Staphylococcus aureus*. *Arthritis Rheum* 1983;10:5–11.

15. Goldenberg D, Reed J: Bacterial arthritis. *N Engl J Med* 1985;312:764–771.

16. Ang-Fonte G, Rozboril M, Thompson G: Changes in non-gonococcal septic arthritis: Abuse and methicillin-resistant *Staphylococcus aureus*. *Arthritis Rheum* 1985;28:210–213.

17. Small C, Slater L, Lowy F, et al: Group B streptococcal arthritis in adults. *Am J Med* 1984;76:367–375.

18. Hall B, Rosenblatt J, Fitzgerald R: Anaerobic septic arthritis and osteomyelitis. *Orthop Clin North Am* 1984;15:505–516.

19. Haley R, Culver D, Morgan W, et al: Identifying patients at high risk of surgical wound infection. *Am J Epidemiol* 1985;121:206–215.

20. Schumacher H, Klippel J, Robinson D: *Primer on the Rheumatic Diseases*, 9th ed. Atlanta, Arthritis Foundation, 1988.

21. Mitchell D: Epidemiology of rheumatoid arthritis, in Utsinger P (ed): *Rheumatoid Arthritis: Etiology, Diagnosis, Management.* Philadelphia, JB Lippincott, 1985, pp 133–150.

22. Harris E: Pathogenesis of rheumatoid arthritis, in Kelley W, Harris E, Ruddy S, Sledge C (eds): *Textbook of Rheumatology.* Philadelphia, WB Saunders, 1985, pp 886–903.

23. Zvaifler N: Immunopathology of joint inflammation in rheumatoid arthritis. *Adv Immunol* 1973;16:265–336.

24. Schumacher H: Synovial membrane and fluid morphologic alterations in early rheumatoid arthritis: Microvascular injury and virus-like particles. *Ann NY Acad Sci* 1975;256:39–64.

25. Ishikawa H, Ziff M: Electron microscopic observations of immunoreactive cells in the rheumatoid synovial membrane. *Arthritis Rheum* 1976;19:1–14.

26. Jasin H: Autoantibody specificities of immune complexes sequestered in articular cartilage of patients with rheumatoid arthritis and osteoarthritis. *Arthritis Rheum* 1985;28:241–248.

27. Weissmann G: Activation of neutrophils and the lesions of rheumatoid arthritis. *J Lab Clin Med* 1983;100:322–333.

28. Alarcon-Segovia D: The pathogenesis of immune dysregulation in systemic lupus erythematosus: A troika. *J Rheumatol* 1984;11:588–590.

29. Kaplan D: The onset of disease in twins and siblings with systemic lupus erythematosus. *J Rheumatol* 1984;11:648–652.

30. Green J, Montassei M, Woodrow J: The association of the HLA-linked genes with systemic lupus erythematosus. *Am Hum Genet* 1986;50:93–96.

31. DeHoratius R, Pillarisetty R, Messner R, et al: Antinucleic acid antibodies in systemic lupus erythematosus patients and their families: Incidence and correlation with lymphocytotoxic antibodies. *J Clin Invest* 1975;56:1149–1154.

32. Alarcon-Segorra D, Kraus A: Drug-related lupus syndrome, in Lemgerger L, Reidenberg M (eds): *Proceedings of the Second World Conference on Clinical Pharmacology and Therapeutics.* Bethesda, American Society of Pharmacology and Experimental Therapeutics, 1984, pp 187–206.

33. Roberts J, Hayashi J: Exacerbation of SLE with alfalfa ingestion. *N Engl J Med* 1983;308:1357–1361.

34. Lahita R: Sex steroids and the rheumatic diseases. *Arthritis Rheum* 1985;28:121–126.

35. Raveche E, Tjio J, Boegel W, et al: Studies on the effects of sex hormones on autosomal and X-linked genetic control on induced and spontaneous antibody production. *Arthritis Rheum* 1971;22:1177–1187.

36. Hughes G: Central nervous system lupus: Diagnosis and treatment. *J Rheumatol* 1980;7:405–411.

37. Medsger TA: Systemic sclerosis (scleroderma), eosinophilic fascitis, and calcinoses, in McCarty D (ed): *Arthritis and Allied Conditions*, 10th ed. Philadelphia, Lea & Febiger, 1985, pp 994–1036.

38. Young EA, Steen V, Medsger TA Jr: Systemic sclerosis without Raynaud's phenomenon. *Arthritis Rheum* 1986;29(suppl 4): S51. Abstract.

39. Masi A, Rodnan G, Medsger T, et al: Preliminary criteria for the classification of systemic sclerosis (scleroderma). *Arthritis Rheum* 1980;23:581–590.

40. Rodman G, Medsger T: The rheumatic manifestations of progressive systemic sclerosis (scleroderma). *Clin Orthop* 1968;57:81–93.

41. Lopez-Ovejero J, Saal S, D'Angelo W, et al: Reversal of vascular and renal crisis of scleroderma by oral angiotensin-converting-enzyme blockade. *N Engl J Med* 1979;300:1417–1419.

42. Salter R: *Textbook of Disorders and Injuries of the Musculoskeletal System*, 2nd ed. Baltimore, Williams & Wilkins, 1984, pp 201–204.

43. Calin A, Fries J: Striking prevalence of ankylosing spondylitis in "healthy" W27 positive males and females: A controlled study. *N Engl J Med* 1975;293:835–839.

44. Russel M: Ankylosing spondylitis: The case of the underestimated female. *J Rheumatol* 1985;12:1–5.

45. Marks S, Barnett M, Calin A: Ankylosing spondylitis in women and men: A case-control study. *J Rheumatol* 1983;10:624–628.

46. Gran J, Ostensen M, Husby G: A clinical comparison between males and females with ankylosing spondylitis. *J Rheumatol* 1985;12:126–130.

47. Medsger T, Dawson W, Masi A: The epidemiology of polymyositis. *Am J Med* 1970;48:715–723.

48. Arnett F, McClusky O, Schacter B: Incomplete Reiter's syndrome: Discriminating features and HLA-W27 in diagnosis. *Ann Intern Med* 1976;84:8–12.

49. Neuwelt C, Borenstein D, Jacobs R: Reiter's syndrome: A male and female disease. *J Rheumatol* 1982;9:266–272.

50. Paronen I: Reiter's disease: A study of 344 cases observed in Finland. *Acta Med Scand* 1948;212(suppl):1–114.

51. Lerisalo M, Skylv G, Kousa M: Follow-up study on patients with Reiter's disease and arthritis, with special reference to HLA-B27. *Arthritis Rheum* 1985;25:249–259.

52. Bismo A: The rise and fall of rheumatic fever. *JAMA* 1985;254:538–541.

53. Markowitz M: The decline of rheumatic fever: Role of medical intervention. *J Pediatr* 1985;254:545–550.

54. Barnert A, Terry E, Persellin R: Acute rheumatic fever in adults. *JAMA* 1975;232:925–928.

55. McDonald E, Weisman M: Articular manifestations of rheumatic fever in adults. *Ann Intern Med* 1978;89:917–920.

56. Krause R: Acute rheumatic fever: An elusive enigma. *J Allergy Clin Immunol.* 1986;77:282–290.

57. Steere A, Grodzicki R, Kornblatt A, et al: The spirochetal etiology of Lyme disease. *N Engl J Med* 1983;308:733–740.

58. Schmid G: The global distribution of Lyme disease. *Rev Infect Dis* 1985;7:41–50.

59. Steere A, Bartenhagen N, Craft J, et al: The early clinical manifestations of Lyme disease. *Ann Intern Med* 1983;99:76–82.

60. Steere A, Schoen R, Taylor E: The clinical evolution of Lyme arthritis. *Ann Intern Med* 1987;107:725–731.

61. Pachner A, Steere A: The triad of neurologic manifestations of Lyme disease: Meningitis, cranial neuritis, and radiculoneuritis. *Neurology* 1985;35:47–53.

62. Marcus L, Steere A, Duray P, et al: Fatal pancarditis in a patient

with coexistent Lyme disease and babesiosis: Demonstration of spirochetes in the heart. *Ann Intern Med* 1985;103:374–376.

63. Wright V: Seronegative polyarthritis: A unified concept. *Arthritis Rheum* 1978;21:619–632.

64. Lambert J, Wright V: Psoriatic spondylitis: A clinical and radiological description of the spine in psoriatic arthritis. *Q J Med* 1979;184:411–425.

65. Kruger G, Bergstresser P, Lowe N, et al: Psoriasis. *J Am Acad Dermatol* 1984;11:937–947.

66. Lambert J, Wright V: Eye inflammation in psoriatic arthritis. *Ann Rheum Dis* 1976;35:354–356.

67. Moll J: Inflammatory bowel disease. *Clin Rheum Dis* 1985; 11:87–111.

68. Oppenheimer D, Jones H: Hypertrophic osteoarthropathy in chronic inflammatory bowel disease. *Skeletal Radiol* 1982; 9:109–113.

69. Nugent F, Glasser D, Fernandez-Herlihy L: Crohn's colitis associated with granulomatous bone disease. *N Engl J Med* 1976; 294:262–263.

70. Menard D, Haddad H, Blain J, et al: Granulomatous myositis and myopathy associated with Crohn's colitis. *N Engl J Med* 1976;295:818–819.

71. Greenstein A, Janowitz H, Sachar D: The extra-intestinal complications of Crohn's disease and ulcerative colitis: A study of 700 patients. *Medicine* 1976;55:401–412.

72. Goslin J, Graham W, Lazarus G: Cutaneous polyarteritis nodosa: A report of a case associated with Crohn's disease. *Arch Dermatol* 1983;119:326–329.

73. Brower A, Allman R: The neuropathic joint: A neurovascular bone disorder. *Radiol Clin North Am* 1981;19(4):571–580.

74. Katz I, Rabinowitz J, Dziadiw R: Early changes in Charcot's joints. *Am J Roentgenol* 1961;86:965–974.

75. Arnold W, Hilgartner M: Hemophilic arthropathy: Current concepts of pathogenesis and management. *J Bone Joint Surg [Am]* 1977;59:287–305.

76. Mainardi C, Levine P, Werb Z, et al: Proliferative synovitis in hemophilia: Biochemical and morphologic observations. *Arthritis Rheum* 1978;21:137–144.

77. Kim H, Klein K, Hirsch J, et al: Arthroscopic synovectomy in the treatment of hemophilic synovitis. *Scand J Haematol* 1984;33(suppl 40):271–279.

78. Wyngaarden J, Kelley W: *Gout and Hyperuricemia.* New York, Grune & Stratton, 1976.

79. Boss G, Seegmiller J: Hyperuricemia and gout: Classification, complications, and management. *N Engl J Med* 1979;300: 1459–1468.

80. Seegmiller J: Disease of purine and pyrimidine metabolism, in Bondy P, Rosenburg L (eds): *Metabolic Control and Disease,* 8th ed. Philadelphia, WB Saunders, 1980, p 777.

81. Agudelo C, Weinberger A, Schumacher H, et al: Definitive diagnosis of gout arthritis by identification of urate crystals in asymptomatic metatarsophalangeal joint. *Arthritis Rheum* 1979;22:559–560.

82. Allard C, Goulet C: Serum uric acid not a discriminator of coronary heart disease in men and women. *Can Med Assoc J* 1973;109:986–988.

83. Bywater G: Still's disease in the adult. *Ann Rheum Dis* 1971;30:121–133.

84. Bujak J, Aptekar R, Decker J, et al: Juvenile rheumatoid arthritis presenting in the adult as fever of unknown origin. *Medicine* 1973;52:431–444.

85. Medsger T, Christy W: Carpal arthritis with ankylosis in late onset Still's disease. *Arthritis Rheum* 1976;19:232–242.

86. Esdaile J, Tannenbaum H, Lough J, et al: Hepatic abnormalities in adult onset of Still's disease. *J Rheumatol* 1979;6:673–679.

87. Troum O, Mohler J, Koss M, et al: Pulmonary abnormalities in adult onset Still's disease. *Arthritis Rheum* 1985;28(suppl 4): S78. Abstract.

88. Bank I, Marboe C, Redberg R, et al: Myocarditis in adults Still's disease. *Arthritis Rheum* 1985;28:452–454.

89. Ansell B: *Rheumatic Disorders in Children.* Boston, Butterworth, 1980, pp 1–199.

90. Calabro J: Soft tissue rheumatism, in Gershwin M, Robbins D (eds): *Musculoskeletal Diseases in Children.* New York, Grune & Stratton, 1983, pp 57–71.

91. Biro F, Gewanter H, Baum J: The hypermobility syndrome. *Pediatrics* 1983;72:801–806.

92. Petty RE: Epidemiology and genetics of the rheumatic diseases of childhood, in Cassidy J (ed): *Textbook of Pediatric Rheumatology.* New York, John Wiley & Sons, 1982, pp 15–45.

93. Berstein B, Stobie D, Singsen B, et al: Growth retardation in juvenile rheumatoid arthritis (JRA). *Arthritis Rheum* 1977; 20(suppl):212–216.

94. Hanson V, Kornreich H, Berstein B, et al: Prognosis of juvenile rheumatoid arthritis. *Arthritis Rheum* 1977;20(suppl):279–284.

95. Ciccone C: *Pharmacology in Rehabilitation.* Philadelphia, FA Davis, 1990, pp 174–185.

96. Granberry G: Orthopedic management, in Brewer E, Giannini E, Person D (eds): *Juvenile Rheumatoid Arthritis,* 2nd ed. Philadelphia, WB Saunders, 1982, pp 229–285.

97. Donatelli R, Owens-Burkhart H: Effects of immobilization on the extensibility of periarticular connective tissue. *J Orthop Sports Phys Ther* 1981;3:67–72.

98. Vallbona C: Bodily responses to immobilization, in Kottke F, Stillwell K, Lehmann J (eds): *Krusen's Handbook of Physical Medicine and Rehabilitation.* Philadelphia, WB Saunders, 1982, pp 963–976.

BIBLIOGRAPHY

Alarcon-Segovia D: The pathogenesis of immune dysregulation in systemic lupus erythematosus: A troika. *J Rheumatol* 1984; 11:588–590.

Ansell B: *Rheumatic Disorders in Children.* Boston, Butterworth, 1980.

Boss G, Seegmiller J: Hyperuricemia and gout: Classification, complications, and management. *N Engl J Med* 1979;300:1459–1468.

Calabro J: Soft tissue rheumatism, in Gershwin M, Robbins D (eds): *Musculoskeletal Diseases of Children.* New York, Grune & Stratton, 1983, pp 57–71.

Granberry G: Orthopedic management, in Brewer E, Giannini E, Person D (eds): *Juvenile Rheumatoid Arthritis,* 2nd ed. Philadelphia, WB Saunders, 1982, pp 229–285.

Greenstein A, Janowitz H, Sachar D: The extra-intestinal complications of Crohn's disease and ulcerative colitis: A study of 700 patients. *Medicine* 1976;55:401–412.

Hall B, Rosenblatt J, Fitzgerald R: Anaerobic septic arthritis and osteomyelitis. *Orthop Clin North Am* 1984;15:505–516.

Harris E: Pathogenesis of rheumatoid arthritis, in Kelley W, Harris E, Ruddy S, Sledge C (eds): *Textbook of Rheumatology.* Philadelphia, WB Saunders, 1985, pp 886–903.

Hoaglund FT, Shiba R, Newberg AH, Leung KY: Diseases of the hip: A comparative study of Japanese oriental and American white patients. *J Bone Joint Surg* 1985;67:1376–1388.

Jasin H: Autoantibody specificities of immune complexes sequestered in articular cartilage of patients with rheumatoid arthritis and osteoarthritis. *Arthritis Rheum* 1985;28:241–248.

Lane N, Bloch D, Jones H, et al: Long-distance running, bone density, and osteoarthritis. *JAMA* 1986;255:1147–1151.

Lerisalo M, Skylv G, Kousa M: Follow-up study on patients with Reiter's disease and arthritis, with special reference to HLA-B27. *Arthritis Rheum* 1985;25:249–259.

Mitchell D: Epidemiology of rheumatoid arthritis, in Utsinger P (ed): *Rheumatoid Arthritis: Etiology, Diagnosis, Management.* Philadelphia, JB Lippincott, 1985, pp 133–150.

Salter R: *Textbook of Disorders and Injuries of the Musculoskeletal System,* 2nd ed. Baltimore, Williams & Wilkins, 1984.

Schumacher H, Klippel J, Robinson D: *Primer on the Rheumatic Disease,* 9th ed. Atlanta, Arthritis Foundation, 1988.

Steere A, Bartenhagen N, Craft J, et al: The early clinical manifestations of Lyme disease. *Ann Intern Med* 1983;99:76–82.

Steere A, Grodzicki R, Kornblatt A, et al: The spirochetal etiology of Lyme disease. *N Engl J Med* 1983;308:733–740.

Vallbona C: Bodily responses to immobilization, in Kottke F, Stillwell K, Lehmann J (eds): *Krusen's Handbook of Physical Medicine and Rehabilitation.* Philadelphia, WB Saunders, 1982, pp 963–976.

Young EA, Steen V, Medsger TA Jr: Systemic sclerosis without Raynaud's phenomenon. *Arthritis Rheum* 1986;29(suppl 4): S51. Abstract.

UNIT XV

Alterations in the Integument

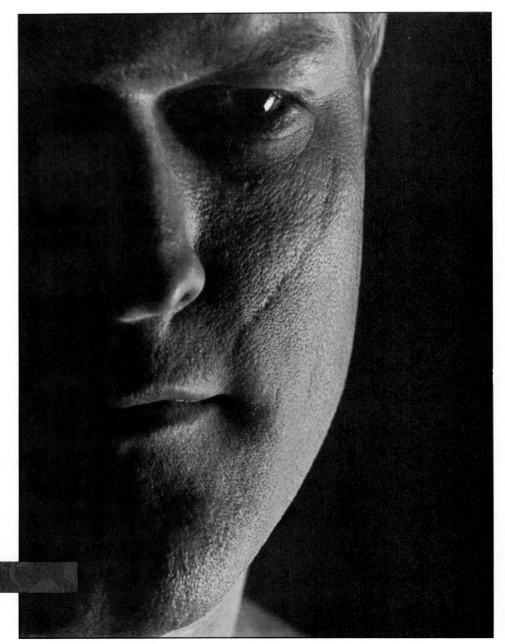

*Facial scarring is an example of
altered skin integrity.*

Photo by Kathleen Kelly

A Boston University School of Medicine study reports that care for chronic wounds costs up to $4 billion a year. These are not the wounds that heal quickly, may or may not leave a scar, and lead to quick recovery and a dimming memory of an accident or a surgery. Chronic wounds are the painful and dangerous afflictions of cancer patients, patients with diabetes, patients confined to bed for long periods, the elderly, or those whose immune systems have been compromised, whose wounds may be prone to serious infection.

Most wounds heal by themselves, perhaps with some timely help from medical professionals. The wound occurs, and almost immediately the specialized cells that contribute to coagulation rush to the site, attracted by chemical signals. Unusually rapid cell proliferation begins, and the process of healing starts. For patients troubled by slowly healing or unhealing wounds, physicians and nurses have been able to provide some relief through treatment and watchful care. But researchers assume that additional help is needed, and they are finding that the understanding of growth factors provides a direction toward better therapy in healing.

For some time researchers have known that endogenous growth factors, released at the location of the wound, are conducive to wound healing. Each of the four major families of angiogenic growth factors can induce soft tissue vascularization, promoting healing. Clinical trials in humans have accelerated epidermal regeneration in cutaneous wounds.

It appears that some growth factors are active at every stage of wound healing. It has been assumed that key growth factors are missing or wrongly combined in slow-healing wounds. Research intended to confirm the assumption has been inconclusive, but scientists have had some success applying, in clinical situations, a combination of growth factors and other molecules that mimic the natural healing process.

Scientists have long known that the first response to a wound is the formation of a fibrin clot by a protein called fibrinogen, which circulates in the bloodstream and in an emergency seals damaged blood vessels. Fibronectin, another protein in the clot, makes a connection with the extracellular matrix as a bridge between the clot and surrounding tissue.

But it appears that the extracellular matrix, a structure consisting of proteins and polysaccharides which is said to govern the geometry of tissues, does more than stabilize the clot. After an injury cellular responses, including production of growth factors, originate in the matrix. Basic fibroblast growth factor and signal cells originating in the matrix, as well as other growth factors produced during healing, cause cell proliferation.

Among its other precisely calibrated healing functions, the matrix, one researcher says, "choreographs the process." Molecules such as collagen, fibronectin, and heparin, which make up the matrix, bind growth factors to prevent them from inducing cell division where acceleration might be harmful.

"Without this binding," biochemist Michael Pierschbacher observed, "wound healing would be a systemic response, not the local one it needs to be."

FRONTIERS OF RESEARCH
Wounds and Wound Healing
Michael J. Kirkhorn

If this sounds as though there is a universal process in wound healing, there is, but it is strongly affected by the age, condition, and habits of the patients seeking care.

Age is a consideration in wound healing. Aged patients heal more slowly than younger patients, but the outcome is likely to be the same if the requirements of age are taken into account. Aged skin is more fragile, and the aged are less able to defend themselves against infection. They may be poorly nourished, and decreased perfusion may slow down the healing process. Chronic disease, medications, motivation, and social habits are other factors that skilled healers such as nurses take into account as they observe the healing process.

Partly because it decreases capillary and arteriolar flow to the skin, perhaps damaging connective tissues, cigarette smoking is a consideration in wound healing. Medical professionals find in their practices that cigarette smoke, which contains nicotine, carbon monoxide, and hydrogen cyanide, hinders healing among smokers. Nicotine reduces blood flow to the skin, carbon monoxide reduces oxygen transport and metabolism, and hydrogen cyanide inhibits metabolism and oxygen transport at the cellular level. Smokers who undergo plastic or reconstructive surgery heal less satisfactorily and have more complications following breast surgery.

Wounds caused by violence and aggravated by poverty are attracting the attention of dermatologists, who see patients with injuries or unhealed lesions caused by physical abuse, intravenous drug use, and sexually transmitted diseases.

CHAPTER 52
Structure and Function of the Integumentary System

LEE-ELLEN C. COPSTEAD

KEY TERMS

hair: Keratinized, threadlike outgrowth of the skin that covers most of the body.

hair follicle: Slender, cylindrical tube in which hair grows.

integument: Covering; refers to the skin.

integumentary system: The skin and its appendages, including the hair and nails.

keratin: Tough, water-repellant protein produced by keratinocytes and found in hair, nails, and horny tissue.

melanin: Dark pigment found in melanocytes that gives color to hair and skin.

nails: Appendages of the skin composed of keratinized epidermal cells.

sebaceous gland: Oil- or serum-producing gland that anoints hair and skin.

skin: A relatively flat membrane composed of an outer, thinner layer (epidermis) and an inner, thicker layer (dermis).

stratum: Layer.

sweat gland: Most numerous of the skin glands. Sweat glands are of two types, apocrine and eccrine.

*B*ecause skin forms a barrier between the internal organs and the external environment, it is uniquely subjected to noxious external agents and is also a sensitive reflection of internal disease. **Integument** is another name for skin, and **integumentary system** is a term used to denote skin and its appendages—hair, nails, and skin glands.

The integumentary system is the largest system of the human body. It is composed of tissue that grows, differentiates, and renews itself constantly. An understanding of the complex interplay between this system and the external environment begins with an overview of structure and function. Normal histology is described in this chapter as a basis for understanding diseases of the skin, described in Chapter 53.

The skin as an organ has many functions. It acts as a barrier against noxious agents, prevents the loss of vital fluids and electrolytes, and regulates body temperature. The cutaneous sensory nerve makes the skin's vast surface area an important sensory organ. The skin has a role in vitamin D synthesis. A less well-known property of the skin may be its ability to store glycogen and contribute to glucose metabolism.[1] The skin also has a psychosocial function. Emotions such as shame, anger, and fear can be expressed cutaneously. Because skin is a visible envelope covering the body, it is also an important component of body image. Table 52–1 summarizes the functions of the skin. All of these functions are important. Without the protection of the skin, the external environment could not be endured.

Structure and Function of Skin

The **skin** is a thin, somewhat flat organ classified as a membrane, the *cutaneous membrane.* Two main layers compose it: an outer, thinner layer, termed the **epidermis,** and an inner, thicker layer, termed the **dermis.**

The cellular epidermis is an epithelial layer derived from the ectodermal germ layer of the embryo. By the 17th week of gestation, the epidermis of the developing fetus has all the essential characteristics of the adult.[2]

The deeper dermis is a relatively dense and vascular connective tissue layer that may average just over 4 mm thick in some body areas.[3] The specialized area where the cells of the epidermis meet the connective tissue cells of the dermis is called the **dermoepidermal junction.**

Epidermis

The epidermis of the skin is composed of stratified squamous epithelium. "Thin skin," which covers most of the body surface, the outer epidermis is less than 0.17 mm thick (1/200th of an inch) in most areas.[4] Exceptions are body surfaces chronically exposed to pressure or friction, such as the soles of the feet and the palms of the hands, where the epidermis is appreciably thicker (1–1.3 mm).[5] Figure 52–1 shows regional variations in skin layers.

Cell Types

The epidermis consists of several types of epithelial cells. **Keratinocytes** are able to synthesize DNA and produce a tough, fibrous protein called **keratin.** Keratin is capable of absorbing vast quantities of water. This quality may be readily apparent after a long bath, when the skin of the palms and soles becomes white and swollen. Keratinocytes, arranged in distinct **strata,** or layers, are by far the most important cells in the epidermis. They comprise over 90 percent of the epidermal cells and form the principal structural element of the outer skin.[6] **Melanocytes** contribute color to the skin and serve to filter ultraviolet light. Although they may comprise over 5 percent of the epidermal cells, melanocytes may be completely absent from the skin in certain nonlethal conditions.[7] Another cell type, **Langerhans' cells,** are thought to play a limited role in immunologic reactions that affect the skin and may serve as a defense mechanism for the body. Research suggests that Langerhans' cells may serve as a possible source of prostaglandins.[8] **Merkel's cells** consist of free nerve endings attached to modified epidermal cells. Their origin remains unknown, and they are the least densely populated cells of the epidermis. It is generally agreed that Merkel's cells function as touch receptors.[9]

Cell Layers

Five layers define the epidermis over most of the body (Fig. 52–2). The outermost layer—the *stratum corneum,* or *horny layer*—is composed of flat, compact cells that have lost their nuclei. This layer, which may vary in thickness, is the skin's first line of defense.

The *stratum lucidum,* or *lucid layer,* is next and appears as a translucent line of flat cells. This layer of the skin is present only on the palms and the soles. The lucid layer and the granular layers make up the transitional layer of the epidermis and act as a barrier to the inward transfer of noxious substances and outward loss of water.

The third layer is the *stratum granulosum,* or *granular layer.* Here the cells are flatter and contain protein granules, called *keratohyaline granules.* Normal oral mucosa does not have a granular layer or horny layer.[10]

Fourth is the *stratum spinosum,* or *prickle cell layer.* Composed of upwardly migrating and maturing keratinocytes, this layer forms the bulk of the epidermis over most of the body.

Keratinocytes originate in the *stratum germinativum,* or *basal cell layer,* a line of cuboidal cells that marks the lowest boundary of the epidermis and divides it from the dermis.

TABLE 52–1. Functions of the Skin

Function	Epidermis	Dermis	Subcutaneous Tissue
Protection	Keratin provides protection from injury by corrosive materials Inhibits proliferation of microorganisms because of dry external surface Mechanical strength through intracellular bonds	Provides fibroblasts for wound healing Provides mechanical strength Collagen fibers Elastin fibers Ground substance Lymphatic and vascular tissues respond to inflammation, injury, and infection	Mechanical shock absorber
Homeostasis (water balance)	Low permeability to water and electrolytes prevents systemic dehydration and electrolyte loss		
Temperature regulation	The eccrine sweat glands allow dissipation of heat through evaporation of sweat secreted onto skin surface	Cutaneous vasculature, through dilation or constriction, promotes or inhibits heat conduction from skin surface	
Sensory organ	Transmits a variety of sensations through neuroreceptor system	Encloses extensive network of free and encapsulated nerve endings for relaying sensations to the brain	Contains large pressure receptors
Vitamin synthesis	7-Dehydrocholesterol present in large concentrations in malpighian cells; photoconversion to vitamin D takes place		
Psychosocial	Body image alterations result with many epidermal diseases, such as generalized psoriasis	Body image alterations seen with many dermal diseases, such as scleroderma	

From Rosen T, Lanning MB, Hill MJ: Cutaneous anatomy and physiology, in Rosen T, Lanning MB, Hill MJ (eds): *Nurse's Atlas of Dermatology.* Published by Little, Brown and Company, Boston, 1983, p 4. Reproduced with permission.

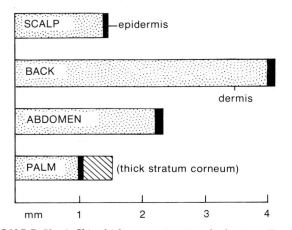

FIGURE 52–1. Skin thicknesses at various body sites. (From Jacob SW, Francone CA: *Elements of Anatomy and Physiology,* 2nd ed. Philadelphia, WB Saunders, 1989, p 38. Reproduced with permission.)

Pigmentation

Pigmentation in human skin is due to **melanin,** a chemical derivative of the amino acid tyrosine. Melanin is produced within melanocytes, which are specialized cells of neural origin. Pigment-producing melanocytes are also scattered along the basal layer.

Within the melanocytes are membrane-bound, enzyme-rich structures called melanosomes. These organelles are responsible for melanin synthesis. Melanocytes are situated along the basal cell layer of the epidermis. They extend branching outpouchings (dendrites) to encircle adjacent keratinocytes in the prickle cell layer (Fig. 52–3). The presence of melanin within the epidermis is necessary for protection against the adverse effects of ultraviolet radiation (exposure to the sun).

Epidermal melanocytes have an average density of about 1,500 to 1,600/mm, with regional variation.[11]

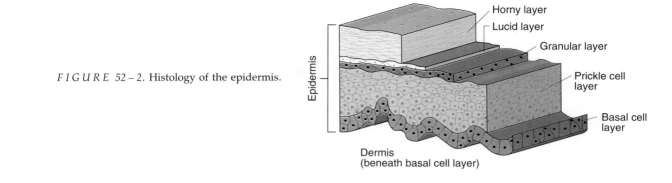

FIGURE 52–2. Histology of the epidermis.

Two to three times more melanocytes are found in forehead skin than in abdominal skin. There are no racial differences in the relative number of melanocytes: increased pigmentation in dark-skinned individuals is due to the presence of larger, more active melanocytes and melanosomes, which produce greater quantities of melanin. With advancing age, melanocytes may decrease in number, but the remaining melanocytes increase in size. Because of the smaller number of active melanocytes, aging skin appears paler and more translucent.

Control of melanocyte function is complex. Genes determine basic skin color by controlling the amount of melanin synthesized and deposited in the epidermis. But many other factors also play a role. Melanosomes (containing melanin) are transferred from melanocytes to keratinocytes and therein to the upper layers of the epidermis. Exposure to sunlight stimulates melanin production and melanosome transfer in the skin (suntan), as does low-grade cutaneous inflammation. Hormones such as melanocyte-stimulating hormone (MSH) from the pituitary gland promote pigment production. Estrogenic hormones (e.g., birth control pills or the hormonal production during pregnancy) may also stimulate melanin production, especially in sun-exposed areas such as the face (Fig. 52–4).

Growth and Repair

Turnover and *regeneration time* describe the time period required for a population of cells to mature and repro-

duce. As the surface cells of the stratum corneum are lost, replacement of keratinocytes by mitosis must occur. New cells must be formed at the same rate that old keratinized cells flake off from the stratum corneum to maintain a constant thickness of the epidermis. Cells push upward from the basal layer into each successive layer, die, become keratinized, and eventually desquamate (fall away), as did their predecessors.

Research suggests that the regeneration time required for the completion of mitosis, differentiation, and movement of new keratinocytes from the basal layer to the surface of the epidermis is about 3 or 4 weeks.[12] The process can be accelerated by abrasion of the skin surface, which tends to peel off a few of the cell layers of the stratum corneum. The result is an intense stimulation of mitotic activity in the basal layer and a shortened turnover period. If abrasion continues over a prolonged period of time, the increase in mitotic activity and shortened turnover time will result in an abnormally thick stratum corneum and the development of calluses at the point of friction or irritation. Although callus formation is a normal and protective response of the skin to friction, skin disease (i.e., psoriasis) is also characterized by an abnormally high mitotic activity in the epidermis (see Chap. 53). In psoriasis, the thickness of the corneum is dramatically increased. As a result, scales accumulate and skin lesions develop.

Normally about 10 percent to 12 percent of all cells in the basal layer enter mitosis each day.[13] Cells migrating to the surface proceed upward in vertical

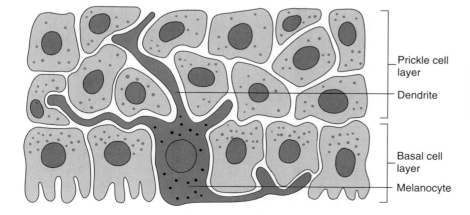

FIGURE 52–3. Melanocytes are located along the basal cell layer of the epidermis. Dendrites extend from melanocytes to encircle adjacent keratinocytes in the prickle cell layer.

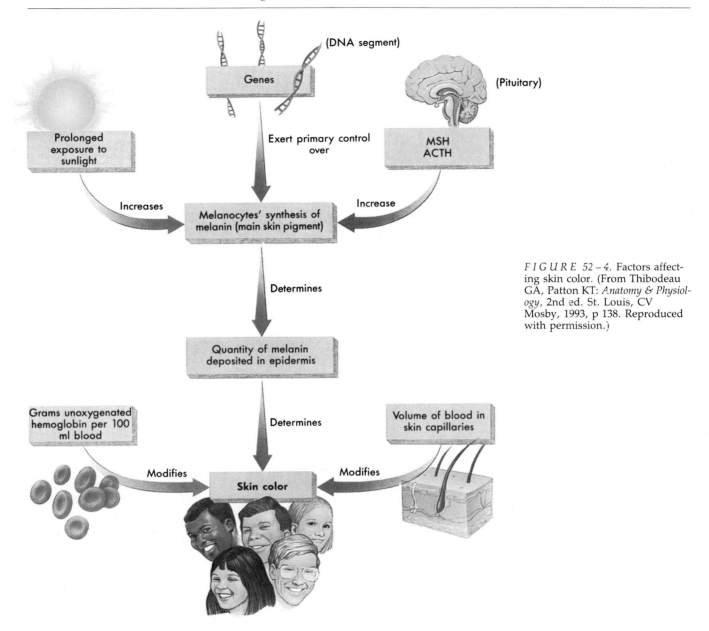

FIGURE 52–4. Factors affecting skin color. (From Thibodeau GA, Patton KT: *Anatomy & Physiology,* 2nd ed. St. Louis, CV Mosby, 1993, p 138. Reproduced with permission.)

columns from discrete groups of eight to ten of these basal cells that are undergoing mitosis. Each group of active basal cells, together with its vertical columns of migrating keratinocytes, is called an **epidermal proliferating unit** (EPU). Keratinization proceeds as the cells migrate toward the stratum corneum. As mitosis continues and new basal cells enter the column and migrate upward, fully cornified "dead" cells are sloughed off at the skin surface (Fig. 52–5).

Surface Film

The ability of the skin to act as a protective barrier against environmental influences is also due, in no small measure, to the proper functioning of a thin film of emulsified material spread over its surface. **Surface film** is produced by the mixing of residue and secretions from sweat and sebaceous glands with the epithelial cells that are constantly being cast off from the epidermis. The shedding of epithelial elements from the skin surface is called **desquamation.**

The functions of surface film include antibacterial and antifungal activity, lubrication, hydration of the skin surface, buffering of caustic irritants, and blockade of many toxic agents.

The chemical composition of the surface film includes amino acids, sterols, and complex phospholipids from the breakdown of sloughed epithelial cells; fatty acids, triglycerides, and waxes from sebum; and water, ammonia, lactic acid, urea, and uric acid from sweat.[14]

The specific chemical composition of surface film varies considerably; samples taken from skin covering one body area will often have a completely different

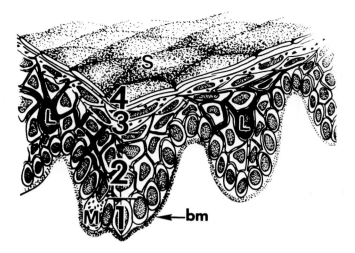

FIGURE 52–5. Cells composing normal epidermis. The majority are keratinocytes that undergo progressive upward maturation from ovoid cells of the basal layer cell (1) that rest on the basement membrane (BM), to more polyhedral stratum spinosum cells (2), then to flattened stratum granulosum (granular) cells (3), and finally to anucleate cells of the epidermal surface(s), the stratum corneum (4). Dendritic melanocytes (M) and Langerhans' cells (L) are interspersed in relatively low numbers within the epidermal layer. (From Murphy GF, Mihm MC: The skin, in Cotran RS, Kumar V, Robbins SL (eds): *Robbins Pathologic Basis of Disease,* 4th ed. Philadelphia, WB Saunders, 1989, p 1278. Reproduced with permission.)

composition from film covering skin in another area. This difference helps explain the unique and localized distribution patterns of certain skin diseases (discussed in Chap. 53) and why the skin covering one area of the body is sometimes more susceptible to attack by certain bacteria or fungi.

Dermoepidermal Junction

Electron microscopy and histochemical studies of the skin have demonstrated the existence of a gel-like amorphous matrix that serves to cement the superficial epidermis to the dermis below. This specialized junction functions to "glue" the two layers together and to provide a mechanical support for the epidermis, which is attached to its upper surface. It serves as a partial barrier to the passage of some cells and large molecules such as dyes and certain chemicals, and prevents separation of the two skin layers, even when they are subjected to relatively high shear forces. Nevertheless, the dermoepidermal junction is thought to play only a limited role in preventing passage of harmful disease-causing organisms through the skin from the external environment.[15]

Dermis

Under the basal layer of the epidermis lies the **dermis.** Composed mainly of collagen, it gives the skin its strength. In addition to protecting against mechanical injury and compression, this layer of the skin provides a reservoir for water and important electrolytes. A specialized network of nerves and nerve endings in the dermis also processes sensory information such as pain, pressure, touch, and temperature. At various levels of the dermis, there are muscle fibers, hair follicles, sweat and sebaceous glands, and many blood vessels (Fig. 52–6). The rich vascular supply of the dermis plays a critical role in regulation of body temperature.

Cell Types

The cells of the dermis are of three groups—a *reticulohistiocytic group,* a *myeloid group,* and a *lymphoid group.*[16] Under pathologic conditions, the potentiality of these cells can change.

The reticulohistiocytic group consist of fibroblasts, histiocytes, and mast cells. Immature cells of the reticulohistiocytic group are called reticulum cells.

Fibroblasts form collagen fibers, which compose the bulk of the dermis. Fibroblasts may be the progenitors of all other connective tissue cells. **Histiocytes** normally are present in small numbers around blood vessels, but in pathologic conditions they can migrate in the dermis as tissue monocytes. They can also form abundant reticulum fibers. When they phagocytize bacteria and particulate matter, they are known as macrophages.

Histiocytes, under special pathologic conditions, can also change into epithelioid cells, which in turn can develop into so-called giant cells. **Mast cells** are also called histiocytic cells. Mast cells have intracytoplasmic basophilic metachromatic granules containing heparin and histamine.[17] The normal skin contains relatively few mast cells, but their number is increased in many different skin conditions, particularly the itching dermatoses.

Plasma cells, rarely seen in normal skin secretions, occur in small numbers in most chronic inflammatory diseases of the skin and in larger numbers in granulomas. The origin of plasma cells is unknown, but they are thought to arise from reticulum cells.

In the myeloid group of cells, the **polymorphonuclear leukocyte** (PMN) and the **eosinophilic leukocyte** occur quite commonly with various dermatoses, especially those with an allergic etiology.[18]

In the lymphoid group, the **lymphocyte** is commonly found in inflammatory lesions of the skin. The myeloid and the lymphoid groups of cells are also found in specific neoplasms of the skin.[19]

Cell Layers

The dermis, or corium, is sometimes called the true skin. It is composed of a thin papillary layer and a thicker reticular layer. The **papillary layer** is made of bumps (papillae) that project into the epidermis (see Fig. 52–6). Papillae are made essentially of loose connective tissue elements and a fine network of thin collagenous and elastic fibers. The thin epidermal layer of the skin conforms tightly to the ridges of

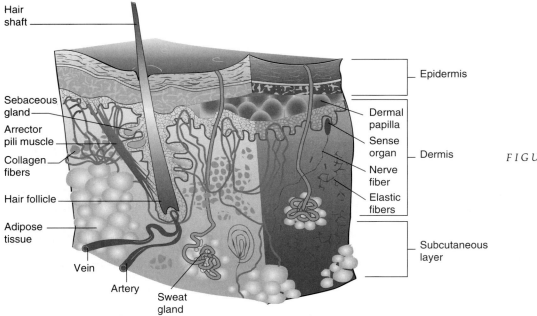

Hair
shaft

Sebaceous
gland

Arrector
pili muscle

Collagen
fibers

Hair follicle

Adipose
tissue

Vein

Artery

Sweat
gland

Epidermis

Dermal
papilla

Sense
organ

Nerve
fiber

Elastic
fibers

Dermis

Subcutaneous
layer

FIGURE 52–6. Dermis.

dermal papillae. As a result, the epidermis also has characteristic ridges on its surface. Epidermal ridges are especially well defined on the tips of the fingers and toes.

The thick **reticular layer** of the dermis consists of a more dense reticulum (network) of fibers than the papillary layer above it. The reticular layer is made of collagen and elastin and contains skeletal (voluntary) and smooth (involuntary) muscle fibers.

Growth and Repair

Unlike the epidermis, the dermis does not continually shed and regenerate itself. It does maintain itself, but rapid degeneration of connective tissue in the dermis occurs only during unusual circumstances, as in the healing of wounds (Fig. 52–7).

Wound healing is a dynamic process by which the body repairs damage or creates a new covering for the damaged area—a scar. Following injury, a blood clot forms. At the same time, the intact blood vessels undergo a reflex vasodilation that allows plasma to leak into the injured area.[20]

Within several hours of injury, dermal cells start to migrate into the area, beginning with PMNs. These cells are the first line of defense against bacteria and debris. The second important cell type in wound healing is the monocyte. These cells aid in phagocytizing bacteria and debris and release certain substances that stimulate fibroblastic activity and angiogenesis.[21]

Within a day of wounding, reepithelization begins. Epithelial cells from the surrounding non-wounded skin as well as from any remaining adnexal structures move into the wound. When the migration of epithelial cells is completed, the base of the wound has been covered by a moist layer under the clot. Then they resume their normal upward proliferation and differentiation into normal keratinocytes.[22]

During reepithelialization, healing progresses within the dermis. Proliferating fibroblasts start to synthesize collagen and restore strength to the tissue. After 10 to 14 days of collagen production, remodeling and strengthening of the scar begins. This process is generally completed after 6 months.

Wound contraction, beginning several days after the initial wound, decreases the diameter of the wound. The process is assisted by the myofibroblasts.[23]

In the healing of a wound such as a surgical incision, fibroblasts in the dermis quickly reproduce and begin forming an unusually dense mass of new connective tissue fibers. If this dense mass is not replaced by normal tissue, it remains as a scar.

The dense bundles of white collagenous fibers that characterize the reticular layer of the dermis tend to orient themselves in patterns that differ in appearance from one body area to another. The result is formation of patterns called Langer's lines, or cleavage lines (Fig. 52–8).[24] If surgical incisions are made parallel to the cleavage lines, the resulting wound will have less tendency to gape open and will tend to heal with a thinner and less noticeable scar.

The rate at which wound healing takes place depends on several factors other than those directly associated with the process of healing. Good oxygenation in tissue promotes healing.[25] Several vitamins, mainly C, A, K, and B, have also been shown to play a role in enhancing wound healing.

On the other hand, infection, hypothermia, protein deficiency, and diabetes impair healing.[26] Delayed healing in an elderly person may be due to factors such as circulatory changes, a poor nutritional state, or lowered resistance to infection.

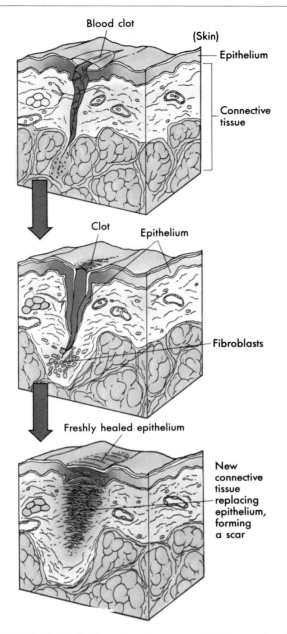

FIGURE 52–7. Healing of a minor wound. When a minor injury damages a layer of epithelium and the underlying connective tissue (as in a minor skin cut), both the epithelial tissue and the connective tissue can repair itself. (From Thibodeau GA, Patton KT: *Anatomy & Physiology*, 2nd ed. St. Louis, CV Mosby, 1993, p 119. Reproduced with permission.)

If the elastic fibers in the dermis are stretched too much—for example, by a rapid increase in the size of the abdomen during pregnancy or as a result of obesity—they will weaken and tear. The initial result is formation of pinkish or slightly bluish depressed furrows with jagged edges. These tiny linear markings (stretch marks) are really tiny tears. When they heal and lose their color, the striae (furrows) that remain appear as glistening, silver-white scar lines.

Subcutaneous Tissue

Beneath the dermis lies a loose subcutaneous layer rich in fat and areolar tissue. It is sometimes called the **hypodermis,** or **superficial fascia.** The fat content of the hypodermis varies with the state of nutrition and in obese individuals may exceed 10 cm in thickness in certain areas.[27] The density and arrangement of fat cells and collagen fibers in this area determine the relative mobility of the skin. Deeper hair follicles and the sweat glands originate in this layer.

Although the subcutaneous layer is not part of the skin itself, it serves as a receptacle for the formation and storage of fat, is a locus of highly dynamic lipid metabolism, and supports the blood vessels and the nerves that pass from the tissues beneath to the dermis above.

The epidermis, dermis, and subcutaneous tissue layers are also supported by an underlying network of collagen fibers and associated elastin fibers. The collagen fibers attach the skin to the underlying tissues and the elastin fibers give the skin flexibility, elasticity, and strength.

Vascular and Neural Supply

Vessels

A continuous meshwork of arteries and veins perforates the subcutaneous tissues and extends into the dermis. Blood vessels of varying sizes are present in all levels and all planes of the skin tissue and appendages. In fact, the vascularization is so intensive that it has been suggested that its primary function is to regulate heat and blood pressure of the body, with the nutrition of the skin as a secondary function.[28,29]

Nerves

The nerve supply of the skin consists of sensory nerves and motor nerves.

Sensory Nerves. Millions of specialized nerve endings called *receptors* are located in the dermis of all skin areas. They permit the skin to serve as a sense organ, transmitting sensations of pain, pressure, touch, and temperature. Millions of terminal nerve endings function to specify skin sensation.

Itching is one of the most important dermal sensations and is actually a mild pain experience that differs from pain in having a lower impulse frequency.[30] The release of proteinases may be responsible for the sensation.[31] Itching may range on a continuum from prickling to burning and can vary in intensity from individual to individual. One authority has suggested that abnormally sensitive persons may be termed "itchish," analogous to the term "ticklish."[32] Itching can occur with or without clinical manifestations of skin disease, or from circulating allergens, or from local superficial contactants.

Motor Nerves. Involuntary sympathetic motor nerves control the sweat glands, the arterioles, and the smooth muscles of the skin. Each hair follicle has

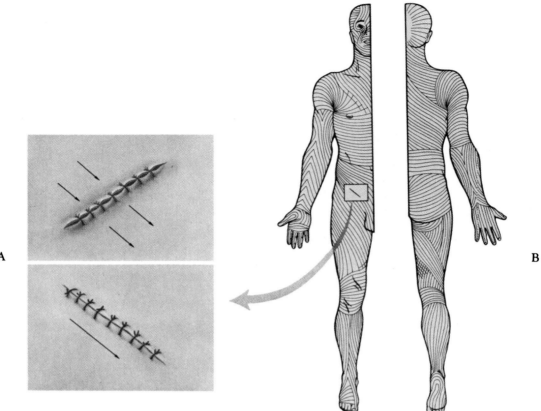

FIGURE 52–8. Langer's cleavage lines. **A,** If an incision cuts across cleavage lines, stress tends to pull the cut edges apart and may retard healing. **B,** Surgical incisions that are parallel to cleavage lines are subjected to less stress and tend to heal more rapidly. (From Thibodeau GA, Patton KT: *Anatomy & Physiology,* 2nd ed. St. Louis, CV Mosby, 1993, p 137. Reproduced with permission.)

a small bundle of involuntary muscles attached to it. Adrenergic fibers carry impulses to the arrectores pilorum muscles, which produce "goose bumps" when they are stimulated. This is due to traction of the muscle on the hair follicles to which it is attached.

In the dermis of the scrotum and in the pigmented skin called the areolae surrounding the nipples, smooth muscle cells form a loose network. Contraction of these smooth muscle cells will wrinkle the skin and cause elevation of the testes or erection of the nipples.

Appendages of the Skin

Hair, nails, and sweat glands are considered to be appendages of the skin. All of the appendages are derived from specialized cells of the epidermis and receive essential nutrients and innervation from the dermis.

Hair

Hair is composed of tightly fused keratinized epidermal cells. Layers of the hair may be depicted schematically (Fig. 52–9). Since no new hair follicles are formed

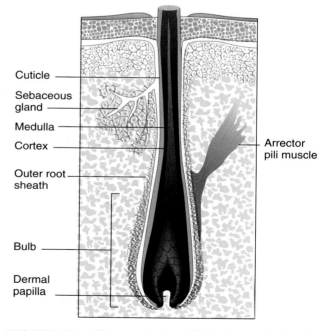

Cuticle

Sebaceous gland

Medulla

Cortex

Outer root sheath

Bulb

Dermal papilla

Arrector pili muscle

FIGURE 52–9. Diagram of a hair follicle showing layers of the hair schematically.

after birth, the different types of body hairs are manifestations of the effect of location and of internal and external stimuli.[33] Hair is found on all body surfaces except the palms and soles.

Types of Hair. There are two main types of hair, *terminal* and *vellus.* *Terminal* hairs are long, coarse, thick, and visible. The *vellus* hairs are tiny and almost unnoticeable (Fig. 52–10). Terminal hair is easily visible on the scalp, beard, moustache, axillae, and pubis. By comparison, vellus hair—downy or lanugo hair—is only visible on close inspection. It covers the whole body, except on the palms and soles.

Distribution of Hair. The distribution of hair over the body warrants careful observation. Scalp hair, eyebrows, eyelashes, and downy hair of the body are present in both sexes. After puberty, coarse body hair located in the axillary and genital areas, evolves in distinct male and female patterns (Fig. 52–11).

Hair Growth. Hormones are the most important internal stimulus influencing the various types of hair growth. Hair goes through two main phases, the *anagen,* or growing phase, and the *telogen,* or resting phase. Hair in different regions of the body has a different growth cycle. Scalp hair grows about 2 mm weekly, and the growing phase of any one hair is 2 to 3 years.[34] Resting hairs make up 5 to 15 percent of the total of 100,000 hairs on the human scalp.[35] The resting phase occurs every few months to a few years.[36] Terminal hairs elsewhere on the body have a shorter growing phase than those on the scalp.

Because hair is an adornment for many men and women, its loss or excess often provokes embarrassment and anxiety and conflicts with the person's self-image of masculinity or femininity. Awareness and sensitivity to this issue are important.

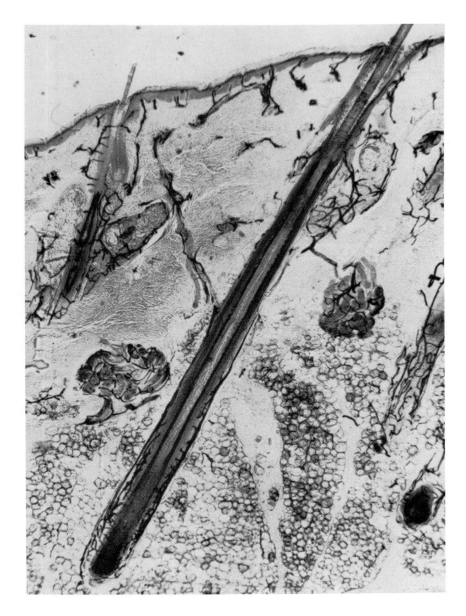

FIGURE 52–10. Thick, frozen section of skin from the scalp of a 12-year-old boy, with a vellus follicle on the left and a terminal follicle on the right. The preparation has been treated with alkaline phosphatase staining to show blood vessels. (From Montagna W, Parakkal PF: *The Structure and Function of Skin,* 3rd ed. New York, Academic Press, 1974, p 246. Reproduced with permission.)

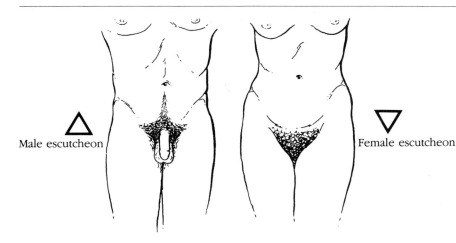

F I G U R E 52 – 11. Normal hair distribution in adult men and women. Changes may signal hormonal abnormalities. (From Judge RD, Zuidema GD, Fitzgerald FT (eds): *Clinical Diagnosis: A Physiologic Approach*, 4th ed. Published by Little, Brown and Company, Boston, 1982, p 37. Reproduced with permission.)

The normal scalp sheds about 20 to 100 hairs per day.[37] To determine whether any complaints of hair loss are noteworthy, instruct the concerned party to collect and count the hairs on a comb or hairbrush the day before washing the head, after washing, and on 2 succeeding days—4 days in all. An average daily loss of over 100 hairs is abnormal.[37]

Lubrication. Another pertinent feature relating to the hair is its amount of lubrication. Sebum from sebaceous glands anoints the hair and keeps it from drying and becoming brittle by limiting the amount of absorption and evaporation of water from the surface. The sebaceous glands are most numerous over the face and scalp. Assessing these areas gives the best indication regarding the amount of skin oiliness.

Nails

Nails are specialized epidermal structures composed of keratinized cells cemented together. The visible part of each nail is called the nail body. The rest of the nail, namely the root, lies in a groove hidden by a fold of skin called the cuticle. The nail body nearest the root has a crescent-shaped white area known as the lunula, or "little moon." Under the nail lies a layer of epithelium called the nail bed. Because it contains abundant blood vessels, it appears pink in color through the translucent nail bodies (Fig. 52–12).

Normal fingernails grow about 0.1 mm per day, while toenails grow approximately 0.05 mm per day.[38] Like hair, nails grow more rapidly during the warmer months of the year and more slowly with advancing age.

Normal nails are transparent, with pink nail beds and translucent white tips at the point of separation of the nail from the nail bed. Surface longitudinal ridges and flecks of white spots in the nail are within normal limits.

Glands

Three types of glands arise from specialized invaginations of the epidermis: **sebaceous** (oil), **apocrine sweat,** and **eccrine sweat glands.** Sebaceous and apocrine sweat glands discharge their products onto the skin through the **hair follicle** (hair pore), whereas the eccrine sweat glands open directly onto the skin surface (Fig. 52–13).

Sebaceous Glands. **Sebaceous glands** are most numerous on the face, scalp, upper chest, and back; they are sparse on the extremities and absent on the palms and soles. Despite their presence in profuse numbers,

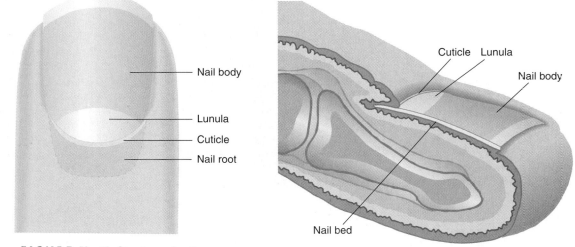

FIGURE 52 – 12. Structure of nails.

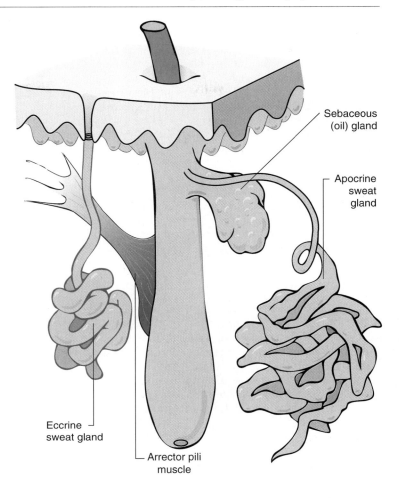

FIGURE 52–13. Relationship of hair follicle, eccrine and apocrine sweat glands, and sebaceous glands.

Sebaceous (oil) gland

Apocrine sweat gland

Eccrine sweat gland

Arrector pili muscle

sebaceous glands are not grossly visible except when they occur in aberrant clusters on the oral mucosa. Sebaceous glands produce a constant, imperceptible flow of a complex lipid mixture known as *sebum* onto the skin surface, which acts as a lubricant. The secretion of sebaceous glands is hormone (androgen) dependent.

Apocrine Sweat Glands. **Apocrine sweat glands** are located deep in the subcutaneous layer of the skin in the armpit (axilla), the areola of the breast, and the pigmented skin areas around the anus. They are much larger than eccrine glands and often have secretory units that reach 5 mm or more in diameter.[39] They are connected with hair follicles and are classified as simple, branched tubular glands. Apocrine glands enlarge and begin to function at puberty, producing a more viscous and colored secretion than eccrine glands. In the female, apocrine gland secretions show cyclic changes that are linked to the menstrual cycle. Odor, often associated with apocrine gland secretion, is not caused by the secretion itself. Rather, odor is caused by contamination and decomposition of the secretion by skin bacteria.

Ceruminous Glands. **Ceruminous glands** are a special variety or modification of apocrine sweat glands. Histologically they appear as simple coiled tubular glands with excretory ducts that open onto the free surface of the skin in the external ear canal or with sebaceous glands into the necks of hair follicles in this area. The mixed secretions of sebaceous and ceruminous glands form a brown waxy substance called **cerumen.** Although it serves a useful purpose in protecting the skin of the ear canal from dehydration, excess cerumen can harden and cause blockage in the ear, resulting in loss of hearing. This can be especially problematic in the elderly.

Eccrine Sweat Glands. By far the most numerous, important, and widespread sweat glands in the body, **eccrine sweat glands** are quite small, with a secretory portion less than 0.4 mm in diameter.[40] Eccrine sweat glands are distributed over the total body surface with the exception of the lips, ear canal, glans penis, and nail beds. Eccrine sweat glands are a simple coiled tubular type of gland. They function throughout life to produce a transparent watery liquid (perspiration, or sweat) rich in salts, ammonia, uric acid, urea, and other wastes. In addition to elimination of waste, sweat plays a critical role in helping the body maintain a constant core temperature. Histologists estimate that a single square inch of skin on the palms of the hands contains about 3,000 sweat glands.[41] Eccrine sweat glands are also very numerous on the soles of the feet, forehead, and upper torso.

Regulation of Body Temperature

Regulation of body temperature is important for maintenance of health and homeostasis. To maintain an even temperature, the body must balance heat loss with gain. If this does not occur, if increased heat loss does not closely follow increased heat production, body temperature will climb steadily upward.

If body temperature *increases* above normal for any reason, the skin plays a critical role in restoring normalcy. Blood vessels in the dermis dilate and sweat secretion increases. More heat is therefore lost by radiation from the larger volume of blood in the skin and by evaporation of sweat on the skin's surface. Together these changes return blood temperature back to its normal level.

If blood temperature *decreases* below normal, skin blood vessels constrict and sweat secretion decreases. The physical phenomena of evaporation, radiation, conduction, and convection help explain the skin's ability to regulate temperature.

Evaporation

Evaporation of water is one method by which heat is lost from the skin. Evaporation, or the change from liquid form to vapor, is significant at high environmental temperatures when it is the only method by which heat can be lost from the skin.

A humid atmosphere slows the process of evaporation and therefore lessens its cooling effect—the reason why the same degree of temperature seems hotter in humid climates than in dry ones. At moderate temperatures, evaporation accounts for about half as much heat loss as does radiation.

Radiation

Radiation is the transfer of heat through space or matter from the surface of one object to that of another without actual contact between the two. Heat radiates from the body surface to nearby objects that are cooler than the skin, and radiates to the skin from objects that are warmer than the skin. This explains the principle of heating and cooling systems. In cool environmental temperatures, radiation accounts for a greater percentage of heat loss from the skin than both conduction and evaporation combined. However, in hot environments, no heat is lost by radiation but instead may be gained by radiation from warmer surfaces to the skin.

Conduction

Conduction means the transfer of heat to any substance actually in contact with the body, such as clothing or jewelry, or even cold foods or liquids that have been ingested. Cool compresses applied to the skin can enhance heat loss by conduction.

Convection

Convection is the transfer of heat away from a surface by movement of heated air or fluid particles. Usually convection causes very little heat loss from the body's surface. But, under certain conditions, it can account for considerable heat loss, such as when one steps from a warm bath into slightly moving air from an open window or electric fan.

KEY CONCEPTS

- Skin consists of two layers, an outer epidermal layer and a deeper dermal layer. A subcutaneous tissue layer lies under the skin and supports blood and nerve supply to the skin. Accessory structures of the dermis include hair follicles, nails, and glands.
- The epidermis is composed of stratified squamous epithelial cells. Keratinocytes are the predominant cell type; they produce the tough structural protein keratin. Keratinocytes develop in the basal cell layer and migrate to the outer layers of the skin as they mature. The outermost region of the epidermis consists of old cells that have lost their nuclei. These cells continuously flake away as new cells migrate upward. The epidermis also contains small numbers of melanocytes, which manufacture pigment (melanin) important for filtering ultraviolet light. Small numbers of immune cells and sensory touch receptors are present in the epidermis.
- The skin surface is covered by a surface film composed of old epithelial cells, sweat, sebum, and other chemicals. The composition of the surface film varies with body location. It functions to keep skin from drying and has antimicrobial properties.
- The cellular elements of the dermis include various immune cells (histiocytes, granulocytes, lymphocytes, mast cells) and fibroblasts, which produce collagen, the primary component of dermis. The dermis is an important line of defense against microbial invasion and an important structure for cutaneous wound healing.
- The skin is supplied with an extensive capillary network, far exceeding that required to meet nutritive needs. A primary function of the skin blood flow is to regulate body temperature. Skin is also richly innervated with sensory afferent fibers and sympathetic efferent fibers. Sympathetic fibers regulate skin blood flow, sweat glands, and piloerection.
- Hair distribution and growth rate are a reflection of hormonal regulation and the adequacy of perfusion and nutrition of hair follicles. Poor perfusion is often accompanied by hair loss.
- Three types of glands are distributed within the skin: (1) oil-secreting sebaceous glands, (2) sweat-producing apocrine glands in hair follicles, and (3) sweat-producing eccrine glands. Sebaceous glands are stimulated to produce oil by androgenic hormones. Apocrine glands lubricate hair shafts and produce ear wax (cerumen). Eccrine sweat glands are numerous and widely distributed. Sweating eliminates wastes and plays an important role in temperature regulation.
- The skin plays a critical role in body temperature regulation. Alteration of skin blood flow can con-

serve heat (constriction) or dissipate heat (dilation) through altering radiant, convective, and conductive heat loss. Evaporative heat loss can be increased significantly by sympathetically mediated increases in eccrine gland secretion.

Age-Related Changes

The skin undergoes dramatic changes from birth through the mature years. Healthy infants and young children have relatively smooth and unwrinkled skin characterized by elasticity and flexibility. Because skin tissues are in an active phase of new growth, healing of skin injuries is often rapid and efficient. Young children and elderly persons have fewer sweat glands than adults, so their bodies rely more on increased blood flow to maintain a normal body temperature.

As adulthood begins, at puberty, hormones stimulate the development and activation of sebaceous glands and sweat glands. After the sebaceous glands become active, especially during the initial years, they may overproduce sebum and thus give the skin an unusually oily appearance. Sebaceous ducts may become clogged or infected and form acne pimples or other blemishes on the skin. Activation of apocrine sweat glands during puberty causes increased sweat production—an ability needed to maintain an adult body properly—and also the possibility of increased "body odor." Body odor is caused by wastes produced by bacteria that feed on the organic compounds found in apocrine sweat and on the surface of the skin.

Past early adulthood and into middle age, the sebaceous and sweat glands become less active. Although this can provide a relief to those who suffer from acne or other problems associated with overactivity of these glands, it can affect the normal function of the body. For example, the reduction in sebum production can cause the skin and hair to become less resilient.

Changes in the appearance and function of the skin, perhaps more than in any other organ, reflect the continual aging process. One need only look at a person to determine an approximate age. Evidence of advancing age includes wrinkles, sagging skin, gray hair, and baldness. Aging changes are also linked to environmental influences, genetic makeup, and other bodily changes.

Exposure to sunlight is one of the greatest factors in age-related skin changes.[42] The result of such exposure can be seen in people who work outdoors in sunlight. Results are also evident when skin exposed to sunlight is compared with nonexposed skin. Skin that is usually covered shows little change with age. Blue-eyed, fair-skinned individuals are more susceptible to solar skin damage than people with darker, more heavily pigmented skin.

Epidermis

The epidermis shows a generalized thinning with advancing age, although there may be some thickening in sun-exposed areas. Although there is an increased variation in epidermal thickness, the average number of cell layers remains unchanged. The prickle cells of the inner layer of the epidermis show greater variation in nuclear and cytoplasmic size with a less orderly arrangement of cells.[43] Cells reproduce more slowly and are larger and more irregular; however, exposed epidermal cells may divide more frequently than unexposed cells.[44]

Dermis and Subcutaneous Tissue

The dermis contains blood vessels, nerves, hair follicles, and sebaceous glands, but the major portion is made up of collagen and elastin. The elasticity of the skin is largely due to dermal elastin. Decreased skin strength and elasticity with aging are attributed to a decreased amount of elastin and a proportionate increase in the collagen : elastin ratio. Collagen fibers change with age, becoming cross-linked and rearranged into thicker bundles. This condition is called *elastosis* and is closely associated with exposure to sunlight (*solar elastosis*). It produces a weather-beaten or tanned appearance.

Aging also produces a decrease in the vascularity of the dermal skin, as evidenced by decreasing numbers of epithelial cells and blood vessels. There is greater vascular fragility, leading to the frequent appearance of hemorrhages (senile purpura), cherry angiomas, venous stasis, and venous lakes on the ears, face, lips, and neck. The decreased vascularity and circulation in the dermis and the underlying subcutaneous tissue also has an effect on drug absorption. Drugs administered subcutaneously are absorbed more slowly, thus prolonging their half-life. The amount of subcutaneous fat tissue also decreases, especially in the extremities, so that arms and legs appear to be thinner.

Broadly speaking, with advancing age, the skin becomes folded, lined, and wrinkled and has diminished ability to maintain body temperature and homeostasis.

Appendages

Hair

The most obvious change in aging hair is its color. Half of the population over age 50 has at least 50 percent gray body hair, regardless of sex or hair color.[45] Gray hair is determined by an autosomal dominant gene and results from a decreased rate of melanin production by the hair follicle. Hair color generally darkens with age, but this process is reversed with the onset of graying. Graying usually begins at the temples of the head and extends to the vertex of the scalp. It may not occur in the axilla, especially in women, and occurs to a lesser extent in the presternum, or pubis.

Changes in hair growth and distribution are also associated with aging. The amount and distribution of hair are determined by racial, genetic, and sex-linked factors; however, almost all older people have a diminution of body hair except on the face. Adults develop a full terminal hair pattern by age 40, and this is followed by a progressive loss of hair in reverse order of development.[46] Postmenopausal white women lose trunk hair first, then pubic and axillary hair. Unopposed adrenal androgens produce coarse facial hair in 50 percent of white women over 60, especially on the chin and around the lips.[47]

While men also show a general thinning of hair distribution, with the hairs of the eyebrows, ears, and nose become longer and coarser. Baldness is often a concern, particularly in aging men, although women also tend to show some thinning of scalp hair. Frontal recession of the hairline occurs in 80 percent of older women and 100 percent of older men.[48] Baldness in men is inherited from the mother and occurs only in the presence of testosterone. Onset is variable and is manifested by an M-shaped pattern of hair loss on either side of the midline or by a thinning patch over the vertex.

In general, both men and women change from darker, thicker, more numerous hairs to lighter, thinner, and less numerous hairs with aging. Hair changes begin in midlife and become highly noticeable in later life, especially after age 60. Women seem to manifest more hair loss on the trunk and extremities, while men have greater hair loss on the head.

Nails

With aging, nails become dull, brittle, hard, and thick. Most nail changes are due to a diminished vascular supply to the nail bed. There is approximately a 30 to 50 percent decrease in the growth rate of fingernails, from 0.1 mm per day in 30-year-olds to 0.07 mm per day in 90-year-olds.[49] Aging nails show an increase in longitudinal striations, which can cause splitting of the nail surface.

Toenails are particularly prone to thickening, perhaps as a result of constant trauma and pressure from shoe coverings.

Glands

Sebaceous glands show little atrophy or histologic change with age; however, their function tends to diminish, as evidenced by a decrease in sebum secretion. In men the decrease is minimal, but in women there is a gradual diminution in sebum secretion after menopause with no significant changes after the seventh decade. There are fewer sebaceous glands in older people, which appears related to the loss of hair follicles. The decrease in sebum secretion and in the number of sebaceous glands results in the dryer, coarser skin associated with aging.

Sweat glands generally decrease in size, number, and function with age. In the eccrine glands, the secretory epithelial cells become uneven in size, ranging from normal to small, and there is a progressive accumulation of lipofuscin in the cytoplasm.[50] In the very

old, the secretory coils of many eccrine glands are replaced by fibrous tissue, which drastically diminishes their capacity to produce sweat. The thermal threshold for sweating is raised, so that the amount of sweat output at a body temperature of 38°C decreases.[51] This may be due to the fact that there are fewer blood vessels and nerve cells around the glands that enable the body to respond to temperature changes. Apocrine glands do not decrease in number or size, but they do decrease in function. An accumulation of lipofuscin has also been noted in apocrine glands. The diminished functioning of sweat glands in the elderly greatly impairs the ability to maintain body temperature homeostasis.

Table 52–2 summarizes the morphologic features of aging human skin, and Figure 52–14 summarizes the histologic changes associated with aging in normal human skin.

KEY CONCEPTS

- The glandular function of skin varies considerably with age. Young children and elderly adults have fewer functional sweat glands and therefore less efficient evaporative heat loss capabilities. Sebaceous glands are particularly active during puberty, predisposing to acne, then become less active with age, predisposing to dry skin.
- The epidermis and dermis undergo degenerative changes with aging. The epidermis thins, the dermis becomes less elastic and less vascular. Subcutaneous fat decreases. Exposure to sunlight is an important factor in the development of aged skin.
- Graying of hair results from decreased melanin production by the hair follicle. After age 40, progressive hair loss occurs. Male pattern balding is an inherited trait that is mediated by testosterone.

Evaluation of the Integumentary System

A careful history and evaluation of the skin should focus on the age of the individual, past conditions

TABLE 52–2. Morphologic Features of Aging Human Skin

Epidermis	Dermis	Appendages
Flat dermoepidermal junction	Atrophy	Graying of hair
Variable thickness	Fewer fibroblasts	Loss of hair
Variable cell size and shape	Fewer blood vessels	Conversion of terminal to vellus hair
Occasional nuclear atypia	Shortened capillary loops	Abnormal nail plates
Loss of melanocytes	Abnormal nerve endings	Fewer glands

From Gilchrest BA: Skin, in Rowe JW, Besdine RW (eds): *Health and Disease in Old Age.* Published by Little, Brown and Company, Boston, 1982, p 383. Reproduced with permission.

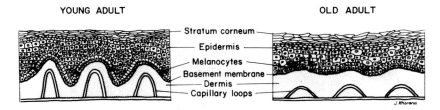

FIGURE 52 – 14. Histologic changes associated with aging in normal human skin. Note flattening of the dermoepidermal junction and shortening of capillary loops in older skin. Variability in size and shape of epidermal cells, irregular stratum corneum, and loss of melanocytes are also apparent. Age-associated loss of dermal thickness and subcutaneous fat is not shown, since the diagram includes only the epidermis and superficial or papillary dermis. (From Gilchrest BA: Skin, in Rowe JW, Besdine RW (eds): *Health and Disease in Old Age.* Published by Little, Brown and Company, Boston, 1982, p 383. Reproduced with permission.)

and systemic diseases, drug use, nutrition, conditions of the environment, the color, temperature, texture, and thickness of the skin, and any lesions or abnormalities. The essential elements of a skin assessment are described in Table 52–3.

Careful visual *inspection* of the skin yields valuable information about general health. *Palpation* is used

TABLE 52 – 3. Skin Assessment

History

Past and present *skin conditions:*
 Onset, development, pattern, duration, symptoms
Past and present *systemic diseases:*
 History and treatment
Drug history:
 Topical, systemic, prescription, nonprescription, allergies
Nutrition:
 Malnourished, obese, diet and eating habits
Functional status:
 Mobility, mental status, activities of daily living capacity
Environment:
 Physical (temperature, climate, use of soaps or other drying agents)
 Social (support systems, work, family interactions)

Physical Assessment

Color:
 Red, jaundiced, brown, gray, cyanotic, pale, blotchy
Temperature:
 Hot, warm, cool
Moisture:
 Dry, oily, or combination of both; moist, clammy
Texture:
 Rough, smooth, scaly, flaky
Edema:
 Location, extent
Thickness:
 Differences among various parts of the body, relationship to itching or redness
Mobility and turgor:
 Supple, pliable, flexible, creases and folds
Lesions:
 Color, size, texture, identifying characteristics, distribution
Hair:
 Amount, distribution, texture, color, dandruff or scaling, odor
Nails:
 Color, length, cleanliness, thickness, splitting, swelling, accumulations

---

Data from Bates B: *Guide to Physical Examination and History Taking,* 5th ed. Philadelphia, JB Lippincott, 1991.

to validate further the data that are gathered from inspection and to ascertain other qualities such as texture, temperature, hydration, and turgor.

Texture

The character of the skin's surface (i.e., fineness, coarseness) and the feel of deeper portions are its texture. The presence or absence of such textures as rough, dry, smooth, or velvety is best ascertained by stroking the volar surface of the forearm with the dorsal side of the fingers.

Temperature

Although skin temperature is an inadequate measure of the body's internal temperature, it gives valuable information about the patient's functional status.

Of the total body heat produced, 85 percent is lost through the skin by conduction, convection, radiation, and evaporation.[52] Cooling of the body by evaporation, through sweating, is of various types and has many etiologies. Identification of the type of sweating often helps in differentiating normal from abnormal body functioning. The eccrine sweat glands, which are found over the entire body, respond principally to thermal and emotional stimuli. Most sweating due to emotion occurs on the palms, soles, and axillae, whereas most thermal sweating is seen on the fingers, arms, forehead, and axillae. Factors that may raise body temperature and induce thermal sweating include a high activity level, an elevated room temperature, a hot bath or shower, some medications, or the ingestion of highly spiced foods. Eating highly spiced foods may cause gustatory sweating, indicated by sweat on the forehead, upper lip, scalp, and back of the neck. Sweating primarily on the palms and soles may be evidence of fear or anxiety.

The apocrine sweat glands are less numerous than the eccrine sweat glands and are found in hair-bearing areas. They do not play a role in thermoregulation but respond instead to emotional and sensory stimuli.

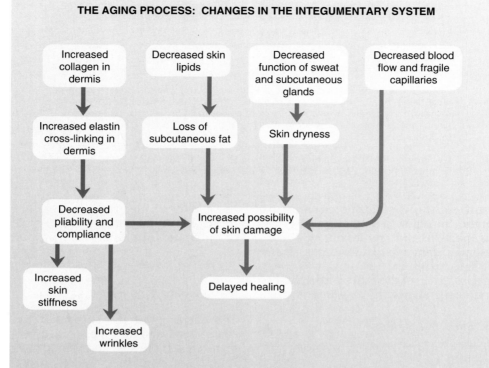

THE AGING PROCESS: CHANGES IN THE INTEGUMENTARY SYSTEM

With aging, the skin's protective functions decline. The function of the water and chemical barriers in the stratum corneum is reduced even though the thickness of the stratum corneum remains the same. In the epidermis, mitosis decreases and cellular variation increases. The thickness of the epidermis is unchanged. Melanocytes decrease in Caucasians, with declining function. The melanocytes are less efficient and lack uniformity in pigment production with sun exposure.

In the dermis, there is a decrease in thickness and subcutaneous fat. There is an increase in collagen and elastin with cross-linking and calcification of elastin fibers. These changes cause a loss of skin pliability, compliance, and resiliency. There is an accompanying rise in skin stiffness and an increase in skin wrinkles. Sebaceous and sweat gland function declines, resulting in drier, less oily skin. The number of sensory nerves and blood vessels in the skin declines, resulting in decreased sensation and loss of effective vasoactivity by dermal arterioles.

Nail and hair growth declines. The nails may become yellowed and thickened. Graying of the hair is due to the loss of melanocytes at the hair follicle base. The degree and pattern of hair loss is affected by genetic and endocrine factors. Body hair patterns change, with thinning of leg, axillary, and pubic hair.

The cumulative effect of these skin changes is loss of the regulatory, secretory, and excretory properties of the skin. The skin becomes injured more easily, and once injured, the skin heals more slowly.

Faith Young Peterson

Hydration and Turgor

Other skin qualities useful to assess are hydration and turgor. The state of hydration of the skin and mucous membranes helps to indicate body fluid balance. Skin turgor (tension) can be assessed by picking up and releasing the skin, particularly on the dorsum of the hands or forearms. Normal skin usually snaps back immediately into its resting position. With aging, there is a loss of elasticity.

Pigmentation

Normal color distribution patterns vary from person to person and race to race. For example, dark-skinned people like those of Mediterranean origin may have very blue lips, unrelated to cyanosis. Blotchy or bluish pigmentation of the gums and brown melanin deposits in the scleras, nail beds, or both are often normal findings in very dark-skinned individuals. In the dark-skinned person, the areas of lighter melanization (abdomen, buttocks, and volar surface of the forearm) allow more accurate evaluation of pigmentation.

KEY CONCEPTS

- **Most pathophysiologic conditions have associated skin manifestations. Careful history taking and physical examination of the skin are necessary to assess primary skin problems and those occurring secondary to other disease processes.**
- **Skin assessment includes assessment of color, texture, temperature, hydration, turgor, hair distribution, pigmentation, and the presence of lesions.**

Summary

Human skin comes in a wide assortment of colors and performs a variety of critically important functions. Without its protection, heat, chemicals, and radiant energy would be overwhelming, traumatic forces. The ability to regulate heat, water, and mineral balance would be upset by excessive evaporation.

The skin is a large organ that contains highly developed appendages and receptors that are specialized for receiving stimuli and displaying emotions. Nerve endings in the skin permit perception of touch, pain, pressure, heat, and cold. Emotions such as shame, anger, fear, and anxiety can be expressed cutaneously because the skin is responsive to internal and external stimuli.

Structurally, skin is composed of epidermis and dermis. Keratinocytes and melanocytes are two major types of cells in the epidermis. The dermis is composed primarily of collagen, which gives the skin its strength. Subcutaneous tissue contains appendages of the skin and fat. The aging process profoundly affects the integumentary system and exerts visible effects on skin, hair, and nails.

REFERENCES

1. Arndt KA, Jick H: Rates of cutaneous reactions to drugs. *JAMA* 1976;235(9):918–923.
2. Arey LB: The integumentary system, in Arey LB (ed): *Human Histology: A Textbook in Outline Form.* Philadelphia, WB Saunders, 1974, pp 186–189.
3. Jacob SW, Francone CA: Tissues and the skin, in Jacob SW, Francone CA (eds): *Elements of Anatomy and Physiology,* 2nd ed. Philadelphia, WB Saunders, 1989, pp 33–41.
4. Pinkus H, Mehregan AH: Normal structure of skin, in Pinkus H, Mehregan AH (eds): *A Guide to Dermatohistopathology,* 3rd ed. New York, Appleton-Century-Crofts, 1981, pp 5–38.
5. Holbrook KA, Odland GF: Regional differences in the thickness (cell layers) of the human stratum corneum: An ultrastructural analysis. *J Invest Dermatol* 1974;62(4):415–422.
6. Sober AJ, Fitzpatrick TB: Hair and nails, in Sober AJ, Fitzpatrick TB (eds): *Year Book of Dermatology.* St. Louis, CV Mosby, 1990, pp 153–160.
7. Mosher DB, Pathak MA, Fitzpatrick TB: Vitiligo: Etiology, pathogenesis, diagnosis, and treatment, in Fitzpatrick TB, Eisen AZ, Wolff K, Freedburg IM, Austin KF (eds): *Update: Dermatology in General Medicine.* New York, McGraw-Hill, 1983, pp 205–225.
8. Berman, B: Langerhans cells, in Stone J: *Dermatologic Immunology and Allergy.* St. Louis, CV Mosby, 1985, pp 217–236.
9. Hartschuh W, Grube D: The Merkel cell—a member of the APUD cell system: Fluorescence and electron microscopic contribution to the neurotransmitter function of the Merkel cell granules. *Arch Dermatol Res* 1979;265(2):115–122.
10. Sauer GC: Structure of the skin, in Sauer GC (ed): *Manual of Skin Diseases,* 4th ed. Philadelphia, JB Lippincott, 1980, pp 1–7.
11. Berardesca E, de-Rigal J, Leveque JL, Maibach HI: In vivo biophysical characterization of skin physiological differences in races. *Dermatologica* 1991;182(2):89–93.
12. Murphy GF, Kwan TH, Mihm MC Jr: The skin, in Robbins SL, Cotran RS, Kumar V: *Pathologic Basis of Disease,* 3rd ed. Philadelphia, WB Saunders, 1984, pp 1275, 1279, 1298.
13. Dobson RL, Abele DC: Common viral infections, in Dobson RL, Abele DC (eds): *The Practice of Dermatology.* New York, Harper & Row, 1985, pp 213–225.
14. Kligman AM, Leyden J: The interaction of fungi and bacteria in the pathogenesis of athlete's foot, in Maibach HI, Aly R (eds): *Skin Microbiology: Relevance to Clinical Infection.* New York, Springer-Verlag, 1981, pp 203–219.
15. Dobson RL: Acne, in Theirs BH, Dobson RL (eds): *Pathogenesis of Skin Disease.* New York, Churchill Livingstone, 1986, pp 35–40.
16. Katz SI, Tamaki K, Sachs DH: Epidermal Langerhans cells are derived from cells originating in bone marrow. *Nature* 1979;282:324–327.
17. Ebertz JM, Hirshman CA, Kettlkamp NS, Uno H, Hanifin JM: Substance P-induced histamine release in human cutaneous mast cells. *J Invest Dermatol* 1987;88:682–685.
18. Slaven RG, Ducomb DF: Allergic contact dermatitis. *Hosp Pract* 1989;24(7):39–51.
19. Goopman J: Neoplasms in the acquired immune deficiency syndrome: The multidisciplinary approach. *Semin Oncol* 1987;14(2)(suppl 3):1–6.
20. Pollack SV: Wound healing: A review. I. The biology of wound healing. *J Dermatol Surg Oncol* 1979;5(5):389–393.
21. Leibovich SJ, Ross R: The role of the macrophage in wound repair: A study with hydrocortisone and antimacrophage serum. *Am J Pathol* 1975;78(1):71–100.
22. Cooper DM: Acute surgical wounds, in Bryant RA (ed): *Acute and Chronic Wounds.* St. Louis, Mosby–Year Book, 1992, pp 91–100.
23. Ryan GB, Cliff WJ, Gabbiani G, et al: Myofibroblasts in human granulation tissue. *Hum Pathol* 1974;5(1):55–67.
24. Wysocki AB: Skin, in Bryant RA (ed): *Acute and Chronic Wounds.* St. Louis, Mosby–Year Book, 1992, pp 1–25.
25. Fischer B: Topical hyperbaric oxygen treatment of pressure sores and skin ulcers. *Lancet* 1969;2:405–409.
26. Fischer B: Wound healing: A review. III. Nutritional factors affecting wound healing. *J Dermatol Surg Oncol* 1979;5(8):615–619.

27. Wright S: Essential fatty acids and the skin. Br J Dermatol 1991;125(6):503–515.
28. Payne PA: Measurement of properties and function of skin. *Clin Phys Physiol Meas* 1991;12(2):105–129.
29. Jaszczak P: Blood flow rate, temperature, oxygen tension and consumption in the skin of adults measured by a heated microcathode oxygen electrode. *Dan Med Bull* 1988;5(4):322–334.
30. Church MK, el-Lati S, Okayama Y: Biological properties of human skin mast cells. *Clin Exp Allergy* 1991;21(suppl 3):1–9.
31. Greco PJ, Ende J: An office-based approach to the patient with pruritus. *Hosp Prac* 1992;27:121–128.
32. Banov CH, Epstein JH, Grayson LD: When an itch persists. *Patient Care* 1992;26(5):75–81, 84–88, and 90.
33. Stenn KS: The molecular and structural biology of hair: Introduction. *Ann NY Acad Sci* 1991;642:xi–xiii.
34. Reynolds AJ, Jahoda CA: Inductive properties of hair follicle cells. *Ann NY Acad Sci* 1991;642:226–41.
35. Powell DB, Nesci A, Rogers GE: Regulation of keratin gene expression in hair follicle differentiation. *Ann NY Acad Sci* 1991;642:1–20.
36. Janniger CK, Bryngil JM: Hair in infancy and childhood. *Cutis* 1993;51(5):336–338.
37. Paus R, Link RE: The psoriatic epidermal lesion and anagen hair growth may share the same "switch-on" mechanism. *Yale J Biol Med* 1988;61(5)467:476.
38. Johnson M, Comaish JS, Shuster S: Nail is produced by the normal nail bed: A controversy resolved. *Br J Dermatol* 1991;125(1):27–29.
39. Sauer GC: Structure of the skin, in Sauer GC (ed): *Manual of Skin Diseases*, 4th ed. Philadelphia, JB Lippincott, 1980, pp 10–13.
40. Lever WF, Schaumberg-Lever G: Histology of the skin, in Lever WF, Schaumberg-Lever G (eds): *Histopathology of the Skin*, 7th ed. Philadelphia, JB Lippincott, 1989, pp 20–25.
41. Murphy GF, Mihm MC Jr: The skin, in Cotran RS, Kumar V, Robbins SL (eds): *Robbins Pathologic Basis of Disease*, 4th ed. Philadelphia, WB Saunders, 1989, pp 1277–1313.
42. Bates BB: The skin, in *A Guide to Physical Examination and History Taking*, 5th ed. Philadelphia, JB Lippincott, 1991, pp 139–154.
43. Cerimele D, Celleno L, Serri F: Physiological changes in aging skin. *Br J Dermatol* 1990;122(suppl 35):13–20.
44. Raab WP: The skin surface and stratum corneum. *Br J Dermatol* 1990;122(suppl 35):37–41.
45. Ortonne JP: Pigmentary changes of the ageing skin. *Br J Dermatol* 1990;122(suppl 35):21–28.
46. Lapiere CM: The ageing dermis: The main cause for the appearance of old skin. *Br J Dermatol* 1990;122(suppl 35):5–11.
47. Kligman AM: Psychological aspects of skin disorders in the elderly. *Cutis* 1989;43:498–501.
48. Beauregard S, Gilchrest BA: A survey of skin problems and skin care regimens in the elderly. *Arch Dermatol* 1987;123:1638–1643.
49. Jemec GB, Agner T, Serup J: Transonychial water loss: Relation to sex, age and nail-plate thickness. *Br J Dermatol* 1989;121(4):443–446.
50. Stuttgen G, Ott A: Senescence in the skin. *Br J Dermatol* 1990;122(suppl 35):43–48.
51. Montagna W, Carlisle K: Structural changes in ageing skin. *Br J Dermatol* 1990;122(suppl 35):61–70.
52. Phillips RJ, Dover JS: Recent advances in dermatology. *N Engl J Med* 1992;326:167–178.

BIBLIOGRAPHY

Baker BI: The role of melanin-concentrating hormone in color change. *Ann NY Acad Sci* 1993;680:279–289.

Berardesca E, Maibach HI: Sensitive and ethnic skin: A need for special skin-care agents? *Dermatol Clin* 1991;9(1):89–92.
Berardesca E, Maibach H: Transcutaneous CO_2 and O_2 diffusion. *Skin Pharmacol* 1993;6(1):3–9.
Bolognia J: Aging skin, epidermal and dermal changes. *Prog Clin Biol Res* 1989;320:121–135.
Caughman SW, Li LJ, Degitz K: Human intercellular adhesion molecule-1 gene and its expression in the skin. *J Invest Dermatol* 1992;98(suppl 6):61S–65S.
Dalziel KL: Aspects of cutaneous ageing. *Clin Exp Dermatol* 1991;16(5):315–323.
Emerit I: Free radicals and aging of the skin. *EXS* 1992;62:328–341.
Fowler JR Jr: Dermatology in space: The final frontier. *Dermatology* 1991;6:73–81.
Gilchrest BA, Yaar M: Ageing and photoageing of the skin: Observations at the cellular and molecular level. *Br J Dermatol* 1992;127(suppl 41):25–30.
Grando SA: Physiology of endocrine skin interrelations. *J Am Acad Dermatol* 1993;28(6):981–992.
Grove GL: Physiologic changes in older skin. *Clin Geriatr Med* 1989;5(1):115–125.
Haake AR, Polakowska RR: Cell death by apoptosis in epidermal biology. *J Invest Dermatol* 1993;101(2):107–112.
Kenney JA: Black dermatology. *Cutis* 1983;32(4):310–392.
Klymkowsky MW: Intermediate filaments: Getting under the skin. *Nature* 1991;354:264–265.
Leveque JL, et al: In vivo studies of the evolution of physical properties of the human skin with age. *Int J Dermatol* 1984;23:322–329.
Lynn CJ, Saidi IS, Oelberg DG, Jacques SL: Gestational age correlates with skin reflectance in newborn infants of 24–42 weeks gestation. *Biol Neonate* 1993;64(2–3):69–75.
McDonald CJ: Some thoughts on differences in black and white skin. *Int J Dermatol* 1976;15:427–430.
Michel L, Dubertret L: Leukotriene B4 and platelet-activating factor in human skin. *Arch Dermatol Res* 1992;284(suppl 1):S12–S17.
O'Donoghue MN: Cosmetics for the elderly. *Dermatol Clin* 1991;9(1):29–34.
Oriba HA, Elsner P, Maibach HI: Vulvar physiology. *Semin Dermatol* 1989;8(1):2–6.
Parmley T, O'Brien TJ: Skin changes during pregnancy. *Clin Obstet Gynecol* 1990;33(4):713–717.
Paus R: Does prolactin play a role in skin biology and apthology? *Med Hypotheses* 1991;36(1):33–42.
Polla BS: Heat (shock) and the skin. *Dermatologica* 1990;180(3):113–117.
Rosen T, Martin S: *Atlas of Black Dermatology*. Boston, Little, Brown & Co, 1981.
Rossman I: *Clinical Geriatrics*, 3rd ed. Philadelphia, JB Lippincott, 1986.
Rutter N: The immature skin. *Br Med Bull* 1988;44(4):957–970.
Ruzicka T: The physiology and pathophysiology of eicosanoids in the skin. *Eicosanoids* 1988;1(2):59–72.
Smith L: Histopathologic characteristics and ultrastructure of aging skin. *Cutis* 1989;43(5):414–424.
Swerlick RA: Cytokines in dermatology. *Semin Dermatol* 1991;10(3):260–267.
Tamaki K, Stingl G, Katz SI: The origin of Langerhans cells. *J Invest Dermatol* 1980;74:309–311.
Uitto J, Olsen DR, Frazio MJ: Extracellular matrix of the skin: 50 years of progress. *J Invest Dermatol* 1989;2(4 suppl):61S–77S.
van-Rappard JH, Sonneveld GJ, Borghouts JM: Histologic changes in soft tissues due to tissue expansion (in animal studies and humans). *Facial Plast Surg* 1988;5(4):280–286.
Weiss JS, Ellis CN, Headington JT, et al: Topical retinoin improves photoaged skin. *JAMA* 1988;259:527–532.
Zitelli JA: Synthetic skin. *Adv Dermatol* 1989;4:325–341.

CHAPTER 53
Alterations in the Integument

LEE-ELLEN C. COPSTEAD

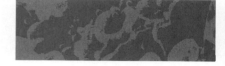

actinic keratosis: A horny, keratotic premalignancy caused by excessive exposure to sunlight.

albinism: Partial or total absence of pigment in skin, hair, and eyes.

alopecia: Loss of hair; baldness.

cyanosis: Blueness of skin.

dermatitis: Inflammation of the skin.

dermatosis: Any disorder of the skin.

erythema: A form of macula characterized by diffuse redness of skin.

hirsutism: Excessive growth of the hair or presence of hair in unusual places.

hyperkeratosis: Horny overgrowth, such as callus formation.

hypertrichosis lanuginosa: Excessive hair growth over the entire body.

jaundice: Yellowness of skin.

leukoderma: Patch of depigmentation, also called **vitiligo.**

neoplasia: New and abnormal tissue formation, such as tumor or growth.

nevi: Congenital discoloration of a circumscribed area of the skin, commonly called **moles** or **birthmarks.**

onycholysis: Separation of the nail from its bed.

primary lesions: Injuries that originate in the skin.

pruritus: Itching of the skin.

seborrheic keratosis: Benign skin tumor common in the elderly, composed of immature epithelial cells.

secondary lesions: Injuries modified by normal progress over time or by such external agents as scratching.

strawberry hemangioma: A soft, vascular nevus usually present on the face or neck, occurring at birth or shortly afterward.

strawberry tongue: Bright red, papillated tongue, characteristic of scarlet fever.

verrucae: Circumscribed elevations of the epidermis, commonly called **warts.**

*I*n systemic diseases, the color, texture, and composition of the skin mirror and participate in widespread pathophysiologic events. For example, internal disease states such as acquired immunodeficiency syndrome (AIDS), collagen diseases such as scleroderma and dermatomyositis, diabetes, gout, malignancies, neurologic diseases, liver disease, muscle weakness, and vascular, inflammatory, and metabolic disorders all exhibit cutaneous manifestations. Because the skin mirrors the interior condition of the body, it is important in the diagnosis of disease. Cutaneous manifestations may be caused by bodily changes such as pregnancy or obesity. They may also be caused by external factors such as climate, industrial contamination, indoor heating systems, clothing, plant life, and toxic or allergic reactions to drugs and cosmetics.

This chapter focuses on altered structure and function of the integumentary system. The etiology,

pathogenesis, clinical manifestations of selected skin disorders, and general considerations regarding treatment modalities and their therapeutic application are described.

Categorization and Description of Skin Lesions

A careful examination of the skin yields valuable information that may aid in identifying a systemic disease or a specific problem of the skin or appendages. Diagnostic evaluations include a careful history, and Table 53–1 provides a general guide. A proper skin examination also describes the objective signs of dermatologic disease, including all types of lesions and their distribution.

TABLE 53-1. Summary of Key Assessment Items

Assessment Item	Purpose and Relevant Questions to Ask
Family history	Some skin diseases are familial or hereditary. When this is ascertained, one may have the opportunity both to correct misconceptions and allay fears about the presence, absence, or prognosis of disease. What are the current familial dermatologic diseases?
Personal history	Age at onset of problem? How has the patient adjusted to the problem? By social withdrawal? Cosmetic coverup? Withdrawal from school athletic activities that require showers (e.g., football, tennis)? Does the problem threaten patient's self-image of masculinity or femininity? What is race or ethnic origin? (Some skin diseases are more common in certain ethnic groups.)
Geographic origin and present abode	Length of time spent living in each area? Some skin diseases are indigenous. This may be important because of increased exposure. Occasionally, a contact of only 5 minutes is all that is necessary for acquisition of a disease.
Season	Seasonal occurrence of problem? Pollen? Sunlight?
Occupation	Type of work? Skin contact material (e.g., chemicals, dusts, gases); excessive heat and abnormal lighting; unhygienic surroundings; possible infected insects; other family members' occupational exposures?
Leisure activities	Does the problem occur only on weekends? After yard activities? Painting? Woodworking? Camping? Fishing? Hiking? Associated with children's play habits?
Accompanying diseases	Collagen disease? Drug therapy for collagen disease? Other diseases and their drug therapy?
Previous treatment	Self-treatment? Other drugs prescribed?
Special history	Onset of skin lesion (abnormality)? Remissions, exacerbations, or recurrences? Site of onset? Character of lesions? Original character and subsequent changes? Course or extension? Symptoms? Itching? Ability to perform duties? Topical therapy? Self-treatment? Psychological factors? What does the patient associate with exacerbations of the problem (e.g., stress of a family argument, tax time, report time)?

Data from Rosen T, Lanning, MB, Hill MJ (eds): *Nurse's Atlas of Dermatology.* Boston, Little, Brown & Co, 1983.

Primary and Secondary Lesions

Physical descriptions should include the lesions and their classification, generally **primary** (original appearance) or **secondary** (appearance modified by normal progress over time or by such external agents as scratching). Figure 53–1 shows clinical examples of primary and secondary lesions.

Lesion Descriptors

After a skin lesion has been classified as primary or secondary, other features should be noted, particularly color, number, and distribution. Skin lesions may assume a wide range of colors—red–salmon pink, brown-black, blue-purple, bone white–slate gray, and yellow, to name a few. Each color suggests certain diagnoses. Skin lesions may be solitary, few in number, or profuse. When more than one lesion is present, the distribution pattern may be quite important in suggesting the diagnosis. Look for these common patterns: symmetric (affecting mirror image portions of the body); sun-exposed (affecting skin sites that routinely receive solar irradiation); intertriginous (affecting warm, moist apposed skin sites); and flexor or extensor predominance. Additional descriptors are often used to further characterize and describe

a skin lesion or the relationship between various skin lesions. Table 53–2 lists common morphologic and configurational terms.

KEY CONCEPTS

- Skin lesions may be categorized as primary or secondary. Primary lesions retain their original appearance, unmodified by time and external processes such as scratching. Secondary lesions are those whose appearance has been modified over time; they may look quite dissimilar to the original lesion. The differentiation of primary from secondary lesions aids in establishing a correct diagnosis.

- A description of lesion color, shape, number, and distribution is helpful in determining the etiology of a lesion.

Integumentary Manifestations of Systemic Disease

The skin reflects the status of many organ systems. For example, the endocrine, cardiovascular, renal, respiratory, and hepatic systems all have possible dermal manifestations. Metabolic disorders and internal

NONPALPABLE
PRIMARY LESIONS (Original Appearance)

NONPALPABLE

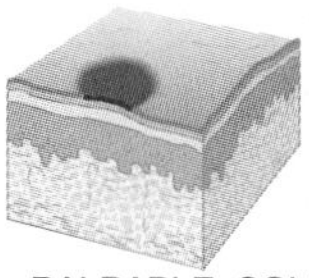

Macule: A spot, circumscribed, up to 1 cm; not palpable; not elevated above or depressed below surrounding skin surface; hypopigmented, hyperpigmented, or erythematous. **Example:** freckles. Referred to as **patch** if greater than 1 cm. **Examples:** café au lait spots, mongolian spots.

PALPABLE, SOLID

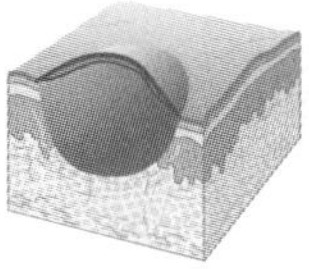

Papule: A bump, palpable and circumscribed, elevated and less than 5 mm in diameter; may be pigmented, erythematous, or flesh-toned. **Example:** elevated nevus (mole).

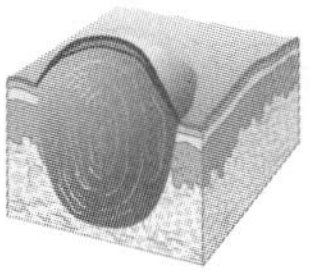

Nodule: A lesion similar to a papule, with a diameter of 5 mm to 2 cm; may have a significant palpable dermal component. **Examples:** fibroma, xanthoma, intradermal nevi.

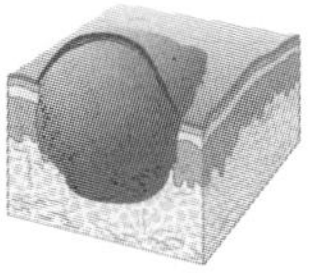

Tumor: Any mass lesion; generally larger than a nodule; may be either malignant or benign. **Example:** lipoma.

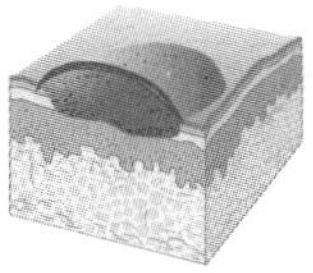

Plaque: Usually well-circumscribed lesion with large surface area and slight elevation.
Examples: psoriasis, lichen planus.

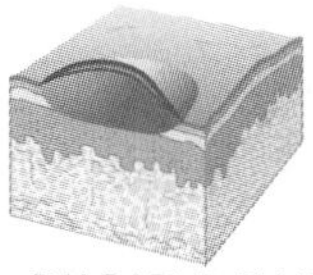

Wheal: An elevation in the skin, with a smooth surface, sloping borders, and (usually) light pink color; caused by acute areas of edema in the skin; may appear, disappear, or change form abruptly within minutes or hours; size ranges from 3 mm to 20 cm. **Example:** mosquito bite.

PALPABLE, FLUID-FILLED

Vesicle: A small blister (up to 5 mm in diameter); fluid collection may be subcorneal, intraepidermal, or subepidermal.
Example: herpes simplex (early stages).

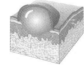

Bulla: A blister larger than 5 mm; fluid may be located at various levels. **Examples:** pemphigus, pemphigoid.

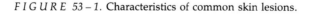

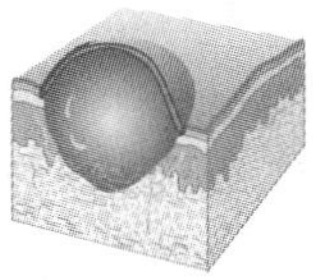

Pustule: An elevated, well-circumscribed lesion containing purulent exudate.
Example: acne vulgaris.

FIGURE 53–1. Characteristics of common skin lesions.

SECONDARY LESIONS (Modification of Original Appearance)

DAMAGED OR DIMINISHED SKIN SURFACE   AUGMENTED OR INCREASED SKIN SURFACE

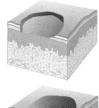

Erosion: Loss of epidermis that does not extend into dermis. **Example:** ruptured chicken pox vesicle.

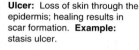

Crust: A collection of serous exudate and debris on the surface of damaged or absent outer skin layers. **Example:** impetigo.

Ulcer: Loss of skin through the epidermis; healing results in scar formation. **Example:** stasis ulcer.

Scale: A compact portion of desquamating stratum corneum; may vary in size, thickness, and consistency. **Examples:** psoriasis scale (compact and thick), pityriasis rosea scale (thin and small).

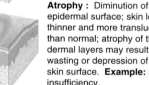

Fissure: A split in all epidermal layers of skin **Example:** athlete's foot.

Lichenification: Epidermal thickening and roughening of the skin with increased visibility of skin surface furrows. **Example:** chronic atopic dermatitis.

Atrophy : Diminution of epidermal surface; skin looks thinner and more translucent than normal; atrophy of the dermal layers may result in wasting or depression of the skin surface. **Example:** arterial insufficiency.

Scar : A collection of fibrous tissue that forms to replace lost epidermal and dermal tissue. **Examples:** surgical scar, acne scar.

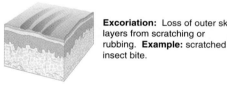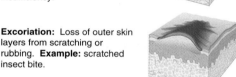

Excoriation: Loss of outer skin layers from scratching or rubbing. **Example:** scratched insect bite.

Keloid: Augmentation of scar tissue, creating a significant elevation on the skin surface after healing. **Examples:** postsurgical scar, post-acne scar.

FIGURE 53–1 Continued

malignancies also cause cutaneous alterations. Certainly manifestations of internal malignancy in the skin can be obvious. The late-appearing features of **cachexia** (wasting), pallor, and cutaneous metastases are obvious signs of malignancy. Abnormalities of endocrine function also produce a myriad of cutaneous changes. (See Chapters 40 and 41, describing endocrine and metabolic disorders.) In general, systemic disease states are expressed through altered color, sensation, texture, and temperature of the skin; altered growth, texture, color, and lubrication of the hair; and changes in nail shape, color, and texture.

Skin

Color

Color changes in the skin can signal the existence of systemic disease. The entire color spectrum (red, orange, yellow, green, blue, indigo, and violet) is represented through possible coloration changes in the skin.

Redness (**erythema**) may be generalized, as with carbon monoxide poisoning, or may be generalized or localized, as in rashes or on the palms. Although erythema is often visible in lighter-skinned persons,

it may be less apparent in those whose skin is dark; however, the affected part may become an even deeper shade of brown. Redness may accompany inflammation.

When inflammation is suspected in the dark-skinned person, other parameters can be assessed by palpation, among them increased skin temperature, tight skin suggestive of edema, induration of deep tissue or blood vessels, and tenderness. Because the dorsal skin surface of the fingers is more sensitive to subtle skin temperature differences than the palmar surface, the examiner should use the dorsal portion of the fingers to move from one skin area to another for comparison. The patient's family and friends are also helpful in validating color change, particularly when it has occurred gradually.

Orange discoloration can occur from the deposition of carotene. Protein-calorie malnutrition can cause hypopigmentation in African-American children, causing the hair and skin to appear orange.

Yellow discoloration can occur locally when lipids are deposited in skin secondary to a metabolic defect in blood lipids. More commonly, a generalized yellow (jaundiced) appearance arises because of liver disease. Bilirubin accumulates in blood and saturates the tissues. **Jaundice** is observed in the usual sites (e.g.,

T A B L E 53 – 2. Lesion Descriptors

Term	Definition
Confluent	Blending together
Discrete	Remaining separate although close together
Diffuse	Generalized or widespread
Eczematous	Vesicles with oozing crust
Herpetiform	Closely grouped vesicles (herpeslike)
Linear	Set in a straight line
Localized	Found only in one area
Pedunculated	On a stalk
Reticulate(d)	Netlike array
Round lesions	Annular (ring-shaped, active edge, clear center)
	Arcuate (arc-shaped, incomplete circle)
	Circinate (circular)
	Guttate (small-dropletlike)
	Iris (concentric circles, such as a bull's eye)
	Nummular (coin shaped)
	Ovoid (oval shaped)
Serpiginous	Wandering, snakelike
Telangiectatic	Characterized by dilated surface vessels
Verrucous	Rough, wartlike surface
Zosteriform	Similar to shingles, following along a nerve root dermatome

Data from Sauer GC: *Manual of Skin Diseases*, 6th ed. Philadelphia, JB Lippincott, 1991.

mucous membranes, nail beds). Because many factors can alter these findings, one single positive finding should not be held as conclusive. Other parameters, such as environmental temperature, drugs, smoking, amount of hemoglobin, and the color of urine or stools, can support a description of cyanosis or jaundice. Both in the dark-skinned and light-skinned person, yellow scleras may indicate jaundice, but other factors can cause yellow scleral pigmentation; fatty deposits that contain carotene are a common finding in dark-skinned people. To determine whether the yellow scleras signify jaundice, observe the hard palate in bright daylight. Jaundice can be detected there quite early (i.e., when serum bilirubin is 2 to 4 mg/100 mL) if the palate does not have heavy melanin pigmentation.[1] If the hard palate does not show jaundice when the scleras are yellow, the pigmentation may be due to some other factor, such as carotene accumulation. All these factors support the importance of repeated observations and accurate descriptions of what is seen. As often as possible, the same person should perform the entire examination and should confirm specific findings in one area with additional data from other areas.

When jaundice is severe, **biliverdin** also accumulates. A person with obstructed bile ducts can become green-yellow due to biliverdin.

Blueness of the skin (**cyanosis**) often occurs on the tips of the fingers, toes, nose, and lips in people with cardiac or respiratory problems that prevent oxygenation of blood. Localized blueness with pain of the fingers on exposure to cold is termed Raynaud's disease. It frequently arises from cryoglobulins, which solidify in the cold, and is also associated with disorders of the immune system, such as lymphoma and AIDS.[2]

Indigo discoloration occurs locally, as in gangrene of the toes from severe generalized arteriosclerosis. The skin can darken from increased melanin synthesis, as in chronic adrenal insufficiency. Also, silver poisoning can make the skin dusky. Violet-colored palms (palmar erythema) can be seen in some persons with liver diseases and occasionally in pregnant women as a response to hyperestrogenism.

Shades of violet occur in the legs from vascular insufficiency or when cardiopulmonary function is compromised.

The primary sites for assessing skin **pallor** are the nail beds, lips, and conjunctivae. When observing the lower eyelid (inferior palpebral conjuntiva) for pallor, the examiner should lower the lid sufficiently to see not only the conjunctiva near the outer canthus but also the inner canthus, since the former is often darker in color. Greater perception is necessary in assessing the darkly pigmented individual for pallor, because the changes are subtle. There may be an absence of red tones; the brown-skinned person may appear more yellowish brown, and the black-skinned person may appear ash-gray. This supports the need for accurate baseline data for comparison.

Sensation

Sensory innervation is generally responsible for the itching (**pruritis**) and **pain** that accompany most skin diseases. *Itching* is often the presenting symptom in such conditions as atopic eczema, allergic contact dermatitis, scabies, dermatophytosis, psoriasis, and varicella. It can also be associated with systemic disorders, including carcinoma, diabetes, thyroid disease, uremia, and obstructive biliary disease. Other dermatologic conditions, for instance herpes simplex, aphthous stomatitis, herpes zoster, furuncles, and cellulitis, produce considerable *pain*.

Texture

Normal aging produces an alteration in the texture of skin (see Chap. 52). Loose and wrinkled skin that lacks tone may also indicate **dehydration,** an abnormal finding. Dehydration may also be apparent through inspection of the oral cavity. On inspection, a dry, leathery appearance of the tongue is *not* a reliable indicator of dehydration, since mouth breathing frequently makes the tongue look dry even when the individual is well hydrated. A more reliable method of assessing hydration of the oral cavity is to palpate the mucous membranes along the area of the gum and cheek where the membranes approximate. If the membranes are dry and the finger does not slide easily, dehydration is evident.

To evaluate **fluid excess,** palpate the skin over the hands, feet, ankles, and sacrum. If the skin is firm and indents easily (pitting edema) on moderate pressure from the fingertips, fluid excess is present.

Feeling the deeper portions of the skin may reveal areas of **induration** (hardness) such as those resulting from multiple intramuscular or subcutaneous administrations of medication. **Lipodystrophies** consist of smooth, large depressions in the skin that indicate atrophy of the subcutaneous fat layer, which is of a spongy consistency. Both induration and lipodystrophies are often seen at sites of repeated insulin injections.

Temperature

If the skin feels warm and dry in a person who is febrile (feverish), the blood temperature is probably rising, an indication that the thermoregulatory mechanism of sweating may not be functioning. Likewise, if the skin is warm and wet, the temperature can be expected to fall, owing to the cooling mechanism of sweating.

Sweating can also occur when there is a rapid fall in blood glucose with a resultant rise in the blood epinephrine level. **Hypoglycemic sweating** can usually be distinguished from other causes of sweating because of the additional symptoms of weakness, tachycardia, hunger, headache, and "inward nervousness"—mental irritability and confusion.

Because skin temperature depends on the amount of blood circulating through the dermis, decreased localized blood flow (resulting in coolness), often to the feet, may indicate a **peripheral vascular dysfunction.** Generalized skin coolness may indicate **decreased metabolism** such as that occurring after general anesthesia. If the temperature is very low, signs of **shock** may be evident.

On the other hand, an increase in skin temperature may indicate a **hypermetabolic state,** such as that occurring in hyperthyroidism and after sun exposure or sunburn.

Hair

Disturbances in body function are often reflected in changes in growth pattern, amount, texture, color, and lubrication of the hair. (See Chapter 52 for a description of the normal changes that occur during the aging process.)

Growth

The high speed of growth of the scalp hair makes it more susceptible to damage from systemic disease, toxic drugs, radiation, and stress. The rate of growth varies with general health and age. Hair growth is dependent on circulating hormonal factors (primarily testicular or adrenal androgens). Thus, hormonal imbalances or shifts (e.g., those accompanying childbirth) may also result in disturbances in the hair growth cycle. Nutritional factors, although often promoted in nonmedical literature, have little effect on hair growth except in cases of severe malnutrition.

Amount

Alterations in the amount of body hair can be extremely anxiety-provoking for both males and fe-males. In the female with hypertrichosis or **hirsutism,** hair growth is intensified on the upper lip, chin, cheeks, chest, around the nipples, and from the pubic crest to the umbilicus (along the linea alba); the downy hair on the arms, legs, and back becomes coarse. The pubic hair often takes on the upright triangular distribution typical of the male as opposed to the female's usual inverted triangle (see Fig. 52–11 for normal hair distribution patterns). An endocrine malfunction such as excess androgen production may sometimes be associated with hirsutism, but ethnic background (Mediterranean groups predominantly) may also be responsible for the excessive hair growth. This is especially true of the hair on the arms, legs, back, and blooded African-American female and male Native American rarely have facial hair. Distribution of the hair in family members and ethnic background are thus important considerations in ascertaining hair growth.

Hypertrichosis lanuginosa is typically a congenital, autosomal dominant disorder in which there is excessive hair distributed over the entire body throughout life. The condition is usually associated with other congenital anomalies, such as spina bifida.[3] In some cases, such as with certain internal carcinomas, hypertrichosis lanuginosa is acquired; the degree of hairiness is variable and usually involves the face.

Color

Perhaps the most common color change in the hair is generalized graying that accompanies the aging process. This age-related change is discussed in Chapter 52 as a normal variant.

Texture

Normal aging also produces a decrease in hair thickness (see Chap. 52).

Disturbances of the thickness of scalp hair are common. Baldness (**alopecia**) or thinning of the hair that is generalized or creates a receding hairline often is genetically determined (Fig. 53–2). Some rare genetic defects in the hair shaft itself may produce breaking of the hairs and may be erroneously diagnosed as alopecia. Generalized and localized baldness may result from treatment modalities such as radiation therapy or chemotherapy. In addition, various types of scalp diseases (e.g., fungal, lupus) and telogen effluvium (transient hair loss occurring 2 to 3 months after general anesthesia, febrile illness, or giving birth) can cause hair loss. Other traumatic types of hair loss may occur from pulling of the hair because of a nervous habit, hair styles such as tight braids or ponytails, or wearing constrictive apparel such as a hat.

Lubrication

Hyperfunction of the sebaceous glands is associated with androgen stimulation such as occurs with the excessive scalp oiliness and facial acne in adolescence. Dry, brittle hair is commonly the result of excessive

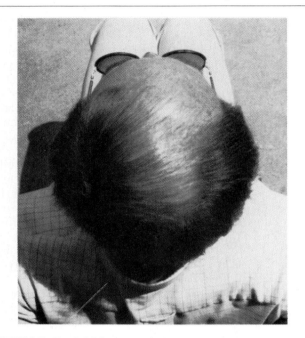

FIGURE 53–2. Male pattern baldness. (From Thibodeau GA, Patton KT: *Anatomy and Physiology,* 2nd ed. St. Louis, CV Mosby, 1993, p 140. Reproduced with permission.)

washing or the application of chemical agents (coloring, bleach, or detergent shampoos) to the hair.

In addition to direct observation of the scalp and face, correlation of the findings with the data from the patient history helps to determine dysfunctional states of health.

Nails

Because nails derive from a highly active tissue, they may be affected by any serious systemic illness. More-over, any local skin disease that affects the epidermis may also affect the nail matrix (epidermal cells that give rise to the nail plate), leading to an abnormal (**dystrophic**) nail. By measuring the distance between abnormalities (pits, grooves, and lines) and the proximal nail border, one may estimate the time of initial illness.

Shape

Transverse furrows (**Beau's lines**) in the nail indicate that nail growth has been disturbed. This can result from infection, systemic disease, or injury. Nails with a concave curve are known as spoon nails, or **koilonychia.** They may signal a form of iron deficiency anemia, and they are also associated with other disorders such as coronary disease, syphilis, or the use of strong soaps. Destruction of the nails (**onycholysis**) may accompany hyperthyroidism, fungal nail infection or psoriasis. **Splinter hemorrhages** may be linked to bacterial endocarditis and trichinosis. These red or brown splinters or streaks run parallel to the finger in the nail bed (Fig. 53–3). **Clubbing** of the fingers is characterized by a flattening of the angle of the base of the nail (see Fig. 20–3). It may occur in association with cardiovascular disease, subacute bacterial endocarditis, and pulmonary disease.

Color

Nail color indicates the amount of blood oxygenation. Bluish or purplish discoloration of the nail beds occurs with **cyanosis,** whereas **pallor** often indicates anemia. To compare color of the nail beds, apply slight pressure on the free edge of the second or third fingernail. The blanching that results is then compared to the normal color of the nail. The rate of color return

Beau's lines

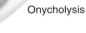

Onycholysis

FIGURE 53–3. Nail alterations.

Koilonychia (Spoon nails)

Splinter hemorrhages

also indicates the quality of peripheral vasomotor function.

Texture

Thickening of the nail may result from nutritional disturbances, repeated trauma, inflammation, and local infection. Along with thickening, toenails may become discolored and grooved, and debris may accumulate under the nail. This condition may be exacerbated as the distal portion of the nail works free from the underlying nail bed, accumulating more debris; fungal infections may also follow. Treatment usually consists of periodic debridement of the nail plate; however, a return to normal nail structure rarely occurs after thickening. (See Chapter 52 for age-related alterations in the nails.)

KEY CONCEPTS

- Many systemic diseases are associated with alterations in skin, hair, and nails. Skin reflects systemic inflammation and fever as erythema. A rising fever is evidenced as warm, dry skin, whereas warm, moist skin indicates a fever beginning to decline. Poor oxygenation and circulation may be manifest with cyanosis, pallor, or coolness. Jaundice indicates altered bilirubin metabolism, usually due to liver or biliary disease. Fluid balance may be evidenced in the skin as decreased turgor or edema. Sympathetic activation may be evidenced as cool, pale, diaphoretic skin.

- Hair growth, strength, texture, and color are affected by systemic diseases such as endocrine abnormalities, extreme malnutrition, and drugs. Excessive androgen may result in hirsutism. Alopecia may result from chemotherapeutic drugs or radiation therapy.

- Abnormalities of nail growth (pits, grooves, lines) occur as a result of nearly any serious systemic illness. Certain nail defects are characteristic of particular diseases: spoon nails may indicate iron deficiency anemia; clubbing is associated with cardiopulmonary disease. Nail color is commonly assessed to determine the adequacy of oxygenation and perfusion.

Age-Related Disorders

The skin and the skin problems of special groups warrant consideration. Certain skin problems are seen only in infants and children (e.g., cradle cap and diaper rash). Other dermatoses are seen in both children and in adults, but in children these dermatoses may appear different from the adult counterpart. Still other dermatoses affect primarily older persons.

Infancy

Infancy connotes soft, flawless skin. In general, this is a true image. Several congenital skin lesions, such as mongolian spots, hemangiomas, and nevi (moles), are nevertheless associated with the early neonatal period.

Mongolian spots are caused by selective pigmentation. They usually occur on the buttocks or sacral area and are commonly seen in Asians or blacks.

Hemangiomas are vascular disorders of the skin. Two types of hemangiomas are commonly seen in infants and small children: bright red, raised *strawberry hemangiomas,* and flat, reddish-purple *port wine stain hemangiomas.* Strawberry hemangiomas begin as small red lesions shortly after birth. They may remain as small superficial lesions or extend to involve subcutaneous tissue. Strawberry hemangiomas usually disappear before the child reaches 5 to 7 years of age without leaving an appreciable scar.[4] Port wine stain hemangiomas are rare, usually occur on the face and neck, and can be quite disfiguring. They do not disappear with age and there is no satisfactory medical treatment, although laser surgery may be effective in some cases. Coverage using cosmetic makeup such as Derma Blend may sufficiently conceal their disfiguring effects.

Nevi may vary in shape or size, and they may be present at birth or develop later in life.

Infant skin is also exquisitely sensitive to irritation, injury, and extremes of temperature. Prolonged exposure to a warm humid environment can lead to **prickly heat,** and too frequent bathing can cause excessive dryness. Soiled diapers, left unchanged, can lead to **contact dermatitis** and bacterial infections. **Cradle cap** occurs in response to infrequent or inadequate washing of the scalp. Figure 53–4 illustrates common skin problems of the infant and small child.

The primary factor in preventing infant skin disorders is careful and meticulous skin care. Baby lotions are helpful in maintaining skin moisture, whereas baby powder acts as a drying agent. Both are helpful aids when used selectively and according to the nature of the skin problem (excessive moisture or dryness).

Baby powders containing talc can cause serious respiratory problems if inhaled; therefore, containers should be kept out of the reach of small children. Corn starch is preferable to talc, and baby powders containing corn starch are readily available. Unnecessary bathing should be avoided, and clothing should be comfortable and appropriate for environmental conditions.

Diaper rash results from the ammonia and alkali by-products of urine breakdown. Disposable diapers or diapers washed in gentle detergent and thoroughly rinsed to remove all traces of ammonia and alkali help prevent diaper rash. Treatment includes frequent diaper changes with careful cleansing of any irritated areas. This is especially important in hot weather. Exposing irritated areas to air is also helpful. Use of plastic pants should be discouraged.

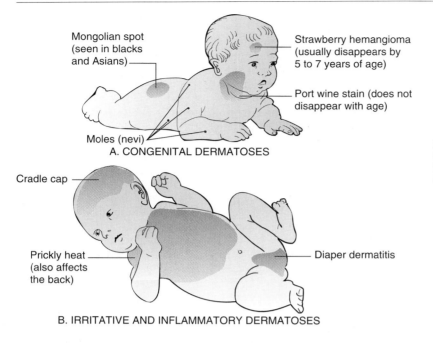

Mongolian spot
(seen in blacks
and Asians)

Strawberry hemangioma
(usually disappears by
5 to 7 years of age)

Port wine stain (does not
disappear with age)

Moles (nevi)

A. CONGENITAL DERMATOSES

Cradle cap

Prickly heat
(also affects
the back)

Diaper dermatitis

B. IRRITATIVE AND INFLAMMATORY DERMATOSES

F I G U R E 53 – 4. Sites of common dermatoses of the infant and small child. **A,** Congenital dermatoses. **B,** Irritative and inflammatory dermatoses.

Prickly heat results from prolonged exposure to a warm and humid environment, leading to midepidermal obstruction and rupture of the sweat glands. Treatment includes removal of excessive clothing, cooling with warm water baths, drying with powders, and avoiding hot, humid environments.

Cradle cap is usually treated by mild shampooing and gentle combing to remove the scales.

Childhood

As infants grow and develop into active young children, they become susceptible to the many skin disorders affecting people of all age groups who encounter environmental agents. Children, because of their physiologic development and playful nature, may also be more prone to accidents that result in major skin trauma, such as lacerations or burns. (See Chapter 55 for a further discussion of burn injury.) Careful activity supervision helps to prevent such accidental traumas.

Besides interacting with the environment, children are frequently in close contact with other children. As a result, communicable diseases such as head lice, tinea capitis, and impetigo are more frequently seen in children (Fig. 53–5). Epidemiologically, the incidence of rubella, roseola, rubeola (measles), chickenpox, and scarlet fever is also highest in this age group.

Rubella

Rubella (3-day measles, German measles) is a childhood disease caused by the rubella virus. It is characterized by a diffuse punctate, macular rash that begins on the trunk and spreads to the arms and legs. Mild febrile states occur; generally the fever is less than 100°F.[4] Postauricular, suboccipital, and cervical lymph node adenopathy is common. Coldlike symptoms usually accompany the disease in the form of cough, congestion, and coryza (profuse nasal mucous membrane discharge). Treatment is symptomatic.

Rubella generally has no long-lasting sequelae; however, transmission of the disease to pregnant women early in the gestation period may result in severe teratogenic effects in the unborn fetus. Among the teratogenic effects are cataracts, microcephaly, mental retardation, deafness, patent ductus arteriosus, glaucoma, purpura, and bone defects.[4] Most states require immunization to prevent the transmission of rubella to pregnant women. Immunization is with a live virus vaccine. The vaccination is called MMR (measles, mumps, rubella). One injection during infancy is followed by one booster dose as the child enters kindergarten or first grade, or as the child enters middle school or junior high school. Administration of these two injections is considered adequate to prevent rubella. Cases of rubella in immunized children are rare.

Roseola Infantum

Roseola infantum is a contagious viral disease that generally affects children under 4 and usually children about 1 year of age.[4] It produces a characteristic maculopapular rash covering the trunk and spreading to the appendages. A rapid rise in temperature to 105°F and coldlike symptoms accompany the disease.[4] Unlike rubella, no cervical or postauricular lymph node adenopathy occurs. The symptoms usually subside within 3 to 5 days.[4] Roseola infantum is frequently mistaken for rubella. Rubella can usually be ruled out by the age of the child as well as by the absence of

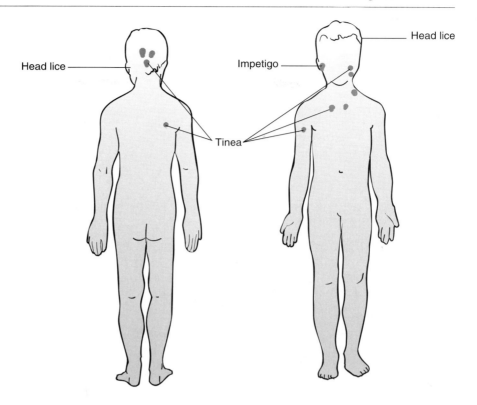

FIGURE 53–5. Sites of selected common communicable dermatoses affecting children.

lymph node adenopathy. Generally, children less than 6 to 9 months do not develop rubella because of maternal antibodies.[4] Blood antibody titers may be assayed to determine the actual diagnosis. In most cases there are no long-term effects from this disease.

Treatment for roseola infantum is palliative. As with rubella, antipyretic drugs such as acetaminophen (Tylenol) and cooling baths are used to reduce the fever. Rest and fluid are recommended for recuperation and body rehydration. Pruritis may accompany the other symptoms, but this is rare. If severe, pruritis can be treated with topical lotions such as Caladryl.

Measles

Hard **measles** or 7-day measles (rubeola) is a communicable viral disease caused by the morbillivirus. The characteristic rash is macular and blotchy (Fig. 53–6); sometimes the macules become confluent. The rubeola rash usually begins on the face and spreads to the appendages. There are several accompanying symptoms: a fever of 100°F or greater, Koplik's spots (small irregular red spots with a bluish white speck in the center) on the buccal mucosa, and mild to severe photosensitivity.[5] Coldlike symptoms and general malaise and myalgia are often present. In severe cases the macule may hemorrhage into the skin tissue or to another body surface. This is called *hemorrhagic measles*. Measles is more severe in malnourished children. Complications include otitis media, pneumonia, and encephalitis.

Measles is preventable by vaccine (MMR), and immunization is required by law in most states. Im-

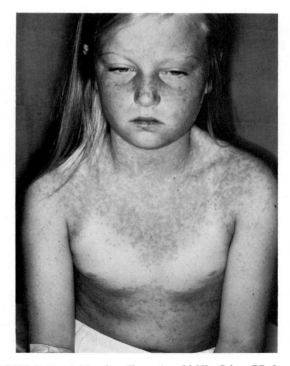

FIGURE 53–6. Measles. (From Arnold HL, Odom RB, James WD: *Andrews' Diseases of the Skin: Clinical Dermatology*, 8th ed. Philadelphia, WB Saunders, 1990, p 466. Reproduced with permission.)

munization is accomplished by the MMR schedule (see discussion under Rubella).

For a positive diagnosis, most states require antibody titer determination. Blood titers are usually determined during the disease process and 6 weeks after the symptoms have resided.

The treatment of measles is symptomatic. Children are kept in darkened rooms. Antipyretic medications are given to reduce the fever, and rest and fluids are encouraged.

Chickenpox

Chickenpox is a common communicable childhood disease. It is caused by the herpes zoster virus, which is also the causative agent in shingles. The characteristic skin lesion occurs in three stages: macule, vesicle, and granular scab. The macular stage is characterized by the rapid development (within hours) of macules over the trunk of the body, spreading to the limbs, buccal mucosa, scalp, axillae, upper respiratory tract, and conjunctivae. During the second stage, the vacules versiculate (blister) and may become depressed or umbilicated (raised blisters with depressed centers). The vesicles break open, and a scab forms during the third stage. Crops of lesions occur successively, so that all three forms of the lesion are usually visible by the third day of the illness. Mild to extreme pruritus accompanies these lesions and can be a complicating factor by leading to scratching and the subsequent development of secondary bacterial infection. Other symptoms that accompany chickenpox are coldlike symptoms, including cough, coryza, and sometimes photosensitivity. Mild febrile states usually occur. Side effects such as pneumonia, septic complications, and encephalitis are rare.[4]

Treatment is symptomatic. Antipyretic drugs such as acetaminophen are given for fever reduction; they may also relieve local discomfort. Pruritus is relieved with lukewarm baths. Oral administration of Benadryl or other antihistamines may be prescribed to alleviate itching. Application of topical antipruritics such as Caladryl lotion is also helpful. However, in young children, care must be taken to avoid topical preparations of Caladryl containing diphenhydramine (Benadryl) in order to avoid possible overdose of this agent through systemic absorption of Benadryl. (This is an especially important consideration if the young child is also taking oral Benadryl.) Home remedies such as baking soda baths also relieve itching. Rest and fluids are important in recuperation and rehydration. Some authorities recommend acyclovir, an antiviral agent, in the treatment of chickenpox.[6]

Varicella-zoster immune globulin (VZIG) provides passive immunity against chickenpox and is recommended following exposure, especially for high-risk groups. A vaccine against chickenpox that will provide active immunity is likely to be available for widespread use in the near future. Currently, vaccination is available for children with acute lymphocytic leukemia for compassionate use only.[7]

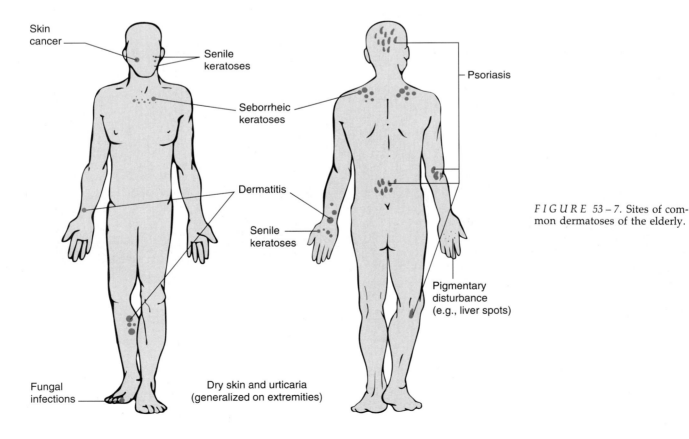

Skin cancer

Senile keratoses

Seborrheic keratoses

Dermatitis

Senile keratoses

Fungal infections

Dry skin and urticaria (generalized on extremities)

Psoriasis

Pigmentary disturbance (e.g., liver spots)

F I G U R E 53 – 7. Sites of common dermatoses of the elderly.

Scarlet Fever

Scarlet fever is a systemic reaction to the toxins produced by the Group A β-hemolytic streptococci. It occurs when the person is sensitized to the toxin-producing variation of streptococci. It frequently occurs in association with streptococcal sore throat (strep throat); but it may also be associated with a wound, skin infection, or puerperal infection. Scarlet fever is characterized by a pink punctate skin rash on the neck, chest, axillae, groin, and thighs. When palpated, the rash feels like fine sandpaper. There is flushing of the face with circumoral pallor. Other symptoms include high fever, nausea and vomiting, strawberry tongue, raspberry tongue, and skin desquamation. Complications of scarlet fever include otitis media, peritonsillar abscess, rheumatic fever, acute glomerulonephritis, and cholera. Penicillin is the drug of choice for treatment.

Adolescence and Young Adulthood

The most common disorder of adolescence and young adulthood is **acne vulgaris.** The increased production of sex hormones and oils contributes to the development of acne. Childhood diseases are less common in adolescence; however, chronic skin diseases may be exacerbated.

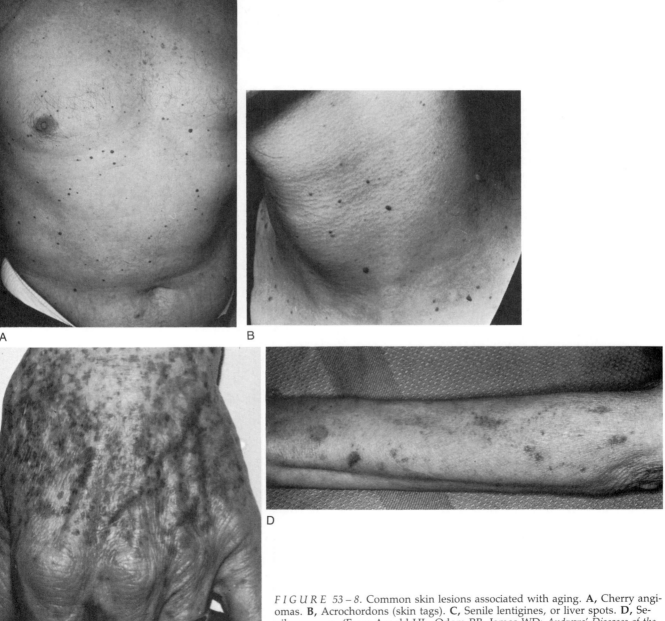

FIGURE 53-8. Common skin lesions associated with aging. **A,** Cherry angiomas. **B,** Acrochordons (skin tags). **C,** Senile lentigines, or liver spots. **D,** Senile purpura. (From Arnold HL, Odom RB, James WD: *Andrews' Diseases of the Skin: Clinical Dermatology,* 8th ed. Philadelphia, WB Saunders, 1990, pp 689 (**A**), 719 (**B**), 809 (**C**), 954 (**D**). Reproduced with permission.)

Geriatric Considerations

Skin disorders are so common in elderly people that it is difficult to distinguish normal from abnormal. More than 90 percent of all older people have some kind of skin disorder (Fig. 53–7, page 1056).[8,9] The most common skin disorders in the elderly are **keratoses** and **skin cancers,** followed by **fungal infections, dermatitis, pigmentary disturbances, psoriasis,** and **urticaria.** Other skin disorders frequently seen in the elderly are comedones (blackheads), asteoses (scaling), cherry angiomas (small, red, benign tumors) nevi (moles), skin tags (pedunculated fleshy growths), and lentigines ("liver spots"). In addition, the incidence of senile purpura and senile warts (papillomata) significantly increases, especially among the very old. Senile purpura is related to the loss of subcutaneous tissue, which supports the skin capillaries. Minor trauma can cause small bruises or ecchymotic lesions, which largely occur on the extensor surface of the forearms. Forty percent of older men and 77 percent of older women show evidence of senile purpura.[10] Senile papillomata are small yellow, brown, or black warts located on the trunk, limbs, and face. Sixty-three percent of all older people have some senile papillomata.[11]

Figure 53–8 (page 1057) illustrates several of the common skin lesions associated with aging. Most of these lesions are considered normal concomitants of aging and cause little discomfort. The greatest concern regarding body image is the appearance of the skin, which tends to look mottled and spotty. Disorders of the skin that tend to cause the most physical discomfort are pruritus, keratoses, epitheliomas, malignant melanomas, herpes zoster, psoriasis, and pressure sores.

KEY CONCEPTS

- Certain skin disorders are more common in particular age groups. Infants are prone to irritation lesions, including prickly heat, contact dermatitis, and cradle cap. Altered areas of pigmentation are first noticed in infancy, including mongolian spots, hemangiomas, and nevi.
- Children are prone to skin injuries and communicable diseases. A number of viral infections, including rubella, roseola, measles, and chickenpox, are associated with characteristic skin rashes. Fever and malaise are usually present. Treatment is symptomatic. Vaccinations are available to prevent rubella and measles. Scarlet fever is due to a bacterial infection and is treated with antibiotics.
- Children are often exposed to superficial infections and infestations, including head lice, ringworm, scabies, and impetigo.
- Acne is the most common skin disorder of adolescents.
- Elderly skin is prone to a number of problems, including psoriasis, angiomas, and skin tags. Cancerous and precancerous lesions are common, requiring careful screening examination.

Selected Examples of Skin Disorders

Major pathogenic processes affecting the skin include infectious processes, inflammatory conditions, allergic reactions, parasitic infestations, overexposure or hypersensitivity to sunlight, ulcers and tumors, and malignant neoplasms. Although many of these disorders are not life-threatening, they can affect the quality of life.

Infectious Processes

Viral Infections

Verrucae, or warts (Fig. 53–9), are common benign papillomas caused by DNA-containing papoviruses. Although warts vary in appearance, depending on their location, the histology of all lesions is similar. The wart is actually an exaggeration of normal skin composition. There is an irregular thickening of the stratum corneum. The human papillomaviruses (HPVs), the subgroup of papoviruses that cause human warts, are not found in animals and invade only the skin and mucous membrane of humans.

Warts resolve spontaneously when immunity to the virus develops. The immune response may be delayed for years. After 5 years, 95 percent of warts left untreated will have disappeared.[12] Current surgical treatment may be directed at removal of the wart using laser. Liquid nitrogen or acid chemicals, cryotherapy, and salicyclic acid paint or plasters have also been effective medical treatments.

Herpes simplex virus (HSV) infections of the skin and mucous membranes are common (Fig. 53–10). Two types of herpesviruses infect humans, type 1 and type 2. Most of the HSV 1 infections occur above the waist.[13] HSV 1 may result when external infection is

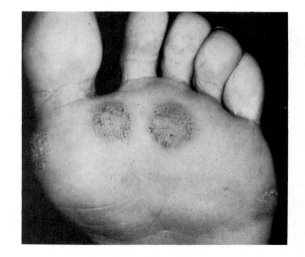

FIGURE 53–9. Plantar warts. (From Arnold HL, Odom RB, James WD: *Andrews' Diseases of the Skin: Clinical Dermatology,* 8th ed. Philadelphia, WB Saunders, 1990, p 470. Reproduced with permission.)

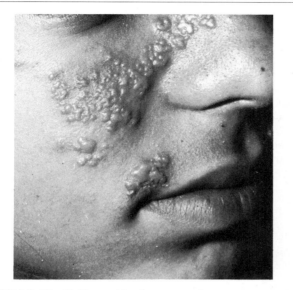

FIGURE 53-10. Herpes simplex, unusually extensive. (From Arnold HL, Odom RB, James WD: *Andrews' Diseases of the Skin: Clinical Dermatology*, 8th ed. Philadelphia, WB Saunders, 1990, p 437. Reproduced with permission.)

spread to the other parts of the body through the occupational hazards that exist in professions such as dentistry and medicine, and some athletics. HSV 2 is responsible for most infections in the genital region.[13] (See Chapter 34 for a further discussion of sexually transmitted diseases.)

Herpesvirus lesions usually begin with a burning or tingling sensation. Vesicles and erythema follow and progress to pustules, ulcers, and crusts before healing. The lesion is most common on the lips, face, and mouth. Pain is common, and healing takes place within 10 to 14 days.[14] After the initial infection, the herpesvirus persists in latent form in the trigeminal and other ganglia. Recurrent lesions are common in a small percentage of people; precipitating factors may be stress, sunlight exposure, menses, or injury.[15]

There is no cure for herpes simplex. Most treatment measures are palliative. Lidocaine (Xylocaine) or diphenhydramine (Benadryl) application and aspirin help relieve pain. Cold compresses help in the acute stages. Severe forms have been treated with idoxuridine (IDI, Stoxil), which prevents certain aspects of DNA synthesis and thereby inhibits viral reproduction without causing cell injury. Some authorities recommend acyclovir (Zovirax), an antiviral agent.

Herpes zoster (*shingles*) is an acute localized inflammatory disease of a dermatomal segment of the skin (Fig. 53-11). It is caused by the same herpesvirus that causes chickenpox, varicella-zoster. It is believed to be the result of reactivation of a latent varicella-zoster virus that has been present in the sensory dorsal ganglia since childhood infection. During an attack of shingles, the reactivated virus travels from the ganglia to the skin of the corresponding dermatome.

The clinical manifestations of shingles include the eruption of vesicles with erythematous bases that are restricted to skin areas supplied by sensory neurons

of a single or associated group of dorsal root ganglia. Eruptions are generally unilateral and occur on the thorax, trunk, and face. In immunosuppressed persons, the lesions may extend beyond the dermatome. New crops of vesicles erupt for 3 to 5 days along the nerve pathway.[13] Lesions are deeper and more confluent than those of chickenpox. The vesicles dry, form crusts, and eventually fall off. Lesions usually clear in 2 to 3 weeks.[13] Severe pain and paresthesis are common. In the elderly, herpes-zoster is a particularly serious condition that may be long lasting. Pain reports from elderly individuals indicate an increased severity and lengthy episodes of up to 1 year.[13]

Postherpetic neuralgia is the most important complication occurring in people over the age of 50.[13] Eye involvement can result in permanent blindness.

Treatment for shingles includes acyclovir (Zovirax). Topical agents such as Burrow's compresses or aqueous alcohol shake lotions may also be used. Pain medication may be indicated in severe cases. Systemic corticosteroids have also been effective in healthy persons over 50 years old with severe pain, but their use remains controversial. High doses of interferon, an antiviral glycoprotein, have been used in persons with cancer when the herpetic lesions are limited to the dermatome.[16]

Superficial Fungal Infections

Three general classifications of **fungi** (**dermatophytes**) commonly infect human skin: *Microsporum, Trichophyton,* and *Epidermophyton*. These organisms can cause infection termed **tinea** in any cutaneous area, including the hair and nails. Infections in different locations are named after the location: tinea capitis (scalp), tinea barae (beard), tinea faciale (face), tinea corporis

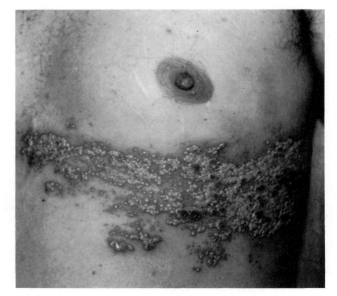

FIGURE 53-11. Herpes zoster. (From Arnold HL, Odom RB, James WD: *Andrews' Diseases of the Skin: Clinical Dermatology*, 8th ed. Philadelphia, WB Saunders, 1990, p 447. Reproduced with permission.)

(trunk), tinea manus (hand), tinea cruris (groin), and tinea pedis (foot).

The clinical signs of superficial fungal infections vary depending on the physical location and the hosts's response to the invading organism (Fig. 53–12). Often fungal infections present as erythematous macules or plaques with peripheral scaling and some central clearing. Vesicular lesions often accompany the dry scaling on the feet. Because of the variability of presentation, superficial dermatophytosis must be considered in evaluating even a weeping, crusted area more suggestive of eczema or impetigo.

Dermatophyte infection of the nails, or onychomycosis, usually presents as a white or yellow opaque discoloration that often progresses to a thickened, crumbed, or deformed nail (see Fig. 53–12).

Topical treatment of localized superficial dermatophyte infections is very effective. Among the topical antifungal preparations available in cream and solution form are miconazole nitrate, clotrimazole, econazole nitrate, ciclopirox olamine, and terbinafine; a 4-week course of twice daily applications will usually clear symptoms. For more extensive infections involving the hair, nails, or resistant organisms, systemic

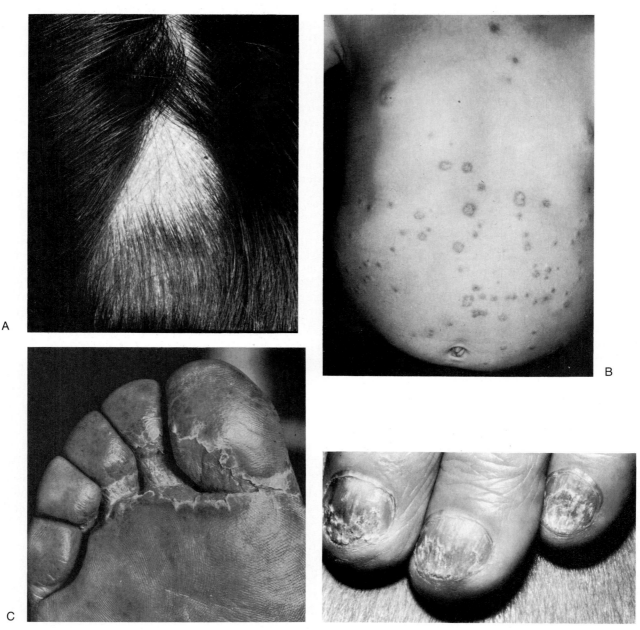

F I G U R E 53 – 12. Tinea. **A,** Tinea capitis, localized patch, caused by *Trichophyton tonsurans.* **B,** Tinea corporis in a child, caused by *Microsporum canis.* **C,** Tinea pedis showing interdigital scalping (*Trichophyton mentagrophytes*). **D,** Onychomycosis. (From Arnold HL, Odom RB, James WD: *Andrews' Diseases of the Skin: Clinical Dermatology,* 8th ed. Philadelphia, WB Saunders, 1990, pp 319 (**A**), 327 (**B**), 332 (**C**), 337 (**D**). Reproduced with permission.)

therapy (griseofulvin or ketoconazole) is required. The treatment duration ranges from 3 to 4 weeks (tinea corporis) to 12 months (onychomycosis).

Yeast Infections

The yeast *Candida albicans* is another frequent source of superficial infection (Fig. 53–13). It is manifested in newborns as the white lesions of **thrush,** in infants and bedridden patients as **intertrigo,** and in immunoimpaired persons as the systemic disorder **mucocutaneous candidiasis.**

Localized yeast infections, such as oral candidiasis (thrush), may be treated with nystatin mouth rinse or clotrimazole troches (throat lozenges). The topical antifungal medications mentioned above may also be used in the treatment of localized yeast infections. Widespread or systemic infections respond well to oral ketoconazole or fluconazole (Diflucan).

Bacterial Infections

Impetigo is an acute, contagious skin disease characterized by the formation of vesicles, pustules, and yellowish crusts (Fig. 53–14). It is the most common cause of infection of the skin and is caused by staphylococci or streptococci bacteria. Approximately 5 percent of persons sustain *Staphylococcus* infections each year of a severity sufficient to require medical attention.[17] Approximately 20 percent of adults are chronic carriers of the bacterium, *Staphlococcus aureus,* and another 60 percent are intermittent carriers.[17] The bacte-

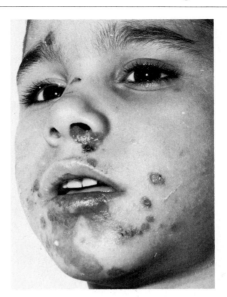

FIGURE 53–14. Impetigo. (From Arnold HL, Odom RB, James WD: *Andrews' Diseases of the Skin: Clinical Dermatology,* 8th ed. Philadelphia, WB Saunders, 1990, p 275. Reproduced with permission.)

rium is carried in the nasal area and may pass onto the skin, producing disease. Staphylococcal infections are a special problem for hospitalized patients, who may become infected from the infected staff of the hospital.

Treatment for impetigo includes topical application of 2 percent mupirocin ointment (Bactroban). If a large area of skin is involved or if the person is febrile, impetigo may be treated systemically using oral dicloxacillin, cephalexin, or erythromycin.

A variety of sexually transmitted diseases caused by bacteria can infect the genitalia. The most serious is **syphilis.** Syphilis is caused by *Treponema pallidum.* If untreated, three stages can occur. In primary syphilis, a chancre (ulcer) generally occurs as a single lesion of the genitalia; the spirochetal microorganism that causes syphilis can be seen in a scraping of the chancre. Secondary syphilis is characterized by a disseminated rash that cannot be clearly distinguished from other rashes. Both the primary and secondary stages of syphilis are contagious. Studies to detect serum antibodies against syphilis (such as the VDRL) and examination of the pustules for the spirochete are required to achieve a diagnosis. Penicillin is very effective in eradicating syphilis in the primary and secondary stages, but unfortunately, damage caused by tertiary syphilis to the cardiovascular and central nervous systems is permanent.

Leprosy is a chronic infectious disease of the skin caused by the intracellular bacillus *Mycobacterium leprae.* Approximately 11 million people worldwide have leprosy.[17] The diagnosis is made with a skin biopsy. Leprosy has a low rate of infectivity and is usually responsive to sulfone drugs like dapsone. For chronic deformities, corrective orthopedic surgery may be required.

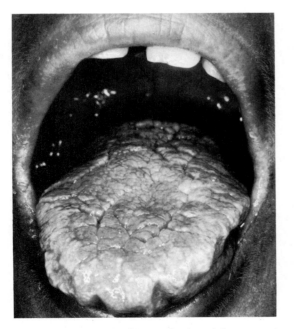

FIGURE 53–13. Candida albicans infection of the tongue in chronic mucocutaneous candidiasis. (From Arnold HL, Odom RB, James WD: *Andrews' Diseases of the Skin: Clinical Dermatology,* 8th ed. Philadelphia, WB Saunders, 1990, p 341. Reproduced with permission.)

TABLE 53–3. Comparison of Chronic Discoid Lupus Erythematosus (LE) With Systemic Lupus Erythematosus (SLE)

Parameter	Chronic Discoid LE	Systemic LE
Primary lesions	Red, scaly, thickened, well-circumscribed patches with enlarged follicles and elevated border.	Red, mildly scaly, diffuse, puffy lesions. Purpura also seen.
Secondary lesions	Atrophy, scarring, and pigmentary changes.	No scarring. Mild hyperpigmentation.
Distribution	Face, mainly in "butterfly" area, but also on scalp, ears, arms, and chest. May not be symmetric.	Face in "butterfly" area, arms, fingers, and legs. Usually symmetric.
Course	Very chronic, with gradual progression; slow healing under therapy; no effect on life.	Acute onset with fever, rash, malaise, and joint pains. Most cases respond rather rapidly to steroid and supportive therapy, but the prognosis for life is poor.
Season	Aggravated by intense sun exposure or radiation therapy.	Same.
Sex incidence	Almost twice as common in females.	Same.
Systemic pathology	None obvious.	Nephritis, arthritis, epilepsy, pancarditis, hepatitis, etc.
Laboratory findings	Biopsy characteristic in classic case. LE cell test negative, as are other laboratory tests.	Biopsy less useful. LE cell test usually positive. Leukopenia, anemia, albuminuria, increased sedimentation rate, positive antinuclear antibody test, and biologic false-positive serologic test for syphilis.

From Sauer GC: *Manual of Skin Diseases*, 6th ed. Philadelphia, JB Lippincott, 1991, p 253. Reproduced with permission.

Inflammatory Conditions

Lupus Erythematosus

Lupus erythematosus (LE) is an inflammatory disease that has cutaneous manifestations. Systemic LE and chronic discoid LE are clinically dissimilar but basically related diseases. The two diseases differ in regard to characteristic skin lesions, subjective complaints, other organ involvement, LE cell test findings, response to treatment, and eventual prognosis. A comparison of the two conditions is found in Table 53–3. Figure 53–15 illustrates characteristic skin lesions of both conditions.

Seborrheic Dermatitis

Seborrheic dermatitis (Fig. 53–16) is a papulosquamous skin disease manifested by various degrees of scaling and erythema in areas of high oil gland concentration such as the scalp, eyebrows, glabellae, eyelids, nasolabial folds, pinna and posterior sulcus of the ears, sternum, axillae, umbilicus, and anogenital area. Common manifestations of this disease are cradle cap in newborns and dandruff in adolescents and adults.

Although seborrheic dermatitis is not curable, it may be controlled with topical medication. The regular use of tar shampoos often clears the symptoms and signs of seborrheic dermatitis in the scalp; mild topical corticosteroids (e.g., 1 percent hydrocortisone) clear the lesions on the face and ears.

Psoriasis

Psoriasis is a common chronic skin disease characterized by papules and plaques with an overlying silvery scale. The disease may affect, with varying degrees of severity, people of all ages. Lesions can appear on any area of the body; however, they seem to have a predilection for the knees, elbows, lower back, scalp, and nails (Fig. 53–17). Disease progression is unpredictable, and the patient may periodically experience spontaneous exacerbations or remission.

There is no known cure for psoriasis. Treatments, both topical and systemic, are directed at clearing and controlling the lesions. Therapies include topical corticosteroids (most commonly used), a vitamin D derivative (calcipotriene ointment, Dovonex), ultraviolet light exposure, topical tar preparations, and combinations of ultraviolet light with topical tar or systemic psoralen. Systemic therapies with methotrexate and hydroxyurea are also effective in clearing psoriasis but carry considerable risk of toxicity.

Lichen Planus

Lichen planus is a relatively common, chronic, pruritic disease involving inflammation and papular

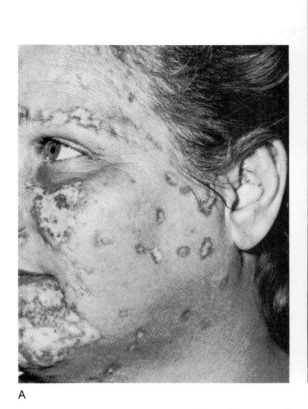

A

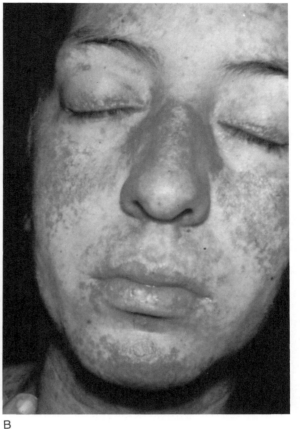

B

FIGURE 53–15. **A,** Disseminated discoid lupus erythematosus. **B,** Acute cutaneous lupus erythematosus (systemic lupus erythematosus with skin lesions). (From Arnold HL, Odom RB, James WD: *Andrews' Diseases of the Skin: Clinical Dermatology*, 8th ed. Philadelphia, WB Saunders, 1990, pp 162 (**A**), 166 (**B**). Reproduced with permission.)

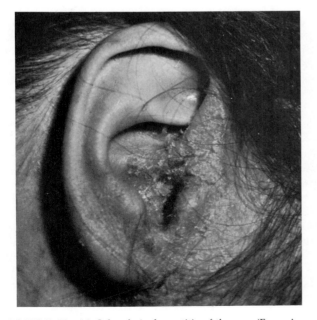

FIGURE 53–16. Seborrheic dermatitis of the ear. (From Arnold HL, Odom RB, James WD: *Andrews' Diseases of the Skin: Clinical Dermatology*, 8th ed. Philadelphia, WB Saunders, 1990, p 195. Reproduced with permission.)

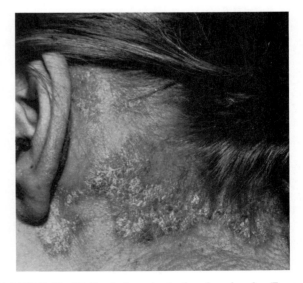

FIGURE 53–17. Psoriasis on back of neck and scalp. (From Arnold HL, Odom RB, James WD: *Andrews' Diseases of the Skin: Clinical Dermatology*, 8th ed. Philadelphia, WB Saunders, 1990, p 200. Reproduced with permission.)

eruption of the skin and mucous membranes. Idiopathic lichen planus is of unknown etiology but can be stimulated by a variety of drugs and chemicals in susceptible persons. The characteristic lesion is a shiny, white-topped, purply polygonal papule. Lesions appear on the wrist, ankles, and trunk (Fig. 53–18). Mucous membrane lesions are white and lacy and may become bullous. Pruritus is severe, and new lesions develop as a result of scratching. Nails are affected in approximately 10 percent of people with lichen planus.[18]

In the majority of people, lichen planus is a self-limiting disease. Treatment measures include discontinuing all medications, followed by topical corticosteroids and occlusive dressings. Systemic corticosteroids may be indicated in severe cases. Antipruritic agents are helpful in reducing the itch.

Pityriasis Rosea

Pityriasis rosea is a rash of unknown origin that primarily affects young adults. The incidence is highest in spring and fall. It has been speculated to be viral in origin, but to date no virus has been isolated. The

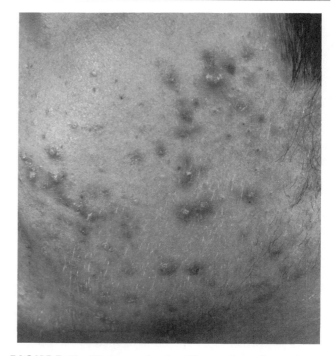

FIGURE 53–19. Acne vulgaris, with papules and pustules, on the cheek. (From Arnold HL, Odom RB, James WD: *Andrews' Diseases of the Skin: Clinical Dermatology,* 8th ed. Philadelphia, WB Saunders, 1990, p 251. Reproduced with permission.)

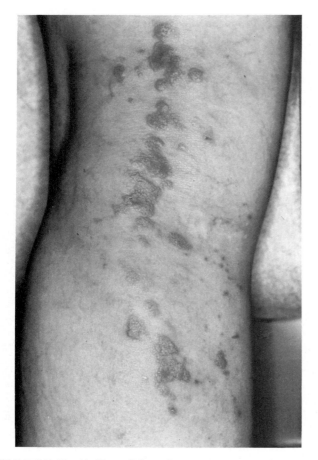

FIGURE 53–18. Linear lichen planus. (From Arnold HL, Odom RB, James WD: *Andrews' Diseases of the Skin: Clinical Dermatology,* 8th ed. Philadelphia, WB Saunders, 1990, p 244. Reproduced with permission.)

characteristic lesion is a macule or papule with surrounding erythema. The lesion spreads with central clearing, much like tinea corporis. This initial lesion is a solitary lesion, called the herald patch, and is usually on the trunk or neck. As the lesion enlarges and begins to fade away (2–10 days), successive crops of lesions appear on the trunk and neck.[19] The extremities, face, and scalp may be involved, and mild to severe pruritis may occur. The disease is self-limiting and usually disappears within 6 to 8 weeks.[19] Treatment is palliative and includes topical steroids, antihistamines, and colloid baths. Systemic corticosteroids may be indicated in severe cases.

Acne Vulgaris

Acne, an extremely common disease of the pilosebaceous unit, affects up to 90 percent of all individuals, producing unsightly lesions and sometimes permanent scarring and disfigurement (Fig. 53–19).[20] Etiologically, acne involves multiple factors such as sex hormones, heredity, bacterial flora of the skin, stress, mechanical occlusion, and cosmetics use. Acne arises from the sludging of sebaceous oils and the deposition of loose epithelial cells, causing an obstruction of the follicular canal. Continued oil production and bacterial growth in this obstructed follicle may cause rupture of the wall or sebaceous gland, resulting in an inflamed lesion.

There is no cure for acne. Treatment modalities are directed toward clearing the lesions and maintaining

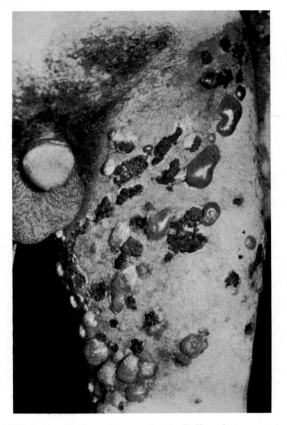

FIGURE 53–20. Pemphigus vulgaris. Bullous lesions arising from apparently normal skin surface, with crusts. (From Arnold HL, Odom RB, James WD: *Andrews' Diseases of the Skin: Clinical Dermatology*, 8th ed. Philadelphia, WB Saunders, 1990, p 535. Reproduced with permission.)

a clear complexion. Topical therapy works for most patients. Such medications are designed to cause increased peeling of the stratum corneum and loosening of the follicular plugs.

Many products are available to achieve this goal. Soaps, lotions, and gels containing sulfur, resorcinol, salicylic acid, or benzoyl peroxide all enhance drying and peeling. Astringents, liquids primarily composed of alcohol with acetone, are used as solvents to remove the surface lipid and loose skin cells as well as to enhance drying. Another effective topical preparation is retinoic acid, a derivative of vitamin A.[14] A peeling agent, it is very useful in dealing with open comedones and papules. Topical antibiotics are also available, the most effective being liquid preparations of erythromycin and clindamycin (Cleocin T) with an alcohol base.

For cases characterized by inflammatory lesions, pustules, or nodules, systemic therapy can be useful. Antibiotics, especially tetracycline and erythromycin, have long been used in such treatments. In resistant cases, minocycline, sulfamethoxazole-trimethoprim, and sulfones are occasionally used. Isotretinoin, a vitamin A derivative, is effective in the treatment of nodular and cystic acne.[14] Birth control pills, especially the estrogen-dominant type, can be of value in treating severe recalcitrant acne in females. However, an-

drogen-dominant contraceptives can aggravate or precipitate acne.

As with any medication regimen, both systemic and topical acne treatments can produce unwanted side effects in sensitive patients. Systemic tetracycline may cause gastrointestinal upset, nausea, diarrhea, and vaginal *Monilia* overgrowth. Tetracycline should not be used in children because their unerupted teeth may be severely and permanently discolored. Topical antibiotics can cause irritant or allergic contact dermatitis.

Other useful acne treatments include ultraviolet light, controlled sunlight exposure, corticosteroid injection into cysts and nodules, and surgery, which involves extraction of the comedones and drainage of fluctuant cystic lesions.[15]

Pemphigus

A group of related disorders (**pemphigus group** of vulgaris, vegetans, foliaceus, and erythematous) is characterized by bullous eruptions (blister). These disorders are thought to be caused by autoimmune reactions. Patients show antibodies against keratinocytes and basement membranes. The autoantibodies perhaps cause the keratinocytes to separate from one another to form blisters. Of the group of related diseases, **pemphigus vulgaris** has the worst prognosis (Fig. 53–20). Bullae can erupt on the skin and mucous membranes (e.g., esophagus), and toxemia and infection can cause death if proper treatment (cortisone) is not administered.

Allergic Skin Responses

Atopic Dermatitis

Atopy, or **allergy,** is indicated by a personal and sometimes family history of asthma, allergic rhinitis,

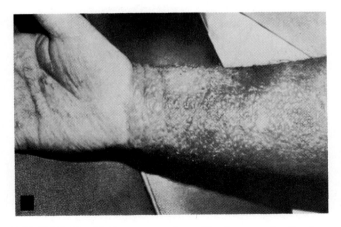

FIGURE 53–21. Eczematous dermatitis. In an acute allergic contact dermatitis, numerous vesicles appear at the site of antigen exposure (in this case, laundry detergent). (From Murphy GF, Mihm MC: The skin, in Cotran RS, Kumar V, Robbins SL (eds): *Robbins Pathologic Basis of Disease*, 5th ed. Philadelphia, WB Saunders, 1994, p 1194. Reproduced with permission.)

or—the most commonly seen manifestation—eczematous dermatitis (Fig. 53–21). The highest incidence of atopic dermatitis occurs in children, with most cases developing before age 5.[21] The characteristic presentation depends on the age at onset but is always pruritic. In infants, the disease characteristically appears on the face, scalp, or extensor surfaces of the extremities; the predominant lesion is an oozing, crusting, coalescent papule. The disease in children is most often seen as erythema, papules, and lichenification of the flexor surfaces of the extremities, especially the antecubital and popliteal areas, the wrists, and the nape of the neck (Fig. 53–22). In older children and young adults there is thickening of the skin or lichenification, along with fine, dry scaling and some papules. These changes are again seen on the flexor surfaces of the extremities, the scalp, face, and upper chest. Retrospective studies show that in nearly half of all patients presenting with childhood atopic dermatitis, the disease improves or clears with age.[22]

Treatment of atopic dermatitis is usually carried out on an outpatient basis. The most important considerations are moisturization of the skin and prevention of continued drying and water loss. The drying and scaling that are characteristic features of atopic dermatitis impair the skin's ability not only to retain moisture but also to repel such external invaders as chemical irritants and surface bacteria. Milder cases of atopic eczema can be treated conservatively by decreasing the frequency of bathing, using of tepid water in baths, eliminating alkaline soaps, and using moisturizing creams (especially after baths and washing). In more severe cases that involve an inflammatory response to skin breakdown, topical steroids are an important part of therapy. Short courses of systemic antibiotics such as erythromycin have also been helpful in controlling the severity of atopic eczema by reducing the concentration of cutaneous bacterial flora. Even after all these measures have been executed, some patients with severe atopic dermatitis are hospitalized for continuous wet dressings and topical steroids.

An important feature of all atopic dermatitis that must be dealt with is pruritus. The topical treatments previously mentioned are helpful in reducing itch. If additional measures are needed, systemic antihistamines (e.g., hydroxyzine and diphenhydramine) are effective.

Contact Dermatitis

Contact dermatitis is a cutaneous reaction to either topical irritation or allergy. Irritant contact dermatitis develops in any person exposed to a sufficiently high concentration of the irritating agent. Some of the more active irritants are acids, alkalis, and hydrocarbons.

Allergic contact dermatitis indicates delayed acquired hypersensitivity to a specific allergin. Dermatologic problems may appear after years of asymptomatic exposure to the precipitating agent. Chromates, nickel, ethylenediamine, paraphenylenediamine, neomycin, formaldehyde, and lanolin components may cause allergic contact dermatitis.

Aside from reactions to various industrial chemicals, the most common type of allergic contact dermatitis is to plants. **Rhus dermatitis** encompasses allergy to poison ivy, poison oak, and poison sumac. Clinically, rhus dermatitis begins within 48 hours of contact. The first symptom is pruritus, followed by erythema and vesicle formation, sometimes in linear fashion (Fig. 53–23). As long as the allergin remains on the surface of the skin, it can be spread to nonexposed areas. Therefore, thorough washing can help prevent spread by hand contact. Exposure to blister fluid does not spread poison ivy lesions.

Contact dermatitis from exposure to poison ivy can range from mild to severe. For the mildest cases, application of topical steroids or cooling shake lotions of camphor and menthol may effectively decrease discomfort. Severe cases may require hospitalization for cooling baths and wet dressings, which dry the lesions and decrease the tense, pruritic blisters. Discomfort and generalized edema often respond to administration of systemic steroids over a 10- to 14-day period.

Drug Eruptions

Adverse or undesirable reactions to medically administered drugs are common, yet cutaneous reactions

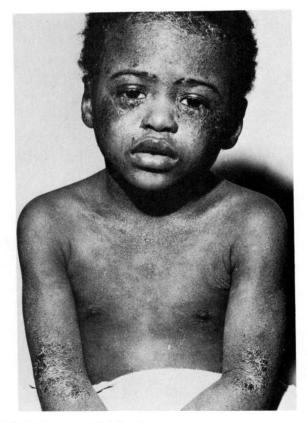

FIGURE 53–22. Childhood atopic dermatitis. Lichenification and some scarring have occurred. (From Arnold HL, Odom RB, James WD: *Andrews' Diseases of the Skin: Clinical Dermatology*, 8th ed. Philadelphia, WB Saunders, 1990, p 69. Reproduced with permission.)

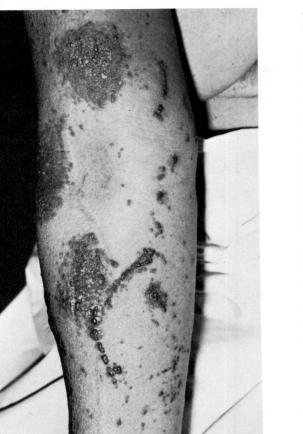

FIGURE 53 – 23. Rhus dermatitis with characteristic linear groups of vesicles. (From Arnold HL, Odom RB, James WD: *Andrews' Diseases of the Skin: Clinical Dermatology,* 8th ed. Philadelphia, WB Saunders, 1990, p 95. Reproduced with permission.)

are uncommon (0.1 percent) within the overall prescription-taking population.[23] Cutaneous reactions to medication usually begin within a week of drug exposure, although reactions to the penicillins may occur later. Women experience more cutaneous drug eruptions than men. The drugs that most frequently result in adverse cutaneous eruptions are ampicillin, penicillin, cephalosporins, and barbiturates. Blood transfusions also occasionally produce cutaneous reactions identical to a drug eruption.

The most common type of adverse cutaneous drug eruption is an erythematous maculopapular exanthem (rash). These often pruritic lesions are usually widely dispersed and clearing is gradual, continuing for several weeks after the drug is discontinued. Other common drug reactions include urticaria, erythema multiforme (including Stevens-Johnson syndrome),

exfoliative dermatitis, photosensitivity, vasculitis, and fixed drug eruption.

Exanthem-type eruptions can be caused by such medications as barbiturates, griseofulvin, penicillin, thiazides, and sulfonamides. Urticarial eruptions may result from the use of barbiturates, penicillin, chloramphenicol, phenolphthalein, salicylates, sulfonamides, or tetracycline. Erythema multiforme is seen with erythromycin, penicillin, phenolphthalein, salicylate, diphenylhydantoin, and thiazide. Exfolitative dermatitis can be caused by barbiturates, gold, penicillin, phenothiazides and sulfonamides, and photosensitivity is seen with chlordiazepoxide, fluoroquinolones, griseofulvin, phenothiazines, sulfonamides, tetracycline, and thiazides. Cutaneous vasculitis may be triggered by iodines, erythromycin, penicillin, quinidine, sulfonamides, and thiazides. Another effect of fixed drug eruption is a round to oval, violaceous macule or slightly palpable plaque that is often recurrent, especially in previously affected sites, on reexposure to the irritating medication. This effect can be caused by barbiturates, gold, phenolphthalein, sulfonamides, and tetracycline. (These drug lists are not inclusive, and several substances are known to cause multiple adverse cutaneous reactions.[24]) The treatment of drug eruptions includes discontinuation of the offending drug and administration of oral antihistamines and/or antipruritic lotions of hydrocortisone, menthol, camphor, or other proven substances for relief of pruritus. For more severe eruptions a 2- to 3-week course of systemic corticosteroids should be considered. In addition, the patient should be counseled regarding use of the offending medication and an appropriate notation should be placed in the patient's medical record.

Vasculitis

When antigen and antibody react in blood vessels in the skin, severe **necrotizing inflammation (vasculitis)** can appear. This can occur from drug allergies, disorders such as systemic lupus erythematosus, rheumatoid arthritis, glomerulonephritis, and certain infectious diseases such as hepatitis B. **Polyarteritis nodosum** is a form of systemic vasculitis that can cause inflamed arteries in visceral organs, brain, and skin.

Immunofluorescent studies will reveal antibodies and serum immunoglobulins trapped in the wall of the blood vessel that is inflamed by neutrophils. Acute vasculitis can cause damage not only to skin but also to the brain and visceral organs. When vasculitis is severe, systemic cortisone may be administered in high doses.

Parasitic Infestations

Scabies

Sarcoptes scabiei is a mite, and infestations with this mite in humans are called **scabies.** Scabies begins with eggs laid in the stratum corneum. These eggs hatch into larvae within 3 to 4 days and grow to adulthood within 2 months. Scabies is usually contracted after close personal contact with an infested individual.

Clinically, scabies lesions are small (1–4 mm) erythematous papules, some with an overlying dry scale or crust (Fig. 53–24). In some cases, linear burrows are seen. Scabies mites have a predilection for the finger webs, wrists, umbilicus, and groin area. The history related by most patients is of an intensely pruritic eruption that spreads over a period of weeks from a single area of the body to other areas.

Scabies treatment consists of topical permethrin cream (Elimite), gamma benzene hexachloride (lindane), or crotamiton (Eurax). For infants, 5 to 6 percent precipitated sulfur in petrolatum applied twice daily for a week is usually adequate.

Fleas

Three types of flea commonly bite and cause cutaneous reactions in humans—the human flea (*Pulex irritans*), the cat flea (*Ctenocephalides felis*), and the dog flea (*Ctenocephalides canis*). Flea bites may present as small erythematous macules, erythematous papules, wheals, or a vesicle.

Diethyltoluamide or pyrethrin insect repellents are effective in preventing flea infestation. Indoor carpeting, an ideal environment for fleas, should be treated with an appropriate insecticide.

The milder papular form of flea bites can be treated with soothing shake lotions of menthol and camphor or with topical steroids. More severe reactions (e.g., vesicles or bullae) may require a course of systemic steroids.

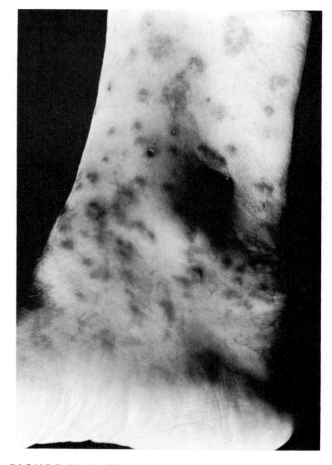

F I G U R E 53 – 25. Chigger bites. (From Arnold HL, Odom RB, James WD: *Andrews' Diseases of the Skin: Clinical Dermatology*, 8th ed. Philadelphia, WB Saunders, 1990, p 529. Reproduced with permission.)

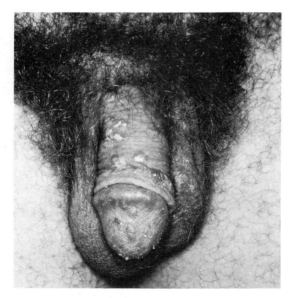

F I G U R E 53 – 24. Scabies. Note lesions on glans penis. (From Arnold HL, Odom RB, James WD: *Andrews' Diseases of the Skin: Clinical Dermatology*, 8th ed. Philadelphia, WB Saunders, 1990, p 523. Reproduced with permission.)

Lice

Phthirius pubis (crab lice), *Pediculus humanis var. capitis* (head lice), and *Pediculus humanis var. corporis* (body lice) are the types of lice most often found on humans. They are surface-dwelling, unlike the burrowing scabies mite, and can usually be seen without magnification. Control and eradication are possible with gamma benzene hexachloride (lindane) shampoo or lotion, permethrin cream rinse, or pyrethrins and piperonyl butoxide liquid, gel, or shampoo.

Chiggers

Chiggers are mites that reside in grasses and bushes. They are common in the southern United States but can be found as far north as Canada. The mite punctures the skin to obtain nourishment, producing pruritic papules commonly seen wherever it encounters resistance, such as the top of socks, at the belt line, or around the neckband area (Fig. 53–25). Secondary lesions are excoriations from scratching that have become infected by bacteria. Treatment is palliative, and insect repellent is encouraged for prevention.

Ticks

Ticks are insects that live in woods and underbrush. They attach to human and animal hosts and burrow in the epidermis, where they feed on blood. The tick bite itself is not problematic, but the infectious bacteria or viruses that ticks carry to human hosts create problems. There are many tick-borne illnesses, including Central European encephalitis, Q fever, babesiasis, relapsing fever, Rocky Mountain spotted fever, and Lyme disease. Both Rocky Mountain spotted fever and Lyme disease are relatively common in the United States.

Rocky Mountain spotted fever (RMSF) is caused by a tick that carries *Rickettsia rickettsii*. RMSF used to be localized to the Rocky Mountain area, but by 1982 most states had reported a case of RMSF.[17]

The initial tick bite appears as a papule or macule, with or without a central punctate area. The tick burrows in and enlarges as it feeds. The tick must be attached to the human host for 4 to 6 hours before the rickettsiae are activated by the blood.[17] Rickettsiae are found in the tick feces and body parts. The rickettsiae then enter the bloodstream and multiply in the body tissues. Within 4 to 8 days the patient experiences fever, headache, muscle aches, nausea, and vomiting.[17] A rash then starts on the wrist or ankle. The characteristic rash is a macular or maculopapular rash that spreads to the rest of the body. Other symptoms include generalized edema, conjunctivitis, petechial lesions, photophobia, lethargy, confusion, and cranial nerve deficits.

Treatment for RMSF requires hospitalization and antibiotic therapy. The most important measure is to prevent tick bites by using insect repellents while engaged in activities in the woods. Once a tick has attached itself, it is important to remove all the body parts to limit the possibility of infection. Ticks may be removed by slowly pulling them, dousing them with mineral oil or alcohol before removing them with tweezers, or applying a hot match to the end of the tick. The latter method is not the most effective, as the tick may regurgitate into the open wound.

Lyme disease is caused by the bite of a tick that carries the spirochete *Borrelia burgdorferi*. White-tailed deer and white-footed mice are the main reservoirs of this disease-causing spirochete. Lyme disease causes multiple symptoms affecting the skin, nervous system, heart, and musculoskeletal system. The disease has three clinical stages. Stage I usually occurs in the summer and early fall with single or multiple erythematous papules that may itch, sting, or burn. The thighs, groin, and axillae are particularly common sites of involvement. This disease is often accompanied by flulike symptoms (fatigue, headache, chills, fever, sore throat, stiff neck, nausea, myalgias, and arthralgias). If the disease remains untreated, stage II Lyme disease appears weeks to months later. This

stage is characterized by meningitis, cranial nerve palsies, and peripheral neuropathy; occasionally, there is cardiac involvement. In stage III, oligoarticular arthritis occurs. In early Lyme disease, treatment includes antibiotic therapy such as doxycycline or amoxicillin or erythromycin for 10 to 21 days. Neurologic disease, arthritis, or cardiac disease is treated with doxycycline or amoxicillin for 1 month or with intravenous penicillin for 10 to 14 days.

Bedbugs

The common bedbug, *Cimex lectularius*, is a reddish brown insect, 3 to 6 mm long, that turns purple after feeding. Like most parasites, bedbugs feed on human blood. Importantly, they can also alternate between human and animal hosts, and they live up to and sometimes beyond 1 year.[17] When not feeding, bedbugs stay hidden in the cracks and crevices of furniture, mattresses, wallpaper, picture frames, baseboards, flooring, door locks, or any darkened area. Unless their source is eliminated, recurrence is inevitable. Professional extermination is advised because of their many hiding places. Bedbugs have been known to feed on animal populations when forced from their living quarters. On rehabitation in the same quarters, the bedbug can easily return to human hosts.

They are nocturnal feeders, and when squashed, they emit a foul odor. The bedbug bite is painless and produces a pruritic oval or oblong wheal with a small hemorrhagic punctum at the center. Bullous lesions are not uncommon. Usually, lesions are multiple and arranged in rows or clusters on the face, neck, hands, and arms. No area is exempt. The wheal is probably a type I sensitivity reaction to the anticoagulant saliva of the bedbug. Secondary excoriation and bacterial infections may occur.

The diagnosis depends on the time of the day when the lesions appear. Because of the painless bite, it is not uncommon for the victim to awake with one or several pruritic papules. Topical antipruritics are used in the treatment.

Mosquitoes

Most people have experienced mosquitoes and are familiar with their bites. The typical lesion is a raised wheal on an erythematous base, accompanied by pruritus within 45 minutes of the bite. A second type of reaction is the delayed response. Eight to 12 hours after the bite, the lesion becomes raised, erythematous, and indurated, with extensive pruritus or pain. This reaction peaks 24 hours to 72 hours after the bite.[18] The saliva of the mosquito is believed to be the source of the skin reaction. Although severe skin reactions are possible, they are rare. Insect repellents are encouraged for prevention; local antipruritics are used for treatment.

Blood Flukes

Bathers in the freshwater lakes of Wisconsin, Michigan, and Minnesota are prone to periodic attacks of inflammatory, papular, urticarial, and vesicular eruptions on the uncovered areas of the body, mainly the legs. This pruritic eruption, commonly called "swimmer's itch," usually subsides within a week and is caused by the invasion of the skin by the cercariae (larvae) of the schistosomes (worms) of ducks and mammals. The life cycle of these various species of schistosomes includes the snail as an intermediate host. On invasion of the abnormal definitive host, the human skin, the cercariae die, and the resulting skin eruption is the skin's reaction in ridding itself of the foreign bodies. Repeated attacks are met with stronger resistance, and the dermatitis becomes increasingly more severe. Secondary infection, edema, and lymphangitis can occur.

Swimmer's itch is best prevented by destruction of the snails through careful addition of a combination of copper sulfate and hydrated lime to the lake water. Rapid drying of the swimmer with a towel apparently prevents penetration of the cercariae. Active therapy is directed toward the relief of the itching and preventing secondary infection.

Scleroderma

Other disorders of the dermis include **scleroderma,** in which there is massive collagen deposition with fibrosis, accompanied by inflammatory reactions and vascular changes in the capillary network (see Chap. 51).

There are two forms of scleroderma that are clinically dissimilar except for some common skin histopathology. Localized scleroderma (morphea) is a benign disease. Diffuse scleroderma (progressive systemic sclerosis) is serious, progressive, and fatal.

Localized Scleroderma

This condition has unknown etiology, no systemic involvement, and no known treatment. Disability is confined to the area involved. Lesions tend to involute (shrivel) slowly and spontaneously. Relapses are rare. Primary skin lesions are single or multiple, violet-colored, firm, inelastic macules and plaques that enlarge slowly. The progressing border retains a violet hue, while the center becomes whitish and slightly depressed beneath the skin surface. Bizarre lesions occur, such as long linear bands on extremities, "saber-cut" lesions in scalp, or lesions involving one side of the face or the body. Secondary lesions include mild or severe scarring after healing, permanent hair loss due to scalp lesions, and, rarely, ulceration. The trunk, extremities, and head are most frequently involved (Fig. 53–26).

Diffuse Scleroderma

This rare systemic collagen disease of unknown etiology is characterized by a long course of progressive

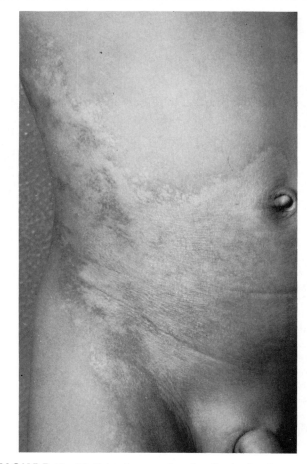

FIGURE 53–26. Extensive morphea (localized scleroderma). (From Arnold HL, Odom RB, James WD: *Andrews' Diseases of the Skin: Clinical Dermatology,* 8th ed. Philadelphia, WB Saunders, 1990, p 177. Reproduced with permission.)

disability due to lack of mobility of the areas and the organs that are affected. The skin becomes hardened like hide, the esophagus and the gastrointestinal tract semirigid, the lungs and the heart fibrosed, the bones resorbed, and the overlying tissue calcified. Figure 53–27 illustrates the "hidelike" skin on the face of a woman with diffuse scleroderma.

Another rare collagen disorder, **dermatomyositis** is characterized by the acute or insidious onset of muscle pain, weakness, fever, arthralgia, and, in some cases, a puffy erythematous eruption that is usually confined to the face and the eyelids. Progression of the disease results in muscle atrophy and contractures, skin telangiectasiae (vascular lesions formed by blood vessel dilation) and atrophy, and generalized organ involvement. Death occurs in 50 percent of cases.[25,26]

Sunburn and Photosensitivity

Effects of Sunlight

Sunlight is an extremely harmful environmental agent because it produces the short ultraviolet wavelength that is responsible for sunburn, thickening of the stra-

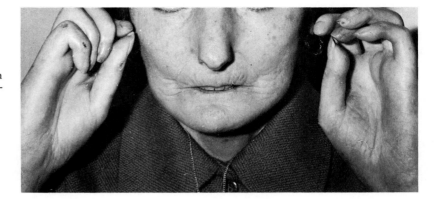

FIGURE 53–27. Hide-like skin on the face of a woman with diffuse scleroderma (progressive systemic sclerosis). (From Arnold HL, Odom RB, James WD: *Andrews' Diseases of the Skin: Clinical Dermatology*, 8th ed. Philadelphia, WB Saunders, 1990, p 176. Reproduced with permission.)

tum corneum, suntan, and increased melanin production. Sunlight produces direct local effects on the skin in the form of elastotic syndromes, keratoacanthomas, premalignant diseases, basal cell epitheliomas, and squamous cell epitheliomas. Both indirect and direct effects can produce malignant melanomas.[27]

Sunburn initially manifests with erythema, pain, heat, and occasionally blistering, edema, and tenderness. In severe sunburn these symptoms may also be accompanied by constitutional symptoms of chills, fever, nausea, and generalized discomfort.

The most effective treatment is to avoid or limit exposure to sunlight. Wearing protective clothing is effective; sunscreens are also quite useful in preventing sunburn and the chronic solar changes of the skin. Para-aminobenzoic acid (PABA) is the most widely used sunscreen. People sensitive to PABA may use cinnamates and benzophenones as substitutes. Opaque screens such as zinc oxide and titanium dioxide also work well. However, these white preparations are not cosmetically elegant. Recently, titanium dioxide has been incorporated into foundation makeup for women.

Sunburn can be treated symptomatically with cold water baths or compresses; topical steroids are often effective in relieving the discomfort of localized severe burns. For widespread sunburn a 10- to 14-day course of systemic steroids may suppress the symptoms.

Ulcers

An unfortunate problem for the bedridden person may be development of **pressure sores** or **decubitus ulcers.** Thinning epithelial cells and blood vessels have a slower rate of repair, resulting in a higher and more severe incidence of decubitus ulcers and slower healing of damaged skin among the elderly.

Pressure sores are localized areas of cellular necrosis resulting from prolonged pressure between any bony prominence and an external object, such as a bed or wheelchair. The tissues are deprived of blood supply and eventually die. Areas frequently affected in older persons include the heels, greater trochanter, sacrum, dorsal spine (especially in thin kyphotic persons), scapular spine, and elbows. Long-term pressure increases vulnerability to decubitus ulcer development. High pressure maintained for a short time is less dangerous than low pressure continued for a long time. Predisposing factors include poor nutrition, aging, immobility, superficial sensory loss, and disturbed autonomic function (loss of bowel and bladder control).[28] Older people with dementia are particularly likely to develop pressure sores because of arteriosclerotic changes in the vessels, loss of subcutaneous tissue and tissue elasticity, and clouding of the sensorium.[28]

There are two types of pressure sores, superficial (benign) and deep (malignant). Superficial sores are reddened areas involving only the outer skin layers. They are less dangerous than deep sores and are caused by friction, shearing stresses, trauma, infection, and saturation with urine or other wet agents. The lesions are frequently painful but are easily treated and prevented. Treatment consists of keeping the area clean, dry, and free from infection or further pressure; a covering with a nonstick dressing also promotes healing. Measures such as frequent turning (every 2 hours), getting the person moving—out of bed and into a chair, keeping the vulnerable areas clean and dry, and keeping the weight of the bedcovers off the feet are most effective in warding off superficial pressure sores.

Deep sores develop quickly as a result of thrombosis of the vessels in deep tissue overlying the bony prominences. The muscle and fat layers are more vulnerable than the dermis, causing deep, large ulcers. The sore begins as a reddening of the skin with unobservable necrosis in the deep underlying tissues. In 1 to 2 days the lesion bursts through the skin like an abscess, revealing a deep cavity full of black or infected slough, which may go through to the bone.[28] There is a large area of skin loss, resulting in extensive scarring. The appearance of deep pressure sores with an illness can delay recovery and may even be fatal.

Prevention is more difficult with deep pressure sores, especially in the elderly. The risk of developing these lesions is greatest during the 10 days after the onset of illness or admission to the hospital, which coincides with the period of greatest immobility.[28] A deep sore that develops early and penetrates deeply is most dangerous to the older person. Early signs of deterioration include apathy, loss of appetite, and

TABLE 53–4. Preventing Deep Pressure Sores

1. Change position every 2 hr
2. Do not over- or undersedate
3. Avoid or correct malnutrition
4. Avoid dehydration; maintain blood pressure and cardiac output
5. Use an alternating-pressure air bed or waterbed

Data from Rosen T, Lanning MB, Hill MJ (eds): *Nurse's Atlas of Dermatology.* Boston, Little, Brown & Co, 1983.

incontinence. Some measures that can help prevent deep pressure sores are described in Table 53–4.

Treatment consists primarily of reinforcing preventive measures, including maintenance of fluid and protein stores that are lost through serous and purulent discharge; repair of tissues by giving vitamin supplements; avoidance of general infections, such as pneumonia or cystitis; and remediation of anemia. The lesions should be cleaned and dressed, taking care to treat local infection. To promote granulation and healing, the wound should be irrigated with warm saline every day. Irrigation washes out the debris, lowers the growth of anaerobes, promotes the separation of the slough, and decreases the pocketing of infection in deeper tissues. Infection must be eradicated and the slough must separate before healing can take place.

Altered Cell Growth

Epidermal Proliferation

The keratinocyte produces keratin. Rare, inherited defects in the keratinocytes can occur. The inherited disease **congenital ichthyosis** is characterized by an excessive growth of keratinocytes and keratin, giving the skin a fishscale appearance (Fig. 53–28).

Corns and **calluses** result from **hyperkeratosis.** Stimulation of the epidermis by intermittent pressure elicits hyperkeratosis (corn and callus formation). By contrast, *atrophy* of the epidermis can arise from a decreased blood supply.

Benign or malignant **neoplasms** commonly arise from keratinocytes. **Warts** (verrucae), for instance, are caused by a virus that provokes a benign proliferation of keratinocytes. **Squamous cell carcinomas** (arising from keratinocytes) often occur in areas of skin excessively exposed to sunlight.

Tumors

Each cell type of the skin can give rise to either benign or malignant tumors. Benign tumors, including squamous papillomas, arise from keratinocytes, common moles (**nevi**) arise from melanocytes, lipomas from adipose cells, vascular tumors (hemangiomas) from blood vessels, dermatofibromas from fibroblasts, and neuromas from nerves.

Kaposi's sarcoma arises from reticulocytes and is multifocal, metastastizing, and malignant. Kaposi's

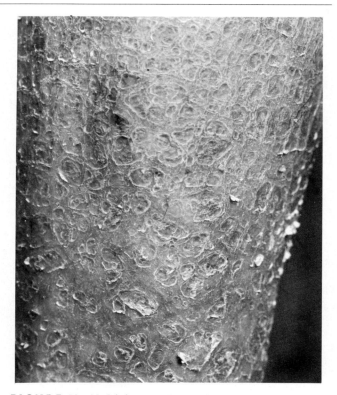

FIGURE 53–28. Ichthyosis. (From Johnson ML: Skin diseases, in Wyngaarden JB, Smith LH (eds): *Cecil Textbook of Medicine,* 17th ed. Philadelphia, WB Saunders, 1985, p 2251. Reproduced with permission.)

sarcoma is classified as an opportunistic neoplasm because it occurs in persons with preexisting immunodeficiency, for example, in persons with primary immunodeficiency, in those who undergo therapeutic immunosuppression, and in persons with HIV infection. Figures 53–29 and 53–30 show some of the cutaneous diseases associated with HIV infection. (See also Figures 10–16, 10–17, and 10–18 on Color Plate I.)

Cancer

Cancer of the skin is common. Most skin cancers are trivial, but certain types can be lethal. Excessive exposure to sunlight in a person with fair skin often leads to skin cancer. Besides sunlight, exposure to irritating chemicals, recurrent trauma, and irradiation is associated with a high risk of skin cancer.

Basal cell carcinomas are the commonest skin tumors and the most benign (Fig. 53–31).[29] Squamous cell carcinomas are the next most common malignancy (Fig. 53–32).[29] They can occasionally metastasize. By contrast, malignant melanoma is rare but can be highly malignant (Fig. 53–33). Melanoma is notoriously unpredictable; however, the prognosis is based on the size, the depth of invasion of the tumor, and the presence of metastasis.[30] Lumps that increase rapidly in size, change color, ulcerate, or bleed should be biopsied and examined microscopically to rule out

FIGURE 53-29. Some of the cutaneous diseases associated with HIV infection. **A,** Molluscum contagiosum. Numerous large, umbilicated waxy papules have coalesced to form crusted plaques. They may be seen on other body parts as well. (From Friedman-Kien AE: *Color Atlas of AIDS*. Philadelphia, WB Saunders, 1989, p 99. Reproduced with permission.) **B,** Classic Kaposi's sarcoma, nodular stage. Coalescing brown to violet, plaque to nodular lesions with overlying adherent hyperkeratotic scales. (From Friedman-Kien AE: *Color Atlas of AIDS*. Philadelphia, WB Saunders, 1989, p 17. Reproduced with permission.)

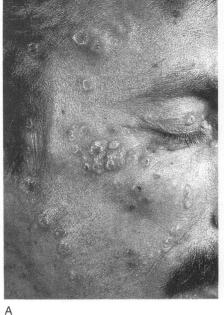

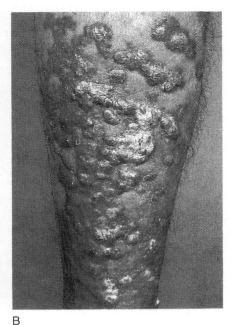

A   B

A   B

FIGURE 53-30. Some of the cutaneous diseases associated with HIV infection. **A,** Herpes zoster in AIDS. (From Arnold HL, Odom RB, James WD: *Andrews' Diseases of the Skin: Clinical Dermatology*, 8th ed. Philadelphia, WB Saunders, 1990, p 481. Reproduced with permission.) **B,** Seborrheic dermatitis. Pinkish red scaly and crusted plaques are seen in the malar areas but also in other locations. (From Friedman-Kien AE: *Color Atlas of AIDS*. Philadelphia, WB Saunders, 1989, p 113. Reproduced with permission.)

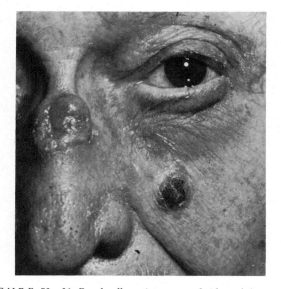

FIGURE 53-31. Basal cell carcinomas on bridge of the nose and left cheek of an 80-year-old woman. (From Arnold HL, Odom RB, James WD: *Andrews' Diseases of the Skin: Clinical Dermatology*, 8th ed. Philadelphia, WB Saunders, 1990, p 765. Reproduced with permission.)

malignancy. Complete surgical excision is the treatment of choice for skin cancers.

Pigmentation

Special Characteristics of Dark Skin

There are a number of disorders of the skin that exclusively affect people with dark skin. Pigmentary disturbances from many causes, both hypopigmentation and hyperpigmentation, are common. Postinflammatory hyperpigmentation, for example, may occur in African-American individuals when melanocytes are

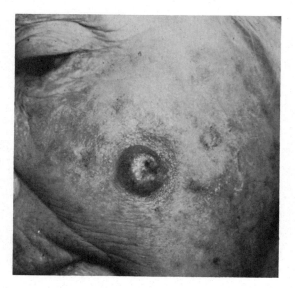

FIGURE 53-32. Squamous cell carcinoma. Note the dome shape of the tumor. (From Arnold HL, Odom RB, James WD: *Andrews' Diseases of the Skin: Clinical Dermatology*, 8th ed. Philadelphia, WB Saunders, 1990, p 778. Reproduced with permission.)

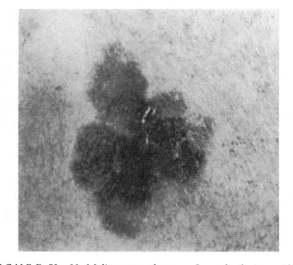

FIGURE 53-33. Malignant melanoma. Irregular lesion with varying pigmentation and early central thickening. (From Moschella SL, Hurley JH: *Dermatology*, 2nd ed. Philadelphia, WB Saunders, 1985, p 1576. Reproduced with permission.)

stimulated by inflammation. Hyperpigmentation in any person with dark skin can occur after traumatic injury, skin infection, or inflammatory skin disease. Patchy areas of depigmentation known as **vitiligo** are more noticeable in persons with dark skin because of the color contrast. Some lesions, such as those causing erythema, may show no visible color change in darkly pigmented individuals. Petechiae, for example, which cause pinpoint purplish red lesions, are usually observable only on the oral mucosa or conjunctiva.

Disorders such as seborrheic dermatitis and keloids are seen with greater frequency in African-Americans.[31] The custom of tightly plaiting the hair or using hot oil and tension on the scalp leads to gradual damage to the hair follicles, hair thinning, and eventually hair loss. Known as **traumatic alopecia,** this condition is also seen with greater frequency in African-Americans.

Conversely, many skin disorders such as squamous cell or basal cell carcinoma, senile keratoses, and psoriasis that affect light-skinned people only rarely affect darker-skinned persons.

Psoriasis is rare among the African-American population. If present, it may be difficult to detect. The typical bright red color is not present. The plaques assume a blue or violet hue because of stimulation of melanocytes. The characteristic silvery scale is often absent.

Literature related specifically to abnormalities of dark skin is also rare. Normal variants, such as the mongolian spot in infants, Futcher's or Voight's line, and linear nail pigmentation, are frequently mistaken for disorders. Table 53–5 presents tips for assessing dark skin.

Vitiligo

Vitiligo (leucoderma) is a condition in which pigment disappears from a patch of skin. The onset is sudden

TABLE 53–5. Tips for Assessing Dark Skin

1. Skin color should be observed in the sclerae, conjunctivae, buccal mucosa, tongue, lips, nail beds, palms, and soles.
2. Inspection should be accompanied by palpation, especially if inflammation or edema is suspected.
3. Findings should always be correlated with the patient's history to arrive at a diagnosis.
4. *Pallor* in brown-skinned patients may present as a yellowish brown tinge to the skin. In a black-skinned patient the skin will appear ash-gray. It can be difficult to determine. Pallor in dark-skinned individuals is characterized by absence of the underlying red tones in the skin.
5. *Jaundice* may be observed in the sclera but should not be confused with the normal yellow-pigmented sclera of the dark-skinned black patient. The best place to inspect is in the portion of the sclera that is observable when the eye is open. If jaundice is suspected, the posterior portion of the hard palate should also be observed for a yellowish cast. This is most effective when done in bright daylight.
6. The *oral mucosa* of dark-skinned individuals may have a normal freckling of pigmentation that may also be evident in the gums, the borders of the tongue, and the lining of the cheeks.
7. The gingiva normally may have a dark blue color that may appear blotchy or be evenly distributed.
8. *Petechiae* are best observed over areas of lighter pigmentation—the abdomen, gluteal areas, and volar aspect of the forearm. They may also be seen in the palpebral conjunctiva and buccal mucosa.
9. To differentiate petechiae and ecchymosis from erythema, remember that pressure over the area will cause erythema to blanch but will not affect either petechiae or ecchymosis.
10. *Erythema* usually is associated with increased skin temperature, so palpation should also be used if an inflammatory condition is suspected.
11. *Edema* may reduce the intensity of the color of an area of skin because of the increased distance between the external epithelium and the pigmented layers. Therefore, darker skin would appear lighter. On palpation the skin may feel "tight."
12. *Cyanosis* can often be difficult to determine in dark-skinned individuals. Familiarity with the precyanotic color is often helpful. However, if this is not possible, close inspection of the nail beds, lips, palpebral conjunctiva, palms, and soles should show evidence of cyanosis.
13. *Skin rashes* may be assessed by palpating for changes in skin texture.

Data from Rosen T, Martin S: *Atlas of Black Dermatology.* Boston, Little, Brown & Co, 1981.

and may be associated with pernicious anemia, hyperthyroidism, and diabetes mellitus.

Vitiligo is a concern to darkly pigmented people of all races. It also affects light-skinned persons, but not as often. The lesion is a depigmented macular patch with definite borders on the face, axillae, neck, or extremities (Fig. 53–34). The borders are smooth. Size varies from small to large macules involving great skin surfaces. The large macular type is much more common. Depigmented areas, which burn in sunlight, appear bone-colored or sometimes grayish blue.

Vitiligo appears at any age, in men and women alike, and usually occurs before the age of 21.[32] Its incidence has been increasing in India, Pakistan, and Far Eastern countries.[32] Although the etiology is unknown, inheritance and autoimmune factors have been implicated. Affected areas spread over time. Treatment is experimental and consists of psoralen administration in conjunction with ultraviolet radiation (PUVA). Cosmetics such as Derma Blend may be used to camouflage the areas of depigmentation.

Albinism

Melanocytes produce melanin. A partial or total absence of melanin arises as an inborn error in metabolism in persons with **albinism.** Albinism, also termed oculocutaneous albinism, is characterized by a generalized lack of pigmentation of the skin and the hair.

In addition, the eyes may show nystagmus and a lack of pigmentation of the fundi and translucent irises. The condition is recessively inherited. Biochemically, albinism occurs because of impaired or absent melanin synthesis. The long-term consequences of albinism may include solar keratoses and basal and squamous cell cancers.

Education regarding the use of sunscreens and clothing for protection against ultraviolet light–induced damage is indicated. Sunglasses and magnifiers are beneficial for the ocular symptoms.

KEY CONCEPTS

- **Skin infections may be caused by viral, fungal, or bacterial organisms. Viruses are associated with warts, human papillomavirus, cold sores (herpes simplex), and shingles (herpes zoster). Warts are painless. They may be surgically removed but often resolve spontaneously. Herpes simplex lesions are painful, may be treated symptomatically, and often recur in times of stress. Herpes zoster inhabits sensory dorsal ganglia neurons and causes pain along a dermatome.**

- **Superficial fungal infections (tinea, ringworm) often present with central clearing and peripheral scaling. They may be effectively treated with topical antifungals. Yeast infections tend to occur in moist areas such as mucous membranes and are treated with sys-**

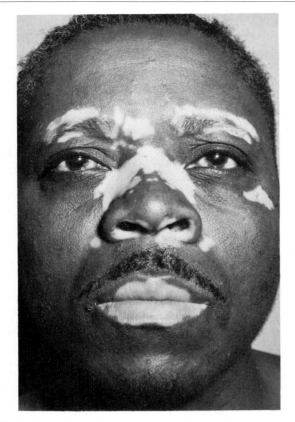

FIGURE 53–34. Vitiligo. (From Arnold HL, Odom RB, James WD: *Andrews' Diseases of the Skin: Clinical Dermatology*, 8th ed. Philadelphia, WB Saunders, 1990, p 1001. Reproduced with permission.)

temic and/or topical drugs. Impetigo is caused by staphylococcal or streptococcal infection and is characterized by yellowish pustules and crusts. It responds to antibiotic therapy.

- The etiology of noninfectious inflammatory diseases is usually unknown. Lupus, seborrheic dermatitis, psoriasis, lichen planus, pityriasis rosea, and acne are in this category. Treatment is aimed at reducing inflammation rather than cure. Antibiotics may be used to prevent or treat lesion superinfections.
- Skin allergies are associated with substances that cause erythema and itching. Atopic dermatitis (eczema), commonly seen in young children, is due to contact with substances to which the individual is allergic. Contact dermatitis occurs in anyone coming in contact with a certain substance. Drug reactions are allergic responses manifested as widely dispersed, often pruritic rashes. Antigen-antibody reactions within cutaneous blood vessels can result in severe necrotizing vasculitis.
- The skin is subject to invasion by a number of different bugs, ticks, and parasites. Lesions tend to be singular or grouped and in areas exposed to the particular pest. Scabies commonly occurs on the hands and wrists and may appear as linear burrows. Bites from fleas, mites, bedbugs, and mosquitoes are often pruritic macules or papules. Tick bites are usually painless but may be problematic, because ticks

may carry diseases such as Rocky Mountain spotted fever and Lyme disease.

- Scleroderma is a collagen disease of unknown etiology. It may be localized to the skin or produce systemic involvement. The skin is discolored, thick, and hardened.
- Utraviolet rays in sunlight are associated with acute damage to the skin (sunburn) as well as increasing the long-term risk of skin cancer.
- Pressure ulcer is a significant problem of immobility due to prolonged pressure on bony prominences. Superficial sores are reddened areas involving outer skin layers. Deep sores are due to thrombosis of vessels deep in the tissue. Deep sores may be unnoticed initially, then burst through the skin like an abscess.
- Abnormalities of skin cell growth may result in such benign processes as corns and calluses, or the more serious consequence, cancer. Basal cell and squamous cell carcinomas are slowly progressive and generally amenable to surgical excision. Malignant melanoma is more prone to metastasis and carries a poorer prognosis.
- Abnormal pigmentation may occur in response to skin injury, infection, or inflammation, or may be genetically determined. Albinism is due to lack of melanin production. Vitiligo is a depigmented patch of skin that is most noticeable in dark-skinned persons. The etiology is unknown.

Treatment

A distinct advantage in treating the skin is the ease of direct observation of the pathology and the effects of treatment. Culture, scrape, or biopsy also facilitate diagnosis. Correct diagnosis can help prevent complications from improper therapy, but it does not lessen the importance of choosing an appropriate delivery system.

Topical Treatment

Wet Dressings

Wet dressings, the application of a liquid in compress form, are a very important part of the dermatologic therapy delivery system. The applied liquid can be plain water or water with additives (e.g., sodium, magnesium, or aluminum salts).

Wet dressings are a versatile, even paradoxical therapeutic approach, able to dry or hydrate as necessary. Intermittently applied, they serve as an effective astringent for the weeping, oozing lesions that accompany stasis and decubitus ulcers and impetigo. Vesicular lesions, including those seen in dyshydrotic eczema, herpes zoster, and pemphigus, also respond nicely to treatment with intermittent wet dressings. By drying disease-related lesions, intermittent dressings help speed recovery.

Continuous wet dressings, on the other hand, are effective in rapidly hydrating the skin. This technique, used most often in severe cases of atopic eczema, normally requires hospitalization. Wet dressings of gauze soaked in tap water are applied directly to the skin and covered with an insulating agent such as towels, large thick gauze pads, or even long underwear to prevent evaporation. It is very important that dressings remain moist. Therefore, they must be resoaked and changed every 3 hours around the clock throughout the course of treatment. Once the desired state residue of hydration has been achieved, the dressings can be discontinued and emollient creams used to prevent redrying of the treated area.

Lotions

Lotions are mixtures of small, highly suspended particles in a liquid vehicle. They are homogeneous suspensions and generally do not separate into their component parts. When it is necessary to cover large surface areas with a thin film of medication, lotions are often the treatment of choice. They are also useful around the fingernails and toenails, as well as in hairy or exposed areas where other preparations are not as convenient or cosmetically pleasing.

Some lotions contain large amounts of water or alcohol in their base preparations and can dry the skin. A base composed primarily of an oil eliminates that problem but may feel greasy and stain clothing.

Gels

Most gels are clear, colorless, volatile substances. They generally penetrate better than creams. They are very convenient to use on wet lesions because of their astringent tendencies. Since they do not leave the white or oily residue of creams and ointments, they are appropriate for use on scalp lesions.

Creams

Creams are most widely used dermatologic delivery system. Many different bases are used in creams, but the "vanishing" type is most common and allows application with no surface residue. Creams penetrate well and do have some moisturizing capability. They are used most frequently in treating dry to slightly moist dermatoses.

Ointments

The medication in most ointments is carried in a petrolatum-type base, which facilitates penetration into the upper skin layers. Ointments are frequently used on skin lesions that have overlying dry scaling and crusting, but they are also very effective on severe dermatoses requiring increased medication dosage. Ointments are semiocclusive and often are not appropriate for use on lesions that are oozing and discharging a transudate or exudate.

Aerosols

Aerosols, fine particle sprays of medication usually delivered by gas under pressure, are a cosmetically elegant way of treating dermatoses, especially on hairy areas of the body.

Intralesional Injection

Intralesional injection is the deposition of medication directly into the lesion. This can be done with a conventional needle and syringe or with an instrument (Dermajet) that injects fine particles of medication through the skin with air pressure. This delivery form is especially useful in delivering higher concentrations of corticosteroids to lesions (usually with deep dermal components) that do not respond to topical medication.

Selection of a Delivery System

Delivery system selection depends on the disease being treated, the type of lesions clinically present, and the practitioner's preferred medication routine. For instance, weeping exudative lesions require drying (wet dressings) and perhaps corticosteroids. Initial delivery as a gel would increase the drying tendency; as the lesion dries, a cream may be used to prevent overdrying and fissure formation.

In a disease state such as chronic atopic eczema with a lichenoid or thickened skin presentation, the prescriber may choose an ointment to enhance penetration of the medication into the lesion. The ointment's occlusive nature reduces moisture loss from the skin.

Seborrhea and psoriasis in the scalp may be treated with aerosols, which are quick, easy to use, and have a high degree of patient compliance. Patients often find them cosmetically superior to the identical medication in cream form. Keloids, which require highly concentrated medication to be delivered to a small area, are ideal candidates for intralesional injection of corticosteroids.

Corticosteroids

Corticosteroids are a very important part of the practice and treatment of dermatologic disease. Dermatologists administer steroids systemically and topically. Steroids may be characterized as short-acting (cortisone, hydrocortizone); intermediate-acting (prednisone, prednisolone, methylprednisolone, or triamcinolone); or long-acting (dexamethasone or betamethaxone).

Systemic Steroids

Administration of systemic steroids in dermatologic disease is usually oral. Intermediate-acting steroids (prednisone, prednisolone, methylprednisolone) are used most often; intermediate-acting steroids (triamcinolone) are used occasionally. The greatest benefit of oral administration is the ability to adjust dosage schedules quickly if required. Once daily doses, divided daily dosage, or alternate-day regimens are all effective.

Intramuscular administration of corticosteroids is also common. Preparations such as triamcinolone acetonide are used most often. These drugs, which may reduce inflammation for more than 4 weeks, ensure that an unreliable patient will receive appropriate doses of medication.

Systemic corticosteroids are generally used for relatively short periods of time. Therefore, the complications commonly associated with corticosteroid use are not usually seen in dermatologic treatment. However, the long-term use of corticosteroids in diseases such as pemphigus and lupus erythematosus often results in side effects such as a round, puffy face, "buffalo hump," fatigue and weakness, acne, swelling of the feet and abdomen, gastrointestinal bleeding, and infection.

Topical Steroids

Corticosteroids can also be applied topically to suppress inflammation. Although this does not cure the disease, the reduction in erythema, edema, and pruritis promotes healing. Topical steroids are available in a variety of forms. Based on their capacity to cause cutaneous vasoconstriction, the topical steroids are divided into five groups, from group 1, the most potent (Diprolene and Temovate) to group 5, the least potent (1 percent hydrocortisone).

KEY CONCEPTS

- **Selection of topical treatment depends largely on whether the desired effect is to moisturize or dry the affected area. Continuous wet dressings, lotions, creams, and ointments tend to be moisturizing. Intermittent wet dressings and gels tend to be astringents for weeping, oozing lesions.**
- **Corticosteroids are commonly administered to reduced inflammation. They may be given topically, intralesionally, or systemically.**

Summary

The integumentary system—the skin and its appendages—envelopes the body and mirrors its state of health. In systemic diseases, the color, texture, and composition of the skin may also be affected.

Diseases of the skin are divisible into two broad etiologic categories: inflammatory/infectious, and proliferative/neoplastic. Inflammatory disorders of the skin often occur in individuals who have hypersensitivity reactions to substances in the environment. Infectious agents ranging from viruses to insects may infect the skin. Proliferative conditions include psoriasis, seborrheic keratosis, cysts, warts, and papillomas. Other benign tumors arise from other cells in the skin: nevi, lipomas, dermatofibromas, neuromas, and hemangiomas. Kaposi's sarcoma is a malignant, opportunistic neoplasm that occurs in persons with preexisting immunodeficiency.

Skin cancer is the most common malignancy in the United States, but, except for malignant melanoma and a few squamous carcinomas, skin cancers are not life-threatening. Ultraviolet light damages sun-exposed skin and is a major factor in causing skin cancer.

A distinct advantage in treating the skin is the ability to observe the pathology and the effects of treatment. In addition to a careful history, a culture, scrape, or biopsy provides good diagnostic information. A correct diagnosis can help prevent complications from improper therapy, but it does not lessen the importance of choosing an appropriate delivery system.

REFERENCES

1. Rosen T, Martin S: Variants of normal skin in blacks, in Rosen T, Martin S (eds): *Atlas of Black Dermatology.* Boston, Little, Brown & Co, 1981, pp 1–16.
2. Ackerman AB, Cockerell CJ: Cutaneous lesions: Correlations from microscopic to gross morphologic features. *Cutis* 1986;37:137–138.
3. Arnold ML, Odam RB, James WD: Diseases of the skin appendages, in Arnold ML, Odam RB, James WD (eds): *Andrew's Diseases of the Skin: Clinical Dermatology,* 7th ed. Philadelphia, WB Saunders, 1982, pp 936–985.
4. Cohen S: Programmed instruction: Skin rashes in infants and children. *Am J Nurs* 1978;78:1–32.
5. Johnson ML: Skin diseases, in Wyngaarden JB, Smith LH Jr (eds): *Cecil Textbook of Medicine,* 17th ed. Philadelphia, WB Saunders, 1985, pp 2227–2276.
6. Dunkle LM, Arvin AM, Whitley RJ, et al: A controlled trial of acyclovir for chickenpox in normal children. *N Engl J Med* 1991;325(22):1539–1544.
7. Hardy I, Gershon, AA, Steinberg SP, et al, for the Varicella Vaccine Collaborative Study Group: The incidence of zoster after immunization with live attenuated varicella vaccine: A study in children with leukemia. *N Engl J Med* 1991; 325(22):1545–1550.
8. Lombardo PC: Dermatologic disorders in the elderly, in Rossman I (ed): *Clinical Geriatrics,* 2nd ed. Philadelphia, JB Lippincott, 1979, pp 338–351.
9. Goldman R: Decline in organ function with aging, in Rossman I (ed): *Clinical Geriatrics,* 2nd ed. Philadelphia, JB Lippincott, 1979, pp 23–52.
10. Smith L: Histopathologic characteristics and ultrastructure of aging skin. *Cutis* 1989;43:414–424.
11. Cerimele D, Celleno L, Serri F: Physiological changes in ageing skin. *Br J Dermatol* 1990;122(suppl 35):13–20.
12. Spanos NP, Williams V, Gwynn MI: Effects of hypnotic, placebo, and salicylic acid treatments on wart regression. *Psychosom Med* 1990;52:109–114.
13. Dobson RL, Abele DC: Common viral infections, in Dobson RL, Abele DC (eds): *Practice of Dermatology.* New York, Harper & Row, 1985, pp 213–225.
14. Dicken CH: Retinoids: A review. *J Am Acad Dermatol* 1984; 11(4):541–552.
15. Epstein JH: Phototherapy and photochemistry. *N Engl J Med* 1990;322:1149–1151.
16. Goopman J: Neoplasms in the acquired immune deficiency syndrome: The multidisciplinary approach. *Semin Oncol* 1987;14(2)(suppl 3):1–6.
17. Benenson AS (ed): *Control of Communicable Diseases in Man,* 15th ed. Washington, D.C., American Public Health Association, 1990.
18. Ackerman AB, Cockerell CJ: Papules. *Cutis* 1986;37:242–245.
19. Herndon JH: Pruritus, in Moschella SL (ed): *Dermatology Update.* New York, Elsevier, 1982, pp 185–196.
20. Strauss JS: Biology of the sebaceous gland and the pathophysiology of acne vulgaris, in Soter NA, Baden HP (eds): *Pathophysiology of Dermatologic Diseases.* New York, McGraw-Hill, 1984, pp 159–173.

21. Sober AJ, Fitzpatrick TB: Atopic dermatitis, in Sober AJ, Fitzpatrick TB (eds): *Year Book of Dermatology*. St. Louis, CV Mosby, 1990, pp 63–70.
22. Roth H, Kierland R: The natural history of atopic dermatitis. *Arch Dermatol* 1964;89:209–214.
23. Wintroub B, Stern R, Arndt K: Cutaneous reactions to drugs, in Fitzpatrick TB, Eisen AZ, Wolff K, Freedburg IM, Austen KF (eds): *Dermatology in General Medicine*, 3rd ed. New York, McGraw-Hill, 1987, pp 1353–1366.
24. Sober AJ, Fitzpatrick TB: Adverse drug reactions, in Sober AJ, Fitzpatrick TB (eds): *Year Book of Dermatology*. St. Louis, CV Mosby, 1990, pp 109–120.
25. Callen JP: The value of malignancy evaluation in patients with dermatomyositis. *J Am Acad Dermatol* 1982;6(2):253–259.
26. Rockerbie NR, Woo TY, Callen JP, et al: Cutaneous changes of dermatomyositis precede muscle weakness. *J Am Acad Dermatol* 1989;20(4):629–632.
27. Gilchrest BA, Yaar M: Ageing and photoageing of the skin: Observations at the cellular and molecular level. *Br J Dermatol* 1992;127(suppl 41):25–30.
28. Bryant RA, Shannon ML, Pieper B, Braden BJ, Morris DJ: Pressure ulcers, in Bryant RA (ed): *Acute and Chronic Wounds*. St. Louis, Mosby–Year Book, 1992, pp 105–163.
29. Friedman RJ, Reigel DS, Berson DS, et al: Skin cancer: Basal cell and squamous cell carcinoma, in Holleb AI, Fink DJ, Murphy GP (eds): *Clinical Oncology*, 7th ed. New York, American Cancer Society, 1991, pp 290–303.
30. Sherman CD, McCune CS, Rubin P: Malignant melanoma, in Rubin P (ed): *Clinical Oncology*, 6th ed. New York, American Cancer Society, 1983, p 190.
31. Berardesca E, Maibach HI: Sensitive and ethnic skin: A need for special skin-care agents? *Dermatol Clin* Jan 1991;9(1):89–92.
32. Mosher DB, Pathak MA, Fitzpatrick TB: Vitiligo: Etiology and pathology, in Fitzpatrick TB, Eisen AZ, Wolff K, Freedburg IM, Austin KF (eds): *Update: Dermatology in General Medicine*. New York, McGraw-Hill 1983, pp 205–225.

BIBLIOGRAPHY

Abel E: *Photochemotherapy in Dermatology*. New York, Igaku-Shoin, 1992.
Arbeter A, Starr SE, Plotkin SA: Varicella vaccine studies in healthy children and adults. *Pediatrics* 1986;78(suppl):748–756.
Arlian LG, Estes SA, Vyszenski-Moher DL: Prevalence of *Sarcoptes scabiei* in the homes and nursing homes of scabietic patients. *J Am Acad Dermatol* 1988;19(5 pt 1):806–811.
Balch CM, Houghton AN, Milton GW, et al: *Cutaneous Melanoma*, 2nd ed. Philadelphia, JB Lippincott, 1992.
Banov CH, Epstein JH, Grayson LD: When an itch persists. *Patient Care* 1992;26(5):75–81, 84–88, and 90.
Beauregard S, Gilchrest BA: A survey of skin problems and skin care regimens in the elderly. *Arch Dermatol* 1987;123:1638–1643.
Benenson AS: *Control of Communicable Diseases in Man*. Washington, D.C., American Public Health Association, 1990.
Brunnel PA: Chickenpox: Examining our options. *N Engl J Med* 1991;325:1577–1579.
Callen JP: Systemic lupus erythematosus in patients with chronic cutaneous (discoid) lupus erythematosus. *J Am Acad Dermatol* 1985;12:278–288.
Cunliffe WJ: Evolution of a strategy for treatment of acne. *J Am Acad Dermatol* 1987;16:591–599.
Davis B: Drug eruptions, in Garcia R (ed): *Diagnosis and Therapy of Common Skin Diseases*. Buffalo, Westwood Pharmaceuticals, 1980.
Doughty DB: Principles of wound healing and wound management, in Bryant RA (ed): *Acute and Chronic Wounds*. St. Louis, Mosby–Year Book, 1992, pp 31–61.
Fischer B: Topical hyperbaric oxygen treatment of pressure sores and skin ulcers. *Lancet* 1969;2:405–409.
Fitzpatrick TB: Trends in dermatology: Ozone depletion and the dermatologist: Need we prepare for the consequences of a UVB "holocaust" in the next decades? in Sober AJ, Fitzpatrick

TB (eds): *Year Book of Dermatology*. St. Louis, CV Mosby, 1990, pp xiii–xxii.
Gip L, Molin L: Skin diseases in geriatrics. *Cutis* 1970;6:771–775.
Greco PJ, Ende J: An office-based approach to the patient with pruritus. *Hosp Prac* 1992;27:121–128.
Herrero C, Bielsa I, Font J, et al: Subacute cutaneous lupus erythematosus: Clinicopathologic findings in thirteen cases. *J Am Acad Dermatol* 1988;19:1057–1062.
Hilliard GW: Growth factors in plastic surgery. *Perspect Plast Surg* 1992;5:41–53.
Kligman AM: Psychological aspects of skin disorders in the elderly. *Cutis* 1989;43:498–501.
Koh HK: Cutaneous melanoma. *N Engl J Med* 1991;325:171–182.
Kreig T, Meurer M: Systemic scleroderma. *J Am Acad Dermatol* 1988;18(3):457–481.
Leibovich SJ, Ross R: The role of the macrophage in wound repair: A study with hydrocortisone and antimacrophage serum. *Am J Pathol* 1975;78(1):71–100.
Leveque JL, Corcuff P, DeRigal J, Agache P: In vivo studies of the evolution of physical properties of the human skin with age. *Int J Dermatol* 1984;23:322–329.
Lo JS, Berg RE, Tomecki KJ: Treatment of discoid lupus erythematosus. *Int J Dermatol* 1989;28(8):497–507.
Lowe NJ: Systemic treatment of severe psoriasis. *N Engl J Med* 1991;324:33–34.
Maibach HI, Aly R: *Skin Microbiology: Relevance to Clinical Infection*. New York, Springer-Verlag, 1981, pp 203–219.
Malloy BM, Perez-Wood RC: Neonatal skin care: Prevention of skin breakdown. *Pediatr Nurs* 1991;17(1):41–48.
Marzulli FN, Maibach HI: Contact allergy: Predictive testing in humans, in Marzulli FN, Maibach HI (eds): *Dermatotoxicology* 3rd ed. New York, Hemisphere, 1987, pp 319–337.
Murphy GF, Mihm MC Jr (eds): The skin, in Robbins SL, Cotran RS, Kumar V: *Pathologic Basis of Disease*, 5th ed. Philadelphia, WB Saunders, 1993, pp 1173–1211.
NIH Consensus Conference: Diagnosis and treatment of early melanoma. *JAMA* 1992;268(10):1314–1319.
Parish LC, Witokowski JA, Cohen HB: Clinical picture of scabies, in Parish LC, Nutting WB, Schwartzman RM (eds): *Cutaneous Infestations of Man and Animal*. New York, Praegar, 1983, pp 70–78.
Pathak MA, Fitzpatrick TB, Greiter F, Kraus EW: Preventive treatment of sunburn, dermatoheliosis, and skin cancer with sun protective agents, in Fitzpatrick TB, Eisen AZ, Wolf K, Austen KF (eds): *Dermatology in Medicine: Textbook and Atlas*. New York, McGraw-Hill, 1987, pp 1507–1522.
Phillips RJ, Dover JS: Recent advances in dermatology. *N Engl J Med* 1992;326:167–178.
Poikolainen K, Reunala T, Karvonen J, Lauharanta J, Karkkainin P: Alcohol intake: A risk factor for psoriasis in young and middle aged men? *Br Med J* 1990;300:780–783.
Pollack SV: Wound healing: A review. I. The biology of wound healing. *J Dermatol Surg Oncol* 1979;5(5):389–393.
Pollack SV: Wound healing: A review. III. Nutritional factors affecting wound healing. *J Dermatol Surg Oncol* 1979;5(8):615–619.
Rajka G: *Essential Aspects of Atopic Dermatitis*. London, Springer Verlag, 1991.
Rook A, Dawber R: *Diseases of the Hair and Scalp*. Oxford, Blackwell Scientific Publications, 1991.
Roth H, Kierland R: The natural history of atopic dermatitis. *Arch Dermatol* 1964;89:209–214.
Ryan GB, Cliff WJ, Gabbiani G, et al: Myofibroblasts in human granulation tissue. *Hum Pathol* 1974;5(1):55–67.
Slaven RG, Ducomb EF: Allergic contact dermatitis. *Hosp Pract* 24(7):39–51.
Sober AJ, Rhodes AR, Day CL, Fitzpatrick TB, Mihm MC: Primary melanoma of the skin: Recognition of precursor lesions and estimation of prognosis in stage I, in Fitzpatrick TB, Eisen AZ, Wolff K, Freedburg IM, Austen KF (eds): *Update: Dermatology in General Medicine*. New York, McGraw-Hill, 1983, pp 98–112.
Stern RS, Weinstein MC, Baker SG: Risk reduction for nonmelanoma skin cancer with childhood sunscreen use. *Arch Dermatol* 1986;122:537–545.

UNIT XVI
Selected Multisystem Alterations and Considerations in Critical Illness

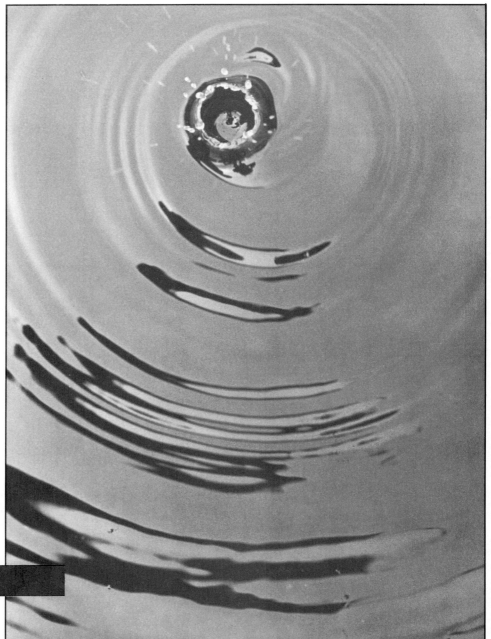

Just as one body system affects another, a single water droplet initiates a chain reaction.

Photo by Kathleen Kelly

We begin with the cell and end with the organism, and that is very much like beginning and ending in the same place on a different scale. Whenever we read new molecular research we are reminded that the cell is a tiny universe of activity—infinitesimal and infinite. The organism consists of cells organized in systems. The systems communicate with one another through their cells. Critical illness may be seen as a violation of the relationships between the body's systems.

Health is the desirable condition for cell, organ, system, and organism that allows us to realize the promise of life. Disease is the attack from within or without that challenges the pursuit of health.

Disease is inevitable, pervasive, insistent. We accept it philosophically. In the immune system we observe the complicated exchanges between antigen and defense and marvel at the refined adjustments to the threat of disease that we have inherited from, among others, early invertebrates that would scare us to death if we met them on the street.

But in daily practice we find it unacceptable and struggle against it. While those who suffer diseases often make useful, rich, even astonishing contributions—sometimes because disease challenges them to excel—illness restricts. Life usually ends with the success of disease or of complications associated with disease.

Recent decades have seen the emergence, in laboratories as well as in the popular mind, of diseases that attack a number of bodily systems at once or in succession. The persistence of diseases that are not easily confined suggests that it is important to recognize the threat to health of multisystem disorders.

About 1 million Americans have been infected with human immunodeficiency virus (HIV), which causes AIDS. One of the multisystem diseases associated with AIDS is *Cryptococcus neoformans*, which, after *Pneumocystis carinii*, cytomegalovirus, and mycobacteria, is the most common life-threatening fungal infection in AIDS patients. It can infect the lungs, skin, mucous membranes, bones, and other organs, and when it penetrates the central nervous system, which it does in 90 percent of cases, it causes cryptococcal meningitis.

Other medical calamities invite us to consider the body's total or systemic involvement. Critical injury is one.

Each year 12,000 Americans die from burns, 100,000 are hospitalized with burns, and more than 2.5 million suffer serious burns. Any burn will damage the skin, but a bad burn can reach the bone. When a burn causes such harm it damages more than one body system. The diagnosis and treatment of multisystem disease or injury must respond to threats or damage to organs and systems and to the relationships between them.

Medical professionals who care for critically ill patients recognize the danger of common and often fatal multiple organ failure accompanying critical illness or injury. Acknowledgment of the danger of multiple organ dysfunction syndrome (MODS) is a current concern resulting from a sequence of studies that goes back to the recognition of "sequential system failure" in the early 1970s. MODS is the leading cause of death after burns, trauma, and sepsis for patients admitted to critical care units.

Those who care for the critically ill or injured also are alarmed by a related condition called systemic inflammatory

FRONTIERS OF RESEARCH
Complex Care Challenges and Opportunities

Michael J. Kirkhorn

response syndrome (SIRS), which is found in most patients admitted to a critical care unit because it is a response to tissue injury. The SIRS-MODS combination further troubles medical professionals because, as the authors of one article observe, researchers do not yet understand the syndromes well enough to "halt the overall process once it has begun."

Research of the kind that is directed to SIRS-MODS involves the study of a number of body systems. Here the body is seen as a combination of interactions, some clearly understood, others still mysterious. But in medical research today the specific findings often also contribute to a perception of continuous life, of seamlessness. This continuity extends from the single cell, the tiny universe in itself, to the visible systems of the organism.

A person may survive damage to a number of bodily systems. Then, for the survivor, life goes on, as it does, for example, in a person recovering from a stroke, but the valuable cooperation between systems has been damaged—the circulation and molecular circuitry of the brain, for example, from its speech center, or the ability to walk or lift objects or perceive distinctions. Or a burn victim may lose skin or suffer organ impairment, then face the psychological challenge of recovering as fully as possible or accepting impairment.

The helping or caring professional, whether a nurse attending the patient or the hospital social worker who must find suitable nursing home care for a disabled patient, must know all that it is possible to know about the connections between one system and another. The caregiver has a primary responsibility for that person's ability to function, which often means to overcome impairment, recover from illness, regain the functioning relationship between systems, and live as wholly as possible.

CHAPTER 54
Cardiogenic, Hypovolemic, Septic, Anaphylactic, and Neurogenic Shock

GAIL SUMMERS

KEY TERMS

afterload: The strain or stress on the venticle at peak systole.

anaphylactic shock: A shock state resulting from an antigen/antibody reaction resulting in circulatory alterations.

cardiac index: A measurement of the heart's pumping ability taking into account body surface area.

cardiac output: The amount of blood the heart pumps in 1 minute.

cardiogenic shock: A shock state resulting from severe ventricular dysfunction resulting in inadequate cardiac output.

hypovolemic shock: A shock state resulting from a significant loss of circulating blood volume.

oxygen consumption: The amount of oxygen used by the tissues in 1 minute.

oxygen delivery: The amount of oxygen delivered to the tissues each minute.

oxygen extraction ratio: A comparison of oxygen consumption in relation to the amount of oxygen delivered.

preload: The amount of stretch in the ventricle at the end of diastole.

septic shock: A shock state secondary to sepsis resulting in maldistribution of blood volume.

shock: A life-threatening circulatory condition resulting in an imbalance between oxygen supply and oxygen demand at the cellular level.

---

*I*n 1895, John Collins Warren described shock as a momentary pause in the act of death.[1] Despite advances in the understanding and treatment of this clinical syndrome, shock still has associated with it a high mortality. Because this life-threatening syndrome may develop in any patient, it is imperative that nurses have a thorough understanding of the pathophysiology of shock and be able to recognize it clinically so that therapeutic measures may be implemented as soon as possible. This chapter presents an overview of shock, outlining the pathophysiology, clinical signs and symptoms, and treatment modalities currently in use for the major types of shock.

Circulatory Shock

Definition of Shock

Shock is complex and is not just a single physiologic entity; rather, it represents a widely diverse group of life-threatening circulatory conditions.[2] Shock is not always associated with hypotension, just as hypotension does not always result in shock.

Circulatory shock (failure to maintain perfusion of vital organs) is characterized by an imbalance between oxygen supply and oxygen demand at the cellular level. The common denominator of shock, regardless of its cause, is reduced or inadequate oxygen consumption.[3-5] When the cell does not have adequate amounts of oxygen and nutrients, it is unable to meet its metabolic demands. When oxygen consumption is reduced or inadequate to meet cellular needs, cellular hypoxia develops.[5] Functional impairment of cells, tissues, organs, and body systems can ultimately develop if the shock state progresses.[6]

Hemodynamic Principles

To fully understand the pathophysiology and presentation of shock, one must understand hemodynamic forces and oxygen transport principles. These are reviewed briefly here before further discussion of the physiology of shock.

Cardiac Output

Cardiac output reflects the amount of blood the heart pumps in 1 minute. Cardiac output is calculated by multiplying the heart rate by stroke volume (CO = HR × SV). The normal value for cardiac output is 4 to 8 L/min. The heart has the ability to respond to the metabolic needs of the body and adjust the cardiac output by altering either heart rate or stroke volume.

Heart rate is under the influence of the autonomic nervous system. **Sympathetic innervation** results in an increased heart rate, whereas **parasympathetic innervation** results in a decreased heart rate. Increasing the heart rate will increase the cardiac output by up to three times normal in a healthy individual. For a person with ischemic heart disease, increasing the heart rate beyond a critical level can actually decrease the cardiac output, as the increased heart rate results in decreased diastolic filling time and increased myocardial oxygen demand.

Stroke volume is the amount of blood ejected by the ventricle with each heart beat. The normal value is 70 mL per beat. Stroke volume is influenced by three major factors: preload, contractility, and afterload (Fig. 54–1).

Preload is the amount of stretch in the ventricle at the end of diastole. The amount of stretch in the ventricle at the end of diastole determines the pressure on the walls of the ventricle. In the left ventricle the amount of pressure is referred to as the **left ventricular end-diastolic pressure.** In the right ventricle it is referred to as the **right ventricular end-diastolic pressure.** The fundamental control mechanism of preload is the **Frank-Starling law.**[7] As volume is returned to the ventricle, the ventricle distends, myocardial fibers stretch, and contractility increases.

The normal left ventricle distends and accepts increases in diastolic volume without significant increases in ventricular filling pressures (end-diastolic pressure) to a certain point. Further increases in filling pressure beyond the maximum length-tension relationship results in end-diastolic pressures rising rapidly.[7]

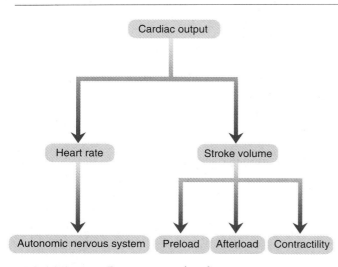

FIGURE 54–1. Determinants of cardiac output.

The major **determinants of preload** are compliance and volume. For example, if venous return is decreased, there will be less stretch in the ventricle, resulting in a decreased preload and decreased stroke volume. If the ventricle is stiff and filling pressures are high, preload will be increased but stroke volume may actually decrease.

Afterload is the strain or stress on the ventricle at peak systole. The degree of resistance the ventricle faces in ejecting its contents is determined by the arterial resistance it meets. Left ventricular afterload is determined by the **systemic vascular resistance.** Right ventricular afterload is determined by the **pulmonary vascular resistance.** As resistance to left ventricular ejection increases, stroke volume will decrease. Conversely, as resistance falls, stroke volume will increase.[8]

Contractility is influenced by myocardial ischemia and necrosis, underlying heart disease, and certain drugs. The ability of the heart to contract and respond to alterations in preload and afterload affects cardiac output.

Oxygen Transport Principles

The common denominator of shock is a reduced or inadequate oxygen consumption.[5] **Oxygen consumption** ($\dot{V}o_2$) refers to the amount of oxygen actually used by the tissues per minute.[9,10] Oxygen consumption is important because it is a measure of the body's total overall metabolism.[11] A reduction in oxygen consumption can be caused by several factors, including (1) decreased cardiac output, as with hypovolemic shock or cardiogenic shock; (2) an uneven distribution of blood flow, as with sepsis; and (3) increases in metabolic demands that create an imbalance between the amount of oxygen available and the amount required to meet the increased need.[2,3,5]

Oxygen delivery ($\dot{D}o_2$) refers to the amount of oxygen delivered to the tissues each minute.[9,10] Oxygen delivery is a product of blood flow and oxygen content and reflects the ability of the circulatory system to deliver nutrients to the cell.[5,12] Oxygen delivery can be manipulated by (1) increasing the cardiac output, (2) increasing the hemoglobin level, or (3) increasing arterial oxygen saturation.[13] Both oxygen delivery and oxygen consumption can be calculated from data obtained with a pulmonary artery catheter (Table 54–1).

Information regarding the supply and demand of oxygen can be obtained by calculating the **oxygen extraction ratio** (O_2ER), which compares oxygen consumption to the total amount of oxygen delivered.[14] Normal oxygen extraction is 25 percent. Oxygen extraction will increase when oxygen consumption increases or when oxygen delivery decreases (see Table 54–1).

A final variable that compares oxygen supply and demand is **mixed venous oxygen saturation** ($S\bar{v}o_2$). Random samples to determine mixed venous oxygen saturation can be obtained from the distal port of a pulmonary artery catheter. Continuous monitoring of $S\bar{v}o_2$ saturation is possible by utilizing a fiber-optic pulmonary artery catheter. The normal range of $S\bar{v}o_2$ is 60 to 80 percent. A finding of less than 60 percent may indicate anemia, low cardiac output, arterial oxy-

TABLE 54–1. Calculation of Oxygen Transport Variables

Variable	Calculation	Normal Value
Arterial oxygen content (CaO_2)	CaO_2 = hemoglobin × arterial oxygen saturation × 1.36	16–20 vol%
Oxygen delivery ($\dot{D}o_2$)	$\dot{D}o_2$ = arterial oxygen content × cardiac index × 10	520–720 mL/min/m^2
Atriovenous oxygen content difference [$C(a - \bar{v})o_2)$]	$C(a - \bar{v})o_2$ = arterial oxygen content − venous oxygen content	4–5.5 mL/100 mL
Oxygen consumption ($\dot{V}o_2$)	$\dot{V}o_2 = C(a - \bar{v})o_2$ × cardiac index × 10	100–180 mL/min/m^2
Venous oxygen content ($C\bar{v}o_2$)	$C\bar{v}o_2$ = hemoglobin × venous oxygen saturation × 1.36	12–15 vol%
Oxygen extraction ratio (O_2ER)	$O_2ER = (CaO_2 - C\bar{v}o_2)/CaO_2$	22–30%

Adapted from Summers G: The clinical and hemodynamic presentation of the shock patient. *Crit Care Nurs Clin North Am* 1990;2(2):162. Reproduced with permission.

gen desaturation, or an increase in oxygen consumption. A common cause of an $S\bar{v}o_2$ greater than 80 percent is sepsis.[10,12] The $S\bar{v}o_2$ does not always guarantee a normal balance between oxygen supply and oxygen delivery. If cardiac output is increased as a compensatory measurement, $S\bar{v}o_2$ may be normal even though there is an imbalance between oxygen supply and demand.[10] $S\bar{v}o_2$ monitoring must be taken in context with the other oxygen transport variables.

Stages of Shock

Shock can be divided into different stages. Each stage of shock represents pathologic changes that result from the underlying cause and history of the shock state. The shock state will progress if not interrupted and corrected. Each stage does not occur over a specific time period but varies with the individual's response to the shock state. The **three stages of shock** used in this discussion are (1) the compensatory stage, (2) the progressive stage, and (3) the irreversible stage.

Compensatory Stage

In the **compensatory stage** of shock there is a decrease in cardiac output that results from the shock state. In response to this decrease in cardiac output, compensatory mechanisms are activated in an attempt to augment the cardiac output.

The **determinants of blood pressure** are cardiac output and resistance to flow. Decreased cardiac output results in a decreased blood pressure. Pressoreceptors situated in the arterial walls within the aorta and carotid sinuses sense this decrease in pressure and transmit a signal to the vasomotor center in the medulla. The autonomic nervous system is activated, resulting in **sympathetic nervous stimulation.**[15] The adrenal medulla releases increased amounts of the catecholamines epinephrine and norepinephrine. In the heart β_1 receptors respond by increasing the heart rate and force of contraction in an attempt to increase cardiac output. The coronary arteries vasodilate in response to β_2 receptors, resulting in increased blood flow to the myocardium to meet the increased oxygen needs of the heart. Stimulation of β_2 receptors in the lung causes bronchodilation. The rate and depth of respirations are increased. Alpha receptor stimulation causes vasoconstriction, which reduces flow through the capillary bed. This decreases the hydrostatic pressure in the capillaries and results in a shifting of fluid out of the interstitial spaces into the capillary vascular beds in an attempt to increase venous return and cardiac output. Blood vessels in the skin, kidneys, and gastrointestinal tract constrict and shunt blood to the heart and brain.[15] Contraction of the radial muscle of the iris causes the pupils to dilate. The activity of sweat glands increases, resulting in a cool, clammy skin. The liver responds by breaking down stores of glycogen to increase available amounts of glucose for energy production.

The decreased cardiac output and the vasoconstriction in the kidneys decrease renal perfusion, resulting in renal ischemia. The renal ischemia stimulates the release of **renin** by the juxtaglomerular apparatus. The circulating renin reacts with angiotensinogen that is produced in the liver, resulting in the production of angiotensin I. A converting enzyme in the lungs converts angiotensin I to angiotensin II. **Angiotensin II** is a potent peripheral vasoconstrictor.[15] This increases blood pressure and venous return. In addition, angiotensin II stimulates the release of **aldosterone** from the adrenal cortex. Aldosterone increases reabsorption of sodium and water in the kidneys. This reabsorption of water also increases venous return to the heart.

Pulmonary blood flow is decreased as a result of the decreased cardiac output. Even though at this point there is adequate ventilation, the decrease in pulmonary blood flow results in **decreased exchange of oxygen and carbon dioxide** between the alveoli and capillaries, and a ventilation/perfusion mismatch occurs.[15] Chemoreceptors in the aorta and carotid arteries respond to the decreased arterial oxygen tensions, and the respiratory center in the brain responds by increasing the rate and depth of respirations in an attempt to compensate for the decreased oxygen tension.[15]

Clinical findings associated with the compensatory phase of shock include

- A normal blood pressure that is often associated with a narrow pulse pressure
- Sinus tachycardia, with heart rates exceeding 100 beats/min
- Fast and deep respirations
- Decreased urinary output due to the effects of aldosterone and increased levels of antidiuretic hormone
- Increased urine-specific gravity
- Cool, clammy skin
- Altered sensorium
- Dilated pupils
- Increased blood sugar
- Respiratory alkalosis with hypoxemia

Progressive Stage

In the **progressive stage** of shock the compensatory mechanisms can no longer compensate for the decreased cardiac output and are unable to maintain normal blood pressure. If the shock state is not corrected, deleterious effects of cellular hypoxia are observed.

Hypotension and arteriolar vasoconstriction result in **decreased oxygen delivery** to the cells. Cellular hypoxia results. This causes a shift from aerobic to anaerobic metabolism. Production of adenosine triphosphate (ATP) is decreased. Metabolic processes in the cell are reduced owing to lack of energy stores. The net result is a **decrease in oxygen consumption.** Glycolysis results in pyruvate being converted to lactate, as it cannot enter the citric acid cycle. Lactate levels increase and pH falls, resulting in a metabolic acidosis.

The decrease in available ATP causes the sodium/potassium pump to fail. Active transport of sodium and potassium across the cell membrane is reduced. Sodium ions accumulate inside the cell and potassium ions escape from the cell. Swelling occurs inside the cell as a result of the influx of the sodium ions and the increased retention of water inside the cell. Organelles inside the cell begin to swell, and their function deteriorates. The alteration of sodium and potassium ion concentrations causes the resting membrane potential to become more positive. The combination of a more positive resting membrane potential and a metabolic acidosis leads to arrhythmia formation. In addition, depolarization and repolarization times are prolonged, allowing for conduction disturbances and arrhythmia formation.

Capillary fluid dynamics are altered. The metabolic acidosis causes the precapillary sphincters to relax, but postcapillary vasoconstriction is maintained. Flow into the capillaries is unimpaired, but because the flow still faces resistance in the venules, the flow rates are reduced. The **capillary hydrostatic pressures increase,** and the net movement of fluid is out of the capillary vascular bed and into the interstitial space. Interstitial edema develops. The movement of fluid out of the vascular beds results in decreased blood volume and decreased venous return.

Myocardial contractility is decreased because of the effects of ongoing ischemia and acidosis. Cardiac output decreases further, thus potentiating cellular hypoxia.

Capillary flow rates are decreased, resulting in the formation of microemboli, which increase the risk of **disseminated intravascular coagulation.**

Clinical findings associated with the progressive stage of shock include

- Decreased blood pressure, with a narrow pulse pressure
- Continued increase in heart rate
- Fall in urine output owing to renal ischemia
- Decrease in specific gravity and in creatinine clearance; increase in creatinine and blood urea nitrogen (BUN) levels because of acute renal failure
- Decrease in cerebral blood flow, resulting in altered level of consciousness
- Increase in respiratory rates
- Audible crackles in the lungs on auscultation as a result of interstitial pulmonary edema
- Development of peripheral edema
- Development of metabolic and respiratory acidosis with hypoxemia

Irreversible Stage

The **irreversible stage** is the last stage of shock. The body becomes refractory to all therapeutic measures. The patient cannot recover, and death is inevitable.

TABLE 54–2. Classification of Shock

Cardiogenic
Hypovolemic
Vasogenic
  Septic
  Anaphylactic
  Neurogenic

Classification of Shock

There are **three major types of shock:** (1) cardiogenic, (2) hypovolemic, and (3) vasogenic. **Cardiogenic shock** reflects an inability of the heart to pump. **Hypovolemic shock** represents a significant reduction in circulating blood volume. **Vasogenic shock** results from alterations in the vascular system. Maldistribution of blood volume results, with altered capillary permeability. There are three types of vasogenic shock: **septic, anaphylactic,** and **neurogenic** (Table 54–2).[6] Cardiogenic, hypovolemic, and septic shock are the three most common forms of shock.

KEY CONCEPTS

- Shock represents a diverse group of life-threatening circulatory conditions. The commonality among all types of shock is cellular hypoxia and impaired cellular oxygen utilization (consumption). Inadequate cellular oxygenation may result from decreased cardiac output, maldistribution of blood flow, reduced blood oxygen content, and increased metabolic demands.

- Normally, about 25 percent of the oxygen in arterial blood is extracted by the tissues, resulting in a mixed venous oxygen saturation ($S\overline{v}O_2$) of approximately 75 percent. Low cardiac output may result in a greater oxygen extraction and lower $S\overline{v}O_2$; maldistribution of flow (sepsis) may result in less oxygen extraction and a higher $S\overline{v}O_2$.

- During the compensatory stage of shock, homeostatic mechanisms are able to maintain adequate tissue perfusion despite a reduction in cardiac output. Manifestations of sympathetic nervous system activation are predominant: elevated heart rate, increased myocardial stimulation, bronchodilation, vasoconstriction, cool, clammy skin, dilated pupils, renin release, decreased urine output, and increased serum glucose. Blood pressure is maintained even though cardiac output has fallen.

- During the progressive stage of shock, compensatory mechanisms begin to fail, resulting in hypotension and progressive tissue hypoxia. Cells shift to anaerobic metabolism, resulting in lactate production and metabolic acidosis. Lack of cellular ATP production leads to cellular swelling, dysfunction, and death. Cardiac arrhythmias, poor cardiac output, and microvascular failure may ensue.

- Irreversible shock is refractory to treatment and results in death.

Hemodynamic Monitoring of the Patient in Shock

The nurse caring for the patient in shock must continuously assess the patient's **physiologic status.** The goal of therapy is to increase oxygen delivery and oxygen consumption. **Hemodynamic monitoring** is necessary to accurately measure a variety of hemodynamic pressures, both direct and derived; to assess the need for intervention; to select the appropriate intervention; and to assess the efficacy of that intervention.[16]

Central Venous Pressure Monitoring

Central venous pressure (CVP) **monitoring** should be used to assess right heart function only. When properly positioned, the CVP catheter gives direct information about **right atrial pressure.** In diastole, the tricuspid valve is open. As a result, there is open communication between the right atrium and the right ventricle. Therefore the pressure recorded by the CVP catheter in diastole will reflect the pressure in the right ventricle at the end of diastole. For accurate assessment of right ventricular end-diastolic pressure, or **right ventricular preload,** there can be no incidence of tricuspid valve disease.

The CVP catheter should *not* be used to assess left ventricular function.

Pulmonary Artery Catheter Monitoring

A flow-directed **pulmonary artery catheter** allows assessment of both left- and right-sided intracardiac pressures.[17,18]

The typical balloon-tipped flow-directed catheter used for hemodynamic monitoring has at least three lumina (Fig. 54–2). When the catheter is properly positioned in the pulmonary artery, the proximal lumen lies in the right atrium and the distal lumen lies in the pulmonary artery.

The proximal lumen in the right atrium allows measurement of right atrial pressure (Fig. 54–3). By monitoring the right atrial pressure in the absence of tricuspid valve disease, right ventricular end-diastolic pressure can be assessed.

The distal lumen in the pulmonary artery allows measurement of **pulmonary artery pressures** (Fig. 54–4). The **pulmonary artery systolic pressure** reflects right ventricular systolic pressure in the absence of pulmonic valve disease. In systole, the pulmonic valve is open; therefore, the pressure measured in systole in the pulmonary artery reflects the systolic pressure in the right ventricle.[16,19,20]

In diastole, the pulmonic valve closes. The **pulmonary artery diastolic pressure** will therefore not be influenced by right ventricular events. The pulmonary artery diastolic pressure will, however, be influenced by left-sided events. In diastole, the mitral valve is open. As there are no valves between the pulmonary artery and the left atrium, the pulmonary artery catheter looks forward into the left atrium and directly reflects left atrial pressure. Because the mitral valve is open in diastole, the pressure in the left atrium is a reflection of the pressure in the left ventricle. In the absence of mitral valve disease, left atrial pressure is an indication of left ventricular end-diastolic pressure, or left ventricular preload. The pulmonary artery diastolic pressure will therefore be an **indirect measurement of left ventricular end-diastolic pressure** or a measurement of left ventricular function.[16,19,20]

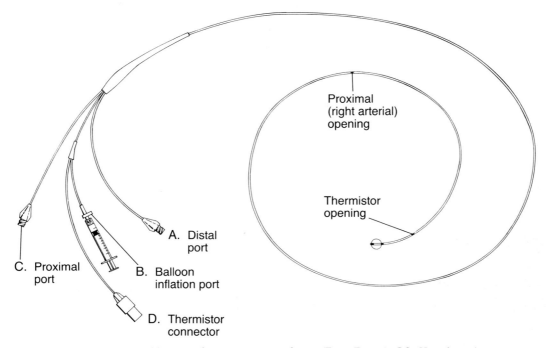

FIGURE 54–2. Thermodilution pulmonary artery catheter. (From Darovic GO: *Hemodynamic Monitoring.* Philadelphia, WB Saunders, 1987, p 140. Reproduced with permission.)

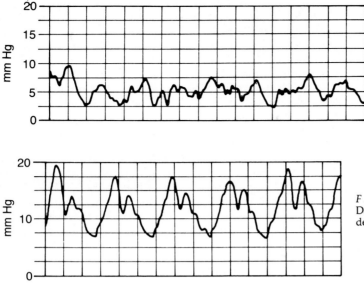

FIGURE 54–3. Right atrial pressure waveform. (From Darovic GO: *Hemodynamic Monitoring.* Philadelphia, WB Saunders, 1987, p 148. Reproduced with permission.)

FIGURE 54–4. Pulmonary artery pressure waveform. (From Darovic GO: *Hemodynamic Monitoring.* Philadelphia, WB Saunders, 1987, p. 149. Reproduced with permission.)

When the balloon is blown up, the catheter migrates into a small pulmonary artery and wedges itself there. A **pulmonary artery wedge pressure** will be recorded (Fig. 54–5). The pulmonary artery wedge pressure will also indirectly reflect left ventricular end-diastolic pressure. The pulmonary artery wedge pressure is usually 1 to 5 mm Hg lower than the pulmonary artery diastolic pressure. If the gradient between the pulmonary artery diastolic pressure and the pulmonary artery wedge pressure is less than 5 mm Hg, there is a good correlation between the two parameters, and the pulmonary artery diastolic pressure can be used to assess left ventricular function. If the gradient is greater than 5 mm Hg, then the pulmonary artery wedge pressure must be used to assess left ventricular function. If significant pulmonary disease is present, the pulmonary artery diastolic pressure will reflect the higher pressures associated with the pulmonary disease and will no longer be a true indicator of left ventricular function.[16,19,20]

Cardiac output may be measured directly by the pulmonary artery catheter by use of a thermodilution technique. A thermistor is located at the distal end of the catheter. A room-temperature solution is injected into the right atrial port. The thermistor records the change in fluid temperature (the body is much warmer than fluid at room temperature) and notes the time until the temperature returns to the first reading. The time required to return the fluid temperature to room temperature is inversely proportional to the cardiac output. If cardiac output is high, the temperature will return to normal quickly; if cardiac output is low, it will take much longer. In effect, right-sided cardiac output is being measured, but normally, right- and left-sided cardiac output are equal.[16]

To assess the pumping ability of the heart more accurately, the **cardiac index** should be calculated. Cardiac output does not take into account the size of the person. For example, a large person may have a cardiac output of 4 L/min, which is within the range of normal, but that value may be suboptimal for a person with a large body mass. Cardiac index takes body surface area into account and gives a more accurate measurement of the heart's pumping ability.

Afterload, or the resistance the ventricle faces to eject its contents, can be calculated using data obtained from the pulmonary artery catheter. Left ventricular afterload is obtained by calculating systemic vascular resistance, and right ventricular afterload is obtained by calculating the pulmonary vascular resistance.

The normal values and the necessary calculations for the derived data are shown in Table 54–3. In conjunction with the oxygen transport variables, these hemodynamic parameters allow **total assessment** of the physiologic response of the body to shock and allow one to assess the efficacy of therapeutic interventions.

FIGURE 54–5. Pulmonary artery wedge pressure waveform. (From Darovic GO: *Hemodynamic Monitoring.* Philadelphia, WB Saunders, 1987, p. 150. Reproduced with permission.)

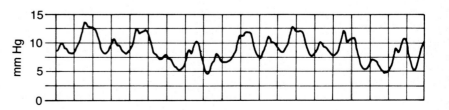

TABLE 54–3. Normal Hemodynamic Values and Calculations

Variable	Calculation	Normal Value
Right atrial pressure (RAP)	Direct measurement	2–6 mm Hg
Right ventricular pressure (RVP)	Direct measurement	20–30/0–5 mm Hg
Pulmonary artery pressure (PAP)	Direct measurement	20–30/8–12 mm Hg
Mean pulmonary artery pressure (PAP)	Direct measurement	11–15 mm Hg
Pulmonary artery wedge pressure (PAWP)	Direct measurement	4–12 mm Hg
Cardiac output (CO)	Direct measurement	4–8 L/min
Systemic vascular resistance (SVR)	$\dfrac{\text{Mean arterial pressure} - \text{RAP}}{\text{CO}} \times 80$	900–1,400 dynes/sec/cm^{-5}
Pulmonary vascular resistance (PVR)	$\dfrac{\text{PAP} - \text{PAWP}}{\text{CO}} \times 80$	100–200 dynes/sec/cm^{-5}
Cardiac index (CI)	CO/Body surface area	2.5–3.5 L/min/m^2
Mixed venous oxygen saturation S$\bar{v}o_2$	Direct measurement	60–80%

Adapted from Summers G: The clinical and hemodynamic presentation of the shock patient. *Crit Care Nurs Clin North Am* 1990;2(2):163. Reproduced with permission.

KEY CONCEPTS

- **Hemodynamic monitoring during shock states is helpful for assessing cardiac output, volume status, oxygen delivery and oxygen consumption. Usual pressures monitored include right atrial pressure, pulmonary artery pressure, left atrial pressure (usually estimated by pulmonary artery wedge pressure), and arterial blood pressure.**
- **Cardiac output may be measured using a thermodilution technique. Cardiac index, derived by dividing cardiac output by body surface area, may better reflect the adequacy of cardiac performance.**
- **Measured pressures and outputs are used to derive estimates of pulmonary and systemic vascular resistance. Resistances indicate the afterload against which the right or left ventricle must pump.**

Cardiogenic Shock

Etiology

Cardiogenic shock occurs primarily as a result of severe left and/or right ventricular dysfunction that results in inadequate cardiac pumping.[21,22] The **most common cause** of cardiogenic shock is myocardial infarction resulting in a significant loss (greater than 40 percent) of left ventricular myocardium.[5,22–24] Other causes of cardiogenic shock include right ventricular myocardial infarction, end-stage cardiomyopathy, papillary muscle dysfunction, free wall rupture, and ventricular septal defects (Table 54–4).[25]

Decreased contractility results in decreased cardiac output. The low cardiac output state results in decreased forward flow and tissue perfusion. The high left ventricular diastolic filling pressure signifies both reduced myocardial compliance and increased diastolic volume.[26]

The high left ventricular filling pressures result in the movement of fluid out of the pulmonary vascular beds and into the pulmonary interstitial space, resulting in initially interstitial pulmonary edema and later alveolar pulmonary edema (Fig. 54–6).

The sympathetic nervous system is stimulated as a compensatory mechanism in an attempt to increase cardiac output. The result is an increase in heart rate, contractility, and systemic vascular resistance. The increase in systemic vascular resistance makes it even more difficult for the heart to pump. Activation of the renin-angiotensin system results in further increases in resistance and an increased venous return. The increase in venous return further increases left ventricular filling pressures. The net result of the activation of compensatory mechanisms is **to decrease cardiac output further and to increase myocardial oxygen demand.**

Clinical Manifestations

Sympathetic nervous stimulation increases heart rate and force of contraction. Initially this compensatory mechanism maintains blood pressure and is adequate to perfuse vital organs.

As compensatory mechanisms fail, the systolic blood pressure falls and the diastolic pressure in-

TABLE 54–4. Causes of Cardiogenic Shock

Large myocardial infarction
Multiple small myocardial infarctions
Right ventricular myocardial infarction
End-stage cardiomyopathy
Papillary muscle dysfunction
Free wall rupture
Ventricular septal defect

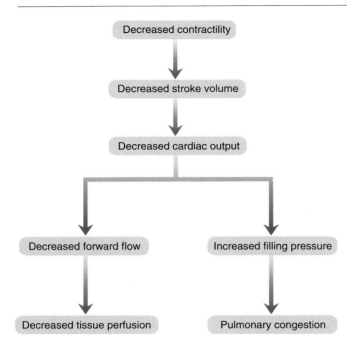

F I G U R E 54 – 6. Pathophysiology of cardiogenic shock.

creases (as a result of the sympathetic stimulation), causing a **narrowed pulse pressure.** Heart rates increase above 100 beats/min. Peripheral vasoconstriction occurs, resulting in cool, clammy skin.

Respirations are rapid and deep. The increased rate and depth of respirations can lead to a respiratory alkalosis. Auscultation of the lungs reveals coarse crackles resulting from the increased left ventricular filling pressures. A summation gallop may be audible over the left apex as a result of increased pressure in the left ventricle and decreased compliance.

Urine output decreases initially because of reabsorption of sodium and water as a result of aldosterone secretion. The urine becomes concentrated as a result of water reabsorption. As the shock state progresses, renal ischemia increases and renal function deteriorates. Urine output falls below 20 mL/hr, BUN and creatinine levels rise, and creatinine clearance decreases.

The patient's level of consciousness is altered. Initially the patient may be restless and confused. If cerebral hypoperfusion increases, the patient may become lethargic and unresponsive (Table 54–5).[5,27]

Hemodynamic Manifestations

In cardiogenic shock the underlying pathology results in decreased contractility that is manifested by a **decreased cardiac output and cardiac index.** Pulmonary artery pressures are increased, with the pulmonary artery wedge pressure typically being greater than 18 mm Hg. When the pulmonary artery wedge pressure is greater than 18 mm Hg, pulmonary congestion develops as a result of the high left ventricular end-diastolic pressure.

TABLE 54–5. Presentation of Cardiogenic Shock

Parameter	Alteration
Blood pressure	↓
Heart rate	↑
Respiratory rate	↑
Urine output	↓
Temperature	Normal
Skin	Cool
Color	Pale
Cardiac output	↓
Cardiac index	↓
Pulmonary artery pressure	↑
Pulmonary artery wedge pressure	↑
Systemic vascular resistance	↑
Mixed venous oxygen saturation	↓

Vasoconstriction is evidenced by the **elevated systemic vascular resistance.** Decreased oxygen delivery to the tissues results in decreased oxygen consumption. Oxygen extraction increases in an attempt to compensate for the decreased oxygen delivery. Mixed venous blood samples show a decreased venous oxygen saturation because of increased oxygen extraction by the tissues. Arterial blood gas values initially demonstrate a respiratory alkalosis secondary to hyperventilation. As the shock state progresses, metabolic and respiratory acidosis with hypoxemia result because of alveolar hypoventilation[5] (see Table 54–5).

Treatment

The best treatment of cardiogenic shock is preventative. If no contraindications exist, a patient experiencing myocardial infarction should immediately be treated with a **thrombolytic agent** in the emergency department as soon as the diagnosis is made. The three most widely used agents to date are streptokinase, tissue-type plasminogen activator (t-PA), and anisoylated plasminogen streptokinase activator complex (APSAC). All three agents **activate the fibrinolytic system** and have the potential to break down a fresh thrombus and restore forward flow in the occluded coronary artery, thereby reducing the size of the infarct. Recent clinical trials have shown that thrombolytic drugs cause a significant reduction in mortality following myocardial infarction.[28–31]

Current treatment of cardiogenic shock can be achieved both pharmacologically and mechanically. The goal of treatment is to decrease myocardial oxygen demands, increase myocardial oxygen delivery, and increase cardiac output.

Examples of **positive inotropic drugs** used in the treatment of cardiogenic shock include dobutamine and dopamine. Both drugs have the ability to increase contractility, increase cardiac output, and increase tissue perfusion. Dobutamine increases contractility by stimulating β_1 receptors. The major effect of dobutamine is on contractility, not on heart rate or blood vessels. Dobutamine should not be used as a vasopressor to increase blood pressure, as it does not cause vasoconstriction.[32]

Dopamine stimulates dopaminergic, beta and alpha receptor sites. Dopaminergic activation results in increased mesenteric and renal blood flow. Beta-adrenergic stimulation results in increased contractility and heart rate. Alpha-adrenergic stimulation results in increased systemic vascular resistance. All of the effects are dose dependent. Dopamine instead of dobutamine should be used when hypotension is present. Dopamine increases myocardial oxygen demands more than dobutamine does; therefore, if blood pressure is greater than 90 mm Hg, dobutamine should be used.

Vasodilators may be used to decrease the work load of the heart by decreasing resistance to flow. Examples of commonly used vasodilators include nitroprusside and nitroglycerin. Nitroprusside causes both venous and arterial vasodilation. As a result, nitroprusside decreases afterload by decreasing systemic vascular resistance, increases cardiac output, decreases preload, and decreases myocardial oxygen demand.[22] Nitroprusside, because of its vasodilating effects, has a tendency to produce hypotension. To maintain arterial perfusion, the blood pressure should be at least 110 mm Hg before initiating nitroprusside use.

Nitroglycerin is a venovasodilator and a coronary artery vasodilator. Nitroglycerin is used to increase coronary artery blood flow and to decrease pulmonary congestion by decreasing venous return and left ventricular preload. Nitroglycerin also has a tendency to lower blood pressure; therefore, blood pressure must be stable prior to administration of nitroglycerin.

Another group of pharmacologic agents used in the treatment of cardiogenic shock are the **phosphodiesterase inhibitors.** Phosphodiesterase inhibitors act by inhibiting cyclic adenosine monophosphate (cAMP) phosphodiesterase, leading to increased levels of cAMP and increased activity of cAMP-dependent protein kinases. These enzymes cause an increase in intracellular levels of calcium (Fig. 54–7).[33] Amrinone is an example of a phosphodiesterase inhibitor. Amrinone increases myocardial contractility and causes both arterial and venous vasodilation. As a result, amrinone decreases both preload and afterload, resulting in increased cardiac output.

If hemodynamic stability cannot be restored pharmacologically, **intra-aortic balloon counterpulsation** may be indicated for temporary circulatory assistance.[34] A polyurethane balloon is percutaneously inserted through the femoral artery and is positioned just distal to the left subclavian artery. The balloon is connected to a console that triggers the balloon to inflate in diastole and deflate in systole. The overall effects of counterpulsation are increased cardiac output, increased coronary perfusion, decreased preload, decreased afterload, and decreased myocardial work and oxygen consumption.[34]

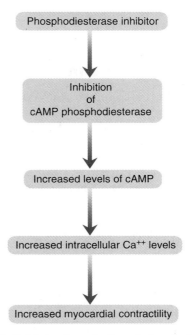

FIGURE 54–7. Mechanism of action of phosphodiesterase inhibitors.

KEY CONCEPTS

- Cardiogenic shock is usually a result of severe ventricular dysfunction associated with myocardial infarction. Other causes include cardiomyopathy, ventricular rupture, and ventricular septal defect.

- Diagnostic features of cardiogenic shock include decreased cardiac output due to left ventricular dysfunction, accompanied by elevated left ventricular end-diastolic pressure. Extra heart sounds, S_3 and S_4, and pulmonary edema result. Sympathetic activation leads to increased heart rate, vasoconstriction, and a narrow pulse pressure.

- Low cardiac output leads to reduced oxygen delivery to tissues. Tissues extract a greater percentage of oxygen from the delivered blood, leading to reduced $S\bar{v}O_2$.

- Therapy is aimed at improving cardiac output and myocardial oxygen delivery while reducing cardiac work load. Pharmacologic treatment often includes the use of inotropic agents (dopamine, dobutamine, amrinone), afterload-reducing agents (alpha antagonists, direct vasodilators), and preload reducing agents (venodilators, diuretics). Intra-aortic balloon counterpulsation may be used to reduce afterload and improve coronary artery perfusion.

Hypovolemic Shock

Etiology

Hypovolemic shock results when there is an inadequate circulating plasma volume associated with a blood volume deficit of at least 15 to 25 percent.[35]

The **blood volume deficit** may be the result of either internal or external losses.

Internal losses can result from internal hemorrhage, fracture of long bones, or leakage of fluid into third spaces.[6] **External losses** can result from external hemorrhage, burns, or dehydration. External hemorrhage is the most common cause of hypovolemic shock.

Pathogenesis

The decreased intravascular volume leads to a decrease in venous return, which causes a decrease in cardiac output. The decrease in cardiac output results in decreased tissue perfusion and decreased oxygen delivery (Fig. 54–8).

The posterior pituitary gland responds to the decrease in the circulating blood volume by increasing the secretion of antidiuretic hormone, resulting in increased retention of water by the kidneys.[35] The anterior pituitary gland releases increased amounts of adrenocorticotropic hormone, which, through the production of glucocorticoids, stimulates glucose production.

Sympathetic innervation dominates, and norepinephrine and epinephrine are released. Peripheral vasoconstriction results, causing decreased capillary hydrostatic pressure, which allows for the movement of fluid from the interstitial space into the vascular bed in an attempt to increase intravascular volume.

Hemorrhagic Shock

The American College of Surgeons classifies hemorrhagic shock according to the percentage of blood volume lost.[36] The four classifications are briefly described in the following subsections.

Class I Hemorrhagic Shock

Class I hemorrhage indicates a mild blood loss, up to 15 percent of the total body volume, or 750 mL. Compensatory mechanisms maintain cardiac output, and the patient's signs and symptoms remain within normal range.[37] If the lost volume is to be replaced, a crystalloid solution is used following the **3 : 1 rule** (replace three times the initial amount lost).[36]

Class II Hemorrhagic Shock

Class II hemorrhage represents a moderate blood loss, from 15 to 30 percent of total body volume (750–1,500 mL). The patient becomes anxious and restless. The blood pressure remains normal but the pulse pressure is narrowed. The heart rate is between 100 and 120 beats/min. The respiratory rate is normal. Urine output is between 20 and 30 mL/hr. The **capillary blanch test** is positive. The capillary blanch test is performed by depressing a patient's fingernail and observing how long after release the skin color takes to return to normal. The normal time is less than 2 seconds, the time required to say the words "capillary blanch."[37] Lost fluid should be replaced with crystalloid solutions, following the 3 : 1 rule.[36]

Class III Hemorrhagic Shock

Class III hemorrhage indicates a major blood loss, from 30 to 40 percent of total body volume (1,500–2,000 mL). The patient is anxious and confused. The blood pressure is decreased, with a narrow pulse pressure. The heart rate is greater than 120 beats/min. Respiratory rates are between 30 and 40 respirations/min. Urine output is 5 to 15 mL/hr. The capillary blanch test is positive. Lost fluid should be replaced with crystalloid solutions and blood products, following the 3 : 1 rule, or until hemodynamically stable.[36]

Class IV Hemorrhagic Shock

Class IV hemorrhage represents a severe blood loss, with greater than 40 percent of total body volume lost (2,000 mL or more). The patient is lethargic and has severe hypotension with a narrow pulse pressure.[37] The heart rate exceeds 140 beats/min, and the respiratory rate is greater than 35 respirations/min. Urine output is negligible. The capillary blanch test is positive. Lost fluid should be replaced with crystalloid solutions and blood products, following the 3 : 1 rule, or until hemodynamically stable.[36]

The clinical presentation of other forms of hypovolemic shock is similar to the presentation of the patient in hemorrhagic shock, although they are not grouped into different classes (Table 54–6).

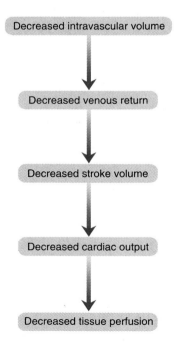

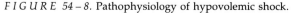

F I G U R E 54–8. Pathophysiology of hypovolemic shock.

TABLE 54–6. Presentation of Hypovolemic Shock

Parameter	Alteration
Blood pressure	↓
Heart rate	↑
Respiratory rate	↑
Urine output	↓
Temperature	Normal
Skin	Cool
Color	Pale
Cardiac output	↓
Cardiac index	↓
Pulmonary artery pressure	↓
Pulmonary artery wedge pressure	↓
Systemic vascular resistance	↑
Mixed venous oxygen saturation	↓

Hemodynamic Manifestations

Cardiac output and cardiac index are decreased. **Pulmonary artery pressures and the pulmonary artery wedge pressures are decreased** because of the **decreased preload.** Systemic vascular resistance is increased as a result of sympathetic innervation. S$\overline{\text{v}}$o$_2$ saturation is decreased owing to decreased oxygen delivery and increased oxygen extraction (Table 54–6).

Treatment

The **first intervention** for hypovolemic shock is an attempt to control the source of blood loss and to replace the intravascular losses with appropriate fluid. There are **three types of fluid therapy:** colloids, crystalloids, and blood products.[37]

Colloids are solutions that increase the serum colloid osmotic pressure within the vascular compartment. The net effect is the movement of fluid into the vascular space. The advantage in administering colloid solutions is that only small amounts need to be given to restore the vascular volume. A potential disadvantage to their administration is the leakage of fluid out of the vascular compartment into the interstitial space if there is increased capillary permeability. Examples of colloid solution are normal human serum albumin, dextran, and hetastarch.

Crystalloids are solutions that contain electrolytes. Isotonic solutions such as lactated Ringer's solution or normal saline solution are the two most commonly used crystalloid solutions. A disadvantage to volume replacement with crystalloid solutions is the potential for pulmonary edema to develop because of the large volumes of fluid required to restore the intravascular volume.

The ideal way to restore whole blood losses is with **blood products.** Whole blood contains all blood components. Packed red blood cells have most of the plasma volume removed and as a result have no clotting factors. Plasma contains clotting factors but no platelets. In hypovolemic shock, whole blood or packed red blood cells with plasma and platelets may be given to restore blood loss.

Dopamine may be administered initially in conjunction with fluid therapy to restore arterial pressure.

KEY CONCEPTS

- Hypovolemic shock results from inadequate circulating blood volume precipitated by hemorrhage, burns, dehydration, or leaking of fluid into third spaces.

- The classic features of hypovolemic shock are the result of low cardiac output and low intracardiac pressures. Manifestations are due primarily to sympathetic nervous system activation: elevated heart rate, vasoconstriction, and increased myocardial contractility.

- The severity of symptoms of hemorrhagic shock correlates with the amount of blood loss:

  Class I: 15 percent blood loss; mild symptoms, cardiac output near normal.

  Class II: 15 to 30 percent blood loss; blood pressure normal, but heart rate and vascular resistance are elevated.

  Class III: 30 to 40 percent blood loss; blood pressure falls, heart rate is >120 beats/min, urine output falls.

  Class IV: >40% blood loss; severe hypotension and tachycardia (>140 beats/min) result, oliguria is seen.

- Therapy for hypovolemic shock is aimed at fluid replacement and controlling the source of volume loss. Colloids, crystalloids, and blood may be used as replacement fluids.

Septic Shock

Etiology

Septic shock is the most common cause of death in intensive care units in the United States. The incidence of the disease continues to increase, with most cases being nosocomial.[38] Patients are at greater risk of developing septic shock because of the advent of invasive technology, the use of chemotherapy, and the use of immunosuppressive drug therapy. The patient who is elderly is at greater risk of infection.[38,39] The **mortality** associated with septic shock ranges from 40 percent to 85 percent.[40,41]

Definitions

To understand the pathogenesis of septic shock, one must understand the terminology related to different clinical states.[42] **Bacteremia** refers to the presence of bacteria in the blood.[42] A simple cut results in bacteremia; however, the body's defense systems effectively destroy the bacteria. **Septicemia** implies the presence of microorganisms in the blood associated with a systemic infection.[42] **Septic shock** is a syndrome secondary to sepsis that results in hemodynamic alteration caused by **maldistribution of blood volume.**

Risk Factors

Risk factors for the development of septic shock can be either patient related or treatment related. The patients at risk of septic shock are those under 1 year of age or those over 65 years of age.[39,42] Patients in these age groups are less likely to be able to destroy an invading microorganism.[42] Patients who are debilitated, malnourished, and have chronic health problems are also at risk.[39,42]

Treatment-related factors that predispose a patient to septic shock include the use of invasive lines and catheters, invasive procedures, and surgical procedures; treatment for traumatic wounds or burns; and immunosuppression.[39,42]

Causative Microorganisms

Escherichia coli is the organism most likely to induce sepsis and septic shock.[40] Other common gram-negative bacteria include *Klebsiella pneumoniae, Enterobacter aerogenes, Serratia marcescens, Pseudomonas aeruginosa,* and *Proteus* species.[40,42,43] Gram-negative bacteria are responsible for the majority of cases of septic shock. Gram-positive organisms are less prevalent, with the most common organism being *Staphylococcus aureus.*[43] Viruses, fungi, and rickettsiae can also cause septic shock, although the incidence is less.[42]

The most common portal of entry is the genitourinary tract. Other entry sites include the gastrointestinal tract, the respiratory tract, and the skin.[40]

Pathogenesis

Gram-negative bacteria have within their cell walls a lipopolysaccharide or **endotoxin.** It is composed of an O antigen side chain, an R core, and an inner lipid A, which is the toxic component of the endotoxin.[42,44] Endotoxins are released into the blood during bacterial cell lysis and initiate a chain of pathophysiologic events.[38,40,45-47] **Macrophages** are phagocytic cells found in the lung interstitium and alveoli, liver sinuses, and other tissue sites.[47] Macrophages are activated by the endotoxin to release the cytokines **tumor necrosis factor, interleukin-1,** and **interleukin-2.**[47] Tumor necrosis factor is thought to be a major endogenous toxin in the pathogenesis of septic shock.[46]

The endotoxin activates **granulocytes,** which release many toxic mediators such as platelet-activating factor, oxygen-derived free radicals, and proteolytic enzymes.[47] Endotoxins activate the **arachidonic acid cascade** resulting in prostaglandin, leukotriene, thromboxane, and prostacyclin release, all of which have profound effects on vascular smooth muscle.[46,47] Increased levels of **thromboxane A_2** and **B_2** produce pulmonary vasoconstriction, mediate bronchoconstriction, and act as a potent platelet aggregator.[47] **Prostaglandin E_2** and **prostacyclin** levels are elevated.

Prostacyclin is a very potent vasodilator and may be responsible for the development of hypotension.[47]

The **complement system** is activated with release of C5a and C3a, which produce microemboli and endothelial cell destruction.[42] **Histamine,** a potent vasodilator, is released by the mast cells. Histamine also increases capillary permeability, which allows for the movement of fluid out of the vascular bed. Beta-endorphins are released and may contribute to the development of hypotension.[38] **Myocardial depressant factor** is released from the pancreas and significantly decreases contractility in the heart. The coagulation system is activated and may enhance the development of microemboli.[42,46] The **kinin system** is activated and bradykinin is released, which results in vasodilation and increased capillary permeability (Fig. 54–9).[42]

Hemodynamic Alterations

Septic shock causes profound **peripheral vasodilation.** The systemic vascular resistance is decreased, and despite an increased cardiac output, blood pressure falls. The veins also dilate, and intravascular pooling occurs in the venous capacitance system.[48]

There is **maldistribution of blood flow** so that some tissues are underperfused and some are overperfused. Excessive flow to areas of low metabolic demand limits oxygen extraction, which accounts for a narrowing in the difference between arterial and venous oxygen content.[41]

Initially there is an increase in cardiac output, but the increase is insufficient to maintain oxygen delivery. Even though cardiac output is increased, the **ejection fraction** is usually decreased. Ejection fraction is the percent of the diastolic volume that is ejected in systole. As such, it is an excellent indicator of cardiac function. In septic shock, the decreased ejection fraction indicates that there is depressed myocardial contractility despite an increased cardiac output.[49-51] Right ventricular dysfunction is also common and is likely the result of pulmonary hypertension and myocardial depression.[52,53]

Increased capillary permeability results in fluid movement out of the vascular beds and into the interstitial space. Generalized soft tissue edema results and can interfere with tissue oxygenation and organ function (Fig. 54–10).[48]

Venous return is decreased as a result of the pooling of blood volume in the venous capacitance system and the increased capillary permeability.

Microembolization occurs in the microcirculation and results in sluggish flow. The decreased flow rates decrease oxygen utilization and increase the risk of developing disseminated intravascular coagulation.

Clinical Manifestations— Hyperdynamic Phase

The initial manifestation of septic shock is a hyperdynamic state, which may progress to a hypodynamic state.

In the **hyperdynamic state** blood pressure falls because of the decreased systemic vascular resistance

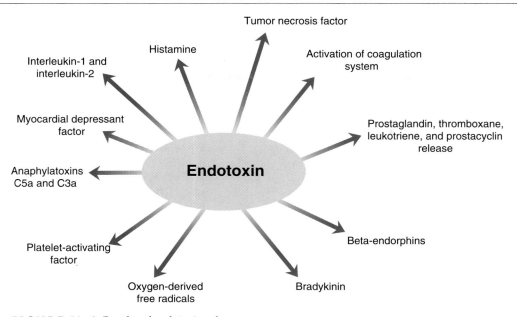

FIGURE 54–9. Results of endotoxin release.

and decreased venous return. The diastolic pressure falls because of a lack of sympathetic tone, resulting in a widened pulse pressure. Heart rates increase in an attempt to increase cardiac output further to compensate for the decreased blood pressure.

Pulmonary blood flow decreases, pulmonary vascular resistance increases, and increased capillary permeability results in pulmonary congestion. Impaired gas exchange results.[42] Respiratory rate and depth increase, which may result in an early respiratory alkalosis. Crackles may be audible on auscultation as a result of the interstitial pulmonary edema.[5]

The patient is usually febrile and may have associated chills. The skin is pink and warm to the touch as a result of peripheral vasodilation. Level of consciousness may be altered as a result of cerebral ischemia (Table 54–7).

Hemodynamic Manifestations— Hyperdynamic Phase

In this phase cardiac output and cardiac index are often abnormally high owing to the decreased systemic vascular resistance. Pulmonary artery pressures and the pulmonary artery wedge pressure are below normal because of decreased venous return.

Unlike cardiogenic or hypovolemic shock, in septic shock $S\bar{v}o_2$ levels are above normal because of the maldistribution of blood flow. Oxygen consumption is decreased (see Table 54–7).

Clinical Manifestations— Hypodynamic Phase

Not all patients in septic shock progress to the **hypodynamic phase.** The hypodynamic phase is characterized by decreased cardiac output and sympathetic nervous stimulation.

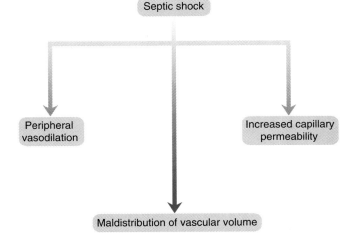

FIGURE 54–10. Hemodynamic alterations in septic shock.

TABLE 54–7. Presentation of Septic Shock

Parameter	Alteration
Blood pressure	↓
Heart rate	↑
Respiratory rate	↑
Urine output	↑ then ↓
Temperature	↑ then ↓
Skin	Warm then cool
Color	Flushed then pale
Cardiac output	↑ then ↓
Cardiac index	↑ then ↓
Pulmonary artery pressure	↓ then ↑
Pulmonary artery wedge pressure	↓ then ↑
Systemic vascular resistance	↓ then ↑
Mixed venous oxygen saturation	↑ then ↓

Peripheral vasoconstriction results in a narrowing of the pulse pressure and cool, clammy skin. Profound hypotension occurs because of the increased afterload and decreased contractility.[5]

Respirations are rapid and shallow. Crackles and wheezes are audible owing to the pulmonary congestion. Urine output decreases as a result of renal hypoperfusion. The patient may become lethargic (see Table 54–7).

Hemodynamic Manifestations— Hypodynamic Phase

In this phase the systemic vascular resistance is increased. Cardiac output and cardiac index are decreased owing to severe myocardial depression. Pulmonary artery pressures and the pulmonary artery wedge pressure are elevated (see Table 54–7). Arterial blood gases reveal a metabolic and respiratory acidosis with hypoxemia.

Treatment

The primary treatment goal in septic shock is **fluid administration** to restore an adequate ventricular preload. The pulmonary artery wedge pressure should be maintained at 12 mm Hg.[54] Controversy remains as to whether crystalloid or colloid solutions should be administered. Colloids offer the advantage of rapid volume replacement; however, the increased capillary permeability associated with septic shock and colloid administration may lead to the movement of fluid into the interstitial space.

Appropriate **antibiotic therapy** must be started as soon as septic shock is suspected and should not be delayed until blood cultures become positive. **Positive blood cultures** should only narrow the antibiotic regimen to cover the specific microbes.[43] Treatment is begun with a third-generation cephalosporin plus an aminoglycoside, or with either a carbapenem or a selected third-generation cephalosporin alone.[43]

If fluid administration does not restore hemodynamic stability, treatment should be started with either dopamine, dobutamine, or epinephrine in an attempt to increase oxygen delivery.[55,56]

Corticosteroid therapy is no longer indicated in the treatment of septic shock. Several clinical trials have shown no beneficial effects of high-dose corticosteroids in septic shock.[57–60]

Anti-endotoxin drugs are currently being developed and investigated. HA-1A is a human IgM antibody that binds to the lipid A domain of the endotoxin and has been shown to decrease mortality significantly in patients with septic shock and gram-negative bacteremia.[61]

KEY CONCEPTS

- Septic shock results from systemic infection (septicemia). **Gram-negative bacteria, particularly *E. coli*, are responsible for most cases of septic shock. Endo-** toxins in bacterial cell walls stimulate massive immune system activation. Immune cells release a large number of mediators (cytokines), resulting in widespread inflammation. The clotting cascade, complement system, and kinin systems are activated as part of the immune response.
- Widespread inflammation leads to profound peripheral vasodilation with hypotension, maldistribution of blood flow with cellular hypoxia, and increased capillary permeability with edema formation. Activation of the clotting cascade increases the risk of microemboli formation and disseminated intravascular coagulation.
- Initially, septic shock is characterized by abnormally high cardiac output resulting from inflammatory vasodilation and sympathetic activation of the heart. The patient is usually febrile, pink, and warm. Even though cardiac output is high, cellular hypoxia is present because of maldistribution of blood flow. Reduced cellular oxygen utilization is manifested as a high $S\bar{v}O_2$.
- Therapy for septic shock is aimed at improving distribution of blood flow and treating infection with antibiotics. Administration of fluid and drugs to increase cardiac performance is done to improve distribution of blood flow.

Anaphylactic and Neurogenic Shock

Etiology

Normally, the body produces antibodies that protect it against foreign substances (antigens). Repeated exposure to an antigen can cause the immune system to overreact.[62] A **type I anaphylactic reaction** involves an antigen/IgE antibody reaction.[62–64] IgE antibodies are produced in response to an antigen. The IgE antibodies then attach themselves to receptor sites on mast cells and basophils, where they remain.[62] The next exposure to that antigen causes the antigen/antibody reaction that mediates a host of vasoactive reactions. Histamines, leukotrienes, bradykinins, eosinophilic chemotactic factor, platelet-activating factor, kinins, and prostaglandins are released.[62,64] These substances result in bronchoconstriction, massive peripheral vasodilation, and increased capillary permeability.

Neurogenic shock is the least common of the shock states and is often transitory in nature. Neurogenic shock may result from depression of the vasomotor center in the medulla or from interruption of sympathetic nerve fibers.

The loss of sympathetic tone leads to profound peripheral vascular vasodilation of both arterioles and veins.[6,65] Systemic vascular resistance is decreased secondary to vasodilation in the arterioles. Venous return is decreased, leading to decreased left ventricular filling pressures and cardiac output.

Pathogenesis

The most frequently reported cases of anaphylactic shock result from **antibiotic therapy,** in particular the **penicillins** and **cephalosporins.**[64] Other common causes include other drugs, contrast media, food, insect stings, and snake bites.

Causes of neurogenic shock include brain injury that results in depression of the vasomotor center in the medulla, spinal cord injury, high spinal anesthesia, and drug overdose.[6,65]

Clinical Manifestations of Anaphylactic Shock

Onset of symptoms is usually within 20 minutes of exposure. The earlier the onset of the symptoms, the more severe the reaction.[62] Urticaria, pruritus, and angioedema develop. Often the patient has a sense of "impending doom." Bronchoconstriction causes wheezing and cyanosis. Laryngeal edema results in hoarseness and stridor.[5,62,64]

Venous return is severely impaired as a result of massive peripheral vasodilation and increased capillary permeability, resulting in a shift of fluid into the interstitial spaces. Significant hypotension develops. Initially the patient appears very anxious, with an increased heart rate and respiratory rate.

Treatment of Anaphylactic Shock

The initial therapy is directed toward **airway management.** Intubation and ventilation may be needed. Bronchodilators, such as epinephrine and aminophylline, are used to treat the bronchospasm.

Fluid therapy is critical to restore the intravascular volume and improve the cardiac output. A vasopressor such as dopamine or epinephrine is given for vascular support. **Steroids** are given for their anti-inflammatory action.[62] **Antihistamines** are administered to block the effects of histamine release and block the increased capillary permeability.[62]

KEY CONCEPTS

- Anaphylactic and neurogenic shock are characterized by excessive vasodilation and peripheral pooling of blood. Cardiac output is reduced because of inadequate preload.
- Anaphylactic shock is a result of excessive mast cell degranulation in response to antigen. Mast cell degranulation is mediated by IgE antibodies. Mast cell degranulation releases vasodilatory mediators such as histamine into the circulation, resulting in severe hypotension. Urticaria, bronchoconstriction, stridor, wheezing, and itching are usually present. Treatment includes maintenance of airway patency and the use of antihistamines, vasopressors, and fluids to restore blood pressure.
- Neurogenic shock results from loss of sympathetic activation of arteriolar smooth muscle. Medullary

depression (brain injury, drug overdose) or lesions of sympathetic nerve fibers (spinal cord injury) are the usual causes.

Complications of Shock

The pathology of the shock state and the effects on other organs may precipitate life-threatening complications. The patient may survive the shock state only to succumb to a resulting complication. **Complications** associated with shock include adult respiratory distress syndrome, disseminated intravascular coagulation, acute renal failure, and multiple organ failure.

Adult Respiratory Distress Syndrome

Adult respiratory distress syndrome (ARDS), a form of respiratory failure, is most commonly associated with **septic shock.** ARDS is characterized by the development of refractory hypoxemia, decreased pulmonary compliance, and radiologic evidence of pulmonary edema associated with normal pulmonary artery wedge pressures.[66] Acute lung injury causes increased capillary permeability, pulmonary interstitial edema, and intra-alveolar edema.[67] The mortality associated with ARDS ranges from 50 percent to 90 percent.

Acute Renal Failure

The most common cause of **acute renal failure** as a result of shock is **acute tubular necrosis.** In shock, the kidneys undergo prolonged periods of hypoperfusion. Vasoconstriction of the afferent arteriole causes decreased glomerular blood flow, decreased glomerular hydrostatic pressure, and decreased glomerular filtration rates.[68] Cellular damage results.

Acute tubular necrosis is commonly associated with decreased creatinine clearance, high urinary sodium, low specific gravity, low osmolality, high BUN and creatinine levels, and decreased urine output.[68]

A return to normal renal function is possible with appropriate treatment.

Disseminated Intravascular Coagulation

In **disseminated intravascular coagulation** (DIC) the coagulation system is overstimulated by an acute illness. Septic shock is the most common cause of DIC. Sluggish blood flow, endothelial damage, and microemboli place the patient at risk for developing DIC.

In DIC, large quantities of both thrombin and plasmin are found in the circulation.[69] The thrombin acts on fibrinogen to make fibrin clots. Large numbers of clots are produced and are deposited in the microcirculation.[69] These clots further reduce blood flow and oxygen delivery to the tissues.

The large amount of plasmin present in the circulation breaks down fibrin. **Fibrin degradation products** are released when fibrin is broken down, and these products act as anticoagulants. Hemorrhage develops when the patient is unable to form a stable clot.[69] The net result of DIC is that clots are formed where they are not needed and are unable to be formed where they are needed.

The patient with DIC has the capacity to bleed from anywhere in the body. Hematuria, hemoptysis, and gastrointestinal bleeding may be present. The skin may be cold and mottled.

Multiple Organ Failure

The patient may survive the shock state, recover, and appear to do well, only to die days or weeks later of **multiple organ failure** (MOF). Despite resuscitation from a shock state, microcirculatory hypoxia during the shock phase places the patient at risk for MOF.[70]

Following the shock state, the patient becomes hypermetabolic and hyperglycemic.[71] Lactate, bilirubin, and creatinine levels rise. Oxygen consumption increases.[71] Some patients survive this hypermetabolism without developing MOF; others go on to develop it. The mortality associated with MOF is 40 percent to 100 percent.[71]

KEY CONCEPTS

- Shock states result in reduced or inadequate cellular oxygen consumption and may affect all organs and systems in the body. Complications of shock can be viewed as inflammatory in nature. Inflammation is triggered by hypoxic injury to cells, by antigen, or by endotoxin. Excessive or inappropriate inflammation leads to leaky capillaries; damage from proteolytic enzymes; and systemic activation of the clotting, complement, and kinin systems.

- Respiratory and kidney failure are commonly associated with shock. Inappropriate activation of the clotting cascade may result in DIC. Multiple organ failure may occur with widespread cellular hypoxia and necrosis.

Summary

Shock is a life-threatening syndrome associated with high mortality. Early recognition of clinical signs and symptoms and initiation of therapeutic measures may decrease the risk for the development of shock. Fundamental to the recognition and successful treatment of shock is a thorough understanding of the underlying pathophysiology.

ACKNOWLEDGMENTS

My sincere thanks to the Library Staff at Centenary Health Centre for their ongoing enthusiasm and support of this project.

REFERENCES

1. Warren JC: *Surgical Pathology and Therapeutics.* Philadelphia, WB Saunders, 1895.
2. Shoemaker WC, Kram HB, Appel PL: Therapy of shock based on pathophysiology, monitoring, and outcome prediction. *Crit Care Med* 1990;18(1):S19–S25.
3. Shoemaker WC: A new approach to physiologic monitoring and therapy of shock states. *World J Surg* 1987;11(2):133–146.
4. Shoemaker WC: Pathophysiology, monitoring, outcome prediction, and therapy of shock states. *Crit Care Clin* 1987;3(2):307–357.
5. Summers G: The clinical and hemodynamic presentation of the shock patient. *Crit Care Nurs Clin North Am* 1990;2(2):161–166.
6. Rice V: Shock, a clinical syndrome: An update. Part 1. *Crit Care Nurse* 1991;11(4):20–27.
7. Weeks LN: Cardiovascular physiology, in Weeks LN (ed): *Advanced Cardiovascular Nursing.* Boston, Blackwell Scientific Publications, 1986.
8. Meehan AA: Hemodynamic assessment using the automated physiologic profile. *Crit Care Nurse* 1986;6(1):29–46.
9. Aberman AA: Fundamentals of oxygen transport physiology in a hemodynamic monitoring context, in Fahey PJ (ed): *Continuous Measurement of Blood Oxygen Saturation in The High Risk Patient.* San Diego, Beach International, 1985, vol 2.
10. Mims BC: Physiologic rationale of $S\overline{v}O_2$ monitoring. *Crit Care Nurs Clin North Am* 1989;1(3):619–628.
11. Shoemaker WC: Circulatory mechanisms of shock and their mediators. *Crit Care Med* 1987;15(8):787–794.
12. Hardy GH: $S\overline{v}O_2$ continuous monitoring techniques. *Dimens Crit Care Nurse* 1988;7(1):8–17.
13. Barone JE, Snyder AB: Treatment strategies in shock: Use of oxygen transport measurements. *Heart Lung* 1991;20(1):81–86.
14. Rutherford KA: Advances in the treatment of oxygen disturbances. *Crit Care Nurs Clin North Am* 1989;1(4):659–667.
15. Rice V: Shock, a clinical syndrome. Part II: The stages of shock. *Crit Care Nurse* 1981;1(4):4–14.
16. Halfman-Franey M, Bergstrom D: Clinical management using direct and derived parameters. *Crit Care Nurs Clin North Am* 1989;1(3):547–561.
17. Forrester JS, Ganz W, Diamond G, McHugh T, Chonette DW, Swan HJ: Thermodilution cardiac output determination with a single flow-directed catheter. *Am Heart J* 1972;83(3):306–311.
18. Swan HJ, Ganz W, Forrester J, Marcus H, Diamond G, Chonette D: Catheterization of the heart in man with use of a flow-directed balloon-tipped catheter. *N Engl J Med* 1970;283(9):447–451.
19. Darovic GO: *Hemodynamic Monitoring.* Philadelphia, WB Saunders, 1987.
20. Daily EK, Schroeder JS: *Techniques in Bedside Hemodynamic Monitoring.* St. Louis, CV Mosby, 1985.
21. Daily EK: Use of hemodynamics to differentiate pathophysiology causes of cardiogenic shock. *Crit Care Nurs Clin North Am* 1989;1(3):589–602.
22. Roberts SL: Cardiogenic shock: Decreased coronary artery tissue perfusion. *Dimens Crit Care Nurs* 1988;7(4):196–208.
23. Ayres SM: The prevention and treatment of shock in acute myocardial infarction. *Chest* 1988;93(1):17S–21S.
24. Resnekov L: Cardiogenic shock. *Chest* 1983;83(6):893–898.
25. Schreiber TL, Miller DH, Zola B: Management of myocardial infarction: Current status. *Am Heart J* 1989;117(2):435–443.
26. Messines FC, Hager WD: Hemodynamic complications of acute myocardial infarction. *Hosp Pract* 1989;24(8):147–166.
27. Rice V: Shock, a clinical syndrome. Part III: The nursing care. Prevention and patient assessment. *Crit Care Nurse* 1981;1(5):36–47.
28. Gruppo Italiano per lo Studio della Sopravvivenza nell'Infarto miocardio. GISSI-2: A factorial randomized trial of alteplase versus streptokinase and heparin versus no heparin among 12,490 patients with acute myocardial infarction. *Lancet* 1990;336:65–71.
29. ISIS-2 (Second International Study of Infarct Survival) Collaborative Group: Randomized trial of intravenous streptokinase, oral aspirin, both, or neither among 17,187 cases of suspected myocardial infarction: ISIS-2. *Lancet* 1988;2:349–360.
30. ISIS-3 (Third International Study of Infarct Survival) Collaborative Group: ISIS-3: A randomized comparison of streptokinase vs tissue plasminogen activator vs anistreplase and of aspirin plus heparin vs aspirin alone among 41,299 cases of suspected acute myocardial infarction. *Lancet* 1992;339:753–770.

31. The GUSTO Investigators (Global Utilization of Streptokinase and Tissue Plasminogen Activator for Occluded Coronary Arteries): An international randomized trial comparing four thrombolytic strategies for acute myocardial infarction. *N Engl J Med* 1993;329(10):673–682.

32. Burns KM: Vasoactive drug therapy in shock. *Crit Care Nurs Clin North Am* 1990;2(2):167–178.

33. Chatterjee K: Newer oral inotropic agents: Phosphodiesterase inhibitors. *Crit Care Med* 1990;18(1):S34–S38.

34. Schott KE: Intra-aortic balloon counterpulsation as a therapy for shock. *Crit Care Nurs Clin North Am* 1990;2(2):187–193.

35. Niedringhaus L: Hypovolemic shock, in Perry AG, et al (eds): *Shock: Comprehensive Nursing Management.* St. Louis, CV Mosby, 1983.

36. American College of Surgeons, Committee on Trauma: *Advanced Trauma Life Support Course for Physicians.* Chicago, American College of Surgeons, 1984.

37. Sommers MS: Fluid resuscitation following multiple trauma. *Crit Care Nurse* 1990;10(10):74–81.

38. Parrillo JE: The cardiovascular pathophysiology of sepsis. *Annu Rev Med* 1989;40:469–485.

39. Wahl SC: Septic shock: How to detect it early. *Nursing* 1989;19(1):52–59.

40. Mostow SR: Management of gram-negative septic shock. *Hosp Pract* 1990;25(10):121–130.

41. Rackow EC, Astiz ME, Weil MH: Cellular oxygen metabolism during sepsis and shock. *JAMA* 1988;259(13):1989–1992.

42. Rice V: The clinical continuum of septic shock. *Crit Care Nurse* 1984;5:84–109.

43. Roach AC: Antibiotic therapy in septic shock. *Crit Care Nurs Clin North Am* 1990;2(2):179–186.

44. Luce JM: Pathogenesis and management of septic shock. *Chest* 1987;91(6):883–888.

45. Danner RL, Elin RJ, Hosseini JM, Wesley RA, Reilly JM, Parillo JE: Endotoxemia in human septic shock. *Chest* 1991;99(1):169–175.

46. Natanson C: The mediators of the common pathway of injury, in Parrillo JE (moderator): Septic shock in humans. *Ann Intern Med* 1990;113(3):227–242.

47. Stroud M, Swindell B, Bernard GR: Cellular and humoral mediators of sepsis syndrome. *Crit Care Nurs Clin North Am* 1990;2(2):151–160.

48. Thijs LG, Schreider AJ, Groeneveld ABJ: The hemodynamics of septic shock. *Intensive Care Med* 1990;16(suppl 3):S182–S186.

49. Parker MM, Shelhamer JH, Bacharach SL, et al: Profound but reversible myocardial depression in patients with septic shock. *Ann Intern Med* 1984;100(4):483–490.

50. Parrillo JE, Burch C, Shelhamer JH, Parker MM, Natanson C, Schuette W: A circulating myocardial depressant substance in humans with septic shock: Septic shock patients with a reduced ejection fraction have a circulatory factor that depresses in vitro myocardial cell performance. *J Clin Invest* 1985;76(4):1539–1553.

51. Suffredini AF, Fromm RE, Parker MM, et al: The cardiovascular response of normal humans to the administration of endotoxin. *N Engl J Med* 1989;321(5):280–287.

52. Reuse C, Frank N, Contempre B, Vincent JL: Right ventricular function in septic shock. *Intensive Care Med* 1988;14(suppl 2):486–487.

53. Vincent JL: Right ventricular dysfunction in septic shock: Assessment by measurement of right ventricular ejection fraction using the thermodilution technique. *Acta Anaesthesiol Scand* 1989;33:34–38.

54. Schremmer B, Dhainaut JF: Heart failure in septic shock: Effects of inotropic support. *Crit Care Med* 1990;18(1):S49–S55.

55. Bollaert PE, Bauer P, Audibert G, Lambert H, Larcan A: Effects of epinephrine on hemodynamics and oxygen metabolism in dopamine-resistant septic shock. *Chest* 1990;98(4):949–953.

56. Vincent JL, Van der Linden P, Domb M, Blecic S, Azimi G, Bernard A: Dopamine compared to dobutamine in experimental septic shock: Relevance to fluid administration. *Anesth Analg* 1987;66(6):565–571.

57. Bone RC, Fisher CJ Jr, Clemmer TP, Slotman GJ, Metz CA, Balk RA: A controlled clinical trial of high-dose methylprednisolone in the treatment of severe sepsis and septic shock. *N Engl J Med* 1987;317(11):653–658.

58. Putterman C: Corticosteroids in sepsis and septic shock: Has the jury reached a verdict? *Isr J Med Sci* 1989;25(6):332–338.

59. Sprung CL: The effects of high-dose corticosteroids in patients with septic shock. *N Engl J Med* 1984;311(18):1139–1143.

60. The Veterans Administration Systemic Sepsis Cooperative Study Group: Effect of high-dose glucocorticoid therapy on mortality in patients with clinical signs of systemic sepsis. *N Engl J Med* 1987;317(11):659–665.

61. Ziegler EJ: Treatment of gram-negative bacteremia and septic shock with HA-1A human monoclonal antibody against endotoxin. *N Engl J Med* 1991;324(7):429–436.

62. Black NL, Shaffer MA: Systemic anaphylaxis. *Top Emerg Med* 1988;9(4):19–32.

63. Ellis C: Allergic and immune reactions. *Practitioner* 1990;234:1054–1058.

64. Haupt MT, Carlson RW: Anaphylactic and anaphylactoid reactions, in Shoemaker WC, Ayres S, Grenvik A, Holbrook PR, Thompson WL (eds): *Textbook of Critical Care.* Philadelphia, WB Saunders, 1984, pp 72–81.

65. Niedringhaus L: Classification of shock, in Perry AG, et al (eds): *Shock: Comprehensive Nursing Management.* St. Louis, CV Mosby, 1983.

66. Murray JF, Mathay MA, Luce JM, Flick MR: An expanded definition of the adult respiratory distress syndrome. *Am Rev Respir Dis* 1988;138(3):720–723.

67. Vaughan P, Brooks C: Adult respiratory distress syndrome. *Crit Care Nurs Clin North Am* 1990;2(2):235–253.

68. Lancaster L: Renal response to shock. *Crit Care Nurs Clin North Am* 1990;2(2):221–233.

69. Bell TN: Disseminated intravascular coagulation and shock. *Crit Care Nurs Clin North Am* 1990;2(2):255–268.

70. Cerra FB: The systemic septic response: Concepts of pathogenesis. *J Trauma* 1990;30(suppl 12):S169–S174.

71. Lekander BJ, Cerra FB: The syndrome of multiple organ failure. *Crit Care Clin* 1990;2(2):331–342.

BIBLIOGRAPHY

Alpert JS, Becker RC: Cardiogenic shock: elements of etiology, diagnosis, and therapy. *Clin Cardiol* 1993;16(3):182–190.

Alpert JS, Becker RC: Mechanisms and management of cardiogenic shock. *Crit Care Clin* 1993;9(2):205–218.

Astiz ME, Rackow EC: Assessing perfusion failure during circulatory shock. *Crit Care Clin* 1993;9(2):299–312.

Astiz ME, Rackow EC, Weil MH: Pathophysiology and treatment of circulatory shock. *Crit Care Clin* 1993;9(2):183–203.

Barron RL: Pathophysiology of septic shock and implications for therapy. *Clin Pharm* 1993;12(11):829–845.

DeGent GE, Greenbaum DM: Mechanical ventilatory support in circulatory shock. *Crit Care Clin* 1993;9(2):377–393.

Domsky MF, Wilson RF: Hemodynamic resuscitation. *Crit Care Clin* 1993;9(4):715–726.

Gould SA, Sehgal LR, Sehgal HL, Moss GS: Hypovolemic shock. *Crit Care Clin* 1993;9(2):239–259.

Imm A, Carlson RW: Fluid resuscitation in circulatory shock. *Crit Care Clin* 1993;9(2):313–333.

Prewitt RM: Thrombolytic therapy in patients where hypotension or cardiogenic shock complicate myocardial infarction. *Can J Cardiol* 1993;9(2):155–157.

Urban N: Integrating the hemodynamic profile with clinical assessment. *AACN Clin Issues Crit Care Nurs* 1993;4(1):161–179.

CHAPTER 55
Burn Injuries

MELVA KRAVITZ

KEY TERMS

autograft: Surgical procedure to move skin from one area of the body to an area of injury. The purpose is to provide permanent skin coverage to the injured area.

circumferential burn: Injury wraps completely around an extremity or the trunk. Loss of elasticity of skin results in a tourniquet effect, compromising circulation to distal tissues or respiratory expansion of chest. Escharotomy or fasciotomy is necessary.

deep partial thickness burn: The destruction of entire dermis, leaving only epidermal skin appendages, marks this second-degree burn. All physiologic functions of skin are absent. Such burns heal in about 30 days. The preferred treatment is autografting to diminish scarring.

eschar: Burn tissue.

escharotomy: A surgical incision through eschar of a circumferential extremity burn for the purpose of restoring distal blood flow, or through eschar of the chest to restore respiratory expansion.

first-degree burn: Superficial tissue destruction in the outermost layers of the epidermis. All physiologic functions of the skin remain intact.

full-thickness burn: Also called a third-degree burn, this thermal injury is marked by destruction of epidermis, dermis, and underlying tissue. All physiologic functions of the skin are absent. This burn will not heal and requires autografting.

inhalation injury: Cellular injury to lung tissue as a result of inhalation of toxic smoke. Associated smoke inhalation significantly increases the morbidity and mortality from burn injury.

superficial partial thickness burn: Marked by destruction of the epidermis and dermis, a superficial partial thickness burn is also a second-degree burn. The water vapor barrier is absent, but tactile and pain sensors are intact.

---

*T*hermal injury may occur as a result of exposure to heat, cold, chemicals, or electricity. The depth of injury determines the method of wound closure; the extent of injury determines morbidity and mortality. Small burn injuries result in local tissue destruction, an accompanying inflammatory reaction, and activation of the healing process. Extensive burn injury produces systemic changes at the cellular level that result in death without appropriate medical intervention.

Magnitude of the Thermal Injury Problem

Incidence and Mortality

Thermal injury is the second most common cause of death by accident in the United States.[1] Nearly 6,000 people per year are killed in the United States by fire, with the home being the location of the incident in 93 percent of all episodes. House fires kill at the same rate in the general population as they did 50 years ago (2 per 100,000).[2] Burns in the elderly carry a significant mortality rate because of the patient's general pre-injury disability, age-related immunosuppression, and impaired healing mechanisms. A mortality of over 50 percent occurs in the elderly with burns of only 10 to 14 percent of total body surface area (TBSA). This figure increases to 75 percent with a 30 percent TBSA burn.[2]

The type of injury is age related, with scald injury commonly occurring in two populations: children less than 5 years old and adults more than 65 years old.[3] Indications are that these injuries occur to children left in bathtubs without adult supervision. Scald burns in elderly persons appear to be related to balance problems, which result in inadvertent changes in water temperature as the person reaches for the faucet handle to regain balance. Failing eyesight and the need to shower while not wearing corrective lenses, in combination with the sensory losses that occur in the frail elderly, compound the problem. Burn injury is the fourth leading cause of accidental death in the 65-year-old and older age group, with 50 percent of the injuries caused by flames, 19 percent by scalding, and 10 percent by flammable liquids.[2] In a group of 247 women admitted to a burn center between 1983 and 1988, cooking-related injuries were the cause in 27 percent of women older than 59 years, with the primary mode of injury due to reaching across a cooking

stove to adjust burners. Manufacturers have recognized this problem, and newer stoves have controls located in front or side panels, but many stoves with rear-panel controls remain in use.[4]

Preexisting disease also contributes to the incidence and mortality of burn injury. Heart disease is a major health problem in the United States, and its presence has been shown to significantly alter the morbidity and mortality of surgical patients. The stress of a burn injury results in an increased cardiac work load and may exceed cardiac capabilities. A study of 2,477 consecutive burn admissions revealed that 257 patients (10.4 percent) had either a history of cardiac disease before the burn injury or an in-hospital cardiac event. The cardiac history group had a mean age of 58.3 years and a mean burn size of 18.4 percent TBSA. Nearly half of the patients with a history of previous cardiac disease manifested cardiac dysfunction, most commonly an arrhythmia disturbance, during hospitalization for burn injury. The mortality was 30 percent for the group, but death was not directly related to cardiac events in each case. A second group consisted of 142 patients with no previous history of cardiac disease who experienced an in-hospital cardiac event. Their mean age was 43.2 years, the mean burn size was 38.6 percent TBSA, and the most common event was arrhythmia (31 percent).[5]

High-Risk Populations

Certain factors have been identified as increasing the risk of accidental burn injury, among them alcohol or drug abuse, neurologic disorders, psychiatric disorders, and immobilizing physical disabilities. One study found that 3.25 percent of patients admitted to a burn unit had both thermal injury and neurologic disorders, with seizures the most common finding.[6] Burns in children also occurred at an alarming rate, with child abuse, neglect, or both often found as a contributing factor. The occurrence of burns during pregnancy is rare but often results in fetal death, even with relatively small maternal TBSA burns, because of the psychologic adaptive mechanisms that identify the gravid uterus and fetal-placental circulation as low priority in the presence of diminished circulating blood volume such as occurs with burn injury.[7]

Environmental and life-style factors also influence the frequency and magnitude of burn injury. The fire loss record in the United States is the worst in the industrialized world, with the fire death rate double that of most countries on a per capita basis. Ignition of upholstered furniture and mattresses by cigarettes is the single leading cause of fire death. In 1984, 67,000 cigarette-initiated fires were reported, resulting in 1,570 deaths and 7,000 serious injuries.[8] A new problem has recently been identified as fires and burns associated with misuse of disposable butane lighters. Maley[9] reported an estimated 2,970 emergency room visits in 1984 associated with cigarette lighters; 2,250 of these injuries were thermal burns, with 25 percent (563) occurring in children under 5 years of age. Additionally, 200 deaths per year are associated with fires started by cigarette lighters which led to the deaths of 125 children under 5 years of age.

Electrical injury usually accounts for less than 2 percent of admissions to burn facilities, but injury from electricity has been increasing in the United States in recent years.[10] Electrical injuries are classified as high-voltage (1,000 volts or greater) or low-voltage. Household currents of 120 and 220 volts typically cause low-voltage electrical injury. High-voltage injuries are frequently due to high-tension sources, which commonly carry from 7,200 to 19,000 volts but may involve from 100,000 to 1,000,000 volts.[11] Major electrical injury occurs almost exclusively in men who work with electricity or in farm workers who move irrigation pipe.

Burn facilities serving rural areas tend to have a higher percentage of electrical injury admissions than those serving urban areas. Few of these injuries are the result of household accidents, although toddlers occasionally insert metal objects, usually keys, into electrical outlets and are subsequently injured. Teething infants tend to chew on electrical cords and may sustain electrical burns to the mouth,[12,13] but these are not "true" electrical injuries because the entry and exit wound both tend to be in the mouth and the electrical current rarely passes through the body.

Lightning injuries kill between 150 and 300 people per year in the United States.[11] Lightning is direct current of 100 million or more volts and up to 200,000 amps, which can injure either by a direct strike or by a side flash as a result of the flow of current between a person and a nearby object struck by lightning.

KEY CONCEPTS

- **Thermal injury is the second most common cause of accidental death in the United States. Fire within the home results in 93 percent of all burn episodes.**
- **Other sources of burn injuries include scalding, flammable liquids, electrical shock, and cooking mishaps.**
- **The risk of burn injury is increased in situations of alcohol or drug abuse; neurologic, psychological, or debilitating disorders; child abuse; and cigarette smoking.**

Structure and Function of Skin

The skin, the largest organ of the body, constitutes about 20 percent of total body weight and is composed of three layers (Fig. 55–1): the **epidermis, dermis,** and **hypodermis** (or **subcutaneous layer**). The epidermis contains two main types of cells: **melanocytes** and **keratinocytes.** Melanocytes are scattered through the basal layer (stratum germinativum) and produce melanin, a pigment that shields deeper structures of the skin from sunlight. With burn injury, healing occurs in advance of the formation of new melanocytes and

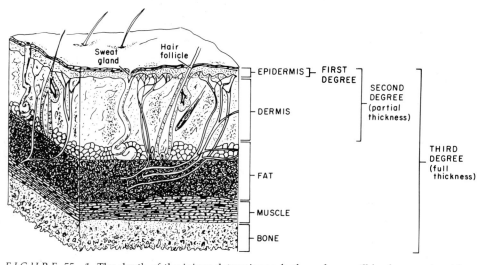

F I G U R E 55 – 1. The depth of the injury determines whether a burn will heal or require skin grafting. First- and second-degree burns will heal because they are partial thickness injuries; thus, the elements necessary to generate new skin remain. Full-thickness injury destroys all dermal appendages and requires skin grafting to achieve coverage. (From Kravitz M: Thermal injuries, in Cardona VD, Hurn PD, Mason PJ, Scanlon-Schlipp AM, Veise-Berry SW (eds): *Trauma Nursing: From Resuscitation Through Rehabilitation.* Philadelphia, WB Saunders, 1988, p 709. Reproduced with permission.)

provides a light pink or reddish layer of new skin, with color restored at a later time. Keratinocytes develop from cells in the basal layer of the epidermis and progress upward from the stratum germinativum to the stratum corneum over about 14 days. The epidermis is a thin, avascular layer nourished by diffusion from blood vessels in the dermis. Epidermal appendages include the hair, nails, and glands (apocrine, eccrine, and sebaceous). Although these appendages originate from the epidermal layer, they are anatomically located in both the epidermis and dermis. Hair destroyed as a result of burn injury will grow back at about 1 cm per month unless the depth of the burn has destroyed the hair follicle, in which case alopecia results. Nails grow from the nail matrix and will often be shed following a deep hand or foot burn, with gradual regrowth if the burn is not destructive to the matrix. New nail formation is often irregular and of abnormal thickness following nail regrowth.

Two types of sweat glands are found in the skin. Apocrine glands, the large sweat glands, are rudimentary structures with no known useful purpose. They respond to autonomic nervous rather than thermal stimulation to produce an odorless, viscous, milklike droplet from the hair shaft. Apocrine glands are greater in number in women and are located in the axilla, areola of nipples, groin, perineum, perianal, and periumbilical regions. Eccrine glands are small sweat glands distributed over the body to act as true secretory glands that produce sweat responsible for heat regulation. At environmental temperatures above 31° or 32°C (90°F), sweating occurs over the entire body; at lower temperatures, microscopically visible droplets are secreted periodically as part of total insensible water loss from the body. The function of sweat glands is severely altered in areas of thermal injury following healing, and they become hypersecretory. Sweat normally provides skin with an acid mantle (average pH, 5.7 to 6.4), which retards growth of the many bacteria that reside in the keratin layer, glands, and hair follicles.

Sebaceous glands secrete sebum, a complex mixture of lipids, which is emptied into the hair shaft. The rate of production of sebum and its location depend on the male hormone androgen, which initiates and continues production. During the hypermetabolic state that follows major thermal injury, all hormones are decreased, and low production of sebum contributes to the dry skin conditions commonly found following recovery.

Normal physiologic functions of the skin are lost with burn injury. The extent of the injury determines whether this is a localized problem or a systemic pathophysiology. The depth of burn injury describes the local tissue damage and is largely a factor of length of exposure and the temperature or destructive potential of the agent causing the damage. Studies have shown that most water heaters in homes are set at about 140°F. A full-thickness injury can occur in 5 seconds at this temperature. Temperatures between 140° and 130°F increase the time to full-thickness in-

jury to 30 seconds. At 120°F, a serious burn injury can occur in about 5 minutes.

KEY CONCEPTS

- The skin provides several essential functions that are lost with burn injury. These include immunologic defense, fluid conservation, and temperature regulation.
- Important elements of skin include melanocytes (which pigment the skin and hair) and glands. Sweat-producing exocrine glands may become hypersecretory in healed areas after thermal injury.

Burn Injury

Depth Classification

In clinical areas, classification of the depth of burn injury is based on criteria established by the American Burn Association.[14] Depth of injury is divided into four classifications (Table 55–1): **first degree, superficial and deep partial thickness** (**second degree**), and **full-thickness** (**third degree**). The International Classification of Diseases by the U.S. Department of Health and Human Services describes burn injury as including abrasion or friction burns, whereas sunburn is coded as contact dermatitis due to solar radiation.[15] Both classification systems agree that loss of skin function is the major pathophysiology.

First-Degree Burns

First-degree burns involve only superficial tissue destruction in the outermost layers of the epidermis. All physiologic functions of the skin remain intact (Table 55–2). First-degree burns are not included in estimates of the percentage of TBSA burned because the skin does not lose its ability to function as a water vapor and bacterial barrier. Local pain and erythema develop and may be followed by blister formation over the following 24-hour period. Erythema, a dermal vascular response that occurs in first-degree burns in the absence of direct trauma to the dermis, is probably related to the release of tissue contents into the superficial circulation. Extensive first-degree burns may result in mild to absent systemic responses that are usually limited to headache, chills, local discomfort, nausea, and vomiting. The injury needs no treatment except in large burns of an infant or elderly person, when fluid losses into the blisters, especially in combination with nausea and vomiting, may lead to systemic dehydration. Treatment is aimed at rehydration, possibly with administration of intravenous fluids. The injury heals in 3 to 5 days without scarring. Sunburn is the typical example of a first-degree burn, although exposure to low-intensity heat sources over sufficient time or brief exposure to high-intensity heat can produce this superficial tissue destruction. Treatment of first-degree burns focuses on comfort mea-

TABLE 55–1. Depth of Injury

Characteristic	First Degree	Second Degree Superficial Partial Thickness	Second Degree Deep Partial Thickness	Third Degree Full-Thickness
Morphology	Destruction of epidermis only	Destruction of epidermis and some dermis	Destruction of epidermis and dermis, leaving only skin appendages	Destruction of epidermis, dermis, and underlying subcutaneous tissue
Skin function	Intact	Absent	Absent	Absent
Tactile and pain sensors	Intact	Intact	Intact but diminished	Absent
Blisters	Present only after first 24 hr	Present within minutes, thin-walled, fluid-filled	May or may not appear as fluid-filled blisters; often is layer of flat, dehydrated "tissue paper" that lifts off in sheets	Blisters rare; usually is layer of flat, dehydrated "tissue paper" that lifts off easily
Appearance of wound after initial debridement	Skin peels at 24 to 48 hr, normal or slightly red underneath	Red to pale ivory, moist surface	Mottled with areas of waxy white, dry surface	White, cherry red, or black; may contain visible thrombosed veins; dry, hard, leathery surface
Healing time	3–5 days	21–28 days	30 days–many months	Will not heal; may close from edges as secondary healing if wound is small
Scarring	None	Present, influenced by genetic predisposition	Highest because slow healing rate increases scar tissue development, influenced by genetic predisposition	Skin graft scarring is minimized by early excision and grafting, influenced by genetic predisposition

From Kravitz M: Thermal injuries, in Cardona VD, Hurn PD, Mason PJ, Scanlon-Schlipp AM, Veise-Berry SW (eds): *Trauma Nursing: From Resuscitation Through Rehabilitation.* Philadelphia, WB Saunders, 1988, p 709. Reproduced with permission.

sures. Previously healthy persons with extensive first-degree burns will have symptoms relieved with aspirin (for adults) or acetaminophen (for children) every 4 hours in age-appropriate dosages for the first 24 hours following injury. Frequent application of water-soluble lotions also promotes comfort.

Superficial Partial Thickness Burns

Second-degree burns are subdivided into superficial and deep partial thickness injury, a classification that defines the anatomic and physiologic effects of the depth of injury. **Superficial partial thickness injury** involves the epidermis and dermis and appears red to pale ivory in color. The formation of moist, thin-walled blisters occurs within minutes of the injury. Pain is a major clinical feature of this depth of injury because the tactile and pain sensors remain intact (see Table 55–2). The injury will heal in 21 to 28 days in previously healthy people in the absence of wound infection. The amount of scarring that follows is a genetically determined trait, with some groups of people tending to scar excessively (blacks and people with red hair) or minimally (Native American and Asian groups). Hair follicles remain intact and will regrow hair in the area of injury. Hair usually reappears 7 to 10 days following superficial partial thickness injury.

Deep Partial Thickness Burns

Deep partial thickness burns may involve the entire dermis, leaving only the epidermal skin appendages

located in hair follicles. The area of injury has a mottled appearance, with large areas of waxy-white tissue surrounded by light pink or red tissue. The surface is dry, and blisters tend to resemble flat, dry tissue-paper rather than the fluid-filled raised areas seen with superficial partial thickness injury. Tactile and pain sensors are either absent or greatly diminished in the area of deepest tissue destruction, but this area is usually surrounded by margins of lesser depth of injury in which pain and tactile sensors are intact. Deep partial thickness injury is visually and clinically indistinguishable from full-thickness injury at the time of injury. These wounds will heal spontaneously in previously healthy people and in the absence of infection in about 30 days. In some patients, these wounds are allowed to heal if the patient is not a candidate for surgical treatment because of preexisting disease or if large areas of full-thickness injury require skin grafting as a priority for survival. However, wounds that require a longer time for healing also result in significantly more scar formation later, so current therapy indicates excision of the wound followed by skin grafting to diminish scarring and to achieve early wound closure. (See the section on wound management in Emergent Phase, later in this chapter.)

Full-Thickness Burns

Third-degree full-thickness burns involve the epidermis, dermis, and underlying subcutaneous tissue. Immediately following the injury, the area appears

TABLE 55-2. Normal Physiologic Functions of the Skin Altered or Lost Following Thermal Injury

Protection

Barrier between internal organs and external environment. Continuous with mucous membrane at external openings of organs of digestive, respiratory, and urogenital systems. Acidic skin (pH, 4.2–5.6) and perspiration protect against bacterial invasion. Thickened skin of palms and soles provides padding.

Percutaneous Absorption

Epidermis relatively impermeable to most chemical substances; some may be absorbed through epidermis or orifices of hair follicles.

Sensory Processing

Receptor skin nerve endings allow constant monitoring of the environment by sensing warm and cold temperature, pain, touch, and pressure.

Production

Endogenous production of vitamin D_3, necessary for synthesis of vitamin D.

Barrier

Skin prevents water and electrolyte loss, maintains moist subcutaneous tissues, and prevents water absorption during immersion.

Thermoregulation

Body continuously produces heat as cellular metabolism by-product; heat is dissipated through skin. Internal body temperature is regulated by radiation, conduction, or convection. Rate of heat loss depends primarily on surface temperature of skin, which is a function of skin blood flow.

Immunologic

Major site of immune complexes is dermal-epidermal junction and dermal vessels of skin. Monocyte/macrophage system mobilized by local tissue mediators.

Circulatory

Skin temperature depends on rate of blood flow through skin; circulatory system distributes pharmacologic agents to local tissues.

Aesthetic

Provides individual identity of a person.

---

white, cherry red, or black. Deep blisters may be present under a dry, tissue-paper layer of dehydrated skin. Superficial blood vessels coagulated by the heat of injury may be visible through the skin as thrombosed veins. One of the physiologic characteristics of the skin that is lost (see Table 55–2) is the elasticity of the dermis; this results in a wound with a dry, hard, leathery texture. The massive edema that accompanies major burn injury (see discussion under Acute Injury), combined with the loss of elasticity, may result in a tourniquet-like effect when the injury includes a circumferential limb or torso burn. Release of the constriction which may accompany **circumferential burns** is accomplished by a surgical cut through the burn **eschar (escharotomy)** or, if this does not restore distal circulation, an incision to the **fascia (fasciotomy)**. Full-thickness burns are painless to touch because all superficial nerve endings in the skin have been destroyed. However, as with the partial thickness injuries, rarely are burn injuries totally uniform, and an area of lesser injury, in which pain and tactile sensors are intact, is usually located on the margins. Full-thickness injury areas larger than 1.5 to 2 inches in diameter require skin grafting with the patient's own skin (**autograft**) because all dermal elements have been destroyed and cannot regenerate. Small injuries will heal by forming new dermal elements on the margins of the wound and closing from the edges toward the center, a process that requires many weeks even in small wounds.

Severity Criteria

Severity of burn injury is determined by the extent to which the physiologic functions of the skin are disrupted beyond the body's normal ability to respond with compensatory mechanisms. The American Burn Association[14] classifies burn injury as minor, moderate uncomplicated, and major (Table 55–3). The severity of burn injury and the eventual morbidity and mortality associated with it are related to a combination of factors, including the patient's age, medical history, extent and depth of burn, body area involved, and the presence of concomitant trauma sustained at the time of the burn.

TABLE 55–3. American Burn Association: Definitions of Injury Extent

Minor Burn Injury	Moderate Uncomplicated Burn Injury	Major Burn Injury
Second-degree burn of less than 15% TBSA in adults or less than 10% TBSA in children	Second-degree burns of 15%–25% TBSA in adults or 10%–20% in children	Second-degree burns of greater than 25% TBSA in adults or 20% TBSA in children
Third-degree burn of less than 2% TBSA not involving special care areas (eyes, ears, face, hands, feet, perineum)	Third-degree burns of less than 10% TBSA not involving special care areas	All third-degree burns of 10% TBSA or greater
Excludes electrical injury, inhalation injury, complicated injury (fractures), all poor-risk patients (e.g., at extremes of age, with intercurrent disease)	Excludes electrical injury, complicated injury (fractures), inhalation injury, all poor-risk patients (e.g., at extremes of age, with intercurrent disease)	All burns involving hands, face, eyes, ears, feet, perineum
		All inhalation injury, electrical injury, complicated burn injury involving fractures or other major trauma
		All poor-risk patients

From Kravitz M: Thermal injuries, in Cardona VD, et al (eds): *Trauma Nursing: From Resuscitation Through Rehabilitation.* Philadelphia, WB Saunders, 1988, p 711. Reproduced with permission. TBSA, total body surface area.

Most burn injuries are small in size and minor in effect, resulting only in mild discomfort to the patient until the wound begins to heal in 3 to 5 days. However, major burn injury can result in death if appropriate intervention is not initiated and continued using state-of-the-art knowledge by a team of burn experts with access to the latest technology and resources to support the healing process. Major burn injury produces both localized skin pathology related to loss of skin function (see Table 55–2) and systemic response related to loss of circulating cardiovascular fluids from the cardiovascular system. Burn shock occurs in adult patients with 25 percent TBSA burn or greater and in children with 10 to 15 percent TBSA burn. The magnitude of burn shock is directly related to the extent of TBSA burn involvement.

Extent of Injury

Extent of injury refers to the percentage of TBSA burned. Estimates can be calculated using the rule of nines (Fig. 55–2) or the Lund and Browder chart (Fig. 55–3). The rule of nines is commonly used in prehospital settings and emergency departments, whereas the Lund and Browder chart or a variation of it is used in burn centers. Burns greater than 25 percent TBSA in adults or 20 percent TBSA in children are major burn injuries requiring therapeutic interventions by health care providers to ensure survival and optimal functional recovery. In general, people with minor burn injury are treated as outpatients either in a physician's office, clinic, or hospital physical therapy department.

Treatment

Therapy is aimed at promoting wound healing and providing analgesia for patient comfort as indicated. Tetanus immunization status is determined and updated as needed. Patients with moderate, uncomplicated burn injury will be initially admitted to a hospital for acute management, followed by teaching sessions for the patient and family focusing on the required dressing changes, pain management, and nutritional support needed for home care following discharge. Discharge to a suitable environment is possible within 5 to 7 days, but this time frame will be greatly prolonged in the absence of suitable home caregivers. Patients with major burn injury face prolonged periods in intensive care in a hospital followed by weeks or months of emergency and rehabilitative care. The hospital course is frequently stormy, as the patient

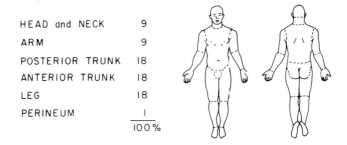

HEAD and NECK	9
ARM	9
POSTERIOR TRUNK	18
ANTERIOR TRUNK	18
LEG	18
PERINEUM	1
	100%

FIGURE 55–2. The rule of nines is a commonly used assessment tool that permits timely and useful estimate of the percentage of the total body surface area burned. (From Kravitz M: Thermal injuries, in Cardona VD, et al. (eds): *Trauma Nursing: From Resuscitation Through Rehabilitation.* Philadelphia, WB Saunders, 1988, p 710. Reproduced with permission.)

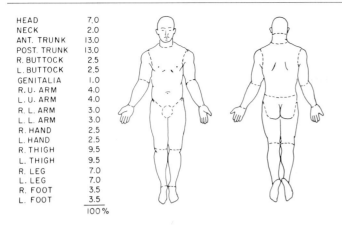

HEAD	7.0
NECK	2.0
ANT. TRUNK	13.0
POST. TRUNK	13.0
R. BUTTOCK	2.5
L. BUTTOCK	2.5
GENITALIA	1.0
R.U. ARM	4.0
L.U. ARM	4.0
R.L. ARM	3.0
L.L. ARM	3.0
R. HAND	2.5
L. HAND	2.5
R. THIGH	9.5
L. THIGH	9.5
R. LEG	7.0
L. LEG	7.0
R. FOOT	3.5
L. FOOT	3.5
	100%

FIGURE 55–3. The Lund and Browder chart. The areas of the body are presented in section, which permits a more accurate estimation of burn size. (From Kravitz M: Thermal injuries, in Cardona VD et al (eds): *Trauma Nursing: From Resuscitation Through Rehabilitation.* Philadelphia, WB Saunders, 1988, p 710. Reproduced with permission. Originally adapted from Lund CC, Browder NC: *Surg Gynecol Obstet* 1944;79:352–358. By permission of Surgery, Gynecology, and Obstetrics.)

faces repeated operative procedures to achieve wound coverage. Infection, either of the burn wound itself or related to pulmonary complications or systemic sepsis, remains a potential risk until wound closure is achieved over 80 percent of the body surface area. Burn injury with an associated inhalation injury carries a much higher mortality than an equal burn injury alone. Survival from burn injury is significantly more likely when patients are treated in a burn center.

The American Burn Association has developed a set of Burn Center Referral Criteria[14] to assist local hospitals in appropriate triage (Table 55–4). In addition to burn depth and extent, factors such as anatomic location of the burn, electrical injury, inhalation injury, concurrent trauma, and preexisting medical disease are recognized as contributing to the morbidity and mortality of the burn injury. Improvements

TABLE 55–4. Advanced Burn Life Support Triage Criteria for Referral to a Burn Center

Second- and third-degree burns greater than 10% total body surface area (TBSA) in patients under 10 or over 50 years of age
Second- and third-degree burns with serious threat of functional or cosmetic impairment that involve face, hands, feet, genitalia, perineum, and major joints
Third-degree burns greater than 5% TBSA in any age group
Electrical burns, including lightning injury
Chemical burns that seriously threaten functional or cosmetic impairment
Inhalation injury with burn injury
Age group extremes. Hospitals without qualified personnel or equipment for the care of children should transfer burned children to a burn center with these capabilities
Preexisting medical conditions
Associated trauma

From *Advanced Burn Life Support Course Instructor's Manual,* Lincoln, Nebraska Burn Institute; 1987, pp III-61–III-62. Reproduced with permission.

in burn care have resulted in an expected survival rate of 50 percent for previously healthy individuals with deep burns involving 50 pecent TBSA in the absence of associated inhalation injury.

KEY CONCEPTS

- First-degree burns destroy only superficial layers of skin (epidermis). Physiologic functions of the skin remain intact. Manifestations include local pain, blistering, and erythema. The injury heals in 3 to 5 days without scarring. For large burns, hydration and symptom relief with aspirin-like analgesics may be recommended.
- Second-degree burns include two subtypes: superficial, and deep partial thickness. Superficial partial thickness burns involve the epidermis and dermis. Pain and blistering occur. The burn heals in 21 to 28 days, and scarring may occur, depending on genetic tendency. Hair follicles remain intact. Deep partial thickness burns involve the entire dermis. The injury is mottled, has dry blisters, and is relatively painless. Healing occurs in about 30 days spontaneously.
- Third-degree full-thickness burns involve the epidermis, dermis, and underlying subcutaneous tissue. Skin is charred and may appear black, white, or cherry red. The wound is painless to touch. Skin grafting is indicated for wounds greater than 2 inches in diameter.
- The severity of burn injury is related to the depth and extent of burn. Burns covering greater than 25 percent of TBSA in adults and 20 percent in children are classified as major burns requiring intensive intervention. Burns greater than 25 percent of TBSA are usually associated with burn shock.

Initial Interventions

Eliminate Source of Burn and Treat

People whose clothing is on fire tend to run; this leads to more extensive burns, compounded by inhalation injury as they breathe the flaming gases rising about their face. A national campaign to educate the public, the "Stop, Drop and Roll" campaign, has been enormously successful in decreasing the extent of flame burns associated with clothing fires. If the patient with flaming clothes already knows, "Stop, Drop and Roll," hearing someone say the phrase may initiate the action. During the event is not the time to teach someone the maneuver, so, if the desirable action does not occur, stop the person from running and attempt to get him or her horizontal to the ground to keep flames away from the face and airway. The ideal method to extinguish flame is with water, because this eliminates the source of the heat immediately and cools the skin underneath. The water does not need to be sterile or even clean; the objective is to put out the fire. If water is not available, flames may be smothered with a blanket, coat, or other available covering that will deprive the flames of oxygen required for continued combustion. Then remove the cover so that the heat can escape from the body and its clothing, thereby reducing the depth of injury. Scald injury is also best treated immediately with cool water, which will immediately decrease the temperature of the scalding liquid and the skin underneath. If water is not available, remove the clothing. Chemicals causing contact burns of the skin are treated by removing the clothing, dusting off any powdered chemicals, followed by diluting the chemicals by flushing the area with copious amounts of water. Do not attempt to neutralize chemicals on the skin because neutralization is a heat-producing chemical reaction that will leave the patient with a chemical and a thermal injury.

Chemical accidents tend to occur in industrial settings or in military actions; personnel in both settings are familiar with initial treatment, and shower heads are located at strategic intervals whenever conditions allow. If the patient is stable and has no other injuries, place in a shower or under a hose spray for 15 to 20 minutes to flush chemical from skin contact. If the eyes are involved, flush each eye with at least 1 liter of solution. When available, Ringer's lactate solution or other sterile intravenous infusion solutions may be flushed through intravenous tubing, which is used as a small hose to direct the flow of the solution into the eye. Chemical burns to the eye are very painful, but early intervention may save vision later. Phosphorus burns are an unusual occurrence limited mainly to military conflicts or terrorist attacks. Phosphorus demonstrates continuous burning when exposed to ambient oxygen; thus, phosphorus burns should initially be treated by irrigation with water or saline and then by soaked occlusive dressings until the patient arrives in a hospital.[16] Anhydrous ammonia is a frequent source of chemical injury in agricultural areas of the country. Because it is 82 percent nitrogen, it is good fertilizer, but its unplanned release into the environment releases the liquid chemical plus ammonia gas. The highly alkaline ammonia quickly degrades epidermal fats and breaches the barrier to enter the more hydrophilic dermis, followed by denaturing of tissue proteins. Inhalation of ammonia gases can cause coughing, edema of the glottic region, and laryngospasm resulting in respiratory arrest and death. Irrigation with water to dilute and remove ammonia liquid from the skin is accomplished after removing the patient from areas of ammonia fumes. Ocular injuries are common and occur within 5 to 10 seconds of exposure.[17]

Tar, asphalt, and melted plastic are frequent agents of injury in certain parts of the United States. Initial intervention is aimed at decreasing the temperature of the material rapidly using water; if no water is available, the material will cool to room temperature within 2 to 3 minutes, but the time lapse will extend the depth of injury. The cooled material becomes a sterile dressing, and no attempt should be made at the scene to remove the material unless the patient's airway is compromised.

Electrical injury occurs under a variety of conditions that may also put the rescuer at risk. Initial care at the scene must be delivered in a manner that ensures rescuer safety, because contact with a patient who remains in contact with the electrical source will result in an electrical injury to both. Rescuers will move the patient, not the wires, away from the area and then assess the patient for cardiopulmonary arrest secondary to electrical current disrupting normal heart rhythm. Cardiopulmonary resuscitation is initiated as indicated, using standard protocols. After airway and circulatory support have been established, the patient is stabilized using a cervical collar and spinal board. Electrical current passing through the body causes severe muscle contraction and may result in compression and/or dislocation fracture of the spine. As current passes through the body, sustained muscle contractions prevent the patient from maintaining an effective airway because the muscles of respiration are also in sustained contraction, as is the heart muscle. Patients may have a cardiac arrest related to electrical disruption of cardiac muscle and a respiratory arrest related to tetanic contractions. Alternating current, even at low voltages, produces muscle contractions, making self-extrication impossible; household alternating current of 120 volts can result in death if assistance is not nearby. Direct current of low voltage is not as dangerous because it does not produce muscle contractions. Current greater than 500 volts may be fatal because it tends to produce ventricular fibrillation or cardiac standstill.[18]

KEY CONCEPTS

- **Elimination of the source of burn is the first priority. Water is the best element to extinguish flame, dilute chemical burn, and cool scald injury. In the absence of water, flames may be extinguished by rolling the victim or by smothering the flames with a blanket or other cover.**
- **Electrical injury is associated with intense muscle contraction and cardiac dysrhythmia. Cardiopulmonary resuscitation and spinal cord stabilization are indicated.**

Major Burns

Acute Phase

Two different but simultaneous mechanisms occur in cases of major burns: local wound pathophysiology related to the loss of skin integrity, and systemic pathophysiology related to sequelae of burn injury. The most immediate systemic change is identified as burn shock and includes pathophysiologic changes in the cardiovascular system that are profound, systemic, and lethal without timely and appropriate medical intervention to support the patient's failing cardiovascular system.

Shock

Within minutes of the burn injury, the cardiovascular system, which is normally a closed, semipermeable system, becomes an open system through which the patient's circulating volume leaves the circulatory system. The phenomenon, known as "capillary leak," occurs within just a few minutes of injury and continues for approximately 24 hours before closure occurs. The mechanism of burn shock is unknown but its sequence is known, and therapy is aimed at supporting the patient through the burn shock by restoring the circulating volume using intravenous fluids at an infusion rate equal to the rate fluid is being lost.

Burn shock is not a phenomenon localized to the burn area but occurs throughout the body and results in profound hypovolemia and death if not treated. The capillary leak (Fig. 55–4) occurs not just in the area of burn but also in the capillary system throughout the body; fluid lost in the area of the burn will leak through the burn into the environment, while fluid lost internally will collect in nearby tissues and produce extensive edema (Fig. 55–5). As the plasma and fluids leak from the capillaries, the red blood cells and white blood cells remain because they are too large to leak out; thus, the hematocrit is initially elevated and may reach values as high as 60 percent as burn shock progresses.

Fluid Resuscitation

The rate and volume of fluid lost are related directly to the extent of burn injury; therefore, formulas for the resuscitation of burn shock have been developed.

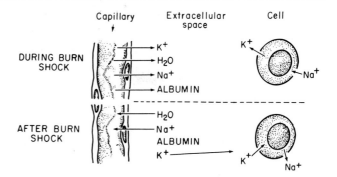

FIGURE 55–5. Direction of fluid and electrolyte shifts associated with burn shock. (From Kravitz M: Thermal injuries, in Cardona VD, et al. (eds): *Trauma Nursing: From Resuscitation Through Rehabilitation.* Philadelphia, WB Saunders, 1988, p 712. Reproduced with permission.)

Fluid must be administered at a rate to maintain urine output at 30 mL/hr in adults or 1 cc/kg/hr in children. Systemic circulatory pressures sufficient to perfuse the kidneys and produce this amount of urine are known to be adequate to ensure tissue perfusion throughout the body. Renal failure is not a component of burn shock, but the kidneys will cease production of urine in order to preserve circulating volume if perfusion pressures are too low to preserve adequate systemic pressure.

The most widely used formula for fluid resuscitation of burn shock is the Parkland formula (Table 55–5). This formula predicts the amount of intravenous fluid required during the first 24 hours after burn injury to restore the fluid being lost. The formula is a guideline for fluid administration, but urine output

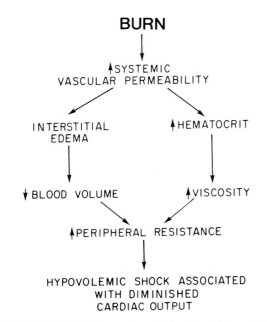

BURN

↑SYSTEMIC
VASCULAR PERMEABILITY

INTERSTITIAL EDEMA   ↑HEMATOCRIT

↓BLOOD VOLUME   ↑VISCOSITY

↑PERIPHERAL RESISTANCE

HYPOVOLEMIC SHOCK ASSOCIATED
WITH DIMINISHED
CARDIAC OUTPUT

FIGURE 55–4. Cardiovascular effects of major burn injury during burn shock. (From Kravitz M: Thermal injuries, in Cardona VD, et al. (eds): *Trauma Nursing: From Resuscitation Through Rehabilitation.* Philadelphia, WB Saunders, 1988, p 711. Reproduced with permission.)

TABLE 55–5. Parkland Formula of Fluid Resuscitation for Burn Shock

During the first 24 hr after a burn, administer intravenous lactated Ringer's solution at the following rate:

4 mL lactated Ringer's/% TBSA burn/kg body weight

where

- Time is calculated from time of burn injury
- TBSA is total body surface area
- Half of total fluid is administered in the first 8 hr after burn
- One-fourth of total is administered in the second 8 hr
- One-fourth of total is administered in the third 8 hr or in quantities to maintain adult urine output at 30 mL/hr or child urine output at 1 mL/kg/hr

Example of formula calculation in a 70-kg patient with a 50% TBSA burn:

4 mL × 70 kg × 50% TBSA burn = 14,000 mL or 14 L of lactated Ringer's in 24 hr

- Administer 7,000 mL in first 8 hr at 875 mL/hr
- Administer 3,500 mL in second 8 hr at 437 mL/hr
- Administer 3,500 mL in third 8 hr at 437 mL/hr

Data from Baxter CR: Guidelines for fluid resuscitation. *J Burn Care & Rehabilitation* 1981;2:279–286.

is the clinical parameter that defines the amount of fluid actually administered. Some patients will require more than the predicted 4 mL/kg/percent TBSA burn, and a few will require less. Patients expected to need more fluid than predicted are those with accompanying inhalation injury, deep burns into muscle, and those whose fluid resuscitation was delayed. Approximately 24 hours after the burn, the patient's capillary seal will be spontaneously regained and the cardiovascular integrity restored. At this time, plasma will be administered according to a formula (Table 55–6) to replace the plasma that has been lost during burn shock.

If burn shock resuscitation does not occur in a timely manner and at a rate to restore circulating volume, the patient progresses through hypovolemic shock to death as the circulating volume is lost through capillary leakage. Administration of plasma before restoration of the capillary seal is contraindicated because the fluid will leak out and be of no benefit. After capillary integrity has been restored, administered plasma will remain in the circulatory volume. Electrolyte imbalances will not occur in burn patients resuscitated with Ringer's lactate solution because it closely approximates the fluid being lost to the circulation (Table 55–7). Resuscitation with nonelectrolyte intravenous fluids will produce profound hyponatremia and hypokalemia within a few hours; resuscitation with normal saline will increase the serum sodium content but not to an excessive level. *Fluid replacement is the prime objective of initial burn treatment.*

One of the major functions of intact skin is to serve as a barrier to evaporative water loss from the body. With major burn injury, this ability of the skin to regulate evaporative water loss is totally disrupted. In a classic study done in 1962, Moncrief and Mason[19] attempted to determine the magnitude of such a loss and found that daily evaporative water loss was in the range of 20 times normal in the early phase of burn injury, with gradual decreases as wound closure was achieved. Further studies revealed that the insen-

TABLE 55–6. Plasma Requirements and Evaporative Water Loss Following Burn Injury

Colloid Replacement

Twenty percent of blood volume given as fresh frozen plasma or plasma expander
    Adult males = 20% (5 mL/kg body weight)
    Adult females and children = 20% (8 mL/kg)

Maintenance Fluids Until Wound Closure Is Achieved

Basal fluid requirements
    1,500 mL fluid/m² TBSA = 24-hr requirement
Evaporative water loss from burn wound until healed
    Adults = (25 + % TBSA burn) m² BSA = mL/hr requirement
    Children = (35 + % TBSA burn) m² BSA = mL/hr requirement
Maintenance fluids = basal fluid requirements plus evaporative water loss; may be administered intravenously, orally, or by nasogastric or jejunal tube, according to patient need

TABLE 55–7. Electrolyte Content of Lactated Ringer's Solution and Extracellular Fluid

Electrolyte	Extracellular Fluid (mEq/L)*	Lactated Ringer's Solution (mEq/L)†
Sodium	135–145	130
Potassium	3.2–4.5	4
Chloride	95–105	109
Lactate (bicarbonate)	24–28	28

*Normal values may differ slightly between laboratories.
†Plus 80–100 mL free water/L solution.

sible water loss through burned skin is not from evaporation of water from sweat glands but rather from water vapor formed within the body and lost through the skin.[20,21] The amount of evaporative water loss through the burn wound is calculated using the following formula:

(25 + percent TBSA burn) (square meter body surface area) = mL/hr evaporative water loss

Thus, a 70-kg patient with a 50 percent TBSA burn requires an additional 3,000 mL of free water per day just to replace evaporative water loss. These losses continue until the wound heals or is surgically closed. Replacement of the losses is mandatory to prevent dehydration followed by hypovolemic shock and severe electrolyte imbalances.

Cardiovascular Dysfunction

Cardiovascular dysfunction is also a component of major burn injury. Burn shock is accompanied by a sudden precipitous drop in cardiac output that does not parallel the gradual reduction in blood volume. Furthermore, infusion of intravenous fluids in amounts to restore the circulating volume does not return the cardiac output to preburn levels.[22,23] The consistent burn shock finding of inappropriately low cardiac output in the presence of vigorous intravenous fluid resuscitation and massive catecholamine release has led to the suggestion of a specific myocardial depressant factor.[24,25] Although there is agreement that myocardial dysfunction is present with all major burn injuries, the cause of the depression remains to be described except in the most general terms. There appears to be no simple, specific myocardial depressant factor but rather a cascade of events that is generally termed the cellular response to burn injury and includes both metabolic and immunologic factors. These factors initiate the cardiovascular sequence of loss of capillary seal and subsequent hypovolemic shock.

Respiratory Dysfunction

The acute phase of burn injury is also a time when the patient's airway and pulmonary system may become compromised. Three types of respiratory risks are present: airway obstruction related to edema of the upper airway; hypoxia related to smoke inhalation and its accompanying edema and acute respiratory distress syndrome (ARDS); and hypoxia related to carbon monoxide poisoning. Although all three conditions can occur simultaneously in the same person, each is discussed separately.

The massive body edema that accompanies major burn injury is partly related to the patient's loss of body fluid into the tissues but is mainly related to iatrogenic complications from the administration and subsequent leakage of intravenous fluids used to support the cardiovascular system through burn shock. Burns to the head and neck area increase the incidence of airway obstruction, but extensive burns without head and neck involvement also carry a risk. On occasion, burns to the oral cavity and upper airway occur as superheated air is breathed or hot water enters the mouth. The pulmonary system is extremely efficient at dissipating heat and prevents the inhalation of superheated air beyond the bronchi, but live steam may actually be breathed into the lungs.

Edema and subsequent airway obstruction can occur within the first hour after a burn but tend to occur within 2 to 4 hours after injury as burn shock resuscitation fluids accumulate to form tissue edema. Endotracheal intubation is performed prophylactically when impending airway obstruction is identified. The nasal-pharyngeal route of intubation is most comfortable for the patient but, on occasion, oral-pharyngeal intubation is performed. Tracheostomy is avoided whenever possible because of its known increase in morbidity and mortality in burn patients related to pulmonary infection and sepsis. Tape will not adhere to burn wounds; therefore, the endotracheal tube is secured using cotton twill tape which is released and retied frequently to allow for the increase in head and face circumference related to increasing, massive edema.

The patient's eyes will also swell shut secondary to edema formation, and hearing will be impaired as edema forms in the auditory canals. The combination of not being able to speak, see, or hear is extremely frightening for the patient and requires special patient reassurance measures until the edema subsides, 3 to 5 days following injury. As the external, visible edema subsides, so does the internal airway edema resolve; therefore, a clinical guide for extubation of patients intubated for airway edema alone is the patient's ability to open the eyes.

Smoke inhalation injury greatly increases the morbidity and mortality of any size of burn; the most common cause of death following burn injury is complications related to smoke inhalation injury. Inhalation of the products of combustion leads to an acute hypoxia that cannot be corrected by the administration of oxygen. The more profound damage occurs as a result of the chemical denaturing of the pulmonary tissue by the smoke. As the tissue is irritated, edema forms to compound the problem by increasing the distance across which oxygen must diffuse to the capillaries. Within 24 to 48 hours of inhalation injury, ARDS develops and follows its predicted clinical course (see Chapter 23 for a discussion of ARDS). The presence of high levels of bacteria in the burn wounds greatly increases the risk of pulmonary infection and sepsis following inhalation injury. Treatment consists of intubation and support with a mechanical ventilator to provide adequate tissue oxygenation until the lungs recover from the sequelae of ARDS.

Carbon monoxide poisoning occurs relatively frequently with smoke inhalation but varies depending on the products of combustion produced in a particular fire. The initial treatment of all patients with suspected smoke inhalation injury is oxygen, and this treatment will dilute carbon monoxide, taking it out of the system fairly quickly. Neurologic changes related to carbon monoxide inhalation will be noted when carbon monoxide levels reach certain parameters.

Metabolic Changes

Acute burn injury results in changes in the body's metabolism related to the massive release of catecholamines into the general circulation as part of the "fight or flight reaction" that accompanies major trauma. The metabolic response to the stress of a major burn injury involves the response of the sympathetic nervous system and other homeostatic regulators. Catecholamines are found in increased amounts in both the serum and urine of burn patients. The sustained heart rate increases to about 120 to 140 beats/min, and oxygen consumption increases to about 150 percent of normal.

The hypermetabolism of burn injury persists until the burn wound is reduced to less than 20 percent TBSA and is a major challenge in medical management because of the increased caloric and oxygen needs during a prolonged period. In addition, the body's internal temperature set point is increased upward so that the body strives to achieve a core body temperature of about 38.5°C. Wilmore et al.[26] described the hypermetabolic state of 20 burn patients with persistent elevation of core body temperatures as unrelated to ambient temperature. The metabolic rate increases in relation to burn size in a curvilinear relationship until oxygen consumption reaches, but rarely exceeds, 2.5 times basal levels.

Evaporative water loss and surface cooling are not the primary stimulus for the hypermetabolic state; rather, the hypermetabolism is related to an increase and resetting of the thermal regulatory set point. A reflex arc mobilizes neural and/or hormonal afferent stimuli to the hypothalamus, producing a catecholamine response clinically manifested as hypermetabolism, hyperthermia, and hyperglycemia. Glucose and lactate kinetics are also altered after burn injury. Although tissue hypoxia produces lactic acidosis, its persistence in the presence of adequate tissue perfusion suggests an increased rate of glycogenolysis.[27] An absolute or relative insulin deficiency in combination with an excess of glucocorticoid, glucagon, and/or catecholamine are the signals that promote gluconeogenesis.

Gastrointestinal Changes

Gastrointestinal changes that occur immediately after burn injury include adynamic ileus accompanied by vomiting unless the stomach is decompressed by means of a nasogastric tube connected to low suction. During burn shock, circulating blood volume is preferentially shunted to vital organs such as the brain, hepatorenal circulation, and lungs. The ileus will persist for about 3 days following injury.

Evidence of hepatic response to burn injury is characterized by alteration in the clotting factors. A hypercoagulable state develops as manifested by an elevated plasma fibrinogen concentration in the presence of shortened prothrombin and activated partial thromboplastin times.[28]

Cellular Changes

Major burn injury affects the entire body, but survival ultimately depends on its effect at the cellular level. The cellular response to burn injury occurs as a metabolic pathophysiology and as an immunologic pathophysiology. The basic pathology, named the "sick cell syndrome" by Welt in 1967,[29] is a cell membrane transport defect related to an alteration in the steady-state composition and characterized by high intracellular concentrations of sodium. Entry of sodium into the intracellular space occurs simultaneously with entry of water, which leads to cellular edema and, possibly, rupture of the cell wall. Trunkey et al.[30] found a marked decrease in primate muscle extracellular water and an increase in intracellular sodium and water during burn shock. An associated decrease in resting membrane potential occurs as the transmembrane potential is disrupted, resulting in a decrease in amplitude of the action potential and a prolongation of the repolarization and depolarization time, as described by other investigators.[31,32] As sodium and water enter the cell, the sodium-potassium pump is disrupted and potassium moves out, thus further exacerbating the electrolyte imbalance intracellularly. Calcium channel transport is disrupted, along with a loss of intracellular magnesium and phosphate[33] and an increase in serum lactic dehydrogenase levels.[34] The cascade of events that occurs at the level of the cell membrane suggests impairments of basic cellular function as the underlying cause of the diminished membrane potentials. Although the pathophysiology has not been completely described, data suggest a decrease in the efficiency of the sodium-potassium pump, a change that can be reversed over time by adequate fluid resuscitation that reverses burn shock.

Evidence suggests that the burn wound itself at least partially mediates the physiologic response to burn injury at both the local and systemic level. Burn tissue inflammation can lead to vasodilation, increased capillary permeability, and edema—which would be normal conditions that promote wound healing.[35-38] Despite profound redistribution of the peripheral circulation following burn injury, both heat and glucose are preferentially transported to the wound. The energy cost of attempts to heal the burn wound become maladaptive with massive injury and result in increased metabolic demands and consumption of inflammatory mediators by the wound when, in actuality, the priority for survival would be transport of these substrates to healthy tissue.

The extensive evaporative water loss that accompanies burn injury is a heat-consuming process, with the energy need met in part by increased visceral heat production. The physiologic mechanism for this response is unknown; individuals whose wounds have been denervated by previous spinal cord injury also exhibit similar metabolic responses to burn injury. Hypothalamic function alterations result in elevated serum human growth hormone levels even in the presence of hyperglycemia, a finding opposite to normal states.[39] The hypermetabolic rate is not decreased during rest, sleep, external warmth, or even induction of anesthesia. The increased oxygen consumption cannot be accounted for on the basis of elevated body temperature alone; thus, an increased basal metabolic rate, not a thermoregulatory drive, is responsible for the increased heat production.[40]

Immune Response

The immune response to burn injury is immediate, prolonged, and severe. The end result in individuals surviving burn shock is immunosuppression with increased susceptibility to potentially fatal systemic burn wound and/or pulmonary sepsis. The role of circulating factors has been intensely studied, and the findings clearly demonstrate that serum from burned animals will induce burn shock in unburned animals and that burn serum has immunosuppressive qualities in vitro. Leukocyte chemotactic studies in vitro revealed a decrease in leukocyte migration, with the decrease inversely correlated with burn size.[41] Placing the burn-suppressed leukocytes into serum obtained from healthy donors returned the levels to 107 percent of normal activity.[42] Ninnemann[43] reported the participation of both a serum-borne factor and a specific subset of B-lymphocytes in the generation of suppressor cells.

The white blood cells are also altered at a time when they are vitally needed to inhibit microbacterial proliferation. Normally, opsonin renders bacteria susceptible to phagocytosis, but burn injury triggers a consumptive opsoninopathy. Burn serum contains an inhibitor of C3 conversion that leads to decreased opsonization and polymorphonuclear neutrophil dysfunction.[44,45]

A host of chemicals found in burn plasma in altered concentrations may also play a role in burn shock. These include vasoactive amines (histamine, serotonin), products of complement activation (C3a,

C5a), prostaglandins, kinins, endotoxin, and the metabolic hormones (catecholamines, glucocorticoids). A decrease in the complement components C3a and C5a in the circulation after burn injury suggests a nonspecific activation of the complement system. Activation of the complement system in injured tissue results in an inflammatory response caused by the release of histamine and serotonin by C3a and C5a. Because both histamine and serotonin alter capillary permeability, some investigators propose this as a cause for burn shock, as these vasoactive amines initiate the inflammatory response along with kinin polypeptides and other chemical mediators. As a result of these vascular changes, fluid and fibrinogen leave the dilated, permeable vessels. Prostaglandins function in the inflammatory process by regulating the metabolism of the cells of inflammation.

Electrical Injury

The pathophysiology of electrical injury is related to the subsequent tissue damage as electrical energy is converted to heat. Arcing electricity produces surface heat, which may produce clothing fire and superficial tissue destruction, but internal damage is absent; this injury is actually a flame or thermal injury and not electrical. These injuries are properly classified as heat injuries, for which the treatment plan is identical to that for other heat injuries.[46] True electrical injury occurs as electrical current enters the body, traverses some area of the body, and exits at another body site. Electrical injuries are usually deeper than full-thickness skin injury and are often classified as **fourth-degree injury.** The extent of damage is influenced by voltage, type of current (direct or alternating), and length of contact.[47] Each true electrical injury produces an entrance wound and at least one exit wound, with the most extensive damage commonly occurring at the exit point. Electrical current follows the path of least resistance: in humans, this path is through blood vessels, nerves, tendons, and bone. Skin has high resistance; thus, the current enters through the skin but goes deeper to travel the path of least resistance until it exits the body. The current rarely produces direct visceral damage, but severe injuries to the extremities are common. The amputation rate following electrical injury exceeds 90 percent; the pathophysiology, in addition to direct tissue destruction, involves heat coagulation of blood vessels, which leaves distal areas without blood supply. Electrical injuries produce both systemic and local pathophysiologic alterations. The systemic changes produce three common complications during the acute period: arrhythmias or cardiac arrest, metabolic acidosis, and myoglobinuria.[48] Locally, electrical injury produces direct cellular denaturation as areas of healthy tissue are devascularized as a result of heat coagulation of arteries and veins. These events are followed 48 to 72 hours after injury by gross tissue necrosis and subsequent gangrene resulting from lack of blood flow. Amputation is required early in electrical injury to prevent the development of clinical gangrene and sepsis leading to death.

Once the patient is in the health care system, airway management is the primary focus of concern; patients with major electrical injury often require endotracheal intubation to ensure a patent airway. A condition similar to burn shock develops within a few minutes of major electrical injury and requires similar fluid resuscitation measures. No formula exists to predict fluid requirements for electrical injury shock because often the only apparent damage is the entrance and exit wound, and no assessment of internal damage is possible. The adult patient is given a 1-liter bolus of Ringer's lactate solution intravenously within the first 15 minutes following intravenous line placement; children are given a smaller, size-appropriate amount. Thereafter fluid is infused at a rate to produce a urine volume of 100 mL/hr in adults and 2 mL/kg/hr in children. Adult patients frequently require 1 to 2 liters of fluid per hour to support the cardiovascular system.

The potential for cardiac arrhythmias and arrest remains high for 24 hours following injury. The patient's electrocardiogram will reveal abnormal complex configurations which resemble those seen with acute myocardial infarction, but the pattern will be restored toward normal over a period of weeks. Measured cardiac enzymes will initially reveal elevated values, also suggesting acute myocardial damage, but in these patients these findings are not indicative of cardiac pathology.[49]

Electrical injury also produces a profound, potentially lethal metabolic acidosis. Electrically injured patients often have initial serum pH values of 6.8 to 7.2 on admission to emergency departments; pH levels of less than 7.0 are incompatible with survival. Treatment consists of intravenous administration of sodium bicarbonate in amounts to return the values toward normal. The metabolic acidosis is a recurring problem requiring ongoing treatment until the problem resolves at 24 to 48 hours after injury. The pathophysiology is related to the release of intracellular contents into the general circulation from the areas of tissue damage and to the lactic acidosis that accompanies hypotensive shock states.

Myoglobinuria follows electrical injury as the myoglobin, a component of muscle tissue, is released from muscles damaged by electrical current and enters systemic circulation. Myoglobin is a large protein that mechanically obstructs renal tubules and leads to acute tubular necrosis unless the accumulation is prevented by maintaining urine output at 100 mL/hr in adults and 2 mL/kg/hr in children until the urine clears. Mannitol, an osmotic diuretic, is administered along with large volumes of intravenous fluids to prevent the development of acute tubular necrosis, a totally preventable sequela of electrical injury with proper management.

Local effects of electrical injury are related to alterations in tissue perfusion. Surgical decompression of areas of electrical burn is accomplished for the purpose of releasing any increased compartment pressures that may be compromising blood flow. Surgical amputation may be required during the initial surgery for devascularized areas. Because of the continued presence of necrotic tissue, areas of surgical decompression or initial amputation are not closed surgically.[50] Surgical decompression is performed as soon as the patient is adequately ventilated, has a serum pH level corrected to near normal, has had complete physical and radiographic examinations to identify and treat any concurrent injuries, has an intravenous access site established and volume administered to establish adequate urine output, has had a nasogastric tube inserted to decompress the stomach and drain gastric contents, and as soon as an operating room and surgical team are available.[51]

Central nervous system alterations will be noted in all patients with major electrical injury. The typical patient has no short-term memory: events prior to the injury are remembered clearly, but hour-to-hour memory deficits occur for many weeks. The condition improves slowly over time and is usually resolved by 4 to 6 weeks after injury. The patient may not remember the initial hospital course and may experience daily emotional distress because the visual impact of the extensive physical damage is perceived as *new* information with each dressing change. Rarely does the patient have immediate perceptions of altered body image; thus, an abrupt crisis may occur as the extent of change is eventually realized. Another complication of the short-term memory loss is the patient's inability to remember visitors, which may lead to anger and charges of abandonment toward family members and health care personnel because the patient does not remember who was present earlier. Other central nervous system deficits following electrical injury include ataxia and gait alterations accompanied by sensory deficits. These alterations may improve or remain constant over time.

KEY CONCEPTS

- Burn shock is a life-threatening process that occurs in the acute phase after major burn injury. Massive fluid leak from capillaries results in intravascular hypovolemia, extensive edema, hemaconcentration, and reduced urine output. Capillary leak resolves about 24 hours after injury. Fluid replacement is the primary treatment objective during burn shock.
- Major burn injury is associated with alterations in organs and systems throughout the body, such as the following.
  1. Cardiovascular. Low cardiac output may occur in response to unknown myocardial depressant factors.
  2. Respiratory. Inhalation injury can cause airway obstruction, carbon monoxide poisoning, and hypoxia. Acute respiratory distress syndrome is a serious complication of burn injury characterized by refractory hypoxemia.
  3. Metabolic. Release of catecholamines in response to burn stress is associated with increased heart rate, increased oxygen consumption, and increased serum glucose. A hypermetabolic state is maintained by hypothalamic thermoregulation.
  4. Gastrointestinal. Adynamic ileus lasts for about 3 days following burn. The liver may increase production of clotting factors.
  5. Cellular. Dysfunction of energy-requiring cellular processes, such as pumping of ions, results in widespread cellular swelling and altered membrane potentials.
  6. Immune. Inflammation is initiated by burned tissue, resulting in release of cytokines that mediate increased capillary permeability and vasodilation. In general, immune system depression is predominant with decreased leukocyte migration and poor opsonization.
- Electrical shock is associated with injury deep within the body, particularly involving low-resistance tissues such as blood vessels and nerves. Cardiac arrest, coagulation of blood within the vessels, and renal damage secondary to myoglobinuria are serious consequences of electrical injury. Severe short-term memory loss, ataxia, and sensory deficits may occur as a result of neuronal damage.

Emergent Phase

The emergent phase of burn care refers to the time between the end of burn shock and closure of the burn wound to less than 20 percent TBSA. There are three essential elements for survival of a major burn injury: meticulous wound management, adequate nutritional support to establish positive nitrogen balance, and early surgical excision and grafting of full-thickness wounds. Burn recovery is long and stormy—with complications as the rule rather than the exception. The goal of burn management is wound closure in a manner to promote survival. Recovery from a major burn is never assured but will usually occur once the burn wound is reduced to less than 20 percent TBSA.

Meticulous Management of Wound

Meticulous wound management consists of measures to limit bacterial proliferation on the wound and adjacent tissues. The body's first line of defense, the skin, has been destroyed by the burn injury. Initially burn wounds are sterile because of the heat that caused the burn, but bacterial flora soon reestablish colonies on the burn eschar. This medium is favorable for pathogenic growth because of the necrotic tissue and warm environment that exist within the burn wound dressing. Benign microorganisms normally found on skin, in the gastrointestinal tract, and in the pulmonary system become lethal as they colonize the burn wound, and invasive sepsis occurs. Once established, invasive burn wound sepsis carries a 75 percent mortality rate. The goals of wound care are to cleanse and debride the wound of necrotic tissue and debris that promote bacterial growth, minimize further destruction to viable tissue, preserve body heat and energy, and promote patient comfort. Patients do not die from burn wound infections but, rather, from systemic invasion by burn organisms; thus, a great deal of time is required to clean the wound, prevent cross-contamination from other patients, and limit environmental contaminants. The most common source of burn wound bacteria is the patient's own hair follicles, sweat glands, pulmonary tract, and gastrointestinal system, although poor hand-washing techniques by staff members can establish infection through cross-contamination from other patients. Infected partial thickness burn wounds convert to full-thickness injury immediately.

Wound care consists of daily observation and management, which includes bathing the patient two or three times daily in a cleansing solution. Some of the more commonly used agents include chlorhexidine gluconate (Hibiclens), providone-iodine (Betadine), or diluted chlorine bleaches. Burn wounds are washed to remove accumulated bacteria, debride necrotic tissue, and remove previously applied ointments. The cleansing of burn wounds is the most stressful and painful event burn patients endure; unfortunately, because of the rapid rate of wound recolonization, the procedure must occur every 8 to 12 hours. Pain medication diminishes the pain only marginally because the most effective analgesics, morphine and meperidine, work most effectively on visceral or deep pain rather than pain at superficial skin nerve endings.

After the wound is clean, topical antibacterial agents are applied and covered with a light dressing (Table 55–8). Systemic antibiotics are not helpful in controlling burn wound flora because there is no blood supply to the burn eschar, and therefore no delivery of the antibiotic to the wound. Topical burn agents penetrate the eschar, thereby inhibiting bacterial invasion of the wound.[52] Systemic antibiotics are administered when the patient demonstrates signs of systemic infection and prophylactically at times of surgical procedures. Appropriate antibiotic selection is based on laboratory cultures of the patient's wound tissue in order to identify and deliver antibiotics to which the bacteria are sensitive.

Healing of burn wounds begins when white blood cells have surrounded the burn wound and phagocytosis begins. Necrotic tissue begins to slough. Fibroblasts begin to lay down matrices of the collagen precursors that eventually form granulation tissue. Kept free from infection, a partial thickness burn will heal from the edges and from below in a process that occurs over a 14- to 21-day period. Full-thickness burn injury requires autografting to achieve wound closure because there are no dermal elements to form new skin.

Nutritional Support for Positive Nitrogen Balance

Healing occurs only in a state of positive nitrogen balance. Hypermetabolism characterizes the metabolic response to thermal injury; the magnitude of the physiologic alteration is related to the extent of burn injury. One of the most significant advances in recent burn management is recognition of the critical importance of nutrition to the wound healing process. The magnitude of nutritional support required by burn patients depends on two factors: the patient's preburn nutritional status, and the extent of the TBSA burn. Patients with minor burns need no nutritional support beyond a regular diet. However, patients with moderate burns need a high-calorie, high-protein diet, while patients with major burn injury must receive additional nutritional support to survive. Patients with poor preburn nutritional status are classified as having a critical injury regardless of burn size because of the body's decreased ability to resist infection, heal the burn, and tolerate required operative procedures. The most easily recognized and documented finding in the absence of adequate nutritional support following burn injury is the massive loss of body weight that occurs. Maintenance of body protein appears to be critical for survival. Loss of one fourth to one third of the protein mass from the body is predictably fatal; this degree of negative nitrogen balance in humans is associated with a 40 to 50 percent body weight loss.

Patients with greater than 40 percent TBSA burn demonstrate the maximal stress response within predictable ranges of body mass. In these hypermetabolic patients, providing early protein and caloric support of at least the predicted energy requirement is necessary for optimal outcome and may be essential for survival. Weight loss following thermal injury is not an obligatory component of the response to trauma but, rather, a reflection of the difference between the total energy requirements of the patient versus the ability to provide these requirements in the form of adequate caloric intake. With the early initiation of vigorous nutritional support, usually within 2 to 4 days following injury as the adynamic ileus resolves, erosion of the total body mass and subsequent starvation leading to immunologic alteration are not inevitable in the massively burned patient.

Hypermetabolism in burn patients directly correlates with the extent of the burn injury; therefore, the caloric requirement also varies with size of the burn injury. General formulas are used to estimate the caloric requirements of burn patients, all of which are based on either preburn body weight and percentage TBSA burn or square meters of body surface area and percentage TBSA burn. The two most widely used formulas are the Curreri formula for adult patients and the Polk formula for pediatric patients. Curreri et al.[53] demonstrated caloric requirements in adult burn patients can be expressed by the following formula:

$$(25 \times \text{body weight [kg]}) + (40 \times \text{percent TBSA burn})$$
$$= \text{24-hr caloric needs.}$$

The requirements in children[54] are predicted as:

$$(60 \times \text{body weight [kg]}) + (36 \times \text{percent TBSA burn})$$
$$= \text{24-hr caloric needs.}$$

It is important to emphasize that these formulas represent more than just total caloric intake; they are used to predict positive nitrogen balance for each pa-

TABLE 55-8. Topical Antibiotic Therapy for Thermal Injury Wounds

Drug	Indications for Use	Advantages	Disadvantages	Method of Use
Bacitracin	Bland ointment with minimal antibiotic properties used to promote comfort in patients with minor injury (<25% TBSA)	Prevents drying of wound, keeps eschar soft and pliable, economical, works well on facial burns to promote healing and patient comfort without facial dressings, painless upon application	No major antibiotic properties; oil based, so is difficult to wash away	1. Apply to cleansed wound twice daily, cover with Adaptic and Kerlix 2. Apply to facial burns twice daily 3. Apply to recently grafted or healed areas twice daily, wrap with Adaptic and Kerlix
Silver sulfadiazine (Silvadene)	Partial and/or full-thickness thermal injury (>25% TBSA); small wounds, such as frostbite, that require topical antibiotic therapy	Wide-spectrum bacteriostatic action and painless upon application. Organisms resistant to silver nitrate are usually sensitive to silver sulfadiazine. Eschar remains soft and pliable. Water-miscible base promotes ease of removal.	Not effective against fungal organisms, can cause leukopenia, expensive; sulfa component can produce allergic reactions in sensitive patients; resistant organisms can occur with prolonged use	Apply to cleansed wound one to three times daily; may leave wound open or cover with light dressing
Silver nitrate	Partial and/or full-thickness burns (>25% TBSA), fungal infections, patients with sulfa allergy	Wide-spectrum bacteriostatic action, effective against fungal infections, comfortable, economical, no sensitivity reported, painless on application, no resistant organisms	Can cause severe electrolyte imbalances (hyponatremia and hypochloremia), which are corrected with oral and IV NaCl; poor penetration into wound; requires bulky dressing, thereby severely limiting motion; messy and time-consuming to use; stains everything it contacts grayish-black	0.5% solution in distilled water applied to wet dressing every 2 hours, dressing changes twice daily
Mafenide acetate (Sulfamylon)	Electrical injury, ear burns, wounds colonized with organisms resistant to other topical agents. Most effective of all topicals because it penetrates eschar more deeply	Wide-spectrum bacteriostatic action; active penetration allows delayed therapy to be effective; requires no dressing, thereby promoting motion; resistant organisms do not develop with prolonged use; drug of choice for all electrical wounds and wounds colonized with organisms resistant to other topical agents	Causes severe metabolic alterations within 72 hours when used on > 20% TBSA wounds; carbonic anhydrase inhibition with HCO_3^- excretion and chloride retention; compensation is by hyperventilation with subsequent CO_2 decrease or depletion; only treatment is to discontinue the drug until metabolic balance is restored; drug can be resumed in about 3–5 days; pain is severe upon application and for 20–30 minutes thereafter; sulfa component can produce allergic reaction in sensitive patient	Apply to cleansed wound one to two times daily; leave open because wrapping produces maceration

From Kravitz M: Thermal injuries, in Cardona VD, et al (eds): *Trauma Nursing: From Resuscitation Through Rehabilitation.* Philadelphia, WB Saunders, 1988, p 723. Reproduced with permission.
Abbreviations: TBSA, total body surface area; IV, intravenous; NaCl, saline; HCO_3^-, bicarbonate ion; CO_2, carbon dioxide.

tient. Thus, if the patient is losing tremendous amounts of nitrogen or is not absorbing glucose, the net caloric utilization will be much less than the intake, even though the adult patient may be receiving as much as 5,000 calories per day. Monitoring of daily nitrogen balance using indirect calorimetry is essential throughout the course of burn treatment to ensure a positive nitrogen balance.

The routes for initiating caloric support following major burn injury are either enteral or parenteral. Any patient with a functioning gastrointestinal tract should receive enteral nutrition either orally, by tube feeding, or by a combination of both. In some burn patients, enteral feeding may not be possible, and intravenous hyperalimentation may become the only method available for providing nutritional support.

Surgical Excision and Skin Grafting

The third element essential to survival following major burn injury is the surgical excision of burn eschar followed by skin grafting with the patient's own skin (autograft). Current medical management of burn wounds involves early removal of the necrotic tissue followed by split-thickness autograft. This therapy has changed the management of burn care in the past 20 years from one of daily bathing and mechanical debridement of necrotic tissue for months following burn injury to one of early surgical removal of the burn wound and a dramatic reduction in hospitalization time. In the past, patients with major burns had low rates of survival because healing and wound coverage took so long that death from infection usually occurred before healing. Now, mortality and morbidity are greatly decreased as a result of early surgical intervention.

The two types of surgical excision are **tangential excision** and **full-thickness excision.** With tangential excision, eschar is removed in thin layers using an instrument called a dermatome until viable tissue is visible. The procedure is usually done 2 to 7 days after injury. Full-thickness excision using surgical knives removes eschar to fascia. After bleeding has been controlled in the area of excision, application of an autograft, skin substitutes, or dressings follows. To establish optimal conditions for autografting, some surgeons cover the area with wet dressings soaked in antibiotic solutions for 24 hours and perform autografting the following day. Both tangential and full-thickness excision procedures involve massive blood loss, requiring red blood cell transfusion to restore hemoglobin levels to normal.

Several temporary biological dressing are available for use in patients with extensive burns that do not permit initial autografting. Products available for temporary coverage include homograft (skin harvested from cadavers), xenograft (skin harvested from pigs), synthetic skin (a variety of products for temporary coverage), and amnion (amniotic lining of human placenta harvested from afterbirth following human delivery). These dressings promote patient comfort while partially restoring the water vapor barrier and some antibacterial properties to the wound until an autograft is available. The unburned area of the patient from which skin is harvested in a paper-thin sheet is referred to as the donor site. Donor sites heal in about 5 to 7 days in the presence of adequate nutritional support and the absence of infection and can be reharvested at that time. Donor sites can be harvested as many times as necessary to achieve wound coverage, a fact which permits survival in some patients with TBSA injury as large as 90 percent. To expand the surface area a sheet of autograft will cover, skin is cut in a manner which resembles a net or mesh using an instrument called a skin mesher. The skin may then be expanded, depending on the size of the mesh, to cover two, three, four or more times its original size. This combination of repeated harvesting and meshing allows autografting of massive burn injuries over a period of a few weeks. Following grafting, the areas must be protected from infection, pressure, shearing, and trauma, which produces bruising or bleeding under the graft. Bulky dressings are used the first few days, followed by use of wraps and elastic bandages to protect extremity or trunk grafts. Patients are returned to the operating room about once a week until grafting procedures are complete.

Surgical wound management in elderly burn patients is determined by the philosophy of the burn center. Elderly patients do not generally tolerate any surgical procedure as well as younger patients; this knowledge has been applied to the treatment of burn wounds in some patients, and conservative, nonsurgical wound management for weeks after injury has produced acceptable survival rates in elderly patients.[55] Others[56] report that early excision of eschar and early wound closure are associated with increased survival and decreased length of stay for older patients with burns. Children under the age of 2 years have a high mortality rate with major burn injury, but older children recover at a high rate with proper medical management.

Electrical Injury

Electrical injury patients are treated in the same manner as other burn patients during the acute phase. Wound closure may be delayed for several weeks until areas of demarcation are clearly defined and amputation accomplished, with retention of as much limb length as possible. Wound closure is accomplished using full- or split-thickness skin grafts and primary closure. Nutritional support of the magnitude previously discussed is required by electrical injury patients also. The neurologic deficits will persist but should diminish over a few weeks.

Rehabilitation Phase

The rehabilitation phase is defined as beginning when the burn size is reduced to less than 20 percent TBSA and the patient is capable of assuming some self-care.[57] This can occur as early as 2 weeks or as long as 2 to 3 months following the burn and, when there is major debilitating or disfiguring injury, may last many years. Goals for this period are to assist the patient in resuming a functional role in society and to accomplish functional and cosmetic reconstruction.

Wound Healing

During the rehabilitation phase the pathophysiology of hypermetabolism and impaired immunology are restored toward normal, although some changes will persist beyond discharge from the hospital. The major pathophysiology of this phase is related to the dysfunctional results of wounds healing in a manner that results in flexor contractures, excessive scarring, and keloid formation. The burn wound has healed either by primary intention or by autografting. Layers of epithelization begin building back the tissue structure destroyed by the burn injury. Collagen fibers present in the new scar tissue help healing and add strength to weakened areas. After healing, the new skin appears flat and pink, even in dark-skinned people.

In approximately 4 to 6 weeks, the area becomes raised and hyperemic. If adequate range of motion is not instituted early in the hospital course, the new tissue will shorten, causing contracture. Mature healing is reached in 6 months to 1 year, when suppleness has returned and the pink or red color has faded to a slightly lighter hue than the surrounding unburned tissue. It takes longer for darker skin to regain its color because many of the melanocytes were destroyed, and often the skin never regains its original color. The mesh pattern in meshed autograft fades with time, but in the larger expansions such as 4:1 or greater, the pattern may persist.

Scarring has two components: the first is discoloration, the second is contour. The discoloration of scars fades with time and can be covered with makeup on visible body surface areas. However, scar tissue tends to develop altered contours; that is, the skin is no longer flat but becomes raised above the contours of the surrounding area. Areas of the face tend to scar in an even plane, deleting the natural contours around the nose, chin, and mouth and thus greatly altering a patient's appearance. Scarring on the cheeks can contract and pull the lower eyelid down sufficiently to prevent closure and protection of the eye normally afforded by the eyelid, a condition named ectropion. Burns to the eyelid can also result in ectropion, a condition corrected by reconstructive surgery. Pressure can help to keep a scar flat if the pressure is slightly greater than capillary pressure and is continuous during the healing process. This knowledge led to the development of burn garments, which are custom-made for each patient to contour with pressure over the area of burn for about 1 year following burn. Except for bath times, the garments must be worn continuously; patient compliance often becomes an issue.

Excessive and sometimes debilitating discomfort from itching occurs in the healing burn wound and persists for many months. The exact pathophysiology is not known but is related to the absence of sebaceous glands in the area and to the hyperactivity of sweat glands. Topical lotions and orally administered antihistamines partially relieve symptoms, but patients develop tolerance to the drugs and often require a series of different medications over time. The newly formed skin is extremely sensitive to trauma, and blisters form following very slight pressure or friction. The newly healed areas may be hypersensitive or hyposensitive to cold, heat, or touch. Ward et al.[58] studied loss of cutaneous sensibility after grafting in 60 patients and found that 97 percent demonstrated markedly diminished or absent responses to sharp/dull, hot/cold, and light touch stimuli over the grafted areas. Grafted areas are more likely to be hyposensitive until peripheral nerve regeneration occurs, although donor sites harvested several times will show all the same healing pathology as healed burn wounds.

Scarring is a genetically inherited trait. Some people will have minimal scarring while others, especially black people and those with red hair, tend to have significant scarring and keloid formation in which the scar tissue actually outgrows the bounds of the original wound. Healed burn wounds must be protected from direct sunlight for 1 year to prevent hyperpigmentation.

The most common complications during the rehabilitation phase are related to formation of skin and joint contractures. Because of pain associated with movement, the patient will want to assume the position of comfort, which is with all extremities flexed, but this position predisposes to contracture formation. To minimize contracture formation, positioning in extension, splinting in the position of function, and active range of motion are initiated on admission and continue throughout the course of treatment. The areas most subject to contracture formation include the anterior and lateral neck areas, axillae, antecubital fossae, fingers, groin areas, popliteal fossae, and ankles. Not only does the skin develop contractures but also the underlying tissues such as ligaments and tendons have a tendency to shorten during the healing process. Therapy is aimed at extension of body parts to assure that flexors are stronger than extensors.

Electrical Injury

Electrical injury patients have all the problems of rehabilitation plus possible adjustments to amputation and gait instability related to central nervous system impairment. Skin grafting in areas adjacent to amputation presents challenging prosthetic problems that may delay independent ambulation and restoration of self-care abilities.[59] In general, patients with electrical injury experience longer rehabilitation periods than thermally injured patients.

A unique complication of electrical injury is the formation of corneal cataracts,[60] the cause of which is unknown. The cataracts may be detected upon ophthalmic examination as early as 1 month or as late as 12 months after injury and may occur in one or both eyes. The electrical injury does not have to be on or near the head for the condition to develop. Progression is rapid, causing a completely opaque cornea within a matter of months. Ophthalmic examinations should be performed monthly for the first year and then every 3 months during the second year after injury to identify this pathology early. The patient will usually complain of blurring vision, but young children may not mention blurring because they do not know the concept. Treatment consists of corneal transplants.

KEY CONCEPTS

- The emergent phase is the time between the end of burn shock and closure of the wound to less than 20 percent TBSA. Wound management, nutritional support, and surgical grafting of full-thickness wounds are the priorities of treatment during the emergent phase.

- Wound management is necessary to prevent bacterial colonization of the wound and subsequent septicemia. Early surgical wound management is essential. Topical antibiotics are used because systemic antibiotics cannot reach the wound because of lack of blood supply.

- Nutritional requirements after burn injury are high. A high-calorie, high-protein diet is needed. Persons with major burns cannot usually ingest sufficient nutrients and require parenteral and enteral supplementation. A positive nitrogen balance is essential for healing.

- Early surgical excision and skin grafting is the treatment of choice for deep burns. Excision procedures result in significant blood loss, requiring blood transfusions. Skin grafts are taken from a healthy portion of the patient's own skin and may be reharvested every 5 to 7 days. Temporary grafts (e.g., cadaver skin, synthetic, pig skin) may be used to cover the wound until an autograft can be completed.

- The rehabilitation phase begins when the burn is reduced to less than 20 percent TBSA. Problems during this phase include skin contracture and excessive scarring. Healing is complete at 6 months to 1 year. Positioning in extension and range of motion are important to prevent contracture.

Summary

Severity of burn injury is determined by depth and extent of injury. Depth of injury determines the method of wound closure; extent of injury determines morbidity and mortality. Minor burns heal in a few days with only mild discomfort to the patient. Moderate burn injury requires meticulous wound management and adequate nutrition to avoid infection and promote healing. Major burn injury is a life-threatening event requiring major medical intervention to promote survival. Burn shock develops within minutes of major burn injury and requires infusion of massive amounts of intravenous fluid to sustain systemic circulation for the first 24 to 36 hours following burn injury. Smoke inhalation associated with flames significantly increases mortality and requires intubation and ventilatory support through the subsequent acute respiratory distress syndrome episode. Full-thickness burns do not heal, and require autografting of the patient's own skin to achieve wound coverage. Surgical removal of the eschar and autograft application are performed as soon as possible to diminish the risk of systemic sepsis. Pain relief is a major component of burn therapy. Recovery from burn injury requires many months of patient care focusing on physical therapy, nutritional support, and psychosocial adaptation. Nurses interact with the patient and family to achieve optimal rehabilitation.

REFERENCES

1. Artz CP: Epidemiology, causes and prognosis, in Artz CP, Moncrief JA, Pruitt BA Jr (eds): *Burns: A Team Approach*. Philadelphia, WB Saunders, 1979, pp 17–22.
2. Jerrard DA, Cappadoro K: Burns in the elderly patient. *Emerg Med Clin North Am* 1990;8(2):421–428.
3. Maley MP: Scald burns associated with tap water. *J Burn Care Rehabil* 1989;10(2):172–173.
4. Turner DG, Leman CJ, Jordan MH: Cooking-related burn injuries in the elderly: Preventing the "granny gown" burn. *J Burn Care Rehabil* 1989;10(4):356–359.
5. Goff DR, Purdue GF, Hunt JL, Cochran RP: Cardiac disease and the patient with burns. *J Burn Care Rehabil* 1990;11(4):305–307.
6. Larson CM, Braun S, Sullivan J, Saffle JR: Complications of burn care in patients with neurologic disorders. *J Burn Care Rehabil* 1988;9(5):482–484.
7. Deitch EA, Wrightmire DA, Clothier J, Blass N: Management of burns in pregnant women. *Surg Gynecol Obstet* 1985;161(1):1–4.
8. Achauer BM, McGuire A: Fire safe cigarettes: An update. *J Burn Care Rehabil* 1989;10(2):173–174.
9. Maley MP: Children under age five and butane cigarette lighters. *J Burn Care Rehabil* 1988;9(4):423–424.
10. Artz CP: Electrical injury, in Artz CP, Moncrief JA, Pruitt BA Jr (eds): *Burns: A Team Approach*. Philadelphia, WB Saunders, 1979, pp 351–362.
11. Nebraska Burn Institute: *Advanced Burn Life Support Course. Instructor's Manual*. Lincoln, Nebraska Burn Institute, 1987, p III–44.
12. Leake JE, Curtin JW: Electrical burns of the mouth in children. *Clin Plast Surg* 1984;11:669–683.
13. Port RM, Cooley RO: Treatment of electrical burns of the oral and perioral tissues in children. *J Am Dent Assoc* 1986;112:352.
14. American Burn Association: *American Burn Association Committee on Specific Optimal Criteria for Hospital Resources for Care of Patients with Burn Injury*. San Antonio, Tex, American Burn Association, 1976.
15. Hendricks WM: The classification of burns. *J Am Acad Dermatol* 1990;22(5 pt 1):838–839.
16. Kaufman T, Ullmann Y, Har-Shai Y: Phosphorus burns: A practical approach to local treatment. *J Burn Care Rehabil* 1988;9(5):474–475.
17. Millea TP, Kucan JO, Smoot EC: Anhydrous ammonia injuries. *J Burn Care Rehabil* 1989;10(5):448–453.
18. Bingham H: Electrical burns. *Clin Plast Surg* 1986;13:75–85.
19. Moncrief JA, Mason AD: Water vapor loss in the burned patient. *Surg Forum* 1962;13:38–41.
20. Moncrief JA: Burns, in Schwartz SI, Shires GT, Spencer FC, Husser WC (eds): *Principles of Surgery*, 2nd ed. New York, McGraw-Hill, 1974, pp 253–274.
21. Roe CF, Kinney JM: Water and heat exchange in third-degree burns. *Surgery* 1964;56:212–220.
22. Aikawa N, Martyn JAJ, Burke JF: Pulmonary artery catheterization and thermodilution cardiac output determination in the management of critically burned patients. *Am J Surg* 1978;135:811–817.
23. Dobson EL, Warner GF: Factors concerned in the early stages of thermal shock. *Circ Res* 1957;5:69–74.
24. Baxter CR, Cook WA, Shires GT: Serum myocardial depressant factor of burn shock. *Surg Forum* 1966;17:1–4.
25. Lefer AM, Martin J: Origin of myocardial depressant factor in shock. *Am J Physiol* 1970;218:1423–1427.
26. Wilmore DW, Long JM, Mason AD Jr, Skreen RW, Pruitt BA Jr: Catecholamines: Mediators of the hypermetabolic response to thermal injury. *Ann Surg* 1974;180(4):653–669.
27. Wilmore DW, Aulick HL, Goodwin CW: Glucose metabolism following severe injury. *Acta Chir Scand* 1979;498:43–47.

28. McManus WF, Eurenius K, Pruitt BA Jr: Disseminated intravascular coagulation in burned patients. *J Trauma* 1973; 13:416–422.
29. Welt LG: Membrane transport defect: The sick cell. *Trans Assoc Am Physicians* 1967;80:217–226.
30. Trunkey DD, Illner H, Wagner IY, Shires GT: The effect of hemorrhagic shock on intracellular muscle action potentials in the primates. *Surgey* 1973;74(2):241–250.
31. Cunningham JN Jr, Shires GT, Wagner Y: Changes in intracellular sodium and potassium content of red blood cells in trauma and shock. *Am J Surg* 1971;122:650–654.
32. Rosenthal SM, Tabor H: Electrolyte changes and chemotherapy in experimental burn and traumatic shock and hemorrhage. *Arch Surg* 1945;51:244–252.
33. Turinsky J, Gonnerman WA, Loose LD: Impaired mineral metabolism in postburn muscle. *J Trauma* 1981;21:417–423.
34. Deets DK, Glaviano VV: Plasma and cardiac lactic dehydrogenase activity in burn shock. *Proc Soc Exp Biol Med* 1973; 142:412–416.
35. Gump FE, Price JB Jr, Kinney JM: Blood flow and oxygen consumption in patients with severe burns. *Surg Gynecol Obstet* 1970;130:23–28.
36. Wilmore DW, Aulick LH, Mason AD Jr, Pruitt BA Jr: Influence of the burn wound on local and systemic responses to injury. *Ann Surg* 1977;186(4):444–458.
37. Wilmore DW, Goodwin GW, Aulick LH, Powanda MC, Mason AD Jr, Pruitt BA Jr: Effect of injury and infection on visceral metabolism and circulation. *Ann Surg* 1980;192(4):491–504.
38. Wilmore DW, Aulick LH: Metabolic changes in burned patients. *Surg Clin North Am* 1978;58:1173–1187.
39. Wilmore DW, Orcutt TW, Mason AD Jr, Pruitt BA: Alterations in hypothalamic function following thermal injury. *J Trauma* 1975;15(8):697–703.
40. Aulick LH, Hander EH, Wilmore DW, Mason AD Jr, Pruitt BA Jr: The relative significance of thermal and metabolic demands on burn hypermetabolism. *J Trauma* 1979;19(8):559–560.
41. Warden GD, Mason AD Jr, Pruitt BA Jr: Evaluation of leukocyte chemotaxis in vitro in thermally injured patients. *J Clin Invest* 1974;54:1001–1004.
42. Warden GD, Mason AD Jr, Pruitt BA Jr: Suppression of leukocyte chemotaxis in vitro by chemotherapeutic agents used in the management of thermal injuries. *Ann Surg* 1975;181:363–369.
43. Ninnemann JL: Immunosuppression following thermal injury through a B cell activation of suppressor T cells. *J Trauma* 1980;20:206–213.
44. Alexander JW, McClellan MA, Ogle CK, Ogle JD: Consumptive opsoninopathy: Possible pathogenesis in lethal and opportunistic infections. *Ann Surg* 1976;184(6):672–678.
45. Bjornson AB, Altemeier WA, Bjornson HS: Changes in humoral components of host defense following burn trauma. *Ann Surg* 1977;186:96–99.
46. Rouse RG, Dimick AR: The treatment of electrical injury compared to burn injury: A review of pathophysiology and comparison of patient management protocols. *J Trauma* 1978;18:43–47.
47. Luce EA, Gottlieb SE: "True" high-tension electrical injuries. *Ann Plast Surg* 1984;12:321–326.
48. Hunt JL, Sato RM, Baxter CR: Acute electrical burns. *Arch Surg* 1980;115:434–438.
49. Housinger TA, Green L, Shahangian S, Saffle JR, Warden GD: A prospective study of myocardial damage in electrical injuries. *J Trauma* 1985;25(2):122–124.
50. Robson MC, Murphy RC, Heggers JP: A new explanation for the progressive tissue loss in electrical injuries. *Plast Reconstr Surg* 1984;73:431–437.
51. Holliman CJ, Saffle JR, Kravitz M, Warden GD: Early surgical decompression in the management of electrical injuries. *Am J Surg* 1982;144(6):733–739.
52. Bull JP: Current trends in research on burns. *Proc R Soc Med* 1972;65:27–30.
53. Curreri PW, Richmond D, Marvin J: Dietary requirements of patient with major burns. *J Am Diet Assoc* 1974;65:415.
54. Haynes BW Jr: The management of burns in children. *J Trauma* 1965;5:267.
55. Housinger T, Saffle J, Ward F, Warden G: Conservative approach to the elderly patient with burns. *Am J Surg* 1984;148(6):817–820.
56. Slater AL, Slater H, Goldfarb IW: Effect of aggressive surgical treatment in older patients with burns. *J Burn Care Rehabil* 1989;10(6):527–530.
57. Feller I, Archambeault-Jones C: *Nursing the Burn Patient.* Ann Arbor, Institute for Burn Medicine, 1973.
58. Ward RS, Saffle JR, Schnebly WA, Hayes-Lundy C, Reddy R: Sensory loss over grafted areas in patients with burns. *J Burn Care Rehabil* 1989;10(6):536–538.
59. Ward RS, Hayes-Lundy C, Schnebly WA, Saffle JR: Prosthetic use in patients with burns and associated limb amputations. *J Burn Care Rehabil* 1990;11(4):361–364.
60. Saffle JR, Crandall A, Warden GD: Cataracts: A long-term complication of electrical injury. *J Trauma* 1985;25:17–21.

BIBLIOGRAPHY

Carrougher GJ: Inhalation injury. *AACN Clin Issues Crit Care Nurs* 1993;4(2):367–377.

Faldmo L, Kravitz M: Management of acute burns and burn shock resuscitation. *AACN Clin Issues Crit Care Nurs* 1993; 4(2):351–366.

Heink NR: Fluid resuscitation and the role of exchange transfusion in pediatric burn shock. *Crit Care Nurse* 1992;12(7):50–56.

Helvig E: Pediatric burn injuries. *AACN Clin Issues Crit Care Nurs* 1993;4(2):433–442.

Kravitz M: Immune consequences of burn injury. *AACN Clin Issues Crit Care Nurs* 1993;4(2):399–413.

Kravitz M: Thermal Injuries, in Cardona VD, Hurn PD, Mason PJB, Scanlon-Schilpp AM, Veise-Berry SW (eds): *Trauma Nursing: From Resuscitation Through Rehabilitation.* Philadelphia, WB Saunders, 1988, p 707–745.

Marvin J: Burn nursing history: The history of burn care. *J Burn Care Rehabil* 1993;14(2):252–256.

McLaughlin EG: *Critical Care of the Burn Patient: A Case Study Approach.* Rockville, Md, Aspen, 1990.

Molter NC: When is the burn injury healed? Psychosocial implications of care. *AACN Clin Issues Crit Care Nurs* 1993;4(2):424–432.

Richard RL, Staley, MJ: *Burn Care and Rehabilitation: Principles and Practice.* Philadelphia, FA Davis, 1994.

Rieg LS: Metabolic alterations and nutritional management. *AACN Clin Issues Crit Care Nurs* 1993;4(2):388–398.

Rylah LT: *Critical Care of the Burned Patient.* Cambridge, England, Cambridge University Press, 1992.

Trofino RB: *Nursing Care of the Burn-injured Patient.* Philadelphia, FA Davis, 1991.

Walter PH: Burn wound management. *AACN Clin Issues Crit Care Nurs* 1993;4(2):378–387.

Wardrope J, Smith JA: *Management of Wounds and Burns.* New York, Oxford University Press, 1992.

Weber JM, Tompkins DM: Improving survival: Infection control and burns. *AACN Clin Issues Crit Care Nurs* 1993;4(2):414–423.

CHAPTER 56
Nutritional Alterations in Critical Illness

KAREN GROTH

KEY TERMS

anemia: A decrease in the quantity of hemoglobin, hematocrit, and/or red blood cells.

anthropometric: Measurements of the body or body parts such as height and weight.

basal energy expenditure (BEE): A term used to describe the calculated basal metabolic rate.

basal metabolic rate (BMR): The least amount of energy required for an individual to maintain vital processes such as respiration, digestion, and circulation.

branched-chain amino acids: A group of amino acids that includes valine, leucine, and isoleucine which are mainly metabolized in the muscle.

cachexia: A combination of symptoms including anorexia, weight loss, muscle wasting, and weakness that is associated with the severe malnutrition of chronic disease such as cancer.

catabolism: The process of converting large molecules of carbohydrate, protein, and fat into smaller molecules to be utilized for energy.

essential amino acids: The amino acids that must be supplied in the diet because the body cannot manufacture them.

fatty acid: An organic acid with a long straight hydrocarbon chain that is a fundamental component of lipids. Some fatty acids are manufactured by the body, others are essential and must be supplied in the diet.

glycogen: A carbohydrate consisting of branched chains of glucose produced by the muscle and liver as a storage form of glucose.

glycogenesis: The synthesis of glycogen from glucose.

glycolysis: The anaerobic degradation of glucose to pyruvate or lactate in order to form ATP.

immunosuppression: An inability to produce an immune response to an antigen, resulting in reduced resistance to infection.

kilocalorie: The unit of measure for energy value of foods.

metabolism: The chemical and physical processes needed to change the organic constituents (foods eaten) into energy needed for body processes (catabolism) and for building up of tissues (anabolism).

nutritional screening: A quick determination of the nutritional status of an individual from a selected group of anthropometric and biochemical tests.

nutritional status: The state of an individual's nutrition resulting from the consumption and utilization of nutrients.

respiratory quotient: The ratio of volume of carbon dioxide exhaled to the volume of oxygen absorbed in the alveoli.

urea: Substance produced in the liver from the breakdown of protein and excreted in the urine.

vitamin: A group of organic substances that are essential in the diet and are required for the body's utilization of energy-containing nutrients.

Most physicians and nurses working in critical care agree that malnutrition impedes or complicates patient recovery. Yet nutritional deficiencies in this setting are commonplace. Bistrain[1] in 1976 suggested that malnutrition was a major cause of increased mortality and morbidity in hospitalized patients. A significant degree of malnutrition currently exists in intensive care units.[2] Even with recent advances in nutritional support, malnutrition results in prolonged hospitalization and subsequent increased costs. As many as half of hospitalized patients are malnourished, and the nutritional status of as many as 75 percent worsens during hospitalization.[2]

Many critically ill patients experience a significant degree of physiologic stress and multiple organ involvement, both of which increase specific and general nutritional needs. Additionally, the critically ill patient incurs an increased nutritional risk from treatment modalities, altered intake, and altered mobility. As a result, malnutrition in the critically ill patient is often iatrogenic and could be prevented if nutritional assessment and therapy were started earlier during the hospitalization. Some of the practices in hospitals that contribute to malnutrition are listed in Table 56–1.

Establishing scientifically a link between a patient's nutritional status and clinical outcome is difficult.[3] In general, adequate nutrition is needed for growth, organ function, activity, repair of injury, and resistance to infection. The multisystem effect of malnutrition combined with the effect of a disease process frequently reduces the accuracy with which researchers can predict the effect of nutrition on clinical outcome. Lack of a firm scientific basis can lead to a lack of aggressiveness in providing nutritional therapy to the critically ill patient.

Nutritional assessment is a complex process involving the integration of data gathered from the patient's dietary and medical history, anthropometric measures, biochemical analysis, and clinical observation. Nutritional assessment is best accomplished using a team approach, with utilization of the expertise of the nurse, dietitian, physician, and pharmacist in a collaborative process. A complete nutritional assessment will give the health care team parameters by which to identify patients at risk from nutritional factors and to monitor nutritional support.[4] Early assessment and treatment of potentially life-threatening problems is now becoming standard in the critical care unit. The focus of this chapter is on the essential nutritional information required to provide that care.

Health care professionals in general, and nurses in particular, have an integral part in the incorporation of nutritional goals into care planning. An understanding of nutritional assessment parameters, nutritional requirements, and effects of specific physiologic stressors on nutritional status is necessary when working with critically ill adults. The professional nurse must assume more responsibility in providing

TABLE 56-1. Factors Influencing Nutritional Status in the Critically Ill Patient

Inadequate Monitoring and Assessment of Nutritional Status

Infrequent assessment of weight
Failure to monitor fluid status
Inadequate understanding of biochemical analysis
Failure to use anthropometric measures
Delay in recognizing clinical symptoms of nutritional deficiency

Assessment Equipment Not Available

Inadequate Nutritional Support

Prolonged "nothing by mouth" status
Failure to adjust therapy based on assessed needs
Prolonged use of crystalloid intravenous fluids
Delay in starting nutritional support
Inadequate support in preoperative and postoperative care
Failure to respond to moderate to severe depletion

Inadequate Nutritional Knowledge of Health Care Providers

Lack of awareness of the role of nutrition in preventing complications
Lack of awareness of the role of nutrition in recovery
Lack of knowledge regarding nutritional assessment and monitoring
Lack of knowledge regarding nutritional needs of a critically ill patient
Lack of knowledge regarding nutritional support available for general and specialized needs

Inadequate Nutritional Support Team

Poor collaboration between health care providers: dietician, nurses, pharmacists, physicians
Lack of nutritional professionals skilled in care of critically ill patient
Line insertion and care as major focus of support team

nutritional care to the critically ill patient through collaboration with other team members.

Nutritional Assessment

Nutritional assessment allows the health care professional to measure the degree to which the patient's physiologic need for nutrients is being met. For optimal patient nutrition, a balance exists between nutrient intake and nutrient requirements. An acute illness can tip that balance to either side. Such imbalances result in inability of the patient to meet his or her particular nutritional requirements. The initial assessment of the critically ill patient in terms of this balance allows the nurse to establish a baseline for serial monitoring of nutritional status and treatment.

A second reason for obtaining a thorough nutritional assessment is to identify a patient at risk for nutritional complications of the disease process, treatment modalities, and healing process. Early recognition of problems will afford the health care team an opportunity to initiate early preventive treatment.

The measurement and analysis of data to determine nutritional status are not a simple task.[5] A variety of tools and skills should be used. Four types of data are gathered in a clinical nutritional assessment: history, anthropometric measurements, biochemical analysis, and signs and symptoms of nutrient deficiency (Fig. 56-1). Whether the assessment is done to gain information on general nutritional status or the status of a specific nutrient, data from all four areas will be used. A single test does not allow adequate clinical assessment of nutritional status. The implications of results of specific assessments in the critically ill patient may not be clear unless all available resources are used.

History

Although a dietary history and medical history are integral parts of the nutritional assessment, the critically ill patient often cannot provide these data. The nurse may have to rely on family or other significant persons in the patient's life as well as past medical records to obtain the information. If the nurse can obtain a thorough history, this information will allow an approximation of the patient's prehospitalization nutritional status. For example, by assessing gaps in consumption of the five food groups, the nurse can evaluate the potential for nutrient deficiency (Table 56-2). If the patient does not eat—or has minimal access to—fruits and vegetables, potential deficiencies in vitamins A, C, and B complex should be considered.

The history obtained should also include chronic disease states and medication use, as both of these can have an impact on specific nutrient utilization (Table 56-3). Previous gastrointestinal (GI) surgery or disease can have a major effect on nutrient digestion and absorption. Details regarding GI surgery or disease will give the nurse information about potential defects in secretion of GI hormones and enzymes that affect absorption of nutrients. This information is prerequisite to certain types of nutritional support and is valuable when decisions are made regarding methods of nutritional support.

Knowledge of a patient's current dietary modification, either professionally prescribed or self-prescribed, is essential when taking a dietary history. Again, this information can prove useful in determining nutritional risk. A history of recent weight changes can indicate a preexisting change in supply or demand for energy and may have a significant impact on the current disease process. Food allergy, including intolerances and sensitivities, is another important aspect of a nutritional history. Because nutritional therapy is a *treatment* just as is drug therapy, this information allows identification of any potential for allergic reactions before treatment begins.

The historical data base will have an immediate impact on planning the nutritional care of the critically ill patient. Further data obtained from a patient's history and profile will have a greater significance in the recovery and discharge planning phases of patient care. Table 56-4 summarizes the information obtained

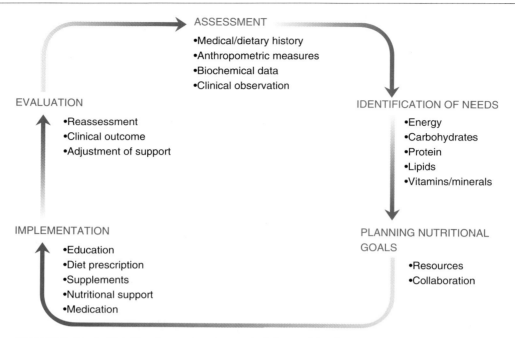

FIGURE 56–1. Nutritional assessment as part of the nutritional care process.

from a medical and dietary history that will affect nutritional care.

Part of the history used later in the patient's course of hospitalization includes socioeconomic and cultural factors, which often affect food consumption. These factors can be income, involvement in federal food programs, ethnic and cultural background, meal patterns, and availability of assistance for meal preparation. Discharge planning needs to incorporate socioeconomic and cultural information into the plan of care.

During recovery and resumption of oral intake, a knowledge of appetite history is needed. Changes in taste and appetite can frequently be caused by prescribed drugs, such as respiratory inhalants for obstructive lung disease. A history of the effect that dental and oral health has had on food consumption will also need to be available when the patient resumes oral intake. Physical activity limitations need to be addressed in terms of overall energy requirements.

In summary, a detailed medical and dietary history is used throughout the care of the critically ill

TABLE 56–2. Nutrients Provided by the Five Food Groups (1992 Food Guide Pyramid)

Milk Group (2–3 Servings)	Meat Group (2–3 Servings)	Vegetable Group (3–5 Servings) and Fruit Group (2–4 Servings)	Bread, Cereal, Rice, and Pasta Group (6–11 Servings)
Calcium*	Protein*	Vitamin A*	Thiamine
Protein*	Niacin*	Vitamin C*	Niacin
Riboflavin*	Thiamine*	Folic acid	Iron
Vitamin B_6*	Iron*	Fiber	Protein
Vitamin B_{12}*	Zinc*	Vitamin E	Zinc
Vitamin A*	Vitamin B_{12}*	Calcium†	Vitamin B_6
Vitamin D‡	Riboflavin*	Iron†	Vitamin E
Magnesium	Fatty acids	Magnesium†	Calcium
Phosphorus	Magnesium	Riboflavin†	Magnesium
Zinc	Phosphorus	Vitamin B_6†	Phosphorus
		Carbohydrate	

From U.S. Department of Agriculture: *Food Guide Pyramid.* Leaflet no. 572. Washington, D.C., Human Nutrition Information Service, 1992.
Number of servings refers to the required daily intake from each food group that will provide a balanced diet.
*Major nutrients in each group.
†Found in dark green vegetables.
‡Found in fortified milk.

TABLE 56–3. Potential Nutrient Deficiency Associated With Chronic Disease or Medication Usage

Nutrient	Chronic Disease or Medication
Vitamin A	Conditions associated with fat malabsorption
	Use of antilipidemics, neomycin, mineral oil
Vitamin D	Conditions associated with fat malabsorption or renal insufficiency
	Use of anticonvulsants, neomycin, mineral oil, corticosteroids, antilipidemics, sedatives/hypnotics
Vitamin K	Conditions associated with fat malabsorption, alteration of gastrointestinal microflora, or liver failure
	Use of aspirin, anticonvulsants, tetracycline, neomycin, mineral oil, antilipidemics, coumarin derivatives
Vitamin E	Conditions associated with fat malabsorption or long-term deficiency in calories
Vitamin B group	Alcoholism, conditions associated with small bowel dysfunction or alteration of gastrointestinal microflora
	Use of antacids, anticonvulsants, neomycin, chloramphenicol, sulfonamides, antineoplastics, antiparkinsonian drugs, antitubercular drugs, diuretics, corticosteroids, antilipidemics, uricosurics, antihypertensives, oral contraceptives
Vitamin C	Cigarette smoking
	Use of aspirin, tetracycline, antiparkinsonian drugs, corticosteroids, oral contraceptives, sedatives/hypnotics
Calcium	Conditions associated with fat malabsorption
	Vitamin D deficiency, cancer, renal disease, phosphorus imbalance
	Use of anticonvulsants, antidepressants, tetracycline, neomycin, antineoplastics, diuretics, mineral oil, antilipidemics, uricosurics
Magnesium	Conditions associated with fat malabsorption, alcoholism
	Use of anticonvulsants, antidepressants, tetracycline, diuretics, oral contraceptives, uricosurics
Phosphorus	Alcoholism, chronic acidosis, renal disease, hyperparathyroidism, vitamin D deficiency, calcium imbalance
	Use of antacids, mineral oil, corticosteroids, uricosurics
Iron	Conditions associated with blood loss or with gastrointestinal inflammation
	Use of antacids, antimicrobials, antitubercular drugs, antilipidemics
Zinc	Conditions associated with fat malabsorption
	Dialysis, diabetes mellitus, burns, or liver dysfunction
	Use of tetracycline, corticosteroids, oral contraceptives, diuretics

patient. Initially, the history may be limited to data from past medical records and information given by the patient, family, or others. However, the nurse adds to the data base continually during hospitalization to facilitate discharge planning.

Anthropometric Measurements

Anthropometric measurements are used to assess growth, weight change, available fat stores, and muscle mass as an indicator of protein reserve.[6] By using direct measurements or calculations, an analysis can be made of three body compartments—bone, lean tissues, and fat. This information can be used in evaluating changes in energy and protein metabolism. Anthropometry is simple to perform, but skill is needed to minimize error in measurement. The main advantages of these techniques are that they are simple, safe, inexpensive, and can be used by the nurse at the bedside. In addition to technical skill in assessment, selection and maintenance of equipment such as scales and skin thickness calipers are important.

Changes in body compartments—as a result of age, edema, or decreased muscle tone—alter the reliability of many of the anthropometric measurements because the standards used in comparisons do not reflect these changes. Variation in repeated measurements made by one nurse or in measurements made by different nurses may result in inability to use the measurements accurately. Poor equipment maintenance can be a source of further error. Proper training and equipment upkeep will maximize the accuracy. Also, if the nurse understands the technical limitations of these measurements, such as hydration, clinical application of this data will be improved. Although specificity and sensitivity are limited, anthropometric measurements provide additional data for the overall

TABLE 56–4. Medical and Diet History Data to Be Obtained

Food allergies
Ethnic and cultural impact on food habits
Appetite
Ability to obtain and prepare food
Community resources currently used
Amount and type of physical activity
Chronic disease requiring dietary modification
Gastrointestinal disease
Vitamin, mineral, or food supplementation used
Weight patterns
Dietary concerns of the patient
Dental and oral health
Medications that have nutritional implications

nutritional assessment that are relevant to the management of nutrition in the critically ill patient.

Because the nurse often obtains or assists the hospital nutritionist in obtaining anthropometric data, it is important for the nurse to understand how anthropometric measurements will be used. Is estimation adequate, or is an exact measurement needed? Usually, if an estimated measure can be verified by direct measurement, it should be done. A comparison of current measurements with previous measurements is more valuable if direct data are used on a routine basis.

Height and Weight

Typically the critically ill patient cannot stand upright to be measured for height. This does not eliminate the need for or opportunity to obtain an accurate height measurement. Some biochemical tests and nutritional therapy require a height measurement, so it is important to obtain one directly. Various methods have been researched to determine height using long bone measurements.[7] Long bone measurement may be preferable in the elderly patient with age-related height changes, but complete standards are not available, so that clinical application is currently limited.

One method for determining the height of a bed-confined patient is, with the patient and bed flat, to mark the top of the head and the heel on the sheet, then roll the patient over and measure the length between these marks. A second approach is to measure the patient in parts (head to shoulder, shoulder to hip, hip to knee, and so forth), then add the measurements for a total height. This technique is very useful when a patient is unable to lie flat. An adaptation of this technique is to stretch a string from the top of the patient's head and move it along the body parts to the heel, then measure the total string length. An estimated height is often quite inaccurate, so if an accurate height is not known, it is essential that the nurse directly measure the patient's height and document it on the permanent medical record.

Weight is easily obtained for even the most critically ill patient. Because weight trends are important in nutritional monitoring, it is important that an accurate measurement be recorded at patient admission to serve as a baseline for future comparisons. It is also imperative to note the assessed fluid status at the time the admission weight is determined, for better comparison of weight changes can be made as the patient's fluid status changes during hospitalization. The usual weight that the patient maintains is another piece of data needed for weight assessment. The present weight can be compared with the usual weight, and recent changes noted on the medical chart.

The use of a chair and bed scales is routine in most critical care units. The addition of critical care beds with built-in scales has made obtaining daily weights on the critically ill patient even easier. The balance-type scale is best for accuracy but needs regular calibration. Weight is frequently used in calcula-

tions of both drug dosage and nutritional requirements; thus, factors that can alter an accurate weight need to be considered in the measurement and calculation process. These factors include fluid imbalance, prosthesis or cast, loss of a limb, and tumor mass. For example, if the patient has 2 liters of excess fluid, an increase in weight of 2 kg could be expected (1 liter = 1 kg; or 454 mL = 1 pound). When determining energy requirements or drug dosage, the nurse does not want to provide calories or drugs for this water weight.

Measuring weight preoperatively and postoperatively is helpful in identifying a patient at risk for a catabolic state. If the postoperative weight is less than the preoperative weight, the patient may be at nutritional risk or may need fluid volume replacement. If the postoperative weight exceeds the preoperative weight, then fluid retention associated with surgical stress is most likely the cause. A postoperative weight gain of 0.5 to 5 kg above preoperative weight will usually be eliminated through the renal system within 24 to 48 hours; however, when the postoperative gain is 5 kg or more, fluid restriction may be required.

Daily weight determination is an important nursing order in the critical care unit, especially if the disease or treatment requires monitoring of fluid and nutritional status. Weight can be a misleading indicator of a catabolic state if water weight is replacing fat and muscle loss. The nurse needs to assess the percentage of weight lost over time. Percent weight loss is calculated using the following formula:

$$\% \text{ Weight loss} = \frac{\text{Usual weight} - \text{Present weight}}{\text{Usual weight}} \times 100.$$

For example, a patient who had very poor nutritional intake over the past 6 months weighed 188 pounds (85.5 kg) prior to his illness. His current weight, according to the in-bed scale, is 127 pounds (57.7 kg). The nurse can now calculate the percent weight loss from the formula:

$$\frac{188 - 127}{188} \times 100 = 32.4.$$

This calculation tells the nurse that this patient has lost over 32 percent of his usual weight in 6 months, a severe weight loss that puts him at nutritional risk.

A large weight change over a short period is more significant than a small change over a longer period in terms of nutritional status (Table 56–5). A large percent weight change over a short period may indicate a decreased ability of the patient to meet current metabolic demands.

Comparison of a patient's weight with established norms from various tables has limited use in critical care. It does, however, allow the general categorization of a patient as obese (20 percent above ideal body weight for height) or nutritionally at risk (20 percent below ideal body weight for height).

The critically ill patient should not have significant weight gain or loss (as defined in Table 56–7) during hospitalization. Some loss of weight is common in

TABLE 56–5. Evaluation of Weight Change Over Time

Time	Significant Weight Loss (%)	Severe Weight Loss (%)
1 wk	1–2	> 2
1 mo	5	> 5
3 mo	7.5	> 7.5
6 mo	10	> 10

critically ill patients as intake is frequently poor and catabolism is often present. Prevention of weight loss is a goal that can be accomplished by early intervention with appropriate nutritional support. Overfeeding must also be avoided. Further complications of overfeeding are discussed later in this chapter in the section on Overnutrition.

Weight measurements of critically ill patients provide a crucial tool for the nurse in assessing nutritional status and fluid status and monitoring nutritional support. It is the nurse's responsibility to ensure that accurate weights are obtained and recorded on the permanent medical record for use as an assessment parameter.

Determination of Body Fat and Muscle Mass

One method used to determine fat stores or caloric reserve is the skin fold thickness measurement. For this technique, pressure-sensitive calipers are used to measure subcutaneous fat from four muscle sites: triceps, biceps, suprailiac, and subscapular. A single individual measurement or the mean of three measurements can be compared with age-, sex-, and race-specific charts, allowing the patient to be classified within a percentile.[8] If the patient is in the tenth percentile or less, there is a risk of malnutrition, as this reflects a depletion of caloric reserves. Changes in skin fold thickness measurements usually occur over time, making skin fold thickness of limited usefulness in the short-term care of the critically ill patient. Individual trends in skin fold thicknesses are more relevant for long-term care of critically ill patients.

A measurement to determine fat and protein reserves is the midarm circumference measurement (a measure of the circumference of the arm at midpoint). The available somatic protein reserves can be calculated using the triceps skin fold measurement and the midarm circumference to provide an estimation of the midarm muscle circumference (AMC). Although formulas are available for determining the AMC, the quickest and easiest way to determine this measurement is from established nomograms. Intepretation is made by comparison with available standards. A low percentile is indicative of protein-energy malnutrition and increases the patient's nutritional risk. The measurement must be done by someone who is trained, must be accurate, and must be interpreted

with caution. In addition, the limb used must be in a normal state, not injured or edematous. For example, a 66-year-old man has been hospitalized in the critical care unit for 2 months with a long-term illness. During this time his metabolic needs have been high as a result of fever, infection, and rapid respiration. The dietician measures his tricep skin fold measurement at 8 mm and his midarm circumference at 25 cm. By comparison with an established age-based nomogram, the AMC is estimated to be 22.5 cm. This is then compared with percentiles for estimation of upper arm muscle area. For a 66-year-old man, an AMC of 22.5 cm is in the 5th percentile. This low percentile indicates that the patient is experiencing protein-calorie malnutrition and has an increased nutritional risk associated with this critical illness.

Creatinine-Height Index

The creatinine-height index is used to assess skeletal muscle mass as an indication of somatic protein reserves. It has the advantage of being less affected by the patient's hydration status than is muscle mass. A 24-hour urinary excretion of creatinine is divided by a predicted value based on the height of the patient, then multiplied by 100 to get a percentage value for creatinine-height index (CHI):

$$\% \text{ CHI} = \frac{\text{Actual 24-hr urinary creatinine}}{\text{Predicted 24 hr urinary creatinine}} \times 100.$$

A percentage less than 60 is an indication of moderate protein depletion. Because many factors can affect this test, such as liver disease, kidney disease, protein intake, age, trauma, infection, and stress, use in the critically ill patient is limited.

Muscle Function

Measurement of skeletal muscle function is a newer measurement of skeletal muscle mass as an indication of protein reserves.[9] Because malnutrition decreases muscle contraction force and increases muscle fatigue, it is thought that changes in function could precede changes in composition of tissue. Patients are asked to demonstrate simple muscle contraction, such as using a handgrip with a graded scale reflecting the pressure applied. This tool may prove useful in bedside determination of protein reserves.

Although anthropometric measurements have limited use in the short-term critical care patient, they may be useful in long-term patients. The measurements can be valuable in gross analysis of nutritional status by indicating levels that are adequate or insufficient. They also play a role in adding data to other measurements available to the nurse. Weight is the most important anthropometric parameter in assessment of nutritional and fluid status in the critical care setting and needs to be carefully and regularly monitored and recorded by the nurse. Analysis of weight variation needs to be done in collaboration with activities of the patient's other primary caregivers.

Biochemical Data

Biochemical data determinations range from simple and routine measurements to complex and rarely available testing. Specimens assayed may include blood, urine, cerebrospinal fluid, hair, and nails.

Serum Albumin

One area of nutritional assessment subject to routine biochemical analysis is visceral protein.[10] Because much of visceral protein is albumin, serum albumin (SA) levels (3.5–5.0 g/100 mL) are used to extrapolate a patient's protein status. However, the half-life of albumin is long (about 17–20 days); therefore, detection of significant changes that may be due to malnutrition are often delayed if one relies solely on SA measurements. Also, the nurse needs to remember that factors other than malnutrition can significantly change SA levels. These factors include fluid status, liver disease, renal disease, stress, trauma, and administration of albumin.

One important consideration in the use of SA as a nutritional parameter is fluid volume. A patient with an increased intravascular fluid volume, often reflected in a low serum sodium value, may also have an SA level that appears low. This decrease in serum sodium and albumin levels is a dilutional reflection of fluid status. A determination of protein status and protein needs should not be based on an SA value that is inaccurate. Generally an SA level less than 3.0 g/dL in the absence of the other factors mentioned indicates protein malnutrition. This laboratory test is still a key factor in nutritional assessment, even with its limitations.

Transferrin

A serum component more sensitive for assessing visceral protein is transferrin (200–400 mg/dL). Transferrin is an iron transport protein with a half-life of 7 to 10 days. Because its half-life is shorter than that of albumin, changes in nutritional status can be determined earlier than with SA results. If transferrin levels are low (less than 150 mg/dL) depletion of visceral protein stores is suspected. Transferrin levels are affected by iron stores such that a decrease in iron stores (as with chronic anemia) causes an increase in transferrin. Its level can also be affected by blood transfusions, infection, fluid status, and trauma. Transferrin can be easily calculated from total iron-binding capacity, which is a laboratory value often obtained in chemistry profiles.

Prealbumin

A test for prealbumin is more sensitive in protein assessment than either SA or transferrin values and is very useful clinically.[11] Prealbumin has a half-life of about 2 days. In addition to the high turnover rate, there is minimal pooling of this protein. Thus, changes in protein status from malnutrition can be detected much more quickly.

Prealbumin is a protein involved in the transport of thyroxine. A value less than 16 mg/dL indicates visceral protein depletion. As with the previous laboratory tests, stress, infection, and trauma will decrease the level of prealbumin. This is because the liver responds to stress by making acute phase protein (such as lymphocytes) rather than other visceral proteins. Prealbumin is often utilized to confirm suspected low protein reserves. If a patient with a low SA value of 3.0 mg/dL has also gained 10 pounds (4.5 kg) over 48 hours and has a serum sodium value of 130 mEq/L, the albumin may not be a true reflection of protein reserve because of the complication of suspected fluid volume overload. The total iron binding capacity of 241 mg/dL from 2 days ago is available on the chart. An estimated serum transferrin value can be calculated at 166 mg/dL for this patient. This value is low; however, the biochemical assessment of the visceral protein status remains difficult because of the questionable SA value and the borderline transferrin value. A prealbumin level can confirm that the patient is experiencing an acute protein deficit. A prealbumin level of 16 mg/dL would indicate that the patient's current visceral protein status is depleted.

Immune Function

The nurse can also assess visceral protein status through biochemical changes related to immunity.[12] Lymphocytes are formed from proteins, so malnutrition can markedly decrease the number and function of lymphocytes. A total lymphocyte count (TLC) less than 1,500 mg indicates a decreased ability of the body to respond to an infection and also indicates a potentially decreased visceral protein reserve. The TLC is determined by using the following formula:

$$\frac{\% \text{ Lymphocytes} \times \text{WBC}}{100} = \text{TLC}.$$

Because biochemical tests for the percentage of lymphocytes and the number of white blood cells (WBCs) are frequently done on critically ill patients, the nurse will have no difficulty calculating the TLC.

Skin Tests

Other factors can decrease lymphocyte numbers, such as drugs and cancer treatment modalities. Cellular immunity can be used as a clinical tool for assessment of visceral protein. To test cellular immunity, the nurse may administer skin tests involving recall antigens (antigens to which the patient has previously been sensitized) to elicit a positive response. A positive response would be expected within 48 hours to recall antigens used (e.g., a challenge dose of mumps) if the patient has a functioning immune system with the capacity to make needed immune system proteins. Absence of a positive response is interpreted as diminished capacity to form essential proteins.

TABLE 56–6. Evaluation of Visceral Protein Status

Value	Degree of Malnutrition		
	Mild	Moderate	Severe
Serum albumin (g/dL)	2.8–3.5	2.1–2.7	< 2.1
Serum transferrin (mg/dL)	150–200	100–150	< 100
Total lymphocyte count (no./mm³)	1,200–2,000	800–1,199	< 800

Urinary Nitrogen

Alternatively, a measure of protein catabolism is obtained from the 24-hour urinary urea nitrogen measurement. The measured urinary urea is increased by 4 grams to account for the nonurinary loss of nitrogen each day. This value is then compared to the nitrogen intake, which is determined by dividing the protein intake by 6.25. If excretion is significantly higher than intake, a negative nitrogen balance is present that is caused by increased protein breakdown, decreased intake, or both. As with the creatinine-height index, reliance on an accurate 24-hour urine output and 24-hour protein intake analysis is critical to the reliability of this test. If renal function is normal, blood urea nitrogen (BUN) and serum creatinine values can also be used as indicators of protein catabolism. Increased levels potentially indicate increased breakdown of protein.

An assessment of the degree of protein depletion using values for SA, transferrin, and TLC is seen in Table 56–6. The nurse will often have access to these biochemical tests directly or through calculation. This will allow the nurse to make an estimation of the degree of malnutrition a patient may be experiencing.

Prognostic Nutritional Index

A tool called the Prognostic Nutritional Index (PNI)[13] combines a number of biochemical tests to predict operative complication risk. The higher the PNI value, the greater the risk of postoperative complications caused by nutritional factors. Frequently, acutely or critically ill patients require surgery that is not urgent.

The health care team, including the nurse, can use the PNI to assess the risk versus benefit of a surgical procedure at a given time in the course of an illness. For example the question could be asked: given the current nutritional risk and potential for complications based on the PNI, would a few days of nutritional intervention be better for the patient than going to surgery immediately? The PNI is determined using the following formula:

$$PNI = 158 - 16.6 \text{ (serum albumin [g/dL])}$$
$$- 0.78 \text{ (triceps skin fold [mm])}$$
$$- 0.2 \text{ (serum transferrin [mg/dL])}$$
$$- 5.8 \text{ (delayed hypersensitivity)}$$

where delayed hypersensitivity is graded as follows: 0, nonreactive; 1, <5 mm reactivity; 2, >5 mm reactivity.

This index uses a variety of parameters to measure fat and protein reserves to determine whether surgical candidates are in need of nutritional support before surgery or immediately after surgery. For example, a patient at surgical risk secondary to poor nutritional status would undergo a variety of tests before surgery. The health care team would use these data to determine the PNI to determine the best surgical nutrition approach. If a patient's PNI was high, preoperative nutrition would be indicated to decrease surgical risk as well as postoperative complications.

Hemoglobin/Red Blood Cell Indices

Hemoglobin values and red blood cell (RBC) indices can be used to assess nutritional anemias. If the hemoglobin is less than normal (values for women are 12–16 g/dL; for men, 13–18 g/dL), the nurse can assess the available patient history and the RBC indices to determine if the existing anemia has a nutritional basis. In Table 56–7 the common causes and RBC indices associated with various anemias are contrasted.

An anemia frequently seen with malnutrition is caused by folate deficiency. This occurs because the body has a low storage capability for folate. Therefore a short time of poor intake can result in a clinically observable deficiency. Folate deficiency causes a megaloblastic anemia similar to vitamin B_{12} deficiency. Other laboratory tests more specific for particular causes of anemia (such as serum iron, serum vitamin

TABLE 56–7. Nutritional Deficiencies Associated With Anemia

Anemia Type	Red Blood Cell Indices*	Common Causes
Macrocytic-megaloblastic	MCV decreased and MCHC decreased	Folate deficiency, vitamin B_{12} deficiency, drugs
Microcytic-hypochromic	MCV increased and MCHC increased	Iron deficiency, chronic blood loss
Normocytic-normochromic	MCV normal and MCHC normal	Acute blood loss; overexpansion of blood volume; aplastic anemia; renal, liver, or endocrine disease

*MCV, mean corpuscular volume (80–94 μ^3); MCHC, mean corpuscular hemoglobin concentration (32%–36%).

T A B L E 56–8. Blood Tests Used to Document Iron Deficiency Anemia

Blood Test	Iron Depletion	Iron Deficiency	Iron Anemia
Serum iron	Normal	Decreased	Decreased
Total iron-binding capacity	High normal	Increased	Increased
Transferrin	Low normal	Decreased	Decreased
Ferritin	Decreased	Decreased	Decreased

B_{12}, or serum folate) can further differentiate the cause of anemia. In iron deficiency anemia, the change in hemoglobin value occurs late in the course of disease; therefore, more sensitive blood tests are used such as serum iron, total iron-binding capacity, transferrin, and ferritin (Table 56–8). Transferrin, total iron-binding capacity, and ferritin show the earliest changes, as these values represent changes in iron transport and stores.

Other Biochemical Tests

Assessment of electrolytes and vitamin status is also a part the biochemical data available to the nurse. Most tests for serum vitamin levels are expensive and not routinely available or necessary. Frequently other tests involving metabolites of vitamin breakdown or enzymes used during vitamin utilization are performed to assess vitamin status. Measurements of electrolytes are routinely available; however, alterations are typically caused by disease or treatment modalities rather than solely by nutritional deficiencies.

One relationship important in critical care is the effect of albumin levels on serum calcium (normal levels are 8.5–10.5 mg/100 mL). Because 80 percent of calcium is carried by albumin, a low level of albumin could result in a falsely low value for serum calcium. And as serum calcium alterations are common in many disease states, such as renal disease and cancer, it is important that serum calcium levels be corrected based on SA levels. A corrected calcium level can be calculated using all the following formulas in the given steps:

1. Normal albumin − actual albumin = A; then
2. $A \times 0.8 = Y$; then
3. Serum calcium + Y = adjusted calcium.

For example, a patient with a current serum calcium level of 7.2 mg/dL and an SA of 2.1 g/dL would have a corrected serum calcium level of 8.72 mg/dL, which is within normal limits. A more specific test that directly measures ionized calcium would also indicate more accurately the calcium status.

To control health care costs, it is necessary to be selective in biochemical analysis, particularly in ordering expensive tests. The nurse and other members of the health care team must examine the need for further nutritional biochemical assessment by monitoring the frequently available tests with the knowledge

that their sensitivity is limited. An initial dietary and medical history, physical examination, and understanding of current physiologic stressors as related to nutritional status are factors that contribute to determining whether, and what, additional biochemical tests will be necessary. Biochemical changes occur

T A B L E 56–9. Frequently Used Nutritional Biochemical Assessment Tests

Nutrient	Test*
Carbohydrate	Plasma glucose*
Fat	Serum cholesterol*
	Serum triglyceride*
Protein	Total protein*
	Serum albumin*
	Serum transferrin
	Total iron-binding capacity*
	Prealbumin
	Total lymphocytic count*
	Skin tests
	Urinary nitrogen
	Serum creatinine*
	Blood urea nitrogen*
Vitamin A	Serum vitamin A
	Serum carotene
Vitamin D	Plasma 25-hydroxycholecalciferol
	Serum alkaline phosphatase*
	Phosphorus*
Vitamin E	Plasma vitamin E
Vitamin K	Prothrombin time*
Vitamin C	Serum ascorbic acid
Thiamine	Red blood cell (RBC) transketolase activity
	Thiamine phosphatase effect
	Urinary thiamine
Riboflavin	Serum or plasma riboflavin
	RBC glutathione reductase
Niacin	Urinary 2-pyridone
	RBC nicotinamide mononucleotide
Vitamin B_6	Plasma or RBC pyridoxal phosphate
	Tryptophan load test
Vitamin B_{12}	Serum or RBC vitamin B_{12}
	Schilling test
Folic acid	RBC or serum folate
Iron	Hemoglobin and hematocrit*
	Ferritin
	Total iron-binding capacity*
	Transferrin
	Serum iron*
Sodium	Serum sodium*
Calcium	Serum calcium*
Potassium	Serum potassium*
Phosphorus	Serum phosphorus*
Zinc	Serum and plasma zinc*
Magnesium	Serum magnesium*

*Routinely used and available.

prior to the clinical signs and symptoms of nutritional deficiency, and therefore can be important analytic tools for the nurse in nutritional assessment. A summary chart of the laboratory tests frequently used in nutritional assessment is shown in Table 56–9.

Physical Examination

The clinical observation of the patient will aid in determination of nutritional status. The nurse should examine the patient in terms of both potential nutrient deficiency and non-nutritional problems. If a particular tissue is abnormal in appearance or function, nutritional causes should be considered along with disease or treatment causes. The tissues commonly showing signs of nutrient deficiencies are hair, eyes, skin, mucous membranes, skeleton, muscles, and nervous system (Table 56–10). For example, changes in the appearance of the tongue and lips are often related to vitamin B deficiencies. In addition, vitamin B deficiency can also cause neurologic changes. Clinical signs and symptoms of suspected deficiencies should be confirmed with the medical history and with anthropometric or biochemical analyses. Recall that signs and symptoms occur last in the sequence of nutrient deficiency and that signs and symptoms of nutrient deficiencies are similar to specific disease symptoms or side effects of treatment modalities. Because of these similarities, it is often easy for the health care providers to overlook or underestimate nutrient deficiency as a potential cause of observable signs and symptoms.

Energy Expenditure Measurement

Knowledge of the critically ill patient's current energy expenditure is needed to provide adequate nutritional support in terms of calorie requirements. Assessment of energy expenditure is accomplished by calorimetry, the measure of heat production. A technique to measure energy expenditure, called indirect calorimetry, can be used at the bedside and also in mechanically ventilated patients.

Indirect calorimetry measures oxygen consumption ($\dot{V}o_2$) and carbon dioxide production ($\dot{V}co_2$) as a reflection of resting energy expenditure. The relationship of carbon dioxide produced to oxygen consumed is called the **respiratory quotient** (RQ). The RQ depends on the type of diet consumed. A mixed normal diet has an RQ of 0.8. This means that more oxygen is consumed during metabolism of nutrients than carbon dioxide is produced, because RQ = $\dot{V}co_2/\dot{V}o_2$. The RQ can also be used to differentiate among the energy sources, such as carbohydrates, protein, or fat, that are being utilized to meet energy requirements (Table 56–11).

The RQ for carbohydrate is 1.0, which means that oxygen consumed is equal to carbon dioxide produced. Because fat metabolism consumes more oxygen with less carbon dioxide produced, the RQ for fat is 0.7, which is less than the RQ for carbohydrate. If the RQ is over 1.0, excessive kilocalories will cause lipogenesis (conversion of glucose to fatty acids). Using the concept of the RQ, the nurse can understand why excessive carbohydrate intake in a respiratory patient results in high production of carbon dioxide,

T A B L E 56–10. Physical Signs Indicative or Suggestive of Malnutrition

Site	Signs Associated With Malnutrition	Possible Disorder or Nutrient Deficiency
Hair	Lack of natural shine, dull and dry, thin and fine, dyspigmented	Kwashiorkor or marasmus (less common)
Eyes	Pale	Anemia (iron)
	Red membranes, Bitot's spots, dryness, corneal dullness, keratomalacia	Vitamin A
	Redness and fissuring of eyelids	Riboflavin, pyridoxine
	Corneal arcus (white ring), xanthelasma (yellow lumps)	Hyperlipidemia
Lips	Angular cheilosis (white or pink lesions at corner of mouth)	Riboflavin
Tongue	Red or scarlet color	Nicotinic acid
	Magenta (purple) color	Riboflavin
	Atrophy or hypertrophy of filiform papillae	Folic acid
Gums	Spongy, bleeding, or receding gums	Vitamin C
Glands	Thyroid enlargement	Iodine
	Parotid enlargement	Starvation, bulimia
Skin	Dryness, follicular hyperkeratosis	Vitamin A
	Petechiae	Vitamin C
	Excessive bruising	Vitamin K
	Fat deposits under skin	Hyperlipidemia
Nervous system	Mental confusion	Thiamine, nicotinic acid
	Depression, sensory loss, motor weakness, loss of position sense, hyporeflexia in lower extremities, paresthesia	Pyridoxine, vitamin B_{12}
	Dementia	Niacin, vitamin B_{12}

Adapted with permission from Mahan LK, Arlin MT: *Krause's Food, Nutrition and Diet Therapy*, 8th ed. Philadelphia, WB Saunders, 1992, p 304.

TABLE 56–11. Respiratory Quotients for Carbohydrate, Protein, and Fat

Nutrient Source	Respiratory Quotient	Energy Produced for 1 L of O_2 (kcal)
Carbohydrate	1.0	5.0
Fat	0.7	4.7
Protein	0.8	4.6

which can be detrimental to that patient's respiratory status. Providing supplemental calories to the respiratory patient with obstructive pulmonary disease in the form of carbohydrate would add to the carbon dioxide load and potentially complicate the underlying respiratory disease process.

Various calculations are available to determine basal energy expenditure (BEE). Using indirect calorimetry, the liters of oxygen consumed is divided by 5 to determine energy needs (5 is the approximate energy produced by each nutrient to consume 1 liter of oxygen). A less exact measurement of BEE can be calculated using standard formulas. The Harris-Benedict formula is commonly used to calculate BEE[14]:

$$BEE \text{ (women)} = 655.096 + 9.563 \text{ (weight in kg)}$$
$$+ 1.85 \text{ (height in cm)}$$
$$- 4.676 \text{ (age in years)}$$
$$BEE \text{ (men)} = 66.473 + 13.752 \text{ (weight in kg)}$$
$$+ 5.003 \text{ (height in cm)}$$
$$- 6.755 \text{ (age in years)}$$

To determine the BEE for a 40-year-old man who weighs 188 pounds (85.5 kg) and is 6 feet (182.8 cm) tall, these numbers are used:

$$66.473 + 13.752 \,(85.5) + 5.003 \,(182.8)$$
$$- 6.755 \,(40) = 1886.6 \text{ kcal.}$$

Once the parameters of height, age, and weight are known, nomograms for the Harris-Benedict equation are available for use at the bedside. The BEE measurement provides a base kilocalorie need. Additional kilocalories are needed for other significant energy requirements of the critically ill patient, such as treatment and disease process.

Understanding energy expenditure concepts allows the nurse to better appreciate the percentage of calories needed from the various nutrient sources (carbohydrate, fat, or protein) to meet energy requirements. It is critical that determination of the patient's needs be an individual assessment, especially given the consequences of underfeeding and overfeeding the critically ill patient. The nutritional effect of physiologic stress and the consequences of malnutrition are discussed in the following sections.

KEY CONCEPTS

- Nutritional assessment is based on four types of data: history, anthropometric measurements, biochemical analysis, and physical signs and symptoms. Nutritional assessment enables identification of nutritional requirements and prediction of nutritional complications.
- Nutritional assessment begins with history taking. Questions regarding preadmission dietary habits, chronic disease states, medications, recent weight change, allergies, previous GI operations, appetite, and social, economic, and cultural factors that affect nutritional intake may reveal actual or potential nutritional problems.
- Anthropometric measurements are used to assess growth, weight, body fat, and muscle composition. Height and weight should be measured, not estimated. Acute changes in weight usually reflect changes in fluid volume (1 kg = 1 liter). Weight can be a misleading indicator of catabolic state when fat and muscle losses are replaced by water weight. Computation of percent weight gain or loss is useful for determining weight change.
- Fat and protein stores may be estimated using anthropoetric measures, including skin fold thickness, arm circumference, creatinine-height index, and muscle strength.
- Biochemical tests that assess protein metabolism are routinely performed in the clinical setting. Low serum albumin, transferrin, and prealbumin levels are indicative of poor protein intake or poor utilization of protein by the liver. Red and white blood cells are particularly sensitive to poor nutrition because of rapid turnover. Anemia (iron, vitamin B_{12}, or folate deficiency) and decreased immune function (protein deficiency) may result. Increased body protein catabolism may be apparent from elevated BUN and serum creatinine levels as well as from increased excretion of urinary nitrogen.
- Calculation of energy expenditure is important in critically ill individuals whose nutritional requirements may be high due to stress, fever, trauma, and abnormal losses (burns). Indirect calorimetry measures oxygen consumption and carbon dioxide production to determine the respiratory quotient (RQ = V_{O_2}/V_{CO_2}). The respiratory quotient reflects the substrate being used for energy metabolism. Pure carbohydrate utilization yields an RQ of 1.0, pure fat an RQ of 0.7. The basal energy expenditure can also be calculated from sex, age, height, and weight using the Harris-Benedict formula.

Nutritional Effect of Physiologic Stress

Metabolic Response to Physiologic Stress

There is an important difference between the response of the body to starvation and to physiologic stress.[15] Starvation is a gradual process in which there is a decrease in the metabolic rate and exhaustion of carbohydrate reserves. As insulin levels decrease, free fatty acids are stimulated to be released for energy use. Despite the available free fatty acids, protein is used for energy by means of gluconeogenesis, as the body's tissues prefer glucose as an energy source. This creates a negative nitrogen balance. As starvation continues there is an overall reduction in energy needs and the tissues that usually require glucose for function adapt by using ketones for energy. Then lipolysis provides the source of needed energy, decreasing the use of protein as an energy source. This is a adaptive response through which the body strives to conserve lean body mass. Overall the result is a minimal depletion of the body's protein. The starvation state is characterized by decreased glucose and urinary nitrogen excretion along with elevation in ketones and free fatty acids. Fasting (starving) alone is not associated with a high mortality unless it is on a long-term basis, such as in anorexia nervosa. Figure 56–2 provides a summary of the physiologic effect of starvation.

With physiologic stress, the response is quite different, and conservation of lean body mass does not occur. Metabolic rate increases rather than decreases, resulting in a high sustained rate of catabolism (breakdown of protein to meet energy needs). Protein is used as an energy source by gluconeogenesis through release of muscle stores of amino acids. This quickly results in a negative nitrogen balance. There is a redistribution of cell mass in response to the stressor, with an increase in the production of acute phase proteins. The degree of hypermetabolism, hypercatabolism, and negative nitrogen balance associated with a physi-

ologic stress depends on the type, duration, and severity of the stressor present.

Typically, the catabolic response to stress is seen in two phases: the immediate phase, lasting 5 to 8 days; and the adaptive phase, occurring after the immediate response. The physiologic effects of each phase are summarized in Figures 56–3 and 56–4.

The immediate phase of catabolism is characterized by high sympathetic nervous system stimulation with release of glucagon, glucocorticoids, and catecholamines. Resultant decreased production and circulation of insulin causes a pseudodiabetic state. The patient develops hyperglycemia from decreased circulating insulin and decreased utilization of glucose by muscle and other tissues (insulin resistance).

An energy deficit is created, and alternative mechanisms of glucose production need to be used. The oxidation of branched-chain amino acids occurs for two reasons: to meet energy requirements, and for the amino acids to provide the liver a substrate for synthesis of acute phase proteins (immunoglobulins, lymphocytes, and leukocytes). As the amino acids are mobilized to meet energy needs, alanine is formed (ammonia plus pyruvate), which stimulates gluconeogenesis. Sodium and water are retained secondary to an increase in aldosterone, which results in potassium loss. The mineralocorticoid aldosterone is released secondary to the stimulation of the sympathetic nervous system. During this phase fat is not well utilized as an energy source because there is some level of insulin present, which has a antilipolytic action.

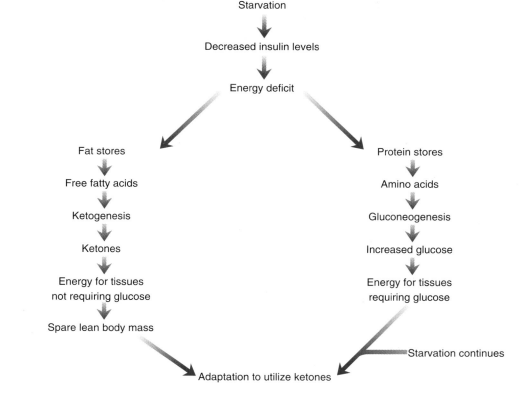

FIGURE 56–2. Catabolic response to starvation.

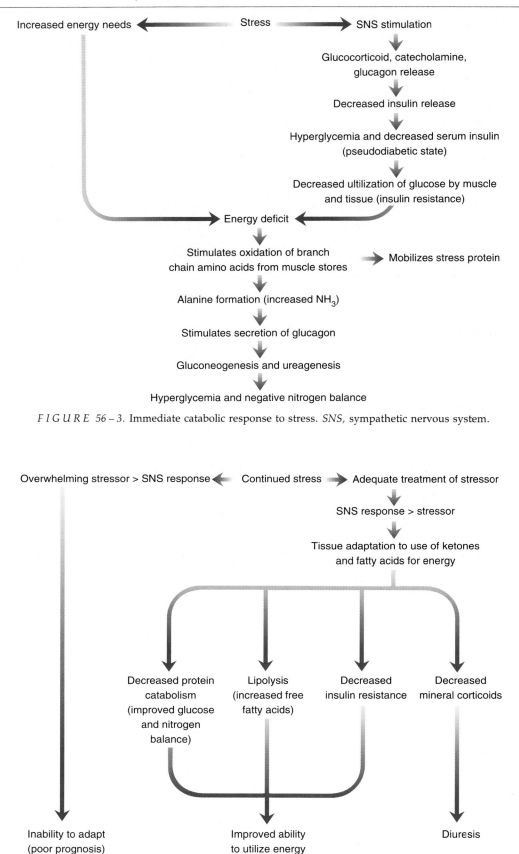

F I G U R E 56 – 3. Immediate catabolic response to stress. *SNS*, sympathetic nervous system.

F I G U R E 56 – 4. Adaptive phase of catabolic response to stress. *SNS*, sympathetic nervous system.

The nutritional result of the immediate phase to stress on the body is hyperglycemia, negative nitrogen balance, and retention of fluid and sodium. This protective mechanism utilizes skeletal muscle to meet energy requirements and protects the rest of the body's tissue from breaking down during periods of high energy need. There is an overall loss of nitrogen and other electrolytes, including magnesium, phosphorus, and zinc.

The adaptive phase occurs if the sympathetic nervous system response can selectively keep up with the stressors present. If the stressors are so great as to overwhelm the body's response system, there will be a negative effect on prognosis. In the adaptive phase the body begins to utilize ketones and fatty acids (lipolysis) for energy, conserving proteins. As the sympathetic nervous system response lessens, there is a decrease in the insulin resistance, and the utilization of glucose will improve. In addition, aldosterone levels return to normal, resulting in diuresis. The overall result is an improvement in negative nitrogen balance as the serum glucose improves. This phase is similar to the response of the body during starvation, when fat is utilized to meet energy requirements. Recall that chronic conditions such as diabetes, liver disease, or renal disease have an extreme impact on the body's ability to move into the adaptive phase during physiologic stress. Chronic system failure or inadequate support of the current disease process complicate the course of recovery for the patient. Nutritional support is used more efficiently by the body's tissue during the adaptive phase than during the immediate phase. It is in this phase that nutrition can play a vital role in recovery. The combination of starvation (fasting) and a physiologic stress increases the risk for morbidity and mortality. A compromised nutritional status at the time of a physiologic stress decreases the body's ability to best respond. In addition, the ability to mobilize the immune response is decreased with cell-mediated immunity, humoral immunity, and alteration of the tissue barriers to infection.

Nutrient Requirements During Physiologic Stress

Energy and Protein Requirements

Energy is obtained from three sources: carbohydrate, protein, and fat. A healthy adult has variable energy needs, with an average between 25 and 30 kcal/kg/day, or about 1,800 to 2,500 calories each day, depending on height, weight, and activity.[14] The carbohydrate intake in a typical American diet usually accounts for about 50 percent of the total calories, protein accounts for 10 to 20 percent, and fat accounts for 30 to 40 percent. About 4 kcal is produced from 1 gram of carbohydrate. Protein also produces about 4 kcal/g, while fat produces about 9 kcal/g.

Most calories are obtained from carbohydrate because it is an efficient source of energy and, when metabolized, has protein-sparing and antiketogenic effects. Carbohydrate intake must be at least 100 to 150 g/day. Carbohydrate is stored as glycogen in the liver for immediate use during stress, but it can be depleted within 24 hours. Inadequate carbohydrate results in gluconeogenesis to form glucose from other sources (amino acids). Excess carbohydrate (above glycogen storage capacity) is converted to triglyceride for storage in adipose tissue.

Stress alters carbohydrate metabolism. Because circulating glucose is high and serum insulin is low, glucose is not utilized efficiently during the immediate phase of stress. Even though the need for glucose is increased with stress, because of the poor glucose utilization excessive carbohydrate intake (greater than 400–700 g/day) could result in carbohydrate being stored as fat. In addition, high intake of carbohydrates causes an increase in RQ, resulting in increased carbon dioxide production. This increase in carbon dioxide may be detrimental to the patient's respiratory function.

The energy needs of a patient with physiologic stress are best determined by calorimetry. Energy needs have also been related to urinary urea (as a degree of catabolism), as seen in Table 56–12. Most patients undergoing a significant physiologic stress need a 20 to 50 percent increase in calories above BEE to prevent catabolism. This requirement can increase even more for severely traumatized or burn patients. An average total calorie intake of 40 to 45 kcal/kg ideal body weight/day is needed during acute physiologic stress. This represents a 20 percent increase in calories above BEE.

Protein is not stored in the body, but rather is functional. It is needed for growth, tissue maintenance and repair, and enzyme and hormone production. For every 6.25 grams of protein intake, 1 gram of nitrogen is produced. Nitrogen balance occurs when

TABLE 56–12. Degree of Catabolism Related to Urinary Urea Loss

Clinical Situation	Degree of Catabolism	Increase in Metabolic Rate over BMR (%)	Total Energy Requirement (kcal)
Bedridden	Normal	None	1,800
Surgery	Mild	0–20	1,800–2,200
Trauma	Moderate	20–50	2,200–2,700
Burns	Severe	50–125	2,700–4,000

Adapted with permission from Mahan LK, Arlin MT: *Krause's Food, Nutrition and Diet Therapy*, 8th ed. Philadelphia, WB Saunders, 1992, p 493; and from Rutten P, Blackburn GL, Flatt JP, Hollowell E, Cochran D: Determination of optimal hyperalimentation infusion rate. *J Surg Res* 1975;18:477–483.

normal protein intake and breakdown of protein to nitrogen are in equilibrium. The recommended intake of protein is 0.8 g/kg/day. Protein can be available as an energy source. Amino acids are highly utilized for energy during the immediate phase of physiologic stress, when glucose and fat utilization is decreased.

Physiologic stress increases the need for protein. Protein is needed for synthesis of acute phase proteins, wound repair, energy, and replacement of renal and wound losses. Protein intake should be 16 percent of the total energy needs. Assuming a nitrogen-to-kilocalorie ratio of 1:150, protein needs can be calculated by dividing total energy requirement by 24. Therefore, if total energy needs were 3,120 kcal/day, protein intake should be 130 g/day. Another method to determine protein need is to use a range of 1.0 to 2.5 g/kg/day based on degree of stress (Table 56–13). A 70-kg patient with multiple trauma would have a stress level of 2. This patient would require 40 kcal/kg/day (2,800 kcal per day). The protein needs based on this stress level would utilize 2.0 g/kg/day or 140 g/day.

It is important to have an accurate record of patient weight when weight-based formulas need to be calculated. The nurse must make an assessment of fluid status, as initial weight gain following initiation of nutritional support is often attributable to fluid retention. With maximum nutritional support, a weight increase of about 0.25 kg/day would be expected. Increases greater than 0.25 kg/day are usually the result of fluid retention.

Protein sources need to be easily digestible and utilized. Because of this, the use of amino acids in commercial nutritional supplements has increased. Selective amino acids are now placed in specialized nutritional formulas to provide better utilized protein sources for specific diseases. Branched-chain amino acids are placed into formulas for patients with liver disease, and only essential amino acids are placed into formulas for patients with renal disease.

Fat is needed for energy, transport of vitamins, provision of essential fatty acids, and cell membrane structure. When fat is used to meet energy needs, metabolites such as ketones can build up, resulting in a metabolic acidosis. Some glucose-dependent tissues such as the brain and kidney require a constant level of glucose to meet energy needs. These tissues do not utilize other energy sources well and can show symptoms when glucose is not available as a substrate for energy production.

The use of fat in nutritional support of an acute illness, in addition to providing additional kilocalories, is to prevent fatty acid deficiency. Using only carbohydrate and protein as an energy source can contribute to the development of fatty liver, cholestasis, and increased carbon dioxide production. To avoid these complications of overfeeding with carbohydrate, fat is used to provide kilocalories as a replacement for a certain percentage of carbohydrate calories. The use of fat as an additional energy source depends on the degree of stress and the type of stress, each of which affects energy needs. For example, a patient with respiratory impairment may need a higher percentage of kilocalories from fat to avoid the increase in carbon dioxide production associated with high carbohydrate loads.

Vitamin and Mineral Requirements

There is a high degree of individual variance in regard to vitamin and mineral requirements during critical illness. Typically, vitamin deficiencies do not occur suddenly. However, borderline nutritional status at the time of an acute illness may increase the risk that deficiencies will rapidly develop. Overall, vitamin requirements generally increase during physiologic stress. Water-soluble vitamins such as vitamin C and the B vitamins have limited body storage, which requires daily replenishment. Fat-soluble vitamins such as vitamins A, D, E, and K are stored in the body longer and will not need immediate replenishment, if the patient's nutrition had been adequate prior to hospital admission. Vitamin supplementation will need to be part of the nutritional support given during a critical illness.

Electrolytes, minerals, and trace minerals also must be replenished during physiologic stress. Electrolytes and minerals should be assayed routinely with biochemical testing and replaced as needed. Both a previous history of poor intake, such as seen with chronic alcohol abuse, and the potential for nutrient loss, such as draining wound, need to be considered in the assessment and treatment of deficiencies.

TABLE 56–13. Relationship of Stress Level to Energy Needs

Stress Level	Kcal Need (total kcal/kg/day)	Calorie to Nitrogen Ratio	Percent of Total Kcal		
			AA	CHO	Fat
0	28	150:1	15	60	25
1	32	100:1	20	50	30
2	40	100:1	25	40	35
3	50	80:1	30	70	0

Adapted with permission from Lang CE (ed): *Nutritional Support in Critical Care.* Rockville, MD, Aspen, 1987, p 74; and from *Nutritional Support Services Magazine* 1985;5(1); 26–27. Copyright January 1985, Creative Age Publications.
Abbreviations; kcal, kilocalorie; AA, amino acids; CHO, carbohydrate.

Drug therapy can further deplete or alter the vitamin and mineral balance in the body. For example, the antibiotic neomycin can cause a deficiency of fat-soluble vitamins. Anticonvulsants such as phenytoin increase the metabolism of vitamins D and K. Phosphate and calcium deficiency are associated with the long-term use of antacids. Knowledge of the effect of treatment modalities on nutritional status guides the critical care nurse to make needed observations in the early detection of potential deficiencies.

Current knowledge of trace mineral requirements during physiologic stress is limited. Replacement of trace minerals is necessary with long-term illnesses and can be easily provided. Guidelines for safe dosages of vitamins and minerals are available in medical and nutritional texts.

Patients at Nutritional Risk

The patients who will be at predictable risk for nutritional complications of current disease process must be identified quickly so that nutritional status can be assessed and current requirements determined. These patients usually need additional nutritional support in their treatment plan. The nurse plays a major role in identifying the patient at risk for nutritional complications and in communicating this assessment to other health care providers.

Overnutrition

Overnutrition in the form of obesity is a major health concern. Obesity is defined as a weight measurement that is 20 percent or more over ideal body weight for height and build. Health risks associated with obesity have been associated more often with the *distribution* of body fat rather than with total body fat. Upper body obesity is an identified risk for diabetes and atherosclerosis. Central obesity is a risk factor for coronary artery disease. Thus, measurements such as the waist-hip ratio and the waist-thigh ratio become important in determining fat distribution and health risk. The nurse is often involved in obtaining such measurements. A waist-hip ratio greater than 0.8 for women and 1.0 for men can indicate higher cardiovascular risk. Other conditions associated with obesity and increased body fat include congestive heart failure, hypertension, gout, cancer of the breast, endometriosis, and cholelithiasis.

Weight gain is often accompanied by increases in blood pressure, blood lipids, and serum glucose levels. Insulin resistance is a common problem associated with obesity. Additionally, the increase in blood volume can adversely affect cardiac output and the regulating sympathetic activity.

The debate concerning the major factors influencing the development of obesity continues, with experts on both sides of the genetic versus environmental theories. Additionally, the concepts of thermic effect of food, overfeeding, and exercise intertwine both theories.

Fat cells, or adipocytes, increase in size when excess energy is provided. It is believed that the number of fat cells in the body does not diminish with weight loss, but rather that cell size decreases. This may contribute to the weight fluctuations experienced with repeated diets. Additionally, enzyme levels or activity alter with weight change. The enzyme adipose lipoprotein lipase determines fat uptake rates. This enzyme is elevated in obesity and may increase activity during weight loss, thus adding to the difficulty of weight maintenance.

When obtaining anthropometric measures in the obese patient, it is important to remember that fat stores do not indicate adequate protein, vitamin, or mineral status. Frequently, there is delay in providing nutritional support to obese patients because health care providers believe there is adequate storage of fuel to support to patient's nutritional needs. This can often lead to a problem in protein-energy malnutrition, even in a seemingly well-nourished patient.

Protein-Energy Malnutrition

Protein-energy malnutrition is classified into three categories: marasmus, kwashiorkor, and marasmus-kwashiorkor. The differences between kwashiorkor and marasmus are in the type of protein lost (visceral or somatic) and the cause of the deficiency (decreased protein intake and stress or decreased calorie intake). Marasmus occurs because of inadequate caloric intake, resulting in the use of fat and protein for energy. It usually develops slowly and reflects a loss of somatic protein with preservation of visceral proteins. The clinical consequences of marasmus usually are not significant, as there is preservation of the body's ability to respond to short-term stress. Patients with marasmus do not have a significant increase in mortality. Because somatic protein is lost, clinical signs and symptoms can be seen in anthropometric measures: a body weight less than 80 percent of ideal body weight, a creatinine-height index less than 80 percent of standard, a decreased midarm circumference, and a decreased tricep skin fold measurement. Patients with marasmus often appear emaciated.

Although marasmus is not life-threatening, an intense or long-term physiologic stress will cause the patient to develop a mixed marasmus-kwashiorkor type of protein-calorie malnutrition that is associated with increases in mortality. Kwashiorkor is a primary deficit in protein without calorie deficit and is associated with presence of a physiologic stressor. It develops more quickly than marasmus and reflects a loss of visceral protein. The clinical consequences include decreased wound healing, susceptibility to infection, decreased cellular immunity, and high mortality. Because visceral protein is lost, assessment is made on the basis of biochemical data. The changes include decreased SA, decreased serum transferrin, decreased serum prealbumin, decreased TLC, and nonreactive skin tests. The patient often appears well nourished and to have normal anthropometric measures. Recall that SA is the major protein contributing to osmotic pressure. It is this pressure that prevents the accumulation of fluid in the interstitial space. In the patient with kwashiorkor, enough protein can be lost that the osmotic pressure is decreased and edema develops.

The two types of protein-energy malnutrition may not be different entities but rather different responses to a decrease in energy and protein. Marasmus presents as an adaptive response to the physiologic stress of inadequate intake, while kwashiorkor is a maladaptive response resulting from the added physiologic stress of illness. A combination of the two protein-energy malnutrition categories is often seen in critically ill patients, in whom decreased intake and physiologic stress are both present. There is loss of both somatic and visceral protein, with changes seen in both anthropometric and biochemical parameters.

Malnutrition (inability to meet protein and calorie needs) in the critically ill patient can be related to increased basal metabolism secondary to the illness, to iatrogenic starvation, and to alteration of nutrient metabolic pathways. The resulting loss of tissue, the decreased organ function, and the decreased work capacity of the malnourished patient lead to further diminishment in the ability to respond to stress. Acute stress produces strains on the existing or remaining energy reserve. The malnourished patient will benefit from carefully selected nutritional support aimed at energy and nitrogen balance. Rebuilding of tissue (anabolism) is most effective during the adaptive phase of the catabolic response, when the patient is capable of more efficient use of nutrition supplied.

Effect of Malnutrition on Specific Systems

Cardiovascular System

The cardiovascular system is not spared the effects of malnutrition. Deficiencies in thiamine and selenium can directly cause cardiomyopathy. Protein-energy malnutrition as seen in the acutely ill patient can result in visceral protein loss and decreases in myocardial function.[16] A decrease in heart size and atrophy of cardiac muscle could result in decreased cardiac output. The increase in extracellular fluid commonly associated with physiologic stress could further compromise cardiac output. In compensation, the cardiac muscle fibers lengthen in response to increased work load. This compensation, together with a decreased oxygen demand secondary to decreased intake, curtails the development of cardiac failure. However, if the cardiac muscle is diseased, malnutrition will contribute to uncompensated heart failure.

Even though heart failure in the malnourished patient can be compensated, heart failure is common even in the healthy heart when starvation is corrected by refeeding. Refeeding increases the metabolism of the stressed state, resulting in increased cardiac output to meet oxygen demands. This added stress could lead to heart failure. In addition, providing a high-carbohydrate diet (RQ = 1) during the refeeding period would increase carbon dioxide production, re-

sulting in an increased work of breathing. This places further demand on the heart. It is necessary to provide some of the energy needs with fat to decrease the carbon dioxide production. The patient needs to resume feeding with caution and must be carefully monitored for signs and symptoms of cardiac failure. Additionally, rapid weight loss secondary to malnutrition has been associated with ventricular dysfunction and dysrhythmias, so that cardiac monitoring is an essential component in care of the patient.

Cardiac cachexia associated with chronic congestive heart failure promotes malnutrition. The mechanisms involved in cardiac cachexia are shown in Figure 56–5. A vicious cycle exists, with congestive heart failure causing malnutrition and malnutrition contributing further to the congestive heart failure.

Respiratory System

Malnutrition affects the ability of the lungs to function. It decreases the structure of the lung parenchyma, as protein is used for energy and an overall decrease in protein synthesis occurs. This structural alteration can cause increased lung compliance (stiff lungs), resulting in an increased work of breathing.[17] Respiratory muscle function is decreased as a result of visceral protein loss, affecting both endurance and contractility.

Patients with malnutrition often present with decreased vital capacity and decreased respiratory muscle strength. If vital capacity and muscle strength fall below 50 percent of predicted norms, respiratory failure is likely, owing to retention of carbon dioxide. Malnutrition also decreases the immune response within the lung. Surfactant stability is decreased, contributing to decreased lung compliance and microatelectasis. The result of an alteration in immune function and structural changes is an increase in respiratory tract infections. Infections develop easily and are not controlled by the protein-based immune system. The consequences of energy deficit in lung disease are summarized in Figure 56–6. When a patient has respiratory distress and increased work of breathing, the caloric requirement for breathing alone can increase 10 times normal. Inadequate intake and increased utilization contribute further to the effects of malnutrition on the respiratory system.

Immune System

An increased rate of infection seen in malnourished patients secondary to the depression of the immune system and defense mechanisms is caused by nutrient deficiency. Changes in the immune system vary according to the type of nutrient lacking (Table 56–14). For example, lack of protein can impair the immune response differently from that of other nutrients.[18] As previously mentioned cellular immunity (delayed cutaneous hypersensitivity), which is needed for reaction to an antigen in skin testing, is often depressed in the undernourished patient. In addition, TLC decreases. Thus the normal reaction that occurs with

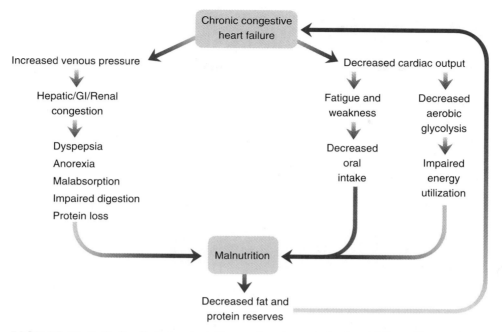

FIGURE 56–5. Cyclic effect of malnutrition on chronic congestive heart failure. GI, gastrointestinal.

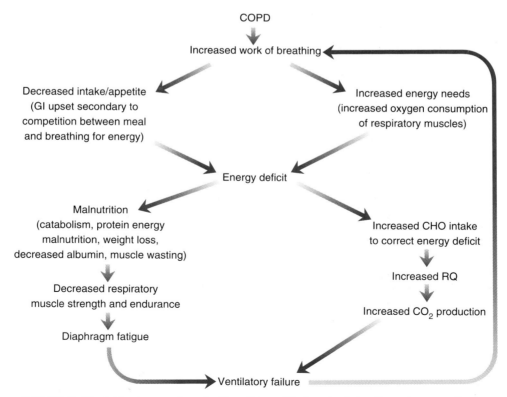

FIGURE 56–6. The increased work of breathing with chronic obstructive pulmonary disease (COPD). CHO, carbohydrate; RQ, respiratory quotient; CO_2, carbon dioxide; GI, gastrointestinal.

TABLE 56–14. Effects of Deficiency of Selected Nutrients on Immunity

Deficient Nutrient	Immune System Change
Vitamin C	Decreased mobility of neutrophils
Vitamin A	Lymphoid tissue atrophy
Vitamin B group	Lymphoid tissue atrophy
Amino acids	Decreased immunoglobulins, interferons, and acute phase proteins
Fatty acids	Impaired lymphocyte function
Iron	Decreased bactericidal activity of phagocytes
Zinc	Lymphoid tissue atrophy
Selenium	Decreased antibody production

antigen stimulation is absent or decreased in malnutrition secondary to both a decreased synthesis of immune system cells and a decrease in the antibody response to stimulation (humoral immunity).

Malnutrition also causes a decrease in lymphoid mass, a decrease in circulating T- and B-lymphocytes, depression of phagocytic function, and a decrease in complement activity. The overall result is a decrease in resistance and increased infection rate. In the critical care setting the number of invasive procedures and indwelling lines is high, increasing the potential for infection and complicating the patient's recovery.

KEY CONCEPTS

- Acute physiologic stress results in activation of the sympathetic nervous system. The immediate phase is characterized by a high metabolic rate, sustained catabolism, hyperglycemia, and salt and water retention. The sympathetic response promotes use of protein stores for gluconeogenesis, resulting in negative nitrogen balance. Fat stores are poorly utilized.

- After 5 to 7 days of acute physiologic stress, the body may enter an adaptive phase, which more closely resembles the normal response to starvation. Ketones and fatty acids from lipolysis of fat stores are used for energy, and body proteins are conserved. Glucose utilization improves and hyperglycemia resolves. Aldosterone secretion diminishes and edema resolves. During the adaptive phase, nutrients supplied to the body are used more efficiently than during the immediate phase.

- Physiologic stress increases energy and protein requirements. An increase in needed calories of 20 to 50 percent above baseline is typical. Because glucose is poorly utilized during the immediate phase, carbohydrate intake is managed to avoid exacerbation of hyperglycemia and excessive carbon dioxide production. Protein should supply about 16 percent of total energy needs. Fats are given to fill the remaining caloric requirements. Vitamin and mineral replacement may also be required.

- Obesity is defined as a weight 20 percent or more above ideal weight for height and build. Upper body obesity increases the risk for diabetes and ath-erosclerosis. Weight gain is associated with increased blood pressure, blood lipids, and serum glucose levels. Excessive fat stores may mask protein-energy malnutrition.

- Protein-energy malnutrition may result from inadequate caloric intake (marasmus), from physiologic stress (kwashiorkor), or from a combination of the two. Marasmus results in loss of somatic protein and fat stores with preservation of visceral protein. It can be detected best by anthropometric measurements (e.g., body weight less than 80 percent of ideal). Kwashiorkor is associated with loss of visceral protein and is best assessed by biochemical tests (e.g., decreased blood proteins and lymphocyte function). A combination of protein malnutrition types is common in critically ill individuals, in whom physiologic stress is associated with poor nutrient intake.

- The cardiovascular, respiratory, and immune systems are particularly susceptible to the effects of malnutrition. Cardiac atrophy and reduced cardiac output may be associated with heart failure, particularly during refeeding, which increases the myocardial work load. Respiratory muscle atrophy and fatigue and deficient surfactant production impair effective respiration. Immune system depression is associated with an increased risk of infection.

Effects of Physiologic Stressors on Nutritional Requirements

Infection, Sepsis, and Fever

A complex interaction exists between the development of infection, the immune system, and nutritional intake.[19] Malnutrition contributes to the infectious process by directly depressing the immune system. This depression impairs the patient's defense mechanism, opening the path for infection to grow unchecked. Infection then potentiates malnutrition through a variety of mechanisms.

Fever is a common symptom accompanying infection. Fever increases metabolic needs by 7 percent for each 1°F increase (13 percent for each 1°C increase). Energy requirements can increase by 40 percent when a high fever (above 104°C) is present. The metabolic response to fever is both anabolic and catabolic, which greatly increases nutrient requirements.

It is known that peptide mediators stimulated by macrophages initiate the metabolic alterations associated with infection. The mediator-stimulated response is summarized in Figure 56–7. This process is complex, with the need for protein synthesis requiring the availability of amino acids.[20] Although catabolism may be detrimental in some aspects, it is also a protective mechanism that provides needed substrates for activation of the immune response to infection. Nutritional support is often aimed at decreasing catabolism, but it is also important to provide substrate (amino

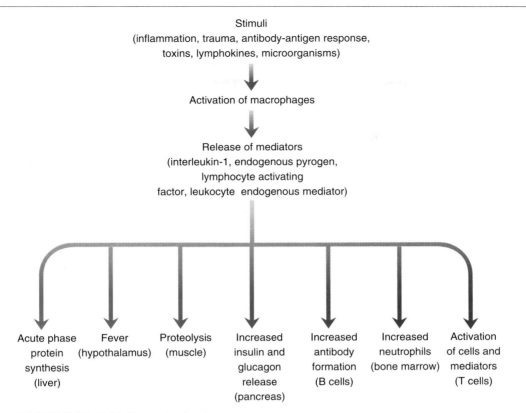

Stimuli
(inflammation, trauma, antibody-antigen response,
toxins, lymphokines, microorganisms)

↓

Activation of macrophages

↓

Release of mediators
(interleukin-1, endogenous pyrogen,
lymphocyte activating
factor, leukocyte endogenous mediator)

| Acute phase protein synthesis (liver) | Fever (hypothalamus) | Proteolysis (muscle) | Increased insulin and glucagon release (pancreas) | Increased antibody formation (B cells) | Increased neutrophils (bone marrow) | Activation of cells and mediators (T cells) |

FIGURE 56-7. Mediator-stimulated response.

acids) for the protective mechanisms that catabolism supports.

Infection is a stressor that increases energy expenditure as a result of fever, increased immune cell demand, and catabolism. The body's metabolic response to the infection is to increase available glucose. Often the demand is too great for the body to manage, considering that sepsis can increase the energy expenditure 20 percent to 60 percent above basal energy requirements. Nutritional support is needed to supply additional energy and the necessary substrates so that body stores are not totally depleted.

Surgery

Ensuring nutritional adequacy before and after surgery promotes wound healing, decreases complications, prevents infection, and decreases mortality. It is critical to get a patient in the most positive nutritional status possible before surgery.[21] A common cause of malnutrition in the postoperative patient is starvation. The combination of poor presurgical nutritional status with postoperative starvation can result in increased nutritional risk, with increased complications postoperatively, such as wound dehiscence. The addition of the stressor, surgery, to a poor nutritional status and postoperative starvation results in both increased metabolism and inability to meet the patient's energy needs.

Nutritional needs in the postoperative period depend on the extent and type of surgery, as well as the presurgical nutritional status. The postoperative energy requirement can increase from 10 to 35 percent above the basal metabolic rate. Frequently postoperative oral intake is delayed in critically ill patients well beyond the return of bowel function. This combination of increased need with decreased intake can have a major impact on wound healing. The functions of various nutrients in wound healing have been long established and are listed in Table 56–15. In addition, nitrogen loss through wounds can be large, establishing a greater need for increased protein intake. A protein intake sufficient to replace losses and to promote anabolism will be required, together with nonprotein calories for energy requirements. As with every patient, individual assessment and determination of exact needs are required.

Trauma

The general catabolic response to stress is also seen in the trauma patient.[22] Energy expenditure is increased by 15 to 30 percent. Increased carbohydrate intake will be needed, but the nurse must watch for complications of high carbohydrate intake. Nitrogen loss can be high secondary to catabolism and cellular damage. Circulating hormones in the immediate phase have an anti-insulin effect that decreases glucose utilization; therefore, gluconeogenesis is increased to meet energy needs. As with other stress states, the catabolism of protein provides a source of amino acids for acute phase protein synthesis. Be-

T A B L E 56 – 15. Role of Nutrients in Wound Healing

Nutrient	Role in Wound Healing
Proteins (amino acids and albumin)	Maintain osmotic pressure to decrease edema; maintain cell-mediated immune responses; cellular proliferation, including neurovascular components, lymphocytes, and fibroblasts
Carbohydrates (glucose)	Meet energy requirements of cells involved in healing process and prevention of infection
Fats (essential fatty acids)	Components of cellular membranes; building blocks for prostaglandins, which regulate cellular function
Vitamins	Roles in cellular function, including capillary function and formation, enzyme cofactors, immune cell function, clotting mechanism, calcium and phosphorus metabolism, collagen synthesis
Minerals	Roles in cellular function, including oxygen transport, immune cell function, collagen synthesis, cellular proliferation

cause trauma is a sudden stress, catabolism is much greater than anabolism because there is no time for replenishment of proteins lost. This results in excessive negative nitrogen balance and significant loss of skeletal muscle, which will be a problem in posttrauma rehabilitation.

With other physiologic stress, fatty acids cannot be used as a source of energy. In the trauma patient, however, it is thought that fatty acids can be utilized because of extremely high levels of catecholamines, which mobilize fat through the stimulation of lipases. In addition, if glycogen stores are intact, an initial source of glucose and free fatty acids is available. Glucose utilization is maintained in the trauma patient so that glucose is an effective source of energy during the immediate phase. These differences in the nutritional effect of physiologic stress in the trauma patient stem from both the suddenness of the stress and the usually healthy state of the patient prior to admission.

Burns

A burn is an extreme physiologic stressor, resulting in significant hypermetabolism.[23] In addition, loss of the skin barrier increases energy expenditure through evaporative heat loss. The energy needs of the burn patient increase 50 percent to 100 percent from the basal metabolic requirement. Because of individual variations such as preburn nutritional status, other physiologic stresses present, activity level, stage of burn, and age, indirect calorimetry would be the best method for determination of individual needs.

As with other stressors, negative nitrogen balance is contributed to by catabolism and by the use of amino acids in formation of stress proteins. In addition, burn wounds contribute directly to protein loss. Elevation of fatty acids also occurs in response to the release of stress hormones and breakdown of lipoproteins. The ability of the burn patient to utilize this available energy source in the immediate phase is unclear.

Cancer

An increasing number of cancer patients receive support in critical care units over periods of marked physi-

ologic stress during treatment. The nutritional effects of cancer can be severe, resulting in what is commonly termed **cancer cachexia**.[24] Cachexia is associated with the end stage of cancer but can also develop earlier. The cause of cachexia is a decrease in nutritional intake relative to energy requirements. It results in significant weight loss, muscle weakness, and anorexia. A major cause of cachexia is anorexia associated with the malignancy and with the treatment. Sensory changes such as changes in smell or taste can be associated with cancer treatment and malnutrition. These changes can contribute significantly to the anorexia experienced during cancer treatment. Thus, the cancer patient often enters the critical care environment with mild to severe malnutrition.

Beyond the anorexia and sensory changes, abnormalities of intermediate metabolism in cancer promote tissue loss. The normal response to decreased intake is a decreased resting metabolic rate. The abnormalities in substrate metabolism in cancer increase total energy expenditure and raise the resting metabolic rate. The tumor also requires energy for growth—often using anaerobic metabolism, which increases the lactic acid production and promotes an increase in gluconeogenesis. The metabolism of vitamins, minerals, and enzymes is also thought to be altered. Because both nutrient intake and substrate metabolism are altered, nutritional support is difficult to achieve and frequently ineffective in reversing the existing cachexia.

Immobility

The mobility of patients in the critical care unit is restricted, with most patients on total bed rest. The main nutritional effect of immobilization is loss of calcium from nonstressed bone. This can elevate serum calcium and phosphorus levels. This demineralization is best treated with weight bearing as early as possible rather than with calcium supplementation. The physical therapist needs to be consulted early to assist in prevention of demineralization. Because the negative calcium balance can increase in a catabolic state, serum calcium levels need to be monitored and abnormalities treated.

A second effect of immobilization is nitrogen loss, as tissue mass is decreased from disuse atrophy. This loss can total 2 to 3 g/day, requiring up to 10 to 15 grams of protein to replenish the daily loss. This further emphasizes the need for early physical therapy and aggressive range-of-motion exercises.

KEY CONCEPTS

- Infection is associated with fever and an increased metabolic rate. For each 1°F increase in body temperature, metabolic needs increase 7 percent. The synthesis of acute phase proteins and immune factors requires sufficient amino acid substrates.

- A major nutritional problem in postoperative patients is starvation. In addition, nitrogen loss through wounds may be significant.

- Major trauma is associated with a 15 to 30 percent increase in energy expenditure. Glucose utilization is maintained. Trauma victims are usually in good nutritional health prior to admission.

- Major burns are extreme physiologic stressors that result in an increase in energy expenditure of 50 to 100 percent above baseline. Protein loss from burned areas is high.

- Cancer cachexia is a result of several factors, including anorexia, poor intake, and nutrient utilization by tumor cells.

- Immobility is associated with muscle atrophy and bone demineralization.

Summary

Physiologic stress is accompanied by changes in metabolism that alter nutrient utilization and increase nutrient requirements. The degree to which this happens varies with the type and severity of the particular stress. If the patient is not provided with adequate nutrition when one or more stressors are present, the hypermetabolism, hypercatabolism, and negative nitrogen balance associated with the physiologic stress will have detrimental effects on recovery.

Health care professionals must be aware of the impact of stressors on the nutritional status of the body as well as the impact of nutrition on the well-being of body systems. If this is well understood, appropriate interventions can be taken to prevent some of the complications that can develop when nutritional support is inadequate. Most well-nourished patients can tolerate a short time of inadequate intake (about 5 days) without untoward effects. The critically ill patient, however, requires early nutritional support because of the magnitude and intensity of the stressors. Identification of the various risk factors and the nutritional needs of patients is an essential part of nursing care for the critically ill patient. Overfeeding of the patient is also to be avoided, as specific complications can develop with inappropriate nutritional support as well. The nurse must also understand nutritional interventions in critical care so that decisions regarding nutritional support for the patient can be based on specific nutritional assessments and knowledge of individual needs.

REFERENCES

1. Bistrain B: Prevalence of malnutrition in general medical patients. *JAMA* 1976;235:1567–1570.
2. Hills SW: Nutritional aspects of critical care, in Emanuelsen KL, Rosenlicht JM (eds): *Handbook of Critical Care Nursing.* New York, Wiley, 1986.
3. Dempsey DT: The link between nutritional status and clinical outcome: Can nutritional intervention modify it? *Am J Clin Nutr* 1988;47:352–356.
4. Dionigi R: Diagnosing malnutrition. *Gut* 1986;27:(suppl 1):5–8.
5. Bozzetti R: Nutritional assessment from the perspective of a clinician. *JPEN J Parenter Enteral Nutr* 1987;11(suppl 5):115–121.
6. Heymsfield S, Casper K: Anthropometric assessment of the adult hospitalized patient. *JPEN J Parenter Enteral Nutr* 1987;11(55):36–41.
7. Mitchell CO, Lipschitz DA: Arm length measurement as an alternative to height in nutritional assessment in the elderly. *JPEN J Parenter Enterol Nutr* 1982;6(3):226–229.
8. Blackburn GL, Thornton PA: Nutritional assessment of the hospitalized patient. *Med Clin North Am* 1979;63(5):1103.
9. Heymsfield S: Muscle mass: Reliable indicator of protein-energy malnutrition severity and outcome. *Am J Clin Nutr* 1982;35:1192–1199.
10. Blazey ME: Nutritional assessment of protein status. *Dimens Crit Care Nurs* 1986;5(6):328–332.
11. Winkler MF, Gerrior SA, Pomp A, Albina JE: Use of retinol binding protein and prealbumin as indicators of the response to nutritional therapy. *J Am Diet Assoc* 1989;89(5):684–687.
12. Salmond SW: How to assess the nutritional status of acutely ill patients. *Am J Nurs* 1980;80(5):922–923.
13. Buzby GP: Prognostic nutrition index in gastrointestinal surgery. *Am J Surg* 1980;134:160.
14. Krause MV, Mahan LK: *Food, Nutrition, and Diet,* 7th ed. Philadelphia, WB Saunders, 1984.
15. Kinney J, Weissman C: Forms of malnutrition in stressed and unstressed patients. *Clin Chest Med* 1986;7(1):19–28.
16. Webb JG, Keiss MC, Chan-Yan CC: Malnutrition and the heart. *Can Med Assoc J* 1986;135:753–757.
17. Openbrier D, Covey M: Ineffective breathing pattern related to malnutrition. *Nurs Clin North Am* 1987;22(1):225–247.
18. Beisel W: Role of nutrition in immune system diseases. *Compr Ther* 1987;13(1):13–19.
19. Keusch G, Farthing M: Nutrition and infection. *Annu Rev Nutr* 1986;6:131–154.
20. Pomposelli J: Role of biochemical mediators in clinical nutrition and surgical metabolism. *JPEN J Parenter Enteral Nutr* 1988;12(2):212–218.
21. Bellanton R: Preoperative parenteral nutrition in the high risk surgical patient. *JPEN J Parenter Enteral Nutr* 1988;12(2):115–121.
22. Anderson B: The metabolic needs of head trauma victims. *J Neurosci Nurs* 1987;19(4):211–215.
23. Lang CE: *Nutritional Support in Critical Care.* Gaithersburg, Md, Aspen, 1987.
24. Kern K, Norton J: Cancer cachexia. *JPEN J Parenter Enteral Nutr* 1988;12(3):286–298.

BIBLIOGRAPHY

Abbott W, Blackburn GL: Nutritional support in hospitalized patients, in Zschoche DA (ed): *Comprehensive Review of Critical Care.* St. Louis, CV Mosby, 1986, pp 254–267.
Berger R, Adams L: Nutritional support in the critical care setting (part 1). *Chest* 1989;96(1):139–150.
Berger R, Adams L: Nutritional support in the critical care setting (part 2). *Chest* 1989;96(2):372–380.
Bower R: Nutrition and immune fraction. *Nutr Clin Pract* 1990;5(5):189–195.

Curtas S: Evaluation of nutritional status. *Nurs Clin North Am* 1989;24(2):301–313.

Davis J, Sherer K: *Applied Nutrition and Diet Therapy for Nurses,* 2nd ed. Philadelphia, WB Saunders, 1994.

Harwood A: Malnourishment in the ICU. *Intensive Care Nurs* 1990;6(4):205–208.

Hennessy K: Nutritional support and gastrointestinal disease. *Nurs Clin North Am* 1989;24(2):373–382.

Kirpatrik JR: *Nutrition and Metabolism in the Surgical Patient.* Mount Kisco, NY, Futura, 1983.

Knox LS: Ethical issues in nutritional support nursing: Withholding and withdrawing nutritional support. *Nurs Clin North Am* 1989;24(2):427–436.

Mahan LK, Arlin MT: *Krause's Food, Nutrition and Diet Therapy,* 8th ed. Philadelphia, WB Saunders, 1992.

Marvin JA: Nutritional support of the critically injured patient. *Crit Care Nurs Q* 1988;11(2):21–34.

Mattox T, Teasley-Strausburg KM: Overview of biochemical markers for nutrition support. *Drug Intelligence and Clinical Pharmacology (The Annals of Pharmacotherapy)* 1991;25(3):265–271.

Michelsen CB, Askanazi T: The metabolic response to injury: Mechanisms and clinical implications. *J Bone Joint Surg [Am]* 1986;68-A(5):782–787.

Poleman CM, Peckenpaugh NJ: *Nutrition: Essentials and Diet Therapy.* Philadelphia, WB Saunders, 1991.

Schlichtig R, Ayres S: *Nutritional Support of the Critically Ill.* Chicago, Year Book Medical Publishers, 1988.

Weinsier RL, Butterwork CE: *Handbook of Clinical Nutrition,* 2nd ed. St. Louis, CV Mosby, 1989.

CHAPTER 57
Human System Response to Special Care Units

BARBARA BARTZ

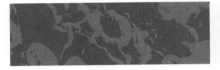

KEY TERMS

intensive care unit psychosis: A transient and reversible episode of psychological impairment occurring during hospitalization in an intensive care unit.

sensory deprivation: Loss of usual sensory input, such as the patient's normal daily routine and contact with family members and the community.

sensory overload: Excessive exposure to unfamiliar environmental stimulation in the hospital such as noise, light, sleep interruptions, and painful experiences.

sleep deprivation: Loss of the usual quantity and quality of sleep; lack of normal progression through sleep stages.

transfer anxiety: Anxiety occurring in reaction to an anticipated move to another unit, for example, a move from the intensive care unit to an acute care unit.

Admission to a critical care unit is invariably associated with psychosocial as well as physiologic problems. The patient, family, and friends must cope with an often unexpected admission to an environment where critical illness is the norm and death is a possible outcome. Intensive care units (ICUs) are designed to facilitate frequent monitoring and treatment of critically ill individuals. While necessary, these functions are usually in conflict with the needs of the patient for rest and social support. Health care professionals are in a position to decrease the negative impact of the critical care environment on patients and their visitors and to assist patients, families, and others in coping with the psychosocial as well as the physiologic aspects of having a severe illness or injury.

This chapter presents information about potential psychosocial responses to a severe illness or sudden traumatic event. Environmental stressors of the critical care environment are discussed. Finally, the impact of critical illness on those who care for these patients is described. Chapter 7 of this text also presents helpful information about human responses to stress and the role of homeostasis.

Psychosocial Responses to Severe Illness or Trauma

Factors Affecting Psychosocial Responses

Psychosocial responses to injury or illness are affected by such factors as the patient's personal background, reason for hospitalization, social support system, and medical therapies, and are unique to each patient. One important factor in determining psychosocial response to a special care unit is whether the admission has been planned or is unplanned. The response when a patient is admitted after a planned surgery is likely to be far different than when the admission results from an unexpected illness or trauma (Fig. 57–1).[1] Other factors affecting the psychosocial response include length of stay and the adequacy of the family's financial resources. The age and developmental level of the patient greatly influence the response to hospitalization.[2] Another factor in determining the reaction of both patient and family to a severe illness is the usual role of the patient in the family. Careful assessment of the individual patient and the family unit is necessary to determine the psychosocial response to critical illness and appropriate interventions. Factors for the nurse to consider in assessing psychological reactions to critical illness are shown in Table 57–1.

Emotional Responses to Critical Illness

Usual emotional responses to illness may be intensified when hospitalization in a special care unit is required. Emotions such as fear and anxiety, and feelings of isolation, powerlessness, and helplessness are

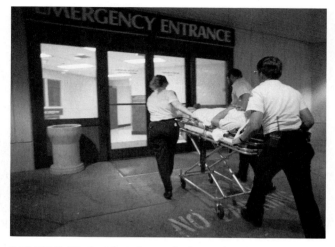

FIGURE 57–1. Admission to the hospital and the special care unit is frequently unexpected and the result of sudden illness or trauma. (Photograph courtesy of St. Elizabeth Medical Center, Yakima, Wash.)

frequently experienced. In the case of a sudden trauma or unexpected illness, patients admitted to the critical care unit frequently have sustained a major loss of some kind. Denial, anger, guilt, depression, and sadness may be seen as part of their gradual adaptation to this loss. Finally, hope is a potential positive response to critical illness. Potential emotional responses to severe illness or injury are summarized in Table 57–2.

Fear and Anxiety

Fear and anxiety are very common responses to critical illness and may result not only from being in a life-threatening situation, but also from anticipation of painful procedures.[1] Manifestations of fear and anxiety may include poor concentration, restlessness, and

TABLE 57–1. Factors Affecting Psychosocial Responses to Critical Illness

Situational Factors

Whether admission is planned or unplanned
Type of illness or injury
Length of stay in special care unit
Previous admissions to special care units

Sociological Factors

Financial resources and insurance status
Role of patient in family or social group
Social support available

Personal Factors

Age and developmental level
Spiritual belief system
Intellectual abilities
Ability to communicate
Level of consciousness
Sensory alterations

TABLE 57-2. Emotional Responses to Severe Illness or Injury

Emotional Response	Intervention
Fear and anxiety	Be available to patient and family Conduct preoperative teaching Educate patient and family about procedures Facilitate pain control Encourage family visits Provide hope for the future Prepare carefully for transfer from unit
Isolation	Establish flexible visiting hours Encourage family visits Include family in patient care Encourage the presence of family pictures and personal possessions Provide telephone, if possible Use newspapers and television to maintain contact with normal events
Powerlessness and helplessness	Encourage independence in some aspects of care Include patient and family in decision-making Provide structured situations for decision-making
Denial	Allow denial as defense from unbearable anxiety Reinforce need for care and activity restrictions Reflect inaccurate patient statements back to patient Monitor for potentially harmful behaviors
Anger	Listen to and acknowledge expressions of anger Avoid defending staff, physicians, and hospital Assist family members when anger is directed toward them Acknowledge reasons for anger and make changes if possible
Guilt	Recognize feelings of guilt Explain that illnesses are multifactorial, not due to just one cause
Depression	Acknowledge feelings of depression Encourage family visits Provide hope for future
Sadness	Acknowledge feelings of sadness Accept crying or other expressions of sadness Provide hope for future
Hope	Convey positive expectations to patient Encourage family visits Assist patient and family in setting realistic short-term goals Allow patient control over decisions

irritability, as well as verbalized statements of fear. Physiologic signs such as tachycardia, sweating, and a dry mouth may also indicate anxiety. A common psychological reaction to an anxiety-provoking situation is denial of the seriousness of the condition. **Transfer anxiety** may develop when the patient is discharged from the special care unit to an area where there is less monitoring and nurse–patient contact.[3,4] A patient with transfer anxiety may state that he or she does not feel ready to move out of the ICU or may even develop physiologic symptoms such as arrhythmias or chest pain as transfer becomes imminent.

Isolation

Isolation of the patient from significant persons and things and from the events of normal life may result in intense feelings of loneliness (Fig. 57–2). The patient may appear withdrawn and quiet or may call the nurse into the room frequently for minor requests.[1,5]

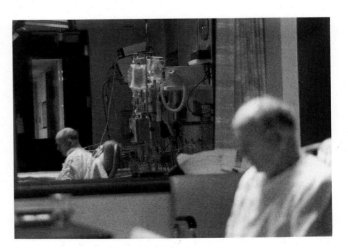

FIGURE 57–2. Isolation from the normal events of daily life and from interactions with one's family or other significant persons can cause intense feelings of loneliness in the critically ill patient. (Photographer: Elizabeth Green, Seattle, Wash.)

Helplessness and Powerlessness

Feelings of helplessness and powerlessness may be seen, related to the patient's dependence on others for even basic aspects of daily life. Behaviors seen in the patient who is feeling powerless may include lack of motivation, a low level of learning, and statements indicating feelings of victimization, fatalism, and incapability.[6]

Adaptation to Loss

Many types of physical or psychosocial loss may occur during severe acute illness. Patients may have lost their self-image as healthy persons, or permanent loss of function or of a body part may have occurred. If the patient is an infant or child, the parents may have lost their image of an expected happy outcome to pregnancy or healthy child. Adaptation to loss has been described as occurring in four, somewhat sequential stages: (1) shock and disbelief, (2) development of awareness, (3) restitution, and (4) resolution.[7]

Shock and Disbelief

During the phase of shock and disbelief, the most frequently utilized coping mechanism is denial. Anxiety is the underlying cause of this reaction; the patient's anxiety is so great that it can be dealt with only by denying that there is cause for fear. Patients and significant others may appear numb and uncomprehending. Alternative explanations to the illness may be presented. For example, a patient who has suffered a myocardial infarction may state that the pain was due to indigestion. The patient is unable to absorb the implications of the illness, so that behaviors detrimental to the patient's health, such as insisting on getting out of bed, may occur.[7,8]

Development of Awareness

As denial becomes less effective as a defense mechanism, patients begin to develop an awareness of the illness. "Why me?" is a question that the patient confronts. Depression occurs as the reality of the illness or injury is accepted. Depression may be seen as sadness or withdrawal; irritability may also be a sign of depression. Anger and guilt are frequent reactions as the reality of the loss is absorbed. Anger may be directed internally, and guilt may be expressed relative to behaviors that may have contributed to the illness or injury. Anger may also be directed at caregivers or significant others.[7,8]

Restitution

Restitution is characterized by beginning acceptance of the illness and the resultant changes in life-style. Sadness is a dominant emotional response during this phase. Individuals may spend a great deal of time talking about the illness or injury and about fears for the future.[7]

Resolution

During the phase of resolution, the patient comes to terms with any permanent limitations or life-style changes that have resulted from the injury or illness and incorporates these changes into a new self-image.[7]

The final stages of adaptation to loss are usually seen after the patient is discharged from the ICU. However, it must be emphasized that adaptation to loss is accomplished in a unique way by each individual and family and does not necessarily occur in linear fashion. Patients may adapt to different aspects of their loss at different times; thus, behaviors typical of several stages may be present simultaneously.

Positive Emotional Responses in Special Care Units

Patients may also have positive psychological responses to critical care units. In a recent study by Rowe and Weinert,[9] patients indicated that some aspects of the coronary care unit environment were reassuring and comforting. The authors speculated that the equipment and treatment gave patients the sense of being cared for and closely monitored.[9] Another response that may be seen in critically ill patients is hope.[10,11] Caregivers can foster hope through conveying positive expectations to patients, encouraging family visitation, assisting patients in setting achievable goals, and allowing patients control over decisions when possible. The coping mechanism of denial may allow the patient to be hopeful.[11]

Psychosocial Responses in Children

An important factor to consider in hospitalized children is the developmental level of the child, which will affect the response to the hospital setting (Fig. 57–3). Psychological, social, motor, and cognitive development must be considered when assessing and planning care for children and adolescents. Young children may not have the cognitive ability to understand the reason for hospitalization or that hospitalization is a temporary situation. The loss for them is likely to be more immediate; separation from family members and inability to do their normal activities will be stressful to them.[12] Older children and adolescents, while better able to understand the reasons for hospitalization, may be more affected by potential changes in body image and separation from peers.[2] Developmental tasks and characteristics, the potential impact of intensive care, and some suggestions for addressing psychosocial issues in children and adolescents are described in Table 57–3.

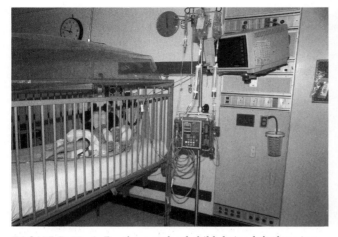

FIGURE 57–3. For the preschool child, being left alone is a major stressor associated with hospitalization. Familiar toys can be used to assist in decreasing the child's anxiety when parents cannot be with the child. (Photograph courtesy of St. Elizabeth Medical Center, Yakima, Wash.)

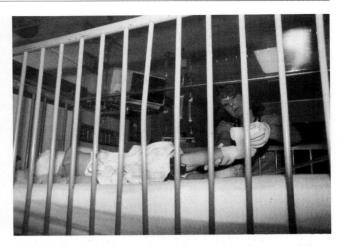

FIGURE 57–4. Play can be used to teach and prepare children for procedures such as dressing changes. (Photograph courtesy of St. Elizabeth Medical Center, Yakima, Wash.)

TABLE 57–3. Developmental Aspects in the Care of Critically Ill Children

Developmental Tasks and Characteristics	Potential Impact of Special Care Unit	Interventions
Preterm Infant or Low-Birth-Weight Infant		
Task: Physical, motor, and nervous system development to normal neonate level *Characteristics:* Vary according to gestational age Limp posture Jerky, irregular movements Energy used for growth Vital sign changes, behavioral changes are indicators of stress	Stress due to excessive tactile, visual, and auditory stimulation Parental feelings of anxiety, helplessness, incompetence	Assess response to gentle touch Minimize noise levels, artificial lighting Provide rest periods between caregiving activities Modify care routines according to individual reaction to procedures Update parents on infant's status frequently Encourage parental involvement in care Teach parents assessment and caretaking skills
Neonate (birth (gestational age ≥ 37 wk) to 1 mo)		
Task: Parent-infant bonding Sibling-infant bonding *Characteristics:* Crying a major form of communication Little tolerance for delayed gratification	Loss of normal parental caretaking role Loss of sibling contact Inability to cry if intubated	Encourage parental involvement in care Encourage sibling visits Individualize visiting hours to parent needs Assess intubated neonate for signs of distress other than crying
Infant (1–12 mo)		
Task: Development of trusting relationship with the parent or primary caregiver *Characteristics:* Crying, then cooing, babbling for verbal communication Rapid motor and cognitive development Stranger anxiety at about 8 months	Separation from parents and family life Monitoring equipment, therapies may decrease mobility and ability to learn about own body Isolation from typical stimulants to growth and development	Encourage parental involvement in care Flexible visiting hours Restrain infant as little as possible with equipment Incorporate age-appropriate toys in care (mirrors, mobiles, tapes of parent and sibling voices)

Table continued on following page

TABLE 57–3. Developmental Aspects in the Care of Critically Ill Children Continued

Developmental Tasks and Characteristics	Potential Impact of Special Care Unit	Interventions
Toddler (12 mo–3 yr)		
Task: Development of sense of autonomy *Characteristics:* Verbal abilities grow from one word to short phrases Negativism Rituals important Toilet training at end of this period Separation anxiety	Regression from prehospitalization toilet training, language, and self-care skills Despair due to separation from parents Loss of usual rituals	Flexible visiting hours Encourage parental involvement in care Use transitional objects like familiar blankets or toys to reduce separation anxiety Observe rituals child has used at home Reassure parents and child that regression is not unusual or permanent Use play for teaching (Fig. 57–4) Encourage independence with feeding, dressing as possible Allow control over some aspects of care Incorporate toys such as videotapes, audiotaped stories, talking toys
Pre-Schooler (3–6 yr)		
Task: Development of sense of initiative *Characteristics:* Vocabulary increases Ask many questions Enjoy imitative play Fears of pain, dark, being left alone Separation anxiety decreases Conscience begins to develop	Threats to bodily integrity from procedures Anticipation and fear of painful procedures Anxiety because of being left alone May view hospitalization as punishment	Give concrete answers to questions Use play to demonstrate procedures, talk about fears Encourage consistent visiting pattern by parents Stay with patient, or arrange care so patient is not alone Leave at least one light on
School Age (6–11 yr)		
Task: Development of a sense of industry and competence *Characteristics:* Increasing ability to use language Perception of time maturing Focus still on present Concrete thinking Peer relationships become important Privacy becoming important	Loss of opportunities for accomplishment Separation from peers and normal social activities Unable to conceptualize discharge from intensive care Lack of privacy is distressing	Use drawings, toys, and verbal explanations for teaching Maintain contact with school and social activities Maintain privacy as much as possible Provide opportunities to successfully learn and demonstrate new skills
Adolescent (12–18 yr)		
Task: Development of sense of identity and self-concept *Characteristics:* Well-developed cognitive abilities Able to think beyond present Rapid physical growth, including sexual maturity Preoccupation with body image Conflict with parents frequently occurs Peers very important Emotionally labile	Changes in appearance or body function Separation from peers and usual social activities Anxiety and anger regarding body-revealing procedures	Have adolescent use own clothing Provide opportunities for grooming Tape player for music of choice Oral and written explanations can be understood Discuss teaching, options for care with adolescent independently from parents Provide telephone and privacy for conversations with peers

Family Responses to Critical Illness

The responses of family members are similar to those of patients. Typical emotional reactions include anxiety and fear, shock and denial, helplessness, anger and hostility, guilt, depression, grief, withdrawal, and hope (Fig. 57–5).[4,13,14] Adaptation to loss occurs in family members as well as patients, although the perceived loss will be different. For example, family members may experience the loss of the patient as wage earner, head of household, or caregiver, depending on which roles the patient has filled in the family. Again, the experience is unique to each family, and individualized assessment is necessary to provide appropriate assistance to families of critically ill patients. Progression through the stages of adaptation to loss can occur at different times in the family and the patient.

Family members may experience anticipatory grieving if they perceive that the patient is likely to

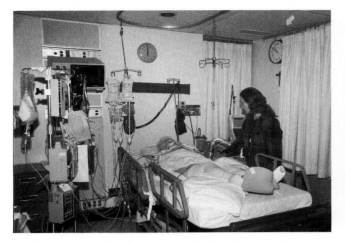

FIGURE 57 – 5. The array of technical equipment in intensive care may be intimidating to visitors. The health care professional can decrease this anxiety by assisting visitors to find a place at the bedside where they can be near the patient. (Photograph courtesy of St. Elizabeth Medical Center, Yakima, Wash.)

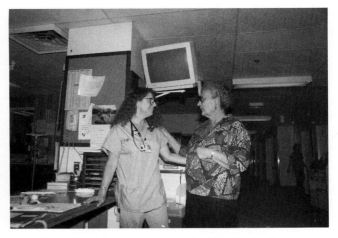

FIGURE 57 – 6. Important needs identified by family members of critically ill patients include the need for information about the patient, the need for hope, and the need to feel that staff members care about the patient. (Photograph courtesy of St. Elizabeth Medical Center, Yakima, Wash.)

die. These painful feelings may cause family members to cease visiting or to withdraw from emotional contact with the patient—although the patient may have a strong emotional need to visit with family.

Recent nursing research indicates that the most important perceived needs of family members include the need to feel hope, the need for information about the patient's prognosis and treatment, the need to feel that the patient is receiving optimal care, and the need to feel that the staff cares about the patient (Fig. 57–6).[15] Other family needs are frequent visits with the patient and the opportunity to talk with the patient's physician daily.[16] When the patient is a parent, the ages and developmental levels of the children must be considered in assessing family needs.

In addition to the usual stresses associated with the admission of a family member to a special care unit, additional anxieties arise when the patient is a child. Parents of pediatric patients frequently indicate that alterations in the parenting role are the most stressful aspect of having a critically ill child (Fig. 57–7). Other major stressors for parents include the child's appearance, emotional status, and behaviors.[17]

KEY CONCEPTS

- The psychosocial response to hospitalization in a critical care unit is affected by length of stay, financial resources, and whether the treatment is planned or unplanned. Age and developmental level of both the patient and visitors affect the response to hospitalization.

- Common emotional responses to critical illness are fear, anxiety, and feelings of helplessness and powerlessness. Frequent painful procedures, the potential for imminent death, and dependence on others for nearly all aspects of daily life perpetuate these emotions.

- Critically ill individuals may progress through four phases of grieving during hospitalization. These stages are (1) shock and disbelief, (2) development of awareness, (3) restitution, and (4) resolution. Depression, anger, guilt, and sadness may be expressed during the grieving process.

- Separation anxiety may be the predominant emotion in young children separated from parents during critical illness.

- Families experience emotions and grieving responses similar to the patient's. The primary needs expressed by families of critically ill patients are (1) to feel hope, (2) to visit freely, (3) to receive information, and (4) to know that the patient is receiving optimal treatment from a caring staff.

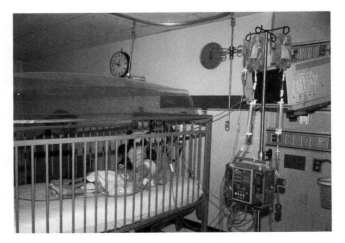

FIGURE 57 – 7. A major stressor described by parents of critically ill children is the alteration in the parenting role. It is essential to both parent and child that the parents be encouraged to participate actively in caring for the child. (Photograph courtesy of St. Elizabeth Medical Center, Yakima, Wash.)

Stressors Within the Critical Care Environment

In addition to the stress associated with severe illness, the environment of an ICU produces iatrogenic stress. Patients may suffer from **sensory overload,** as they are almost constantly exposed to a variety of new and unpleasant experiences. **Sensory deprivation** may also occur owing to isolation from usual stimuli. Stressors intrinsic to the ICU include environmental factors such as noise levels, frequent interruptions for observation or therapy, and the presence of unfamiliar surroundings and equipment.[11,18,19] Other stressors are pain and discomfort, social isolation from significant others, and the administration of multiple pharmacologic interventions with a high potential for drug interactions that may affect cognitive and emotional function.[11,19,20]

These factors, together with the almost constant presence of artificial light and the lack of natural light, cause a marked decline in both the quantity and quality of sleep, and **sleep deprivation,** a major stressor.[19,21–23] Fatigue and confusion are common in these patients due to the interruptions of normal day-night cycling and sleep loss. The phenomenon known as **intensive care unit psychosis** results in many patients partly as a reaction to the environmental haz-ards in critical care areas of the hospital.[19,20] These are discussed further later in this chapter. Potential environmental stressors associated with critical care units are described in Table 57–4, and some helpful interventions are suggested.

Noise

Sound intensity or loudness is measured in decibel (dB) units. An increase in intensity of 10 dB is perceived as approximately twice as loud by the human ear. A whisper represents about 30 dB, normal conversation registers at 50 dB, and a radio at full volume registers 60 dB.[24] The International Noise Council has recommended constant noise levels of no greater than 45 dB during the day and 20 dB at night. Research has consistently found hospital noise levels to be greater than recommended levels.[3,18]

Hilton studied noise levels in a variety of ICU settings.[18] Microphones placed at the head of patient beds recorded average continuous noise levels ranging from 48.5 to 68.5 dB in large open ICUs and from 32.5 to 57 dB in smaller units with private rooms. The noise levels of such constantly functioning equipment as oxygen delivery systems, chest tube bubbling, and ventilators ranged from 49 to 70 dB. Intermittent events such as raising and lowering bed rails regis-

TABLE 57–4. Suggested Interventions to Alleviate Stressors Within the Special Care Unit Environment

Stressor	Intervention
Noise	Avoid unnecessary talk among staff members Avoid calling or shouting Choose equipment that makes minimal noise Use architectural devices (carpet, curtains, insulation) to reduce noise Use noise-producing supplies away from the bedside, if possible
Frequent interruptions	Cluster patient care Evaluate need to disturb patient
Unfamiliar surroundings	Educate patient about unit equipment and procedures Encourage family visits Encourage family to bring photographs and personal belongings
Isolation	Encourage visits by family members Use television, newspapers, and radio for sensory stimuli Individually assess need for telephone Comforting touch may be helpful Use alternative means of communication if the patient is unable to communicate orally or verbally
Polypharmacy	Assess drug interactions, especially in elderly patients Monitor for potential medication side effects and interactions Promote sleep and relaxation with nonpharmaceutical interventions
Lack of sleep	Cluster care when possible Maintain normal day-night lighting and activity levels Provide adequate pain control Minimize noise levels, especially at night
Pain	Assess frequently for adequate pain control Minimize treatments that produce discomfort Premedicate for potentially painful treatments Use nonpharmaceutical interventions (music, relaxation techniques, comforting touch) Decrease noise levels Assess for and intervene to reduce anxiety Enhance opportunities for sleep

tered levels as high as 92 dB. Talking by staff, visitors, and patients was determined to be louder than necessary, with over half of all conversation occurring at levels of 60 dB or more.[18] As a small decrease in decibel level causes a relatively large change in noise as perceived by the human ear, even minor changes in conversation and equipment noise can affect patient comfort dramatically.

Frequent Interruptions for Monitoring and Treatment

It is implicit in the term *intensive care* that patients in an ICU require frequent or even constant monitoring and adjustments to therapy. The average time between interruptions in adult ICU areas has been found to range from 20 to 50 minutes.[3,19] A study of contacts experienced by 16 neonates in an ICU documented a mean of 93.5 direct contacts per infant over a 2-hour time period.[25] In a pediatric ICU, a mean of 53.75 direct contacts was experienced per child over a 3-hour period.[26] It is clear that uninterrupted rest is not a likelihood in either adult or pediatric intensive care settings; however, essential care should be scheduled to allow as much time as possible between interruptions.

Unfamiliar Surroundings and Equipment

The strangeness of the physical environment and equipment in the critical care area is frequently mentioned as a potential stressor.[11,19,20] Interestingly, there is not a consensus about this issue. Some patients identify the unfamiliarity of the surroundings as one of the most stressful factors of being in the ICU, whereas others do not appear to find this particularly

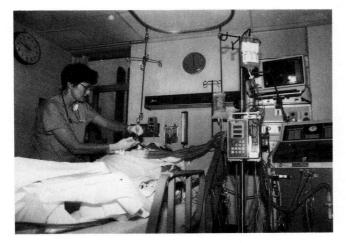

FIGURE 57-8. Careful preparation of the patient for procedures and assessment of the need for analgesics prior to procedures can help minimize discomfort associated with necessary treatments, such as suctioning. (Photograph courtesy of St. Elizabeth Medical Center, Yakima, Wash.)

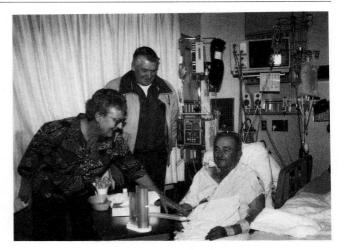

FIGURE 57-9. Encouraging the family visits is an important means of decreasing many of the adverse psychosocial reactions to critical illness. (Photograph courtesy of St. Elizabeth Medical Center, Yakima, Wash.)

stressful.[9,11] It seems that at least for some individual patients, being in an unfamiliar setting is highly stressful.

Pain and Discomfort

Many elements of critical illness may cause patient discomfort. Pain may result from incisions, trauma, and disease. Therapies such as endotracheal intubation, intravenous medications, and dressing changes also cause distress (Fig. 57-8). Finally, the forced immobility that results from placement of monitoring lines, casts, and restraints is a source of discomfort. Recent surveys of both children and adults describe pain as the most frequently mentioned stressor in the critical care setting.[27,28] Pain perception is increased by anxiety, high noise levels, and sleeplessness, and in turn contributes to sleeplessness and anxiety in a vicious circle.[1] Control of pain is an essential intervention in the critically ill.

Social Isolation

When a patient is admitted to the ICU there are a myriad of reasons to feel isolated from significant persons in their normal lives. These include restrictions on visitation, inability to communicate because an endotracheal tube or other device has been placed in the oropharynx, aphasia resulting from cerebral injury, or the use of paralytic medications. Visitors may feel inhibited from touching or even speaking to a patient who is connected to many technical-looking pieces of equipment (Fig. 57-9). Health care professionals can mitigate a patient's loneliness and isolation by encouraging frequent visits by significant others, discussing the events of life outside the hospital, and using alternative means of communication for patients who are unable to communicate verbally.

Pharmaceutical Interventions

Many medications used in the treatment of critically ill patients have potential psychological side effects. These medications include not only those with obvious central nervous system side effects such as narcotics and sedatives, but also such frequently administered medications as antiarrhythmics, antihypertensives, antibiotics, bronchodilators, anticonvulsants, and corticosteroids.[20] The effects of these drugs may be synergistic and may contribute to the patient's feelings of confusion, depression, and psychosis.[20,29] In addition, commonly administered medications may have detrimental effects on sleep and may indirectly affect psychosocial functioning.[29]

Sleep Deprivation

The combination of physiologic and psychological responses to severe illness and the intensive care environment frequently leads to **sleep deprivation.** Sleep has been studied using electroencephalography (EEG), electromyography (EMG), and electrooculography (EOG) to monitor brain wave activity, muscle activity, and eye movement during sleep. Two general categories of activity in sleep have been documented. These are characterized as non–rapid eye movement (NREM) and rapid eye movement (REM). Stages and characteristics of NREM and REM sleep are listed in Table 57–5.

During a normal sleep cycle, individuals progress from stage 1 through stage 4 NREM sleep, then return through stage 3 and stage 2 sleep and move into REM sleep. Subsequent sleep cycles are similar but omit stage 1, the sleep stage closest to waking. Each cycle takes about 90 to 110 minutes to complete, and approximately four to six cycles occur per sleep period.[30]

T A B L E 57 – 5. Phases of Sleep

Non–Rapid Eye Movement (NREM)

Stage 1
    Electroencephalogram (EEG) shows relatively low voltage
    Easily arousable
    Fair amount of muscle tone
Stage 2
    Sleep spindles and K complexes appear on EEG
    More difficult to arouse
    Slight decrease in muscle tone
Stage 3
    EEG shows 20%–30% delta waves (slow wave)
    Difficult to arouse
    Low level of muscle activity
Stage 4
    EEG shows >50% delta waves
    Very difficult to arouse
    Low level of muscle activity
    Stages 3 and 4 ("deep sleep")

Rapid Eye Movement (REM)

EEG is of mixed frequency, similar to the awake state
EOG shows rapid eye movements
Arousability is variable
Presence of dreams
Suppression of muscle tone

Sleep is essential for optimal psychological and mental functioning. When individuals are experimentally deprived of total sleep or selectively deprived of REM sleep, symptoms ranging from fatigue and confusion to hallucinations may occur. When subjects are allowed to sleep after total sleep deprivation, the "recovery sleep" consists initially of stages 3 and 4 (deep sleep) and then of REM sleep. It is theorized that these are the categories of sleep most essential to psychological (and perhaps physiologic) health.[23]

As interruptions are likely to occur in the ICU before an entire sleep cycle can take place, it is not surprising that decreased quality and quantity of sleep has been consistently found in intensive care patients.[19,21,22,27] Fontaine[21] studied nocturnal sleep patterns in 20 critically ill trauma patients and documented an increase in stage 1 sleep and a decrease in stages 2, 3, 4, and REM sleep. The mean number of awakenings per night was 32. Reasons for sleep disturbance in this study were stated as the severity of illness and concomitant pain; a crowded, noisy environment; and frequent interruptions. In addition, all patients were receiving narcotics and sedatives, which have the potential to decrease sleep quality.[21] The consequences of the critical care milieu are likely to be a decrease in the sleep stages that are most important for psychological well-being, as well as a decrease in total sleep time. Sleep quality and quantity can be maximized by thoughtful planning of care so that 90- to 120-minute periods of rest are possible.

Intensive Care Unit Psychosis

Intensive care unit psychosis is a transient, reversible period of psychological impairment that occurs in the setting of an ICU. Generally, the period of impairment occurs after 2 to 5 days of lucidity and resolves within 48 hours after transfer from the ICU. The reported incidence ranges from 14 percent to 72 percent of critically ill patients.[19]

Possible contributing factors include predisposing patient factors such as preexisting psychiatric illness, drug or alcohol addiction, chronic illness, and metabolic or hemodynamic abnormalities. The polypharmaceutical interventions used for many patients are frequently cited as a contributing factor. Sleep deprivation and the effects of the physical environment in the special care unit are probably major contributors to this phenomenon.[19,20,31] A recent comprehensive review found little report of delirium in patients less than 25 years old.[20] In the elderly, there was an increased likelihood of acute confusion.[19,31]

Varying degrees of impairment, ranging from disorientation to more dramatic symptoms such as feelings of paranoia and visual hallucinations, are exhibited by patients. Some common themes of patients' experiences are the perception of being tied down and held captive, being forced to take drugs, being tortured, and being used as a sex object. It is rare for a patient to experience a pleasant hallucination.[20] In a setting in which patients may be immobilized by casts, dressings, intravenous lines, and monitoring

THE AGING PROCESS: CHANGES IN SLEEP PATTERNS

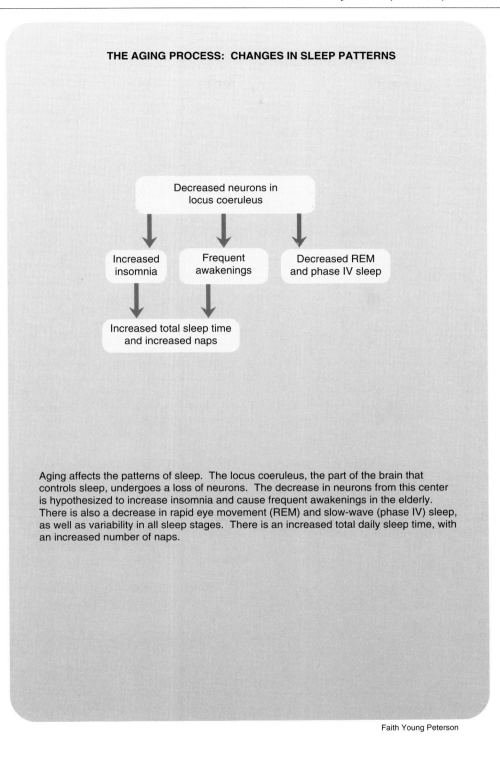

Aging affects the patterns of sleep. The locus coeruleus, the part of the brain that controls sleep, undergoes a loss of neurons. The decrease in neurons from this center is hypothesized to increase insomnia and cause frequent awakenings in the elderly. There is also a decrease in rapid eye movement (REM) and slow-wave (phase IV) sleep, as well as variability in all sleep stages. There is an increased total daily sleep time, with an increased number of naps.

Faith Young Peterson

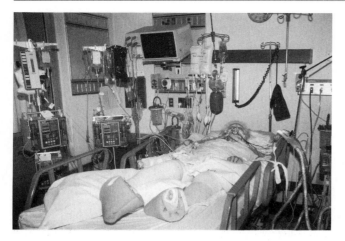

F I G U R E 57 – 10. The elderly patient is at high risk for the adverse psychosocial impact of the special care unit environment. (Photograph courtesy of St. Elizabeth Medical Center, Yakima, Wash.)

equipment, may be given a variety of medications, may be subjected to uncomfortable procedures, and may be physically exposed while strangers care for them in intimate ways, it is not difficult to imagine that misinterpretation of these experiences may easily occur.

Special Considerations in the Elderly

The elderly patient appears especially vulnerable to cognitive and psychological impairment while hospitalized. Factors implicated in this increased vulnerability include impaired visual and auditory sensory input, the presence of multiple chronic illnesses, and an increased likelihood that the patient is receiving multiple medications (Fig. 57–10). Poor nutrition and altered physiology, leading to greater metabolic instability, probably also influence the response to illness and hospitalization.[29,31,32] In addition, the sleep patterns of elderly individuals are generally more fragmented than those of younger adults and may be more sensitive to the disruptive potential of the intensive care environment.[29]

KEY CONCEPTS

- The critical care unit is associated with many environmental stressors including high noise levels, frequent interruptions, unfamiliar equipment, and abnormal light-dark cycles. Sensory overload from these unfamiliar environmental stimuli and sensory deprivation resulting from social isolation are common problems in the critical care unit.

- Sleep deprivation is a frequent problem in critically ill patients. A normal sleep cycle requires about 90 minutes to complete. Deep sleep and REM sleep are particularly important for psychological health. Frequent interruptions result in a poor quantity and quality of sleep. Narcotics and sedatives may also contribute to poor-quality sleep.

- Sleep deprivation, drugs, social isolation, and sensory overload may predispose the patient to ICU psychosis. Two to 5 days in the intensive care setting, particularly in the elderly, is often sufficient to precipitate psychosis. Mental impairment usually resolves within 48 hours after transfer from the unit. Manifestations include paranoia, disorientation, and hallucinations.

Health Professionals in Critical Care Units

The experience of critical illness also affects health care professionals who work with critically ill patients and their families in special care units. The nature of critical illness requires that staff must take responsibility for rapid decision-making, deal frequently with issues of death and dying, and have intense contact with patients and families with many psychosocial needs. In addition, ICU staff are exposed to some of the same environmental hazards as patients (although on a more time-limited basis). Constant artificial lighting, high noise levels, frequent interruptions, and dependence on technical equipment with a potential for malfunction are stressors for staff as well as patients and families (Fig. 57–11). Finally, the nature of critical care nursing and medicine is one of frequent improvement and change; thus, working with critically ill patients requires ongoing formal and informal education.

Soon after the development of intensive care and coronary care units, research into the psychological impact of working in these areas began. Initially, research indicated that critical care units were more stressful to work in than general medical-surgical units. However, some recent studies indicate that it may in fact be less stressful to work in special care areas.[33]

Norbeck used a questionnaire to study the relationships among perceived job stress, job satisfaction,

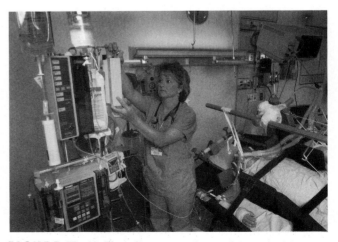

F I G U R E 57 – 11. The reliance on noise-producing, highly technical equipment is potentially stressful for both the patient and the health care professional. (Photograph courtesy of St. Elizabeth Medical Center, Yakima, Wash.)

and psychological symptoms in 180 critical care nurses from eight different hospitals.[34] Factors most frequently rated as stressful were the number of rapid decisions that had to be made, the work load and amount of physical work, cardiac arrest procedures, death of a patient, and the amount of knowledge needed to work in critical care. However, of these factors, only work load had an effect on job satisfaction. The other four factors were stated by Norbeck to be intrinsic to the nature of critical care nursing and may describe the qualities that some nurses seek in choosing this specialty area (Fig. 57–12). The physical setup of the unit, dealing with the psychological needs of the family, the noise level of the unit, physical injury to the nurse, numerous pieces of equipment, and communication problems among nurses all correlated significantly with decreased job satisfaction or psychological symptoms in this study.[34]

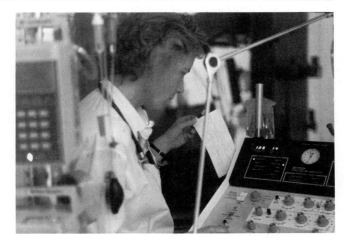

FIGURE 57–12. The challenge of working in an area requiring specialized knowledge and rapid decision-making may attract some health care providers to critical care units. (Photographer: Elizabeth Green, Seattle, Wash.)

TABLE 57–6. Research in Psychosocial Response to Special Care Units

Study	Findings
Family Needs	
Norris LO, Grove S: Investigation of selected psychosocial needs of family members of critically ill adult patients. *Heart Lung* 1986;15:194–199	Questionnaires were used to study needs perceived by family members of critically ill patients. The most important needs identified were (1) to be assured that the best possible care was being given to the patient, (2) to have questions answered honestly, (3) to feel that hospital personnel cares about the patient, and (4) to feel there was hope.
Environmental Stressors	
Fontaine DK: Measurements of nocturnal sleep patterns in trauma patients. *Heart Lung* 1989;18:402–410	Nocturnal sleep patterns were studied in critically ill trauma patients. An increase in stage 1 NREM sleep and number of awakenings was present; decreases in stages 2, 3, and 4 NREM and REM sleep were noted.
Hilton BA: Noise in acute patient care areas. *Res Nurs Health* 1985;8:283–291	Noise levels in intensive care (ICU) and general units were studied. Continuous high noise levels (48.5–68.5 dB) were found in open recovery room and ICU. Lower levels (32.5–57 dB) were found in small, private room ICUs. Intermittent dB levels caused by equipment were as high as 92 dB.
Orsuto J, Corbo B: Approaches of health caregivers to young children in a pediatric intensive care unit. *Matern Child Nurs J* 1988;16:157–175	The frequency of direct and indirect health care giver contacts with critically ill pediatric patients was studied. Mean number of direct contacts per child was 53.75 over a 3-hour period.
Pohlman S, Beardslee C: Contacts experienced by neonates in intensive care environments. *Matern Child Nurs J* 1988;16:207–226	Direct contacts experienced by critically ill neonates were studied. Mean number of direct contacts was 93.5 per child during a 2-hour period.
Simpson TF, Armstrong S, Mitchell P: American Association of Critical-Care Nurses demonstration project: Patients' recollections of critical care. *Heart Lung* 1989;18:325–332	Open-ended questions were used to determine patients' recollections of critical care 24–48 hours after transfer from the unit. Forty-four percent described the experience as neutral or positive. Pain and sleeplessness were identified most frequently as problems.
Tichy AM, et al: Stressors in pediatric intensive care units. *Pediatr Nurs* 1988;14:40–42	An interview was conducted with children and parents within 48 hours after transfer from the pediatric ICU to determine perceived stressors of these groups. Children identified invasive procedures causing pain and discomfort as the worst stressors. Parents described environmental and physical stressors as equally important.
Reactions of Health Care Professionals	
Norbeck J: Perceived job stress, job satisfaction, and psychological symptoms in critical care nursing. *Res Nurs Health* 1985;8:253–259	Relationships between job stress, job satisfaction, and psychological symptoms were studied. Four of five top-ranked stressors were not associated with decreased job satisfaction or psychological symptoms. It was proposed that positive stressors are present for nurses working with critically ill patients.

Summary

The intensive care environment can be described as stressful whether the individual is a patient, a family member, or a health care professional working with critically ill patients. It is important to remember that the psychosocial response to the critical care areas will be unique to each individual. Ongoing assessments of patients and families are necessary if truly helpful interventions are to occur. Health care personnel working with critically ill patients need insight about their own stressors and stress levels in order to care effectively for patients, families, and themselves. Some recent research about potential stressors in the intensive care environment are summarized in Table 57–6 (page 1157).

REFERENCES

1. Fontaine DK: Physical, personal, and cognitive responses to trauma. *Crit Care Nurs Clin North Am* 1989;1(1):11–22.
2. Whaley LF, Wong DL: *Nursing Care of Infants and Children,* 4th ed. St. Louis, Mosby–Year Book, 1991.
3. Dracup K: Are critical care units hazardous to health? *Appl Nurs Res* 1988;1(1):14–21.
4. Urban N: Response to the environment, in Kinney MR, Packa DR, Dunbar SB (eds): *AACN's Clinical Reference for Critical Care Nursing,* 2nd ed. New York, McGraw-Hill, 1988, pp 96–112.
5. Buchda VL: Loneliness in critically ill adults. *Dimens Crit Care Nurs* 1987;6:335–340.
6. Boeing MH, Mongera CO: Powerlessness in critical care patients. *Dimens Crit Care Nurs* 1989;8:274–279.
7. Hudak CM, Gallo BM, Benz JJ: *Critical Care Nursing: A Holistic Approach.* Philadelphia, JB Lippincott, 1990, pp 11–14.
8. Burke LE, Scalzi CC: Behavioral responses of the patient and family: Myocardial infarction and coronary artery bypass surgery, in Underhill SL, Woods SL, Froelicher ESS, Halpenny CJ (eds): *Cardiac Nursing,* 2nd ed. Philadelphia, JB Lippincott, 1989, pp 692–703.
9. Rowe MA, Weinert C: The CCU experience: Stressful or reassuring? *Dimens Crit Care Nurs* 1987;6:341–348.
10. Miller JF: Hope-inspiring strategies of the critically ill. *Appl Nurs Res* 1989;2:23–29.
11. O'Malley PA, Menke E: Relationship of hope and stress after myocardial infarction. *Heart Lung* 1988;17:184–190.
12. Wilson T, Broome ME: Promoting the young child's development in the intensive care unit. *Heart Lung* 1989;18:274–281.
13. Etzler CA: Parents' reactions to pediatric critical care settings: A review of the literature. *Issues Compr Pediatr Nurs* 1984; 7:319–331.
14. Kleeman KM: Families in crisis due to multiple trauma. *Crit Care Nurs Clin North Am* 1989;1:23–31.
15. Norris LO, Grove SK: Investigation of selected psychosocial needs of family members of critically ill adult patient. *Heart Lung* 1986;15:194–199.
16. Dracup K, Clark S: Challenges in critical care nursing: Helping patients and families cope. *Crit Care Nurse* 1993 Aug; supplement: 1–22, 23–24.
17. Philichi LM: Supporting the parents when the child requires intensive care. *Focus Crit Care* 1988;15(2):34–38.
18. Hilton BA: Noise in acute patient care areas. *Res Nurs Health* 1985;8:283–291.
19. Wilson VS: Identification of stressors related to patients' physiologic responses to the surgical intensive care unit. *Heart Lung* 1987;16:267–273.
20. Easton C, MacKenzie F: Sensory-perceptual alterations: Delirium in the intensive care unit. *Heart Lung* 1988;17:229–235.
21. Fontaine DK: Measurement of nocturnal sleep patterns in trauma patients. *Heart Lung* 1989;18:402–410.
22. Richards KC, Bairnsfather L: A description of night sleep patterns in the critical care unit. *Heart Lung* 1988;17:35–42.
23. Sanford SJ: Sleep and the critically ill patient, in Kinney MR, Packa DR, Dunbar SB (eds): *AACN's Clinical Reference for Critical-Care Nursing,* 2nd ed. New York, McGraw-Hill, 1988, pp 399–413.
24. Woods N, Falk SA: Noise stimuli in the acute care area. *Nurs Res* 1974;23:144–150.
25. Pohlman S, Beardslee C: Contacts experienced by neonates in intensive care environments. *Matern Child Nurs J* 1988; 16:207–226.
26. Orsuto J, Corbo B: Approaches of health caregivers to young children in a pediatric intensive care unit. *Matern Child Nurs J* 1988;16:157–175.
27. Simpson TF, Armstrong S, Mitchell P: American Association of Critical-Care Nurses demonstration project: Patients' recollections of critical care. *Heart Lung* 1989;18:325–332.
28. Tichy AM, Braam CM, Meyer TA, Rattan NS: Stressors in pediatric intensive care units. *Pediatr Nurs* 1988;14(1):40–42.
29. Davis-Sharts J: The elder and critical care: Sleep and mobility issues. *Nurs Clin North Am* 1989;24:755–767.
30. Carskadon MA, Dement WC: Normal human sleep: An overview, in Kryger MH, Roth T, Dement WC (eds): *Principles and Practice of Sleep Medicine.* Philadelphia, WB Saunders, 1989, pp 3–13.
31. Foreman MD, Gilles DA, Wagner D: Impaired cognition in the critically ill elderly patient: Clinical implications. *Crit Care Nurs Q* 1989;12:61–73.
32. Williams MA: Physical environment of the intensive care unit and elderly patients. *Crit Care Nurs Q* 1989;12:52–60.
33. Harris RB: Reviewing nursing stress according to a proposed coping-adaptation framework. *Adv Nurs Sci* 1989;11(2):12–28.
34. Norbeck JS: Perceived job stress, job satisfaction, and psychological symptoms in critical care nursing. *Res Nurs Health* 1985;8:253–259.

BIBLIOGRAPHY

Bokinskie J: Family conferences: A method to diminish transfer anxiety. *J Neurosci Nurs* 1992;24(3):129–133.
Boumans NPG, Landeweerd JA: Working in an intensive or non-intensive care unit: Does it make any difference? *Heart Lung* 1994;23(1):71–79.
Doll-Speck L, Miller B, Rohrs K: Sibling education: Implementing a program for the NICU. *Neonatal Network* 1993;12(4):49–52.
Dracup K, Bryan-Brown CW: An open door policy in ICU. *Am J Crit Care* 1992;1(2):16–18.
Edwards GB, Schuring LM: Sleep protocol: A research-based practice change. *Crit Care Nurs* 1993;13(2):84–88.
Gaw-Ens B: Informational support for families immediately after CABG surgery. *Crit Care Nurs* 1994;14(1):41–50.
Harvey MA, Ninos NP, Adler DC, Goodnough-Hanneman SK, Kaye WE, Nikas DL: Results of the consensus conference on fostering more humane critical care: Creating a healing environment. *AACN Clin Issues Crit Care Nurs* 1993;4(3):484–507.
Kaiser K: Assessment and management of pain in the critically ill trauma patient. *Crit Care Nurs Q* 1992;15(2):14–34.
Kirchhoff KT, Pugh E, Calame RM, Reynolds N: Nurses' beliefs and attitudes toward visiting in adult critical care settings. *Am J Crit Care* 1993;2(3):238–245.
Kleinpell R, Powers M: Needs of family members of intensive care unit patients. *Appl Nurs Res* 1992;5(1):2–8.
LaMontagne LL, Hepworth JT, Pawlak R, Chiafery M: Parental coping and activities during pediatric critical care. *Am J Crit Care* 1992;1(2):76–80.
Lekander B, Lehmann S, Lindquist R: Therapeutic listening: Key intervention for several nursing diagnoses. *Dimens Crit Care Nurs* 1993;12(1):24–29.
Miller D, Holditch-Davis D: Interactions of parents and nurses with high-risk preterm infants. *Res Nurs Health* 1992;15(3):187–197.
Oehler JM, Davidson MG: Job stress and burnout in acute and nonacute pediatric nurses. *Am J Crit Care* 1992;1(2):81–90.
Williams M, Murphy J: Noise in critical care units: A quality assurance approach. *J Nurs Quality Assurance* 1991;6(1):53–59.

Bibliography for Frontiers of Research

Unit I: Central Concepts of Pathophysiology

Cheever MA, Chen W, Disis ML, Takahashi M, Peace DJ: T cell immunity to oncogenic proteins including mutuated *ras* and chimeric bcr-abl, in Bystryn JC, Ferrone S, Livingston P (eds): *Specific Immunotherapy of Cancer with Vaccines.* New York, New York Academy of Sciences, 1993, pp 110–112.

Cheever MA, Greenberg P, Fefer A: Specific adopted therapy of established leukemia with syngeneic lymphocytes sequentially immunized in vivo and in vitro and nonspecifically expanded by culture with interleukin-2. *J Immunol* 1981;126: 1318–1322.

Cheever MA, Thompson D, Klarnet J, Greenberg P: Antigen-driven long-term cultured T cells proliferate in vivo, distribute widely, mediate specific tumor therapy and persist long-term as functional memory T cells. *J Exp Med* 1986;163:1100–1112.

Clendening L: *Source Book on Medical History.* New York, Dover Publications, 1960.

Disis ML, Calenoff E, McLaughlin G, et al: Existent T cell and antibody immunity to HER-2/*neu* protein in patients with breast cancer. *Cancer Res* 1994;54:16–20.

Disis ML, Smith JW, Murphy AE, Chen W, Cheever MA: In vitro generation of human cytotoxic T cells specific for peptides derived from the HER-2/*neu* proto-oncogene protein. *Cancer Res* (in press).

Thomas L: *The Lives of a Cell: Notes of a Biology Watcher.* New York, Viking Press, 1974.

Unit II: Alterations in Cellular Function

Caskey CT: Presymptomatic diagnosis: A first step toward genetic health care. *Science* 1993;262:48.

Collins F, Galas D: A new five-year plan for the U.S. human genome project. *Science* 1993;262:43–46.

Holzman D: A tool for all seasons. *Mosaic* 1992;23(2):2–11.

Posner MI: Seeing the mind. *Science* 1993;262:673.

Unit III: Alterations in Defense

Cancer vaccines get a shot in the arm. *Science* 1993;262:841.

McGinnis JM, Foege WH: Actual causes of death in the United States. *JAMA* 1993;270(18):2207–2211.

Morsy M, Mitani K, Clemens P, Caskey CT: Progress toward gene therapy. *JAMA* 1993;270(19):2338–2345.

Special issue on the immune system. *Sci Am* 1993;269(3):52–144.

Unit IV: Alterations in Oxygen Transport, Blood Coagulation, Blood Flow, and Blood Pressure

Black HR: Treatment of mild hypertension. *JAMA* 1993;270(6): 757–759. Editorial.

Erickson D: Life in the blood. *Sci Am* 1991;264(2):126–127.

Golde DW, Gasson JC: Hormones that stimulate the growth of blood cells. *Sci Am* 1988;259(1):62–71.

Markovitz JH, Matthews KA, Kannell WB, et al: Psychological predictors of hypertension in the Framingham Study: Is there tension in hypertension? *JAMA* 1993;270(20):2439–2443.

Morsy M, Mitani K, Clemens P, Caskey CT: Progress toward human gene therapy. *JAMA* 1993;270(19):2338–2345.

Unit V: Alterations in Cardiac Function

American Heart Association: Abstracts from the 66th Scientific Sessions, Atlanta, Georgia, November 8–11, 1993. *Circulation* 1993;88(4, pt 2):I1–827.

Cochrane BL: Acute myocardial infarction in women. *Crit Care Nurs Clin North Am* 1992;4(2):279–289.

Gore JM, Dalen JE: Cardiovascular disease. *JAMA* 1993;270(2): 190–192.

Williams RB, Chesney MA: Psychosocial factors and prognosis in established coronary artery disease. *JAMA* 1993;270(15): 1860–1861. Editorial.

Unit VI: Alterations in Respiratory Function

Beal AL, Cerra FB: Multiple organ failure syndrome in the 1990s. *JAMA* 1994;271(3):226–233.

Gattinoni L, Bombino M, Pelosi P, et al: Lung structure and function in different stages of severe adult respiratory distress syndrome. *JAMA* 1994;271(22):1772–1779.

Hunter FC, Mitchell S: Managing ARDS. *RN* 1993;53–57.

Morsy MA, Mitani K, Clemens P, Caskey CT: Progress toward human gene therapy. *JAMA* 1993;270(19):2338–2345.

Unit VII: Alterations in Fluid, Electrolyte, and Acid-Base Homeostasis

Cullen L: Interventions related to fluid and electrolyte balance. *Nurs Clin North Am* 1992;27(2):569–594.

Kositzke JA: A question of balance: Dehydration in the elderly. *J Gerontol Nurs* 1990;16(5):4–11, 40–41.

Rapoport J: The importance of drinking. *Isr J Med Sci* 1993; 29(2–3):109–110.

Terry J: The other electrolytes: Magnesium, calcium and phosphorus. *J Intraven Nurs* 1991;14(3):167–175.

Unit VIII: Alterations in Intra- and Suprarenal Function

Golde DW, Gasson JC: Hormones that stimulate the growth of blood cells. *Sci Am* 1988;259(1):62–71.

Shipway KH: Bartter's syndrome: A chronic electrolyte losing syndrome. *ANNA* 1992;19(6):559–565.

Unit IX: Alterations in Genitourinary Function

Aral SO, Holmes KK: Sexually transmitted diseases in the AIDS era. *Sci Am* 1991;264(2):62–69.

Sidransky D, Von Eschenbach A, Tsai YC, et al: Identification of p53 gene mutations in bladder cancers and urine samples. *Science* 1991;252:706–708.

Unit X: Alterations in Gastrointestinal Function

Carey WD, Achtar E: Colon polyps and cancer in 1994. *Am J Gastroenterol* 1994;89(6):823–825.

Dixon M: Acid, ulcers, and *H. pylori. Lancet* 1993;342:384–385.

Dixon M: Advances in the management of hepatic disease: Clarifying the issues. Proceedings of a symposium. *Am J Med* 1994; 96(suppl 1A):15–605.

Fernandez-del Castillo C, Rattner DW, Warshaw L: Acute pancreatitis. *Lancet* 1993;342:475–478.

Goodwin CS: Gastric cancer and *Helicobacter pylori*: The whispering killer? *Lancet* 1993;342:507–508.

Morsy MA, Mitani K, Clemens P, Caskey CT: Progress toward human gene therapy. *JAMA* 1993;27(19):2338–2344.

Ondrusek RS: Cholecystectomy: An update. *RN* 1993;561(1):28–33.

Unit XI: Alterations in Endocrine Function and Metabolism

Newgard CB: Cellular engineering and gene therapy strategies for insulin replacement in diabetes. *Diabetes* 1994;43:341–349.

Porth CM, Erickson M: Physiology of thirst and drinking: Implication for nursing practice. *Heart Lung* 1992;21(3):273–282.

Rubin RJ, Altman WM, Mendelson DN: Health care expenditures for people with diabetes mellitus, 1992. *J Clin Endocrinol Metab* 1994;78:809A–809E.

Sullivan SJ, Maki T, Borland KM, et al: Biohybrid artificial pancreas: Long-term implantation studies in diabetic, pancreatectomized dogs. *Science* 1991;252:718–721.

Unit XII: Alterations in Neural Function

Cancer Pain Guideline Panel: Management of cancer pain: Adults. *Am Fam Physician* 1994;49(8):1853–1868.

Ferrell BR, McCaffery M, Ropchan R: Pain management as a clinical challenge for nursing administration. *Nurs Outlook* 1992;40(6): 263–268.

Koshland DE Jr: Frontiers in neuroscience. *Science* 1993;262:635.

Posner MI: Seeing the mind. *Science* 1993;262:673.

Unit XIII: Alterations in Neuropsychological Function

Brumback RA: Is depression a neurologic disease? *Neurol Clin* 1993;11:79–104.

Goldstein M, Deutch AY: Dopaminergic mechanisms in the pathogenesis of schizophrenia. *FASEB J* 1992;6(7):2413–2421.

Pickar D, Litman RE, Konicki PE, et al: Neurochemical and neural

mechanisms of positive and negative symptoms in schizophrenia." *Mod Probl Pharmacopsychiatry* 1990;24:124–151.

Risch SC, Nemeroff CB: Neurochemical alterations of serotonergic neuronal systems in depression. *J Clin Psychiatry* 1992; 53(suppl):3–7.

Rothchild JA: Biology of depression. *Med Clin North Am* 1988; 72(4):765–790.

Siever LJ, Kalus OF, Keefe RS: The boundaries of schizophrenia. *Psychiatr Clin North Am* 1993;16(2):217–244.

Unit XIV: Alterations in Musculoskeletal Support and Movement

Lloyd T, Andon MB, Rollings SN, et al: Calcium supplementation and bone mineral density in adolescent girls. *JAMA* 1993;270(7):841–844.

Morsy MA, Mitani K, Clemens P, Caskey CT: Progress toward human gene therapy. *JAMA* 1993;270(19):2338–2344.

Unit XV: Alterations in the Integument

Hom DB, Maisel RH: Angiogenic growth factors: Their effects and potential in soft tissue wound healing. *Ann Otol Rhinol Laryngol* 1992;101(4):349–354.

Jones PL, Millman A: Wound healing and the aged patient. *Nurs Clin North Am* 1990;25(1):263–277.

Mo JA, Sanchez MR: The cutaneous manifestations of violence and poverty. *Arch Dermatol* 1992;128(6):829–839.

Silverstein P: Smoking and wound healing. *Am J Med* 1992; 31:22S–24S.

Skerrett PJ: 'Matrix algebra' heals life's wounds. *Science* 1991; 252:1064–1066.

Wokalek H, Ruh H: Time course of wound healing. *J Biomater Appl* 1991;514:337–362.

Unit XVI: Selected Multisystem Alterations and Considerations in Critical Illness

Beal AL, Cerra FB: Multiple organ failure syndrome in the 1990s, systemic inflammatory response and organ dysfunction. *JAMA* 1994;271(3):226–233.

Calistro AM: Burn care basics and beyond. 1993;56(3):26–31.

Roccograndi JF, Clements KS: Managing AIDS-related meningitis. *RN* 1993;56(11):36–39.

Bibliography for Aging Process Boxes

Andresen GP: A fresh look at assessing the elderly. *RN* 1989;28–39.

Bachman DL: Sleep disorders with aging: Evaluation and treatment. *Geriatrics* 1992;47(9):53–61.

Bell JE, Dixon L, Sehy YA: Physical assessment: The breast and the pulmonary, cardiovascular, gastrointestinal, and genitourinary systems, in Chenitz WC, Stone JT, Salisbury SA (eds): *Clinical Gerontological Nursing: A Guide to Advanced Practice.* Philadelphia, WB Saunders, 1991, pp 51–69.

Burggraf V, Donlon B: Assessing the elderly. *Am J Nurs* 1985;85(9):974–984.

Burrage RL: Physical assessment: Musculoskeletal and nervous systems, in Chenitz WC, Stone JT, Salisbury SA (eds): *Clinical Gerontological Nursing: A Guide to Advanced Practice.* Philadelphia, WB Saunders, 1991, pp 71–89.

Burrage RL, Dixon L, Sehy YA: Physical assessment: An overview with sections on the skin, eye, ear, nose and neck, in Chenitz WC, Stone JT, Salisbury SA (eds): *Clinical Gerontological Nursing: A Guide to Advanced Practice.* Philadelphia, WB Saunders, 1991, pp 27–49.

Felver L: Speed of response and oxygenation in healthy aged. *Washington State Journal of Nursing* 1981;53:19–24.

Frantz RA, Ferrell-Torry A: Physical impairments in the elderly population. *Adv Clin Nurs Res* 1993;28(2):363–371.

Foyt MM: Impaired gas exchange in the elderly. *Geriatric Nursing* 1992;262–268.

Gawlinski A, Jensen GA: The complications of cardiovascular aging. *Am J Nurs* 1991;91(11):26–30.

Gennis V, Garry PJ, Haaland KY, Yeo RA, Goodwin JS: Hearing and cognition in the elderly. *Arch Intern Med* 1991;151:2259–2264.

Gioiella EC, Bevil CW: *Nursing Care of the Aging Client: Promoting Healthy Adaptation.* Norwalk, Conn, Appleton-Century-Crofts, 1985.

Kohn RR: Aging and age-related diseases: Normal processes, in Johnson HA (ed): *Relations Between Normal Aging and Disease.* New York, Raven Press, 1985.

Morgan S: Effects of age on cardiovascular functioning. *Geriatric Nursing* 1993;14(5):249–251.

Morris JC, McManus DQ: The neurology of aging: Normal versus pathologic change. *Geriatrics* 1991;46(8):47–54.

Mooradian AD, Morley JE, Korenman SG: Endocrinology in aging, in Bone RC (ed.): *Disease-a-Month.* Chicago, Ill, Year Book Medical Publishers, 1988.

Phillips SK, Bruce SA, Newton D, Woledge RC: The weakness of old age is not due to failure of muscle activation. *J Gerontol* 1992;47(2):M45–49.

Rousseau P, Fuentevilla-Clifton A: Urinary incontinence in the aged, part 1: Patient evaluation. *Geriatrics* 1992;47(6):22–34.

Russell RM: Changes in gastrointestinal function attributed to aging. *Am J Clin Nutr* 1992;55:1203S–1207S.

Rusting RL: Why do we age? *Sci Am* 1992;130–141.

Saul RL, Gee P, Ames BN: Free radicals, DNA damage, and aging, in Warner HR, et al (eds): *Modern Biological Theories of Aging.* New York, Raven Press, 1987.

Selkoe DJ: Aging brain, aging mind. *Sci Am* 1992;135–142.

Siskind GW: Aging and the immune system, in Warner HR, et al (eds): *Modern Biological Theories of Aging.* New York, Raven Press, 1987.

Stevens JC: Aging and spatial acuity of touch. *J. Gerontol* 1992;47(1):35–40.

Verbeken EK, Cauberghs M, Mertens I, Clement J, Lauweryns JM, Van de Woestijine KP: The senile lung. *Chest* 1992; 101(3):800–809.

Wei JY: Age and the cardiovascular system. *N Engl J Med* 1992;327(24):1735–1739.

Weksler MC: Protecting the aging immune system to prolong quality of life. *Geriatrics* 1990;45(7):72–76.

Appendix: 1994 Chromosome Maps

It is projected that by the year 2000, the genes of an entire human genome will be mapped to specific chromosome locations. Already the gene loci associated with nearly 1000 human disorders have been mapped. The 1994 chromosome maps are included here to emphasize the central role that genetics plays in many human disorders.

Mapping genes to specific chromosome locations, however, is only a beginning and should not lead to the assumption that the role these genes play in human function is understood. Indeed, it will take many years to clone, identify, and ascribe function to the great majority of these genes after they are mapped. The potential benefits that drive this enormous mapping endeavor include a better understanding of human development and the possibility of manipulating genes to prevent or treat genetic diseases.

Key	
▭	Allelic disorders
[ ]	"Nondisease"
*	Neoplasm with specific chromosomal change and/or relation to oncogene or anti-oncogene and/or loss of heterozygosity in tumor (selected samples)
•	Malformation syndrome with restricted chromosomal change
?	Confirmation of the gene or locus is in limbo
{ }	Specific susceptibility or resistance with single-gene basis
italics	Genes recently repositioned on chromosomes – January 1994 to June 1994
bold	Recently located disorders – January 1994 to June 1994

The chromosome maps and key are from The human genome 1994: Human genetic disorders. *J NIH Res* 1994;6(8):115–134. Reprinted with permission from *The Journal of NIH Research*, Washington, DC. Information on the gene defects mapped on the following pages was obtained from *Mendelian Inheritance in Man* (11th edition, Johns Hopkins University Press, Baltimore, 1994) by Victor A. McKusick of Johns Hopkins University in Baltimore.

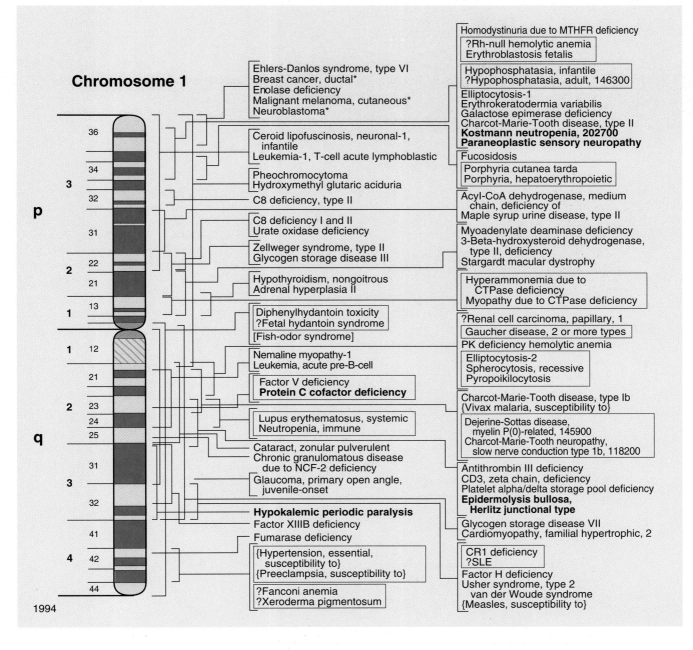

Chromosome 1

Ehlers-Danlos syndrome, type VI
Breast cancer, ductal*
Enolase deficiency
Malignant melanoma, cutaneous*
Neuroblastoma*

Ceroid lipofuscinosis, neuronal-1,
 infantile
Leukemia-1, T-cell acute lymphoblastic

Pheochromocytoma
Hydroxymethyl glutaric aciduria

C8 deficiency, type II

C8 deficiency I and II
Urate oxidase deficiency

Zellweger syndrome, type II
Glycogen storage disease III

Hypothyroidism, nongoitrous
Adrenal hyperplasia II

Diphenylhydantoin toxicity
?Fetal hydantoin syndrome

[Fish-odor syndrome]

Nemaline myopathy-1
Leukemia, acute pre-B-cell

Factor V deficiency
Protein C cofactor deficiency

Lupus erythematosus, systemic
Neutropenia, immune

Cataract, zonular pulverulent
Chronic granulomatous disease
 due to NCF-2 deficiency
Glaucoma, primary open angle,
 juvenile-onset

Hypokalemic periodic paralysis
Factor XIIIB deficiency
Fumarase deficiency

{Hypertension, essential,
 susceptibility to}
{Preeclampsia, susceptibility to}

?Fanconi anemia
?Xeroderma pigmentosum

Homodystinuria due to MTHFR deficiency
?Rh-null hemolytic anemia
Erythroblastosis fetalis

Hypophosphatasia, infantile
?Hypophosphatasia, adult, 146300

Elliptocytosis-1
Erythrokeratodermia variabilis
Galactose epimerase deficiency
Charcot-Marie-Tooth disease, type II
Kostmann neutropenia, 202700
Paraneoplastic sensory neuropathy

Fucosidosis
Porphyria cutanea tarda
Porphyria, hepatoerythropoietic

Acyl-CoA dehydrogenase, medium
 chain, deficiency of
Maple syrup urine disease, type II
Myoadenylate deaminase deficiency
3-Beta-hydroxysteroid dehydrogenase,
 type II, deficiency
Stargardt macular dystrophy

Hyperammonemia due to
 CTPase deficiency
Myopathy due to CTPase deficiency

?Renal cell carcinoma, papillary, 1
Gaucher disease, 2 or more types
PK deficiency hemolytic anemia

Elliptocytosis-2
Spherocytosis, recessive
Pyropoikilocytosis

Charcot-Marie-Tooth disease, type Ib
{Vivax malaria, susceptibility to}

Dejerine-Sottas disease,
 myelin P(0)-related, 145900
Charcot-Marie-Tooth neuropathy,
 slow nerve conduction type 1b, 118200

Antithrombin III deficiency
CD3, zeta chain, deficiency
Platelet alpha/delta storage pool deficiency
Epidermolysis bullosa,
 Herlitz junctional type

Glycogen storage disease VII
Cardiomyopathy, familial hypertrophic, 2

CR1 deficiency
?SLE
Factor H deficiency
Usher syndrome, type 2
 van der Woude syndrome
{Measles, susceptibility to}

1994

Chromosome 2

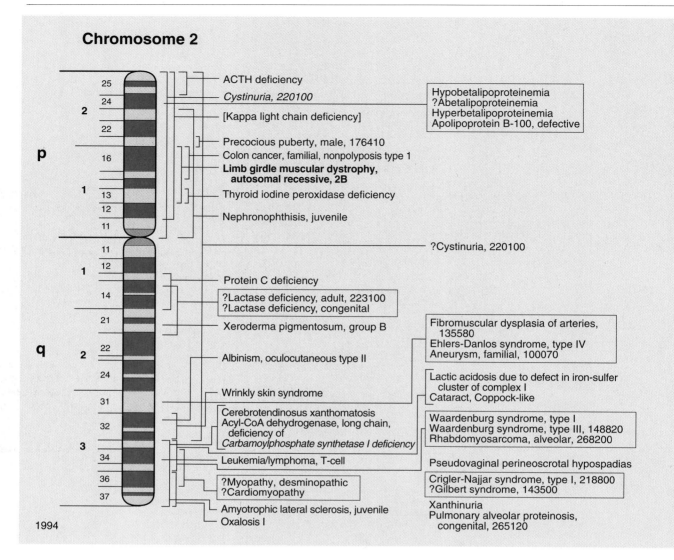

ACTH deficiency

Cystinuria, 220100

[Kappa light chain deficiency]

Hypobetalipoproteinemia
?Abetalipoproteinemia
Hyperbetalipoproteinemia
Apolipoprotein B-100, defective

Precocious puberty, male, 176410

Colon cancer, familial, nonpolyposis type 1

Limb girdle muscular dystrophy, autosomal recessive, 2B

Thyroid iodine peroxidase deficiency

Nephronophthisis, juvenile

?Cystinuria, 220100

Protein C deficiency

?Lactase deficiency, adult, 223100
?Lactase deficiency, congenital

Xeroderma pigmentosum, group B

Fibromuscular dysplasia of arteries, 135580
Ehlers-Danlos syndrome, type IV
Aneurysm, familial, 100070

Albinism, oculocutaneous type II

Lactic acidosis due to defect in iron-sulfer cluster of complex I
Cataract, Coppock-like

Wrinkly skin syndrome

Cerebrotendinosus xanthomatosis
Acyl-CoA dehydrogenase, long chain, deficiency of
Carbamoylphosphate synthetase I deficiency

Waardenburg syndrome, type I
Waardenburg syndrome, type III, 148820
Rhabdomyosarcoma, alveolar, 268200

Leukemia/lymphoma, T-cell

Pseudovaginal perineoscrotal hypospadias

?Myopathy, desminopathic
?Cardiomyopathy

Crigler-Najjar syndrome, type I, 218800
?Gilbert syndrome, 143500

Amyotrophic lateral sclerosis, juvenile

Oxalosis I

Xanthinuria
Pulmonary alveolar proteinosis, congenital, 265120

1994

Chromosome 3

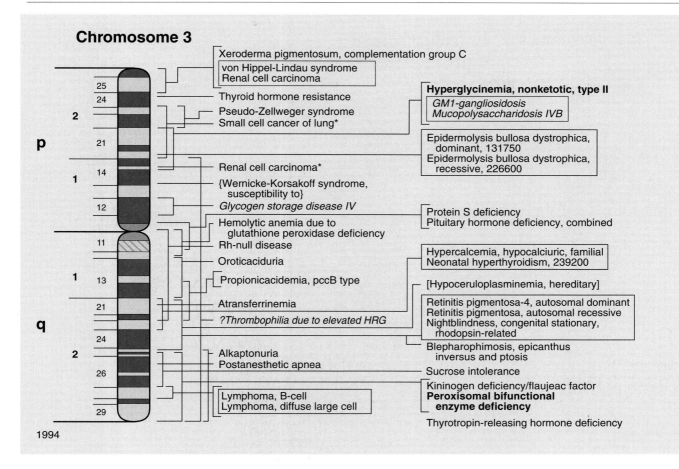

Xeroderma pigmentosum, complementation group C

von Hippel-Lindau syndrome
Renal cell carcinoma

Thyroid hormone resistance

Pseudo-Zellweger syndrome
Small cell cancer of lung*

Hyperglycinemia, nonketotic, type II

GM1-gangliosidosis
Mucopolysaccharidosis IVB

Epidermolysis bullosa dystrophica,
dominant, 131750
Epidermolysis bullosa dystrophica,
recessive, 226600

Renal cell carcinoma*

{Wernicke-Korsakoff syndrome,
susceptibility to}

Glycogen storage disease IV

Protein S deficiency
Pituitary hormone deficiency, combined

Hemolytic anemia due to
glutathione peroxidase deficiency

Rh-null disease

Oroticaciduria

Hypercalcemia, hypocalciuric, familial
Neonatal hyperthyroidism, 239200

Propionicacidemia, pccB type

[Hypoceruloplasminemia, hereditary]

Atransferrinemia

Retinitis pigmentosa-4, autosomal dominant
Retinitis pigmentosa, autosomal recessive
Nightblindness, congenital stationary,
rhodopsin-related

?Thrombophilia due to elevated HRG

Blepharophimosis, epicanthus
inversus and ptosis

Alkaptonuria
Postanesthetic apnea

Sucrose intolerance

Kininogen deficiency/flaujeac factor
**Peroxisomal bifunctional
enzyme deficiency**

Lymphoma, B-cell
Lymphoma, diffuse large cell

Thyrotropin-releasing hormone deficiency

1994

Chromosome 4

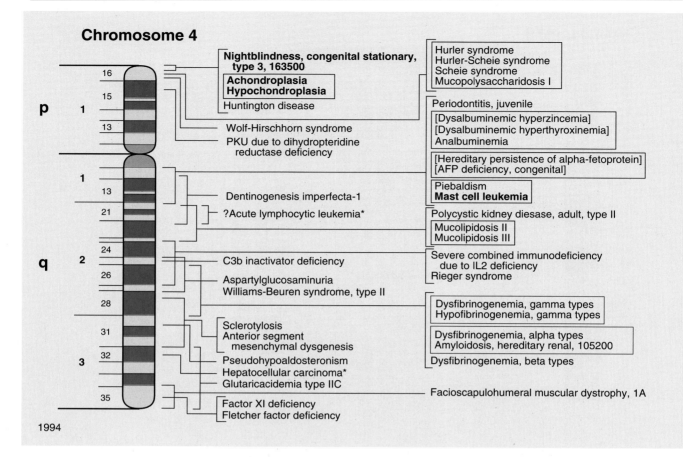

Nightblindness, congenital stationary, type 3, 163500

Achondroplasia
Hypochondroplasia

Huntington disease

Wolf-Hirschhorn syndrome
PKU due to dihydropteridine reductase deficiency

Hurler syndrome
Hurler-Scheie syndrome
Scheie syndrome
Mucopolysaccharidosis I

Periodontitis, juvenile

[Dysalbuminemic hyperzincemia]
[Dysalbuminemic hyperthyroxinemia]
Analbuminemia

[Hereditary persistence of alpha-fetoprotein]
[AFP deficiency, congenital]

Piebaldism
Mast cell leukemia

Dentinogenesis imperfecta-1

?Acute lymphocytic leukemia*

Polycystic kidney diesase, adult, type II

Mucolipidosis II
Mucolipidosis III

C3b inactivator deficiency

Severe combined immunodeficiency
due to IL2 deficiency
Rieger syndrome

Aspartylglucosaminuria
Williams-Beuren syndrome, type II

Dysfibrinogenemia, gamma types
Hypofibrinogenemia, gamma types

Sclerotylosis
Anterior segment
mesenchymal dysgenesis

Dysfibrinogenemia, alpha types
Amyloidosis, hereditary renal, 105200

Pseudohypoaldosteronism
Hepatocellular carcinoma*
Glutaricacidemia type IIC

Dysfibrinogenemia, beta types

Facioscapulohumeral muscular dystrophy, 1A

Factor XI deficiency
Fletcher factor deficiency

1994

Chromosome 5

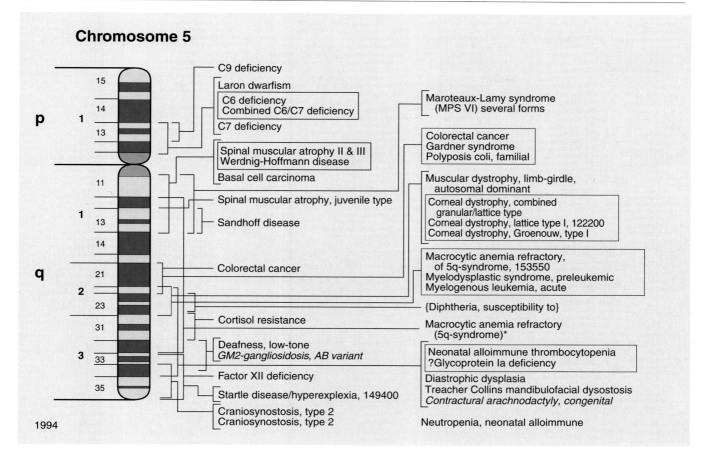

1994

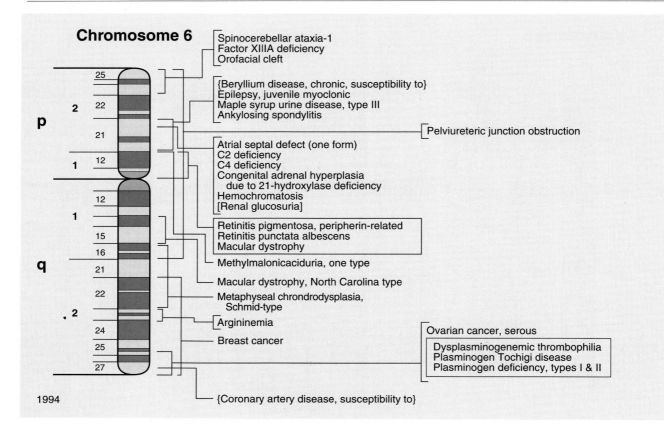

Chromosome 6

Spinocerebellar ataxia-1
Factor XIIIA deficiency
Orofacial cleft

{Beryllium disease, chronic, susceptibility to}
Epilepsy, juvenile myoclonic
Maple syrup urine disease, type III
Ankylosing spondylitis

Pelviureteric junction obstruction

Atrial septal defect (one form)
C2 deficiency
C4 deficiency
Congenital adrenal hyperplasia
  due to 21-hydroxylase deficiency
Hemochromatosis
[Renal glucosuria]

Retinitis pigmentosa, peripherin-related
Retinitis punctata albescens
Macular dystrophy

Methylmalonicaciduria, one type

Macular dystrophy, North Carolina type

Metaphyseal chrondrodysplasia,
  Schmid-type

Argininemia

Breast cancer

Ovarian cancer, serous

Dysplasminogenemic thrombophilia
Plasminogen Tochigi disease
Plasminogen deficiency, types I & II

1994

{Coronary artery disease, susceptibility to}

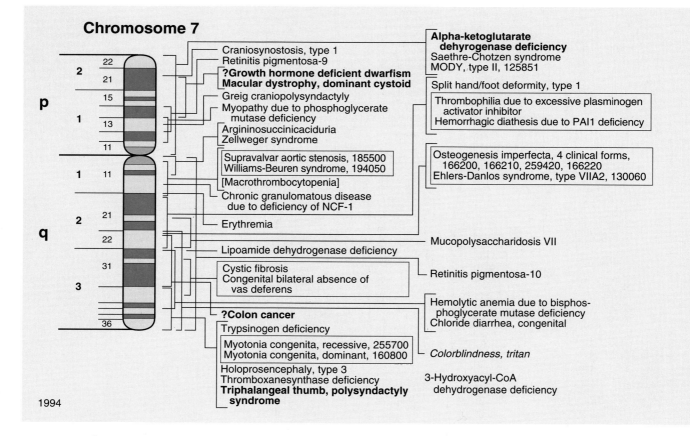

Chromosome 7

Craniosynostosis, type 1
Retinitis pigmentosa-9
?Growth hormone deficient dwarfism
Macular dystrophy, dominant cystoid
Greig craniopolysyndactyly
Myopathy due to phosphoglycerate
  mutase deficiency
Argininosuccinicaciduria
Zellweger syndrome

Supravalvar aortic stenosis, 185500
Williams-Beuren syndrome, 194050

[Macrothrombocytopenia]
Chronic granulomatous disease
  due to deficiency of NCF-1

Erythremia

Lipoamide dehydrogenase deficiency

Cystic fibrosis
Congenital bilateral absence of
  vas deferens

?Colon cancer
Trypsinogen deficiency

Myotonia congenita, recessive, 255700
Myotonia congenita, dominant, 160800

Holoprosencephaly, type 3
Thromboxanesynthase deficiency
Triphalangeal thumb, polysyndactyly
  syndrome

Alpha-ketoglutarate
  dehyrogenase deficiency
Saethre-Chotzen syndrome
MODY, type II, 125851

Split hand/foot deformity, type 1

Thrombophilia due to excessive plasminogen
  activator inhibitor
Hemorrhagic diathesis due to PAI1 deficiency

Osteogenesis imperfecta, 4 clinical forms,
  166200, 166210, 259420, 166220
Ehlers-Danlos syndrome, type VIIA2, 130060

Mucopolysaccharidosis VII

Retinitis pigmentosa-10

Hemolytic anemia due to bisphos-
  phoglycerate mutase deficiency
Chloride diarrhea, congenital

Colorblindness, tritan

3-Hydroxyacyl-CoA
  dehydrogenase deficiency

1994

Chromosome 8

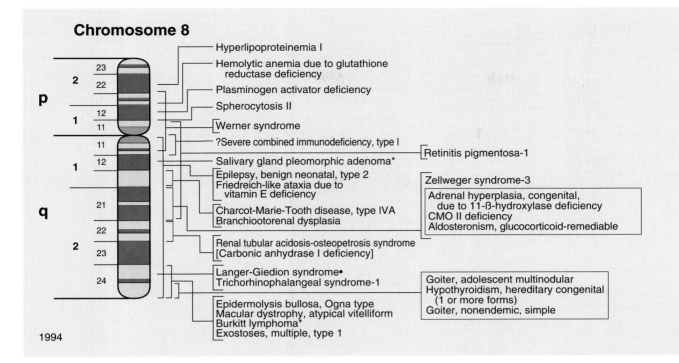

- Hyperlipoproteinemia I
- Hemolytic anemia due to glutathione reductase deficiency
- Plasminogen activator deficiency
- Spherocytosis II
- Werner syndrome
- ?Severe combined immunodeficiency, type I
- Salivary gland pleomorphic adenoma*
  - Retinitis pigmentosa-1
- Epilepsy, benign neonatal, type 2
- Friedreich-like ataxia due to vitamin E deficiency
- Charcot-Marie-Tooth disease, type IVA
- Branchiootorenal dysplasia
  - Zellweger syndrome-3
    - Adrenal hyperplasia, congenital, due to 11-ß-hydroxylase deficiency
    - CMO II deficiency
    - Aldosteronism, glucocorticoid-remediable
- Renal tubular acidosis-osteopetrosis syndrome [Carbonic anhydrase I deficiency]
- Langer-Giedion syndrome•
- Trichorhinophalangeal syndrome-1
  - Goiter, adolescent multinodular
  - Hypothyroidism, hereditary congenital (1 or more forms)
  - Goiter, nonendemic, simple
- Epidermolysis bullosa, Ogna type
- Macular dystrophy, atypical vitelliform
- Burkitt lymphoma*
- Exostoses, multiple, type 1

1994

Chromosome 9

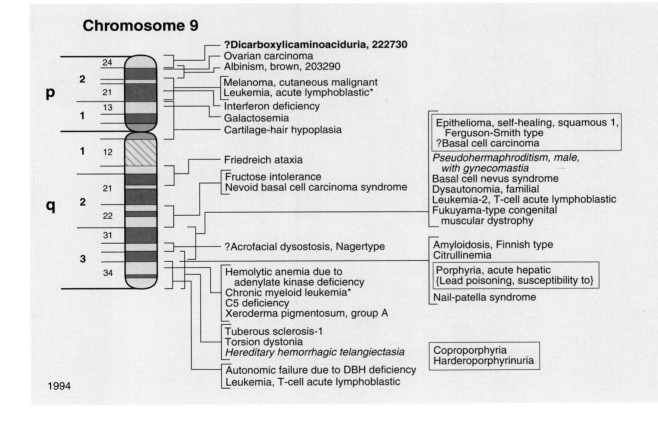

- **?Dicarboxylicaminoaciduria, 222730**
- Ovarian carcinoma
- Albinism, brown, 203290
- Melanoma, cutaneous malignant
- Leukemia, acute lymphoblastic*
- Interferon deficiency
- Galactosemia
- Cartilage-hair hypoplasia
  - Epithelioma, self-healing, squamous 1, Ferguson-Smith type
  - ?Basal cell carcinoma
- Friedreich ataxia
- Fructose intolerance
- Nevoid basal cell carcinoma syndrome
  - *Pseudohermaphroditism, male, with gynecomastia*
  - Basal cell nevus syndrome
  - Dysautonomia, familial
  - Leukemia-2, T-cell acute lymphoblastic
  - Fukuyama-type congenital muscular dystrophy
- ?Acrofacial dysostosis, Nagertype
  - Amyloidosis, Finnish type
  - Citrullinemia
- Hemolytic anemia due to adenylate kinase deficiency
- Chronic myeloid leukemia*
- C5 deficiency
- Xeroderma pigmentosum, group A
  - Porphyria, acute hepatic {Lead poisoning, susceptibility to}
  - Nail-patella syndrome
- Tuberous sclerosis-1
- Torsion dystonia
- *Hereditary hemorrhagic telangiectasia*
  - Coproporphyria
  - Harderoporphyrinuria
- Autonomic failure due to DBH deficiency
- Leukemia, T-cell acute lymphoblastic

1994

Chromosome 10

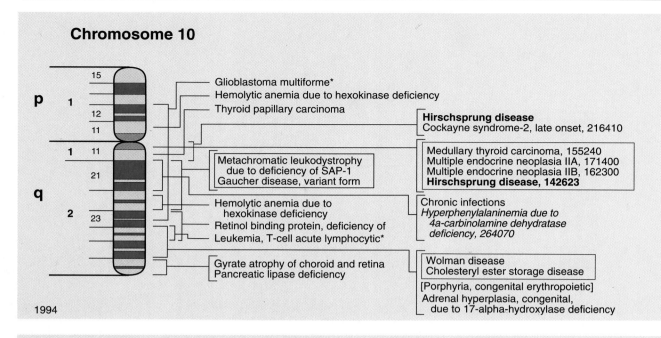

Glioblastoma multiforme*
Hemolytic anemia due to hexokinase deficiency
Thyroid papillary carcinoma

Hirschsprung disease
Cockayne syndrome-2, late onset, 216410

Metachromatic leukodystrophy
   due to deficiency of SAP-1
Gaucher disease, variant form

Medullary thyroid carcinoma, 155240
Multiple endocrine neoplasia IIA, 171400
Multiple endocrine neoplasia IIB, 162300
Hirschsprung disease, 142623

Hemolytic anemia due to
   hexokinase deficiency
Retinol binding protein, deficiency of
Leukemia, T-cell acute lymphocytic*

Chronic infections
Hyperphenylalaninemia due to
   4a-carbinolamine dehydratase
   deficiency, 264070

Gyrate atrophy of choroid and retina
Pancreatic lipase deficiency

Wolman disease
Cholesteryl ester storage disease

[Porphyria, congenital erythropoietic]
Adrenal hyperplasia, congenital,
   due to 17-alpha-hydroxylase deficiency

1994

Chromosome 11

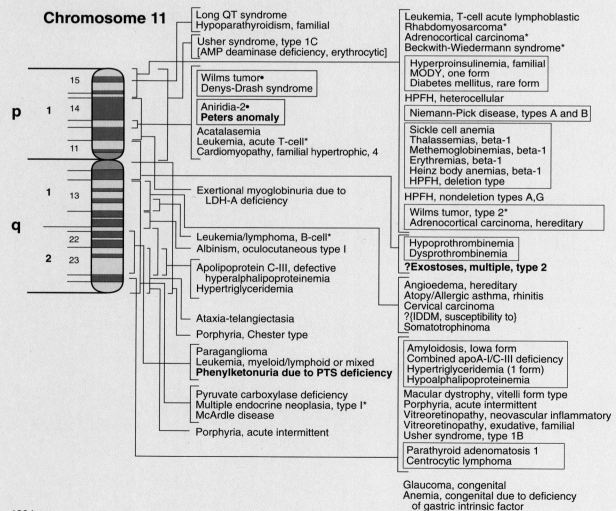

Long QT syndrome
Hypoparathyroidism, familial

Usher syndrome, type 1C
[AMP deaminase deficiency, erythrocytic]

Leukemia, T-cell acute lymphoblastic
Rhabdomyosarcoma*
Adrenocortical carcinoma*
Beckwith-Wiedermann syndrome*

Wilms tumor•
Denys-Drash syndrome

Hyperproinsulinemia, familial
MODY, one form
Diabetes mellitus, rare form

Aniridia-2•
Peters anomaly

HPFH, heterocellular

Niemann-Pick disease, types A and B

Acatalasemia
Leukemia, acute T-cell*
Cardiomyopathy, familial hypertrophic, 4

Sickle cell anemia
Thalassemias, beta-1
Methemoglobinemias, beta-1
Erythremias, beta-1
Heinz body anemias, beta-1
HPFH, deletion type

Exertional myoglobinuria due to
   LDH-A deficiency

HPFH, nondeletion types A,G

Wilms tumor, type 2*
Adrenocortical carcinoma, hereditary

Leukemia/lymphoma, B-cell*
Albinism, oculocutaneous type I

Hypoprothrombinemia
Dysprothrombinemia

Apolipoprotein C-III, defective
   hyperalphalipoproteinemia
Hypertriglyceridemia

?Exostoses, multiple, type 2

Angioedema, hereditary
Atopy/Allergic asthma, rhinitis
Cervical carcinoma
?{IDDM, susceptibility to}
Somatotrophinoma

Ataxia-telangiectasia

Porphyria, Chester type

Paraganglioma
Leukemia, myeloid/lymphoid or mixed
Phenylketonuria due to PTS deficiency

Amyloidosis, Iowa form
Combined apoA-I/C-III deficiency
Hypertriglyceridemia (1 form)
Hypoalphalipoproteinemia

Pyruvate carboxylase deficiency
Multiple endocrine neoplasia, type I*
McArdle disease

Macular dystrophy, vitelli form type
Porphyria, acute intermittent
Vitreoretinopathy, neovascular inflammatory
Vitreoretinopathy, exudative, familial
Usher syndrome, type 1B

Porphyria, acute intermittent

Parathyroid adenomatosis 1
Centrocytic lymphoma

Glaucoma, congenital
Anemia, congenital due to deficiency
   of gastric intrinsic factor
CD59 deficiency

1994

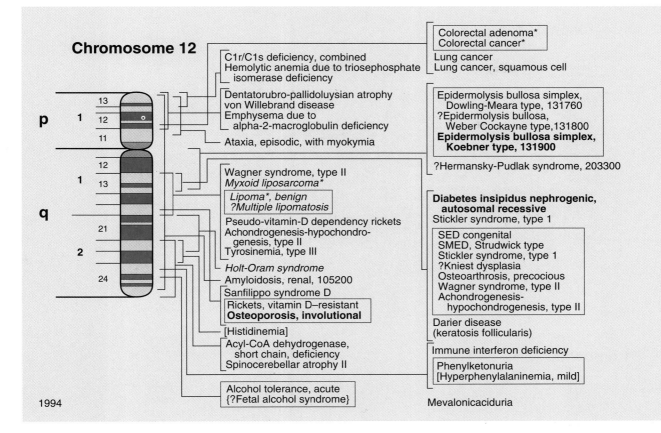

Chromosome 12

C1r/C1s deficiency, combined
Hemolytic anemia due to triosephosphate
  isomerase deficiency

Dentatorubro-pallidoluysian atrophy
von Willebrand disease
Emphysema due to
  alpha-2-macroglobulin deficiency

Ataxia, episodic, with myokymia

Wagner syndrome, type II
*Myxoid liposarcoma**

Lipoma, benign*
?Multiple lipomatosis

Pseudo-vitamin-D dependency rickets
Achondrogenesis-hypochondro-
  genesis, type II
Tyrosinemia, type III

Holt-Oram syndrome
Amyloidosis, renal, 105200

Sanfilippo syndrome D
Rickets, vitamin D–resistant
Osteoporosis, involutional

[Histidinemia]

Acyl-CoA dehydrogenase,
  short chain, deficiency
Spinocerebellar atrophy II

Alcohol tolerance, acute
{?Fetal alcohol syndrome}

Colorectal adenoma*
Colorectal cancer*
Lung cancer
Lung cancer, squamous cell

Epidermolysis bullosa simplex,
  Dowling-Meara type, 131760
?Epidermolysis bullosa,
  Weber Cockayne type,131800
**Epidermolysis bullosa simplex,
  Koebner type, 131900**

?Hermansky-Pudlak syndrome, 203300

**Diabetes insipidus nephrogenic,
  autosomal recessive**
Stickler syndrome, type 1

SED congenital
SMED, Strudwick type
Stickler syndrome, type 1
?Kniest dysplasia
Osteoarthrosis, precocious
Wagner syndrome, type II
Achondrogenesis-
  hypochondrogenesis, type II

Darier disease
(keratosis follicularis)

Immune interferon deficiency

Phenylketonuria
[Hyperphenylalaninemia, mild]

Mevalonicaciduria

1994

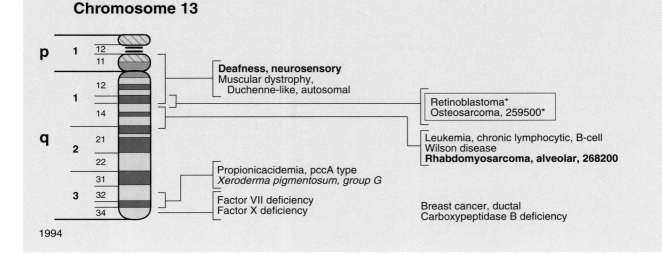

Chromosome 13

Deafness, neurosensory
Muscular dystrophy,
  Duchenne-like, autosomal

Propionicacidemia, pccA type
Xeroderma pigmentosum, group G

Factor VII deficiency
Factor X deficiency

Retinoblastoma*
Osteosarcoma, 259500*

Leukemia, chronic lymphocytic, B-cell
Wilson disease
Rhabdomyosarcoma, alveolar, 268200

Breast cancer, ductal
Carboxypeptidase B deficiency

1994

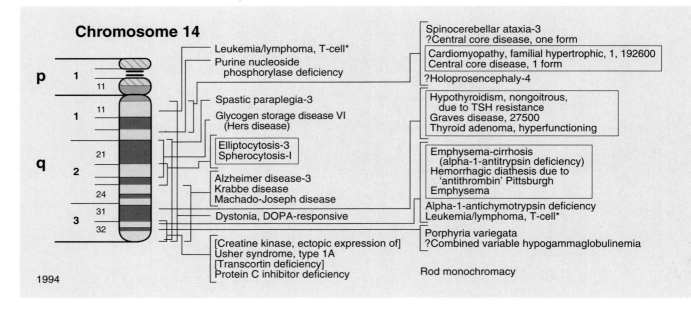

Chromosome 14

p 1 11

1 11

q 2 21

24

2

31 3

32

1994

Leukemia/lymphoma, T-cell*
Purine nucleoside
   phosphorylase deficiency

Spastic paraplegia-3
Glycogen storage disease VI
   (Hers disease)

Elliptocytosis-3
Spherocytosis-I

Alzheimer disease-3
Krabbe disease
Machado-Joseph disease

Dystonia, DOPA-responsive

[Creatine kinase, ectopic expression of]
Usher syndrome, type 1A
[Transcortin deficiency]
Protein C inhibitor deficiency

Spinocerebellar ataxia-3
?Central core disease, one form

Cardiomyopathy, familial hypertrophic, 1, 192600
Central core disease, 1 form

?Holoprosencephaly-4

Hypothyroidism, nongoitrous,
   due to TSH resistance
Graves disease, 27500
Thyroid adenoma, hyperfunctioning

Emphysema-cirrhosis
   (alpha-1-antitrypsin deficiency)
Hemorrhagic diathesis due to
   'antithrombin' Pittsburgh
Emphysema

Alpha-1-antichymotrypsin deficiency
Leukemia/lymphoma, T-cell*

Porphyria variegata
?Combined variable hypogammaglobulinemia

Rod monochromacy

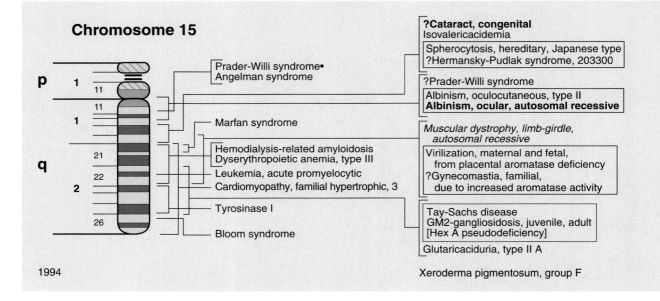

Chromosome 15

p 1 11

11

1

q 2 21

22

2

26

1994

Prader-Willi syndrome•
Angelman syndrome

Marfan syndrome

Hemodialysis-related amyloidosis
Dyserythropoietic anemia, type III
Leukemia, acute promyelocytic
Cardiomyopathy, familial hypertrophic, 3

Tyrosinase I

Bloom syndrome

?Cataract, congenital
Isovalericacidemia

Spherocytosis, hereditary, Japanese type
?Hermansky-Pudlak syndrome, 203300

?Prader-Willi syndrome

Albinism, oculocutaneous, type II
Albinism, ocular, autosomal recessive

Muscular dystrophy, limb-girdle,
*   autosomal recessive*

Virilization, maternal and fetal,
   from placental aromatase deficiency
?Gynecomastia, familial,
   due to increased aromatase activity

Tay-Sachs disease
GM2-gangliosidosis, juvenile, adult
[Hex A pseudodeficiency]

Glutaricaciduria, type II A

Xeroderma pigmentosum, group F

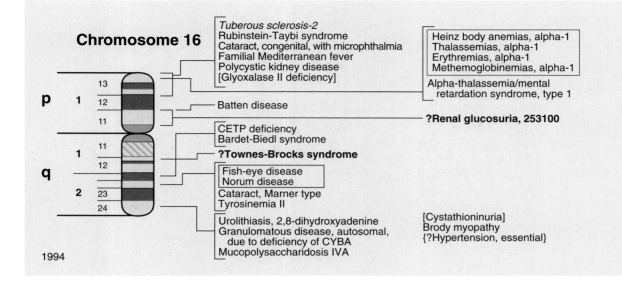

Chromosome 16

p	1	13
		12
		11
q	1	11
		12
	2	23
		24

1994

Tuberous sclerosis-2
Rubinstein-Taybi syndrome
Cataract, congenital, with microphthalmia
Familial Mediterranean fever
Polycystic kidney disease
[Glyoxalase II deficiency]

Heinz body anemias, alpha-1
Thalassemias, alpha-1
Erythremias, alpha-1
Methemoglobinemias, alpha-1

Alpha-thalassemia/mental
retardation syndrome, type 1

Batten disease

?Renal glucosuria, 253100

CETP deficiency
Bardet-Biedl syndrome

?Townes-Brocks syndrome

Fish-eye disease
Norum disease

Cataract, Marner type
Tyrosinemia II

Urolithiasis, 2,8-dihydroxyadenine
Granulomatous disease, autosomal,
due to deficiency of CYBA
Mucopolysaccharidosis IVA

[Cystathioninuria]
Brody myopathy
{?Hypertension, essential}

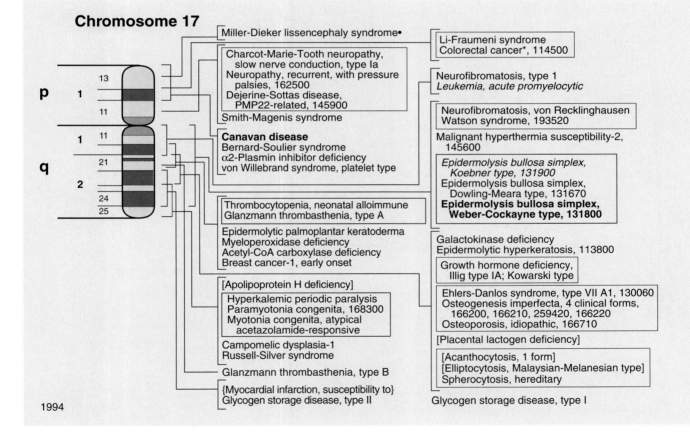

Chromosome 17

p	1	13
		11
q	1	11
		21
	2	
		24
		25

1994

Miller-Dieker lissencephaly syndrome•

Li-Fraumeni syndrome
Colorectal cancer*, 114500

Charcot-Marie-Tooth neuropathy,
slow nerve conduction, type Ia
Neuropathy, recurrent, with pressure
palsies, 162500
Dejerine-Sottas disease,
PMP22-related, 145900
Smith-Magenis syndrome

Neurofibromatosis, type 1
Leukemia, acute promyelocytic

Neurofibromatosis, von Recklinghausen
Watson syndrome, 193520

Malignant hyperthermia susceptibility-2,
145600

Canavan disease
Bernard-Soulier syndrome
α2-Plasmin inhibitor deficiency
von Willebrand syndrome, platelet type

*Epidermolysis bullosa simplex,
Koebner type, 131900*
Epidermolysis bullosa simplex,
Dowling-Meara type, 131670
**Epidermolysis bullosa simplex,
Weber-Cockayne type, 131800**

Thrombocytopenia, neonatal alloimmune
Glanzmann thrombasthenia, type A

Epidermolytic palmoplantar keratoderma
Myeloperoxidase deficiency
Acetyl-CoA carboxylase deficiency
Breast cancer-1, early onset

Galactokinase deficiency
Epidermolytic hyperkeratosis, 113800

Growth hormone deficiency,
Illig type IA; Kowarski type

[Apolipoprotein H deficiency]

Hyperkalemic periodic paralysis
Paramyotonia congenita, 168300
Myotonia congenita, atypical
acetazolamide-responsive

Ehlers-Danlos syndrome, type VII A1, 130060
Osteogenesis imperfecta, 4 clinical forms,
166200, 166210, 259420, 166220
Osteoporosis, idiopathic, 166710

Campomelic dysplasia-1
Russell-Silver syndrome

[Placental lactogen deficiency]

Glanzmann thrombasthenia, type B

[Acanthocytosis, 1 form]
[Elliptocytosis, Malaysian-Melanesian type]
Spherocytosis, hereditary

{Myocardial infarction, susceptibility to}
Glycogen storage disease, type II

Glycogen storage disease, type I

Chromosome 18

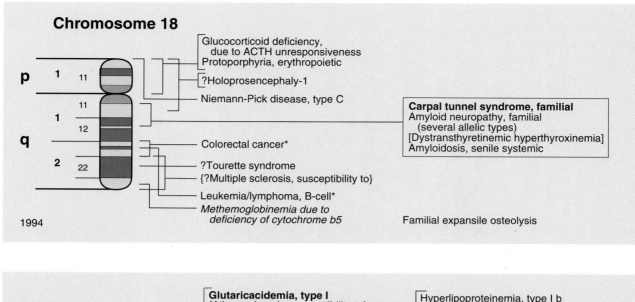

Glucocorticoid deficiency,
   due to ACTH unresponsiveness
Protoporphyria, erythropoietic
?Holoprosencephaly-1
Niemann-Pick disease, type C

Carpal tunnel syndrome, familial
Amyloid neuropathy, familial
   (several allelic types)
[Dystransthyretinemic hyperthyroxinemia]
Amyloidosis, senile systemic

Colorectal cancer*
?Tourette syndrome
{?Multiple sclerosis, susceptibility to}
Leukemia/lymphoma, B-cell*
*Methemoglobinemia due to
   deficiency of cytochrome b5*

Familial expansile osteolysis

1994

Chromosome 19

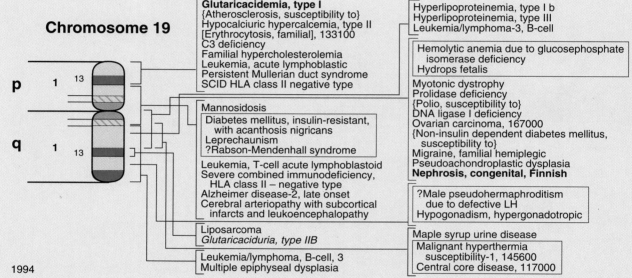

Glutaricacidemia, type I
{Atherosclerosis, susceptibility to}
Hypocalciuric hypercalcemia, type II
[Erythrocytosis, familial], 133100
C3 deficiency
Familial hypercholesterolemia
Leukemia, acute lymphoblastic
Persistent Mullerian duct syndrome
SCID HLA class II negative type

Mannosidosis

Diabetes mellitus, insulin-resistant,
   with acanthosis nigricans
Leprechaunism
?Rabson-Mendenhall syndrome

Leukemia, T-cell acute lymphoblastoid
Severe combined immunodeficiency,
   HLA class II – negative type
Alzheimer disease-2, late onset
Cerebral arteriopathy with subcortical
   infarcts and leukoencephalopathy

Liposarcoma
Glutaricaciduria, type IIB

Leukemia/lymphoma, B-cell, 3
Multiple epiphyseal dysplasia

Hyperlipoproteinemia, type I b
Hyperlipoproteinemia, type III
Leukemia/lymphoma-3, B-cell

Hemolytic anemia due to glucosephosphate
   isomerase deficiency
Hydrops fetalis

Myotonic dystrophy
Prolidase deficiency
{Polio, susceptibility to}
DNA ligase I deficiency
Ovarian carcinoma, 167000
{Non-insulin dependent diabetes mellitus,
   susceptibility to}
Migraine, familial hemiplegic
Pseudoachondroplastic dysplasia
Nephrosis, congenital, Finnish

?Male pseudohermaphroditism
   due to defective LH
Hypogonadism, hypergonadotropic

Maple syrup urine disease
Malignant hyperthermia
   susceptibility-1, 145600
Central core disease, 117000

1994

Chromosome 20

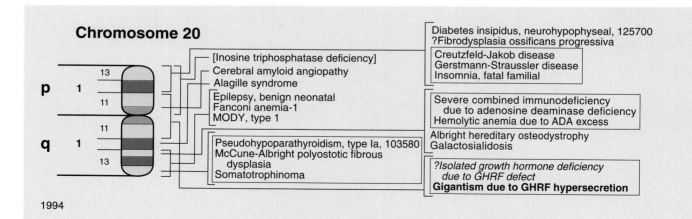

[Inosine triphosphatase deficiency]
Cerebral amyloid angiopathy
Alagille syndrome
Epilepsy, benign neonatal
Fanconi anemia-1
MODY, type 1

Pseudohypoparathyroidism, type Ia, 103580
McCune-Albright polyostotic fibrous
   dysplasia
Somatotrophinoma

Diabetes insipidus, neurohypophyseal, 125700
?Fibrodysplasia ossificans progressiva
Creutzfeld-Jakob disease
Gerstmann-Straussler disease
Insomnia, fatal familial

Severe combined immunodeficiency
   due to adenosine deaminase deficiency
Hemolytic anemia due to ADA excess

Albright hereditary osteodystrophy
Galactosialidosis

?Isolated growth hormone deficiency
   due to GHRF defect
Gigantism due to GHRF hypersecretion

1994

Chromosome 21

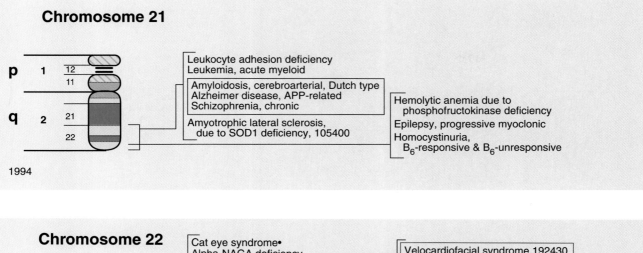

Leukocyte adhesion deficiency
Leukemia, acute myeloid

Amyloidosis, cerebroarterial, Dutch type
Alzheimer disease, APP-related
Schizophrenia, chronic

Amyotrophic lateral sclerosis,
    due to SOD1 deficiency, 105400

Hemolytic anemia due to
    phosphofructokinase deficiency
Epilepsy, progressive myoclonic
Homocystinuria,
    B$_6$-responsive & B$_6$-unresponsive

1994

Chromosome 22

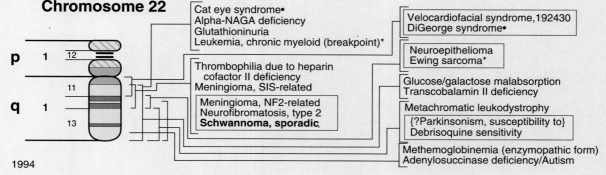

Cat eye syndrome•
Alpha-NAGA deficiency
Glutathioninuria
Leukemia, chronic myeloid (breakpoint)*

Thrombophilia due to heparin
    cofactor II deficiency
Meningioma, SIS-related

Meningioma, NF2-related
Neurofibromatosis, type 2
Schwannoma, sporadic

Velocardiofacial syndrome,192430
DiGeorge syndrome•

Neuroepithelioma
Ewing sarcoma*

Glucose/galactose malabsorption
Transcobalamin II deficiency

Metachromatic leukodystrophy

{?Parkinsonism, susceptibility to}
Debrisoquine sensitivity

Methemoglobinemia (enzymopathic form)
Adenylosuccinase deficiency/Autism

1994

Chromosome Y

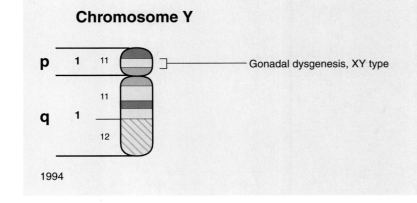

Gonadal dysgenesis, XY type

1994

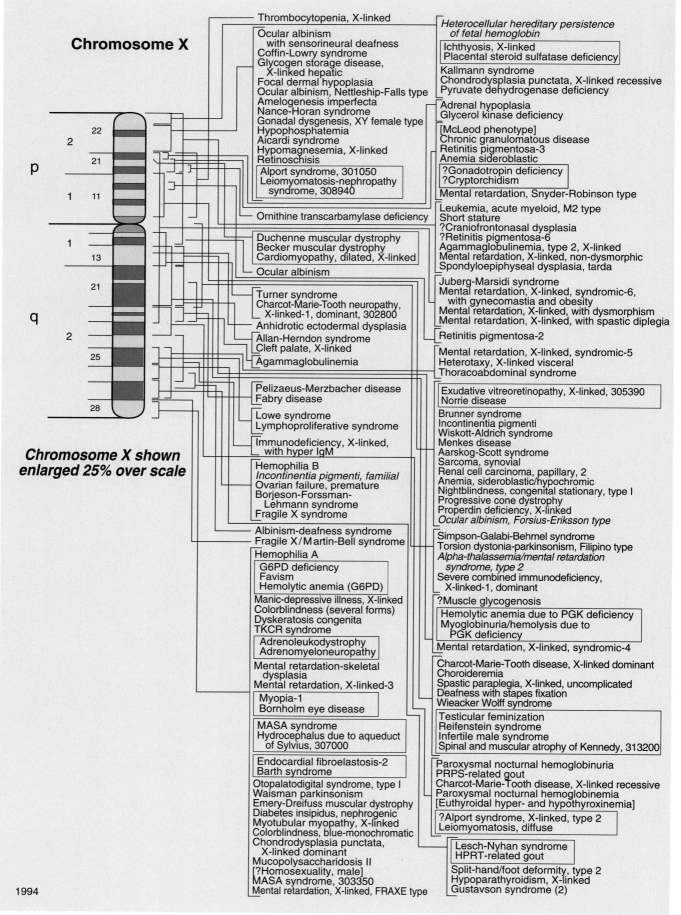

Chromosome X

Chromosome X shown enlarged 25% over scale

1994

1176

Index

Note: Page numbers followed by *f* refer to figures; numbers followed by *t* refer to tables.

Calculus/calculi, bladder. See *Bladder calculus*
   renal. See *Bladder calculus; Renal calculi*
   urinary tract, definition of, 570
Calices, renal, 550, 550*f*, 613, 614*f*
Calluses, 1072
Callus formation, in fracture healing, 998
Calmodulin, 88
Calymmatobacterium granulomatis, 695
cAMP. See *Cyclic AMP*
Campylobacter, sexual transmission, 696
Canalicular period, of lung development, 429–430
Canals of Lambert, 436
Cancer, 23. See also *Malignant tumor; Neoplasia; Tumor(s)*
   biology, principles of, 118–123
   bladder. See *Bladder cancer*
   breast. See *Breast cancer*
   causes of, 114
   cervical, 678
   colon. See *Colon cancer*
   cure rate for, 126
   deaths, by site and sex, 128, 129*f*–130*f*
   effects, on host, 125–126
     on inflammation and healing, 197
   endometrial, 678
   epidemiology of, 128, 129*f*
   esophageal, 738
   gastric, 699, 738
   immune response to, 123–124
   immunodepressive effects, 124–125
   immunotherapy for, 127–128
   incidence of, by site and sex, 129*f*
   in liver transplant recipient, 775
   leukemia. See *Leukemia(s)*
   liver, 772
   loss of growth control in, 115–116
   lymphoma. See *Lymphoma(s)*
   nutritional requirements with, 1142
   nutrition and, 131
   of female reproductive tract, 677–679
   ovarian, 678
   penile, 640
   prostate, 645
   risk factors, 128
   skin, 1072–1073, 1074*f*
   surgery for, 126
   testicular, 642–643
   tobacco use and, 128–131
   treatment of, 126–128. See also *Chemotherapy; Radiation therapy*
   lymphedema secondary to, 323, 323*f*
   vaginal, 678
   vulvar, 678–679
Cancer pain, 125, 847, 931
Candidate hormones, 779
Candidiasis, 24*f*, 161*t*
   chronic mucocutaneous, 212, 212*t*
   oral, 1061
   superficial, 1061
   vulvovaginitis caused by, 674–675
CAP (catabolite activator protein), 81
Capacitance vessels, 309
Capacitation, of spermatozoa, 631
Capillaries, 302
   anatomy of, 305, 306*f*
Capillary bed. See *Microcirculation*
Capillary fluid dynamics, in shock, 1086
Capillary fluid pressure, 309–310
Capillary fragility test, 292*t*
Capillary hydrostatic pressure, 526
   increased, 530
Capillary hydrostatic pressures, in shock, 1086

Capillary leak, 309, 1109
Capillary osmotic pressure, 526. See also *Colloid osmotic pressure, glomerular capillary*
   decreased, 530
Capillary permeability, 305, 437
Capillary pressure gradient, 309*f*, 309–310
Capsid, viral, 158
Capsule, renal, 549, 550*f*
Carbaminohemoglobin, 266, 441
Carbohydrate(s), absorption, 719
   digestion, 717*t*, 717–718
   in diabetic diet, 836–837
   metabolism, 789–790, 790*f*, 791*t*
Carbon dioxide, diffusion, 439–440, 440*f*
   partial pressure, definition of, 538
     in arterial blood, 265*t*, 475, 475*t*, 539–540
     in venous blood, 265*t*
   transport, 262, 265–266, 441
Carbonic acid, 265–266, 441
   acid-base homeostasis and, 539–540
   buffering function, 539
   deficit. See *Respiratory alkalosis*
   definition of, 538
   excess. See *Respiratory acidosis*
   excretion, 539–540
   formation, in kidney, 559
Carbonic anhydrase, 253, 262, 265–266, 441, 559
Carbonic anhydrase inhibitors, 595
Carbon monoxide, cellular injury caused by, 69
   lung disease and, 515*t*
   poisoning, with burn injury, 1111
Carbon tetrachloride, 69
Carboxypeptidase, activity of, 718
Carcinogen(s), 118
   definition of, 113
Carcinogenesis, multistep nature of, 122–123
Carcinoma. See also *Cancer*
   definition of, 114
Cardia, gastric, 704, 704*f*
   Mallory-Weiss syndrome and, 729–730
Cardiac catheterization, 368, 371–374
Cardiac cycle, 350–352, 351*f*
   aortic events in, 352
   atrial events in, 351–352
   isovolumic contraction phase, 351
   isovolumic relaxation phase, 351
   pulmonary artery events in, 352
   ventricular ejection phase, 351
Cardiac function, alterations of, 375–402
Cardiac function curve, 367, 367*f*
Cardiac function tests, 368–374
Cardiac glycosides, for heart failure, 410*t*, 411
   mechanism of action, 411, 412*f*
Cardiac index, 365, 1088
   calculation, 1089*t*
   definition of, 1082
   normal, 1089*t*
Cardiac muscle, 87, 88*f*, 347, 349*f*
   calcium imbalances and, 533–534
   cells, 354. See also *Myocyte(s), cardiac*
   contractile apparatus. See also *Thick filaments; Thin filaments*
     structure of, 355–356, 356*f*
   contractility, 367, 1084
     definition of, 403, 411
     impaired (diminished), 404
     management, in heart failure, 411–413, 412*f*
   contraction, 366–367, 367*f*
     molecular basis of, 357–359

excitability, 354
   potassium imbalances and, 532–533
Cardiac output, 265, 328–329, 1083–1084, 1084*f*, 1088
   age-related changes in, 373
   calculation, 1089*t*
   definition of, 325, 346, 1082
   determinants of, 328, 364–368
   in heart failure, 404, 405*f*, 405–406
   in pregnancy, 662
   normal, 365, 1089*t*
Cardiac reserve, 405
Cardiac tamponade, 392–393
   definition of, 375
Cardiac work, 368
   increased, 404
Cardinal ligaments, alterations in, 670–671
Cardiogenic shock, 405, 1086, 1089–1091
   clinical features of, 1089–1090, 1090*t*
   definition of, 1082
   etiology of, 1089, 1089*t*
   hemodynamic manifestations, 1090, 1090*t*
   pathophysiology of, 1089, 1090*f*
   treatment of, 1090–1091
Cardiomyopathy, 390
   definition of, 375, 391
   dilated (congestive), 391
   hypertrophic, 391
   peripartum, 391
   primary, 391–392
   restrictive, 391–392
   secondary, 391–392, 392*t*
Cardiopulmonary arrest, mixed acid-base imbalance with, 544
Cardiovascular disease, effects on inflammation and healing, 197
   epidemiology of, 17
Cardiovascular response(s), impaired, orthostatic (postural) hypotension due to, 341–342
Cardiovascular system, age-related changes in, 73*t*
   in malnutrition, 1138
Carina, 433
   definition of, 428
Carotid endarterectomy, 888
Carrier(s), definition of, 209
   disease, definition of, 91
Carrier protein(s), 47–48, 48*f*. See also *Calcium pump(s); Sodium ion/potassium ion pump*
   transmembrane movement, 48, 48*f*
Carrion's disease. See *Bartonellosis*
Cartilage, 86
   age-related changes in, 985
Cartilage cells, 984
Cartilage-hair hypoplasia, 212*t*
Caseous necrosis, 65, 67*f*
Cast(s), urinary, 564–565
   definition of, 548, 570
Catabolism, 43–44, 788–789
   definition of, 43, 778, 1121
   degree of, related to urinary urea, 1135, 1135*t*
   in physiologic stres, 1132–1135, 1133*f*–1134*f*
Catalase, 41
Cataract(s), 922–923
Catatonic posturing, 953*f*
Catecholamine(s), actions, 789, 791, 791*t*, 793*t*, 800*t*
   definition of, 826
   for respiratory disease, 456*t*
   in glucose metabolism, 828
   in stress response, 143*f*, 143–144